A Practice of Anesthesia
for Infants and Children

A Practice of Anesthesia for Infants and Children

Third Edition

Charles J. Coté, MD
Professor of Anesthesiology and Pediatrics
Northwestern University Medical School
Vice Chairman and Director of Research
Department of Pediatric Anesthesiology
The Children's Memorial Hospital
Chicago, Illinois

I. David Todres, MD
Professor of Pediatrics (Anaesthesia)
Harvard Medical School
Pediatrician and Anesthetist
Massachusetts General Hospital
Boston, Massachusetts

John F. Ryan, MD
Associate Professor of Anaesthesia
Harvard Medical School
Anesthetist
Massachusetts General Hospital
Boston, Massachusetts

Nishan G. Goudsouzian, MD
Professor of Anaesthesia
Harvard Medical School
Anesthetist
Massachusetts General Hospital
Boston, Massachusetts

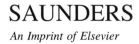

SAUNDERS
An Imprint of Elsevier

SAUNDERS
An Imprint of Elsevier
The Curtis Center
Independence Square West
Philadelphia, PA 19106

Library of Congress Cataloging-in-Publication Data

A practice of anesthesia for infants and children—3rd ed./edited by Charles J. Coté—[et al.].

p.   cm.

Includes bibliographical references and index.

ISBN-13: 978-0-7216-7286-1   ISBN-10: 0-7216-7286-8

1. Pediatric anesthesia.   I. Coté, Charles J.
   [DNLM: 1. Anesthesia—Child.   2. Anesthesia—Infant.   WO 440 P895
   2001]

RD139.P73 2001   617.9′6798—dc21

00–030776

ISBN-13: 978-0-7216-7286-1
ISBN-10: 0-7216-7286-8

Acquisitions Editor: Allan Ross
Production Manager: Norman Stellander
Illustration Specialist: Robert Quinn
Book Designer: Gene Harris

A PRACTICE OF ANESTHESIA FOR INFANTS AND CHILDREN

Printed in the United States of America.

Last digit is the print number: 9   8   7   6

Contributors

Charles B. Berde, MD, PhD
Professor of Anaesthesia (Pediatrics), Harvard Medical School; Director, Pain Treatment Services, and Senior Associate, Anesthesia, Children's Hospital, Boston, Massachusetts
Postoperative Pain Management

Bruno Bissonnette, MD, FRCPC
Professor of Anaesthesia, University of Toronto Faculty of Medicine; Staff Anesthesiologist, Director of Neurosurgical Anaesthesia, and Cross-Appointment Critical Care Medicine, The Hospital for Sick Children, Toronto, Ontario, Canada
Temperature Regulation: Normal and Abnormal (Malignant Hyperthermia)

Frederick A. Burrows, MD, MEd
Professor of Anesthesiology and Pediatrics, University of Arkansas School for Medical Sciences; Staff Anesthesiologist, Arkansas Children's Hospital, Little Rock, Arkansas
Anesthesia for Children Undergoing Heart Surgery

Stephen Campo, MD
Instructor in Anaesthesia, Harvard Medical School; Assistant in Anesthesia, Massachusetts General Hospital, Boston, Massachusetts
Pediatric Emergencies

Charles J. Coté, MD
Professor of Anesthesiology and Pediatrics, Northwestern University Medical School; Vice Chairman and Director of Research, Department of Pediatric Anesthesiology, The Children's Memorial Hospital, Chicago, Illinois
The Practice of Pediatric Anesthesia, Preoperative Evaluation of Pediatric Patients, Pediatric Airway, Pharmacokinetics and Pharmacology of Drugs in Children, Premedication and Induction of Anesthesia, Strategies for Blood Product Management and Transfusion Reduction, Anesthesia for Children with Burn Injuries, Anesthesia Outside the Operating Room, Pediatric Sedation for Diagnostic and Therapeutic Procedures Outside the Operating Room, Pediatric Regional Anesthesia, Pediatric Equipment, Procedures

Jonathan H. Cronin, MD
Assistant Professor of Pediatrics, Harvard Medical School; Associate Chief, Neonatology Unit, Massachusetts General Hospital for Children, Massachusetts General Hospital, Boston, Massachusetts
Growth and Development; Neonatal Emergencies

Peter J. Davis, MD
Professor of Anesthesiology, Critical Care Medicine and Pediatrics, University of Pittsburgh School of Medicine; Anesthesiologist-in-Chief, Children's Hospital of Pittsburgh, Pittsburgh, Pennsylvania
Anesthesia for Organ Transplantation

Alberto J. de Armendi, MD, AM
Assistant Professor of Anesthesiology, University of Tennessee School of Medicine, Memphis; Chief of Anesthesia, St. Jude Children's Research Hospital, Memphis, Tennessee
Postanesthesia Care Unit

William T. Denman, MB ChB FRCA
Assistant Professor of Anaesthesia, Harvard Medical School; Assistant in Anesthesia, Massachusetts General Hospital, Boston, Massachusetts
Pediatric Emergencies

Richard M. Dsida, MD
Assistant Professor of Anesthesiology, Northwestern University Medical School; Attending Anesthesiologist, Department of Pediatric Anesthesiology, The Children's Memorial Hospital, Chicago, Illinois
Strategies for Blood Product Management and Transfusion Reduction

Elizabeth A. Eldredge, MD
Instructor in Anaesthesia, Harvard Medical School; Assistant in Anesthesia, Children's Hospital, Boston, Massachusetts
Pediatric Neurosurgical Anesthesia

Erich A. Everts Jr, MD
Chairman, Department of Anesthesia, St. Mary Medical Center, Langhorne, Pennsylvania
Anesthesia for Organ Transplantation

Lynne R. Ferrari, MD
Associate Professor of Anaesthesia, Harvard Medical School; Medical Director Perioperative Services and Senior Associate in Anesthesia, Children's Hospital, Boston, Massachusetts
Anesthesia for Otorhinolaryngology Procedures, Anesthesia for Ophthalmology

Marla S. Gendelman, MD
Assistant Professor, Hahnemann University Medical College of Pennsylvania/Allegheny University of Health Sciences; Staff Anesthesiologist, Allegheny General Hospital, Pittsburgh, Pennsylvania
Anesthesia for Organ Transplantation

Nishan G. Goudsouzian, MD
Professor of Anaesthesia, Harvard Medical School;
Anesthetist, Massachusetts General Hospital, Boston,
Massachusetts
*The Practice of Pediatric Anesthesia, Preoperative Evaluation
of Pediatric Patients, Muscle Relaxants in Children*

Steven C. Hall, MD
Professor of Anesthesiology, Northwestern University
Medical School, Anesthesiologist-in-Chief, Arthur C. King
Professor of Pediatric Anesthesia, Department of Pediatric
Anesthesiology, The Children's Memorial Hospital,
Chicago, Illinois
Pediatric Trauma

Raafat S. Hannallah, MD
Professor of Anesthesiology and Pediatrics, The George
Washington University Medical Center; Chairman of
Anesthesiology, Children's National Medical Center,
Washington, DC
Outpatient Anesthesia

Paul R. Hickey, MD
Professor of Anaesthesia, Harvard Medical School;
Anesthesiologist-in-Chief, Children's Hospital, Boston,
Massachusetts
Anesthesia for Children Undergoing Heart Surgery

Zeev N. Kain, MD
Associate Professor of Anesthesiology, Child Psychiatry
and Pediatrics, Yale University School of Medicine; Chief,
Section of Pediatric Anesthesia, Yale–New Haven
Children's Hospital, New Haven, Connecticut
Perioperative Behavioral Stress Response in Children

Richard F. Kaplan, MD
Professor of Anesthesiology and Pediatrics, The George
Washington University Medical Center; Attending
Anesthesiologist, Children's National Medical Center,
Washington, DC
*Pediatric Sedation for Diagnostic and Therapeutic Procedures
Outside the Operating Room*

Letty M. P. Liu, MD
Professor, Department of Anesthesiology, Director of
Pediatric Anesthesiology, University of Medicine and
Dentistry of New Jersey–New Jersey Medical School,
Newark, New Jersey
Premedication and Induction of Anesthesia

Ralph A. Lugo, PharmD
Associate Professor of Pharmacy Practice, University of
Utah College of Pharmacy; Adjunct Assistant Professor,
University of Utah School of Medicine; Clinical Pharmacy
Specialist, Pediatric Intensive Care Unit, Primary
Children's Hospital, Salt Lake City, Utah
Pharmacokinetics and Pharmacology of Drugs in Children

J. A. Jeevendra Martyn, MD
Professor of Anaesthesia, Harvard Medical School;
Anesthetist, Massachusetts General Hospital; Associate
Director of Anesthesia, Shriners Burns Hospital, Boston,
Massachusetts
Anesthesia for Children with Burn Injuries

Linda C. Mayes, MD
Arnold Gesell Associate Professor of Child Development,
Pediatrics and Psychology, Yale Study Center, New Haven,
Connecticut
Perioperative Behavioral Stress Response in Children

Aleksandra J. Mazurek, MD
Assistant Professor of Anesthesiology, Northwestern
University Medical School; Attending Anesthesiologist,
Department of Pediatric Anesthesiology, The Children's
Memorial Hospital, Chicago, Illinois
Pediatric Trauma

Francis X. McGowan Jr, MD
Associate Professor of Anaesthesia, Harvard Medical
School; Senior Associate in Anesthesia, Co-Director,
Cardiac Anesthesia Services, Children's Hospital, Boston,
Massachusetts
Cardiac Physiology and Pharmacology

Michael L. McManus, MD
Assistant Professor of Anaesthesia, Harvard Medical
School; Associate Director, Multidisciplinary Intensive
Care Unit, Senior Associate in Anesthesia, Children's
Hospital, Boston, Massachusetts
Pediatric Fluid Management

Leila Mei Pang, MD
Associate Professor of Anesthesiology and Pediatrics,
College of Physicians and Surgeons of Columbia
University; Associate Attending Anesthesiologist, Columbia
Presbyterian Medical Center, New York Presbyterian
Hospital, New York, New York
Premedication and Induction of Anesthesia

David M. Polaner, MD
Associate Professor of Anesthesiology, University of
Colorado School of Medicine; Attending Anesthesiologist,
The Childrens Hospital, Denver, Colorado
*Pediatric Regional Anesthesia, Postoperative Pain
Management*

Mateen Raazi, MBBS
Clinical Assistant Professor, University of Saskatchewan
College of Medicine; Staff Anesthesiologist, Department of
Anesthesia, Royal University Hospital, Saskatoon,
Saskatchewan, Canada
Anesthesia for Organ Transplantation

Robert W. Reid, MD
Assistant Professor of Anesthesiology, University of
Missouri School of Medicine, Kansas City, Missouri; Staff
Anesthesiologist, International Children's Heart Foundation,
Memphis, Tennessee
Anesthesia for Children Undergoing Heart Surgery

Jesse D. Roberts Jr, MD, MS
Assistant Professor of Anaesthesia (Pediatrics), Harvard
Medical School; Assistant Anesthetist and Pediatrician,
Massachusetts General Hospital, Massachusetts General
Hospital for Children, Boston, Massachusetts
Neonatal Emergencies

Mark A. Rockoff, MD
Professor of Anaesthesia, Harvard Medical School;
Associate Anesthesiologist-in-Chief, Children's Hospital,
Boston, Massachusetts
Pediatric Neurosurgical Anesthesia

John F. Ryan, MD, MEd
Associate Professor of Anaesthesia, Harvard Medical
School; Anesthetist, Massachusetts General Hospital,
Boston, Massachusetts
*The Practice of Pediatric Anesthesia, Preoperative Evaluation
of Pediatric Patients, Temperature Regulation: Normal and
Abnormal (Malignant Hyperthermia)*

Charles L. Schleien, MD
Professor of Pediatrics and Anesthesiology, College of
Physicians and Surgeons of Columbia University; Medical
Director, Division of Pediatric and Critical Care Medicine,
Columbia Presbyterian Medical Center, New York
Presbyterian Hospital, New York, New York
Cardiopulmonary Resuscitation

Robert L. Sheridan, MD
Associate Professor of Surgery, Harvard Medical School;
Assistant Chief-of-Staff, Shriners Burns Hospital; Associate
Visiting Surgeon, Massachusetts General Hospital, Boston,
Massachusetts
Anesthesia for Children with Burn Injuries

Sulpicio G. Soriano, MD, MSEd
Associate Professor of Anaesthesia, Harvard Medical
School; Associate in Anesthesia, Children's Hospital,
Boston, Massachusetts
Pediatric Neurosurgical Anesthesia

James M. Steven, MD
Associate Professor of Anesthesia and Pediatrics,
University of Pennsylvania School of Medicine; Associate
Anesthesiologist-in-Chief, The Children's Hospital of
Philadelphia, Philadelphia, Pennsylvania
Cardiac Physiology and Pharmacology

Maureen A. Strafford, MD
Associate Professor of Anesthesia and Pediatrics, Tufts
University School of Medicine; Associate Professor of
Anesthesiology and Pediatrics, New England Medical
Center, Boston, Massachusetts
*Management of the Patient with Repaired or Palliated
Congenital Heart Disease, Pediatric Sedation for Diagnostic
and Therapeutic Procedures Outside the Operating Room*

Santhanam Suresh, MD
Assistant Professor of Anesthesiology, Northwestern
University Medical School; Attending Anesthesiologist,
Co-Director, Pain Management Service, Department of
Pediatric Anesthesiology, The Children's Memorial
Hospital, Chicago, Illinois
Pediatric Regional Anesthesia

S. K. Szyfelbein, MD
Associate Professor of Anaesthesia, Harvard Medical
School; Anesthetist, Assistant in Surgery, Massachusetts
General Hospital; Chief of Anesthesia, Shriners Burns
Hospital, Boston, Massachusetts
Anesthesia for Children with Burn Injuries

I. David Todres, MD
Professor of Pediatrics (Anaesthesia), Harvard Medical
School; Pediatrician and Anesthetist, The Massachusetts
General Hospital for Children, Massachusetts General
Hospital, Boston, Massachusetts
*The Practice of Pediatric Anesthesia, Growth and
Development, Preoperative Evaluation of Pediatric Patients,
Ethical Issues in Pediatric Anesthesiology, Pediatric Airway,
Cardiopulmonary Resuscitation, Neonatal Emergencies,
Pediatric Emergencies, Postanesthesia Care Unit, Procedures*

Robert D. Truog, MD, MA
Professor of Anaesthesia and Medical Ethics, Harvard
Medical School; Director, Multidisciplinary Intensive Care
Unit, Senior Associate in Anesthesia, Children's Hospital,
Boston, Massachusetts
Ethical Issues in Pediatric Anesthesiology

Susan A. Vassallo, MD
Assistant Professor of Anaesthesia, Harvard Medical
School; Assistant Anesthetist, Massachusetts General
Hospital, Boston, Massachusetts
*Anesthesia for Otorhinolaryngology Procedures, Anesthesia for
Ophthalmology*

David B. Waisel, MD
Instructor in Anaesthesia, Harvard Medical School;
Assistant in Anesthesia, Children's Hospital, Boston,
Massachusetts
Ethical Issues in Pediatric Anesthesiology

Robert M. Ward, MD
Professor of Pediatrics and Director, Pediatric
Pharmacology Program, University of Utah School of
Medicine; Attending Neonatologist, Primary Children's
Medical Center, Salt Lake City, Utah
Pharmacokinetics and Pharmacology of Drugs in Children

Melissa Wheeler, MD
Assistant Professor of Anesthesiology, Northwestern
University Medical School; Attending Anesthesiologist,
Co-Director, Chronic Pain Service, Department of Pediatric
Anesthesiology, The Children's Memorial Hospital,
Chicago, Illinois
Pediatric Airway

Myron Yaster, MD
Professor of Anesthesiology, Critical Care Medicine and
Pediatrics, Johns Hopkins University School of Medicine,
Baltimore, Maryland
*Pediatric Sedation for Diagnostic and Therapeutic Procedures
Outside the Operating Room*

Maurice S. Zwass, MD
Professor of Anesthesia and Pediatrics, University of
California, San Francisco, School of Medicine; Associate
Director, Pediatric Critical Care Medicine, University of
California San Francisco Moffitt-Long Hospitals, San
Francisco, California
Postoperative Pain Management

Preface

The third edition of *A Practice of Anesthesia for Infants and Children* has taken a new direction. The editors and contributors, instead of coming primarily from one institution, now come from many institutions in the United States and North America and represent a broader view of the practice of pediatric anesthesiology.

This edition expands the chapter on pharmacology to include the input of a neonatal pharmacologist and a Doctor of Pharmacy. The resuscitation chapter has a markedly expanded discussion of the pathophysiology of resuscitation and the unique aspects of resuscitation in the operating room. We have added chapters on the psychological development of the child, on ethical issues related to pediatric anesthesiology, as well as a chapter dedicated to outpatient anesthesia practice.

Another important addition is the chapter on anesthesia for children with repaired congenital heart disease written by an anesthesiologist who is also a pediatric cardiologist.

There are few data collated in the literature to guide the trainee and practitioner who occasionally treat these children. A chapter on trauma has been included that emphasizes the important problem of child abuse. Illustrations of classic examples of cutaneous manifestations that an anesthesiologist might encounter are included. All chapters of the textbook have undergone extensive revision with the addition of new illustrations, algorithms, and tables.

The editors of *A Practice of Anesthesia for Infants and Children* have purposefully continued to include a discussion of many older medications and techniques, recognizing that some of the newer medications and techniques may not be available to all practicing anesthesiologists throughout the world.

We trust this textbook will provide a framework for learning for students in pediatric anesthesiology as well as for seasoned practitioners and will assist in providing for the safe care of pediatric patients everywhere.

Acknowledgments

We wish to thank the Chairpersons of the Departments of Anesthesiology who supported the academic endeavors of their staff and thus made it possible for them to contribute to the third edition of *A Practice of Anesthesia for Infants and Children.* In particular, Dr. Coté wishes to thank Dr. Steven C. Hall and members of the Department of Anesthesiology at the Children's Memorial Hospital for the support that was required to bring this book to fruition. We also wish to thank Mr. Paul Andriesse for his outstanding drawings and illustrations and Ms. Corri Hefner, RN, Ms. Eva Panzera, and Ms. Carmen Torres for their wonderful support and assistance in this endeavor.

NOTICE

Anesthesiology is an ever-changing field. Standard safety precautions must be followed, but as new research and clinical experience broaden our knowledge, changes in treatment and drug therapy may become necessary or appropriate. Readers are advised to check the most current product information provided by the manufacturer of each drug to be administered to verify the recommended dose, the method and duration of administration, and the contraindications. It is the responsibility of the treating physician, relying on experience and knowledge of the patient, to determine the dosages and the best treatment for each individual patient. Neither the Publisher nor the editor assumes any liability for any injury and/or damage to persons or property arising from this publication.

THE PUBLISHER

Contents

Chapter 1
The Practice of Pediatric Anesthesia 1
Charles J. Coté, I. David Todres, John F. Ryan, and
Nishan G. Goudsouzian

Chapter 2
Growth and Development 5
I. David Todres and Jonathan H. Cronin

Chapter 3
Perioperative Behavioral Stress Response
in Children 25
Zeev N. Kain and Linda C. Mayes

Chapter 4
Preoperative Evaluation of Pediatric Patients 37
Charles J. Coté, I. David Todres, John F. Ryan, and
Nishan G. Goudsouzian

Chapter 5
Outpatient Anesthesia 55
Raafat S. Hannallah

Chapter 6
Ethical Issues in Pediatric Anesthesiology 68
David B. Waisel, I. David Todres, and Robert D. Truog

Chapter 7
Pediatric Airway 79
Melissa Wheeler, Charles J. Coté, and I. David Todres

Chapter 8
Pharmacokinetics and Pharmacology of Drugs
in Children 121
Charles J. Coté, Ralph A. Lugo, and Robert M. Ward

Chapter 9
Premedication and Induction of Anesthesia 172
Leila Mei Pang, Letty M. P. Liu, and Charles J. Coté

Chapter 10
Muscle Relaxants in Children 196
Nishan G. Goudsouzian

Chapter 11
Pediatric Fluid Management 216
Michael L. McManus

Chapter 12
Strategies for Blood Product Management and
Transfusion Reduction 235
Charles J. Coté and Richard M. Dsida

Chapter 13
Cardiopulmonary Resuscitation 265
Charles L. Schleien and I. David Todres

Chapter 14
Neonatal Emergencies 294
Jesse D. Roberts Jr, Jonathan H. Cronin, and
I. David Todres

Chapter 15
Pediatric Emergencies 315
Stephen Campo, William T. Denman, and
I. David Todres

Chapter 16
Pediatric Trauma 334
Aleksandra J. Mazurek and Steven C. Hall

Chapter 17
Cardiac Physiology and Pharmacology 353
Francis X. McGowan, Jr, and James M. Steven

Chapter 18
Anesthesia for Children Undergoing
Heart Surgery 391
Robert W. Reid, Frederick A. Burrows, and
Paul R. Hickey

Chapter 19
Management of the Patient with Repaired or
Palliated Congenital Heart Disease 415
Maureen A. Strafford

Chapter 20
Anesthesia for Otorhinolaryngology Procedures 461
Lynne R. Ferrari and Susan A. Vassallo

Chapter 21
Anesthesia for Ophthalmology 479
Susan A. Vassallo and Lynne R. Ferrari

Chapter 22
Pediatric Neurosurgical Anesthesia 493
Elizabeth A. Eldredge, Sulpicio G. Soriano, and
Mark A. Rockoff

Chapter 23
Anesthesia for Children with Burn Injuries 522
S. K. Szyfelbein, J. A. Jeevendra Martyn,
Robert L. Sheridan, and Charles J. Coté

C h a p t e r 2 4

Anesthesia for Organ Transplantation 544
*Marla S. Gendelman, Mateen Raazi, Peter J. Davis,
and Erich A. Everts, Jr*

C h a p t e r 2 5

Anesthesia Outside the Operating Room 571
Charles J. Coté

C h a p t e r 2 6

Pediatric Sedation for Diagnostic and Therapeutic
Procedures Outside the Operating Room 584
*Richard F. Kaplan, Myron Yaster, Maureen A. Strafford,
and Charles J. Coté*

C h a p t e r 2 7

Temperature Regulation: Normal and Abnormal
(Malignant Hyperthermia) 610
Bruno Bissonnette and John F. Ryan

C h a p t e r 2 8

Pediatric Regional Anesthesia 636
*David M. Polaner, Santhanam Suresh, and
Charles J. Coté*

C h a p t e r 2 9

Postoperative Pain Management 675
*Maurice S. Zwass, David M. Polaner, and
Charles B. Berde*

C h a p t e r 3 0

Postanesthesia Care Unit 698
Alberto J. de Armendi and I. David Todres

C h a p t e r 3 1

Pediatric Equipment 715
Charles J. Coté

C h a p t e r 3 2

Procedures 739
I. David Todres and Charles J. Coté

Index 757

The Practice of Pediatric Anesthesia

Charles J. Coté, I. David Todres, John F. Ryan, *and* Nishan G. Goudsouzian

Preoperative Evaluation and Management

Informed Consent

Operating Room and Monitoring

Induction and Maintenance of Anesthesia

Clinical Monitors

Airway and Ventilation

Fluids

Conduct of Anesthesia Team

Recovery Room

Postoperative Visit

Conclusion

This chapter outlines the basis of our collective practice of pediatric anesthesia. These basic principles of practice can be applied regardless of the circumstances; they provide the foundation for safe anesthesia.

Preoperative Evaluation and Management

Anesthesiologists must assume an active role in the preoperative assessment of children. Ideally, the anesthesiologist performing the preoperative evaluation will also anesthetize the patient. A complete medical and surgical history, family history, chart review, and physical examination are performed on every patient to be anesthetized (see Chapter 4). When appropriate, the child should receive preoperative medical therapy to optimize his or her condition or conditions before receiving anesthesia (e.g., patients with seizure disorders or reactive airway disease). In addition, the emotional state of the child and family must be considered and appropriate psychological and, if necessary, pharmacologic support provided. The anesthesia team, working in concert with surgical colleagues and nursing and child life specialists, must find appropriate and creative techniques (e.g., videotapes, booklets, hospital tours, and trained paramedical personnel) to prepare the child and family. The marked increase in outpatient surgical procedures has reduced the

time available for interaction between the anesthesiologist and the family and patient (see Chapter 5). Despite this reduced contact time, these support techniques should not be neglected.

Familiarity with a child's clinical and psychological status is essential. Meeting a child for the first time in the operating room and then proceeding impersonally with the anesthetic procedure is potentially hazardous and unfair to the child and family. The anesthetic experience itself is unique for a child, and proper rapport among child, anesthesiologist, and family is crucial for success. This relationship must carry through to the postoperative phase, and special attention should be given to the relief of pain and anxiety. Anesthesiologists can provide valuable assistance in this respect because of their understanding of the pharmacology of sedative and narcotic drugs, as well as their ability to perform nerve blocks (see Chapters 28 and 29).

Anesthesiologists must always understand a proposed surgical or investigative procedure to facilitate the planning of an appropriate level of monitoring and selection of anesthetic drugs and technique. The anesthesiologist must anticipate a surgeon's needs regarding patient positioning and muscle relaxation, as well as a patient's need for fluid, blood, opioids, and analgesics. For complex cases, the anesthesiologist and surgeon should formulate a plan preoperatively and explain the plan to the parents and child. If any important medical issues require further clarification, this consultation should be a part of the preoperative evaluation and planning process. It is useful to discuss your concerns with the consultant so as to focus his or her attention on the specific issue of interest. Consultant recommendations must be carefully reviewed and ideally should reflect the consultant's understanding of the anesthesia process and what it is you need from him or her regarding management issues.

Appropriate preoperative abstinence from food and fluid should always be ordered. Infants must receive special consideration; prolonged abstinence may lead to dehydration or hypoglycemia (see Chapter 11). Children may surreptitiously circumvent the preoperative fasting order. One must always be on guard for the possibility of a full stomach and its sequelae. For example, the risk for pulmonary aspiration of gastric contents is increased in some patients (e.g., those with obesity, previous esophageal surgery, difficult intubation, hiatal hernia). This risk may be reduced by a prophylactic regimen against acid aspiration as part of the preoperative plan.

Preoperative consideration must be given to proper psychological support, appropriate premedication, and the timing of the premedication (see Chapters 3, 4, and 9). Premedication may be omitted because of the critical nature of a child's illness or because a child is especially cooperative. Psychological support of the child and parents must never be neglected, no matter how calm they might appear. Premedication may be administered on the ward or in the room adjacent to the operating room. Once any medication is administered, a child must be monitored for changes in cardiopulmonary function. The transport of a medicated child to the operating room must be undertaken with caution and with appropriate monitoring (see Chapter 16). A critically ill patient must be accompanied by skilled staff who will ensure continued infusion of vasoactive medications and who are skilled in the management of any emergencies that could arise during transport.

The possible need for postoperative intensive care, including assisted ventilation, should be anticipated and fully discussed with the parents and child (if the child is of an appropriate age). It is also important to discuss postoperative pain management and therapeutic options, such as patient-controlled analgesia, continuous caudal or epidural anesthesia, or single shot caudal or regional nerve blocks (see Chapters 28 and 29).

Informed Consent

The risks and benefits of the anesthetic procedure must be presented in clear, easily understood terms. A simple explanation to the parents of what the anesthesiologists will be doing to ensure good care and safety for their child should provide the information necessary to relieve preoperative anxiety. During this explanation, reference should be made to the anesthesiologist's careful monitoring of parameters such as temperature (e.g., use of special heating blankets); heart rate and breath sounds (e.g., electrocardiogram and stethoscope); and continuous oxygen saturation and expired carbon dioxide/anesthetic agent monitoring. Whenever invasive monitoring devices are to be applied, the parents and child should be assured that in most cases these will be placed after induction of anesthesia to avoid causing discomfort and that they will be removed as soon as the child's postoperative condition permits. An explanation of the information obtained by these monitors and how they help improve the safety of anesthesia also helps relieve anxiety. This is especially important because of the apprehension parents feel about the adequacy of oxygenation during surgery. Emphasizing the information provided by pulse oximetry helps to relieve parental anxiety regarding oxygenation of their child. Details should not be recited in a cold and technical manner but with dialogue that responds to the parents' and child's questions and concerns. This dialogue is frequently given too little time, leaving the parents and child insecure and unnecessarily apprehensive. Body language is especially important during this preoperative interview. The anesthesiologist who never sits down, talks rapidly, and has one foot pointed toward the door presents a

very different picture from the anesthesiologist who sits down, talks slowly and clearly, takes the time to answer questions, and does not seem to be in a rush. If the family speaks a different language than the anesthesiologist, then help should be sought through an interpreter.

It is important to reassure the parents and child that the anesthesiologist is in constant attendance and is responsible for the medical well-being of the child while the surgeon undertakes the necessary operation. This explanation provides reassurance and also emphasizes our role as physicians in the operating room. The anesthesiologist who exhibits a high profile postoperatively on the ward and in the intensive care unit makes important contributions to this phase of a patient's care. Our special training in coping with rapid changes in physiologic status, as well as our increasing role in the management of postoperative pain, should be emphasized. In discussing the procedure with the child, the child's age and level of understanding determine how to present the concept of anesthesia, surgery, and postoperative care. Children require reassurance that *they will not wake up during the procedure and that they will awaken at the conclusion.* Many children are fearful of not awakening (see Chapter 4). The possibility of postoperative pain and the relief the child will receive in the form of nerve blocks and analgesics must be clearly presented to the parents and child.

Operating Room and Monitoring

For the anesthesiologist to successfully carry out a proposed anesthetic plan, the patient's chart must be re-examined prior to induction of anesthesia for pertinent information that may have been added at the last moment. It is most important that the patient's identification bracelet be checked, especially if the anesthetizing team is different from the preoperative evaluation team. All equipment for induction and maintenance of anesthesia, including suction and all necessary monitoring devices, must be functioning and reliable (see Chapter 31). *Equipment must be checked by the anesthesia team taking care of the child.* Too often it is presumed that particular equipment is functioning when other personnel have checked it.

The degree of monitoring must be adjusted according to a child's underlying clinical condition and the planned surgical procedure. In every situation, basic monitoring is essential; to this are added special monitoring devices as they become necessary. The basic monitors are the anesthesiologist's eyes, ears, and hands, which confer the ability to observe a patient's color and chest movements, to listen for heart tones and breath sounds, and to palpate the arterial pulse and temperature of the skin. A precordial or esophageal stethoscope should be placed on every child as part of basic monitoring. All children, except those undergoing the briefest noninvasive procedures, should have an intravenous line inserted to allow for fluid replacement and provide a route for rapid and predictable administration of drugs. Fluid replacement is particularly important in children who have undergone prolonged fasting or who have ongoing third-space losses. Continuous monitoring of the electrocardiogram, temperature, inspired oxygen concentration, oxygen saturation, expired carbon dioxide, and intermittent blood pressure determination are considered routine. Expired carbon dioxide monitors (especially those that display the waveform) and pulse oximetry are extremely important in the early detection of potential anesthetic-related events that, if undetected, could result in serious morbidity or mortality. Monitoring of the anesthetic agent is also helpful but not necessary. The role of bispectral electroencephalographic analysis in pediatrics is yet to be defined.

Invasive cardiovascular monitoring (e.g., direct arterial blood pressure, central venous pressure, or pulmonary artery occlusion pressure) may be required for major surgery if extensive blood loss or major fluid shifts are anticipated or if a patient is medically unstable. A urinary catheter provides indirect data about intravascular volume status and organ perfusion. Monitoring urinary output is particularly useful for long operations, procedures involving severe blood loss, those in which there is the potential for rapid or massive blood loss, those in which wide variations in blood pressure and fluid balance can be anticipated, or during induced hypotensive anesthesia.

If a particular variable would be monitored in an adult, then a child deserves the same approach. Invasive monitoring procedures are sometimes forsaken in a child because of the anesthesiologist's inexperience with pediatric techniques; the need for invasive monitoring is thus dismissed as being "excessive." These monitors, however, allow the accurate measurement of blood pressure, cardiac output, filling pressures, and cardiac and pulmonary function. In turn, they provide a safe mechanism for assessing the response to pharmacologic interventions, as well as the responses to administration of blood products, fluids, and vasoactive medications.

A cautionary note: With increased sophistication in monitoring, anesthesiologists have become more distanced than ever from their patients. Relying totally on mechanical monitoring devices to detect clinical abnormalities is dangerous. *The focus must always be on the child and the surgical field. Monitors may fail, and if the anesthesiologist focuses attention on the monitor in an effort to interpret it, rather than attending directly to the patient, the patient may suffer.* This is the reason that a precordial stethoscope is so useful; strong heart tones in the face of failed monitors provides assurance that the child is likely not in severe trouble.

Induction and Maintenance of Anesthesia

Significant differences in the physiology and behavior of a child, especially a newborn, in comparison with an adult, mandate that the anesthesiologist not consider a child as merely a small adult. In an infant, the rate of uptake of inhalation anesthetic agents is more rapid than in an adult. An infant's response to most oral and intravenous medications is also different; therefore, changes made in concentration of an inspired inhalation agent should be more gradual and the doses of medication diluted and carefully titrated.

The approach to an anesthetic procedure in a child is in principle similar to that in an adult. In practice, however, it is often advisable to modify the sequence of application of monitoring devices. In a relatively stable child, anesthesia induction may proceed with a precordial stethoscope and pulse oximeter, with the remaining monitors applied after anesthesia is induced. This sequence often avoids a prolonged preparation phase during which a child may have more time to become upset. In a critically ill child, however, while attempting always to approach a child in the least threatening way, establishing monitoring must not be compromised. Thus, therapeutic interventions in very sick children and adults proceed along similar pathways. Obviously in a struggling, upset child, some but not all monitors may be successfully applied. The pulse oximeter may not function until the child's finger or toe is relaxed.

Clinical Monitors

In children as in adults, monitoring begins with the basic observations of a patient's general condition, the heart rate, blood pressure, respirations, and temperature. The most important aspect of basic monitoring consists of using the senses of sight, hearing, and touch to integrate all the data provided by patient observations and the monitors.

Sight

Constantly observing a patient's chest excursions (depth and symmetry), the color of the nail beds, oral mucosa, and capillary refill provides vital information about ventilation and perfusion. Observation of the surgical field provides immediate input about fluid shifts, blood loss, the color of the blood in the surgical field, muscle relaxation, depth of anesthesia, and any technical problems related to surgery (e.g., surgical retraction causing venous obstruction).

Hearing

Constantly listening to the quality of the heart tones and breath sounds through a precordial or esophageal stethoscope gives instant feedback about heart rate and rhythm, cardiac output (changes in intensity of heart sounds), and ventilation (wheezing, stridor, laryngeal spasm, no air exchange). This information is particularly helpful in diagnosing arrhythmias, hypovolemia, anesthetic overdose, and airway obstruction. Listening to the sounds of surgery may also be helpful, such as the sudden change in the noise of the suction device with rapid blood loss or the surgeon's comments regarding technical difficulties with the procedure.

Touch

Intermittently examining a patient—especially palpating peripheral pulses and feeling the skin—provides information confirming the auditory input about heart rate, cardiac output, blood pressure, perfusion, and temperature.

Airway and Ventilation

The most important consideration in the safe practice of pediatric anesthesia is attention to the airway. Obstruction occurs readily because of the unique characteristics of an infant's and a child's airway (see Chapter 7). Thus, the anesthesiologist must maintain constant vigilance over the airway to ensure that it remains clear at all times. Airway obstruction leads to hypoventilation, but the causes of hypoventilation may be central (narcotics or inhalation agents) or peripheral (muscle relaxants) in origin. Thus, anesthesiologists must always place emphasis and attention on constantly monitoring the adequacy of ventilation, particularly during anesthesia managed by face mask, because the accuracy of expired carbon dioxide monitoring in this circumstance is often marginal. Although it is desirable to ventilate optimally and maintain an arterial carbon dioxide pressure of approximately 40 mm Hg, rarely at the operating table is an infant or child harmed by mild to moderate overventilation; underventilation has far more serious consequences.

Constant monitoring of inspired oxygen concentrations, expired carbon dioxide concentrations, and oxygen saturation is a valuable adjunct to the senses of sight, hearing, and touch. *Failure to ventilate adequately is probably the most important factor in the morbidity and mortality of children undergoing anesthesia.*

Fluids

Intraoperative fluid management is especially important in infants and children (see Chapter 11). Rapid development of hypovolemia with what may appear to be a trivial amount of blood loss or fluid shifts may occur in infants because of their relatively small blood volume. Replacement of lost blood and basic fluid administration must be carefully titrated (using rate-limiting devices), because overhydration is easily produced. The anesthesiologist should therefore have a clear plan of fluid administration. Preoperative calculation of maintenance, deficit, and potential third-space losses helps in formulating this fluid management plan. A well-planned outline results in a rational and safe approach to correction of fluid deficit, maintenance, and losses (see Chapter 11).

Conduct of the Anesthesia Team

The anesthesiologist must maintain full concentration throughout the procedure; the child's safety is in his or her hands, and any inattention may place the child's life in jeopardy. Should members of the anesthesia team need to replace each other during the anesthetic procedure, it is essential that the "baton" of responsibility be passed in a smooth and coordinated manner. A clear dialogue between team members must be established about the nature of the surgery, the child's underlying conditions, anesthetic agents and other medications, fluid and blood product management, and any special problems. Drugs on the anesthesia machine must be clearly labeled by name and dosage.

Ongoing communication between the anesthesiologist and surgeon is always important, to allow the anesthesiologist to anticipate potential changes in a child's physiologic status due to surgical manipulations and thus to deal with them immediately, appropriately, and more effectively.

The conclusion of an anesthetic procedure is fraught with potential problems. Therefore, the anesthesiologist should not be alone or relax vigilance while a patient is awakening and being transferred to the recovery room or intensive care unit. It is during this stage that patients are most likely to have problems with postanesthetic excitement, vomiting, or airway obstruction (see Chapter 30).

Records of an anesthetic procedure must be accurate and complete; however, anesthesiologists must avoid the compulsion to complete these during the procedure if a child's condition warrants special attention.

Recovery Room

The anesthesiologist's responsibility to a child continues into the recovery room. Transport to the recovery room must be carried out with appropriate monitoring, attention to a clear airway, and adequate ventilation and perfusion. If necessary, battery-powered infusion pumps should be used to maintain accurate infusion of vasopressors. If there is need, oxygen should be administered and oxygen saturation monitored during transport. Oxygen administration is generally advisable in unconscious patients. A clear summary of the medical and surgical problems of the child and of the anesthetic procedure is given to recovery room personnel who will continue to monitor the child. Appropriate resuscitation equipment must be at hand. Vital signs (temperature, heart rate, blood pressure, respirations, and oxygen saturation) are recorded. Special instructions are given relating to fluid management, oxygen administration, drug therapy, analgesics, blood tests (e.g., hematocrit, blood gases, electrolytes, coagulation profile), and radiographs.

Postoperative Visit

The anesthesiologist should visit the child and family postoperatively to assess the postanesthetic clinical course and discuss their reaction to the anesthetic procedure. A note should be placed in the child's record. All too often the anesthesiologist is a "nonperson" in the eyes of the family. If the public is to understand and respect the profession of anesthesiology as a medical specialty, close interaction and trust among parents, child, and anesthesiologist are essential. A follow-up phone call from the nursing staff is also useful in managing anesthetia-related postoperative issues.

Conclusion

This introductory chapter has outlined the fundamentals of pediatric anesthesia practice. The chapters that follow elaborate on these principles, which our collective experience has shown to guide practicing anesthesiologists. We reiterate specific points throughout to emphasize their importance and to present several different perspectives on those issues.

Growth and Development

I. David Todres *and* Jonathan H. Cronin

Normal and Abnormal Growth
  Gestational Age Assessment
  Weight and Length
  Head Circumference
  Face
  Teeth
  Body Composition
Development of Organ Systems
  Development of Airways and Lungs
  Transition to Air Breathing
Mechanics of Breathing
  Chest Wall and Respiratory Muscles
  Elastic Properties of the Lung
  Static Lung Volumes
  Total Lung Capacity
  Functional Residual Capacity
  Closing Capacity
Airway Dynamics
  Resistance and Conductance
  Distribution of Resistance
  Inspiratory and Expiratory Flow Limitation
Gas Exchange
  Regulation of Breathing
  Normal Respiratory Parameters
Cardiovascular System
  Heart Rate
  Blood Pressure
  Cardiac Output
  Normal Electrocardiographic Findings from Infancy to Adolescence
Renal System
Hepatic System
  Physiologic Jaundice
Gastrointestinal Tract
  Swallowing

  Gastroesophageal Reflux
  Meconium
Pancreas
Hematopoietic System
  Coagulation in the Infant
Neurologic Development
  Mental Handicap

We acknowledge the contribution of Ronald Gore, M.D., from the second edition.

As an infant matures, vital changes occur that affect the child's response to disease, drugs, and the environment. Growth is an increase in physical size, and development is an increase in complexity and function. An overview of the subject is presented so that anesthesiologists can appreciate the uniqueness of developing children from both the physical and psychological perspectives. We discuss the respiratory organ system in depth because of its primary considerations for anesthesiologists; however, it is necessary to integrate *all* the organ systems so that a child is treated as a whole.

Normal and Abnormal Growth

Prenatal growth is the most important phase, comprising organogenesis in the first 8 weeks (embryonic growth), followed by the development of organ systems function and maturation of the fetus to full term (fetal growth). Rapid growth occurs particularly in the second trimester; a major increase in weight from subcutaneous tissue and muscle mass occurs in the third trimester. The duration of gestation and the weight of an infant have an important relationship (Table 2–1); deviations from this relationship may be associated with (1) inadequate maternal nutrition (malnutrition or placental insufficiency); (2) significant maternal disease (pregnancy-induced hypertension, diabetes, collagen disorders); (3) maternal toxins (tobacco, alcohol, drugs); (4) fetal infections (toxoplasmosis, rubella, cytomegalovirus, syphilis); (5) genetic abnormalities (trisomy 21, 18, 13); and (6) fetal congenital malformations.

The term *prematurity* has conventionally been applied to infants weighting less than 2500 g at birth; but the designation *preterm infant* is more appropriate and is defined as one born before 37 completed weeks of gestation. A *term infant* is one born after 37 and before 42 completed weeks of

Table 2–1. The Relationship of Gestational Age to Weight

Gestation (weeks)	Mean Weight	
	Grams	*Pounds*
28	1050	2 pounds 4 ounces
32	1700	3 pounds 8 ounces
36	2500	5 pounds 4 ounces
40 (full-term)	3400	7 pounds 8 ounces

gestation. *Postterm infant* refers to an infant born after 42 completed weeks of gestation.

Preterm infants are further classified according to their actual birth weight. A low birth weight infant (LBW) is one weighing less than 2500 g irrespective of the duration of the pregnancy. A very low birth weight (VLBW) infant weighs less than 1500 g, and an extremely low birth weight infant weighs less than 1000 g. In addition, infants weighing less than 750 g are now being called micropremies; there is little published information regarding the anesthetic management of this vulnerable subpopulation.

An infant may also be classified as small for gestational age (SGA), large for gestational age (LGA), or appropriate for gestational age (AGA) depending on where the infant's birth weight plots out on a fetal growth curve. SGA infants (those whose weight is below the 10th percentile at any gestational age) have usually been affected by intrapartum factors that have led to intrauterine malnutrition, such as toxemia and placental insufficiency. Other known causes include intrauterine infections, chromosomal abnormalities, and congenital malformations.[1] SGA infants are particularly prone to hypoglycemia, hypocalcemia, polycythemia, poor temperature regulation, and, potentially, mental and physical handicaps. Problems associated with length of gestation and body weight are summarized in Table 2–2.

Infants classified as LGA (those whose weight is above the 90th percentile at any gestational age) are usually born to mothers whose pregnancy has been complicated by diabetes. The increased weight is the result of organomegaly and excessive deposition of subcutaneous fat secondary to increased fetal insulin produced in response to maternal hyperglycemia. With improved control of maternal diabetes with home blood glucose monitoring, these infants are less likely to be LGA, and therefore are at less risk for hypoglycemia, polycythemia, birth trauma, hyaline membrane disease, and congenital malformations.[2, 3]

Gestational Age Assessment

The gestational age of an infant may be assessed in one of three ways. The most accurate means of assessing gestational age is by measuring the crown-rump length of the fetus during a first trimester ultrasonographic examination. Another method involves calculating gestational age from the first day of the mother's last menstrual period, but this is commonly inaccurate, leading to errors in estimation. Finally, the Dubowitz scoring system is a well-accepted method combining neurologic and physical criteria of the infant to provide an accurate assessment of gestational age.[4, 5] A summary of the more significant neurologic and physical signs of maturity is presented in Table 2–3.

Weight and Length

Assessment of growth is measured by changes in weight, length, and head circumference. Percentile charts are valuable for monitoring the child's growth and development. Deviation from growth within the same percentile for a child of any age is of greater significance than any single

Table 2–2. Common Neonatal Problems with Respect to Weight and Gestation

Gestation	Relative Weight	Neonatal Problems at Increased Incidence
Preterm (<37 weeks)	SGA	Hyaline membrane disease
		Apnea
		Perinatal depression
		Hypoglycemia
		Polycythemia
		Hypocalcemia
		Hypomagnesemia
		Hyperbilirubinemia
		Viral infection
		Thrombocytopenia
		Congenital anomalies
		Maternal drug addiction
		Fetal alcohol syndrome
	AGA	Hyaline membrane disease
		Apnea
		Hypoglycemia
		Hypocalcemia
		Hypomagnesemia
		Hyperbilirubinemia
	LGA	Hyaline membrane disease
		Hypoglycemia: infant of a diabetic mother
		Apnea
		Hypocalcemia
		Hypomagnesemia
		Hyperbilirubinemia
Normal (37–42 weeks)	SGA	Congenital anomalies
		Viral infection
		Thrombocytopenia
		Maternal drug addiction
		Perinatal depression
		Hypoglycemia
	AGA	—
	LGA	Birth trauma
		Hyperbilirubinemia
		Hypoglycemia: infant of a diabetic mother
Postmature (>42 weeks)	SGA	Meconium aspiration syndrome
		Congenital anomalies
		Viral infection
		Thrombocytopenia
		Maternal drug addiction
		Perinatal depression
		Aspiration pneumonia
		Hypoglycemia
	AGA	—
	LGA	Birth trauma
		Hyperbilirubinemia
		Hypoglycemia: infant of a diabetic mother

AGA, appropriate for gestational age; LGA, large for gestational age; SGA, small for gestational age.

Table 2–3. Neurologic and External Physical Criteria to Assess Gestational Age

Physical Exam	Preterm (<37 weeks)	Term (≥37 weeks)
Ear	Shapeless, pliable	Firm, well formed
Skin	Edematous, thin skin	Thick skin
Sole of foot	Creases on anterior third	Whole foot creased
Breast tissue	Less than 1 mm diameter	More than 5 mm diameter
Genitalia		
Male	Scrotum poorly developed	Scrotum rugated
	Testes undescended	Testes descended
Female	Large clitoris, gaping labia majora	Labia majora developed
Limbs	Hypotonic	Tonic (flexed)
Grasp reflex	Weak grasp	Can be lifted by reflex grasp
Moro reflex	Complete but exhaustible (>32 weeks)	Complete
Sucking reflex	Weak	Strong, synchronous with swallowing

measurement (Figs. 2–1 and 2–2). Weight is a more sensitive index of well-being, illness, or poor nutrition than length or head circumference and is the most commonly used measurement of growth. Change in weight reflects changes in muscle mass, adipose tissue, skeleton, and body water and thus is a nonspecific measure of growth. Measurement of length provides the best indicator of skeletal growth because it is not affected by changes in adipose tissue or water content.

Term infants may lose 5 to 10% of their body weight during the first 24 to 72 hours of life from loss of body water. Birth weight is usually regained in 7 to 10 days. A daily increase of 30 g (210 g/wk) is satisfactory for the first 3 months. Thereafter, weight gain slows so that at 10 to 12 months of age it is 70 g each week. For full-term infants, birth weight is approximately doubled at 6 months and tripled at 1 year (Table 2–4).

Preterm infants may lose up to 15% of their body weight during the first 7 to 10 days of life. This significant weight loss is secondary to the fact that premature infants have a higher percentage of total body water per unit weight than term infants do (Table 2–5). Regaining birth weight is very variable, depending on the infant's gestational age and medical problems. Whereas healthy LBW infants can regain birth

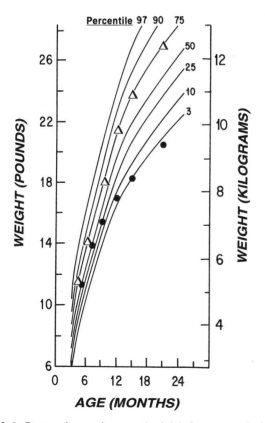

Figure 2–1. Postnatal growth curve (weight) for term male infants. This figure represents normal growth curves. Triangles indicate a normal child. Circles demonstrate failure to thrive in a child with severe renal failure.

Figure 2–2. Postnatal growth curve (weight) for preterm infants. This figure represents normal growth curves for preterm infants. Triangles indicate a normal preterm infant. Circles demonstrate failure to thrive in an infant with bronchopulmonary dysplasia.

Table 2–4. The Relationship of Age to Weight

Age (years)	Weight (kg)
1	10
3	15
5	19
7	23

weight in approximately 10 to 14 days, VLBW and smaller infants may take as long as 3 to 4 weeks. Preterm infants gain weight more slowly than term infants (20 g/day) in general, but it is common for them to have significant growth spurts during the first year of life. When plotting the weight of a premature infant on a growth chart, it is common to use the infant's corrected gestational age instead of his or her chronologic age during the first 2 years of the infant's life so as to correct for prematurity.

Knowledge of the average weight at various ages is helpful in judging whether an infant possibly has a growth-limiting illness. Anesthesiologists should recognize an infant or child whose weight deviates from normal. Failure to thrive indicates that a serious underlying disorder that could significantly affect the anesthetic procedure may be present (Table 2–6).

Head Circumference

Head size reflects growth of the brain and correlates with intracranial volume and brain weight. Changing head circumference reflects head growth and is a part of the total body growth process; it may or may not indicate underlying involvement of the brain. The mean expected head circumference for preterm and full-term newborns is presented in Table 2–7. An abnormally large or small head may indicate abnormal brain development, which must alert the anesthesiologist to possible underlying neurologic problems. A large head may indicate a normal variation, familial feature, or pathologic condition (e.g., hydrocephalus or increased intracranial pressure), whereas a small head may indicate a normal variant, a familial feature, or pathologic condition such as craniostenosis or failure of brain development and mental subnormality.

During the first year of life, head circumference normally increases 10 cm, and 2.5 cm in the second year. By 9 months of age, head circumference reaches 50% of adult size, and by 2 years it is 75%. For the first 6 months of life, the circumference of the head is greater than that of the thorax. After 2 years of age, the head circumference increases much less rapidly (i.e., 2 to 3 cm during the next 10 years). Head

Table 2–6. Common Causes of Failure to Thrive

Genetic: parental size, chromosomal disorders
Nutritional: inadequate or inappropriate intake, malabsorption, diarrhea, vomiting, cystic fibrosis, celiac disease, carbohydrate intolerance, milk protein allergy
Malformations: especially cardiac or urinary tract
Infections: pulmonary, renal, hepatic, enteral, congenital infections
Metabolic/endocrine disorders: hypothyroidism, renal tubular acidosis
Preterm and small-for-gestational-age infants
Malignancy
Bronchopulmonary dysplasia

circumference is closely followed on standard percentile growth curves. As with weight, deviations of growth of the head within the same percentile are more significant than a single measurement; head circumference must be correlated with a child's body weight.

The anterior fontanelle should be palpated to assess whether it is sunken (dehydration) or bulging abnormally, which suggests increased intracranial pressure (hydrocephalus, infection, hemorrhage, increased carbon dioxide tension [$Paco_2$]). If it is bulging, the sutures should be palpated for abnormal separation due to increased intracranial pressure. The anterior fontanelle closes between 9 and 18 months of age; the posterior fontanelle closes by about 4 months of age. Premature synostosis of sutures (craniosynostosis) can result in an abnormal head shape and may retard brain growth and development. The head may be abnormal in shape as a result of genetic and not necessarily pathologic causes. Cranial molding is seen particularly in LBW infants and is usually of no clinical importance.

Face

Although the cranial vault increases rapidly in size, the face and base of the skull develop at a slower rate. At birth, the mandible is small, but as a child develops, forward growth occurs, reducing the obliquity of the mandibular angle. Failure of prenatal development of the mandible may be associated with severe congenital defects (e.g., Pierre Robin, Treacher Collins, or Goldenhar syndrome). These syndromes often have other associated anomalies. After 2 years of age, although the cranial vault increases relatively little in size, a significant change in facial configuration occurs. The upper jaw grows rapidly to accommodate the developing teeth. In addition, the frontal sinuses develop by 2 to 6 years of age, and the maxillary, ethmoidal, and sphenoidal sinuses appear after 6 years of age.

Table 2–5. Relationship of Age to Total Body Water

Age	Body Water (%)
Fetus	90
Preterm	80
Full-term	70
6–12 months	60

Table 2–7. Relationship of Gestational Age to Head Circumference

Gestation (weeks)	Head Circumference (cm)
28	25
32	29
36	32
40 (full-term)	35

Teeth

The first tooth, usually a lower incisor, erupts at approximately 6 months of age (deciduous dentition). Eruption of all deciduous teeth is usually complete by 28 months of age. Permanent teeth appear at 6 years, with the shedding of the deciduous teeth; this process takes place during the next 6 to 8 years. Poor nutrition and chronic illness may interfere with calcification of deciduous and permanent teeth. *Loose teeth should be sought in any child between the ages of 5 and 10 years* or when severe dental caries occur as a result of poor dental hygiene and infection. Care must be taken when placing an oral airway and performing laryngoscopy in children with loose teeth. Abnormally developed teeth occur with hereditary disturbances, Down syndrome, cerebral palsy, and nutritional defects. Premature infants may show severe enamel hypoplasia in their primary dentition.[6] Tetracycline administration during the period of calcification in children leads to permanent discoloration.

Body Composition

The more immature an infant, the greater the relative water content (see Table 2–5). Serial measurements of the extracellular volume of VLBW infants (<32 weeks of gestation) show a postnatal reduction of the extracellular volume with natriuresis in the first 2 weeks of life. This represents a physiologic reduction of the expanded extracellular volume of a fetus. Hyponatremia occurring after the first 2 weeks of life may be an indication of excessive sodium loss and extracellular volume depletion.[7] Total body water decreases at the expense of the extracellular compartment, with adult levels attained at 1 year of age.[8] This finding has implications for drug dosage and distribution in the infant (see Chapter 8). Males have a higher percentage of water, whereas females have a slightly higher percentage of fat. The percentage decrease in extracellular volume is greater than the decrease in total body water because of the simultaneous increase in intracellular water.

Development of Organ Systems

Development of Airways and Lungs

Neonatal respiratory dysfunction is common because the process of lung development is protracted and differentiation of anatomic structures for gas exchange occurs late in gestation. The limit of viability is around the 24th week, when the lungs develop a gas exchanging surface and surfactant production begins. Thereafter, survival increases markedly.

Laws of Lung Development

Normal lung growth is governed by three "laws" that describe the temporal development of the conducting airways, alveoli, and pulmonary vessels.[9]

1. *Airways*: The bronchial tree down to and including the terminal bronchioles forms by the 16th week of gestation. The acinus, consisting of all the airway structures distal to the terminal bronchiole and the entire gas exchanging apparatus, develops throughout the remainder of gestation.

2. *Alveoli*: Alveoli develop mainly after birth, increasing in number until approximately 8 years of life and in size until growth of the chest wall ceases.

3. *Pulmonary vessels*: Arteries and veins accompanying the bronchial tree form by the 16th week of gestation. Those vessels lying within the acinus follow the development of the alveoli. The appearance and growth of arterial smooth muscle lags behind the sprouting of new vessels and is not completed until late adolescence.

Embryology of the Lungs

The lung bud appears as a diverticulum of the embryonic foregut around day 26 of gestation,[10] elongating to form the primordial trachea and branching to form the bronchial tree and the epithelial lining of the lungs, including the alveoli. By day 52, the segmental bronchi are present and the diaphragm is complete, marking the end of the embryonic phase of development, which is succeeded by three stages of fetal tissue differentiation.[11]

1. The *glandular stage* (7–16 weeks) includes formation of intrasegmental airways and associated vessels. Differentiation of cartilage begins in the trachea and mainstem bronchi at 10 weeks, reaching the smallest bronchi at term.

2. The *canalicular stage* (16–24 weeks) involves growth of the liquid-filled airways, forming new branches that constitute the first vestiges of the acinus. By the end of this stage, two milestones are achieved: A viable gas exchanging surface forms, and surfactant production begins.[12, 13] At 24 weeks, the distance separating the capillaries from the potential air spaces is roughly two to three times the adult value, and the type II pneumocytes begin producing surfactant.[14] Infants born at this gestational age may survive even though their lungs are very primitive and the surface area available for gas exchange is at an order of magnitude less than at term.[15]

3. The *terminal saccule* or *alveolar stage* (24 weeks to term) involves further intra-acinar branching of the airway epithelium, forming alveolar ducts and sacs.[16] The surface area available for gas exchange increases exponentially, and its thickness decreases.[15] From 30 to 36 weeks, surfactant secretion into the amniotic fluid increases, providing a clinically useful indicator of lung maturity.[17] The incidence of respiratory distress syndrome declines rapidly during this period and is very low after 35 to 36 weeks of gestation.

Development of the Pulmonary Vessels

The main pulmonary artery and veins develop with the heart and secondarily link up with the lungs. The main pulmonary artery, its first-degree branches, and the ductus arteriosus are derived from the right sixth branchial arch artery (its companion on the left side involutes). The four main pulmonary veins are derived from a vessel that sprouts from the left side of the embryonic atrium.

By the third week of gestation, the heart tube forms and connects with the arterial and venous systems at its cranial and caudal ends. Early in gestation, the heart is located ventrally in the pharyngeal region; it later moves into the thorax. The ventral aorta links with right and left dorsal aortas (which fuse caudally) via the paired branchial cleft arteries, which appear during the fifth week. The sixth arch arteries give off branches that connect with a pre-existing vascular plexus in the lung bud. A few days later, the ventral aorta divides so that only blood from the right ventricle enters the lungs. Around this time, paired segmental branches of the dorsal aortas also supply the lungs. In normal development, these are lost; true bronchial arteries develop between weeks 9 and 12.

The main pulmonary veins develop a few days later than the pulmonary arteries. Venous blood initially drains into the systemic vessels of the foregut. A capillary outgrowth from the left side of the atrium connects with the lung vessels. The primitive pulmonary vein bifurcates several times, but the first two branches are later incorporated into the wall of the atrium, which is then perforated by four separate venous channels. By the seventh week, the typical fetal pattern of blood flow is established, that is, into the lungs via the main pulmonary artery, directly into the aorta via the larger ductus arteriosus, and from the lungs to the left atrium via the pulmonary veins.[10] Although intrapulmonary vessels develop at the same time as the epithelial elements with which they are associated (namely, all preacinar arteries form in the first 16 weeks of gestation), their branching pattern is more complicated than that of the airways because they are more numerous.[18, 19]

In fetuses and adults, arterial wall structure changes in an orderly sequence along each arterial pathway from the hilum to the periphery.[20] The large proximal vessels have an elastic structure. Distally they are replaced by smaller muscular arteries. In smaller vessels, the continuous layer of medial smooth muscle gives way to a spiral that incompletely envelops the arterial wall; these are called *partially muscular arteries*. The smallest vessels just proximal to the capillary bed lack a muscle layer and are called *nonmuscular arteries*.

Although the structural sequence is the same in fetuses and adults, important age-related differences are noted.[18] In a fetus, elastic tissue is less differentiated than in an adult, especially before 12 weeks, and mature smooth muscle is not present before 23 weeks. The zone of transition from the elastic to the muscular structure gradually extends peripherally during the first half of gestation, reaching the seventh generation (the same as in an adult) by the 19th week. The transition from muscular to partially muscular and from partially muscular to nonmuscular arteries occurs more proximally in a fetus than in an adult. At birth, no muscular arteries are found beyond the level of the terminal bronchiole, whereas in an adult, fully muscular arteries are found even in the walls of alveoli.[20] The fetal pulmonary circulation may be said to be less muscular than the adult circulation. However, fetal pulmonary arteries are more muscular; for muscularized vessels of a given external diameter, the muscle layer is thicker in a fetus than in an adult.[11]

Circulation of blood through the fetal pulmonary circuit is limited by vessel diameter, vessel number, and vasoconstriction.[21] In fetal lambs, during the second half of gestation, pulmonary blood flow increases from 3.5% to 10% of the combined output of the right and left ventricles, reflecting growth of the pulmonary vascular bed.[22] The increase in pulmonary blood flow occurring after birth is a consequence of rapid arterial dilation and the closure of extrapulmonary

shunt pathways. Growth of the pulmonary vascular bed may be disturbed in many conditions, particularly those involving lung hypoplasia such as congenital diaphragmatic hernia (see Chapter 14). In cases of severe lung hypoplasia, the size and number of vessels may be so reduced that the pulmonary circulation cannot accommodate the cardiac output at normal pressure, even with maximal dilation.

The pattern of muscularization of pulmonary arteries may be disturbed prenatally, most strikingly in persistent pulmonary hypertension of the newborn. In this condition, muscularization of peripheral arteries is exaggerated; affected infants are born with smooth muscle down to the level of the alveolar wall, as found in adults.[23] Clinically, infants with persistent pulmonary hypertension of the newborn demonstrate increased pulmonary vascular reactivity, leading to episodic pulmonary hypertension and right-to-left shunting with resultant hypoxemia.[24]

Postnatal Lung Growth

Around birth, shallow indentations (primordial alveoli) appear in the walls of the terminal saccules.[25, 26] Mature alveoli are seen around 5 weeks of age; alveolar multiplication continues until the age of 8 years.[9, 26] Full-term newborns have approximately 20 million gas-exchanging saccules, compared with 300 million in adults.[26] For the first 3 years, alveolar numbers increase but size remains relatively constant. Thereafter, size increases progressively until full stature is achieved. The increase in alveolar number and size produces an increase in alveolar surface area from about 1.8 m^2 at birth to between 40 m^2 and 120 m^2 in adults.[27] The increase in surface area is greatest in the first 5 years of life, paralleling the period of rapid alveolar multiplication.

As alveoli increase in number, so do the number of intra-acinar vessels (arteries and veins). The number of arteries per unit area of lung increases in the first 3 years of life but decreases after about 5 years as alveolar diameter increases.[26, 28] Arterial structure also changes throughout childhood as there is a gradual peripheral extension of the smooth muscle layer.[9] There are no fully muscular arteries in the gas-exchanging region at birth. Fully muscular arteries are observed at the alveolar duct level by 10 years, but not until 19 years are they seen at the level of the alveolar wall. Postnatal proliferation and muscularization of the pulmonary vessels may be disturbed in any condition with abnormal pulmonary blood flow, most notably in association with congenital heart lesions with increased or decreased pulmonary blood flow (see Chapters 17 and 18).

Although airway number does not increase after the 16th week of gestation, growth in length and size continue throughout childhood. Comparisons of airway diameter at different levels and various ages indicate that growth is symmetrical in different parts of the bronchial tree, from the mainstem bronchi downward.[29]

Transition to Air Breathing

Fetal breathing movements have been detected as early as 11 weeks of gestational age; they are interspersed with long periods of apnea and produce little tidal movement of lung fluid.[30, 31] The critical event in the change from placental to pulmonary gas exchange is the first inspiration, which initiates pulmonary ventilation, promotes the clearance of lung fluid, and triggers the change from the fetal to the neonatal pattern of circulation.

In late gestation, the volume of lung fluid approximates postnatal functional residual capacity (30 mL/kg).[32] During normal birth, a portion of this fluid is squeezed out through the upper airway as the thorax is compressed in the birth canal; elastic recoil of the chest wall helps to inflate the lungs. These events are not a necessary prelude to the first breath, as most babies born by cesarean section have no difficulty clearing the fluid from their lungs.[33] The first breath is a gasp that generates a transpulmonary distending pressure of 40 to 80 cm H_2O.[34] This moves the tracheal fluid (100 times more viscous than air), overcomes surface forces that develop as the air/fluid interface reaches the small airways, and overcomes tissue resistance. As the lung fills with air, inspiration becomes less forceful. Lung fluid is expelled through the airway or absorbed into the lung interstitium, where it is drawn into the circulation by oncotic forces or carried away as increased lymph flow.[35] In some children, the removal of lung fluid may be delayed, producing the syndrome called *transient tachypnea of the newborn*.[36] Tachypnea lasts for 24 to 72 hours and is associated with a characteristic chest radiographic appearance consisting of increased perihilar markings, fluid in the interlobar fissures, and streaky linear opacities in the parenchyma.

With the onset of pulmonary ventilation, pulmonary blood flow sharply increases. Decreased pulmonary vascular resistance (PVR) and increased peripheral systemic vascular resistance (loss of the umbilical circulation) are the two crucial events involved in the immediate transition from the fetal circulation to the normal postnatal pattern (see Chapter 17). The increase in systemic afterload causes an immediate closure of the flap valve mechanism of the foramen ovale and reverses the direction of shunt through the ductus arteriosus. Until these fetal shunt pathways close anatomically, the pattern of circulation is unstable. Increased pulmonary vascular reactivity in response to hypoxia and acidosis may precipitate a reversal to right-to-left shunting.

The decrease in PVR may be produced in part by mechanical stretching of small arteries or by the secretion of vasoactive substances triggered by lung inflation; however, the major factor is the sudden increase in oxygen in the pulmonary vessels with the onset of ventilation.[21, 37] In addition to the immediate change in PVR that occurs in the first few hours of life, a slower increase occurs in the compliance of small muscular pulmonary arteries during the first few days of life, further contributing to a decline in pulmonary artery pressure and augmentation of pulmonary blood flow.[20]

In the first few minutes of life, a state of "normal" asphyxia exists as a result of impairment of placental blood flow during labor. The arterial oxygen tension (Pao_2) and pH are low, whereas $Paco_2$ is high immediately after birth, but these parameters change rapidly in the first hour of life. Extrapulmonary shunting through fetal channels and intrapulmonary shunting, probably through unexpanded regions of the lung, persist for some time after birth, so that in newborns the physiologic right-to-left shunt is about three times that in adults.[38]

Mechanics of Breathing

Chest Wall and Respiratory Muscles

The accessory muscles of inspiration are relatively ineffective in infants compared with those of adults because of an unfavorable anatomic rib configuration. In infancy, the ribs extend horizontally from the vertebral column, moving little with inspiration.[39] Furthermore, the chest wall is easily deformed, tending to move inward on inspiration. These factors increase the work load on the diaphragm. Consequently, and in contrast with an adult, thoracic cross-sectional area is fairly constant throughout the breathing cycle, and inspiration occurs almost entirely as a result of diaphragmatic descent. After assuming an upright posture, a young child gradually acquires the caudal slant and downward rotation of the ribs that are characteristic of an adult.

The chest wall of a newborn infant is floppy because it has a high content of cartilage, its musculature is poorly developed, and the ribs are incompletely calcified.[40] Intercostal muscle tone stabilizes the chest wall of a term neonate, who usually exhibits retractions only during rapid eye movement sleep when these muscles are inhibited.[41] Chest wall stiffness varies directly with gestational age; therefore, preterm infants have more severe retractions, which occur in all stages of the sleep-wake cycle.[42] Paradoxic chest wall movement commonly occurs in young children after infancy whenever there is an increase in respiratory effort. It frequently occurs under general anesthesia as a consequence of upper airway obstruction but may also be caused by depression of intercostal muscle tone. Inward movement of the rib cage opposes the inspiratory action of the diaphragm. As its severity increases, diaphragmatic displacement must also increase to maintain tidal volume. The increased work load may lead to diaphragmatic fatigue and respiratory failure or apnea, especially in premature infants.[43, 44]

The tendency to respiratory muscle fatigue is the result of the metabolic characteristics of the diaphragm, which has a low content of type I (slow twitch, high oxidative capacity) muscle fibers. Before 37 weeks of gestational age, fatigue-resistant fibers make up less than 10% of the total.[45] A high proportion of type I fibers confers fatigue resistance. Type I muscle fibers constitute about 50% of the fibers in an adult's diaphragm but only 25% of the diaphragm in a term infant (see Fig. 7–11).

Elastic Properties of the Lung

Changes in the static pressure-volume relationship of the lungs during growth are caused by increases in volume and changes in the elastic properties of lung tissue. Volume is the principal factor that determines lung compliance, which increases throughout childhood. To make comparisons that are less dependent on size, compliance is frequently indexed to some parameter of growth such as functional residual capacity (FRC) or total lung capacity (TLC). The resultant indexed value is called *specific compliance* to distinguish it from the raw value. Specific lung compliance remains relatively constant throughout childhood.[46] In contrast, specific compliance of the chest wall declines throughout childhood and adolescence, reflecting the progressive calcification of the ribs and the increasing bulk of the thoracic muscles. Specific compliance of the entire respiratory system also declines because of the changes in the chest wall.[47, 48]

Elastic recoil pressure (the recoil pressure of the lung at a specified reference volume) increases throughout childhood, reaches a peak in late adolescence, and declines thereafter. Structural studies indicate that the period of increasing elastic recoil coincides with an increase in the pulmonary content

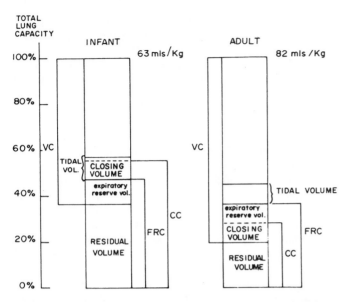

Figure 2–3. Lung volumes in infants and adults. Note that in infants, tidal volume breathing occurs at the same volume as closing volume. (From Nelson NM: Respiration and circulation after birth. In Smith CA, Nelson NM (eds): The Physiology of the Newborn Infant, p 207. Springfield, IL, Charles C Thomas, 1976.)

of elastic fibers, whereas the phase of decreasing elastic recoil coincides with the gradual deterioration of these fibers with aging.[49, 50] Elastic recoil is an important determinant of static lung volume.

Static Lung Volumes

Figure 2–3 summarizes the major differences in static lung volumes between infants and adults. TLC in relation to body weight is indicated for each, and other volumes are shown as fractions of TLC. More detailed information expressing static lung volumes on the basis of body weight are detailed in Table 2–8.

Total Lung Capacity

Adults have a markedly greater TLC than infants. This difference reflects the fact that TLC is an effort-dependent parameter, depending on the strength and efficiency of the inspiratory muscles, which can be estimated by the maximum inspiratory pressure at FRC. An adult can generate pressures in excess of 100 cm H_2O; inspiratory pressures as high as 70 cm H_2O have been recorded for neonates, a surprisingly high value in view of their underdeveloped musculature and highly compliant chest wall. This may be a consequence of the small radius of curvature of an infant's rib cage, which by the Laplace relationship converts a small tension into a large pressure difference.[49]

Functional Residual Capacity

Functional residual capacity (FRC) is similar on a per kilogram basis at all ages, but the mechanical factors on which it is based are different in infants and adults.[51] In adults, FRC is the same as the volume at which the elastic forces generated by the passive recoil of the chest wall are balanced by the recoil of the lung (Fig. 2–4); this is the volume attained at end-expiration with an open glottis.

In an infant, the elastic recoil of the chest is exceedingly small, and the recoil pressure of the lung is less than an adult's. An analysis of these forces reveals that if they are brought into equilibrium, a value for FRC around 10% of TLC is predicted instead of the observed value of slightly less than 40%.[52] Thus, the FRC in an infant is set by a cessation of exhalation at a lung volume in excess of its relaxation volume, so-called laryngeal braking, that is, prolongation of the expiratory time constant.[53] This observation is confirmed by the fact that apneic lung volume is less than

Table 2–8. Age-Dependent Respiratory Variables

	NB	6 mo	12 mo	3 yr	5 yr	12 yr	Adult	Units
F	50 ± 1	30 ± 5	24 ± 6	24 ± 6	23 ± 5	18 ± 5	12 ± 3	Breaths/min
TV	21	45	78	112	270	480	575	mL
	6–8						6–7	mL/kg
V_E	1.05	1.35	1.78	2.46	5.5	6.2	6.4	L/min
	200–260						90	mL/kg/min
V_A	665		1245	1760	1800	3000	3100	mL/min
	100–150						60	mL/kg/min
V_D/V_T	0.3						0.3	
VO_2	6–8						3–4	mL/kg/min
VC	120			870	1160	3100	4000	mL
FRC	80			490	680	1970	3000	mL
	30						30	mL/kg
TLC	160			1100	1500	4000	6000	mL
	63						82	mL/kg
pH	7.3–7.4		7.35–7.45				7.35–7.45	
PaO_2	60–90		80–100				80–100	mm Hg
$PaCO_2$	30–35		30–40				37–42	mm Hg

F, frequency; FRC, functional residual capacity; $PaCO_2$, arterial carbon dioxide tension; PaO_2, arterial oxygen tension; TLC, total lung capacity; TV, tidal volume; V_A, alveolar ventilation; V_D/V_T, dead space/tidal volume; V_E, minute ventilation; VC, vital capacity; VO_2, oxygen consumption.

Modified from O'Rourke PP, Crone RK: The respiratory system. In: Gregory GA, ed: Pediatric Anesthesia, 2nd ed. New York: Churchill Livingstone, 1989.

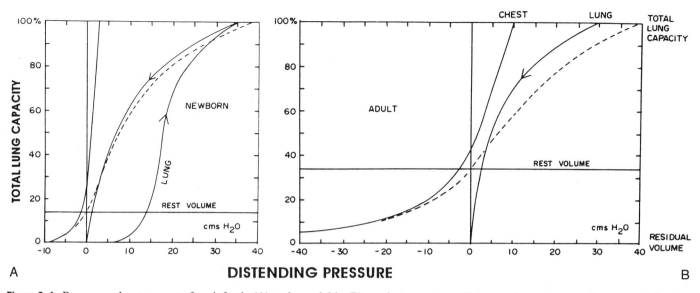

Figure 2–4. Pressure-volume curves of an infant's (A) and an adult's (B) respiratory system. Note that the passive recoil accounted for by the chest is significantly less in newborns than in adults. Theoretically, the resting volume should be less in an infant than in an adult; however, other factors offset the effects of elastic recoil (see text for details). (From Nelson NM: Respiration and circulation after birth. In Smith CA, Nelson NM (eds): The Physiology of the Newborn Infant, p 205. Springfield, IL, Charles C Thomas, 1976.)

FRC in an infant. This volume is close to the collapse volume of the lungs because intrapleural pressure is nearly equal to atmospheric pressure in an apneic infant whose chest wall elastic recoil pressure is so low. In fact, the major factor preventing complete collapse of the lungs is airway closure, which is directly related to lung elastic recoil.[49] It is unknown at what age FRC ceases to be determined by dynamic rather than passive factors.

An important clinical implication of the dynamic control of FRC is that an apneic infant has a disproportionately smaller store of intrapulmonary oxygen on which to draw than a similarly affected adult. This is one of the reasons hypoxemia develops rapidly if control of the airway is lost in an anesthetized infant.

Closing Capacity

As exhalation proceeds to completion, small airways in dependent regions of the lung close, leading to air trapping in the affected areas. Closing capacity is closely related to age, declining throughout childhood and adolescence and increasing thereafter throughout adult life. This pattern of change has been related to the development and deterioration of lung elastic tissue and its effect on recoil pressure. The latter is the principal determinant of transmural pressure and therefore patency of the smallest airways, which lack intrinsic stability because they contain no cartilage.

Closing volume is within the range of tidal breathing in some adults older than 40 years and some children younger than 10 years. It is not possible to measure closing volume in children younger than 5 years, but because elastic recoil pressure decreases to very low levels in infancy, it is likely that some airways remain closed throughout tidal breathing. This conclusion is supported by the finding that infants have a large "trapped gas volume" that is not in free communication with the conducting airways. Age-related changes in PaO_2, which parallel the changes in the difference

between FRC and closing volume, may also be related to airway closure.[49]

Airway Dynamics

Resistance and Conductance

Airway resistance declines markedly with growth from 19 to 28 cm H_2O/L/sec in newborns to less than 2 cm H_2O/L/sec in adults.[51, 54] Airway resistance is higher in preterm than in full-term infants. On the other hand, specific airways conductance (reciprocal of resistance) is higher in preterm infants, and it continues to decline throughout the first 5 years of life, probably reflecting disproportionate growth of the gas-exchanging region of the lungs.[55, 56]

Distribution of Resistance

The distribution of airways resistance changes markedly around the age of 5 years. Airway resistance per gram of lung tissue is constant at all ages in the "central airways" (trachea to the 12th to 15th bronchial generation), whereas it decreases markedly around the age of 5 years in the "peripheral airways" (12th to 15th generation to the alveoli). These data explain why young children with inflammation of the small airways (bronchiolitis) suffer a severe impairment of respiratory function, whereas older children and adults with similar pathology have a milder illness.[57]

Inspiratory and Expiratory Flow Limitation

Tracheal compliance in newborns is twice that of adults; it is even greater in preterm infants and appears to be a consequence of cartilaginous immaturity. The functional importance of this finding is that dynamic collapse of the trachea may occur with inspiration and expiration (see Fig. 7–10).

Gas Exchange

Pulmonary gas exchange occurs by diffusion and has the same underlying mechanism for all ages. Of all the factors affecting pulmonary diffusing capacity, the one that changes most in childhood is the surface area of the alveolar-capillary membrane. Total diffusing capacity at term is similar to that of adults when referenced to oxygen consumption or alveolar ventilation, which has been interpreted to mean that gas exchange is flow limited rather than diffusion limited. This is not too surprising in view of the similarity of the thickness of the anatomic barrier to gas exchange in term infants and in adults. On the other hand, it must be borne in mind that the gas-exchanging surface area is smaller in relation to body size in infancy than in adulthood, suggesting that the physiologic reserve for diffusion is reduced in newborns.

Throughout growth and development, diffusing capacity increases linearly with height, which in turn is closely related to lung growth. The range of values at all ages is comparable to adult measurements when allowance is made for height. It is unknown whether diffusion limitation occurs in preterm infants, but the relationship of gestational age to both the thickness of the blood-gas barrier and its surface area suggests that the margin for diffusion limitation declines at earlier gestational ages. Despite the presumed absence of diffusion limitation, the alveolar-arterial oxygen difference ($AaDO_2$) is much higher in full-term neonates than in adults. Not surprisingly, it is even higher in preterm infants. The precise point in infancy at which adult values are reached is not known.

Venous admixture in infants is higher than in adults. The shunt fraction is estimated at 10 to 20% of cardiac output, with values at the upper end of the range occurring immediately postnatally, whereas the resting shunt fraction in adults is 2 to 5%. Intrapulmonary anatomic shunting, perhaps around the mouths of shallow developing alveoli, is a major cause of venous admixture. The nature of ventilation/perfusion imbalance in infants may be different from that in adults, arising from opening and closing of individual lung units rather than from decreased ventilation of open units.[38] Extrapulmonary right-to-left shunting contributes to $AaDO_2$ in the first few hours of life but only episodically thereafter in association with transient reversal of the pressure gradient between the right and left atrium. Episodic shunting may continue up to the time of anatomic closure of the foramen ovale.

Regulation of Breathing

In neonates as in adults, PaO_2, $PaCO_2$, and pH control pulmonary ventilation, with PaO_2 acting mainly through peripheral chemoreceptors in the carotid and aortic bodies and $PaCO_2$ and pH acting on central chemoreceptors in the medulla. Infants respond to an increase in $PaCO_2$ with an increase in alveolar ventilation just as adults; that is, they increase tidal volume and respiratory rate. The strength of the response is directly related to gestational and postnatal age, the principal change being an increase in the slope of the response rather than a change in the apneic threshold.[46, 58] Unlike an adult, an infant's response to hypercapnia is not potentiated by hypoxia. In fact, hypoxia may depress the hypercapnic ventilatory response in term and preterm infants.[59]

High concentrations of oxygen depress newborn respiration, whereas low concentrations stimulate it. The hypoxic response is not sustained. However, sustained hypoxia leads first to a return to baseline ventilation and then to ventilatory depression. This pattern persists longer in preterm infants. This pattern of response persists in normal term infants for the first week of life, after which the response to sustained hypoxia is replaced by a sustained increase in ventilation.[60]

Relatively nonspecific factors such as blood glucose level, hematocrit, and temperature also affect breathing in infants. Hypoglycemia and anemia may limit substrate availability, especially in the presence of increased metabolic demand. Cold stress decreases ventilatory drive through an unknown mechanism.[61]

The Hering-Breuer reflex, consisting of induced apnea in response to lung inflation, appears to be operative in the first few weeks of life. This reflex does not appear to have a role in an adult's respiration.

Periodic breathing commonly occurs in newborn infants. It is characterized by recurrent pauses in ventilation lasting no more than 5 to 10 seconds, alternating with bursts of respiratory activity (Fig. 2–5). Such episodes are not associated with any obvious physiologic impairment. This pattern of breathing is related to gestational age and to the sleep state. It is more common in preterm infants than in term infants and also occurs more frequently during rapid eye movement sleep. Periodic breathing should be distinguished from clinical apnea, which occurs in as many as 25% of all preterm infants but especially the most premature. Apnea of prematurity may be a life-threatening condition. Ventilatory pauses are prolonged and are associated with desaturation of arterial oxygen, bradycardia, and loss of muscle tone (Fig. 2–6). Apneic episodes may be terminated by tactile stimulation but in severe cases may require a resuscitative effort with bag-mask ventilation. Many factors have been implicated in the etiology of apnea of prematurity. These include brainstem immaturity, as reflected in decreased hypercarbic and hypoxic responses or in impulse conduction delays through the brainstem as assessed by auditory evoked poten-

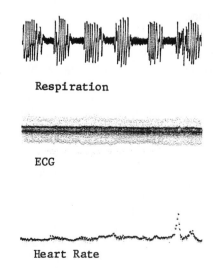

Respiration

ECG

Heart Rate

Figure 2–5. Pneumogram of a normal preterm infant, demonstrating the periodic type of respiratory pattern that is common in premature infants. Note that there are no changes in the heart rate. (Courtesy of Dr. Dorothy Kelly.)

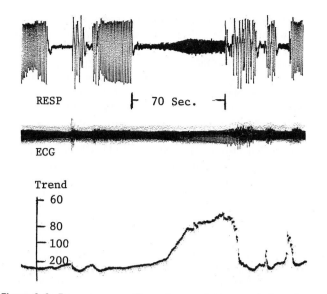

RESP |— 70 Sec. —|

ECG

Trend
|— 60
|— 80
|— 100
|— 200

Figure 2–6. Pneumogram of an abnormal preterm infant demonstrating apnea/bradycardia spells after general anesthesia. Note that severe bradycardia accompanies the apnea. (Courtesy of Dr. Dorothy Kelly.)

tials.[62] Respiratory fatigue precipitated by chest wall distortion has also been strongly implicated.[43] Treatment is directed at increasing the central drive to ventilation (theophylline or caffeine), stabilizing the chest wall (positive end-expiratory pressure), or stimulation by rocking and stroking.

Prematurity is an important risk factor that increases the chance of life-threatening apnea in infants undergoing general anesthesia.[63] The risk of postanesthetic respiratory depression is inversely related to gestational age. It has been stated that infants may be at risk up to 60 weeks postconception[64–66]; however, the greatest risk is in infants 55 weeks or less postconception. Children considered at risk should be monitored in an environment where resuscitative equipment and trained personnel skilled in neonatal resuscitation are readily available (see Chapters 4 and 14).

Normal Respiratory Parameters

The stimulus driving pulmonary ventilation is metabolic demand. The resting oxygen consumption of infants is twice that of adults (see Table 2–8), and this in turn leads to a doubling of alveolar ventilation on a per kilogram basis.[67] Infants increase alveolar ventilation primarily by increasing respiratory rate rather than increasing tidal volume, the latter bearing a constant relationship to body size throughout life. It has been postulated that respiratory rate at different ages is set to minimize the sum of elastic and resistive work of breathing.

Static lung volume (including TLC, vital capacity, FRC, and residual volume) is linearly related to the logarithm of height. A divergence of lung growth between males and females begins in early childhood and produces persistent differences between the sexes in adult life.[68] Part of the increase in the so-called effort-dependent lung volumes (e.g., TLC, vital capacity) is related to the development and efficiency of the diaphragm and other inspiratory muscles. One

measure of the role of muscle strength is the maximum inspiratory pressure at FRC. Maximum inspiratory pressure increases slightly throughout childhood and to a greater extent in adolescence, especially in males.

During the first few hours of life, PaO_2 and $PaCO_2$ change rapidly as an infant recovers from the relative "asphyxia" associated with birth, and a regular pattern of ventilation and stable lung volumes are established. Thereafter, these values remain fairly constant for the first week of life. PaO_2 continues to be depressed in neonates. The lower PaO_2 of neonates is compensated by a higher oxygen-carrying capacity due to high hemoglobin levels, which decline during the first several weeks of life. At birth, the hemoglobin content of the blood is made up of 50% fetal hemoglobin, which has an in vivo oxygen-dissociation curve that is shifted to the left in comparison with normal adult hemoglobin. The position of the whole blood oxygen-dissociation curve depends on the ratio of adult to fetal hemoglobin. It shifts to the right during the course of the first week of life, reflecting a switch from fetal to adult hemoglobin formation.[46]

Normal $PaCO_2$ and pH are somewhat lower in the neonatal period than in later infancy (see Table 2–8). They are even lower in premature infants. Immediately after birth, some degree of metabolic acidosis may be present along with an increase in blood lactate. Another factor of importance is the relatively large extracellular volume of an infant, leading to dilution of blood bicarbonate. The threshold for renal bicarbonate excretion is also reduced in premature infants.

The range of normal values for arterial pH, PaO_2, and $PaCO_2$ is stable from late infancy throughout adult life. However, average PaO_2 gradually increases throughout childhood, with a peak in late adolescence and a gradual decline thereafter throughout adult life. This pattern has been related to lung closing capacity, which is high in infancy, declines throughout childhood to late adolescence, and rises throughout adulthood. Newborn infants and older adults share the characteristic of closure of some airways during tidal ventilation.

Cardiovascular System

An understanding of cardiovascular development is important for anesthesiologists. This section briefly considers developmental changes in heart rate, blood pressure, cardiac output, and the electrocardiogram (ECG); a more detailed description is found in Chapter 17.

Heart Rate

Autonomic control of the heart in utero is mediated predominantly through the parasympathetic nervous system. It is only shortly after birth that sympathetic control appears. In newborn infants, the heart rate may have a wide variation that is within normal limits. In 50% of apparently healthy newborns, 24-hour ECG recordings have shown rhythm changes resembling complete, two-to-one, or Wenckebach sinoatrial block.[69]

In older children, a significant number of arrhythmias and conduction abnormalities are also encountered, with marked fluctuations in heart rate due to variations in autonomic tone. The mean heart rate in newborns in the first 24 hours of life

Table 2–9. The Relationship of Age to Heart Rate

Age	Mean Heart Rate (beats/min)
0–24 hours	120
1–7 days	135
8–30 days	160
3–12 months	140
1–3 years	125
3–5 years	100
8–12 years	80
2–16 years	75

is 120 beats per minute (bpm). It increases to a mean of 160 bpm at 1 month, after which it gradually decreases to 75 bpm at adolescence (Table 2–9).[69]

Blood Pressure

Mean systolic blood pressure in neonates and infants rises from 65 mm Hg in the first 12 hours of life to 75 mm Hg at 4 days and 95 mm Hg at 6 weeks. There is little change in mean systolic pressure between 6 weeks and 1 year of age; between 1 year and 6 years, there is only a slight change, followed by a gradual rise.[70, 71] These measurements apply to infants and children who are awake and quiet. The blood pressure of preterm infants in the first 12 hours is lower than in full-term infants; a gradual rise in blood pressure occurs after birth—68/43 mm Hg on day 1 of life compared with 90/55 mm Hg on day 70 of life (Table 2–10).[72] It has also been noted that infants with birth asphyxia and those on ventilators have lower blood pressures.[73]

Cardiac Output

Myocardial performance may be seriously impaired in a critically ill infant or child. Measurement of cardiac output is a valuable indicator of myocardial contractility and may be superior to the traditional monitors of hemodynamic performance such as capillary refill, heart rate, blood pressure, and urine output. Determination of cardiac output and blood pressure allows calculation of systemic vascular resistance. It provides important information relating to the left ventricular afterload and allows rational application of pressor agents (vasoconstrictor, vasodilator) and inotropic drugs. Measurement of cardiac output may be carried out by the Fick method (using oxygen extraction) or thermodilution using a pulmonary artery flow-directed catheter. In neonates, the latter technique is rarely used, because shunts at the atrial and ductal level introduce errors in interpreting the results.

Pulsed Doppler determinations of cardiac output appear to provide reasonable noninvasive estimates of cardiac output for clinical application in newborns. Cardiac output increases linearly with increasing birth weight. An upper limit of 325 mL/min/kg and lower limit of 200 mL/min/kg are appropriate for clinical use.[74, 75] This resting cardiac output is two to three times adult values. The relatively large cardiac output may reflect the higher metabolic rate and oxygen consumption compared with adults. This higher oxygen consumption may be related in part to the loss of body heat, which is relatively greater in newborns because of the larger surface area in relation to body mass. Pulsed Doppler estimation of cardiac output has been found helpful in assessing left ventricular myocardial dysfunction in neonates from perinatal asphyxia and acidosis and its response to therapy.[76] An excellent review of this topic as well as fetal, transesophageal, intravascular, and three-dimensional echocardiography has been written.[77]

Normal Electrocardiographic Findings from Infancy to Adolescence

Electrocardiographic findings undergo changes with age. Normal patterns in infants are distinctly abnormal if observed at a later stage of growth. The P wave reflects atrial depolarization and varies little with age. The PR interval increases with age (mean value for the first year is 0.10 sec, increasing to 0.14 sec at 12–16 years). The duration of the QRS complex increases with age, but prolongation greater than 0.10 seconds is abnormal at any age.

At birth, the QRS axis is right-sided, reflecting the predominant right ventricular intrauterine development. It moves leftward in the first month as left ventricular muscle hypertrophies. Thereafter, the QRS follows a gradual change away from the initial marked right-sided axis.

At birth, T waves are upright in all chest leads. Within hours, they become isoelectric or inverted over the left chest; by the seventh day, the T waves are inverted in V4R, V1, and across to V4; from then on, the T waves remain inverted over the right chest until adolescence, when they become upright over the right chest again. Failure of T waves to become inverted in V4R and V1 to V4 by 7 days may be the earliest ECG evidence of right ventricular hypertrophy.[78, 79]

Studies of the ECG of premature infants at 1 year of age show that for those without a history of bronchopulmonary dysplasia, the ECG findings are generally similar to the published norms for healthy 1-year-olds. However, in those with residual lung disease, right ventricular hypertrophy is very prevalent. Thus, the ECG may be useful in the follow-up and assessment of infants with chronic residual lung disease.[80]

Renal System

In utero, the kidneys are active organs, producing a large volume of urine and helping to maintain amniotic fluid volume. Potter syndrome, consisting of a disfigured face,

Table 2–10. The Relationship of Age to Blood Pressure

Age	Normal Blood Pressure (mm Hg)	
	Mean Systolic	*Mean Diastolic*
0–12 hours (preterm)	50	35
0–12 hours (full-term)	65	45
4 days	75	50
6 weeks	95	55
1 year	95	60
2 years	100	65
9 years	105	70
12 years	115	75

pulmonary hypoplasia, and skeletal deformities, is a result of lack of amniotic fluid secondary to renal agenesis. In utero, the fetus maintains its metabolic homeostasis thorough the placenta, and it is only after birth that the kidneys assume responsibility for metabolic function. More than 90% of newborns will have voided urine within the first 24 hours after birth. All normal infants should have voided within 48 hours after birth.[81]

At birth, glomerular filtration rate is 15 to 30% of normal adult values but reaches 50% of adult values on the fifth to tenth day and gradually attains adult values at the end of the first year of life.[82] Low glomerular filtration rate significantly affects the neonate's ability to excrete saline and water loads, as well as drugs. Tubular function develops rapidly after 34 weeks of gestation.[83] An infant's immature kidneys respond to stress with changes in their capacity to function; however, a neonate's kidneys do not have the reserve to deal with the stress of serious illness.

The so-called physiologic acidemia of infancy is largely due to a diminished renal tubular threshold for bicarbonate.[84] An infant's kidneys concentrate urine to a maximum of 200 to 800 mOsm/L. This reflects some renal immaturity (fewer and shorter loops of Henle) but is in large part due to the low level of production and excretion of urea by a growing infant. An infant can dilute its urine (to a minimum of 50 mOsm/L) as can an older child; however, the rate of excretion of a water load is less. An infant's urea production is reduced as a result of growth, and thus "immature kidneys" are able to maintain a normal blood urea nitrogen level. Elevated blood urea nitrogen, however, signifies renal failure, excessive dietary intake of protein (blood in the gastrointestinal tract, e.g., necrotizing enterocolitis), or interference with growth due to disease while intake of food has been maintained.

Growth of renal length and cross-sectional area can be related to height or age. Capacity for growth extends into adulthood. For example, if one kidney is removed or destroyed, the remaining normal kidney hypertrophies; most compensatory growth occurs within 6 weeks and is usually complete within 6 months.

Serious renal malfunctioning is usually associated with growth retardation. When this occurs, a child's rate of growth may be below the third percentile for chronologic age (see Fig. 2–1).

Hyperkalemia (defined as a serum potassium concentration of ≥ 6.8 mEq/L) has been noted in preterm infants weighing less than 1000 g and associated with significant ECG dysrhythmias. Hyperkalemia appears to be partly related to immature distal tubule function and a relative hypoaldosteronism.[85]

Hepatic System

Development of the liver and bile ducts begins as an outgrowth of the foregut; by 10 weeks of gestation, the biliary tract has completed its development. The vitelline veins give rise to the portal and hepatic veins. Hepatic sinusoids form the ductus venosus, the bridge between the hepatic vein and the inferior vena cava. Most umbilical venous blood from the placenta passes through the ductus venosus to the inferior vena cava. The remainder passes via the portal vein through the liver to the hepatic veins. The portal venous drainage to the left lobe is less than to the right lobe, leading to a relative underdevelopment of the left lobe. The ductus venosus closes soon after birth.

At 12 weeks of gestation there is evidence of gluconeogenesis and protein synthesis; at 14 weeks, glycogen is found in liver cells. Although by late gestation liver cell morphology is similar to that of adults, the functional development of the liver is immature in newborns, and more so in preterm infants. The liver has a major role in metabolism, controlling carbohydrate, protein, and lipid delivery to the tissues. Toward the end of pregnancy, large amounts of glycogen appear in the liver, and as a result preterm and SGA infants with smaller stores of glycogen are liable to develop hypoglycemia. Bile acid secretion in newborns is depressed, and malabsorption of fat occurs.

The liver is the site for the synthesis of proteins; this process is active in fetal and neonatal life. In fetal life, the main serum protein is alpha-fetoprotein. This protein first appears at 6 weeks of gestation and reaches a peak at 13 weeks. Albumin synthesis starts at 3 to 4 months of gestation and approaches adult values at birth; in preterm infants, the level is lower. Proteins involved in clotting are also formed in the liver and are at a lower level than normal in preterm and full-term neonates for the first few days of life. Hematopoiesis occurs in the fetal liver, with peak activity at 7 months of gestation. After 6 weeks of age, hematopoiesis is confined to the bone marrow except under pathologic conditions, such as hemolytic anemia.

The capacity to enzymatically break down proteins is depressed at birth. This is particularly important in preterm infants, when high protein intake can lead to dangerous levels of serum amino acid concentrations. In the first weeks of life, drug metabolism is less efficient than in later life. In addition to less effective hepatic metabolism, altered drug binding by serum proteins and immature renal function contribute to the problem (see Chapter 8).

Physiologic Jaundice

Hyperbilirubinemia is an especially important problem in neonates. The mechanisms for producing jaundice are outlined in Table 2–11.[86] Increased concentrations of indirect bilirubin usually occur in the first few days of life. In term infants, bilirubin levels of 6 to 8 mg/100 mL are commonly seen within the first 3 days of life. In preterm infants, the peak level of 10 to 12 mg/100 mL occurs on the fifth to seventh day of life. After this period, levels gradually decrease to adult values of less than 2 mg/100 mL in 1 to 2 months for both term and preterm infants. The cause of nonhemolytic physiologic hyperbilirubinemia is excessive bilirubin production from breakdown of red blood cells and increased enterohepatic circulation of bilirubin with deficient

Table 2–11. Causes of Jaundice in Neonates

Excess bilirubin production
Impaired uptake of bilirubin
Impaired conjugation of bilirubin
Defective bilirubin excretion
Increased enterohepatic circulation of bilirubin

hepatic conjugation due to depressed glucuronyl transferase activity. The relationship between breast-feeding and hyperbilirubinemia has been well documented. It is usually delayed in onset (after the third day of life), its cause remains unclear, and it occurs in about 1% of breast-feeding infants. An earlier hypothesis ascribing it to inhibition of glucuronyl transferase by 3-alpha, 20 beta-pregnanediol activity has not been substantiated.

Important pathologic causes of jaundice in newborns are presented in Table 2–12. Once the distinction between physiologic and hemolytic hyperbilirubinemia has been made, the underlying cause can then be treated and efforts can be directed at preventing bilirubin encephalopathy (kernicterus) by the use of phototherapy and, in selected cases, exchange transfusions. Sick preterm infants are especially at risk for kernicterus and are more aggressively treated at lower bilirubin levels than full-term infants.[87] Increasingly common is a form of cholestatic jaundice in LBW infants receiving prolonged hyperalimentation. Its mechanism is unclear, but it may be due to inhibition of bile flow by amino acids.[88] Future therapy for hyperbilirubinemia in LBW infants may include the use of tin-mesoporphyrin, which inhibits the production of bilirubin.[89]

Gastrointestinal Tract

In a fetus, the digestive tract consists of the developing foregut and hindgut. These rapidly elongate so that a loop of gut is forced into the yolk sac. At 5 to 7 weeks, this loop twists around the axis of the superior mesenteric artery and returns to the abdominal cavity. Maturation occurs gradually from the proximal to the distal end. Blood vessels and nerves (Auerbach and Meissner plexus) are developed by 13 weeks of gestation, and peristalsis begins. Parotid, sublingual, and submandibular salivary glands arise from the oral mucosa. The pancreas arises from two outgrowths of the foregut; a diverticulum of the foregut gives rise to the liver.

Enzyme levels of enterokinase and lipase increase with gestational age but are lower at birth than in older children. Nevertheless, newborn and preterm infants are able to handle proteins reasonably well. Preterm infants, however, are unable to tolerate large protein loads. Fat digestion is limited, particularly in preterm infants, who absorb only 65% of adult levels. Neonatal duodenal motility undergoes marked maturational changes between 29 and 32 weeks of gestation. This is one factor limiting tolerance of enteral feeding before 29 to 30 weeks of gestation. Central nervous system abnormalities will delay these maturational changes.[90]

Anomalies arising from maldevelopment of the gut may

Table 2–12. Pathologic Causes of Jaundice in Newborns

Antibody-induced hemolysis (Rh and ABO)
Hereditary red blood cell disorders, e.g., glucose-6-phosphate dehydrogenase deficiency, which gives rise to hemolysis from drugs or infection
Infections, e.g., neonatal hepatitis, sepsis, severe urinary tract infections
Hemorrhage into the body, e.g., intracerebral
Biliary atresia
Metabolic, e.g., hypothyroidism, galactosemia

be appreciated from an understanding of normal development.

- *Esophageal atresia and tracheoesophageal fistula.* This anomaly occurs when the respiratory tract fails to separate completely from the foregut at 4 weeks of gestation. Failure of separation may be seen as a laryngeal cleft. In its extreme form, the cleft may extend from the glottis to the carina.
- *Intestinal atresia and stenosis.* These anomalies are common causes of obstruction in newborns, particularly in the duodenal region; this lesion is frequently associated with Down syndrome. The cause may be a failure of recanalization in utero as a result of a vascular accident (intussusception, volvulus, or thrombosis).
- *Duplication and diverticulum.* These may be blind pouches or may communicate with the intestinal lumen. The mucosa frequently is gastric and liable to hemorrhage. Other complications include obstruction, perforation, and infection. Meckel diverticulum is relatively common and is due to persistence of the vitellointestinal duct.
- *Hirschsprung disease.* Hirschsprung disease is due to failure of development of the Meissner and Auerbach plexus.
- *Peritoneal bands.* These bands, which cause obstruction, result from faulty rotation and fixation of the gut, most commonly at the duodenojejunal junction.
- *Omphalocele and gastroschisis.* In these conditions, intestine protrudes from the abdominal wall as a result of failure of closure of the rectus muscles (omphalocele) at 8 weeks of gestation or herniation of the intestine through a para-umbilical defect (gastroschisis) (see Chapter 14).

Swallowing

Swallowing is a complex procedure that is under central and peripheral control. The reflex is initiated in the medulla, through cranial nerves to the muscles that control the passage of food through the pharyngoesophageal sphincter. In the process, the tongue, soft palate, pharynx, and larynx all are smoothly coordinated. Any pathologic condition of these structures can interfere with normal swallowing. Neuromuscular incoordination, however, is more likely to be responsible for any dysfunction. This is particularly evident when the central nervous system has sustained damage either before or during delivery. With swallowing, pressure in the pharynx rises, the pharyngoesophageal sphincter opens, and peristaltic waves in the upper esophagus carry the bolus of food downward. Peristaltic waves are absent in the lower esophagus in infants, although present in adults. With the immaturity of the pharyngoesophageal sphincter, frequent regurgitation or "spitting" of gastric contents is observed in healthy infants.

Gastroesophageal Reflux

Approximately 40% of newborn infants in the first few days of life regurgitate their food.[91] Lower esophageal pressures are low and take approximately 3 to 6 weeks to achieve adult levels. Symptoms of reflux include persistent vomiting, failure to thrive, and in severe cases hematemesis and anemia, occasionally complicated by stricture formation. These symptoms are also found with hiatal hernia. Gastroesophageal reflux is one of a number of conditions associated with apnea and bradycardia in premature infants.[92]

Meconium

Meconium is the material contained in the intestinal tract before birth. It consists of desquamated epithelial cells from the intestinal tract and bile, pancreatic and intestinal secretions, and water (70%). Meconium is usually passed in the first few hours after birth; virtually all term infants pass their first stool by 48 hours. However, passage of the first stool is usually delayed in LBW infants. Infants weighing less than 1500 g at birth may take up to 6 to 7 days, probably because of immaturity of the motility and lack of gut hormones due to delayed enteral feeding. This normal developmental delay should be appreciated, because late passage of the first stool raises the suspicion of a pathologic condition such as meconium ileus, meconium plug syndrome, or intestinal atresia.[93] Meconium ileus occurs in 10% of children with cystic fibrosis. The meconium is inspissated and causes intestinal obstruction. Newborns who fail to pass meconium may also be suffering from Hirschsprung disease; reduced colonic activity results in increased water absorption and inspissation of the meconium. Meconium in the amniotic fluid may indicate intrauterine asphyxia. Aspiration of meconium may have serious effects on pulmonary function, leading to pneumonia, pneumothorax, and persistent pulmonary hypertension (persistent fetal circulation).[94, 95]

Pancreas

The placenta is impermeable to both insulin and glucagon. The islets of Langerhans in the fetal pancreas, however, secrete insulin from the 11th week of fetal life; the amount of insulin secretion increases with age. After birth, insulin response is related to gestational and postnatal age and is more mature in term infants.

Maternal hyperglycemia, particularly when uncontrolled, results in hypertrophy and hyperplasia of the fetal islets of Langerhans. This leads to increased levels of insulin in the fetus, affecting lipid metabolism and giving rise to a large, overweight infant characteristic of a mother with poorly controlled diabetes. Hyperglycemia alone is not instrumental in this effect; it may also be the result of an increase in serum amino acids found in diabetic mothers. Meticulous control of a mother's diabetes during pregnancy and delivery has led to a reduction in morbidity and mortality of the infants of diabetic mothers. Hyperinsulinemia of the fetus persists after birth and may lead to rapid development of serious hypoglycemia. In addition to severe hypoglycemia, the infant has an increased incidence of congenital anomalies.

Infants who are SGA are frequently hypoglycemic, and this may be the result of malnutrition in utero. Some of these infants secrete inappropriately large amounts of insulin in response to glucose and for this reason may suffer from serious hypoglycemia. In addition, hepatic glycogen stores are inadequate, and deficient gluconeogenesis exists. Preterm infants may be hypoglycemic without demonstrable symptoms, therefore necessitating close monitoring of blood glucose levels.

Full-term neonates undergo a metabolic adjustment after birth with regard to glucose. Studies have defined values for glucose levels below which there should be concern: plasma glucose less than 35 mg/100 mL in the first 3 hours of life; less than 40 mg/100 mL between 3 and 24 hours; and less than 45 mg/100 mL after 24 hours.[96] Others have defined hypoglycemia in full-term infants as a serum glucose concentration of less than 30 mg/100 mL in the first day of life or less than 40 mg/100 mL in the second day of life.[97] It is important to appreciate that infants, although showing no symptoms, may develop serious hypoglycemia leading to irreversible central nervous system damage. Other infants may present with convulsions, but signs may also be subtle (e.g., lethargy, somnolence, and jitteriness).

Hyperglycemia (plasma glucose $\geq$150 mg/100 mL) occurs in stressed neonates, particularly LBW infants infused with glucose-containing solutions. Hyperglycemia has been associated with increased morbidity and mortality. Hyperglycemia commonly occurs in infants undergoing elective surgery under general anesthesia; infusion of glucose-containing solutions may aggravate the tendency to become hyperglycemic. Thus it is advisable that intraoperative glucose levels be monitored. Replacement of blood, "third-space," and deficit fluid losses should be carried out with dextrose-free solutions. Maintenance fluid requirements may be replaced with glucose-containing solutions administered with a constant-infusion pump to avoid bolus glucose administration. A study in infants undergoing surgery under general anesthesia showed that postsurgical plasma glucose values were significantly higher than postinduction values; insulin changes were minimal.[98] The risk of hyperglycemia is considerably greater in infants weighing less than 1000 g compared with infants of 2000 g or more.[99] Hyperglycemia may be due to multiple causes, such as exogenous glucose solutions, lipid infusions, hypoxemia, sepsis, surgical procedures, and drugs such as theophylline. Hyperglycemia may also lead to osmotic diuresis and dehydration and has been associated with an increased incidence of intraventricular hemorrhage and handicap.

The mechanism of glucose intolerance in a neonate depends on the underlying cause. Hypoxemia stimulates alpha-adrenergic receptors and release of catecholamines while diminishing the insulin response.[100–102] Careful titration of glucose according to an infant's needs as measured by plasma blood glucose levels is required. Administration of 3 to 4 mg/kg/min dextrose in infants weighing less than 1000 g is a useful starting point.[103] Adjustments are made according to the infant's needs. Dextrose should be decreased in the infusate should plasma glucose levels exceed 150 mg/100 mL. If this maneuver is inadequate to achieve lower and safer blood glucose levels (i.e., levels are > 250–300 mg/kg), a continuous insulin drip (0.05–0.2 U/kg/hr) can be administrated intravenously and titrated to achieve normoglycemia.[104]

Hematopoietic System

The blood volume of a full-term newborn infant is dependent on the time of cord clamping, which modifies the volume of placental transfusion. Blood volume is 93 mL/kg when cord clamping is delayed after delivery, compared with 82 mL/kg with immediate cord clamping.[105, 106] Within the first 4 hours after delivery, however, fluid is lost from the blood and the plasma volume contracts by as much as 25%. The larger the placental transfusion, the larger this loss of fluid in the first few hours after birth, with resultant hemoconcentration. The blood volume in preterm infants is higher (90 to 105 mL/kg) than in full-term infants because of increased plasma volume.[105]

The normal hemoglobin range is between 14 g/100 mL and 20 g/100 mL. The site of sampling must be considered, however, when interpreting these values for the diagnosis of neonatal anemia or hyperviscosity syndrome. Capillary sampling (e.g., heel stick) gives higher values, as much as 6 g/100 mL, because of stasis in peripheral vessels leading to loss of plasma and hemoconcentration; thus a venipuncture is preferred. In 1% of infants, fetal-maternal transfusion occurs and may be responsible for some of the "lower normal" hemoglobin values reported.

Erythropoietic activity from the bone marrow decreases immediately after birth in both full-term and preterm infants. The cord blood reticulocyte count of 5% persists for a few days and declines below 1% by 1 week. This is followed by a slight increase to 1 to 2% by the 12th week, where it remains throughout childhood. Premature infants have higher reticulocyte counts (up to 10%) at birth. Abnormal reticulocyte values reflect hemorrhage or hemolysis.

In term infants, the hemoglobin concentration falls during the ninth to 12th week to reach a nadir of 10 to 11 g/100 mL (hematocrit 30 to 33%) and then rises. This decrease in hemoglobin concentration is due to a decrease in erythropoiesis and to some extent due to a shortened life span of the red blood cells. In preterm infants, the decrease in the hemoglobin level is greater and is directly related to the degree of prematurity; also, the nadir is reached earlier (4–8 weeks).[107] In infants weighing 800 to 1000 g, the decrement may reach a low of 8 g/100 mL. This "anemia" is a normal physiologic adjustment to extrauterine life. Despite the reduction in hemoglobin, the oxygen delivery to the tissues may not be compromised because of a shift of the oxygen-hemoglobin dissociation curve (to the right), secondary to an increase of 2,3-diphosphoglycerate.[108] In addition, fetal hemoglobin is replaced by adult-type hemoglobin, which also results in a shift in the same direction. In neonates, especially preterm infants, low hemoglobin levels may be associated with apnea and tachycardia.[109] Vitamin E administration does not prevent anemia of prematurity; no significant difference was noted between vitamin E–supplemented and unsupplemented groups in terms of hemoglobin concentration, reticulocyte and platelet counts, or erythrocyte morphology in infants at 6 weeks of age.[110] Infants with anemia of prematurity have been found to have an inadequate production of erythropoietin (the primary regulator in erythropoiesis). Some centers are now using recombinant human erythropoietin in VLBW infants to stimulate erythropoiesis and decrease the need for multiple transfusions.[111]

After the third month, the hemoglobin level stabilizes at 11.5 to 12.0 g/100 mL, until about 2 years of age. The hemoglobin values of full-term and preterm infants are comparable after the first year. Thereafter follows a gradual increase to mean levels at puberty of 14.0 g/100 mL for females and 15.5 g/100 mL for males.

The white blood cell count may normally reach 21,000/mm³ in the first 24 hours of life and 12,000/mm³ at the end of the first week, with the number of neutrophils equaling the number of lymphocytes. It then decreases gradually, reaching adult levels at puberty. At birth, neutrophil granulocytes predominate but rapidly decrease in number so that during the first week of life and through 4 years, the lymphocyte is the predominant cell. After the fourth year, the values approximate an adult's. Neonates have an increased susceptibility to bacterial infection, which is related in part to immaturity of leukocyte function. Sepsis may be associated with a minimal leukocyte response or even with leukopenia. Spurious increases in the white blood cell content may be due to drugs (e.g., epinephrine).

Thrombocytopenia occurs frequently in preterm infants suffering from hyaline membrane disease. Mechanical ventilation has been associated with a significant decrease in the platelet count in newborns.[112] There appears to be an inverse correlation between gestational age or birth weight and the severity of platelet reduction. A study of neonatal thrombocytopenia and its impact on hemostatic integrity showed that thrombocytopenic infants are at greater risk for bleeding than equally sick nonthrombocytopenic infants.[113]

Neonatal polycythemia (central hematocrit > 65%) occurs in 3 to 5% of full-term newborns.[114] In studies of animals, hyperviscosity with a hematocrit exceeding 70% is associated with an increase in systemic and pulmonary vascular resistance and decreased cardiac output.[115] Using M-mode echocardiography, a study of neonates demonstrated an increase in PVR with hyperviscosity.[116] Partial exchange transfusion to lower the hematocrit and decrease the blood viscosity improves systemic and pulmonary blood flow and oxygen transport. The increased organ blood flow should prevent the cardiovascular and neurologic symptoms associated with the hyperviscosity syndrome.[117]

Coagulation in the Infant

At birth, vitamin K–dependent factors (i.e., II, VII, IX, and X) are at levels of 20 to 60% of adult values; in preterm infants, the values are even less. The result is prolonged prothrombin times, normally encountered in full-term and preterm infants. Synthesis of vitamin K–dependent factors occurs in the liver, which, being immature, leads to relatively lower levels of the coagulation factors, even with the administration of vitamin K. It takes several weeks for the levels of coagulation factors to reach adult values; the deficit is even more pronounced in premature infants. Vitamin K prophylaxis has been re-evaluated.[118] The findings show that the majority of cases of neonatal vitamin K deficiency occur in normal newborns. Thus, all newborns should receive prophylactic vitamin K soon after birth to prevent hemorrhagic disease of the newborn. Its omission could lead to serious and life-threatening consequences, especially if surgery is undertaken. Infants of mothers who have received anticonvulsant drugs during pregnancy may develop a serious coagulopathy similar to that encountered with vitamin K deficiency.[119] Vitamin K_1 administered to newborns usually reverses this bleeding tendency, but death has occurred despite therapy. Other risk factors include maternal use of drugs such as warfarin, rifampin, and isoniazid. Breast-feeding may also be associated with severe vitamin K deficiency.

Table 2–13. Relationship of Motor Milestones to Age

Motor Milestone	Age
Supports head	3 months
Sits alone	6 months
Stands alone	12 months
Balances on one foot	3 years

Table 2–15. Relationship of Language Milestones to Age

Language Milestones	Age
Squeals	1.5–3.0 months
Turns to voice	6 months
Combines two words	1.5 years
Composes short sentences	2 years
Gives entire name	3 years

Neurologic Development

Reduction of perinatal mortality during the past decade has not resulted in the expected reduction in the prevalence of cerebral palsy. The strongest predictors of cerebral palsy appear to be congenital anomaly, LBW, low placental weight, or abnormal fetal position before labor and delivery and not perinatal complications such as perinatal asphyxia.[120]

An infant's normal mental development depends on maturation of the central nervous system. This development may be affected by physical illness or by inadequate psychosocial support. Delay in development in preterm infants, however, may be normal, depending on the degree of prematurity.

The rate of brain growth is different from the growth rate of other body systems. The brain has two growth spurts—neuronal cell multiplication between 15 and 20 weeks of gestation and glial cell multiplication—commencing at 25 weeks and extending into the second year of life. Myelination continues into the third year. Malnutrition during this phase of neural development may have profound handicapping effects. Knowledge of the normal pattern of a child's development allows one to evaluate the development of an individual child.

Normal brain development may be impaired by events leading to damage of the blood-brain barrier, particularly in an immature brain. The endothelial cells of the brain microvascular structure form tight junctions as a result of an interaction between the astrocytes of the brain and endothelial cells.[121] Plasma membrane transport selectively promotes the passage of essential substrates such as glucose, organic acids, and amino acids across the blood-brain barrier. Hypoxemia and ischemia may lead to a breakdown in this barrier, with resulting edema and increased intracranial pressure. Injury to the blood-brain barrier may be on the basis of abnormal entry of calcium or formation of free radicals. Further studies of the mechanism of this breakdown will lead to rational approaches to therapy. In premature infants stressed by hypoxia, the blood-brain barrier may become particularly permeable to the water-soluble bilirubin, with possible damage to the brain.[122]

Normal newborns show various primitive reflexes, which include the Moro response and grasp reflex. Milestones of development are useful indicators of mental development and possible deviations from normal. It should be appreciated, however, that these milestones represent the *average,* and infants can vary in their rates of maturation of different body functions and still be within the normal range.[123] The Denver developmental screening test is a useful scheme for assessing these milestones. The test focuses on four areas: (1) gross motor function, (2) fine motor and adaptive skills, (3) language, and (4) personal and social skills. Developing infants acquire motor skills. For effective movement, an infant needs postural control, which develops in a cephalocaudal direction. It starts with head control and progresses to sitting, standing, walking, and finally running (Table 2–13).

Adaptive skills are performed through well-coordinated fine motor movements (Table 2–14). Abnormal development may be reflected in a delay in appearance of a particular milestone or in its pathologic persistence with maturation in a child. For example, at 20 weeks, a child reaches and retrieves objects, frequently placing them in his or her mouth. As an infant matures, however, this behavior pattern usually ceases at 12 to 13 months of age; in infants with a mental abnormality, this practice may continue much longer.

Language development correlates closely with cognitive skills (Table 2–15). Personal and social skills are modified by environmental factors and cultural patterns (Table 2–16). Development of walking, speech, and sphincter control are most important. For appropriate evaluation consider familial patterns, level of intelligence, and physical illness. Deafness may cause delayed speech.

Mental Handicap

Children with a mental handicap are late in *all* aspects of development. Smiling, vocalization, sitting, walking, speech, and sphincter control are delayed. When there is a delay in the eye following an object and the head turning in response to sound, blindness and deafness may erroneously be diagnosed. Drooling, common in young infants, is frequently prolonged for years in mentally abnormal children. Initially, a mentally handicapped infant appears to be inactive and

Table 2–14. Relationship of Fine Motor/Adaptive Milestones to Age

Fine Motor/Adaptive Milestones	Age
Grasps rattle	3 months
Passes cube hand to hand	6 months
Pincer grip	1 year
Imitates vertical line	2 years
Copies circle	3 years

Table 2–16. Relationship of Personal-Social Milestones to Age

Personal-Social Milestones	Age
Smiles spontaneously	3 months
Feeds self crackers	6 months
Drinks from cup	1 year
Plays interactive games	2 years

Table 2–17. Causes of Mental Handicaps

Infections, e.g., meningitis, encephalitis
Head injury
Hypoxemia, e.g., near drowning, carbon monoxide poisoning
Metabolic, e.g., severe hypoglycemia, hypernatremia,
    hypothyroidism, phenylketonuria, chronic malnutrition
Lead poisoning, addicting drugs
Degenerative disease of the nervous system
Cerebral tumor, vascular accident (intraventricular hemorrhage)
Congenital malformation
Prematurity

may be seen as a "good child." The child later demonstrates constant and sometimes uncontrollable overactivity. In diagnosing mental abnormality, anesthesiologists must be aware of possible pitfalls:

- Infants born prematurely will be delayed and should be assessed in terms of their conceptual age.
- Infants with cerebral palsy or sensory deficits (auditory and visual) may have normal mental development, but the handicap may interfere with assessment of mental status.
- The effects of drugs should be considered (e.g., barbiturates for epilepsy).

Mental handicaps may be due to a wide range of causes, among which those listed in Table 2–17 should be considered.

REFERENCES

1. Lugo G, Cassady G: Intrauterine growth retardation: Clinicopathologic findings in 233 consecutive infants. Am J Obstet Gynecol 1971;109:615–622.
2. Kitzmiller JL, Cloherty JP, Younger MD, et al: Diabetic pregnancy and perinatal morbidity. Am J Obstet Gynecol 1978;131:560–580.
3. Hertel J, Kuhl C: Metabolic adaptations during the neonatal period in infants of diabetic mothers. Acta Endocrinol Suppl (Copenh) 1986;277:136–140.
4. Dubowitz LM, Dubowitz V, Goldberg C: Clinical assessment of gestational age in the newborn infant. J Pediatr 1970;77:1–10.
5. Narayanan I, Dua K, Gujral VV, et al: A simple method of assessment of gestational age in newborn infants. Pediatrics 1982;69:27–32.
6. Moylan FM, Seldin EB, Shannon DC, et al: Defective primary dentition in survivors of neonatal mechanical ventilation. J Pediatr 1980;96:106–108.
7. Shaffer SG, Bradt SK, Meade VM, et al: Extracellular fluid volume changes in very low birth weight infants during first 2 postnatal months. J Pediatr 1987;111:124–128.
8. Friis-Hansen B: Body composition during growth: in vivo measurements and biochemical data correlated to differential anatomical growth. Pediatrics 1971;47:264–274.
9. Reid L: 1976 Edward B.D. Neuhauser lecture. The lung: Growth and remodeling in health and disease. AJR 1977;129:777–788.
10. Charnock EL, Doershuk CF: Developmental aspects of the human lung. Pediatr Clin North Am 1973;20:275–292.
11. Boyden EA: Development and growth of the airways. In: Hodson WA, ed: Development of the Lung, pp 3–36. New York: Marcel Dekker; 1977.
12. Bucher HU, Reid LM: The pattern of branching and development of cartilage at various stages of intrauterine life. Thorax 1961;16:207–218.
13. Hislop A, Reid L: Lung development in relation to gas exchange capacity. Bull Physiopathol Respir 1973;9:1317–1343.
14. Campiche MA, Gautier A, Hernandez EI, et al: An electron microscope study of the fetal development of the human lung. Pediatrics 1963;32:976–994.
15. Langston C, Kida K, Reed M, et al: Human lung growth in late gestation and in the neonate. Am Rev Respir Dis 1984;129:607–613.
16. Hislop A, Reid L: Development of the acinus in the human lung. Thorax 1974;29:90–94.
17. Gluck L, Kulovich MV: Lecithin-sphingomyelin ratios in amniotic fluid in normal and abnormal pregnancy. Am J Obstet Gynecol 1973;115:539–546.
18. Hislop A, Reid L: Intra-pulmonary arterial development during fetal life-branching pattern and structure. J Anat 1972;113:35–48.
19. Hislop A, Reid L: Fetal and childhood development of the intrapulmonary veins in man: Branching pattern and structure. Thorax 1973;28:313–319.
20. Reid LM: The 1978 J. Burns Amberson Lecture. The pulmonary circulation: Remodeling in growth and disease. Am Rev Respir Dis 1979;119:531–546.
21. Cassin S, Dawes GS, Mott JC, et al: The vascular resistance of the foetal and newly ventilated lung of the lamb. J Physiol 1964;171:61–79.
22. Rudolph AM, Heymann MA: Circulatory changes during growth in the fetal lamb. Circ Res 1970;26:289–299.
23. Murphy JD, Rabinovitch M, Goldstein JD, et al: The structural basis of persistent pulmonary hypertension of the newborn infant. J Pediatr 1981;98:962–967.
24. Walsh-Sukys MC: Persistent pulmonary hypertension of the newborn. The black box revisited. Clin Perinatol 1993;20:127–143.
25. Dunnill MS: Postnatal growth of the lung. Thorax 1962;17:329–333.
26. Davies G, Reid L: Growth of the alveoli and pulmonary arteries in childhood. Thorax 1970;25:669–681.
27. Thurlbeck WM: Postnatal human lung growth. Thorax 1982;37:564–571.
28. Hislop A, Reid L: Pulmonary arterial development during childhood: Branching pattern and structure. Thorax 1973;28:129–135.
29. Hislop A, Muir DC, Jacobsen M, et al: Postnatal growth and function of the pre-acinar airways. Thorax 1972;27:265–274.
30. Boddy K, Dawes GS: Fetal breathing. Br Med Bull 1975;31:3–7.
31. Maloney JE, Alcorn D, Bowes G, et al: Development of the future respiratory system before birth. Semin Perinatol 1980;4:251–260.
32. Avery ME: The J. Burns Amberson Lecture. In pursuit of understanding the first breath. Am Rev Respir Dis 1969;100:295–304.
33. Johnson JWC: A study of fetal intrathoracic pressures during labor and delivery. Am J Obstet Gynecol 1962;84:15–19.
34. Karlberg P, Adams FH, Geubele F, et al: Alteration of the infant's thorax during vaginal delivery. Acta Obstet Gynecol Scand 1962;41:223–229.
35. Bland RD, McMillan DD, Bressack MA, et al: Clearance of liquid from lungs of newborn rabbits. J Appl Physiol 1980;49:171–177.
36. Avery ME, Gatewood OB, Brumley G: Transient tachypnea of newborn: Possible delayed resorption of fluid at birth. Am J Dis Child 1966;111:380–385.
37. Hall SM, Haworth SG: Normal adaptation of pulmonary arterial intima to extrauterine life in the pig: Ultrastructural studies. J Pathol 1986;149:55–66.
38. Hodson WA, Alden ER: Gas exchange in the developing lung. In: Hodson WA, ed. Development of the Lung. New York: Marcel Dekker; 1977.
39. Takahashi E, Atsumi H: Age differences in thoracic form as indicated by thoracic index. Hum Biol 1955;27:65–74.
40. Gerhardt T, Bancalari E: Chestwall compliance in full-term and premature infants. Acta Paediatr Scand 1980;69:359–364.
41. Knill R, Andrews W, Bryan AC, et al: Respiratory load compensation in infants. J Appl Physiol 1976;40:357–361.
42. Davi M, Sankaran K, Maccallum M, et al: Effect of sleep state on chest distortion and on the ventilatory response to CO_2 in neonates. Pediatr Res 1979;13:982–986.
43. Heldt GP, McIlroy MB: Distortion of chest wall and work of diaphragm in preterm infants. J Appl Physiol 1987;62:164–169.
44. Heldt GP: Development of stability of the respiratory system in preterm infants. J Appl Physiol 1988;65:441–444.
45. Keens TG, Bryan AC, Levison H, et al: Developmental pattern of muscle fiber types in human ventilatory muscles. J Appl Physiol Resp 1978;44:909–913.
46. Godfrey S: Growth and development of the respiratory system: Functional development. In: Davies JA, Dobbing J, eds: Scientific Foundations of Paediatrics, pp 432–450. Baltimore: University Press; 1982.
47. Motoyama EK: Pulmonary mechanics during early postnatal years. Pediatr Res 1977;11:220–223.

48. Sharp JT, Druz WS, Balagot RC, et al: Total respiratory compliance in infants and children. J Appl Physiol 1970;29:775–779.

49. Bryan AC, Mansell AL, Levison H: Development of the mechanical properties of the respiratory system. In: Hodson WA, ed. Development of the Lung. New York: Marcel Dekker; 1977.

50. Turner JM, Mead J, Wohl ME: Elasticity of human lungs in relation to age. J Appl Physiol 1968;25:664–671.

51. Taussig LM, Harris TR, Lebowitz MD: Lung function in infants and young children: Functional residual capacity, tidal volume, and respiratory rates. Am Rev Respir Dis 1977;116:233–239.

52. Agostoni E, Mead J: Statics of the respiratory system. In: Fenn WO, Rahn H, eds: Handbook of Physiology. Washington: American Physiologic Society; 1964.

53. Olinsky A, Bryan MH, Bryan AC: Influence of lung inflation on respiratory control in neonates. J Appl Physiol 1974;36:426–429.

54. Karlberg P, Koch G: Development of mechanics of breathing during the first week of life: A longitudinal study. Acta Paediatr Scand 1962;51:121–129.

55. Stocks J, Godfrey S: Specific airway conductance in relation to post-conceptional age during infancy. J Appl Physiol 1977;43:144–154.

56. Doershuk CF, Downs TD, Matthews LW, et al: A method for ventilatory measurements in subjects 1 month–5 years of age: Normal results and observations in disease. Pediatr Res 1970;4:165–174.

57. Hogg JC, Williams B, Richardson JB, et al: Age as a factor in the distribution of lower-airway conductance and in the pathologic anatomy of obstructive lung disease. N Engl J Med 1970;282:1283–1287.

58. Rigatto H, Brady JP, De La Torre Verduzco R: Chemoreceptor reflexes in preterm infants: II. The effect of gestational and postnatal age on the ventilatory response to inhaled carbon dioxide. Pediatrics 1975;55:614–620.

59. Rigatto H, De La Torre Verduzco R, Gates DB: Effects of O_2 on the ventilatory response to CO_2 in preterm infants. J Appl Physiol 1975;39:896–899.

60. Rigatto H, Brady JP, De La Torre Verduzco R: Chemoreceptor reflexes in preterm infants: I. The effect of gestational and postnatal age on the ventilatory response to inhalation of 100% and 15% oxygen. Pediatrics 1975;55:604–613.

61. Brady JP, Ceruti E: Chemoreceptor reflexes in the new-born infant: Effects of varying degrees of hypoxia on heart rate and ventilation in a warm environment. J Physiol (Lond) 1966;184:631–645.

62. Henderson-Smart DJ, Pettigrew AG, Campbell DJ: Clinical apnea and brain-stem neural function in preterm infants. N Engl J Med 1983;308:353–357.

63. Steward DJ: Preterm infants are more prone to complications following minor surgery than are term infants. Anesthesiology 1982;56:304–306.

64. Liu LM, Coté CJ, Goudsouzian NG, et al: Life-threatening apnea in infants recovering from anesthesia. Anesthesiology 1983;59:506–510.

65. Kurth CD, Spitzer AR, Broennle AM, et al: Postoperative apnea in preterm infants. Anesthesiology 1987;66:483–488.

66. Coté CJ, Zaslavsky A, Downes JJ, et al: Postoperative apnea in former preterm infants after inguinal herniorrhaphy. A combined analysis. Anesthesiology 1995;82:809–822.

67. Cross KW, Flynn DM, Hill JR: Oxygen consumption in normal newborn infants during moderate hypoxia in warm and cool environments. Pediatrics 1966;37:565–576.

68. DeMuth GR, Howatt WF, Hill BM: Lung volumes. Pediatrics 1965;35:162–176.

69. Southall DP, Richards JM, Johnstone PGB, et al: Study of cardiac rhythm in healthy newborn infants. Br Heart J 1979;41:382–382.

70. de Swiet M, Fayers P, Shinebourne EA: Systolic blood pressure in a population of infants in the first year of life: The Brompton study. Pediatrics 1980;65:1028–1035.

71. Southall DP, Johnston F, Shinebourne EA, et al: 24-hour electrocardiographic study of heart rate and rhythm patterns in population of healthy children. Br Heart J 1981;45:281–291.

72. Tan KL: Blood pressure in very low birth weight infants in the first 70 days of life. J Pediatr 1988;112:266–270.

73. Hegyi T, Anwar M, Carbone MT, et al: Blood pressure ranges in premature infants: II. The first week of life. Pediatrics 1996;97:336–342.

74. Alverson DC, Eldridge M, Dillon T, et al: Noninvasive pulsed Doppler determination of cardiac output in neonates and children. J Pediatr 1982;101:46–50.

75. Walther FJ, Siassi B, Ramadan NA, et al: Pulsed Doppler determina-

tions of cardiac output in neonates: Normal standards for clinical use. Pediatrics 1985;76:829–833.

76. Walther FJ, Siassi B, Ramadan NA, et al: Cardiac output in newborn infants with transient myocardial dysfunction. J Pediatr 1985;107:781–785.

77. Rice MJ, McDonald RW, Reller MD, et al: Pediatric echocardiography: Current role and a review of technical advances. J Pediatr 1996;128:1–14.

78. Southall DP, Vulliamy DG, Davies MJ, et al: A new look at the neonatal electrocardiogram. Br Med J 1976;2:615–618.

79. Rautaharju PM, Davignon A, Soumis F, et al: Evolution of QRS-T relationship from birth to adolescence in Frank-lead orthogonal electrocardiograms of 1492 normal children. Circulation 1979;60:196–204.

80. Walsh EP, Lang P, Ellison RC, et al: Electrocardiogram of the premature infant at 1 year of age. Pediatrics 1986;77:353–356.

81. Clark DA: Times of first void and first stool in 500 newborns. Pediatrics 1977;60:457–459.

82. Leake RD, Trygstad CW, Oh W: Inulin clearance in the newborn infant: Relationship to gestational and postnatal age. Pediatr Res 1976;10:759–762.

83. Arant BSJ: Developmental patterns of renal functional maturation compared in the human neonate. J Pediatr 1978;92:705–712.

84. Edelmann CMJ, Spitzer A: The maturing kidney: A modern view of well-balanced infants with imbalanced nephrons. J Pediatr 1969;75:509–519.

85. Gruskay J, Costarino AT, Polin RA, et al: Nonoliguric hyperkalemia in the premature infant weighing less than 1000 grams. J Pediatr 1988;113:381–386.

86. Oski FA: Jaundice. In: Avery ME, Taeusch HW Jr, eds. Schaffer's Diseases of the Newborn, 5th ed. Philadelphia: WB Saunders; 1984.

87. Seligman JW: Recent and changing concepts of hyperbilirubinemia and its management in the newborn. Pediatr Clin North Am 1977;24:509–527.

88. Touloukian RJ, Downing SE: Cholestasis associated with long-term parenteral hyperalimentation. Arch Surg 1973;106:58–62.

89. Valaes T, Petmezaki S, Henschke C, et al: Control of jaundice in preterm newborns by an inhibitor of bilirubin production: studies with tin-mesoporphyrin. Pediatrics 1994;93:1–11.

90. Morriss FHJ, Moore M, Weisbrodt NW, et al: Ontogenic development of gastrointestinal motility: IV. Duodenal contractions in preterm infants. Pediatrics 1986;78:1106–1113.

91. Winter HS, Grand RJ: Gastroesophageal reflux. Pediatrics 1981;68:134–136.

92. Shannon DC, Gotay F, Stein IM, et al: Prevention of apnea and bradycardia in low-birthweight infants. Pediatrics 1975;55:589–594.

93. Jhaveri MK, Kumar SP: Passage of the first stool in very low birth weight infants. Pediatrics 1987;79:1005–1007.

94. Levin DL, Gregory GA: The effect of tolazoline on right-to-left shunting via a patent ductus arteriosus in meconium aspiration syndrome. Crit Care Med 1976;4:304–307.

95. Wiswell TE, Bent RC: Meconium staining and the meconium aspiration syndrome: Unresolved issues. Pediatr Clin North Am 1993;40:955–981.

96. Srinivasan G, Pildes RS, Cattamanchi G, et al: Plasma glucose values in normal neonates: A new look. J Pediatr 1986;109:114–117.

97. Heck LJ, Erenberg A: Serum glucose levels in term neonates during the first 48 hours of life. J Pediatr 1987;110:119–122.

98. Kennealy JA, McLennan JE, Loudon RG, et al: Hyperventilation-induced cerebral hypoxia. Am Rev Respir Dis 1980;122:407–412.

99. Srinivasan G, Jain R, Pildes RS, et al: Glucose homeostasis during anesthesia and surgery in infants. J Pediatr Surg 1986;21:718–721.

100. Cowett RM, Wolfe RR: Glucose and lactate kinetics in the neonate. J Dev Physiol 1991;16:341–347.

101. Cowett RM, Andersen GE, Maguire CA, et al: Ontogeny of glucose homeostasis in low birth weight infants. J Pediatr 1988;112:462–465.

102. Cowett RM: Pathophysiology, diagnosis, and management of glucose homeostasis in the neonate. Curr Probl Pediatr 1985;15:1–47.

103. Pildes RS: Neonatal hyperglycemia. J Pediatr 1986;109:905–907.

104. Collins JW Jr, Hoppe M, Brown K, et al: A controlled trial of insulin infusion and parenteral nutrition in extremely low birth weight infants with glucose intolerance. J Pediatr 1991;118:921–927.

105. Usher R, Lind J: Blood volume of the newborn premature infant. Acta Paediatr Scand 1965;54:419–431.

106. Usher R, Shephard M, Lind J: The blood volume of the newborn

infant and placental transfusion. Acta Paediatr Scand Suppl 1963;52:497–512.

107. O'Brien RT, Pearson HA: Physiologic anemia of the newborn infant. J Pediatr 1971;79:132–138.

108. Delavoria-Papadolpulos M, Roncevic N, Oski FA: Postnatal changes in oxygen transport of term, premature and sick infants: The role of red cell, 2,3-diphosphoglycerate and adult hemoglobin. Pediatr Res 1971;5:235–245.

109. Ross MP, Christensen RD, Rothstein G, et al: A randomized trial to develop criteria for administering erythrocyte transfusions to anemic preterm infants 1 to 3 months of age. J Perinatol 1989;9:246–253.

110. Zipursky A, Brown EJ, Watts J, et al: Oral vitamin E supplementation for the prevention of anemia in premature infants: A controlled trial. Pediatrics 1987;79:61–68.

111. Shannon KM, Keith JF, III, Mentzer WC, et al: Recombinant human erythropoietin stimulates erythropoiesis and reduces erythrocyte transfusions in very low birth weight preterm infants. Pediatrics 1995;95:1–8.

112. Andrew M, Castle V, Saigal S, et al: Clinical impact of neonatal thrombocytopenia. J Pediatr 1987;110:457–464.

113. Ramamurthy RS, Brans YW: Neonatal polycythemia: I. Criteria for diagnosis and treatment. Pediatrics 1981;68:168–174.

114. Fouron JC, Hebert F: The circulatory effects of hematocrit variations in normovolemic newborn lambs. J Pediatr 1973;82:995–1003.

115. Murphy DJJ, Reller MD, Meyer RA, et al: Effects of neonatal polycythemia and partial exchange transfusion on cardiac function: An echocardiographic study. Pediatrics 1985;76:909–913.

116. Swetnam SM, Yabek SM, Alverson DC: Hemodynamic consequences of neonatal polycythemia. J Pediatr 1987;110:443–447.

117. Shannon KM, Naylor GS, Torkildson JC, et al: Circulating erythroid progenitors in the anemia of prematurity. N Engl J Med 1987;317:728–733.

118. Shapiro AD, Jacobson LJ, Armon ME, et al: Vitamin K deficiency in the newborn infant: prevalence and perinatal risk factors. J Pediatr 1986;109:675–680.

119. Mountain KR, Hirsh J, Gallus AS: Neonatal coagulation defect due to anticonvulsant drug treatment in pregnancy. Lancet 1970;1:265–268.

120. Torfs CP, van den Berg B, Oechsli FW, et al: Prenatal and perinatal factors in the etiology of cerebral palsy. J Pediatr 1990;116:615–619.

121. Illingworth RS: Development of the Infant and Young Child, Normal and Abnormal, 9th ed. New York: Churchill Livingstone; 1987.

122. Goldstein GW, Robertson P, Betz AL: Update on the role of the blood-brain barrier in damage to immature brain. Pediatrics 1988;81:732–734.

123. Levine RL, Fredericks WR, Rapoport SI: Entry of bilirubin into the brain due to opening of the blood-brain barrier. Pediatrics 1982;69:255–259.

3

The Perioperative Behavioral Stress Response in Children

Zeev N. Kain *and* Linda C. Mayes

Overview

Developmental Issues

    Social Interaction

    Attachment

    Temperament

Preoperative Anxiety: Risk Factors

Preoperative Anxiety: Interventions

    Behavioral Interventions

    Pharmacologic Interventions

Preoperative Anxiety: Outcomes

Summary

Overview

Anxiety in children undergoing anesthesia and surgery is characterized by feelings of tension, apprehension, and nervousness.[1] This response is attributed to separation from parents, loss of control, uncertainty about the anesthesia, and uncertainty about the surgery and its outcome.[1] Some children verbalize their fears explicitly, whereas for others anxiety is expressed only by changes in behavior. Children may look scared, look agitated, breathe deeply, tremble, stop talking or playing, and start to cry. Some may wet or soil themselves, have increased motor tone, and actively attempt to escape from medical personnel.[2] These behaviors may give children some sense of control in the situation and thereby diminish the damaging effects of a sense of helplessness.[1, 2] Unfortunately, these negative behavioral manifestations are not limited to the *preoperative* period. A number of studies have indicated that up to 60% of all children undergoing outpatient surgery may develop negative *postoperative* behavioral changes within 2 weeks following surgery.[3–5] These negative postoperative behaviors may include sleep and eating disturbances, separation anxiety, apathy, withdrawal, and new onset enuresis.[6, 7] In fact, some children may develop long-lasting psychological effects that will have

an impact on their responses to subsequent medical care. Interference with normal development has also been described.[8]

In addition to the behavioral manifestations detailed here, several studies have documented that anxiety prior to surgery is associated with neuroendocrinologic changes, such as increased serum cortisol, epinephrine, growth hormone, and adrenocorticotropin hormone levels and increased natural killer cell activity.[9–11] Significant correlations between heart rate, blood pressure, and behavioral ratings of anxiety have also been reported.[12, 13] In adults, increased preoperative anxiety has been shown to correlate with increased postoperative pain, increased postoperative analgesic requirements, and prolonged recovery and hospital stay.[14–16] Further, although reports are conflicting, preoperative anxiety has been suggested to delay gastric emptying and increase gastric acidity and is considered by some anesthesiologists to be a risk factor for pulmonary aspiration of gastric contents.[17, 18] In children, however, there are data to indicate that there is no association between preoperative anxiety and the amount of gastric residual volume.[19, 20] The gastric residual volume of children who are anxious preoperatively is not higher compared with the gastric residual volume of children who are calm preoperatively. Thus one might not expect a higher incidence of pulmonary aspiration of gastric contents in highly anxious children.

Developmental Issues

Coping with separation is a lifelong challenge, not only inevitable but necessary for a child's normal development.[21] Separation experiences such as saying good-bye at the door of school or sleeping overnight at a friend's house facilitate normal childhood psychological growth and personality organization by mobilizing opportunities for learning and adaptation. Other separation experiences, especially those occurring in the context of loss, illness, or other stressors, precipitate states of confusion, anger, and anxiety. Separation distress (separation anxiety) refers to a child's response to being separated from the parent or other primary caretaker. Between these two extremes, there are many separation experiences with varying degrees of psychological and psychobiologic stress. Adaptive and defensive mechanisms are called into play with varying degrees of effectiveness; feelings of mastery or helplessness are aspects of these responses. Brief separations are most stressful for infants, toddlers, and preschool-aged children. Indeed, for school-aged children, responses to separation may reflect, in part, response patterns established early in the preschool years.[21]

The impact of separations, brief or prolonged, on the developing infant, toddler, and preschool child has been an issue of concern to child professionals for many years. Indeed, the impetus for studying both the nature of early parent-child relations and the impact of briefer but early separations came from findings demonstrating pervasive, severe, and enduring effects of institutional and hospital care on infants and young children.[21–23] The extent to which separations are traumatic and produce overwhelming feelings of anxiety or evoke adaptive responses reflects an individual child's genetics, personality, parenting, and life experiences.

Separation cannot be regarded as an event that has a predictable outcome or effect on a child's later development. Any one separation experience is given weight by the developmental age and competency of the child, by the previous history of loss and separation for the child and family, and by how the family or responsible adults respond to the particular experience vis-à-vis themselves and the child. For example, separations occurring in the early preschool years have a potentially greater developmental impact than those that occur later. For children with biologically based vulnerabilities, such as a sensitivity to novelty and transitions, even expected separations may impose a greater degree of stress than for less sensitive children.[21] Similarly, for children with specific or general developmental delays, age-expected separations, such as entry into preschool, may be experienced with a degree of anxiety, and developmental stress more like that experienced by a younger child. From the environmental side, how parents and caring adults help the child mediate a separation experience plays a crucial role in the child's acute and long-term responses. In the extreme, the adult most responsible for the child may be unable to mediate the experience for the child because of psychological and functional limitations including depression, severe anxiety, or substance abuse. Situations of profound family disruption, such as occur when families are displaced from their homes, in cases of divorce, or when one parent is acutely ill, impose not only the potential loss of cared for persons but also the loss of familiar, comforting surroundings. How well children have been cared for up to the time of the separation also influences their response to the stressor at the time. Children from chronically depriving or chaotic homes are at much greater risk for increased stress in response to separations, even when brief. Thus, the response to separation is a multi-determined event based on developmental age, parenting experiences, genetic endowment, and environmental stability. Three areas of development—social interaction, attachment, and reactivity to novelty (as measured by temperament)—are, however, *most* influential in determining a child's response to a separation experience. It is important to note that studies have found, through both behavioral and physiologic responses, that induction of anesthesia is the most stressful event the child experiences during the perioperative period.[1, 24]

Social Interaction

In the first weeks of life, infants are able to discriminate among people, but will usually accept care and comfort from adults other than their parents.[25] By 3 months of age, infants begin to respond differently to familiar and unfamiliar people. Older infants smile more at familiar people and may even try to engage their attention over that of strangers.[26, 27] Separation anxiety often begins around 5 to 6 months of age and may peak around the child's first birthday. In part, separation anxiety represents the infant's acquisition of a new cognitive ability defined as object permanence. Object permanence means that the baby holds a mental image of the object for a long enough period of time to search for it when it is no longer visible. After obtaining object permanence, the baby can think about and remember his or her parents even in their absence but cannot understand where they have gone or when they will return. Separation anxiety declines with age, largely because with increasing cognitive sophistication and memory capacity, older children are able to understand that although their parents are gone, they will return. Unfortunately, this increase in memory capacity and cognitive sophistication does not immunize toddlers and preschoolers against the stress and distress of separation.

Attachment

Separation anxiety is an indicator of an infant's attachment to its parents. Attachment develops as a function of a very young infant's emotional experiences and manifests behaviorally in the way in which infants look at their parents, move toward or away from them, smile, and become distressed with separation.[26, 27] Through interactions with the mother, an infant develops a sense of trust and security in the reliability and predictability of their relationship and the world.[26, 27] This sense of security and basic trust is important to the development of autonomy and independence, and to the child's security in exploring novel environments such as the operating room. Children may be "securely attached," "insecurely attached," and "anxiously attached" to their parents.

Infants who are more securely attached to their parents deal more adaptively with the stress of brief separation and with the novelty of the hospital experience. These infants are more willing to explore their world and respond positively to their mother's return, using her as a secure, stable base from which to approach strangers and new situations.[25, 28] As preschoolers, securely attached children are often more socially mature and interactive with same-age peers. In contrast, toddlers classified as anxiously attached to their mother tend to be distressed in unfamiliar situations even when their mother is with them. When their mother returns after brief separations, these infants tend to be angry and distressed and to avoid physical contact. Other forms of insecure attachment include avoidance. Avoidant children do not explore their surroundings as much as securely attached infants do and tend to ignore their mother. They rarely show distress upon separation and avoid interactions with their mother when she returns. Conversely, insecurely attached infants are

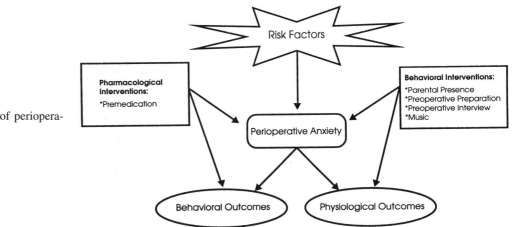

Figure 3–1. Operational overview of perioperative anxiety.

more easily distressed by even brief separations and spend more time trying to stay close to their parents. More anxious about novelty and separation, they are less likely to explore and less likely to adapt positively to new situations.

Temperament

Response to the stress of separation in infancy and preschool years reflects in part the child's relationships with parents *as well as* the child's temperament. Temperament refers to emotional responses that are characteristic of individual infants and young children. Clusters of related characteristics may constitute a temperament type. While conceptually related to personality, temperament characteristics in children are presumed to have a primarily genetic basis.[29–31] Later personality characteristics, such as adulthood characteristics, presumably reflect the interaction between temperament traits, arising in early childhood, and environmental influences. Some authors find that it is useful to classify infants on three main dimensions: emotionality, activity, and sociability.[32] *Emotionality* refers to the ease with which an infant becomes aroused or anxious, especially in situations that might lead to fear, such as perioperative settings. *Activity* refers to the infant's customary level of energy and intensity of behavior. *Sociability* reflects the infant's tendency to approach or avoid others. These behavioral dimensions of temperament are also reflected in physiologic responses related to anxiety.[33] For example, measures of heart rate variability are closely related to infants' reactivity and lability in the first year of life.[23] Infants with less variability in heart rate (presumably reflecting increased sympathetic relative to parasympathetic influence on heart rate) are more labile and reactive to novelty. Infants who have a tendency to avoid novelty cry more easily and are less active in contrast to those who readily approach the unfamiliar. In long-term studies, infants who are inhibited in the face of novelty continue to be so through early school age.[34] Thus, temperament as a behavioral descriptor appears to characterize an enduring cluster of traits reflecting reactivity and anxiety regulation in the face of novelty.

Preoperative Anxiety: Risk Factors

Anxiety along with distress prior to surgery is a clinically important phenomenon and it should be treated as any other

clinical phenomenon or disease. In epidemiologic terms, *all* diseases are characterized operationally by risk factors, interventions, and outcomes; preoperative anxiety is no exception. In the rest of this chapter we review the phenomenon of preoperative anxiety using the classic epidemiologic model of a disease (Fig. 3–1).

Identifying risk factors for preoperative anxiety is important because the routine use of pharmacologic and behavioral interventions may carry with them important disadvantages. Routine administration of sedative premedicants, for example, may result in increased indirect pharmacy costs, additional nursing staff, and increased need for appropriately monitored bed space in the preoperative holding area. Delayed discharge in children undergoing extremely short outpatient procedures may also occur. Similarly, behavioral preparation programs administered preoperatively are associated with increased hospital operational costs. Thus, identifying children who are at a particularly high risk for developing extreme anxiety and distress prior to surgery would be very useful in helping to guide the use of limited resources in the most beneficial directions.

Variation in children's behavioral responses to the perioperative experience has its origin in at least four domains:

1. Age and developmental maturity
2. Previous experience with medical procedures and illness
3. Individual capacity for affect regulation and trait anxiety (baseline anxiety)
4. Parental state (situational) and trait (baseline) anxiety

Studies examining behavioral responses to induction of anesthesia in children have paid attention to each of these factors.[6, 35–37] To date, several demographic and personality-related variables have been identified as predictors for preoperative anxiety in children (Table 3–1). Children between the ages of 1 and 5 years are at greatest risk for developing

Table 3–1. Demographic and Personality Factors Predictive of Preoperative Anxiety

Age	Social adaptability
Parental anxiety	Coping style
Temperament	Lack of premedication
Previous experience	

extreme anxiety and distress. This is not surprising, as separation anxiety often does not peak until 1 year, and children over the age of 5 can more easily cope with new and unpredictable situations. A history of prior stressful medical encounters, such as in the pediatrician's office, the dentist's office, with previous surgery, or with previous hospitalization, colors how a child reacts to new medical encounters and has been reported as an important risk factor for preoperative anxiety. Children who are shy and inhibited, as identified by temperament tests, have been reported to be at increased risk for developing anxiety and distress prior to surgery. In addition, children who lack good social adaptive abilities are likewise at greater risk to develop severe anxiety prior to surgery.[38]

Finally, parental characteristics have a strong influence on the child's behavior during the perioperative experience. Children of parents who are more anxious, children of parents who use avoidance coping mechanisms, and children of separated or divorced parents all appear to be at high risk for developing preoperative anxiety. Since children of anxious parents are more likely to experience high levels of preoperative anxiety, it is important to identify predictors for increased *parental* preoperative anxiety. Gender of the parent (mothers are more anxious than fathers), age of the child less than 1 year, repeated hospital admissions, and baseline temperament of the child are predictors of parental preoperative anxiety.[39-41] Once one identifies children and parents who are at the highest risk for developing anxiety and distress prior to surgery, one can then take steps to treat this at-risk population.

Preoperative Anxiety: Interventions

Both pharmacologic interventions, such as administration of premedications, and behavioral interventions, such as psychological preparation programs, are used to treat preoperative anxiety and distress in children and their parents.[42]

Behavioral Interventions

Preoperative Preparation Programs

Psychological preparation for children undergoing anesthesia and surgery has been advocated, and currently the majority of large children's hospitals offer behavioral preoperative programs to children and their parents.[43] These preparation programs may provide narrative information, an orientation tour of the operative facility, role rehearsal using dolls, modeling using videotapes or a puppet show, child life preparation, or coping education and relaxation skills.[44-46]

Although there is general agreement in the medical community about the desirability of such programs, recommendations regarding the content of behavioral preoperative preparation programs differ widely. Preparation programs in the 1960s were information-oriented and designed to facilitate emotional expression and trust between the medical staff, the child, and the parent.[47] Modeling techniques in which children and parents indirectly experienced anesthesia and surgery by viewing a video or a puppet show emerged in the 1970s.[48] This form of preparation was augmented in the late 1980s with child life preparation and coping skills education.[45] Child life specialists are trained individuals who

facilitate development of coping skills and the adjustment of children and parents to the perioperative environment by providing play experiences, presenting information about events and procedures, and establishing supportive relationships with children and parents.[46] In making information accessible to children, child life specialists incorporate descriptions of the sensations children will experience, provide opportunities to examine and manipulate equipment to be used in their care, and encourage rehearsal with dolls. Currently, development of coping skills is considered the most effective preoperative intervention, followed by modeling, play therapy, operating room tour, and printed material.[43] Interestingly, when development of coping skills preparation was compared with lower rated techniques, such as providing information and modeling, the highly rated coping skills preparation technique with child life specialists was associated with less anxiety in the holding area on the day of surgery and upon separation from parents upon entry to the operating room.[49] In contrast, no differences were found among the various techniques during induction of anesthesia, in the recovery room period, or at 2 weeks postoperatively. Thus, from a cost-effectiveness point of view, one must decide whether the additional cost associated with child life specialists is justified by reduction of anxiety *only* during the preoperative period.

It is important that these preparation programs are tailored to the individual, age-appropriate needs of each child. Several variables have been identified as influencing the response of children to preparation programs.[40] For example, children who are 6 years old and older benefit most if they participate in a preparation program more than 5 days prior to the scheduled surgery and benefit least if the program is given only 1 day prior to surgery. In fact, older children prepared a week in advance showed an *increase* in anxiety level during and immediately after the preparation, but demonstrated a gradual decrease in anxiety during the 5 days before the time of surgery.[50] To avoid increasing excessive anticipatory anxiety, older children should be given enough time to process the new information and to rehearse newly acquired coping skills. It is also important to realize that there may be a *negative* effect of a preparation program on children younger than 3 years of age. This may be a result of their inability to distinguish fantasy from reality.[51] A reality-based preparation program may do little to calm young children and may even exacerbate anxiety or sensitize the young child to the surgery. From age 3 to 6 years, children demonstrate an increasing ability to distinguish fantasy from reality and by the age of 6 this distinction is usually accomplished.[51] The need to consider the age of the child who will most benefit from such programs thus relates to both the amount of anxiety such exposure might generate and the length of time over which they can deal with knowing what will happen.

In addition to age and timing, previous experience in a hospital setting also influences the effectiveness of a preparation program. A child who was previously hospitalized is more likely to develop an exaggerated emotional response to a behavioral preoperative preparation program and the perioperative experience.[40, 50, 52, 53] Information about what will occur as demonstrated by sensory expectation and doll-play does *not* provide new information for these children. Further, if the child has had a previous negative medical experience, the routine preparation may increase anxiety by triggering negative memories. In this case, alternative behavioral interventions, such as extensive individualized coping skills training combined with desensitization and actual practice may be better suited and indicated.[52] Since increased parental preoperative anxiety has been shown to result in increased preoperative anxiety in their children, preparation programs for surgery should also be directed at parents.[6] While various interventions are routinely used to reduce a child's anxiety, there is a paucity of information regarding interventions directed toward reducing parental anxiety.[54] One study has demonstrated that parental preoperative anxiety decreased after viewing an educational videotape.[55] More interventions such as these need to be developed. In conclusion, most studies to date suggest that preoperative preparation programs for children reduce preoperative anxiety and enhance coping.[45, 50, 56] It is important, however, to consider these variables before implementing such programs.

Parental Presence During Induction of Anesthesia

It is well established that most parents and children prefer to stay together during procedures such as immunization, bone marrow aspiration, and dental treatment.[57, 58] Several survey studies have also indicated that most parents prefer to be present during induction of anesthesia regardless of the child's age or previous surgical experience.[59, 60] Further, a majority of parents believe that they are of some help to their child and the anesthesiologist during the anesthesia induction process.[60] Over 90% of parents, however, report some degree of anxiety during the anesthesia induction process.[61] The most upsetting factors are seeing the child go limp during induction and then having to leave the child.[61] An interesting finding is that 32% of the parents in one report decided not to be present during induction if their child was adequately sedated preoperatively.[59]

There is also significant variability in the practice and attitudes about parental presence between anesthesiologists and surgeons from different parts of the world.[62–65] Recent survey studies found that, overall, anesthesiologists from Great Britain support and allow parental presence during induction of anesthesia significantly more often than anesthesiologists from the United States. Although most Great Britain respondents (84%) allow parental presence in more than 75% of their cases, the majority of anesthesiologists in the United States (59%) *never* have parents present during induction. Twenty-three percent of United States anesthesiologists allow parents to be present during induction in less than 25% of cases and only 10% of United States anesthesiologists have parents present during induction in more than 75% of cases (Fig. 3–2). The reasons for these differences in practice between anesthesiologists from the United States and those from Great Britain may include the use of different induction techniques (mask induction in the United States versus intravenous induction in Great Britain), less concern about legal ramifications in Great Britain, and a stronger demand for parental presence in Great Britain. The reported prevalence of practice also varied widely among the different geographic locations within the United States. The lowest prevalence of allowing parental presence during anesthetic

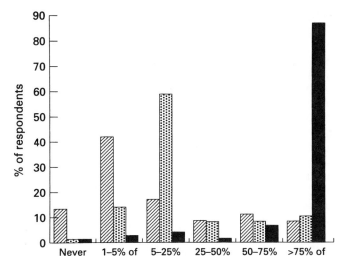

Figure 3–2. Reported frequency of parental presence in the operating room: practice in the United States and Great Britain. Striped bars represent data from the United States Society for Pediatric Anesthesia; dotted bars, United States Section on Anesthesiology, American Academy of Pediatrics; solid bars, Great Britain. (From Kain ZN, Ferris CA, Mayes LC, Rimar S: Parental presence during induction of anaesthesia: Practice differences between the United States and Great Britain. Paediatr Anaesth 1996;6:187–193.)

induction was in the south-central region and the highest in the northwest and northeast regions of the United States.[63]

Potential benefits from parental presence include minimizing the need for premedication and avoiding the screaming and struggling of the child that may result upon separation from the parents. Other benefits, such as decreasing the child's anxiety during induction and potentially decreasing the long-term behavioral effects of surgery, remain controversial. Common objections to parental presence include concern about disruption of the operating room routine, compromising operative sterility, crowded operating rooms, and a possible adverse reaction of the parent. In addition, parental anxiety in the operating suite can result in increased child anxiety, prolonged induction, and additional stress on the anesthesiologist, especially if an anesthetic complication develops. For some children, their behavioral response to stress may be more negative when a parent is present than when the parent is absent.[66] Several reports indicate that parental presence may result in disruptive behavior, parents failing to leave the room when requested, and even removal of a child from the operating room by a grandmother during the second stage of anesthesia.[67, 68] However, one report has described a 4-year experience with 3086 children in a free-standing ambulatory surgery center in which no parent needed to be escorted from the operating room because of undue anxiety, and only two parents developed syncope, with prompt recovery.[69]

The experimental evidence to date does not clearly support the routine use of parental presence during induction of anesthesia.[62, 70–72] Although early studies suggested reduced anxiety and increased cooperation if parents were present during induction,[73, 74] later investigations indicate that routine parental presence may *not* always be beneficial.[62, 70, 71] One study demonstrated that only children who are over 4 years of age, who also have a "calm" baseline personality, or have a parent with a "calm" baseline personality have been found to benefit from parental presence during induction of anesthesia.[62] When interpreting the results of these studies, however, several factors should be considered. First, the design of a randomized controlled study, while considered a gold standard in research, may *not* reflect the practice of *all* anesthesiologists. That is, although a randomized controlled study is applicable to centers that offer parental presence for *all* parents, it may not be applicable to centers in which each request for parental presence is considered individually based on personality characteristics of each child and parent. Such centers may have different results with parental presence than were demonstrated in experimental studies. Second, allowing a parent into an operating room without adequate preparation of the parent may be counterproductive. Some parent behaviors, such as criticism, excessive reassurance, and commands, are associated with greater distress.[75] Research interests in this area should shift toward an emphasis on what parents actually do during induction of anesthesia, rather than simply on their presence. Blount et al.[76] reported that among children undergoing immunizations, parents who were taught to be active in distracting the child through conversation and reading or in reassuring them through touch and eye contact were able to reduce the child's distress. It may be that effective methods of training and educating parents as to what to expect and how they can be most helpful to their child can be developed for enhancing the value of parental presence during induction of anesthesia.

There may also be important legal implications to parental presence during induction. Lewyn[77] described a lawsuit in which a mother was invited by a nurse to accompany her son into an emergency treatment room. According to the court, the mother fainted in the treatment room and suffered an injury to the head as a result of the fall. In its verdict, the Illinois Supreme court stated that a hospital that *allows* a "non-patient" to accompany a patient during treatment does not have a duty to protect the non-patient from fainting. However, if medical personnel *invite* the non-patient to participate in the treatment, then the hospital has a legal responsibility toward the non-patient. Since this is a unique individual state ruling, this concern may not apply in all situations or in all states. Each patient must be considered individually regarding the question of parental presence during induction of anesthesia.

The Preoperative Interview

Although most anesthesiologists may not realize it, the preoperative interview is a behavioral intervention that is being routinely administered to *all* patients undergoing anesthesia and surgery.[78] It is clear that anesthesiologists have an ethical and legal responsibility to disclose to patients detailed anesthetic risk information when obtaining informed consent, but how far this disclosure must extend remains controversial. A common reason given for not providing detailed anesthetic risk information is that it may result in increasing the patient's preoperative anxiety. Comparative studies investigating anxiety levels in patients given a limited amount of information versus more detailed information concerning procedural and anesthetic risks report conflicting results. An

early study found that although the majority of patients were satisfied when they received more detailed information about the risks of angiography, up to 35% of patients were made uncomfortable by the information.[79] Similarly, adult patients who were given extensive information preoperatively were found to be more tense, depressed, and uncomfortable.[80] Conversely, no increase in preoperative anxiety was demonstrated in a study of British and Scottish men undergoing elective herniorrhaphy when presented with detailed risk information.[81] Several studies performed in the United States and Australia have shown that patients and parents who received detailed information, including numerical estimates of anesthesia-related complications, were no more anxious than those given minimal information regarding risks (Fig. 3–3).[82–84] Furthermore, parents have indicated that they would like to have as much perioperative information about their child's surgery as possible.[83] Thus, the presentation of very detailed anesthetic information of what might go wrong does not increase parental or patient anxiety and has the advantage of allowing for fully informed choices. It should be emphasized, however, that anesthesiologists should note the particular coping style of the parent. Parents use different strategies to cope or handle difficult, unclear, or unpleasant life experiences, such as a child undergoing surgery. While some parents try to avoid information about unpleasant or unclear situations ("avoidance behavior"), others may seek any available information ("monitoring behavior").[12] While a "monitor" parent will benefit from a large amount of perioperative information, an "avoidance" parent may react to the information with increased anxiety and distress. Thus,

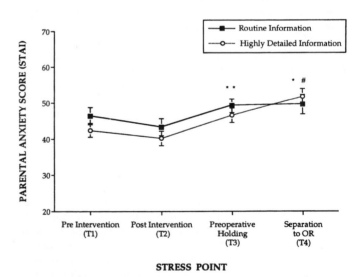

STRESS POINT

Figure 3–3. Changes in parental anxiety over the four time points (T1–T4) are shown. The difference between groups was not significant by one-way repeated-measures analysis of covariance [F(1,45) = 0.6, P = 0.4]. The interaction between time and group assignment was also not significant [F(3,135) = 1.66, P = 0.18]. For the control group: ★T4 is significantly different from T1 and T2, P < 0.01. For the study group: ★★T3 is significantly different from T1 and T2, P < 0.01; #T4 is significantly different from T3, P < 0.01. STAI, State Trait Anxiety Inventory state subscale; OR, operating room. Data are mean ± SEM. (From Kain ZN, Wang SM, Caramico LA, et al: Parental desire for perioperative information and informed consent: A two-phase study. Anesth Analg 1997;84:299–306.)

the amount of information provided should be tailored to the needs of the individual parent.

Pharmacologic Interventions

Overview

Sedation before surgery is an effective method for decreasing anxiety.[42] The primary goals of administering a premedication to children are to facilitate an anxiety-free separation from their parents and to facilitate a smooth, stress-free induction of anesthesia. Other effects that may be achieved by pharmacologic preparation of the child include amnesia, anxiolysis, prevention of physiologic stress, such as avoiding tachycardia in patients with cyanotic congenital heart disease, and analgesia (see Chapter 9).

The reported rate of use of sedative premedications in the United States varies widely among age groups and geographic locations.[63] Premedicant sedative drugs are least often prescribed for children younger than 3 years of age and most often prescribed for adults under 65 years of age (25 vs. 75%). When analyzed by geographic location, sedative premedicants are used least often in the southwest and northeast regions and most often in the southeast region ($P = 0.001$) (Fig. 3–4). Interestingly, when the frequency of premedication in children is examined against Health Maintenance Organization (HMO) penetration (i.e., HMO enrollment by total population) in the various geographic regions, correlation coefficients (r) ranged from -0.96 to -0.85.[63] It appears that physicians who practice in areas that are highly penetrated by HMOs are significantly less likely to premedicate children undergoing surgery. It is also reported that anesthesiologists who are younger in age, in practice fewer years, and spend a lower percentage of their time anesthetizing outpatients premedicated more of their patients. Currently, the most commonly used sedative premedicant in the preoperative holding area is midazolam ($\sim$80%), followed by ketamine (4%), transmucosal fentanyl (3%), and meperidine (2%) (Fig. 3–5). When data of several survey studies were reviewed, it was noted that United States anesthesiologists who allowed parental presence the *least* used sedative premedication the *most,* and vice versa.[63–65] Thus, most anesthesiologists in the United States use either parental presence or sedative premedication to treat preoperative anxiety in children.

Pharmacologic Interventions Versus Behavioral Interventions

When pharmacologic interventions are directly compared with behavioral interventions, children receiving a sedative are less anxious and more compliant than those accompanied into the operating room by a parent (Fig. 3–6).[71] Interestingly, parental anxiety is also lower when the child has received a premedication. One study examined whether a combination of parental presence and sedative premedication is more effective than sedative premedication alone for reducing the anxiety of children and their parents and for improving parental satisfaction.[85] The investigators found that parental presence during induction of anesthesia has no additive anxiolytic effects for children who receive a sedative preoperatively. However, parents who accompany their sedated children into the operating rooms are significantly less anxious and more satisfied both with the separation process and with the overall anesthetic, nursing, and surgical care provided.

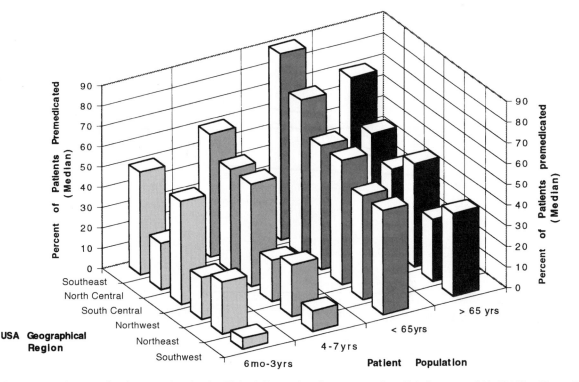

Figure 3–4. Frequency of premedication practice in the United States (medians; range for all values was 0%–100%). (From Kain ZN, Mayes LC, Bell C, et al: Premedication in the United States: A status report. Anesth Analg 1997;84:427–432.)

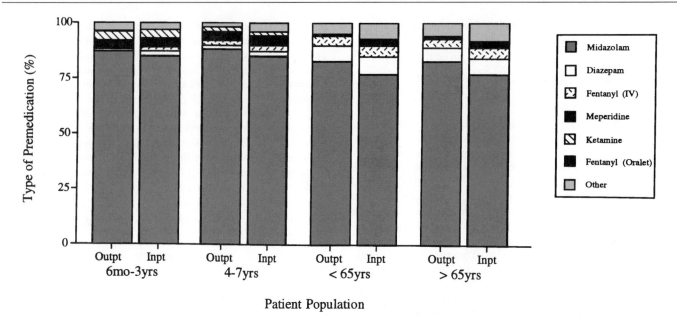

Figure 3–5. Types of premedicants used in the preoperative holding area. (From Kain ZN, Mayes LC, Bell C, et al: Premedication in the United States: A status report. Anesth Analg 1997;84:427–432.)

In conclusion, although sedative premedicants are effective for treatment of preoperative anxiety in children, they should *not* routinely be used in all children undergoing surgery. Their use should be directed to children who are at high risk for the development of preoperative anxiety. Variables such as length of surgery and potential recovery delays should also be considered. However, it is important to not withhold premedication if that premedication would likely be of benefit to a selected child. Even if the scheduled

procedure is brief, if a particular child is highly anxious, then that child will likely benefit from a premedication regardless of the negative effects on recovery and discharge.

Preoperative Anxiety: Outcomes

Four decades ago, Janis[86] proposed that moderate levels of preoperative anxiety in adult patients were associated with

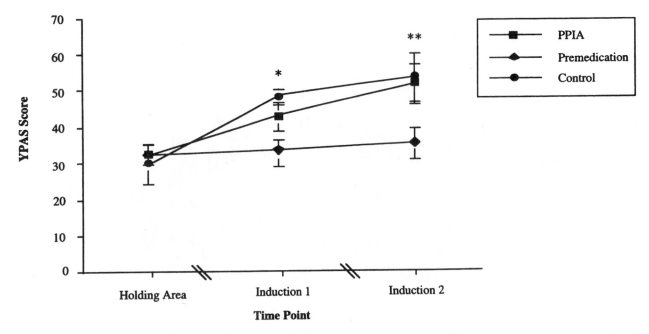

Figure 3–6. Anxiety of the child during the perioperative period. As can be seen, anxiety of the premedication group was significantly lower during both induction 1 ($\star P = 0.0171$) and induction 2 ($\star\star P = 0.0176$) than anxiety of the parental presence during induction of anesthesia (PPIA) of control group. Induction 1 is entrance to the operating room; induction 2 is introduction of the anesthesia mask to the child. YPAS, Yale Preoperative Anxiety Scale. (From Kain ZN, Mayes LC, Wang SM, et al: Parental presence during induction of anesthesia versus sedative premedication: Which intervention is more effective? Anesthesiology 1998;89:1147–1156.)

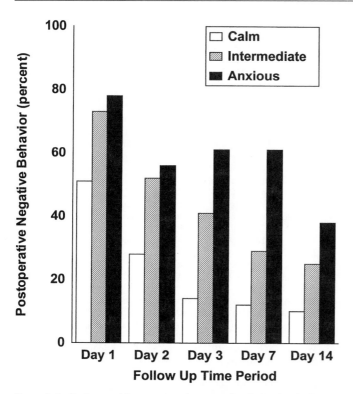

Figure 3–7. Patients with postoperative negative behavioral changes as a function of both postoperative time and anxiety during the induction of anesthesia. (From Kain ZN, Wang SM, Mayes LC, et al: Distress during the induction of anesthesia and postoperative behavioral outcomes. Anesth Analg 1999;88:1042–1047.)

good postoperative behavioral recovery, whereas low and high levels of preoperative anxiety were associated with poor behavioral recovery. Although Janis's theory is intriguing, his studies were based on descriptive data from nonrandom, limited samples and retrospective reports of questionable validity. Subsequent studies have been critical of Janis's methodology and have reported a linear rather than a curvilinear relationship between anxiety level and postoperative behavioral recovery.[87–90] That is, low levels of preoperative anxiety are associated with good postoperative behavioral recovery, whereas moderate and high levels of preoperative anxiety are associated with poor postoperative behavioral recovery. The assumption that low preoperative anxiety is predictive of good postoperative outcomes underlies many interventions in which the aim is to reduce preoperative anxiety. To date, preoperative preparation studies in adult patients have used diverse postoperative outcome measures, including intensity of pain, analgesic requirements, postsurgical complications, length of hospital stay, patient satisfaction, blood cortisol levels, changes in blood pressure and heart rate, and behavioral indices of recovery.[16, 89, 91–100] Reviews of this research, while critical of the methodology, have concluded that psychologically prepared adult patients may have improved postoperative recovery.[14–16, 93, 94]

As indicated earlier, a significant number of children may demonstrate new negative behaviors postoperatively, such as new onset of general anxiety, nighttime crying, enuresis, separation anxiety, temper tantrums, and sleep or eating disturbances. These behaviors may occur in up to 44% of

children 2 weeks following surgery; about 20% of these children continue to demonstrate negative behaviors 6 months postoperatively.[6] The postoperative negative behavioral changes are likely the result of an interaction between the distress the child experiences during the perioperative period and the individual personality characteristics of the child. Previously, variables such as the age and temperament of the child and the state and trait anxiety of the parent have been identified as predictors for the occurrence of negative postoperative behavioral changes.[6] There is a paucity of data, however, regarding a possible association between the distress the child experiences during induction of anesthesia and the occurrence of these negative postoperative behavioral changes. One investigation concluded that extreme anxiety, such as with a stormy induction of anesthesia, was associated with an *increased* incidence of postoperative negative behavioral changes (Fig. 3–7).[101] The investigators recommend that anesthesiologists advise parents of children who are anxious during induction of anesthesia of the increased likelihood that their children will develop postoperative negative behavioral changes, such as nightmares, separation anxiety, and aggression toward authority.[101]

Since the anxiety level of the child and mother in the preoperative holding area predicts the occurrence of negative postoperative behavioral problems,[6] it can be hypothesized that if sedative premedicants lower anxiety of the child and the parents in the preoperative holding area, they may also have an effect on negative postoperative behavioral outcomes.[75] One investigation of premedicated children found a significantly lower incidence of negative behavioral changes during the first week after surgery (Fig. 3–8).[102] This study

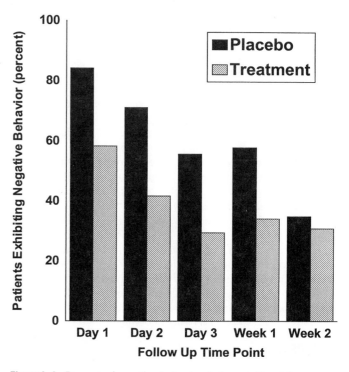

Figure 3–8. Percent of negative behavioral changes found in groups receiving treatment or placebo across the postoperative follow-up period. (From Kain ZN, Mayes LC, Wang SM, Hofstadter MB: Postoperative behavioral outcomes in children: Effects of sedative premedication. Anesthesiology 1999;90:758–765.)

suggests that reducing anxiety in the holding area had a beneficial effect not only on the preoperative behavior of the child but also on the immediate postoperative period.[102]

It is also commonly believed that increased anxiety prior to surgery is associated with increased intraoperative anesthetic requirements.[100, 103] This belief, however, is based on early studies with questionable scientific validity,[13, 104, 105] many of which did not use validated scales to measure anxiety or control for potential confounding variables like sedative premedication and the surgical procedure.[13] One investigation indicated that high baseline (i.e., trait) anxiety is associated with increased intraoperative anesthetic requirements. The investigators in this study controlled for the surgical procedure, used bispectral electroencephalographic analysis (the bispectral index) monitoring to ensure the same anesthetic depth in all patients, and used a total intravenous anesthetic technique to ease the calculation of the anesthetics used.[106] While further research is needed to make clear the relationship between preoperative anxiety and personality characteristics to postoperative clinical recovery, it does seem clear that a high baseline, or trait, anxiety is associated with increased intraoperative anesthetic requirements.

Several review articles suggest that increased anxiety prior to undergoing surgery and anesthesia is associated with postoperative nausea and vomiting.[107, 108] Experimental data suggest that children's anxiety in the preoperative holding area is not predictive of postoperative nausea and vomiting either in the postanesthesia care unit or at home.[109]

SUMMARY

Approximately three million children undergo anesthesia and surgery in the United States every year. It is reported that 40 to 60% of these children develop behavioral stress prior to their surgery. Multiple interventions have been suggested to treat the preoperative behavioral stress response in children. Currently, however, there is a trend towards *reduction* in both behavioral and pharmacologic preoperative interventions aimed at children. A possible reason may be that some physicians feel that reduction of parental anxiety during the preoperative period is a surrogate outcome. Perhaps rather than evaluating the effects of various preoperative interventions on the transient preoperative behavior, we should concentrate on research directed at demonstrating that reduction of preoperative anxiety can change postoperative outcomes. It is well established that low levels of preoperative anxiety are associated with good postoperative behavioral recovery, whereas moderate and high levels of preoperative anxiety are associated with poor postoperative behavioral recovery. A far more intriguing question is the possible association between preoperative anxiety and the postoperative clinical recovery; valid research needs to be developed in this area of postoperative clinical recovery and preoperative anxiety.

REFERENCES

1. Kain ZN, Mayes LC: Anxiety in children during the perioperative period. In: Borestein M, Genevro J, eds: Child Development and Behavioral Pediatrics. Mahwah, NJ: Lawrence Erlbaum Associates; 1996:85–103.
2. Burton L: Anxiety relating to illness and treatment. In: Verma V, ed: Anxiety in Children. London: Methuen Croom Helm; 1984:151–171.
3. Kotiniemi LH, Ryhanen PT, Moilanen IK: Behavioural changes following routine ENT operations in two-to-ten-year-old children. Paediatr Anaesth 1996;6:45–49.
4. Kotiniemi LH, Ryhanen PT, Moilanen IK: Behavioural changes in children following day-case surgery: A 4-week follow-up of 551 children. Anaesthesia 1997;52:970–976.
5. Kotiniemi LH, Ryhanen PT, Valanne J, et al: Postoperative symptoms at home following day-case surgery in children: A multicentre survey of 551 children. Anaesthesia 1997;52:963–969.
6. Kain ZN, Mayes LC, O'Connor TZ, et al: Preoperative anxiety in children: Predictors and outcomes. Arch Pediatr Adolesc Med 1996;150:1238–1245.
7. Kotiniemi LH, Ryhanen PT: Behavioural changes and children's memories after intravenous, inhalation and rectal induction of anaesthesia. Paediatr Anaesth 1996;6:201–207.
8. Vernon DT, Schulman JL, Foley JM: Changes in children's behavior after hospitalization. Some dimensions of response and their correlates. Am J Dis Child 1966;111:581–593.
9. Ramsay MA: A survey of pre-operative fear. Anaesthesia 1972;27:396–402.
10. Fell D, Derbyshire DR, Maile CJ, et al: Measurement of plasma catecholamine concentrations: An assessment of anxiety. Br J Anaesth 1985;57:770–774.
11. Tonnesen E: Immunological aspects of anaesthesia and surgery—with special reference to NK cells. Dan Med Bull 1989;36:263–281.
12. Williams JG, Jones JR: Psychophysiological responses to anesthesia and operation. JAMA 1968;203:415–417.
13. Williams JG, Jones JR, Williams B: A physiological measure of preoperative anxiety. Psychosom Med 1969;31:522–527.
14. Wallace LM: Pre-operative state anxiety as a mediator of psychological adjustment to and recovery from surgery. Br J Med Psychol 1986;59:253–261.
15. Johnston M: Pre-operative emotional states and post-operative recovery. Adv Psychosom Med 1986;15:1–22.
16. Martinez-Urrutia A: Anxiety and pain in surgical patients. J Consult Clin Psychol 1975;43:437–442.
17. Haavik PE, Soreide E, Hofstad B, et al: Does preoperative anxiety influence gastric fluid volume and acidity? Anesth Analg 1992;75:91–94.
18. Nygren J, Thorell A, Jacobsson H, et al: Preoperative gastric emptying. Effects of anxiety and oral carbohydrate administration. Ann Surg 1995;222:728–734.
19. Coté CJ, Goudsouzian NG, Liu LM, et al: Assessment of risk factors related to the acid aspiration syndrome in pediatric patients—gastric pH and residual volume. Anesthesiology 1982;56:70–72.
20. Patel RI, Hannallah RS, Verghese ST: Preoperative anxiety and gastric fluid secretion in healthy children scheduled for outpatient surgery. Paediatr Anaesth 1994;4:319–322.
21. Provence SA, Mayes LC: Separation and deprivation. In: Lewis M, ed. Child and Adolescent Psychiatry: A Comprehensive Textbook. Philadelphia: Williams & Wilkins; 1996:382–394.
22. Skodak M, Skeels HM: A final follow-up study of one hundred adopted children. J Genetic Psych 1949;75:85–125.
23. Stifter CA, Fox NA: Infant reactivity: Physiological correlates of newborn and 5-month temperament. Dev Psych 1990;26:582–588.
24. Schwartz BH, Albino JE, Tedesco LA: Effects of psychological preparation on children hospitalized for dental operations. J Pediatr 1983;102:634–638.
25. Bretherton I: Open communication and internal working models: Their role in the development of attachment relationships. In: Thompson R, ed: Nebraska Symposium on Motivation, 1988: Socioemotional Development. Current Theory and Research in Motivation. Lincoln, NE: University of Nebraska Press; 1990:57–113.
26. Lamb M: Qualitative aspects of mother-infant and father-infant attachment. Infant Behav Develop 1978;1:265–275.
27. Lamb ME, Hwang C-P, Frodi AM, et al: Security of mother and father infant attachment and its relation to sociability with strangers in traditional and nontraditional Swedish families. Infant Behav Develop 1982;5:355–367.
28. Belsky J, Lerner RM, Spanier GB: The Child in the Family. Reading, MA: Addison-Wesley Publishing Co; 1984.
29. Chess S, Thomas A: Temperament and its functional significance. In: Greenspan SI, Pollock GH, eds: The Course of Life, Vol 2: Early Childhood. Madison, CT: International Universities Press; 1989:163–228.

30. Chess S, Thomas A: Temperamental individuality from childhood to adolescence. J Am Acad Child Psychiatry 1977;16:218–226.

31. Thomas A, Chess S: Temperament and development. New York: Brunner/Mazel; 1977.

32. Buss AH, Plomin R: Temperament: Early Developing Personality Traits. Hillsdale, NJ: Lawrence Erlbaum Associates; 1984.

33. Strelau J: Emotion as a key concept in temperament research. J Res Personal 1987;21:510–528.

34. Kagan J, Snidman N: Temperamental factors in human development. Am Psychol 1991;46:856–862.

35. Vetter TR: The epidemiology and selective identification of children at risk for preoperative anxiety reactions. Anesth Analg 1993;77:96–99.

36. Brophy CJ, Erickson MT: Children's self-statements and adjustment to elective outpatient surgery. J Dev Behav Pediatr 1990;11:13–16.

37. Lumley MA, Melamed BG, Abeles LA: Predicting children's presurgical anxiety and subsequent behavior changes. J Pediatr Psychol 1993;18:481–497.

38. Sparrow SS, Balla DA, Cichetti DV: Manual for the Vineland Adaptive Behavior Scales. Circle Pines, MN: American Guidance Service; 1984.

39. Litman RS, Berger AA, Chhibber A: An evaluation of preoperative anxiety in a population of parents of infants and children undergoing ambulatory surgery. Paediatr Anaesth 1996;6:443–447.

40. Kain ZN, Mayes LC, Caramico LA: Preoperative preparation in children: A cross-sectional study. J Clin Anesth 1996;8:508–514.

41. Shirley PJ, Thompson N, Kenward M, et al: Parental anxiety before elective surgery in children. A British perspective. Anaesthesia 1998;53:956–959.

42. Zuckerberg AL: Perioperative approach to children. Pediatr Clin North Am 1994;41:15–29.

43. O'Byrne KK, Peterson L, Saldana L: Survey of pediatric hospitals' preparation programs: Evidence of the impact of health psychology research. Health Psychol 1997;16:147–154.

44. Pruitt SD, Elliott CH: Paediatric procedures. In: Johnston M, Wallace L, eds: Stress and Medical Procedures. Oxford: Oxford University Press; 1990:157–174.

45. Melamed BG, Ridley-Johnson R: Psychological preparation of families for hospitalization. J Dev Behav Pediatr 1988;9:96–102.

46. American Academy of Pediatrics Committee on Hospital Care: Child life programs. Pediatrics 1993;91:671–673.

47. Vernon DTA, Foley JM, Sipowicz RR, et al: The Psychological Responses of Children to Hospitalizations and Illness: A Review of the Literature. Springfield, IL: Charles C Thomas; 1965.

48. Melamed BG, Siegel LJ: Reduction of anxiety in children facing hospitalization and surgery by use of filmed modeling. J Consult Clin Psychol 1975;43:511–521.

49. Kain ZN, Caramico LA, Mayes LC, et al: Preoperative preparation programs in children: A comparative examination. Anesth Analg 1998;87:1249–1255.

50. Melamed BG, Siegel LJ: Psychological preparation for hospitalization. In: Franks CM, Evans JA, eds: Behavioral Medicine: Practical Applications in Health Care. New York: Springer Publishing; 1980:307–355.

51. Piaget J: The Language and Thought of the Child, 3rd ed. New York: The Humanities Press; 1955.

52. Melamed BG, Dearborn M, Hermecz DA: Necessary considerations for surgery preparation: age and previous experience. Psychosom Med 1983;45:517–525.

53. Faust J, Melamed BG: Influence of arousal, previous experience, and age on surgery preparation of same day of surgery and in-hospital pediatric patients. J Consult Clin Psychol 1984;52:359–365.

54. Kain ZN: Perioperative information and parental anxiety: the next generation. Anesth Analg 1999;88:237–239.

55. Cassady JF Jr, Wysocki TT, Miller KM, et al: Use of a preanesthetic video for facilitation of parental education and anxiolysis before pediatric ambulatory surgery. Anesth Analg 1999;88:246–250.

56. Saile H, Burgmeier R, Schmidt LR: A meta-analysis of studies on psychological preparation of children facing medical procedures. Psychol Health 1988;2:107–132.

57. Bouchner H, Vinci R, Waring C: Pediatric procedures: Do parents want to watch? Pediatrics 1989;84:907–909.

58. Henderson MA, Baines DB, Overton JH: Parental attitudes to presence at induction of paediatric anaesthesia. Anaesth Intens Care 1993;21:324–327.

59. Braude N, Ridley SA, Sumner E: Parents and paediatric anaesthesia: A prospective survey of parental attitudes to their presence at induction. Ann R Coll Surg Engl 1990;72:41–44.

60. Ryder IG, Spargo PM: Parents in the anaesthetic room: A questionnaire survey of parents' reaction. Anaesthesia 1991;46:977–979.

61. Vessey JA, Bogetz MS, Caserza CL, et al: Parental upset associated with participation in induction of anaesthesia in children. Can J Anaesth 1994;41:276–280.

62. Kain ZN, Mayes LC, Caramico LA, et al: Parental presence during induction of anesthesia. A randomized controlled trial. Anesthesiology 1996;84:1060–1067.

63. Kain ZN, Mayes LC, Bell C, et al: Premedication in the United States: A status report. Anesth Analg 1997;84:427–432.

64. Kain ZN, Fernandes LA, Touloukian RJ: Parental presence during induction of anesthesia: The surgeon's perspective. Eur J Pediatr Surg 1996;6:323–327.

65. Kain ZN, Ferris CA, Mayes LC, et al: Parental presence during induction of anaesthesia: Practice differences between the United States and Great Britain. Paediatr Anaesth 1996;6:187–193.

66. Shaw EG, Routh DK: Effect of mother presence on children's reaction to aversive procedures. J Pediatr Psychol 1982;7:33–42.

67. Bowie JR: Parents in the operating room? Anesthesiology 1993;78:1192–1193.

68. Schofield NM, White JB: Interrelations among children, parents, premedication, and anaesthetists in paediatric day stay surgery. Br Med J 1989;299:1371–1375.

69. Gauderer MW, Lorig JL, Eastwood DW: Is there a place for parents in the operating room? J Pediatr Surg 1989;24:705–706.

70. Bevan JC, Johnston C, Haig MJ, et al: Preoperative parental anxiety predicts behavioral and emotional responses to induction of anaesthesia in children. Can J Anaesth 1990;37:177–182.

71. Kain ZN, Mayes LC, Wang SM, et al: Parental presence during induction of anesthesia versus sedative premedication: which intervention is more effective? Anesthesiology 1998;89:1147–1156.

72. Hickmott KC, Shaw EA, Goodyer I, et al: Anaesthetic induction in children: the effects of maternal presence on mood and subsequent behaviour. Eur J Anaesthesiol 1989;6:145–155.

73. Hannallah RS, Rosales JK: Experience with parents presence during anesthesia induction in children. Can Anaesth Soc J 1983;30:287–290.

74. Schulman JL, Foley JM, Vernon DT, et al: A study of the effect of the mother's presence during anesthesia induction. Pediatrics 1967;39:111–114.

75. Dahlquist LM, Gil KM, Armstrong FD, et al: Preparing children for medical examinations: the importance of previous medical experience. Health Psychol 1986;5:249–259.

76. Blount RL, Bachanas PJ, Powers SW, et al: Training children to cope and parents to coach them during routine immunizations: Effects on child, parent, and staff behaviors. Behav Ther 1992;23:689–705.

77. Lewyn MJ: Should parents be present while their children receive anesthesia? Anesth Malpract Protect 1993;56–57.

78. Egbert LD, Battit GE, Turndorf H, et al: The value of a preoperative visit by an anesthetist: A study of doctor-patient rapport. JAMA 1963;185:553–555.

79. Alfidi RJ: Informed consent: A study of patient reaction. JAMA 1971;216:1325–1329.

80. Miller SM, Mangan CE: Interacting effects of information and coping style in adapting to gynecologic stress: Should the doctor tell all? J Pers Soc Psychol 1983;45:223–236.

81. Kerrigan DD, Thevasagayam RS, Woods TO, et al: Who's afraid of informed consent? Br Med J 1993;306:298–300.

82. Kain ZN, Kosarussavadi B, Hernandez-Conte A, et al: Desire for perioperative information in adult patients: A cross-sectional study. J Clin Anesth 1997;9:467–472.

83. Kain ZN, Wang SM, Caramico LA, et al: Parental desire for perioperative information and informed consent: A two-phase study. Anesth Analg 1997;84:299–306.

84. Inglis S, Farnill D: The effects of providing preoperative statistical anaesthetic-risk information. Anaesth Intensive Care 1993;21:799–805.

85. Kain ZN, Mayes LC, Wang SM, et al: Parental presence and sedative premedicants for children undergoing surgery: A hierarchical study. Anesthesiology 1998;89:1147–1156.

86. Janis IL: Stress: Psychoanalytic and Behavioral Studies of Surgical Patients. New York: Wiley; 1958.

87. Johnson JE, Leventhal H, Dabbs JM Jr: Contribution of emotional and instrumental response processes in adaptation to surgery. J Pers Soc Psychol 1971;20:55–64.

88. Johnston M, Carpenter L: Relationship between pre-operative anxiety and post-operative state. Psychol Med 1980;10:361–367.
89. Newman S: Anxiety, hospitalization, and surgery. In: Fitzpatrick R, Hinton J, Newman S, et al., eds: The Experience of Illness. London: Tavistock Publications; 1984:132–153.
90. Pick B, Molloy A, Hinds C, et al: Post-operative fatigue following coronary artery bypass surgery: Relationship to emotional state and to the catecholamine response to surgery. J Psychosom Res 1994;38:599–607.
91. Lindeman CA, Stetzer SL: Effect of preoperative visits by operating room nurses. Nurs Res 1973;22:4–16.
92. Egbert LD, Battit GE, Welch CE, et al: Reduction of postoperative pain by encouragement and instruction of patients. N Engl J Med 1964;270:825–827.
93. George JM, Scott DS, Turner SP, et al: The effects of psychological factors and physical trauma on recovery from oral surgery. J Behav Med 1980;3:291–310.
94. Johnson JE, Dabbs JM Jr, Leventhal H: Psychosocial factors in the welfare of surgical patients. Nurs Res 1970;19:18–29.
95. Johnson JE, Rice VH, Fuller SS, et al: Sensory information, instruction in a coping strategy, and recovery from surgery. Res Nurs Health 1978;1:4–17.
96. Ray C, Fitzgibbon G: Stress arousal and coping with surgery. Psychol Med 1981;11:741–746.
97. Taenzer P, Melzack R, Jeans ME: Influence of psychological factors on postoperative pain, mood and analgesic requirements. Pain 1986;24:331–342.
98. Scott LE, Clum GA, Peoples JB: Preoperative predictors of postoperative pain. Pain 1983;15:283–293.
99. Lim AT, Edis G, Kranz H, et al: Postoperative pain control: Contribution of psychological factors and transcutaneous electrical stimulation. Pain 1983;17:179–188.
100. Parris WC, Matt D, Jamison RN, et al: Anxiety and postoperative recovery in ambulatory surgery patients. Anesth Prog 1988;35:61–64.
101. Kain ZN, Wang SM, Mayes LC, et al: Distress during the induction of anesthesia and postoperative behavioral outcomes. Anesth Analg 1999;88:1042–1047.
102. Kain ZN, Mayes LC, Wang SM, Hofstadter MB: Postoperative behavioral outcomes in children: Effects of sedative premedication. Anesthesiology 1999;90:758–765.
103. Johnston M: Impending surgery. In: Fisher S, Reason J, eds: Handbook of Life Stress. New York: John Wiley & Sons; 1988:79–100.
104. Williams JGL, Jones JR, Workhoven MN, et al: The psychological control of preoperative anxiety. Psychophysiology 1975;12:50–54.
105. Goldmann L, Ogg TW, Levey AB: Hypnosis and daycase anaesthesia. A study to reduce pre-operative anxiety and intra-operative anaesthetic requirements. Anaesthesia 1988;43:466–469.
106. Maranets I, Kain ZN: Preoperative anxiety and intraoperative anesthetic requirements. Anesth Analg 1999;89:1346–1351.
107. Watcha MF, White PF: Postoperative nausea and vomiting: Its etiology, treatment, and prevention. Anesthesiology 1992;77:162–184.
108. Lerman J: Surgical and patient factors in postoperative nausea and vomiting. Br J Anaesth 1992;69:24S–32S.
109. Wang SM, Kain ZN: Preoperative anxiety and postoperative nausea and vomiting in children: Is there an association? Anesth Analg 2000;90:571–575.

4 Preoperative Evaluation of Pediatric Patients

Charles J. Coté, I. David Todres, John F. Ryan, *and* Nishan Goudsouzian

Psychological Preparation of Children for Surgery

History of Present Illness

Past Medical History

Family History

Physical Examination

Laboratory Data

Special Problems

    Fasting

    Full Stomach

    Anemia

    Upper Respiratory Tract Infection (URI)

    Fever

    Sickle Cell Disease

    Mentally Handicapped Children

    Retinopathy of Prematurity

    Post-Anesthesia Apnea in Former Preterm Infants

    Bronchopulmonary Dysplasia

    Diabetic Children

    Seizure Disorders

    Hyperalimentation

    Asthma and Reactive Airway Disease

The preoperative evaluation and preparation of pediatric patients are basically similar to those of adults from a physiologic standpoint. However, the psychological preparation of infants and children is different (see Chapter 3). A child does not have the experience to place a hospital, with its overwhelming size, odors, and noise levels, in perspective. Children fear pain, threat of needles, and separation from parents and may have difficulty in comprehending the need for hospitalization or surgery. A specific child-oriented approach by the anesthesiologist, surgeon, nurses, and parents is required. Preoperative evaluation is usually simplified once the basic concepts of how to evaluate a child are understood.

Psychological Preparation of Children for Surgery

Many hospitals have either an open house or a brochure to describe the preoperative programs available to parents before their child's admission.[1] Anesthesiologists are encouraged to participate in the design of these programs so that they accurately reflect the anesthetic practice of the institution.

The preoperative anesthetic experience begins at the time parents are first informed that their child is to have surgery or a procedure requiring general anesthesia. This is the most appropriate time to introduce the parents to preparative programs, rather than waiting for a hasty and often inadequate last-minute discussion with nervous and preoccupied parents. The greater understanding and amount of information that the parents have, the less their anxiety will be; this attitude in turn will be reflected in the child. Being prepared enables parents to answer their child's questions and thus paves the way for a smooth preanesthetic course. Inadequate preparation of children and their families often makes the anesthetic induction traumatic and difficult for both the child and the anesthesiologist, with the possibility of postoperative psychological disturbances.[2]

Special aspects of a child's perception of anesthesia should be anticipated; children often have the same fears as adults but are unable to articulate those fears. It is important to reassure children that anesthesia is a type of *deep sleep*, not the same as the usual nightly sleep, but rather *a special type during which they will feel no pain from surgery and from which they will very definitely awaken.* Many children fear the possibility that they will wake up in the middle of the anesthetic and surgical process. They should be reassured that they will awaken *only* when the operation is completed. The reason and need for a surgical procedure should also be carefully explained to the child.

The words the anesthesiologist uses to describe what can be anticipated must be carefully chosen, because children think concretely and tend to interpret literally. Examples of this are presented by the following anecdotes:

A 4-year-old child was informed that in the morning she would receive a "shot" that would "put her to sleep." That night, a frantic call was received from the mother, describing a very upset child; the child thought she was going to be "put to sleep" like the veterinarian had "put to sleep" her sick pet.

A 5-year-old child was admitted to the hospital for elective inguinal herniorrhaphy. He received heavy premedication and was sleeping upon arrival in the operating room. After discharge, the parents frequently discovered him wandering about the house at night. On questioning, the child stated that he was "protecting" his family. He stated: "I don't want anyone sneaking up on you and operating while you are sleeping."

In the first example, the child's concrete thought processes misunderstood the anesthesiologist's choice of words. The second case represents a problem of communication; the child was never told he would have an operation.

The importance of proper psychological preparation for surgery should not be underestimated.[3–6] Often, little has been explained to either patient or parents. Anesthesiologists can have a key role in alleviating fear of the unknown if they understand a child's age-related perception of anesthesia and surgery (see Chapter 3). They can convey their understanding by presenting a calm and friendly face (smiling, looking at the child and making eye contact), offering a warm introduction, touching the patient in a reassuring manner (holding a child's or parent's hand), and being completely honest. Children respond positively to an honest description of exactly what they can anticipate. This includes informing them of the slight discomfort of starting an intravenous line or giving an intramuscular premedication, the possible bitter taste of an oral premedication, or a mask induction for anesthesia. The anesthesiologist who condescendingly tells a child that there will be no pain loses credibility when the child does experience pain. The child then becomes more frightened and distrustful.

The postsurgical process, from the operating room to the recovery room and the onset of postoperative pain, should be described. Encourage the patient and family to ask any questions they may have. The patient and family should be told that everything possible will be done to maintain comfort, such as the use of postoperative long-acting local anesthetics, nerve blocks, continuous caudal or epidural blocks, patient-controlled, nurse-controlled, or parent-controlled analgesia or epidural analgesia, or intermittent narcotics.

A very important feature of the preoperative process is preparation not only for this unique experience in a child's life but also for possible future anesthetic or surgical procedures. Close cooperation between the anesthesiologist and the parents in preparing a child is vital to a favorable outcome. While focusing on the preparation of the child, it is crucial to appreciate that the most favorable outcome depends on preparation of the whole family unit: the child, siblings, and parents. In certain circumstances, parents will want to accompany their child to the operating room environment. If this is judged to be in the child's best interest, the anesthesiologist should support the parents' decision. What eases the parents calms their child, and this can only enhance patient care. Allowing a favorite security blanket or teddy bear to accompany a child to the operating room may provide a great source of emotional comfort.

Before surgery, it is essential to discuss anesthetic risks in clear terms. This should be carried out in a reassuring manner by describing to the parents exactly what measures will be taken to closely monitor the safety of their child. Mentioning specific details and the purpose of the various monitoring devices helps diminish the parents' anxiety by demonstrating to them that their child will be anesthetized with the utmost safety and care. A blood pressure cuff will "check the blood pressure," electrocardiographic monitors will "watch the heartbeat," a stethoscope will help us "to continuously listen to the heart sounds," a pulse oximeter will "measure the oxygen in the bloodstream," a carbon dioxide analyzer will "monitor the breathing," an anesthetic agent monitor will "accurately measure the level of anesthesia," and an intravenous catheter will be placed "to administer fluid and medications as needed." Parents should be given ample opportunity to ask questions during this preoperative preparation.

Children often return home after an anesthetic-surgical experience and then relive unpleasant memories in the form of nightmares. In addition, some children exhibit psychosomatic manifestations of this experience, such as the development of tics, agitation, lack of concentration, or bed-wetting. It is for these reasons that attention toward reducing anxiety and unpleasant experiences is most important. Fortunately, many of these problems resolve after a short time.[7]

History of Present Illness

The medical history of a pediatric patient begins in utero; problems that may have been present during gestation and birth may still be relevant in the neonatal period (Table 4–1). This history is especially important for a neonate who requires an urgent surgical procedure. The problems expected in a full-term baby of normal birth weight are different from those anticipated in a full-term baby who is small for gestational age. These considerations are magnified for a premature baby of appropriate weight and are markedly intensified for a baby who is both premature and small for gestational age (see Chapters 2 and 14). A careful neonatal and gestational history often enables the anesthesiologist to anticipate problems that could prove potentially dangerous during or following anesthesia. Several scoring systems for both physical characteristics and neurologic examination provide reasonable estimates of gestational age.[8–12] By plotting gestational age against birth weight, general categories of neonates can be defined, each with its own risk for associated neonatal problems. For example, a 2000 g baby with characteristics of a 29-week gestation would be large for gestational age, whereas at 35 weeks of gestation the weight would be appropriate for gestational age. The same weight in a child of 40 weeks of gestation would be considered small for gestational age. Thus, weight alone is not the sole criterion for determining maturity. The maternal medical and pharmacologic history (therapeutic, drug abuse) may also provide valuable data for the management of a neonate requiring surgery.

In most situations, the history of the present illness is described to physicians by the parents. If the child is old enough, it is helpful to obtain the child's corroboration. The history should focus on the following aspects:

■ The relevant organ systems involved.
■ Medications related to and taken before the present illness.
■ Previous surgical and hospital experiences related to the current problem.

Table 4–1. Maternal History with Commonly Associated Neonatal Problems

Maternal History	Commonly Expected Problems with Neonate
Rh-ABO incompatibility	Hemolytic anemia, hyperbilirubinemia, kernicterus
Toxemia	SGA and its associated problems (see Table 2–2), muscle relaxant interaction with magnesium therapy
Hypertension	SGA and its associated problems (see Table 2–2)
Drug addiction	Withdrawal, SGA
Infection	Sepsis, thrombocytopenia, viral infection
Hemorrhage	Anemia, shock
Diabetes	Hypoglycemia, birth trauma, LGA, SGA and associated problems (see Table 2–2)
Polyhydramnios	Tracheoesophageal fistula, anencephaly, multiple anomalies
Oligohydramnios	Renal hypoplasia, pulmonary hypoplasia
Cephalopelvic disproportion	Birth trauma, hyperbilirubinemia, fractures
Alcoholism	Hypoglycemia, congenital malformation, fetal alcohol syndrome, SGA and associated problems (see Table 2–2)

LGA, large for gestational age; SGA, small for gestational age.

- Additionally, the past history of other medical problems unrelated to the present illness. For example, in young infants, a history of prematurity or apnea may significantly alter the routine postoperative course.[13]
- The time of last oral intake and its relation to the illness or injury, time of last urination (wet diaper), or time of vomiting and diarrhea. It is essential to appreciate that decreased gastrointestinal motility often begins with the illness or injury. A child who has had an accident within several hours of eating should be considered to have a full stomach, even though the surgical procedure may be planned for many hours after the accident.
- Review of all other body systems should also be made (Table 4–2), with special emphasis on a history of a recent upper respiratory tract infection (URI), history of croup, allergic reactions, bleeding tendencies (bruising), fever, anemia, seizures, diarrhea, and vomiting. Vomiting and fever are particularly important concerns in young infants because of the rapid fluid turnover and increased risk of hypovolemia.
- Family history of anesthesia-related complications, particularly any history of death or high fever in the perioperative period (malignant hyperthermia) or history of prolonged neuromuscular blockade (pseudocholinesterase deficiency).

Past Medical History

Past medical history should include a history of previous hospitalizations (medical or surgical), immunizations, childhood illnesses, past medication history (particularly important for children who have had chemotherapy, which may have resulted in cardiac toxicity),[14–17] and possible contacts with infectious diseases. A history of prematurity and apnea or bradycardic spells is highly significant. A history of croup may warn of potential post-intubation croup. A history of intubation in the neonatal period may be later associated with subglottic stenosis.

Examination of previous medical, surgical, and anesthetic records assists in planning the anesthetic procedure. Special note should be taken of any difficulties previously encountered before, during, and after surgery. Specific attention should be paid to airway problems, tracheal intubation, venous access, hypotension, bradycardia, oxygen saturation, agitation, and the response to or need for a premedication. Sometimes this review reveals the need for greater than normal amounts of premedication or the success of intramuscular compared with oral premedication.

Family History

It is important to inquire about a family history of (1) prolonged paralysis associated with anesthesia (pseudocholinesterase deficiency), (2) unexpected deaths (sudden infant death syndrome, malignant hyperthermia), (3) genetic defects, (4) familial medical conditions such as muscular dystrophy, cystic fibrosis, sickle cell disease, bleeding tendencies (hemophilia, von Willebrand disease), (5) allergic reactions, and (6) drug addiction (drug withdrawal, human immunodeficiency virus carrier).

Physical Examination

A great deal of information can be gained during the physical examination by observing how children interact with their parents, nurses, and physicians. While observing a child and talking to the family, we are gaining the child's acceptance. We can also readily determine the anxiety level of parents and child; in so doing, we can begin to formulate appropriate premedication or induction techniques. A child is not examined in the same way as an adult. Examination begins with careful, nonthreatening observations and proceeds to the physical examination according to the child's interaction with the anesthesiologist.

While looking at a patient, observe the skin and facies for pallor, cyanosis, sweating, jaundice, apprehension, pain, or signs of previous operations. Does the child have an obvious upper respiratory tract infection? Is the child having respiratory difficulty (nasal flaring, grunting respirations, stridor, retractions, or wheezing)? Is there abdominal distension? Are there congenital abnormalities? It is important to be alert to any unusual features, because these may represent a specific syndrome. *When a child has one congenital malformation, the likelihood of another is increased.*

Table 4–2. Review of Systems: Anesthetic Implications

System	Questions to Ask	Possible Anesthetic Implications
Respiratory	Cough, asthma, recent cold	Irritable airway, bronchospasm, medication history, atelectasis, infiltrate
	Croup	Subglottic narrowing
	Apnea/bradycardia	Postoperative apnea/bradycardia
Cardiovascular	Murmur	Septal defect, avoid air bubbles in intravenous line
	Cyanosis	Right-to-left shunt
	History of squatting	Tetralogy of Fallot
	Hypertension	Coarctation, renal disease
	Rheumatic fever	Valvular heart disease
	Exercise intolerance	Congestive heart failure, cyanosis
Neurologic	Seizures	Medications, metabolic derangement
	Head trauma	Intracranial hypertension
	Swallowing incoordination	Aspiration, esophageal reflux, hiatus hernia
	Neuromuscular disease	Neuromuscular relaxant drug sensitivity, malignant hyperpyrexia
Gastrointestinal/hepatic	Vomiting, diarrhea	Electrolyte imbalance, dehydration, full stomach
	Malabsorption	Anemia
	Black stools	Anemia, hypovolemia
	Reflux	Treat like full stomach
	Jaundice	Drug metabolism/hypoglycemia
Genitourinary	Frequency	Urinary tract infection, diabetes, hypercalcemia
	Time of last urination	State of hydration
	Frequent urinary tract infections	Evaluate renal function
Endocrine/metabolic	Abnormal development	Endocrinopathy, hypothyroidism, diabetes
	Hypoglycemia, steroid therapy	Hypoglycemia, adrenal insufficiency
Hematologic	Anemia	Need for transfusion
	Bruising, excess bleeding	Coagulopathy, thrombocytopenia, thrombocytopathy
	Sickle cell disease	Hydration, possible transfusion
Allergies	Medications	Possible drug interaction
Dental	Loose, carious teeth	Aspiration of loose teeth, subacute bacterial endocarditis prophylaxis

Devices that are attached to the child may provide important clues to underlying conditions and ongoing therapy, such as an endotracheal tube, a ventilator, intravenous lines, a venous port, a peripherally inserted central line, infusions of medications (vasopressors), urinary catheter, nasogastric tube, or respiratory and cardiac monitors.

Having talked with the parents and observed the child, the examiner proceeds in a manner similar to that used for an adult, with some special differences. It is important to warm the stethoscope and the examining hands. The examination of children is an examination of opportunity. With the child quiet, begin with the less painful areas; listen to the heart and lungs and defer the throat examination and potentially painful examinations to the end. Special points of interest are (1) fever; (2) missing or loose teeth (possible dislodgment during laryngoscopy); (3) micrognathia (difficult intubation); (4) nasal speech or mouth breathing (hypertrophied adenoids or tonsils, difficult induction, potential bleeding with nasogastric tube or nasotracheal intubation, sleep apnea, pulmonary artery hypertension); (5) heart murmurs (take care to avoid air bubbles in intravenous lines, make certain that the cause of the murmur has been defined by echocardiogram); (6) abdominal distension (full stomach, impeded respirations); (7) the child's neurologic status (increased intracranial pressure, loss of the gag reflex, control of the airway and breathing, seizure disorder); and (8) edema (congestive heart failure, nephrotic syndrome, hypoproteinemia, renal failure). Special emphasis must be paid to hydration, because fluid turnover is much more rapid in infants than in adults (dry mouth, loss of tears, tenting of the skin, sunken fontanelle and eyeballs, mottled skin) (see Chapter 11).

In very young infants, one must avoid causing possibly dangerous hypothermia due to prolonged periods of undress during the physical examination. The anesthesiologist can readily evaluate an infant in an incubator. A rapid assessment of gestational age can be made by examining specific physical and neurologic characteristics (see Table 2–3).[9–12]

Laboratory Data

The amount of laboratory data gathered should be appropriate to the history, illness, and surgical procedure. Routine hemoglobin or urinalysis is no longer required for most elective procedures in children; the value of even these tests is questionable when the surgical procedure will not involve clinically important blood loss. We do not insist that every pediatric patient have a preoperative hemoglobin determination.[18] We request a hemoglobin determination only for patients who will undergo procedures with the potential for blood loss, those with specific risk factors for a hemoglobinopathy, former preterm infants, and those under 6 months of age. In general, routine chest radiography is not necessary; studies have confirmed that routine chest radiographs are not cost-effective in children.[19–21] A room air pulse oximeter measure of oxygen saturation is very helpful. A baseline saturation of 95% or less is suggestive of clinically important pulmonary or cardiac compromise and warrants further investigation. If major reconstructive surgery is contemplated, a bleeding profile (platelet count, prothrombin time, and partial thromboplastin time) may be indicated; a bleeding time may be useful for children taking medications containing aspirin or other antiplatelet drugs. Special laboratory tests, such as electrolyte and blood glucose determinations, renal function tests, blood gas analysis, seizure medication levels, digoxin levels, electrocardiography, echocardiography, liver function tests, computed tomography or magnetic resonance imaging scan, or pulmonary function tests, should be performed when appropriate.

Finally, the patient's history, physical examination, medications, and laboratory data must be synthesized into an anesthetic plan that combines the psychological needs of the patient and the anesthesiologist's concerns for the patient's safety with optimal operating conditions for the surgeon.

Special Problems

Fasting

Patients are ordered to fast from ingesting liquids and solids to minimize the dangers of pulmonary aspiration of gastric contents. Fasting protects against aspiration of particulate matter but may not protect against gastric fluid aspiration. The period of time that a child can safely fast is variable and usually is dependent on a child's age, weight, and nutritional status. One of the major concerns is the possibility of hypoglycemia; this is unlikely in a routine healthy pediatric patient but is possible in a debilitated, poorly nourished child or in a child with metabolic dysfunction.[22–25] There is no need for excessive preoperative fasting.[26] Clear liquids are very rapidly absorbed from the stomach with a half-life of approximately 15 minutes (Fig. 4–1). Breast milk, which can cause significant pulmonary injury if aspirated,[27] has a very high and variable fat content (determined by maternal diet), which will delay gastric emptying. Breast milk is not considered a clear liquid.[28]

In the past, as a general rule, most pediatric anesthesiologists would request an 8-hour period free of milk, solids, and liquids for children older than 3 years; an 8-hour fast from milk and solids but 6 hours for liquids for children 6 months to 3 years of age; and a 4-hour fast from milk and solids for infants 6 months of age or younger, with neonates allowed clear liquids until 2 hours before induction. A number of studies have demonstrated that the need to fast from *clear liquids* is considerably less than previously recommended.[29–35] All of these studies have found no significant difference in gastric residual volume or pH in children who were allowed to have *clear liquids* until 2 to 3 hours before surgery, compared with control populations with standard preoperative fasting. In accordance with these data, it is still reasonable to order all children to fast from milk and solids as in the past, but all patients are now encouraged to have clear liquids *ad libitum* until 3 hours before induction. Three hours of fasting from clear liquids provides flexibility in the operative schedule should the procedure occur up to 1 hour earlier than expected. Premature infants and infants up to 6 months of age have small glycogen stores and therefore should be offered clear liquids (apple juice, sugar water, water) up to 2 hours before surgery. This fasting regimen has made the preoperative fast a much more humane process for both children and their parents. Possible benefits may be

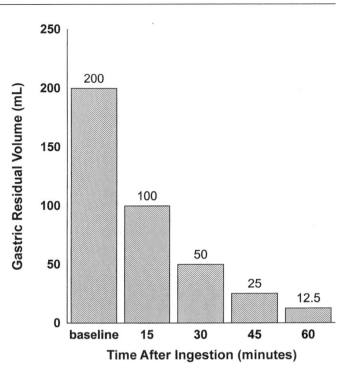

Figure 4–1. Clear liquids are rapidly absorbed from the stomach with a half-life of approximately 15 minutes. In this figure, for example, 200 mL of apple juice would be reduced to 12.5 mL after 60 minutes. (Data abstracted from Hunt JN, MacDonald M: The influence of volume on gastric emptying. J Physiol 1954;126:459–474.)

a lower incidence of anesthetic-induced hypotension due to relative hypovolemia and the avoidance of the need for glucose-containing solutions during routine cases (see Chapter 11).[26] A scheduled operation on a premature infant or neonate may occasionally be delayed, thus extending the period of fasting to a point that may be potentially dangerous (hypoglycemia or hypovolemia). In this circumstance, we recommend that an intravenous line be started and appropriate fluids administered before induction of anesthesia. Alternatively, if the period of delay is known, an infant is offered clear fluids until 2 hours before induction.

It is important to explain to older children why they must not eat or drink for the prescribed time before anesthesia. When children are told of the risk of vomiting and aspiration into the lungs, they then become motivated to follow the anesthesiologist's directives. Nevertheless, partially digested food is frequently discovered in the stomach of pediatric patients even though they are instructed to fast.

A study of children anesthetized for elective surgery found that even with strict abstinence from fluids and solids, 75% had a gastric residual volume greater than 0.4 mL/kg and a gastric pH less than 2.5. These are factors that at the time were believed to place children at risk for acid aspiration (Mendelson syndrome).[36] The data from the original article that established the conditions needed to cause Mendelson syndrome for rhesus monkeys were never published in a peer-reviewed journal.[37] The majority of articles on this subject also make the assumption that every milliliter of gastric fluid is "magically" funneled directly into the trachea and lungs. This obviously is not what occurs in real life, and in fact, the incidence of pulmonary aspiration in routine elective pediatric or adult cases without known risk factors is low (4:10,000 for adults and 10:10,000 for children).[38-41] Furthermore, one published study found that 0.8 mL/kg of aspirated fluid (pH 1[AU1]) is necessary to cause Mendelson syndrome in rhesus monkeys.[42] It appears that many of our concerns about this anesthetic complication are unwarranted and most of the previously published reports have made incorrect assumptions. It is for these reasons that we feel reassured that the changes in fasting are reasonable and safe. If a child has known risk factors (e.g., gastroesophageal reflux, previous esophageal surgery, a difficult airway, extreme obesity), then this patient may benefit from the full retinue of acid aspiration prophylaxis.[26] Cimetidine (7.5 mg/kg) reduces both gastric residual volume and acid content in children.[43] Metoclopramide and clear antacid may also be indicated. Even when aspiration does occur, morbidity and mortality are rare for elective surgical procedures and generally reflect underlying American Society of Anesthesiologists (ASA) physical status; that is, both the incidence and sequelae are more severe with ASA 3 and 4 patients. Most ASA 1 or 2 patients who aspirate clear gastric contents generally have minimal or no sequelae.[40, 41]

Full Stomach

A full stomach is probably the most common problem in pediatric anesthesia. Children can never be trusted to fast. Therefore, anesthesiologists must always be suspicious and ask children just prior to induction if they have eaten or drunk anything (although the veracity of the answer is questionable). It is not unusual to find bubble gum, candy, or other food in a child's mouth. When the anesthesiologist suspects a full stomach, induction of anesthesia must be managed appropriately. The preferred method under these circumstances is rapid intravenous induction. Before this is undertaken, the anesthesiologist must ensure that the proper equipment is at hand: two functioning laryngoscope blades and handles (should a bulb or contact fail, a spare is available), two suctions (should the suction be blocked by vomitus or blood, a second is available), appropriate drugs, a leak-free anesthesia circuit, endotracheal tubes of appropriate sizes, and stylet. All monitors should be properly functioning, and at a minimum, the pulse oximeter, blood pressure cuff, and precordial stethoscope applied (in a crying, struggling child the pulse oximeter may not function properly until after anesthetic induction). After an intravenous line is started, the child is given atropine (0.02 mg/kg body weight IV) and is denitrogenated with 100% oxygen ("preoxygenated") for several breaths. Studies of adult patients have demonstrated that oxygen saturation remains greater than 95% for 6 minutes despite only four vital capacity breaths of 100% oxygen.[44] Similar studies have not been performed in cooperative or uncooperative pediatric patients; however, after induction of anesthesia it is clear that younger patients will desaturate more rapidly than older patients.[45, 46] One study has shown a more rapid rise in inspired oxygen concentrations in infants compared with older patients, suggesting that preoxygenation can be accomplished in a shorter time.[47] Even with a crying child, it is possible to increase the arterial oxygen tension (Pao_2) by enriching the immediate environment with high flows of oxygen. Preoxygenation

should not be carried out in such a way that it upsets a child. It is important to preoxygenate patients to avoid positive-pressure ventilation before intubation because positive-pressure ventilation might result in distension of an already full stomach, with possible regurgitation and aspiration. After preoxygenation, the child is given thiopental (5 to 6 mg/kg)[48] or propofol (3 mg/kg) IV,[49, 50] followed immediately by 1 to 2 mg/kg succinylcholine. Succinylcholine is still the agent of choice for rapid onset and short duration; however, should duration of paralysis be less of a concern, one study has shown equivalent intubating conditions 30 seconds following rocuronium administration (1.2 mg/kg).[51] In that study, the mean time to return of 25% twitch was 46.3 ± 23.4 minutes (range, 30–72) for rocuronium compared with 5.8 ± 3.3 minutes (range, 1.5–8.25) for succinylcholine. It appears that high-dose rocuronium may be used as an alternate muscle relaxant should there be a concern about using succinylcholine.

If a child's fluid volume status is marginal, then a smaller dose of thiopental or propofol is advised or, alternatively, ketamine (1–2 mg/kg IV) may be administered. The child should have cricoid pressure (Sellick maneuver) applied as he or she falls asleep, and pressure should be maintained until an endotracheal tube is safely inserted and the lungs inflated.[52, 53] Evidence suggests that the gastric residual volume in children undergoing emergency surgery is greater if a child is anesthetized within 4 hours of hospital admission (1.1 mL/kg). However, if surgery can be delayed for at least 4 hours, then the mean gastric residual volume is on average much less (0.51 mL/kg) (Fig. 4–2).[54] This gastric residual volume is in fact similar to that observed in children who have fasted for routine surgical procedures.[36] This does not imply that these patients should not be regarded as having a full stomach; rather, the risk may be somewhat reduced if surgery can be delayed several hours. In addition, there is evidence to suggest that the size of the gastric residual volume (mL/kg) in emergency cases is in part related to the time between last food ingestion and the time of the injury. Patients who last ate more than 4 hours prior to injury, as a group, have a gastric residual volume similar to patients who have had a standard fast (Fig. 4–3). *There is some comfort in these numbers, but one should never consider such patients as not having a full stomach but rather as having a less full stomach.* Additionally, the possible value of H_2-blocking agents, metoclopramide, and clear antacids may be considered in these patients. Neonates may be intubated awake if indicated; this may provide a greater margin of safety because it preserves spontaneous ventilation as well as laryngeal reflexes. Skillfully performed awake intubation in neonates is not generally associated with significant adverse cardiovascular responses.[55]

Anemia

Few data designate the minimum hematocrit necessary to ensure adequate oxygen transport and delivery in pediatric patients. It is recognized that patients with chronic anemia, such as those with renal failure, do not need to be transfused for minor procedures because of compensatory mechanisms such as increased 2,3-diphosphoglycerate, increased oxygen extraction, and cardiac output. Elective surgery on an anemic pediatric patient is controversial. Consideration must be

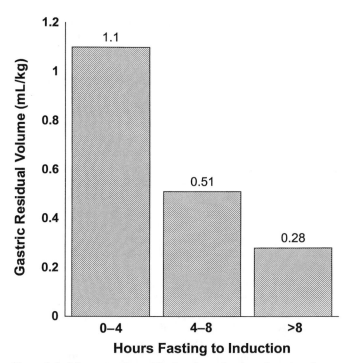

Figure 4–2. Mean gastric residual volume is plotted against hours of fasting prior to anesthetic induction in emergency pediatric cases. These data suggest that a 4-hour fast, if it does not compromise patient safety, may reduce gastric residual volume and therefore reduce (but not eliminate) risk for aspiration. (Data abstracted from Schurizek BA, Rybro L, Boggild-Madsen NB, Juhl B: Gastric volume and pH in children for emergency surgery. Acta Anaesthesiol Scand 1986;30:404–408.)

given to the type of operation planned and how urgent it is. Most pediatric anesthesiologists would recommend a hematocrit greater than 25%, but under special circumstances (e.g., physiologic anemia between 2 and 4 months of age, renal failure), a lower value may be acceptable. If significant blood loss is anticipated and the surgery is elective, then the cause of anemia should be investigated and treated and the surgery postponed until the hematocrit is restored to the normal range. *Children should not receive blood transfusions for elective surgery to bring their hematocrit up to 30%* because of the potential risk of contracting hepatitis and human immunodeficiency virus infection. Early studies of pediatric morbidity found a strong association between a hematocrit of less than 30% and cardiac arrest; no similar data are available for modern pediatric anesthesia practice. One survey found only one anesthetic death in 40,000 pediatric cases; obviously, the level of anesthesia care has improved markedly in the past 25 years.[39, 56] Anemic former premature infants represent a special category of anemic patients who require careful postoperative monitoring for apnea.[13, 57]

Upper Respiratory Tract Infection (URI)

Another common problem faced by pediatric anesthesiologists is the safety of electively anesthetizing a child who has or is recovering from a URI. Allergic rhinitis needs to be distinguished from a URI. Allergic rhinitis tends to be sea-

sonal in character, and patients have a clear nasal discharge and no fever. It probably poses no higher incidence of intraoperative anesthetic complications and is not a contraindication to general anesthesia. One study found no correlation between postintubation croup in children who had an active URI compared with noninfected patients. This study was flawed because the entire study population was not evaluated through appropriate statistical analysis and because it included a number of patients who were allowed to have "tight-fitting" endotracheal tubes.[58] It is unclear how many patients in each group had a tight-fitting endotracheal tube that could have skewed the data in either direction. A retrospective study described a series of intraoperative complications such as atelectasis and cyanosis in children with a history of a recent URI; this study was flawed because of its retrospective nature and the lack of a control population.[59] This report does point out that very severe complications are occasionally associated with the administration of anesthesia in the presence of recently infected airways. Tait and Knight[60] retrospectively examined their experience with 3585 children, 122 of whom had had a recent URI and 133 who fulfilled their criteria for a URI at the time of the surgical procedure. They did not observe an increased incidence of intraoperative complications in those with an active URI, even in those patients managed with endotracheal intu-

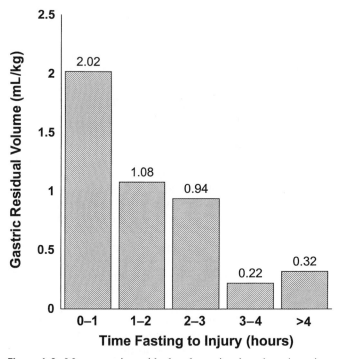

Figure 4–3. Mean gastric residual volume is plotted against time from last food ingestion to time of injury. These data suggest that the longer the time from ingestion to injury, the lower the risk for pulmonary aspiration of gastric contents. These data suggest that if more than 4 hours have elapsed between the time of last food ingestion and time of injury, the risk is similar to that for patients with routine fasting. However, even with a 4-hour fasting time period, these patients must still be treated as though they have a full stomach. (Data abstracted from Bricker SRW, McLuckie A, Nightingale DA: Gastric aspirates after trauma in children. Anaesthesia 1989;44:721–724.)

bation. Interestingly, they found a higher incidence of respiratory complications in those patients who had recently had a URI; unfortunately, this study is flawed because of the pitfalls inherent in a retrospective review of patients' symptoms and complications. These same workers reported their prospective experience with 489 children who were to undergo myringotomy for tube placement; they were randomly assigned to a group having surgery and a group whose surgery was postponed. Of the 244 patients undergoing anesthesia and surgery, 78 fulfilled the criteria of a URI, 81 were symptom free, and 84 were "symptomatic" but did not fulfill their criteria of a URI. No difference in the incidence of laryngospasm was noted, and the investigators reported a *shorter* period of URI symptoms in the patients who had the surgical procedure.[61] The major flaw with this study is that none of the patients was managed with endotracheal intubation, and it is expected that a number of patients would improve once the fluid buildup in the ear had been drained. It is difficult to evaluate this study because bronchospasm would not be expected without endotracheal intubation.[62, 63] In a study of pulse oximetry, we found an increased incidence of bronchospasm in patients who were intubated (3/196 versus 0/206), but the incidence was higher in patients with a URI (2/15 versus 1/181).[63] Olsson,[62] in a study of approximately 24,500 children 9 years of age or younger, reported a 10-fold increase in the incidence of bronchospasm in children with a URI (41:1000); mechanical stimulation of the airway appeared to be an important contributory factor. Olsson and Hallen[65] reported a fivefold higher incidence of laryngospasm in children with a URI (96:1000) compared with those without a URI (17:1000). These larger studies are consistent with our observations in a much smaller population. Our oximetry study also examined the incidence of intraoperative desaturation events in children with a URI compared with those without; a higher incidence of minor but not major desaturation events was observed.[63] In another large series of patients, children with a URI were examined and an overall increase in respiratory related adverse events was found, but this was only significant when all respiratory events were lumped into one category.[64] This increased incidence in adverse respiratory events was further exacerbated in patients who both had a URI and required endotracheal intubation.

It appears, when one combines the findings of all these studies, that a child with a mild URI that is not of acute onset may be safely anesthetized for minor surgical procedures; if an endotracheal tube is inserted, then there is propensity toward bronchospasm, laryngospasm, and desaturation events.[58, 60–65] It also appears that most such events are not associated with significant morbidity; that is, the severity of oxygen desaturation is no worse in this population than in patients without a URI.[63] Such patients may also be more susceptible to mild episodes of oxygen desaturation in the recovery room; again, these episodes are readily treated with supplemental oxygen administration.[66] All of these studies, however, have deleted those patients with acute-onset URIs and those who were clinically "ill." It is our practice to postpone surgery on patients with an active infection, such as those with fever, a recent onset of purulent nasal discharge, or "wet" cough, because this may represent a prodrome of a more serious or infectious illness (chickenpox, measles). If a child is recovering from a URI, findings on

physical examination should be nearly normal (clear nasal discharge, mild cough without rales or rhonchi, no fever); in this situation, we would generally proceed with anesthesia. However, it is up to an individual clinician's judgment and experience whether to proceed with or postpone elective surgery should the child require prolonged endotracheal intubation.[62, 63, 65, 67, 68] The bottom line is that we have the medications needed to treat the complications associated with URIs: albuterol and inhalation agent to treat bronchospasm, succinylcholine to treat laryngospasm, and oxygen to treat mild hypoxemia. The very worse case of laryngospasm one author (CJC) has seen occurred following endotracheal intubation in a child without a prior history of reactive airway disease or an active URI.

The next practical question is, once the decision has been made to postpone surgery, how long should one wait? Bronchial hyperreactivity is associated with a URI, and spirometric changes have been documented as late as 7 weeks after a URI.[67, 69] These studies suggest that surgery should be postponed for at least 7 weeks after resolution; this plan is not particularly practical because most children will already be infected with a new URI within that period of time. Postponing surgery until 2 weeks after resolution of symptoms is a common but as yet unproven safety measure. In fact, there are some scientific data to suggest that the incidence of adverse respiratory events is just as high in this population as in those who were anesthetized during the acute phase of the URI.[70, 71]

Fever

It is common for a child to have a low-grade fever before elective surgery; it is nearly always a dilemma whether to proceed with anesthesia. In general, if a child has only 0.5°C to 1.0°C of fever and no other symptoms, this degree of fever is not a contraindication to general anesthesia. If, on the other hand, the fever is associated with a recent onset of rhinitis, pharyngitis, otitis media, dehydration, or any other sign of impending illness, one must consider postponing the procedure. On occasion, it is necessary to anesthetize a child with fever, and in this situation an effort should be made to reduce the fever before induction of anesthesia, primarily to reduce oxygen demands. Reduction of the fever should not include aspirin, because it may interfere with platelet function. Acetaminophen is rapidly absorbed orally with a blood level achieved within several minutes[72]; rectal administration requires at least 60 minutes to achieve a significant blood level.[73, 74] There is no evidence that an existing fever predisposes a patient to malignant hyperthermia.[75] Anesthetic agents do, however, blunt the febrile response to pyrogens.[76] Thermoregulation is considered in greater detail in Chapter 27.

Sickle Cell Disease

Whenever sickle cell disease (HgbSS) or trait (HgbSs) is a possibility, the anesthetic and postanesthetic management is modified.[77–101] It is important to obtain a complete family history and a sickle cell preparation if the patient has not been previously tested. If the sickle cell preparation is positive and the surgery is elective, then a formal hemoglobin electrophoresis is indicated to more carefully delineate the severity of the hemoglobinopathy. It must be emphasized that the status of hydration and oxygenation is critical in all patients with sickle cell disease or trait. Thus a secure intravenous route with hydration of at least one and a half times maintenance is recommended well into the postoperative period, especially after procedures in which ileus may result (third-space losses). Meticulous attention to details to ensure a stable cardiovascular and ventilatory status establishes adequate oxygenation to prevent sickling. Pulse oximetry is of particular value in managing these patients by providing an early warning of developing desaturation. Children with hemoglobin SC are especially at risk because they have a relatively normal hemoglobin level yet are extremely vulnerable to the complications of sickle cell crisis.[79, 97] It appears that children with hemoglobin SC undergoing abdominal surgery will benefit from preoperative transfusion therapy, whereas those undergoing a minor procedure such as a myringotomy do not require such management.[97] Children with sickle cell disease must have hematologic consultation regarding prophylactic preoperative transfusion. A large multi-institution study found a lower incidence of sickle cell–related complications in children who were transfused to a hemoglobin value of 10 g/100 mL.[84, 101] Thus single-unit transfusions or partial exchange transfusions appear to be as effective as exchange transfusions.[87, 101–103]

Several papers have pointed out the slight inaccuracy of pulse oximetry in patients with sickle cell disease.[104, 105] This relates to shifts of the oxygen hemoglobin dissociation curve and other factors not accounted for in the algorithm of the oximeter. Nevertheless, pulse oximetry is very useful for trending and to determine the effectiveness of therapy. One should not disregard lower than expected oximetry readings in this population simply because they have sickle cell disease on the theory that the oximeter may not be completely accurate.

Mentally Handicapped Children

Mentally handicapped children may be challenging patients to anesthetize because one of our most important tools, our ability to explain procedures and reassure a patient, may be compromised. A bad hospital experience can greatly magnify the difficulties of future admissions. Therefore, the care of these children requires the utmost in patience, understanding, preparation, and cooperation among the family, pediatrician, surgeon, anesthesiologist, and nursing staff. These patients often have extensive medical and surgical histories and may be transported from a chronic-care facility. Often these patients are wards of the state and require special consent for surgery; similar planning is required if a caudal, epidural, or local block is planned for pain relief. It is vital to obtain the medical records to become familiar with underlying present and past medical conditions. It is also important to continue medications up to and beyond the surgical or anesthetic procedure (e.g., seizure medications). One does not wish to discover the presence of a seizure disorder when a patient has a seizure because medications have not been continued.

Sedating such a child before surgery is often indicated and may be accomplished with oral midazolam (0.25–0.75 mg/kg)[106] or rectal methohexital.[107] Oral premedication with a combination of ketamine, midazolam, and atropine may

also be indicated in this patient population.[108–110] Mentally handicapped children are often limited in their ability to relate to people outside the family. In these situations, we try to have a family member with the child for induction of anesthesia, if appropriate, and when he or she awakens in the recovery room. Traditional exclusion of the parents at this time may not be in a child's best interests. If such a child is so frightened of the medical environment that he or she is combative, a combination of intramuscular ketamine (3–4 mg/kg) combined with atropine (0.02 mg/kg) and midazolam (0.05–0.1 mg/kg) may be indicated.

Retinopathy of Prematurity

Multicenter studies have shown that retinopathy of prematurity (ROP) occurs most frequently in sick low birth weight infants (less than 1000 g) who were exposed to oxygen therapy for a prolonged period. No significant correlation has been shown with specific levels of Pao_2 and the development of ROP even when oxygen therapy is tightly controlled.[111–122] Retinopathy of prematurity has been associated with a wide variety of factors, including candidal sepsis, blood transfusions, fluctuating levels of carbon dioxide, hyperoxia, hypoxia, and a number of others.[112, 113, 115, 119, 122–128] This condition has appeared in stillborn infants and infants with cyanotic congenital heart disease who never received oxygen therapy.[129] The incidence of ROP is increasing with advances in neonatology.[113, 130–132] The role of intraoperative oxygen administration in producing ROP is questionable, particularly because the infants at greatest risk are also those most likely to require surgery.[132–137] This does not imply that anesthesiologists should no longer be concerned with this complication.[115] However, because ROP is multifactorial in origin, it is unlikely that any one factor such as intraoperative hyperoxia can be entirely responsible.[133] Anesthesiologists are still faced with the dilemma of balancing the administration of oxygen during anesthesia to provide an adequate concentration to the vital organs, the brain and heart, while avoiding possible damaging effects of hyperoxia on the immature retina. An infant's retina does not mature until 42 to 44 weeks of gestation.[138] This would suggest that it might be advisable to delay *elective* surgery until after retinal maturation, that is, after 44 weeks of gestation. Pulse oximetry has greatly facilitated the management of oxygen therapy during anesthesia in low birth weight infants who require surgery; by maintaining the oxygen saturation at 93 to 95%, one may avoid hyperoxia.[139]

Post-Anesthesia Apnea in Former Preterm Infants

The former preterm infant may have a multitude of residual problems due to intensive care therapy, prolonged intubation, and still maturing organogenesis. The incidence of subglottic stenosis is increased in this population. These infants are highly prone to develop perioperative respiratory complications.[140] At the time surgery is scheduled, these infants may or may not continue to have intermittent apnea spells and often appear normal for their age. Since the original descriptions of this subgroup of patients, a number of prospective studies have attempted to define the population at greatest risk for postoperative apnea.[57, 140–149] One paper pooled the

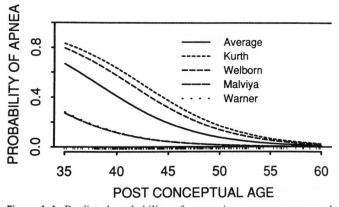

Figure 4–4. Predicted probability of apnea in recovery room and post-recovery room by weeks of postconceptual age for all patients for each investigator. Bottom marks indicate the number of data points versus postconceptual age. The curves are nearly identical for the Kurth et al. and Welborn et al. studies in the upper range and for the Malviya et al. and Warner et al. studies in the lower range. There was significant institution-to-institution variability. The reasons for this may represent differences in monitoring technology as well as patient populations, because the studies with the highest rate of apnea were also those that used continuous recording devices. (From Coté CJ, Zaslavsky A, Downes JJ, et al: Postoperative apnea in former preterm infants after inguinal herniorrhaphy: A combined analysis. Anesthesiology 1995;82:807–808.)

original data from eight published prospective papers from four institutions carried out over 6 years.[13] The incidence of apnea is inversely related to both gestational and post-conceptual age (Fig. 4–4).[13] For example, if two infants are now 45 weeks post-conceptual age and one was born at 28 weeks but the other at 32 weeks, the 28-week-gestational-age infant would be at nearly twice the risk for postoperative apnea (Fig. 4–5).[13] Likewise, if two infants were anesthetized and one was 45 weeks post-conceptual age and the other 50 weeks post-conceptual age, the younger infant would be at greater risk for apnea.

The diagnosis of apnea in the postoperative period is dependent upon the type of monitor used to follow the infants; that is, simple observation and impedance pneumography are less able to make the diagnosis than continuous recording devices.[13, 150, 151] Preterm infants with anemia (hematocrit < 30%) are more prone to apnea and the incidence is unrelated to post-conceptual or gestational age (see Fig. 4–5).[13, 57] It appears that the risk for apnea does not fall below 1% with statistical certainty until approximately 55 weeks of post-conceptual age if one excludes anemic infants and those with obvious apnea in the recovery room. This risk is approximately 5% with statistical certainty at approximately 48 weeks post-conceptual age (Fig. 4–6). Each clinician must decide the balance between risk for unrecognized apnea and the benefit in terms of cost savings and not hospitalizing the infant for overnight monitoring.[152] It should be noted that the multivariate analysis described is limited in terms of the number of patients over 45 weeks postconceptual age and the number of these patients who did not have the obvious risk factors of apnea in recovery or anemia (1/77). There was extreme institution to institution variability and within institution variability in the incidence of apnea. Despite these limitations, these are the best available data, and the prudent practitioner may use this information to justify post-surgical hospitalization to the insurance carrier. The easiest guideline to follow is not to specifically use anemia or apnea in the recovery room as an admission criterion. It is simpler to admit and monitor all former preterm infants of less than 60 weeks of post-conceptual age, with the further insight that infants who have apnea in recovery or who are anemic are more likely to have multiple and ongoing apnea after anesthesia and surgery. This avoids confusing our surgical colleagues with rules for admission and monitoring.

If a child is receiving theophylline preoperatively, this therapy should be continued into the postoperative period.

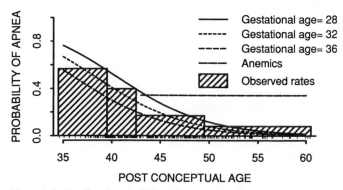

Figure 4–5. Predicted probability of apnea for all patients, by gestational age and weeks of postconceptual age. Patients with anemia are shown as the horizontal hatched line. Bottom marks indicate the number of data points by post-conceptual age. The shaded boxes represent the overall rates of apnea for infants within that gestational age range. The probability of apnea was the same regardless of postconceptual age or gestational age for infants with anemia (horizontal hatched line). (From Coté CJ, Zaslavsky A, Downes JJ, et al: Postoperative apnea in former preterm infants after inguinal herniorrhaphy: A combined analysis. Anesthesiology 1995;82:807–808.)

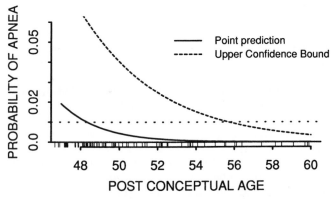

Figure 4–6. Predicted probability of apnea after leaving recovery room by weeks of postconceptual age for infants who did not have apnea in recovery room or anemia. Bottom marks indicate the number of data points by postconceptual age. The risk does not fall below 1% with 95% statistical confidence until 56 weeks' postconceptual age. (From Coté CJ, Zaslavsky A, Downes JJ, et al: Postoperative apnea in former preterm infants after inguinal herniorrhaphy: A combined analysis. Anesthesiology 1995; 82:807–808.)

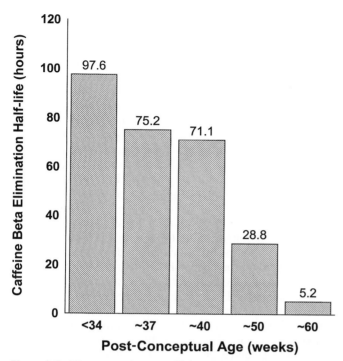

Figure 4–7. The approximate caffeine beta elimination half-life (hours) is plotted against weeks of postconceptual age. Note that there is rapid maturation of the ability to excrete caffeine and that by 60 weeks of postconceptual age the half-life is only about 5 hours. One should not expect a single dose of caffeine to completely eliminate the potential for apnea in former preterm infants. (Data abstracted from Pia DeCarolis M, Romagnoli C, Muzil U, et al: Pharmacokinetic aspects of caffeine in premature infants. Dev Pharmacol Ther 1991;16:117–122.)

A serum concentration of 10 to 15 µg/mL is considered to be a standard therapeutic level.[153] If a child is not receiving theophylline at the time of surgery, then we do not administer aminophylline, because no studies have indicated efficacy in this circumstance. We have, however, observed several infants who had been weaned from theophylline develop recurrence of their apnea after a surgical procedure. Several small series suggest that caffeine (10 mg/kg) may prevent postoperative apnea spells in high-risk infants.[148, 149] The pharmacokinetics of caffeine in premature and term newborns suggest a clinical effect that may last several days after a single dose of caffeine; however, the kinetics of caffeine in this older age group is far different and therefore the duration of therapeutic blood levels far shorter (Fig. 4–7).[154] There is also a great deal of patient to patient variability. Further studies are needed in older patients before dose recommendations can be made because age-related kinetics have shown that in infants of 60 weeks post-conceptual age, the half-life of caffeine is only about 5 hours.[154] Larger well-controlled studies are indicated before advocating that all such infants be routinely treated with caffeine. In particular, the age-related pharmacokinetics must be carefully defined to develop scientific recommendations regarding dose, frequency of administration, and duration of treatment after surgery and anesthesia. *One should not administer caffeine and then discharge the infant home assuming that the caffeine is preventative.*

Apnea may be related to many causes (Fig. 4–8). The most common following an operative procedure, however, relate to metabolic derangements, pharmacologic effects, or central nervous system immaturity. Metabolic causes of apnea such as hypothermia, hypoglycemia, hypocalcemia, acidosis, and hypoxemia can be avoided by meticulous attention to the details of the anesthetic management of neonates (see Chapter 14). Pharmacologic effects cannot be avoided, because administering anesthesia requires the use of drugs, and most drugs used in anesthesia affect the respiratory system either directly or indirectly. Most inhalation agents, narcotics, and sedatives depress the central response to carbon dioxide in adults in a dose-related fashion.[155] Few studies have examined this problem in neonates. Such respiratory depression, however, is probably more likely to occur in neonates who have an immature respiratory center. Studies of adults have demonstrated both ablation of the response to hypoxia and potentiation of that response by hypercarbia in the presence of halothane in concentrations as low as 0.1%; thus, residual anesthetic action may contribute to the development of apnea in infants.[156] In addition, most pharmacologic agents used in anesthesia decrease muscle tone of the upper airway, thus contributing to the development of upper airway obstruction, more labored breathing, fatigue, and apnea. One study has demonstrated that pharyngeal airway obstruction frequently contributes to the apnea associated with general anesthesia.[146] Potent inhalation anesthetic agents decrease intercostal muscle tone, thus reducing functional residual capacity and therefore increasing the propensity to develop hypoxemia.[157] Figure 4–9 presents several possible sequences of events leading to the development of apnea.

Regional anesthesia has been described as reducing the propensity for postoperative apnea spells compared with general anesthesia. Regional techniques may offer an advantage, but these studies are too small to conclude definitively that regional anesthesia is safer, especially because apnea has also been associated with regional anesthesia techniques.[142, 158, 159] One study found a reduced incidence of desaturation and bradycardia but not a reduced incidence of apnea in a series comparing spinal anesthesia with general

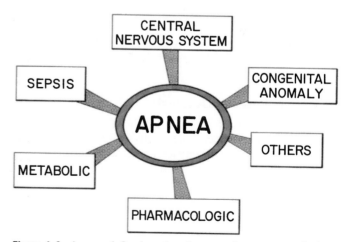

Figure 4–8. Apnea, defined as the absence of movement of air at the mouth or nose, may have many causes. Those that anesthesiologists are most often involved with are of metabolic, pharmacologic, or respiratory origins.

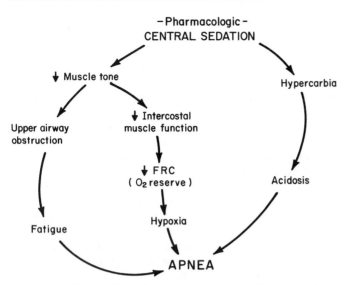

Figure 4–9. Pharmacologic interventions may result in several sequences of events leading to apnea. FRC = functional reserve capacity.

anesthesia.[160] The bottom line is that these infants must not be anesthetized as outpatients even when a regional technique has been utilized; they still require postoperative monitoring for apnea.

There does not appear to be an "ideal" anesthetic technique for former preterm infants. These infants should therefore be cared for only in a facility that has the capability to provide continuous postoperative cardiorespiratory monitoring. This monitoring should be continued until the child has been free of apnea for 12 to 24 hours. The preoperative evaluation of these patients requires discussion with the pharmacy regarding the availability of intravenous caffeine, discussion with the intensive care unit regarding availability of beds and monitoring equipment, and discussion with the family regarding the risks of anesthesia and apnea in this age group.

To further add to the confusion regarding the problem of postoperative apnea, several reports have described full-term infants who have developed apnea after an apparently uneventful general anesthetic procedure.[161–163] Thus, if an infant of less than 44 weeks of post-conceptual age, although a full-term infant, demonstrates any abnormality of respiration after anesthesia, it is reasonable to admit the infant for further evaluation.

Bronchopulmonary Dysplasia

Bronchopulmonary dysplasia is a form of chronic lung disease associated with prolonged mechanical ventilation (barotrauma) and oxygen toxicity in a premature neonate with hyaline membrane disease. Infants with bronchopulmonary dysplasia suffer from chronic hypoxemia, hypercarbia, abnormal functional airway growth, tracheomalacia, bronchomalacia, an abnormal response to hypoxemia, an increased incidence of reactive airway disease, propensity toward atelectasis and pneumonia, an increased pulmonary vascular resistance, and an abnormally shaped chest.[164–172] They may also have cor pulmonale and congestive heart failure. Pulmonary interstitial edema increases the possibility of respiratory

failure; these infants frequently are on diuretic therapy.[173–175] In evaluating these infants for anesthesia and surgery, adequate preoperative preparation must be carried out (in some cases for several days) to optimize oxygenation and myocardial function. Many of these patients also suffer neurodevelopmental problems and seizures due to intraventricular hemorrhage or hypoxic insults.[176] Pulmonary function abnormalities, including a reduced functional residual capacity, reduced forced expiratory volumes at one second, airway obstruction, reduced diffusion capacity, abnormal response to hyperoxia (abnormal chemoreceptors), and reduced exercise tolerance (desaturation), may persist into the school-age years.[177–185] Many of these children are discharged home on oxygen therapy and will require oxygen for transport into the operating room.[186, 187] Some of these children will have electrolyte abnormalities due to chronic diuretic administration.[175, 188–190] Others may have a cardiomyopathy due to steroid therapy in the neonatal period or the combination of steroid therapy and intercurrent viral infection.[191–193] Some of these patients will have systemic hypertension.[194, 195] These children therefore require special attention to fluid and electrolyte balance and careful titration of intraoperative fluids. In addition, chronic air trapping should alert the anesthesiologist to the potential dangers of nitrous oxide.[196] It is also important to *allow adequate expiratory time* and to *avoid excessive positive-pressure ventilation.* The avoidance of endotracheal intubation by using a laryngeal mask airway (LMA) may offer some advantage in reducing the incidence of coughing, coughing-related desaturation, wheezing, and hoarseness; the LMA should only be used for minor procedures.[197] The incidence of sudden infant death syndrome is increased several-fold in these patients, possibly related to an abnormal response to hypoxemia, which would suggest the possible need for postoperative apnea monitoring.[170, 198, 199] For some procedures (e.g., inguinal hernia repair), spinal anesthesia may provide an acceptable alternative technique, avoiding the need for endotracheal intubation.

Diabetic Children

Diabetes is a relatively common childhood disease, and when diabetic patients come to surgery, careful management of their insulin therapy must be continued. Knowledge of insulin schedule, normal serum glucose curves, and time of glucosuria is important. A patient's normal diet and insulin regimen should be maintained up to and including the day before surgery. In general, an attempt should be made to schedule a diabetic patient as the first case of the day. An intravenous infusion containing 5% glucose, administered at maintenance rate, should be started on the ward to avoid dangerous hypoglycemia. We usually administer half the normal insulin dosage the morning of surgery *after* the intravenous infusion is started; 5% glucose at maintenance rates is continued throughout the surgical procedure. Serum glucose levels should be monitored both intraoperatively and postoperatively until the child is back on a routine schedule.[200]

An alternative to this regimen is to use a continuous infusion of glucose and insulin. Few published studies have addressed the use of continuous insulin infusions for patients undergoing elective surgery, especially children. One study of adults found better control of glucose levels, but it was necessary to alter the infusions to prevent hypoglycemia.[201]

Emergency surgery (e.g., appendectomy) and the resultant stress on diabetic patients may lead to marked alteration in glucose-insulin response and acid-base status.[202] Hydration and efforts to correct hyperglycemia and ketoacidosis should be made before induction of general anesthesia.[203] Serum glucose and potassium levels must be closely monitored (usually on an hourly basis) and appropriate doses of insulin administered until they are stable.[204] Rapid or inappropriate correction of ketoacidosis can lead to cerebral edema.[205, 206]

Two methods for correction of ketoacidosis are generally accepted. The first is the standard loading dose of insulin, half intravenously and half subcutaneously, with increments given every 1 to 2 hours as indicated. The second method uses a loading dose of insulin followed by a constant infusion. The latter method purportedly provides a smoother correction; however, no studies have proved one method superior to the other. Both methods require meticulous attention to glucose and potassium levels; the latter method may have a lower incidence of these problems.[207–211]

Seizure Disorders

Management of a child with a seizure disorder requires knowledge of the medication the child is taking, the medication schedule, and possible interaction between the patient's medications and anesthetic drugs.[212–218] The stress of surgery and anesthesia may alter the seizure threshold and result in increased seizure activity. We continue seizure medications until the immediate time of elective surgery, allowing a child to take the medications with a sip of water the morning of surgery. For emergency procedures, missing one or two doses usually does not result in serious alteration of pharmacologic drug levels; however, if the medications are to be interrupted for a longer period of time, intravenous or intramuscular therapy must be instituted. Blood levels of anticonvulsant drugs should be monitored to ensure proper therapeutic effect.[219–221] Some patients will have what are considered subtherapeutic blood levels but will have been seizure-free for a year or more. It is also important to know what type of seizure disorder a child has to avoid medications that might precipitate a seizure (e.g., methohexital can exacerbate temporal lobe epilepsy).[222] Consultation with the child's neurologist will help in determining the optimal approach for each patient.

Hyperalimentation

Intravenous alimentation is frequently used as a means of life support and to prepare patients for surgery.[223] It is important for anesthesiologists to know the composition and rate of administration of these fluids so that potential intraoperative complications can be avoided. Most of these solutions are hypertonic, have a high glucose content, and must be administered through a centrally placed intravenous route.

Basic principles of care are as follows:

1. Avoid contaminating the line. Do not puncture it for administering medications or changing fluids without first communicating with the managing physicians. If a line change at the end of surgery is appropriate, then the existing line may be used intraoperatively.

2. Do not suddenly stop the hyperalimentation fluid, because this would leave a child in a relative hyperinsulinemic state, which might result in profound hypoglycemia, the signs of which might be masked by general anesthesia.

3. Use an infusion device at all times so that the rate of infusion is constant. Accidental rapid infusion of large amounts of hyperalimentation fluid may cause hypertonic nonketotic coma.[223] We generally decrease the infusion rate by 33 to 50% during surgical procedures. This avoids hyperglycemia resulting from a reduced metabolic rate due to the effects of anesthetic agents and a reduced body temperature.

4. Perioperative and intraoperative monitoring of serum levels of glucose, potassium, sodium, and calcium, as well as acid-base status, is important.

5. A preoperative check of correct intravascular line placement (x-ray film or aspiration of blood) is important to avoid intraoperative complications such as hydrothorax or hemothorax.

Asthma and Reactive Airway Disease

Patients with reactive airway disease or asthma undergoing elective surgery should be free of significant wheezing.[224, 225] A history of prior emergency room visits and hospitalizations should be obtained.[226–228] Specific information sought should include current and recent medication history[229–233] and a history of pneumothorax, respiratory arrests, steroid therapy, and bronchodilator drug overdose. All medications should be maintained up to and including the morning of surgery so that the patient is receiving optimal bronchodilator treatment.[234–237] It is helpful for these patients to visit their allergist just prior to scheduled surgery so as to optimize therapy; some patients benefit from short-term oral corticosteroid therapy for several days prior to surgery.[234, 238] If the patient is on theophylline, levels should be in the range of 10 to 20 μg/mL for optimal therapeutic effect.[239–241] A baseline electrocardiograph and chest radiograph may be of value for a severely asthmatic patient who may have chronic air trapping, pulmonary hypertension, pulmonary blebs, or pneumonitis. Some institutions routinely administer treatment with albuterol or other bronchodilator prior to induction of anesthesia; there is, however, no scientific evidence demonstrating a reduction in intraoperative airway reactivity. Since reaction to an endotracheal tube is a major cause of bronchospasm, it may make sense in some cases to attempt to avoid intubation and use an LMA. An LMA should not be used, however, if complete control of the airway is an important aspect of anesthetic and surgical management. When elective or emergent surgery is required, a means for administering a bronchodilator through the endotracheal tube or LMA must be available. Specific adaptors allow the interface of metered dose inhalers with the intact anesthesia circuit. These adapters are particularly helpful for timing delivery of drug during inspiration and much more effective in drug delivery than simply spraying the drug down an endotracheal tube but without the special adapter.

Emergency surgery may result in the need for anesthesia despite the presence of continued bronchospasm. In this situation, the urgency of the operation must be balanced against the severity of the bronchospasm. Some control of bronchospasm should ideally be instituted before induction of anesthesia (oxygen administration, hydration, subcutaneous epinephrine, aminophylline infusion, beta$_2$-agonist therapy, steroids, and antibiotics). Baseline blood gas analysis may be critical to differentiate moderate from severe airway obstruction. Any asthmatic patient with an arterial carbon dioxide value greater than 45 mm Hg must be considered to have incipient respiratory failure.[242] Some patients may require intraoperative infusions of isoproterenol.[243] Postoperative mechanical ventilation, when indicated, is generally well tolerated.[244]

REFERENCES

1. Karl HW, Pauza KJ, Heyneman N, et al: Preanesthetic preparation of pediatric outpatients: The role of a videotape for parents. J Clin Anesth 1990;2:172–177.
2. Payne KA, Coetzee AR, Mattheyse FJ, et al: Behavioral changes in children following minor surgery: Is premedication beneficial? Acta Anaesthesiol Belg 1992;43:173–179.
3. Azarnoff P: Parents and siblings of pediatric patients. Curr Probl Pediatr 1984;14:1–40.
4. Azarnoff P, Woody PD: Preparation of children for hospitalization in acute care hospitals in the United States. Pediatrics 1981;68:361–368.
5. Egbert LD, Battit GE, Turndorf H, et al. The value of a preoperative visit by an anesthetist: A study of doctor-patient rapport. JAMA 1963;185:553–555.
6. Kain ZN, Mayes LC, Caramico LA: Preoperative preparation in children: A cross-sectional study. J Clin Anesth 1996;8:508–514.
7. Kain ZN, Mayes LC, O'Connor TZ, et al: Preoperative anxiety in children: Predictors and outcomes. Arch Pediatr Adolesc Med 1996;150:1238–1245.
8. Battaglia FC, Lubchenco LO: A practical classification of newborn infants by weight and gestational age. J Pediatr 1967;71:159–163.
9. Farr V, Kerridge DF, Mitchell RG: The value of some external characteristics in the assessment of gestational age at birth. Dev Med Child Neurol 1966;8:657–660.
10. Farr V, Mitchell RG, Neligan GA, et al: The definition of some external characteristics used in the assessment of gestational age in the newborn infant. Dev Med Child Neurol 1966;8:507–511.
11. Dubowitz LM, Dubowitz V, Goldberg C: Clinical assessment of gestational age in the newborn infant. J Pediatr 1970;77:1–10.
12. Narayanan I, Dua K, Gujral VV, et al: A simple method of assessment of gestational age in newborn infants. Pediatrics 1982;69:27–32.
13. Coté CJ, Zaslavsky A, Downes JJ, et al: Postoperative apnea in former preterm infants after inguinal herniorrhaphy: A combined analysis. Anesthesiology 1995;82:809–822.
14. Grenier MA, Lipshultz SE: Epidemiology of anthracycline cardiotoxicity in children and adults. Semin Oncol 1998;25:72–85.
15. Krischer JP, Epstein S, Cuthbertson DD, et al: Clinical cardiotoxicity following anthracycline treatment for childhood cancer: The Pediatric Oncology Group experience. J Clin Oncol 1997;15:1544–1552.
16. Ali MK, Ewer MS, Gibbs HR, et al: Late doxorubicin-associated cardiotoxicity in children: The possible role of intercurrent viral infection. Cancer 1994;74:182–188.
17. Steinherz LJ, Graham T, Hurwitz R, et al: Guidelines for cardiac monitoring of children during and after anthracycline therapy: Report of the Cardiology Committee of the Childrens Cancer Study Group. Pediatrics 1992;89:942–949.
18. Patel RI, DeWitt L, Hannallah RS: Preoperative laboratory testing in children undergoing elective surgery: analysis of current practice. J Clin Anesth 1997;9:569–575.
19. Alario AJ, McCarthy PL, Markowitz R, et al: Usefulness of chest radiographs in children with acute lower respiratory tract disease. J Pediatr 1987;111:187–193.
20. Sane SM, Worsing RA Jr, Wiens CW, et al: Value of preoperative chest X-ray examinations in children. Pediatrics 1977;60:669–672.
21. Wood RA, Hoekelman RA: Value of the chest X-ray as a screening test for elective surgery in children. Pediatrics 1981;67:447–452.
22. Aun CS, Panesar NS: Paediatric glucose homeostasis during anaesthesia. Br J Anaesth 1990;64:413–418.
23. Jensen BH, Wernberg M, Andersen M: Preoperative starvation and blood glucose concentrations in children undergoing inpatient and outpatient anaesthesia. Br J Anaesth 1982;54:1071–1074.
24. van der Walt JH, Carter JA: The effect of different pre-operative feeding regimens on plasma glucose and gastric volume and pH in infancy. Anaesth Intensive Care 1986;14:352–359.
25. Welborn LG, McGill WA, Hannallah RS, et al: Perioperative blood glucose concentrations in pediatric outpatients. Anesthesiology 1986;65:543–547.
26. Coté CJ: NPO after midnight for children: A reappraisal. Anesthesiology 1990;72:589–592.
27. O'Hare B, Lerman J, Endo J, et al: Acute lung injury after instillation of human breast milk or infant formula into rabbits' lungs. Anesthesiology 1996;84:1386–1391.
28. Litman RS, Wu CL, Quinlivan JK: Gastric volume and pH in infants fed clear liquids and breast milk prior to surgery. Anesth Analg 1994;79:482–485.
29. Schreiner MS, Treibwasser A, Keon TP: Ingestion of liquids compared with preoperative fasting in pediatric outpatients. Anesthesiology 1990;72:593–597.
30. Sandhar BK, Goresky GV, Maltby JR, et al: Effect of oral liquids and ranitidine on gastric fluid volume and pH in children undergoing outpatient surgery. Anesthesiology 1989;71:327–330.
31. Splinter WM, Stewart JA, Muir JG: The effect of preoperative apple juice on gastric contents, thirst and hunger in children. Can J Anaesth 1989;36:55–58.
32. Meakin G, Dingwall AE, Addison GM: Effects of fasting and oral premedication on the pH and volume of gastric aspirate in children. Br J Anaesth 1987;59:678–682.
33. Splinter WM, Schaefer JD: Clear fluids three hours before surgery do not affect the gastric fluid contents of children. Can J Anaesth 1990;37:498–501.
34. Splinter WM, Stewart JA, Muir JG: Large volumes of apple juice preoperatively do not affect gastric pH and volume in children. Can J Anaesth 1990;37:36–39.
35. Splinter WM, Schaefer JD: Ingestion of clear fluids is safe for adolescents up to 3 h before anaesthesia. Br J Anaesth 1991;66:48–52.
36. Coté CJ, Goudsouzian NG, Liu LM, et al: Assessment of risk factors related to the acid aspiration syndrome in pediatric patients—gastric pH and residual volume. Anesthesiology 1982;56:70–72.
37. Roberts RB, Shirley MA: Reducing the risk of acid aspiration during cesarean section. Anesth Analg 1974;53:859–868.
38. Olsson GL, Hallen B, Hambraeus-Jonzon K: Aspiration during anaesthesia: A computer-aided study of 185,358 anaesthetics. Acta Anaesthesiol Scand 1986;30:84–92.
39. Tiret L, Nivoche Y, Hatton F, et al: Complications related to anaesthesia in infants and children: A prospective survey of 40240 anaesthetics. Br J Anaesth 1988;61:263–269.
40. Warner MA, Warner ME, Weber JG: Clinical significance of pulmonary aspiration during the perioperative period. Anesthesiology 1993;78:56–62.
41. Borland LM, Sereika SM, Woelfel SK, et al: Pulmonary aspiration in pediatric patients during general anesthesia: Incidence and outcome. J Clin Anesth 1998;10:95–102.
42. Raidoo DM, Marszalek A, Brock-Utne JG: Acid aspiration in primates (a surprising experimental result). Anaesth Intensive Care 1988;16:375–376.
43. Goudsouzian NG, Coté CJ, Liu LM, et al: The dose-response effects of oral cimetidine on gastric pH and volume in children. Anesthesiology 1981;55:53–56.
44. Gambee AM, Hertzka RE, Fisher DM: Preoxygenation techniques: Comparison of three minutes and four breaths. Anesth Analg 1987;66:468–470.
45. Xue FS, Luo LK, Tong SY, et al: Study of the safe threshold of apneic period in children during anesthesia induction. J Clin Anesth 1996;8:568–574.
46. Kinouchi K, Fukumitsu K, Tashiro C, et al: Duration of apnoea in anaesthetized children required for desaturation of haemoglobin to 95%: Comparison of three different breathing gases. Pediatr Anaesth 1995;5:115–119.
47. Morrison JEJ, Collier E, Friesen RH, et al: Preoxygenation before laryngoscopy in children: How long is enough? Pediatr Anaesth 1998;8:293–298.
48. Coté CJ, Goudsouzian NG, Liu LM, et al: The dose response of intravenous thiopental for the induction of general anesthesia in unpremedicated children. Anesthesiology 1981;55:703–705.
49. Hannallah RS, Baker SB, Casey W: Propofol: Effective dose and induction characteristics in unpremedicated children. Anesthesiology 1991;74:217–219.

50. Aun CS, Short SM, Leung DH, et al: Induction dose-response of propofol in unpremedicated children. Br J Anaesth 1992;68:64–67.
51. Mazurek AJ, Rae B, Hann S, et al: Rocuronium versus succinylcholine: Are they equally effective during rapid-sequence induction of anesthesia? Anesth Analg 1998;87:1259–1262.
52. Sellick BA: Cricoid pressure to control regurgitation of stomach contents during induction of anaesthesia. Lancet 1961; 404–406.
53. Salem MR, Wong AY, Fizzotti GF: Efficacy of cricoid pressure in preventing aspiration of gastric contents in paediatric patients. Br J Anaesth 1972;44:401–404.
54. Schurizek BA, Rybro L, Boggild-Madsen NB, Juhl B: Gastric volume and pH in children for emergency surgery. Acta Anaesthesiol Scand 1986;30:404–408.
55. Lindgren L, Saarnivaara L: Cardiovascular responses to tracheal intubation in small children: Effects of the induction of anaesthesia with halothane. Br J Anaesth 1985;57:1183–1187.
56. Salem MR, Bennett EJ, Schweiss JF, et al: Cardiac arrest related to anesthesia: Contributing factors in infants and children. JAMA 1975;233:238–241.
57. Welborn LG, Hannallah RS, Luban NLC, et al: Anemia and postoperative apnea in former preterm infants. Anesthesiology 1991;74:1003–1006.
58. Koka BV, Jeon IS, Andre JM, et al: Postintubation croup in children. Anesth Analg 1977;56:501–505.
59. McGill WA, Coveler LA, Epstein BS: Subacute upper respiratory infection in small children. Anesth Analg 1979;58:331–333.
60. Tait AR, Knight PR: Intraoperative respiratory complications in patients with upper respiratory tract infections. Can J Anaesth 1987;34:300–303.
61. Tait AR, Knight PR: The effects of general anesthesia on upper respiratory tract infections in children. Anesthesiology 1987;67:930–935.
62. Olsson GL: Bronchospasm during anaesthesia: A computer-aided incidence study of 136,929 patients. Acta Anaesthesiol Scand 1987;31:244–252.
63. Rolf N, Coté CJ: Frequency and severity of desaturation events during general anesthesia in children with and without upper respiratory infections. J Clin Anesth 1992;4:200–203.
64. Cohen MM, Cameron CB: Should you cancel the operation when a child has an upper respiratory tract infection? Anesth Analg 1991;72:282–288.
65. Olsson GL, Hallen B: Laryngospasm during anaesthesia: A computer-aided incidence study in 136,929 patients. Acta Anaesthesiol Scand 1984;28:567–575.
66. DeSoto H, Patel RI, Soliman IE, et al: Changes in oxygen saturation following general anesthesia in children with upper respiratory infection signs and symptoms undergoing otolaryngological procedures. Anesthesiology 1988;68:276–279.
67. Empey DW, Laitinen LA, Jacobs L, et al: Mechanisms of bronchial hyperreactivity in normal subjects after upper respiratory tract infection. Am Rev Respir Dis 1976;113:131–139.
68. Tait AR, Reynolds PI, Gutstein HB: Factors that influence an anesthesiologist's decision to cancel elective surgery for the child with an upper respiratory tract infection. J Clin Anesth 1995;7:491–499.
69. Collier AM, Pimmel RL, Hasselblad V, et al: Spirometric changes in normal children with upper respiratory infections. Am Rev Respir Dis 1978;117:47–53.
70. Tait AR, Knight PR: The effects of general anesthesia on upper respiratory tract infections in children. Anesthesiology 1987;67:930–935.
71. Levy L, Pandit UA, Randel GI, et al: Upper respiratory tract infections and general anaesthesia in children. Anaesthesia 1992;47:678–682.
72. Wheeler M, Tobin MJ, Birmingham PK, Coté CJ, Henthorn TK, Kennedy-Mooney SH: Pharmacokinetics and dose response for oral acetaminophen in children. Anesthesiology 1997;87:A1054.
73. Birmingham PK, Tobin MJ, Henthorn TK, et al: Twenty-four-hour pharmacokinetics of rectal acetaminophen in children: An old drug with new recommendations. Anesthesiology 1997;87:244–252.
74. Birmingham PK, Tobin MJ, Henthorn TK, et al: "Loading" and subsequent dosing of rectal acetaminophen in children: A 24 hour pharmacokinetic study of new dosing recommendations. Anesthesiology 1996;85:A1105.
75. Steward DJ: Malignant hyperthermia: The acute crisis. Int Anesthesiol Clin 1979;17:1–9.
76. Lenhardt R, Negishi C, Sessler DI: Perioperative fever. Acta Anaesthesiol Scand Suppl 1997;111:325–328.
77. Esseltine DW, Baxter MR, Bevan JC: Sickle cell states and the anaesthetist. Can J Anaesth 1988;35:385–403.
78. Dobson MB: Anesthesia for patients with hemoglobinopathies. Int Anesthesiol Clin 1985;23:197–211.
79. Rockoff AS, Christy D, Zeldis N, et al: Myocardial necrosis following general anesthesia in hemoglobin SC disease. Pediatrics 1978;61:73–76.
80. Konotey-Ahulu FI: Anaesthetic deaths and the sickle-cell trait. Lancet 1969;1:267–268.
81. Oduntan SA, Isaacs WA: Anaesthesia in patients with abnormal haemoglobin syndromes: A preliminary report. Br J Anaesth 1971;43:1159–1166.
82. Browne RA: Anaesthesia in patients with sickle-cell anemia. Br J Anaesth 1965;37:181–188.
83. McGarry P, Duncan C: Anesthetic risks in sickle cell trait. Pediatrics 1973;51:507–512.
84. Adams RJ, McKie VC, Hsu L, et al: Prevention of a first stroke by transfusions in children with sickle cell anemia and abnormal results on transcranial Doppler ultrasonography. N Engl J Med 1998;339:5–11.
85. Baxter MR, Bevan JC, Esseltine DW, et al: The management of two pediatric patients with sickle cell trait and sickle cell disease during cardiopulmonary bypass. J Cardiothorac Anesth 1989;3:477–480.
86. Bunn HF: Pathogenesis and treatment of sickle cell disease. N Engl J Med 1997;337:762–769.
87. Cohen A: Management issues for collaborative study in hematology. Sickle cell anemia, hemophilia, and ITP. Clin Pediatr (Phila) 1987;26:615–619.
88. Davies SC, Olatunji PO: Blood transfusion in sickle cell disease. Vox Sang 1995;68:145–151.
89. Davies SC, Roberts-Harewood M: Blood transfusion in sickle cell disease. Blood Rev 1997;11:57–71.
90. Davies SC, Oni L: Management of patients with sickle cell disease. Br Med J 1997;315:656–660.
91. Griffin TC, Buchanan GR: Elective surgery in children with sickle cell disease without preoperative blood transfusion. J Pediatr Surg 1993;28:681–685.
92. Gross ML, Schwedler M, Bischoff RJ, et al: Impact of anesthetic agents on patients with sickle cell disease. Am Surg 1993;59:261–264.
93. Halvorson DJ, McKie V, McKie K, et al: Sickle cell disease and tonsillectomy: Preoperative management and postoperative complications. Arch Otolaryngol Head Neck Surg 1997;123:689–692.
94. Hatley RM, Crist D, Howell CG, et al: Laparoscopic cholecystectomy in children with sickle cell disease. Am Surg 1995;61:169–171.
95. Kittner SJ, Adams RJ: Stroke in children and young adults. Curr Opin Neurol 1996;9:53–56.
96. Koshy M, Weiner SJ, Miller ST, et al: Surgery and anesthesia in sickle cell disease. Cooperative Study of Sickle Cell Diseases. Blood 1995;86:3676–3684.
97. Neumayr L, Koshy M, Haberkern C, et al: Surgery in patients with hemoglobin SC disease. Preoperative Transfusion in Sickle Cell Disease Study Group. Am J Hematol 1998;57:101–108.
98. Scott-Conner CE, Brunson CD: The pathophysiology of the sickle hemoglobinopathies and implications for perioperative management. Am J Surg 1994;168:268–274.
99. Shulman G, McQuitty C, Vertrees RA, et al: Acute normovolemic red cell exchange for cardiopulmonary bypass in sickle cell disease. Ann Thorac Surg 1998;65:1444–1446.
100. Styles LA, Vichinsky EP: New therapies and approaches to transfusion in sickle cell disease in children. Curr Opin Pediatr 1997;9:41–45.
101. Vichinsky EP, Haberkern CM, Neumayr L, et al: A comparison of conservative and aggressive transfusion regimens in the perioperative management of sickle cell disease. The Preoperative Transfusion in Sickle Cell Disease Study Group. N Engl J Med 1995;333:206–213.
102. Charache S: Treatment of sickle cell anemia. Annu Rev Med 1981;32:195–206.
103. Alavi JB: Sickle cell anemia. Pathophysiology and treatment. Med Clin North Am 1984;68:545–556.
104. Weston Smith SG, Glass UH, Acharya J, et al: Pulse oximetry in sickle cell disease. Clin Lab Haematol 1989;11:185–188.
105. Pianosi P, Charge TD, Esseltine DW, et al: Pulse oximetry in sickle cell disease. Arch Dis Child 1993;68:735–738.
106. Suresh S, Cohen IJ, Matuszczak M, et al: Dose ranging, safety, and efficacy of a new oral midazolam syrup in children. Anesthesiology 1998;89:A1313.

107. Liu LMP, Goudsouzian NG, Liu P: Rectal methohexital premedication in children: A dose comparison study. Anesthesiology 1980;53:343–345.

108. Gutstein HB, Johnson KL, Heard MB, et al: Oral ketamine preanesthetic medication in children. Anesthesiology 1992;76:28–33.

109. Rosenberg M: Oral ketamine for deep sedation of difficult-to-manage children who are mentally handicapped: Case report. Pediatr Dent 1991;13:221–223.

110. Warner DL, Cabaret J, Velling D: Ketamine plus midazolam, a most effective paediatric oral premedicant. Paediatr Anaesth 1995;5:293–295.

111. Bancalari E, Flynn J, Goldberg RN, et al: Influence of transcutaneous oxygen monitoring on the incidence of retinopathy of prematurity. Pediatrics 1987;79:663–669.

112. Ben Sira I, Nissenkorn I, Kremer I: Retinopathy of prematurity. Surv Ophthalmol 1988;33:1–16.

113. Bossi E, Koerner F: Retinopathy of prematurity. Intensive Care Med 1995;21:241–246.

114. Phelps DL: Retinopathy of prematurity. Pediatr Clin North Am 1993;40:705–714.

115. Saito Y, Omoto T, Cho Y, et al: The progression of retinopathy of prematurity and fluctuation in blood gas tension. Graefes Arch Clin Exp Ophthalmol 1993;231:151–156.

116. Hoon AH, Jan JE, Whitfield MF, et al: Changing pattern of retinopathy of prematurity: A 37-year clinic experience. Pediatrics 1988;82:344–349.

117. Purohit DM, Ellison RC, Zierler S, et al: Risk factors for retrolental fibroplasia: Experience with 3,025 premature infants. National Collaborative Study on Patent Ductus Arteriosus in Premature Infants. Pediatrics 1985;76:339–344.

118. Avery GB, Glass P: Light and retinopathy of prematurity: What is prudent for 1986? Pediatrics 1986;78:519–520.

119. Glass P, Avery GB, Subramanian KN, et al: Effect of bright light in the hospital nursery on the incidence of retinopathy of prematurity. N Engl J Med 1985;313:401–404.

120. James S, Lanman JT: History of oxygen therapy and retrolental fibroplasia. Prepared by the American Academy of Pediatrics, Committee on Fetus and Newborn with the collaboration of special consultants. Pediatrics 1976;57(2):591–642.

121. Phelps DL: Retinopathy of prematurity: An estimate of vision loss in the United States—1979. Pediatrics 1981;67:924–925.

122. Gunn TR, Easdown J, Outerbridge EW, et al: Risk factors in retrolental fibroplasia. Pediatrics 1980;65:1096–1100.

123. Avery GB, Glass P: Retinopathy of prematurity: What causes it? Clin Perinatol 1988;15:917–928.

124. Bancalari E, Flynn J, Goldberg RN, et al: Transcutaneous oxygen monitoring and retinopathy of prematurity. Adv Exp Med Biol 1987;220:109–113.

125. Hesse L, Eberl W, Schlaud M, et al: Blood transfusion: Iron load and retinopathy of prematurity. Eur J Pediatr 1997;156:465–470.

126. Holmes JM, Duffner LA, Kappil JC: The effect of raised inspired carbon dioxide on developing rat retinal vasculature exposed to elevated oxygen. Curr Eye Res 1994;13:779–782.

127. Holmes JM, Zhang S, Leske DA, et al: Carbon dioxide-induced retinopathy in the neonatal rat. Curr Eye Res 1998;17:608–616.

128. Mittal M, Dhanireddy R, Higgins RD: Candida sepsis and association with retinopathy of prematurity. Pediatrics 1998;101:654–657.

129. Kalina RE, Hodson WA, Morgan BC: Retrolental fibroplasia in a cyanotic infant. Pediatrics 1972;50:765–768.

130. Bardin C, Zelkowitz P, Papageorgiou A: Outcome of small-for-gestational age and appropriate-for-gestational age infants born before 27 weeks of gestation. Pediatrics 1997;100:E4.

131. Dobson V, Quinn GE: Retinopathy of prematurity. Optom Clin 1996;5:105–124.

132. Flynn JT: Retinopathy of prematurity: Perspective for the nineties. Acta Ophthalmol Scand Suppl 1995;214:12–14.

133. Flynn JT: Oxygen and retrolental fibroplasia: Update and challenge. Anesthesiology 1984;60:397–399.

134. Lucey JF, Dangman B: A reexamination of the role of oxygen in retrolental fibroplasia. Pediatrics 1984;73:82–96.

135. Valentine PH, Jackson JC, Kalina RE, et al: Increased survival of low birth weight infants: Impact on the incidence of retinopathy of prematurity. Pediatrics 1989;84:442–445.

136. Gobel W, Richard G: Retinopathy of prematurity: Current diagnosis and management. Eur J Pediatr 1993;152:286–290.

137. Keith CG, Doyle LW: Retinopathy of prematurity in extremely low birth weight infants [see comments]. Pediatrics 1995;95:42–45.

138. Quinn GE, Betts EK, Diamond GR, et al: Neonatal age (human) at retinal maturation. Anesthesiology 1981;55:S326.

139. Bucher HU, Fanconi S, Baeckert P, et al: Hyperoxemia in newborn infants: Detection by pulse oximetry. Pediatrics 1989;84:226–230.

140. Steward DJ: Preterm infants are more prone to complications following minor surgery than are term infants. Anesthesiology 1982;56:304–306.

141. Liu LM, Coté CJ, Goudsouzian NG, et al: Life-threatening apnea in infants recovering from anesthesia. Anesthesiology 1983;59:506–510.

142. Welborn LG, Rice LJ, Hannallah RS, et al: Postoperative apnea in former preterm infants: Prospective comparison of spinal and general anesthesia. Anesthesiology 1990;72:838–842.

143. Welborn LG, Ramirez N, Oh TH, et al: Postanesthetic apnea and periodic breathing in infants. Anesthesiology 1986;65:658–661.

144. Kurth CD, Spitzer AR, Broennle AM, et al: Postoperative apnea in preterm infants. Anesthesiology 1987;66:483–488.

145. Warner LO, Teitelbaum DH, Caniano DA, et al: Inguinal herniorrhaphy in young infants: Perianesthetic complications and associated preanesthetic risk factors. J Clin Anesth 1992;4:455–461.

146. Kurth CD, LeBard SE: Association of postoperative apnea, airway obstruction, and hypoxemia in former premature infants. Anesthesiology 1991;75:22–26.

147. Malviya S, Swartz J, Lerman J: Are all preterm infants younger than 60 weeks postconceptual age at risk for postanesthetic apnea? Anesthesiology 1993;78:1076–1081.

148. Welborn LG, De Soto H, Hannallah RS, et al: The use of caffeine in the control of post-anesthetic apnea in former premature infants. Anesthesiology 1988;68:796–798.

149. Welborn LG, Hannallah RS, Fink R, et al: High-dose caffeine suppresses postoperative apnea in former preterm infants. Anesthesiology 1989;71:347–349.

150. Muttitt SC, Finer NN, Tierney AJ, et al: Neonatal apnea: Diagnosis by nurse versus computer. Pediatrics 1988;82:713–720.

151. Brouillette RT, Morrow AS, Weese-Mayer DE, et al: Comparison of respiratory inductive plethysmography and thoracic impedance for apnea monitoring. J Pediatr 1987;111:377–383.

152. Fisher DM: When is the ex-premature infant no longer at risk for apnea? Anesthesiology 1995;82:807–808.

153. Kelly DH, Shannon DC: Treatment of apnea and excessive periodic breathing in the full-term infant. Pediatrics 1981;68:183–186.

154. Le Guennec JC, Billon B, Paré C, et al: Maturational changes of caffeine concentrations and disposition in infancy during maintenance therapy for apnea of prematurity: Influence of gestational age, hepatic disease, and breast-feeding. Pediatrics 1985;76:834–840.

155. Kafer ER, Marsh HM: The effects of anesthetic drugs and disease on the chemical regulation of ventilation. Int Anesthesiol Clin 1977;15:1–38.

156. Knill RL, Gelb AW: Ventilatory responses to hypoxia and hypercapnia during halothane sedation and anesthesia in man. Anesthesiology 1978;49:244–251.

157. Tusiewicz K, Bryan AC, Froese AB: Contributions of changing rib cage: Diaphragm interactions to the ventilatory depression of halothane anesthesia. Anesthesiology 1977;47:327–337.

158. Watcha MF, Thach BT, Gunter JB: Postoperative apnea after caudal anesthesia in an ex-premature infant. Anesthesiology 1989;71:613–615.

159. Desparmet JF: Total spinal anesthesia after caudal anesthesia in an infant. Anesth Analg 1990;70:665–667.

160. Krane EJ, Haberkern CM, Jacobson LE: Postoperative apnea, bradycardia, and oxygen desaturation in formerly premature infants: Prospective comparison of spinal and general anesthesia. Anesth Analg 1995;80:7–13.

161. Tetzlaff JE, Annand DW, Pudimat MA, et al: Postoperative apnea in a full-term infant. Anesthesiology 1988;69:426–428.

162. Coté CJ, Kelly DH: Postoperative apnea in a full-term infant with a demonstrable respiratory pattern abnormality. Anesthesiology 1990;72:559–561.

163. Noseworthy J, Duran C, Khine HH: Postoperative apnea in a full-term infant. Anesthesiology 1989;70:879–880.

164. Calder NA, Williams BA, Smyth J, et al: Absence of ventilatory responses to alternating breaths of mild hypoxia and air in infants who have had bronchopulmonary dysplasia: Implications for the risk of sudden infant death. Pediatr Res 1994;35:677–681.

165. De Boeck K, Smith J, Van Lierde S, et al: Flat chest in survivors of bronchopulmonary dysplasia. Pediatr Pulmonol 1994;18:104–107.

166. Wauer RR, Maurer T, Nowotny T, et al: Assessment of functional residual capacity using nitrogen washout and plethysmographic techniques in infants with and without bronchopulmonary dysplasia. Intensive Care Med 1998;24:469–475.

167. Moylan FM, Shannon DC: Preferential distribution of lobar emphysema and atelectasis in bronchopulmonary dysplasia. Pediatrics 1979;63:130–134.

168. Miller RW, Woo P, Kellman RK, et al: Tracheobronchial abnormalities in infants with bronchopulmonary dysplasia. J Pediatr 1987;111:779–782.

169. Tepper RS, Morgan WJ, Cota K, et al: Expiratory flow limitation in infants with bronchopulmonary dysplasia. J Pediatr 1986;109:1040–1046.

170. Garg M, Kurzner SI, Bautista D, et al: Hypoxic arousal responses in infants with bronchopulmonary dysplasia. Pediatrics 1988;82:59–63.

171. Goodman G, Perkin RM, Anas NG, et al: Pulmonary hypertension in infants with bronchopulmonary dysplasia. J Pediatr 1988;112:67–72.

172. Berman W Jr, Yabek SM, Dillon T, et al: Evaluation of infants with bronchopulmonary dysplasia using cardiac catheterization. Pediatrics 1982;70:708–712.

173. Engelhardt B, Elliott S, Hazinski TA: Short- and long-term effects of furosemide on lung function in infants with bronchopulmonary dysplasia. J Pediatr 1986;109:1034–1039.

174. Moylan FM, O'Connell K, Todres ID, et al: Edema of the pulmonary interstitium in infants and children. Pediatrics 1975;55:783–787.

175. Kao LC, Durand DJ, Phillips BL, et al: Oral theophylline and diuretics improve pulmonary mechanics in infants with bronchopulmonary dysplasia. J Pediatr 1987;111:439–444.

176. Gray PH, Burns YR, Mohay HA, et al: Neurodevelopmental outcome of preterm infants with bronchopulmonary dysplasia. Arch Dis Child Fetal Neonatal Ed 1995;73:F128–F134.

177. Gross SJ, Iannuzzi DM, Kveselis DA, et al: Effect of preterm birth on pulmonary function at school age: A prospective controlled study. J Pediatr 1998;133:188–192.

178. Chernick V: Long-term pulmonary function studies in children with bronchopulmonary dysplasia: An ever-changing saga. J Pediatr 1998;133:171–172.

179. Mitchell SH, Teague WG: Reduced gas transfer at rest and during exercise in school-age survivors of bronchopulmonary dysplasia. Am J Respir Crit Care Med 1998;157:1406–1412.

180. Giacoia GP, Venkataraman PS, West-Wilson KI, et al: Follow-up of school-age children with bronchopulmonary dysplasia. J Pediatr 1997;130:400–408.

181. Baraldi E, Filippone M, Trevisanuto D, et al: Pulmonary function until two years of life in infants with bronchopulmonary dysplasia. Am J Respir Crit Care Med 1997;155:149–155.

182. Cano A, Payo F: Lung function and airway responsiveness in children and adolescents after hyaline membrane disease: A matched cohort study. Eur Respir J 1997;10:880–885.

183. Hakulinen AL, Jarvenpaa AL, Turpeinen M, et al: Diffusing capacity of the lung in school-aged children born very preterm, with and without bronchopulmonary dysplasia. Pediatr Pulmonol 1996;21:353–360.

184. Parat S, Moriette G, Delaperche MF, et al: Long-term pulmonary functional outcome of bronchopulmonary dysplasia and premature birth. Pediatr Pulmonol 1995;20:289–296.

185. Katz-Salamon M, Jonsson B, Lagercrantz H: Blunted peripheral chemoreceptor response to hyperoxia in a group of infants with bronchopulmonary dysplasia. Pediatr Pulmonol 1995;20:101–106.

186. Baraldi E, Carra S, Vencato F, et al: Home oxygen therapy in infants with bronchopulmonary dysplasia: A prospective study. Eur J Pediatr 1997;156:878–882.

187. Voter KZ, Chalanick K: Home oxygen and ventilation therapies in pediatric patients. Curr Opin Pediatr 1996;8:221–225.

188. Kazzi NJ, Morbach CA, Brans YW: Effects of thiazide diuretics on the lipid profile of infants with bronchopulmonary dysplasia. Biol Neonate 1992;61:318–325.

189. Brem AS: Electrolyte disorders associated with respiratory distress syndrome and bronchopulmonary dysplasia. Clin Perinatol 1992;19:223–232.

190. Giacoia GP, Pineda R: Diuretics, hypochloremia, and outcome in bronchopulmonary dysplasia patients. Dev Pharmacol Ther 1991;16:212–220.

191. Anwar M, Marotta F, Fort MD, et al: The ventilatory response to carbon dioxide in high risk infants. Early Hum Dev 1993;35:183–192.

192. Haney I, Lachance C, van Doesburg NH, et al: Reversible steroid-induced hypertrophic cardiomyopathy with left ventricular outflow tract obstruction in two newborns. Am J Perinatol 1995;12:271–274.

193. Farstad T, Brockmeier F, Bratlid D: Cardiopulmonary function in premature infants with bronchopulmonary dysplasia: A 2-year follow up. Eur J Pediatr 1995;154:853–858.

194. Anderson AH, Warady BA, Daily DK, et al: Systemic hypertension in infants with severe bronchopulmonary dysplasia: Associated clinical factors. Am J Perinatol 1993;10:190–193.

195. Alagappan A, Malloy MH: Systemic hypertension in very low-birth-weight infants with bronchopulmonary dysplasia: Incidence and risk factors. Am J Perinatol 1998;15:3–8.

196. Gold MI, Joseph SI: Bilateral tension pneumothorax following induction of anesthesia in two patients with chronic obstructive airway disease. Anesthesiology 1973;38:93–96.

197. Ferrari LR, Goudsouzian NG: The use of the laryngeal mask airway in children with bronchopulmonary dysplasia. Anesth Analg 1995;81:310–313.

198. Werthammer J, Brown ER, Neff RK, et al: Sudden infant death syndrome in infants with bronchopulmonary dysplasia. Pediatrics 1982;69:301–304.

199. Garg M, Kurzner SI, Bautista DB, et al: Clinically unsuspected hypoxia during sleep and feeding in infants with bronchopulmonary dysplasia. Pediatrics 1988;81:635–642.

200. Milaszkiewicz RM: Diabetes mellitus and anesthesia: What is the problem? Int Anesthesiol Clin 1997;35:35–62.

201. Taitelman U, Reece EA, Bessman AN: Insulin in the management of the diabetic surgical patient: Continuous intravenous infusion vs subcutaneous administration. JAMA 1977;237:658–660.

202. Umpierrez GE, Khajavi M, Kitabchi AE: Review: Diabetic ketoacidosis and hyperglycemic hyperosmolar nonketotic syndrome. Am J Med Sci 1996;311:225–233.

203. Linares MY, Schunk JE, Lindsay R: Laboratory presentation in diabetic ketoacidosis and duration of therapy. Pediatr Emerg Care 1996;12:347–351.

204. Krane EJ: Diabetic ketoacidosis. Biochemistry, physiology, treatment, and prevention. Pediatr Clin North Am 1987;34:935–960.

205. Mel JM, Werther GA: Incidence and outcome of diabetic cerebral oedema in childhood: Are there predictors? J Paediatr Child Health 1995;31:17–20.

206. Krane EJ, Rockoff MA, Wallman JK, et al: Subclinical brain swelling in children during treatment of diabetic ketoacidosis. N Engl J Med 1985;312:1147–1151.

207. Martin AL, Martin MM: Continuous infusion of insulin vs repeated SC injections in the treatment of diabetic ketoacidosis in children. Acta Diabetol Lat 1978;15:81–87.

208. Martin MM, Martin AA: Continuous low-dose infusion of insulin in the treatment of diabetic ketoacidosis in children. J Pediatr 1976;89:560–564.

209. Edwards GA, Kohaut EC, Wehring B, et al: Effectiveness of low-dose continuous intravenous insulin infusion in diabetic ketoacidosis: A prospective comparative study. J Pediatr 1977;91:701–705.

210. Perkin RM, Marks JF: Low-dose continuous intravenous insulin infusion in childhood diabetic ketoacidosis. Clin Pediatr (Phila) 1979;18:540–548.

211. Weber ME, Abbassi V: Continuous intravenous insulin therapy in severe diabetic ketoacidosis: Variations in dosage requirements. J Pediatr 1977;91:755–756.

212. Pellock JM: Status epilepticus in children: Update and review. J Child Neurol 1994;9(Suppl):27–35.

213. Morton LD, Rizkallah E, Pellock JM: New drug therapy for acute seizure management. Semin Pediatr Neurol 1997;4:51–63.

214. Fisher R, Kalviainen R, Tanganelli P, et al: Newer antiepileptic drugs as monotherapy: Data on vigabatrin. Neurology 1996;47:S2–S5.

215. Perucca E: Pharmacological principles as a basis for polytherapy. Acta Neurol Scand Suppl 1995;162:31–34.

216. Richens A: Rational polypharmacy. Seizure 1995;4:211–214.

217. Beghi E, Perucca E: The management of epilepsy in the 1990s. Acquisitions, uncertainties and priorities for future research. Drugs 1995;49:680–694.

218. Gilman JT: Developmental principles of antiepileptic drug therapy. J Child Neurol 1994;9:S20–S25.

219. Cascino GD: Epilepsy: Contemporary perspectives on evaluation and treatment. Mayo Clin Proc 1994;69:1199–1211.

220. Bardy AH, Seppala T, Salokorpi T, et al: Monitoring of concentrations of clobazam and norclobazam in serum and saliva of children with epilepsy. Brain Dev 1991;13:174–179.
221. Choonara IA, Rane A: Therapeutic drug monitoring of anticonvulsants. State of the art. Clin Pharmacokinet 1990;18:318–328.
222. Rockoff MA, Goudsouzian NG: Seizures induced by methohexital. Anesthesiology 1981;54:333–335.
223. Blackburn GL, Maini BS, Pierce EC Jr: Nutrition in the critically ill patient. Anesthesiology 1977;47:181–194.
224. Lieu TA, Quesenberry CPJ, Capra AM, et al: Outpatient management practices associated with reduced risk of pediatric asthma hospitalization and emergency department visits. Pediatrics 1997;100:334–341.
225. Carlson CM, O'Connell EJ: Asthma in childhood: A review. Minn Med 1993;76:31–33.
226. LeSon S, Gershwin ME: Risk factors for asthmatic patients requiring intubation: A comprehensive review. Allergol Immunopathol (Madr) 1995;23:235–247.
227. Mielck A, Reitmeir P, Wjst M: Severity of childhood asthma by socioeconomic status. Int J Epidemiol 1996;25:388–393.
228. Schuh S, Johnson D, Stephens D, et al: Hospitalization patterns in severe acute asthma in children. Pediatr Pulmonol 1997;23:184–192.
229. Rowe BH, Keller JL, Oxman AD: Effectiveness of steroid therapy in acute exacerbations of asthma: A meta-analysis. Am J Emerg Med 1992;10:301–310.
230. Konig P, Shaffer J: The effect of drug therapy on long-term outcome of childhood asthma: A possible preview of the international guidelines. J Allergy Clin Immunol 1996;98:1103–1111.
231. Barnes N: Relative safety and efficacy of inhaled corticosteroids. J Allergy Clin Immunol 1998;101:S460–S464.
232. Amirav I, Newhouse MT: Metered-dose inhaler accessory devices in acute asthma: Efficacy and comparison with nebulizers. A literature review. Arch Pediatr Adolesc Med 1997;151:876–882.
233. Davis KC, Small RE: Budesonide inhalation powder: a review of its pharmacologic properties and role in the treatment of asthma. Pharmacotherapy 1998;18:720–728.
234. Zachary CY, Evans R 3d: Perioperative management for childhood asthma. Ann Allergy Asthma Immunol 1996;77:468–472.
235. Nelson DR, Sachs MI, O'Connell EJ: Approaches to acute asthma and status asthmaticus in children. Mayo Clin Proc 1989;64:1392–1402.
236. Siegel SC, Rachelefsky GS: Continuing medical education: Asthma in infants and children: Part 1. J Allergy Clin Immunol 1985;76:1–15.
237. Rachelefsky GS, Siegel SC: Asthma in infants and children: Treatment of childhood asthma. Part II. J Allergy Clin Immunol 1985;76:409–425.
238. Van Asperen PP, Mellis CM, Sly PD: The role of corticosteroids in the management of childhood asthma. The Thoracic Society of Australia and New Zealand. Med J Aust 1992;156:48–52.
239. Weinberger M: Theophylline for treatment of asthma. J Pediatr 1978;92:1–7.
240. Ellis EF: Theophylline toxicity. J Allergy Clin Immunol 1985;76:297–301.
241. Peck CC, Nichols AI, Baker J, et al: Clinical pharmacodynamics of theophylline. J Allergy Clin Immunol 1985;76:292–297.
242. Downes JJ, Wood DW, Striker TW, et al: Arterial blood gas and acid-base disorders in infants and children with status asthmaticus. Pediatrics 1968;42:238–249.
243. Victoria MS, Tayaba RG, Nangia BS: Isoproterenol infusion in the management of respiratory failure in children with status asthmaticus: Experience in a small community hospital and review of the literature. J Asthma 1991;28:103–108.
244. Dworkin G, Kattan M: Mechanical ventilation for status asthmaticus in children. J Pediatr 1989;114:545–549.

5 Outpatient Anesthesia

Raafat S. Hannallah

Patient Selection Criteria
  Patient
  Procedure
  Pediatric Perioperative Environment
Preoperative Requirements
  Preoperative Fasting
  Preoperative Laboratory Testing
  Patient and Family Education and Preparation
Screening
Pre-anesthetic Management
  Pharmacologic Premedication
  Preinduction Techniques
  Parents' Presence During Induction
Anesthetic Agents and Techniques
  Inhalational Techniques
  Intravenous Techniques
  Perioperative Fluid Management
Postoperative Analgesia
Postoperative Nausea and Vomiting
Recovery and Discharge
  Recovery
  Discharge Home
Complications and Admissions
  Complications
  Admissions
  Follow-up
New Challenges and Opportunities
  Fast-Tracking
  Twenty-Three-Hour Recovery Units
  Office-Based Anesthesia

Children are excellent candidates for outpatient (ambulatory or day) surgery. Most children are healthy and most pediatric surgical procedures are simple and associated with prompt recovery. It is not surprising, therefore, that up to 60% of pediatric surgery in the United States is performed on an outpatient basis.[1, 2] The key to the success of this practice lies in careful selection, screening, and preparation of prospective patients. In current practice, many newly introduced anesthetic agents help ensure prompt emergence, fast recovery, and safe discharge with excellent control of postoperative pain and vomiting. These new anesthetic drugs have expanded our ability to care for sicker patients undergoing more complex outpatient procedures than previously possible.

Patient Selection Criteria

The primary factors that must be considered when selecting a child for outpatient surgery are the physical status of the patient and the type of surgical procedure to be performed. These factors must be balanced with the capability of the surgical facility and the ability of its staff to deal with any expected or unexpected complications.

Patient

The child should be in good health; if not, any systemic disease must be well controlled. Many patients with chronic medical conditions present for surgical procedures that are normally considered appropriate for outpatient surgery. In these cases, an understanding of the underlying pathophysiology and thorough preoperative evaluation will help guide the anesthesiologist as to the appropriateness of choosing an outpatient setting for each individual patient. Although the pathophysiology and anesthetic management of some of these conditions are discussed in detail elsewhere in this book, the following is a brief discussion of the implications of scheduling some of these patients on an outpatient basis.

Former Premature Infant

It is generally considered that infants younger than 46 weeks of post-conceptual age and those who have a preoperative history of apnea are at greatest risk for postoperative apnea; however, some authors have reported apnea in infants as old as 60 weeks of post-conceptual age. In an outpatient, apnea that occurs following discharge may go unnoticed long enough to cause death or serious neurologic injury. Many anesthesiologists admit former premature infants who are younger than 50 to 55 weeks of post-conceptual age to a hospital or to a 23-hour recovery facility so that they can be monitored postoperatively for apnea, bradycardia, and oxygen desaturation.[3] If the infant was extremely premature or has bronchopulmonary dysplasia, anemia, or other neonatal problems, this period may need to be extended beyond 55 to 60 weeks of post-conceptual age.[3, 4] It seems prudent to have a high index of suspicion when dealing with these infants, and to err on the side of recommending postoperative inpatient care and monitoring. Infants who develop apnea in the recovery room should also be admitted and monitored (see Chapters 4 and 14).

Child with a Runny Nose

A child who presents with a runny nose may have a completely benign, noninfectious condition, such as seasonal or vasomotor rhinitis, in which case elective surgery may be performed. On the other hand, the runny nose may be a symptom of an upper respiratory tract infection, in which case elective surgery may need to be postponed. Since an estimated 20 to 30% of all children have a runny nose a significant part of the year, every child with a runny nose must be evaluated on an individual basis.

Although the definitive pre-anesthetic assessment of these patients requires a complete history, a physical examination, and occasionally the interpretation of certain laboratory data, the history is the most important element in the differential diagnosis. Specifically, allergic problems should be actively sought. The general assessment of the child (e.g., fever, fatigue, lack of sleep, loss of appetite) can help differentiate an acute illness from a chronic condition. Parents can usually tell whether their child's runny nose is "the usual runny nose" or something different that may require cancellation of elective surgery. Parents of outpatients can be instructed to call the surgical unit on the morning of surgery if the child develops symptoms of upper respiratory infection so that the findings can be reviewed and, if a decision to cancel surgery is made, they are spared a wasted trip to the hospital.

If surgery is postponed because of simple nasopharyngitis, it can usually be rescheduled in 1 to 2 weeks. If a flu-like syndrome that involves both the upper and the lower respiratory tract is present, surgery is generally postponed until at least a month after the child has recovered (see Chapter 4).

Asthma

Asthma is the most common chronic disease of childhood, affecting 5 to 10% of children in the United States, and the incidence is on the rise. It is common for patients with asthma to present for a minor surgical procedure in an outpatient setting. The decision to accept and proceed with surgery depends on the severity and frequency of symptoms and the adequacy of pharmacologic control. A good history, which is an important part of a well-organized screening process, can help establish the severity of asthma. Children with *mild asthma* who have infrequent symptoms and do not require continuous medications are excellent candidates for outpatient surgery. When children with *moderate* a*sthma* (those who require daily medications to control their symptoms) are scheduled for outpatient surgery, they should be instructed to continue their medications until (and including) the morning of surgery.[5] A beta-agonist is generally administered in the preoperative holding area by a nebulizer to young children or by an inhaler if the patient is older. If the patient is wheezing or has co-existing upper respiratory infection, persistent cough, or tachypnea on the day of surgery, it is best to reschedule the procedure. Children with *severe asthma,* who are never wheeze-free, usually require aggressive perioperative medical management and may not be good candidates for outpatient surgery.[6]

The choice of a specific anesthetic technique in an asthmatic child is usually dictated by the nature of the surgical procedure. Most anesthetics have been used successfully in asthmatic patients. If an endotracheal tube must be used, sufficient depth of anesthesia must be established first. Intravenous lidocaine or a beta-agonist inhalant or both may be administered just prior to extubation to blunt the possibility of bronchospasm. Deep extubation should be considered when possible. Patients may leave the facility when the usual discharge criteria are met. Children should not have any signs of wheezing when discharged. Adequate hydration should be ensured.

Other Medical Conditions

Children with well-controlled diabetes, congenital cardiac defects, or hematologic problems are often good candidates for brief outpatient procedures that do not interfere with their medical management. As stated previously, prior consultation with the treating physician and thorough preparation are essential.

Children who are thought to be susceptible to malignant hyperthermia syndrome can be candidates for outpatient anesthesia and surgery as long as nontriggering agents are used. A longer period of postoperative observation may be required before these patients are discharged home.[7]

Procedure

The planned day surgical procedure should be associated with only minimal bleeding and minor physiologic derangements. The length of the procedure is not in itself a significant limitation. Although many experts believe that almost any operation that does not require a major intervention into the cranial vault, abdomen, or thorax can be considered, superficial procedures are the most common.

The five most frequently performed outpatient surgical procedures at Children's National Medical Center (CNMC) during the past 2 years were herniorrhaphy, myringotomy, adenoidectomy with or without myringotomy, circumcision, and eye-muscle surgery.

Performance of adenotonsillectomy as an outpatient procedure remains a debatable issue. Some surgeons are reluctant to perform tonsillectomy on an outpatient basis because of the risk of postoperative hemorrhage. However, experience indicates that outpatient adenotonsillectomy is safe and cost-effective and that there is little benefit in keeping these patients in the hospital more than a few hours after surgery to ensure adequate hydration and absence of bleeding.[8] Children who bleed in the recovery room, however, belong to a high-risk subgroup for recurrent bleeding and may need to be admitted.[8] Chiang and associates[9] reported 40,000 outpatient adenotonsillectomy procedures without a single death. They emphasized careful selection of cases and preoperative evaluation to eliminate patients with bleeding tendencies and cardiopulmonary disease. To decrease the risk of hemorrhage, no patients with allergies were operated on during the pollen season, and no operation was performed until 4 to 5 weeks after an acute attack of tonsillitis.

There have been reports of postoperative apnea or airway obstruction in children after tonsillectomy.[10] Most of those patients were less than 3 years of age and had a documented preoperative history of obstructive sleep apnea syndrome or other obstructive phenomena during sleep. These patients have a diminished ventilatory response to CO_2 rebreathing and are at increased risk for postoperative respiratory compromise.[11] In extreme cases, the airway obstruction can result in pulmonary hypertension and cor pulmonale. Most of these children continue to suffer from the same symptoms in the immediate postoperative period. It is therefore very important that the indication for tonsillectomy (repeated infections versus obstructive symptoms) be carefully reviewed, especially in young patients. Postoperative observation in a 23-hour recovery facility is appropriate for patients with mild obstructive symptoms. Inpatient care or even admission to the intensive care unit for airway support may be indicated in those with documented obstructive sleep apnea syndrome.[12] Management of post-tonsillectomy pain and vomiting continues to be a clinical challenge and is discussed later in this chapter.

Pediatric Perioperative Environment

A publication by the Section on Anesthesiology of the American Academy of Pediatrics introduced specific guidelines for patient care facilities and their medical staff who wish to provide pediatric anesthesia care.[13] This document emphasizes important facility-based issues such as the experience and training of the health-care team and the resources committed to the care of infants and children throughout the perioperative period, including the postoperative period. Competency by the staff in addressing such issues as airway management, fluid administration, temperature regulation, monitoring, vascular catheter insertion, and postoperative pain are as important as the skill and experience of the individual anesthesiologist in determining the type of patient to be selected and procedure to be performed in any specific outpatient facility.

Preoperative Requirements

Preoperative Fasting

The need for prolonged fasting before elective surgery in healthy pediatric outpatients has been challenged.[14] Studies have shown that children who are allowed to drink clear liquids until 2 hours prior to induction of anesthesia do not have an increase in gastric volume or acidity compared with those who fast overnight.[15] Although there is still no uniform fasting practice for children before elective surgery in the United States and Canada,[16] most pediatric anesthesiologists have liberalized preoperative fasting requirements for otherwise healthy patients.[16–18] Solid food is still not generally allowed on the day of surgery. Some children will have unintentionally ingested varying amounts and types of solid foods; the decision to proceed after waiting an appropriate period of time is made on a case-by-case basis. Children

may drink clear liquids until 2 hours of the scheduled surgical time. Breast-fed infants are allowed to nurse up to 4 hours preoperatively (see Table 11–6). The main advantage of these liberal guidelines is that children are not thirsty and irritable while waiting for surgery. Other possible benefits include a decreased incidence of perioperative hypotension and hypoglycemia. Unfortunately, many pediatric outpatients still arrive to the facility on the morning of surgery with unnecessarily long periods of starvation. This is more frequently seen in those scheduled for morning surgery. In this case, meeting the fasting guidelines requires the parent to awaken the child to offer clear fluids.[19]

Preoperative Laboratory Testing

Until rather recently, most children scheduled for surgery were required at minimum to have a hemoglobin level or hematocrit determination as well as a urinalysis. Most anesthesiologists will not request urinalysis unless there is a specific history of genitourinary disease that warrants it. Studies have shown that the incidence of anemia in healthy children is extremely low[20, 21] and does not usually require modification in the anesthetic management.[21] Accordingly, most anesthesiologists request preoperative hemoglobin or hematocrit testing only when the medical history suggests that significant anemia may be present, such as in infants or adolescent females or in the presence of chronic disease.[21]

Patient and Family Education and Preparation

The practice of outpatient anesthesia is synonymous with speed and efficiency. Patients arrive as close to the time of scheduled surgery as possible. The time available for orientation and preoperative counseling on the day of surgery is often very brief and may not allow for a detailed explanation of the proposed procedures. Most outpatient surgical facilities, therefore, have a preoperative information and preparation program for children awaiting surgery. Typically, these programs are offered 1 or 2 weeks before the day of surgery and provide reading material to the family, allow for telephone counseling, and may organize visits to the facility a few days before the scheduled day of surgery. The program at CNMC starts by having the admitting office contact the parents as soon as possible after the procedure is scheduled. A mailing is sent that includes a coloring book depicting some basic information about surgery, anesthesia, and being a patient in a hospital. The parents are invited to bring their children to the hospital for a preoperative preparation visit on the Sunday preceding the day of surgery, or earlier if they wish. Often these preoperative visits are also mentioned and promoted by the surgeons when they counsel the parents about surgery in the first place.

Volunteer staff, under the direction of child life specialists, conduct the actual visit. The script is reviewed by many health-care professionals, including the anesthesiologist. During the visit, the children and their parents are told what to expect on the day of surgery. They are shown the areas of the hospital where they will be arriving (AM Surgical Admission Center), and waiting for surgery (the preoperative playroom). They are allowed to see and handle anesthesia equipment such as a face mask and breathing circuit and are shown the recovery areas where they will reunite with their parents. At CNMC, a video is shown to reinforce the ideas presented in person. Videotape viewing has been shown to facilitate preoperative preparation and lessen preoperative anxiety.[22, 23]

Children respond psychologically to the prospect of surgery in a variable and age-dependent manner,[24] and although most practitioners believe that preoperative preparation programs are valuable in allaying the child's anxiety, there exists little evidence that they are indeed useful. Rosen et al.[25] attempted to objectively examine the effect of the preparation program at CNMC on the children's behavior during induction of anesthesia. They found that children who participated in a preoperative preparation program were more likely to be cooperative during induction than those who did not. However, these investigators also found that only a small percentage of the parents who were invited to bring their children to the tour did in fact participate. Most of the families who toured the facility were extremely motivated parents who admitted to having prepared their children in many other ways. In addition, parents of very young children and of children who were coming for repeat surgery were less likely to come for the tour. These are the children who are at the highest risk for being upset during induction.[25] Kain,[26] on the other hand, found that 2- to 12-year-old children who received an extensive behavioral preparation program prior to outpatient surgery were less anxious in the preoperative holding area, but not during the induction of anesthesia or postoperatively (see Chapter 3).

The value of the preoperative visit with the anesthesiologist in allaying the fears of the child and parents cannot be overemphasized, especially for the outpatient who does not have enough time to get familiar with the surgical routine. A full explanation of the anesthetic plan must be offered to the parents *and* the child as appropriate for his or her age.[24] Although a brief discussion of the risks associated with anesthesia and surgery is appropriate, and often desired by the parents,[27] this should not be presented in a way that adds to the inevitable apprehension of awaiting surgery for one's child.

Screening

Most outpatient surgical units actively participate in the preoperative screening of their patients. The degree of involvement varies from a simple telephone call to the parents a day or two prior to surgery to the establishment of a formal screening clinic to "clear" all patients before surgery. At CNMC, the parents are interviewed by telephone shortly after the operation is scheduled. A second call is made 24 hours or less before surgery. During the initial call, the child's medical history is reviewed using a preapproved directed questionnaire format seeking "no" or "yes" answers, and allowing room for explanation. Information is sought concerning past or present risk factors, such as a history of prematurity or cardiac or respiratory problems. This information helps determine whether additional preoperative evaluation or consultation is required prior to the day of surgery. In some cases, it may lead to a re-evaluation of the appropriateness of scheduling the procedure on an outpatient basis. During the second phone call, an assessment of the child's current health is made. Fasting orders are

reinforced, and practical matters related to parking, insurance papers, what to bring to the hospital, and expected duration of stay are explained.

On the day of surgery, all patients are screened for acute illness and fasting status. Vital signs are recorded. Any consultation reports are evaluated, and the need for special preoperative psychological or pharmacologic treatment is considered before the child arrives into the operating room area. Our experience with this method has been extremely favorable, with a lower rate of cancellation for screened patients than for patients who were not screened.[28] Success in contacting more parents by phone can be increased by calling during evening hours and by having the surgeons inform the parents to initiate the calls themselves if they are not easy to reach. Future efforts will undoubtedly be directed toward using the Internet to have the parents answer these questionnaires and get needed information on the Web when it is a convenient time for them.

Although many outpatient units find that having a screening clinic to examine all the patients prior to the day of surgery reduces the time for preoperative evaluation on the morning of surgery, there is no evidence that this method provides better medical evaluation or reduces cancellation compared with telephone or last-minute screening.[29] Potential disadvantages include added staffing costs and the need to have the parents take additional time off work and travel to bring the child for the extra visit.

Pre-Anesthetic Management

Pharmacologic Premedication

The routine use of preoperative sedation in pediatric outpatient surgery has gone a full cycle. When the practice of outpatient surgery first became popular, one of the major modifications to our anesthetic routine at the time was to discontinue the use of preoperative sedation in this patient population. This was thought to be necessary because the most popular premedicant drugs that were available at the time (e.g., morphine and pentobarbital) were long acting, delayed recovery, and increased the incidence of postoperative vomiting. In addition, most children dreaded the painful intramuscular injection that was required to administer these drugs. Without preoperative sedation, the recovery from anesthesia was fast, and patients were able to leave the facility very soon after the conclusion of surgery. It was an efficient approach that very quickly became the routine in most institutions.

Of late, however, anesthesiologists became more concerned by the number of unpremedicated young children who were uncooperative during induction of anesthesia. It became clear that quite often we were compromising the psychological welfare of many children for the sake of efficiency.[30] The search started for new drugs that can result in preoperative sedation without delaying recovery and discharge from the facility. The "discovery" of oral midazolam premedication is the main reason pharmacologic sedation is now again popular in pediatric anesthesia, even in outpatients.[31] Midazolam, which is now available as a commercial syrup preparation, can be administered orally in a dose of 0.25 to 0.5 mg/kg (max 20 mg) 20 to 45 minutes before induction of anesthesia to facilitate separation from the parents and improve the cooperation with anesthesia induction.[32, 33] Some authors have even suggested that children can be separated from their parents as early as 10 minutes after receiving oral midazolam.[34] Higher doses of midazolam (0.75 and 1 mg/kg) appear to not offer any additional benefits and may cause more side effects.[35] Although most investigators report no delayed recovery with this technique, some have shown that early recovery as well as hospital discharge are somewhat longer in children premedicated with oral midazolam after brief sevoflurane anesthetics compared with placebo.[36] Children who received midazolam, however, experienced less disturbed sleep at home during the night following surgery.

Preinduction Techniques

Low-dose (2 mg/kg) intramuscular ketamine can be used as a preinduction technique in young children who do not cooperate with other methods of induction. The onset time is short (2–3 minutes), and recovery from anesthesia is not prolonged. When ketamine is followed by an inhaled technique, there is minimal likelihood of delirium or bad dreams during recovery.[37]

Rectal administration of methohexital is sometimes used in preschool children. A dose of 25 mg/kg (10% solution) has an onset time of 6 to 10 minutes and produces enough sedation to peacefully separate an upset child from his or her parents.[38] Rectal midazolam (1 mg/kg) has the same onset time, improves separation from parents, and does not generally delay discharge home.[39] Intranasal administration of intravenous midazolam formulation (0.2 mg/kg) has also been reported to produce anxiolysis and sedation in preschool-aged children with a rapid onset (5–10 minutes) and no evidence of delayed recovery, but it stings.[40]

Parents' Presence During Induction

One of the main reasons for administering routine premedication, or having to resort to using a preinduction technique, is to facilitate separation of the child from the parents. Some anesthesiologists find that they can reduce or even eliminate the need for such agents by allowing the parents to stay with the child during the induction of anesthesia.[41] Although still controversial,[42] this approach is gaining a lot of supporters and is being requested by many parents. Some institutions have separate induction rooms where the parents can accompany their children without having to wear special operating room attire. Others allow selected parents to wear a cover-all gown or scrubs and walk with the child into the operating room. Studies have shown that children are less upset when the parents are present.[41] Parent selection and education are essential for the success of this approach, since anxious parents can make their children even more upset.[43] It is therefore important to explain in detail what parents might observe during anesthetic induction. They should be warned that they may observe their child's eyes rolling up, may hear noises from their child's throat (airway obstruction), and observe movement (excitement) from the anesthetic agent's effects on the brain. They should be assured that although these events may be upsetting to observe, they are expected normal events during a gaseous induction to anesthesia.

Anesthetic Agents and Techniques

The choice of an anesthetic technique for the pediatric outpatient should ensure smooth induction, quick emergence at the end of surgery, prompt recovery in the post-anesthesia care unit (PACU), and rapid discharge with no or minimal pain and postoperative nausea and vomiting (PONV). Although many of the newer agents and techniques that were developed to meet these goals in outpatients are now the standard for most patients and are familiar to all anesthesiologists, it is important to review and understand the rationale for their selection.

Inhalational Techniques

Children and pediatric anesthesiologists have long favored inhalation induction. For over three decades, halothane has been the standard inhalational induction agent in pediatrics. It offered reasonably fast onset with minimal airway irritation. Despite some concerns over its tendency to slow the heart rate and, in the presence of hypercarbia and light anesthesia, to predispose the child to develop arrhythmias,[44] it continued to be the gold standard against which other inhalational agents had to be compared. With the recent introduction of sevoflurane in the United States, after years of experience in Japan, this preference is changing.

Sevoflurane has solubility characteristics closer to those of desflurane and nitrous oxide than to halothane or isoflurane. The drug has a relatively pleasant smell and is the least irritating inhalational induction agent available.[45] Sevoflurane can be used for both induction and maintenance of anesthesia in children. Clinical experience with sevoflurane has shown the drug to result in smooth induction with no or minimal airway irritation, and faster emergence and recovery when compared with halothane.[46] Sevoflurane undergoes metabolic breakdown in the body that results in release of free fluoride ions. The clinical importance of this breakdown appears to be negligible, especially in children undergoing brief outpatient surgical procedures. Sevoflurane considerably improves the ease of inhalation induction in pediatric outpatients, although improved speed of induction has not been consistently borne out in clinical trials that mandated a gradual increase in anesthetic concentration during induction.[47] In a multicenter comparative study, the time to loss of eyelash reflex with sevoflurane was only 0.3 minutes faster than with halothane.[48] In practice, however, patients will readily accept an 8% inspired sevoflurane concentration once they are comfortable with face mask application. The anesthetic uptake and loss of consciousness are extremely rapid (15–20 seconds) with no or minimal resistance or irritation. There is a lower incidence of bradycardia or arrhythmias than with halothane. There is no question that the availability of sevoflurane has reduced the need for preoperative sedation or for the use of alternate induction techniques in pediatric outpatients.

Recovery following sevoflurane anesthesia was reported to be 33% more rapid than with halothane.[48] The time to discharge from the hospital, however, was similar for both anesthetics. This may be due to the fact that the incidence of agitation attributable to sevoflurane was almost threefold greater than that attributable to halothane, therefore necessitating more frequent use of sedation during recovery. The more rapid recovery advantage of sevoflurane over halothane, however, was not shown in a different study that compared sevoflurane with both halothane and desflurane.[49] Patients who received desflurane anesthesia (following halothane induction) had faster emergence and recovery than those who received halothane or sevoflurane. Halothane and sevoflurane emergence and recovery were not significantly different. Again, the times to discharge from the hospital were essentially similar for the three agents. It is the author's conclusion that sevoflurane is the clear choice for inhalational induction in the frequently unpremedicated pediatric outpatient. If predictably rapid emergence is desired, such as with ear, nose, and throat surgery, then desflurane maintenance (in a low-flow gas mixture to save on the cost) is preferable.

Desflurane has chemical and physical characteristics that are potentially attractive for outpatient surgical patients. Desflurane's low blood-gas partition coefficient (0.42) should theoretically result in rapid alveolar uptake. However, early experience with desflurane in pediatric patients indicates that it results in an unacceptably high incidence of airway irritation, moderate-to-severe coughing, and laryngospasm that results in arterial oxygen desaturation. Desflurane is not, therefore, indicated for the induction of anesthesia in children.[50] Desflurane can be easily introduced following other induction agents, however, typically sevoflurane or halothane. Welborn et al.[51] found that a brief period of halothane induction, followed by administration of desflurane, resulted in the same rapid emergence and recovery as when desflurane was used for both induction and maintenance of anesthesia. In addition, desflurane maintenance resulted in significantly faster emergence and recovery when compared with halothane. This approach is particularly useful in patients undergoing ear, nose, and throat procedures such as tonsillectomy or adenoidectomy when the timing of the end of surgery cannot be accurately predicted, and when rapid emergence and return of airway reflexes is desirable. Recovery following unsupplemented desflurane (and to a slightly lesser degree, sevoflurane) anesthesia has been associated with a higher incidence of excitement than when halothane is used.[52] Attempts to modify the emergence agitation that is frequently seen with these agents have not been completely successful. Attention must be given to ensuring adequate analgesia in these patients. Even in the absence of pain, as usually seen in children who have a functional regional block, agitation still occurs. Recent experience indicates that a dose of 2 to 3 μg/kg of fentanyl is effective in reducing this emergence phenomenon without delaying emergence or discharge when desflurane or sevoflurane is used in pediatric ear, nose, and throat patients.[53]

Intravenous Techniques

Intravenous induction is the method of choice in many older children, especially when EMLA (eutectic mixture of local anesthetics, a lidocaine/prilocaine cream) is used to facilitate a painless venipuncture. The use of EMLA in outpatients requires careful planning, since at least 1 hour of contact time under an occlusive dressing is required for full effect.[54, 55] Efforts to have EMLA applied at home by parents should be encouraged, especially with the current availability of a prepackaged EMLA patch. In most cases, EMLA should be applied to two potential intravenous sites to have a back-up site available in case the first venipuncture is not successful.

When *thiopental sodium* is used in healthy unpremedicated children, a relatively large dose (5–6 mg/kg) may be required to ensure smooth and rapid transition to general inhalational anesthesia.[56, 57] Children who receive a barbiturate induction tend to be sleepier and require more airway support for the first 15 minutes of recovery than those who have received halothane alone. This difference disappears by 30 minutes.[58]

Studies of the use of *propofol* in children indicate that it results in a smooth induction with a lower incidence of side effects and faster recovery than thiopental. Propofol can be used in a dose of 2.5 to 3.5 mg/kg for induction of anesthesia in children who accept a venipuncture. Pain on injection can be minimized or even prevented by using the large antecubital veins for drug administration. If the hand veins must be used, lidocaine can be mixed with propofol (1–2 mg lidocaine /1 mL of propofol) immediately prior to its injection, with excellent results. Alternatively, a propofol infusion can be started following a brief inhalational induction and establishment of intravenous access. Because of their higher volume of distribution and increased clearance, children require a higher infusion rate (125–250 μg/kg/min) than adults. This is especially true for younger children and during the early part of maintenance.

Propofol anesthesia has been consistently shown to be associated with an extremely low incidence of postoperative vomiting, even following surgical procedures that normally result in vomiting, such as strabismus surgery[59] or when combined with ondansetron for tonsillectomy.[60] The absence of vomiting has been shown to result in a faster discharge home time when compared to halothane.[58]

Perioperative Fluid Management

The need for routine administration of intravenous fluids during pediatric outpatient anesthesia is controversial. Children undergoing very brief surgical procedures, such as myringotomies, may not receive any parenteral fluid administration as long as they are not excessively starved preoperatively and are expected to be able to ingest and retain oral fluids soon after they are awake. For most other children, intraoperative maintenance fluid administration can be calculated based on the child's body weight according to standard formulas (see Chapter 11).

Intravenous fluid therapy during and after surgery is specifically indicated in longer operations, in procedures known to be associated with a high incidence of postoperative nausea and vomiting, such as strabismus surgery, and in young children who have been fasting for a prolonged period of time. If continuing postoperative loss through vomiting or inability to tolerate oral intake is anticipated, it is advisable to start making up that anticipated deficit early on so that it is ensured that the child is well hydrated when ready to go home. This will avoid delaying discharge while "catch-up" fluid administration is instituted. Adequate parenteral hydration also obviates the need for forcing children to ingest oral fluids before they are allowed to go home. Children who are forced to drink before leaving the facility have a higher incidence of vomiting, and are discharged home later, than children who are allowed to drink only when they are thirsty enough to request a drink.[61]

Postoperative Analgesia

The need for analgesics following surgery depends on the nature of the procedure and the pain threshold of the patient. It does not depend on whether the child is an outpatient or an inpatient. Regional blocks or local infiltration should be used whenever possible to supplement general anesthesia and to limit the need for narcotics during recovery. Postoperative pain or discomfort can be managed by one or a combination of the following methods.

Acetaminophen is the most commonly used mild analgesic for pediatric outpatients. For young children, the initial dose is often administered rectally (up to 45 mg/kg) prior to awakening from anesthesia.[62–65] Supplemental doses are given orally (10 mg/kg every 4 hours or 20 mg/kg every 6 hours and not "as needed") or rectally (20 mg/kg every 6 hours) to maintain adequate blood levels and therefore effective analgesia.[63, 64, 66] The total 24-hour dose should not exceed 100 mg/kg. Acetaminophen can be combined with codeine for more effective control of moderately severe pain and discomfort. Acetaminophen with codeine elixir contains 120 mg acetaminophen and 12 mg codeine per 5 mL. The usual dose is 5 mL for children 3 to 6 years of age, and 10 mL for the 7- to 12-year-old age group. It is important to advise parents to start analgesics prior to a regional block or local infiltration wearing off.

Nonsteroidal anti-inflammatory drugs (NSAIDs) have proved effective in relieving postoperative pain following minor operations in children. Ketorolac is an efficacious NSAID. Early administration immediately following induction seems to provide optimal postoperative analgesia. Several studies have demonstrated the analgesic and opioid-sparing effects of ketorolac, which may reduce the incidence of opioid-related adverse effects such as respiratory depression, nausea, and vomiting. Ketorolac, however, like many other NSAIDs, has some troubling side effects. These include instances of decreased bone repair after osteotomy, bronchospasm, acute renal failure, and possibly increased surgical bleeding secondary to altered platelet function.[67–70] Several papers reported an increased incidence of postoperative hemorrhage in tonsillectomy patients who received ketorolac.[71, 72] Some, however, did not find increased bleeding when ketorolac was given at the end of the procedure.[73] More studies are required to determine the optimal dose and route of administration of ketorolac, as well as its efficacy as an analgesic following more painful outpatient surgical procedures in children. It would seem prudent to administer the ketorolac at the end of the procedure after hemostasis has been obtained. It is expected that parenteral preparations of newer NSAIDs will soon be available that will selectively block pain receptors with minimal side effects, especially antiplatelet effects. These newer agents should be extremely valuable in the care of pediatric outpatients.

Potent narcotic analgesics may be indicated in the recovery period; when they are, a short-acting drug is generally chosen. Intravenous use allows more accurate titration of the dose and avoids the use of "standard" dosages based on weight, which may lead to a relative overdose. If remifen-tanil is used intraoperatively, planning for postoperative analgesia must be started prior to the patient's awakening. Fentanyl, up to a dose of 2.0 μg/kg, is this author's drug of choice for intravenous use in outpatients. Meperidine (0.5 mg/kg) and codeine (1.0–1.5 mg/kg) can be used intramuscularly if an intravenous route is not established. Intramuscular codeine tends to result in less vomiting than other opioids, especially morphine.[74] Nasal administration of fentanyl has been shown to result in an analgesic blood level comparable to that following intravenous use,[75] which makes it useful for children who do not have, or have lost, intravenous access.[76]

Regional anesthesia can be combined with light general anesthesia to provide excellent postoperative pain relief and early ambulation, with minimal or no need for opioids (see Chapter 28). By placing the block before surgery starts but after the child is asleep, one can reduce the requirement for general anesthetic agents during surgery, which in turn may result in a more rapid recovery, earlier discharge, more rapid return of normal appetite, and less nausea and vomiting. Only the skill and interest of the anesthesiologist limit the types of blocks that can be used safely in the pediatric surgical outpatient. Generally, the techniques chosen should be simple to perform, have minimal or no side effects, and not interfere with motor function and early ambulation (see Chapters 28 and 29).

An *ilioinguinal and iliohypogastric nerve block* can be performed by infiltration of 0.25% bupivacaine solution (in doses up to 2 mg/kg) in the region medial to the anterior superior iliac spine. This block has been successfully used to provide excellent postoperative analgesia for pediatric outpatients following elective inguinal herniotomy or orchiopexy.[77, 78]

A *dorsal nerve block of the penis* can be performed by simple injection of 1 to 4 mL of 0.25% bupivacaine *without epinephrine* deep to Buck's fascia 1 cm from the midline. This has been shown to provide over 6 hours of analgesia following circumcision.[79–81] Alternate approaches to penile block are a midline injection or subcutaneous infiltration (ring block), which presumably blocks the nerve after it has traversed into the subcutaneous tissue. Topical application of lidocaine on the incision site at the conclusion of surgery has also been shown to be effective.[82]

A *caudal block* provides excellent postoperative analgesia following a wide variety of surgical procedures such as circumcision, hypospadias repair, orchiopexy, and herniorrhaphy. With the use of bupivacaine 0.25% solution in a dose of 0.5 to 0.7 mL/kg, no motor paralysis is produced. If a larger volume (1–1.5 mL/kg) is indicated, the use of 0.125% bupivacaine or 0.2% ropivacaine is recommended to avoid motor weakness.[83] Caudal block has been extensively used in our outpatient surgical unit, with most children discharged home free of pain between 1 and 2 hours postoperatively. Analgesia (as measured by subsequent need of a mild oral analgesic) lasts 4 to 6 hours with this technique. Although voiding may be slightly delayed in children who receive a caudal block, catheterization is rarely needed, and children can be allowed to go home before voiding.

Pain management after tonsillectomy remains a considerable clinical problem in children. The ideal analgesic should be effective, safe, easy to administer, and free from associated respiratory depression. Although systemic opioids have been extensively used to treat post-tonsillectomy pain, there is an increased incidence of vomiting, and the risks of respiratory depression and airway obstruction are constant concerns. This is especially true in the younger patients in whom preoperative airway obstruction is the main indication for surgery. The use of local anesthetic techniques is not consistently effective in these patients. A recent study concluded that post-tonsillectomy infiltration of bupivacaine 0.5% with 1:200,000 epinephrine reduced immediate postoperative pain in children compared with a similar concentration of bupivacaine administered by spray, or with placebo.[84] Unfortunately, the clinical analgesic effect of the infiltrated bupivacaine was limited to less than 1 hour. The authors speculated that the short analgesic effect in their patients was due to the fact that the local anesthetic infiltration was performed after the surgical stimulation. This prevented the potential for any pre-emptive blockade of the release of nociceptive neuromediators that may be responsible for the maintenance of postoperative pain. An earlier study in which 0.25% bupivacaine infiltration was performed *before* surgical incision still concluded that postoperative analgesic requirements were not modified by the local anesthetic infiltration.[85] Tonsillectomy can be performed in adults with only local anesthetic infiltration and minimal intravenous sedation, but a similar technique in anesthetized children fails to produce adequate or sustained postoperative pain relief. It is possible that post-tonsillectomy pain is multifactorial in nature. Factors such as the excessive muscle stretching resulting from the use of a mouth gag, compression of the tongue, trauma to other pharyngeal structures, and so on are not modified by the local anesthetic infiltration of the peritonsillar fossa.

Attempts to use currently available NSAIDs in tonsillectomy/adenoidectomy patients have also been controversial: In one study subjects received either 1.5 mg/kg codeine IM or 1 mg/kg ketorolac IV before the commencement of surgery.[71] The study had to be terminated after only 64 patients were enrolled because interim analysis of the data concluded that the patients who received ketorolac were at an undue risk for excessive bleeding without beneficial effects. Other investigators, however, did not find increased bleeding when ketorolac was given at the end of the procedure.[73] In general, these studies and individual clinical experience have dissuaded many practitioners, both anesthesiologists and surgeons, from using ketorolac for tonsillectomies.[70]

There is increasing evidence that the use of a single dose of dexamethasone (0.5–1 mg/kg IV, maximum 20 mg) during anesthesia has many desirable effects in these patients, including decreased pain and swelling and a cost-effective way of reducing PONV.[86–88]

Postoperative Nausea and Vomiting

Postoperative nausea and vomiting can be a significant problem in pediatric outpatients. Contributing factors include the type of surgical procedure, the presence of pain, the use of opioid analgesics, a history of motion sickness, and sudden movement. Certain surgeries are particularly emesis prone: tonsillectomy, strabismus repair, orchiopexy, hernia repair, ear surgery, and laparoscopy. Tramer et al.[89] reviewed 27 randomized clinical trials involving a total of 2033 children undergoing strabismus surgery and found an average 54% incidence of early (<6 hours) and 59% incidence of late (up to 24 hours) emesis when prophylaxis was not administered.

A multicenter trial of 429 children concluded that intravenous ondansetron prophylaxis (0.1 mg/kg; maximum 4 mg) was more effective than placebo in preventing postoperative vomiting in children during both the 0- to 2-hour and 0- to 24-hour study periods (89 vs. 70% and 68 vs. 39%, respectively).[90] Intravenous ondansetron (0.1 mg/kg) was also found to be effective in treating established postoperative emesis in another multicenter trial of 2720 pediatric outpatients.[91]

Although intravenous ondansetron is an effective prophylactic antiemetic, many authors continue to compare it to other less expensive alternatives. Davis et al.[92] compared the effects of ondansetron (0.1 mg/kg), droperidol (75 μg/kg), and placebo on the incidence of emesis in children undergoing dental surgery in whom anesthesia was maintained with N_2O/O_2 and alfentanil. The 24-hour incidence of emesis was significantly less with ondansetron (9%) than with placebo (35%) or droperidol (32%). Ondansetron-treated patients also had significantly shorter hospital stay than the droperidol-treated patients.

Rose et al. conducted two prospective, randomized, double-blind, placebo-controlled studies evaluating PONV after tonsillectomy.[93, 94] Preoperative oral ondansetron 0.15 mg/kg decreased both the incidence of vomiting in the 24-hour postoperative period and the number of vomiting episodes per patient, whereas a 0.075 mg/kg dose was no better than placebo. The time to discharge was not significantly different among the groups evaluated.[93] In a different study, Rose[94] also found that two doses of either metoclopramide 0.25 mg/kg IV or ondansetron 0.15 mg/kg IV (one dose preoperatively, and a second dose 1 hour postoperatively) were more effective than a single dose of either drug in reducing vomiting after tonsillectomy in children who have received either isoflurane or propofol anesthesia. As indicated previously, the combination of propofol and ondansetron has been found extremely effective in reducing the incidence of vomiting following tonsillectomy in children.[60] A meta-analysis of published randomized clinical trials concluded that ondansetron and droperidol were more effective than metoclopramide in preventing postoperative vomiting.[95] However, whereas ondansetron and droperidol were equally effective in adults, ondansetron was more effective than droperidol in preventing vomiting in children.[95]

Dimenhydrinate, an H_1-receptor antagonist, has been used to both prevent and treat postoperative vomiting in children for several decades. In a prospective randomized study of children undergoing strabismus surgery, Vener et al.[96] concluded that, compared with placebo, dimenhydrinate (0.5 mg/kg IV) decreased postoperative vomiting both in hospital and for 24 hours after discharge (10 and 39% vs. 38 and 65%, respectively), without prolonged sedation or other adverse effects. The study suggests that dimenhydrinate's efficacy stems from actions on the vestibular/inner ear system, decreasing the development of late or delayed vomiting during and after the car ride home in outpatients.

Granisetron is a selective 5-HT3–receptor antagonist that has a more potent and longer activity against vomiting associated with chemotherapy than ondansetron. In a randomized, double-blind study of 97 pediatric outpatients, Cieslak et al.[97] found that 40 μg/kg intravenous granisetron decreased postoperative vomiting from 42 to 9% when compared with a placebo. Although this dose is much higher than the dose recommended for chemotherapy-induced emesis, a lower dose (10 μg/kg) was not effective. Fujii[98] found the same dose of granisetron (40 μg/kg) to be more effective than metoclopramide (0.25 mg/kg) or placebo in preventing vomiting after strabismus and tonsillectomy surgery in children without an increase in side effects. This study, performed in Japan, noted granisetron to be 59 times as expensive as droperidol and 167 times the cost of metoclopramide. The same authors also found that a combination antiemetic therapy, such as granisetron 40 μg/kg plus droperidol 50 μg/kg, was superior (97% effective) to each antiemetic alone in children undergoing general anesthesia for tonsillectomy.[99]

The fact that there are many approaches to the management of PONV would indicate that there is no one answer to the problem.[100] It appears, however, that a combination antiemetic regimen, possibly combined with the intraoperative use of dexamethasone is as close to being the most effective as one can possibly get. It is probably fair to say, however, that even now, many anesthesiologists continue to base their choice of antiemetics on personal experience and anecdotal evidence. Even when scientific data strongly suggest that one drug, or a combination of drugs, is superior to all others, the cost factor must be taken into consideration. What price tag one can put on patients' comfort and satisfaction, however, is beyond the scope of this discussion. Nevertheless, it is expected that any new treatment modality of PONV in the future will have to prove pharmacoeconomic as well as pharmacodynamic superiority to existing protocols.

For patients with persistent postoperative vomiting, our current approach is to stop any attempt at offering oral fluids and ensure adequate intravenous hydration. Intravenous metoclopramide 0.15 to 0.2 mg/kg or ondansetron 0.1 mg/kg is administered. In the absence of an intravenous line, or if vomiting occurs after the intravenous line is removed, ondansetron can be placed over the tongue for quick absorption without the need for swallowing. Occasionally, rectal promethazine 0.5 mg/kg (Phenergan 12.5–25 mg) or prochlorperazine 0.1 mg/kg (Compazine 2.5–5 mg) is administered in the hospital or given to the parents to use at home, or both.

Recovery and Discharge

Recovery

The key to understanding the reasoning behind the selection, modification, or avoidance of certain anesthetic agents and techniques in outpatient surgery is related to recovery. Rapid recovery and early ambulation are major objectives in pediatric outpatient surgery. When we deal with outpatients, we must guarantee safe discharge not only from the recovery room but also from the hospital. There is no second opportunity to transfer care of the outpatient to other medical or paramedical personnel, and there is no further period of observation, monitoring, and treatment.[101]

Facilities for postoperative care vary among institutions. Patients in some centers go to the main recovery room and then to a short-stay area from which they are discharged home. Others are discharged home directly from the recovery room. In freestanding units, the patient goes directly to the short-stay recovery area until discharged, whereas in many office practices the child may have to go home directly from the operating area.

Many parents want to be with their children as soon as the operation is terminated. In addition to confirming that the child has indeed survived the procedure, parents believe that the child relates to them better than to other unfamiliar faces at a time when anxiety could result from separation (see Chapters 3 and 9). Unfortunately, most recovery rooms are not large enough or properly designed to enable parents to participate in this aspect of care. In addition, some recovery room nurses fear that participation of the parents at this level may be detrimental to the care of their child and perhaps that of other children as well. Parent participation in recovery of extremely anxious or handicapped children has proved useful in our institution in selected cases, especially for deaf, blind, or mentally delayed children whose ability to communicate with anyone other than the parent or guardian is compromised. Parents should not have access to the recovery room until the child's vital signs have stabilized, airway obstruction is no longer a threat, and awakening has begun. The parents must understand that should the child's condition deteriorate or should it for any reason seem prudent to request them to leave the unit at any time, they must do so promptly and without argument.

On the other hand, parents are encouraged or may even be required to participate in the child's care in the short-stay, post-recovery unit. Parents can care for and hold, cuddle, and feed the child, and their involvement helps reduce the need for a high nurse-to-patient ratio. It also helps to prepare them to care for the child at home.

Discharge Home

Discharge of the child from the hospital cannot be based on criteria used for adults, such as ability to make decisions. The patient, however, must at least have reached a maximum on the recovery room scoring system, appear to be fully awake and back to baseline, and have no evidence of surgical or anesthetic complications.

In an effort to provide uniform care, and to ensure a complete legal record, most institutions have developed discharge criteria. Unlike a scoring system, all criteria must be met. At CNMC, discharge from the short-stay unit is guided by, but not necessarily limited to, the following:

1. Attainment of a state of consciousness appropriate to the developmental level.
2. Appropriateness and stability of vital signs.
3. Absence of respiratory distress.
4. Ability to ambulate consistent with the developmental age levels.
5. Ability to swallow oral fluids and cough or demonstrate a gag reflex.
6. Absence of nausea, vomiting, and dizziness.

In our institution, the attending physician may write a discharge order in advance so that, provided specific discharge criteria are met, the patient is authorized to be released without further evaluation by a physician at the time of discharge. A registered nurse documents the status of the patient, acts only as an observer to document that all criteria are met, and makes no decisions independently.

Every child, whatever his or her age, must have an escort

home.[102] The journey preferably should be by private car or taxicab, and the escort should be provided with written instructions as to the home care of the child and be provided with a telephone number to call for further advice or to report complications. In addition to counseling the parent of each child about postoperative care, most units have designed handouts that specify the care to be provided and the signs that might herald a complication. For convenience, the handout is usually limited to postoperative instructions for a specific operative procedure.

Complications and Admissions

Complications

Although life-threatening complications after outpatient anesthesia are rare, discomfort that prolongs or complicates recovery is common.[102, 103] The most commonly reported complications before discharge are sore throat, headache, muscle pains, nausea and vomiting, and postoperative pain. Sore throat is related to endotracheal intubation and its incidence has been reported to be as high as 59%.[102] Sore throat has also been observed in 24% of patients in whom an oropharyngeal airway has been used, compared with 6% in whom it was not.[102] Headache has been reported in 12% of children after surgery. Both sore throat and headache are usually treated easily and successfully with non-narcotic analgesics.

Admissions

Complications that result in unplanned admission of the patient to a hospital are usually the same types of problems discussed previously, but they occur with either greater frequency or greater severity. In a well-formulated program in a modern institution, the admission rate is usually less than 2%. At our institution, the unplanned admission rate for surgical outpatients has dropped from 0.9 to 0.3%.[103] The most common reasons for admission of the patients operated on in our unit are shown in Table 5–1.[103] These can be subgrouped into anesthetic (e.g., protracted vomiting or severe croup), surgical, and social/administrative reasons.

Severe postoperative vomiting is the most common anes-

Table 5–1. Reasons for Unplanned Admission to the Hospital at Children's National Medical Center*

Reason	Number of Patients (%)
Protracted vomiting	30 (33)
Complicated surgery	15 (17)
Croup	8 (9)
Parental request	6 (7)
Fever	6 (7)
Bleeding	3 (3)
Sleepiness	2 (2)
Others	20 (22)
Total	90 (100)

*Overnight hospital admission rate: 90 of 10,000 patients (0.9%).
Data from Patel RI, Hannallah RS: Anesthetic complications following pediatric ambulatory surgery: A 3-year study. Anesthesiology 1988;69:1009–1012.

Table 5–2. Post-hospitalization Complications Reported by Parents*

Complications	Number of Patients (%)
Vomiting (frequency)	
1–2 times	359 (7.2)
3–4 times	64 (1.2)
>4 times	24 (0.5)
Vomiting (total)	447 (8.9)
Cough	324 (6.5)
Sleepiness	297 (5.9)
Sore throat	257 (5.1)
Fever	235 (4.7)
Hoarseness/mild croup	168 (3.4)
Total	1728 (34.5)

*N = 4998.
Data from Patel RI, Hannallah RS: Anesthetic complications following pediatric ambulatory surgery: A 3-year study. Anesthesiology 1988;69:1009–1012.

thesia-related reason for unanticipated overnight admission after outpatient surgery in our hospital and most others. As mentioned previously, forcing children to drink after surgery may induce vomiting, which may even result in an overnight admission.[61] We currently admit patients who continue to vomit spontaneously in spite of withholding oral fluids and administration of aggressive antiemetic therapy. Patients who vomit only when challenged to drink are allowed to go home NPO as long as they have been adequately hydrated intravenously.

Although croup is now uncommon after endotracheal intubation of pediatric patients, it does occur. Fortunately, croup that is severe enough to cause respiratory distress almost always occurs during the recovery phase rather than after discharge. Treatment of croup with racemic epinephrine is highly effective. Nevertheless, we do not recommend discharge home unless the physician believes that the croup is mild; the parents have observed this problem in their child previously and are not alarmed; the parents live close to the hospital; and the child no longer requires racemic epinephrine to alleviate symptoms. In general, the smaller the child, the more likely is the possibility of admission. Croup can be a life-threatening complication. If any doubt exists concerning its severity and course, admission to the hospital is indicated.

Surgery-related reasons for admission can be the result either of an unexpected complication, such as postoperative bleeding after tonsillectomy, or of more extensive surgery than originally scheduled. Unplanned overnight admission may also be necessary if it becomes apparent that the parents are unable or cannot be relied on to care for the child at home.

Follow-up

Telephone or mailed questionnaires are necessary to determine the frequency of post-hospitalization problems. A large percentage of parents have reported that the child has continued to have an upset stomach, sleepiness, and other problems after their return home (Table 5–2).[103] Fortunately, most of the complications reported are mild and require no treatment.

A questionnaire should be designed not only to detect problems in the child but also to determine whether the parents were satisfied with the care received, and, if not, to request suggestions for improvement.

Any outpatient unit should collect and analyze data for trends that might indicate ways to correct deficiencies and eventually to improve patient care. Design and modification of policy are better done by prospective review rather than by reacting to mishaps. The former method leads to more uniform, safer care and minimizes the potential for medicolegal actions.

New Challenges and Opportunities

Fast-Tracking

With the availability of anesthetic agents and techniques that allow more rapid emergence, it has been possible to have patients completely awake in the operating room and transferred directly to a phase-2 recovery, thus completely bypassing the PACU. The PACU bypass rate for adult patients who received general anesthesia has been reported to vary from 14 to 42% in one study.[104] Experience with fast-tracking in children is still limited. Patel[105] reported success in bypassing the PACU in children undergoing a limited variety of procedures including myringotomies and hernia repair. Parents were extremely satisfied with the earlier union with their children. The children were discharged home faster, had less need for analgesics, and experienced less PONV than those who had the traditional stay in the PACU.

Twenty-Three-Hour Recovery Units

Many patients continue to need a prolonged period of observation in spite of meeting the traditional discharge criteria of the outpatient facility. An example is the child who needs aggressive management of PONV. Many institutions are now offering these patients, and their insurance carriers, the option of staying in an otherwise vacant hospital bed that is appropriately staffed and monitored for 23 hours or less until the child is medically fit for discharge home. Since the child is in the hospital less than 24 hours, the facility gets reimbursed at an outpatient rate as if the child had gone home from the outpatient facility directly.

The economics of this practice vary among institutions. Most of the time, however, these patients are "loss leaders" since they get the use of a room without having the hospital reimbursed for its expenses. If this arrangement extends the capability of the institution to perform more complex cases and to compete with freestanding surgical centers for these cases, then the extra cost may be economically justified.

Office-Based Anesthesia

Since office-based anesthesia is an extension of freestanding outpatient practice, all appropriate management guidelines should apply equally to both practice locations. One of the major requirements for safe management in either location is the anesthesiologist's high level of comfort, based on training and experience with the child's age, medical condition, and proposed surgical procedure. Another requirement is the availability of an environment that is designed and equipped to cater to the special needs of children both operatively and postoperatively.

Since most procedures in children require general anesthesia, or a deep level of sedation, and since most children prefer a technique that does not involve "a needle" when they are awake, the availability of an anesthesia machine is an important factor in determining the type of pediatric procedures that can be readily performed in the office (e.g., bilateral myringotomy and tube placement).

The child should be in good health; if not, any systemic disease must be under good control. An understanding of the underlying pathophysiology and thorough preoperative evaluation will help guide the anesthesiologist as to the appropriateness of choosing the office setting in each individual patient.

Although an absolute minimal age for otherwise healthy infants undergoing outpatient surgery cannot be suggested, it is probably prudent to limit the selection of office procedures to infants who have successfully transitioned from the neonatal period, that is, age 3 to 6 months for full-term babies.

The planned surgical procedure should be associated with only minimal bleeding and minor physiologic derangements. Brief and superficial procedures such as herniorrhaphy, myringotomy, and circumcision are selected most often. In scheduling children in an office setting, the need to send the children home quickly must be balanced with the desire to have the anesthesiologist leave soon after the last patient recovers. This may mandate that patients who have longer procedures or who may need longer observation be scheduled earlier so that their recovery coincides with the anesthetic management of the last quick cases on the schedule.

Preoperative screening and preparation is usually done in association with the surgeon and his or her office staff. It is very desirable to have the anesthesiologist contact the parents in advance of the day of surgery by phone or any other convenient way to introduce himself or herself, get a good history, explain the need for preoperative fasting, and discuss the anesthetic and recovery plans.

REFERENCES

1. Hannallah RS: General anesthesia techniques. In: White PF, ed: Ambulatory Anesthesia and Surgery: An International Prospective. London: WB Saunders; 1997:573–582.
2. Hannallah RS, Patel RI: Pediatric considerations. In: Twersky RS, ed: The Ambulatory Anesthesia Handbook. St. Louis: Mosby; 1995:145–170.
3. Coté CJ, Zaslavsky A, Downes JJ, et al: Postoperative apnea in former preterm infants after inguinal herniorrhaphy: A combined analysis. Anesthesiology 1995;82:809–822.
4. Welborn LG, Hannallah RS, Luban NLC, et al: Anemia and postoperative apnea in former preterm infants. Anesthesiology 1991;74:1003–1006.
5. Lindeman KS: Anesthesia, airways, and asthma. Semin Anesth 1995;14:221–225.
6. Zachary CY, Evans R 3d: Perioperative management for childhood asthma. Ann Allergy Asthma Immunol 1996;77:468–472.
7. Yentis SM, Levine MF, Hartley EJ: Should all children with suspected or confirmed malignant hyperthermia susceptibility be admitted after surgery? A 10-year review. Anesth Analg 1992;75:345–350.
8. Rakover Y, Almog R, Rosen G: The risk of postoperative haemorrhage in tonsillectomy as an outpatient procedure in children. Int J Pediatr Otorhinolaryngol 1997;41:29–36.
9. Chiang TM, Sukis AE, Ross DE: Tonsillectomy performed on an

outpatient basis: Report of a series of 40,000 cases performed without a death. Arch Otolaryngol 1968;88:307–310.

10. Tom LWC, DeDio RM, Cohen DE, et al: Is outpatient tonsillectomy appropriate for young children? Laryngoscope 1992;102:277–280.

11. Strauss SG, Lynn AM, Bratton SL, et al: Ventilatory response to CO_2 in children with obstructive sleep apnea from adenotonsillar hypertrophy. Anesth Analg 1999;89:328–332.

12. Patel R, Hannallah R: Ambulatory tonsillectomy. Amb Surg 1993;1:89–92.

13. Section on Anesthesiology, American Academy of Pediatrics: Guidelines for the pediatric perioperative anesthesia environment. Pediatrics 1999;103:512–515.

14. Coté CJ: NPO after midnight for children: A reappraisal. Anesthesiology 1990;72:589–592.

15. Schreiner MS, Treibwasser A, Keon TP: Ingestion of liquids compared with preoperative fasting in pediatric outpatients. Anesthesiology 1990;72:593–597.

16. Ferrari LR, Rooney FM, Rockoff MA: Preoperative fasting practices in pediatrics. Anesthesiology 1999;90:978–980.

17. Splinter WM, Schreiner MS: Preoperative fasting in children. Anesth Analg 1999;89:80–89.

18. American Society of Anesthesiologist Task Force on Preoperative Fasting: Practice guidelines for preoperative fasting and the use of pharmacologic agents to reduce the risk of pulmonary aspiration: Application to healthy patients undergoing elective procedures. Anesthesiology 1999;90:896–905.

19. Norden JM, Hannallah RS: Compliance with the new fasting guidelines for children: Does it depend on the time of surgery? Anesth Analg 1997;84:S447.

20. Steward DJ: Screening tests before surgery in children. Can J Anaesth 1991;38:693–695.

21. Roy WL, Lerman J, McIntyre BG: Is preoperative haemoglobin testing justified in children undergoing minor elective surgery? Can J Anaesth 1991;38:700–703.

22. Cassady JF Jr, Wysocki TT, Miller KM, et al: Use of a preanesthetic video for facilitation of parental education and anxiolysis before pediatric ambulatory surgery. Anesth Analg 1999;88:246–250.

23. Karl HW, Pauza KJ, Heyneman N, et al: Preanesthetic preparation of pediatric outpatients: The role of a videotape for parents. J Clin Anesth 1990;2:172–177.

24. McGraw T: Preparing children for the operating room: Psychological issues. Can J Anaesth 1994;41:1094–1103.

25. Rosen DA, Rosen KR, Hannallah RS: Anaesthesia induction in children: Ability to predict cooperation. Paediatr Anaesth 1993;3:365–370.

26. Kain ZN, Caramico LA, Mayes LC, et al: Preoperative preparation programs in children: A comparative examination. Anesth Analg 1998;87:1249–1255.

27. Litman RS, Perkins FM, Dawson SC: Parental knowledge and attitudes toward discussing the risk of death from anesthesia. Anesth Analg 1993;77:256–260.

28. Patel RI, Hannallah RS: Preoperative screening for pediatric ambulatory surgery: Evaluation of a telephone questionnaire method. Anesth Analg 1992;75:258–261.

29. Pollard JB, Olson L: Early outpatient preoperative anesthesia assessment: Does it help to reduce operating room cancellations? Anesth Analg 1999;89:502–505.

30. Kain ZN, Mayes LC, Wang SM, et al: Postoperative behavioral outcomes in children: Effects of sedative premedication. Anesthesiology 1999;90:758–765.

31. Kain ZN, Mayes LC, Bell C, et al: Premedication in the United States: A status report. Anesth Analg 1997;84:427–432.

32. Weldon BC, Watcha MF, White PF: Oral midazolam in children: Effect of time and adjunctive therapy. Anesth Analg 1992;75:51–55.

33. Suresh S, Cohen IJ, Matuszczak M, et al: Dose ranging, safety, and efficacy of a new oral midazolam syrup in children. Anesthesiology 1998;89:A1313.

34. Levine MF, Spahr-Schopfer IA, Hartley E, et al: Oral midazolam premedication in children: The minimum time interval for separation from parents. Can J Anaesth 1993;40:726–729.

35. McMillan CO, Spahr-Schopfer IA, Sikich N, et al: Premedication of children with oral midazolam. Can J Anaesth 1992;39:545–550.

36. Viitanen H, Annila P, Viitanen M, et al: Premedication with midazolam delays recovery after ambulatory sevoflurane anesthesia in children. Anesth Analg 1999;89:75–79.

37. Hannallah RS, Patel RI: Low-dose intramuscular ketamine for anesthesia pre-induction in young children undergoing brief outpatient procedures. Anesthesiology 1989;70:598–600.

38. Goresky GV, Steward DJ: Rectal methohexitone for induction of anaesthesia in children. Can Anaesth Soc J 1979;26:213–215.

39. Spear RM, Yaster M, Berkowitz ID, et al: Preinduction of anesthesia in children with rectally administered midazolam. Anesthesiology 1991;74:670–674.

40. Karl HW, Keifer AT, Rosenberger JL, et al: Comparison of the safety and efficacy of intranasal midazolam or sufentanil for preinduction of anesthesia in pediatric patients. Anesthesiology 1992;76:209–215.

41. Hannallah RS: Who benefits when parents are present during anaesthesia induction in their children? Can Anaesth Soc J 1994;41:271–275.

42. Kain ZN, Mayes LC, Wang SM, et al: Parental presence during induction of anesthesia versus sedative premedication: Which intervention is more effective? Anesthesiology 1998;89:1147–1156.

43. Bevan JC, Johnston C, Haig MJ, et al: Preoperative parental anxiety predicts behavioural and emotional responses to induction of anaesthesia in children. Can J Anaesth 1990;37:177–182.

44. Rolf N, Coté CJ: Persistent cardiac arrhythmias in pediatric patients: Effects of age, expired carbon dioxide values, depth of anesthesia, and airway management. Anesth Analg 1991;73:720–724.

45. Doi M, Ikeda K: Airway irritation produced by volatile anaesthetics during brief inhalation: comparison of halothane, enflurane, isoflurane and sevoflurane. Can J Anaesth 1993;40:122–126.

46. Greenspun JC, Hannallah RS, Welborn LG, et al: Comparison of sevoflurane and halothane anaesthesia in children undergoing outpatient ear, nose, and throat surgery. J Clin Anesth 1995;7:398–402.

47. Goresky GV, Muir J: Inhalation induction of anaesthesia. Can J Anaesth 1996;43:1085–1089.

48. Lerman J, Davis PJ, Welborn LG, et al: Induction, recovery, and safety characteristics of sevoflurane in children undergoing ambulatory surgery. A comparison with halothane. Anesthesiology 1996;84:1332–1340.

49. Welborn LG, Hannallah RS, Norden JM, et al: Comparison of emergence and recovery characteristics of sevoflurane, desflurane, and halothane in pediatric ambulatory patients. Anesth Analg 1996;83:917–920.

50. Zwass MS, Fisher DM, Welborn LG, et al: Induction and maintenance characteristics of anesthesia with desflurane and nitrous oxide in infants and children. Anesthesiology 1992;76:373–378.

51. Welborn LG, Hannallah RS, McGill WA, et al: Induction and recovery characteristics of desflurane and halothane anaesthesia in paediatric outpatients. Paediatr Anaesth 1994;4:359–364.

52. Davis PJ, Cohen IT, McGowan FXJ, et al: Recovery characteristics of desflurane versus halothane for maintenance of anesthesia in pediatric ambulatory patients. Anesthesiology 1994;80:298–302.

53. Cohen IT, Hannallah RS, Finkel J, et al: The effect of fentanyl on the emergence following desflurane or sevoflurane anesthesia in children. Anesth Analg 2000;90:S353.

54. Bjerring P, Arendt-Nielsen L: Depth and duration of skin analgesia to needle insertion after topical application of EMLA cream. Br J Anaesth 1990;64:173–177.

55. Steward DJ: Eutectic mixture of local anesthetics (EMLA): What is it? What does it do? J Pediatr 1993;122:S21–S23.

56. Coté CJ, Goudsouzian NG, Liu LM, et al: The dose response of intravenous thiopental for the induction of general anesthesia in unpremedicated children. Anesthesiology 1981;55:703–705.

57. Brett CM, Fisher DM: Thiopental dose-response relations in unpremedicated infants, children, and adults. Anesth Analg 1987;66:1024–1027.

58. Hannallah RS, Britton JT, Schafer PG, et al: Propofol anaesthesia in paediatric ambulatory patients: A comparison with thiopentone and halothane. Can J Anaesth 1994;41:12–18.

59. Martin TM, Nicolson SC, Bargas MS: Propofol anesthesia reduces emesis and airway obstruction in pediatric outpatients. Anesth Analg 1993;76:144–148.

60. Barst SM, Leiderman JU, Markowitz A, et al: Ondansetron with propofol reduces the incidence of emesis in children following tonsillectomy. Can J Anaesth 1999;46:359–362.

61. Schreiner MS, Nicolson SC, Martin T, et al: Should children drink before discharge from day surgery? Anesthesiology 1992;76:528–533.

62. Montgomery CJ, McCormack JP, Reichert CC, et al: Plasma concentrations after high-dose (45 mg.kg^{-1}) rectal acetaminophen in children. Can J Anaesth 1995;42:982–986.

63. Birmingham PK, Tobin MJ, Henthorn TK, et al: Twenty-four-hour pharmacokinetics of rectal acetaminophen in children: an old drug with new recommendations. Anesthesiology 1997;87:244–252.

64. Birmingham PK, Tobin MJ, Henthorn TK, Kennedy-Mooney SH, Coté CJ: "Loading" and subsequent dosing of rectal acetaminophen in children: A 24 hour pharmacokinetic study of new dosing recommendations. Anesthesiology 1996;85:A1105.

65. Houck CS, Sullivan LJ, Wilder RT, Rusy LM, Burrows FA: Pharmacokinetics of a higher dose of rectal acetaminophen in children. Anesthesiology 1995;83:A1126.

66. Anderson BJ, Holford NH, Woollard GA, et al: Perioperative pharmacodynamics of acetaminophen analgesia in children. Anesthesiology 1999;90:411–421.

67. Buckley MMT, Brogden RN: Ketorolac: A review of its pharmacodynamic and pharmacokinetic properties, and therapeutic potential. Drugs 1990;39:86–109.

68. Forrest JB, Heitlinger EL, Revell S: Ketorolac for postoperative pain management in children. Drug Saf 1997;16:309–329.

69. Gillis JC, Brogden RN: Ketorolac: A reappraisal of its pharmacodynamic and pharmacokinetic properties and therapeutic use in pain management. Drugs 1997;53:139–188.

70. Hall SC: Tonsillectomies, ketorolac, and the march of progress. Can J Anaesth 1996;43:544–548.

71. Splinter WM, Rhine EJ, Roberts DW, et al: Preoperative ketorolac increases bleeding after tonsillectomy in children. Can J Anaesth 1996;43:560–563.

72. Judkins JH, Dray TG, Hubbell RN: Intraoperative ketorolac and post-tonsillectomy bleeding. Arch Otolaryngol Head Neck Surg 1996;122:937–940.

73. Agrawal A, Gerson CR, Seligman I, et al: Postoperative hemorrhage after tonsillectomy: Use of ketorolac tromethamine. Otolaryngol Head Neck Surg 1999;120:335–339.

74. Semple D, Russell S, Doyle E, et al: Comparison of morphine sulphate and codeine phosphate in children undergoing adenotonsillectomy. Paediatr Anaesth 1999;9:135–138.

75. Galinkin JL, Watcha MF, Chiavacci RM, Kurth CD, Shah U: Blood levels of fentanyl after intranasal administration in children undergoing bilateral myringotomy and tube placement (BMT). Anesthesiology 1999;91:A1279.

76. Finkel JF, Hannallah RS, Hummer KA, et al: The effect of intranasal fentanyl on the emergence characteristics following sevoflurane anesthesia in children undergoing surgery for bilateral myringotomy and tube (BMT) placement. Anesthesiology 2000; in press.

77. Hannallah RS, Broadman LM, Belman AB, et al: Comparison of caudal and ilioinguinal/iliohypogastric nerve blocks for control of post-orchiopexy pain in pediatric ambulatory surgery. Anesthesiology 1987;66:832–834.

78. Casey WF, Rice LJ, Hannallah RS, et al: A comparison between bupivacaine instillation versus ilioinguinal/iliohypogastric nerve block for postoperative analgesia following inguinal herniorrhaphy in children. Anesthesiology 1990;72:637–639.

79. Soliman MG, Tremblay NA: Nerve block of the penis for postoperative pain relief in children. Anesth Analg 1978;57:495–498.

80. Chhibber AK, Perkins FM, Rabinowitz R, et al: Penile block timing for postoperative analgesia of hypospadias repair in children. J Urol 1997;158:1156–1159.

81. Kirya C, Werthmann MWJ: Neonatal circumcision and penile dorsal nerve block: A painless procedure. J Pediatr 1978;92:998–1000.

82. Taddio A, Stevens B, Craig K, et al: Efficacy and safety of lidocaine-prilocaine cream for pain during circumcision. N Engl J Med 1997;336:1197–1201.

83. Da Conceicao MJ, Coelho L, Khalil M: Ropivacaine 0.25% compared with bupivacaine 0.25% by the caudal route. Paediatr Anaesth 1999;9:229-233.

84. Wong AK, Bissonnette B, Braude BM, et al: Post-tonsillectomy infiltration with bupivacaine reduces immediate postoperative pain in children. Can J Anaesth 1995;42:770–774.

85. Broadman LM, Patel RI, Feldman BA, et al: The effects of peritonsillar infiltration on the reduction of intraoperative blood loss and post-tonsillectomy pain in children. Laryngoscope 1989;99:578–581.

86. Pappas AL, Sukhani R, Hotaling AJ, et al: The effect of preoperative dexamethasone on the immediate and delayed postoperative morbidity in children undergoing adenotonsillectomy. Anesth Analg 1998;87:57–61.

87. Splinter WM, Roberts DJ: Dexamethasone decreases vomiting by children after tonsillectomy. Anesth Analg 1996;83:913–916.

88. Splinter W, Roberts DJ: Prophylaxis for vomiting by children after tonsillectomy: dexamethasone versus perphenazine. Anesth Analg 1997;85:534–537.

89. Tramer M, Moore A, McQuay H. Prevention of vomiting after paediatric strabismus surgery: a systematic review using the numbers-needed-to-treat method. Br J Anaesth 1995;75:556–561.

90. Patel RI, Davis PJ, Orr RJ, et al: Single-dose ondansetron prevents postoperative vomiting in pediatric outpatients. Anesth Analg 1997;85:538–545.

91. Khalil S, Rodarte A, Weldon BC, et al: Intravenous ondansetron in established postoperative emesis in children. S3A–381 Study Group. Anesthesiology 1996;85:270–276.

92. Davis PJ, McGowan FX Jr, Landsman I, et al: Effect of antiemetic therapy on recovery and hospital discharge time: A double-blind assessment of ondansetron, droperidol, and placebo in pediatric patients undergoing ambulatory surgery. Anesthesiology 1995;83:956–960.

93. Rose JB, Brenn BR, Corddry DH, et al: Preoperative oral ondansetron for pediatric tonsillectomy. Anesth Analg 1996;82:558–562.

94. Rose JB, Martin TM: Posttonsillectomy vomiting: Ondansetron or metoclopramide during pediatric tonsillectomy: are two doses better than one? Paediatr Anaesth 1996;6:39–44.

95. Domino KB, Anderson EA, Polissar NL, et al: Comparative efficacy and safety of ondansetron, droperidol, and metoclopramide for preventing postoperative nausea and vomiting: a meta-analysis. Anesth Analg 1999;88:1370–1379.

96. Vener DF, Carr AS, Sikich N, et al: Dimenhydrinate decreases vomiting after strabismus surgery in children. Anesth Analg 1996;82:728–731.

97. Cieslak GD, Watcha MF, Phillips MB, et al: The dose-response relation and cost-effectiveness of granisetron for the prophylaxis of pediatric postoperative emesis. Anesthesiology 1996;85:1076–1085.

98. Fujii Y, Toyooka H, Tanaka H: Antiemetic efficacy of granisetron and metoclopramide in children undergoing ophthalmic or ENT surgery. Can J Anaesth 1996;43:1095–1099.

99. Fujii Y, Toyooka H, Tanaka H: A granisetron-droperidol combination prevents postoperative vomiting in children. Anesth Analg 1998;87:761–765.

100. Baines D: Postoperative nausea and vomiting in children. Paediatr Anaesth 1996;6:7–14.

101. Epstein BS: Recovery from anesthesia. Anesthesiology 1975;43:285–288.

102. Steward DJ: Outpatient pediatric anesthesia. Anesthesiology 1975;43:268–276.

103. Patel RI, Hannallah RS: Anesthetic complications following pediatric ambulatory surgery: A 3-year study. Anesthesiology 1988;69:1009–1012.

104. Apfelbaum JL, Grasela TH, Walawander CA, and the S.A.F.E. study team. Bypassing the PACU: A new paradigm in ambulatory surgery. Anesthesiology 1997;87:A32.

105. Patel R, Hannallah R, Verghese S, et al: Fast-tracking (bypassing phase 1 recovery unit) in children undergoing short surgical procedures. Anesthesiology 1998;89:A53.

Ethical Issues in Pediatric Anesthesiology

David B. Waisel, I. David Todres, *and* Robert Truog

Informed Consent
    Informed Consent Process for Pediatric Patients
    Special Situations in Pediatric Informed Consent
Forgoing Life-Sustaining Treatment
    Do-Not-Resuscitate Orders in the Operating Room
    Concept of Futility
    Withdrawing Care
Pediatric Issues in Clinical Anesthesia Practice
    Pain Management
    Special Requirements for Pediatric Research
    Confidentiality for Adolescents
    Acquired Immunodeficiency Syndrome
    Suspicion of Child Abuse
    Practicing Procedures on Deceased Children
    Production Pressure
    Ethics Consultation Service
Summary

Ethical dilemmas occur in the practice of pediatric anesthesiology. Can parents refuse resuscitation for their 2-year-old with terminal cancer? Should a hysterical 14-year-old be held down for an intramuscular injection of ketamine to subdue him for anesthesia? Can we practice intubation skills on deceased children? What factors matter in making these determinations? Bioethics is designed to help the motivated physician identify and resolve dilemmas such as these. This chapter seeks to provide a framework for thinking about these issues.

Informed Consent

The doctrine of informed consent centers on the belief that patients have a right to self-determination. Physicians facilitate this right by explaining to the patient the risks, benefits, and alternatives to the procedure, and by obtaining from the patient an active, voluntary, informed authorization to perform a specific plan.[1] Components of the informed consent process include competence and decision-making capacity, disclosure, and autonomy (Table 6–1).

All adult patients are considered to be competent to make decisions unless ruled otherwise by a judge. Decision-making capacity, on the other hand, refers to the ability to participate in health-care decisions and may vary, depending on the patient's age, situation, and level of risk in the decision. For example, a patient who normally has decision-making capacity may have a decrement in that capacity following sedation. The patient then may be capable of making decisions involving lesser risks but not greater risks.

Table 6–1. Elements of Consent and Assent as Defined by the American Academy of Pediatrics Committee on Bioethics

Consent

1. Adequate provision of information including the nature of the ailment or condition, the nature of the proposed diagnostic steps or treatment, and the probability of their success; the existence and nature of the risks involved; and the existence, potential benefits, and risks of recommended alternative treatments (including the choice of no treatment).
2. Assessment of the patient's understanding of the above information.
3. Assessment, if only tacit, of the capacity of the patient or surrogate to make the necessary decisions.
4. Assurance, insofar as it is possible, that the patient has the freedom to choose among the medical alternatives without coercion or manipulation.

Assent

1. Helping the patient achieve a developmentally appropriate awareness of the nature of his or her condition.
2. Telling the patient what he or she can expect with tests and treatment.
3. Making a clinical assessment of the patient's understanding of the situation and the factors influencing how he or she is responding (including whether there is inappropriate pressure to accept testing or therapy).
4. Soliciting an expression of the patient's willingness to accept the proposed care.

From Community on Bioethics, American Academy of Pediatrics: Informed consent, parental permission, and assent in pediatric practice. Pediatrics 1995;95:314–317.

A patient gives evidence of decision-making capacity by being able to appreciate his or her situation, to understand the proposed procedure and the alternatives, and to communicate a decision based on internally coherent reasoning.

It is often difficult to know what information to disclose to a patient. Two legal approaches are used throughout most localities in the United States: the professional practice standard and the reasonable person standard.[1] The professional practice standard holds the extent of disclosure to be determined by the practices of other professionals in the community. The reasonable person standard requires disclosure to be to the level that would be desired by the hypothetical reasonable person. Neither of these approaches, however, defines exactly what information should be given. Some suggest that a third approach, the subjective person standard, may be more successful at fulfilling the spirit of informed consent.[1] This standard holds that informed consent should be matched to the wants and needs of the individual person giving consent. Although this may be considered the ideal form of disclosure, its greater ambiguity makes it difficult to use as a legal standard.

Although no definite list exists of what should be included in a specific disclosure, the following guidelines may be helpful. Events relevant to anesthesia practice, such as complications of airway management, invasive monitoring, and the risks and benefits of the possible anesthetic plans, should be discussed.[2] Dornette[3] has proposed that relevant risks be defined as those events that have a 10% incidence of temporary complication or a 0.5% incidence of permanent sequelae. Listing less relevant risks clutters the informed consent process and should be avoided unless specifically requested.[4] Perhaps the best way to determine the optimal extent of disclosure is to provide certain relevant information and then ask patients if they wish to know more.[5-7]

The informed consent process should conclude with the autonomous authorization of the patient to have the specific procedure performed. This in part gives evidence that the patient freely chose to proceed. This desire to have the patient voluntarily pick the course of action does not preclude the anesthesiologist from offering suggestions. In fact, the communication of the anesthesiologist's opinion along with an explanation of the supporting reasons is a critical part of the informed consent process. With this information, the patient is better able to determine which anesthetic provides the most desired benefits. Persuasion, the act of using argument and reason to influence a patient's decision, is appropriate. Coercion, the outright use of a credible threat, or manipulation, the use of misleading information, is not appropriate.[1] The freedom to choose may also be usurped by rushing the informed consent process, thereby limiting the time for patients to consider their options and formulate questions.

Two common misunderstandings exist in the process of obtaining informed consent. The first is the belief that the requirements for informed consent must be achieved fully and perfectly for the consent to be valid. As a corollary, some clinicians feel that if an ideal quality of informed consent cannot be attained, then the entire concept is meaningless and should be abandoned. *Mandating such an unobtainable level is unrealistic and destructive to the goals of informed consent.*[8] Simply because the requirements cannot be totally achieved, however, does not mean that they cannot

be successfully and sufficiently accomplished. Few, if any, can achieve the idealized requirements of informed consent. Many, however, can reach an adequate level to achieve substantial self-determination.

The second misunderstanding is the belief that an anesthesiologist successfully fulfills the obligation to obtain informed consent by completing the legal requirements. Informed consent has both a legal and an ethical sense. The legal sense is defined by institutional policies, which may require completing a form or writing a progress note as defined by local statutes and hospital regulations. Fulfilling such policies does not necessarily achieve the goals of informed consent, nor does it provide protection against liability. The anesthesiologist can best achieve both the ethical and legal senses of informed consent by making the patient a full partner in decision-making and actively seeking to fulfill the patient's informed consent needs.[2]

Informed Consent Process for Pediatric Patients

Informed Permission

Parents have traditionally acted as the surrogate decision-makers for their children, and legally they or other appointed surrogates give consent for the pediatric patient. But this consent does not fulfill the spirit of consent, which is based on obtaining an individualized autonomous decision from the patient receiving the treatment. As such, the American Academy of Pediatrics has suggested that the proper role for the surrogate decision-maker is to provide informed permission.[9] Informed permission has the same requirements as informed consent, but it recognizes that the doctrine of informed consent cannot apply. Throughout the discussion that follows, we use the term "parent" to describe the individual who provides informed permission for the child. Whenever this term is used, however, it should be understood that parents may not always be the legal surrogate decision-makers (as when a child is in the custody of the state), and that the authority of the parents may be limited in older children and adolescents (as when a minor is legally judged to be "mature" or "emancipated," as described later).

Parents and physicians primarily use the concept of best interests to guide their decision-making about health care for minors. The best interests standard acknowledges that the cornerstone of informed consent, the right to self-determination, is not applicable when it is impossible to know or even surmise from previous interactions what a patient's preference would be. Instead, this standard requires the decision-maker to select the care that is objectively the best. Using this standard, then, requires determining (1) who will make the decision and (2) what is the best care. The difficulties arise in assuming that there is always one best choice, because if there is, it should not matter who makes the decision. However, in today's heterogeneous and multicultural society, there is a wide latitude of what constitutes acceptable decision-making, particularly in complex decisions about informed consent, end-of-life issues, and confidentiality.[10, 11] Traditionally, parents who are present and capable of participating in the decision-making process are well suited to be the primary decision-makers for their children. This is in part due to society's respect for the concept of the family, and the assumption that parents care greatly for their children. Although we can never know what a child would decide if he or she were capable of participating in the decision-making process, it is reasonable to assume that the child will incorporate some of the parents' values as he or she grows and matures, making the values of the parents a good first approximation for the future values of the child.[12] For these reasons, parents have extensive leeway in determining what is in a child's best interests.

One way to decide what is in the best interests of the child is to define what choices fall outside the range of acceptable decision-making. Criteria to make this determination include the amount of harm to the child by the intervention or its absence, the likelihood of success, and the overall risk-to-benefit ratio.[13] In the classic Baby Doe case, a child was born with Down syndrome and duodenal atresia and was permitted to die without intervention.[14] Public discussion ensued, and it was felt that not repairing a correctable lesion was outside the bounds of acceptable undertreatment. In fact, this spurred the "Baby Doe regulations," which define what care must be given to certain infants.[15] In this effort to avoid unacceptable undertreatment, some believe that such regulations cause unacceptable overtreatment of patients, primarily because regulations are a crude instrument for dissecting complex clinical situations.[16, 17]

The continuum between unacceptable and acceptable treatment in the practice of anesthesiology provides clear extremes, but an ambiguous gray zone. For example, it is nearly always considered unacceptable undertreatment for Jehovah's Witnesses to refuse a life-sustaining blood transfusion for their child. On the other hand, parents may decline to have an epidural placed in their child for postoperative pain management, depriving the child of an optimal source of pain control. This is not considered unacceptable undertreatment, in part because the harm is limited by other adequate methods of pain control.

The anesthesiologist's sole responsibility is to the patient. Parents and surrogates may not always make decisions that are in the child's best interests.[18] Although anesthesiologists must respect the diversity of values in society and the relationship between the parent and the child, decision-making that imperils the health of a child needs to be challenged. The anesthesiologist who believes that the parent is choosing an unacceptable treatment should determine the basis of this judgment, address the specific concerns, and involve other caregivers, both to offer an assessment of the appropriateness of care and to engage the parents in discussion.[19] Charging a parent of not acting in the child's best interests is serious and can have significant social, fiscal, and familial ramifications. If, however, after exhausting other options, the anesthesiologist believes the parent has chosen unacceptable treatment, he or she should report the situation to proper child welfare authorities for possible legal action.

Assent: Role of the Patient

Although most pediatric patients cannot legally consent to medical care (see exceptions discussed later), pediatric patients can and should share in decision-making to the extent their development permits (see Table 6–1). The participation of children should increase as they grow older and depends

on both the patient's maturity and the consequences involved in the decision.

Anesthesiologists should attempt to achieve both informed permission from the parent or surrogate and assent as appropriate from the pediatric patient.[9, 20] The Rule of Sevens provides a useful way to think about pediatric patients' decision-making capacities. The Rule of Sevens comes from British Common Law, which held that children under the age of 7 years were incapable of criminal intent, children between the ages of 7 and 14 years were unlikely to be capable of criminal intent, and children over the age of 14 were capable of criminal intent.[22, 23] These ages continue to have importance today, and they correspond loosely with developmental milestones as describe by Piaget.[23, 24]

The *preoperational period* occurs from ages 2 to 7 years.[23, 24] A child of this age uses associative thinking, which is based on linked ideas, phenomena, and magical explanations and not on reasoning and cause-and-effect. An example of such thinking may be that the sun stays in the sky because it is round. The *concrete operational period* then follows from ages 7 to 12 years.[23, 24] Children of this age are capable of using logic and reason and are able to define and relate multiple aspects of a situation. Younger children in this period tend to be more rigid and absolute in applying rules. For these children, "do's and don'ts" are very important, and breaking rules, even with good reason, can lead to harsh rebukes and loss of trust. Around age 10, children tend to develop the flexibility to understand motives and different situations. In early adolescence, the *formal operational period* begins.[23, 24] These adolescents have the ability to use abstract thought, apply complex reasoning, foresee outcomes, and understand concepts such as probability. The critical ability to simultaneously evaluate multiple options evolves at this time. Indeed, the development of formal operational thought is considered to be the "ideal level of cognition." Anesthesiologists should recognize that although some adolescents may have cognitive abilities similar to those of adults, these abilities do not necessarily translate into good decision-making skills, because adolescents may be hindered by other limitations such as insufficient emotional development.[23, 25]

Since infants and young children have no decision-making capacity, assent is not a viable option, and anesthesiologists should obtain informed permission from the parent. School-aged children are developing decision-making capacity, so anesthesiologists should seek both informed permission from the parent and assent and participatory decision-making from the patient. Such situations may include whether to sedate a 6-year-old prior to an inhalation induction, to use an inhalation or intravenous induction of anesthesia in an 8-year-old, or to place an epidural for postoperative analgesia in a 12-year-old. Some adolescents and young adults over 14 years will have developed decision-making capacity, and anesthesiologists should try to fulfill the ethical requirements of consent while obtaining assent. Examples may include obtaining consents from a 14-year-old for anesthesia for scoliosis surgery and from a 16-year-old for an awake thoracic epidural placement for a pectus repair.

Informed Refusal

The requirements to achieve an informed refusal of a procedure are similar to the requirements for informed consent in that the patient should be substantially well versed about the risks, benefits, and alternatives before declining. When parents refuse what caregivers believe is necessary care for a minor who cannot participate in the decision-making process, caregivers may invoke the best interests standard as described earlier. This situation is more complicated when the minor expresses significant decision-making capacity and refuses a nonemergent procedure. Anesthesiologists should respect the right of pediatric patients not to assent to a procedure and should go out of their way to avoid coercing or forcibly making the child have the procedure. Achieving the patient's assent may necessitate further discussions with the patient, parents, and other providers, and such discussions may best take place away from the operating room. In cases in which the parent and child disagree, clinicians should seek the assistance of others experienced in conflict resolution to help resolve the dispute with a minimum of rancor.[21] For example, consider a 15-year-old girl who arrives in the preoperative holding area for an elective knee arthroscopy. The day before she had given assent and her parents had given informed permission for anesthesia and surgery. In the holding area, she starts crying and refuses to cooperate. Rather than forcibly or surreptitiously sedating her, the anesthesiologist should try to discuss her concerns. If she is unable to discuss the issues, the anesthesiologist should consider physically removing her from the area and giving her time to regain composure before readdressing the situation. Often such simple actions will allow the situation to be resolved. If the withdrawal of assent was in part related to anxiety, the patient may assent to receiving ample premedication prior to returning to the holding area to permit her to receive the operation. It would be important to obtain her assent prior to administering the sedation, however, and not to simply assume that forceful or surreptitious administration is justified. These simple interventions should also be used in most urgent cases, in which a trivial delay can often permit communication sufficient to obtain the patient's assent.

Special Situations in Pediatric Informed Consent

Emancipated Minor Status and Mature Minor Doctrine

Some patients under 18 years have the legal right to consent to treatment.[22, 26] The term *emancipated minor* refers to minors who have been given the global right to make their own health-care decisions. This status is generally awarded to patients who are married, minor-aged patients who are parents, those in the military, and those who are economically independent, and may also include patients who are pregnant. The mature minor doctrine holds that minors who have decision-making capacity are legally and ethically capable of giving informed consent in specific situations as determined by a court. Although particulars vary by state, the mature minor doctrine in general requires patients to be at least 14 years old and tends to permit decisions of lesser risk. The nearer the child is to majority (usually an age of 18 years), the more likely the court is to grant the child the ability to consent.[27]

Pregnant Pediatric Patients and Abortion

Even though pediatric patients who are pregnant may be considered emancipated, many states require some form of parental involvement such as parental consent or notification prior to an elective abortion in an adolescent.[28-30] If a state requires parental involvement, the ability of the minor to circumvent this regulation by seeking relief from a judge, known as judicial bypass, must be available. Requirements and enforcement of statutes vary from state to state.[31] The need for parental involvement in minor abortions is not always legally straightforward, and it may be best to consult with hospital counsel in determining these issues. Although this is clearly an area in which honorable people disagree, it is worth noting that both the American Academy of Pediatrics and the American Medical Association have issued statements affirming the rights of adolescents to confidentiality when contemplating an abortion.[31, 32]

Children of Jehovah's Witnesses

Jehovah's Witnesses interpret biblical scripture as prohibiting blood transfusions because blood holds the "life force" and that anyone who takes blood will be "cut off from his people" and not earn eternal salvation.[33, 34] The courts have fairly consistently upheld the rights of nonpregnant adults who are not sole providers to refuse blood transfusions.[35] The presumption is that they are making an informed decision about the risks and benefits of receiving blood. The courts, however, have uniformly intervened under the legal doctrine of *parens patriae,* the obligation of the state to protect the interests of incompetent patients, when Jehovah's Witnesses have refused blood transfusions on behalf of their children in both emergent and elective cases.[27, 35-37]

Obtaining informed permission and assent for the care of a ward of a Jehovah's Witness should squarely address the transfusion issue. The patient and family should be informed that attempts will be made to limit the need to give a blood transfusion, and the anesthesiologist should clarify which interventions are acceptable.[38] Deliberate hypotension, deliberate hypothermia, and hemodilution are often acceptable techniques. Synthetic colloid solutions, dextran, erythropoietin, desmopressin, and preoperative iron are usually acceptable. Some Jehovah's Witnesses will accept blood removed and returned in a continuous loop, such as cell-saver blood. The family should know, however, that in a life-threatening situation, the anesthesiologist will seek a court order authorizing the administration of life-sustaining blood. Anesthesiologists should be familiar with the local mechanism (such as contacting hospital counsel) for obtaining a court order authorizing transfusion. In cases in which the likelihood of requiring blood is high, or the local judiciary is not that familiar with case law for Jehovah's Witnesses, the anesthesiologist may choose to obtain the court order prior to the operation.

In elective procedures that may be safely delayed, the patient and family may also consider postponing the procedure until the child is of sufficient age and maturity to decide about transfusion therapy. The problem lies in whether the delay may increase the risk or decrease the likelihood of a good outcome. This decision requires the same balancing act as discussed in determining the best interests for a child. Questions that affect the decision include the quantitative change in risk or benefit, the quality of the risk or benefit, and the clinical importance of the risk or benefit. For example, it may be easier to postpone a procedure that is purely cosmetic (although it would still be difficult) than to postpone a procedure that may lead to permanent injury or a shortened life.

Emergency Care

In modern society, children are frequently without their parents or surrogate decision-makers for a portion of each day.[26] As such, it is likely that an anesthesiologist will at some point need to perform an emergent anesthetic for a minor who does not have a parent available to give legal consent or informed permission. In an emergency situation, the presumption is that necessary therapy is desirable and should be given.[26] It is reasonable to attempt to contact the parents or surrogate, but that should not delay necessary treatment. Emergencies include problems that could cause death, disability, and the increased risk of future complications.

This situation becomes more complex when a minor near majority refuses assent for emergency care that the parent desires. The right of the minor to refuse treatment turns on the minor's decision-making capacity and the resulting harm from the refusal of care.[21, 39] If the harm is significant, and the patient's rationale is decidedly short term or filled with misunderstanding, it is necessary to question the minor's decision-making capacity. At this point one may revert to asking what is in the best interests of the minor. For example, a 15-year-old football player suffers a cervical fracture. He is brought to the preoperative holding area where he refuses emergency stabilization, stating that he does not want to live life without football. Most would hold that his conclusion implies less than full decision-making capacity, especially in light of the suddenness of the injury, and that he should receive emergency treatment. If, however, 12 months later this same patient was quadriplegic and was continuing to refuse interventions to sustain life, then the clinicians caring for him would have to give serious weight to his requests.

Forgoing Life-Sustaining Treatment

Do-Not-Resuscitate Orders in the Operating Room

Do-not-resuscitate (DNR) orders are predicated on the idea that patients may forgo certain procedures and their possible benefits because they choose not to undertake the associated burdens. The burdens may be related to the resuscitation attempt itself, or to the decrement in functional or cognitive capacity that would likely follow from even a successful attempt at resuscitation. This individualized weighing of the risk-to-benefit ratios of resuscitative procedures is as valid in the operating room as on the ward.[40] For this reason, both the American Society of Anesthesiologists and the American College of Surgeons recommend mandatory re-evaluation of the DNR order before transporting the patient to the operating room.[41, 42]

Re-evaluation of the DNR order requires clarifying the patient's goals for the proposed surgery and end-of-life care. For pediatric patients, the anesthesiologist needs to involve the patient, surrogates, and other caregivers such as surgeons, intensivists, and pediatricians in determining what is in the best interests of the child. Although it is immensely difficult to define what is a benefit and what is a burden, it is helpful to consider the guidelines set forth by the American Academy of Pediatrics. Benefits include prolongation of life under certain circumstances, improved quality of life (such as reduction of pain or the ability to leave the hospital), and increased enjoyment of life. Burdens include intractable pain and suffering, disability, and events that cause a decrement in the quality of life, as viewed by the patient.[43] These guidelines may be helpful in considering short- and long-term goals, and putting into appropriate context specific fears such as long-term ventilatory dependency, pain, and suffering. Decision-makers also should be educated about the differences between resuscitation on the ward and in the operating room. For example, anesthesia routinely brings about conditions such as apnea and hemodynamic instability that normally would require resuscitation when the patient is on the ward. Surgical interventions may also increase the likelihood of needing resuscitation. Outcomes from a witnessed arrest such as one that would occur in the operating room, however, are likely to be better than from an unwitnessed arrest.[44, 45] By considering these issues, the anesthesiologist and appropriate parties can determine the desired extent of resuscitation by using either a procedure-directed approach or goal-directed approach.[41, 46]

The procedure-directed approach replicates successful mechanisms used to document DNR orders on the ward. A checklist of specific interventions is presented, and the decision-makers choose which interventions may be used. Anesthesiologists can advise their patients based on the benefit and burden of each intervention, as well as the likelihood of that intervention allowing the patient to achieve desired goals. Interventions frequently on such lists are tracheal intubation or other airway management, postoperative ventilation, chest compressions, defibrillation, vasoactive drugs, and invasive monitoring.[41, 46] The strength of procedure-directed orders is that they are unambiguous and clearly define which procedures are desired. This important feature is necessary for ward medicine, where a patient may have multiple caregivers throughout his or her stay. Procedure-directed orders, however, do not allow for clinical subtleties that may be difficult to precisely document and define.[47, 48]

The goal-directed approach permits patients to guide therapy by prioritizing outcomes rather than procedures. After defining desirable outcomes, decision-makers have the caregivers use clinical judgment to determine how specific interventions will affect achieving the goals. Predictions about the success of interventions that are made by the anesthesiologist at the time of the resuscitation are likely to be more accurate than predictions made preoperatively, when the quality and nature of the problems are not known. Therapy may be guided by goals rather than specific procedures because patients in the operating room are cared for by dedicated providers for a short period of time. This allows these caregivers to have the necessary discussions with the decision-makers to be able to understand and therefore implement the specific plans. It is helpful to define a goal-directed approach on three axes: the burden the patient is willing to accept, the benefit the patient wants, and the likelihood of success. For example, one patient may wish to undertake a significant burden of resuscitation if the likelihood of leaving the hospital is high but not if it is low. Another patient may choose to accept only minor burdens in the form of pain and suffering and only if the likelihood of returning to his or her preoperative function is very high.

In practice, both methods may be used to facilitate discussion before completing documentation in accordance with institutional policies. An important part of the re-evaluation is determining postoperative plans. A patient may want therapy continued for a limited time before withdrawing it. This expresses the patient's belief that a burden (a few days of ventilatory support) may be worth a benefit (extubation of the trachea), but at some point the increasing burden may not be worth the decreasing likelihood of the benefit. Indeed, it is well accepted that withholding and withdrawing life-sustaining treatments are conceptually equivalent actions and the considerations in making the decisions should be the same.[49] Nonetheless, some physicians may feel uncomfortable with withdrawing care after its initiation, mistakenly believing that starting a treatment requires them to continue it, or that withdrawing implies that they have failed in their duties. By recasting the purpose of postoperative ventilation as a trial of therapy to achieve a specific goal, physicians may be psychologically more comfortable with withdrawing care. In fact, the act of withholding therapy requires more certainty that the therapy will fail than the act of withdrawing unsuccessful therapy.

Concept of Futility

When caregivers believe the likelihood of success of a certain intervention is low, they often label the procedure as futile. To be fair to parents and other decision-makers, judgments about futility must carefully take into account both qualitative and quantitative considerations. The qualitative aspects define the goals of the treatment, and the quantitative aspects state the likelihood of achieving the defined result. For example, the act of intubation may have a high likelihood of achieving the goal of successful ventilation, but it may have a low likelihood of leading to the patient's discharge from the hospital and an even lower likelihood of the patient being able to leave the hospital in "good" condition, as the patient defines it. When the likelihood of success increases, the burdens a patient would be willing to undergo may increase. Therefore, it is important to be as precise as possible when advising a patient that a therapy has a low likelihood of achieving a certain success. In one study, a majority of physicians defined a treatment to be futile if it had a 1% to 10% probability of success, but 19% of physicians defined a procedure to be futile if it had a 20% or higher probability of success, and 4% of physicians defined it as futile with even a 50% probability of success.[50] At least in this study, some physicians seemed much more likely to judge treatments as being futile than would seem justified by the common understanding of the term in our language. Further, when offering these percentages of success, physicians should be clear as to the quality of the information used to form the estimation: is it from intuition, clinical experience, or rigorous scientific studies?

Some hospital policies allow for physicians to unilaterally withhold or withdraw care they consider to be futile.[51] These policies tend to define as futile those therapies undertaken in specific disease states, such as certain types of cancer, or therapies that have particularly low rates of success.[52, 53] The trend is away from such absolute definitions, because these judgments do not take into account patient-defined parameters such as the willingness to undertake significant burdens and the value of relatively small benefits.[54] A simple example would be the patient who is willing to undergo significant hardships for a few days to be able to see a sibling one more time. After seeing the sibling, the patient may then choose to reject previously accepted interventions that involve significant burdens.

Withdrawing Care

When care is being withdrawn, most notably when the child is being disconnected from mechanical ventilation, family members may request that the patient receive sedation. The criteria of benefits to burdens should be applied when determining the appropriateness of sedation. In most cases, the benefit of administering sedation is minimized discomfort and suffering, while the only burden associated with giving sedation is the decreased likelihood of the presumably already remote possibility of survival. Physicians may indeed feel uncomfortable that they are causing death. When faced with this problem, some appeal to the principle of double effect, which assesses the rightness of the action based on its intent, which is to minimize pain and suffering, rather than on its foreseeable but unintended side effect (double effect), which is to hasten the child's death.[1] If anesthesiologists are uncomfortable providing analgesia and sedation in these circumstances, they should decline to provide care and consider finding a suitable replacement.[55]

Pediatric Issues in Clinical Anesthesia Practice

Pain Management

For years, it was thought that newborns had immature neurologic pathways that did not respond to pain and that if they did have pain, they did not remember.[56, 57] Indeed, myths such as these led to the "Liverpool technique," in which newborns received muscle relaxants and minimal anesthesia for surgery. Older children have also had their pain undertreated.[58–61] Reasons for this undertreatment included limited training and knowledge about pediatric pain, the difficulty in doing pain research on children, and the mistaken belief that children are more prone to addiction and respiratory depression.[56, 57]

Aside from the humanitarian imperative to control pain, children do in fact have a physiologic response to pain, and adequate pain control may lead to less morbidity and mortality.[62] Comfortable children are more capable of achieving the goals of assent and are more cooperative with care. The obligation to provide postoperative pain management requires anesthesiologists to minimize pain in the least objectionable ways. Limitations to achieving successful analgesia after surgery include inadequate postoperative care facilities, inexperience, and no designated pain service.[63]

Components of pain management include analgesia and elimination of fear, which often includes obliteration of awareness, anxiolysis, and perhaps amnesia. Amnesia and anxiolysis without adequate pain control, particularly for a procedure that will be repeated like sampling bone marrow, does not wholly fulfill the humanitarian and physiologic goals and should not be confused with adequate pain management. In the same vein, control of pain without sufficient management of awareness and fear is not desirable care.

The concept of suffering deserves special note. Suffering is an intensely personal feeling that can be defined as "the state of severe distress associated with events that threaten the intactness of the person."[64] Suffering should be considered when evaluating pain control, and adequate steps should be taken to find and alleviate sources of suffering. Factors that may contribute to a patient's suffering include not knowing the origin or meaning of the pain, inability to influence important aspects of care such as pain management, and a belief that the pain will never be relieved.[64] This is especially true in children, who often interpret pain as punishment for something that they have done wrong. Anesthesiologists can help minimize suffering by clearly communicating about these issues with patients and affording patients as much control of their care as possible.

Special Requirements for Pediatric Research

The anesthesiologist Henry K. Beecher was one of the first to propose different requirements for pediatric research as compared with adult research.[65] Most proposed pediatric research is closely examined both because children may be incapable of understanding and consenting to experiments and because they are vulnerable to abuse and at risk for long-term harm.[65] Federal guidelines give four categories of pediatric research, with each ascending category requiring greater scrutiny of the risk-to-benefit ratio, especially in research without therapeutic benefit for the subject (Table 6–2). Although obtaining the assent of the child whenever possible is important for therapeutic medical procedures (as discussed earlier), it is absolutely essential in the context of research, along with the informed permission of the parents.

Informed consent and assent for research requires the decision-makers to be fully educated about the risks, benefits, and alternatives of the proposed research. In addition, patients must be informed that they are free to withdraw from the study at any time without prejudice. Other ethical requirements of research hold. A study must provide quality care for the subject and legitimate options for the non-participant. The investigator should have good reason to

Table 6–2. Federal Classifications for Pediatric Research

1. Research not involving greater than minimal risk.*
2. Research involving greater than minimal risk by presenting the prospect of direct benefit to the individual subjects.
3. Research involving greater than minimal risk and no prospect of direct benefit to individual subjects, but likely to yield generalizable knowledge about the subject's disorder or condition.
4. Research not otherwise approvable that presents an opportunity to understand, prevent, or alleviate a serious problem affecting the health or welfare of children.

*Minimal risk means that the probability and magnitude of harm or discomfort anticipated in the research are not greater in and of themselves than those ordinarily encountered in daily life or during the performance of routine physical or psychological examinations or tests.
From U.S. Department of Health and Human Services: Additional protection for children involved as subjects in research. 45 CFR 46 Subpart D Federal Register; 1995.

believe the study will sufficiently benefit the subject or science as a whole with respect to the incurred risk. A poorly conducted study wastes resources and places subjects at risk, and if published may affect treatment decisions and harm other patients. Institutional review boards help ensure that these principles are met by monitoring and safeguarding the quality of the research as well as the informed consent processes.

Pediatric caregivers need to ensure that pediatric patients are not underserved by the research being performed. One area in which pediatric patients have often been overlooked is in drug therapy. For example, a 1991 survey found that more than 80% of common drugs were not fully researched in children.[66] Those with official and unofficial authority have a responsibility to ensure that agencies and companies perform such research.[67] As such, and in response to the Food and Drug Administration Modernization Act of 1997, the FDA in 1998 determined that all drugs that are "approved for use in adults for indications that occur in the pediatric population" should undergo additional study in pediatric patients. The FDA prioritized study in drugs that were commonly used and drugs that present unique opportunities to improve health care in the pediatric population. As an indication of how widespread the problem is, as of 1998, the following medications were included on the list: ketamine, propofol, isoflurane, sevoflurane, fentanyl, remifentanil, morphine, vecuronium, cis-atracurium, bupivacaine, ropivacaine, ondansetron, and furosemide.[68]

Confidentiality for Adolescents

The obligation to maintain confidentiality requires physicians to protect patient information from unauthorized and unnecessary disclosure. Confidentiality is necessary for the development of a patient-physician relationship that supports an open and uncensored flow of information and concerns. A trusting alliance is particularly important in the care of adolescents who are more likely to defer needed treatment because they are concerned about confidentiality.[69–73] Emancipated and mature minors have a right to complete confidentiality. For other adolescents, if the knowledge is of minimal harm to the health of the patient, physicians should encourage the patient to be forthright with the parents but respect their decision not to be. If, on the other hand, withholding the information may result in serious harm to the patient, the physician is ethically justified in notifying the parents.[69] Possible exceptions to the principle of confidentiality are notifications required by law such as reporting statutes and notifying parents, and when a patient makes a credible threat to harm another person.

The quality of the information obtained in the preoperative interview may be directly affected by the adolescent's trust of the anesthesiologist. The anesthesiologist can enhance this trust by interviewing the adolescent in private, acknowledging the adolescent's concerns about confidentiality, and following through on any promises made. Unintended breeches of confidentiality are as harmful as intentional ones; anesthesiologists should be aware that many disclosures take place unwittingly in public spaces or social situations.[74, 75]

Acquired Immunodeficiency Syndrome

Up to half of surveyed physicians report they would not care for patients with acquired immunodeficiency syndrome if they had a choice.[76, 77] Physicians may not, however, decline to provide care for a patient solely because the patient is infected with human immunodeficiency virus (HIV). Discrimination is inappropriate and illegal.[78] Many states require a formal specific informed consent for HIV testing of patients.[79] Even if not required, testing should be done only after proper counseling because of the stunning personal and professional ramifications of being seropositive.[80] In some states, patients may be tested for HIV without their consent in certain circumstances, such as when a health-care worker is significantly exposed to the body fluids of a patient.[81] Anesthesiologists can decrease the perceived need for both consensual and nonconsensual testing by the consistent use of universal precautions, which will not only protect physicians but may also reduce the need and desire to define which patients are seropositive. Similar to other groups of physicians, however, anesthesiologists do not reliably follow this requirement.[82] Seventy-five percent of anesthesiologists do not use universal precautions for a "low-risk" patient, and 12% do not use universal precautions when caring for a seropositive patient.[83]

Of particular interest to the pediatric anesthesiologist may be whether newborns should be tested for HIV. HIV testing in the newborn examines only for the presence of maternal antibodies, and the majority of newborns with seropositive mothers do not become infected with the virus. However, a seropositive newborn does confirm an infected mother, bringing forth complex issues of confidentiality. Current policy in most jurisdictions is to inform the mother of the availability of testing and to seek her informed consent or refusal for the procedure.[84]

Suspicion of Child Abuse

Approximately 2% to 3% of children are abused each year.[85] Child abuse includes acts of physical abuse, sexual abuse, emotional abuse, and neglect. Anesthesiologists are in a unique position to recognize some forms of physical abuse given their more than usual attention to patients' hands, arms, ankles, and faces. Anesthesiologists should be particularly sensitive to bruises or burns in the shape of objects, injuries to soft tissue areas such as upper arms, unexplained mouth and dental injuries, fractures in infants, and height and weight less than the fifth percentile (see Fig. 16–5).[85–88] Children who have physical or mental handicaps are particularly prone to abuse.[89] Amazingly, child abuse occurs in the hospital and even while a child is undergoing diagnostic or therapeutic care.[90] Anesthesiologists, as all physicians, are legally required to report the suspicion of child abuse or neglect to appropriate authorities. Indeed, in most jurisdictions, a physician can be criminally prosecuted if found liable for failing to report suspected child abuse.[13, 87]

Practicing Procedures on Deceased Children

Practicing procedures on newly deceased patients may allow junior caregivers an opportunity to gain valuable experiences under controlled circumstances with no risk.[91] Such procedures should be undertaken with respect, however. Physicians should obtain permission to practice procedures, just as they would obtain permission for autopsies or the procurement of organs. Although each institution has to determine appropriate policy, we believe that consent is best obtained and documented by oral discussion with the parents and by a written note in the medical record. An additional form for this rare event seems cumbersome and unnecessarily stressful to the parents; adding a statement about the procedure to forms discussing autopsy seems like an inappropriate combination of activities. Procedures should be non-mutilating, such as tracheal intubation. Only those caregivers who have a legitimate need to learn should be permitted to perform the technique. This group is not necessarily limited to physicians, as others, such as emergency medical technicians and nurses, may need this skill. The procedure should be performed under supervision and after proper preparation. This groundwork legitimates the exercise as an educational experience while fulfilling the obligation to treat the body and its donation with respect.

Production Pressure

Anesthesiologists are prone to production pressure, which has been defined as "the internal or external pressure on the anesthetist to keep the operating room schedule moving along speedily. . . ."[91] Indeed, nearly half of surveyed anesthesiologists reported seeing what they considered unsafe anesthetic practices in response to this production pressure.[93] As a consequence, anesthesiologists may not want to take the time to allow a child to ask questions about the anesthetic, to adequately premedicate an anxious child, or to engage the parents in a lengthy discussion about postponing the surgery because their child has a mild upper respiratory infection.[94, 95]

Anesthesiologists should also be cognizant of their level of skill in providing anesthesia. For example, the "routine" tonsillectomy may be beyond some anesthesiologists' ability in the child with multiple congenital deficits. Anesthesiologists have an obligation to the patient and themselves to provide care only within their skills, and to recognize when economic and administrative pressures may induce them to do otherwise.

Another source of production pressure may be from managed care organizations (MCOs). Managed care in and of itself is neither good nor bad. At its best, managed care can encourage preventative care, continuing patient-physician relationships, collaborative relationships among primary care clinicians and specialists, and cost-effective and good performance improvement programs. At its worst, managed care can result in a mercurial bureaucratic system that prioritizes magnifying short-term cost-containment, developing a young and predominantly healthy customer population, and using time to avoid paying for expensive care.[96] MCOs accomplish these goals by "managing" or controlling physician and patient behavior through the use of case managers to coordinate care, financial and administrative incentives to encourage physicians to conserve resources, gate-keeping devices to control access to specialty care, and practice guidelines to limit imaging tests, expensive drugs, and longer hospital stays. Physicians have the obligation to participate in managed care to ensure that it is performed well and should participate in legislative initiatives to curb potential abuses, work with MCOs to design systems that minimize conflicts of interest, and actively fight abuses on an individual level. Anesthesiologists need to closely examine any MCO contract for inherent problems. Problems to look for in an MCO contract include compensation through financial incentives, plans that do not have a reasonable or responsive appeals process, and policies that have an undefined physician termination procedure.[97-99]

Ethics Consultation Service

The ethical dilemmas that occur in the practice of anesthesiology may be difficult for the practitioner to resolve alone. The Joint Commission on Accreditation of Healthcare Organizations requires hospitals to have institutional mechanisms to address ethical conflicts and many fulfill this mandate by having ethics committees and ethics consultation services.[100] Ethics committees and their consulting services act in an advisory role to help caregivers, patients, and families amicably resolve ethical dilemmas.[101] Anesthesiologists may find ethics consultation helpful with questions about informed consent, decision-making capacity, and resuscitation decisions, and in resolving disagreements among patients, families, and caregivers.[102-104] Following consultations, clinicians feel greater satisfaction in managing cases with ethical conflicts, not only because of their heightened awareness of the expert consulting services available but also because of their increased knowledge and comfort in dealing with these issues.[104-106] Ethics committees are also available to consult on policy development and to organize continuing educational programs.

Summary

Ethical issues in the care of children tend to center on questions about decision-making capacity. Infants and children are often incapable of successfully "speaking for themselves" and may be in need of supervision and protection. This protection is generally well-executed by the parents, but at times is not, and the state, through caregivers and the legal system, must sometimes seek to ensure proper care for children by balancing the "natural rights" of the parents with the obligation of the state to protect the child.[13] Those caring for adolescents need to incorporate the increasingly accepted concept of children as active participants in determining their care.[107] Many anesthesiologists who are uncomfortable with this approach become even more threatened when they realize that there are different categories of decision-making, which require considerations of the child and the situation. Finally, there is the problem of defining what criteria should be used to determine what is in the best interests of the minor. Decisions such as these may appear difficult at best and insurmountable at worst. Anesthesiologists can help themselves and their patients by utilizing available resources such as ethics consultation services for guidance and conflict resolution.

REFERENCES

1. Beauchamp TL, Childress JF: Principles of Biomedical Ethics, 4th ed. New York: Oxford University Press; 1994.

2. Hirsh HL: A visitation with informed consent and refusal. In: Wecht CH, ed: Legal Medicine. Charlottesville,VA: Michie; 1995:147–204.

3. Dornette WH: Informed consent and anesthesia. Anesth Analg 1974;53:832–837.

4. Foley HT, Dornette WHL: Consent and informed consent. In: Dornette WHL, ed: Legal Issues in Anesthesia Practice. Philadelphia: F.A. Davis; 1991:81–92.

5. Lonsdale M, Hutchison GL: Patients' desire for information about anaesthesia: Scottish and Canadian attitudes. Anaesthesia 1991;46:410–412.

6. Litman RS, Perkins FM, Dawson SC: Parental knowledge and attitudes toward discussing the risk of death from anesthesia. Anesth Analg 1993;77:256–260.

7. Waisel DB, Truog RD: The benefits of the explanation of the risks of anesthesia in the day surgery patient. J Clin Anesth 1995;7:200–204.

8. Beauchamp TL: Informed consent. In: Veatch RM, ed: Medical Ethics, 2nd ed. Sudbury MA: Jones and Bartlett; 1997:185–208.

9. Committee on Bioethics, American Academy of Pediatrics: Informed consent, parental permission, and assent in pediatric practice. Pediatrics 1995;95:314–317.

10. Orr RD, Marshall PA, Osborn J: Cross-cultural considerations in clinical ethics consultations. Arch Fam Med 1995;4:159–164.

11. Barker JC: Cultural diversity: Changing the context of medical practice. West J Med 1992;157:248–254.

12. President's Commission for the Study of Ethical Problems in Medicine and Biomedical and Behavioral Research: Deciding to forgo life-sustaining treatment. Washington D.C.: U.S. Government Printing Office; 1983.

13. McMenamin JP, Bigley GL: Children as patients. In: Sanbar SS, Gibofsky A, Firestone MH, et al., eds: Legal Medicine, 3rd ed. Baltimore: Mosby; 1995:456–487.

14. Pless JE: The story of Baby Doe: N Engl J Med 1983;309:664.

15. U.S. Department of Human Services: Services and treatment for disabled infants. Federal Register 45 CFR 1340.15. 1999.

16. Kopelman LM, Irons TG, Kopelman AE: Neonatologists judge the "Baby Doe" regulations. N Engl J Med 1988;318:677–683.

17. Todres ID, Guillemin J, Grodin MA, et al: Life-saving therapy for newborns: A questionnaire survey in the state of Massachusetts. Pediatrics 1988;81:643–649.

18. Harth SC, Johnstone RR, Thong YH: The psychological profile of parents who volunteer their children for clinical research: a controlled study. J Med Ethics 1992;18:86–93.

19. Anderson B, Hall B: Parents' perceptions of decision making for children. J Law Med Ethics 1995;23:15–19.

20. Midwest Bioethics Center Task Force on Health Care Rights for Minors: Health care treatment decision-making guidelines for minors. Bioethics Forum 1995;11:7–12.

21. Strong C: Respecting the health care decision-making capacity of minors. Bioethics Forum 1995;11:7–12.

22. Sigman GS, O'Connor C: Exploration for physicians of the mature minor doctrine. J Pediatr 1991;119:520–525.

23. Committee on Child Psychiatry, Group for the Advancement of Psychiatry: How old is enough? The age of rights and responsibilities. New York: Brunner/Mazel Publishers; 1989: Report 126, 1–117.

24. Sahler OJZ, Wood BL: Theories and concepts of development as they relate to pediatric practice. In: Hoekelman RA, Friedman SB, Nelson NM, et al., eds: Primary Pediatric Care, 3rd ed. St. Louis: Mosby-Year Book; 1997:581–601.

25. Gardner W, Scherer D, Tester M: Asserting scientific authority: Cognitive development and adolescent legal rights. Am Psychol 1989;44:895–902.

26. Tsai AK, Schafermeyer RW, Kalifon D, et al: Evaluation and treatment of minors: Reference on consent. Ann Emerg Med 1993;22:1211–1217.

27. Green. 292 A.2d 387 (1972).

28. Wheeler M, Coté CJ: Preoperative pregnancy testing in a tertiary care children's hospital: A medico-legal conundrum. J Clin Anesth 1999;11:56–63.

29. Worthington ELJ, Larson DB, Lyons JS, et al: Mandatory parental involvement prior to adolescent abortion. J Adolesc Health 1991;12:138–142.

30. Crosby MC, English A: Mandatory parental involvement/judicial bypass laws: Do they promote adolescents' health? J Adolesc Health 1991;12:143–147.

31. Council on Ethical and Judicial Affairs, American Medical Association: Mandatory parental consent to abortion. JAMA 1993;269:82–86.

32. Committee on Adolescence American Academy of Pediatrics: The adolescent's right to confidential care when considering abortion. Pediatrics 1996;97:746–751.

33. Leviticus 7:27.

34. Watch Tower Bible and Tract Society of Pennsylvania: How can blood save your life? Brooklyn, NY: Watchtower Bible and Tract Society of New York, and International Bible Students Association; 1990.

35. Rothenberg DM: The approach to the Jehovah's witness patient. Anesth Clin N Am 1990;8:589–607.

36. Sampson v. Taylor. 29N.Y.2d 900 (1972).

37. Wallace v. Labrenz. 104 N.E.2d 769 (1952).

38. Benson KT: The Jehovah's Witness patient: Considerations for the anesthesiologist. Anesth Analg 1989;69:647–656.

39. Sullivan DJ: Minors and emergency medicine. Emerg Med Clin North Am 1993;11:841–851.

40. Clemency MV, Thompson NJ: Do not resuscitate orders in the perioperative period: Patient perspectives. Anesth Analg 1997;84:859–864.

41. American Society of Anesthesiologists: Ethical guidelines for the anesthesia care of patients with do-not-resuscitate orders or other directives that limit treatment. American Society of Anesthesiologists Standards, Guidelines, and Statements. Park Ridge, IL: American Society of Anesthesiologists; 1998:400–401.

42. Statement of the American College of Surgeons on Advance Directives by Patients: "Do not resuscitate" in the operating room. Am Col Surg Bull 1994;79:29.

43. American Academy of Pediatrics Committee on Bioethics: Guidelines on foregoing life-sustaining medical treatment. Pediatrics 1994;93:532–536.

44. Peatfield RC, Sillett RW, Taylor D, et al: Survival after cardiac arrest in hospital. Lancet 1977;1:1223–1225.

45. Taffet GE, Teasdale TA, Luchi RJ: In-hospital cardiopulmonary resuscitation. JAMA 1988;260:2069–2072.

46. Truog RD, Waisel DB, Burns JP: DNR in the OR: A goal-directed approach. Anesthesiology 1999;90:289–295.

47. Mittelberger JA, Lo B, Martin D, et al: Impact of a procedure-specific do not resuscitate order form on documentation of do not resuscitate orders. Arch Intern Med 1993;153:228–232.

48. Heffner JE, Barbieri C, Casey K: Procedure-specific do-not-resuscitate orders: Effect on communication of treatment limitations. Arch Intern Med 1996;156:793–797.

49. Council on Ethical and Judicial Affairs, American Medical Association: Decisions near the end of life. JAMA 1992;267:2229–2233.

50. Van McCrary S, Swanson JW, Youngner SJ, et al: Physicians' quantitative assessments of medical futility. J Clin Ethics 1994;5:100–105.

51. Waisel DB, Truog RD: The cardiopulmonary resuscitation-not-indicated order: Futility revisited. Ann Intern Med 1995;122:304–308.

52. Schneiderman LJ, Jecker NS, Jonsen AR: Medical futility: Its meaning and ethical implications. Ann Intern Med 1990;112:949–954.

53. Murphy DJ, Finucane TE: New do-not-resuscitate policies: A first step in cost control. Arch Intern Med 1993;153:1641–1648.

54. Tomlinson T, Czlonka D: Futility and hospital policy. Hastings Cent Rep 1995;25:28–35.

55. Truog RD, Berde CB, Mitchell C, et al: Barbiturates in the care of the terminally ill. N Engl J Med 1992;327:1678–1682.

56. Schechter NL, Berde CB, Yaster M: Pain in infants, children, and adolescents: An overview. In: Schechter NL, Berde CB, Yaster M, eds: Pain in Infants, Children, and Adolescents. Baltimore: Williams & Wilkins; 1993:3–9.

57. Nolan K: Ethical issues in pediatric pain management. In: Schechter NL, Berde CB, Yaster M, eds: Pain in Infants, Children, and Adolescents. Baltimore: Williams & Wilkins; 1993:123–132.

58. Quinn M, Carraccio C, Sacchetti A: Pain, punctures, and pediatricians. Pediatr Emerg Care 1993;9:12–14.

59. Schechter NL, Bernstein BA, Beck A, et al: Individual differences in children's response to pain: Role of temperament and parental characteristics. Pediatrics 1991;87:171–177.

60. Beyer JE, DeGood DE, Ashley LC, et al: Patterns of postoperative analgesic use with adults and children following cardiac surgery. Pain 1983;17:71–81.

61. Mather L, Mackie J: The incidence of postoperative pain in children. Pain 1983;15:271–282.

62. Anand KJS, Hickey PR: Halothane-morphine compared with high-dose sufentanil for anesthesia and postoperative analgesia in neonatal cardiac surgery. N Engl J Med 1992;326:1–9.

63. de Lima J, Lloyd-Thomas AR, Howard RF, et al: Infant and neonatal pain: Anaesthetists' perceptions and prescribing patterns. Br Med J 1996;313:787.

64. Cassell EJ: The nature of suffering and the goals of medicine. N Engl J Med 1982;306:639–645.

65. Curran WJ, Beecher HK: Experimentation in children: A reexamination of legal ethical principles. JAMA 1969;210:77–83.

66. Gilman JT, Gal P: Pharmacokinetic and pharmacodynamic data collection in children and neonates: A quiet frontier. Clin Pharmacokinet 1992;23:1–9.

67. Committee on Drugs American Academy of Pediatrics: Guidelines for the ethical conduct of studies to evaluate drugs in pediatric populations. Pediatrics 1995;95:286–294.

68. Centers for Drug Evaluation and Research and Food and Drug Administration: List of approved drugs for which additional pediatric information may produce health benefits in the pediatric population. Docket No. 98N-0056. 1998.

69. Council on Scientific Affairs, American Medical Association: Confidential health services for adolescents. JAMA 1993;269:1420–1424.

70. Hofmann AD: A rational policy toward consent and confidentiality in adolescent health care. J Adolesc Health Care 1980;1:9–17.

71. Chamie M, Eisman S, Forrest JD, et al: Factors affecting adolescents' use of family planning clinics. Fam Plan Perspect 1982;14:126–139.

72. Marks A, Malizio J, Hoch J, et al: Assessment of health needs and willingness to utilize health care resources of adolescents in a suburban population. J Pediatr 1983;102:456–460.

73. Cheng TL, Savageau JA, Sattler AL, et al: Confidentiality in health care: A survey of knowledge, perceptions, and attitudes among high school students. JAMA 1993;269:1404–1407.

74. Benrubi GI: Confidentiality in the age of AIDS. J Reprod Med 1992;37:969–972.

75. Ubel PA, Zell MM, Miller DJ, et al: Elevator talk: Observational study of inappropriate comments in a public space. Am J Med 1995;99:190–194.

76. Gerbert B, Maguire BT, Bleecker T, et al: Primary care physicians and AIDS: Attitudinal and structural barriers to care. JAMA 1991;266:2837–2842.

77. Shapiro MF, Hayward RA, Guillemot D, et al: Residents' experiences in, and attitudes toward, the care of persons with AIDS in Canada, France, and the United States. JAMA 1992;268:510–515.

78. Council on Ethical and Judicial Affairs: Ethical issues involved in the growing AIDS crisis. JAMA 1988;259:1360–1361.

79. Brennan TA: Transmission of the human immunodeficiency virus in the health care setting: Time for action. N Engl J Med 1991;324:1504–1509.

80. Council on Ethical and Judicial Affairs: HIV Testing. Opinion 2.23, 61–62. In: Code of Medical Ethics: Current Opinions with Annotations. Chicago: American Medical Association; 1997.

81. Derse AR: HIV and AIDS: Legal and ethical issues in the emergency department. Emerg Med Clin North Am 1995;13:213–223.

82. Hwang PH, Tami TA, Lee KC, et al: Attitudes, knowledge, and practices of otolaryngologists treating patients infected with HIV. Otolaryngol Head Neck Surg 1995;113:733–739.

83. Tait AR, Tuttle DB: Prevention of occupational transmission of human immunodeficiency virus and hepatitis B virus among anesthesiologists: A survey of anesthesiology practice. Anesth Analg 1994;79:623–628.

84. Working Group on HIV Testing of Pregnant Women and Newborns: HIV infection, pregnant women, and newborns: A policy proposal for information and testing. JAMA 1990;264:2416–2420.

85. Wissow LS: Child abuse and neglect. N Engl J Med 1995;332:1425–1431.

86. Johnson CF, Kaufman KL, Callendar C: The hand as a target organ in child abuse. Clin Pediatr (Phila) 1990;29:66–72.

87. Johnson CF: Inflicted injury versus accidental injury. Pediatr Clin North Am 1990;37:791–814.

88. McClelland CQ, Heiple KG: Fractures in the first year of life: A diagnostic dilemma. Am J Dis Child 1982;136:26–29.

89. Newberger EH: Child physical abuse. Prim Care 1993;20:317–327.

90. Southall DP, Plunkett MC, Banks MW, et al: Covert video recordings of life-threatening child abuse: Lessons for child protection. Pediatrics 1997;100:735–760.

91. Burns JP, Reardon FE, Truog RD: Using newly deceased patients to teach resuscitation procedures. N Engl J Med 1994;331:1652–1655.

92. Gaba DM, Fish DM, Howard SK: Crisis Management in Anesthesiology, 1st ed. New York: Churchill Livingstone; 1994.

93. Gaba DM, Howard SK, Jump B: Production pressure in the work

environment: California anesthesiologists' attitudes and experiences. Anesthesiology 1994;81:488–500.

94. Frader J: Minors and health care decisions: Broadening the scope. Bioethics Forum 1995;11:13–16.

95. McGraw T: Preparing children for the operating room: psychological issues. Can J Anaesth 1994;41:1094–1103.

96. Anders G: Health Against Wealth: HMOs and the Breakdown of Medical Trust. New York: Houghton Mifflin; 1996.

97. Committee on Medical Liability American Academy of Pediatrics: Liability and managed care. Pediatrics 1996;98:792–794.

98. Howe EG: Managed care: "New moves," moral uncertainty, and a radical attitude. J Clin Ethics 1995;6:290–305.

99. Pearson SD, Sabin JE, Emanuel EJ: Ethical guidelines for physician compensation based on capitation. N Engl J Med 1998;339:689–693.

100. Joint Commission on Accreditation of Healthcare Organizations: Comprehensive Accreditation Manual for Hospitals. Oakbrook Terrace; 1999.

101. Singer PA, Pellegrino ED, Siegler M: Ethics committees and consultants. J Clin Ethics 1990;1:263–267.

102. Simpson KH: The development of a clinical ethics consultation service in a community hospital. J Clin Ethics 1992;3:124–130.

103. La Puma J, Stocking CB, Darling CM, et al: Community hospital ethics consultation: Evaluation and comparison with a university hospital service. Am J Med 1992;92:346–351.

104. La Puma J, Stocking CB, Silverstein MD, et al: An ethics consultation service in a teaching hospital: Utilization and evaluation. JAMA 1988;260:808–811.

105. Pellegrino ED, Hart RJJ, Henderson SR, et al: Relevance and utility of courses in medical ethics: A survey of physicians' perceptions. JAMA 1985;253:49–53.

106. White BD, Zaner RM: Clinical ethics training for staff physicians: Designing and evaluating a model program. J Clin Ethics 1993;4:229–235.

107. Bartholome WG: Hearing children's voices. Bioethics Forum 1995;11:3–6.

Pediatric Airway

Melissa Wheeler, Charles J. Coté, *and* I. David Todres

The Larynx
 Anatomy
 Function
Developmental Anatomy of the Airway
 Tongue
 Position of Larynx
 Epiglottis
 Vocal Folds
 Subglottis
Physiology of the Respiratory System
 Obligate Nasal Breathing
 Tracheal and Bronchial Function
 Work of Breathing
 Airway Obstruction During Anesthesia
Evaluation of the Airway
 Clinical Evaluation
 Diagnostic Testing
Airway Management: The Normal Airway
 Mask Ventilation
 Tracheal Intubation
 Laryngeal Mask Airway
 Other Airway Devices
Airway Management: The Abnormal Airway
 Classifying the Abnormal Pediatric Airway
 Management Principles
 Special Techniques for Ventilation
 Special Techniques for Intubation

The differences between a child's airway and an adult's dictate differences in anesthetic management techniques. Knowledge of normal developmental anatomy and physiologic function is required to understand and manage both the normal and the pathologic airways of infants and children. Techniques and principles to assist in this management are reviewed in this chapter.

The Larynx

The classic works by Negus, Eckenhoff, and Fink and Demarest form the foundation of our knowledge about the structure and function of the pediatric and adult airway.[1-3]

Anatomy

Structure

The larynx is composed of one bone (hyoid) and a series of cartilages (the single thyroid, cricoid, and epiglottis and the paired arytenoid, corniculate, and cuneiform cartilages). These are suspended by ligaments from the base of the skull. The body of the cricoid cartilage articulates posteriorly with the inferior cornu of the thyroid cartilage. The paired triangular arytenoid cartilages rest on top of and articulate with the superior posterior aspect of the cricoid cartilage. The arytenoid cartilages are protected by the thyroid cartilage (Fig. 7–1).

These cartilages are covered by tissue folds and muscles. Contraction of the intrinsic laryngeal muscles alters the position and configuration of these tissue folds, thus influencing laryngeal function during respiration, forced voluntary glottic closure (Valsalva maneuver), reflex laryngospasm, swallowing, and phonation (Fig. 7–2A, B).

The laryngeal tissue folds consist of the following:

1. Paired aryepiglottic folds extending from the epiglottis posteriorly to the superior surface of the arytenoids (the paired cuneiform and corniculate cartilages lie within for support and reinforcement).
2. Paired vestibular folds (false vocal cords) extending from the thyroid cartilage posteriorly to the superior surface of the arytenoids.
3. Paired vocal folds (true vocal cords) extending from the posterior surface of the thyroid plate to the anterior projection or vocal process of the arytenoids.
4. A single interarytenoid fold (composed of the interarytenoid muscle covered by tissue) bridging the arytenoid cartilages.
5. A single thyrohyoid fold extending from the hyoid bone to the thyroid cartilage.

Histology

The highly vascular mucosa of the mouth is continuous with that of the larynx and trachea. This mucosa consists of

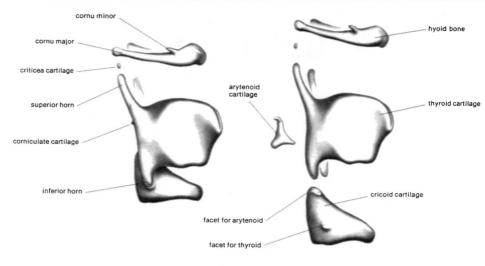

Figure 7–1. Laryngeal cartilages. The natural positions of the laryngeal cartilages are presented on the left, with the individual cartilages separated on the right. (From Fink BR, Demarest RJ: Laryngeal Biomechanics. Cambridge, MA, Harvard University Press, © 1978 by the President and Fellows of Harvard College.)

squamous, stratified, and pseudostratified ciliated epithelium. The vocal cords are covered with stratified epithelium. The mucosa and submucosa are rich in lymphatic vessels and seromucous-secreting glands, which lubricate the laryngeal folds. The submucosa consists of loose fibrous stroma; therefore, the mucosa is loosely adherent to the underlying structures in most areas. However, the submucosa is scant on the laryngeal surface of the epiglottis and the vocal cords; therefore, the mucosa is tightly adherent in these areas.[4, 5] For this reason, most inflammatory processes of the airway above the level of the vocal cords are limited by the barrier formed by the firm adherence of the mucosa to the vocal cords.[5] For example, epiglottitis is usually limited to the supraglottic structures, and the loosely adherent mucosa explains the ease with which localized swelling occurs (see Fig. 15–2A–C). In a similar manner, an inflammatory process of the subglottic region (laryngotracheobronchitis) results in significant subglottic edema in the loosely adherent mucosa of the airway below the vocal cords, but it does not usually spread above the level of the vocal cords (see Fig. 15–3A–C).[4]

Sensory and Motor Innervation

Two branches of the vagus nerve, the recurrent laryngeal and the superior laryngeal supply both sensory and motor innervation to the larynx. The sensory innervation of the supraglottic larynx is derived from the recurrent laryngeal nerve, whereas the internal branch of the superior laryngeal nerve innervates the infraglottic region. The external branch of the superior laryngeal nerve supplies motor innervation to the cricothyroid muscle. The recurrent laryngeal nerve supplies motor innervation to all other laryngeal muscles.[5, 6] Local anesthetic agents injected to block the superior laryngeal nerve result in anesthesia of the supraglottic region down to the inferior margin of the epiglottis and motor blockade of the cricothyroid muscle, which results in relaxation of the vocal cords. Transtracheal injection of local anesthetic or a specific recurrent laryngeal nerve block is required for infraglottic and tracheal anesthesia.[7–9]

Blood Supply

Laryngeal branches of the superior and inferior thyroid arteries provide the blood supply to the larynx. The recurrent

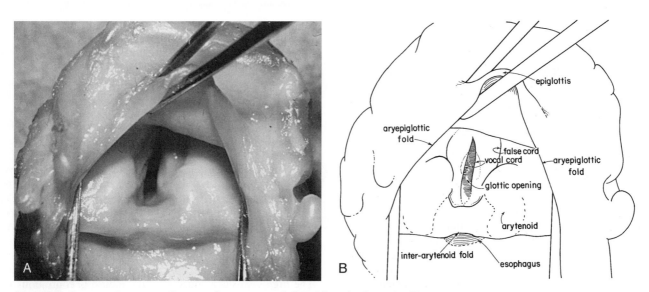

Figure 7–2. Laryngeal anatomy. Larynx of a premature infant (*A*) and schematic (*B*).

laryngeal nerve and artery lie in close proximity to each other, thus accounting for the occasional vocal cord paresis following attempts to control bleeding during thyroidectomy.[10]

Function

Inspiration

With inspiration, the larynx is pulled downward by the negative intrathoracic pressure generated by the descent of the diaphragm and contraction of the intercostal muscles. Longitudinal stretching of the larynx results, thus increasing the distance between the aryepiglottic and vestibular folds as well as the distance between the vestibular and vocal folds. Contraction of the intrinsic muscles within the larynx results in lateral movement and posterior displacement of the arytenoids (rocking backwards), causing an increase in the interarytenoid distance and separation as well as stretching of the paired aryepiglottic, vestibular, and vocal folds. Overall, inspiration results in enlargement of the laryngeal opening, both longitudinally and laterally, allowing free passage of air.

Expiration

At the end of expiration, the larynx reverts to its resting position, with longitudinal shortening of the distance between the aryepiglottic, vestibular, and vocal folds. The arytenoids return simultaneously to their resting position by rotating medially and rocking forward, thus decreasing the interarytenoid distance and reducing the tension on the paired aryepiglottic, vestibular, and vocal folds and causing them to thicken.

Forced Glottic Closure and Laryngospasm

Glottic closure during forced expiration (forced glottic closure or Valsalva maneuver) is voluntary laryngeal closure and is physiologically similar to involuntary laryngeal closure (laryngospasm). Forced glottic closure occurs at several levels. Contraction of intrinsic laryngeal muscles results in (1) marked reduction in the interarytenoid distance; (2) anterior rocking and medial movement of the arytenoids, causing apposition of the paired vocal, vestibular, and aryepiglottic folds; (3) longitudinal shortening of the larynx, obliterating the space between the aryepiglottic, vestibular, and vocal folds. Contraction of an extrinsic laryngeal muscle, the thyrohyoid, pulls the hyoid bone downward and the thyroid cartilage upward, leading to further closure.[1, 3, 11–15]

Closure of the larynx during laryngospasm is similar, but not identical to, that described for voluntary forced glottic closure. There are two important differences. First, laryngospasm is accompanied by an inspiratory effort, which separates longitudinally the vocal from the vestibular folds. Second, during laryngospasm, contraction of the thyroarytenoid and thyrohyoid muscles does not occur; thus apposition of the aryepiglottic folds and median thyrohyoid folds is minimal. During mild laryngospasm, therefore, the upper part of the larynx may be left partially open, resulting in the typical high-pitched inspiratory stridor.[1, 11] Anterior and upward displacement of the mandible (a "jaw thrust") separates longi-

tudinally the base of the tongue, the epiglottis, and the aryepiglottic folds from the vocal folds, helping to relieve laryngospasm.[12]

Swallowing

Glottic closure during swallowing is also similar to that which occurs with forced glottic closure. Protection of the glottic opening is accomplished primarily by apposition of the laryngeal folds and secondarily by upward movement of the larynx. The upward movement of the larynx brings the thyroid cartilage closer to the hyoid bone, resulting in folding of the epiglottis over the glottic opening.[1, 11, 13, 14] With loss of consciousness or deep sedation, the normal protective mechanism of the larynx may be lost or obtunded, thus predisposing to pulmonary aspiration of pharyngeal contents.

Phonation

Phonation is accomplished by alteration of the angle between the thyroid and cricoid cartilages (the cricothyroid angle) and by medial movement of the arytenoids during expiration.[1, 6, 15] These movements result in fine alterations in vocal fold tension during movement of air, causing vibration of the vocal folds. Lesions or malfunction of the vocal folds, such as inflammation, papilloma, or paresis, therefore affect phonation. Phonation is the only laryngeal function that alters the cricothyroid angle.[1] Thus, despite significant airway obstruction during inspiration, it may be possible to phonate.

Developmental Anatomy of the Airway

The five major anatomic differences between the neonatal and adult airway are discussed in the following sections.[2, 3, 16]

Tongue

An infant's tongue is relatively large in proportion to the rest of the oral cavity and thus more easily obstructs the airway, especially in a neonate. The tongue is more difficult to manipulate and stabilize with a laryngoscope blade.

Position of Larynx

An infant's larynx is higher in the neck (C3–4) than is an adult's (C4–5) (Fig. 7–3). Because the larynx is more rostral (higher) in the neck of an infant, the distances between the tongue, hyoid bone, epiglottis, and roof of the mouth are shorter than in an older child or adult. Thus, the tongue is closer to the roof of the mouth and easily obstructs the airway. The proximity of the tongue to the more superior larynx also makes visualization of laryngeal structures more difficult because it produces a more acute angulation between the plane of the tongue and the plane of the glottic opening. Therefore, the infant tongue is more likely to obstruct the view of the larynx. It is for this reason that a straight laryngoscope blade, which more completely elevates the tongue from the field of view during laryngoscopy, facilitates visualization of an infant's larynx. Thus, the larynx of an infant is not "anterior" (a common misnomer) but rather is "high," "rostral," or "superior" in the neck com-

GLOTTIC OPENING RELATIVE
TO CERVICAL VERTEBRA (C)

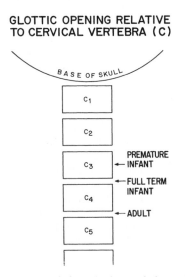

Figure 7–3. In a premature infant, the larynx is located at the middle of the third cervical vertebra (C3); in a full-term infant, at the C3-4 interspace; and in an adult, at the C4-5 interspace. (Adapted from Negus VE: The Comparative Anatomy and Physiology of the Larynx. Oxford, Butterworth-Heinemann, 1949.)

pared with that in the older child or adult. This anatomic relationship is further exaggerated in the Pierre Robin syndrome and other syndromes associated with mandibular hypoplasia, thus making direct visualization of the glottis difficult and sometimes impossible (Fig. 7–4). The reason for this difficulty is that with mandibular hypoplasia, the entire larynx is positioned more *posteriorly* than normal; the result is an even greater acute angulation between the plane of the tongue and the plane of the laryngeal inlet (often 90 degrees) (Fig. 7–5A–D). In this situation, conventional rigid laryngoscopy results in direct visualization of the esophageal inlet

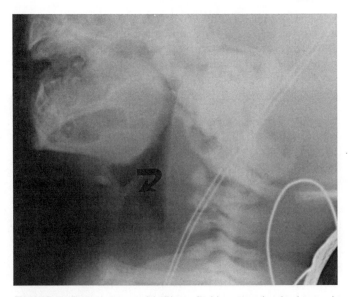

Figure 7–4. In a neonate with Pierre Robin anomaly, the larynx is located high in the neck (C3-4) and in a posterior position. Acute angulation between the laryngeal inlet (arrow) and the base of the tongue results. (Courtesy of Donna J Seibert, M.D., and John A. Kirkpatrick, Jr, M.D.)

rather than of the laryngeal inlet. In these patients, special equipment or special techniques may be required for successful endotracheal intubation.

Epiglottis

An adult's epiglottis is broad, and its axis is parallel to that of the trachea (Fig. 7–6A, B). An infant's epiglottis is narrower and angled away from the axis of the trachea (Fig. 7–7A, B). It is therefore more difficult to lift the infant's epiglottis with the tip of a laryngoscope blade.

Vocal Folds

An infant's vocal folds (cords) have a lower attachment anteriorly than posteriorly, whereas in an adult, the axis of the vocal folds is perpendicular to the trachea. This anatomic feature occasionally leads to difficulty in intubation, especially with the nasal approach; the tip of the endotracheal tube may be held up at the anterior commissure of the vocal folds.

Subglottis

The narrowest portion of an infant's larynx is the cricoid cartilage; in an adult, it is the rima glottidis (Fig. 7–8A, B). In an adult, therefore, an endotracheal tube that traverses the glottis passes freely into the trachea because the airway beyond is of larger diameter. In a child, however, an endotracheal tube might easily pass through the vocal folds but not through the subglottic region (Fig. 7–8B). The cricoid is the only complete ring of cartilage in the laryngotracheobronchial tree and is therefore nonexpandable. A tight-fitting endotracheal tube that compresses the tracheal mucosa at this level may cause edema and result in a clinically important increase in airway resistance at the time of extubation. Because the subglottic region of an infant is smaller than in an adult, the same degree of airway edema is more compromising in the infant. For example, assuming the diameter of the infant trachea to be approximately 4 mm and the diameter of the adult trachea to be approximately 8 mm, if 1 mm of circumferential edema forms, the cross-sectional area of the infant trachea is decreased by 75%, whereas the adult cross-sectional area is decreased by only 44%. Similarly, the proportional increase in resistance to airflow will also be greater in the infant (Fig. 7–9).[2] As a child matures, at approximately 10 to 12 years of age, the cricoid and thyroid cartilages have grown, eliminating both the angulation of the vocal cords and the narrow subglottic area.

Physiology of the Respiratory System

Obligate Nasal Breathing

Infants are generally described as obligate nasal breathers.[17, 18] Obstruction of the anterior or posterior nares (nasal congestion, stenosis, choanal atresia) may cause asphyxia.[19–21] Immaturity of coordination between respiratory efforts and oropharyngeal motor/sensory input accounts in part for obligate nasal breathing.[22] Furthermore, because the larynx is higher in the neck of an infant and oropharyngeal structures are closer together during quiet respiration, the tongue rests

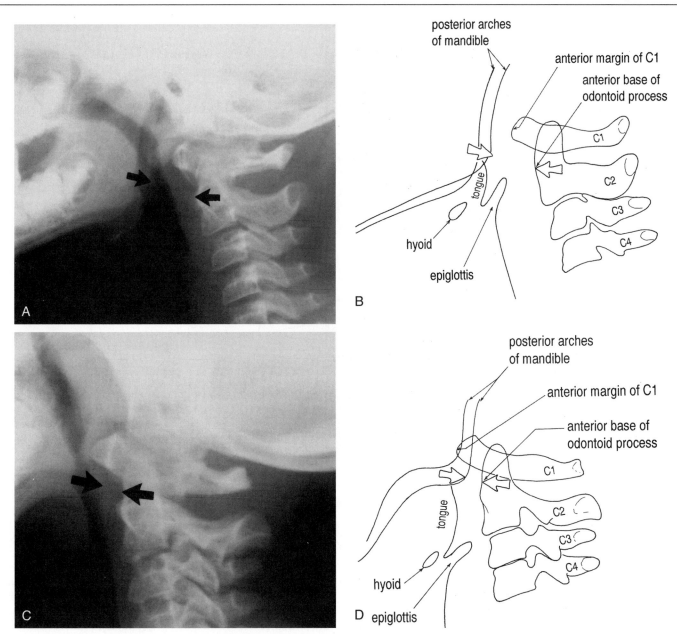

Figure 7–5. The larynx in children with mandibular hypoplasia is located more posteriorly than in children with normal anatomy. (A) A lateral radiograph of the upper airway including the base of the skull and cervical spine of a normal 7-year-old child; the arrows denote the posterior border of the ramus of the mandible and the anterior border of the second cervical vertebra. (B) A diagrammatic representation of the normal anatomy shown in part A. (C) The same radiographic projection in a 6-year-old child with Treacher Collins syndrome; the arrows again denote the posterior border of the ramus of the mandible and the anterior margin of the second cervical vertebra. (D) A diagrammatic representation of the anatomy shown in part C. Note the significantly smaller space between the ramus of the mandible and the second cervical vertebra; the anterior margin of the first cervical vertebra overlaps the posterior margin of the mandible. This extreme posterior location of the tongue and larynx makes direct visualization of the laryngeal inlet nearly impossible in many children with this anomaly because of the acute angulation between the base of the tongue and the laryngeal inlet. (Radiographs courtesy of Donna J. Seibert, M.D., John A. Kirkpatrick, Jr, M.D., and Robert H. Cleveland, M.D.)

against the roof of the mouth, resulting in oral airway obstruction.[18] Multiple sites of pharyngeal airway obstruction may also contribute to airway obstruction when attempting to breathe against a partially obstructed upper airway.[23–27] As an infant matures, the ability to coordinate respiratory and oral function develops; the larynx enlarges and moves down lower in the neck as the cervical spine lengthens, and the infant is now able to breathe adequately through the mouth.

This maturation occurs by age 3 to 5 months. Studies have found that the ability to breathe through the mouth when the nares are obstructed is age dependent. Only 8% of premature infants at 31 to 32 weeks of postconceptual age were able to breathe through the mouth in response to nasal occlusion, whereas in this same group of infants at 35 to 36 weeks of postconceptual age 28% were able to breathe through the mouth.[28] In a second study completed by these same investi-

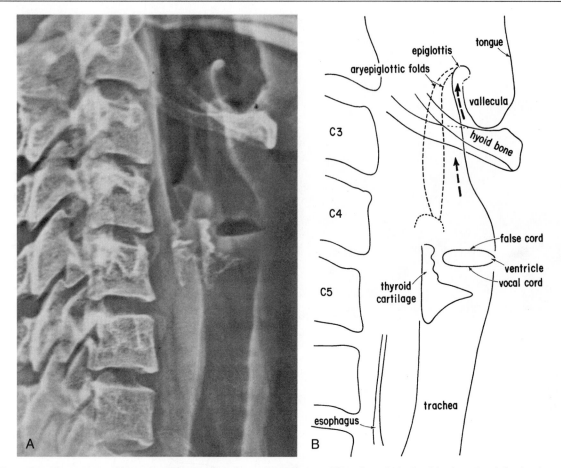

Figure 7–6. Lateral neck xerogram (A) and schematic (B) of an adult's larynx. Note the relatively thin, broad epiglottis, the axis of which is parallel to the trachea. The hyoid bone "hugs" the epiglottis; there is no subglottic narrowing.

gators, approximately 40% of full-term infants demonstrated the ability to switch from nasal to oral breathing.[29] However, more recent data are contradictory. Slow and fast nasal occlusion was applied to 17 healthy preterm infants (gestational age 32 ± 1 week, postnatal age 12 ± 2 days). All demonstrated the ability to switch from nasal to oral breathing. These authors attribute the difference in findings to the longer observation period in their study (> 15 sec).[30]

Tracheal and Bronchial Function

Tracheal and bronchial diameters are a function of elasticity and of distending or compressive forces (Fig. 7–10A–D). An infant's larynx, trachea, and bronchi are highly compliant compared with an adult's and therefore more subject to distending and compressing forces.[17, 31, 32] The intrathoracic trachea is subject to stresses that are different from those in the extrathoracic portion.[31] On expiration, intrathoracic pressure remains slightly negative, thus maintaining patency of the intrathoracic trachea and bronchi (Fig. 7–10B). On inspiration, a greater negative intrathoracic pressure dilates and stretches the *intrathoracic* trachea.[33] The *extrathoracic* trachea is slightly narrowed by dynamic compression resulting from the differential between intratracheal pressures and atmospheric pressures; patency is maintained by the cartilages of the trachea and by the muscles and soft tissues of the neck (Fig. 7–10A). Obstruction of the extrathoracic

upper airway that can occur with epiglottitis, laryngotracheo-bronchitis, or a foreign body, alters normal airway dynamics. Inspiration against an obstruction results in the development of a more negative intrathoracic pressure, thus dilating the intrathoracic airways to a greater degree. Clinically, the result is an increased tendency toward dynamic collapse of the extrathoracic trachea below the level of the obstruction. This collapse is greatest at the thoracic inlet, where the highest pressure gradient exists between negative intratracheal and atmospheric pressures. As a result, inspiratory stridor is prominent (Fig. 7–10C).[31–38] With intrathoracic tracheal obstruction, such as a foreign body or vascular ring, stridor may occur during both inspiration and expiration.[39–42] In lower airway obstruction, such as asthma or bronchiolitis, significant intrathoracic tracheal and bronchial collapse may occur as a result of the prolonged expiratory phase and greatly increased positive extraluminal pressure (Fig. 7–10D).[43] In addition, because a child's airways are highly compliant, they may be more susceptible to closure during bronchial smooth-muscle contraction, such as with reactive airway disease. Preterm and term infants may experience airway closure even during quiet respirations.

Avoiding dynamic airway collapse is particularly important. The highly compliant trachea and bronchi of an infant or child are very susceptible to collapse, particularly at the extremes of transluminal pressures that may occur when a child is crying. For this reason, it is most important

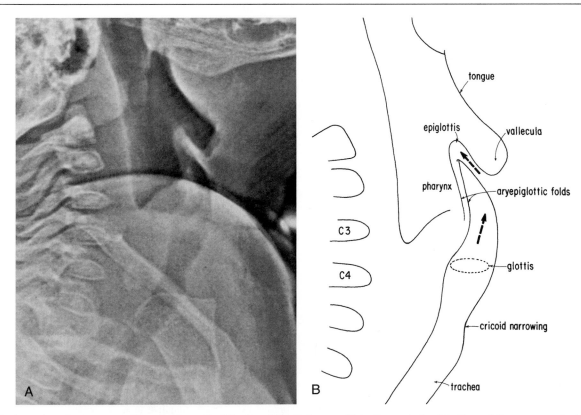

Figure 7–7. Lateral neck xerogram (A) and schematic (B) of an infant's larynx. Note the angled epiglottis and the narrow cricoid cartilage.

to keep children with airway obstruction calm. Skill and understanding are required on the part of the parents, nursing staff, and physicians. *The use of sedatives and narcotics before control of the airway (endotracheal tube inserted) may result in significant morbidity or mortality, because the life-sustaining voluntary efforts to breathe are depressed.* The susceptibility of a child to these dynamic forces on the airway is inversely related to age, with premature infants most susceptible and adults least susceptible.[44]

Work of Breathing

Work may be defined as pressure times volume; therefore, the work of breathing may be analyzed by plotting transpulmonary pressure against tidal volume. The work of breathing

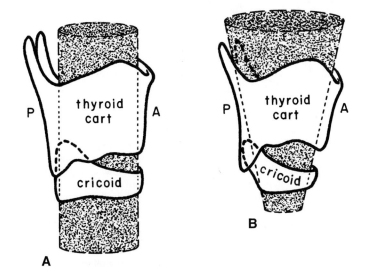

Figure 7–8. Configuration of the larynx of an adult (A) and an infant (B). Note the cylinder shape of an adult's larynx; an infant's larynx is funnel-shaped because of the narrow, undeveloped cricoid cartilage.

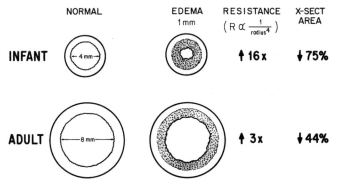

Figure 7–9. Relative effects of airway edema in an infant and an adult. The normal airways of an infant and an adult are presented on the left, edematous airways (1 mm circumferential) on the right. Note that resistance to air flow is inversely proportional to the radius of the lumen to the fourth power for laminar flow, and to the radius of the lumen to the fifth power for turbulent flow. The net result in an infant is a 75% reduction in cross-sectional area and a 16-fold increase in resistance to airflow, compared with a 44% reduction in cross-sectional area and a three-fold increase in resistance to air flow in an adult.

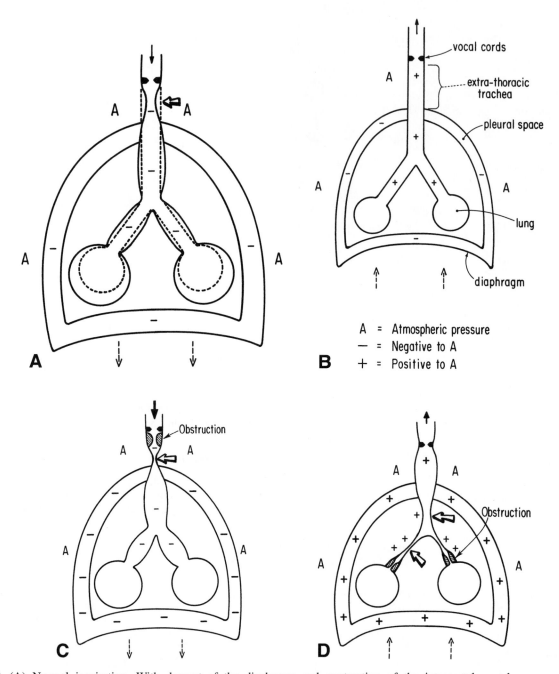

Figure 7–10. (A) Normal inspiration. With descent of the diaphragm and contraction of the intercostal muscles, a greater negative intrathoracic pressure relative to intraluminal and atmospheric pressure is developed. The net result is longitudinal stretching of the larynx and trachea, dilatation of the intrathoracic trachea and bronchi, movement of air into the lungs, and some dynamic collapse of the extrathoracic trachea (arrow). The dynamic collapse is due to the highly compliant trachea and the negative intraluminal pressure in relation to atmospheric pressure. (B) Normal expiration. The normal sequence of events at end-expiration is a slight negative intrapleural pressure stenting the airways open. In infants, the highly compliant chest does not provide the support required; thus, airway closure occurs with each breath. Intraluminal pressures are slightly positive in relation to atmospheric pressure, resulting in air being forced out of the lungs. (C) Obstructed extrathoracic airway during inspiration. Note the severe dynamic collapse of the extrathoracic trachea below the level of obstruction. This collapse is greatest at the thoracic inlet, where the largest pressure gradient exists between negative intratracheal pressure and atmospheric pressure (arrow).[31] (D) Obstructed intrathoracic trachea or airways during expiration. Note that breathing against an obstructed lower airway (e.g., bronchiolitis, asthma) results in greater positive intrathoracic pressures, with dynamic collapse of the intrathoracic airways (prolonged expiration or wheezing [arrows]).

for each kilogram of body weight is similar in infants and adults. However, the oxygen consumption of a full-term newborn (4 to 6 mL/kg/min) is twice that of an adult (2 to 3 mL/kg/min).[45] This greater oxygen consumption in infants accounts for the increased respiratory frequency. In premature infants, the oxygen consumption related to breathing is three times that in adults.[46]

The source of airway resistance differs between infants and adults. The nasal passages account for 25% of the total resistance to airflow in a neonate, compared with 60% in an adult.[18, 47] In infants, most resistance to airflow occurs in the bronchial and small airways. This is because airway diameters are relatively smaller and because the supporting structures of the trachea and bronchi are more compliant.[17, 48, 49] In particular, the chest wall of a neonate is highly compliant; the ribs provide less support to maintain negative intrathoracic pressure. This lack of negative intrathoracic pressure combined with the high compliance of the bronchi can lead to functional airway closure with every breath.[50–52] In infants and children, therefore, small-airway resistance accounts for most of the work of breathing, whereas in adults the nasal passages provide the major proportion of flow resistance.[18, 50, 51, 53–58] In the presence of increased airway resistance or decreased lung compliance, an increased transpulmonary pressure is required to produce a given tidal volume and thus the work of breathing is increased. Any pathologic alteration of the airway that increases the work of breathing may lead to respiratory failure. Recall that the resistance component of respiratory work is inversely proportional to the radius of the lumen increased by the power of four. Because infants have smaller airways than adults, pathologic airway narrowing has greater adverse effects on the work of breathing. Increase in the work of breathing may also occur with a long endotracheal tube of small diameter, an obstructed endotracheal tube, or a narrowed airway. These situations all result in increased oxygen consumption, which in turn increases oxygen demand.[59] The increased oxygen demand is initially met by an increase in respiratory rate, but the increased work of breathing may not be able to be sustained and may result in exhaustion, leading to respiratory failure (carbon dioxide retention and hypoxemia).

The difference in histology of the diaphragm and intercostal muscles of premature and term infants compared with older children also contributes to the infant's increased susceptibility to respiratory fatigue or failure. Type I muscle fibers permit prolonged repetitive movement (e.g., long-distance runners through repeated exercise increase the proportion of type I muscle fibers in their legs). Fewer type I muscle fibers are present in the diaphragm and intercostal muscles of premature than term infants, and term infants have fewer type I muscle fibers than 2-year-old children (Fig. 7–11). Thus, any condition that increases the work of breathing in neonates and infants may easily fatigue the respiratory muscles and result in respiratory failure.[60–62]

Airway Obstruction During Anesthesia

A classic teaching of anesthesiologists is that airway obstruction during anesthesia or loss of consciousness is primarily due to apposition of the tongue to the posterior pharyngeal wall. Studies of adults now suggest that airway obstruction may be primarily related to loss of muscle tone of pharyn-

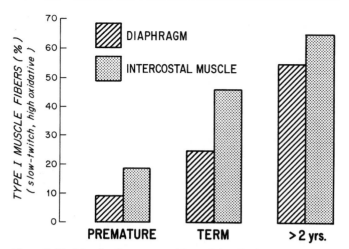

Figure 7–11. Muscle fiber composition of the diaphragm and intercostal muscles related to age. Note that a premature infant's diaphragm and intercostal muscles have fewer type I fibers compared with term newborns and older children. The data suggest a possible mechanism for early fatigue in premature and term infants when the work of breathing is increased. (Data from Keens TG, Bryan AC, Levison H, et al: Developmental pattern of muscle fiber types in human ventilatory muscles. J Appl Physiol 1978; 44:909–913.)

geal structures.[23, 24, 63, 64] Loss of pharyngeal and laryngeal muscle tone results in airway obstruction at the level of the soft palate and the epiglottis; forceful inspiration with partial upper airway obstruction results in multiple sites of pharyngeal collapse and obstruction.[23, 24, 63] Extension of the head at the atlanto-occipital joint with anterior displacement of the cervical spine results in improved hypopharyngeal airway patency but does not necessarily result in change in the position of the tongue.[25–27] It has been proposed that progressive loss of tone in the tongue muscle as well as in other pharyngeal muscles with deepening of anesthesia results in progressive airway obstruction.[27, 65, 66] Pharyngeal airway obstruction has been demonstrated to occur during obstructive sleep apnea in infants and adults.[22, 67] It appears that upper airway obstruction during loss of consciousness has multiple causes, including mechanical obstruction by the tongue, soft palate, and epiglottis.

Evaluation of the Airway

A history and physical examination with specific reference to the airway should be performed in all pediatric patients requiring sedation or anesthesia. In special situations, radiologic and laboratory studies are required to further evaluate and clarify a disorder revealed by the history and physical examination. Although many methods exist for evaluating and predicting the difficult airway in adults,[68–72] no studies have been published that assess the use of any of these techniques in children.[73, 74] Instead, routine airway evaluation of all children followed by correlation with any airway problems occurring during anesthetic management helps to develop experience. This experience then may be used to identify patients who might have airway difficulties during or following anesthesia.

Clinical Evaluation

The *medical history* (both present and past) should investigate the following signs and symptoms. A positive history should alert the practitioner to the potential problems that are noted in parentheses.

- Presence of an upper respiratory tract infection (predisposition to coughing, laryngospasm, bronchospasm, and desaturation during anesthesia or to postintubation subglottic edema or postoperative desaturation)[75–79]
- Snoring or noisy breathing (adenoidal hypertrophy, upper airway obstruction, obstructive sleep apnea)
- Presence and nature of cough ("croupy" cough may indicate subglottic stenosis or previous tracheoesophageal fistula repair; productive cough may indicate bronchitis or pneumonia; chronicity affects the differential diagnosis, e.g., the sudden onset of a persistent cough may indicate foreign body aspiration)
- Past episodes of croup (postintubation croup, subglottic stenosis)
- Inspiratory stridor, usually high-pitched (subglottic narrowing, laryngomalacia, macroglossia, laryngeal web, extrathoracic foreign body, or extrathoracic tracheal compression)
- Hoarse voice (laryngitis, vocal cord palsy, papillomatosis, granuloma)
- Asthma and bronchodilator therapy (bronchospasm)

- Repeated pneumonias (incompetent larynx with aspiration, gastroesophageal reflux, cystic fibrosis, bronchiectasis, residual tracheoesophageal fistula, pulmonary sequestration, immune suppression, congenital heart disease)
- History of foreign body aspiration (increased airway reactivity, airway obstruction, impaired neurologic function)
- Previous anesthetic problems, particularly related to the airway (difficult intubation or extubation or difficulty with mask ventilation)
- Atopy, allergy (increased airway reactivity)
- History of a congenital syndrome (many are associated with difficult airway management)

The *physical examination* should include the following observations:

- Facial expression
- Presence or absence of nasal flaring
- Presence or absence of mouth breathing
- Color of mucous membranes
- Presence or absence of retractions (suprasternal, intercostal, subcostal)
- Respiratory rate
- Presence or absence of voice change
- Mouth opening (Fig. 7–12A)
- Size of mouth
- Size of tongue and its relationship to other pharyngeal structures (Mallampati)[71]

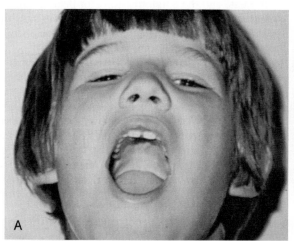
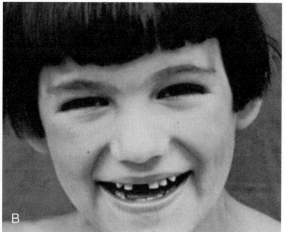
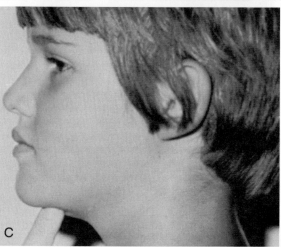

Figure 7–12. (A) How far can a child open his or her mouth? Are there any abnormalities of the mouth, tongue, palate, or mandible? (B) Are any teeth loose or missing? (C) Is the mandible of normal configuration? How much space is there between the genu of the mandible and the thyroid cartilage? This space is an indication of the extent of the superior and posterior displacement of the larynx; there should normally be at least one finger's breadth in a newborn and three fingers' breadths in an adolescent.

- Loose or missing teeth (Fig. 7–12B)
- Size and configuration of palate
- Size and configuration of mandible
- Location of larynx (Fig. 7–12C)
- Presence of stridor and if present:
    Is stridor predominantly inspiratory, suggesting an upper airway (extrathoracic) lesion?
    Is stridor both inspiratory and expiratory, suggesting an intrathoracic lesion (foreign body, vascular ring, or large esophageal foreign body)?
    Is the expiratory phase prolonged or stridor predominantly expiratory, suggesting lower airway disease?
- Baseline oxygen saturation in room air
- Global appearance:
    Are there congenital anomalies that may fit a recognizable syndrome? *The finding of one anomaly mandates a search for others.* If a congenital syndrome is diagnosed, specific anesthetic implications must be considered (see Appendix 7–1).

Diagnostic Testing

Routine evaluation of the airway usually requires only a careful history and physical examination. With airway pathology, however, laboratory and radiologic evaluation may be extremely valuable. Radiographs of the upper airway (anteroposterior and lateral films and fluoroscopy) may provide evidence about the site and cause of airway obstruction. When necessary, magnetic resonance imaging and computed tomography provide more detailed information.[80–95] *Radiologic airway examination in a child with a compromised airway must be undertaken only when there is no immediate threat to the child's safety and only in the presence of skilled and appropriately equipped personnel able to manage the airway.* Securing the airway through endotracheal intubation must not be postponed to obtain a radiologic diagnosis when a patient has severely compromised air exchange. Blood gas analysis is occasionally of value in assessing the degree of physiologic compromise, especially with chronic airway obstruction and compensated respiratory acidosis. Performing an arterial puncture for blood gas analysis, although providing helpful information, is often upsetting to a child and runs the risk of aggravating the underlying airway obstruction through dynamic airway collapse. Candidates for blood gas analysis therefore must be carefully selected, and the procedure skillfully performed.

Endoscopic evaluation (flexible fiberoptic endoscopy) can be useful in infants and in older cooperative children for evaluation prior to intubation when glottic pathology is suspected or when glottic visualization is anticipated to be difficult.

Airway Management: The Normal Airway

Mask Ventilation

Technique

Face masks are available in many sizes. We commonly use the disposable, clear plastic masks with an inflatable rim. The inflatable rim helps provide an atraumatic seal. The clear plastic allows visualization of the airway to monitor for secretions, vomitus, or cyanosis. The appropriately sized mask should rest on the bridge of the nose (avoiding the eyes) and extend to the chin. The most common error in technique is to cause obstruction of the airway by compressing the pharyngeal space by placing the fingers below the mandibular ridge and squeezing too tightly. Minimal pressure is required and the fingers should rest on the mandible. A hand should be on the ventilating bag at all times during spontaneous ventilation to help monitor effectiveness of ventilation and to provide continuous positive airway pressure if needed to maintain airway patency.

Guidelines from the American Heart Association and the American Academy of Pediatrics[96, 97] caution against extreme positions of an infant's head during bag or mask ventilation because stretching of the highly compliant infant trachea may cause narrowing and airway obstruction. One study showed this to be untrue. After induction of anesthesia, 18 healthy full-term infants who were less than 4 months of age had their tracheas videotaped in each of three head positions: neutral, flexed, and extended. Video images, analyzed by an investigator blinded to head position, showed that there was no statistical change in tracheal dimension with change in head position.[98] Thus stretching of the trachea does not result in tracheal lumen narrowing. However, this study did not examine the effects of these head positions on the supraglottic airway. It is possible that these maneuvers (head extension) may result instead in supraglottic airway obstruction.

Oropharyngeal Airways

An infant's tongue is relatively large in proportion to the oropharynx and often obstructs the airway during induction of anesthesia or loss of consciousness due to any cause. It is important, therefore, to select an oropharyngeal airway of appropriate size to achieve unobstructed air exchange. By holding the airway as shown in Figure 7–13A and B, one can estimate the appropriate size; airways one size larger and one size smaller should be readily available. Airway insertion is facilitated with a tongue depressor to prevent folding of the tongue, which may cause impaired venous and lymphatic drainage, macroglossia, and airway obstruction. If the airway extends too deeply, its tip may push the epiglottis down, causing traumatic epiglottitis, or the tip may impinge on the uvula, causing uvular swelling and airway obstruction (Fig. 7–13C, D).[99, 100] If the airway is too short, it rests against the base of the tongue, forcing it posteriorly and thus further aggravating airway obstruction (Fig. 7–13E, F). Care must be taken to avoid trauma to the lips and tongue, which may be caught between the teeth and the airway. An oral airway is also used to protect an oral endotracheal tube from compression by a child's teeth and it can facilitate oropharyngeal suctioning.

Nasopharyngeal Airways

Nasopharyngeal airways are occasionally of value in pediatric patients; the distance from the nares to the angle of the mandible approximates the proper length. Commercial airways are available in size 12F to 36F (Rüsch Inc., Duluth, GA). Some have an adjustable flange that enables manipulation of the airway to the appropriate length. Alternatively,

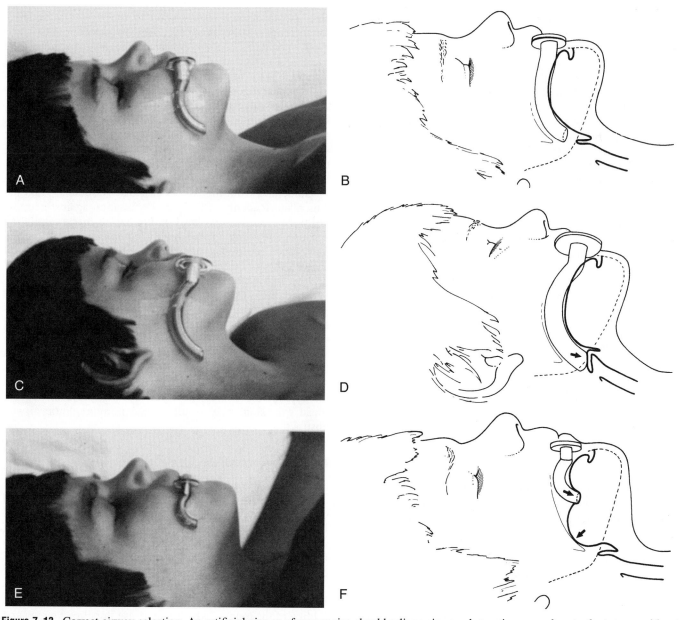

Figure 7–13. Correct airway selection. An artificial airway of proper size should relieve airway obstruction secondary to the tongue without damaging laryngeal structures. The appropriate size can be estimated by holding the airway against the child's face; the tip of the airway should end just cephalad to the angle of the mandible (A). This should result in proper alignment with the glottic opening (B). If too large an oral airway is inserted, the tip lines up posterior to the angle of the mandible (C) and obstructs the glottic opening by pushing the epiglottis down (D, arrow). If too small an oral airway is inserted, the tip lines up well above the angle of the mandible (E); airway obstruction is thus exacerbated by kinking the tongue (F, arrows).

for infants and small children, a shortened endotracheal tube may be used. The nasopharyngeal airway may be better tolerated in the lightly anesthetized patient than is the oropharyngeal airway. Under most circumstances, however, nasopharyngeal airways are avoided to prevent trauma to and bleeding from hypertrophied adenoids.

Tracheal Intubation

Technique

Because of differences in anatomy, there are important differences in techniques for intubating the trachea of infants and children compared with adults.[1–3, 12–15, 84, 101, 102] The trachea of older children (6 years of age and older) and adults is most easily intubated when a folded blanket or pillow is placed beneath the occiput of the head (5–10 cm elevation), resulting in anterior displacement of the cervical spine.[103] Extension of the head at the atlanto-occipital joint produces the classic "sniffing" position.[84, 104, 105] These movements result in alignment of the axes of the structures of the mouth, oropharynx, and trachea and permit more direct visualization of laryngeal structures. They also result in improved hypopharyngeal patency.[25, 27, 63, 104, 105] Figure 7–14A–F demonstrates maneuvers for positioning the head during airway management. In infants and younger children, it is usually

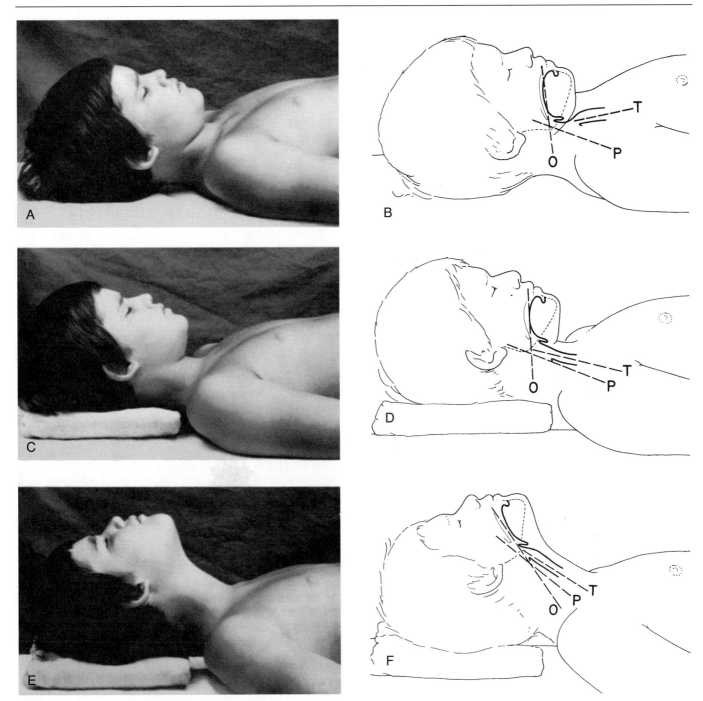

Figure 7–14. Correct positioning for ventilation and tracheal intubation. With a patient flat on the bed or operating table (A), the oral (**O**), pharyngeal (**P**), and tracheal (**T**) axes pass through three divergent planes (B). A folded sheet or towel placed under the occiput of the head (C) aligns the pharyngeal (**P**) and tracheal (**T**) axes (D). Extension of the atlanto-occipital joint (E) results in alignment of the oral (**O**), pharyngeal (**P**), and tracheal (**T**) axes (F).

unnecessary to elevate the occiput because the head is large in proportion to the trunk; head extension at the atlanto-occipital joint alone aligns the airway axes. When the occiput is elevated excessively, exposure of the glottis may actually be hindered. In newborns, it is helpful for an assistant to hold the shoulders flat on the operating room table with the head slightly extended.

Laryngoscopy can be performed with a patient awake, anesthetized, and breathing spontaneously, or with a combi-

nation of anesthesia and neuromuscular blockade. Most intubations in children who are awake are performed in neonates, an approach not feasible or humane in older awake and uncooperative children. Awake intubation in a neonate is generally well tolerated and, if performed smoothly, is not associated with significant hemodynamic changes.[106] However, data suggest that even neonates and preterm infants are better managed with sedation and paralysis.[107–109] Preterm infants in particular may be at risk for intraventricular hemorrhage if intubation is performed awake without sedation or anesthesia because of adverse hemodynamic responses.[109]

Selection of Laryngoscope Blade

A straight blade is generally more suitable in infants and young children than a curved blade because it facilitates lifting the base of the tongue and exposing the glottic opening. One technique consists of advancing the blade into the esophagus, with laryngeal visualization achieved during withdrawal of the blade. *This maneuver may result in laryngeal trauma when the tip of the blade scrapes the arytenoids and aryepiglottic folds.* Our preferred technique consists of advancing the blade under constant vision along the surface of the tongue and placing the tip of the blade directly in the vallecula. This avoids trauma to the laryngeal structures. One can thus lift the base of the tongue, which in turn lifts the epiglottis, exposing the glottic opening. If this technique is unsuccessful, one may then directly lift the epiglottis with the tip of the blade. Care must be taken to avoid using the laryngoscope as a fulcrum with pressure on the teeth or alveolar ridge. Curved blades are satisfactory in older children. The blade size chosen depends on the body mass of the patient and the preference of the anesthesiologist. Table 7–1 presents the sizes commonly used.

Endotracheal Tubes

The selection of a proper size endotracheal tube depends on the *individual* patient.[110] The only size requirement for manufacturers is that they standardize the internal diameter (ID) of an endotracheal tube. The external diameter may vary, depending on the material from which the endotracheal tube is constructed and its manufacturer. This diversity in external diameter mandates the need to check for proper endotracheal tube size and leak around the endotracheal tube. An appropriately sized uncuffed endotracheal tube may be approximated according to the patient's age (Table 7–2).[111] In children younger than 8 years, in general, it is desirable to select an uncuffed tube that would result in an air leak around the tube at 20 to 35 cm H_2O peak inflation pressure. This pressure is believed to approximate capillary pressure of the adult tracheal mucosa. If lateral wall pressure exceeds this amount, ischemic damage to the subglottic mucosa may occur.[112] An uncuffed endotracheal tube also allows insertion of an endotracheal tube of larger ID, resulting in less airway resistance.[113] In addition, an uncuffed endotracheal tube with an air leak exerts minimal pressure

Table 7–1. Laryngoscope Blades Used in Infants and Children

| Age | Blade Size | | |
	Miller	Wis-Hippel	Macintosh
Premature	0	—	—
Neonate	0	—	—
Neonate–2 years	1	—	—
2–6 years	—	1.5	2
6–12 years	2	—	2
Over 12 years	2–3	—	3

Table 7–2. Endotracheal Tubes Used in Infants and Children

Age	Size (mm ID)
Preterm	
1000 g	2.5
1000–2500 g	3.0
Neonate–6 months	3.0–3.5
6 months–1 year	3.5–4.0
1–2 years	4.0–5.0
Beyond 2 years	(age in years + 16)/4

ID, internal diameter.

on the internal surface of the cricoid cartilage and thus poses potentially less risk for postextubation edema (croup). If a cuffed endotracheal tube is passed, an endotracheal tube with a smaller ID must be selected to compensate for the endotracheal tube cuff. Inflation of the cuff should be adjusted so as to still provide a leak between 20 and 35 cm H_2O peak inflation pressure.[114] This air leak must be re-evaluated during the anesthetic procedure if nitrous oxide is used, because the gas may diffuse into the cuff, producing excessive tracheal mucosal pressure.[114, 115]

We select the endotracheal tube size according to Table 7–2 and have available endotracheal tubes of half ID size above and below the selected size. Following intubation and stabilization of the child, should there be no leak below 35 cm H_2O peak inflation pressure, the endotracheal tube is changed to the next half size smaller. Be aware, however, that if a child is intubated without the aid of muscle relaxants, laryngospasm around the endotracheal tube may prevent any gas leak and mimic a tight-fitting endotracheal tube. Once the level of anesthesia has been deepened, then an air leak should become evident.

Endotracheal Tube Insertion Distance

The length of the trachea (vocal cords to carina) in neonates and children up to 1 year of age varies from 5 to 9 cm.[33] In most infants 3 months to 1 year of age, if the 10 cm mark of the endotracheal tube is placed at the alveolar ridge, the tip of the tube rests above the carina. In premature or term infants, the distance is less. In children 2 years old, 12 cm is usually appropriate. An easy way to remember this is **10** for a newborn, **11** for a 1-year-old, and **12** for a 2-year-old. After this age, the correct length of insertion (in centimeters) for oral intubation may be approximated by formulas based on age or weight (Table 7–3)[116–118]:

Age (years)/2 + 12 or weight (kilograms)/5 + 12.

After the endotracheal tube is inserted and the first strip of adhesive tape is applied to secure it, one must observe for symmetry of chest expansion and auscultate for equality of breath sounds high in the axillae and apices. A CO_2 monitor confirms intratracheal positioning.[119] It is also important to auscultate over the stomach and to observe for cyanosis. Once satisfactory position is achieved, a second strip of tape ensures secure fixation (Fig. 7–15A–C). We have observed a number of patients whose endotracheal tube moved into a mainstem bronchus after initial correct position

Table 7–3. Distance for Insertion of an Endotracheal Tube by Patient Age

Age	Approximate Distance of Insertion (cm) Even with Alveolar Ridge
Preterm <1000 g	6
Preterm <2000 g	7–9
Term newborn	10
1 year	11
2 years	12
6 years	15
10 years	17
16 years	18
20 years	20

during positioning for the surgical procedure; this manifested as a slight but persistent decrease in oxygen saturation, such as changing from 100% to 93% to 95%. *When a small but persistent change in oxygen saturation is noted, rather than increase the inspired oxygen concentration (FIO$_2$) by reflex, one must first reassess the position of the endotracheal tube.*[120]

Complications of Endotracheal Intubation

Postintubation Croup. The reported incidence of perioperative postintubation croup in children ranges from 0.1 to 1%.[121, 122] Factors associated with increased risk of croup are too large an endotracheal tube (no leak at > 25 cm H$_2$O pressure),

change in patient position during the procedure, patient position other than supine, repeated attempts at intubation, traumatic intubation, patient age between 1 and 4 years, duration of surgery greater than 1 hour, coughing on the endotracheal tube, and previous history of croup.[121, 122] Concurrent upper respiratory infection has been variously reported both to be a risk factor and to be unrelated.[75, 122] Treatment consists of humidified mist, nebulized racemic epinephrine, and dexamethasone administered intravenously or by nebulizer. The rationale for these treatments is drawn primarily from experience with the treatment of infectious croup in children.[123–130] It is obvious that these two types of croup are not identical processes and efficacy of any of these interventions for the treatment of postintubation croup has not been proven in a controlled trial. Studies examining the effect of dexamethasone given prior to extubation in patients who have had prolonged intubation are contradictory; some support the use of dexamethasone to reduce stridor and others do not.[131–133]

Laryngotracheal (Subglottic) Stenosis. Ninety percent of acquired subglottic stenoses are the result of endotracheal intubation, particularly prolonged intubation.[134–137] Preterm infants and neonates may have a lower incidence after prolonged intubation because of the relative immaturity of the cricoid cartilage. At this age, the cartilage structure is hypercellular and the matrix has a high fluid content, making the structures more resilient and less susceptible to ischemic injury.[138]

The pathogenesis of acquired subglottic stenosis results from ischemic injury secondary to lateral wall pressure from the endotracheal tube. Ischemia results in edema, necrosis, and ulcerations of the mucosa. Secondary infection results

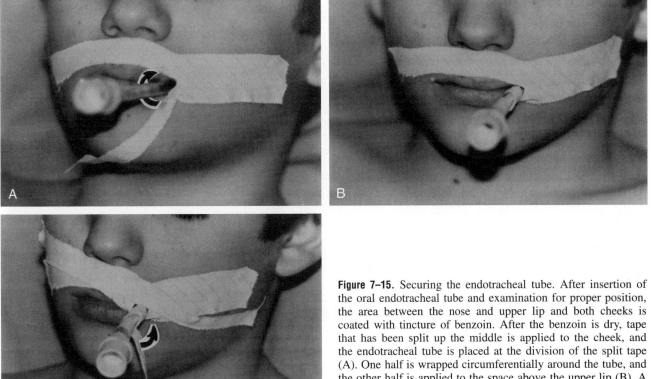

Figure 7–15. Securing the endotracheal tube. After insertion of the oral endotracheal tube and examination for proper position, the area between the nose and upper lip and both cheeks is coated with tincture of benzoin. After the benzoin is dry, tape that has been split up the middle is applied to the cheek, and the endotracheal tube is placed at the division of the split tape (A). One half is wrapped circumferentially around the tube, and the other half is applied to the space above the upper lip (B). A second piece of tape is applied in similar fashion from the opposite direction (C). A nasal endotracheal tube may also be secured with this technique.

in exposure of the cartilage. Within 48 hours, granulation tissue begins to form within these ulcerations. Eventually, scar tissue forms, resulting in narrowing of the airway (Fig. 7–16A–C).[139, 140]

Factors that predispose to subglottic stenosis are intubation with too large an endotracheal tube, laryngeal trauma (traumatic intubation, chemical or thermal inhalation, external trauma, surgical trauma, gastric reflux), prolonged intubation (particularly greater than 25 days), repeated intubation, sepsis and infection, chronic illness, and chronic inflammatory disease.[137, 141, 142]

Laryngeal Mask Airway

The laryngeal mask airway (LMA) has become a standard alternative for airway management during general anesthe-sia.[143–148] The LMA is made of medical-grade silicon and consists of a large-bore tubular structure (barrel), which has a 15 mm adapter at its proximal end and an elliptical mask-like device that fits over the laryngeal inlet at its distal end (Fig. 7–17). The mask is inflated via a valved pilot tube and balloon. The LMA is available in seven sizes. Guidelines for selecting the appropriate mask for pediatric applications are based on weight (Table 7–4).

The LMA has been described for use in virtually all types of surgical cases.[149] Some authors suggest that the LMA can be used for any case in which spontaneous ventilation is appropriate or any case that might reasonably be managed by face mask. The advantage of the LMA over the face mask is that it frees the anesthesiologist's hands for other tasks and may be associated with a lesser amount of op-

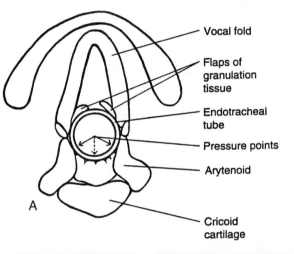

Vocal fold

Flaps of granulation tissue

Endotracheal tube

Pressure points

Arytenoid

Cricoid cartilage

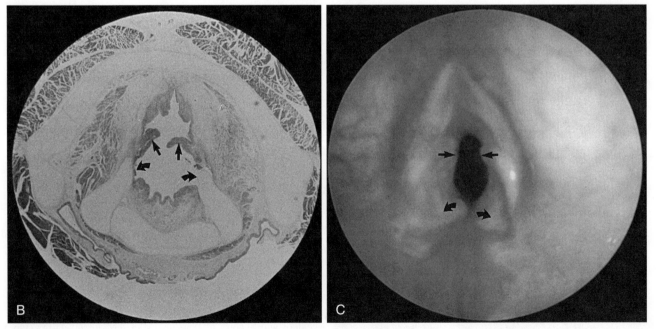

Figure 7–16. The pathogenesis of intubation injuries. (A) Schemata of a cross section through the glottis. Pressure necrosis causes ulcerations at the vocal processes of the arytenoids with exposed cartilage. Flaps of granulation tissue are present anterior to these ulcerations. (B) Cross section of the glottis at this same level; straight arrows indicate flaps of granulation tissue and curved arrows the absence of mucosa and ulcerations with exposed cartilage on the vocal processes of the arytenoids. (C) Intubation injury to a 2-month-old infant; straight arrows indicate granulation tissue and curved arrows indicate area of ulcerations (white area). It should be noted that the most severe area of injury is generally at the level of the cricoid cartilage, resulting in subglottic stenosis. (From Holinger LD, Lusk RP, Green CG: Pediatric Laryngology and Bronchoesophagology. Philadelphia: Lippincott-Raven; 1997.)

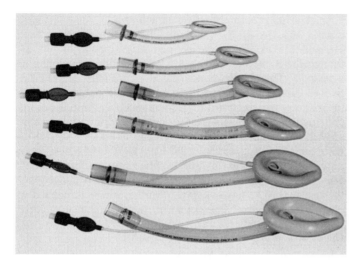

Figure 7–17. The laryngeal mask airway is available in seven sizes; see Table 7–4 for size versus age match.

erating room pollution compared with mask ventilation.[150, 151] The use of controlled ventilation with the LMA has been described[152, 153]; however, this practice is more controversial than the use of the LMA in spontaneously breathing patients because of concerns about possible air insufflation into the stomach and resultant regurgitation.[154–156] Air insufflation into the stomach is more likely if high ventilating pressures are used or required (pressures greater than the pressure that produces an audible air leak).[152, 157] Flexible bronchoscopy, radiotherapy, radiologic procedures, ear, nose, and throat surgeries, and ophthalmologic procedures are the most commonly described pediatric indications for the LMA.[148, 149, 158, 159] The LMA is associated with no increase in intraocular pressure, in contrast to endotracheal intubation.[160] The advantage of the LMA for flexible bronchoscopy is that it allows for oxygenation and ventilation while allowing a larger bronchoscope to be used than can be passed through an age-appropriate endotracheal tube.[159, 161, 162] It also allows visualization and evaluation of the laryngeal structures. For children requiring frequent anesthetics over a short period of time, as in radiotherapy, the LMA provides a secure airway without the trauma of repeated intubation.[148] The LMA has also been advocated for use in place of intubation in patients who are at increased risk of bronchial airway reactivity, that is, patients with upper respiratory infection and patients with a history of reactive airway disease.[163–165] Caution is required,

however, particularly in children with upper respiratory infection, because the risk of laryngospasm is still present. The LMA has also become an important tool in the management of the difficult airway (see discussion under Difficult Airway). However, it should be noted that the LMA is a supraglottic device and as such does not protect against pulmonary aspiration of gastric contents.[154–156]

The recommended insertion technique is the same as is described for adults. The cuff is completely deflated, and the posterior surface of the mask is well lubricated. The patient is placed in the age-appropriate intubating position. Induction may proceed by inhalation of halothane or sevoflurane or by intravenous injection of 3 to 3.5 mg/ kg of propofol.[149, 166] The noninsertion hand is used to extend the head and flex the neck (sniffing position). The laryngeal mask airway is inserted with the mask aperture facing anteriorly (toward the tongue). The index finger of the insertion hand should be placed in the cleft between the mask and the barrel. With the index finger, one pushes the LMA upward and backward toward the top of the patient's head. This will flatten the mask against the palate. Continued backward pressure (toward the top of the patient's head) will guide the LMA along the palate and down into the upper esophageal sphincter. It is essential that pressure be applied to force the LMA against the roof of the mouth. The mask is advanced along the palate until some resistance is felt. At this point, air is injected into the mask cuff (see Table 7–4 for maximum recommended inflation volumes). Inflating the cuff causes the end of the airway to move out of the mouth about 1 cm and forms a loose seal around the esophageal inlet, thus directing gas flow into the trachea. *If no outward movement is observed with inflation of the mask, the LMA is not properly positioned.* Proper position can be ascertained further by auscultation of breath sounds, movement of the anesthesia bag, measurement of expired carbon dioxide, the ability to provide gentle assisted ventilation, and, if necessary, by direct visualization with rigid or fiberoptic laryngoscopy. If the patient cannot be gently ventilated (peak airway pressure < 20 cm H_2O) or no breath sounds are heard, the LMA must be immediately removed because it has not been properly positioned and the patient's airway might be obstructed. When proper placement is confirmed, the LMA should be secured with tape, and a soft bite block, such as a rolled gauze, should be inserted.

Several reports claim that when the traditional insertion technique is used in children, the LMA frequently hangs up in the posterior pharynx, thus making proper positioning

Table 7–4. Selecting Laryngeal Mask Size

Mask Size	Patient's Weight	Maximum Cuff Volume (mL)	Largest Endotracheal Tube (mm ID)
1	Neonate/infants up to 5 kg	4	3.5
1.5	Infants 5–10 kg	7	4.0
2	Infants/children 10–20 kg	10	4.5
2.5	Children 20–30 kg	14	5.0
3	Children/small adults over 30 kg	20	6.0, cuffed
4	Normal and large adolescents/adults	30	6.0, cuffed
5	Large adolescents/adults	40	7.0, cuffed

ID, interior diameter.

difficult.[167, 168] Therefore, other insertion techniques have been described. The rotational or reverse technique for children has been advocated as simpler and more successful than the traditional placement technique. The LMA is placed in the mouth with the cuff facing the hard palate (the opposite of the traditional technique). It is then advanced and rotated into position simultaneously.[167, 168] A partial mask inflation technique has also been advocated as more successful than the traditional (mask deflated) technique.[169] The LMA is left partially inflated to smooth the edges of the mask and then is inserted in the usual manner.[170] A jaw thrust maneuver and the use of a rigid laryngoscope have also been advocated to assist in placement.[171]

Regardless of insertion method, the most common cause of failure is using an LMA that is the wrong size. An LMA that is too large will not pass beyond the posterior pharynx. An LMA that is too small will pass easily but will not seal against the laryngeal inlet. Another common mistake when using the traditional insertion method is to try to press the LMA *down* into the pharynx. Pressure should be directed *back,* toward the pharyngeal wall, so the airway will follow the natural curve of the pharynx and seat correctly in the esophageal sphincter without kinking. Attempting to place the LMA when the patient is inadequately anesthetized may make advancement impossible or result in laryngospasm.

Insertion of an LMA can result in laryngeal injuries.[172, 173] Various studies report that sore throat is as common as with endotracheal intubation.[174, 175] LMA use in infants requires special caution. A review of the use of the size 1 LMA in 50 infants found that the LMA may migrate over time even after apparent correct initial placement (delayed airway obstruction occurred in 12 infants after apparent successful placement).[176] Vigilance is required to prevent loss of the airway. However, the LMA has been used successfully for neonatal resuscitation. Some suggest that this is an easier skill to acquire than bag-mask ventilation.[177, 178]

The timing for removal of the LMA in the pediatric patient is controversial. Experts have advocated both "awake" and "deep" removal.[169, 179–183] Deep removal avoids excessive airway reactivity and potential laryngospasm but may increase the risk of aspiration or airway obstruction. Awake removal ensures return of protective reflexes but with the attendant problems of airway reactivity. One author suggests leaving the cuff inflated until the child begins swallowing or is able to open the mouth upon command as a means of reducing the potential for laryngospasm.[169] Lubrication of the cuff with 2% lidocaine jelly or the addition of intravenous narcotics to the anesthetic may reduce coughing on emergence.[170]

A new prototype laryngeal mask modified specifically for children has been evaluated. This LMA has a second smaller mask that rests against the upper esophageal sphincter. It also has a second cuff to increase the seal pressure of the glottic mask. The dorsal and ventral cuffs communicate, allowing simultaneous inflation by a single pilot balloon. The new LMA is reported to be easy to insert, to allow higher airway pressures with positive pressure ventilation and to provide better protection against gastric insufflation.[184]

Other Airway Devices
Cuffed Oropharyngeal Airway (COPA)

The cuffed oropharyngeal airway (COPA) consists of an oral airway with an integrated inflatable cuff and a 15 mm

adapter at its proximal end for attachment to the anesthesia circuit (Fig. 7–18).[185, 186] It is available in four sizes: 8, 9, 10, and 11 cm. There are no pediatric sizes available, although the 8 cm size has been used in children as young as 2 years.[187] This device is advocated as a hands-free alternative to airway management in short procedures in which the patient will be breathing spontaneously. Initial reports conclude, however, that many patients require at least one airway intervention during an average anesthetic session to maintain airway patency.[185, 186] The COPA has also been described for use as an aid to fiberoptic intubation.[188–190] There are conflicting reports regarding its advantage over the use of LMA, however.[191–197] Further study is needed to elucidate the role of this device in the airway management of children.

Glottic Aperture Seal Airway

The glottic aperture seal airway is a supraglottic device that is similar to the LMA. It consists of a breathing tube that ends in a foam cushion designed to fit across the surface of the laryngeal inlet. An inflation balloon lies behind the foam cushion. When the device is properly placed and this balloon is inflated, it presses the foam cushion against the laryngeal inlet to create a seal. A preliminary report in adults states that this device is as easy to place as the LMA and capable of allowing higher ventilation pressures.[198] There are no pediatric-sized devices available at this time.

Airway Management: The Abnormal Airway

Classifying the Abnormal Pediatric Airway

It is important to recognize circumstances that may cause airway obstruction or difficult laryngoscopy. Conditions that

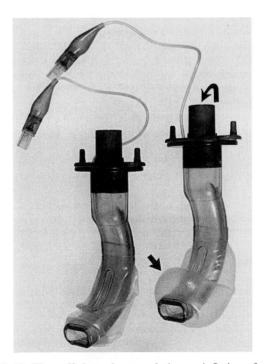

Figure 7–18. The cuffed oropharyngeal airway; inflation of the cuff (straight arrow) seals the airway and a 15 mm connector (curved arrow) allows direct connection to the anesthesia circuit.

Table 7–5. Pediatric Airway Pathology Related to Anatomic Site

Anatomic Site	Etiology	Clinical Condition
Nasopharynx	Congenital	Choanal atresia, stenosis,[19, 20] encephalocele[304]
	Traumatic	Foreign body, trauma
	Inflammatory	Adenoidal hypertrophy,[305] nasal congestion[21]
	Neoplastic	Teratoma
Tongue	Congenital	Hemangioma, Beckwith-Wiedemann syndrome,[306] Down syndrome[307–315]
	Traumatic	Burn, laceration, lymphatic/venous obstruction[99, 100, 316–321]
	Metabolic	Beckwith-Wiedemann syndrome,[322, 323] hypothyroidism, mucopolysaccharidosis,[324–326] glycogen storage disease,[327] gangliosidosis, congenital hypothyroidism
	Neoplastic	Cystic hygroma,[328, 329] cystic teratoma
Mandible/maxilla	Congenital hypoplasia	Pierre Robin syndrome,[330–338] Treacher Collins syndrome,[339–343] Goldenhar syndrome,[344, 345] Apert syndrome,[346] achondroplasia,[347–350] Turner syndrome,[351, 352] Cornelia de Lange syndrome,[353, 354] Smith-Lemli-Opitz syndrome,[355] Hallermann-Streiff syndrome,[356] Crouzan syndrome[357]
	Traumatic	Fracture,[358] neck burn with contractures
	Inflammatory	Juvenile rheumatoid arthritis[359–363]
	Neoplastic	Tumors, cherubism[364]
Pharynx/larynx	Congenital	Laryngomalacia (infantile larynx),[365] Freeman-Sheldon syndrome (whistling face),[366, 367] laryngeal stenosis,[368] laryngocele,[365] laryngeal web
	Traumatic	Dislocated/fractured larynx,[369–375] foreign body,[39, 40, 376–384] inhalation injury (burn),[316–321] postintubation edema/granuloma/stenosis,[385–395] swelling of uvula,[99] soft palate trauma, epidermolysis bullosa[396–398]
	Inflammatory	Epiglottitis,[35–37, 399–414] acute tonsillitis,[305] peritonsillar abscess,[415, 416] retropharyngeal abscess, diphtheritic membrane, laryngeal polyposis[417–419]
	Metabolic	Hypocalcemic laryngospasm[32]
	Neoplastic	Tumors
	Neurologic	Vocal cord paralysis, Arnold-Chiari malformation[420–423]
Trachea	Congenital	Vascular ring,[41, 42] tracheal stenosis,[424] tracheomalacia[365, 368, 395, 403]
	Inflammatory	Laryngotracheobronchitis (viral),[34, 37, 38, 122, 425–427] bacterial tracheitis
	Neoplastic	Mediastinal tumors: neurofibroma,[428] paratracheal nodes (lymphoma)

predispose to airway problems may be grouped according to anatomic location and may result from congenital, inflammatory, traumatic, metabolic, or neoplastic disorders. Tables 7–5 and 7–6 list the more common pediatric airway problems according to anatomic location. Appendix 7–1 lists the more common pediatric syndromes and associated anesthetic considerations; more complete information may be obtained elsewhere.[199, 200]

Management Principles

For any laryngoscopy, but especially for a difficult airway, the proper array of equipment must always be available. We advocate the creation of a difficult airway cart stocked with equipment useful in the management of the difficult airway for pediatric patients of all sizes and ages. Suggestions for contents are listed in Table 7–7. The approach to a difficult airway, as described earlier, must include a careful history and physical examination and, when indicated, radiologic evaluation. In the past, lateral neck xerograms have been useful in delineating anatomic aberrations; however, magnetic resonance imaging and computed tomography have largely replaced this modality.[80–95] In addition to the airway pathology, the pathophysiology of the congenital syndrome or associated disease process must be fully evaluated.

Table 7–6. Cervical Spine Anomalies*

Etiology	Clinical Condition
Congenital	Down syndrome,[310–315, 429] Klippel-Feil malformation,[430] Goldenhar syndrome,[344, 345] torticollis
Traumatic	Fracture, subluxation,[369–373, 431] neck burn contracture
Inflammatory	Juvenile rheumatoid arthritis[359–363]
Metabolic	Mucopolysaccharidosis (Morquio syndrome)[324–326, 432–437]

*Abnormalities of the cervical spine may limit extension and flexion, thus contributing to the difficulties of airway management; a significant percentage of Down syndrome infants have atlantoaxial instability.[314, 315]

Table 7–7. Suggested Equipment for Difficult Airway Cart

Laryngoscope blades and handles (spares), Oxyscope*
Endotracheal tubes of various sizes
Stylets and endotracheal tube guides
Fiberoptic intubation equipment
Retrograde intubation equipment
Laryngeal mask airways (all sizes)
Dilational percutaneous cricothyrotomy kits
Jet ventilation stylets
Equipment for jet ventilation
Endotracheal tube exchangers
Exhaled CO_2 detector
Oral and nasopharyngeal airways (variety of sizes)

*Foregger, Langhorne, PA.

The safest approach to managing a difficult airway is to formulate a plan and have skilled help available, especially a surgeon experienced in performing pediatric bronchoscopy and tracheostomy. To maximize success and safety, a skilled assistant should help position the patient, facilitate airway management, and help observe the monitors and the patient's vital signs. To direct an assistant, there should be clear communication about the airway management plan and specific details about maneuvers needed to facilitate the process. Familiarity with difficult airway algorithms and difficult airway management reviews can help the practitioner formulate a reasonable plan and ensure that no viable management options are missed.[201–206]

Certain general principles apply to the management of any patient in whom difficulty with airway management is anticipated. In most circumstances, an awake or awake but sedated approach would be the primary management strategy for the anticipated difficult airway if airway concerns were considered in isolation. However, often the practitioner who is caring for a child is restricted from choosing an awake approach because of difficulty with patient cooperation. Assisted spontaneous ventilation during general anesthesia is the preferred technique when abnormal airway anatomy is present and difficulty with patient cooperation is anticipated; it provides adequate oxygenation while the airway is evaluated for the appropriate approach to tracheal intubation. Thus the first choice for management of a potentially difficult airway is to maintain spontaneous ventilation whether the patient is sedated or under general anesthesia.[84, 201, 206–209] There are two reasons for maintaining spontaneous gas exchange. First, should neuromuscular blockade be administered to facilitate intubation, total airway obstruction can result because the muscle tone of the tongue, pharyngeal and laryngeal muscles, and suspensory ligaments is lost; this obstruction may not be easily alleviated with manual ventilation of the lungs. If airway obstruction or the potential for airway obstruction exists, neuromuscular blockade should not be used.[27] Second, if a patient is paralyzed, the loss of spontaneous breath sounds eliminates a valuable guide to locating the glottis. For example, in patients with Goldenhar, Pierre Robin, and Treacher Collins syndromes or with cervical burn contracture, one may be able to visualize only the tip of the epiglottis with rigid laryngoscopy. By shaping the endotracheal tube tip into a 90-degree angle with a stylet, placing the tip behind the epiglottis, and then listening for breath sounds with the ear in proximity to the proximal end of the tracheal tube, one is often able to "blindly" locate the glottic opening and trachea (Fig. 7–19).

If a patient is able to cooperate with an awake, sedated method of airway management, there are several options. Opioids are often used in combination with benzodiazepines. The opioid blunts airway reactivity and decreases discomfort while the benzodiazepine provides anxiolysis and amnesia. Benzodiazepine-opioid combinations, particularly fentanyl and midazolam, are effective for sedation of adolescents and mature preteens.[210] For pediatric usage, dosing is based on weight, but also guided by clinical parameters, including pre-existing medical conditions that may affect sensitivity to these medications. For younger and less cooperative patients, the addition of small doses of droperidol adds a neuroleptic dimension and may improve success with this technique.

However, it is important to keep in mind that droperidol, unlike a benzodiazepine or opioid, has no reversal agent.

For an already frightened young child, benzodiazepine-opioid sedation may be difficult; sufficient sedation to ensure compliance with securing the airway may be too much to preserve adequate spontaneous ventilation. Alternatively, ketamine, which provides both hypnosis and analgesia, can be used alone or in conjunction with midazolam for infants, young children, or older children or adolescents who are intellectually impaired.[210] Ketamine usually preserves adequate spontaneous ventilation while providing anesthesia to prevent laryngeal reactions to airway manipulation. Ketamine and midazolam should be slowly titrated to effect so as to avoid oversedation and apnea.[211] It should be recalled that midazolam takes nearly 5 minutes to achieve peak electroencephalographic effects, therefore necessitating adequate time between incremental doses (see Fig. 9–2).[212, 213] Ketamine is generally titrated in doses of 0.25 to 0.5 mg/kg every 2 minutes. Although there is a high incidence of psychomimetic emergence reactions in adults, these reactions are less common in children, particularly if combined with midazolam. Ketamine can cause increased secretions that may increase airway reactivity and interfere with fiberoptic airway management. Administration of an antisialagogue prior to ketamine and pre-endoscopy suctioning of the airway is recommended so as to minimize this problem.

Topical anesthesia can be used in conjunction with sedation or general anesthesia to blunt airway reactivity in those patients in whom spontaneous ventilation is preserved. For children, useful methods to provide topical anesthesia to the airway include (1) nebulized lidocaine; (2) topical application of local anesthetic sprays, jellies, or ointments; (3) translaryngeal delivery of lidocaine; (4) "spray as you go" with lidocaine injected onto the surface of the larynx and vocal cords through the channel of a fiberoptic scope usually used for suctioning or administering oxygen; and (5) superior laryngeal nerve block.[210] Caution is required to avoid delivering a toxic dose of local anesthetic. Maximum doses of the local anesthetic are based on the patient's weight and should be calculated in advance. Lidocaine seems to have the best safety profile; we limit our maximum dose to 5 mg/kg. We do not recommend the use of Cetacaine spray in children weighing less than 40 kg, since it is associated with methemoglobinemia and it is difficult to titrate or limit the dose administered.[73, 214] An antisialagogue decreases secretions that can interfere with the effectiveness of topically administered local anesthesia and with flexible fiberoptic techniques. In addition, the anticholinergic effect of atropine or glycopyrrolate will blunt the reflex bradycardia that can occur with airway manipulation.

Many techniques and devices for managing a difficult airway have been recommended. These techniques and devices are reviewed in detail below. Previous experience in normal airways can render these devices valuable adjuncts in difficult airway management.

Finally, if one is unable to intubate the airway, it is important to recognize the limits of one's ability. In this circumstance, the anesthesiologist should not hesitate to seek assistance from a colleague or request the surgeon to perform a tracheostomy or bronchoscopy. As an alternative, the child can be awakened and referred to a major pediatric center. In an urgent life-threatening situation, LMA placement or

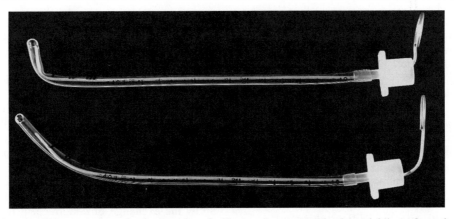

Figure 7–19. A stylet placed within an endotracheal tube often facilitates placement ("hockey-stick" configuration, bottom). In children with midfacial hypoplasia syndromes, in which the anatomic relation of the base of the tongue to the laryngeal inlet is abnormal, a stylet with a 90-degree bend 1 to 2 cm from the tip allows placement of the endotracheal tube behind the epiglottis and at the laryngeal inlet (top). Breath sounds audible at the 15 mm connector confirm appropriate location; maintaining the position of the stylet while advancing the endotracheal tube frequently allows successful "blind" endotracheal intubation even without the use of special airway equipment.

percutaneous cricothyroidotomy may be life-saving (see Unexpected Difficult Intubation).[145, 159, 161, 162, 215–217]

Documentation

Documentation of the difficult airway is essential to providing useful information for the next time that the child requires sedation or anesthesia. A note in the anesthesia record should clearly address the following issues:

1. Whether or not mask ventilation was attempted and if so, if there was any difficulty.
2. Special maneuvers that were required for successful mask ventilation.
3. Special maneuvers that were not helpful with mask ventilation.
4. Any difficulty with intubation.
5. Special techniques that were required for successful intubation.
6. Special techniques that were not helpful for intubation.
7. Grade of laryngoscopic view of laryngeal structures during rigid laryngoscopy (Fig. 7–20).

In addition to discussion with the family and patient (when age-appropriate), a letter should be written to the family and patient outlining the difficulties and referring them to the Medic Alert registry.[218] This should be copied and circulated to the medical record and the Medic Alert registry. In the United States, the Medic Alert registry for difficult airway or difficult intubation can be reached at 1(800)432-5378. Similar registries are also being formed internationally.[219] The Medic Alert registration form asks for clinical details about the type of airway difficulty, maneuvers that were successful in management, and those that were not. Any practitioner who provides airway management to the registered patient can update this information at any time. Despite the fact that scoring systems used in adults[68–72] have not been thoroughly investigated in children,[73] it is nevertheless useful to describe in detail the view of the larynx one was able to achieve and how it was achieved (e.g., blade type, size, external cricoid pressure) (see Fig. 7–20).

Unexpected Difficult Intubation

With careful preoperative evaluation and planning, the unexpected difficult pediatric airway should be a rare event. However, the practitioner should always be prepared for this potentially life-threatening event. Because the unexpected difficult airway occurs after beginning an anesthetic procedure, many of the management decisions required for the anticipated difficult airway have been made. Of primary importance is maintaining adequate oxygenation while a

Grade I   Grade II   Grade III   Grade IV

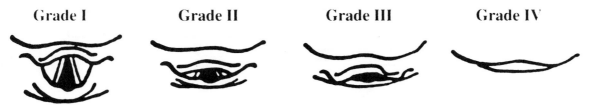

Figure 7–20. The laryngoscopic grading system of Cormack and Lehane offers a reasonable means of describing visualization of the larynx. It is useful to grade the degree of visualization during laryngoscopy and how that visualization was achieved, such as external cricoid pressure or laryngeal manipulation, the size and configuration of the laryngoscope blade, and so on. This provides useful information for the next person attempting laryngoscopy so that they have some degree of knowledge regarding what to expect. Grade I is visualization of the complete laryngeal opening; grade II, visualization of just the posterior area; grade III, visualization of just the epiglottis; and grade IV, visualization of just the soft palate. (From Cormack RS, Lehane J: Difficult tracheal intubation in obstetrics. Anaesthesia 1984;39:1105–1111.)

definitive course of action is pursued. A reasonable decision tree, based on the American Society of Anesthesiologists' difficult airway algorithm is presented in Figure 7–21. An important difference between infants and adults should be noted in this scenario. Because infants have an increased metabolic rate and decreased functional residual capacity, the time between the loss of the airway and resultant hypoxemia with secondary neurologic injury is significantly diminished compared with adults.[220] Approximate time to zero oxygen saturation from an inspired oxygen concentration of 90% is 4 minutes in a 10 kg child, whereas the same event in a healthy 70 kg adult takes almost 10 minutes.[221]

Extubation of the Child with the Difficult Airway

Unless a child in whom airway management is difficult requires a tracheostomy for long-term management, he or she will require extubation. Preparation for extubation begins shortly after the airway is secured. Equipment used to secure the airway should be rechecked, quickly returned to functional status, and then left in the operating room until successful extubation. Patients who had prolonged attempts at intubation or who will have procedures that may lead to airway edema may benefit from a dose of dexamethasone

(0.5–1 mg/kg). If significant airway edema is suspected either because of airway management or the type of surgery, one should consider leaving the patient intubated postoperatively until this resolves. The patient must be fully awake and have full return of strength and adequate ventilatory effort before extubation is attempted. Consideration should be given to extubation over a ventilating stylet (Airway exchanger, Rapi-Fit, Cook Inc., Bloomington, IN). The ventilating stylet is a hollow plastic guide with holes on its distal end and an adapter on its proximal end that allows the placement of either a Luer-lock connector for connection to a jet-ventilator or a 15 mm adapter for connection to standard anesthesia ventilating systems. It is available in four sizes to allow the exchange of endotracheal tubes greater than 3, 4, 5, or 6 mm ID. It can be used for oxygenation and ventilation and as a guide to reinsert the endotracheal tube if the patient's ventilatory efforts are inadequate or if airway obstruction occurs.[222] Caution is required when using this device for jet ventilation, however, as significant barotrauma has been reported.[223, 224] In circumstances in which the patient will remain intubated for a prolonged period of time following surgery, it is advisable to have the patient return to the operating room for extubation. Both a surgeon who is prepared to perform rigid bronchoscopy or tracheostomy and

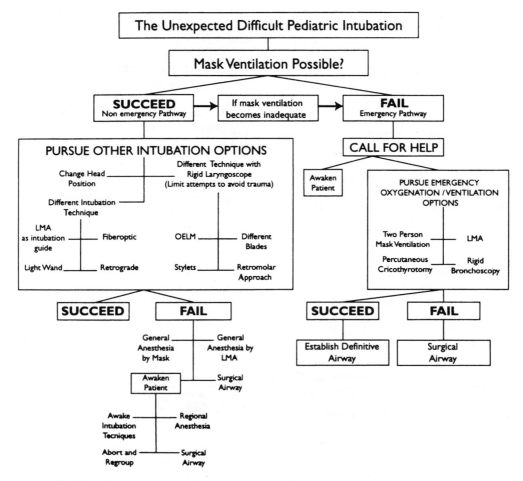

Figure 7–21. A suggested algorithm for management of the unexpected difficult pediatric airway. LMA, laryngeal mask airway; OELM, optimal external laryngeal manipulation. (From Wheeler M: Management strategies for the difficult pediatric airway. Anesth Clin North Am 1998;16:743–761.)

an anesthesiologist who is familiar with the techniques used for the previously successful airway management should be in attendance.

Special Techniques for Ventilation

Multihanded Mask Ventilation Techniques

Multihanded mask ventilation techniques can provide an effective temporizing measure until the airway is secured or the patient awakened. One person uses both hands to maintain an adequate mask fit and a second person compresses the ventilation bag (Fig. 7–22). A single person using two hands to optimize the mask fit and the anesthesia ventilator to provide ventilation can replicate this technique.[225] Occasionally, a second person must assist by performing a jaw thrust with one hand while compressing the anesthesia bag with the other. Rarely, a third person may be required to compress the anesthesia bag with two hands (so as to generate a higher peak inflation pressure) while the first person holds the mask with two hands and a second person performs a two-handed jaw thrust.

Laryngeal Mask Airway

The LMA has revolutionized difficult airway management in children. Numerous case reports and extensive clinical experience attest to the value of the LMA for establishing an airway when both ventilation and intubation are extremely difficult or impossible.[203, 226–229] The LMA has been described as a tool for use in both the non-emergency (can ventilate/cannot intubate) and the emergency pathway (cannot ventilate/cannot intubate) of the American Society of Anesthesiologists' difficult airway algorithm.[201, 203] Use has been described in the awake patient (LMA insertion in awake infants

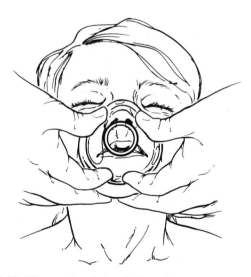

Figure 7–22. The two-handed technique for mask ventilation may be useful to improve mask fit and therefore ventilation when the traditional technique is inadequate. One person holds the mask while a second person squeezes the ventilation bag. Occasionally a third person is required to perform a two-handed jaw thrust (see text). (Reproduced with permission from American Academy of Pediatrics: Pediatric Advanced Life Support. Elk Grove Village, IL: © American Heart Association, 1994.)

with Pierre Robin syndrome)[227] and in the anesthetized patient with known or suspected difficult airway. It can be used as the definitive airway in some circumstances, as a conduit for intubation, or as a temporizing airway while other options are pursued, such as a surgical airway.

Percutaneous Needle Cricothyrotomy

In children, percutaneous needle cricothyrotomy is recommended over surgical cricothyrotomy because there is less risk of injury to vital structures such as the carotid arteries or jugular veins. In addition, most practitioners can more rapidly perform the percutaneous procedure. However, the cricothyroid membrane is of small width in infants and children. Attempts at cricothyrotomy may readily damage cricoid and thyroid cartilages, resulting in subsequent laryngeal stenosis and permanent damage to the speech mechanism. Therefore, this procedure should be reserved for use only under emergency circumstances.[230–234] A schema of this procedure is presented in Figure 7–23A–H. A commercial product called Jet-Ventilation-Catheter (VBM Medizintechnik GmBH, Sulz am Neckar, Germany) is available in three sizes: 18 gauge, 14 gauge, and 13 gauge. It consists of slightly curved puncture needle within a Teflon, kink-resistant cannula (Fig. 7–24). This cannula has two lateral eyes at its distal end and a combined Luer-lock and 15 mm adapter at its proximal end. It also has a fixation flange and foam neck tape to secure the airway. *Percutaneous needle cricothyrotomy provides only a means for oxygen insufflation and does not reliably provide the means for adequate ventilation.* In the spontaneously breathing patient, simple delivery of intratracheal oxygen may be sufficient in the short term because hypercarbia is generally well tolerated by healthy children.[231, 232] A number of children with arterial CO_2 values well above 150 mm Hg survived neurologically intact when adequate oxygenation was maintained.[235] Thus, simple oxygenation without attempts at ventilation may be all that is required to sustain life. For the child without respiratory effort, there is a need to provide ventilation in addition to oxygenation. An Ambu bag with the pop-off valve closed can provide some ventilation through a percutaneous catheter. Extremely high ventilating pressures are required, but midtracheal pressures are significantly lower (10–16 mm Hg).[232] A percutaneous cricothyrotomy catheter can also be used with a jet ventilation system. Jet ventilation via a catheter passed through a narrow glottic opening has also been described.[236–239] Be aware that if upper airway obstruction is present (for example after multiple unsuccessful attempts at rigid laryngoscopy), there will be a limited pathway for egress of air and oxygen and barotrauma may result from insufflation of oxygen or attempts at ventilation. Very serious morbidity and mortality may result from massive subcutaneous emphysema or tension pneumothorax.[240, 241] Thus, jet ventilation must be used with extreme caution in infants and children.[242]

A commercial kit is available for percutaneous dilation cricothyrotomy. A staged technique is used, similar to the Seldinger technique used for placement of central venous catheters, to place a larger airway. A percutaneous needle cricothyrotomy is performed and a guidewire is passed through the needle. The needle is removed, leaving the wire within the trachea. A scalpel blade is used to make a small

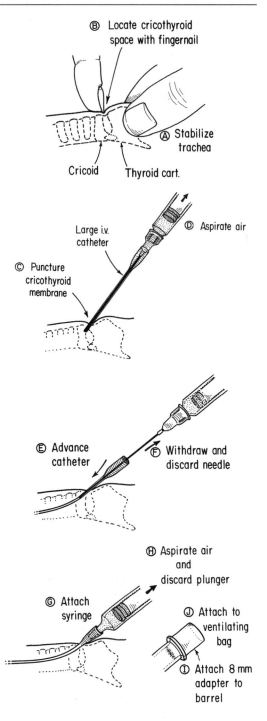

Figure 7–23. Percutaneous cricothyroidotomy. Extend the head in the midline with a rolled towel or folded sheet beneath the shoulders; standing to the left of the patient, stabilize trachea with the right hand (A). The cricothyroid membrane is located with the index fingertip of the left hand between the thyroid and cricoid cartilages (B). This space is so narrow (1 mm) in an infant that only a fingernail can discern it. The trachea is then stabilized between the middle finger and thumb of the left hand while the fingernail of the index finger marks the cricothyroid membrane. A large intravenous catheter (12- to 14-gauge) is then inserted through the cricothyroid membrane (C), and air is aspirated (D). The catheter is advanced into the trachea through the membrane (E), and the needle is discarded (F); intraluminal position is reconfirmed by attaching a 3 mL syringe (G) and aspirating for air (H). A 3 mm adapter from a pediatric endotracheal tube can be attached to any intravenous catheter (G). Ventilation is accomplished by attaching to a breathing circuit with a standard 22 mm connector. An alternative would be to leave the barrel of the 3 mL syringe attached to the intravenous catheter, insert an 8 mm endotracheal tube adapter to the syringe barrel (I) and then attach to a ventilating system with a standard 22 mm adapter (J). (From Coté CJ, Eavey RD, Todres ID, et al: Cricothyroid membrane puncture: Oxygenation and ventilation in a dog model using an intravenous catheter. Crit Care Med 16:615–619; © Williams & Wilkins, 1988.)

skin incision around the wire and a dilator is passed over the guidewire. The dilator is removed, leaving the wire within the trachea. The cricothyrotomy tube is passed over the dilator and both are threaded over the wire into the trachea. The dilator and guidewire are removed, leaving the airway in place. The Arndt Emergency Cricothyrotomy Set (Cook Critical Care, Bloomington, IN) provides a 3.0 mm ID airway that is sufficient for ventilation as well as oxygenation (Fig. 7–25). There is limited experience with this device in children, however, particularly infants. Other similar devices are available, also with limited pediatric use[243]; kits designed to place a full-sized tracheostomy are associated with significant morbidity.[244, 245] Direct large needle

cricothyrotomy kits, such as Nu-Trake (International Medical Devices, Inc., Northridge, CA) or Abelson (Gilbert Surgical Instruments, Inc., Bellmawr, NJ) may potentially cause tracheal/laryngeal injury in small patients because of the relatively large size of the needle, but again little experience in children is available.

Laryngeal Mask Airway Versus Percutaneous Needle Cricothyroidotomy and Transtracheal Jet Ventilation

The LMA has proven to be an extremely useful device in airway emergencies.[145, 159, 161, 162, 203, 215, 216, 227–229, 246] In contrast to percutaneous needle cricothyrotomy, it is an effective device for ventilation as well as a conduit for intubation. The LMA is easily inserted and requires a relatively low level of skill, as demonstrated in numerous studies that compare this technique to other airway management skills (e.g., mask ventilation, endotracheal intubation).[177, 178, 247–250] Also, in contrast to transtracheal jet ventilation, the complication rate is low.[251] However, this is a supraglottic device. If glottic or subglottic obstruction to ventilation is present, it will be ineffective and transtracheal jet ventilation via percutaneous needle cricothyrotomy is still the emergency technique of choice. Since the introduction of the LMA, clinical experience suggests that if glottic or subglottic pathology is not suspected, LMA placement to establish ventilation may be appropriately attempted first.[203]

Surgical Airway

Establishing a surgical airway emergently requires great technical skill. It is difficult to perform quickly and other methods to provide oxygenation should be pursued first. In nonemergent airway management for children, a tracheostomy is preferred to a cricothyrotomy because of fewer long-term complications and better results with later decannulation of the airway.[252]

Anterior Commissure Scope and Rigid Ventilating Bronchoscope

Two pieces of equipment used by otolaryngologists that can assist in visualizing the larynx and providing a method of ventilation are the anterior commissure scope and rigid ventilating bronchoscope. The anterior commissure scope is a rigid tubular straight blade laryngoscope with a light at the tip. The technique to place the anterior commissure scope

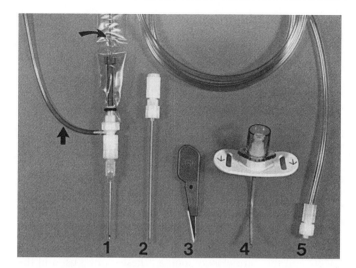

Figure 7–25. Percutaneous dilation cricothyrotomy uses a staged technique, similar to the Seldinger technique used for placement of central venous catheters, to place a secure airway. A percutaneous needle cricothyrotomy is performed and negative pressure via a syringe and side port (straight arrow) confirm aspiration of air. A guidewire (curved arrow) is then passed through the needle (1). The needle is removed, leaving the wire within the trachea. A scalpel (3) is used to puncture the skin. A dilator (2) is passed over the guidewire and removed, leaving the wire within the trachea. The cricothyrotomy tube (4) is passed over the dilator and both together are threaded over the guidewire into the trachea. The dilator and guidewire are removed, leaving the cricothyrotomy tube (airway) in place. The Arndt Emergency Cricothyrotomy Set (Cook Critical Care, Bloomington, IN) provides a 3 mm inside diameter airway that is sufficient for ventilation as well as oxygenation. A connection for jet ventilation is also provided (5). There is limited experience with this device in children, particularly infants.

and the advantages for visualization are similar to those described for the straight blade used with the retromolar approach.[253, 254]

Special Techniques for Intubation
Rigid Laryngoscopy

The rigid laryngoscope is the most familiar and most universally available piece of airway equipment; therefore, it is critical to be skillful in its use and to know a variety of techniques. Some suggestions are reviewed below. It is reasonable to take a second look with the rigid laryngoscope after an unexpected failed intubation; however, a good rule is to always change something about the approach that may improve visualization. Awake rigid intubation is also a traditional approach to the problematic infant airway. However, some anatomic features are completely unfavorable for success with the rigid laryngoscope, regardless of technique. Repeated unsuccessful attempts should be avoided because this can lead to airway trauma and edema. Since infants and children already have smaller airway structures, they are uniquely susceptible to a rapid progression from the "can ventilate/cannot intubate" to the "cannot ventilate/cannot intubate" scenario.

Tips and Techniques

Whether approaching a patient with a normal airway or a patient with an abnormal airway, it is essential to ensure

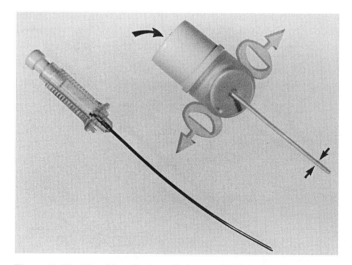

Figure 7–24. The Ventilation-Catheter (VBM, Medizintechnik GmBH, Sulz am Neckar, Germany) is available in three sizes: 18 gauge, 14 gauge, and 13 gauge. It consists of slightly curved puncture needle within a Teflon, kink-resistant cannula. This cannula has two lateral eyes (small arrows) at its distal end and a combined Luer-lock and 15 mm adapter (surrounding the Luer lock) at its proximal end (curved arrow), thus allowing both jet and standard ventilation. It also has a fixation flange and foam neck tape to secure the airway.

correct patient positioning and to use age-appropriate equipment. The following maneuvers have been found to be helpful in successful intubation of the patient with a difficult airway.

Optimal External Laryngeal Manipulation (OELM). This is pressure applied externally to the larynx during the intubation to maximize visualization.[255] OELM is particularly helpful for children with immobile or shortened necks and for infants. Either an assistant or the laryngoscopist can perform OELM. When the laryngoscopist performs the maneuver, either the assistant can pass the endotracheal tube into the glottis while the laryngoscopist maintains OELM or OELM can be assumed by the assistant to allow the laryngoscopist to pass the endotracheal tube.[255]

Intubation Guides. These include plastic coated flexible metal stylets and the gum elastic bougie. These can be used in the blind placement of the endotracheal tube under the epiglottis. A flexible stylet is placed inside the endotracheal tube and preformed to shape the endotracheal tube tip to one that will optimize intubation success (see Fig. 7–19). A hockey-stick configuration is frequently useful, particularly when only the epiglottis or the most posterior portion of the glottis can be visualized. The gum elastic bougie has a preformed angled tip. It is placed alone and then the endotracheal tube is threaded over it and into the trachea.

Oxyscope. The Oxyscope (Foregger, Langhorne, PA) is a Miller 1 laryngoscope blade with an insufflation channel along its length so that it may be attached to an oxygen source. An Oxyscope provides increased F_{IO_2} and is particularly useful for intubation in a conscious neonate whose oxygen consumption is high and in whom desaturation may rapidly develop (Fig. 7–26A, B).[256]

Dental Mirror. The authors of one report used a short-handled dental mirror (#3, Stortz Instrument Company, Manchester, MT, England) to assist in the indirect visualization of the larynx of a 10-week-old infant. Laryngoscopy was impossible with a Miller #1 blade. Therefore, the patient was returned to spontaneous ventilation and a Macintosh #1 blade was used to expose the pharynx and the mirror used to visualize the larynx. A styletted endotracheal tube was then passed into the glottis under indirect vision.[257]

Retromolar, Paraglossal, or Lateral Approach Using a Straight Blade. This technique may allow glottic visualization when the classic rigid intubation technique fails, particularly when the difficulty is secondary to a large tongue or small mandible (Fig. 7–27).[253, 254] With the head turned slightly to the left, a Miller blade is introduced into the extreme right side of the mouth. It is advanced in the space between the tongue and the lateral pharyngeal wall; the tongue is swept completely to the left and is essentially bypassed. It is very helpful to have an assistant pull back the right corner of the mouth with a small retractor, such as a Senn, to increase the space for endotracheal tube placement. The blade is advanced while staying to the right, overlying the molars, until the epiglottis or the glottis is visualized. If the epiglottis is seen, it is elevated with the blade tip to expose the glottis. At this point, it may be possible to bring the proximal end of the blade toward the midline to increase room for endotracheal tube placement and manipulation. If the glottis is not visualized, the head can be rotated further to the left and the blade can be kept lateral to improve visualization. The endotracheal tube should be styletted and formed into a 90-degree bend configuration to assist in placement (see Fig. 7–19), particularly if the view of the glottis is only partial. A shorter length blade, usually a Miller #1 even in older children, than that used in the traditional midline approach is chosen because the distance to the glottis with this method is greatly shortened.

Several mechanisms are responsible for the improved view of the glottis with the retromolar approach to laryngoscopy. First, there is a reduced need for soft tissue displacement and compression because the lateral placement of the blade bypasses the tongue. This mechanism for improved glottic visualization is particularly useful for the patient with

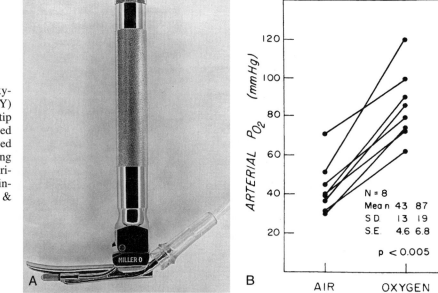

Figure 7–26. Modified laryngoscope. The Oxyscope (Olympus America, Inc., Melville, NY) delivers oxygen and anesthetic agent at the tip of the blade during laryngoscopy (A). Increased levels of arterial oxygen tension were achieved during laryngoscopy of spontaneously breathing infants (B). (From Todres ID, Crone RK: Experience with a modified laryngoscope in sick infants. Crit Care Med 9:544–545; © Williams & Wilkins, 1981.)

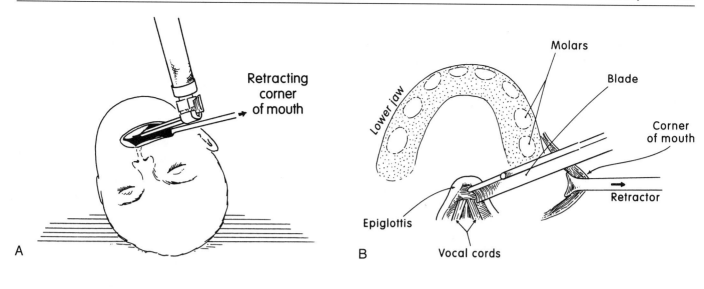

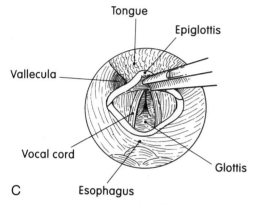

Figure 7–27. The retromolar, paraglossal, or lateral approach to rigid laryngoscopy utilizing a straight blade. Note that the patient's head is turned to the left (A) and that the laryngoscope blade is inserted over the molars (B) toward the glottic opening (C) (see text for details).

micrognathia. With this anomaly, there is reduced space for the tongue displacement that is required in the traditional midline approach to rigid laryngoscopy. Second, there is a lowered proximal end of the line of view because the incisors and maxillary structures are bypassed by lateral blade placement and by shifting the head to the left. Finally, the use of a straight blade avoids the possible intrusion of a curved blade into the line of view.[254]

Fiberoptic Laryngoscopy

Equipment. Fiberoptic bronchoscopes with directable tips are available in various sizes; the smallest is 2.2 mm in diameter (Olympus model LFP, Olympus America, Inc., Melville, NY) and can fit through a 2.5 mm ID endotracheal tube with the 15 mm adapter removed. However, unlike most of the larger fiberoptic bronchoscopes, this scope has no channel for suctioning or administration of oxygen or topical anesthesia (working channel). Newer fiberoptic bronchoscopes with the light source incorporated into the body of the scope are now available. These increase the portability of the instrument, making its use both outside and inside the operating room more simple and convenient.

Ancillary Equipment. Endoscopy masks can be used to provide oxygen to the spontaneously breathing patient and to ventilate the paralyzed patient during fiberoptic laryngoscopy. The Frei endoscopy mask (Fig. 7–28) and the Patil-Syracuse

endoscopy masks are commercially available.[258, 259] The Patil-Syracuse masks are available in a child size but are too large for most children under the age of 4 years.[73] The Frei mask configuration allows the fiberoptic bronchoscope to be placed in a central position, overlying the nose and mouth, which is more favorable for intubation. Alternatively, a disposable face mask can be combined with a bronchoscopic swivel adapter.[260] The fiberoptic scope can then be passed through the diaphragm of the adapter while ventilation is maintained via the anesthesia circuit. Two types of adapters are commercially available. One type is designed to be attached directly to an anesthesia mask. The other type is designed for placement on an endotracheal tube and can be modified to fit on the anesthesia mask by using a 15 mm to 22 mm adapter.

Commercial intubating oral airways are available for use in pediatric patients (IMD Inc., Park City, UT); however, there are only three sizes (infant, child, and adult) and no studies have evaluated their usefulness in assisting fiberoptic intubation in children. Guedel airways can also be modified for use as an oral intubation guide.[260] A strip is cut from the convex surface of the airway to create a channel for placement of the fiberoptic bronchoscope. This modified airway may be used to maintain a midline approach to the glottis, but it is ineffective as a bite block.

Direct Technique. The optimal position of the patient for fiberoptic bronchoscopy is different than the position for rigid

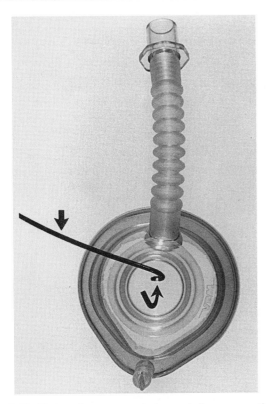

Figure 7–28. Frei endoscopy mask is used for oxygenation and ventilation of a patient; the fiberoptic laryngoscope (straight arrow) with a softened endotracheal tube of appropriate size (presoaked in warm sterile water but not shown) is passed through a membrane opening (curved arrow) in the mask. This allows maintenance of a constant depth of anesthesia and continuous oxygenation while visualizing the airway with the fiberscope.

laryngoscopy. The head should be flat on the table and slightly extended at the atlanto-occipital joint to prevent the epiglottis from obstructing a view of the glottic opening.[261] If an oral approach is selected, it is vital that the fiberoptic bronchoscope be passed in the midline. A nasal approach may make midline placement simpler and avoids the risk of a patient biting the fiberoptic bronchoscope or endotracheal tube. However, advantages of the oral over the nasal approach are that the potential problems of shearing adenoid tissue or causing nasal bleeding are avoided. The oral approach may also be less stimulating and better tolerated than the nasal approach. If nasal intubation is chosen in a young child, a topical vasoconstrictor may be administered to ease placement and reduce the potential for bleeding. An assistant should perform a jaw thrust to open the posterior pharyngeal space. Alternatively, a bite block or intubating airway may be used. Occasionally, the best view is obtained by direct traction on the tongue, which optimally opens the posterior pharynx. The tip of the bronchoscope should be introduced behind the tongue and gradually advanced in the midline under direct vision until a recognizable structure is observed. It is essential that the flexible bronchoscope be kept rigid so that when the direction of the tip is altered it remains in the same plane as the handle of the bronchoscope. When the bronchoscope is rotated, the tip should be slightly bent to provide a panoramic view. Generally, the tip of the bronchoscope is passed into the trachea before any attempts are

made at passing the endotracheal tube through the nose or oropharynx. Because the airway distances in children are shorter, the most common initial error in attempting this technique is to advance the fiberoptic scope too deeply and into the esophagus. To avoid this pitfall, the fiberoptic bronchoscope should only be advanced toward identifiable airway structures. The depth of anesthesia or sedation as well as oxygen saturation (pulse oximetry) must be carefully monitored throughout the procedure. Arrhythmias may be avoided by providing an adequate depth of analgesia or anesthesia and ensuring a patent airway.

Fiberoptic laryngoscopy techniques should be perfected on models and patients with normal anatomy before such techniques are attempted on patients with pathologic airway anatomy.[262–268] One study compared the time to intubation and complications between 20 normal infants intubated conventionally using a rigid Miller #1 laryngoscope and 20 normal infants intubated by using an Olympus LFP fiberoptic bronchoscope. Time to intubation was 13.6 ± 0.9 seconds in the conventional group and 22.8 ± 1.7 seconds in the fiberoptic group. There was no difference in complications. It was concluded that the routine use of the fiberoptic bronchoscope for intubation in normal infants is a safe and reasonable method to gain skills with this technique.[269]

Staged Techniques. Staged methods of fiberoptic intubation can be used in infants and small children when the available fiberoptic bronchoscopes are too large to pass through the appropriately sized endotracheal tube.[270] One method requires a fiberoptic bronchoscope with a working channel and a cardiac catheter with guide wire. The cardiac catheter guide wire is passed through the working channel of the fiberoptic bronchoscope to within 1 inch of its tip. The fiberoptic bronchoscope is then introduced into the mouth and positioned above the vocal cords. The guide wire is advanced under direct observation through the glottis into the trachea. The fiberoptic bronchoscope is removed, leaving the guide wire in place. The patient is ventilated by mask while an assistant passes the cardiac catheter over the guide wire (used to stiffen the guide wire to facilitate passing the endotracheal tube). The endotracheal tube is threaded over the catheter/guide wire combination, which is then removed, leaving the endotracheal tube in place.[270–272] Some authors have found that threading of the cardiac catheter over the guide wire is unnecessary. A modification of this technique when the fiberoptic bronchoscope has no working channel has also been described.[273] The authors used an 8F red rubber catheter attached by waterproof tape to the insertion cord of the fiberoptic bronchoscope proximal to the flexible tip. The larynx was visualized with the fiberoptic bronchoscope and a guide wire was threaded through the rubber catheter into the trachea. With the guide wire in position, the fiberoptic bronchoscope (with the red rubber catheter) was withdrawn and an endotracheal tube was passed over the guide wire into the trachea.

Another alternative for intubation when the fiberoptic bronchoscope is too large to pass through the appropriately sized endotracheal tube is intubation under fiberoptic observation.[274, 275] The fiberoptic bronchoscope is introduced through one of the nares to visually aid the placement of the endotracheal tube that is passed through the other of the nares and manipulated into the glottis. Alternatively, if the observed endotracheal tube is not easily passed into the glottis, a small catheter may be more easily manipulated into the glottis to be used as a stylet to pass the endotracheal tube into the trachea. Spontaneous ventilation is preserved and oxygen can be administered via the endotracheal tube during the intubation. This technique was used successfully in two neonates, one with congenital fusion of the jaws and the other with Dandy-Walker syndrome associated with Klippel-Feil, micrognathia, hypoplasia of the soft palate, and anteversion of the uvula.[274, 275]

If the available fiberoptic bronchoscope is both too large and lacks a working channel, another staged fiberoptic intubation technique can be used. The fiberoptic bronchoscope is loaded with an endotracheal tube that is larger than the larynx of the infant. The larynx is visualized with the fiberoptic bronchoscope and the endotracheal tube is advanced and positioned just above the vocal cords. The fiberoptic bronchoscope is then removed and an endotracheal tube changer or catheter is advanced into the trachea through the larger endotracheal tube. The larger endotracheal tube is then removed and the appropriately sized endotracheal tube for the child is threaded over the tube changer or catheter into the trachea. This technique was used successfully in a 6-month-old infant whose operation had been previously canceled because of failure to intubate.[276]

Advantages. Intubation with the flexible fiberoptic scope does not require extensive head or neck manipulation and is therefore useful in patients who have cervical inflexibility (Klippel-Feil syndrome) or instability (Down syndrome, achondroplastic dwarfism, trauma). The technique is very versatile because the flexible instrument conforms to a variety of abnormal airways; it is well tolerated by the awake, the sedated, and the spontaneously breathing patient.[210]

Disadvantages. Because the fiberoptic bundle that allows visualization is small and provides only a limited field of vision, the presence of blood or copious secretions may render the fiberoptic bronchoscope useless. In addition, the use of the fiberoptic bronchoscope requires extensive experience and practice in normal airways first. Our experience suggests that each size of available fiberoptic bronchoscope should be used in at least 20 normal airways before use is attempted in an abnormal airway. Practice with all available sizes of fiberoptic bronchoscopes is important because the manual skills required for each differ to a degree. Also, fiberoptic bronchoscopes are fragile and expensive. Great care must be taken when using and storing the fiberoptic bronchoscopes to prevent breakage of the fiberoptic bundles and of the adjustable tip mechanism. They must also be thoroughly cleaned between uses so as to maintain the patency of the working channel and clear, bright vision through the fiberoptic bundles.

Lighted Stylet

A lighted stylet ("light wand") is a useful adjunct in managing a difficult pediatric airway.[277–280] This device is essentially a malleable stylet with a high-intensity light at the tip; it is bent into a curve similar to that anticipated for successful passage into the laryngeal inlet (90–120 degrees). To begin, an endotracheal tube is passed over a well-lubricated light wand. The tip of the light wand should remain within the tip of the tube to minimize the potential for airway trauma. The light wand is then introduced into the mouth, following the curvature of the tongue. If the tip of the light wand is not in the proper position, that is, in the esophagus, a diffuse light or no light is observed on the surface of the neck. Proper position is usually ensured when a sharp, well-defined, bright circle of light is observed transilluminating the neck directly in the midline at the level of the cricothyroid membrane. Dimming the room lights may be helpful in identifying this light. Once proper position is ensured, the endotracheal tube is gently advanced and the stylet removed.[281] In general, this technique is useful in those patients in whom there is no intrinsic laryngeal or airway pathology, but in whom visualization is anticipated to be difficult. The light wand may also be of value in patients with a fracture of the cervical spine, because tracheal intubation can be accomplished without movement of the neck.[278] The hemodynamic response to intubation with this technique is similar to that with rigid laryngoscopy.[279] The limitations of this technique are that it is a blind technique and that it may require multiple attempts; however, the success rate markedly increases with experience.[281] The most common cause of difficulty is hanging up on the epiglottis. When this occurs, one should withdraw the light wand and slightly adjust its position more posterior so as to allow passage behind and beyond the epiglottis. Our advice for using this technique is similar to that for bronchoscopy; it should be used in children with normal anatomy to gain the necessary experience required for managing children with abnormal airway anatomy.

Bullard Laryngoscope

The Bullard laryngoscope is an instrument for direct visualization of the laryngeal inlet in patients with airway pathology (Fig. 7–29). It is available in three sizes: adult, pediatric, and pediatric long. This instrument combines fiberoptic techniques and mirrors; the fiberoptic bundles are contained within an instrument that functions and is positioned within the larynx like a laryngoscope blade. It is designed to provide visualization around a 90-degree bend at the tip. This configuration may be helpful for direct visualization of the larynx in children with mandibular hypoplasia syndromes, such as Pierre Robin, Treacher-Collins, and Goldenhar, or cervical fracture restricting motion, when the acute angulation of the base of the tongue to the glottic opening is exaggerated. Once the laryngeal inlet is visualized, a styletted endotracheal tube, with a bent configuration similar to the curve of the Bullard laryngoscope (see Fig. 7–19), is inserted just to the side of the Bullard laryngoscope blade and advanced under direct vision into the trachea. Success with this instrument is also directly proportional to the experience of the anesthesiologist, because the perspective seen through this laryngoscope and the method of visualization are so different from those of a standard laryngoscope. The endotracheal tube can partially obstruct the view of the larynx during insertion and this instrument can be used only for oral intubation.[282]

Retrograde Wire-Guided Intubation

This technique uses transtracheal passage of an intravenous catheter through the cricothyroid membrane into the larynx

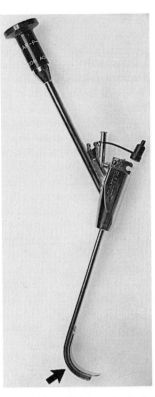

Figure 7–29. The Bullard laryngoscope is available in three sizes: adult, pediatric, and pediatric long. This instrument combines fiberoptic techniques and mirrors; the fiberoptic bundles are contained within an instrument that functions and is positioned within the larynx like a laryngoscope blade. It is designed to provide visualization around a 90-degree bend at the tip (arrow). This configuration may be helpful for direct visualization of the larynx in children with mandibular hypoplasia syndromes, such as Pierre Robin, Treacher-Collins, Goldenhar, or cervical fracture restricting motion, when the acute angulation of the base of the tongue to the glottic opening is exaggerated. Once the laryngeal inlet is visualized, a styletted endotracheal tube, with a bent configuration similar to the curve of the Bullard laryngoscope (see Fig. 7–19), is inserted just to the side of the Bullard laryngoscope blade and advanced under direct vision into the trachea.

and retrograde passage of a guide wire from a Seldinger vascular cannulation set to create a guide for intubation.[283–290] A commercial kit is available for use with endotracheal tubes that are 5 mm ID or larger (Cook Critical Care, Bloomington, IN).

Sight Wands

Sight wands consist of a malleable metal stylet containing a fiberoptic illumination fiber and a fiberoptic vision fiber that is then connected to an eyepiece. The light source may be external or attached to the housing at the base of the eyepiece.[291, 292] These are described for use either with or without rigid laryngoscopy. Sight wands that accommodate a 3.0 mm ID endotracheal tube are available.[291]

Laryngeal Mask Airway as a Conduit for Intubation

Numerous case reports affirm the usefulness of the LMA as a conduit for intubation.[216] Several methods for placing the endotracheal tube through the LMA have been described: blind, fiberoptic-assisted, stylet- or bougie-assisted, and retrograde-assisted.[216, 247, 293–297] Because of the high occurrence in children of the epiglottis overlying the laryngeal inlet,[298] even with apparently correct placement as judged by ability to ventilate, a visual technique for endotracheal tube placement, that is, fiberoptic-assisted, may be the best method. The largest endotracheal tube that will pass through each size of LMA is listed in Table 7–4.

Combined Techniques

Retrograde Wire and the Flexible Fiberoptic Scope. A case series reports the use of this technique in 20 children ages 1 day to17 years.[299] Equipment required is a ventilating endoscopic mask, equipment for retrograde wire intubation, a fiberoptic bronchoscope with a working channel, and grabbing forceps. The technique begins similarly to that of retrograde wire-guided intubation. A venous cannula is passed through the cricothyroid membrane in a cephalad manner. The needle is removed and lidocaine is injected to provide topical anesthesia. One must remember to aspirate first: detection of air confirms correct placement of the cannula within the lumen of the trachea. A guide wire of suitable length is passed through the cannula and advanced cephalad into the pharynx until it can be retrieved with the forceps from the mouth. The wire is then passed into the working channel of a fiberoptic bronchoscope in a retrograde manner starting at the tip of the fiberoptic bronchoscope (some fiberoptic bronchoscopes may require removal of tip components to allow the wire to pass). An endotracheal tube should already be threaded onto the fiberoptic bronchoscope. The fiberoptic bronchoscope is then advanced along the wire while the laryngoscopist looks for familiar anatomic structures. When placement of the fiberoptic bronchoscope tip below the vocal cords is confirmed, the wire is removed in the caudad direction from the cannula. The fiberoptic bronchoscope is advanced to mid-trachea and the endotracheal tube is threaded into place. Tips for success with the technique are to preserve spontaneous ventilation and to remove the guide wire in the caudad direction, as this will tend to pull the fiberoptic bronchoscope further into the airway rather than out of the airway, which might occur if it is removed in the opposite direction. This technique may improve success over retrograde technique alone, because the fiberoptic bronchoscope allows direct visualization and is a stiffer guide for the endotracheal tube than the wire alone. It also may improve success over the fiberoptic bronchoscope alone because the glottis is more readily found, even in the presence of blood or secretions.

Rigid Laryngoscopy and the Flexible Fiberoptic Scope. The rigid laryngoscope blade can be used to facilitate exposure so that a fiberoptic bronchoscope can be used to visualize the larynx.[300]

Flexible Fiberoptic Scope Used in a Retrograde Manner. This technique was used in a 4-year-old child with Nager syndrome who presented for tracheocutaneous fistula closure after decannulation of a tracheostomy. After failed attempts at rigid and direct fiberoptic endotracheal tube placement, a fiberoptic scope was placed in a retrograde fashion, using direct vision, through the fistula, past the vocal cords, into the nasopharynx, and out the nares. It was then used as a stylet for endotracheal tube placement.[301] The clinical scenario is unusual, but the technique was successful for this child.

REFERENCES

1. Fink BR, Demarest RJ: Anatomical background. In: Fink BR, Demarest RJ, eds: Laryngeal Biomechanics. Cambridge, MA: Harvard University Press; 1978:1–14.
2. Eckenhoff JE: Some anatomic considerations of the infant larynx influencing endotracheal anesthesia. Anesthesiology 1951;12:401–410.
3. Negus VE: The Comparative Anatomy and Physiology of the Larynx. New York: Grune & Stratton; 1949.
4. Jones HM: Acute epiglottitis: A personal study over twenty years. Proc R Soc Med 1970;63:706–712.
5. Ballenger JJ: Anatomy of the larynx. In: Ballenger JJ, ed: Diseases of the Nose, Throat, and Ear, 12th ed. Philadelphia: Lea & Febiger; 1977.
6. Pressman JJ, Kelemen G: Physiology of the larynx. Physiol Rev 1955;35:506–554.
7. Canuyt G: Les injections intratracheales par la voie intercricothyroidienne. Soc De Med Et Chir Bordeaux 1920; 249–259.
8. Harken DE, Salzberg AM: Transtracheal anesthesia for bronchoscopy. N Engl J Med 1948;239:383–385.
9. Bonica JJ: Transtracheal anesthesia for endotracheal intubation. Anesthesiology 1949;10:736–738.
10. Vandam LD: Functional anatomy of the larynx. Week Anesth Update 1977;1:2–6.
11. Fink BR: The mechanism of closure of the human larynx. Trans Am Acad Ophthalmol 1956;60:117–129.
12. Fink BR: The etiology and treatment of laryngeal spasm. Anesthesiology 1956;17:569–577.
13. Ardran GM, Kemp FH: The mechanism of the larynx. I. The movements of the arytenoid and cricoid cartilages. Br J Radiol 1966;39:641–654.
14. Ardran GM, Kemp FH: The mechanism of the larynx. II. The epiglottis and closure of the larynx. Br J Radiol 1967;40:372–389.
15. Cavagna GA, Margaria R: An analysis of the mechanics of phonation. J Appl Physiol 1965;20:301–307.
16. Wilson TG: Some observations on the anatomy of the infantile larynx. Acta Otolaryngol 1953;43:95–99.
17. Polgar P: Airway resistance in the newborn infant. J Pediatr 1961;59:915–921.
18. Polgar P, Kong GP: Nasal resistance of newborn infants. J Pediatr 1965;67:557–567.
19. Hobolth N, Buchmann G, Sandberg LE: Congenital choanal atresia. Acta Paediatr Scand 1967;56:286–294.
20. Maniglia AJ, Goodwin WJ Jr: Congenital choanal atresia. Otolaryngol Clin North Am 1981;14:167–173.
21. Passy V, Newcron S, Snyder S: Rhinorrhea with airway obstruction. Laryngoscope 1975;85:888–895.
22. Kurth CD, LeBard SE: Association of postoperative apnea, airway obstruction, and hypoxemia in former premature infants. Anesthesiology 1991;75:22–26.
23. Hudgel DW, Hendricks C: Palate and hypopharynx: Sites of inspiratory narrowing of the upper airway during sleep. Am Rev Respir Dis 1988;138:1542–1547.
24. Nandi PR, Charlesworth CH, Taylor SJ, et al: Effect of general anaesthesia on the pharynx. Br J Anaesth 1991;66:157–162.
25. Morikawa S, Safar P, DeCarlo J: Influence of the head–jaw position upon upper airway patency. Anesthesiology 1961;22:265–279.
26. Galloway DW: Upper airway obstruction by the soft palate: Influence of position of head, jaw, and neck. Br J Anaesth 1990;64:383–384.
27. Drummond GB: "Keep a clear airway." Br J Anaesth 1991;66:153–156.
28. Miller MJ, Carlo WA, Strohl KP, et al: Effect of maturation on oral breathing in sleeping premature infants. J Pediatr 1986;109:515–519.
29. Miller MJ, Martin RJ, Carlo WA, et al: Oral breathing in newborn infants. J Pediatr 1985;107:465–469.
30. deAlmeida VL, Alvaro RA, Haider Z, et al: The effect of nasal occlusion on the initiation of oral breathing in preterm infants. Pediatr Pulm 1994;18:374–378.
31. Wittenborg MH, Gyepes MT, Crocker D: Tracheal dynamics in infants with respiratory distress, stridor, and collapsing trachea. Radiology 1967;88:653–662.
32. Wilson TG: Stridor in infancy. J laryngol Otol 1952;66:437–451.
33. Fearon B, Whalen JS: Tracheal dimensions in the living infant (preliminary report). Ann Otol Rhinol Laryngol 1967;76:965–974.
34. Maze A, Bloch E: Stridor in pediatric patients. Anesthesiology 1979;50:132–145.
35. Lazoritz S, Saunders BS, Bason WM: Management of acute epiglottitis. Crit Care Med 1979;7:285–290.
36. Schloss MD, Hannallah R, Baxter JD: Acute epiglottitis: 26 years' experience at the Montreal Children's Hospital. J Otolaryngol 1979;8:259–265.
37. Davis HW, Gartner JC, Galvis AG, et al: Acute upper airway obstruction: Croup and epiglottitis. Pediatr Clin North Am 1981;28:859–880.
38. Baker SR: Laryngotracheobronchitis: A continuing challenge in child health care. J Otolaryngol 1979;8:494–500.
39. Cohen SR, Herbert WI, Lewis GB Jr, et al: Foreign bodies in the airway: Five-year retrospective study with special reference to management. Ann Otol Rhinol Laryngol 1980;89:437–442.
40. Stark DC, Biller HF: Aspiration of foreign bodies: diagnosis and management. Int Anesthesiol Clin 1977;15:117–145.
41. Mustard WT, Bayliss CE, Fearon B, et al: Tracheal compression by the innominate artery in children. Ann Thorac Surg 1969;8:312–319.
42. Macdonald RE, Fearon B: Innominate artery compression syndrome in children. Ann Otol Rhinol Laryngol 1971;80:535–540.
43. Wohl ME, Stigol LC, Mead J: Resistance of the total respiratory system in healthy infants and infants with bronchiolitis. Pediatrics 1969;43:495–509.
44. Bhutani VK, Rubenstein D, Shaffer TH: Pressure–induced deformation in immature airways. Pediatr Res 1981;15:829–832.
45. Cross KW, Tizard JPM, Trythall DAH: The gaseous metabolism of the newborn infant. Acta Paediatr Scand 1957;46:265–265.
46. Thibeault DW, Clutario B, Awld PA: The oxygen cost of breathing in the premature infant. Pediatrics 1966;37:954–959.
47. Butler J: The work of breathing through the nose. Clin Sci 1960;19:55–62.
48. Briscoe WA, DuBois AB: The relationship between airway resistance, airway conductance, and lung volume in subjects of different age and body size. J Clin Invest 1958;37:1279–1285.
49. Cook CD, Sutherland JM, Segal S, et al: Studies of respiratory physiology in the newborn infant, Part III. Measurements of mechanics of respiration. J Clin Invest 1957;36:440–448.
50. Mansell A, Bryan C, Levison H: Airway closure in children. J Appl Physiol 1972;33:711–714.
51. Anthonisen NR, Danson J, Robertson PC, et al: Airway closure as a function of age. Respir Physiol 1969;8:58–65.
52. Motoyama EK, Brinkmeyer SD, Mutich RL, Walczak SA: Reduced FRC in anesthetized infants: Effect of low PEEP. Anesthesiology 1982;57:A418–A418.
53. Sharp JT, Druz WS, Balagot RC, et al: Total respiratory compliance in infants and children. J Appl Physiol 1970;29:775–779.
54. Lacourt G, Polgar G: Interaction between nasal and pulmonary resistance in newborn infants. J Appl Physiol 1971;30:870–873.
55. Doershuk CF, Mathews LW: Airway resistance and lung volume in the newborn infant. Pediatr Res 1969;3:128–134.
56. Nelson NM, Prod'hom LS, Cherry RB, et al: Pulmonary function in the newborn infant: The alveolar-arterial oxygen gradient. J Appl Physiol 1963;18:534–538.
57. Phelan PD, Williams HE: Ventilatory studies in healthy infants. Pediatr Res 1969;3:425–432.
58. Krieger I: Studies on mechanics of respiration in infancy. Am J Dis Child 1963;105:439–448.
59. Epstein RA, Hyman AI: Ventilatory requirements of critically ill neonates. Anesthesiology 1980;53:379–384.
60. Keens TG, Bryan AC, Levison H, et al: Developmental pattern of muscle fiber types in human ventilatory muscles. J Appl Physiol 1978;44:909–913.
61. Keens TG, Ianuzzo CD: Development of fatigue-resistant muscle fibers in human ventilatory muscles. Am Rev Respir Dis 1979;2:139–141.
62. Keens TG, Chen V, Patel P, et al: Cellular adaptations of the ventilatory muscles to a chronic increased respiratory load. J Appl Physiol 1978;44:905–908.
63. Abernethy LJ, Allan PL, Drummond GB: Ultrasound assessment of the position of the tongue during induction of anesthesia. Br J Anaesth 1990;65:744–748.

64. Mathru M, Esch O, Lang J, et al: Magnetic resonance imaging of the upper airway: Effects of propofol anesthesia and nasal continuous positive airway pressure in humans. Anesthesiology 1996;84:273–279.

65. Drummond GB: Influence of thiopentone on upper airway muscles. Br J Anaesth 1989;63:12–21.

66. Schwartz AR, Smith PL, Wise RA, et al: Induction of upper airway occlusion in sleeping individuals with subatmospheric nasal pressure. J Appl Physiol 1988;64:535–542.

67. Borowiecki B, Pollak CP, Weitzman ED, et al: Fibro-optic study of pharyngeal airway during sleep in patients with hypersomnia obstructive sleep-apnea syndrome. Laryngoscope 1978;88:1310–1313.

68. Frerk CM: Predicting difficult intubation. Anaesthesia 1991;46:1005–1008.

69. Oates JD, MacLeod AD, Oates PD, et al: Comparison of two methods for predicting difficult intubation. Br J Anaesth 1991;66:305–309.

70. Karkouti K, Rose DK, Ferris LE, et al: Inter-observer reliability of ten tests used for predicting difficult tracheal intubation. Can J Anaesth 1996;43:554–559.

71. Mallampati SR, Gatt SP, Gugino LD, et al: A clinical sign to predict difficult tracheal intubation: A prospective study. Can Anaesth Soc J 1985;32:429–434.

72. Samsoon GL, Young JR: Difficult tracheal intubation: A retrospective study. Anaesthesia 1987;42:487–490.

73. Wheeler M: The difficult pediatric airway. In: Hagberg C, ed: Handbook of Difficult Airway Management. New York: Churchill Livingstone; 2000:257–300.

74. Gregory GA, Riazi J: Classification and assessment of the difficult pediatric airway. In: Riazi J, ed: The Difficult Pediatric Airway. Philadelphia: W B Saunders Company; 1998:729–741.

75. Cohen MM, Cameron CB: Should you cancel the operation when a child has an upper respiratory tract infection? Anesth Analg 1991;72:282–288.

76. Empey DW, Laitinen LA, Jacobs L, et al: Mechanisms of bronchial hyperreactivity in normal subjects after upper respiratory tract infection. Am Rev Respir Dis 1976;113:131–139.

77. Empey DW: Effect of airway infections on bronchial reactivity. Eur J Resp Dis-Supplement 1983;128:366–368.

78. Olsson GL: Bronchospasm during anaesthesia: A computer-aided incidence study of 136,929 patients. Acta Anaesthesiol Scand 1987;31:244–252.

79. Olsson GL, Hallen B: Laryngospasm during anaesthesia: A computer-aided incidence study in 136,929 patients. Acta Anaesthesiol Scand 1984;28:567–575.

80. Slovis TL, Haller JO, Berdon WE, et al: Noninvasive visualization of the pediatric airway. Curr Probl Diagn Radiol 1979;8:1–67.

81. Grunebaum M, Adler S, Varsano I: The paradoxical movement of the mediastinum. A diagnostic sign of foreign-body aspiration during childhood. Pediatr Radiol 1979;8:213–218.

82. Kushner DC, Harris GB: Obstructing lesions of the larynx and trachea in infants and children. Radiol Clin North Am 1978;16:181–194.

83. Doust BD, Ting YM: Xeroradiography of the larynx. Radiology 1974;110:727–730.

84. Gordon RA: Anesthetic management of patients with airway problems. Int Anesthesiol Clin 1972;10:37–59.

85. Rosenfield NS, Peck DR, Lowman RM: Xeroradiography in the evaluation of acquired airway abnormalities in children. Am J Dis Child 1978;132:1177–1180.

86. Walner DL, Ouanounou S, Donnelly LF, et al: Utility of radiographs in the evaluation of pediatric upper airway obstruction. Ann Otol Rhinol Laryngol 1999;108:378–383.

87. Rencken I, Patton WL, Brasch RC: Airway obstruction in pediatric patients. From croup to BOOP. Radiol Clin North Am 1998;36:175–187.

88. Contencin P, Gumpert LC, de G, I, et al: Non-endoscopic techniques for the evaluation of the pediatric airway. Int J Pediatr Otorhinolaryngol 1997;41:347–352.

89. Rimell FL, Shapiro AM, Meza MP, et al: Magnetic resonance imaging of the pediatric airway. Arch Otolaryngol Head Neck Surg 1997;123:999–1003.

90. Lee T, Lee SK: Upper airway obstruction in infants and children: Evaluation by tracheobronchography with a non-ionic contrast agent. Pediatr Radiol 1997;27:276–280.

91. Donnelly LF, Strife JL, Bisset GS III: The spectrum of extrinsic lower airway compression in children: MR imaging. AJR Am J Roentgenol 1997;168:59–62.

92. Reed JM, O'Connor DM, Myer CM, III: Magnetic resonance imaging determination of tracheal orientation in normal children: Practical implications. Arch Otolaryngol Head Neck Surg 1996;122:605–608.

93. Mahboubi S, Kramer SS: The pediatric airway. J Thorac Imaging 1995;10:156–170.

94. Simoneaux SF, Bank ER, Webber JB, et al: MR imaging of the pediatric airway. Radiographics 1995;15:287–298.

95. Mahboubi S, Meyer JS, Hubbard AM, et al: Magnetic resonance imaging of airway obstruction resulting from vascular anomalies. Int J Pediatr Otorhinolaryngol 1994;28:111–123.

96. Emergency Cardiac Care Committee and Subcommittees, American Heart Association: Guidelines for cardiopulmonary resuscitation and emergency cardiac care. Part VI. Pediatric advanced life support. JAMA 1992;268:2262–2275.

97. Airway and ventilation. In: Chameides L, Hazinski MF, eds. Pediatric Advance Life Support 2nd ed. Dallas: American Heart Association; 1994:4–1–4–22

98. Wheeler M, Roth AG, Dunham ME, et al: A bronchoscopic, computer-assisted examination of the changes in dimension of the infant tracheal lumen with changes in head position: Implications for emergency airway management. Anesthesiology 1998;88:1183–1187.

99. Haselby KA, McNiece WL: Respiratory obstruction from uvular edema in a pediatric patient. Anesth Analg 1983;62:1127–1128.

100. Moore MW, Rauscher LA: A complication of oropharyngeal airway placement. Anesthesiology 1977;47:526–526.

101. Davenport HT, Rosales JK: Endotracheal intubation in infants and children. Can Anaesth Soc J 1959;6:65–74.

102. Gillespie NA: Endotracheal anaesthesia in infants. Br J Anaesth 1939;17:2–12.

103. Westhorpe RN: The position of the larynx in children and its relationship to the ease of intubation. Anaesth Intensive Care 1987;15:384–388.

104. Reber A, Wetzel SG, Schnabel K, et al: Effect of combined mouth closure and chin lift on upper airway dimensions during routine magnetic resonance imaging in pediatric patients sedated with propofol. Anesthesiology 1999;90:1617–1623.

105. Shorten GD, Armstrong DC, Roy WI, et al: Assessment of the effect of head and neck position on upper airway anatomy in sedated paediatric patients using magnetic resonance imaging. Paediatr Anaesth 1995;5:243–248.

106. Lindgren L, Saarnivaara L: Cardiovascular responses to tracheal intubation in small children: Effects of the induction of anaesthesia with halothane. Br J Anaesth 1985;57:1183–1187.

107. Millar C, Bissonnette B: Awake intubation increases intracranial pressure without affecting cerebral blood flow velocity in infants. Can J Anaesth 1994;41:281–287.

108. Kong AS, Brennan L, Bingham R, et al: An audit of induction of anaesthesia in neonates and small infants using pulse oximetry. Anaesthesia 1992;47:896–899.

109. Friesen RH, Honda AT, Thieme RE: Changes in anterior fontanel pressure in preterm neonates during tracheal intubation. Anesth Analg 1987;66:874–878.

110. Slater HM, Sheridan CA, Ferguson RH: Endotracheal tube sizes for infants and children. Anesthesiology 1955;16:950–952.

111. Corfield HMC: Orotracheal tubes and the metric system. Br J Anaesth 1963;35:34.

112. Dobrin P, Canfield T: Cuffed endotracheal tubes: Mucosal pressures and tracheal wall blood flow. Am J Surg 1977;133:562–568.

113. Glauser EM, Cook CD, Bougas TP: Pressure-flow characteristics and dead spaces of endotracheal tubes used in infants. Anesthesiology 1961;22:339–341.

114. Tu HN, Saidi N, Leiutaud T, et al: Nitrous oxide increases endotracheal cuff pressure and the incidence of tracheal lesions in anesthetized patients. Anesth Analg 1999;89:187–190.

115. Munson ES, Stevens DS, Redfern RE: Endotracheal tube obstruction by nitrous oxide. Anesthesiology 1980;52:275–276.

116. Cole F: Pediatric formulas for the anesthesiologist. Am J Dis Child 1957;94:672–673.

117. Morgan GA, Steward DJ: Linear airway dimensions in children: including those from cleft palate. Can Anaesth Soc J 1982;29:1–8.

118. Morgan GA, Steward DJ: A pre-formed paediatric orotracheal tube designed based on anatomical measurements. Can Anaesth Soc J 1982;29:9–11.

119. Linko K, Paloheimo M, Tammisto T: Capnography for detection of accidental oesophageal intubation. Acta Anaesthesiol Scand 1983;27:199–202.

120. Rolf N, Coté CJ: Diagnosis of clinically unrecognized endobronchial intubation in paediatric anaesthesia: which is more sensitive, pulse oximetry or capnography? Paediatr Anaesth 1992;2:31–35.

121. Litman RS, Keon TP: Postintubation croup in children. Anesthesiology 1991;75:1122–1123.

122. Koka BV, Jeon IS, Andre JM, et al: Postintubation croup in children. Anesth Analg 1977;56:501–505.

123. Sitzman SJ, Fiechtner HB: Treatment of croup with glucocorticoids. Ann Pharmacother 1998;32:973–974.

124. Rizos JD, DiGravio BE, Sehl MJ, et al: The disposition of children with croup treated with racemic epinephrine and dexamethasone in the emergency department. J Emerg Med 1998;16:535–539.

125. Johnson DW, Jacobson S, Edney PC, et al: A comparison of nebulized budesonide, intramuscular dexamethasone, and placebo for moderately severe croup. N Engl J Med 1998;339:498–503.

126. Thomas LP, Friedland LR: The cost-effective use of nebulized racemic epinephrine in the treatment of croup. Am J Emerg Med 1998;16:87–89.

127. Yates RW, Doull IJ: A risk-benefit assessment of corticosteroids in the management of croup. Drug Safety 1997;16:48–55.

128. Kunkel NC, Baker MD: Use of racemic epinephrine, dexamethasone, and mist in the outpatient management of croup. Pediatr Emerg Care 1996;12:156–159.

129. Johnson DW, Schuh S, Koren G, et al: Outpatient treatment of croup with nebulized dexamethasone. Arch Pediatr Adolesc Med 1996;150:349–355.

130. Ledwith CA, Shea LM, Mauro RD: Safety and efficacy of nebulized racemic epinephrine in conjunction with oral dexamethasone and mist in the outpatient treatment of croup. Ann Emerg Med 1995;25:331–337.

131. Anene O, Meert KL, Uy H, et al: Dexamethasone for the prevention of postextubation airway obstruction: A prospective, randomized, double-blind, placebo-controlled trial. Crit Care Med 1996;24:1666–1669.

132. Couser RJ, Ferrara TB, Falde B, et al: Effectiveness of dexamethasone in preventing extubation failure in preterm infants at increased risk for airway edema. J Pediatr 1992;121:591–596.

133. Tellez DW, Galvis AG, Storgion SA, et al: Dexamethasone in the prevention of postextubation stridor in children. J Pediatr 1991;118:289–294.

134. Holinger PH, Kutnick SL, Schild JA, et al: Subglottic stenosis in infants and children. Ann Otol Rhinol Laryngol 1976;85:591–599.

135. Fearon B, Cotton R: Subglottic stenosis in infants and children: the clinical problem and experimental correction. Can J Otolaryngol 1972;1:281–289.

136. Cotton RT, Evans JN: Laryngotracheal reconstruction in children. Five-year follow-up. Ann Otol Rhinol Laryngol 1981;90:516–520.

137. Holinger LD, Lusk RP, Green CG: Pediatric Laryngology and Bronchoesophagology. Philadelphia: Lippincott-Raven; 1997.

138. Hawkins DB: Hyaline membrane disease of the neonate prolonged intubation in management: Effects on the larynx. Laryngoscope 1978;88:201–224.

139. Benjamin B: Prolonged intubation injuries of the larynx: Endoscopic diagnosis, classification, and treatment. Ann Otol Rhinol Laryngol 1993;160:1–15.

140. Liu H, Chen JC, Holinger LD, et al: Histopathologic fundamentals of acquired laryngeal stenosis. Pediatr Pathol Lab Med 1995;15:655–677.

141. Dankle SK, Schuller DE, McClead RE: Risk factors for neonatal acquired subglottic stenosis. Ann Otol Rhinol Laryngol 1986;95:626–630.

142. Sherman JM, Lowitt S, Stephenson C, et al: Factors influencing acquired subglottic stenosis in infants. J Pediatr 1986;109:322–327.

143. Benumof JL: Laryngeal mask airway. Indications and contraindications. Anesthesiology 1992;77:843–846.

144. Brain AI: The laryngeal mask: A new concept in airway management. Br J Anaesth 1983;55:801–805.

145. Brain AI: Three cases of difficult intubation overcome by the laryngeal mask airway. Anaesthesia 1985;40:353–355.

146. Brodrick PM, Webster NR, Nunn JF: The laryngeal mask airway: A study of 100 patients during spontaneous breathing. Anaesthesia 1989;44:238–241.

147. Haynes SR, Morton NS: The laryngeal mask airway: A review of its use in paediatric anaesthesia. Paediatr Anaesth 1993;3:65–73.

148. Grebenik CR, Ferguson C, White A: The laryngeal mask airway in pediatric radiotherapy. Anesthesiology 1990;72:474–477.

149. Ruby RR, Webster AC, Morley-Forster PK, et al: Laryngeal mask airway in paediatric otolaryngologic surgery. J Otolaryngol 1995;24:288–291.

150. Epstein RH, Halmi BH: Oxygen leakage around the laryngeal mask airway during laser treatment of port-wine stains in children. Anesth Analg 1994;78:486–489.

151. O'Hare K, Kerr WJ: The laryngeal mask as an antipollution device. Anaesthesia 1998;53:51–54.

152. Gursoy F, Algren JT, Skjonsby BS: Positive pressure ventilation with the laryngeal mask airway in children. Anesth Analg 1996;82:33–38.

153. Selby IR, Morris P: Intermittent positive ventilation through a laryngeal mask in children: does it cause gastric dilatation? Paediatr Anaesth 1997;7:305–308.

154. Valentine J, Stakes AF, Bellamy MC: Reflux during positive pressure ventilation through the laryngeal mask. Br J Anaesth 1994;73:543–544.

155. Owens TM, Robertson P, Twomey C, et al: The incidence of gastroesophageal reflux with the laryngeal mask: A comparison with the face mask using esophageal lumen pH electrodes. Anesth Analg 1995;80:980–984.

156. Ismail-Zade IA, Vanner RG: Regurgitation and aspiration of gastric contents in a child during general anaesthesia using the laryngeal mask airway. Paediatr Anaesth 1996;6:325–328.

157. Epstein RH, Ferouz F, Jenkins MA: Airway sealing pressures of the laryngeal mask airway in pediatric patients. J Clin Anesth 1996;8:93–98.

158. Webster AC, Morley-Forster PK, Dain S, et al: Anaesthesia for adenotonsillectomy: A comparison between tracheal intubation and the armoured laryngeal mask airway. Can J Anaesth 1993;40:1171–1177.

159. Badr A, Tobias JD, Rasmussen GE, et al: Bronchoscopic airway evaluation facilitated by the laryngeal mask airway in pediatric patients. Pediatr Pulmonol 1996;21:57–61.

160. Watcha MF, White PF, Tychsen L, et al: Comparative effects of laryngeal mask airway and endotracheal tube insertion on intraocular pressure in children. Anesth Analg 1992;75:355–360.

161. Bandla HP, Smith DE, Kiernan MP: Laryngeal mask airway facilitated fibreoptic bronchoscopy in infants. Can J Anaesth 1997;44:1242–1247.

162. Baraka A, Choueiry P, Medawwar A: The laryngeal mask airway for fibreoptic bronchoscopy in children. Paediatr Anaesth 1995;5:197–198.

163. Tait AR, Pandit UA, Voepel-Lewis T, et al: Use of the laryngeal mask airway in children with upper respiratory tract infections: A comparison with endotracheal intubation. Anesth Analg 1998;86:706–711.

164. Ferrari LR, Goudsouzian NG: The use of the laryngeal mask airway in children with bronchopulmonary dysplasia. Anesth Analg 1995;81:310–313.

165. Kim ES, Bishop MJ: Endotracheal intubation, but not laryngeal mask airway insertion, produces reversible bronchoconstriction. Anesthesiology 1999;90:391–394.

166. Martlew RA, Meakin G, Wadsworth R, et al: Dose of propofol for laryngeal mask airway insertion in children: Effect of premedication with midazolam. Br J Anaesth 1996;76:308–309.

167. Chow BF, Lewis M, Jones SE: Laryngeal mask airway in children: Insertion technique. Anaesthesia 1991;46:590–591.

168. McNicol LR: Insertion of laryngeal mask airway in children. Anaesthesia 1991;46:330.

169. Brain AIJ: Removal of the laryngeal mask airway: Airway complications in children anaesthetized versus awake. Paediatr Anaesth 1994;4:271.

170. O'Neill B, Templeton JJ, Caramico L, et al: The laryngeal mask airway in pediatric patients: Factors affecting ease of use during insertion and emergence. Anesth Analg 1994;78:659–662.

171. Yih PS: Laryngoscopy for pediatric laryngeal mask airway insertion. Can J Anaesth 1999;46:617.

172. Figueredo E, Vivar-Diago M, Munoz-Blanco F: Laryngo-pharyngeal complaints after use of the laryngeal mask airway. Can J Anaesth 1999;46:220–225.

173. Lowinger D, Benjamin B, Gadd L: Recurrent laryngeal nerve injury caused by a laryngeal mask airway. Anaesth Int Care 1999;27:202–205.

174. Splinter WM, Smallman B, Rhine EJ, et al: Postoperative sore throat in children and the laryngeal mask airway. Can J Anaesth 1994;41:1081–1083.

175. Rieger A, Brunne B, Hass I, et al: Laryngo-pharyngeal complaints

following laryngeal mask airway and endotracheal intubation. J Clin Anesth 1997;9:42–47.

176. Mizushima A, Wardall GJ, Simpson DL: The laryngeal mask airway in infants. Anaesthesia 1992;47:849–851.

177. Paterson SJ, Byrne PJ, Molesky MG, et al: Neonatal resuscitation using the laryngeal mask airway. Anesthesiology 1994;80:1248–1253.

178. Martens P: The use of the laryngeal mask airway by nurses during cardiopulmonary resuscitation: Results of a multicentre trial. Anaesthesia 1994;49:3–7.

179. Splinter WM, Reid CW: Removal of the laryngeal mask airway in children: Deep anesthesia versus awake. J Clin Anesth 1997;9:4–7.

180. Parry M, Glaisyer HR, Bailey PM: Removal of LMA in children. Br J Anaesth 1997;78:337–338.

181. Varughese A, McCulloch D, Stokes M: Removal of the laryngeal mask airway (LMA) in children: Awake or deep? Anesthesiology 1994;81:A1321–A1321.

182. Laffon M, Plaud B, Dubousset AM, et al: Removal of laryngeal mask airway: Airway complications in children, anaesthetized versus awake. Paediatr Anaesth 1994;4:35–37.

183. Kitching AJ, Walpole AR, Blogg CE: Removal of the laryngeal mask airway in children: Anaesthetized compared with awake. Br J Anaesth 1996;76:874–876.

184. Lopez-Gil M, Brimacombe J, Brain AI: Preliminary evaluation of a new prototype laryngeal mask in children. Br J Anaesth 1999;82:132–134.

185. Brimacombe J, Berry A: The cuffed oropharyngeal airway for spontaneous ventilation anaesthesia. Clinical appraisal in 100 patients. Anaesthesia 1998;53:1074–1079.

186. Asai T, Koga K, Jones RM, et al: The cuffed oropharyngeal airway: Its clinical use in 100 patients. Anaesthesia 1998;53:817–822.

187. Greenberg, RS, 1999, personal communication.

188. Greenberg RS, Kay NH: Cuffed oropharyngeal airway (COPA) as an adjunct to fibreoptic tracheal intubation. Br J Anaesth 1999;82:395–398.

189. Pigott DW, Kay NH, Greenberg RS: The cuffed oropharyngeal airway as an aid to fibreoptic intubation. Anaesthesia 1998;53:480–483.

190. Hawkins M, O'Sullivan E, Charters P: Fibreoptic intubation using the cuffed oropharyngeal airway and Aintree intubation catheter. Anaesthesia 1998;53:891–894.

191. Brimacombe J, Keller C: The cuffed oropharyngeal airway vs. the laryngeal mask airway: a randomized cross-over study of oropharyngeal leak pressure and fibreoptic view in paralyzed patients. Anaesthesia 1999;54:683–685.

192. Voyagis GS, Dimitriou VK, Kyriakis KP: Comparative evaluation of the prolonged use of the cuffed oropharyngeal airway and the laryngeal mask airway in spontaneously breathing anaesthetized patients. Eur J Anaesthesiol 1999;16:371–375.

193. Greenberg RS, Brimacombe J, Berry A, et al: A randomized controlled trial comparing the cuffed oropharyngeal airway and the laryngeal mask airway in spontaneously breathing anesthetized adults. Anesthesiology 1998;88:970–977.

194. Behringer EC: Comparison of the laryngeal mask airway and cuffed oropharyngeal airway: alternative hypotheses. Anesth Analg 1999;88:961–962.

195. Brimacombe JR, Brimacombe JC, Berry AM, et al: A comparison of the laryngeal mask airway and cuffed oropharyngeal airway in anesthetized adult patients. Anesth Analg 1998;87:147–152.

196. van Vlymen JM, Fu W, White PF, et al: Use of the cuffed oropharyngeal airway as an alternative to the laryngeal mask airway with positive-pressure ventilation. Anesthesiology 1999;90:1306–1310.

197. Casati A, Fanelli G, Torri G: Physiological dead space/tidal volume ratio during face mask, laryngeal mask, and cuffed oropharyngeal airway spontaneous ventilation. J Clin Anesth 1998;10:652–655.

198. Benumof JL: The glottic aperture seal airway: A new ventilatory device. Anesthesiology 1998;88:1219–1226.

199. Jones KL: Smith's Recognizable Patterns of Human Malformation, 5th ed. Philadelphia: W.B. Saunders; 1997.

200. Jones AE, Pelton DA: An index of syndromes and their anaesthetic implications. Can Anaesth Soc J 1976;23:207–226.

201. Practice guidelines for management of the difficult airway. A report by the American Society of Anesthesiologists Task Force on Management of the Difficult Airway. Anesthesiology 1993;78:597–602.

202. Crosby ET, Cooper RM, Douglas MJ, et al: The unanticipated difficult airway with recommendations for management. Can J Anaesth 1998;45:757–776.

203. Benumof JL: Laryngeal mask airway and the ASA difficult airway algorithm. Anesthesiology 1996;84:686–699.

204. Cobley M, Vaughan RS: Recognition and management of difficult airway problems. Br J Anaesth 1992;68:90–97.

205. Benumof JL: Management of the difficult adult airway. With special emphasis on awake tracheal intubation. Anesthesiology 1991; 75:1087–1110.

206. Wheeler M: Management strategies for the difficult pediatric airway. 1998;16:743–761.

207. Badgwell JM, McLeod ME, Friedberg J: Airway obstruction in infants and children. Can J Anaesth 1987;34:90–98.

208. Pelton DA, Whalen JS: Airway obstruction in infants and children. Int Anesthesiol Clin 1972;10:123–150.

209. Webster AC: Anesthesia for operations on the upper airway. Int Anesthesiol Clin 1972;10:61–122.

210. Wheeler M, Ovassapian A: Pediatric fiberoptic intubation. In: Ovassapian A, ed: Fiberoptic Endoscopy and the Difficult Airway, 2nd ed. Philadelphia: Lippincott-Raven; 1996:105–116.

211. Smith JA, Santer LJ: Respiratory arrest following intramuscular ketamine injection in a 4-year-old child. Ann Emerg Med 1993;22:613–615.

212. Buhrer M, Maitre PO, Hung O, et al: Electroencephalographic effects of benzodiazepines. I. Choosing an electroencephalographic parameter to measure the effect of midazolam on the central nervous system. Clin Pharmacol Ther 1990;48:544–554.

213. Buhrer M, Maitre PO, Crevoisier C, et al: Electroencephalographic effects of benzodiazepines. II. Pharmacodynamic modeling of the electroencephalographic effects of midazolam and diazepam. Clin Pharmacol Ther 1990;48:555–567.

214. Duncan PG, Kobrinsky N: Prilocaine-induced methemoglobinemia in a newborn infant. Anesthesiology 1983;59:75–76.

215. King CJ, Davey AJ, Chandradeva K: Emergency use of the laryngeal mask airway in severe upper airway obstruction caused by supraglottic oedema. Br J Anaesth 1995;75:785–786.

216. Inada T, Fujise K, Tachibana K, et al: Orotracheal intubation through the laryngeal mask airway in paediatric patients with Treacher-Collins syndrome. Paediatr Anaesth 1995;5:129–132.

217. Cork R, Monk JE: Management of a suspected and unsuspected difficult laryngoscopy with the laryngeal mask airway. J Clin Anesth 1992;4:230–234.

218. Mark LJ, Beattie C, Ferrell CL, et al: The difficult airway: Mechanisms for effective dissemination of critical information. J Clin Anesth 1992;4:247–251.

219. Liban JB: Medic Alert UK should start new section for patients with a difficult airway. Br Med J 1996;313:425.

220. Benumof JL, Dagg R, Benumof R: Critical hemoglobin desaturation will occur before return to an unparalyzed state following 1 mg/kg intravenous succinylcholine. Anesthesiology 1997;87:979–982.

221. Farmery AD, Roe PG: A model to describe the rate of oxyhaemoglobin desaturation during apnoea. Br J Anaesth 1996;76:284–291.

222. Benumof JL: Airway exchange catheters for safe extubation: the clinical and scientific details that make the concept work. Chest 1997;111:1483–1486.

223. Benumof JL: Airway exchange catheters: Simple concept, potentially great danger. Anesthesiology 1999;91:342–344.

224. Baraka AS: Tension pneumothorax complicating jet ventilation via a cook airway exchange catheter. Anesthesiology 1999;91:557–558.

225. Benyamin RM, Wafai Y, Salem MR, et al: Two-handed mask ventilation of the difficult airway by a single individual. Anesthesiology 1998;88:1134.

226. Osses H, Poblete M, Asenjo F: Laryngeal mask for difficult intubation in children. Paediatr Anaesth 1999;9:399–401.

227. Markakis DA, Sayson SC, Schreiner MS: Insertion of the laryngeal mask airway in awake infants with the Robin sequence. Anesth Analg 1992;75:822–824.

228. Nath G, Major V: The laryngeal mask in the management of a paediatric difficult airway. Anaesth Int Care 1992;20:518–520.

229. Castresana MR, Stefansson S, Cancel AR, et al: Use of the laryngeal mask airway during thoracotomy in a pediatric patient with cri-du-chat syndrome. Anesth Analg 1994;78:817.

230. Stinson TW: A simple connector for transtracheal ventilation. Anesthesiology 1977;47:232–232.

231. Frumin MJ, Epstein RM, Cohen G: Apneic oxygenation in man. Anesthesiology 1959;20:789–798.

232. Coté CJ, Eavey RD, Todres ID, et al: Cricothyroid membrane punc-

ture: Oxygenation and ventilation in a dog model using an intravenous catheter. Crit Care Med 1988;16:615–619.

233. Peak DA, Roy S: Needle cricothyroidotomy revisited. Pediatr Emerg Care 1999;15:224–226.

234. Smith RB, Schaer WB, Pfaeffle H: Percutaneous transtracheal ventilation for anaesthesia and resuscitation: A review and report of complications. Can Anaesth Soc J 1975;22:607–612.

235. Goldstein B, Shannon DC, Todres ID: Supercarbia in children: clinical course and outcome. Crit Care Med 1990;18:166–168.

236. Bedger RC Jr, Chang JL: A jet-stylet endotracheal catheter for difficult airway management. Anesthesiology 1987;66:221–223.

237. Ravussin P, Bayer-Berger M, Monnier P, et al: Percutaneous transtracheal ventilation for laser endoscopic procedures in infants and small children with laryngeal obstruction: Report of two cases. Can J Anaesth 1987;34:83–86.

238. Schur MS, Maccioli GA, Azizkhan RG, et al: High-frequency jet ventilation in the management of congenital tracheal stenosis. Anesthesiology 1988;68:952–955.

239. Zornow MH, Thomas TC, Scheller MS: The efficacy of three different methods of transtracheal ventilation. Can J Anaesth 1989;36:624–628.

240. Vivori E: Anaesthesia for laryngoscopy. Br J Anaesth 1980;52:638.

241. Steward DJ: Anaesthesia for laryngoscopy. Br J Anaesth 1981;53:320.

242. Steward DJ: Percutaneous transtracheal ventilation for laser endoscopic procedures in infants and small children. Can J Anaesth 1987;34:429–430.

243. Toursarkissian B, Fowler CL, Zweng TN, et al: Percutaneous dilational tracheostomy in children and teenagers. J Pediatr Surg 1994;29:1421–1424.

244. Suh RH, Margulies DR, Hopp ML, et al: Percutaneous dilatational tracheostomy: Still a surgical procedure. Am Surg 1999;65:982–986.

245. Gopinath R, Murray JM: Percutaneous tracheostomy and Murphy's law: An eye for trouble. Anesth Analg 1999;89:670–671.

246. Tunkel DE, Fisher QA: Pediatric flexible fiberoptic bronchoscopy through the laryngeal mask airway. Arch Otolaryngol Head Neck Surg 1996;122:1364–1367.

247. Brimacombe J, Gandini D: The laryngeal mask airway: Potential applications in neonatal health care. J Obstet Gynecol Neonat Nurs 1997;26:171–178.

248. Brimacombe J: The advantages of the LMA over the tracheal tube or facemask: A meta-analysis. Can J Anaesth 1995;42:1017–1023.

249. Paterson SJ, Byrne PJ: Time required to insert laryngeal mask airway in neonates requiring resuscitation. Anesthesiology 1995;82:318.

250. Pennant JH, Walker MB: Comparison of the endotracheal tube and laryngeal mask in airway management by paramedical personnel. Anesth Analg 1992;74:531–534.

251. Parmet JL, Colonna-Romano P, Horrow JC, et al: The laryngeal mask airway reliably provides rescue ventilation in cases of unanticipated difficult tracheal intubation along with difficult mask ventilation. Anesth Analg 1998;87:661–665.

252. Lim JW, Lerner PK, Rothstein SG: Epiglottic position after cricothyroidotomy: A comparison with tracheotomy. Ann Otol Rhinol Laryngol 1997;106:560–562.

253. Henderson JJ: The use of paraglossal straight blade laryngoscopy in difficult tracheal intubation. Anaesthesia 1997;52:552–560.

254. Bonfils P: Difficult intubation in Pierre-Robin children, a new method: the retromolar route. [in German]. Anaesthesist 1983;32:363–367.

255. Benumof JL, Cooper SD: Quantitative improvement in laryngoscopic view by optimal external laryngeal manipulation. J Clin Anesth 1996;8:136–140.

256. Todres ID, Crone RK: Experience with a modified laryngoscope in sick infants. Crit Care Med 1981;9:544–545.

257. Patil VU, Sopchak AM, Thomas PS: Use of a dental mirror as an aid to tracheal intubation in an infant. Anesthesiology 1993;78:619–620.

258. Wengen DF, Probst RR, Frei FJ: Flexible laryngoscopy in neonates and infants: Insertion through a median opening in the face mask. Int J Pediatr Otorhinolaryngol 1991;21:183–187.

259. Frei FJ, Ummenhofer W: A special mask for teaching fiber-optic intubation in pediatric patients. Anesth Analg 1993;76:458–458.

260. Wilton NC: Aids for fiberoptically guided intubation in children. Anesthesiology 1991;75:549–550.

261. Shorten GD, Ali HH, Roberts JT: Assessment of patient position for fiberoptic intubation using videolaryngoscopy. J Clin Anesth 1995;7:31–34.

262. Taylor PA, Towey RM: The broncho-fiberscope as an aid to endotracheal intubation. Br J Anaesth 1972;44:611–612.

263. Davis NJ: A new fiberoptic laryngoscope for nasal intubation. Anesth Analg 1973;52:807–808.

264. Ovassapian A, Yelich SJ, Dykes MH, et al: Learning fibreoptic intubation: Use of simulators v. traditional teaching. Br J Anaesth 1988;61:217–220.

265. Wood RE, Sherman JM: Pediatric flexible bronchoscopy. Ann Otol Rhinol Laryngol 1980;89:414–416.

266. Labbe A, Dalens B, Lusson JR, et al: Flexible bronchoscopy in infants and children. Endoscopy 1984;16:13–15.

267. Nussbaum E: Usefulness of miniature flexible fiberoptic bronchoscopy in children. Chest 1994;106:1438–1442.

268. Wood RE, Postma D: Endoscopy of the airway in infants and children. J Pediatr 1988;112:1–6.

269. Roth AG, Wheeler M, Stevenson GW, et al: Comparison of a rigid laryngoscope with the ultrathin fibreoptic laryngoscope for tracheal intubation in infants. Can J Anaesth 1994;41:1069–1073.

270. Stiles CM: A flexible fiberoptic bronchoscope for endotracheal intubation of infants. Anesth Analg 1974;53:1017–1019.

271. Howardy-Hansen P, Berthelsen P: Fibreoptic bronchoscopic nasotracheal intubation of a neonate with Pierre Robin syndrome. Anaesthesia 1988;43:121–122.

272. Scheller JG, Schulman SR: Fiber-optic bronchoscopic guidance for intubating a neonate with Pierre-Robin syndrome. J Clin Anesth 1991;3:45–47.

273. Ford RW: Adaptation of the fiberoptic laryngoscope for tracheal intubation with small diameter tubes. Can Anaesth Soc J 1981;28:479–480.

274. Alfery DD, Ward CF, Harwood IR, et al: Airway management for a neonate with congenital fusion of the jaws. Anesthesiology 1979;51:340–342.

275. Gouverneur JM, Veyckemans F, Licker M, et al: Using an ureteral catheter as a guide in difficult neonatal fiberoptic intubation. Anesthesiology 1987;66:436–437.

276. Berthelsen P, Prytz S, Jacobsen E: Two-stage fiberoptic nasotracheal intubation in infants: A new approach to difficult pediatric intubation. Anesthesiology 1985;63:457–458.

277. Katz RL, Berci G: The optical stylet: A new intubation technique for adults and children with specific reference to teaching. Anesthesiology 1979;51:251–254.

278. Ellis DG, Jakymec A, Kaplan RM, et al: Guided orotracheal intubation in the operating room using a lighted stylet: A comparison with direct laryngoscopic technique. Anesthesiology 1986;64:823–826.

279. Knight RG, Castro T, Rastrelli AJ, et al: Arterial blood pressure and heart rate response to lighted stylet or direct laryngoscopy for endotracheal intubation. Anesthesiology 1988;69:269–272.

280. Rehman MA, Schreiner MS: Oral and nasotracheal light wand guided intubation after failed fibreoptic bronchoscopy. Pediatr Anaesth 1997;7:349–351.

281. Holzman RS, Nargozian CD, Florence FB: Lightwand intubation in children with abnormal upper airways. Anesthesiology 1988;69:784–787.

282. Borland LM, Casselbrant M: The Bullard laryngoscope: A new indirect oral laryngoscope (pediatric version). Anesth Analg 1990;70:105–108.

283. Bourke D, Levesque PR: Modification of retrograde guide for endotracheal intubation. Anesth Analg 1974;53:1013–1014.

284. Waters DJ: Guided blind endotracheal intubation for patients with deformities of the upper airway. Anaesthesia 1963;18:158–162.

285. Borland LM, Swan DM, Leff S: Difficult pediatric endotracheal intubation: A new approach to the retrograde technique. Anesthesiology 1981;55:577–578.

286. Duncan JA: Intubation of the trachea in the conscious patient. Br J Anaesth 1977;49:619–623.

287. Rosenberg MB, Levesque PR, Bourke DL: Use of the LTA kit as a guide for endotracheal intubation. Anesth Analg 1977;56:287–288.

288. Roberts KW: New use for Swan-Ganz introducer wire. Anesth Analg 1981;60:67.

289. Cooper CM, Murray-Wilson A: Retrograde intubation. Management of a 4.8-kg, 5-month infant. Anaesthesia 1987;42:1197–1200.

290. Ledbetter JL, Rasch DK, Pollard TG, et al: Reducing the risks of laryngoscopy in anaesthetized infants. Anaesthesia 1988;43:151–153.

291. Shikani AH: New "seeing" stylet-scope and method for the management of the difficult airway. Otolaryngol-Head Neck Surg 1999;120:113–116.

292. Saruki N, Saito S, Sato J, et al: Swift conversion from laryngoscopic

to fiberoptic intubation with a new, handy fiberoptic stylet. Anesth Analg 1999;89:526–528.

293. Chadd GD, Crane DL, Phillips RM, et al: Extubation and reintubation guided by the laryngeal mask airway in a child with the Pierre Robin syndrome. Anesthesiology 1992;76:640–641.

294. Bahk JH, Han SM, Kim SD: Management of difficult airways with a laryngeal mask airway under propofol anaesthesia. Paediatr Anaesth 1999;9:163–166.

295. Walker RW, Allen DL, Rothera MR: A fibreoptic intubation technique for children with mucopolysaccharidoses using the laryngeal mask airway. Paediatr Anaesth 1997;7:421–426.

296. Rabb MF, Minkowitz HS, Hagberg CA: Blind intubation through the laryngeal mask airway for management of the difficult airway in infants. Anesthesiology 1996;84:1510–1511.

297. Heard CM, Caldicott LD, Fletcher JE, et al: Fiberoptic-guided endotracheal intubation via the laryngeal mask airway in pediatric patients: a report of a series of cases. Anesth Analg 1996;82:1287–1289.

298. Goudsouzian NG, Denman W, Cleveland R, et al: Radiologic localization of the laryngeal mask airway in children. Anesthesiology 1992;77:1085–1089.

299. Audenaert SM, Montgomery CL, Stone B, et al: Retrograde-assisted fiberoptic tracheal intubation in children with difficult airways. Anesth Analg 1991;73:660–664.

300. Haas JE, Tsueda K: Direct laryngoscopy with the aid of a fiberoptic bronchoscope for tracheal intubation. Anesth Analg 1996;82:438.

301. Przybylo HJ, Stevenson GW, Vicari FA, et al: Retrograde fibreoptic intubation in a child with Nager's syndrome. Can J Anaesth 1996;43:697–699.

302. Cormack RS, Lehane J: Difficult tracheal intubation in obstetrics. Anaesthesia 1984;39:1105–1111.

303. American Heart Association: Pediatric Advanced Life Support. Elk Grove Village: American Academy of Pediatrics; 1994.

304. Creighton RE, Relton JE, Meridy HW: Anaesthesia for occipital encephalocoele. Can Anaesth Soc J 1974;21:403–406.

305. Meyers EF, Krupin B: Anesthetic management of emergency tonsillectomy and adenoidectomy in infectious mononucleosis. Anesthesiology 1975;42:490–491.

306. Suan C, Ojeda R, Garcia-Perla JL, et al: Anaesthesia and the Beckwith-Wiedemann syndrome. Paediatr Anaesth 1996;6:231–233.

307. Coleman M: Down's syndrome. Pediatr Ann 1978;7:90–103.

308. Clark RW, Schmidt HS, Schuller DE: Sleep-induced ventilatory dysfunction in Down's syndrome. Arch Intern Med 1980;140:45–50.

309. Levine OR, Simpser M: Alveolar hypoventilation and cor pulmonale associated with chronic airway obstruction in infants with Down syndrome. Clin Pediatr (Phila) 1982;21:25–29.

310. Kobel M, Creighton RE, Steward DJ: Anaesthetic considerations in Down's syndrome: Experience with 100 patients and a review of the literature. Can Anaesth Soc J 1982;29:593–599.

311. Pueschel SM: Atlantoaxial instability and Down syndrome. Pediatrics 1988;81:879–880.

312. Williams JP, Somerville GM, Miner ME, et al: Atlanto-axial subluxation and trisomy-21: Another perioperative complication. Anesthesiology 1987;67:253–254.

313. Moore RA, McNicholas KW, Warran SP: Atlantoaxial subluxation with symptomatic spinal cord compression in a child with Down's syndrome. Anesth Analg 1987;66:89–90.

314. Pueschel SM, Moon AC, Scola FH: Computerized tomography in persons with Down syndrome and atlantoaxial instability. Spine 1992;17:735–737.

315. Pueschel SM, Scola FH: Atlantoaxial instability in individuals with Down syndrome: Epidemiologic, radiographic, and clinical studies. Pediatrics 1987;80:555–560.

316. Moylan JA, Chan CK: Inhalation injury: An increasing problem. Ann Surg 1978;188:34–37.

317. Chu CS: New concepts of pulmonary burn injury. J Trauma 1981;21:958–961.

318. Trunkey DD: Inhalation injury. Surg Clin North Am 1978;58:1133–1140.

319. Mellins RB, Park S: Respiratory complications of smoke inhalation in victims in fires. J Pediatr 1975;87:1–6.

320. Fein A, Leff A, Hopewell PC: Pathophysiology and management of the complications resulting from fire and the inhaled products of combustion: review of the literature. Crit Care Med 1980;8:94–98.

321. Hunt JL, Agee RN, Pruitt BA, Jr: Fiberoptic bronchoscopy in acute inhalation injury. J Trauma 1975;15:641–649.

322. Smith DF, Mihm FG, Flynn M: Chronic alveolar hypoventilation secondary to macroglossia in the Beckwith-Wiedemann syndrome. Pediatrics 1982;70:695–697.

323. Combs JT, Grunt JA, Brandt IK: New syndrome of neonatal hypoglycemia. Association with visceromegaly, macroglossia, microcephaly and abnormal umbilicus. N Engl J Med 1966;275:236–243.

324. Jones AE, Croley TF: Morquio syndrome and anesthesia. Anesthesiology 1979;51:261–262.

325. Birkinshaw KJ: Anaesthesia in a patient with an unstable neck. Morquio's syndrome. Anaesthesia 1975;30:46–49.

326. Sjogren P, Pedersen T, Steinmetz H: Mucopolysaccharidoses and anaesthetic risks. Acta Anaesthesiol Scand 1987;31:214–218.

327. Cox JM: Anesthesia and glycogen-storage disease. Anesthesiology 1968;29:221–1225.

328. Weller RM: Anaesthesia for cystic hygroma in a neonate. Anaesthesia 1974;29:588–594.

329. MacDonald DJF: Cystic hygroma: An anaesthetic and surgical problem. Anaesthesia 1966;21:66–71.

330. Fletcher MM, Blum SL, Blanchard CL: Pierre Robin syndrome pathophysiology of obstructive episodes. Laryngoscope 1969;79:547–560.

331. Lapidot A, Rezvani F, Terrefe D, et al: A new functional approach to the surgical management of Pierre Robin syndrome: experimental and clinical report. Laryngoscope 1976;86:979–983.

332. Hawkins DB, Simpson JV: Micrognathia and glossoptosis in the newborn. Surgical tacking of the tongue in small jaw syndromes. Clin Pediatr (Phila) 1974;13:1066–1073.

333. Khouw YH, Kleine JW: A difficult intubation. Acta Anaesthesiol Belg 1975;26:78–80.

334. Cogswell JJ, Easton DM: Cor pulmonale in the Pierre Robin syndrome. Arch Dis Child 1974;49:905–908.

335. Heaf DP, Helms PJ, Dinwiddie R, et al: Nasopharyngeal airways in Pierre Robin Syndrome. J Pediatr 1982;100:698–703.

336. Stern LM, Fonkalsrud EW, Hassakis P, et al: Management of Pierre Robin syndrome in infancy by prolonged nasoesophageal intubation. Am J Dis Child 1972;124:78–80.

337. Lewis MB, Pashayan HM: Management of infants with Robin anomaly. Clin Pediatr (Phila) 1980;19:519–521.

338. Mallory SB, Paradise JL: Glossoptosis revisited: On the development and resolution of airway obstruction in the Pierre Robin syndrome. Pediatrics 1979;64:946–948.

339. MacLennan FM, Robertson GS: Ketamine for induction and intubation in Treacher-Collins syndrome. Anaesthesia 1981;36:196–198.

340. Johnson C, Taussig LM, Koopman C, et al: Obstructive sleep apnea in Treacher-Collins syndrome. Cleft Palate 1981;18:39–44.

341. Divekar VM, Sircar BN: Anesthetic management in Treacher-Collins syndrome. Anesthesiology 1965;26:692–693.

342. Sklar GS, King BD: Endotracheal Intubation and Treacher-Collins syndrome. Anesthesiology 1976;44:247–249.

343. Ross EDT: Treacher-Collins syndrome: An anaesthetic hazard. Anaesthesia 1963;18:350–354.

344. Scholtes JL, Veyckemans F, Van Obbergh L, et al: Neonatal anaesthetic management of a patient with Goldenhar's syndrome with hydrocephalus. Anaesth Intensive Care 1987;15:338–340.

345. Madan R, Trikha A, Venkataraman RK, et al: Goldenhar's syndrome: An analysis of anaesthetic management: A retrospective study of seventeen cases. Anaesthesia 1990;45:49–52.

346. Walts LF, Finerman G, Wyatt GM: Anaesthesia for dwarfs and other patients of pathological small stature. Can Anaesth Soc J 1975;22:703–709.

347. Mather JS: Impossible direct laryngoscopy in achondroplasia: A case report. Anaesthesia 1966;21:244–248.

348. Kalla GN, Fening E, Obiaya MO: Anaesthetic management of achondroplasia. Br J Anaesth 1986;58:117–119.

349. Pauli RM, Gilbert EF: Upper cervical cord compression as cause of death in osteogenesis imperfecta type II. J Pediatr 1986;108:579–581.

350. Allansmith M, Senz E: Chondrodystrophia congenita punctata (Conradi's disease). Am J Dis Child 1960;100:109–116.

351. Noonan JA: Hypertelorism with Turner phenotype: A new syndrome with associated congenital heart disease. Am J Dis Child 1968;116:373–380.

352. Nora JJ, Torres FG, Sinha AK, et al: Characteristic cardiovascular anomalies of XO Turner syndrome, XX and XY phenotype and XO–XX Turner mosaic. Am J Cardiol 1970;25:639–641.

353. Ptacek LJ, Opitz JM, Smith DW, et al: The Cornelia de Lange syndrome. J Pediatr 1963;63:1000–1020.

354. Jervis GA, Stimson CW: De Lange syndrome. The Amsterdam type of mental defect with congenital malformation. J Pediatr 1963;63:634–645.

355. Smith DW, Lemli L, Opitz JM: A newly recognized syndrome of multiple congenital anomalies. J Pediatr 1964;64:210–217.

356. Hoefnagel D, Benirsche K: Dyscephalia mandibulo-oculo-facialis (Hallermann-Streiff syndrome). Arch Dis Child 1998;40:57–61.

357. Poswillo D: The aetiology and pathogenesis of craniofacial deformity. Development 1988;103:207–212.

358. Holinger PH, Schild JA: Pharyngeal, laryngeal and tracheal injuries in the pediatric age group. Ann Otol Rhinol Laryngol 1972;81:538–545.

359. Jacobs JC, Hui RM: Cricoarytenoid arthritis and airway obstruction in juvenile rheumatoid arthritis. Pediatrics 1977;59:292–294.

360. D'Arcy EJ, Fell RH, Ansell BM, et al: Ketamine and juvenile chronic polyarthritis (Still's disease). Anaesthetic problems in Still's disease and allied disorders. Anaesthesia 1976;31:624–632.

361. Jenkins LC, McGraw RW: Anaesthetic management of the patient with rheumatoid arthritis. Can Anaesth Soc J 1969;16:407–415.

362. Edelist G: Principles of anesthetic management in rheumatoid arthritis patients. Anesth Analg 1964;43:227–231.

363. Gardner DL, Holmes F: Anaesthetic and post-operative hazards in rheumatoid arthritis. Br J Anaesth 1961;33:258–264.

364. Hamner JE3, Ketcham AS: Cherubism: An analysis of treatment. Cancer 1969;23:1133–1143.

365. Holinger PH, Brown WT: Congenital webs, cysts, laryngoceles and other anomalies of the larynx. Ann Otol Rhinol Laryngol 1967;76:744–752.

366. Munro HM, Butler PJ, Washington EJ: Freeman-Sheldon (whistling face) syndrome. Anaesthetic and airway management. Paediatr Anaesth 1997;7:345–348.

367. Yamamoto S, Osuga T, Okada M, et al: Anesthetic management of a patient with Freeman-Sheldon syndrome. [in Japanese]. Masui 1994;43:1748–1753.

368. Holinger PH, Johnston KC: Factors responsible for laryngeal obstruction in infants. JAMA 1950;143:1229–1232.

369. Seed RF: Traumatic injury to the larynx and trachea. Anaesthesia 1971;26:55–65.

370. Saletta JD, Folk FA, Freeark RJ: Trauma to the neck region. Surg Clin North Am 1973;53:83–86.

371. Curtin JW, Holinger PH, Greeley PW: Blunt trauma to the larynx and upper trachea: Immediate treatment, complications and late reconstructive procedures. J Trauma 1966;6:493–502.

372. Dalal FY, Schmidt GB, Bennett EJ, et al: Fractures of the larynx in children. Can Anaesth Soc J 1974;21:376–378.

373. Ellis FR: The management of the cut-throat. Anaesthesia 1966;21:253–260.

374. Merritt RM, Bent JP, Porubsky ES: Acute laryngeal trauma in the pediatric patient. Ann Otol Rhinol Laryngol 1998;107:104–106.

375. Gold SM, Gerber ME, Shott SR, et al: Blunt laryngotracheal trauma in children. Arch Otolaryngol Head Neck Surg 1997;123:83–87.

376. Kim IG, Brummitt WM, Humphry A, et al: Foreign body in the airway: A review of 202 cases. Laryngoscope 1973;83:347–354.

377. Steichen FM, Fellini A, Einhorn AH: Acute foreign body laryngotracheal obstruction: A cause for sudden and unexpected death in children. Pediatrics 1971;48:281–285.

378. Chatterji S, Chatterji P: The management of foreign bodies in air passages. Anaesthesia 1972;27:390–395.

379. Baraka A: Bronchoscopic removal of inhaled foreign bodies in children. Br J Anaesth 1974;46:124–126.

380. Baharloo F, Veyckemans F, Francis C, et al: Tracheobronchial foreign bodies: Presentation and management in children and adults. Chest 1999;115:1357–1362.

381. Zerella JT, Dimler M, McGill LC, et al: Foreign body aspiration in children: Value of radiography and complications of bronchoscopy. J Pediatr Surg 1998;33:1651–1654.

382. Hachimi-Idrissi S, Corne L, Vandenplas Y: Management of ingested foreign bodies in childhood: Our experience and review of the literature. Eur J Emerg Med 1998;5:319–323.

383. Halvorson DJ, Merritt RM, Mann C, et al: Management of subglottic foreign bodies. Ann Otol Rhinol Laryngol 1996;105:541–544.

384. Panieri E, Bass DH: The management of ingested foreign bodies in children: A review of 663 cases. Eur J Emerg Med 1995;2:83–87.

385. Allen TH, Steven IM: Prolonged nasotracheal intubation in infants and children. Br J Anaesth 1972;44:835–840.

386. Bain JA: Late complications of tracheostomy and prolonged endotracheal intubation. Int Anesthesiol Clin 1972;10:225–244.

387. Komorn RM, Smith CP, Erwin JR: Acute laryngeal injury with short-term endotracheal anesthesia. Laryngoscope 1973;83:683–690.

388. Markham WG, Blackwood MJ, Conn AW: Prolonged nasotracheal intubation in infants and children. Can Anaesth Soc J 1967;14:11–21.

389. Hatch DJ: Prolonged nasotracheal intubation in infants and children. Lancet 1968;1:1272–1275.

390. Blanc VF, Tremblay NA: The complications of tracheal intubation: A new classification with a review of the literature. Anesth Analg 1974;53:202–213.

391. Joshi VV, Mandavia SG, Stern L, et al: Acute lesions induced by endotracheal intubation. Occurrence in the upper respiratory tract of newborn infants with respiratory distress syndrome. Am J Dis Child 1972;124:646–649.

392. Hawkins DB: Glottic and subglottic stenosis from endotracheal intubation. Laryngoscope 1977;87:339–346.

393. Grillo HC: Surgical treatment of postintubation tracheal injuries. J Thorac Cardiovasc Surg 1979;78:860–875.

394. Morrison MD, Maber BR: Crico-arytenoid joint obliteration following longterm intubation in the premature infant. J Otolaryngol 1977;6:277–283.

395. Othersen HB Jr: Intubation injuries of the trachea in children: Management and prevention. Ann Surg 1979;189:601–606.

396. Kenna MA, Stool SE, Mallory SB: Junctional epidermolysis bullosa of the larynx. Pediatrics 1986;78:172–174.

397. Liu RM, Papsin BC, de Jong AL: Epidermolysis bullosa of the head and neck: A case report of laryngotracheal involvement and 10-year review of cases at the Hospital for Sick Children. J Otolaryngol 1999;28:76–82.

398. Stewart MI, Woodley DT, Briggaman RA: Epidermolysis bullosa acquisita and associated symptomatic esophageal webs. Arch Dermatol 1991;127:373–377.

399. Oh TH, Motoyama EK: Comparison of nasotracheal intubation and tracheostomy in management of acute epiglottitis. Anesthesiology 1977;46:214–216.

400. Baxter JD, Pashley NR: Acute epiglottitis: 25 years' experience in management, The Montreal Children's Hospital. J Otolaryngol 1977;6:473–476.

401. Schuller DE, Birck HG: The safety of intubation in croup and epiglottitis: An eight-year follow-up. Laryngoscope 1975;85:33–46.

402. Travis KW, Todres ID, Shannon DC: Pulmonary edema associated with croup and epiglottitis. Pediatrics 1977;59:695–698.

403. Davison FW: Acute laryngeal obstruction in children: A fifty-year review. Ann Otol Rhinol Laryngol 1978;87:606–613.

404. Phelan PD, Mullins GC, Laundau LI, et al: The period of nasotracheal intubation in acute epiglottitis. Anaesth Intensive Care 1980;8:402–403.

405. Enoksen A, Bryne H, Hoel TM, et al: Epiglottis acuta treated with nasotracheal intubation. Acta Anaesthesiol Scand 1979;23:422–426.

406. Bottenfield GW, Arcinue EL, Sarnaik A, et al: Diagnosis and management of acute epiglottitis: Report of 90 consecutive cases. Laryngoscope 1980;90:822–825.

407. Battaglia JD, Lockhart CH: Management of acute epiglottitis by nasotracheal intubation. Am J Dis Child 1975;129:334–336.

408. Adair JC, Ring WH: Management of epiglottitis in children. Anesth Analg 1975;54:622–625.

409. Milko DA, Marshak G, Striker TW: Nasotracheal intubation in the treatment of acute epiglottitis. Pediatrics 1974;53:674–677.

410. Blanc VF, Weber ML, Leduc C, et al: Acute epiglottitis in children: Management of 27 consecutive cases with nasotracheal intubation, with special emphasis on anaesthetic considerations. Can Anaesth Soc J 1977;24:1–11.

411. Weber ML, Desjardins R, Perreault G, et al: Acute epiglottitis in children—treatment with nasotracheal intubation: Report of 14 consecutive cases. Pediatrics 1976;57:152–155.

412. Gorelick MH, Baker MD: Epiglottitis in children, 1979 through 1992: Effects of Haemophilus influenzae type b immunization. Arch Pediatr Adolesc Med 1994;148:47–50.

413. Ryan M, Hunt M, Snowberger T: A changing pattern of epiglottitis. Clin Pediatr (Phila) 1992;31:532–535.

414. Bonadio WA, Losek JD: The characteristics of children with epiglottitis who develop the complication of pulmonary edema. Arch Otolaryngol Head Neck Surg 1991;117:205–207.

415. Sumner E: Quinsy tonsillectomy: A safe procedure. Anaesthesia 1973;28:558–561.

416. Beeden AG, Evans JN: Quinsy tonsillectomy: A further report. J Laryngol Otol 1970;84:443–448.

417. Kloss J, Petty C: Obstruction of endotracheal intubation by a mobile pedunculated polyp. Anesthesiology 1975;43:380–380.

418. Stein AA, Volk BM: Papillomatosis of trachea and lung. Arch Pathol 1959;68:468–472.

419. Hitz HB, Oesterlin E: A case of multiple papillomata of the larynx with aerial metastases to lungs. Am J Pathol 1932;8:333–339.

420. Fitzsimmons JS: Laryngeal stridor and respiratory obstruction associated with myelomeningocele. Dev Med Child Neurol 1973;15:533–536.

421. Holinger PC, Holinger LD, Reichert TJ, et al: Respiratory obstruction and apnea in infants with bilateral abductor vocal cord paralysis, meningomyelocele, hydrocephalus, and Arnold-Chiari malformation. J Pediatr 1978;92:368–373.

422. Bluestone CD, Delerme AN, Samuelson GH: Airway obstruction due to vocal cord paralysis in infants with hydrocephalus and meningomyelocele. Ann Otol Rhinol Laryngol 1972;81:778–783.

423. Ward SL, Nickerson BG, van der Hal A, et al: Absent hypoxic and hypercapneic arousal responses in children with myelomeningocele and apnea. Pediatrics 1986;78:44–50.

424. Steward DJ: Congenital abnormalities as a possible factor in the aetiology of post-intubation subglottic stenosis. Can Anaesth Soc J 1970;17:388–390.

425. Taussig LM, Castro O, Beaudry PH, et al: Treatment of laryngotracheobronchitis (croup): Use of intermittent positive-pressure breathing and racemic epinephrine. Am J Dis Child 1975;129:790–793.

426. Mitchell DP, Thomas RL: Secondary airway support in the management of croup. J Otolaryngol 1980;9:419–422.

427. Duncan PG: Efficacy of helium-oxygen mixtures in the management of severe viral and post-intubation croup. Can Anaesth Soc J 1979;26:206–212.

428. Bray RJ, Fernandes FJ: Mediastinal tumour causing airway obstruction in anaesthetised children. Anaesthesia 1982;37:571–575.

429. Harley EH, Collins MD: Neurologic sequelae secondary to atlantoaxial instability in Down syndrome: Implications in otolaryngologic surgery. Arch Otolaryngol Head Neck Surg 1994;120:159–165.

430. Gunderson CH, Greenspan RH, Glaser GH, et al: The Klippel-Feil syndrome: Genetic and clinical reevaluation of cervical fusion. Medicine (Baltimore) 1967;46:491–512.

431. Schneider RC: Concomitant craniocerebral and spinal trauma, with special reference to the cervicomedullary region. Clin Neurosurg 1970;17:266–309.

432. Walker RW, Darowski M, Morris P, et al: Anaesthesia and mucopoly-saccharidoses: A review of airway problems in children. Anaesthesia 1994;49:1078–1084.

433. Moores C, Rogers JG, McKenzie IM, et al: Anaesthesia for children with mucopolysaccharidoses. Anaesth Intensive Care 1996;24:459–463.

434. Belani KG, Krivit W, Carpenter BL, et al: Children with mucopolysaccharidosis: Perioperative care, morbidity, mortality, and new findings. J Pediatr Surg 1993;28:403–408.

435. Kulkarni MV, Williams JC, Yeakley JW, et al: Magnetic resonance imaging in the diagnosis of the cranio-cervical manifestations of the mucopolysaccharidoses. Magn Reson Imaging 1987;5:317–323.

436. Myer CM III: Airway obstruction in Hurler's syndrome: Radiographic features. Int J Pediatr Otorhinolaryngol 1991;22:91–96.

437. Tobias JD: Anesthetic care for the child with Morquio syndrome: General versus regional anesthesia. J Clin Anesth 1999;11:242–246.

438. Oberoi GS, Kaul HL, Gill IS, et al: Anaesthesia in arthrogryposis multiplex congenita: Case report. Can J Anaesth 1987;34:288–290.

439. Sobrado CG, Ribera M, Marti M, et al: Freeman-Sheldon syndrome: generalized muscular rigidity after anesthetic induction. [in Spanish]. Rev Esp Anestesiol Reanim 1994;41:182–184.

440. Jones R, Dolcourt JL: Muscle rigidity following halothane anesthesia in two patients with Freeman-Sheldon syndrome. Anesthesiology 1992;77:599–600.

441. Wells DG, Podolakin W: Anaesthesia and Marfan's syndrome: case report. Can J Anaesth 1987;34:311–314.

442. Verghese C: Anaesthesia in Marfan's syndrome. Anaesthesia 1984;39:917–922.

443. Herrick IA, Rhine EJ: The mucopolysaccharidoses and anaesthesia: A report of clinical experience. Can J Anaesth 1988;35:67–73.

444. Gross DM, Williams JC, Caprioli C, et al: Echocardiographic abnormalities in the mucopolysaccharide storage diseases. Am J Cardiol 1988;61:170–176.

445. Nicolson SC, Black AE, Kraras CM: Management of a difficult airway in a patient with Hurler-Scheie syndrome during cardiac surgery. Anesth Analg 1992;75:830–832.

446. Nakayama H, Arita H, Hanaoka K: Anesthesia in a patient with Scheie syndrome. [in Japanese]. Masui 1994;43:1385–1388.

447. Yoskovitch A, Tewfik TL, Brouillette RT, et al: Acute airway obstruction in Hunter syndrome. Int J Pediatr Otorhinolaryngol 1998;44:273–278.

448. Smith GB, Shribman AJ: Anaesthesia and severe skin disease. Anaesthesia 1984;39:443–455.

449. Orr D: Difficult intubation: A hazard in thalassaemia. A case report. Br J Anaesth 1967;39:585–586.

Appendix 7–1. Syndromes and Disease Processes with Associated Airway Difficulties

Syndrome	Airway	Cerebral	Cardiac	Renal	Gastrointestinal	Endocrine Metabolic	Musculoskeletal	Anesthetic Considerations
Achondroplasia[347-350]	Midfacial hypoplasia, small nasal passages and mouth	Megacephaly ± hydrocephalus due to narrow foramen magnum					Dwarfism; odontoid hypoplasia with atlantoaxial instability	Difficult intubation ± Hydrocephalus
Apert syndrome[346]	Maxillary hypoplasia, narrow palate ± cleft palate	Craniosynostosis, flat facies, hypertelorism	± CHD	± Hydronephrosis, ± polycystic kidney	± Esophageal atresia		Syndactyly	Difficult intubation, associated cardiac and renal problems
Arthrogryposis multiplex congenita (multiple congenital contractures)[438]	Associated hypoplastic mandible, cleft palate, Klippel-Feil syndrome, torticollis		± VSD				Thoracolumbar scoliosis	Difficult intubation, associated cardiac disease, minimal muscle relaxant required, ± Malignant hyperthermia
Beckwith-Wiedemann syndrome (visceromegaly)[306, 322, 323]	Macroglossia—regresses with age; may require partial glossectomy	± Mental handicap due to hypoglycemia	Large heart	Enlarged kidneys	Omphalocele, hepatosplenomegaly	Hypoglycemia up to 4 mo of age, polycythemia	Eventration of diaphragm	Difficult intubation, asymptomatic hypoglycemia, omphalocele, neonatal polycythemia
Cherubism (fibrous dysplasia of jaw)[364]	Bilateral painless mandibular and maxillary swelling may progress to airway obstruction							Difficult intubation due to intraoral masses
Cornelia de Lange syndrome[353, 354]	High arch palate, micrognathia, spurs at anterior angle of mandible, large tongue, ± cleft palate, short neck	Mental handicap	± CHD					Difficult intubation, associated cardiac disease
Craniofacial dysostosis of Crouzon[357]	Maxillary hypoplasia with inverted V-shaped palate, ± large tongue	Ocular proptosis due to shallow orbits, craniosynostosis						Difficult intubation, eye injury
Congenital hypothyroid	Large tongue	May be mentally handicapped				Hypothermia, hypometabolic	Umbilical hernia	Difficult intubation, hypothermia, decreased drug metabolism

Table continued on following page

117

Appendix 7–1. Syndromes and Disease Processes with Associated Airway Difficulties *Continued*

Syndrome	Airway	Cerebral	Cardiac	Renal	Gastrointestinal	Endocrine Metabolic	Musculoskeletal	Anesthetic Considerations
Epidermolysis bullosa[396]	Pressure lesions to mouth and airway							Need gentle intubation with small tube, postoperative laryngeal obstruction due to bulla formation
Freeman-Sheldon syndrome (whistling face)[366, 367]	Small mouth, high palate	Hypertelorism, ± increased intracranial pressure, ± mental deficiency, ± microcephaly					Craniocarpotarsal dysplasia, strabismus, kyphoscoliosis, hip/knee contractures	Difficult intubation, ± malignant hyperthermia[439, 440]
Goldenhar syndrome (oculoauriculovertebral syndrome)[344, 345]	Hypoplastic zygomatic arch, mandibular hypoplasia, macrostomia, ± cleft tongue, palate, tracheoesophageal fistula	Hydrocephalus					Occipitalization of atlas, cervical vertebral defects	Difficult intubation, cervical spine defects
Hallerman-Streiff syndrome (oculomandibulo-dyscephaly)[356]	Malar hypoplasia, micrognathia, hypoplasia of rami and anterior displacement of temporomandibular joint, narrow high arch palate							Difficult intubation
Marfan syndrome[441, 442]	Narrow facies with narrow palate		Dissecting aortic aneurysm, aortic insufficiency				Scoliosis, kyphosis	Difficult intubation, associated cardiac and pulmonary disease
Mucopolysaccharido-ses[326, 432-435, 444] Type IH (Hurler)[436]	Coarse facial features, macroglossia, short neck, tonsillar hypertrophy, narrowing of laryngeal inlet and tracheobronchial tree	± Increased intracranial pressure	Severe coronary artery and valvular heart decrease, cardiomyopathy		Hepatosplenomegaly		Joint stiffness, kyphosis, contractures, odontoid hypoplasia and atlantoaxial subluxation	Difficult intubation

Syndrome	Airway/facial features	Neurologic/other features	Cardiac	Hepatosplenomegaly	Musculoskeletal	Anesthetic implications
Type I H/S (Hurler-Scheie)[445]	Macrocephaly, micrognathia	Mild mental deficiency to normal intelligence	± Valvular disease	± Hepato-splenomegaly	Mild joint stiffness	± Difficult intubation
Type IS (Scheie) or Type V[446]	Mandibular prognathism	Normal intelligence, corneal clouding	Aortic insufficiency		Joint stiffness	± Difficult intubation, associated heart disease
Type II (Hunter)[447]	Coarse facial features; tracheomalacia, macrocephaly, macroglossia	Increased intracranial pressure, severe mental deficiency	Valvular heart disease, cardiomyopathy	Hepatosplenomegaly	Joint stiffness, dwarfism, kyphoscoliosis	Difficult intubation
Type III (Sanfilippo)[443]	Mildly coarse facial features	Severe mental deficiency				± Difficult intubation
Type IV (Morquio)[324, 325, 437]	Mildly coarse facial features, prominent mandible, short neck		Late onset aortic regurgitation		Joint laxity, kyphoscoliosis, odontoid hypoplasia with atlantoaxial instability	Difficult intubation, restrictive pulmonary disease, unstable cervical spine, associated heart disease
Nagers syndrome[301]	Micrognathia, cleft palate	Low-set ears, atresia of external auditory canal			Radial limb defects	Difficult intubation
Papillomatosis larynx and trachea	Difficult laryngoscopy					Difficult intubation, care not to seed papilloma into trachea
Pierre Robin syndrome[330–338]	Hypoplastic mandible, pseudomacroglossia, ± high arched and cleft palate					Difficult intubation
Pompe disease (cardiomuscular glycogen storage disease)[327]	Large tongue		Cardiomyopathy		Muscle weakness	Difficult intubation, muscle weakness, sensitive to muscle relaxants, congestive heart failure, sensitive to myocardial depressants
Rheumatoid arthritis[359–363]	Temporomandibular joint mobility limited, hypoplastic mandible, cricoarytenoid arthritis with narrow larynx		Myocarditis, valvular disease, especially aortic insufficiency	Steroid therapy, anemia	Cervical spine subluxation, rigid cervical spine	Difficult intubation, associated heart disease, problems with positioning, steroid therapy

119

Table continued on following page

Appendix 7–1. Syndromes and Disease Processes with Associated Airway Difficulties *Continued*

Syndrome	Airway	Cerebral	Cardiac	Renal	Gastrointestinal	Endocrine Metabolic	Musculoskeletal	Anesthetic Considerations
Rubinstein-Taybi syndrome	Maxillary hypoplasia, narrow palate	Mental handicap	±CHD				Associated cervical vertebral anomalies	Difficult intubation, cervical spine instability, associated cardiac disease
Scleroderma[448]	Extensive scarring of mouth, face, body					Steroid therapy		Difficult intubation, decreased pulmonary compliance, steroid therapy
Smith-Lemli-Opitz syndrome[355]	Micrognathia, ± cleft palate, recurrent pneumonia	Moderate mental handicap, microcephaly	±CHD					Difficult intubation, associated cardiac disease
Stevens-Johnson syndrome	Laryngeal, tracheal, and bronchial bullae, pneumothorax, pleural effusion		Myocarditis	Urethritis	Esophagitis, fluid shifts	Temperature elevations		Difficult intubation, fluid balance, myocarditis, temperature control, avoid intubation if possible
Thalassemia major (Cooley's anemia)[449]	Malar hypoplasia causes relative mandibular hypoplasia		Hemosiderosis					± Difficult intubation, anemia, associated cardiac disease
Treacher-Collins syndrome[339-343]	Malar and mandibular hypoplasia, ± cleft lip, ± choanal atresia, ± macro- or microstomia		±CHD				±Cervical spine deformity	Difficult intubation, associated cardiac disease
Trisomy 21 (Down syndrome)[307-315, 429]	Small mouth, hypoplastic mandible, protruding tongue	Mental handicap	AV communis, VSD, ASD		Duodenal atresia		Hypotonia, cervical spine subluxation	± Difficult intubation, associated cardiac disease, ± less muscle relaxant
Turner syndrome (Noonan syndrome)[351, 352]	Narrow maxilla, small mandible, short neck	Mental handicap	Coarctation of aorta—females, pulmonary artery coarctation—males	Idiopathic hypertension		Hypogonadism		Difficult intubation, associated cardiac disease, hypertension

ASD, atrial septal defect, AV, atrioventricular, CHD, congenital heart disease, VSD, ventricular septal defect.

120

8

Pharmacokinetics and Pharmacology of Drugs in Children

Charles J. Coté, Ralph A. Lugo, *and* Robert M. Ward

Drug Distribution
   Protein Binding
   Body Composition
Metabolism and Excretion
   Hepatic Blood Flow
   Metabolism
   Renal Excretion
Pharmacologic Principles and Calculations
   First-Order Kinetics
   Half-Life
   First-Order Single Compartment Kinetics
   First-Order Multicompartment Kinetics
   Zero-Order Kinetics
   Apparent Volume of Distribution
   Repetitive Dosing and Drug Accumulation
   Steady State
   Loading Dose
Central Nervous System Effects
Drug Approval Process, Package Insert, and Drug Labeling
Inhalation Anesthetic Agents
   Uptake and Distribution
   Halothane (Fluothane)
   Isoflurane (Forane)
   Sevoflurane (Ultane)
   Desflurane (Suprane)
   Nitrous Oxide
   Oxygen
Intravenous Anesthetic Agents
   Barbiturates
   Propofol (Diprivan)

   Ketamine (Ketalar)
   Droperidol (Inapsine)
Narcotics
   Morphine
   Meperidine (Demerol)
   Fentanyl (Sublimaze)
   Alfentanil (Alfenta)
   Sufentanil (Sufenta)
   Remifentanil (Ultiva)
   Butorphanol (Stadol), Nalbuphine (Nubain), and Tramadol (Ultram)
Nonsteroidal Anti-inflammatory Drugs
   Ketorolac (Toradol)
   Acetaminophen (Tylenol)
Sedatives
   Diazepam (Valium)
   Midazolam (Versed)
   Chloral Hydrate
Antihistamines
   Diphenhydramine Hydrochloride (Benadryl)
   Cimetidine (Tagamet) and Ranitidine (Zantac)
   Metoclopramide (Reglan)
   Ondansetron (Zofran)
Anticholinergics
   Atropine and Scopolamine
   Glycopyrrolate (Robinul)

Most medications have different pharmacokinetics and pharmacodynamics when used in pediatric patients, especially neonates, than in adults.[1–6] Pediatric patients respond differently to drugs because of their altered protein binding, larger volume of distribution, smaller proportion of fat and muscle stores, and immature renal and hepatic function.[1, 2, 7–14] These factors may reduce a drug's metabolism or delay elimination, or both. This necessitates modification of the dose and the interval between doses to achieve the desired clinical response and avoid toxicity. In addition, some medications may displace bilirubin from its protein binding sites and possibly predispose an infant to kernicterus.[15–17] The capacity of the end organ, such as the heart or bronchial smooth muscle, to respond to medications may also differ in the pediatric patient compared with the adult. This chapter discusses basic pharmacologic principles as they relate to drugs commonly used by anesthesiologists.

Drug Distribution

Protein Binding

The degree of protein binding is usually less in premature and full-term infants than in adults or older children because of the infants' lower total protein and albumin (Fig. 8–1).[18] In addition, the albumin in preterm and term neonates appears to be qualitatively different from that in older children or adults, resulting in lower binding affinity for many medications. Many drugs that are highly protein bound in adults have less affinity for protein in neonates (Fig. 8–2).[18–22] Lower protein binding results in higher free plasma levels, thus providing more free drug and greater pharmacologic

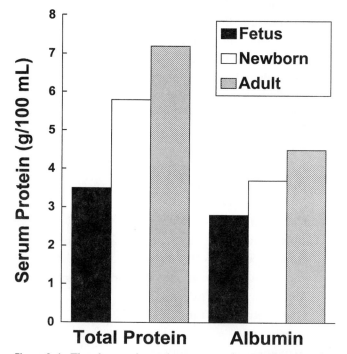

Figure 8–1. The changes in total serum protein and albumin values with maturation. Note that total protein and albumin are less in preterm than term infants and less in term infants than adults. The result may be altered pharmacokinetics and pharmacodynamics for drugs with a high degree of protein binding, because less drug is protein bound and more is available for clinical effect. (Data abstracted from Ehrnebo M, Agurell S, Jalling B, et al: Age differences in drug binding by plasma proteins: Studies on human fetuses, neonates and adults. Eur J Clin Pharmacol 1971;3:189–193.)

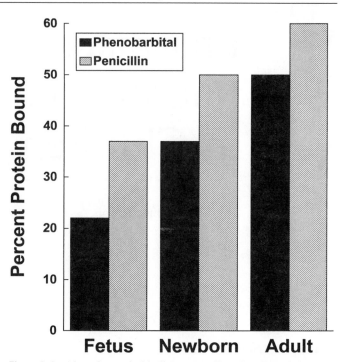

Figure 8–2. Altered protein binding may affect the clinical response to any medication: note the much lower protein binding of phenobarbital and penicillin in the newborn and fetus compared with the adult. This reduced protein binding may partially account for the prolonged pharmacologic effects of barbiturates in newborns because more unbound drug is able to be pharmacologically active. (Data abstracted from Ehrnebo M, Agurell S, Jalling B, et al: Age differences in drug binding by plasma proteins: Studies on human foetuses, neonates and adults. Eur J Clin Pharmacol 1971;3:189–193.)

effect.[1, 2, 7, 9, 12] This effect is more important for drugs that are highly protein bound because lower protein binding results in a proportionally larger unbound fraction (Fig. 8–3). Differences in protein binding may have considerable influence on the response to medications that are acidic and therefore highly protein bound (e.g., phenytoin, salicylate, bupivacaine, barbiturates, antibiotics, theophylline, and diazepam).[12] In addition, some medications, such as phenytoin, salicylate, sulfisoxazole, caffeine, ceftriaxone, diatrizoate (Hypaque), and sodium benzoate, compete with bilirubin for binding to albumin (see Fig. 8–3). If large amounts of bilirubin are displaced, kernicterus may result.[16, 17, 19, 22–24] Hypoxemia and acidosis open the blood-brain barrier and increase the risk of kernicterus. Because these metabolic derangements often occur in sick neonates coming to surgery, special care must be taken in the selection of drugs for these patients.[24] Drugs that are basic (e.g., lidocaine or alfentanil) are generally bound to alpha-1 acid glycoprotein; alpha-1 acid glycoprotein is also lower in preterm and term infants when compared with older children or adults. These medications will also have a higher unbound fraction in preterm and term infants.[25]

Body Composition

Volume of Distribution

Premature and full-term infants have a much greater proportion of body weight in the form of water than do older children and adults (Fig. 8–4).[14] Water-soluble medications will have a greater volume of distribution in these small patients, suggesting the need for a higher initial (loading) dose, based on weight, to achieve the desired serum level and clinical response.[1, 2, 9, 26, 27] A full-term neonate often requires a greater initial loading dose (milligrams per kilogram) for some drugs than an older child; examples of such drugs include digoxin, theophylline, succinylcholine, and many antibiotics such as gentamicin.[26–34] Neonates tend to be sensitive to many medications that affect the respiratory system, the central nervous system, and the cardiovascular system and therefore tend to be more responsive at lower blood levels of these drugs than older patients. Premature infants are usually even more sensitive to central nervous system pharmacologic effects than term neonates and in general require a still lower blood level.[1] Dopamine may increase blood pressure and urine output in term neonates only at doses as high as 50 µg/kg/min. This dose would induce vasoconstriction in adults, suggesting reduced cardiovascular sensitivity in the newborn. *It is important to carefully titrate to response all drugs administered to premature and term infants.*

Fat and Muscle Content

Compared with children and adolescents, premature and full-term neonates have a smaller proportion of body weight in

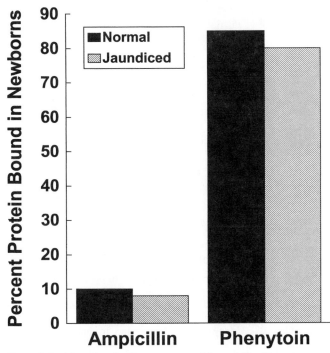

Figure 8–3. Note that in the presence of hyperbilirubinemia, many drugs that are protein bound compete with bilirubin for binding sites, resulting in elevations in both unbound bilirubin and unbound drug. This interaction may lead to an increased propensity for the development of kernicterus as well as more drug available for clinical effect. This effect is particularly important for drugs that normally are highly protein bound (e.g., phenytoin) but would be of minimal importance for drugs that have low protein binding (e.g., ampicillin). (Data abstracted from Ehrnebo M, Agurell S, Jalling B, et al: Age differences in drug binding by plasma proteins: Studies on human foetuses, neonates and adults. Eur J Clin Pharmacol 1971;3:181–193.)

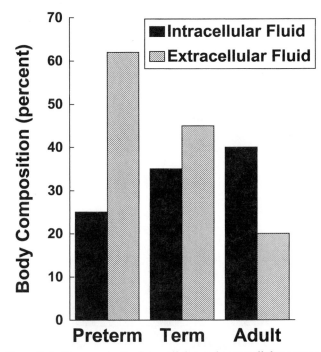

Figure 8–4. Changes in the intracellular and extracellular compartments that occur with maturation. Note the large proportion of extracellular water in preterm and term infants. This large water compartment creates an increased volume of distribution for highly water-soluble medications (e.g., succinylcholine, antibiotics) and may account for the high initial "loading" dose (mg/kg) required for some medications to achieve a satisfactory clinical response. (Data abstracted from Friis-Hansen B: Body composition during growth: In vivo measurements and biochemical data correlated to differential anatomical growth. Pediatrics 1971,47:264–274.)

the form of fat and muscle mass; with growth, the proportion of body weight composed of these tissues increases (Fig. 8–5).[1–3, 14, 32, 33, 35, 36] Drugs that depend on redistribution into muscle and fat probably have a high initial peak blood level, and they may also have a more sustained blood level because neonates have less tissue for redistribution of these drugs. An incorrect dose may result in prolonged undesirable clinical effects; for example, barbiturates and narcotics may cause prolonged sedation and respiratory depression. The possible influence of the small muscle mass on muscle relaxant requirements is exemplified by the effects of curare; neuromuscular blockade is achieved at lower serum levels in infants.[29]

Metabolism and Excretion

Hepatic Blood Flow

The liver is one of the most important organs involved in drug metabolism. Hepatic enzymatic drug metabolism usually converts the drug from a less polar state (lipid soluble) to a more polar, water-soluble compound, as discussed later. Although no categorical statement applies to all drugs and enzymes, the ability to perform these reactions in general is reduced in neonates.[2–6, 11, 28, 37–43] Another important factor influencing hepatic degradation is hepatic blood flow. As an infant matures, a greater proportion of the cardiac output is delivered to the liver, therefore improving drug delivery.

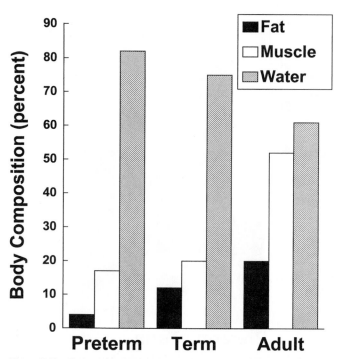

Figure 8–5. Changes in body content for fat, muscle, and water that occur with maturation. Note the small fat and muscle mass in preterm and term infants. These factors may greatly influence the pharmacokinetics and pharmacodynamics of medications that redistribute into fat (e.g., barbiturates) and muscle (e.g., fentanyl) because there is less tissue mass into which the drug may redistribute. (Data abstracted from Friis-Hansen B: Body composition during growth: In vivo measurements and biochemical data correlated to differential anatomical growth. Pediatrics 1971;47:264–274.)

Some drugs are extensively metabolized by the liver or other organs (such as the intestines or lungs) and are referred to as high extraction drugs. This extensive metabolism produces a first-pass effect in which a large proportion of the dose is inactivated as it passes though the organ before reaching the systemic circulation. For certain high extraction drugs, enteral vs intravenous administration has a large effect on how much active drug reaches the circulation.[6] Metabolism via the cytochrome P450 in the intestinal wall may occur during drug absorption. Further metabolism may occur as the portal venous circulation from the small intestine passes through the liver before returning to the heart. In contrast, intravenous administration circulates drug to the liver or intestine for metabolism in proportion to the organ blood flow. Some of the drugs that exhibit extensive first-pass metabolism include propranolol, morphine, and midazolam.[44–51]

The opening or closing of a patent ductus may have profound effects on drug delivery to metabolizing organs in preterm infants.[52, 53] The ability to metabolize and conjugate drugs improves considerably with age as a result of both increased enzyme activity and increased delivery of drug to the liver. Other factors influence the rate of hepatic maturation and metabolism; for example, sepsis and malnutrition may slow maturation while previous exposure to anticonvulsants such as phenytoin or phenobarbital may hasten maturation.[2, 32, 43, 54–58] Diazepam, thiopental, and phenobarbital have markedly increased serum half-lives in infants compared with adults (Fig. 8–6).[7, 21, 59, 60] For diazepam, this effect may

be related in part to the higher protein binding as well as slower hepatic degradation.[59] In general, the half-lives of drugs that are excreted by the liver are prolonged in neonates, are decreased in 4- to 10-year-olds, and reach adult values in older children.

Metabolism

Drug metabolism through biotransformation to more polar forms is required for many drugs before they can be eliminated from the body. The chemical changes designated by phase I reactions make the drug more polar through oxidation, reduction, or hydrolysis, whereas phase II reactions make the drug more polar through conjugation reactions, such as glucuronidation, sulfation, and acetylation.[61, 62] Although the liver is the primary site for biotransformation, other organs are also involved. Hepatic drug metabolism activity appears as early as 9 to 22 weeks of gestation when fetal liver enzyme activity may vary from 2% to 36% of adult activity.[63] It is inaccurate to generalize that the premature newborn can not metabolize drugs. Instead, the specific

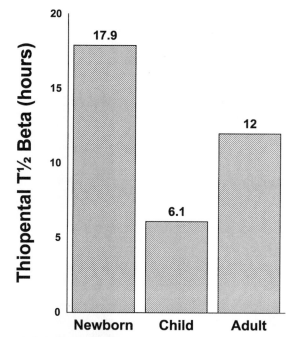

Figure 8–6. Effects of hepatic maturity on thiopental metabolism. Note the markedly prolonged beta elimination half-life for thiopental in newborns compared with children or adults. Also note that children have a shorter beta elimination half-life compared with adults. This effect may in part be related to immature hepatic metabolic pathways in the neonate; a similar effect is observed with most medications metabolized by the liver. This phenomenon may also reflect a smaller proportion of the cardiac output delivered to the liver of a neonate. In the child, this likely reflects a relatively large liver in proportion to body size and a greater proportion of the cardiac output delivered to the liver. (Data abstracted from Christensen JH, Andreasen F, Jansen JA: Pharmacokinetics of thiopental in cesarean section. Acta Anaesthesiol Scand 1981;25:174–179; Ghoneim MM, Van Hamme MJ: Pharmacokinetics of thiopentone: Effects of enflurane and nitrous oxide anaesthesia and surgery. Br J Anaesth 1978;50:1237–1242; Sorbo S, Hudson RJ, Loomis JC: The pharmacokinetics of thiopental in pediatric surgical patients. Anesthesiology 1984;61:666–670.)

pathway or pathways of drug metabolism must be considered.[64] Metabolism of many of the drugs used clinically involves cytochrome P450. Over the past two to three decades, this enzyme system has been divided into multiple forms with different substrate specificities for different drugs.[65] Induction and inhibition of these enzymes by different drugs and chemicals requires a thorough understanding of both the nomenclature of the cytochrome P450 system and the specific isoforms responsible for metabolism of the drugs used frequently in pediatric anesthesia.

Cytochromes P450: Phase I Reactions

Cytochromes P450 are heme-containing proteins that provide most of the phase I drug metabolism for lipophilic compounds in the body.[65] The nomenclature of the cytochrome P450 isozymes begins with CYP. The gene family is designated with an Arabic number, and alphanumeric letters indicate the subfamily of closely related proteins that are numbered within the subfamily.[65] Isozymes that are important in human drug metabolism are found in the CYP1, CYP2, and CYP3 gene families. Table 8–1 outlines the P450 isozymes and their common substrates.

For many drugs, the reduced metabolism by newborns relates to reduced total quantities of cytochrome P450 in hepatic microsomes.[66] Although CYP increases with gestational age, it reaches only 50% of adult values at full term.[66] In neonates, reduced cytochrome P450 decreases clearance and prolongs the half-life for many drugs, including theophylline, caffeine, diazepam, phenytoin, and phenobarbital.[28, 60, 67–69] Although newborns are poor metabolizers of many compounds, specific P450 cytochromes exhibit near adult activity while others produce unique metabolic pathways in the neonatal period that invalidates broad generalizations about neonatal drug metabolism. Table 8–1 outlines important developmental patterns for each enzyme.

Developmental Changes of Specific Cytochromes

Cytochrome P4501A2 (CPY1A2) accounts for much of the metabolism of caffeine (1,3,7-trimethylxanthine)[70, 71] and theophylline (1,3-dimethylxanthine),[72, 73] which are methylxanthines that are frequently used to treat neonatal apnea and bradycardia. CYP1A2 activity is nearly absent in the fetal liver and remains low in the newborn.[74] This limits N-3- and N-7-demethylation of caffeine in the newborn period that prolongs elimination in preterm and term newborns.[71, 75] Adult levels of activity are reached between 4 and 6 months postnatally.[76, 77] A similar pharmacokinetic pattern of reduced metabolism at birth occurs with theophylline in which CYP1A2 catalyzes 3-demethylation and 8-hydroxylation.[72, 73] Theophylline clearance reaches adult levels by 4 to 5 months, coincident with changes in CYP1A2 reflected in urine metabolite patterns.[78]

Other P450 enzymes that are reduced or absent in the fetus include CYP2D6 and CYP2C9.[54, 55, 79] CYP2D6, which is involved in the metabolism of beta-blockers, antiarrhythmics, antidepressants, antipsychotics, and codeine, is absent in the fetal liver and is eventually expressed postnatally (see Table 8–1).[55, 56] In contrast to the slow development of CYP1A2 and CYP2D6, CYP2C9, which is responsible for the metabolism of nonsteroidal anti-inflammatory drugs,

warfarin, and phenytoin, has minimal activity before birth[54] and then develops rapidly after birth.[52, 69]

CYP3A is the most important cytochrome involved in drug metabolism, because of the broad range of drugs that are substrates for these enzymes, and because it comprises the majority of adult human liver cytochrome P450 (see Table 8–1). CYP3A is detectable during embryogenesis as early as 17 weeks, primarily in the form of CYP3A7,[74] and reaches 75% of adult activity by 30 weeks of gestation.[55] In vivo, CYP3A activity appears to be mature at birth[57]; however, there is a poorly understood postnatal transition from the fetal CYP3A7 to the predominant adult isoform CYP3A4.

Phase II Reactions

The other major route of drug metabolism, designated phase II reactions, involves synthetic or conjugation reactions that increase the hydrophilicity of molecules to facilitate renal elimination.[61, 62] The phase II enzymes include glucuronosyltransferase, sulfotransferase, N-acetyltransferase, glutathione S-transferase, and methyl transferase. The phase II enzymes show developmental changes during infancy that influence drug clearance (Table 8–2), but these changes are less well studied than those of the phase I enzymes.

Most conjugation reactions show low activity during fetal development.[80] One of the most familiar synthetic reactions in young infants involves conjugation by uridine diphosphoglucuronosyltransferases (UDP-GT). This enzyme system includes numerous isoforms and is also responsible for glucuronidation of endogenous compounds, such as bilirubin.[80] As occurs with the maturation of bilirubin conjugation, UDP-GT activity is generally limited immediately after birth, and different isoforms appear to mature with different rates postnatally.[81] Dosage adjustments are often needed to avoid toxicity in newborns from drugs that require conjugation by UDP-GT for clearance. Experience with chloramphenicol in the 1960s illustrated this lesson when newborns received standard pediatric doses of chloramphenicol without understanding of the immaturity of UDP-GT and its role in the elimination of chloramphenicol. Infants accumulated chloramphenicol to high concentrations and developed fatal circulatory collapse, a condition known as the Gray Baby Syndrome.[82–84] Although the clearance of chloramphenicol is low during the neonatal period, appropriate dosage adjustments and monitoring allow safe treatment of preterm and full term infants with chloramphenicol.[85]

Morphine, acetaminophen, and lorazepam also undergo glucuronidation. The major steps in the metabolic disposition of morphine in children and adults is glucuronidation in the 3- and 6-position.[44, 86] The limited ability of neonates to glucuronidate morphine necessitates dosage adjustment.[46, 87, 88] Detailed studies have shown that morphine clearance,[46, 89] in particular 3- and 6-glucuronide formation, are low at birth and increase with birthweight,[88] gestational age,[64] and postnatal age.[86, 87] In some studies, morphine clearance approaches adult values by 1 month,[87, 90] although others report that adult clearance is not reached until at least 5 to 6 months.[46, 91] Overall, the maturation of glucuronosyltransferase enzymes varies among isoforms, but in general, adult activity is reached by 6 to 18 months of age.[65]

In contrast to glucuronosyltransferase, the sulfotransferase

Table 8–1. Developmental Patterns and Activities for Important Cytochrome P450 Enzymes (Phase I Reactions) in the Neonate

Enzymes	Selected Substrates	Inducers	Inhibitors	Developmental Changes
CYP1A2	Acetaminophen, caffeine, theophylline, warfarin	Cigarette smoke, charcoal-broiled meat, omeprazole, cruciferous vegetables	α-Naphthoflavone	Not present to an appreciable extent in human fetal liver. Adult levels reached by 4 months of age and may be exceeded in children 1–2 years of age. Inhibited by cigarette smoke, phenobarbital, and phenytoin.
CYP2A6	Coumarin, nicotine	Barbiturates	Tranylcypromine	
CYP2C9	Diclofenac, phenytoin, torsemide, S-warfarin tolbutamide	Rifampin	Sulfaphenazole, sulfinpyrazone	Not apparent in fetal liver. Inferential data using phenytoin disposition as a nonspecific pharmacologic probe suggest low activity during the first week of life, with adult activity reached by 6 months of age and peak activity reached by 3–4 years of age. Metabolism induced by rifampin and phenobarbital and inhibited by cimetidine.
CYP2C19	Phenytoin, diazepam, omeprazole, propranolol	Rifampin	Tranylcypromine	
CYP2D6	Amitriptyline, captopril, codeine, dextromethorphan, fluoxetine, hydrocodone, ondansetron, propafenone, propranolol, timolol	None known	Fluoxetine, quinidine	Low to absent in fetal liver but uniformly present at 1 week of postnatal age. Poor activity (approximately 20% of adult values) at 1 month of postnatal age. Adult competence reached by approximately 3–5 years of age. Metabolism inhibited by cimetidine.
CYP3A4	Acetaminophen, alfentanil, amiodarone, budesonide, carbamazepine, diazepam, erythromycin, lidocaine, midazolam, nifedipine, omeprazole, cisapride, theophylline, verapamil, R-warfarin	Carbamazepine, dexamethasone, phenobarbital, phenytoin, rifampin	Azole antifungals, ethinylestradiol, naringenin, troleandomycin, erythromycin	CYP3A4 has low activity in the first month of life, with approach toward adult levels by 6–12 months postnatally.
CYP3A7	Dehydroepiandrosterone, ethinylestradiol, various dihydropyrimidines	Carbamazepine, rifampin	?Azole antifungals	CYP3A7 is functionally active in the fetus; approximately 30% to 75% of adult levels of CYP3A4. Induced by carbamazepine, dexamethasone, phenobarbital, phenytoin, and rifampin. Enzyme inhibitors include azole antifungals, erythromycin, and cimetidine.

Adapted from Leeder JS, Kearns GL: Pharmacogenetics in pediatrics: Implications for practice. Pediatr Clin North Am 1997;44:55–77.

Table 8–2. Developmental Patterns for Important Conjugation (Phase II) Reactions in the Neonate

Enzymes	Selected Substrates	Developmental Patterns
Uridine diphos-phoglucuronosyl-transferase (UDP-GT)	Chloramphenicol, morphine, acetaminophen, valproic acid, lorazepam	Ontogeny is isoform specific. In general, adult activity is achieved by 6–18 months of age. May be induced by cigarette smoke and phenobarbital.
Sulfotransferase	Bile acids, acetaminophen, cholesterol, polyethylene, glycols, dopamine, chloramphenicol	Ontogeny seems to be more rapid than UDP-GT; however, it is substrate specific. Activity for some isoforms may exceed adult values during infancy and childhood, e.g., that responsible for acetaminophen metabolism.
N-acetyl transferase 2	Hydralazine, procainamide, clonazepam, caffeine, sulfamethoxazole	Some fetal activity present by 16 weeks. Virtually 100% of infants between birth and 2 months of age exhibit the slow metabolizer phenotype. Adult activity present by approximately 1–3 years of age.

Adapted from Leeder JS, Kearns GL: Pharmacogenetics in pediatrics: Implications for practice. Pediatr Clin North Am 1997;44:55–77.

enzyme system is well developed in the newborn, and for some compounds it may compensate for limited glucuronidation. In adults, the primary pathway for acetaminophen metabolism is glucuronidation, yet its half-life is only moderately prolonged in newborns as compared with older infants and adults.[92–94] This occurs because the newborn forms more sulfate than glucuronide conjugate, leading to a greater percent of the dose excreted as the acetaminophen-sulfate conjugate.[93, 94] This metabolic pattern of preferential sulfation of acetaminophen persists into childhood.[93, 95]

Alterations in Biotransformation

Many biotransformation reactions, especially those involving certain forms of cytochrome P450, are inducible before birth through maternal exposure to drugs, cigarette smoke, or other inducing agents. Postnatally, biotransformation reactions may be induced through drug exposure (see Tables 8–1 and 8–2) and may be slowed by hypoxia or asphyxia, organ damage, or illness. Postnatal changes in hepatic blood flow,

protein binding, or biliary function may also alter drug elimination significantly. Additional studies during development from the immature neonate born at 24 weeks through infancy and young childhood are needed to identify the ages and stages of development when drug metabolism changes most rapidly, which will lead to safer and more effective pharmacotherapeutic regimens.

Renal Excretion

The renal function of neonates and premature infants is less efficient than in adults even after adjusting for the differences in body weight. This reduced efficiency is related to the combination of incomplete glomerular development, low perfusion pressure, and inadequate osmotic load to produce full countercurrent effects.[96–101] Premature and full-term newborns have immature glomerular filtration and tubular function; both develop rapidly during the first few months of life. Healthy premature and full-term babies have relatively normal renal drug clearance by 3 to 4 weeks of age. Glomerular filtration and tubular function are nearly mature by 20 weeks of age and fully mature by 2 years of age (Fig. 8–7).[97–101] For these reasons, *drugs that are excreted primarily through glomerular filtration or tubular secretion, for example, aminoglycoside and cephalosporin antibiotics, have a prolonged half-life in neonates* (Fig. 8–8).[102–104]

In the presence of renal failure, one or two doses of renally excreted drugs often achieve and maintain prolonged therapeutic drug levels if there is no alternate pathway of excretion. The first dose may be removed from the circulation by distribution and tissue binding. *Whenever administer-*

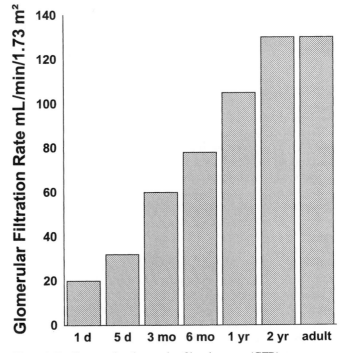

Figure 8–7. Changes in glomerular filtration rate (GFR) versus age. Note the rapid development of glomerular function during the first year of life. Abnormal as well as immature renal function may delay drug excretion. (Data abstracted from Chantler C: Clinical Pediatric Nephrology. Philadelphia: JB Lippincott; 1976.)

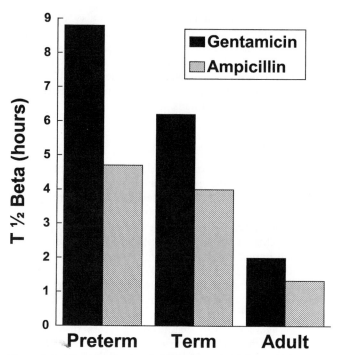

Figure 8–8. Beta elimination half-life for ampicillin and gentamicin versus age. Note the inverse relationship between age and beta elimination half-life; this relationship correlates well with maturing renal function. A similar effect is observed with most medications excreted by glomerular filtration. (Data abstracted from Kaplan JM, McCracken GH Jr, Horton LJ, et al: Pharmacologic studies in neonates given large dosages of ampicillin. J Pediatr 1974;84(4):571–577; McCracken GH Jr: Pharmacological basis for antimicrobial therapy in newborn infants. Am J Dis Child 1974;128(3):407–419; Miranda JC, Schimmel MM, James LS, et al: Gentamicin kinetics in the neonate. Pediatr Pharmacol 1985;5(1):57–61; Merritt GJ, Slade JB: Influence of hyperbaric oxygen on the pharmacokinetics of single-dose gentamicin in healthy volunteers. Pharmacotherapy 1993;13(4):382–385.)

ing a medication to a premature or full-term infant, one must consider what part renal function will play in the termination of its action.

The pharmacokinetics and pharmacodynamics of curare exemplify the complex interaction of increased volume of distribution, smaller muscle mass, and decreased rate of excretion due to immaturity of glomerular filtration. The initial dose of curare needed to achieve neuromuscular blockade is similar in infants and adults.[29] In infants, however, this blockade is achieved at lower serum concentrations than in older children or adults, corresponding to the differences in muscle mass. A larger volume of distribution (total body water) accounts for the equivalent dose for each kilogram of body weight, and the reduced glomerular function in infants compared with older children or adults accounts in part for the longer duration of action.[29] Just as for hepatically excreted drugs, there is a triphasic developmental response to drugs excreted by the kidneys: a prolonged half-life in neonates (immature renal function), a shortened half-life in young children (maturation of the kidneys and increased renal perfusion delivering more drug to the kidneys), and a longer half-life in adolescents and adults (decreased renal function and decreased proportional renal blood flow). Al-

tered protein binding in neonates and premature infants will result in more free drug being delivered to the kidneys and liver for metabolism; however, this also results in a greater amount of drug available to cross biologic membranes. This greater unbound fraction causes more drug to be available to have effect or a greater potential for toxicity.[1, 2, 11, 12]

Pharmacokinetic Principles and Calculations

Changes in drug concentrations within the body with time are referred to as pharmacokinetics. The principles and equations that describe these changes can be used to adjust drug doses rationally to achieve more effective drug concentrations at the site of action.[61, 62, 105–111] The equations in this section are intended for general and practical use, while the more rigorous mathematical intricacies of pharmacokinetics are covered elsewhere.[108–111]

Within the body, a drug may diffuse between several body fluids and tissues at different rates, yet the consistent change in its circulating concentration may be used to characterize its kinetics and to guide dosages. The rate of removal of drug from the circulation usually fits either first-order or zero-order exponential equations. The difference between these two types of rates has important implications for drug treatment.

First-Order Kinetics

Most drugs are cleared from the body with first-order exponential rates in which a constant fraction or constant proportion of drug is removed per unit of time. Because the proportion of drug cleared remains constant, the higher the concentration, the greater the amount of drug removed from the body. Such rates can be described by exponential equations that fit the following form:

$$C = C_0 e^{-kt} \qquad (Eq. 1)$$

where C is the concentration at time t, C_0 is the starting concentration (a constant determined by the dose and distribution volume), and k is the elimination rate constant with units of time^{-1}. First-order indicates that the exponent is raised to the first power ($-kt$ in Eq. 1). Second-order equations are those that are raised to the second power, such as $e^{(z)2}$. First-order exponential equations, such as in Eq. 1, may be converted to the form of the equation of a straight line ($y = mx + b$) by taking the natural logarithm of both sides after which they may be solved by linear regression.

$$\ln C = \ln C_0 + (-kt) \qquad (Eq. 2)$$

If *ln* (i.e., natural logarithm) C is graphed versus time, the slope is $-k$, and the intercept is *ln* C_0. If log (i.e., logarithm base 10) C is graphed versus time, the slope is $-k/2.303$, since ln x equals 2.303 log x. When graphed on linear-linear axes, exponential rates are curvilinear and on semilogarithmic axes, they produce a straight line.

Half-Life

Half-life, the time for a drug concentration to decrease by one half, is a familiar exponential rate used to describe the kinetics of many drugs. Half-life is a first-order kinetic process, since the same proportion or fraction of the drug is removed during equal periods of time. As described earlier, the higher the concentration, the greater the amount of drug removed during each half-life.

Half-life can be determined by several methods. If concentration is converted to the natural logarithm of concentration and graphed versus time, as described in Eq. 2, the slope of this graph is the elimination rate constant, k. For both accuracy and precision, at least three concentration time points should be used to determine the slope, and they should be obtained over an interval during which the concentration decreases at least by half. In clinical practice, for infants and small children, however, k is often estimated from just two concentrations obtained during the terminal elimination phase. With multiple data points, the slope of ln C versus time may be calculated easily by least-squares linear regression analysis. Half-life ($t_{1/2}$) may be calculated from the elimination rate constant, k (time^{-1}), as follows:

$$t_{1/2} = \frac{\text{natural logarithm (2)}}{k} = \frac{0.693}{k} \qquad \text{(Eq. 3)}$$

Graphic techniques may be used to determine half-life from a series of timed measurements of drug concentration. The concentration-time points should be graphed on semilogarithmic axes and used to determine the best-fitting line either visually or by linear regression analysis. This approach is illustrated in Figure 8–9, in which the best-fitting line has been drawn to the concentration-time points and crosses a concentration of 20 at 100 minutes and a concentration of 10 at 200 minutes. The concentration has decreased by one half in 100 minutes so the $t_{1/2}$ is 100 minutes. The elimination rate constant is 0.693/100 min^{-1} or 0.00693 min^{-1}.

First-Order Single Compartment Kinetics

The number of exponential equations required to describe the change in concentration determines the number of compartments. Although a drug may be diffusing among several

tissues and body fluids, its clearance often fits first-order, single-compartment kinetics if it quickly distributes homogeneously within the circulation and is removed rapidly from the circulation through metabolism or excretion. This may be judged visually if a semilogarithmic graph of the change in drug concentration fits a single straight line. Kinetics may appear to be single-compartment, when they are really multiple compartment, if drug concentrations are not measured soon enough after intravenous administration to detect the initial distribution phase (α phase).

First-Order Multicompartment Kinetics

If drug concentrations are measured several times within the first 15 to 30 minutes after intravenous administration as well as during a more prolonged period, more than one rate of clearance is often present. This can be observed as a marked change in slope of a semilogarithmic graph of concentration versus time (Fig. 8–10). The number and nature of the compartments required to describe the clearance of a drug do not necessarily represent specific body fluids or tissues. When two first-order exponential equations are required to describe the clearance of drug from the circulation, the kinetics are described as first-order, two-compartment (for example, central and peripheral compartments) that fit the following equation (see Fig. 8–10)[105]:

$$C = Ae^{-\alpha t} + Be^{-\beta t} \qquad \text{(Eq. 4)}$$

where concentration is *C, t* is time after the dose, *A* is the concentration at time 0 for the distribution rate represented by the broken line graph with the steepest slope, α is the rate constant for distribution, *B* is the concentration at time 0 for the terminal elimination rate, and β is the rate constant for terminal elimination. Rate constants indicate the rate of change in concentration and correspond to the slope of the line divided by 2.303 for logarithm concentration versus time.

Such two-compartment or biphasic kinetics are frequently observed after intravenous administration of drugs that rap-

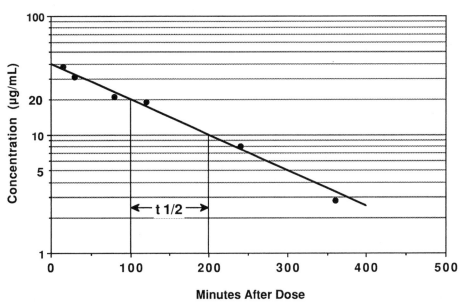

Figure 8–9. Graphic determination of half-life. Half-life can be determined from a series of concentration time points on a semilogarithmic graph if the kinetics are exponential. The concentrations are plotted on semilogarithmic axes; the best-fit line is drawn to the points; convenient concentrations are chosen that decrease in half, such as 20 and 10, as illustrated; and the interval between those concentrations is the half-life, 100 minutes in the illustration.

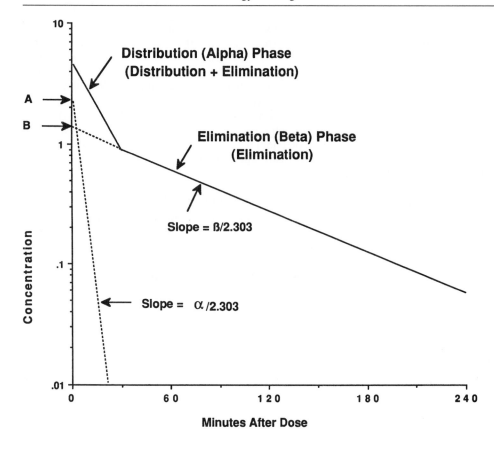

Figure 8–10. Two-compartment kinetics in a semilogarithmic graph. The initial rapid decrease in serum concentration reflects distribution and elimination followed by a slower decrease due to elimination. Subtraction of the initial decrease in concentration due to elimination using the concentrations from the elimination line extrapolated back to time 0 at point B produces the lower line with a steep slope = α (distribution rate constant)/2.303. The terminal elimination phase has a slope = β (elimination rate constant)/2.303.

idly distribute out of the central compartment of the circulation to undergo hepatic metabolism or renal excretion.[105] In such situations, the initial rapid decrease in concentration is referred to as the alpha distribution phase and represents distribution to the peripheral (tissue) compartments in addition to drug elimination. The terminal (beta) phase begins after the inflection point in the line when elimination starts to account for most of the change in drug concentration. To determine the initial change in concentration due to distribution (see Fig. 8–10), the change in concentration due to elimination must be subtracted from the total change in concentration. The slope of the line representing the difference between these two rates is the rate constant for distribution. A more detailed mathematical discussion may be found elsewhere.[108–111]

Although many drugs demonstrate multicompartment kinetics, many studies of kinetics in newborns do not include enough samples shortly after dosing to determine both compartments. For clinical estimates of dose and dosing intervals, it is often not necessary to use multiple compartment kinetics. To minimize cost, limit blood loss, and simplify pharmacokinetic calculations, dose adjustments are often based on only two plasma concentrations (peak and trough) and assume linear, single-compartment kinetics (e.g., gentamicin and vancomycin). Since the elimination rate constant should be determined from the terminal elimination phase, it is important that peak concentrations of multicompartment drugs not be drawn prematurely, that is, during the initial distribution phase. If drawn too early, the concentrations will be higher than those during the terminal elimination phase (see Fig. 8–10), which will overestimate the slope and the terminal elimination rate constant.

Zero-Order Kinetics

The elimination of some drugs occurs with loss of a *constant amount per time, rather than a constant fraction per time.* Such rates are termed zero-order, and since $e^0 = 1$, the change in the amount of drug in the body fits the following equation[108]:

$$-dA/dt = k_0 \qquad \text{(Eq. 5)}$$

where dA is the change in the amount of drug in the body (mg), dt is the change in time, and k_0 is the elimination rate constant with units of amount per time. After solving this equation, it has the following form:

$$A = A_0 - k_0 t \qquad \text{(Eq. 6)}$$

where A_0 is the initial amount of drug in the body and A is the amount of drug in the body (mg) at time t.

Zero-order kinetics may be designated saturation kinetics, because such processes occur when excess amounts of drug saturate the capacity of metabolic enzymes or transport systems. In this situation, only a constant amount of drug is metabolized or transported per unit of time. If kinetics are zero-order, a graph of serum concentration versus time is linear on linear-linear axes and is curved when graphed on linear-logarithmic (i.e., semilogarithmic) axes. Clinically, first-order elimination may become zero-order after administration of excessive doses, after prolonged infusions, or during dysfunction of the organ of elimination. Certain drugs administered to newborns exhibit zero-order kinetics at therapeutic doses and may accumulate to excessive concentrations, including caffeine, chloramphenicol, diazepam, furosemide, indomethacin, and phenytoin.[5] Some drugs, such as phenytoin, may exhibit Michaelis-Menten kinetics—that is, first-order at low concentrations and zero-order after enzymes are saturated at higher concentrations. For these drugs, a small increment in dose may cause disproportionately large increments in serum concentrations (Fig. 8–11).

Apparent Volume of Distribution

The apparent volume of distribution (Vd) is a mathematical term that relates the dose to the circulating concentration observed immediately after administration. It might be viewed as the volume of dilution that can be used to predict the change in concentration after a dose is diluted within the body. Vd does not necessarily correspond to a physiologic body fluid or tissue volume, hence the designation "apparent." For drugs that distribute out of the circulation or bind to tissues such as digoxin, Vd may reach 10 L/kg, a physical impossibility for a fluid compartment in the body. This illustrates the mathematical nature of Vd. The units used to express concentration are amount/volume and may help to remind the reader of the following equation, which expresses the relation between dose in amount/kg and the Vd in volume/kg that dilutes the dose to produce the concentration:

$$\text{Concentration change (mg/L)} = \frac{\text{Dose (mg/kg)}}{\text{Vd (L/kg)}}$$

(Eq.7)

If concentration is expressed with the unconventional units of milligrams per liter rather than micrograms per milliliter (which is equivalent), it is easier to balance the equation. This equation serves as the basis for most of the pharmacokinetic calculations, since it is easily rearranged to solve for Vd and dose. It is also important to note that this equation represents the change in concentration following a rapidly administered intravenous dose of a drug whose elimination is long compared with the time for distribution. Following a mini-infusion, such as with vancomycin or gentamicin, a more complex exponential equation may be required to account for drug elimination during the time of infusion.[108] In neonates, who have relatively slow drug elimination, only a small fraction of drug is eliminated during the time of infusion, and such adjustments can be omitted, whereas more complex equations may be needed in older patients.

Knowledge of the apparent distribution volume is essential for dosage adjustments. The Vd may be calculated by rearranging Eq. 7.

$$\text{Vd (L/kg)} = \frac{\text{Dose (mg/kg)}}{C \text{ (postdose)} - C \text{ (predose) (mg/L)}}$$

(Eq. 8)

The concentration after drug infusion, C (postdose), must be measured after the distribution phase to avoid overestimating the peak concentration that would result in an erroneously low Vd. For the first dose, the predose concentration is 0.

Pharmacokinetic Example

The following example illustrates the application of these pharmacokinetic principles using a four-step approach: (1) calculate Vd; (2) calculate half-life; (3) calculate a new dose and dosing interval based on a desired peak and trough; (4) check the peak and trough of the new dosage regimen.

For example, vancomycin was administered intravenously in a dose of 15 mg/kg over 60 minutes every 12 hours. The following plasma concentrations were measured on the third day of treatment (presumed steady-state). The predose or trough concentration was 12 mg/L; the peak concentration, measured 60 minutes after the *end* of the infusion, was 32 mg/L.

Step 1: Substituting the data into Eq. 8, we calculate Vd.

$$\text{Vd (L/kg)} = \frac{15 \text{ mg/kg}}{32 \text{ mg/L} - 12 \text{ mg/L}} = \frac{15 \text{ mg/kg}}{20 \text{ mg/L}}$$

$$= 0.75 \text{ L/kg}$$

Step 2: At steady-state, peak and trough concentrations reach the same levels after each dose. The time between the peak and trough concentrations is 10 hours, that is, 12 hours minus 1 hour infusion, minus 1 hour to peak concentration. Half-life may be solved by rearranging equation 2 to solve for k (elimination rate constant) and substituting the calculated k into Eq. 3. In this case, the calculated elimination rate constant is 0.098 hours[−1] and the corresponding half-life is 7.1 hours. However, a practical and clinically applicable "bedside" approach may be used without need for logarithmic calculations. For example, the plasma concentration decreased from 32 to 16 mg/L in one half-life, and then from 16 to 12

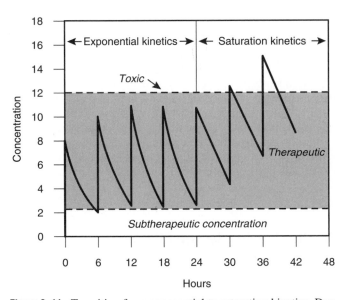

Figure 8–11. Transition from exponential to saturation kinetics. During q6hr dosing, concentrations during the first 24 hours reflect exponential kinetics with a half-life of 3 hours (k = 0.231/hr) followed by a change to saturation kinetics at 24 hours with elimination of 1.0 mg/hr leading to drug accumulation to toxic concentrations.

mg/L in a fraction of the second half-life. At the end of the second half-life, the concentration would have decreased to 8 mg/L. Since 12 mg/L is the midpoint between 1 and 2 half-lives, 1.5 half-lives have elapsed during the 10 hours between the peak and trough. Thus if one assumes a linear decline, the half-life may be estimated as 6.67 hours (10 hours ÷ 1.5 half-lives). Note that the error between the actual half-life of 7.1 hours and the estimated half-life of 6.67 hours is a result of the linear assumptions of this calculation between half-lives. In fact, first-order elimination is a nonlinear process and concentration will actually decline from 32 mg/L to 22.6 mg/L during the first 50% of the first half-life rather than from 32 mg/L to 24 mg/L using this linear approach. The same occurs during subsequent half-lives. However, the small error associated with this method is often acceptable for rapid bedside estimates of pharmacokinetic parameters.

Step 3: A new dosage regimen must be calculated if the concentrations are unsatisfactory. Accordingly, one must decide upon a desired peak and trough concentration. If, for example, the desired vancomycin peak and trough concentrations were 32 mg/L (20–40 mg/L) and 8 mg/L (5–10 mg/L), respectively, then Eq. 8 may be rearranged to solve for the new dose.

$$\text{Dose (mg/kg)} = \text{Vd (L/kg)} \times [\text{C (peak desired)} \\ - \text{C (post desired) (mg/L)}] \qquad \text{(Eq. 9)}$$

$$\text{Dose (mg/kg)} = 0.75 \text{ L/kg} \times (32 \text{ mg/L} - 8 \text{ mg/L})$$

$$\text{Dose (mg/kg)} = 18 \text{ mg/kg}$$

The current dose produces a peak of 32, which is in the recommended therapeutic range, and lengthening the dosing interval to two half-lives (13⅓ hours) after the peak is reached (2 hours after beginning the dose infusion) will produce a trough concentration of 8 mg/L. The dose interval should be increased to 16 hours and the dose increased to 18 mg/kg.

Step 4: Estimating peak and trough concentrations with the new regimen provides a good double check against a mathematical error. Sixteen hours after the 15 mg/kg dose is administered (or approximately two half-lives after the measured peak), the trough should be approximately 8 mg/L. At this time, administration of 18 mg/kg will raise the concentration by 24 mg/L (assuming a volume of distribution of 0.75 L/kg) to a peak concentration of 32 mg/L.

Repetitive Dosing and Drug Accumulation

When multiple doses are administered, the dose is usually repeated before complete elimination of the previous one. In this situation, peak and trough concentrations increase until a steady state concentration (C_{ss}) is reached (see Fig. 8–11). The average C_{ss} can be calculated as follows[106]:

$$\text{Avg } C_{ss} = \frac{1}{\text{Clearance}} \times \frac{f \times D}{\tau} \qquad \text{(Eq. 10)}$$

$$= \frac{1}{k \times Vd_{(area)}} \times \frac{f \times D}{\tau}$$

$$= \frac{1.44 \times t_{1/2}}{Vd_{(area)}} \times \frac{f \times D}{\tau} \qquad \text{(Eq. 11)}$$

In Eq. 10 and Eq. 11, f is the fraction of the dose that is absorbed, D is the dose, τ is the dosing interval in the same units of time as the elimination half-life, k is the elimination rate constant, and 1.44 equals 1/0.693 (see Eq. 3). The magnitude of the average C_{ss} is directly proportional to a ratio of $t_{1/2}/\tau$ and D.[106]

Steady State

Steady state occurs when the amount of drug removed from the body between doses equals the amount of the dose.[107, 111] Five half-lives are usually required for drug elimination and distribution among tissue and fluid compartments to reach equilibrium. When all tissues are at equilibrium, that is, at steady state, the peak and trough concentrations are the same after each dose. However, prior to this time, constant peak and trough concentrations after intermittent doses, or constant concentrations during drug infusions, do not prove that a steady state has been achieved, since drug may still be entering and leaving deep tissue compartments. During continuous infusion, the fraction of steady-state concentration that has been reached can be calculated in terms of multiples of the drug's half-life.[106] After three half-lives, the concentration is 88% of that at steady state. When changing doses during chronic drug therapy, the concentration should usually not be rechecked until several half-lives have elapsed, unless elimination is impaired or signs of toxicity occur. Drug concentrations may not need to be checked if symptoms improve.

Loading Dose

If the time to reach a constant concentration by continuous or intermittent dosing is too long, a loading dose may be used to reach a higher constant concentration more quickly. This frequently is applied to initial treatment with digoxin, which has a 35- to 69-hour half-life in term neonates and an even longer half-life in preterm newborns.[112] Use of a loading dose produces a higher circulating drug concentration earlier in the therapeutic course, but the equilibration to reach a true steady state still requires treatment for five or more half-lives. Loading doses must be used cautiously, since they increase the likelihood of drug toxicity, as has been observed with loading doses of digoxin.[2, 11, 12, 112]

Central Nervous System Effects

Laboratory data have demonstrated the lethal dose in 50% of animals (LD_{50}) for many medications to be significantly lower in newborn than in adult animals.[113, 114] The sensitivity of human newborns to most of the sedatives, hypnotics, and narcotics is clinically well known and may in part be related to increased brain permeability (immature blood-brain barrier) for some medications.[115, 116] Laboratory studies have demonstrated higher brain concentrations of morphine and amobarbital in infant than in adult animals.[117] Incomplete myelination in infants may make it easier for drugs that are not particularly lipid soluble to enter the brain at a greater rate than if the blood-brain barrier were intact.[115–118] When considering the use of any centrally acting medication in children less than 1 year of age and particularly those less than 48 weeks of postconceptual age, one must balance the potential risks and benefits. Dosage must be carefully calculated and titrated to allow the lowest dose that provides the required patient response. Careful monitoring of vital signs is important because prolonged effects or adverse clinical responses may occur in patients of any age, but particularly in infants in whom maturation of the central nervous system may be incomplete.

Drug Approval Process, Package Insert, and Drug Labeling

One area of concern has been the general lack of approval of many medications for populations of pediatric patients. Nearly 80% of currently approved medications have language within the drug label (package insert) that excludes children of varying ages. Many of the drugs we use in the operating room and the intensive care unit have similar language.[119] Common examples of drugs used in our daily practice include bupivacaine (until further experience is gained in children younger than 12 years, administration of Sensorcaine (bupivacaine HCl) Injection is not recommended)[120] and fentanyl (the safety and efficacy of Sublimaze in children under 2 years of age has not been established).[121] Such disclaimers are placed in the package insert because the contents of the package insert must by law be based on adequate, well-controlled studies involving children.[122–124] Any use of a drug that is not specifically described in the package insert is considered "unapproved" or "off label." The reason for the lack of labeling for children is that the appropriate controlled clinical trials were never supported by industry, and the Food and Drug Administration (FDA) did not have the legislative power to force the pharmaceutical companies to perform pediatric studies.[125] In 1994, the FDA passed a new interpretation of the original Food, Drug and Cosmetic Act,[124, 126] which allowed manufacturers to review the published medical literature and submit these data to the FDA to support revised pediatric labeling.[122] Unfortunately, for drugs that are no longer under patent protection, there was no financial incentive to force the issue, so many drugs remain unlabeled for children despite the many papers published describing their use in children of all ages. Recent changes at the FDA (The Food and Drug Administration Modernization Act [FDAMA])[127] and the Final Rule[128] have the potential to further improve drug labeling for children. The FDAMA legislation has empowered the FDA to request at least one pediatric study for drugs currently still under patent protection for which additional pediatric information was deemed necessary. This has resulted in a priority list developed through recommendations from all Sections of the American Academy of Pediatrics, the United States Pharmacopeia, and the National Institutes of Child Health and Human Development. The Secretary of Health now has the power to request pediatric studies, but this legislation will expire in 2001 unless Congress decides to renew it. Unfortunately, the definition of a pediatric study is still somewhat unclear.

It is hoped that the success in developing new information and improved labeling for children will encourage continuance of that legislation. In exchange for studies requested through FDAMA, the manufacturer will be rewarded with 6 months extension of market exclusivity. In some situations, the manufacturer will obtain a further 6 months patent extension in return for developing a new pediatric formulation, e.g., a liquid formulation allowing the drug to be administered to infants and toddlers. This legislation is likely to improve drug availability and labeling for children for drugs that are widely used and have a large market share. It is unlikely to provide adequate incentives for drugs that have a small market share or that will soon be coming off patent before pediatric studies can be completed. The Final Rule legislation has empowered the FDA to require pediatric studies of all new drug applications if there appears to be a pediatric indication. These legislative changes should improve drug therapy for children, but they do not address the issue as it relates to generic drugs that are off patent (no longer patent protected), so the deficiencies in labeling for older drugs are likely to persist.

It is important for the clinician to clearly understand that, despite language on the label regarding use in children, he or she is perfectly within medical and legal rights to use these drugs in children. Unapproved use does not imply an improper use and certainly does not imply an illegal use.[129] The use of a drug in a child is the decision of the individual physician and may be based on the available literature, despite the fact that formal FDA approval and labeling have not been achieved.[123, 124] The Committee on Drugs of the American Academy of Pediatrics is very clear on this issue: Lack of approval for a specific use should not prevent physicians from prescribing an available drug in the best interest of their patients.[129]

Inhalation Anesthetic Agents

The measure of anesthetic potency has traditionally been the minimum alveolar concentration (MAC) or the effective dose in 50% (ED_{50}), that is, the expired concentration at which 50% of patients (or animals) do not move in response to a surgical stimulus. The anesthetic requirements of pediatric patients vary according to age. Early studies of inhalation agents revealed that young infants and adolescents had greater halothane requirements than adults.[130, 131] Newer studies have modified the interpretation of the earlier results, demonstrating that a human neonate from birth to 31 days of age has a lower MAC than an infant 30 to 180 days old (0.87 ± 0.03% versus 1.20 ± 0.06% expired halothane); the ED_{50} for adults is 0.94% (Fig. 8–12).[130–133] Isoflurane has a lower MAC in premature infants than in newborn or older infants.[134] The reasons for the apparently greater anesthetic requirement in infants compared with newborns, premature infants, and adults are unclear.[130–134] Regardless of the mechanism, the clinically important point is that there is nearly a 30% greater anesthetic requirement for all potent anesthetic agents in infants compared with adults to attain a comparable depth of anesthesia. It must be emphasized that there is a smaller margin of safety between adequate anesthesia and

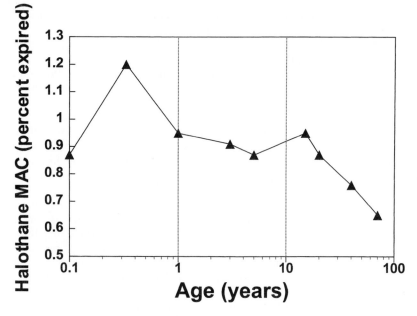

Figure 8–12. The minimum alveolar concentration (MAC) of halothane versus patient age. Note the higher requirements in infants and teenagers. Neonates have lower requirements than infants. (Data abstracted from Gregory GA, Eger EI 2nd, Munson ES: The relationship between age and halothane requirement in man. Anesthesiology 1969;30:488–491; and Lerman J, Robinson S, Willis MM, et al: Anesthetic requirements for halothane in young children 0–1 month and 1–6 months of age. Anesthesiology 1983;59:421–424.)

severe cardiopulmonary depression in infants and children compared with adults. Studies of neonatal rats have confirmed that equianesthetic concentrations of halothane result in greater myocardial depression in neonatal compared with mature animals.[135] Since the cardiac output of neonates is markedly dependent on heart rate, administering vagolytic agents may reverse some of the myocardial depression of the potent inhalation agents.[136] Because premature and term neonates have abnormalities of calcium homeostasis and because some of the myocardial depression caused by potent anesthetic agents is mediated through altered calcium channel activity, it is possible that altered cardiac calcium homeostasis may have a central role in the sensitivity of a premature or newborn infant's heart to potent inhalation agents.[137–139]

A greater depth of anesthesia is required for airway manipulation than for superficial surgical procedures. For this reason, another clinically important concept when anesthetizing children is MAC for endotracheal intubation (MAC_{EI}) (the end-tidal halothane concentration that would allow successful endotracheal intubation with no coughing or movement in 50% of pediatric patients). The MAC_{EI} for children 2 to 6 years of age is 1.33% for halothane.[140] *The anesthetic concentrations necessary for intubation are even closer to those levels that might result in severe cardiopulmonary depression.* The use of neuromuscular blocking agents and short-acting narcotics has greatly improved the safety of general anesthesia in infants, because lower concentrations of potent inhalation agents may be used while providing adequate anesthesia and excellent conditions for endotracheal intubation.

One carefully conducted study examined the contribution of nitrous oxide to MAC.[141] There was a linear relationship with increasing concentrations of nitrous oxide (25% to 75%); 75% nitrous oxide reduced the MAC of halothane from 0.94 ± 0.8% to 0.29 ± 0.06%.

Uptake and Distribution

The uptake and distribution of inhalation agents are more rapid in infants and children than in adults. This effect may

in part be related to their more rapid respiratory rate, increased cardiac index, and the distribution of a larger proportion of the cardiac output to vessel-rich or well-perfused organs.[142–144] These factors result in a more rapid increase in the partial pressure of inhalation agents in mixed venous blood; the more rapid uptake is one of the factors contributing to the ease of producing myocardial depression in infants and children. This more rapid uptake may also account in part for the higher incidence of cardiac arrests in children compared with adults.[145–149]

Ventilation/perfusion mismatch, airway obstruction, and perhaps intracardiac defects (primarily right-to-left shunts) result in a slower rate of uptake and rise in alveolar concentration of the potent inhalation (soluble) agents.[150] More time is required to achieve an adequate plane of anesthesia for safe laryngoscopy and intubation in children with any of the previously mentioned problems. This concept is especially important when inducing anesthesia in a child with airway obstruction, when safe, smooth control of the airway is vital. Nitrous oxide and sevoflurane are insoluble, compared with halothane. Therefore, the effects of respiratory rate, increased cardiac index, and distribution of cardiac output should be of less clinical importance.

The rate of induction and awakening may also be related in part to the type of anesthetic circuit used. A non-rebreathing system produces a more rapid rise in alveolar anesthetic concentration than a similar concentration delivered by a rebreathing (circle) system. With a circle system, it is necessary to consider the volume of the anesthetic tubing, the carbon dioxide absorber, and the humidifier in relationship to the patient's lung volume. With a circle system (volume of 3500 mL), a change in inspired concentration takes longer to equilibrate than a similar change made with a non-rebreathing circuit (volume of 1200 mL). A more rapid induction and perhaps a better control of anesthetic depth may be achieved with a non-rebreathing system. This concept is important in neonatal anesthesia because very small changes in anesthetic concentration rapidly equilibrate with the small lung volume. A non-rebreathing system also allows more rapid elimination of potent inhalation agents. These concerns may be considered when selecting an anesthetic circuit for use in infants and neonates. If very high fresh gas flows are used, a circle system takes on the characteristics of a non-rebreathing system.

Halothane (Fluothane)

Halothane is still commonly used for infants and children because of its acceptance by patients, ease and rapidity of induction, lack of airway irritation, long safety record, and very low cost. It is a relatively poor analgesic and is therefore frequently combined with nitrous oxide or a narcotic. Halothane markedly reduces intercostal muscle function and decreases both minute ventilation and tidal volume, resulting in increased arterial carbon dioxide tension ($PaCO_2$) at increasing concentrations.[151–154] Controlled or assisted ventilation is indicated in small infants and children, bearing in mind the need to reduce the inspired concentration of inhalation agent to avoid overdose. Halothane has weak neuromuscular blocking properties and potentiates the action of nondepolarizing neuromuscular blocking agents. Halothane is a potent bronchodilator and is particularly useful for the management of patients with reactive airway disease because it depresses airway reflexes.[155–157] Halothane is especially useful for bronchoscopic procedures, which require spontaneous ventilation. A disadvantage is that halothane sensitizes the myocardium to the effects of catecholamines; this effect appears to be more of an issue in adults. The combination of halothane anesthesia, high circulating catecholamines, and hypercarbia may occasionally lead to serious arrhythmias.[158, 159]

Because halothane sensitizes the myocardium to arrhythmias secondary to exogenous catecholamines, the total dose of exogenous epinephrine used for vasoconstriction during halothane anesthesia is usually limited. The dose necessary to cause arrhythmias has been demonstrated to be 1.4 to 2.0 μg/kg SC in adults.[160, 161] *Children tolerate higher doses of epinephrine during halothane anesthesia than do adults* (6 to 10 μg/kg); tachycardia and hypertension are more common side effects than arrhythmias.[162–164] It is reasonable to limit the total dose of epinephrine added to local anesthetic or saline to 10 μg/kg/20 min.

Halothane-induced cardiovascular dysfunction appears to be primarily related to direct depression of cardiac contractility with minimal changes in peripheral vascular resistance; some anti-alpha 2-receptor activity has been demonstrated in animal models.[137–139, 165, 166] A neonatal animal's heart is more sensitive to the cardiac depressant effects of halothane than is a more mature heart; this response is similar to that of all potent anesthetic agents.[135] Clinical studies suggest that the incidence of hypotension is similar with halothane and isoflurane but that isoflurane-induced cardiovascular depression is in part mediated by peripheral vascular dilation.[167–169] Studies with sevoflurane have found the greatest reduction in blood pressure to occur with neonates; there is no reflex increase in heart rate in the youngest patients compared with children 3 years of age or older.[170]

Halothane increases cerebral blood flow (CBF) and thus should be used with caution in most patients with increased intracranial pressure (ICP).[171] On some occasions, however, it is almost impossible to secure an intravenous route for an alternative technique. The brief use of halothane in this situation may be indicated on the basis of benefits versus risks (see Chapter 22). An unusual side effect is the development of acute rhabdomyolysis without previous administration of succinylcholine, generally in patients with unrecognized Duchenne muscular dystropy.[172]

Hepatic Toxicity

Although halothane-associated toxicity has been reported, there is little evidence of a clinically important incidence of hepatotoxicity secondary to halothane in the pediatric age group.[173–175] Several retrospective pediatric studies suggest that the incidence of halothane-associated hepatitis ranges from 1 in 82,700 to 1 in 200,155 anesthetic procedures.[176] A prospective examination of 1362 halothane anesthetic procedures in 186 children found minor increases of hepatic enzymes, no cases of jaundice, and several cases of elevated enzyme levels postoperatively in patients with preoperative enzyme abnormalities.[177] Papers reviewing halothane-associated hepatitis have reported a low to nonexistent incidence of "unexplained" hepatitis following exposure to halothane in pediatric patients.[177–179] Despite the very low incidence of halothane-associated hepatitis, the serum of some of these patients was positive for antibodies to rat halothane-sensitized hepatocytes. Out of millions of halothane anesthetics of children, only several pediatric deaths have been reported.[175, 180–183]

Another report summarized the British experience of seven pediatric patients specifically referred with the possible diagnosis of "halothane hepatitis"; one patient died, and the other six recovered uneventfully. The serum from these patients was collected during a 7-year period. Three different tests for halothane antibodies were used to make the presumptive diagnosis.[184] The investigators concluded that repeat exposure to halothane should be avoided in children. A number of concerns about this study question this recommendation. Several of the cases presented were previously reported in other journals, and the case histories differ in part from those in the collected review.[180, 183] Additionally, the specificity of the tests used has been questioned in light of improved enzyme-linked immunosorbent assays using purified trifluoroacetyl halide protein metabolites.[185] Additionally, although evidence suggests that the halothane antibody test has merit, there are still minimal data regarding false-positive test results.[186–195] Thus we do not concur with Kenna's recommendations.[184] Although there is evidence for the existence of "halothane hepatitis" in adults and although animal models have been developed with several postulated mechanisms (hypoxia, toxic metabolites), the true incidence of halothane-associated hepatitis in the pediatric population remains unclear. Because children have fully developed immunologic mechanisms and are capable of metabolizing halothane, the question is: why should the apparent incidence of halothane hepatitis be so much lower in children?[196–198]

The British report's recommendation to avoid repeat halothane administration to children was made without the input from senior pediatric anesthesiologists and is inconsistent with the clinical experience of the majority of the world's major pediatric centers. In fact, there is a higher incidence of fatal hepatic dysfunction in children who have received acetaminophen than in those exposed to halothane.[199]

There are no data to suggest that patients with pre-existing liver disease have an increased propensity to develop halothane-induced hepatic dysfunction. The true incidence of halothane-associated hepatitis in children is unknown; if halothane-associated hepatitis exists in the pediatric age group, the incidence is exceedingly low and significantly lower than it is in adults.[198, 200–204] Because only two or three pediatric patients have been reported to have had fatal "halothane hepatitis" despite many millions of pediatric administrations, the proven efficacy, vast experience, safety, superiority for suppressing airway reflexes for deep intubation with spontaneous respirations in patients with difficult airway anatomy, and ease of acceptance by a patient population that often requires a smooth mask induction to anesthesia, halothane may still be the inhalation agent of choice for many children. The pungent smell of isoflurane, enflurane, and desflurane makes these agents less acceptable to awake pediatric patients, especially those with a compromised airway. The role of sevoflurane compared with halothane in the management of patients with difficult airways is yet to be clearly proven. Anesthesiologists caring for children must use their best medical judgment, not "legal concerns," to dictate the choice of anesthetic agent. Halothane remains one of the safest and smoothest available anesthetic agents for the gaseous induction of anesthesia in children.

Halothane vs. Other Inhalation Agents

One further concern is determining the point at which a child becomes an adult in regard to increased susceptibility to halothane-associated hepatic toxicity. Because halothane-

associated hepatitis is accepted as an entity in the adult population, at what age should patients be considered adults subject to this complication? In general, this decision should be left to the individual practitioner, because the smooth gaseous induction of anesthesia may be just as vital to older as to younger pediatric patients. If an intravenous line is already in place, then a standard intravenous induction, muscle relaxant, or narcotic anesthetic is a satisfactory alternative. It is common practice to use potent anesthetic agents other than halothane in the adolescent population unless there is a severe airway-related problem. One should not substitute sound clinical judgment for fear of halothane-associated hepatic dysfunction, an extremely rare complication.

Isoflurane (Forane)

Isoflurane has a vapor pressure nearly identical to that of halothane.[205] This agent has had the most investigation in terms of MAC; infants 1 to 6 months of age have the highest anesthetic requirement, similar to that for halothane (Fig. 8–13). Isolated heart studies of animal and human tissue have demonstrated less cardiac dysfunction with isoflurane than with halothane.[206–208] Isoflurane has been demonstrated to produce less myocardial depression in children than does halothane using M-mode and pulsed Doppler echocardiography. These data at first glance suggest that isoflurane may be a better choice for the gaseous induction of anesthesia in

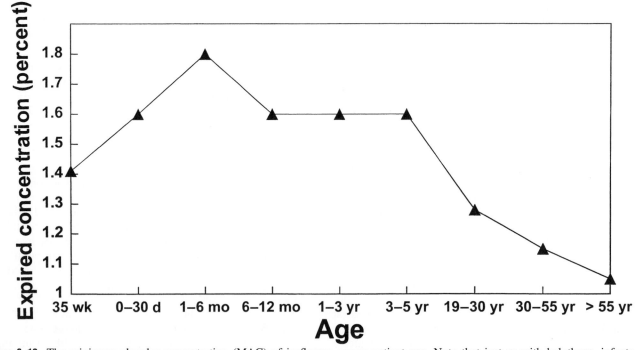

Figure 8–13. The minimum alveolar concentration (MAC) of isoflurane versus patient age. Note that just as with halothane, infants have the highest requirements. This is also one of the few anesthetic agents with data in preterm infants (35 weeks = 35 weeks gestational age). (Data abstracted from Ledez KM, Lerman J: The minimum alveolar concentration (MAC) of isoflurane in preterm neonates. Anesthesiology 1987;67:301–307; Murray DJ, Mehta MP, Forbes RB, Dull DL: Additive contribution of nitrous oxide to halothane MAC in infants and children. Anesth Analg 1990;71:120–124; Cameron CB, Robinson S, Gregory GA: The minimum anesthetic concentration of isoflurane in children. Anesth Analg 1984;63:418–420; and Wade JG, Stevens WC: Isoflurane: An anesthetic for the eighties? Anesth Analg 1981;60:666–682.)

children with compromised cardiovascular function.[169, 209, 210] However, more sophisticated two-dimensional echocardiographic studies combined with pulsed Doppler measurements of blood flow velocity have demonstrated equivalent myocardial depression with halothane and isoflurane.[168] One report suggests that hydration status may be an important variable because the hypotension induced by isoflurane is primarily a result of peripheral vasodilation, whereas with halothane it is primarily a result of myocardial depression.[211] Cardiac output is maintained with isoflurane by an increase in heart rate. In a study of infants free of cardiovascular disease, a decrease in heart rate as well as blood pressure was observed that was similar to halothane.[167] In infants free of cardiovascular disease, it would appear that isoflurane offers no significant cardiovascular advantage compared with halothane; there may be some advantage in children with abnormal cardiac function. Of greater clinical importance is the apparently high incidence of increased secretions and laryngospasm caused by isoflurane compared with halothane[212–216]; this property makes it less useful for the gaseous induction of anesthesia in children.

The attractive properties of isoflurane are the greater potentiation of neuromuscular blockade compared with halothane and less potentiation of cardiac arrhythmias in the presence of epinephrine. To take advantage of these characteristics and circumvent the disadvantages of secretions and laryngospasm, an alternative would be to induce anesthesia with halothane or sevoflurane, administer atropine, intubate the patient, and then change to isoflurane for the remainder of the procedure. Malignant hyperthermia and hepatic necrosis have been associated with isoflurane anesthesia[217–219]; thus, this double exposure of trigger agents may not be desirable. However, if the purported mechanism of halothane-induced hepatic dysfunction relates to breakdown products of halothane, then isoflurane may offer less potential for hepatic toxicity because it undergoes less hepatic biodegradation.[205]

The major purported advantage of isoflurane is its use for neurosurgical procedures. Evidence suggests that isoflurane produces smaller increments in CBF than does halothane and the reversal of this increased CBF by passive hyperventilation is more readily achieved.[205] The cerebral metabolic rate for oxygen ($CMRO_2$) is reduced to a greater degree during isoflurane anesthesia by its direct effect on cortical electrical activity.[220] It is postulated that at deeper planes of isoflurane anesthesia, the reduction in electrical activity may provide some protective effect; this level of anesthesia may often be achieved with isoflurane while maintaining adequate cardiovascular stability. Studies of preterm infants measuring anterior fontanelle pressure found an equivalent but "mild" decrease in anterior fontanelle pressure with both halothane and isoflurane.[221] An animal study examining ICP following cryogenic brain injury found equivalent increases in ICP with both halothane and isoflurane; these increases were not affected by prior hypocapnia.[222] There are minimal scientific data in children to confirm these laboratory observations regarding effects on CBF, ICP, and $CMRO_2$.

One concern regarding isoflurane, which came to light during investigations of desflurane, is the potential to release catecholamines and therefore the development of hypertension and tachycardia when there is a rapid rate of increase of the inspired concentration.[223, 224] One author (CJC) has observed this several times, particularly in teenagers in whom anesthesia was induced with sevoflurane, who received pancuronium, and then were changed to isoflurane. One author (CJC) has also observed several to develop a generalized rash, which passes as the hypertension and tachycardia resolve. This response can be avoided by a more gradual increase in inspired isoflurane concentration. If a patient suddenly develops a marked increase in pulse rate and blood pressure, one should assume first that there was a catecholamine release caused by the rapid increase in inspired isoflurane concentration. One author (CJC) has observed this even in cases in which isoflurane had been used for 30 to 60 minutes but there was a sudden change made because of a perception that the patient was lightly anesthetized. One should also be certain that this effect does not delay the diagnosis of malignant hyperthermia (see Chapter 27); one clue would be the concomitant rise in end-expired carbon dioxide values. Another clue against a diagnosis of malignant hyperthermia would be resolution of the tachycardia as the inspired concentration of isoflurane is reduced. The anesthesiologist's response to isoflurane-associated tachycardia and hypertension is to simply shut off the isoflurane and turn on halothane.

Another potential adverse side effect of isoflurane is its interaction with dry soda lime and the potential for production of carbon monoxide.[225–227] Although this was initially described with desflurane, it has now been shown to also occur with isoflurane.[228] This problem is circumvented by using fresh soda lime; one should avoid using isoflurane for the first case on a Monday morning if someone has left the oxygen running all weekend, since dehydrated Baralyme or dehydrated soda lime is the main offender. A new absorbent that does not contain either sodium hydroxide or potassium hydroxide eliminates the reaction producing carbon monoxide.[229]

Sevoflurane (Ultane)

Sevoflurane has been widely accepted by pediatric anesthesiologists because it provides a rapid induction and awakening, the smell is acceptable to most children, the effects on the cardiovascular system appear to be less than those caused by halothane, and there is less metabolism than with halothane.[170, 230–234] Sevoflurane appears to have more profound effects on respiration when compared with halothane. Both agents produce dose-dependent respiratory depression, but sevoflurane produces both a decrease in tidal volume and a decrease in respiratory rate, whereas halothane produces decreased tidal volume but increased respiratory rate.[235, 236] This observation suggests the need for assisted ventilation rather than spontaneous respirations when using sevoflurane; it is common to observe apnea following induction with high concentrations of sevoflurane.

The effects of sevoflurane on the cardiovascular system differ from those produced by halothane. Sevoflurane is associated with an increase in heart rate, particularly in children older than 3 years of age with no or minimal change in systolic blood pressure, whereas halothane results in a stable heart rate but a fall in systolic blood pressure.[230, 231, 237, 238] As with all inhalation agents, neonates are more susceptible to cardiovascular depression than older patients.[170] One study carefully examined the cardiovascular effects of sevoflurane using a cardiac ultrasonographic system with two-dimensionally directed M-mode and continuous-wave Doppler capability. Pediatric patients with a mean age of approximately 8 years were examined at 1 and 1.5 MAC sevoflurane and halothane. Heart rate did not differ between groups; this finding differs from that of other studies, which have shown a higher heart rate with sevoflurane. Systolic blood pressure decreased in both groups at 1 MAC but increased at 1.5 MAC in both groups. Left ventricular shortening fraction decreased with both agents, but there was a greater degree with halothane. Contractility was felt to fall in the abnormal range with 1.5 MAC halothane but not 1.5 MAC sevoflurane. Systemic vascular resistance decreased with sevoflurane but not with halothane.

The authors believed that the preservation of myocardial performance with sevoflurane was an "attractive alternative" to halothane.[239] Another study examined the echocardiographic effects of sevoflurane compared with halothane in infants and found a decrease in cardiac output with both agents but a lesser reduction with sevoflurane.[240] At least one other study has demonstrated a lower incidence of cardiac arrhythmias associated with sevoflurane compared with halothane anesthesia.[241] These studies suggest that sevoflurane may offer some minor advantage over halothane; however, the high incidence of hypotension in the early clinical trials examining MAC in the youngest, most vulnerable population suggests that the risk for severe myocardial depression is still present with sevoflurane. In fact, perhaps the greatest safety factor with sevoflurane has nothing to do with the drug but rather with the maximal allowable delivered anesthetic concentration in relation to MAC for age. The MAC for sevoflurane in a neonate is 3.3%[170] and the vaporizer limit is 8%, whereas the MAC for halothane in a neonate is 0.87%[133] with the vaporizer limit of 5%. Thus the highest MAC multiple allowable with sevoflurane in a neonate is 2.42 vs. 5.75 for halothane. This difference in MAC multiples is even further exaggerated when using 70% nitrous oxide, since it has been shown that this concentration of nitrous oxide reduces MAC by 70% with halothane but only 20% with sevoflurane.[141, 170] Thus with the capability to deliver several-fold greater MAC concentrations of halothane than sevoflurane, one would not be at all surprised to find a higher incidence of severe cardiovascular depression (Table 8–3). One study examined the cardiovascular responses to incremental induction with halothane or sevoflurane and found a higher incidence of heart rate and blood pressure increases during sevoflurane inductions.[237]

The effects of sevoflurane on the central nervous system are similar to those of isoflurane.[242, 243] As with all inhalation agents, the MAC varies by age, with infants having the

Table 8–3. Minimum Alveolar Concentration (MAC) Multiples for a Neonate Allowed by Current Vaporizers

Agent	Maximum Vaporizer Output (%)	MAC (%)	Maximum Possible MAC Multiples
Halothane	5	0.87	5.75
Isoflurane	5	1.20	4.2
Sevoflurane	8	3.3	2.42
Desflurane	18	9.16	1.96

Table 8–4. Minimum Alveolar Concentration (MAC) for Sevoflurane According to Age

Age	MAC (% Expired)
Neonates (0–30 days)	3.3 ± 0.2
Infants (1–6 months)	3.2 ± 0.1
Infants (6–12 months)	2.5 ± 0.2
Children (1–12 years)	2.5
Adults	2.6
Elderly	1.5

highest MAC (Table 8–4).[170] The MAC for neonates (0–30 days) is slightly higher than for older infants, which is different than most other potent anesthetics. The addition of nitrous oxide 60% reduced MAC to only $2.0 \pm 0.2\%$ (approximately 20% lower) (Fig. 8–14).[170, 231] The MAC in adults (2.6%) is reduced approximately 50% with the addition of nitrous oxide 65%.[244-246]

The major concerns with this agent relate to the theoretic potential for nephrotoxicity due to formation of toxic metabolites and the formation of elevated levels of inorganic fluoride with prolonged administration. Several studies have demonstrated an interaction between sevoflurane and carbon dioxide absorbents, resulting in elimination of hydrogen fluoride from the isopropyl moiety of sevoflurane resulting in the degradation product Compound A [fluoromethyl-2,2-difluoro-1-(trifluoromethyl) vinyl ether].[247-254] Other breakdown products (Compounds B, C, and D) are not apparently produced in sufficient quantity to be of clinical importance.[255] These compounds have been described in pediatric

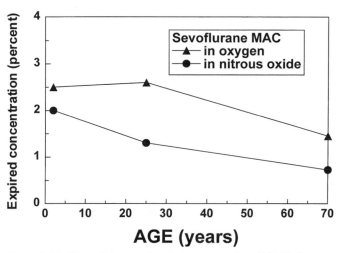

Figure 8–14. The minimum alveolar concentration (MAC) for sevoflurane in 100% oxygen and approximately 67% nitrous oxide. Note that MAC changes with age, as with other potent anesthetic agents. Also note that the proportional reduction in MAC with nitrous oxide is only approximately 20% in toddlers compared with an approximate 50% reduction in adults. The reasons for this pharmacodynamic difference are unclear. (Data abstracted from Fragan RJ, Dunn KL: The minimum alveolar concentration (MAC) of sevoflurane with and without nitrous oxide in elderly versus young adults. J Clin Anesth 1996;8:352–356; and Lerman J, Sikich N, Kleinman S, Yentis S: The pharmacology of sevoflurane in infants and children. Anesthesiology 1994;80:814–824.)

patients.[248] In animal models, compound A produces renal injury.[256] The amount of Compound A produced depends on a number of factors, including the type of absorbent (Baralyme more than soda lime), the amount of water in the circuit (dry absorbent produces more Compound A than wet absorbent),[247] and higher concentrations of sevoflurane. These concerns resulted in a number of studies attempting to define the magnitude of the problem and, because of cost, studies to determine whether low-flow anesthesia resulted in any increase in risk to the patient.[248, 250–253, 257–265] It appears that sevoflurane anesthesia, even at low flow rates does not alter the routine markers of renal function, such as blood urea nitrogen or creatinine.[259, 261] One study in adult volunteers comparing sevoflurane with desflurane has shown *transient injury to (1) the glomerulus, as revealed by postanesthetic albuminuria; (2) the proximal tubule, as revealed by postanesthetic glucosuria and increased urinary α-glutathionine-S-transferase (GST); and (3) the distal tubule, as revealed by postanesthetic increased urinary π-GST.*[262] No such "injury" was found in the desflurane population. A similar study from two other institutions compared sevoflurane with isoflurane in adult volunteers.[259, 261] There was *no significant difference between anesthetic groups in postoperative serum creatinine or blood urea nitrogen, or urinary excretion of protein, glucose, proximal tubular α-GST, or distal tubular π-GST.*[261]

The authors concluded that low-flow sevoflurane (1 L/min) was as safe as low-flow isoflurane anesthesia. How should the practitioner interpret these apparently contradictory findings? One editorial suggests that sevoflurane should be used with caution in patients with known renal impairment.[266] One author's (CJC) interpretation of these data is that sevoflurane is safe for the vast majority of pediatric patients. This author's own practice is to use sevoflurane with a circle system for induction and then change to halothane for maintenance to avoid the entire issue of potential renal toxicity and to save money for the institution. Theoretically, for a very long case, one could then change back to sevoflurane for the end of the case. The introduction of a new carbon dioxide absorbent that does not contain sodium hydroxide or potassium hydroxide (Amsorb, Armstrong Medical Limited, Belfast, Ireland) may completely eliminate concerns regarding Compound A toxicity. This new absorbent would also allow the use of very low fresh gas flow rates that would markedly reduce costs and allow the relatively economical use of sevoflurane, even for long cases.[229, 267–269]

Another potential concern is the release of inorganic fluoride from sevoflurane. Several studies have demonstrated a small and clinically unimportant increase in serum inorganic fluoride values.[260, 270] In children, it appears that the peak inorganic fluoride values are one-half those found in adults with the same MAC hours of exposure.[270] These studies suggest that there should be little concern for fluoride-induced nephrotoxicity, especially since the inorganic fluoride values rapidly decline once anesthesia is discontinued.

Does the use of sevoflurane eliminate anesthetic agent–associated hepatic dysfunction? Approximately 2% to 5% of sevoflurane undergoes hepatic degradation by cytochrome p450 2E1.[255, 271, 272] There are several case reports of sevoflurane-associated hepatic dysfunction.[273–276] Anesthetic-induced hepatic dysfunction is still reported, and it is unclear

whether sevoflurane offers any advantage at all regarding this issue when compared with halothane, especially in pediatric patients. Again as described under halothane, the incidence of anesthetic agent–induced hepatic dysfunction as a fatal complication is so rare that literally millions of anesthetic procedures will need to be administered before a clear estimate of the rate of this severe problem can be derived.

Does sevoflurane have advantages over halothane for the gaseous induction of anesthesia? The ability to perform a smooth gaseous induction in unpremedicated pediatric patients has been described as the best indicator for its use in pediatric anesthesia. However, when the results of several studies are combined, it would seem that there is a similarly low incidence of airway-related events such as laryngospasm, bronchospasm, coughing, breath-holding, and excitement with the use of either agent, even with rapid increases or gradual increases in inspired sevoflurane concentrations (Table 8–5).[170, 230–234, 241, 277–281] At least one study demonstrated less excitement if sevoflurane was combined with nitrous oxide.[231] One other study has found a more rapid loss of lid reflex with 8% sevoflurane combined with 66% nitrous oxide compared with 5% halothane in 66% nitrous oxide (34 ± 12 sec vs. 58 ± 17 sec)[282]; there appears to be no difference in airway-related complications with a rapid 8% induction compared with an incremental sevoflurane induction.[283]

One study has examined the MAC for endotracheal intubation (MAC_{EI}) and the contribution of nitrous oxide in preventing movement in response to intubation in children 1 to 7 years of age.[284] The MAC_{EI} for sevoflurane was 3.54 ± 0.25%; nitrous oxide reduced the MAC_{EI} in a linear and additive fashion. Another study, however, found better intubating conditions with halothane when compared with sevoflurane.[285]

Is there any advantage in terms of rapidity of induction, wake-up, or quality of emergence? Several studies have demonstrated a more rapid induction with sevoflurane, and the difference on average ranged from 20 to 38 seconds.[232–234, 241] Although the magnitude of the difference in rapidity of induction is in reality quite small, in a crying or struggling child, this 20- to 40-second difference assumes a greater clinical importance. Regarding times to awakening, it would appear that the differences between sevoflurane and halothane are quite minimal and may more often relate to clinical experience than to the agents themselves. The time to eye opening in several studies consistently showed sevoflurane patients to awaken more rapidly, and this difference varied on average from 1.8 to 11.6 minutes.[232, 238, 286–289] Time to extubation in most studies is also generally shorter with sevoflurane.[230–232, 287] Some of these studies, however, reflect artifacts created by the study design rather than true clinical practice of anesthesia, in which tapering of inspired anesthetic concentrations begins as clinically indicated rather than as designed by a protocol. If one examines sophisticated measures of recovery such as the Trieger dot test, children do recover more rapidly with sevoflurane compared with halothane.[241] However, this rapid recovery does not necessary translate into an earlier discharge from the hospital, since so many other factors, including the use of premedications, influence this process.[290] Regarding emergence excitement, there appears to be a higher incidence of emergence delirium, particularly in children less than 6 years of

Table 8–5. Problems During Induction: Sevoflurane vs. Halothane

Problem	Sevoflurane			Halothane			Study
	N with Problem	Total	Percent	N with Problem	Total	Percent	
Laryngospasm	21	708	3.0	20	540	3.8	Piat et al.,[230] Sarner et al.,[231] Ariffin et al.,[233] Lerman et al.,[234] Meretoja et al.,[241] Kataria et al.,[277] Sigston et al.[280]
Breath holding	39	649	6.0	46	445	10.3	Sarner et al.,[231] Lerman et al.,[234] Kataria et al.,[277] Black et al.,[278] Sigston et al.[280]
Coughing	20	477	4.2	21	254	8.3	Lerman et al.,[170] Sarner et al.,[231] Epstein et al.,[232] Ariffin et al.,[233] Lerman et al.,[234] Baum et al.[281]
Induction excitement	38	375	10.1	9	211	4.3	Sarner et al.,[231] Epstein et al.,[232] Lerman et al.,[234] Sigston et al.[280]
Bronchospasm	2	544	0.37	2	379	0.53	Sarner et al.,[231] Lerman et al.,[234] Kataria et al.[277]
Emergence excitement	20	239	8.37	51	368	13.86	Epstein et al.,[232] Lerman et al.,[234] Johannesson et al.,[279] Aono et al.,[291] Welborn et al.[311]

age, with sevoflurane anesthesia compared with halothane anesthesia even with adequate analgesia.[234, 279, 291–293] The clinical importance of this would concern the need to administer other medications such as additional opioid or benzodiazepine that in turn may delay recovery.

At least one well-controlled study has found no difference in emergence agitation comparing halothane with sevoflurane for myringotomy tube insertion; the incidence with both agents was reduced with the administration of ketorolac.[294] Another well-controlled study comparing halothane and sevoflurane for longer procedures with both populations receiving caudal analgesia and no opioids or premedication found a higher incidence of emergence agitation for the first 10 minutes of recovery with sevoflurane.[295]

It would appear that sevoflurane is a welcome addition to the care of pediatric patients, particularly in terms of a more rapid induction of anesthesia. There may be a slightly lower incidence of airway-related events with sevoflurane compared with halothane during induction. Whether there is truly an advantage due to a lower incidence of severe hypotension and cardiac arrest with sevoflurane during induction is yet to be and likely never will be proven because one would find it difficult to conduct such a controlled study of a rare event. Another issue is whether the increased cost can be justified in terms of the maintenance of anesthesia and the as yet unresolved questions regarding potential hepatic and renal injury with prolonged exposure to products of sevoflurane metabolism. At the moment, sevoflurane seems to be perfectly safe for brief surgical procedures; with the clinical availability of the new carbon dioxide absorbent, toxicity will be reduced.[229]

Desflurane (Suprane)

Desflurane has a blood/gas partition coefficient similar to that of nitrous oxide (0.42 vs. 0.47).[255, 296] When investigations first began, it was hoped that the potential for rapid induction and awakening would make this the most desired agent for pediatrics. However, the preclinical trial and others

found an unacceptably high incidence of breath holding and laryngospasm during gaseous induction (128/226 = 48%).[297–299] Desflurane is the most pungent in terms of airway irritation, and because of this it is not recommended for the gaseous induction of anesthesia in pediatric patients.[297, 298, 300] Its cardiovascular effects, including interactions with epinephrine, and its effects on cerebral blood flow and intracranial pressure are similar to those of isoflurane.[255, 301–304]

One serious adverse cardiovascular effect of desflurane is sympathetic activation by pulmonary airway irritant receptors causing central excitation of the sympathetic nervous system.[224, 305–307] This sympathetic activation is dependent on the rate of rise of inspired desflurane concentration and may in part be blunted by prior administration of fentanyl.[224, 306]

The MAC for children varies according to age, as with the other potent anesthetic agents (Table 8–6).[308, 309] For infants and all children up to the age of 12 years, the MAC is higher than for adults. In adults 31 to 65 years of age, MAC is 6.0 ± 0.3% (lower in the elderly), but it is higher in young adults 18 to 30 years of age (7.25 ± 0.0%).[308] The addition of nitrous oxide reduces MAC to 2.83 ± 0.6 in 31- to 65-year-olds and to 4.0 ± 0.3 in 18- to 30-year-olds.[308] Just as for sevoflurane, there appears to be a pharmacodynamic difference between adults and children; nitrous oxide

Table 8–6. Minimum Alveolar Concentration (MAC) for Desflurane According to Age

Age	MAC (% Expired)
Neonates (0–30 days)	9.16 ± 0.02
Infants (1–6 months)	9.42 ± 0.006
Infants (6–12 months)	9.98 ± 0.44
Toddlers (1–3 years)	8.72 ± 0.6
Children (3–5 years)	8.62 ± 0.45
Children (5–12 years)	7.98 ± 0.43
Adults	6.0 ± 0.3

60% reduces MAC only approximately 20% to 25% (9.4% to 7.5% for infants 1 to 6 months old and 8.72% to 6.4% for children 1 to 5 years old) (Fig. 8–15).[310]

This agent provides a very stable maintenance period, easily altered depth of anesthesia, and rapid awakening.[298, 299, 311] The ease of altering the depth of anesthesia may translate into the very real potential for anesthetic overdose or cardiovascular depression. The occasional need for multi-MAC concentrations (18%) may lead to dilutional hypoxemia. The use of anesthetic agent analyzers, expired carbon dioxide monitors, and pulse oximetry provides the necessary safety net for closed-circuit or low fresh gas flow anesthesia, which would greatly reduce the cost.

Our experience has been that this agent has induction characteristics similar to those of isoflurane. There is some suggestion that using desflurane in oxygen without nitrous oxide may reduce the severity of airway complications.[299, 309] This agent is not recommended for the gaseous induction of anesthesia in infants. Once induction has been completed with other agents, then desflurane provides a very stable cardiovascular response, and the depth of anesthesia is remarkably easy to control. Awakening from anesthesia with desflurane is more rapid than with halothane or sevoflurane.[246, 263, 311, 312] However, the incidence of emergence delirium is the highest with desflurane when compared with halothane or sevoflurane[311]; as with sevoflurane, the clinical importance of rapid awakening remains to be demonstrated.

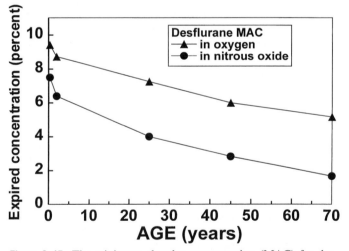

Figure 8–15. The minimum alveolar concentration (MAC) for desflurane in 100% oxygen and approximately 67% nitrous oxide. Note that MAC changes with age, as with other potent anesthetic agents. Also note that the proportional reduction in MAC with nitrous oxide is only approximately 20% in infants and toddlers compared with an approximate 50% reduction in adults. The reasons for this pharmacodynamic difference are unclear, but this same effect was observed with sevoflurane.[170, 244] (Data abstracted from Fisher DM, Zwass MS: MAC of desflurane in 60% nitrous oxide in infants and children. Anesthesiology 1992;76:354–356; Gold MI, Abello D, Herrington C: Minimum alveolar concentration of desflurane in patients older than 65 years. Anesthesiology 1993;79:710–714; Rampil IJ, Lockhart SH, Zwass MS, et al: Clinical characteristics of desflurane in surgical patients: Minimum alveolar concentration. Anesthesiology 1991;74:429–433; Taylor RH, Lerman J: Minimum alveolar concentration of desflurane and hemodynamic responses in neonates, infants, and children. Anesthesiology 1991;75:975–979.)

The impression of one author (CJC) is that nerve blocks performed at the beginning of brief surgical procedures achieve a complete block before the patient awakens, whereas nerve blocks performed near the end occasionally achieve only partial blockade at the time of awakening. The rapid awakening and pain result in a higher level of excitement in the recovery room. It is clear that desflurane will not replace halothane. The blood/gas partition coefficient may offer a significant advantage for rapid awakening from very long surgical procedures, especially neurosurgical procedures; this advantage is less pronounced for brief outpatient procedures.

One additional concern is the apparent interaction between desflurane and dry carbon dioxide absorbant.[225, 226, 228] Just as with isoflurane, the potential for this complication is greater with dry absorbent and greater with soda lime than with Baralyme. One should not run high fresh gas flows though a system for prolonged periods (which would dry out the absorbent) and then administer a desflurane anesthetic. Fortunately with this anesthetic agent, low flow rates are not of any concern; using low flow rates retains exhaled moisture, which reduces the potential for carbon monoxide poisoning and there is no concern for toxic metabolites. Unfortunately, because of the problems with induction, one would have to use either sevoflurane or halothane for induction before changing to desflurane. Since there are a limited number of vaporizer slots on most anesthesia machines, one will have to select from three of the four available. The new absorbent will eliminate concerns regarding carbon monoxide poisoning.[229]

Ideal Inhalation Agent

Nothing is more elusive than finding the "ideal" anesthetic agent, that is, one that has a rapid onset and elimination and is pleasant to smell. In addition, it should have minimal respiratory irritant properties, should not cause cardiovascular and respiratory depression, and should have little effect on cerebral and cardiac blood flow. It should cause reduced cerebral and cardiac oxygen consumption, should have minimal interaction with catecholamines, and should not be metabolized to toxic compounds.[313] Sevoflurane and desflurane solve some of the problems associated with isoflurane and halothane, but they are not yet the ideal agents.

Nitrous Oxide

General Properties

Nitrous oxide is a relatively potent analgesic but a weak anesthetic agent; for these reasons, it should be supplemented with a narcotic, barbiturate, or sedative. As with the potent inhalation agents, the requirement appears to be lower with increasing age.[314] A major advantage is its insolubility. In prolonged surgical procedures, this property enables patients to awaken more rapidly than with the more soluble potent inhalation agents. Other advantages include minimal myocardial and respiratory depression and no serious clinical interaction with exogenous catecholamines; nitrous oxide may cause minimal increases in CBF.[315–317] Nitrous oxide is frequently used alone and as a supplement to general anesthesia when combined with a potent anesthetic agent. Nitrous oxide is usually thought to be additive to the MAC of the potent anesthetic agents. However, it appears that this effect is less pronounced with the less soluble inhalation agents compared with halothane; this lack of effect seems to be more pronounced in younger pediatric patients (Table 8–7).[133, 134, 141, 309, 310]

Nitrous oxide is also used for sedation for various procedures. Nitrous oxide (50%) depresses swallowing reflexes and therefore should be used only when patients have had proper preoperative fasting.[318] The data regarding the effects of nitrous oxide on postoperative nausea and vomiting are conflicting.[319, 320]

Contraindications

The major contraindications to the use of nitrous oxide are the need for a high inspired oxygen concentration or the presence of trapped air in a closed body space. The latter situation is particularly important in pediatric patients. Nitrous oxide is 34 times more soluble than nitrogen. Thus the entry of nitrous oxide is much more rapid than the exit of nitrogen.[321] This differential may lead to a rapid increase in the size of tension pneumothorax and, over a longer period, bowel distension.[322] With 75% nitrous oxide, a twofold increase of intestinal gas can be expected within *3 hours*, and a pneumothorax can double in volume within *10 minutes*.[322] In pediatric patients, the increase in bowel size may be more rapid than in adults because of relatively greater bowel perfusion in children.

Other areas of concern are the rapid increase in ICP following pneumoencephalography, the rupture of tympanic membranes previously infected, the rapid increase in the size of pulmonary lobes in congenital lobar emphysema, and the possibility of pneumothorax in asthmatic patients with evidence of pulmonary blebs.[323–327] Nitrous oxide has been demonstrated to increase pulmonary artery pressure in adult patients. However, a well-controlled study of infants in the intensive care unit (ICU) has demonstrated that nitrous oxide alone has minimal effect on infants with both normal and elevated pulmonary artery pressures.[328, 329]

When equi-MAC combinations of nitrous oxide and either isoflurane or halothane are used, there is equivalent myocardial dysfunction compared with equi-MAC concentrations with either potent agent alone; this response to nitrous oxide is suggestive of mild direct myocardial depression when combined with a potent anesthetic agent.[330] This study suggests that using nitrous oxide with a potent anesthetic agent may have no advantage because the myocardial depression when using a lower inspired concentration of potent agent is offset by the additive effects of nitrous oxide.[330]

Oxygen

The appropriate concentration of oxygen to be delivered for each anesthetic procedure is carefully titrated to an individual's needs. Requirements are monitored by inspired oxygen concentration measurement, oxygen/hemoglobin saturation (pulse oximetry), and arterial blood gas determinations. Oxygen is often liberally administered in excess of a patient's metabolic needs. However, potential dangers in this excess should be noted, particularly in two areas: (1) Pulmonary oxygen toxicity is well documented; despite the fact that it develops slowly, general recommendations are to use an air/oxygen combination for prolonged procedures when nitrous oxide is contraindicated.[331] (2) Of additional concern is the possibility of adverse effects on the immature neonatal retina leading to retinopathy of prematurity (ROP).[332–339]

Retinopathy of Prematurity

Several cases of ROP have been reported in infants whose only known exposure to supplemental oxygen occurred in the operating room; it should be noted that no new cases related to operating room management have been reported since 1981.[340, 341] In the earlier cases of ROP, cardiovascular instability related to the disorder requiring surgery may have been the major factor predisposing to ROP along with prematurity. Many factors contribute to the development of ROP; it has been reported in children with cyanotic congenital heart disease, infants not exposed to exogenous oxygen, and even in stillborn infants.[342, 343] A possible relationship of the development of ROP to arterial carbon dioxide variations, hypercarbia, hypotension, candida sepsis, red blood cell transfusions, and hypoxemia has been suggested.[344–349] Other factors such as exogenous bright light, maternal diabetes, and maternal antihistamine use within 2 weeks of delivery have been found to be risk factors; the evidence for vitamin E deficiency is less convincing.[350–352] The use of continuous transcutaneous oxygen tension monitoring was not found to reduce the risk of ROP in infants weighing less than 1000 g compared with control subjects.[353] It appears that the major risk factor for developing ROP is extreme prematurity; oxygen therapy represents only part of this complex problem.[334, 335, 337] The incidence of ROP is predominantly limited to infants weighing 1000 g or less, but it is a concern in infants with a birthweight less than 1500 g born at less than 28 weeks of gestation.[354–356]

The embryonal development of the retina involves the progressive increase in vascularization of retinal vessels in a nasal to temporal direction. Exposure to high blood oxygen concentrations results in vasoconstriction of retinal vessels, probable occlusion of these vessels by thrombi, development of new vessels (neovascularization), formation of arteriovenous anastomoses, vascularization of the vitreous, and, in some cases, fibrous degeneration and retraction of the scar, as in cicatrization and retinal detachment.[335, 337] This sequence of events apparently does not occur once vascularization of the retina is complete (at about 44 weeks of postconceptual age).[357, 358]

Table 8–7. Percent Minimum Alveolar Concentration (MAC) Reduced in Two-Year-Olds with 60% Nitrous Oxide

Agent	MAC with Oxygen	MAC with 60% Nitrous Oxide	Percent MAC Reduced
Halothane	0.98	0.29	70
Sevoflurane	8.72	6.4	27
Desflurane	2.5	2.0	20

Data abstracted from Lerman et al.,[133] LeDez and Lerman,[134] Murray et al.,[141] Taylor and Lerman,[309] Fisher and Zwass.[310]

The ample evidence implicating hyperoxia as contributing to the development of ROP must be recognized but placed in proper perspective. Anesthesiologists should take practical precautions to protect an infant's retinas from hyperoxemia without unnecessarily endangering the infant. One possibility is to discuss with the surgeon postponement of elective surgery on a neonate of less than 44 weeks of postconceptual age, to allow for further retinal maturation.[358] Obviously, a life-threatening surgical problem must be corrected promptly. Once the decision has been made to proceed with surgery, an ophthalmologic assessment to document possible pre-existing ROP is desirable but often not practical. Postoperative evaluation would help to delineate any possible retinal pathology related to operating room procedures. It is only by this type of careful pre- and postoperative assessment of the retina that some true understanding of the possible anesthetic implications can be achieved. No comprehensive epidemiologic studies have yet examined anesthetic risk factors; many factors are important, anesthesia management being one.[359, 360]

Bearing in mind the possible role of hyperoxia and hypercarbia, intraoperative management must include careful monitoring of inspired oxygen and expired carbon dioxide concentrations. Pulse oximetry allows an anesthesiologist to adjust the inspired concentration of oxygen. Maintaining the oxygen saturation at 93% to 95% results in an arterial oxygen tension (PaO_2) of approximately 70 mm Hg.[336, 361] Unfortunately, individual oximeters may vary considerably in terms of their accuracy, so practitioners must be familiar with their equipment.[362] Most anesthesia machines are equipped with flow ratio valves that prevent the delivery of less than 25% oxygen. The use of air blended with oxygen can be used to further reduce the inspired oxygen concentration.

The accurate measure of expired carbon dioxide concentrations is a problem in small infants, particularly with non-rebreathing circuits. Endotracheal tubes with aspiration ports located at the tip may be of some value; however, the aspiration port often becomes obstructed with secretions or water. An alternative method would be to insert a needle into the side of the endotracheal tube.[363, 364] Whenever significant cardiac or pulmonary disease is present, there may be a large gradient between arterial and expired carbon dioxide concentrations. In this circumstance, the expired carbon dioxide measurement is useful only for trend monitoring.[365] Intermittent blood gas analysis confirms the accuracy of these monitors. Transcutaneous oxygen and carbon dioxide electrodes may provide useful information about the arterial concentrations of oxygen and carbon dioxide. The reality is that not all operating rooms are equipped with transcutaneous monitoring capability, nor should they be. Efforts should be made to maintain the PaO_2 in the range of 60 to 80 mm Hg and the $PaCO_2$ between 35 and 45 mm Hg. A transport system equipped with an air/oxygen blender should be available to continue the titration of oxygen therapy from the operating room to the ICU. While avoiding hyperoxia, one must never lose sight of the importance of *avoiding hypoxemia*; *hypoxemia is life threatening, whereas hyperoxia is not*. One cannot be faulted if ROP should occur, provided a reasonable and safe approach to oxygen administration and ventilation has been made.[336, 366]

Intravenous Anesthetic Agents

The anesthetic effects of intravenous agents are primarily reflected by brain concentrations; to achieve anesthesia, it is necessary to obtain an adequate cerebral blood level. Each drug administered is rapidly redistributed from vessel-rich, well-perfused areas (brain, heart, and kidneys) to muscle and finally to vessel-poor, less well perfused areas (bone, fat).[367] Thus termination of the effect of a single dose is primarily determined by redistribution. Protein binding, volume of distribution, body composition, cardiac output, distribution of cardiac output, metabolism, and excretion may alter the pharmacokinetics and pharmacodynamics of intravenous drugs. Anesthetic level may be altered if a constant cerebral blood level is not maintained. The changes in body composition and the blood-brain barrier that occur during maturation may also greatly affect the duration of action of intravenous drugs, especially in neonates.

Barbiturates

Methohexital (Brevital)

Methohexital is a short-acting barbiturate for the intravenous induction of anesthesia (1–2 mg/kg). Administered intravenously as a 1% solution (10 mg/mL), it produces pain at the injection site; hiccoughs, apnea, and seizure-like activity may also be occasionally observed.[368, 369] Methohexital has minimal effects on cardiovascular function (increased heart rate) in children.[370, 371] Methohexital may be contraindicated in patients with temporal lobe epilepsy.[369] Slow intravenous titration averts apnea. A possible advantage of methohexital over thiopental is that its rate of metabolism is much greater, suggesting a more rapid recovery when high doses have been administered.[372–374]

Rectal methohexital (20 to 30 mg/kg) is a safe and atraumatic method of induction with an acceptable incidence of undesired side effects (hiccoughs 13%, defecation 10%).[375] It is an excellent sedation technique for brief radiologic procedures such as computed tomography (CT) scans, when a single rectal administration of a 10% solution (100 mg/mL given through a well-lubricated catheter) is often sufficient for the 10- to 30-minute procedure.[376, 377] Absorption by this route is quite variable and may account for an occasional child with prolonged or rapid onset of sedation.[372, 378] This technique and dosage have been used safely in children from 3 months to 6 years of age. It is a useful adjunct to induction of anesthesia in older mentally handicapped children or in children who are excessively fearful of the anesthesia mask or an intravenous needle. It is also an alternative for patients who are still in diapers or patients who are not candidates for other premedicants such as midazolam (e.g., patients who are taking erythromycin).[379, 380]

Oxygen desaturation following sedation with rectal methohexital occurs in approximately 4% of cases and is usually related to airway obstruction; this is generally readily corrected by repositioning the head.[375, 381] Although methohexital is an exceedingly safe medication, it should be administered only under the supervision of a physician trained in airway management to ensure adequacy of the airway and ventilation. Blood pressure monitoring and equipment for airway management and ventilation should be readily available, because airway obstruction, seizures, or apnea may rarely occur.[382] Patients must not be left unobserved after administration.

Thiopental (Pentothal)

The induction of anesthesia in healthy, unpremedicated children with intravenous thiopental (2.5%) is generally accomplished with a dose of 5 to 6 mg/kg and then maintained with smaller incremental doses of 0.5 to 2.0 mg/kg as needed.[383–385] It must be recalled that termination of the clinical effect of thiopental is primarily dependent on redistribution rather than metabolism. Children 5 months to 13 years of age, however, are able to metabolize thiopental nearly twice as fast as adults (see Fig. 8–6).[386–388] The longer half-life in neonates is attributed to reduced clearance compared with adults and children.[389, 390] Acute tolerance to thiopental, well demonstrated in adults, may also occur in children.[391] A total intravenous dose of 10 mg/kg is generally the upper limit; however, with this dose, it is common to have a prolonged period of sedation following brief surgical procedures. Thiopental is a weak vasodilator and a direct myocardial depressant; both of these effects may result in significant systemic hypotension in the *hypovolemic* state, such as with dehydration due to prolonged fasting or trauma.[392]

Thiopental in a solution of 10% (20–30 mg/kg) may also be used for induction of anesthesia by rectal instillation when methohexital is contraindicated (temporal lobe epilepsy).[369] The period of sedation may be longer for thiopental than for methohexital, partly because of the slower rate of metabolism.[393]

Thiopental has also been used in the pediatric critical care setting as a continuous high-dose infusion (approximately 2–4 mg/kg/hour) to help control intracranial hypertension. Concentration monitoring may be useful with such therapy to avoid concentrations that depress myocardial function. One study found a longer elimination half-life (similar to adults) than that found with single bolus administration studies (11.7 vs. 6.1 hours).[387, 388] These findings may in part be attributed to the illness of the patients as well as additional drug treatment modalities and a change from first-order to second-order kinetics.[394]

Propofol (Diprivan)

Propofol is a sedative-hypnotic agent useful for both the induction and maintenance of anesthesia. This drug is nearly insoluble in aqueous solution and was initially introduced in a Cremophor EL solvent. Unfortunately, this led to severe anaphylactoid reactions, which necessitated reformulation as an emulsion.[395, 396] Propofol is a highly lipophilic drug that is rapidly distributed into vessel-rich organs, accounting for its rapid onset and usefulness as an induction agent. Termination of effect is determined by the combination of redistribution and rapid hepatic and extrahepatic clearance.[397–399] Propofol undergoes extensive extrahepatic metabolism (lung, kidney), since even patients with biliary atresia have pharmacokinetics similar to those of healthy control subjects.[400] Propofol is conjugated to a water-soluble glucuronide and excreted in the urine.[395] The rapidity of redistribution away from vessel-rich organs accounts for the brief pharmacodynamic action and the need for frequent small boluses or constant infusions to maintain a stable plane of anesthesia and sedation.

In unpremedicated children, a dose of 2.8 to 3.0 mg/kg produces satisfactory induction in most patients, but a higher dose may be required for acceptance of the face mask.[401, 402] Successful insertion of a laryngeal mask airway also requires a higher dose (5.4 mg/kg; 4.7–6.8 mg/kg, 95% confidence interval).[403] The higher induction dose in children may reflect a true pharmacokinetic difference, including a larger volume of distribution at steady state (Vdss) (9.7 L/kg) than that reported in adults, more rapid redistribution, and a clearance (34 mL/min/kg) that is similar to or higher than that reported in adults.[395, 404–406] The varying kinetics of propofol reported in the literature reflect differences in sampling time, pharmacokinetic modeling, and duration of sampling.[406]

Propofol is associated with a reduced blood pressure in approximately 15% of adult patients.[407] A similar observation has been made in children.[402, 404, 408, 409] One study found a greater fall in blood pressure with propofol compared with thiopental[408]; however, other studies found no difference.[409, 410] The incidence of apnea following an induction bolus of propofol compared with thiopental is similar.[402, 408–410] The major clinical drawback in children is pain with injection; this pain can be diminished by injection into a large vein and by combination with small doses of lidocaine (0.5 to 1.0 mg/kg).[401, 402, 404, 409, 410]

Indicators for recovery from anesthesia such as time to eye opening and time to extubation seem to be more rapid in patients induced with propofol when compared with thiopental and in patients whose anesthesia was maintained with propofol.[411–416] Recovery of psychomotor function is more rapid following propofol induction and maintenance of anesthesia compared with thiopental/isoflurane anesthesia.[417] Several studies have reported shortened recovery room stay and an earlier hospital discharge.[412, 413] These advantages have not been consistently observed for all procedures and may reflect local practice variances.

A pharmacodynamic response that may offer patient advantage is the lower incidence of nausea and vomiting with propofol when used as an induction agent or when used for the maintenance of anesthesia.[412, 418–424] There have been conflicting results for particular procedures, however, such as strabismus repair and tonsillectomy and when it is combined with opioids.[425–428] Short-term infusions in the operating room and for a variety of non-operating room procedures demonstrate a clinical advantage in terms of ease in controlling depth of sedation as well as rapidity and quality of recovery.[429–433] Propofol infusions seem particularly well suited for radiologic and oncology procedures. Another major advantage for patients is the reduced incidence of airway irritability compared with thiopental, which translates into a lower incidence of laryngospasm.[410, 434, 435] It appears that insertion of a laryngeal mask airway is better tolerated following propofol when compared with thiopental.[398, 403, 436, 437] An additional advantage may be a better preservation of upper airway patency that is improved further with a chin lift maneuver.[438]

Long-term propofol infusions have also been used in the intensive care environment. Such long-term infusions would result in significant differences in rapidity of wake-up.[397] It appears to be most useful and most economically feasible for short-term (overnight) sedation in the intensive care environment. However, there are a number of concerns regarding infusions of greater than 12 hours. Metabolic acidosis, myocardial failure, and deaths associated with long-term propofol infusions have been reported in children in the critical care environment.[439–442] The clinical importance of these case reports needs to be re-evaluated with more widespread multicenter studies.[443] As with all rapidly acting potent induction agents, the use of propofol should be restricted to individuals trained in its use and having advanced airway management skills.

Ketamine (Ketalar)

Ketamine is a derivative of phencyclidine. Its action is related to central dissociation of the cerebral cortex, and it also causes cerebral excitation. The latter property may be responsible for precipitating seizures in susceptible patients.[444] Ketamine is an excellent analgesic and amnestic; the recommended dose for induction of anesthesia is 1 to 3 mg/kg IV or 5 to 10 mg/kg IM. The duration of action of a single intravenous dose is 5 to 8 minutes, with an alpha elimination half-life of 11 minutes and a beta elimination half-life of 2.5 to 3.0 hours.[445, 446] Further supplementary doses of 0.5 to 1.0 mg/kg are administered when clinically indicated. Atropine or another antisialagogue should usually accompany the initial dose to diminish the production of copious secretions that occur with ketamine.[447] Ketamine may also be administered in very low doses intravenously (0.25–0.5 mg/kg) or intramuscularly (1–2 mg/kg), either alone or in combination with low-dose midazolam (0.05 mg/kg [50 μg/kg]) along with atropine (0.02 mg/kg) for sedation for a variety of procedures such as oncology evaluations, suture of lacerations, or radiologic interventions.[448–452] Bioavailability after intramuscular administration is approximately 93% in adults and even higher in children.[453, 454] If an antisialagogue is not administered, there is a high potential for laryngospasm.[455] It must be understood that higher doses will produce a state of general anesthesia.[456–458] Even with low doses, there is potential for apnea or airway obstruction, particularly when combined with other sedating medications.[456, 459, 460]

Ketamine has also been administered orally, nasally, and rectally both as a premedication prior to general anesthesia and for procedural sedation.[371, 461–474] Bioavailability is approximately 50% following nasal administration and 25% following rectal administration.[475] There are concerns regarding both nasal and rectal drug administration. Rectal ketamine administration can result in very irregular and less predictable times of onset and peak sedation, just as with rectal barbiturates. Nasal drug administration can result in drug entering directly into the central nervous system by tracking along neurovascular tissue of the nasal mucosa (see Fig. 9–1).[476–480] Since the preservative in ketamine has been shown to be neurotoxic, there is the theoretic possibility of central nervous system toxicity due to the preservative.[481, 482] Until better safety information is available, this route of drug administration is not recommended unless preservative-free ketamine is used. Ketamine has also been administered as a means of providing epidural analgesia.[483, 484] The same admonition, and even more importantly, applies here; **epidural ketamine must not be administered unless it is preservative free.**

Ketamine increases heart rate, cardiac index, and systemic blood pressure; it also raises pulmonary artery pressure in adults but has little effect on respiration.[485, 486] In children, there is apparently no effect on pulmonary artery pressure provided that ventilation is controlled.[487] If a child is sedated with ketamine but allowed to breathe spontaneously, elevations in $ETCO_2$ may result in increases in pulmonary artery pressure.[488] Ketamine has negative inotropic effects in patients who are vasopressor dependent.[489] Ketamine appears of have a different effect on upper airway musculature when compared with midazolam; in adults, midazolam has been demonstrated to cause airway obstruction, but ketamine did not produce airway obstruction.[490] This study may explain in part the successful widespread use of this anesthetic by nonanesthesiologists. Ketamine also has been shown to relax airway smooth musculature stimulated by histamine[491]; treatment of acute asthma in subanesthetic doses has not been successful.[492]

The onset of anesthesia is about 30 seconds after an intravenous dose, and this is usually heralded by horizontal or vertical nystagmus.[486, 493] Studies separating equianesthetic doses of ketamine isomers revealed a lower incidence of side effects, more potent analgesia, and fewer cardiovascular effects with the dextroketamine isomer.[486, 494] Acute tolerance to ketamine has been reported.[495] Children require greater doses of ketamine (milligrams per kilogram) than adults because of more rapid degradation; however, there is considerable patient-to-patient variability.[454, 486, 494]

The most common adverse reaction to ketamine is postoperative vomiting, which occurs in 33% of patients.[493] Intraoperative and postoperative dreaming and hallucinations occur more commonly in older than in younger children.[493] The incidence of these latter adverse effects may be reduced when ketamine is supplemented with scopolamine or a benzodiazepine. One clinical report described two children, both 3 years of age, who had recurrent nightmares and abnormal behavior persisting for 10 months after a single ketamine administration.[496]

Indications

Ketamine is a useful agent for children who are developmentally delayed and unable to cooperate or for children who have come to the operating room many times, frightened and combative. Ketamine can be used in very low doses (0.25–0.5 mg/kg) for short-term procedures such as diagnostic spinal punctures, bone marrow aspiration, and in higher doses for radiotherapy, angiography, and cardiac catheterization. Ketamine may be particularly valuable for burn dressing changes, suture removal, induction of anesthesia in hypovolemic patients, patients in whom application of a face mask may prove hazardous such as those with epidermolysis bullosa, and patients who require invasive monitoring before induction of general anesthesia.[167, 486, 494, 497, 498] Ketamine has been successfully used even in neonates with less apparent cardiovascular depression than with halothane or isoflurane.[497]

Contraindications

Ketamine may produce increases in ICP as a result of cerebral vasodilation; it also increases $CMRO_2$. Ketamine may be contraindicated in any patient with central nervous system pathology involving intracranial hypertension.[499, 500] This concern regarding ICP has been challenged; adult patients on controlled mechanical ventilation and sedated with a ketamine infusion demonstrated a decreased ICP following bolus doses of 1.5, 3.0, and 5.0 mg/kg.[501] The caveat here is that these adult patients were already intubated with controlled ventilation and sedated; ketamine is still generally not indicted for emergency airway management of patients with a head injury.

A 30% rise in intraocular pressure has also been noted; thus, ketamine may be potentially dangerous in the presence of a corneal laceration.[502] In children with active upper respiratory tract infections, copious secretions produced by ketamine may well exacerbate an already irritable airway and result in laryngospasm.[447, 455] Ketamine administration may cause an incompetent gag reflex and thus should not be administered to patients with a full stomach without appropriate airway management. Patients with hiatal hernia or gastroesophageal reflux may benefit from appropriate acid aspiration prophylaxis.[503] Ketamine may not be useful as the sole anesthetic agent in any surgical procedure in which total control of the patient's position is necessary, because purposeless movements frequently occur during ketamine anesthesia. Ketamine may be inappropriate in any child with a history of psychiatric or seizure disorder because of its psychotropic and epileptogenic effects.[444, 486, 504]

Although the administration of ketamine appears simple, its side effects are potentially dangerous. *Ketamine must be administered only by physicians experienced with managing a compromised airway.* We urge that it not be used as a premedication unless given in the presence of continuous supervision by properly trained personnel.

Droperidol (Inapsine)

Droperidol is a centrally acting butyrophenone that alters synaptic transmission by causing a buildup of neurotransmitters; consequently it interferes with normal neurohumoral responses and produces a dissociative state of mind.[505] Because its action is primarily in the extrapyramidal areas of the brain, as with haloperidol, the side effects are extrapyramidal: muscle rigidity, visual disturbances, hallucinations, oculogyric crisis, and dysphoria.[506, 507] Droperidol causes a buildup of dopamine and may be contraindicated in patients with endogenous depression, although little has been published about depressed pediatric patients.[508] There has been minimal experience in administering this drug to pediatric patients with metabolic defects or movement disorders that involve the extrapyramidal system. The inhibition of neurotransmitters by dopamine following a low dose of droperidol may be used to advantage for the prevention of nausea and vomiting (50 to 75 μg/kg). However, its efficacy in preventing vomiting in patients recovering from strabismus surgery or tonsillectomy is inconsistent.[505, 509–511]

Adults given droperidol classically appear outwardly calm but feel impending doom or depression and are unable to express this feeling. The plasma half-life of droperidol in adults is about 130 minutes, the duration of action is 6 to 12 hours, and some side effects may last as long as 24 hours. In pediatric patients, the elimination half-life is slightly shorter (101 ± 26 min).[512] Combining droperidol with a narcotic, sedative, or barbiturate reduces the incidence of undesired side effects.[504, 505] The duration of action of all these medications is less than that of high-dose droperidol; therefore, supplemental doses may be required when using high-dose droperidol to cover the full duration of droperidol's effects.[513]

Droperidol is a weak alpha-blocking agent that may cause significant hypotension in hypovolemic patients but has minimal cardiovascular effects in the normovolemic state.[514] It has been demonstrated to oppose epinephrine-induced arrhythmias.[515] Respiratory effects of droperidol include a reduction in functional residual capacity, increased airway resistance, and, when accompanied by fentanyl, an increase in respiratory muscle tone. This increase in tone may mandate greater inflation pressures when no muscle relaxant is administered and may also be an important consideration in patients whose closing volumes are close to functional residual capacity. Droperidol alone has not been demonstrated to cause respiratory depression, although there may be considerable patient-to-patient variation.[516–520]

Advantages and Disadvantages

Alpha-receptor blockade, the antiarrhythmic effect, and the sedative and antiemetic properties of droperidol offer some advantages, especially for awake oral intubation when combined with narcotic and topical anesthetic. The many side effects and prolonged duration of action may pose significant disadvantages. If droperidol is used with large doses of potent narcotics, the threat of respiratory depression combined with the dissociative state it induces may result in airway obstruction, hypoxia, or apnea. In addition, when droperidol is used in patients with increased ICP or hypovolemia, the alpha blockade may result in a lowered systemic pressure and resultant reduction in cerebral perfusion pressure.[521] For these reasons, high doses of droperidol should be limited to selected pediatric situations. The primary use is in low doses as an antiemetic or occasionally for postoperative sedation in children in whom it is desirable to minimize postoperative movement.

Narcotics

Morphine

Morphine is most frequently used in children for postoperative pain management by intermittent bolus, by continuous infusion, or by patient-controlled analgesia (see Chapter 29). The usual initial intravenous dose is 0.1 to 0.2 mg/kg; a lower dose may be indicated in critically ill patients or in patients receiving other supplemental analgesics. The analgesic response to morphine is the standard with which all other opioids are compared. Morphine is rapidly and completely absorbed in adults within 20 minutes of intramuscular injection and has a serum half-life in adults of 2.9 ± 0.5 hours when administered intravenously and 4.5 ± 0.3 hours when administered intramuscularly.[522] Morphine given intramuscularly attains a higher and more sustained level of analgesia than morphine given intravenously, suggesting rapid distribution, metabolism, and excretion.[45] A more rapid decrease occurs in the serum levels of younger adult patients, correlating to some extent with the loss of analgesia. A number of studies have examined the kinetics of intravenous morphine in children.[89, 90, 523–529] The clearance of intravenous morphine tends to be slightly faster in children ranging from 79 to 133 minutes.[523, 528] The half-life can be markedly prolonged (50%) in children requiring pressor support (~400 min).[524] Studies of morphine pharmacokinetics in term and preterm infants have demonstrated very variable and markedly prolonged elimination half-life and diminished clearance.[87, 89, 90, 525, 526, 530, 531] However, morphine clearance markedly increases over time and this maturation of morphine clearance is more rapid in infants undergoing noncardiac surgery compared with infants undergoing cardiac surgery (Fig. 8–16).[46, 529] In infants undergoing noncardiac surgery, clearance increases from 9.2 mL/min/kg during days 1 through 7 of life, to 25 mL/min/kg in infants 31 to 90 days of age, 31 mL/min/kg in infants 91 to 180 days of age, and 49 mL/min/kg in infants 180 to 380 days of age.[529] Adult clearance values are reached at approximately 1 month of age. The metabolism in neonates appears, as in the adult, to have similar contributions by morphine-3 and morphine-6 glucuronide.[525] These observations explain in part the prolonged duration of action in neonates; it also suggests that infants older than 1 month

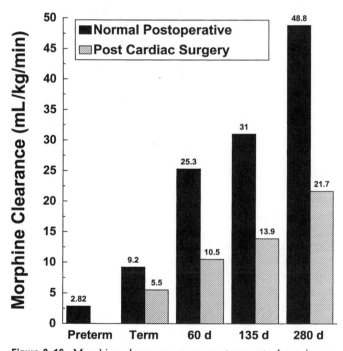

Figure 8–16. Morphine clearance versus postconceptual age in normal postoperative patients and patients undergoing cardiac surgery. Note that there is a rapid increase in an infant's ability to metabolize morphine in the first several weeks of life and that some infants achieve adult values by 1 month of age. Also note that postcardiac surgical patients have a marked impairment of morphine metabolism, which may reflect the use of vasopressors or decreased cardiac output to the liver, or both. There is extreme patient-to-patient variability at all ages; preterm infants have the lowest clearance of any age group. (Data abstracted from Lynn A, Nespeca MK, Bratton SL, et al: Clearance of morphine in postoperative infants during intravenous infusion: The influence of age and surgery. Anesth Analg 1998;86:958–963; Mikkelsen S, Feilberg VL, Christensen CB, Lundstrom KE: Morphine pharmacokinetics in premature and mature newborn infants. Acta Paediatr 1994; 83:1025–1028.)

are able to equal or exceed the reported clearance of morphine in adults.

The major liability for pediatric patients is respiratory depression.[532, 533] Pediatric patients demonstrate adequate postoperative analgesia without the development of hypercarbia at morphine infusion rates of 10 to 30 μg/kg/hr.[527] Ventilatory depression by morphine is a result of diminished tidal volume and ventilatory rate; there are also conflicting data regarding a parallel shift in the carbon dioxide response curve versus a change in slope as well as a shift in the carbon dioxide response. Neonates demonstrate an increased respiratory sensitivity to morphine compared with meperidine.[534] Studies of rats demonstrated a two- to threefold greater brain uptake in neonatal rats than in adult rats.[115] This finding may explain the lower LD_{50} of morphine in neonatal animals, which is five times lower than for adult animals.[113] Because infants have an immature blood-brain barrier, a greater proportion of morphine may cross to the brain in neonates than in adults.[113–115] This immaturity of the blood-brain barrier may account in part for a neonate's apparent increased sensitivity to morphine compared with meperidine or fentanyl, which, because they are much more lipophilic, rapidly cross an adult's or infant's blood-brain barrier; that is, there is essentially no blood-brain barrier for fentanyl.[535, 536] Alternatively, altered pharmacokinetics could lead to drug accumulation in some infants.[90] Another possibility is a maturation of the pharmacodynamic effects on respiration rather than altered pharmacokinetics, that is, a maturation of the sensitivity of the respiratory center to morphine rather than brain equilibrium.[537] Whatever the mechanism, morphine must be used with caution in premature infants and in infants less than 1 month of age. One additional caution is that significant histamine release may follow an intravenous bolus of morphine; it may occasionally, though rarely in children, result in systemic hypotension.[538] Urticaria localized to the path of the vein in which morphine infuses is a local reaction and not equivalent to an allergic reaction. Morphine has been administered orally, rectally, transtracheally, and in the epidural and subarachnoid spaces.[539–546] Rectal administration is generally not recommended because of extremely irregular absorption (6–93% bioavailability)[547] and the potential for delayed respiratory depression.[548]

Meperidine (Demerol)

The principal advantage of meperidine over morphine is the clinical impression that it causes less histamine release. A double-blind study in adult patients questions this observation because histamine release was found most frequently after meperidine.[549] This apparent conflict with previous studies of morphine may be a result of examining lower doses of morphine than in previous reports. The purported benefits of substituting meperidine for morphine when dealing with hypovolemic or asthmatic patients are questionable.

The usual dose of meperidine is 1 to 2 mg/kg; reduced doses should be used in critically ill patients. Meperidine is rapidly absorbed after intramuscular injection and has a serum half-life of 3.7 ± 1.6 hours in adults when administered intravenously.[550] Peak plasma values following intravenous, intramuscular, and rectal administration are 5 ± 1 minutes intravenously, 10 ± 2 minutes intramuscularly, and

60 ± 10 minutes rectally.[551, 552] Rectal administration results in wide variations in systemic blood values (32% to 81% of administered dose) and is thus not recommended.[553] The half-life in children is approximately 3 hours,[553] but the half-life in neonates varies from 3.3 to 59.4 hours.[554]

An infant's respiratory system appears to be less sensitive to meperidine than to morphine.[534] The LD_{50} of a neonatal animal is only 20% lower than adult animal values, corresponding with the human clinical response.[113] This information would seem to suggest that meperidine causes less respiratory depression compared with the equivalent dose of morphine. This difference between morphine and meperidine may be related in part to differences in their ability to cross the blood-brain barrier, which depends on fat solubility. Studies of rats have shown a higher brain concentration of morphine in neonatal rats compared with mature rats,[555] whereas with meperidine, the brain concentration is similar in neonatal compared with mature rats.[115] Since morphine is less fat soluble than meperidine, it may be that proportionally more morphine crosses the immature blood-brain barrier of a neonate than an older patient who has a more developed blood-brain barrier. As with any narcotic, use in very young infants must be accompanied by careful observation for respiratory depression and airway obstruction, because the pharmacokinetics vary considerably in this age group.[554] Since there is concern regarding seizures caused by the buildup of normeperidine,[556] we do not recommend the use of this opioid in the neonatal age group.

One common indication for meperidine has been to reduce postoperative shivering; a study of adult volunteers has found reduced oxygen consumption and carbon dioxide production as a result of decreased shivering.[557] Chronic or high-dose meperidine is generally not recommended for pediatric patients or patients with renal dysfunction due to the possibility of accumulation of normeperidine, which can cause seizures.[558] There are some patients, however, in whom the need to avoid side effects of other opioids will necessitate the use of meperidine. In this situation, the lowest possible dose for the shortest possible time should be utilized.

Fentanyl (Sublimaze)

Fentanyl is the most commonly used opioid supplement to general anesthesia in the pediatric population. This opioid has shown particular efficacy in the care of high-risk premature and term neonates as well as infants and children undergoing cardiac surgical procedures. High doses of fentanyl (10 to 100 μg/kg) are often administered with minimal adverse cardiovascular effects.[559–570] Fentanyl may be administered intravenously, intramuscularly, as a supplement to epidural analgesia, or orally (transoral mucosal absorption), and research is ongoing regarding transdermal iontophoresis.[571] As expected, there are age-dependent effects on pharmacokinetics and pharmacodynamics, particularly in premature and term infants compared with older children. Premature infants have been found to have extremely variable and markedly prolonged clearance (mean beta elimination half-life 17.7 ± 9.3 hr) and longer respiratory depression than term neonates.[559, 572, 573] Term neonates also have a variable ability to clear fentanyl and may have a longer half-life and lower clearance than older infants.[560, 572, 573] Seventy-seven percent of fentanyl is bound to alpha-1-acid glycopro-

tein in preterm infants and 70% in term infants.[25] Older infants (>3 months of age) and children are able to clear a greater amount of drug than adults (clearance 30.6 mL/kg/min versus 17.9 mL/kg/min) and therefore have a shorter beta elimination half-life (68 min versus 121 min).[559, 562, 572–574] Several factors appear to be particularly important in the clearance of fentanyl: hepatic blood flow, hepatic function, and age-dependent changes in volume of distribution.[560, 563, 564, 575] Any factor that decreases hepatic blood flow decreases the amount of fentanyl presented to the liver; infants having repair of omphalocele in particular have been found to have almost no clearance of fentanyl.[560, 563, 564] This observation is not surprising, because animal studies have demonstrated that fentanyl clearance is nearly parallel to hepatic blood flow.[576, 577] One study in neonatal lambs found decreased clearance with increased intra-abdominal pressure, but the mechanism was decreased hepatic function rather than decreased hepatic blood flow from the abdominal pressure.[578]

One additional concern with neonates is the apparent interaction between fentanyl and midazolam. Profound hypotension has been reported following bolus administration of midazolam in infants receiving infusions of fentanyl, and the converse that extreme hypotension may occur with bolus administration of fentanyl in patients receiving infusions of midazolam.[579]

Considerable variability in fentanyl kinetics has also been found in children having cardiac surgical procedures and may in part relate to the type of cardiac surgical defect, the effect this defect has on hepatic blood flow, the volume of distribution, the use of vasopressors, and the age of the patient.[561, 575] Hypothermia has also been demonstrated to significantly alter fentanyl kinetics in both animals and humans.[580] Another population with differing pharmacokinetics is critically ill children receiving long-term infusions; the terminal elimination half-life in this group in general is 21 hours, with a range of 11 to 36 hours.[581] The infusion rates to achieve a similar level of sedation may vary as much as 10-fold.[581] This marked variability in pharmacokinetics and pharmacodynamics strongly emphasizes the need to titrate to effect and to be prepared to provide postoperative ventilatory support. It should be noted that any child who receives an infusion of fentanyl is likely to rapidly develop tolerance and upon discontinuance of the infusion to demonstrate signs of withdrawal. All long-term infusions should be tapered slowly over days rather than abruptly discontinued.[573, 582, 583]

With low-dose fentanyl, the termination of action is primarily a combination of redistribution and rapid clearance by the liver.[573, 584] High-dose fentanyl, on the other hand, accumulates in muscle and fat and is therefore released (recirculated) more slowly, thus accounting in part for the prolonged respiratory depression when high doses are administered. There is no evidence of dose-dependent kinetics; that is, there is no tissue or enzyme saturation in the clinically used ranges.[584] In some respects, this narcotic is very similar to thiopental: with low doses, termination of effect is by redistribution, whereas with high doses, termination of effect requires metabolism.[585–589]

The usual initial dose is 1 to 3 μg/kg, to be supplemented as clinically indicated. Fentanyl is highly lipid soluble and rapidly crosses the blood-brain barrier. This characteristic may in part explain why the LD_{50} for fentanyl in neonatal animals is 90% of that in adult animals; the development of the blood-brain barrier has little effect on the entry of fentanyl (unlike morphine) into brain tissue.[536, 587] Little research has addressed the relationship between blood fentanyl values and ventilatory depression in children. Some data suggest that neonates are no more sensitive to this narcotic than are adults, because the blood-brain barrier should have little effect on the ability of fentanyl to enter the central nervous system.[560, 588] One animal study has shown little in the way of developmental change regarding respiratory depression, which is very different from that found with morphine.[537] Other data suggest that older infants (>3 months) are less sensitive to the respiratory depression of fentanyl than are adults.[576, 588] Continuous operative and postoperative infusions of fentanyl are commonly used in pediatric patients of all ages.[561, 589] Fentanyl is also used to provide patient-controlled analgesia (see Chapter 29).[590, 591]

Chest wall and glottic rigidity has been reported with many of the opioids but most often following fentanyl; the reason for this is not clear.[592-597] Glottic rigidity may account for inability to ventilate by bag and mask following intravenous fentanyl.[595] This adverse pharmacodynamic response can be minimized by slow administration, and it can be reversed with the administration of either a muscle relaxant or naloxone. One other concern is the rare association of increased vagal tone with bolus administration; bradycardia may have profound effects on the cardiac output of neonates. Additionally, fentanyl has been demonstrated to markedly depress baroreceptor reflex control of heart rate in neonates.[598] It is for these reasons that the combination of pancuronium and fentanyl is so popular.

Fentanyl in an oral transmucosal form is one of only several medications currently approved by the FDA for premedication of children. There is relatively rapid absorption of fentanyl through the oral mucosa, which bypasses the liver.[427, 599-604] Approximately half the absorption is gastrointestinal; one study suggests a bioavailability of 33% in children compared with 0.5% in adults.[604] Uptake continues for a period of time after consumption (see Fig. 9–4).[427] The main concerns with this form of fentanyl administration were the apparent high incidence of desaturation and vomiting prior to induction of anesthesia. It appears that at least some of these early concerns were a result of performing studies at high elevations above sea level (low saturations at baseline) and due to the study design (high doses and excessive period for observation allowing for the peak blood levels to occur prior to anesthetic induction).[601, 602] Subsequent studies and personal experience suggest that administration of doses of 10 to 15 μg/kg and induction of anesthesia within a short time of completion (10–20 minutes) markedly reduces or eliminates these potential complications.[427, 604]

The fentanyl patch was developed to provide extended slow drug administration similar to that provided with a continuous intravenous infusion for patients with chronic pain.[605-613] It is important to understand that this formulation was not designed to be administered to treat postsurgical pain but rather for patients who are receiving narcotics chronically. In adults, uptake of fentanyl begins within 1 hour, achieving therapeutic levels within 6 to 8 hours and peak levels at 24 hours.[610, 613, 614] The skin acts as a reservoir, and, even after removal, uptake continues for some hours.

The fentanyl uptake is markedly affected by skin blood flow, skin thickness, and the location of the patch.[615, 616] Alterations in skin blood flow, such as those caused by fever, may increase absorption. The use of this medication should be limited to pain specialists who have familiarity with the unusual pharmacokinetics of this drug delivery system.[617] Children may be particularly vulnerable to the potential for rapid drug absorption compared with adults, because they have thinner skin and better skin blood flow.[476] There is limited experience in pediatric patients; one study examined a population that was mostly teenagers and found the pharmacokinetics to be similar to those described for adults.[618] Further studies are required, however, before this drug formulation can be applied to younger patients.[619]

Alfentanil (Alfenta)

Alfentanil is a fentanyl analogue whose main advantage appears to be lower lipid solubility and much smaller volume of distribution compared with fentanyl.[620] Studies indicate that brain concentrations of alfentanil are seven to nine times lower than brain concentrations of fentanyl, the volume of distribution is four times lower, and protein binding is greater.[621] Alfentanil is more rapidly eliminated than fentanyl, resulting in earlier termination of its effects. An important observation is that pediatric and adult studies demonstrate pharmacokinetics independent of dose, therefore providing a wide margin of safety; that is, *the larger the dose, the greater the amount of drug metabolized*.[621-625] Studies comparing children with adults have found a similar Vdss but a greater clearance (11.1 ± 3.9 mL/kg/min versus 5.9 ± 1.6 mL/kg/min) and therefore a shorter beta elimination phase (63 ± 24 versus 95 ± 20 min).[622-625] Infants 3 to 12 months of age appear to have clearance values, Vdss, and beta elimination half-life similar to those in older children.[624] Clearance is markedly diminished in patients with hepatic disease, so prolonged clinical effects can be expected in any patient with impaired hepatic blood flow, such as premature infants, children with increased intra-abdominal pressure, children on vasopressors, and those with some forms of congenital heart disease.[620, 626, 627] Preterm infants demonstrate a larger volume of distribution (1.0 ± 0.39 vs. 0.48 ± 0.19 L/kg), a smaller clearance (2.2 ± 2.4 vs. 5.6 ± 2.4 ml/min/kg), and a markedly longer and more variable beta elimination half-life (525 ± 305 vs. 60 ± 11 min) compared with older children.[628, 629] Renal failure apparently has little effect on elimination.[630]

Another concern with the use of alfentanil in the preterm infant is the developmental changes in binding to alpha-1 acid glycoprotein. In preterm infants, 65% is bound, whereas in term infants 79% is bound; thus a greater free fraction is available for biologic effect in preterms.[25]

The pharmacokinetics and pharmacodynamics of this medication suggest potential applications for the rapid control of analgesia and the rapid awakening from anesthesia. Alfentanil (10 μg/kg) has been combined with propofol (2.5 mg/kg) for tracheal intubation without addition of a muscle relaxant.[631] High-dose alfentanil is also used for cardiac procedures.

Sufentanil (Sufenta)

Sufentanil is a potent synthetic narcotic that in many respects is similar to fentanyl and alfentanil. The elimination of sufentanil is unaffected by renal failure but markedly altered by factors that influence hepatic blood flow; cirrhosis apparently has little effect on elimination.[620, 632, 633] The majority of pediatric studies of intravenous sufentanil have examined children undergoing cardiac surgical procedures. Pediatric studies have found age-dependent pharmacokinetics; neonates have a larger Vdss, slower clearance, and a longer and more variable beta elimination half-life (Fig. 8–17).[634–636] Significant differences have been found between infants 0 to 7 days of age and the same infants studied at 20 to 28 days of age, suggesting a marked improvement in hepatic blood flow, increased cardiac output, or rapid development of hepatic metabolic pathways.[634] Because the three infants studied over time all had evidence of congestive heart failure and hepatic dysfunction, we cannot be certain which factor is more important; however, hepatic blood flow is most likely the major determinant influencing drug elimination. Elimination may be more rapid in infants without congenital heart disease, as has been described with morphine.[527, 529]

As with most medications, children seem to be able to clear this drug more rapidly than infants or adults. Bradycardia and asystole have been observed with bolus administration, suggesting that the simultaneous administration of a vagolytic agent (atropine, glycopyrrolate, or pancuronium bromide) may be efficacious when this drug giving as a bolus.[637, 638] Transmucosal drug administration via the nasal mucosa has been examined; however, as with any opioid there is always the potential for respiratory depression.[639–641] Several of these studies found better pediatric patient acceptance of nasal sufentanil compared with nasal midazolam; however, there was a higher incidence of vomiting and several children had decreased chest wall compliance after or during induction of anesthesia. It would appear that doses of 2 to 3 μg/kg (nasal) are efficacious.[639, 641]

Remifentanil (Ultiva)

Remifentanil is the newest in the family of synthetic opioids.[642, 643] This opioid is unique because an ester linkage allows rapid metabolism to a carboxylic acid metabolite by blood and tissue esterases.[644] Theoretically this implies that drug metabolism would be unaffected by hepatic or renal function.[645] The active metabolite of remifentanil that is eliminated by the kidneys, however, has approximately 1/300 to 1/1000 the opioid activity of the parent compound and theoretically could lead to drug accumulation and effects in patients with impaired renal function.[646] One study of adults has shown minimal residual opioid effects after a 12-hour infusion in patients with renal failure.[647] Perhaps the most unique property of remifentanil is the very short half-life (10–20 min) and the resultant rapid recovery from a very intense opioid effect to virtually no opioid effect within 10 minutes. Clearance is generally three to four times hepatic blood flow and is dose dependent; that is, clearance increases as more drug is administered.[646]

Unlike all other opioids administered by infusion, there is no increase in the duration of effect with increasing doses or duration of short-term infusions, as during the course of a short or long surgical procedure. If one examines simulations of the time required for a 50% reduction in drug effect, the rate of metabolism is so rapid for remifentanil that the curve is virtually flat (Fig. 8–18).[646] This rapid rate of metabolism has been demonstrated in adults.[643] In one study, despite a 20-fold difference in the rate of infusion, return to spontaneous respirations varied by only 1 to 3 minutes.[645, 648] The concept of biologic half-life, that is, the half-life of clinical effect, is important for this opioid. For opioids, the effect upon respirations is an excellent reflection of pharmacodynamic effects.[649] A study in adults following a

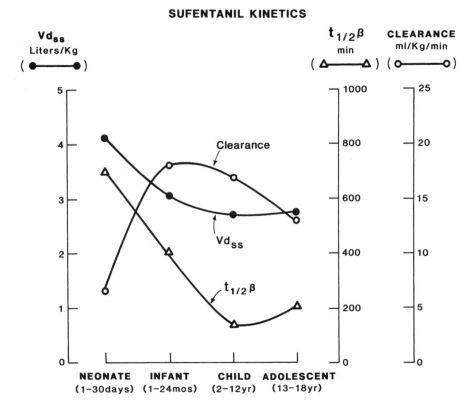

SUFENTANIL KINETICS

Figure 8–17. Pharmacokinetics for sufentanil versus age. Note that the beta elimination half-life and volume of distribution at steady state are inversely related to age; clearance is the lowest in neonates. Pharmacokinetics in children and adolescents is similar to that in adults. (Data abstracted from Greeley WJ, de Bruijn NP, Davis DP: Sufentanil pharmacokinetics in pediatric cardiovascular patients. Anesth Analg 1987;66:1067–1072.)

Figure 8–18. This figure is a simulation of the time required for a 50% reduction in the effective site concentration of remifentanil (solid circles), sufentanil (open circles), alfentanil (solid triangles), and fentanyl (open triangles) after an infusion (duration 0–240 min) designed to maintain a constant effect site concentration. Note that there is a completely flat curve for remifentanil, suggesting that a plateau effect is rapidly reached with remifentanil compared with the other opioids such that even after a long infusion, the time to 50% reduction in effect concentration is still under 4 minutes. (Modified from Westmoreland CL, Hole JF, Sebel PS, et al: Pharmacokinetics of remifentanil (GI87084B) and its major metabolite (GI90291) in patients undergoing elective inpatient surgery. Anesthesiology 1993;79:893–903.)

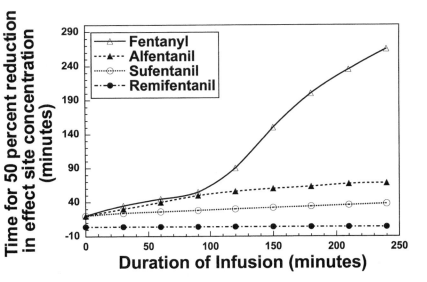

3-hour infusion of alfentanil vs. remifentanil, found that for alfentanil, the pharmacokinetic half-life was 47.3 ± 12 minutes versus 3.2 ± 0.9 minutes for remifentanil. The measured time for 50% return of minute ventilation, the pharmacodynamic effect of opioid, was 54.0 ± 48.1 minutes for alfentanil versus 5.4 ± 1.8 minutes for remifentanil.[649] One possible concern for long-term administration of remifentanil is the acute development of tolerance. In a study of adult volunteers, the analgesic threshold was one fourth of the peak values within 3 hours.[650] This suggests that modification of infusion rates will be required during the course of a remifentanil-based anesthetic to maintain a stable level of analgesia.

These pharmacokinetic and pharmacodynamic effects have important clinical implications because this translates into the ability to rapidly increase or decrease opioid effect. This opioid should be administered only by continuous infusion. If an intravenous line should be shut off, kinked, or disconnected, the patient will very rapidly be without opioid effect. This also means that at the end of a procedure with remifentanil, the anesthetic plan must include a transition to longer acting opioids or the use of a regional block so that the patient wakes up pain free.

Generally, a loading dose of 0.5 to 1.0 μg/kg followed by an infusion of 0.25 to 0.5 μg/kg/min will provide a satisfactory opioid effect. The infusion may be increased as indicated with little fear of producing an "overdose" because of the very favorable pharmacokinetics and pharmacodynamics. Pharmacokinetic data from pediatric patients suggest that the child's response should be similar to the adult's. There is limited information regarding the use of remifentanil in neonates, but one would expect to observe more patient-to-patient variability when compared with older patients. The overall pharmacodynamic profile, however, should still be far superior to that of other opioids in terms of recovery.[651, 652] As with many synthetic opioids, severe bradycardia may occur following bolus administration, especially large doses[653]; the concomitant use of a vagolytic or pancuronium may prevent this adverse cardiac response. This opioid may, with further study, turn out to be the opioid of choice for critically ill infants requiring a surgical procedure but in whom prolonged postoperative ventilation

is not desired. It is important to remember, however, that anesthesia is not produced by opioids alone but that an anxiolytic must also be administered. The half-life of any anxiolytic will far exceed the half-life of remifentanil so that the potential for postoperative respiratory complications would still be present.

Butorphanol (Stadol), Nalbuphine (Nubain), Tramadol (Ultram)

Butorphanol and nalbuphine are synthetic narcotic-agonist-antagonist analgesics.[654–656] The mean elimination half-life of nalbuphine in adults is 2.2 to 2.6 hours[657, 658] but is shorter in children (0.9 hours).[659] The claimed advantage of this family of drugs is adequate analgesia with a ceiling on respiratory depression.[660–662] This family of drugs has had some popularity in pediatric patients.[659, 663–667] The administration of butorphanol by the nasal route has been investigated in adults and may offer some advantage for pediatric patients without intravenous access.[663, 668, 669] What must be remembered is that these agents may reverse mu receptor–mediated analgesic effects of the more potent opioids and should therefore be used as the initial or the sole narcotic.

Tramadol is a relatively new medication, which is a weak opioid with minimal effects on respiration.[670, 671] Tramadol also alters spinal cord pain activation.[671] There is at present little published pediatric information, but at least one study has shown equal efficacy to nalbuphine for postoperative pain relief.[672]

Nonsteroidal Anti-inflammatory Drugs

Ketorolac (Toradol)

Ketorolac is a nonsteroidal anti-inflammatory drug with very potent analgesic properties.[673–676] Ketorolac has been used by itself to treat acute postoperative pain and as a supplement to opioids. Ketorolac has been an important adjuvant to the treatment of postoperative pain, especially in children who require prolonged pain treatment. It is particularly useful for the transition from intravenous to oral therapy. The pharmacokinetics following a single dose is similar in adults and children. The terminal elimination half-life in children 4 to 8 years old is approximately 6 hours according to one study, but the range was 3.5 to 10 hours.[677] Another study found a considerably shorter beta elimination half-life (2.26 ± 1.35 hours) for children 3 to 8 years of age.[678] An additional study found a beta elimination half-life of 3.3 ± 1.9 hours for children 1 to 16 years of age but with a volume of distribution smaller than that reported by other investigators.[677–679] These differences in pharmacokinetics may reflect differences in the duration of sampling times. The analgesic properties of ketorolac are similar to those of low-dose morphine for post-tonsillectomy analgesia.[680] The major use in pediatrics is as an adjuvant to opioid analgesia or for treatment of mild to moderate pain where there is a desire to reduce the potential for respiratory depression or for nausea and vomiting.[675, 681, 682]

One of the major concerns with ketorolac is the inhibition of platelet function through inhibition of cyclooxygenase and the potential for postsurgical bleeding. Ketorolac has been shown to have minimal effect on prothrombin and partial thromboplastin times but has been shown to cause modest increases in bleeding time.[675, 683, 684] It should be noted that the effects of ketorolac on platelet function are different than those of aspirin. With aspirin, the antiplatelet effect lasts for several days after a single administration because of the irreversible acetylation of platelet cyclooxygenase. However, with ketorolac, this effect is reversible and therefore the effect is dependent on the presence of ketorolac within the body.[685] Therefore, the antiplatelet effects of ketorolac are gone when the drug has been excreted. This effect on platelet function has been of most concern in children undergoing adenotonsillectomy.[686–689] In the studies reporting post-tonsillectomy bleeding, most involved administration of the ketorolac during or at the beginning of the surgical procedure before hemostasis was achieved. In addition, the increased incidence of bleeding appears to be primarily during the first 24 hours, which corresponds to the several half-lives it would take to eliminate the ketorolac from the body. The incidence of bleeding after the first 24 hours does not appear to be different. It would therefore be reasonable to not administer this medication until the end of surgery after hemostasis is achieved. Some practitioners prefer to avoid the issue and administer ketorolac only for procedures in which there is less potential for a life-threatening hemorrhage. Concerns regarding the possibility of postoperative hemorrhage appear to be valid, but the true frequency of life-threatening bleeding due exclusively to ketorolac is quite small. The practice of one of the authors (CJC) is to ask the surgeon prior to administration to be certain that it is acceptable to administer this medication and document the conversation in the anesthesia record.

Experience at one institution has been that this is a very potent analgesic with minimal side effects without an increased incidence of bleeding in tonsillectomy patients, provided the drug is administered at the end of surgery after establishment of hemostasis.[690] One other concern is the report of sudden and profound bradycardia following rapid intravenous administration[691]; this would suggest that ketorolac should be administered by slow injection.

Acetaminophen (Tylenol)

Acetaminophen is another analgesic medication useful as an adjunct to opioids.[692] Acetaminophen may be administered orally prior to induction of anesthesia, to have a blood level at the time of wake-up from a brief surgical procedure such as myringotomy and tube insertion. Oral acetaminophen is rapidly absorbed with measurable levels within 5 minutes of oral ingestion (see Fig. 9–5).[693] An oral dose of 10 to 20 mg/kg provides a blood level within the therapeutic range of 10 to 20 μg/mL that has been shown to be the level required for antipyresis; the blood levels for analgesia have not yet been described. For longer procedures, rectal administration at the beginning of surgery will provide a blood level at the time of awakening and before the patient would otherwise be able to take oral medications. Rectal administration, however, is associated with very irregular absorption with peak blood levels achieved 60 to 180 minutes following administration (see Fig. 9–6).[694] It is for this reason that if this medication is to be effective it must be administered at the beginning of surgery rather than upon the patient's admission to the recovery room. Several studies have shown that higher than recommended doses (up to 45 mg/kg) are required to place the patient within the therapeutic range for antipyresis.[694–696] A follow-up study suggests that an initial rectal dose of 40 mg/kg with subsequent rectal doses of 20 mg/kg at 6-hour intervals will produce the desired blood level (Feverall, Upsher-Smith, Minneapolis, MN).[697] This study did not extend beyond 24 hours, nor did it examine other brands of rectal acetaminophen; therefore, no recommendations can be made regarding continued rectal administration beyond 24 hours or administration with other brands. High-dose acetaminophen (40–60 mg/kg) has been demonstrated to be morphine sparing; further study is required before recommending doses higher than 40 mg/kg because of the potential for producing metabolites that are hepatotoxic.[698–700]

Sedatives

Diazepam (Valium)

Diazepam is rapidly absorbed after oral administration, with peak plasma levels at 30 to 90 minutes; the absorption rate has been found to be more rapid in children.[701] Intramuscular administration is painful and results in irregular absorption; plasma levels are only 60% of those obtained with a similar oral dose.[702–704] Oral diazepam is usually administered in a dose of 0.2 to 0.3 mg/kg and has been extensively used for premedication, as an adjunct to balanced anesthesia, for sedation during regional anesthesia, for amnesia, and for control of seizures. Generally the recommended intravenous dose is 0.1 to 0.2 mg/kg. Diazepam has been administered rectally to children in doses ranging from 0.3 to 1.0 mg/kg with satisfactory results.[705–708] One study found a more rapid uptake during the first 2 hours after administration when administered in liquid rather than suppository form; a prolonged, sustained blood level was achieved. However, for brief surgical procedures, it would appear that a lower dose would be more appropriate.[705]

Diazepam is highly plasma bound, with a serum half-life varying from 20 to 80 hours; the half-life is shorter in younger adults and children (approximately 18 hours).[705] This observation probably reflects a greater hepatic blood flow that delivers more drug to the liver for metabolism in younger than in older patients.[68, 709] The liver is the primary site of metabolism, and hepatic disease may decrease the rate of elimination.[709] Studies in neonates who received diazepam transplacentally just before delivery have demonstrated prolonged drug effects and serum half-lives (40–100 hours), probably as a result of immature hepatic excretory mechanisms and low hepatic blood flow (Fig. 8–19).[68, 701, 710] Diazepam is broken down to active metabolites (desmethydiazepam) with similar potency to the parent compound and with half-lives as long or longer than the parent compound, thus emphasizing the importance of not administering this benzodiazepine to neonates.[701, 711, 712]

Another concern is that the preservative (benzyl alcohol) also should be avoided in neonates because of the difficulty in metabolism, the association with kernicterus, and the development of metabolic acidosis.[713] However, the amount of benzyl alcohol administered with the usual doses of diazepam would likely be insufficient to cause harm to the neonate.[714] Diazepam has respiratory depressant effects that are quite variable, especially when combined with narcotics.[715]

Diazepam is a particularly useful oral premedicant in

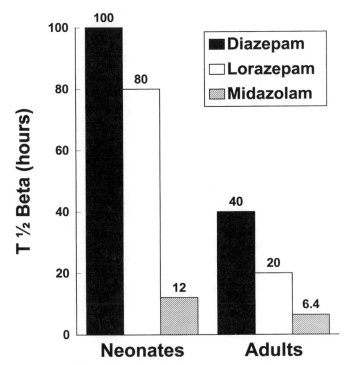

Figure 8–19. Beta elimination half-life of diazepam, lorazepam, and midazolam in neonates compared with adults. Note the excessively long half-lives of diazepam and lorazepam in the neonatal age group. Midazolam has the most favorable pharmacokinetics in the neonate and is the one benzodiazepine approved for use in this age group. (Data abstracted from Jacqz-Aigrain E, Daoud P, Burtin P, et al: Pharmacokinetics of midazolam during continuous infusion in critically ill neonates. Eur J Clin Pharmacol 1992;42:329–332; Abernethy DR, Greenblatt DJ: Effects of desmethydiazepam on diazepam kinetics: A study of effects of a metabolite on drug disposition. Clin Pharmacol Ther 1981;29:757–761; Morselli PL, Principi N, Togononi G, et al: Diazepam elimination in premature and full-term infants and children. J Perinat Med 1973;1:133–141; Greenblatt DJ, Divoll M, Abernethy DR, et al: Clinical pharmacokinetics of the newer benzodiazepines. Clin Pharm 1983;8:233–252; and Greenblatt DJ: Clinical pharmacokinetics of oxazepam and lorazepam. Clin Pharmacokin 1981;6:89–105.)

children (0.2–0.3 mg/kg); its main disadvantage is that it often causes pain when administered intravenously. Prior administration of intravenous lidocaine and slow administration through a rapidly running intravenous line may minimize this pain. Its use as a premedication in newborns or children less than 1 year of age is not indicated because of the prolonged half-life. Diazepam should not be administered intramuscularly because of the pain and irregular absorption.

Midazolam (Versed)

Midazolam is a water-soluble benzodiazepine that offers significant clinical advantages over diazepam. Solubility in water virtually eliminates pain on intravenous and intramuscular injection. A significantly shorter beta elimination half-life (1.7 ± 0.5 hours) compared with diazepam (18 hours in children) may be advantageous when midazolam is used as a premedication, especially for brief surgical or medical procedures. Midazolam is only one of a few medications approved for use in premedicating children and is the only benzodiazepine approved by the FDA for use in neonates. Clearance in adults (1.8–6.4 hours) is slightly slower than in children (1.4–4.0 hours).[716–720] However, clearance is lower in neonates and preterm infants when compared with toddlers and older children (6–12 hours) (see Fig. 8–19).[721, 722] The elimination half-life is still less in preterm infants younger than 32 weeks of gestational age.[573, 721, 722] The recommended infusion rate is 0.5 μg/kg/min for premature infants younger than 32 weeks of gestational age and 1.0 μg/kg/min for infants older than 32 weeks of gestational age. Any factor that impairs hepatic blood flow, such as cardiac surgery with bypass compared with cardiac surgery without bypass, may decrease beta elimination, although cirrhosis has been found to have minimal effect in adults.[723, 724] The elimination half-life may also be prolonged in hypovolemic states and in patients on vasopressors.[724, 725] Midazolam appears to offer the best pharmacokinetic profile for neonates because the active metabolite has a half-life similar to the parent compound but has minimal clinical activity.[573] *Bolus administration to preterm and term neonates has been associated with profound hypotension; the likelihood seems to be greater if the patient is receiving fentanyl.*[579] *Likewise, a neonate receiving a midazolam infusion is more likely to suffer profound hypotension with a bolus of fentanyl.* Rapid intravenous and nasal administration have also been associated with seizure-like activity, although it appears that this is myoclonic rather than true seizure activity.[726]

Midazolam has been administered as a continuous infusion both in the operating room as an adjunct to general anesthesia and in the intensive care unit.[727–729] Prolonged administration does lead to dependency and benzodiazepine withdrawal. Long-term infusions should be tapered over days and patients carefully observed for signs of withdrawal (vomiting, agitation, sweating, bowel distension, seizures, change in neurologic status).[583] Another concern regarding benzodiazepines is the potential to cause benzyl alcohol toxicity with the development of metabolic acidosis and gasping respirations from the preservative. The 24-hour amount of preservative in midazolam if administered according to recommended guidelines should not result in such toxicity.

Midazolam is the most commonly used benzodiazepine

in pediatric anesthesia[730] and has been administered orally, nasally, and rectally as well as intravenously and intramuscularly.[468, 640, 717, 724, 731-744] A commercially prepared oral formulation (2 mg/mL) became only the second medication approved by the FDA for premedication of pediatric patients.[737]

The desired clinical effects include antegrade amnesia (approximately 50%)[745, 746] as well as sedation and anxiolysis before anesthetic induction or a procedure.[468, 731, 732, 735-737, 740, 741] Some evidence suggests that its amnestic properties may be superior to those of diazepam.[747] The clinical end point with this medication may be somewhat different when compared with diazepam. Midazolam produces a general calming effect with minimal sedation and little effect on speech; conversely, diazepam frequently causes very obvious sedation and slurring of speech. It is important to appreciate the subtle difference between these medications to avoid relative overdose, particularly when using midazolam in combination with other potent central nervous system depressants.

When midazolam was first introduced, a number of deaths were attributed to respiratory depression; these deaths were probably a result of using high doses combined with simultaneous administration of other medications, particularly opioids. An important pharmacodynamic effect is that it takes nearly three times longer for midazolam to achieve a peak central nervous system effect (4.8 min) when compared with diazepam (1.5 min) (see Fig. 9–2).[748, 749] This is due to the greater fat solubility of diazepam and therefore a more rapid transit into the central nervous system.[750] It is important, therefore, to wait sufficient time between doses of midazolam (3–5 min) so as to achieve peak central nervous system effect prior to administration of additional drug or other sedating medication.[751] In general, the dose of midazolam is one third to one fifth that of diazepam, especially when combined with a potent narcotic (fentanyl). Whenever this medication is administered, either alone or in combination with other medications, it is vital that the patient be carefully observed for respiratory depression, because midazolam depresses the hypoxic ventilatory response and has been associated with respiratory arrest.[752, 753]

One further concern is the inhibition of the metabolism of midazolam by drugs that alter the cytochrome oxidase system. Examples of this include grapefruit juice, erythromycin, calcium channel blockers, and protease inhibitors.[379, 380, 754-758]

Midazolam has been used as an induction agent but is not as satisfactory as other agents.[717] One author (CJC) has administered as much as 1.0 mg/kg to a child without producing unconsciousness. Commonly used doses and routes of administration are presented in Table 8–8. The nasal route of drug administration has had some proponents.[731] However, the nasal mucosa has a direct connection with the central nervous system (see Fig. 9–1).[476] Since midazolam applied directly to neural tissue has been demonstrated to be neurotoxic,[482] there is the theoretic potential for central nervous system toxicity.[476] An additional fact is that 85% of children who receive nasal midazolam cry.[640, 733] It would seem prudent to avoid this route of administration, since the oral route appears to be just as effective and is less invasive.

Chloral Hydrate

Chloral hydrate is one of the more commonly used sedatives. This drug does not have analgesic properties. The usual dose

Table 8–8. Common Routes and Doses of Midazolam Administration for Infants and Children (Not Neonates)

Route	Dose (mg/kg)	Time of Onset (Minutes)	Time to Peak Effect (Minutes)
Intravenous	0.05–0.15	Immediate	3–5
Intramuscular	0.1–0.2	3–5	10–20
Oral	0.25–0.75	5–30	10–30
Nasal	0.1–0.2	3–5	10–15
Rectal	0.75–1.0	5–10	10–30

is 20 to 75 mg/kg PO or PR. Its primary use in pediatrics is for sedation before noninvasive procedures or as a premedication. Its principal advantage is that it can be administered orally or rectally with excellent absorption and relatively good sedation within 30 to 45 minutes. It also has minimal effects on respiration.[759] It is clear, however, that chloral hydrate can result in airway obstruction, particularly in children with enlarged tonsils.[760-762] Its bitter taste is a disadvantage.[742] Triclofos sodium is a more acceptable oral form and may be administered in a dose of 40 to 70 mg/kg.[763] This drug should not be administered on a chronic basis because of the theoretical concern for potential carcinogenicity with metabolites, concerns for producing severe gastritis possibly related to its metabolism to trichloracetic acid, and the possibility or accumulation of drug metabolites.[764, 765] In addition, its use in neonates is not recommended because of its interference with binding of bilirubin to albumin and the potential accumulation of toxic metabolites leading to metabolic acidosis, renal failure, and hypotonia.[766] The half-life of the active metabolite of chloral hydrate, trichloroethanol, has a half-life of 9.7 ± 1.7 hours in toddlers but 39.8 ± 14.3 hours in preterm infants (see Fig. 9–3).[767] These very long half-lives imply that residual drug effect will be present long after any procedure requiring sedation.[768, 769] It is for this reason that chloral hydrate is not generally recommended for premedication prior to surgery and that a prolonged period of observation is recommended following sedation for a procedure. If nitrous oxide is administered to children who have received chloral hydrate, a state of deep sedation or general anesthesia may occur.[770]

Antihistamines

Diphenhydramine Hydrochloride (Benadryl)

Antihistamines are often used in pediatric anesthesia, both for their H_1-receptor inhibition and for their sedative properties. Diphenhydramine hydrochloride is a commonly used antihistamine; it is rapidly absorbed, and its effects last for 3 to 6 hours. The usual dose is 1.25 mg/kg PO. It is often administered as a premedicant or as an in-hospital sedative. Caution is advised for patients with respiratory problems, because drying of secretions may cause difficulty with expectoration.

Cimetidine (Tagamet) and Ranitidine (Zantac)

Cimetidine and ranitidine are potent, highly hydrophilic, competitive inhibitors of H_2-mediated histamine reactions.

Their use in anesthesia is primarily to reduce gastric acidity before surgery. In children, they reduce the volume of gastric acid and raise the pH above 2.5 when a single dose (cimetidine, 7.5 mg/kg, or ranitidine, 1 mg/kg) is administered orally at least 1 hour before surgery.[771] Cimetidine appears to be ineffective if less than 1 hour or more than 4 hours have elapsed since the patient received the drug. Indications include a history of gastroesophageal reflux, hiatus hernia, previous esophageal surgery, or an anticipated difficult intubation that will require prolonged laryngoscopy, as well as perhaps high-risk patients (American Society of Anesthesiologists classes 3 and 4).

Treatment with H$_2$-blocking agents should include consideration of potential drug-drug interactions. Cimetidine partially inhibits CYP enzymes, which prolongs the half-lives of many drugs, including phenytoin, phenobarbital, theophylline, cyclosporine, carbamazepine, benzodiazepines that do not undergo glucuronidation, calcium channel blockers, propranolol, quinidine, sulfonylureas, mexiletine, warfarin, and tricyclic antidepressants such as imipramine.[772] Part of its effects on other drugs occurs through reduced hepatic blood flow. Although ranitidine also weakly reduces CYP activity, it does not increase the half-life of other medications significantly when administered at the usual therapeutic doses.[773–779] Similarly, famotidine, and nizatidine do not alter drug metabolism.[772, 777–779]

Metoclopramide (Reglan)

Metoclopramide has been used as an antiemetic and to induce pharmacologic gastric emptying.[780] The antiemetic properties result from direct effects on the chemoreceptor trigger zone. Gastric emptying is a result of the antagonism of the neurotransmitter dopamine, which stimulates gastric smooth-muscle activity.[781] A dose of 0.15 mg/kg at the end of surgery has proved efficacious in reducing emesis following strabismus surgery and tonsillectomy.[782]

Ondansetron (Zofran)

Ondansetron is one of a number of selective serotonergic antagonists, which is highly effective in reducing the incidence of nausea and vomiting in children.[783–785] Since the cost of this new family of drugs remains high, most pediatric anesthesiologists limit their routine use to children undergoing procedures known to have a high incidence of nausea and vomiting, such as strabismus repair, tonsillectomy, middle ear surgery, and to children with a known history of motion sickness or previous nausea and vomiting following surgery[786–795] Ondansetron is effective in preventing nausea and vomiting as well as reducing the severity of established nausea and vomiting. The usual recommended dose is 100 to 150 μg/kg every 6 hours. Other agents in this category, such as granisetron, would appear to be equally effective.[794, 796–799] Both ondansetron and granisetron may also be administered orally.[800]

Anticholinergics

Atropine and Scopolamine

Atropine (0.02 mg/kg) and scopolamine (0.01 mg/kg) have central nervous system effects, with the sedating effect of scopolamine being 5 to 15 times greater than that of atropine. Scopolamine is also a two to three times more potent antisialagogue. Atropine and scopolamine decrease the ability to sweat and thus may result in a slight rise in temperature. The normal response to cold stress is also altered, especially in neonates.[801] Atropine and scopolamine appear to have equipotent cardiovascular accelerator properties; however, infants seem to require slightly greater doses per kilogram than adults to achieve this response.[802] Anticholinergics are appropriate in specific situations: to diminish secretions preoperatively, to block laryngeal and vagal reflexes, to treat the bradycardia associated with succinylcholine, and to treat the bradycardia of anesthetic-induced myocardial depression, the muscarinic effects of neostigmine and the oculocardiac reflex. Atropine is painful on intramuscular injection and as a premedicant does not block laryngeal reflexes; it is much more effective for this purpose when given intravenously.

Some data suggest that children with Down syndrome are more susceptible to the cardiac effects of atropine.[803] Our clinical experience and that of others has not demonstrated this.[804, 805] One must be aware, however, that children with Down syndrome frequently have narrow-angle glaucoma, and atropine must be cautiously administered in this situation.[804, 805] Atropine may be administered orally or rectally and is rapidly absorbed when injected into the trachea.[806–809] Oral atropine may be of some value in blunting the hypotensive response to potent inhalation agents during induction of anesthesia in infants less than 3 months of age.[810]

In clinical practice, scopolamine is usually limited to those cases in which its sedative effect, combined with that of morphine, will be most advantageous, such as cardiac surgical patients. It is also very useful as an adjuvant to ketamine anesthesia because of its antisialagogue and central sedative effects. The central sedative effects of both atropine and scopolamine may be reversed with physostigmine. Many centers no longer routinely administer anticholinergic medications as part of the premedication because they are painful, the optimal effect may not coincide with induction of anesthesia, and the modern potent inhalation agents produce fewer secretions. The observation that intravenous atropine rapidly reduces lower esophageal sphincter pressure in infants may have significant implications for children at risk for pulmonary aspiration of gastric contents; further studies are needed to determine the clinical importance of this observation.[811]

Glycopyrrolate (Robinul)

Glycopyrrolate (0.005–0.01 mg/kg) is a synthetic quaternary ammonium compound with potent anticholinergic properties. It offers some advantage over atropine and scopolamine because it minimally penetrates the blood-brain barrier and thus causes few central effects. Several studies have demonstrated glycopyrrolate to be superior to atropine because its anticholinergic effects last for several hours.[812, 813] Minimal change in the heart rate occurs after intravenous administration, and thus the incidence of cardiac arrhythmias is lower.[814, 815] In some children, there appears to be the added advantage of a reduction in gastric volume and acidity.[816, 817]

REFERENCES

1. Besunder JB, Reed MD, Blumer JL: Principles of drug biodisposition in the neonate: A critical evaluation of the pharmacokinetic-pharmacodynamic interface. Part I. Clin Pharmacokinet 1988;14:189–216.

2. Besunder JB, Reed MD, Blumer JL: Principles of drug biodisposition in the neonate: A critical evaluation of the pharmacokinetic-pharmacodynamic interface. Part II. Clin Pharmacokinet 1988;14:261–286.

3. Levy G: Pharmacokinetics of fetal and neonatal exposure to drugs. Obstet Gynecol 1981;58 (Suppl):9S–16S.

4. Ward RM, Mirkin BL: Perinatal/neonatal pharmacology. In: Brody TM, Larner J, Minneman KP, eds: Human Pharmacology: Molecular-to-Clinical, 3rd ed. St Louis: Mosby-Year Book; 1998:873–883.

5. Ward RM: Pharmacologic principles and practicalities. In: Taeusch HW, Ballard RA, eds: Avery's Diseases of the Newborn, 7th ed. Philadelphia: WB Saunders; 1998:404–412.

6. Ward RM, Lugo RA: Drug therapy in the newborn. In: Avery GBN, Fletcher MA, MacDonald M, eds: Neonatology: Pathophysiology and Management of the Newborn, 5th ed. Philadelphia: JB Lippincott; 1999:1363-1406.

7. Somogyi A: Clinical pharmacokinetics and dosing schedules. In: Brody TM, Larner J, Minneman KP, eds: Human Pharmacology Molecular to Clinical, 3rd ed. St Louis: Mosby-Year Book; 1998:47–64.

8. Boreus LO: Principles of Pediatric Pharmacology. New York: Churchill Livingstone; 1982.

9. Brodersen R, Honore B: Drug binding properties of neonatal albumin. Acta Paediatr Scand 1989;78:342–346.

10. Ohning BL: Neonatal pharmacodynamics—basic principles. II: Drug action and elimination. Neonatal Netw 1995;14:15–19.

11. Rane A, Sjoqvist F: Drug metabolism in the human fetus and newborn infant. Pediatr Clin North Am 1972;19:37–49.

12. Wood M: Plasma drug binding: Implications for anesthesiologists. Anesth Analg 1986;65:786–804.

13. Krasner J, Giacoia GP, Yaffe SJ: Drug-protein binding in the newborn infant. Ann N Y Acad Sci 1973;226:101–114.

14. Friis-Hansen B: Body composition during growth: In vivo measurements and biochemical data correlated to differential anatomical growth. Pediatrics 1971;47:264–274.

15. Brodersen R: Bilirubin transport in the newborn infant, reviewed with relation to kernicterus. J Pediatr 1980;96:349–356.

16. Stern L: Drug interactions. II. Drugs, the newborn infant, and the binding of bilirubin to albumin. Pediatrics 1972;49:916–918.

17. Silverman WA, Andersen DH, Blanc WA, et al: A difference in mortality rate and incidence of kernicterus among premature infants allotted to two prophylactic antibacterial regimens. Pediatrics 1956;18:614–625.

18. Ehrnebo M, Agurell S, Jalling B, et al: Age differences in drug binding by plasma proteins: Studies in human foetuses, neonates, and adults. Eur J Clin Pharmacol 1971;3:189–193.

19. Robertson A, Sharp C, Strong WB, et al: Effect of Hypaque injection on bilirubin-albumin binding in newborn infants. J Pediatr 1986;108:138–141.

20. Kanto J, Erkkola R, Sellman R: Distribution and metabolism of diazepam in early and late human pregnancy: Postnatal metabolism of diazepam. Acta Pharmacol Toxicol 1974;35:S49.

21. Christensen JH, Andreasen F, Jansen JA:. Pharmacokinetics of thiopental in caesarean section. Acta Anaesthesiol Scand 1981;25:174–179.

22. Fink S, Karp W, Robertson A: Effect of penicillins on bilirubin-albumin binding. J Pediatr 1988;113:566–568.

23. Rane A, Lunde PK, Jalling B, et al: Plasma protein binding of diphenylhydantoin in normal and hyperbilirubinemic infants. J Pediatr 1971;78:877–882.

24. Hamar C, Levy G: Serum protein binding of drugs and bilirubin in newborn infants and their mothers. Clin Pharmacol Ther 1980;28:58–63.

25. Wilson AS, Stiller RL, Davis PJ, et al: Fentanyl and alfentanil plasma protein binding in preterm and term neonates. Anesth Analg 1997;84:315–318

26. Kaplan JM, McCracken GH Jr, Horton LJ, et al: Pharmacologic studies in neonates given large dosages of ampicillin. J Pediatr 1974;84:571–577.

27. McCracken GH Jr: Pharmacological basis for antimicrobial therapy in newborn infants. Am J Dis Child 1974;128:407–419.

28. Aranda JV, Sitar DS, Parsons WD, et al: Pharmacokinetic aspects of theophylline in premature newborns. N Engl J Med 1976;295:413–416.

29. Fisher DM, O'Keefe C, Stanski DR, et al: Pharmacokinetics and pharmacodynamics of d-tubocurarine in infants, children, and adults. Anesthesiology 1982;57:203–208.

30. Wettrell G, Andersson KE: Clinical pharmacokinetics of digoxin in infants. Clin Pharmacokinet 1977;2:17–31.

31. Perez CA, Reimer JM, Schreiber MD, et al: Effect of high-dose dopamine on urine output in newborn infants. Crit Care Med 1986;14:1045–1049.

32. Morselli PL, Franco-Morselli R, Bossi L: Clinical pharmacokinetics in newborns and infants: Age-related differences and therapeutic implications. Clin Pharmacokinet 1980;5:485–527.

33. Rane A, Wilson JT: Clinical pharmacokinetics in infants and children. Clin Pharmacokinet 1976;1:2–24.

34. Pinsky WW, Jacobsen JR, Gillette PC, et al: Dosage of digoxin in premature infants. J Pediatr 1979;94:639–642.

35. Udkow G: Pediatric clinical pharmacology: A practical review. Am J Dis Child 1978;132:1025–1032.

36. Jusko WJ: Pharmacokinetic principles in pediatric pharmacology. Pediatr Clin North Am 1972;19:81–100.

37. Koch-Weser J, Sellers EM: Binding of drugs to serum albumin (first of two parts). N Engl J Med 1976;294:311–316.

38. Svensson CK, Woodruff MN, Lalka D: Influence of protein binding and use of unbound (free) drug concentrations. In: Evans WE, Schentag JJ, Jusko WJ, eds: Applid Therapeutics: Principles of Therapeutic Drug Monitoring, 2nd ed. Spokane: Applied Therapeutics; 1986:187–219.

39. Evans EF, Proctor JD, Fratkin MJ, et al: Blood flow in muscle groups and drug absorption. Clin Pharmacol Ther 1975;17:44–47.

40. Mirkin BL: Perinatal pharmacology: placental transfer, fetal localization, and neonatal disposition of drugs. Anesthesiology 1975;43:156–170.

41. Krauer B, Draffan GH, Williams FM, et al: Elimination kinetics of amobarbital in mothers and their newborn infants. Clin Pharmacol Ther 1973;14:442–447.

42. Bovill JG, Sebel PS: Pharmacokinetics of high-dose fentanyl: A study in patients undergoing cardiac surgery. Br J Anaesth 1980;52:795–801.

43. Yaffe SJ, Catz CS: Pharmacology of the perinatal period. Clin Obstet Gynecol 1971;14:722–744.

44. Sawe J, Kager L, Svensson Eng JO, et al: Oral morphine in cancer patients: In vivo kinetics and in vitro hepatic glucuronidation. Br J Clin Pharmacol 1985;19:495–501.

45. Brunk SF, Delle M: Morphine metabolism in man. Clin Pharmacol Ther 1974;16:51–57.

46. McRorie TI, Lynn AM, Nespeca MK: The maturation of morphine clearance and metabolism. Am J Dis Child 1992;146:972–976.

47. Nies AS, Shand DG: Clinical pharmacology of propranolol. Circulation 1975;52:6–15.

48. Walle T, Webb JG, Bagwell EE, et al: Stereoselective delivery and actions of beta receptor antagonists. Biochem Pharmacol 1988;37:115–124.

49. Heizmann P, Eckert M, Ziegler WH: Pharmacokinetics and bioavailability of midazolam in man. Br J Clin Pharmacol 1983;16:43S–49S.

50. Reves JG, Fragen RJ, Vinik HR, et al: Midazolam: Pharmacology and uses. Anesthesiology 1985;62:310–324.

51. Garzone PD, Kroboth PD: Pharmacokinetics of the newer benzodiazepines. Clin Pharmacokinet 1989;16:337–364.

52. Bourgeois BF, Dodson WE: Phenytoin elimination in newborns. Neurology 1983;33:173–178.

53. Mirkin BL, Ward RM, Green TP: Disposition of drugs in preterm infants with patent ductus arteriosus: Theoretical and empirical considerations. Pediatr Cardiol 1983;4:85–92.

54. Shimada T, Yamazaki H, Mimura M, et al: Characterization of microsomal cytochrome P450 enzymes involved in the oxidation of xenobiotic chemicals in human fetal liver and adult lungs. Drug Metab Dispos 1996;24:515–522.

55. Jacqz-Aigrain E, Cresteil T: Cytochrome P450-dependent metabolism of dextromethorphan: Fetal and adult studies. Dev Pharmacol Ther 1992;18:161–168.

56. Treluyer JM, Jacqz-Aigrain E, Alvarez F, et al: Expression of CYP2D6 in developing human liver. Eur J Biochem 1991;202:583–588.

57. Vauzelle-Kervroedan F, Rey E, Pariente-Khayat A, et al: Noninvasive in vivo study of the maturation of CYP IIIA in neonates and infants. Eur J Clin Pharmacol 1996;51:69–72.

58. Yaffe SJ, Levy G, Matsuzawa T, et al: Enhancement of glucuronide-conjugating capacity in a hyperbilirubinemic infant due to apparent enzyme induction by phenobarbital. N Engl J Med 1966;275:1461–1466.

59. Kanto J, Erkkola R, Sellman R: Accumulation of diazepam and

N-demethyldiazepam in the fetal blood during the labour. Ann Clin Res 1973;5:375–379.

60. Pitlick W, Painter M, Pippenger C: Phenobarbital pharmacokinetics in neonates. Clin Pharmacol Ther 1978;23:346–350.

61. Benet LZ, Kroetz DL, Sheiner LB: Pharmacokinetics: The dynamics of drug absorption, distribution, and elimination. In: Hardman JG, Limbird LE, Molinoff PB, et al, eds: Goodman & Gilman's the Pharmacological Basis of Therapeutics, 9th ed. New York: McGraw-Hill; 1996:3–27.

62. Hollenberg PF, Brody TM: Absorption, distribution, metabolism, and elimination. In: Brody TM, Larner J, Minneman KP, eds. Human Pharmacology Molecular to Clinical, 3rd ed. St Louis: Mosby-Year Book; 1998:35–46.

63. Pelkonen O, Kaltiala EH, Larmi TK, et al: Comparison of activities of drug-metabolizing enzymes in human fetal and adult livers. Clin Pharmacol Ther 1973;14:840–846.

64. Bhat R, Chari G, Gulati A, et al: Pharmacokinetics of a single dose of morphine in preterm infants during the first week of life. J Pediatr 1990;117:477–481.

65. Leeder JS, Kearns GL: Pharmacogenetics in pediatrics: Implications for practice. Pediatr Clin North Am 1997;44:55–77.

66. Aranda JV, MacLeod SM, Renton KW, et al: Hepatic microsomal drug oxidation and electron transport in newborn infants. J Pediatr 1974;85:534–542.

67. Aldridge A, Aranda JV, Neims AH: Caffeine metabolism in the newborn. Clin Pharmacol Ther 1979;25:447–453.

68. Morselli PL, Principi N, Tognoni G, et al: Diazepam elimination in premature and full-term infants and children. J Perinat Med 1973;1:133–141.

69. Loughnan PM, Greenwald A, Purton WW, et al: Pharmacokinetic observations of phenytoin disposition in the newborn and young infant. Arch Dis Child 1977;52:302–309.

70. Kalow W, Tang BK: The use of caffeine for enzyme assays: A critical appraisal. Clin Pharmacol Ther 1993;53:503–514.

71. Cazeneuve C, Pons G, Rey E, et al: Biotransformation of caffeine in human liver microsomes from foetuses, neonates, infants and adults. Br J Clin Pharmacol 1994;37:405–412.

72. Zhang ZY, Kaminsky LS: Characterization of human cytochromes P450 involved in theophylline 8-hydroxylation. Biochem Pharmacol 1995;50:205–211.

73. Ha HR, Chen J, Freiburghaus AU, et al: Metabolism of theophylline by cDNA-expressed human cytochromes P-450. Br J Clin Pharmacol 1995;39:321–326.

74. Yang HY, Lee QP, Rettie AE, et al: Functional cytochrome P4503A isoforms in human embryonic tissues: Expression during organogenesis. Mol Pharmacol 1994;46:922–928.

75. Aranda JV, Cook CE, Gorman W, et al: Pharmacokinetic profile of caffeine in the premature newborn infant with apnea. J Pediatr 1979;94:663–668.

76. Carrier O, Pons G, Rey E, et al: Maturation of caffeine metabolic pathways in infancy. Clin Pharmacol Ther 1988;44:145–151.

77. Pons G, Carrier O, Richard MO, et al: Developmental changes of caffeine elimination in infancy. Dev Pharmacol Ther 1988;11:258–264.

78. Kraus DM, Fischer JH, Reitz SJ, et al: Alterations in theophylline metabolism during the first year of life. Clin Pharmacol Ther 1993;54:351–359.

79. Ladona MG, Lindstrom B, Thyr C, et al: Differential foetal development of the O- and N-demethylation of codeine and dextromethorphan in man. Br J Clin Pharmacol 1991;32:295–302.

80. Radde IC, Kalow W: Drug biotransformation and its development. In: Radde I, MacLeod S, eds. Pediatric Pharmacology & Therapeutics, 2nd ed. St Louis: Mosby-Year Book; 1993:57–86.

81. Coughtrie MW, Burchell B, Leakey JE, et al: The inadequacy of perinatal glucuronidation: Immunoblot analysis of the developmental expression of individual UDP-glucuronosyltransferase isoenzymes in rat and human liver microsomes. Mol Pharmacol 1988;34:729–735.

82. Weiss CF, Glazko AJ, Weston JK: Chloramphenicol in the newborn infant: A physiologic explanation of its toxicity when given in excessive doses. N Engl J Med 1960;262:787–794.

83. Sutherland JM: Fatal cardiovascular collapse of infants receiving large amounts of chloramphenicol. Am J Dis Child 1959;97:761–767.

84. Burns LE, Hodgeman JE, Cass AB: Fatal and circulatory collapse in premature infants receiving chloramphenicol. N Engl J Med 1959;261:1318–1321.

85. Mulhall A, Berry DJ, de Louvois J: Chloramphenicol in paediatrics: Current prescribing practice and the need to monitor. Eur J Pediatr 1988;147:574–578.

86. Choonara IA, McKay P, Hain R, et al: Morphine metabolism in children. Br J Clin Pharmacol 1989;28:599–604.

87. Pokela ML, Olkkola KT, Seppala T, et al: Age-related morphine kinetics in infants. Dev Pharmacol Ther 1993;20:26–34.

88. Hartley R, Green M, Quinn MW, et al: Development of morphine glucuronidation in premature neonates. Biol Neonate 1994;66:1–9.

89. Mikkelsen S, Feilberg VL, Christensen CB, et al: Morphine pharmacokinetics in premature and mature newborn infants. Acta Paediatr 1994;83:1025–1028.

90. Lynn AM, Slattery JT: Morphine pharmacokinetics in early infancy. Anesthesiology 1987;66:136–139.

91. Olkkola KT, Maunuksela EL, Korpela R, et al: Kinetics and dynamics of postoperative intravenous morphine in children. Clin Pharmacol Ther 1988;44:128–136.

92. Autret E, Dutertre JP, Breteau M, et al: Pharmacokinetics of paracetamol in the neonate and infant after administration of propacetamol chloral hydrate. Dev Pharmacol Ther 1993;20:129–134.

93. Miller RP, Roberts RJ, Fischer LJ: Acetaminophen elimination kinetics in neonates, children, and adults. Clin Pharmacol Ther 1976;19:284–294.

94. Levy G, Khanna NN, Soda DM, et al: Pharmacokinetics of acetaminophen in the human neonate: Formation of acetaminophen glucuronide and sulfate in relation to plasma bilirubin concentration and D-glucaric acid excretion. Pediatrics 1975;55:818–825.

95. Alam SN, Roberts RJ, Fischer LJ: Age-related differences in salicylamide and acetaminophen conjugation in man. J Pediatr 1977;90:130–135.

96. West JR, Smith HW, Chasis H: Glomerular filtration rate, effective renal blood flow, and maximal tubular excretory capacity in infancy. J Pediatr 1948;32:10–18.

97. Guignard JP, Torrado A, Feldman H, et al: Assessment of glomerular filtration rate in children. Helv Paediatr Acta 1980;35:437–447.

98. Fawer CL, Torrado A, Guignard JP: Maturation of renal function in full-term and premature neonates. Helv Paediatr Acta 1979;34:11–21.

99. Guignard JP, Torrado A, Da Cunha O, et al: Glomerular filtration rate in the first three weeks of life. J Pediatr 1975;87:268–272.

100. Leake RD, Trygstad CW, Oh W: Inulin clearance in the newborn infant: Relationship to gestational and postnatal age. Pediatr Res 1976;10:759–762.

101. Leake RD, Trygstad CW: Glomerular filtration rate during the period of adaptation to extrauterine life. Pediatr Res 1977;11:959–962.

102. Eichenwald HF, McCracken GH Jr: Antimicrobial therapy in infants and children. Part I. Review of antimicrobial agents. J Pediatr 1978;93:337–356.

103. Izquierdo M, Lanao JM, Cervero L, et al: Population pharmacokinetics of gentamicin in premature infants. Ther Drug Monit 1992;14:177–183.

104. Miranda JC, Schimmel MM, James LS, et al: Gentamicin kinetics in the neonate. Pediatr Pharmacol (New York) 1985;5:57–61.

105. Greenblatt DJ, Koch-Weser J: Clinical pharmacokinetics (first of two parts). N Engl J Med 1975;293:702–705.

106. Greenblatt DJ, Koch-Weser J: Clinical pharmacokinetics (second of two parts). N Engl J Med 1975;293:964–970.

107. Roberts RJ: Pharmacokinetics: Basic principles and clinical applications. In: Drug Therapy in Infants: Pharmacologic Principles and Clinical Experience. Philadelphia: WB Saunders; 1984:13–24.

108. Galinsky RE: Basic pharmacokinetics. In: Gennaro AR, Chase GD, Mardersonian AD, et al, eds: Remington: The Science and Practice of Pharmacy, 19th ed. Easton: Mack Publishing Co; 1995:724–760.

109. Gibaldi M, Perrier D: Pharmacokinetics, 2nd ed. New York: Marcel Dekker; 1982.

110. Jusko WJ: Guidelines for collection and analysis of pharmacokinetic data. In: Evans WE, Schentag JJ, Jusko WJ, eds: Applied Therapeutics. Principles of Therapeutic Drug Monitoring, 2nd ed. Spokane: Applied Therapeutics; 1986:9–54.

111. Notari RE: Principles of Pharmacokinetics: Biopharmaceutics and Clinical Pharmacokinetics, 3rd ed. 1980:45–106.

112. Roberts RJ: Cardiovascular drugs. In: Drug Therapy in Infants. Pharmacologic Principles and Clinical Experience. Philadelphia: WB Saunders; 1984:138–225.

113. Goldenthal EI: A compilation of LD$_{50}$ values in newborn and adult animals. Toxicol Appl Pharmacol 1971;18:185–207.

114. Done AK: Developmental pharmacology. Clin Pharmacol Ther 1964;5:432–479.

115. Kupferberg HJ, Way HJ: Pharmacologic basis for the increased sensitivity of the newborn to morphine. J Pharmacol Exp Ther 1963;141:105–109.

116. Domek NS, Barlow CF, Roth LJ: An ontogenetic study of phenobarbital-C14 in cat brain. J Pharmacol Exp Ther 1960;130:285–293.

117. Ebert AG, Yim GK: Barbital sensitivity in the young rat. Toxicol Appl Pharmacol 1961;3:182–187.

118. Sanner JH, Woods LA: Comparative distribution of tritium labeled dihydromorphine between maternal and fetal rats. J Pharmacol Exp Ther 1965;148:176–184.

119. White PF, Watcha MF: The practice of anesthesiology and the package insert: Decision-making regarding drug use in anesthesiology. Anesth Analg 1993;76:928–930.

120. Sensorcaine (bupivacaine HCL injection). Package insert. Westborough, MA: Astra USA, Inc.; 1995.

121. Sublimaze (fentanyl citrate) injection. Package insert. Titusville, NJ: Janssen Pharmaceutica; 1992.

122. Department of Health and Human Services, Food and Drug Administration: Federal Register, 64240–64250. 21 CFR Part 201. 1994.

123. Coté CJ, Kauffman RE, Troendle GJ, et al: Is the "therapeutic orphan" about to be adopted? Pediatrics 1996;98:118–123.

124. Coté CJ: Unapproved uses of approved drugs. Paediatr Anaesth 1997;7:91–92.

125. Kauffman RE: Status of drug approval processes and regulation of medications for children. Curr Opin Pediatr 1995;7:195–198.

126. 21 Code of Federal Regulations 312.21 (c). 1938.

127. Food and Drug Administration Modernization Act. Pub. L. 105–115, Section 111 of (21 U.S.C. 355A). 1997.

128. Food and Drug Administration: Regulations requiring manufacturers to assess the safety and effectiveness of new drugs and biological products in pediatric patients. 21 CFR Parts 201, 312, 314, and 601 [Docket No. 97N–0165]. 1998.

129. Committee on Drugs American Academy of Pediatrics: Unapproved uses of approved drugs: The physician, the package insert, and the FDA. Pediatrics 1996;98:143–145.

130. Nicodemus HF, Nassiri-Rahimi C, Bachman L, et al: Median effective doses (ED$_{50}$) of halothane in adults and children. Anesthesiology 1969;31:344–348.

131. Gregory GA, Eger EI, II, Munson ES, et al: The relationship between age and halothane requirements in man. Anesthesiology 1969; 30:488–491.

132. Gregory GA, Wade JG, Beihl DR, et al: Fetal anesthetic requirement (MAC) for halothane. Anesth Analg 1983;62:9–14.

133. Lerman J, Robinson S, Willis MM, et al: Anesthetic requirements for halothane in young children 0–1 month and 1–6 months of age. Anesthesiology 1983;59:421–424.

134. LeDez KM, Lerman J: The minimum alveolar concentration (MAC) of isoflurane in preterm neonates. Anesthesiology 1987;67:301–307.

135. Cook DR, Brandom BW, Shiu G, et al: The inspired median effective dose, brain concentration at anesthesia, and cardiovascular index for halothane in young rats. Anesth Analg 1981;60:182–185.

136. Barash PG, Glanz S, Katz JD, et al: Ventricular function in children during halothane anesthesia: An echocardiographic evaluation. Anesthesiology 1978;49:79–85.

137. Blanck TJ, Runge S, Stevenson RL: Halothane decreases calcium channel antagonist binding to cardiac membranes. Anesth Analg 1988;67:1032–1035.

138. Wheeler DM, Rice RT, Hansford RG, et al: The effect of halothane on the free intracellular calcium concentration of isolated rat heart cells. Anesthesiology 1988;69:578–583.

139. Housmans PR, Murat I: Comparative effects of halothane, enflurane, and isoflurane at equipotent anesthetic concentrations on isolated ventricular myocardium of the ferret. I. Contractility. Anesthesiology 1988;69:451–463.

140. Yakaitis RW, Blitt CD, Angiulo JP: End-tidal enflurane concentration for endotracheal intubation. Anesthesiology 1979;50:59–61.

141. Murray DJ, Mehta MP, Forbes RB, et al: Additive contribution of nitrous oxide to halothane MAC in infants and children. Anesth Analg 1990;71:120–124.

142. Salanitre E, Rackow H: The pulmonary exchange of nitrous oxide and halothane in infants and children. Anesthesiology 1969;30:388–394.

143. Eger EI 2nd, Bahlman SH, Munson ES: The effect of age on the rate of increase of alveolar anesthetic concentration. Anesthesiology 1971;35:365–372.

144. Brandom BW, Brandom RB, Cook DR: Uptake and distribution of halothane in infants: In vivo measurements and computer simulations. Anesth Analg 1983;62:404–410.

145. Culling RD: Frequency of anesthetic cardiac arrest in infants: Effect of pediatric anesthesiologists. J Clin Anesth 1992;4:343–346.

146. Keenan RL, Shapiro JH, Dawson K: Frequency of anesthetic cardiac arrests in infants: Effect of pediatric anesthesiologists. J Clin Anesth 1991;3:433–437.

147. Morray JP, Geiduschek JM, Caplan RA, et al: A comparison of pediatric and adult anesthesia closed malpractice claims. Anesthesiology 1993;78:461–467.

148. Tiret L, Nivoche Y, Hatton F, et al: Complications related to anaesthesia in infants and children: A prospective survey of 40240 anaesthetics. Br J Anaesth 1988;61:263–269.

149. Keenan RL, Boyan CP: Cardiac arrest due to anesthesia: A study of incidence and causes. JAMA 1985;253:2373–2377.

150. Tanner GE, Angers DG, Barash PG, et al: Effect of left-to-right, mixed left-to-right, and right-to-left shunts on inhalational anesthetic induction in children: A computer model. Anesth Analg 1985;64:101–107.

151. Tusiewicz K, Bryan AC, Froese AB: Contributions of changing rib cage-diaphragm interactions to the ventilatory depression of halothane anesthesia. Anesthesiology 1977;47:327–337.

152. Murat I, Delleur MM, MacGee K, et al: Changes in ventilatory patterns during halothane anaesthesia in children. Br J Anaesth 1985;57:569–572.

153. Lindahl SG, Charlton AJ, Hatch DJ: Ventilatory responses to rebreathing and carbon dioxide inhalation during anaesthesia in children. Br J Anaesth 1985;57:1188–1196.

154. Murat I, Chaussain M, Saint Maurice C, et al: Ventilatory responses to carbon dioxide in children during nitrous oxide-halothane anaesthesia. Br J Anaesth 1985;57:1197–1203.

155. Klide AM, Aviado DM: Mechanism for the reduction in pulmonary resistance induced by halothane. J Pharmacol Exp Ther 1967;158: 28–35.

156. Hirshman CA, Edelstein G, Peetz S, et al: Mechanism of action of inhalational anesthesia on airways. Anesthesiology 1982;56:107–111.

157. Shah MV, Hirshman CA: Mode of action of halothane on histamine-induced airway constriction in dogs with reactive airways. Anesthesiology 1986;65:170–174.

158. Rolf N, Coté CJ: Persistent cardiac arrhythmias in pediatric patients: Effects of age, expired carbon dioxide values, depth of anesthesia, and airway management. Anesth Analg 1991;73:720–724.

159. Robertson BJ, Clement JL, Knill RL: Enhancement of the arrhythmogenic effect of hypercarbia by surgical stimulation during halothane anaesthesia in man. Can Anaesth Soc J 1981;28:342–349.

160. Johnston RR, Eger EI, II, Wilson C: A comparative interaction of epinephrine with enflurane, isoflurane, and halothane in man. Anesth Analg 1976;55:709–712.

161. Katz RL, Bigger JT Jr: Cardiac arrhythmias during anesthesia and operation. Anesthesiology 1970;33:193–213.

162. Melgrave AP: The use of epinephrine in the presence of halothane in children. Can Anaesth Soc J 1970;17:256–260.

163. Karl HW, Swedlow DB, Lee KW, et al: Epinephrine-halothane interactions in children. Anesthesiology 1983;58:142–145.

164. Ueda W, Hirakawa M, Mae O: Appraisal of epinephrine administration to patients under halothane anesthesia for closure of cleft palate. Anesthesiology 1983;58:574–576.

165. Nakao S, Hirata H, Kagawa Y: Effects of volatile anesthetics on cardiac calcium channels. Acta Anaesthesiol Scand 1989;33:326–330.

166. Larach DR, Schuler HG, Derr JA, et al: Halothane selectively attenuates alpha 2-adrenoceptor mediated vasoconstriction, in vivo and in vitro. Anesthesiology 1987;66:781–791.

167. Friesen RH, Henry DB: Cardiovascular changes in preterm neonates receiving isoflurane, halothane, fentanyl, and ketamine. Anesthesiology 1986;64:238–242.

168. Murray D, Vandewalker G, Matherne GP, et al: Pulsed Doppler and two-dimensional echocardiography: comparison of halothane and isoflurane on cardiac function in infants and small children. Anesthesiology 1987;67:211–217.

169. Wolf WJ, Neal MB, Peterson MD: The hemodynamic and cardiovascular effects of isoflurane and halothane anesthesia in children. Anesthesiology 1986;64:328–333.

170. Lerman J, Sikich N, Kleinman S, et al: The pharmacology of sevoflurane in infants and children. Anesthesiology 1994;80:814–824.

171. Smith AL, Wollman H: Cerebral blood flow and metabolism: Effects of anesthetic drugs and techniques. Anesthesiology 1972;36:378–400.

172. Rubiano R, Chang JL, Carroll J, et al: Acute rhabdomyolysis following halothane anesthesia without succinylcholine. Anesthesiology 1987;67:856–857.

173. Smith RM: Pediatric anesthesia in perspective. Sixteenth annual Baxter-Travenol Lecture. Anesth Analg 1978;57:634–646.

174. Warner LO, Beach TP, Garvin JP, et al: Halothane and children: The first quarter century. Anesth Analg 1984;63:838–840.

175. Munro HM, Snider SJ, Magee JC: Halothane-associated hepatitis in a 6-year-old boy: Evidence for native liver regeneration following failed treatment with auxiliary liver transplantation. Anesthesiology 1998;89:524–527.

176. Wark HJ: Postoperative jaundice in children: The influence of halothane. Anaesthesia 1983;38:237–242.

177. Wark H, O'Halloran M, Overton J: Prospective study of liver function in children following multiple halothane anesthetics at short intervals. Br J Anaesth 1986;58:1224–1228.

178. Stock JG, Strunin L: Unexplained hepatitis following halothane. Anesthesiology 1985;63:424–439.

179. Carney FM, Van Dyke RA: Halothane hepatitis: A critical review. Anesth Analg 1972;51:135–160.

180. Lewis RB, Blair M: Halothane hepatitis in a young child. Br J Anaesth 1982;54:349–354.

181. Vergani D, Mieli-Vergani G, Alberti A, et al: Antibodies to the surface of halothane-altered rabbit hepatocytes in patients with severe halothane-associated hepatitis. N Engl J Med 1980;303:66–71.

182. Campbell RL, Small EW, Lesesne HR, et al: Fatal hepatic necrosis after halothane anesthesia in a boy with juvenile rheumatoid arthritis: a case report. Anesth Analg 1977;56:589–593.

183. Whitburn RH, Sumner E: Halothane hepatitis in an 11-month-old child. Anaesthesia 1986;41:611–613.

184. Kenna JG, Neuberger J, Mieli-Vergani G, et al: Halothane hepatitis in children. Br Med J (Clin Res Ed) 1987;294:1209–1211.

185. Martin JL, Kenna JG, Pohl LR: Antibody assays for the detection of patients sensitized to halothane. Anesth Analg 1990;70:154–159.

186. Njoku D, Laster MJ, Gong DH, et al: Biotransformation of halothane, enflurane, isoflurane, and desflurane to trifluoroacetylated liver proteins: Association between protein acylation and hepatic injury. Anesth Analg 1997;84:173–178.

187. Bourdi M, Chen W, Peter RM, et al: Human cytochrome P450 2E1 is a major autoantigen associated with halothane hepatitis. Chem Res Toxicol 1996;9:1159–1166.

188. Kharasch ED, Hankins D, Mautz D, et al: Identification of the enzyme responsible for oxidative halothane metabolism: Implications for prevention of halothane hepatitis. Lancet 1996;347:1367–1371.

189. Kitteringham NR, Kenna JG, Park BK: Detection of autoantibodies directed against human hepatic endoplasmic reticulum in sera from patients with halothane-associated hepatitis. Br J Clin Pharmacol 1995;40:379–386.

190. Knight TL, Scatchard KM, Van Pelt FN, et al: Sera from patients with halothane hepatitis contain antibodies to halothane-induced liver antigens which are not detectable by immunoblotting. J Pharmacol Exp Ther 1994;270:1325–1333.

191. Gut J, Christen U, Huwyler J: Mechanisms of halothane toxicity: novel insights. Pharmacol Ther 1993;58:133–155.

192. Kenna JG, Neuberger J, Williams R: Identification by immunoblotting of three halothane-induced liver microsomal polypeptide antigens recognized by antibodies in sera from patients with halothane-associated hepatitis. J Pharmacol Exp Ther 1987;242:733–740.

193. Kenna JG, Neuberger J, Williams R: Specific antibodies to halothane-induced liver antigens in halothane-associated hepatitis. Br J Anaesth 1987;59:1286–1290.

194. Hastings KL, Thomas C, Hubbard AK, et al: Screening for antibodies associated with halothane hepatitis. Br J Anaesth 1991;67:722–728.

195. Pohl LR, Kenna JG, Satoh H, et al: Neoantigens associated with halothane hepatitis. Drug Metab Rev 1989;20:203–217.

196. St. Haxholdt O, Loft S, Clemmensen A, et al: Increased hepatic microsomal activity after halothane anaesthesia in children. Anaesthesia 1986;41:579–581.

197. Wark H, Earl J, Chau DD, et al: Halothane metabolism in children. Br J Anaesth 1990;64:474–481.

198. Walton B: Halothane hepatitis in children. Anaesthesia 1986;41:575–578.

199. Rivera-Penera T, Gugig R, Davis J, et al: Outcome of acetaminophen overdose in pediatric patients and factors contributing to hepatotoxicity. J Pediatr 1997;130:300–304.

200. Pohl LR, Gillette JR: A perspective on halothane-induced hepatotoxicity. Anesth Analg 1982;61:809–811.

201. Adams AP, Campbell D, Clarke RS, et al: Halothane and the liver. Br Med J (Clin Res Ed) 1986;293:1023.

202. Neuberger J, Williams R: Halothane anaesthesia and liver damage. Br Med J (Clin Res Ed) 1984;289:1136–1139.

203. Ray DC, Drummond GB: Halothane hepatitis. Br J Anaesth 1991;67:84–99.

204. Neuberger JM: Halothane and hepatitis: Incidence, predisposing factors and exposure guidelines. Drug Saf 1990;5:28–38.

205. Wade JG, Stevens WC: Isoflurane: An anesthetic for the eighties? Anesth Analg 1981;60:666–682.

206. Frazer MJ, Lynch C 3d: Halothane and isoflurane effects on Ca^{2+} fluxes of isolated myocardial sarcoplasmic reticulum. Anesthesiology 1992;77:316–323.

207. Lynch C 3d: Effects of halothane and isoflurane on isolated human ventricular myocardium. Anesthesiology 1988;68:429–432.

208. Miao N, Frazer MJ, Lynch C 3d: Volatile anesthetics depress Ca^{2+} transients and glutamate release in isolated cerebral synaptosomes. Anesthesiology 1995;83:593–603.

209. Glenski JA, Friesen RH, Berglund NL, et al: Comparison of the hemodynamic and echocardiographic effects of sufentanil, fentanyl, isoflurane, and halothane for pediatric cardiovascular surgery. J Cardiothor Anaesth 1988;2:147–155.

210. Gallagher TM, Shields MD, Black GW: Isoflurane does not reduce aortic peak flow velocity in children. Br J Anaesth 1986;58:1116–1121.

211. Friesen RH, Lichtor JL: Cardiovascular effects of inhalation induction with isoflurane in infants. Anesth Analg 1983;62:411–414.

212. Phillips AJ, Brimacombe JR, Simpson DL: Anaesthetic induction with isoflurane or halothane: Oxygen saturation during induction with isoflurane or halothane in unpremedicated children. Anaesthesia 1988;43:927–929.

213. Kingston HG: Halothane and isoflurane anesthesia in pediatric outpatients. Anesth Analg 1986;65:181–184.

214. Cattermole RW, Verghese C, Blair IJ, et al: Isoflurane and halothane for outpatient dental anaesthesia in children. Br J Anaesth 1986;58:385–389.

215. Fisher DM, Robinson S, Brett CM, et al: Comparison of enflurane, halothane, and isoflurane for diagnostic and therapeutic procedures in children with malignancies. Anesthesiology 1985;63:647–650.

216. McAteer PM, Carter JA, Cooper GM, et al: Comparison of isoflurane and halothane in outpatient paediatric dental anaesthesia. Br J Anaesth 1986;58:390–393.

217. Joseph MM, Shah K, Viljoen JF: Malignant hyperthermia associated with isoflurane anesthesia. Anesth Analg 1982;61:711–712.

218. Carrigan TW, Straughen WJ: A report of hepatic necrosis and death following isoflurane anesthesia. Anesthesiology 1987;67:581–583.

219. Johannesson G, Veel T, Rogstadius J: Malignant hyperthermia during isoflurane anaesthesia: A case report. Acta Anaesthesiol Scand 1987;31:231–232.

220. Newberg LA, Michenfelder JD: Cerebral protection by isoflurane during hypoxemia or ischemia. Anesthesiology 1983;59:29–35.

221. Friesen RH, Thieme RE, Honda AT, et al: Changes in anterior fontanel pressure in preterm neonates receiving isoflurane, halothane, fentanyl, or ketamine. Anesth Analg 1987;66:431–434.

222. Scheller MS, Todd MM, Drummond JC, et al: The intracranial pressure effects of isoflurane and halothane administered following cryogenic brain injury in rabbits. Anesthesiology 1987;67:507–512.

223. Tanaka S, Tsuchida H, Nakabayashi K, et al: The effects of sevoflurane, isoflurane, halothane, and enflurane on hemodynamic responses during an inhaled induction of anesthesia via a mask in humans. Anesth Analg 1996;82:821–826.

224. Weiskopf RB, Moore MA, Eger EI 2d, et al: Rapid increase in desflurane concentration is associated with greater transient cardiovascular stimulation than with rapid increase in isoflurane concentration in humans. Anesthesiology 1994;80:1035–1045.

225. Baum J, Sachs G, v.d.Driesch C, et al: Carbon monoxide generation in carbon dioxide absorbents. Anesth Analg 1995;81:144–146.

226. Fang ZX, Eger EI 2d, Laster MJ, et al: Carbon monoxide production from degradation of desflurane, enflurane, isoflurane, halothane, and sevoflurane by soda lime and Baralyme. Anesth Analg 1995;80:1187–1193.

227. Woehlck HJ, Dunning M 3d, Gandhi S, et al: Indirect detection of intraoperative carbon monoxide exposure by mass spectrometry during isoflurane anesthesia. Anesthesiology 1995;83:213–217.

228. Baxter PJ, Kharasch ED: Rehydration of desiccated Baralyme prevents carbon monoxide formation from desflurane in an anesthesia machine. Anesthesiology 1997;86:1061–1065.

229. Murray JM, Renfrew CW, Bedi A, et al: Amsorb: A new carbon dioxide absorbent for use in anesthetic breathing systems. Anesthesiology 1999;91:1342–1348.

230. Piat V, Dubois MC, Johanet S, et al: Induction and recovery characteristics and hemodynamic responses to sevoflurane and halothane in children. Anesth Analg 1994;79:840–844.

231. Sarner JB, Levine M, Davis PJ, et al: Clinical characteristics of sevoflurane in children: A comparison with halothane. Anesthesiology 1995;82:38–46.

232. Epstein RH, Mendel HG, Guarnieri KM, et al: Sevoflurane versus halothane for general anesthesia in pediatric patients: A comparative study of vital signs, induction, and emergence. J Clin Anesth 1995;7:237–244.

233. Ariffin SA, Whyte JA, Malins AF, et al: Comparison of induction and recovery between sevoflurane and halothane supplementation of anaesthesia in children undergoing outpatient dental extractions. Br J Anaesth 1997;78:157–159.

234. Lerman J, Davis PJ, Welborn LG, et al: Induction, recovery, and safety characteristics of sevoflurane in children undergoing ambulatory surgery: A comparison with halothane. Anesthesiology 1996; 84:1332–1340.

235. Yamakage M, Tamiya K, Horikawa D, et al: Effects of halothane and sevoflurane on the paediatric respiratory pattern. Paediatr Anaesth 1994;4:53–56.

236. Brown K, Aun C, Stocks J, et al: A comparison of the respiratory effects of sevoflurane and halothane in infants and young children. Anesthesiology 1998;89:86–92.

237. Kern C, Erb T, Frei FJ: Haemodynamic responses to sevoflurane compared with halothane during inhalational induction in children. Pediatr Anaesth 1997;7:439–444.

238. Greenspun JC, Hannallah RS, Welborn LG, et al: Comparison of sevoflurane and halothane anesthesia in children undergoing outpatient ear, nose, and throat surgery. J Clin Anesth 1995;7:398–402.

239. Holzman RS, van der Velde ME, Kaus SJ, et al: Sevoflurane depresses myocardial contractility less than halothane during induction of anesthesia in children. Anesthesiology 1996;85:1260–1267.

240. Wodey E, Pladys P, Copin C, et al: Comparative hemodynamic depression of sevoflurane versus halothane in infants: An echocardiographic study. Anesthesiology 1997;87:795–800.

241. Meretoja OA, Taivainen T, Raiha L, et al: Sevoflurane-nitrous oxide or halothane-nitrous oxide for paediatric bronchoscopy and gastroscopy. Br J Anaesth 1996;76:767–771.

242. Scheller MS, Tateishi A, Drummond JC, et al: The effects of sevoflurane on cerebral blood flow, cerebral metabolic rate for oxygen, intracranial pressure, and the electroencephalogram are similar to those of isoflurane in the rabbit. Anesthesiology 1988;68:548–551.

243. Thiel A, Schindler E, Dyckmans D, et al: Transcranial doppler sonography: Effect of sevoflurane in comparison to isoflurane. [German]. Anaesthesist 1997;46:29–33.

244. Fragen RJ, Dunn KL: The minimum alveolar concentration (MAC) of sevoflurane with and without nitrous oxide in elderly versus young adults. J Clin Anesth 1996;8:352–356.

245. Katoh T, Ikeda K: The minimum alveolar concentration (MAC) of sevoflurane in humans. Anesthesiology 1987;66:301–303.

246. Patel SS, Goa KL: Sevoflurane: A review of its pharmacodynamic and pharmacokinetic properties and its clinical use in general anaesthesia. Drugs 1996;51:658–700.

247. Eger EI 2d, Ionescu P, Laster MJ, et al: Baralyme dehydration increases and soda lime dehydration decreases the concentration of compound A resulting from sevoflurane degradation in a standard anesthetic circuit. Anesth Analg 1997;85:892–898.

248. Frink EJ Jr, Green WB Jr, Brown EA, et al: Compound A concentrations during sevoflurane anesthesia in children. Anesthesiology 1996;84:566–571.

249. Munday IT, Ward PM, Foden ND, et al: Sevoflurane degradation by soda lime in a circle breathing system. Anaesthesia 1996;51:622–626.

250. Bito H, Ikeda K: Effect of total flow rate on the concentration of degradation products generated by reaction between sevoflurane and soda lime. Br J Anaesth 1995;74:667–669.

251. Fang ZX, Kandel L, Laster MJ, et al: Factors affecting production of compound A from the interaction of sevoflurane with Baralyme and soda lime. Anesth Analg 1996;82:775–781.

252. Cunningham DD, Huang S, Webster J, et al: Sevoflurane degradation to compound A in anaesthesia breathing systems. Br J Anaesth 1996;77:537–543.

253. Bito H, Ikeda K: Long-duration, low-flow sevoflurane anesthesia using two carbon dioxide absorbents: Quantification of degradation products in the circuit. Anesthesiology 1994;81:340–345.

254. Aldrete JA: Compound A concentrations during sevoflurane anesthesia in children depend on fresh gas flow. Anesthesiology 1996;85:684.

255. Young CJ, Apfelbaum JL: Inhalational anesthetics: Desflurane and sevoflurane. J Clin Anesth 1995;7:564–577.

256. Morio M, Fujii K, Satoh N, et al: Reaction of sevoflurane and its degradation products with soda lime: Toxicity of the byproducts. Anesthesiology 1992;77:1155–1164.

257. Bito H, Ikeda K: Closed-circuit anesthesia with sevoflurane in humans: Effects on renal and hepatic function and concentrations of breakdown products with soda lime in the circuit. Anesthesiology 1994;80:71–76.

258. Baxter AD: Low and minimal flow inhalational anaesthesia. Can J Anaesth 1997;44:643–652.

259. Bito H, Ikeuchi Y, Ikeda K: Effects of low-flow sevoflurane anesthesia on renal function: Comparison with high-flow sevoflurane anesthesia and low-flow isoflurane anesthesia. Anesthesiology 1997;86:1231–1237.

260. Bito H, Ikeda K: Plasma inorganic fluoride and intracircuit degradation product concentrations in long-duration, low-flow sevoflurane anesthesia. Anesth Analg 1994;79:946–951.

261. Kharasch ED, Frink EJ Jr, Zager R, et al: Assessment of low-flow sevoflurane and isoflurane effects on renal function using sensitive markers of tubular toxicity. Anesthesiology 1997;86:1238–1253.

262. Eger EI 2d, Koblin DD, Bowland T, et al: Nephrotoxicity of sevoflurane versus desflurane anesthesia in volunteers. Anesth Analg 1997;84:160–168.

263. Eger EI 2d, Bowland T, Ionescu P, et al: Recovery and kinetic characteristics of desflurane and sevoflurane in volunteers after 8-h exposure, including kinetics of degradation products. Anesthesiology 1997;87:517–526.

264. Liu J, Laster MJ, Eger EI 2d, et al: Absorption and degradation of sevoflurane and isoflurane in a conventional anesthetic circuit. Anesth Analg 1991;72:785–789.

265. Taivainen T, Tiainen P, Meretoja OA, et al: Comparison of the effects of sevoflurane and halothane on the quality of anaesthesia and serum glutathione transferase alpha and fluoride in paediatric patients. Br J Anaesth 1994;73:590–595.

266. Mazze RI, Jamison RL: Low-flow (1 l/min) sevoflurane: Is it safe? Anesthesiology 1997;86:1225–1227.

267. Neumann MA, Laster MJ, Weiskopf RB, et al: The elimination of sodium and potassium hydroxides from desiccated soda lime diminishes degradation of desflurane to carbon monoxide and sevoflurane to compound A but does not compromise carbon dioxide absorption. Anesth Analg 1999;89:768–773.

268. Kharasch ED: Putting the brakes on anesthetic breakdown. Anesthesiology 1999;91:1192–1194.

269. Renfrew CW, Murray JM, Fee JP: A new approach to carbon dioxide absorbents. Acta Anaesthesiol Scand 1998;42:58–60.

270. Levine MF, Sarner J, Lerman J, et al: Plasma inorganic fluoride concentrations after sevoflurane anesthesia in children. Anesthesiology 1996;84:348–353.

271. Kikuchi H, Morio M, Fujii K, et al: Clinical evaluation and metabolism of sevoflurane in patients. Hiroshima J Med Sci 1987;36:93–97.

272. Behne M, Wilke HJ, Harder S: Clinical pharmacokinetics of sevoflurane. Clin Pharmacokinet 1999;36:13–26.

273. Ogawa M, Doi K, Mitsufuji T, et al: Drug-induced hepatitis following sevoflurane anesthesia in a child. [in Japanese]. Masui 1991;40:1542–1545.

274. Shichinohe Y, Masuda Y, Takahashi H, et al: A case of postoperative hepatic injury after sevoflurane anesthesia. [in Japanese]. Masui 1992;41:1802–1805.

275. Schichinohe Y, Masuda Y, Takahashi H, et al: A case of postoperative hepatic injury after sevoflurane anesthesia. Masui 1992;41:1802–1805.

276. Watanabe K, Hatakenaka S, Ikemune K, et al: A case of suspected liver dysfunction induced by sevoflurane anesthesia. Masui 1993;42:902–905.

277. Kataria B, Epstein R, Bailey A, et al: A comparison of sevoflurane to

halothane in paediatric surgical patients: Results of a multicentre international study. Pediatr Anaesth 1996;6:283–292.

278. Black A, Sury MR, Hemington L, et al: A comparison of the induction characteristics of sevoflurane and halothane in children. Anaesthesia 1996;51:539–542.

279. Johannesson GP, Floren M, Lindahl SG: Sevoflurane for ENT-surgery in children: A comparison with halothane. Acta Anaesthesiol Scand 1995;39:546–550.

280. Sigston PE, Jenkins AM, Jackson EA, et al: Rapid inhalation induction in children: 8% sevoflurane compared with 5% halothane. Br J Anaesth 1997;78:362–365.

281. Baum VC, Yemen TA, Baum LD: Immediate 8% sevoflurane induction in children: A comparison with incremental sevoflurane and incremental halothane. Anesth Analg 1997;85:313–316.

282. Agnor RC, Sikich N, Lerman J: Single-breath vital capacity rapid inhalation induction in children: 8% sevoflurane versus 5% halothane. Anesthesiology 1998;89:379–384.

283. Epstein RH, Stein AL, Marr AT, et al: High concentration versus incremental induction of anesthesia with sevoflurane in children: A comparison of induction times, vital signs, and complications. J Clin Anesth 1998;10:41–45.

284. Swan HD, Crawford MW, Pua HL, et al: Additive contribution of nitrous oxide to sevoflurane minimum alveolar concentration for tracheal intubation in children. Anesthesiology 1999;91:667–671.

285. O'Brien K, Kumar R, Morton NS: Sevoflurane compared with halothane for tracheal intubation in children. Br J Anaesth 1998;80:452–455.

286. Michalek-Sauberer A, Wildling E, Pusch F, et al: Sevoflurane anaesthesia in paediatric patients: Better than halothane? Eur J Anaesthesiol 1998;15:280–286.

287. Rieger A, Schroter G, Philippi W, et al: A comparison of sevoflurane with halothane in outpatient adenotomy in children with mild upper respiratory tract infections. J Clin Anesth 1996;8:188–197.

288. Sury MR, Black A, Hemington L, et al: A comparison of the recovery characteristics of sevoflurane and halothane in children. Anaesthesia 1996;51:543–546.

289. Landais A, Saint-Maurice C, Hamza J, et al: Sevoflurane elimination kinetics in children. Paediatr Anaesth 1995;5:297–301.

290. Viitanen H, Annila P, Viitanen M, et al: Premedication with midazolam delays recovery after ambulatory sevoflurane anesthesia in children. Anesth Analg 1999;89:75–79.

291. Aono J, Ueda W, Mamiya K, et al: Greater incidence of delirium during recovery from sevoflurane anesthesia in preschool boys. Anesthesiology 1997;87:1298–1300.

292. Lapin SL, Auden SM, Goldsmith LJ, et al: Effects of sevoflurane anaesthesia on recovery in children: A comparison with halothane. Paediatr Anaesth 1999;9:299–304.

293. Beskow A, Westrin P: Sevoflurane causes more postoperative agitation in children than does halothane. Acta Anaesthesiol Scand 1999; 43:536–541.

294. Davis PJ, Greenberg JA, Gendelman M, et al: Recovery characteristics of sevoflurane and halothane in preschool-aged children undergoing bilateral myringotomy and pressure equalization tube insertion. Anesth Analg 1999;88:34–38.

295. Mazurek AJ, Przybylo HJ, Martini DR, DeMille A, Coté CJ: Emergence patterns following sevoflurane and halothane anesthesia in children. Anesthesiology 1999;91:A1299.

296. Eger EI 2d: New inhaled anesthetics. Anesthesiology 1994;80:906–922.

297. Mannion D, Casey W, Doherty P: Desflurane in paediatric anaesthesia. Paediatr Anaesth 1998;4:301–306.

298. Zwass MS, Fisher DM, Welborn LG, et al: Induction and maintenance characteristics of anesthesia with desflurane and nitrous oxide in infants and children. Anesthesiology 1992;76:373–378.

299. Taylor RH, Lerman J: Induction, maintenance and recovery characteristics of desflurane in infants and children. Can J Anaesth 1992;39: 6–13.

300. Smiley RM: An overview of induction and emergence characteristics of desflurane in pediatric, adult, and geriatric patients. Anesth Analg 1992;75(Suppl):S38–S44.

301. Lutz LJ, Milde JH, Milde LN: The cerebral functional, metabolic, and hemodynamic effects of desflurane in dogs. Anesthesiology 1990;73:125–131.

302. Moore MA, Weiskopf RB, Eger EI 2d, et al: Arrhythmogenic doses of epinephrine are similar during desflurane or isoflurane anesthesia in humans. Anesthesiology 1993;79:943–947.

303. Artru AA: Intracranial volume/pressure relationship during desflurane anesthesia in dogs: Comparison with isoflurane and thiopental/halothane. Anesth Analg 1994;79:751–760.

304. Strebel S, Lam AM, Matta B, et al: Dynamic and static cerebral autoregulation during isoflurane, desflurane, and propofol anesthesia. Anesthesiology 1995;83:66–76.

305. Weiskopf RB: Cardiovascular effects of desflurane in experimental animals and volunteers. Anaesthesia 1995;50(Suppl):14–17.

306. Moore MA, Weiskopf RB, Eger EI 2d, et al: Rapid 1% increases of end-tidal desflurane concentration to greater than 5% transiently increase heart rate and blood pressure in humans. Anesthesiology 1994;81:94–98.

307. Ebert TJ, Muzi M: Sympathetic hyperactivity during desflurane anesthesia in healthy volunteers: A comparison with isoflurane. Anesthesiology 1993;79:444–453.

308. Rampil IJ, Lockhart SH, Zwass MS, et al: Clinical characteristics of desflurane in surgical patients: Minimum alveolar concentration. Anesthesiology 1991;74:429–433.

309. Taylor RH, Lerman J: Minimum alveolar concentration of desflurane and hemodynamic responses in neonates, infants, and children. Anesthesiology 1991;75:975–979.

310. Fisher DM, Zwass MS: MAC of desflurane in 60% nitrous oxide in infants and children. Anesthesiology 1992;76:354–356.

311. Welborn LG, Hannallah RS, Norden JM, et al: Comparison of emergence and recovery characteristics of sevoflurane, desflurane, and halothane in pediatric ambulatory patients. Anesth Analg 1996; 83:917–920.

312. Wolf AR, Lawson RA, Dryden CM, et al: Recovery after desflurane anaesthesia in the infant: Comparison with isoflurane. Br J Anaesth 1996;76:362–364.

313. Heijke S, Smith G: Quest for the ideal inhalation anaesthetic agent. Br J Anaesth 1990;64:3–6.

314. Koblin DD, Lurz FW, Eger EI 2d: Age-dependent alterations in nitrous oxide requirement of mice. Anesthesiology 1983;58:428–431.

315. Henriksen HT, Jorgensen PB: The effect of nitrous oxide on intracranial pressure in patients with intracranial disorders. Br J Anaesth 1973;45:486–492.

316. Todd MM: The effects of $PaCO_2$ on the cerebrovascular response to nitrous oxide in the halothane-anesthetized rabbit. Anesth Analg 1987;66:1090–1095.

317. Wren WS, Allen P, Synnott A, et al: Effects of nitrous oxide on the respiratory pattern of spontaneously breathing children. A reappraisal. Br J Anaesth 1986;58:274–279.

318. Nishino T, Takizawa K, Yokokawa N, et al: Depression of the swallowing reflex during sedation and/or relative analgesia produced by inhalation of 50% nitrous oxide in oxygen. Anesthesiology 1987;67:995–998.

319. Lonie DS, Harper NJ: Nitrous oxide anaesthesia and vomiting: The effect of nitrous oxide anaesthesia on the incidence of vomiting following gynaecological laparoscopy. Anaesthesia 1986;41:703–707.

320. Korttila K, Hovorka J, Erkola O: Nitrous oxide does not increase the incidence of nausea and vomiting after isoflurane anesthesia. Anesth Analg 1987;66:761–765.

321. Tenney SM, Carpenter FG, Rahn H: Gas transfers in a sulfur hexafluoride pneumoperitoneum. J Appl Physiol 1953;6:201–208.

322. Eger EI II, Saidman LJ: Hazards of nitrous oxide anesthesia in bowel obstruction and pneumothorax. Anesthesiology 1965;26:61–66.

323. Blackstock D, Gettes MA: Negative pressure in the middle ear in children after nitrous oxide anaesthesia. Can Anaesth Soc J 1986; 33:32–35.

324. Saidman LJ, Eger EI II: Change in cerebrospinal fluid pressure during pneumoencephalography under nitrous oxide anesthesia. Anesthesiology 1965;26:67–72.

325. Owens WD, Gustave F, Sclaroff A: Tympanic membrane rupture with nitrous oxide anesthesia. Anesth Analg 1978;57:283–286.

326. Perreault L, Normandin N, Plamondon L, et al: Middle ear pressure variations during nitrous oxide and oxygen anaesthesia. Can Anaesth Soc J 1982;29:428–434.

327. Coté CJ: The anesthetic management of congenital lobar emphysema. Anesthesiology 1978;49:296–298.

328. Schulte-Sasse U, Hess W, Tarnow J: Pulmonary vascular responses to nitrous oxide in patients with normal and high pulmonary vascular resistance. Anesthesiology 1982;57:9–13.

329. Hickey PR, Hansen DD, Strafford M, et al: Pulmonary and systemic hemodynamic effects of nitrous oxide in infants with normal and

elevated pulmonary vascular resistance. Anesthesiology 1986;65:374–378.

330. Murray D, Forbes R, Murphy K, et al: Nitrous oxide: Cardiovascular effects in infants and small children during halothane and isoflurane anesthesia. Anesth Analg 1988;67:1059–1064.

331. Winter PM, Smith G: The toxicity of oxygen. Anesthesiology 1972;37:210–241.

332. Dobson V, Quinn GE: Retinopathy of prematurity. Optom Clin 1996;5:105–124.

333. James S, Lanman JT: History of oxygen therapy and retrolental fibroplasia. Prepared by the American Academy of Pediatrics, Committee on Fetus and Newborn with the collaboration of special consultants. Pediatrics 1976;57(2):591–642.

334. Biglan AW, Brown DR, Macpherson TA: Update on retinopathy of prematurity. Semin Perinatol 1986;10:187–195.

335. Ben Sira I, Nissenkorn I, Kremer I: Retinopathy of prematurity. Surv Ophthalmol 1988;33:1–16.

336. DeVoe WM: Prevention of retinopathy of prematurity. Semin Perinatol 1988;12:373–380.

337. Gaynon MW: Retinopathy of prematurity. Pediatrician 1990;17:127–133.

338. Todd DA, Kennedy J, Cassell C, et al: Retinopathy of prematurity in infants <29 weeks' gestation at birth in New South Wales from 1986 to 1992. J Paediatr Child Health 1998;34:32–36.

339. Bossi E, Koerner F: Retinopathy of prematurity. Intensive Care Med 1995;21:241–246.

340. Betts EK, Downes JJ, Schaffer DB, et al: Retrolental fibroplasia and oxygen administration during general anesthesia. Anesthesiology 1977;47:518–520.

341. Merritt JC, Sprague DH, Merritt WE, et al: Retrolental fibroplasia: A multifactorial disease. Anesth Analg 1981;60:109–111.

342. Kalina RE, Hodson WA, Morgan BC: Retrolental fibroplasia in a cyanotic infant. Pediatrics 1972;50:765–768.

343. Adamkin DH, Shott RJ, Cook LN, et al: Nonhyperoxic retrolental fibroplasia. Pediatrics 1977;60:828–830.

344. Wolbarsht ML, George GS, Kylstra J, et al: Speculation on carbon dioxide and retrolental fibroplasia. Pediatrics 1983;71:859–860.

345. Phelps DL, Rosenbaum AL: Effects of marginal hypoxemia on recovery from oxygen-induced retinopathy in the kitten model. Pediatrics 1984;73:1–6.

346. Holmes JM, Zhang S, Leske DA, et al: Carbon dioxide–induced retinopathy in the neonatal rat. Curr Eye Res 1998;17:608–616.

347. Mittal M, Dhanireddy R, Higgins RD: Candida sepsis and association with retinopathy of prematurity. Pediatrics 1998;101:654–657.

348. Hesse L, Eberl W, Schlaud M, et al: Blood transfusion: Iron load and retinopathy of prematurity. Eur J Pediatr 1997;156:465–470.

349. Inder TE, Clemett RS, Austin NC, et al: High iron status in very low birth weight infants is associated with an increased risk of retinopathy of prematurity. J Pediatr 1997;131:541–544.

350. Glass P, Avery GB, Subramanian KN, et al: Effect of bright light in the hospital nursery on the incidence of retinopathy of prematurity. N Engl J Med 1985;313:401–404.

351. Phelps DL, Rosenbaum AL, Isenberg SJ, et al: Tocopherol efficacy and safety for preventing retinopathy of prematurity: a randomized, controlled, double-masked trial. Pediatrics 1987;79:489–500.

352. Avery GB, Glass P: Light and retinopathy of prematurity: what is prudent for 1986? Pediatrics 1986;78:519–520.

353. Bancalari E, Flynn J, Goldberg RN, et al: Influence of transcutaneous oxygen monitoring on the incidence of retinopathy of prematurity. Pediatrics 1987;79:663–669.

354. American Academy of Pediatrics Committee on the Fetus and Newborn and American College of Obstetrics and Gynecology Committee on Obstetric Practice: Guidelines for Perinatal Care, 4th ed. 1997:188–192.

355. Purohit DM, Ellison RC, Zierler S, et al: Risk factors for retrolental fibroplasia: Experience with 3,025 premature infants. National Collaborative Study on Patent Ductus Arteriosus in Premature Infants. Pediatrics 1985;76:339–344.

356. Hoon AH, Jan JE, Whitfield MF, et al: Changing pattern of retinopathy of prematurity: A 37-year clinic experience. Pediatrics 1988;82:344–349.

357. Patz A: Current therapy of retrolental fibroplasia: Retinopathy of prematurity. Ophthalmology 1983;90:425–427.

358. Quinn GE, Betts EK, Diamond GR, et al: Neonatal age (human) at retinal maturation. Anesthesiology 1981;55:S326.

359. Flynn JT: Retinopathy of prematurity: Perspective for the nineties. Acta Ophthalmol Scand Suppl 1995;214:12–14.

360. Lucey JF, Dangman B: A reexamination of the role of oxygen in retrolental fibroplasia. Pediatrics 1984;73:82–96.

361. Bucher HU, Fanconi S, Baeckert P, et al: Hyperoxemia in newborn infants: Detection by pulse oximetry. Pediatrics 1989;84:226–230.

362. Severinghaus JW, Naifeh KH: Accuracy of response of six pulse oximeters to profound hypoxia. Anesthesiology 1987;67:551–558.

363. Badgwell JM, McLeod ME, Lerman J, et al: End-tidal Pco_2 measurements sampled at the distal and proximal ends of the endotracheal tube in infants and children. Anesth Analg 1987;66:959–964.

364. Rich GF, Sullivan MP, Adams JM: Is distal sampling of end-tidal CO_2 necessary in small subjects? Anesthesiology 1990;73:265–268.

365. Burrows FA: Physiologic dead space, venous admixture, and the arterial to end-tidal carbon dioxide difference in infants and children undergoing cardiac surgery. Anesthesiology 1989;70:219–225.

366. Flynn JT: Oxygen and retrolental fibroplasia: Update and challenge. Anesthesiology 1984;60:397–399.

367. Saidman LJ, Eger EI 2d: Uptake and distribution of thiopental after oral, rectal, and intramuscular administration: Effect of hepatic metabolism and injection site blood flow. Clin Pharmacol Ther 1973;14:12–20.

368. Liu LMP, Coté CJ, Goudsouzian NG, et al: Response to intravenous induction doses of methohexital in children. Anesthesiology 1981;55:A330.

369. Rockoff MA, Goudsouzian NG: Seizures induced by methohexital. Anesthesiology 1981;54:333–335.

370. Audenaert SM, Lock RL, Johnson GL, et al: Cardiovascular effects of rectal methohexital in children. J Clin Anesth 1992;4:116–119.

371. Audenaert SM, Wagner Y, Montgomery CL, et al: Cardiorespiratory effects of premedication for children. Anesth Analg 1995;80:506–510.

372. Bjorkman S, Gabrielsson J, Quaynor H, et al: Pharmacokinetics of i.v. and rectal methohexitone in children. Br J Anaesth 1987;59:1541–1547.

373. Breimer DD: Pharmacokinetics of methohexitone following intravenous infusion in humans. Br J Anaesth 1976;48:643–649.

374. Beskow A, Werner O, Westrin P: Faster recovery after anesthesia in infants after intravenous induction with methohexital instead of thiopental. Anesthesiology 1995;83:976–979.

375. Audenaert SM, Montgomery CL, Thompson DE, et al: A prospective study of rectal methohexital: Efficacy and side effects in 648 cases. Anesth Analg 1995;81:957–961.

376. Liu LM, Goudsouzian NG, Liu PL: Rectal methohexital premedication in children: A dose-comparison study. Anesthesiology 1980;53:343–345.

377. Griswold JD, Liu LM: Rectal methohexital in children undergoing computerized cranial tomography and magnetic resonance imaging scans. Anesthesiology 1987;67:A494.

378. Liu LM, Gaudreault P, Friedman PA, et al: Methohexital plasma concentrations in children following rectal administration. Anesthesiology 1985;62:567–570.

379. Olkkola KT, Aranko K, Luurila H, et al: A potentially hazardous interaction between erythromycin and midazolam. Clin Pharmacol Ther 1993;53:298–305.

380. Hiller A, Olkkola KT, Isohanni P, et al: Unconsciousness associated with midazolam and erythromycin. Br J Anaesth 1994;65:826–828.

381. Daniels AL, Coté CJ, Polaner DM: Continuous oxygen saturation monitoring following rectal methohexitone induction in paediatric patients. Can J Anaesth 1992;39:27–30.

382. Yemen TA, Pullerits J, Stillman R, et al: Rectal methohexital causing apnea in two patients with meningomyeloceles. Anesthesiology 1991;74:1139–1141.

383. Coté CJ, Goudsouzian NG, Liu LM, et al: The dose response of intravenous thiopental for the induction of general anesthesia in unpremedicated children. Anesthesiology 1981;55:703–705.

384. Brett CM, Fisher DM: Thiopental dose-response relations in unpremedicated infants, children, and adults. Anesth Analg 1987;66:1024–1027.

385. Jonmarker C, Westrin P, Larsson S, et al: Thiopental requirements for induction of anesthesia in children. Anesthesiology 1987;67:104–107.

386. Burch PG, Stanski DR: The role of metabolism and protein binding in thiopental anesthesia. Anesthesiology 1983;58:146–152.

387. Sorbo S, Hudson RJ, Loomis JC: The pharmacokinetics of thiopental in pediatric surgical patients. Anesthesiology 1984;61:666–670.

388. Russo H, Bressolle F, Duboin MP: Pharmacokinetics of high-dose

thiopental in pediatric patients with increased intracranial pressure. Ther Drug Monit 1997;19:63–70.

389. Garg DC, Goldberg RN, Woo-Ming RB, et al: Pharmacokinetics of thiopental in the asphyxiated neonate. Dev Pharmacol Ther 1988;11:213–218.

390. Russo H, Bressolle F: Pharmacodynamics and pharmacokinetics of thiopental. Clin Pharmacokinet 1998;35:95–134.

391. Toner W, Howard PJ, McGowan WA, et al: Another look at acute tolerance to thiopentone. Br J Anaesth 1980;52:1005–1008.

392. Gelissen HP, Epema AH, Henning RH, et al: Inotropic effects of propofol, thiopental, midazolam, etomidate, and ketamine on isolated human atrial muscle. Anesthesiology 1996;84:397–403.

393. Beekman RP, Hoorntje TM, Beek FJ, et al: Sedation for children undergoing magnetic resonance imaging: Efficacy and safety of rectal thiopental. Eur J Pediatr 1996;155:820–822.

394. Turcant A, Delhumeau A, Premel-Cabic A, et al: Thiopental pharmacokinetics under conditions of long-term infusion. Anesthesiology 1985;63:50–54.

395. Shafer A, Doze VA, Shafer SL, et al: Pharmacokinetics and pharmacodynamics of propofol infusions during general anesthesia. Anesthesiology 1988;69:348–356.

396. Cummings GC, Dixon J, Kay NH, et al: Dose requirements of ICI 35,868 (propofol, "Diprivan") in a new formulation for induction of anaesthesia. Anaesthesia 1984;39:1168–1171.

397. Fulton B, Sorkin EM: Propofol: An overview of its pharmacology and a review of its clinical efficacy in intensive care sedation. Drugs 1995;50:636–657.

398. Bryson HM, Fulton BR, Faulds D: Propofol: An update of its use in anaesthesia and conscious sedation. Drugs 1995;50:513–559.

399. Smith I, White PF, Nathanson M, et al: Propofol: An update on its clinical use. Anesthesiology 1994;81:1005–1043.

400. Raoof AA, van Obbergh LJ, Verbeeck RK: Propofol pharmacokinetics in children with biliary atresia. Br J Anaesth 1995;74:46–49.

401. Patel DK, Keeling PA, Newman GB, et al: Induction dose of propofol in children. Anaesthesia 1988;43:949–952.

402. Mirakhur RK: Induction characteristics of propofol in children: Comparison with thiopentone. Anaesthesia 1988;43:593–598.

403. Martlew RA, Meakin G, Wadsworth R, et al: Dose of propofol for laryngeal mask airway insertion in children: Effect of premedication with midazolam. Br J Anaesth 1996;76:308–309.

404. Valtonen M, Iisalo E, Kanto J, et al: Propofol as an induction agent in children: Pain injection and pharmacokinetics. Acta Anaesthesiol Scand 1989;33:152–155.

405. Kataria BK, Ved SA, Nicodemus HF, et al: The pharmacokinetics of propofol in children using three different data analysis approaches. Anesthesiology 1994;80:104–122.

406. Fisher DM: Propofol in pediatrics: Lessons in pharmacokinetic modeling. Anesthesiology 1994;80:2–5.

407. Hug CC Jr, McLeskey CH, Nahrwold ML, et al: Hemodynamic effects of propofol: Data from over 25,000 patients. Anesth Analg 1993;77:S21–S29.

408. Morton NS, Wee M, Christie G, et al: Propofol for induction of anaesthesia in children: A comparison with thiopentone and halothane inhalational induction. Anaesthesia 1988;43:350–355.

409. Purcell-Jones G, Yates A, Baker JR, et al: Comparison of the induction characteristics of thiopentone and propofol in children. Br J Anaesth 1987;59:1431–1436.

410. Valtonen M, Iisalo E, Kanto J, et al: Comparison between propofol and thiopentone for induction of anaesthesia in children. Anaesthesia 1988;43:696–699.

411. Jones RD, Visram AR, Chan MM, et al: A comparison of three induction agents in paediatric anaesthesia-cardiovascular effects and recovery. Anaesth Intensive Care 1994;22:545–555.

412. Hannallah RS, Britton JT, Schafer PG, et al: Propofol anaesthesia in paediatric ambulatory patients: A comparison with thiopentone and halothane. Can J Anaesth 1994;41:12–18.

413. Kain ZN, Gaal DJ, Kain TS, et al: A first-pass cost analysis of propofol versus barbiturates for children undergoing magnetic resonance imaging. Anesth Analg 1994;79:1102–1106.

414. Runcie CJ, Mackenzie SJ, Arthur DS, et al: Comparison of recovery from anaesthesia induced in children with either propofol or thiopentone. Br J Anaesth 1993;70:192–195.

415. Larsson S, Asgeirsson B, Magnusson J: Propofol-fentanyl anesthesia compared to thiopental-halothane with special reference to recovery and vomiting after pediatric strabismus surgery. Acta Anaesthesiol Scand 1992;36:182–186.

416. Puttick N, Rosen M: Propofol induction and maintenance with nitrous oxide in paediatric outpatient dental anaesthesia: A comparison with thiopentone-nitrous oxide-halothane. Anaesthesia 1988;43:646–649.

417. Schroter J, Motsch J, Hufnagel AR, et al: Recovery of psychomotor function following general anaesthesia in children: A comparison of propofol and thiopentone/halothane. Pediatr Anaesth 1996;6:317–324.

418. Snellen FT, Vanacker B, Van Aken H: Propofol-nitrous oxide versus thiopental sodium-isoflurane-nitrous oxide for strabismus surgery in children. J Clin Anesth 1993;5:37–41.

419. Weir PM, Munro HM, Reynolds PI, et al: Propofol infusion and the incidence of emesis in pediatric outpatient strabismus surgery. Anesth Analg 1993;76:760–764.

420. Splinter WM, Rhine EJ, Roberts DJ: Vomiting after strabismus surgery in children: Ondansetron vs. propofol. Can J Anaesth 1997;44:825–829.

421. Woodward WM, Barker I, John RE, et al: Propofol infusion vs. thiopentone/isoflurane anaesthesia for prominent ear correction in children. Pediatr Anaesth 1997;7:379–383.

422. Standl T, Wilhelm S, von Knobelsdorff G, et al: Propofol reduces emesis after sufentanil supplemented anaesthesia in paediatric squint surgery. Acta Anaesthesiol Scand 1996;40:729–733.

423. Barst SM, Markowitz A, Yossefy Y, et al: Propofol reduces the incidence of vomiting after tonsillectomy in children. Pediatr Anaesth 1995;5:249–252.

424. Martin TM, Nicolson SC, Bargas MS: Propofol anesthesia reduces emesis and airway obstruction in pediatric outpatients. Anesth Analg 1993;76:144–148.

425. Habre W, Sims C: Propofol anaesthesia and vomiting after myringoplasty in children. Anaesthesia 1997;52:544–546.

426. Hamunen K, Vaalamo MO, Maunuksela EL: Does propofol reduce vomiting after strabismus surgery in children? Acta Anaesthesiol Scand 1997;41:973–977.

427. Malviya S, Voepel-Lewis T, Huntington J, et al: Effects of anesthetic technique on side effects associated with fentanyl Oralet premedication. J Clin Anesth 1997;9:374–378.

428. Ved SA, Walden TL, Montana J, et al: Vomiting and recovery after outpatient tonsillectomy and adenoidectomy in children: Comparison of four anesthetic techniques using nitrous oxide with halothane or propofol. Anesthesiology 1996;85:4–10.

429. Vangerven M, Van Hemelrijck J, Wouters P, et al: Light anaesthesia with propofol for paediatric MRI. Anaesthesia 1992;47:706–707.

430. Scheiber G, Ribeiro FC, Karpienski H, et al: Deep sedation with propofol in preschool children undergoing radiation therapy. Paediatr Anaesth 1996;6:209–213.

431. Bloomfield EL, Masaryk TJ, Caplin A, et al: Intravenous sedation for MR imaging of the brain and spine in children: Pentobarbital versus propofol. Radiology 1993;186:93–97.

432. Broennle AM, Cohen DE: Pediatric anesthesia and sedation. Curr Opin Pediatr 1993;5:310–314.

433. Valtonen M: Anaesthesia for computerised tomography of the brain in children: A comparison of propofol and thiopentone. Acta Anaesthesiol Scand 1989;33:170–173.

434. Harling DW, Harrison DA, Dorman T, et al: A comparison of thiopentone-isoflurane anaesthesia vs. propofol infusion in children having repeat minor haematological procedures. Paediatr Anaesth 1997;7:19–23.

435. Schrum SF, Hannallah RS, Verghese PM, et al: Comparison of propofol and thiopental for rapid anesthesia induction in infants. Anesth Analg 1994;78:482–485.

436. Allsop E, Innes P, Jackson M, et al: Dose of propofol required to insert the laryngeal mask airway in children. Paediatr Anaesth 1995;5:47–51.

437. Bandla HP, Smith DE, Kiernan MP: Laryngeal mask airway facilitated fibreoptic bronchoscopy in infants. Can J Anaesth 1997;44:1242–1247.

438. Reber A, Wetzel SG, Schnabel K, et al: Effect of combined mouth closure and chin lift on upper airway dimensions during routine magnetic resonance imaging in pediatric patients sedated with propofol. Anesthesiology 1999;90:1617–1623.

439. Strickland RA, Murray MJ: Fatal metabolic acidosis in a pediatric patient receiving an infusion of propofol in the intensive care unit: Is there a relationship? Crit Care Med 1995;23:405–409.

440. Parke TJ, Stevens JE, Rice AS, et al: Metabolic acidosis and fatal myocardial failure after propofol infusion in children: Five case reports. Br Med J 1992;305:613–616.

441. Bray RJ: Propofol infusion syndrome in children. Paediatr Anaesth 1998;8:491–499.
442. Cray SH, Robinson BH, Cox PN: Lactic acidemia and bradyarrhythmia in a child sedated with propofol. Crit Care Med 1998;26:2087–2092.
443. Miller LJ, Wiles-Pfeifler R: Propofol for the long-term sedation of a critically ill patient. Am J Crit Care 1998;7:73–76.
444. Wilson RD: Current usefulness of ketamine in anesthetic practice. Anesth Analg 1971;50:1057–1058.
445. Pedraz JL, Calvo MB, Lanao JM, et al: Pharmacokinetics of rectal ketamine in children. Br J Anaesth 1989;63:671–674.
446. Wieber J, Gugler R, Hengstmann JH, et al: Pharmacokinetics of ketamine in man. Anaesthetist 1975;24:260–263.
447. Mogensen F, Muller D, Valentin N: Glycopyrrolate during ketamine/diazepam anaesthesia: A double-blind comparison with atropine. Acta Anaesthesiol Scand 1986;30:332–336.
448. Dachs RJ, Innes GM: Intravenous ketamine sedation of pediatric patients in the emergency department. Ann Emerg Med 1997;29:146–150.
449. Marx CM, Stein J, Tyler MK, et al: Ketamine-midazolam versus meperidine-midazolam for painful procedures in pediatric oncology patients. J Clin Oncol 1997;15:94–102.
450. Petrack EM, Marx CM, Wright MS: Intramuscular ketamine is superior to meperidine, promethazine, and chlorpromazine for pediatric emergency department sedation. Arch Pediatr Adolesc Med 1996;150:676–681.
451. Pruitt JW, Goldwasser MS, Sabol SR, et al: Intramuscular ketamine, midazolam, and glycopyrrolate for pediatric sedation in the emergency department. J Oral Maxillofac Surg 1995;53:13–17.
452. Corssen G, Groves EH, Gomez S, et al: Ketamine: Its place for neurosurgical diagnostic procedures. Anesth Analg 1969;48:181–188.
453. Clements JA, Nimmo WS, Grant IS: Bioavailability, pharmacokinetics, and analgesic activity of ketamine in humans. J Pharm Sci 1982;71:539–542.
454. Grant IS, Nimmo WS, McNicol LR, et al: Ketamine disposition in children and adults. Br J Anaesth 1983;55:1107–1111.
455. Gingrich BK: Difficulties encountered in a comparative study of orally administered midazolam and ketamine. Anesthesiology 1994;80:1414–1415.
456. Cotsen MR, Donaldson JS, Uejima T, et al: Efficacy of ketamine hydrochloride sedation in children for interventional radiologic procedures. AJR Am J Roentgenol 1997;169:1019–1022.
457. Parker RI, Mahan RA, Giugliano D, et al: Efficacy and safety of intravenous midazolam and ketamine as sedation for therapeutic and diagnostic procedures in children. Pediatrics 1997;99:427–431.
458. Smith JA, Santer LJ: Respiratory arrest following intramuscular ketamine injection in a 4-year-old child. Ann Emerg Med 1993;22:613–615.
459. Green SM, Rothrock SG: Transient apnea with intramuscular ketamine. Am J Emerg Med 1997;15:440–441.
460. Mitchell RK, Koury SI, Stone CK: Respiratory arrest after intramuscular ketamine in a 2-year-old child. Am J Emerg Med 1996;14:580–581.
461. Diaz JH: Intranasal ketamine preinduction of paediatric outpatients. Pediatr Anaesth 1997;7:273–278.
462. Humphries Y, Melson M, Gore D: Superiority of oral ketamine as an analgesic and sedative for wound care procedures in the pediatric patient with burns. J Burn Care Rehabil 1997;18:34–36.
463. Reinemer HC, Wilson CF, Webb MD: A comparison of two oral ketamine-diazepam regimens for sedating anxious pediatric dental patients. Pediatr Dent 1996;18:294–300.
464. Roelofse JA, Joubert JJ, Swart LC, et al: An evaluation of the effect of oral ketamine and standard oral premedication in the sedation of paediatric dental patients. J Dent Assoc S Afr 1996;51:197–201.
465. Roelofse JA, Joubert JJ, Roelofse PG: A double-blind randomized comparison of midazolam alone and midazolam combined with ketamine for sedation of pediatric dental patients. J Oral Maxillofac Surg 1996;54:838–844.
466. Hollman GA, Perloff WH: Efficacy of oral ketamine for providing sedation and analgesia to children requiring laceration repair. Pediatr Emerg Care 1995;11:399.
467. Warner DL, Cabaret J, Velling D: Ketamine plus midazolam, a most effective paediatric oral premedicant. Pediatr Anaesth 1995;5:293–295.
468. Alderson PJ, Lerman J: Oral premedication for paediatric ambulatory

469. Louon A, Reddy VG: Nasal midazolam and ketamine for paediatric sedation during computerised tomography. Acta Anaesthesiol Scand 1994;38:259–261.
470. Abrams R, Morrison JE, Villasenor A, et al: Safety and effectiveness of intranasal administration of sedative medications (ketamine, midazolam, or sufentanil) for urgent brief pediatric dental procedures. Anesth Prog 1993;40:63–66.
471. Weksler N, Ovadia L, Muati G, et al: Nasal ketamine for paediatric premedication. Can J Anaesth 1993;40:119–121.
472. Beebe DS, Belani KG, Chang PN, et al: Effectiveness of preoperative sedation with rectal midazolam, ketamine, or their combination in young children. Anesth Analg 1992;75:880–884.
473. Gutstein HB, Johnson KL, Heard MB, et al: Oral ketamine preanesthetic medication in children. Anesthesiology 1992;76:28–33.
474. Tobias JD, Phipps S, Smith B, et al: Oral ketamine premedication to alleviate the distress of invasive procedures in pediatric oncology patients. Pediatrics 1992;90:537–541.
475. Malinovsky JM, Servin F, Cozian A, et al: Ketamine and norketamine plasma concentrations after i.v., nasal and rectal administration in children. Br J Anaesth 1996;77:203–207.
476. Committee on Drugs American Academy of Pediatrics: Alternate routes of drug administration: Advantages and disadvantages. Pediatrics 1997;100:143–152.
477. Seki T, Sato N, Hasegawa T, et al: Nasal absorption of zidovudine and its transport to cerebrospinal fluid in rats. Biol Pharm Bull 1994;17:1135–1137.
478. Kida S, Pantazis A, Weller RO: CSF drains directly from the subarachnoid space into nasal lymphatics in the rat: Anatomy, histology and immunological significance. Neuropath Appl Neurobiol 1993;19:480–488.
479. Binhammer RT: CSF anatomy with emphasis on relations to nasal cavity and labyrinthine fluids. Ear Nose Throat J 1992;71:292–294.
480. Sakane T, Akizuki M, Yamashita S, et al: The transport of a drug to the cerebrospinal fluid directly from the nasal cavity: The relation to the lipophilicity of the drug. Chem Pharm Bul 1991;39:2456–2458.
481. Malinovsky JM, Lepage JY, Cozian A, et al: Is ketamine or its preservative responsible for neurotoxicity in the rabbit? Anesthesiology 1993;78:109–115.
482. Malinovsky JM, Cozian A, Lepage JY, et al: Ketamine and midazolam neurotoxicity in the rabbit. Anesthesiology 1991;75:91–97.
483. Semple D, Findlow D, Aldridge LM, et al: The optimal dose of ketamine for caudal epidural blockade in children. Anaesthesia 1996;51:1170–1172.
484. Findlow D, Aldridge LM, Doyle E: Comparison of caudal block using bupivacaine and ketamine with ilioinguinal nerve block for orchidopexy in children. Anaesthesia 1997;52:1110–1113.
485. Tweed WA, Minuck M, Mymin D: Circulatory responses to ketamine anesthesia. Anesthesiology 1972;37:613–619.
486. White PF, Ham J, Way WL, et al: Pharmacology of ketamine isomers in surgical patients. Anesthesiology 1980;52:231–239.
487. Hickey PR, Hansen DD, Cramolini GM, et al: Pulmonary and systemic hemodynamic responses to ketamine in infants with normal and elevated pulmonary vascular resistance. Anesthesiology 1985;62:287–293.
488. Friesen RH, Alswang M: Changes in carbon dioxide tension and oxygen saturation during deep sedation for paediatric cardiac catheterization. Pediatr Anaesth 1996;6:15–20.
489. Christ G, Mundigler G, Merhaut C, et al: Adverse cardiovascular effects of ketamine infusion in patients with catecholamine-dependent heart failure. Anaesth Intensive Care 1997;25:255–259.
490. Drummond GB: Comparison of sedation with midazolam and ketamine: Effects on airway muscle activity. Br J Anaesth 1996;76:663–667.
491. Hirota K, Sato T, Rabito SF, et al: Relaxant effect of ketamine and its isomers on histamine-induced contraction of tracheal smooth muscle. Br J Anaesth 1996;76:266–270.
492. Howton JC, Rose J, Duffy S, et al: Randomized, double-blind, placebo-controlled trial of intravenous ketamine in acute asthma. Ann Emerg Med 1996;27:170–175.
493. Hollister GR, Burn JM: Side effects of ketamine in pediatric anesthesia. Anesth Analg 1974;53:264–267.
494. Reich DL, Silvay G: Ketamine: An update on the first twenty-five years of clinical experience. Can J Anaesth 1989;36:186–197.

495. Byer DE, Gould AB Jr: Development of tolerance to ketamine in an infant undergoing repeated anesthesia. Anesthesiology 1981;54:255–256.

496. Meyers EF, Charles P: Prolonged adverse reactions to ketamine in children. Anesthesiology 1978;49:39–40.

497. Morray JP, Lynn AM, Stamm SJ, et al: Hemodynamic effects of ketamine in children with congenital heart disease. Anesth Analg 1984;63:895–899.

498. LoVerme SR, Oropollo AT: Ketamine anesthesia in dermolytic bullous dermatosis (epidermolysis bullosa). Anesth Analg 1977;56:398–401.

499. Sari A, Okuda Y, Takeshita H: The effect of ketamine on cerebrospinal fluid pressure. Anesth Analg 1972;51:560–565.

500. Crumrine RS, Nulsen FE, Weiss MH: Alterations in ventricular fluid pressure during ketamine anesthesia in hydrocephalic children. Anesthesiology 1975;42:758–761.

501. Albanese J, Arnaud S, Rey M, et al: Ketamine decreases intracranial pressure and electroencephalographic activity in traumatic brain injury patients during propofol sedation. Anesthesiology 1997;87:1328–1334.

502. Yoshikawa K, Murai Y: The effect of ketamine on intraocular pressure in children. Anesth Analg 1971;50:199–202.

503. Carson IW, Moore J, Balmer JP, et al: Laryngeal competence with ketamine and other drugs. Anesthesiology 1973;38:128–133.

504. White PF, Way WL, Trevor AJ: Ketamine: Its pharmacology and therapeutic uses. Anesthesiology 1982;56:119–136.

505. Edmonds-Seal J, Prys-Roberts C: Pharmacology of drugs used in neuroleptanalgesia. Br J Anaesth 1970;42:207–216.

506. Gaal DG, Rice LJ, Hannallah RS: Droperidol-induced extrapyramidal symptoms in an adolescent following strabismus surgery. Middle East J Anesthesiol 1990;10:527–531.

507. Dupre LJ, Stieglitz P: Extrapyramidal syndromes after premedication with droperidol in children. Br J Anaesth 1980;52:831–833.

508. Lassner J, Brown AS, Foldes FF, et al: Symposium on neuroleptanalgesia. Acta Anaesthesiol Scand Suppl 1966;25:251–279.

509. Abramowitz MD, Oh TH, Epstein BS, et al: The antiemetic effect of droperidol following outpatient strabismus surgery in children. Anesthesiology 1983;59:579–583.

510. Hardy JF, Charest J, Girouard G, et al: Nausea and vomiting after strabismus surgery in preschool children. Can Anaesth Soc J 1986;33:57–62.

511. Nicolson SC, Kaya KM, Betts EK: The effect of preoperative oral droperidol on the incidence of postoperative emesis after paediatric strabismus surgery. Can J Anaesth 1988;35:364–367.

512. Grunwald Z, Torjman M, Schieren H, et al: The pharmacokinetics of droperidol in anesthetized children. Anesth Analg 1993;76:1238–1242.

513. Cressman WA, Plostnieks J, Johnson PC: Absorption, metabolism and excretion of droperidol by human subjects following intramuscular and intravenous administration. Anesthesiology 1973;38:363–369.

514. Whitwam JG, Russell WJ: The acute cardiovascular changes and adrenergic blockade by droperidol in man. Br J Anaesth 1971;43:581–591.

515. Long G, Dripps RD, Price HL: Measurement of anti-arrhythmic potency of drugs in man: Effects of dehydrobenzperidol. Anesthesiology 1967;28:318–323.

516. Kallos T, Wyche MQ, Garman JK: The effects of Innovar on functional residual capacity and total chest compliance in man. Anesthesiology 1973;39:558–561.

517. Cottrell JE, Wolfson B, Siker ES: Changes in airway resistance following droperidol, hydroxyzine, and diazepam in normal volunteers. Anesth Analg 1976;55:18–21.

518. Prokocimer P, Delavault E, Rey F, et al: Effects of droperidol on respiratory drive in humans. Anesthesiology 1983;59:113–116.

519. Kay B: Neuroleptanesthesia for neonates and infants. Anesth Analg 1973;52:970–973.

520. McGarry PM: A double-blind study of diazepam, droperidol, and meperidine as premedication in children. Can Anaesth Soc J 1970;17:157–165.

521. Misfeldt BB, Jorgensen PB, Spotoft H, et al: The effects of droperidol and fentanyl on intracranial pressure and cerebral perfusion pressure in neurosurgical patients. Br J Anaesth 1976;48:963–968.

522. Stanski DR, Greenblatt DJ, Lowenstein E: Kinetics of intravenous and intramuscular morphine. Clin Pharmacol Ther 1978;24:52–59.

523. Dahlstrom B, Bolme P, Feychting H, et al: Morphine kinetics in children. Clin Pharmacol Ther 1979;26:354–365.

524. Dagan O, Klein J, Bohn D, et al: Morphine pharmacokinetics in children following cardiac surgery: Effects of disease and inotropic support. J Cardiothorac Vasc Anesth 1993;7:396–398.

525. Barrett DA, Barker DP, Rutter N, et al: Morphine, morphine-6-glucuronide and morphine-3-glucuronide pharmacokinetics in newborn infants receiving diamorphine infusions. Br J Clin Pharmacol 1996;41:531–537.

526. Geiduschek JM, Lynn AM, Bratton SL, et al: Morphine pharmacokinetics during continuous infusion of morphine sulfate for infants receiving extracorporeal membrane oxygenation. Crit Care Med 1997;25:360–364.

527. Lynn AM, Opheim KE, Tyler DC: Morphine infusion after pediatric cardiac surgery. Crit Care Med 1984;123:863–866.

528. Dampier CD, Setty BN, Logan J, et al: Intravenous morphine pharmacokinetics in pediatric patients with sickle cell disease. J Pediatr 1995;126:461–467.

529. Lynn A, Nespeca MK, Bratton SL, et al: Clearance on morphine in postoperative infants during intravenous infusion: The influence of age and surgery. Anesth Analg 1998;86:958–963.

530. Bhat R, Abu-Harb M, Chari G, et al: Morphine metabolism in acutely ill preterm infants. J Pediatr 1992;120:795–799.

531. Kart T, Christrup LL, Rasmussen M: Recommended use of morphine in neonates, infants and children based on a literature review: Part 1. Pharmacokinetics. Paediatr Anaesth 1997;7:5–11.

532. Lynn AM, Nespeca MK, Opheim KE, et al: Respiratory effects of intravenous morphine infusions in neonates, infants, and children after cardiac surgery. Anesth Analg 1993;77:695–701.

533. Weil JV, McCullough RE, Kline JS, et al: Diminished ventilatory response to hypoxia and hypercapnia after morphine in normal man. N Engl J Med 1975;292:1103–1106.

534. Way WL, Costley EC, Way EI: Respiratory sensitivity of the newborn infant to meperidine and morphine. Clin Pharmacol Ther 1965;6:454–461.

535. Meuldermans WE, Hurkmans RM, Heykants JJ: Plasma protein binding and distribution of fentanyl, sufentanil, alfentanil and lofentanil in blood. Arch Int Pharmacodyn Ther 1982;257:4–19.

536. McClain DA, Hug CC Jr: Intravenous fentanyl kinetics. Clin Pharmacol Ther 1980;28:106–114.

537. Bragg P, Zwass MS, Lau M, et al: Opioid pharmacodynamics in neonatal dogs: Differences between morphine and fentanyl. J Appl Physiol 1995;79:1519–1524.

538. Moss J, Rosow CE: Histamine release by narcotics and muscle relaxants in humans. Anesthesiology 1983;59:330–339.

539. Gong L, Middleton RK: Sublingual administration of opioids. Ann Pharmacol 1992;26:1525–1527.

540. Haberkern CM, Lynn AM, Geiduschek JM, et al: Epidural and intravenous bolus morphine for postoperative analgesia in infants. Can J Anaesth 1996;43:1203–1210.

541. Nichols DG, Yaster M, Lynn AM, et al: Disposition and respiratory effects of intrathecal morphine in children. Anesthesiology 1993;79:733–738.

542. Fisher AP, Vine P, Whitlock J, et al: Buccal morphine premedication: A double-blind comparison with intramuscular morphine. Anaesthesia 1986;41:1104–1111.

543. Fisher AP, Fung C, Hanna M: Absorption of buccal morphine: A comparison with slow-release morphine sulphate. Anaesthesia 1988;43:552–553.

544. Westerling D: Rectally administered morphine: Plasma concentrations in children premedicated with morphine in hydrogel and in solution. Acta Anaesthesiol Scand 1985;29:653–656.

545. Chrubasik J, Wust H, Friedrich G, et al: Absorption and bioavailability of nebulized morphine. Br J Anaesth 1988;61:228–230.

546. Bozkurt P, Kaya G, Yeker Y: Single-injection lumbar epidural morphine for postoperative analgesia in children: A report of 175 cases. Reg Anesth 1997;22:212–217.

547. Lundeberg S, Beck O, Olsson GL, et al: Rectal administration of morphine in children: Pharmacokinetic evaluation after a single dose. Acta Anaesthesiol Scand 1996;40:445–451.

548. Gourlay GK, Boas RA: Fatal outcome with use of rectal morphine for postoperative pain control in an infant. Br Med J 1992;304:766–767.

549. Flacke JW, Flacke WE, Bloor BC, et al: Histamine release by four narcotics: A double-blind study in humans. Anesth Analg 1987;66:723–730.

550. Mather LE, Tucker GT, Pflug AE, et al: Meperidine kinetics in

man: Intravenous injection in surgical patients and volunteers. Clin Pharmacol Ther 1975;17:21–30.

551. Jacobsen J, Flachs H, Dich-Nielsen JO, et al: Comparative plasma concentration profiles after I.V., I.M. and rectal administration of pethidine in children. Br J Anaesth 1988;60:623–626.

552. Stambaugh JE, Wainer IW, Sanstead JK, et al: The clinical pharmacology of meperidine: Comparison of routes of administration. J Clin Pharmacol 1976;16:245–256.

553. Hamunen K, Maunuksela EL, Seppala T, et al: Pharmacokinetics of I.V. and rectal pethidine in children undergoing ophthalmic surgery. Br J Anaesth 1993;71:823–826.

554. Pokela ML, Olkkola KT, Koivisto M, et al: Pharmacokinetics and pharmacodynamics of intravenous meperidine in neonates and infants. Clin Pharmacol Ther 1992;52:342–349.

555. Varma RR, Whitesell RC, Iskandarani MM: Halothane hepatitis without halothane: Role of inapparent circuit contamination and its prevention. Hepatology 1985;5:1159–1162.

556. Armstrong PJ, Bersten A: Normeperidine toxicity. Anesth Analg 1986;65:536–538.

557. Macintyre PE, Pavlin EG, Dwersteg JF: Effect of meperidine on oxygen consumption, carbon dioxide production, and respiratory gas exchange in postanesthesia shivering. Anesth Analg 1987;66:751–755.

558. Hagmeyer KO, Mauro LS, Mauro VF: Meperidine-related seizures associated with patient-controlled analgesia pumps. Ann Pharmacother 1993;27:29–32.

559. Collins C, Koren G, Crean P, et al: Fentanyl pharmacokinetics and hemodynamic effects in preterm infants during ligation of patent ductus arteriosus. Anesth Analg 1985;64:1078–1080.

560. Koehntop DE, Rodman JH, Brundage DM, et al: Pharmacokinetics of fentanyl in neonates. Anesth Analg 1986;65:227–232.

561. Koren G, Goresky G, Crean P, et al: Pediatric fentanyl dosing based on pharmacokinetics during cardiac surgery. Anesth Analg 1984;63:577–582.

562. Singleton MA, Rosen JI, Fisher DM: Plasma concentrations of fentanyl in infants, children and adults. Can J Anaesth 1987;34:152–155.

563. Gauntlett IS, Fisher DM, Hertzka RE, et al: Pharmacokinetics of fentanyl in neonatal humans and lambs: Effects of age. Anesthesiology 1988;69:683–687.

564. Yaster M: The dose response of fentanyl in neonatal anesthesia. Anesthesiology 1987;66:433–435.

565. Hickey PR, Hansen DD, Wessel DL, et al: Blunting of stress responses in the pulmonary circulation of infants by fentanyl. Anesth Analg 1985;64:1137–1142.

566. Hickey PR, Hansen DD, Wessel DL, et al: Pulmonary and systemic hemodynamic responses to fentanyl in infants. Anesth Analg 1985;64:483–486.

567. Hansen DD, Hickey PR: Anesthesia for hypoplastic left heart syndrome: Use of high-dose fentanyl in 30 neonates. Anesth Analg 1986;65:127–132.

568. Hickey PR, Hansen DD: Fentanyl- and sufentanil-oxygen-pancuronium anesthesia for cardiac surgery in infants. Anesth Analg 1984;63:117–124.

569. Robinson S, Gregory GA: Fentanyl-air-oxygen anesthesia for ligation of patent ductus arteriosus in preterm infants. Anesth Analg 1981;60:331–334.

570. Anand KJS, Sippell WG, Aynsley-Green A: Randomized trial of fentanyl anaesthesia in preterm babies undergoing surgery: Effects on the stress response. Lancet 1987;1:62–66.

571. Ashburn MA, Streisand J, Zhang J, et al: The iontophoresis of fentanyl citrate in humans. Anesthesiology 1995;82:1146–1153.

572. Santeiro ML, Christie J, Stromquist C, et al: Pharmacokinetics of continuous infusion fentanyl in newborns. J Perinatol 1997;17:135–139.

573. Jacqz-Aigrain E, Burtin P: Clinical pharmacokinetics of sedatives in neonates. Clin Pharmacokinet 1996;31:423–443.

574. Ginsberg B, Howell S, Glass PS, et al: Pharmacokinetic model-driven infusion of fentanyl in children. Anesthesiology 1996;85:1268–1275.

575. Koren G, Goresky G, Crean P, et al: Unexpected alterations in fentanyl pharmacokinetics in children undergoing cardiac surgery: Age related or disease related? Dev Pharmacol Ther 1986;9:183–191.

576. McClain DA, Hug CC Jr: Pharmacodynamics of opiates. Int Anesthesiol Clin 1984;22:75–94.

577. Mather LE: Clinical pharmacokinetics of fentanyl and its newer derivatives. Clin Pharmacokinet 1983;8:422–446.

578. Kuhls E, Gauntlett IS, Lau M, et al: Effect of increased intra-abdominal pressure on hepatic extraction and clearance of fentanyl in neonatal lambs. J Pharmacol Exp Ther 1995;274:115–119.

579. Burtin P, Daoud P, Jacqz-Aigrain E, et al: Hypotension with midazolam and fentanyl in the newborn. Lancet 1991;337:1545–1546.

580. Koren G, Barker C, Goresky G, et al: The influence of hypothermia on the disposition of fentanyl: Human and animal studies. Eur J Clin Pharmacol 1987;32:373–376.

581. Katz R, Kelly HW: Pharmacokinetics of continuous infusions of fentanyl in critically ill children. Crit Care Med 1993;21:995–1000.

582. Katz R, Kelly HW, Hsi A: Prospective study on the occurrence of withdrawal in critically ill children who receive fentanyl by continuous infusion. Crit Care Med 1994;22:763–767.

583. Bergman I, Steeves M, Burckart G, et al: Reversible neurologic abnormalities associated with prolonged intravenous midazolam and fentanyl administration. J Pediatr 1991;119:644–649.

584. Murphy MR, Hug CC Jr, McClain DA: Dose-independent pharmacokinetics of fentanyl. Anesthesiology 1983;59:537–540.

585. Murphy MR, Olson WA, Hug CC Jr: Pharmacokinetics of 3H-fentanyl in the dog anesthetized with enflurane. Anesthesiology 1979;50:13–19.

586. Stoeckel H, Hengstmann JH, Schuttler J: Pharmacokinetics of fentanyl as a possible explanation for recurrence of respiratory depression. Br J Anaesth 1979;51:741–745.

587. Hug CC Jr, Murphy MR: Fentanyl disposition in cerebrospinal fluid and plasma and its relationship to ventilatory depression in the dog. Anesthesiology 1979;50:342–349.

588. Hertzka RE, Gauntlett IS, Fisher DM, et al: Fentanyl-induced ventilatory depression: Effects of age. Anesthesiology 1989;70:213–218.

589. Pathak KS, Brown RH, Nash CL Jr, et al: Continuous opioid infusion for scoliosis fusion surgery. Anesth Analg 1983;62:841–845.

590. Mather LE: Pharmacokinetics and patient-controlled analgesia. Acta Anaesthesiol Belg 1992;43:5–20.

591. Tobias JD, Baker DK: Patient-controlled analgesia with fentanyl in children. Clin Pediatr (Phila) 1992;31:177–179.

592. Sokoll MD, Hoyt JL, Gergis SD: Studies in muscle rigidity, nitrous oxide, and narcotic analgesic agents. Anesth Analg 1972;51:16–20.

593. Askgaard B, Nilsson T, Ibler M, et al: Muscle tone under fentanyl-nitrous oxide anaesthesia measured with a transducer apparatus in cholecystectomy incisions. Acta Anaesthesiol Scand 1977;21:1–4.

594. Scamman FL: Fentanyl-O_2-N_2O rigidity and pulmonary compliance. Anesth Analg 1983;62:332–334.

595. Arandia HY, Patil VU: Glottic closure following large doses of fentanyl. Anesthesiology 1987;66:574–575.

596. Wells S, Williamson M, Hooker D: Fentanyl-induced chest wall rigidity in a neonate: A case report. Heart Lung 1994;23:196–198.

597. Streisand JB, Bailey PL, LeMaire L, et al: Fentanyl-induced rigidity and unconsciousness in human volunteers: Incidence, duration, and plasma concentrations. Anesthesiology 1993;78:629–634.

598. Murat I, Levron JC, Berg A, et al: Effects of fentanyl on baroreceptor reflex control of heart rate in newborn infants. Anesthesiology 1988;68:717–722.

599. Feld LH, Champeau MW, van Steennis CA, et al: Preanesthetic medication in children: A comparison of oral transmucosal fentanyl citrate versus placebo. Anesthesiology 1989;71:374–377.

600. Lind GH, Marcus MA, Mears SL, et al: Oral transmucosal fentanyl citrate for analgesia and sedation in the emergency department. Ann Emerg Med 1991;20:1117–1120.

601. Goldstein-Dresner MC, Davis PJ, Kretchman E, et al: Double-blind comparison of oral transmucosal fentanyl citrate with oral meperidine, diazepam, and atropine as preanesthetic medication in children with congenital heart disease. Anesthesiology 1991;74:28–33.

602. Friesen RH, Lockhart CH: Oral transmucosal fentanyl citrate for preanesthetic medication of pediatric day surgery patients with and without droperidol as a prophylactic anti-emetic. Anesthesiology 1992;76:46–51.

603. Epstein RH, Mendel HG, Witkowski TA, et al: The safety and efficacy of oral transmucosal fentanyl citrate for preoperative sedation in young children. Anesth Analg 1996;83:1200–1205.

604. Dsida RM, Wheeler M, Birmingham PK, et al: Premedication of pediatric tonsillectomy patients with oral transmucosal fentanyl citrate. Anesth Analg 1998;86:66–70.

605. Ridout G, Santus GC, Guy RH: Pharmacokinetic considerations in the use of newer transdermal formulations. Clin Pharmacokinet 1988;15:114–131.

606. Portenoy RK, Southam MA, Gupta SK, et al: Transdermal fentanyl for cancer pain: Repeated dose pharmacokinetics. Anesthesiology 1993;78:36–43.
607. Berner B, John VA: Pharmacokinetic characterization of transdermal delivery systems. Clinical Pharmacokinetics 1994;26:121–134.
608. Calis KA, Kohler DR, Corso DM: Transdermally administered fentanyl for pain management. Clin Pharmacy 1992;11:22–36.
609. Duthie DJR, Rowbotham DJ, Wyld R, et al: Plasma fentanyl concentrations during transdermal delivery of fentanyl to surgical patients. Br J Anaesth 1988;60:614–618.
610. Lehmann KA, Zech D: Transdermal fentanyl: Clinical pharmacology. J Pain Symptom Manage 1992;7(Suppl):S8–S16.
611. Simmonds MA, Richenbacher J: Transdermal fentanyl: Long-term analgesic studies. J Pain Symptom Manage 1992;7:S36–S39.
612. Skaer TL: Management of pain in the cancer patient. Clin Ther 1993;15:638–649.
613. Varvel JR, Shafer SL, Hwang SS, et al: Absorption characteristics of transdermally administered fentanyl. Anesthesiology 1989;70:928–934.
614. Southam MA: Transdermal fentanyl therapy: System design, pharmacokinetics and efficacy. Anti-Cancer Drugs 1995;6(Suppl 3):29–34.
615. Roy SD, Flynn GL: Transdermal delivery of narcotic analgesics: pH, anatomical, and subject influences on cutaneous permeability of fentanyl and sufentanil. Pharm Res 1990;7:842–847.
616. Roy SD, Flynn GL: Transdermal delivery of narcotic analgesics: Comparative permeabilities of narcotic analgesics through human cadaver skin. Pharm Res 1989;6:825–832.
617. Payne R, Chandler S, Einhaus M: Guidelines for the clinical use of transdermal fentanyl. Anti-Cancer Drugs 1995;6(Suppl 3):50–53.
618. Collins JJ, Dunkel IJ, Gupta SK, et al: Transdermal fentanyl in children with cancer pain: Feasibility, tolerability, and pharmacokinetic correlates. J Pediatr 1999;134:319–323.
619. Clotz MA, Nahata MC: Clinical uses of fentanyl, sufentanil, and alfentanil. Clin Pharm 1991;10:581–593.
620. Scholz J, Steinfath M, Schulz M: Clinical pharmacokinetics of alfentanil, fentanyl and sufentanil: An update. Clin Pharmacokinet 1996;31:275–292.
621. Meuldermans W, Van Peer A, Hendrickx J, et al: Alfentanil pharmacokinetics and metabolism in humans. Anesthesiology 1988;69:527–534.
622. Meistelman C, Saint-Maurice C, Lepaul M, et al: A comparison of alfentanil pharmacokinetics in children and adults. Anesthesiology 1987;66:13–16.
623. Roure P, Jean N, Leclerc AC, et al: Pharmacokinetics of alfentanil in children undergoing surgery. Br J Anaesth 1987;59:1437–1440.
624. Goresky GV, Koren G, Sabourin MA, et al: The pharmacokinetics of alfentanil in children. Anesthesiology 1987;67:654–659.
625. Persson MP, Nilsson A, Hartvig P: Pharmacokinetics of alfentanil in total I.V. anaesthesia. Br J Anaesth 1988;60:755–761.
626. Shafer A, Sung ML, White PF: Pharmacokinetics and pharmacodynamics of alfentanil infusions during general anesthesia. Anesth Analg 1986;65:1021–1028.
627. Chauvin M, Bonnet F, Montembault C, et al: The influence of hepatic plasma flow on alfentanil plasma concentration plateaus achieved with an infusion model in humans: Measurement of alfentanil hepatic extraction coefficient. Anesth Analg 1986;65:999–1003.
628. Davis PJ, Killian A, Stiller RL, et al: Pharmacokinetics of alfentanil in newborn premature infants and older children. Dev Pharmacol Ther 1989;13:21–27.
629. Killian A, Davis PJ, Stiller RL, et al: Influence of gestational age on pharmacokinetics of alfentanil in neonates. Dev Pharmacol Ther 1990;15:82–85.
630. Chauvin M, Lebrault C, Levron JC, et al: Pharmacokinetics of alfentanil in chronic renal failure. Anesth Analg 1987;66:53–56.
631. McConaghy P, Bunting HE: Assessment of intubating conditions in children after induction with propofol and varying doses of alfentanil. Br J Anaesth 1994;73:596–599.
632. Davis PJ, Stiller RL, Cook DR, et al: Pharmacokinetics of sufentanil in adolescent patients with chronic renal failure. Anesth Analg 1988;67:268–271.
633. Chauvin M, Ferrier C, Haberer JP, et al: Sufentanil pharmacokinetics in patients with cirrhosis. Anesth Analg 1989;68:1–4.
634. Greeley WJ, de Bruijn NP: Changes in sufentanil pharmacokinetics within the neonatal period. Anesth Analg 1988;67:86–90.
635. Greeley WJ, de Bruijn NP, Davis DP: Sufentanil pharmacokinetics in pediatric cardiovascular patients. Anesth Analg 1987;66:1067–1072.

636. Davis PJ, Cook DR, Stiller RL, et al: Pharmacodynamics and pharmacokinetics of high-dose sufentanil in infants and children undergoing cardiac surgery. Anesth Analg 1987;66:203–208.
637. Spiess BD, Sathoff RH, el-Ganzouri AR, et al: High-dose sufentanil: Four cases of sudden hypotension on induction. Anesth Analg 1986;65:703–705.
638. Starr NJ, Sethna DH, Estafanous FG: Bradycardia and asystole following the rapid administration of sufentanil with vecuronium. Anesthesiology 1986;64:521–523.
639. Zedie N, Amory DW, Wagner BK, et al: Comparison of intranasal midazolam and sufentanil premedication in pediatric outpatients. Clin Pharmacol Ther 1996;59:341–348.
640. Karl HW, Keifer AT, Rosenberger JL, et al: Comparison of the safety and efficacy of intranasal midazolam or sufentanil for preinduction of anesthesia in pediatric patients. Anesthesiology 1992;76:209–215.
641. Henderson JM, Brodsky DA, Fisher DM, et al: Preinduction of anesthesia in pediatric patients with nasally administered sufentanil. Anesthesiology 1988;68:671–675.
642. Thompson JP, Rowbotham DJ: Remifentanil: An opioid for the 21st century. Br J Anaesth 1996;76:341–343.
643. Egan TD: Remifentanil pharmacokinetics and pharmacodynamics: A preliminary appraisal. Clin Pharmacokinet 1995;29:80–94.
644. Egan TD, Lemmens HJ, Fiset P, et al: The pharmacokinetics of the new short-acting opioid remifentanil (GI87084B) in healthy adult male volunteers. Anesthesiology 1993;79:881–892.
645. Rosow C: Remifentanil: A unique opioid analgesic. Anesthesiology 1993;79:875–876.
646. Westmoreland CL, Hoke JF, Sebel PS, et al: Pharmacokinetics of remifentanil (GI87084B) and its major metabolite (GI90291) in patients undergoing elective inpatient surgery. Anesthesiology 1993;79:893–903.
647. Hoke JF, Shlugman D, Dershwitz M, et al: Pharmacokinetics and pharmacodynamics of remifentanil in persons with renal failure compared with healthy volunteers. Anesthesiology 1997;87:533–541.
648. Dershwitz M, Rosow CE: The pharmacokinetics and pharmacodynamics of remifentanil in volunteers with severe hepatic or renal dysfunction. J Clin Anesth 1996;8(Suppl):88S–90S.
649. Kapila A, Glass PS, Jacobs JR, et al: Measured context-sensitive halftimes of remifentanil and alfentanil. Anesthesiology 1995;83:968–975.
650. Vinik HR, Kissin I: Rapid development of tolerance to analgesia during remifentanil infusion in humans. Anesth Analg 1998;86:1307–1311.
651. Lynn AM: Remifentanil: The paediatric anaesthetist's opiate? Pediatr Anaesth 1996;6:433–435.
652. Davis PJ, Lerman J, Suresh S, et al: A randomized multicenter study of remifentanil compared with alfentanil, isoflurane, or propofol in anesthetized pediatric patients undergoing elective strabismus surgery. Anesth Analg 1997;84:982–989.
653. DeSouza G, Lewis MC, TerRiet MF: Severe bradycardia after remifentanil. Anesthesiology 1997;87:1019–1020.
654. Errick JK, Heel RC: Nalbuphine: A preliminary review of its pharmacological properties and therapeutic efficacy. Drugs 1983;26:191–211.
655. Rosow CE: The clinical usefulness of agonist-antagonist analgesics in acute pain. Drug Alcohol Depend 1987;20:329–337.
656. Heel RC, Brogden RN, Speight TM, et al: Butorphanol: A review of its pharmacological properties and therapeutic efficacy. Drugs 1978;16:473–505.
657. Lo MW, Lee FH, Schary WL, et al: The pharmacokinetics of intravenous, intramuscular, and subcutaneous nalbuphine in healthy subjects. Eur J Clin Pharmacol 1987;33:297–301.
658. Lo MW, Schary WL, Whitney CCJ: The disposition and bioavailability of intravenous and oral nalbuphine in healthy volunteers. J Clin Pharmacol 1987;27:866–873.
659. Jaillon P, Gardin ME, Lecocq B, et al: Pharmacokinetics of nalbuphine in infants, young healthy volunteers, and elderly patients. Clin Pharmacol Ther 1989;46:226–233.
660. Gal TJ, DiFazio CA, Moscicki J: Analgesic and respiratory depressant activity of nalbuphine: A comparison with morphine. Anesthesiology 1982;57:367–374.
661. Bowdle TA: Clinical pharmacology of antagonists of narcotic-induced respiratory depression: A brief review. Acute Care 1988;12:70–76.
662. Rosow CE: Butorphanol in perspective. Acute Care 1988;12(Suppl 1):2–7.
663. Tobias JD, Rasmussen GE: Transnasal butorphanol for postoperative

analgesia following paediatric surgery in a Third World country. Pediatr Anaesth 1995;5:63–66.

664. Splinter WM, O'Brien HV, Komocar L: Butorphanol: An opioid for day-care paediatric surgery. Can J Anaesth 1995;42:483–486.

665. Habre W, McLeod B: Analgesic and respiratory effect of nalbuphine and pethidine for adenotonsillectomy in children with obstructive sleep disorder. Anaesthesia 1997;52:1101–1106.

666. Buttner W, Finke W, Schwanitz M: Nalbuphine and piritramid in the postoperative period in young children. 2. External respiration. Anaesthesist 1990;39:258–263.

667. Krishnan A, Tolhurst-Cleaver CL, Kay B: Controlled comparison of nalbuphine and morphine for post-tonsillectomy pain. Anaesthesia 1985;40:1178–1181.

668. Vachharajani NN, Shyu WC, Greene DS, et al: The pharmacokinetics of butorphanol and its metabolites at steady state following nasal administration in humans. Biopharm Drug Dispos 1997;18:191–202.

669. Bennie RE, Boehringer LA, Dierdorf SF, et al: Transnasal butorphanol is effective for postoperative pain relief in children undergoing myringotomy. Anesthesiology 1998;89:385–390.

670. Lehmann KA: Tramadol for the management of acute pain. Drugs 1994;47:19–32.

671. Lee CR, McTavish D, Sorkin EM: Tramadol: A preliminary review of its pharmacodynamic and pharmacokinetic properties, and therapeutic potential in acute and chronic pain states. Drugs 1993;46:313–340.

672. Schaffer J, Piepenbrock S, Kretz FJ, et al: Nalbuphine and tramadol for the control of postoperative pain in children. [in German]. Anaesthetist 1986;35:408–413.

673. Forrest JB, Heitlinger EL, Revell S: Ketorolac for postoperative pain management in children. Drug Saf 1997;16:309–329.

674. Gillis JC, Brogden RN: Ketorolac: A reappraisal of its pharmacodynamic and pharmacokinetic properties and therapeutic use in pain management. Drugs 1997;53:139–188.

675. Houck CS, Wilder RT, McDermott JS, et al: Safety of intravenous ketorolac therapy in children and cost savings with a unit dosing system. J Pediatr 1996;129:292–296.

676. Buckley MMT, Brogden RN: Ketorolac: A review of its pharmacodynamic and pharmacokinetic properties, and therapeutic potential. Drugs 1990;39:86–109.

677. Olkkola KT, Maunuksela EL: The pharmacokinetics of postoperative intravenous ketorolac tromethamine in children. Br J Clin Pharmacol 1991;31:182–184.

678. Gonzalez-Martin G, Maggio L, Gonzalez-Sotomayor J, et al: Pharmacokinetics of ketorolac in children after abdominal surgery. Int J Clin Pharmacol Ther 1997;35:160–163.

679. Dsida RM, Wheeler M, Birmingham PK, et al: Developmental pharmacokinetics of intravenous ketorolac in pediatric surgical patients. Anesthesiology 1997;87:A1055.

680. Watcha MF, Jones MB, Lagueruela RG, et al: Comparison of ketorolac and morphine as adjuvants during pediatric surgery. Anesthesiology 1992;76:368–372.

681. Buck ML: Clinical experience with ketorolac in children. Ann Pharmacother 1994;28:1009–1013.

682. Maunuksela EL, Kokki H, Bullingham RE: Comparison of intravenous ketorolac with morphine for postoperative pain in children. Clin Pharmacol Ther 1992;52:436–443.

683. Spowart K, Greer IA, McLaren M, et al: Haemostatic effects of ketorolac with and without concomitant heparin in normal volunteers. Thromb Haemost 1988;60:382–386.

684. Conrad KA, Fagan TC, Mackie MJ, et al: Effects of ketorolac tromethamine on hemostasis in volunteers. Clin Pharmacol Ther 1988;43:542–546.

685. Camu F, Lauwers MH, Vanlersberghe C: Side effects of NSAIDs and dosing recommendations for ketorolac. Acta Anaesthesiol Belg 1996;47:143–149.

686. Splinter WM, Rhine EJ, Roberts DW, et al: Preoperative ketorolac increases bleeding after tonsillectomy in children. Can J Anaesth 1996;43:560–563.

687. Hall SC: Tonsillectomies, ketorolac, and the march of progress. Can J Anaesth 1996;43:544–548.

688. Gunter JB, Varughese AM, Harrington JF, et al: Recovery and complications after tonsillectomy in children: A comparison of ketorolac and morphine. Anesth Analg 1995;81:1136–1141.

689. Bean-Lijewski JD, Hunt RD: Effect of ketorolac on bleeding time and postoperative pain in children: A double-blind, placebo-controlled comparison with meperidine. J Clin Anesth 1996;8:25–30.

690. Agrawal A, Gerson CR, Seligman I, et al: Postoperative hemorrhage after tonsillectomy: use of ketorolac tromethamine. Otolaryngol Head Neck Surg 1999;120:335–339.

691. Foster PN, Williams JG: Bradycardia following intravenous ketorolac in children. Eur J Anaesthesiol 1997;14:307–309.

692. Rusy LM, Houck CS, Sullivan LJ, et al: A double-blind evaluation of ketorolac tromethamine versus acetaminophen in pediatric tonsillectomy: Analgesia and bleeding. Anesth Analg 1995;80:226–229.

693. Wheeler M, Tobin MJ, Birmingham PK, Coté CJ, Henthorn TK, Kennedy-Mooney SH: Pharmacokinetics and dose response for oral acetaminophen in children. Anesthesiology 1997;87:A1054.

694. Birmingham PK, Tobin MJ, Henthorn TK, et al: Twenty-four-hour pharmacokinetics of rectal acetaminophen in children: An old drug with new recommendations. Anesthesiology 1997;87:244–252.

695. Montgomery CJ, McCormack JP, Reichert CC, et al: Plasma concentrations after high-dose (45 mg.kg-1) rectal acetaminophen in children. Can J Anaesth 1995;42:982–986.

696. Houck CS, Sullivan LJ, Wilder RT, Rusy LM, Burrows FA: Pharmacokinetics of a higher dose of rectal acetaminophen in children. Anesthesiology 1995;83:A1126.

697. Birmingham PK, Tobin MJ, Henthorn TK, Kennedy-Mooney SH, Coté CJ: "Loading" and subsequent dosing of rectal acetaminophen in children: A 24-hour pharmacokinetic study of new dosing recommendations. Anesthesiology 1996;85:A1105.

698. Korpela R, Korvenoja P, Meretoja OA: Morphine-sparing effect of acetaminophen in pediatric day-case surgery. Anesthesiology 1999; 91:442–447.

699. Rumack BH, Peterson RC, Koch GG, et al: Acetaminophen overdose: 662 cases with evaluation of oral acetylcysteine treatment. Arch Intern Med 1981;141:380–385.

700. Rumack BH, Matthew H: Acetaminophen poisoning and toxicity. Pediatrics 1975;55:871–876.

701. Mandelli M, Tognoni G, Garattini S: Clinical pharmacokinetics of diazepam. Clin Pharmacokinet 1978;3:72–91.

702. Gamble JA, Dundee JW, Assaf RA: Plasma diazepam levels after single-dose oral and intramuscular administration. Anaesthesia 1975;30:164–169.

703. Hillestad L, Hansen T, Melsom H, et al: Diazepam metabolism in normal man. I. Serum concentrations and clinical effects after intravenous, intramuscular, and oral administration. Clin Pharmacol Ther 1974;16:479–484.

704. Hillestad L, Hansen T, Melsom H: Diazepam metabolism in normal man. II. Serum concentration and clinical effect after oral administration and cumulation. Clin Pharmacol Ther 1974;16:485–489.

705. Fell D, Gough MB, Northan AA, et al: Diazepam premedication in children: Plasma levels and clinical effects. Anaesthesia 1985;40: 12–17.

706. Sonander H, Arnold E, Nilsson K: Effects of the rectal administration of diazepam. Diazepam concentrations in children undergoing general anaesthesia. Br J Anaesth 1985;57:578–580.

707. Mattila MA, Ruoppi MK, Ahlstrom-Bengs E, et al: Diazepam in rectal solution as premedication in children, with special reference to serum concentrations. Br J Anaesth 1981;53:1269–1272.

708. Haagensen RE: Rectal premedication in children: Comparison of diazepam with a mixture of morphine, scopolamine and diazepam. Anaesthesia 1985;40:956–959.

709. Klotz U, Avant GR, Hoyumpa A, et al: The effects of age and liver disease on the disposition and elimination of diazepam in adult man. J Clin Invest 1975;55:347–359.

710. Morselli PL, Mandelli M, Tognoni G, et al: Drug interactions in the human fetus and in the newborn infant. In: Morselli PL, Cohen SN, Gorattini S, eds: Drug Interactions. New York: Raven Press; 1974:259–270.

711. Meberg A, Langslet A, Bredesen JE, et al: Plasma concentration of diazepam and N-desmethyldiazepam in children after a single rectal or intramuscular dose of diazepam. Eur J Clin Pharmacol 1978; 14:273–276.

712. Kanto J: Plasma concentrations of diazepam and its metabolites after peroral, intramuscular, and rectal administration. Correlation between plasma concentration and sedatory effect of diazepam. Int J Clin Pharmacol Biopharm 1975;12:427–432.

713. Gershanik J, Boecler B, Ensley H, et al: The gasping syndrome and benzyl alcohol poisoning. N Engl J Med 1982;307:1384–1388.

714. American Academy of Pediatrics, Committee on Drugs: "Inactive" ingredients in pharmaceutical products. Pediatrics 1985;76:635–643.

715. Bailey PL, Andriano KP, Goldman M, et al: Variability of the respiratory response to diazepam. Anesthesiology 1986;64:460–465.

716. Smith MT, Eadie MJ, O'Rourke Brophy T: The pharmacokinetics of midazolam in man. Eur J Clin Pharmacol 1981;19:271–278.

717. Salonen M, Kanto J, Iisalo E, et al: Midazolam as an induction agent in children: A pharmacokinetic and clinical study. Anesth Analg 1987;66:625–628.

718. Persson P, Nilsson A, Hartvig P, et al: Pharmacokinetics of midazolam in total I.V. anaesthesia. Br J Anaesth 1987;59:548–556.

719. Rey E, Delaunay L, Pons G, et al: Pharmacokinetics of midazolam in children: Comparative study of intranasal and intravenous administration. Eur J Clin Pharmacol 1991;41:355–357.

720. Payne KA, Mattheyse FJ, Liebenberg D, et al: The pharmacokinetics of midazolam in paediatric patients. Eur J Clin Pharmacol 1989; 37:267–272.

721. Burtin P, Jacqz-Aigrain E, Girard P, et al: Population pharmacokinetics of midazolam in neonates. Clin Pharmacol Ther 1994;56:615–625.

722. Jacqz-Aigrain E, Wood E, Robieux I: Pharmacokinetics of midazolam in critically ill neonates. Eur J Clin Pharmacol 1990;36:191–192.

723. Trouvin JH, Farinotti R, Haberer JP, et al: Pharmacokinetics of midazolam in anaesthetized cirrhotic patients. Br J Anaesth 1988;60:762–767.

724. Mathews HM, Carson IW, Lyons SM, et al: A pharmacokinetic study of midazolam in paediatric patients undergoing cardiac surgery. Br J Anaesth 1988;61:302–307.

725. Adams P, Gelman S, Reves JG, et al: Midazolam pharmacodynamics and pharmacokinetics during acute hypovolemia. Anesthesiology 1985;63:140–146.

726. Grawe G, Ward RM: Seizure-like activity following bolus administration of midazolam to neonates. Clin Res 1994;42:16A.

727. Notterman DA: Sedation with intravenous midazolam in the pediatric intensive care unit. Clin Pediatr (Phila) 1997;36:449–454.

728. Hartvig P, Larsson E, Joachimsson PO: Postoperative analgesia and sedation following pediatric cardiac surgery using a constant infusion of ketamine. J Cardiothorac Vasc Anesth 1993;7:148–153.

729. Tobias JD, Rasmussen GE: Pain management and sedation in the pediatric intensive care unit. Pediatr Clin North Am 1994;41:1269–1292.

730. Kain ZN, Mayes LC, Bell C, et al: Premedication in the United States: A status report. Anesth Analg 1997;84:427–432.

731. Davis PJ, Tome JA, McGowan FX Jr, et al: Preanesthetic medication with intranasal midazolam for brief pediatric surgical procedures: Effect on recovery and hospital discharge times. Anesthesiology 1995;82:2–5.

732. Fosel T, Hack C, Knoll R, et al: Nasal midazolam in children, plasma concentrations and the effect on respiration. Paediatr Anaesth 1995;5:347–353.

733. Karl HW, Rosenberger JL, Larach MG, et al: Transmucosal administration of midazolam for premedication of pediatric patients: Comparison of the nasal and sublingual routes. Anesthesiology 1993;78:885–891.

734. Lejus C, Renaudin M, Testa S, et al: Midazolam for premedication in children: Nasal vs. rectal administration. Eur J Anaesthesiol 1997; 14:244–249.

735. Cray SH, Dixon JL, Heard CM, et al: Oral midazolam premedication for paediatric day case patients. Paediatr Anaesth 1996;6:265–270.

736. Levine MF, Spahr-Schopfer IA, Hartley E, et al: Oral midazolam premedication in children: The minimum time interval for separation from parents. Can J Anaesth 1993;40:726–729.

737. Suresh S, Cohen IJ, Matuszczak M, et al: Dose ranging, safety, and efficacy of a new oral midazolam syrup in children. Anesthesiology 1998;89:A1313.

738. Rita L, Seleny FL, Mazurek A, et al: Intramuscular midazolam for pediatric preanesthetic sedation: A double-blind controlled study with morphine. Anesthesiology 1985;63:528–531.

739. Holm-Knudsen R, Nygard E, Laub M: Rectal induction of anaesthesia in children: A comparison between ketamine-midazolam and halothane for induction and maintenance of anaesthesia. Acta Anaesthesiol Scand 1989;33:518–521.

740. De Jong PC, Verburg MP: Comparison of rectal to intramuscular administration of midazolam and atropine for premedication of children. Acta Anaesthesiol Scand 1988;32:485–489.

741. Taylor MB, Vine PR, Hatch DJ: Intramuscular midazolam premedication in small children. A comparison with papaveretum and hyoscine. Anaesthesia 1986;41:21–26.

742. Saarnivaara L, Lindgren L, Klemola U-M, et al: Comparison of chloral hydrate and midazolam by mouth as premedicants in children undergoing otolaryngological surgery. Br J Anaesth 1988;61:390–396.

743. Wilton NC, Leigh J, Rosen DR, et al: Preanesthetic sedation of preschool children using intranasal midazolam. Anesthesiology 1988;69:972–975.

744. Saint-Maurice C, Landais A, Delleur MM, et al: The use of midazolam in diagnostic and short surgical procedures in children. Acta Anaesthesiol Scand Suppl 1990;92:41–47.

745. Payne KA, Coetzee AR, Mattheyse FJ: Midazolam and amnesia in pediatric premedication. Acta Anaesthesio Belg 1991;42:101–105.

746. Twersky RS, Hartung J, Berger BJ, et al: Midazolam enhances anterograde but not retrograde amnesia in pediatric patients. Anesthesiology 1993;78:51–55.

747. Tolia V, Fleming SL, Kauffman RE: Randomized, double-blind trial of midazolam and diazepam for endoscopic sedation in children. Dev Pharmacol Ther 1990;14:141–147.

748. Buhrer M, Maitre PO, Hung O, et al: Electroencephalographic effects of benzodiazepines. I. Choosing an electroencephalographic parameter to measure the effect of midazolam on the central nervous system. Clin Pharmacol Ther 1990;48:544–554.

749. Buhrer M, Maitre PO, Crevoisier C, et al: Electroencephalographic effects of benzodiazepines. II. Pharmacodynamic modeling of the electroencephalographic effects of midazolam and diazepam. Clin Pharmacol Ther 1990;48:555–567.

750. Arendt RM, Greenblatt DJ, Liebisch DC, et al: Determinants of benzodiazepine brain uptake: Lipophilicity versus binding affinity. Psychopharmacology (Berlin) 1987;93:72–76.

751. Coté CJ: Sedation for the pediatric patient: A review. Pediatr Clin North Am 1994;41:31–58.

752. Alexander CM, Gross JB: Sedative doses of midazolam depress hypoxic ventilatory responses in humans. Anesth Analg 1988;67:377–382.

753. Yaster M, Nichols DG, Deshpande JK, et al: Midazolam-fentanyl intravenous sedation in children: Case report of respiratory arrest. Pediatrics 1990;86:463–467.

754. Gorski JC, Hall SD, Jones DR, et al: Regioselective biotransformation of midazolam by members of the human cytochrome P450 3A (CYP3A) subfamily. Biochem Pharmacol 1994;47:1643–1653.

755. Ameer B, Weintraub RA: Drug interactions with grapefruit juice. Clin Pharmacokinet 1997;33:103–121.

756. Bailey DG, Malcolm J, Arnold O, et al: Grapefruit juice–drug interactions. Br J Clin Pharmacol 1998;46:101–110.

757. Palkama VJ, Ahonen J, Neuvonen PJ, et al: Effect of saquinavir on the pharmacokinetics and pharmacodynamics of oral and intravenous midazolam. Clin Pharmacol Ther 1999;66:33–39.

758. Thummel KE, O'Shea D, Paine MF, et al: Oral first-pass elimination of midazolam involves both gastrointestinal and hepatic CYP3A-mediated metabolism. Clin Pharmacol Ther 1996;59:491–502.

759. Lees MH, Olsen GD, McGilliard KL, et al: Chloral hydrate and the carbon dioxide chemoreceptor response: A study of puppies and infants. Pediatrics 1982;70:447–450.

760. Fishbaugh DF, Wilson S, Preisch JW, et al: Relationship of tonsil size on an airway blockage maneuver in children during sedation. Pediatr Dent 1997;19:277–281.

761. Greenberg SB, Faerber EN: Respiratory insufficiency following chloral hydrate sedation in two children with Leigh disease (subacute necrotizing encephalomyelopathy). Pediatr Radiol 1990;20:287–288.

762. Biban P, Baraldi E, Pettenazzo A, et al: Adverse effect of chloral hydrate in two young children with obstructive sleep apnea. Pediatrics 1993;92:461–463.

763. Lindgren L, Saarnivaara L, Himberg JJ: Comparison of oral triclofos, diazepam and flunitrazepam as premedicants in children undergoing otolaryngological surgery. Br J Anaesth 1980;52:283–290.

764. Steinberg AD: Should chloral hydrate be banned? Pediatrics 1993; 92:442–446.

765. American Academy of Pediatrics, Committee on Drugs, Committee on Environmental Health: Use of chloral hydrate for sedation in children. Pediatrics 1993;92:471–473.

766. Reimche LD, Sankaran K, Hindmarsh KW, et al: Chloral hydrate sedation in neonates and infants: Clinical and pharmacologic considerations. Dev Pharmacol Ther 1989;12:57–64.

767. Mayers DJ, Hindmarsh KW, Sankaran K, et al: Chloral hydrate disposition following single-dose administration to critically ill neonates and children. Dev Pharm Ther 1991;16:71–77.

768. Kao SC, Adamson SD, Tatman LH, et al: A survey of post-discharge side effects of conscious sedation using chloral hydrate in pediatric CT and MR imaging. Pediatr Rad 1999;29:287–290.

769. Coté CJ, Notterman DA, Karl HW, et al: Adverse sedation events in pediatrics: A critical incident analysis of contributory factors. Pediatrics 2000;105:805–814.

770. Litman RS, Kottra JA, Verga KA, et al: Chloral hydrate sedation: The additive sedative and respiratory depressant effects of nitrous oxide. Anesth Analg 1998;86:724–728.

771. Goudsouzian NG, Coté CJ, Liu LM, et al: The dose-response effects of oral cimetidine on gastric pH and volume in children. Anesthesiology 1981;55:53–56.

772. Brunton LL: Agents for control of gastric acidity and treatment of peptic ulcers. In: Hardman JG, Limbird LE, Molinoff PB, et al, eds: Goodman & Gilman's The Pharmacological Basis of Therapeutics, 9th ed. New York: McGraw-Hill; 1996:904–907.

773. Powell JR, Donn KH: Histamine H_2-antagonist drug interactions in perspective: Mechanistic concepts and clinical implications. Am J Med 1984;77:57–84.

774. Somogyi A, Gugler R: Drug interactions with cimetidine. Clin Pharmacokinet 1982;7:23–41.

775. Smith K, Crisp C: Clinical comparison of H_2-antagonists. Conn Med 1986;50:815–817.

776. Eddleston JM, Booker PD, Green JR: Use of ranitidine in children undergoing cardiopulmonary bypass. Crit Care Med 1989;17:26–29.

777. Lopez-Herce Cid J, Albajara Velasco L, Codoceo R, et al: Ranitidine prophylaxis in acute gastric mucosal damage in critically ill pediatric patients. Crit Care Med 1988;16:591–593.

778. Blumer JL, Rothstein FC, Kaplan BS, et al: Pharmacokinetic determination of ranitidine pharmacodynamics in pediatric ulcer disease. J Pediatr 1985;107:301–306.

779. Goresky GV, Finley GA, Bissonnette B, et al: Efficacy, duration, and absorption of a paediatric oral liquid preparation of ranitidine hydrochloride. Can J Anaesth 1992;39:791–798.

780. Olsson GL, Hallen B: Pharmacological evacuation of the stomach with metoclopramide. Acta Anaesthesiol Scand 1982;26:417–420.

781. Albibi R, McCallum RW: Metoclopramide: pharmacology and clinical application. Ann Intern Med 1983;98:86–95.

782. Broadman LM, Ceruzzi W, Patane PS, et al: Metoclopramide reduces the incidence of vomiting following strabismus surgery in children. Anesthesiology 1990;72:245–248.

783. Ang C, Habre W, Sims C: Tropisetron reduces vomiting after tonsillectomy in children. Br J Anaesth 1998;80:761–763.

784. Simpson KH, Hicks FM: Clinical pharmacokinetics of ondansetron: A review. J Pharm Pharmacol 1996;48:774–781.

785. Adams VR, Valley AW: Granisetron: The second serotonin-receptor antagonist. Ann Pharmacother 1995;29:1240–1251.

786. Barst SM, Leiderman JU, Markowitz A, et al: Ondansetron with propofol reduces the incidence of emesis in children following tonsillectomy. Can J Anaesth 1999;46:359–362.

787. Davis A, Krige S, Moyes D: A double-blind randomized prospective study comparing ondansetron with droperidol in the prevention of emesis following strabismus surgery. Anaesth Intensive Care 1995; 23:438–443.

788. Davis PJ, McGowan FX Jr, Landsman I, et al: Effect of antiemetic therapy on recovery and hospital discharge time: A double-blind assessment of ondansetron, droperidol, and placebo in pediatric patients undergoing ambulatory surgery. Anesthesiology 1995;83:956–960.

789. Furst SR, Rodarte A: Prophylactic antiemetic treatment with ondansetron in children undergoing tonsillectomy. Anesthesiology 1994; 81:799–803.

790. Hamid SK, Selby IR, Sikich N, et al: Vomiting after adenotonsillectomy in children: A comparison of ondansetron, dimenhydrinate, and placebo. Anesth Analg 1998;86:496–500.

791. Khalil S, Rodarte A, Weldon BC, et al: Intravenous ondansetron in established postoperative emesis in children. S3A–381 Study Group. Anesthesiology 1996;85:270–276.

792. Litman RS, Wu CL, Lee A, et al: Prevention of emesis after strabismus repair in children: A prospective, double-blinded, randomized comparison of droperidol versus ondansetron. J Clin Anesth 1995;7:58–62.

793. Morton NS, Camu F, Dorman T, et al: Ondansetron reduces nausea and vomiting after paediatric adenotonsillectomy. Pediatr Anaesth 1997;7:37–45.

794. Rose JB, Martin TM: Posttonsillectomy vomiting. Ondansetron or metoclopramide during paediatric tonsillectomy: Are two doses better than one? Pediatr Anaesth 1996;6:39–44.

795. Splinter WM, Rhine EJ, Roberts DW, et al: Ondansetron is a better prophylactic antiemetic than droperidol for tonsillectomy in children. Can J Anaesth 1995;42:848–851.

796. Cieslak GD, Watcha MF, Phillips MB, et al: The dose-response relation and cost-effectiveness of granisetron for the prophylaxis of pediatric postoperative emesis. Anesthesiology 1996;85:1076–1085.

797. Stene FN, Seay RE, Young LA, et al: Prospective, randomized, double-blind, placebo-controlled comparison of metoclopramide and ondansetron for prevention of posttonsillectomy or adenotonsillectomy emesis. J Clin Anesth 1996;8:540–544.

798. Shende D, Mandal NG: Efficacy of ondansetron and metoclopramide for preventing postoperative emesis following strabismus surgery in children. Anaesthesia 1997;52:496–500.

799. Watcha MF, Smith I: Cost-effectiveness analysis of antiemetic therapy for ambulatory surgery. J Clin Anesth 1994;6:370–377.

800. Splinter WM, Baxter MR, Gould HM, et al: Oral ondansetron decreases vomiting after tonsillectomy in children. Can J Anaesth 1995;42:277–280.

801. Shutt LE, Bowes JB: Atropine and hyoscine. Anaesthesia 1979; 34:476–490.

802. Dauchot P, Gravenstein JS: Effects of atropine on the electrocardiogram in different age groups. Clin Pharmacol Ther 1971;12:274–280.

803. Harris WS, Goodman RM: Hyperreactivity to atropine in Down's syndrome. N Engl J Med 1968;279:407–410.

804. Kobel M, Creighton RE, Steward DJ: Anaesthetic considerations in Down's syndrome: Experience with 100 patients and a review of the literature. Can Anaesth Soc J 1982;29:593–599.

805. Wark HJ, Overton JH, Marian P: The safety of atropine premedication in children with Down's syndrome. Anaesthesia 1983;38:871–874.

806. Bejersten A, Olsson GL, Palmer L: The influence of body weight on plasma concentration of atropine after rectal administration in children. Acta Anaesthesiol Scand 1985;29:782–784.

807. Kanto J, Klotz U: Pharmacokinetic implications for the clinical use of atropine, scopolamine and glycopyrrolate. Acta Anaesthesiol Scand 1988;32:69–78.

808. Bray BM, Jones HM, Grundy EM: Tracheal versus intravenous atropine: A comparison of the effects on heart rate. Anaesthesia 1987;42:188–1190.

809. Saarnivaara L, Kautto UM, Iisalo E, et al: Comparison of pharmacokinetic and pharmacodynamic parameters following oral or intramuscular atropine in children: Atropine overdose in two small children. Acta Anaesthesiol Scand 1985;29:529–536.

810. Miller BR, Friesen RH: Oral atropine premedication in infants attenuates cardiovascular depression during halothane anesthesia. Anesth Analg 1988;67:180–185.

811. Opie JC, Chaye H, Steward DJ: Intravenous atropine rapidly reduces lower esophageal sphincter pressure in infants and children. Anesthesiology 1987;67:989–990.

812. Rautakorpi P, Ali-Melkkila T, Kaila T, et al: Pharmacokinetics of glycopyrrolate in children. J Clin Anesth 1994;6:217–220.

813. Ali-Melkkila T, Kaila T, Kanto J: Glycopyrrolate: Pharmacokinetics and some pharmacodynamic findings. Acta Anaesthesiol Scand 1989;33:513–517.

814. Mirakhur RK, Dundee JW, Clarke RS: Glycopyrrolate-neostigmine mixture for antagonism of neuromuscular block: Comparison with atropine-neostigmine mixture. Br J Anaesth 1977;49:825–829.

815. Mirakhur RK: Intravenous administration of glycopyrronium: Effects on cardiac rate and rhythm. Anaesthesia 1979;34:458–462.

816. Warran P, Radford P, Manford ML: Glycopyrrolate in children. Br J Anaesth 1981;53:1273–1276.

817. Salem MR, Wong AY, Mani M, et al: Premedicant drugs and gastric juice pH and volume in pediatric patients. Anesthesiology 1976; 44:216–219.

818. Ghoneim MM, Van Hamme MJ: Pharmacokinetics of thiopentone: Effects of enflurane and nitrous oxide anaesthesia and surgery. Br J Anaesth 1978;50:1237–1242.

819. Chantler C: Newborn Disorders. Clinical Pediatric Nephrology. Philadelphia: JB Lippincott; 1976:310–339.

820. Chantler C: Evaluation of laboratory and other methods of measuring renal function. In: Lieberman E, ed: Clinical Pediatric Nephrology. Philadelphia: JB Lippincott; 1976:510–527.

821. Merritt GJ, Slade JB: Influence of hyperbaric oxygen on the pharmacokinetics of single-dose gentamicin in healthy volunteers. Pharmacotherapy 1993;13:382–385.

822. Cameron CB, Robinson S, Gregory GA: The minimum anesthetic concentration of isoflurane in children. Anesth Analg 1984;63:418–420.

823. Gold MI, Abello D, Herrington C: Minimum alveolar concentration of desflurane in patients older than 65 yr. Anesthesiology 1993;79:710–714.

824. Jacqz-Aigrain E, Daoud P, Burtin P, et al: Pharmacokinetics of midazolam during continuous infusion in critically ill neonates. Eur J Clin Pharmacol 1992;42:329–332.

825. Abernethy DR, Greenblatt DJ: Effects of desmethyldiazepam on diazepam kinetics: A study of effects of a metabolite on parent drug disposition. Clin Pharmacol Ther 1981;29:757–761.

826. Greenblatt DJ, Divoll M, Abernethy DR, et al: Clinical pharmacokinetics of the newer benzodiazepines. Clin Pharmacokinet 1983;8:233–252.

827. Greenblatt DJ: Clinical pharmacokinetics of oxazepam and lorazepam. Clin Pharmacokinet 1981;6:89–105.

9

Premedication and Induction of Anesthesia

Leila Mei Pang, Letty M. P. Liu, *and* Charles J. Coté

Premedication
    General Principles
    Medications
Induction of Anesthesia
    Inhalation Induction
    Intravenous Induction
    Intramuscular Induction
    Rectal Induction
    Rapid-Sequence Induction
    Parental Presence During Induction

The preoperative period can be one of the more stressful experiences of a hospitalized child. Changes in the child's routine, separation from the parents, unfamiliar people and surroundings, uncertainty about the outcome of anesthesia and surgery, and fear of the unknown are just some of the things that produce stress. Eliminating or minimizing stress in the child and the family and providing conditions that will lead to a smooth, atraumatic induction of anesthesia can be accomplished by preparing the child both psychologically and pharmacologically during the preoperative period. Selecting appropriate premedications, which are administered in safe yet effective doses, is a primary responsibility of the anesthesiologist. This chapter focuses on the pharmacologic preparation of the child for anesthesia and anesthetic induction techniques.

Premedication

General Principles

The major objectives of preanesthetic medication are to (1) allay anxiety, (2) block autonomic (vagal) reflexes, (3) reduce airway secretions, (4) produce amnesia, (5) provide prophylaxis against pulmonary aspiration of gastric contents, (6) facilitate the induction of anesthesia, and (7) if necessary, provide analgesia. Premedication may also decrease the stress response to anesthesia and prevent cardiac arrhythmias.[1] The goal of premedication for each patient must be individualized. Light sedation, even though it may not eliminate anxiety, may adequately calm a child so the induction of anesthesia will be smooth and a pleasant experience. In contrast, heavy sedation may be needed for the very anxious patient.

Factors to consider when selecting a drug or a combination of drugs for premedication include the child's age, weight, drug history, and allergic status; underlying medical or surgical conditions and how they might affect the response to premedication or how the premedication might alter anesthetic induction; parent and child expectations; and the child's emotional maturity, personality, anxiety level, cooperation, and physiologic and psychological status. The anesthesiologist should also consider the proposed surgical procedure and the attitudes and wishes of the child and the parents.

Children of different ages vary in their response to the anesthetic experience (see Chapter 3). Predicting whether anxiety will be a problem in the preoperative period is not an easy task. Gender does not seem to make a difference in the degree of anxiety the patient experiences preoperatively; however, age is a predictor of which patients are at risk for anxiety.[2] Infants younger than 6 to 10 months generally tolerate short periods of separation from their parents. They are usually willing to accept a nurse or physician as a parent substitute. Many do not object to an inhalation induction and frequently respond to the smell of the inhalation agents by sucking or licking the mask. These children usually do not need to receive sedative drugs before they enter the operating room. Premedication in this age group is generally limited to medications such as atropine that modify physiologic responses to anesthesia. However, if sedatives are administered to these infants, they should be monitored continuously for possible airway obstruction and for cardiovascular and respiratory depression.

As children mature, they become increasingly aware of their surroundings. Children between 6 months and 6 years frequently cling to their parents. In an unfamiliar environment such as a hospital, preschool children tend to become very anxious, especially if the situation appears threatening. Their anxiety frequently stems from their inability to comprehend why they are in the hospital. This lack of understanding may be why children of this age group appear to have more difficulty adjusting to the hospital environment than older children. Even when parents are present, these children may be very apprehensive. This may occur if they sense that their parents are anxious; thus, efforts to educate the parents to allay their anxiety can be important in reducing the child's anxiety. Increased parental anxiety has been shown to result in increased anxiety in their children.[3] This heightened anxiety response may lead to immediate postoperative maladaptive behavior, such as nightmares, eating disturbances, and new onset enuresis. The percentage of parents of children that appear anxious can be as high as 54%. Viewing an educational videotape about pediatric anesthesia has been shown to lessen parental preoperative anxiety.[4, 5]

Separating preschool children from their parents can be extremely stressful. Compared with other patients, children between 2 and 6 years of age are more likely to exhibit problematic behavior when separated from their parents. The most important predictors of problematic behavior are when the child (1) has not taken a preoperative family tour, (2) has undergone previous surgery, and (3) preoperatively displays a dependent or withdrawn affect. Since the behavior of children can often be predicted, it may not be necessary to routinely sedate all children before anesthesia. Children who display one or more of the predictive risk factors would probably benefit from sedative premedication. In fact, in children 2 to 7 years of age, it was found that oral midazolam premedication resulted in less negative behavioral changes in the first week postoperatively than in placebo-treated control subjects.[6] Children are generally happier if they are with their parents during induction of anesthesia or if they are allowed to fall asleep in their parents' presence in a nonthreatening environment before entering the operating room. In addition, parents are generally more willing to separate from a sleeping child because they realize that their child is unaware of their absence and that their child no longer needs them for comfort.

Children older than 6 years and those who attend preschool or kindergarten are generally more willing to accept short periods of separation from their parents. They tend to be a little more independent than younger children because of their school experience. They are better able to communicate and have a greater understanding of their environment. This enables them to deal with their feelings and fears better than younger children. Their sense of curiosity and interest in new things can be used to elicit their cooperation. Many of these children are very trusting of adults and they can often be persuaded to accept a mask induction of anesthesia, especially if the smell is pleasant. Thus, preoperative sedation may not be necessary for many of these children, and in some cases, sedation may interfere with the child's ability to cooperate.

As children get older, they become more aware of their bodies and may fear mutilation. Some children fear being "put to sleep" like a pet. These patients need to be reassured that the sleep induced by anesthesia is different. They should be told that they will wake up at the end of anesthesia but not before surgery is completed. In addition, they should be reassured that they will not feel any discomfort during the operation and that the anesthesiologist will take good care of them while they are anesthetized. It is also important to emphasize that they will return to their parents when they are awake and that they will be given medication to ease any pain that may result from surgery.

Adolescents frequently appear quite independent and self-confident, but, as a group, they have unique problems. In a moment their mood can change from an intelligent, mature adult to a very immature child who needs support and reassurance. Apprehension about changes that are taking place in their bodies cause them to be quite fragile psychologically. Their self-esteem and body image can be easily altered. Coping with a disability or illness is often very difficult for adolescents. Because they are often comparing their physical appearance with that of their peers, they may become especially anxious when they have a physical problem. Teenagers like to feel that they are in control of their situation, and many dislike being sedated. They often want to know exactly what will transpire during the course of anesthesia and appreciate an honest answer. Their apprehension may be related to the fear that their medical problems might not be corrected, waking up in the middle of the operation, never waking up from anesthesia, or waking up handicapped. Most adolescents can be reasoned with. As a group they are usually cooperative and do not require sedation prior to anesthesia. The occasional overly anxious or rambunctious patient, however, will benefit from preanesthetic medication.

Monitoring the attitude and behavior of a child is very useful. A child who clings to the parents, avoids eye contact, and will not speak is often very anxious. A self-assured, cocky child who "knows it all" may also be apprehensive or frightened. This behavior may be an attempt to mask true emotions, and this child may decompensate just when his or her cooperation is needed. In some cases, nonpharmacologic supportive measures may be effective. In the extremely anxious child, supportive measures alone may be insufficient to reduce anxiety, and premedication may be necessary.

Since Water's classic work in 1938 on premedication of children, numerous reports have addressed this subject.[7] Despite the wealth of studies, no single drug or combination of drugs has been found to be "ideal" for all children. Many drugs used for premedication have similar effects, and a specific drug may have various effects in different children or in the same child under different conditions. The ideal premedicant for children would have the following features:

- allay or minimize anxiety
- produce predictable effects in all patients
- minimal undesirable side effects
- no or minimal adverse cardiovascular or respiratory effects
- rapid onset and recovery
- easy to administer
- painless when administered

The route of administration of premedicant drugs can be very important. Although a drug may be more effective and have a more reliable onset when given intravenously or intramuscularly, most pediatric anesthesiologists refrain from administering parenteral medication to avoid causing children unnecessary pain. They recognize that trauma caused by a needle may outweigh the potential benefit of the drug administered. Many children who are able to verbalize report that receiving a needle puncture was their worst experience in the hospital.[8, 9] Children with this experience frequently become fearful of medical personnel because they associate them with the pain of an injection. In most cases, medication administered without a needle will be more pleasant for patients, their parents, and the medical staff.

Drugs for premedication have been administered by many routes, including the oral, nasal, rectal, buccal, intravenous, and intramuscular routes. Previously, oral administration of drugs for premedication was thought to increase gastric residual volume and consequently increase the risk for pulmonary aspiration. Unless a large volume of fluid is ingested, oral premedication is not associated with aspiration pneumonia.[10] In general, the route of drug administration should depend on the drug chosen, the desired drug effect, and the psychological impact that a given route of administration may have on an individual child. For example, a small dose of oral medication may be sufficient for a relatively calm child, whereas an intramuscular injection, such as ketamine, may be best for an uncooperative, rambunctious, combative, extremely anxious child. Intramuscular medication may be less traumatic for this type patient than forcing him or her to swallow a drug, giving a drug rectally, or forcefully holding an anesthesia mask on the face.[11]

Medications

Several categories of drugs are available for premedicating children before anesthesia (Table 9–1). Selection of drugs for premedication depends on the goal desired. Drug effects should be weighed against potential side effects, and drug interactions should be considered. Premedicant drugs include tranquilizers, sedatives, hypnotics, opioids, antihistamines, anticholinergics, H_2-receptor antagonists, antacids, and drugs that increase gastric motility.

Table 9–1. Doses of Drugs Commonly Administered for Premedication

Drug	Route	Dose (mg/kg)
Barbiturates		
Methohexital 10%	Rectal	20–40
Methohexital 5%	Intramuscular	10
Thiopental 10%	Rectal	20–40
Benzodiazepines		
Diazepam	Oral	0.1–0.3
Midazolam	Oral	0.25–0.75
	Nasal	0.2
	Rectal	0.5–1.0
	Intramuscular	0.1–0.15
Ketamine*	Oral	3–6
	Nasal	3
	Rectal	6–10
	Intramuscular	2–10
Clonidine	Oral	0.004
Narcotics		
Morphine	Intramuscular	0.1–0.2
Meperidine	Intramuscular	1–2
Fentanyl	Oral	0.010–0.015 (10–15 μg/kg)
Sufentanil	Nasal	0.01–0.003 (1–3 μg/kg)

*With atropine 0.02 mg/kg.

Tranquilizers

The major effect of tranquilizers is to allay anxiety, but they also have the potential to produce sedation. This group of drugs includes the benzodiazepines, phenothiazines, and butyrophenones.

Benzodiazepines

Benzodiazepine derivatives are widely used for premedicating children. They are generally given to calm patients, allay anxiety, and diminish recall of perianesthetic events. At low doses, minimal drowsiness and cardiovascular or respiratory depression are produced. Nausea and vomiting are rarely a problem.

Midazolam is a short-acting water-soluble benzodiazepine with an elimination half-life of about 2 hours. It is probably the most widely used benzodiazepine for premedication of children.[12] The major advantage of midazolam over other drugs in its class is its rapid uptake and elimination. It is a water-soluble salt with a pH of less than 4, and it is highly lipophilic at physiologic pH.[13] It can be administered intravenously, intramuscularly, nasally, orally, and rectally with minimal irritation.[14–20] Peak plasma concentrations of midazolam occur approximately 10 minutes after intranasal, 16 minutes after rectal, and 53 minutes after oral administration.[13, 20, 21] The bioavailability of midazolam after different routes of administration is a fraction of the bioavailability after intravenous administration, that is, 0.9 after intramuscular injection, 0.57 after intranasal, 0.4 to 0.5 after rectal, and 0.3 after oral administration.[21, 22] After oral and rectal administration, there is incomplete absorption and extensive hepatic extraction of the drug during the first pass through the liver so systemic bioavailability is not 100%. The decrease in bioavailability of midazolam after oral and rectal administration is a reason why more drug must be given via these routes than via the intravenous or intramuscular routes to achieve the same effect. Most children are adequately sedated after receiving a midazolam dose of 0.025 to 0.1 mg/kg intravenously, 0.1 to 0.2 mg/kg intramuscularly, 0.25 to 0.5 mg/kg orally, 0.2 mg/kg nasally, or 1 mg/kg rectally.

Orally administered midazolam is effective in calming most patients who receive the drug and does not increase gastric pH or residual volume.[23] Children who are premedicated with oral midazolam are calmer than those who are not premedicated, even when parents are present for the induction of anesthesia. Those who receive oral midazolam premedication are less likely to need a rapid 5% halothane induction.[24] Most published studies were carried out using the intravenous formulation, which was then combined with a variety of flavorings, syrups, or medications to mask the bitter taste. A commercially prepared formulation (2 mg/mL) has an acceptable taste for most children. A multicenter study found that even a small oral dose of 0.25 mg/kg resulted in satisfactory sedation and anxiolysis in the majority of the patients within 20 minutes.[25] The availability of a commercially prepared formulation likely has resulted in a more uniform and dependable absorption than that associated with "home formulated" mixtures, which would result in varying concentrations and pH changes that likely would alter the consistency of transmucosal drug absorption. It should be noted, however, that the first pass metabolism can be significantly affected by inhibitors of the cytochrome oxidase system. Grapefruit juice, erythromycin, protease inhibitors, and calcium channel blockers alter (CYP)3A, resulting in unexpectedly high blood levels and prolonged sedation.[26-32] Oral midazolam should be administered in a lower dose or avoided in patients taking these substances.

Although anxiolysis and a mild degree of sedation occur in most children after midazolam, some will become agitated.[33] Adverse behavioral changes in the postoperative period have also been reported. In one study, oral midazolam resulted in less crying during the induction of anesthesia but was associated with greater adverse behavioral changes (nightmares, night terrors, food rejection, anxiety, and negativism) up to 4 weeks postoperatively compared to the placebo-treated group.[34] Another, better controlled, study found fewer negative behavioral changes in the first two postoperative weeks in children who had received midazolam in acetaminophen compared to just acetaminophen.[6]

Anxiolysis and sedation usually occur within 10 minutes after intranasal midazolam.[35] The authors of one study mention that the recommended dose may be less effective in patients with an upper respiratory infection and excessive nasal discharge.[20] Although the drug reduces negative behavior in children during parental separation, it was not well accepted by the patients when given intranasally because it produces irritation and discomfort that may outweigh the sedative effects.[36, 37] Another concern regarding this route of administration is the theoretical potential for neurotoxicity. There are direct connections between the nasal mucosa and the central nervous system (Fig. 9-1). Medications administered nasally can result in a very rapid rise in cerebrospinal fluid drug levels.[38-40] A rapid rise in brain and cerebrospinal fluid concentration of midazolam could occur if the drug is absorbed directly through the cribriform plate.[20] Since midazolam with preservative has been demonstrated to have neurotoxic properties in an animal model, we do not recommend this for the routine route of administration.[41, 42]

Midazolam premedication does not seem to affect the time for recovery from anesthesia or the time it takes to discharge a child from the hospital after anesthesia for surgical procedures lasting at least 10 minutes.[43, 44] When compared with other oral premedicants such as trimeprazine, midazolam was better in terms of sedation during induction, yet the duration and quality of recovery were not significantly different.[45, 46] When oral midazolam was combined with atropine or meperidine, neither adjunct improved the effectiveness of midazolam.

Diazepam is the best-known benzodiazepine derivative. Although it is used to sedate older children, it is rarely used in neonates and infants. In infants and especially preterm neonates, the half-life of diazepam is markedly increased because of immature hepatic function (see Chapter 8). In addition, the active metabolite (desmethydiazepam) has pharmacologic activity equal to the parent compound and a half-life of up to 9 days in adults.[47] Diazepam has a long half-life (43 ± 13 hours in adults).[48] The most effective route of administration is intravenous, followed by oral and rectal. The intramuscular route is not recommended because it is painful and absorption is erratic.[49-53] A rectal solution is more effective and reliable than rectally administered tablets or suppositories.[53, 54] The average oral dose for premedicating healthy children ranges from 0.1 to 0.3 mg/kg; however, doses as high as 0.5 mg/kg have been used.[55] The recommended rectal dose is 1 mg/kg with peak serum concentrations occurring at approximately 20 minutes.[54]

Lorazepam (0.05 mg/kg) orally or intravenously is used primarily in older children.[56, 57] The advantages of lorazepam compared with diazepam are less tissue irritation and more reliable amnesia. It can be administered orally, intravenously, or intramuscularly and is metabolized by the liver to inactive metabolites. Compared with diazepam, its onset of action is slower and its duration of action is longer. These characteristics make it inappropriate for outpatient surgical procedures.

There is another pharmacodynamic difference between benzodiazepines that is important to consider when these drugs are administered intravenously. Entry into the central nervous system is directly related to fat solubility.[58, 59] The higher the fat solubility, the more rapid the transit into the

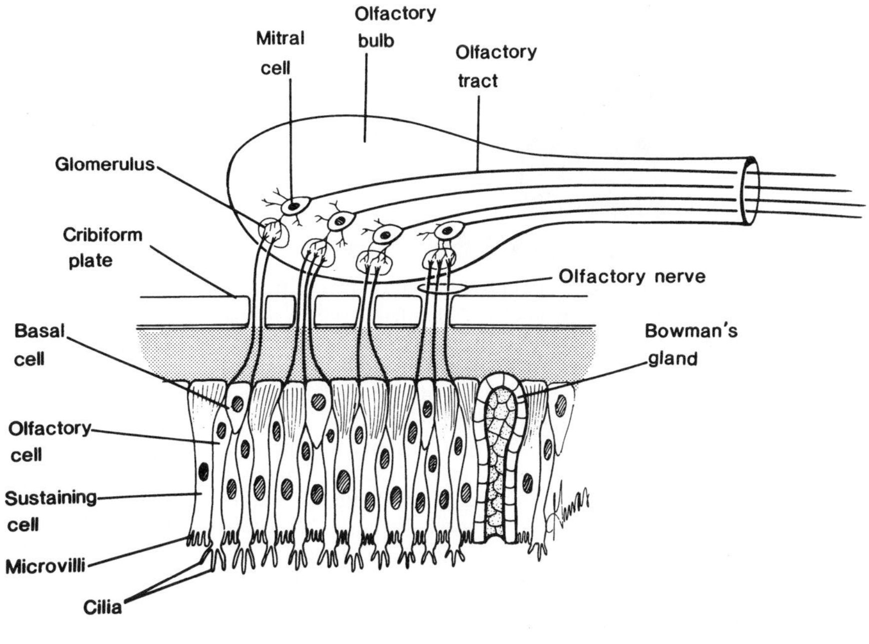

Figure 9-1. Anatomy of the nasal mucosa–cribriform plate interface. The nasal mucosa is the only location in the body that provides a direct connection between the central nervous system and the atmosphere. Drugs administered to the nasal mucosa rapidly traverse through the cribriform plate into the central nervous system by three routes: (1) directly by the olfactory neurons, (2) through supporting cells and the surrounding capillary bed, and (3) directly into the cerebrospinal fluid. (From Hilger PA. Fundamentals of Otolaryngology: A Textbook of Ear, Nose, and Throat Diseases, 6th ed. Philadelphia: WB Saunders; 1989:184.)

central nervous system. It should be noted that the time to peak central nervous system electoencephalographic effect in adults is 4.8 minutes for midazolam but only 1.6 minutes for diazepam (Fig. 9–2). Therefore, when administering intravenous midazolam, it is vital to wait an adequate time between doses to avoid excessive drug administration and unintended oversedation.

Butyrophenones

Droperidol is a major tranquilizer occasionally used for preanesthetic medication. It has ataractic and soporific properties, potentiates the effects of other central nervous system depressants, and produces mild alpha-adrenergic blockade. Its most common use in children is intraoperatively in low doses (50 to 75 μg/kg IV) for its antiemetic effect.[60–66] Although the onset of action after intravenous or intramuscular administration is 3 to 10 minutes, the peak effect may not be apparent until 30 minutes. The drug is rarely administered to infants and young children. When used as a premedicant, the recommended dose for older children ranges from 100 to 150 μg/kg; *this dose may induce anesthesia in some patients.* Sedation and ataraxia after this dose generally last for 2 to 4 hours but may last as long as 12 hours.[67] When droperidol is administered in combination with drugs such as fentanyl or other central nervous system depressants, the

dose of droperidol should be reduced. All children who receive high-dose droperidol should be closely monitored because of the potential complication of apnea. If hypotension develops, relative hypovolemia due to the alpha-adrenergic blockade should be considered in the differential diagnosis. Other side effects include restlessness and extrapyramidal symptoms.[68, 69] Since this is a long-acting medication, it is not generally recommended for outpatient procedures except in the antiemetic dose range.

Phenothiazines

Promethazine is a phenothiazine derivative often used for premedication of children but rarely used prior to anesthesia. It more commonly is used in combination with other medications by nonanesthesiologists for procedural sedation.[70–72] Promethazine produces minimal cardiovascular effects and is metabolized by the liver. In addition to its sedative properties, it is an H_1-blocker and has antiemetic, antihistaminic, anti-motion sickness, and anticholinergic effects. Promethazine is occasionally administered with narcotics 1 hour before anesthesia to control nausea and vomiting. The recommended dose is 0.5 to 1.0 mg/kg. The effects of the drug are apparent within 20 minutes after oral administration and last for 4 to 6 hours. Since this is a long-acting medication, it is not generally recommended for outpatient procedures.[73]

Barbiturates

Barbiturates are among the oldest medications used for premedication. The advantages of barbiturates include sedation, minimal respiratory or cardiovascular depression, anticonvulsant effects, and a very low incidence of nausea and vomiting. The major disadvantage of barbiturates is hyperalgesia. In some cases, a small dose administered to patients with pain may intensify the pain and cause them to become uncooperative. Barbiturates should not be used in patients with porphyria, as this class of drug may cause an acute exacerbation of the disease.

Two short-acting barbituric acid derivatives that were used extensively to premedicate patients are *pentobarbital* and *secobarbital.* Both of these drugs produce effective sedation in most healthy children in 1 to 2 hours after either oral or intramuscular administration of 3 to 5 mg/kg.[74–77] The oral route is preferred because it eliminates the pain of a needle that often persists at the injection site after the drug is administered intramuscularly.[78] Pentobarbital has also been administered by the rectal route (7 mg/kg).[79] Although these drugs are considered to be relatively short acting, they are rarely used for preanesthetic medication of children because their duration of action is frequently longer than the surgical procedure.

Ultrashort-acting barbiturates are more desirable for premedicating children. *Sodium thiopental* was the first of these drugs used for this purpose.[80] Thirty mg/kg produces sleep in about two thirds of the children in 15 minutes.[81–83] *Methohexital* is another ultrashort-acting barbiturate used to premedicate children.[84, 85] Its elimination half-life (3.9 ± 2.1 hours) is shorter than thiopental (9 ± 1.6 hours).[86–90] In some institutions, methohexital is administered rectally to the majority of the patients between 6 months and 6 years

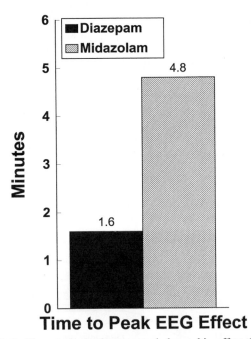

Figure 9–2. Time to peak electroencephalographic effect (EEG) of diazepam versus midazolam in adults. Note that it takes nearly three times longer to achieve a peak EEG effect following intravenous midazolam than diazepam. This is likely due to the difference in fat solubility; since midazolam is less fat soluble than diazepam, midazolam does not cross biologic membranes as easily. The clinical importance of this observation is the need to wait 3 to 5 minutes between intravenous doses of midazolam to avoid stacking of doses and excessive drug effect. (Data abstracted from Buhrer M, Maitre PO, Crevoisier C, Stanski DR: Electroencephalographic effects of benzodiazepines. II. Pharmacodynamic modelling of the electroencephalographic effects of midazolam and diazepam. Clin Pharmacol Ther 1990;48:555–567.)

of age with excellent results.[91] The drug is usually administered in the presence of the parents and the parents are allowed to hold the child until the child falls asleep.

The advantages of rectal methohexital are as follows

- Sedation is achieved without the pain associated with parenteral drug administration
- Separation anxiety is minimized because the child usually falls asleep in the parent's arms
- Parental anxieties are allayed because they are more willing to separate from a sleeping child
- An inhalational induction of anesthesia is facilitated because the patient does not object to the anesthetic mask or the pungent odor of the anesthetic gases
- Environmental pollution by volatile anesthetics is decreased because a better mask fit can be obtained in the sleeping child than the upset combative patient

Methohexital is most often administered as a 10% solution rectally (20–30 mg/kg); the elimination half-life is 150 ± 62 minutes and the bioavailability is about 17%.[92] Approximately 85 to 90% of patients receiving 20 or 30 mg/kg will fall asleep within 15 minutes.[84, 85, 91] Patients undergoing brief surgical procedures are generally given the lower dose to prevent a prolonged recovery from anesthesia. Children sedated for a procedure, such as a computed tomographic scan, who do not require inhalation anesthesia but who require intravenous access are generally given the higher dose. This prevents them from awakening in response to the placement of the intravenous catheter.

Most patients move in response to a needle or strong stimulus but resume quiet sleep after the stimulus subsides. Clinically significant respiratory or cardiovascular depression is rarely a problem, but some children will develop airway obstruction if the head is not maintained in proper position.[93] Children chronically treated with phenobarbital or phenytoin are more resistant to the effects of rectal methohexital, probably because of enzyme induction and neuronal tolerance.[91, 94] The efficacy of sleep in these patients is 32% compared with more than 85% in patients not on these medications.[91] Patients with a myelomeningocele are also less likely to sleep, probably because of leakage of the drug from a patulous anal sphincter.[91] Several other concentrations of rectal methohexital ranging from 1 to 10% have been used rectally.[95–99] A dose of 25 mg/kg as a 10% solution is as effective in producing sleep as 15 mg/kg of a 1% solution.[95] Although sleep is induced faster (5.7 ± 1.9 vs 7.0 ± 2.0 min) after 25 mg/kg of a 1% solution than after the same dose of a 10% solution, recovery time is longer.[99] The longer recovery time can be attributed to the higher plasma concentrations after 1% methohexital. Compared with a 10% solution, a 2% solution does not significantly affect the time to sleep, although it raises plasma methohexital concentration higher than a 10% solution likely because of a larger exposure of rectal mucosa from the larger volume.[96]

Recovery after methohexital is relatively rapid because of the rapid redistribution and metabolism of the drug. A rectal dose of 25 mg/kg does not affect the discharge time from the hospital, but the time to return to full consciousness after a 30-minute or shorter surgical procedures is slightly longer (15 to 30 minutes) in those patients who are premedicated with methohexital rectally compared with those who receive 5 mg/kg of thiopental intravenously for the induction of anesthesia.[100] Higher doses of methohexital can further delay recovery.[94]

The disadvantages of rectal methohexital include the unpredictable systemic bioavailability, defecation after rectal administration (10%), hiccoughs (13%), desaturation to 93% or less (4%), and prolonged recovery after very brief surgical procedures, such as myringotomy.[84, 91, 93, 101, 102] Another disadvantage is that some children strenuously object to any rectal intervention while awake. It is for this reason that most anesthesiologists prefer to administer sedation medications by this route only to children still in diapers. When administered to older patients, some develop the urge to defecate; if the child is still uncomfortable 5 minutes after the drug is administered, we allow the child to use a bedpan. In most patients, a sufficient quantity of drug is absorbed by this time, as many will fall asleep after defecation.

An anesthesiologist or personnel skilled in the airway management of children must monitor the child from the time the drug is administered until recovery from the drug effect, since some patients may develop airway obstruction, apnea, seizures, or an allergic reaction.[93, 103, 104] We have observed each of these complications at least once in our experience with rectal methohexital but careful observation and the immediate availability of emergency airway equipment have prevented major catastrophes.

Contraindications to methohexital include hypersensitivity, temporal lobe epilepsy, and latent or manifest porphyria.[103–105] Rectal methohexital is also contraindicated in patients with rectal mucosal tears or hemorrhoids, as large quantities of the drug can be absorbed, resulting in respiratory or cardiac arrest.

Nonbarbiturate Sedatives

Chloral hydrate and triclofos are orally administered nonbarbiturate drugs that are used to sedate children; both have long onset times and are relatively long acting. They are converted to trichloroethanol, which has a plasma half-life of approximately 9 hours in toddlers (Fig. 9–3).[106] *Chloral hydrate* is frequently used by non-anesthesiologists to sedate children.[107–109] The drug is rarely used by anesthesiologists because it is unreliable in producing sleep, unpleasant to taste, and irritating to the skin, mucous membranes, and gastrointestinal tract. An oral dose (50 to 100 mg/kg) is most effective when administered 1 1/2 to 2 hours before anesthesia (see Chapters 8 and 26). It is not recommended that this drug be used in newborns because of impaired metabolism[110, 111] or administered on a chronic basis because of the theoretical possibility of carcinogenesis.[112, 113]

Opioids

Opioids have been used for many years to premedicate children before anesthesia. They are especially useful for providing analgesia and sedation of patients who have pain preoperatively. Other benefits include a decrease in anesthetic requirement and a smooth awakening from anesthesia because pain from the surgical procedure is attenuated. The major disadvantages of opioids are nausea, vomiting, and respiratory depression. Hypotension, bile duct spasm, dysphoria, and hallucinations are other undesirable side effects of opioids.

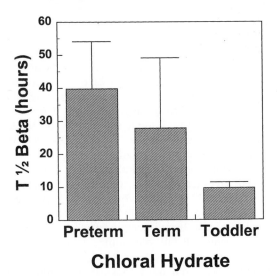

Chloral Hydrate

Figure 9–3. Beta elimination half-life of the active metabolite of chloral hydrate, trichloroethanol, in preterm infants, term infants, and toddlers. Note the extremely long half-lives in all age groups and the large standard deviation. Although often thought of as a short-acting sedative, chloral hydrate can have profoundly long effects. (Data abstracted from Mayers DJ, Hindmarsh KW, Sankaran K, et al: Chloral hydrate disposition following single-dose administration to critically ill neonates and children. Dev Pharm Ther 1991;16:71–77.)

Morphine sulfate is the long-acting opioid against which all others are compared. The recommended dose for preanesthetic medication is 0.1 to 0.2 mg/kg intramuscularly 1 hour before the induction of anesthesia. Morphine is also effective when given orally; rectal administration is not recommended owing to erratic absorption.[114–117] Intravenous administration is common, particularly for children already in pain, such as those with a fracture. In this situation, 0.05 to 0.1 mg/kg will often provide analgesia prior to induction and moving the patient. The major disadvantage of any opioid is the increase in preoperative and postoperative vomiting.[118, 119] Morphine is used more frequently in older than in younger children as a premedicant; it is rarely used to premedicate infants. Neonates are more sensitive to its respiratory depressant effects, although age (>10 days) has little effect on morphine pharmacokinetics.[120–122]

Meperidine is a long-acting synthetic opioid whose onset of action is slightly more rapid than that of morphine; the duration of action is slightly shorter. The usual dose of preanesthetic medication of children is 1 to 2 mg/kg IM 1 hour before the induction of anesthesia. Meperidine premedication can be administered intravenously, intramuscularly, or orally. An oral dose of 1.5 mg/kg in combination with diazepam (0.2 mg/kg) and atropine (0.02 mg/kg) safely sedates patients before anesthesia.[10] The effects and disadvantages of meperidine are very similar to those of morphine. Compared with morphine, meperidine at equianalgesic doses causes less sedation, smooth-muscle spasm, suppression of the cough reflex, and respiratory depression in neonates.[122] Large doses or chronic administration can cause central nervous system excitation (seizures, tremors, muscle twitches) owing to accumulation of the metabolite normeperidine. Meperidine is not recommended for prolonged use in

children but is safe and effective for short-term administration.[123]

Fentanyl is a synthetic opioid that is 80 times more potent than morphine.[48] It has a more rapid onset and shorter duration of action than either morphine or meperidine when administered in low doses. In addition to the intravenous route, fentanyl can be administered to children by dropping the liquid in their mouth or nose with a syringe, or in the form of an oral lozenge, the Fentanyl Oralet. Orally administered fentanyl is most effective when it is absorbed through the oral mucosa; swallowing the drug decreases its effectiveness because the first-pass metabolism through the liver is high. Having children sit upright when licking an Oralet rather than having them lie supine may keep the drug in the mouth longer rather than allowing it to drain to the back of the throat where it is swallowed. The bioavailability of the Fentanyl Oralet is approximately 33% in children.[124] The effect of oral transmucosal fentanyl is dose dependent. Compared with a placebo, oral transmucosal fentanyl effectively sedates children so that they are more willing to separate from their parents.[125] Children begin to show signs of sedation within 10 minutes after receiving a 10 to 15 μg/kg Oralet. Recovery from anesthesia is similar after 10 to 15 μg/kg Oralet compared with an intravenous dose of 2 μg/kg.[124] Desaturation and preoperative nausea seem to be minimized if the patient is brought to the operating room within 10 minutes of completion and if the lower dose (10–15 μg/kg) is used.[124, 126] Higher doses result in an increased incidence of desaturation and nausea and vomiting, as does a prolonged period of time between completion and induction of anesthesia.[125–128] Intravenous droperidol (25 μg/kg) given after the induction of anesthesia does not reduce the incidence of postoperative nausea and vomiting.[127] The high incidence of pruritus, vomiting, and desaturation limits the usefulness of doses greater than 15 μg/kg. It should be noted that the blood levels of fentanyl continue to rise for 10 to 20 minutes after completion of the Oralet (Fig. 9–4).[124] If the patient is anesthetized within 10 minutes of completion, the peak blood level will occur during the operation and thus be more likely to contribute to postoperative analgesia as well as to reduce the incidence of side effects that are related to blood fentanyl level.

Sufentanil is an analgesic that is 10 times more potent than fentanyl. The mean half-life in adults is 2.7 hours.[48] Clearance in infants 0 to 1 months is 6.7 mL/kg/min vs. 13.1 mL/kg/min in children 12 to 16 years, and the half-life is 12.3 hours vs. 3.5 hours for the same ages.[129] After a nasal dose of 1.5 to 3.0 μg/kg, children are usually calm and cooperative, and more than 75% separate easily from their parents.[35, 37] As with any opioid, intranasal sufentanil reduces the intraoperative requirement of inhalational anesthetics and the postoperative requirements for analgesics.[35, 130] There is not a large published experience with this route of premedication, but several children were reported to have reduced chest wall compliance during induction of anesthesia.[35, 37] Prolonged recovery may also be observed compared with midazolam premedication.[37]

Butorphanol is a synthetic opioid agonist-antagonist analgesic with properties similar to those of morphine that can be administered transnasally.[131, 132] It is as effective as equipotent doses of intramuscular meperidine and morphine with an onset of analgesic action in about 15 minutes and

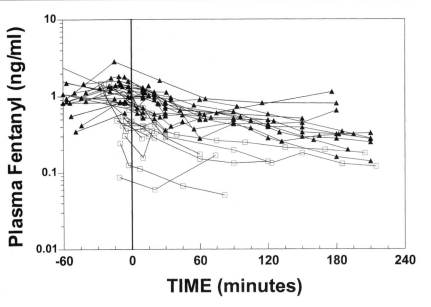

Figure 9–4. Plasma fentanyl concentrations versus time. The solid triangles represent oral transmucosal fentanyl citrate and the open boxes intravenous fentanyl. Time zero represents the time of entry into the recovery room following tonsillectomy. Note that plasma fentanyl concentrations continued to rise after completion of the Fentanyl Oralet and during the surgical procedure. A fairly stable plasma concentration was maintained for several hours. (From Dsida RM, Wheeler M, Birmingham PK, et al: Premedication of pediatric tonsillectomy patients with oral transmucosal fentanyl citrate. Anesth Analg 1998;86:66–70.)

peak activity within 1 or 2 hours in adults. The bioavailability of butorphanol administered transnasally is 60 to 70%. The most frequent side effect is sedation that resolves approximately 1 hour after administration. A dose of 0.025 mg/kg administered one drop at a time on patients' nasal mucosa as they inhaled the inhalational anesthetic resulted in a significantly longer time to oral intake compared with the placebo-treated group, but significantly fewer patients required "rescue" analgesia for myringotomies with tube placement. There was no effect on the incidence of postoperative emesis.[133]

If opioids are used in combination with other sedatives, such as benzodiazepines, the dose of each drug should be appropriately adjusted to avoid serious respiratory depression. For example, if fentanyl is indicated to control pain in a patient who has already received midazolam, the fentanyl dose should be titrated in small increments (0.25–0.5 μg/kg) to prevent hypoxemia and apnea. Fentanyl or other opioids in combination with midazolam produces more respiratory depression than fentanyl or midazolam alone.[134, 135]

Ketamine

Ketamine is a racemic nonbarbiturate cyclohexamine derivative that produces dissociation of the cortex from the limbic system. In infants less than 3 months of age, the volume of distribution is similar to that in older infants, but the elimination half-life is considerably prolonged (185 vs. 65 min).[136] On a milligram per kilogram basis, the amount of ketamine required to prevent gross movement is four times greater in infants under 6 months of age than in 6-year-old children.[137] Ketamine may be administered intravenously, intramuscularly, orally, rectally, and nasally.

One occasionally encounters a very apprehensive or combative child who is uncooperative. When a child refuses a mask induction and will not take oral medication, in whom venous access is difficult, intramuscular ketamine is a reasonable alternative induction technique. A dose of 2 mg/kg is sufficient to adequately calm most uncooperative children in approximately 3 minutes so that they will accept a mask

induction of anesthesia.[11] A larger dose (4 to 5 mg/kg) sedates children within 2 to 4 minutes, and a dose of 10 mg/kg usually produces very deep sedation that lasts from 12 to 25 minutes. After the higher doses, recovery from anesthesia may be prolonged, especially if the surgical procedure is brief. In addition, higher doses are associated with hallucinations, nightmares, vomiting, and an unpleasant emergence from anesthesia.[11, 138] Concomitant administration of benzodiazepines with higher doses will eliminate or attenuate these emergence reactions.[139] The higher doses of intramuscular ketamine are particularly useful for the induction of anesthesia in patients in whom there is a desire to maintain a stable blood pressure and in whom there is no venous access, such as a patient with congenital heart disease. It is recommended that atropine (0.02 mg/kg) be combined with ketamine so as to avoid the copious secretions that can lead to laryngospasm (see Chapters 8 and 26).[140]

Ketamine can also be administered orally; a dose of 6 mg/kg adequately sedates children so that they are calm when separated from their parents.[141] A dose of 5 mg/kg will sedate most children but not as effectively as oral midazolam (0.5 mg/kg), a slightly better sedative and anxiolytic.[142] Oral ketamine (4 mg/kg) in combination with midazolam (0.4 mg/kg) and atropine (0.02 mg/kg) is effective in calmly separating parents and children 100% of the time and allows a smooth mask induction of anesthesia 85% of the time.[143] This oral lytic cocktail may be an effective alternative in patients who previously have not had adequate sedation with oral midazolam alone. The optimal combination for deeper sedation would appear to be 6 to 10 mg/kg oral ketamine combined with 0.25 to 0.5 mg/kg midazolam and 0.02 mg/kg atropine.[141, 143–146]

Rectally (6 mg/kg) and nasally (3 mg/kg) administered ketamine is also effective in sedating children.[147, 148] Intranasal ketamine (6 mg/kg) was more effective than promethazine and meperidine (1 mg/kg, each) intramuscularly.[149] However, as with midazolam, ketamine has been shown to be neurotoxic when applied directly to neural animal tissue. Since it is the preservative that is neurotoxic, preservative-free ketamine would appear to be safe to administer by the nasal route.[41, 150]

Alpha₂-Agonists

Clonidine, an alpha₂-agonist, causes dose-related sedation by its effect in the locus ceruleus by its inhibition of adenylate cyclase.[151] A dose of 3 µg/kg given 45 to 120 minutes before surgery produces sedation that is comparable to that induced by diazepam or midazolam.[152] Clonidine acts both centrally and peripherally to reduce blood pressure and therefore it attenuates the hemodynamic response to intubation.[153] It appears to be relatively free of respiratory depressant properties, even when administered in an overdose.[151] The sedative properties of clonidine reduce the dose of intravenous barbiturate required for induction; when 4 µg/kg was given orally 105 minutes before induction, the dose of thiamylal required to induce anesthesia was reduced.[153] Likewise, clonidine has been shown to reduce the minimum alveolar concentration of sevoflurane for tracheal intubation[154] and the concentration of inhaled anesthetic, as judged by hemodynamic stability intraoperatively, for the maintenance of anesthesia.[155–157] During the first 12 hours after surgery, that same premedicant dose of oral clonidine (4 µg/kg) reduced the postoperative pain scores and the requirement for supplementary analgesics.[158, 159] It also reduced the incidence of vomiting after strabismus surgery compared to (1) a control group, (2) a group that received 2 µg/kg of clonidine, and (3) a group that received 0.4 mg/kg of diazepam.[160] Oral clonidine when given with 0.15 mL/kg of apple juice 100 minutes prior to the induction of anesthesia did not affect the gastric fluid pH and volume in children.[161] Experience with this premedication in children is still somewhat limited, and its role as a premedicant in particular is yet to be defined.

Antihistamines

In the past, antihistamines were often used for premedication. The popularity of these drugs has declined because their sedative side effects are variable. They are rarely given to infants but are occasionally indicated for older children, especially those who are hyperkinetic.

Hydroxyzine is the most common drug in this class that is used for premedication. It is administered mainly for its ataractic properties.[162, 163] Additional benefits may be derived from its antiemetic, antihistaminic, and antispasmodic effects. Minimal respiratory and circulatory changes occur after doses of 0.5 to 1.0 mg/kg. This drug is most commonly administered with other classes of drugs as an intramuscular "cocktail."

Diphenhydramine has antimuscarinic and mild sedative effects and is an H₁-blocker; the incidence of gastrointestinal side effects is low.[164] The dosage for children is 2.5–5 mg/kg/day (maximum dose 300 mg) in four divided doses orally, intravenously, or intramuscularly. Although the duration of action is 4 to 6 hours, it does not appear to significantly interfere with recovery from anesthesia.[48, 165]

Anticholinergic Drugs

Anticholinergic drugs are administered preoperatively to (1) block cholinergic effects of drugs; (2) prevent bradycardia that may result from airway manipulations such as laryngoscopy and intubation, surgical manipulation such as retracting the viscera or extraocular muscles, or anesthetic drugs such as succinylcholine; and (3) reduce secretions. They may also produce sedation and amnesia (scopolamine more so than atropine) and may decrease gastric residual volume and acidity. Undesirable effects of anticholinergics include tachycardia, dry mouth, skin erythema, and hyperthermia due to inhibition of sweating.

The most common anticholinergic drugs used for premedication of children are *atropine, scopolamine,* and *glycopyrrolate.* The recommended dose of atropine or scopolamine is 0.01–0.02 mg/kg. A dose of 0.1 mg intramuscularly or intravenously is generally the lowest administered, except in tiny preterm infants. The maximum single dose for premedication is generally 0.6 mg. Atropine blocks the vagus nerve more effectively than scopolamine, whereas scopolamine is a better sedative, antisialagogue, and amnestic. Both of these drugs cross the blood-brain barrier and cause central nervous system excitement (agitation, confusion, restlessness, ataxia, hallucinations, slurred speech, and memory loss). Anticholinergic overdose may be treated with the centrally active anticholinesterase physostigmine (0.04 mg/kg).

Glycopyrrolate is a synthetic quaternary ammonium compound that does not cross the blood-brain barrier. Thus, it does not produce the restlessness and confusion that may be observed after large doses of atropine and scopolamine. It is twice as potent as atropine in decreasing the volume of secretions, lasts three times longer, and is effective against the bradycardic effects of both neostigmine and pyridostigmine.[166–168] The recommended dose of glycopyrrolate is half the dose of atropine (0.01 mg/kg).

Young children are more prone to bradycardia, because, compared with adults, their parasympathetic tone is greater than their sympathetic tone. Infants and small children who develop bradycardia should be treated promptly. Infants who require atropine should receive it before the decrease in heart rate becomes a problem, because the onset time of the atropine is delayed with bradycardia.[169] If the heart rate is reduced, cardiac output declines and the drug takes longer to reach the postganglionic nerve endings in the heart to produce the cardioaccelerator effect.

Some anesthesiologists routinely prescribe anticholinergic drugs preoperatively to infants and young children. Others administer these drugs only when indicated, such as before intravenous succinylcholine, at the onset of bradycardia, if a patient has a history of bradycardia during intubation or induction of anesthesia, or if a patient is having a procedure that may stimulate vagal reflexes, such as eye surgery. Anticholinergic drugs are often more effective if they are administered just before they are required. If they are given too early, the vagolytic effect may be gone by the time anesthesia is induced. The intravenous route is the most reliable route.[170] They can also be administered intramuscularly, or they can be given orally or rectally to eliminate needle pain. Because mucosal absorption of atropine is rapid and nearly complete, the dose for all routes of administration is the same.

Since most modern inhalation anesthetics do not stimulate secretions, a drying agent is usually not essential. The routine use of an anticholinergic drug for the sole purpose of drying secretions is probably unwarranted, because a dry mouth can be a source of extreme discomfort for a child. It may cause some children to complain before the operation and in some cases even after surgery if the drug effect outlasts the procedure. In one study, more patients who were premedicated with glycopyrrolate reported that they had a sore throat or hoarseness postoperatively than those who did not receive the drug.[171] In some patients, however, an anticholinergic drug may be desirable, such as in patients who drool constantly, patients who receive ketamine as the sole anesthetic drug, patients with a history of anesthetic problems due to excessive secretions, and patients undergoing surgery involving the mouth.

Nonopioid Analgesics

Acetaminophen is the most common nonopioid analgesic administered for postoperative pain relief in the pediatric age group. It can be administered orally preoperatively or rectally immediately after the induction of anesthesia but before the start of surgery. The absorption from the rectal mucosa is quite variable, with a lag time to detectable blood levels of 40 minutes, as opposed to no detectable lag time for the oral administration. The relative bioavailability of the rectal compared with the oral formulation was 0.54.[172] The oral doses of 10 to 15 mg/kg recommended for the antipyretic effect are as effective as ketorolac (1 mg/kg)[173] at 10 or more minutes postoperatively for myringotomies with pressure-equalizing tube placement. Other studies have found that acetaminophen given preemptively may enhance analgesia in the pediatric patient after tonsillectomy surgery.[174] Acetaminophen has opioid-sparing properties.[175] Oral acetaminophen is very rapidly absorbed, with blood levels appearing within several minutes (Fig. 9–5). Acetaminophen and codeine elixir given orally in the preoperative period was found to provide superior analgesia to acetaminophen alone after myringotomy and placement of pressure-equalizing tubes.[176]

The pharmacokinetics of three doses of rectal acetaminophen (10, 20, and 30 mg/kg) were studied in children over a 16-hour period.[177] Peak blood levels occurred at 60 to 180 minutes following administration, emphasizing the importance of administering the rectal acetaminophen immediately following induction so as to have a blood level at the time of awakening. It was found that even with a rectal dose of 30 mg/kg, most patients did not achieve peak or sustained serum values associated with antipyresis (Fig. 9–6). Thus

based on the kinetics, the authors recommended that the initial dose of rectal acetaminophen should be approximately 40 mg/kg followed by 20 mg/kg rectally every 6 hours; a subsequent study confirmed this recommendation.[178] It should be noted that this study involved a specific brand of suppository for the first 24 hours only; these findings may not apply to all brands or for blood levels after the first 24 hours. It should be noted that several other single-dose administration studies have had similar results.[179, 180] Another study took these data a step further by giving tonsillectomy patients an oral preoperative dose of 40 mg/kg plus 20 mg/kg rectally 2 hours later and found that most children achieved a satisfactory pain score for about 8 hours after administration.[172] At higher doses of 40 to 60 mg/kg rectally, given after induction of anesthesia but before a variety of same-day surgical procedures, children required less rescue morphine in the postoperative period and needed less analgesia at home than the children who received either a placebo or 20 mg/kg of acetaminophen rectally.[175] In addition, the patients receiving the higher doses of acetaminophen had less postoperative nausea and vomiting. Since there is concern regarding potential hepatic toxicity, it is advised to obtain a good history of acetaminophen administration prior to anesthesia and to not exceed the 24-hour limits on the drug label.

Ibuprofen is a nonsteroidal anti-inflammatory drug commonly used in children. In a study of children undergoing a variety of surgical procedures, rectal ibuprofen (40 mg/kg/day in divided doses) was given for up to 3 days. In addition, intravenous or intramuscular morphine was given to all children according to clinical need. It was found that the need for additional morphine was less during the 3-day study period for the children who received the rectal ibuprofen.[181] Another study found acetaminophen/codeine to be superior to ibuprofen for analgesia for tonsillectomy, and the ibuprofen-treated patients had a significant increase in bleeding time.[182] Ibuprofen should not be used in patients with impaired renal function or in patients who are hypovolemic due to the increased incidence of renal toxicity.[183, 184]

Ketorolac is a nonsteroidal anti-inflammatory drug that can be administered parenterally and orally and has an opioid-sparing effect, reducing the incidence of adverse effects of opioids such as respiratory depression, nausea, and vom-

Figure 9–5. Oral acetaminophen was administered in four doses to children prior to myringotomy and tube insertion. Oral acetaminophen is rapidly absorbed following oral administration, with the antipyretic range (10–20 μg/mL) reached within 10 minutes following a dose of 20 mg/kg. Compare this to the very slow erratic absorption following rectal drug administration (Fig. 9-6). (From Wheeler M, Tobin MJ, Birmingham PK, et al: Pharmacokinetics and dose response for oral acetaminophen in children. Anesthesiology 1997;87:A1054.)

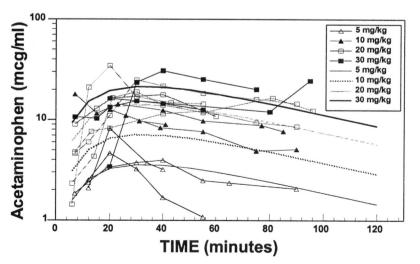

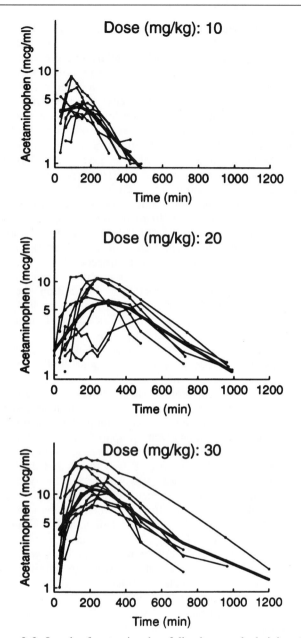

Figure 9–6. Levels of acetaminophen following rectal administration of 10, 20, or 30 mg/kg were recorded. Values for serum concentration of acetaminophen (circles, thin lines) are plotted against time for each patient. Thick lines indicate "average" values. Note that only children who received 30 mg/kg achieved the antipyretic threshold of 10 to 20 μg/mL but that even at this dose that range was not sustained. These data suggest the need to use a higher loading dose (approximately 40 mg/kg) followed by subsequent doses of 20 mg/kg every 6 hours; see text for details. (From Birmingham PK, Tobin MJ, Henthorn TK, et al: Twenty-four-hour pharmacokinetics of rectal acetaminophen: An old drug with new recommendations. Anesthesiology 1997;87:244–252.)

iting. Features that may limit the usefulness of this drug include gastrointestinal irritation and the antiplatelet effects. It diminishes the emergence agitation and pain behavior when given intravenously after induction for myringotomies with pressure-equalization tube insertion.[185] At a dose of 1 mg/kg, there was no significant difference in the pain score of children undergoing tonsillectomy with or without ade-

noidectomy compared with patients who received 35 mg/kg of rectal acetaminophen.[186] At a dose of 1 mg/kg intramuscularly or intravenously given before the onset of tonsillectomy surgery, there was an increase in the intraoperative and postoperative blood loss, as compared with patients who received 1.5 mg/kg of codeine intramuscularly[187] or 0.1 mg/kg morphine intravenously[188, 189] and no difference in awakening time or readiness for discharge between the groups. Ketorolac is a useful adjunct when given intravenously to supplement the local anesthesia infiltrated by the surgeon during inguinal herniorrhaphies.[190] Since ketorolac can increase bleeding time, it is recommended that this drug be administered after completion of surgery and assurance of hemostasis.

Antiemetics

Ondansetron is a selective 5-hydroxytryptamine subtype 3 receptor antagonist that reduces the incidence of vomiting when given prophylactically and when administered to patients with established nausea and vomiting.[191–193] It has been shown to be effective in reducing postoperative vomiting for a variety of procedures known to have a high incidence of vomiting, such as tonsillectomy, strabismus correction, hernia repair, and orchiopexy.[194–199] The usual dose is 0.1 mg/kg IV. It was found to be effective when given intravenously at a lower dose of 0.05 mg/kg for other surgical procedures compared to a higher dose of 0.1 mg/kg.[200] When an intravenous dose of 0.1 mg/kg was compared with droperidol (0.075 mg/kg), it was found that postoperative emesis was similar in the droperidol and placebo groups (32% and 35%), and reduced to 9% in the ondansetron group; the ondansetron group also had a shorter hospital stay than the droperidol-treated group.[201] When an intravenous dose of 0.15 mg/kg was compared with metoclopramide (0.5 mg/kg) or droperidol (0.075 mg/kg), the incidence of post-tonsillectomy emesis was reduced from 62% to 27% in patients who received ondansetron, whereas metoclopramide and droperidol had no effect.[202] Preoperative oral ondansetron has also been found to reduce postoperative vomiting.[192]

Granisetron is a newer, more selective 5-hydroxytryptamine, sub-type 3 antagonist that is also effective in children. At a dose of 0.04 mg/kg intravenously, it reduced the incidence and frequency of postoperative emesis in the immediate postoperative period as well as for the first 24 hours and resulted in a shorter time to discharge readiness compared with the placebo-treated group.[203] Studies similar to those performed with ondansetron have demonstrated its superiority over other antiemetics, such as droperidol and metoclopramide.[204–213]

Droperidol is a useful antiemetic in doses of 25 to 75 μg/kg.[62, 214, 215] When given orally 1 to 1.5 hours preoperatively at a very large dose of 0.3 mg/kg, the incidence of vomiting was reduced from 56% to 27%. Droperidol combined with oral metoclopramide (0.15 mg/kg) or another antiemetic was superior to either drug alone.[206, 216, 217] The combination of drugs was most effective in the period after discharge from the hospital when the incidence of vomiting decreased to 3%, as compared with the placebo-treated group in which the incidence was 20% and the droperidol-treated group in which the incidence was 12%. The effects of the premedication reportedly did not delay discharge from the hospital. Droperidol by itself is not as effective an antiemetic as other more specific medications such as ondansetron or granisetron.[64, 210, 218] When droperidol (0.05 mg/kg) and granisetron (0.04 mg/kg) were administered intravenously after the induction of anesthesia but before the start of tonsillectomy with and without adenoidectomy surgery, the incidence of postoperative emesis was significantly reduced compared with either drug alone.[206, 216, 219]

Dexamethasone is a corticosteroid that has a prolonged antiemetic effect.[220, 221] When given intravenously at a dose of 0.15 mg/kg after induction of anesthesia but before surgery, the incidence of vomiting after a tonsillectomy was reduced from 72% to 40%.[222] A low dose of ondansetron (0.050 mg/kg) plus dexamethasone (0.15 mg/kg) reduced the incidence of postoperative emesis to 9%, whereas the incidence after high-dose ondansetron without dexamethasone was 28%.[223]

Dimenhydrinate is an H_1-receptor antagonist that is a theoclate salt of diphenhydramine and is sold over the counter as Dramamine. An intravenous dose of 0.5 mg/kg was effective in reducing the incidence of in-hospital and overall emesis in pediatric patients undergoing strabismus surgery.[224] At this dose, there was no difference in the time to arousal and discharge from the recovery room and hospital compared with the placebo-treated group. However, when this drug was compared to ondansetron (0.1 mg/kg), the ondansetron group had less vomiting in the first 24 hours.[225]

Perphenazine is a phenothiazine that has moderate anticholinergic effects and weak to moderate sedative effects. The antiemetic effects of dexamethasone were compared with those of perphenazine. Perphenazine reduced the incidence of in-hospital vomiting to 14% compared with the dexamethasone-treated group, which had an incidence of 36%. The incidence of out-of-hospital vomiting was identical for the two groups of patients.[226] When oral perphenazine was compared with oral granisetron given preoperatively 1 hour before surgery, the incidence of postoperative emesis was lower in the granisetron-treated group than in the perphenazine-treated group.[227]

Other Drugs

Other drugs that are administered to children before the induction of anesthesia include steroids, insulin, antibiotics, antacids, H_2-receptor antagonists, and drugs that stimulate gastric motility.

STEROIDS. It is advisable to administer a dose of corticosteroids before anesthesia to prevent symptoms of adrenal cortical insufficiency in patients on chronic corticosteroid therapy and in those who discontinued chronic steroid therapy less than 6 months previously. Children usually receive 1.5 to 2.0 mg/kg of hydrocortisone intramuscularly or intravenously or an equivalent dose of dexamethasone (0.05 to 0.1 mg/kg) approximately 1 hour before the induction of anesthesia or as soon as an intravenous line is established.

INSULIN. Optimal management of diabetic patients undergoing anesthesia entails avoiding hypoglycemia, ketoacidosis, and a hyperosmolar state. Several protocols have been advocated to control diabetic patients. Table 9–2 shows one such protocol.[228] Prolonged starvation should be avoided. Diabetic

Table 9–2. Protocols for Perioperative Insulin Therapy

Regimen	Procedure Morning of Surgery
Classic regimen	Start intravenous infusion of 5% dextrose in 0.45% saline solution at 1500 mL/m² per day
	Administer half of usual morning insulin dose as regular insulin
	Check blood glucose before induction and during anesthesia
Continuous insulin infusion	Start intravenous infusion of 5% dextrose in 0.45% saline solution at 1500 mL/m² per day
	Add 1 to 2 units of insulin per 100 mL of 5% dextrose
	Start insulin dose = 0.02 U/kg/hr
	Check blood glucose before induction and during anesthesia
Insulin- and glucose-free regimen (for operative procedures of short duration)	Withhold morning insulin dose
	If indicated for the procedure: give glucose-free solution (e.g., lactated Ringer's solution) at maintenance rate
	Check blood glucose before induction and during anesthesia

From Maxwell LG, Deshpande JK, Wetzel RC: Preoperative evaluation of children. Pediatr Clin North Am 1994;41:93–110.

children are often administered an intravenous solution containing 5% dextrose early in the morning at a rate equal to their hourly maintenance requirement. Once the solution is started, either insulin is added to the intravenous solution or half of the child's usual morning insulin requirement is administered subcutaneously. Blood glucose, urine glucose, and acetone determinations should be made at frequent intervals during the perianesthetic period, and insulin or glucose administered as indicated. Ideally, these patients should be anesthetized early in the day to achieve the most stable management of blood glucose levels and insulin requirements.

ANTIBIOTICS. Antibiotics are frequently administered preoperatively to prevent or reduce infection in surgical patients. It is recommended that antibiotics be administered as prophylaxis against endocarditis to children with structural heart disease 30 to 60 minutes before the start of anesthesia and surgery; in reality, these antibiotics are administered after induction of anesthesia and after establishment of intravenous access. The preoperative doses recommended by the American Heart Association are presented in Table 17–4.[229]

ANTACIDS, H_2-ANTAGONISTS, AND GASTROINTESTINAL MOTILITY DRUGS. Mendelson first described the syndrome of pulmonary aspiration of gastric contents in anesthetized patients in 1946.[230] A gastric volume greater than 0.4 mL/kg and a gastric fluid pH of less than 2.5 was thought to be critical for the production of pulmonary acid aspiration syndrome (Mendelson syndrome). By these criteria, which were derived from unpublished data of pulmonary aspiration in rhesus monkeys,[231] the majority of children would be at increased risk for this syndrome because 75% of elective surgical pediatric patients have a gastric volume of 0.4 mL/

kg or greater and a pH less than 2.5.[232] The rare incidence of the syndrome ($\sim$ 1:1,000), however, is inconsistent with the number of patients who meet the volume and pH criteria.[233–236] One study of rhesus monkeys found that a greater volume (0.8 mL/kg) was required to produce the syndrome in monkeys.[237] Although most children probably are not at risk for aspiration, certain children, such as those with a hiatus hernia, a history of gastroesophageal reflux, prior esophageal surgery, difficult airway, obesity, or trauma, are prone to gastric reflux and aspiration.

Preanesthetic administration of drugs that reduce gastric volume and acidity may reduce the risk of pulmonary acid aspiration syndrome (Table 9–3).[232, 238, 239] Gastric pH can also be effectively raised by a nonparticulate antacid such as sodium citrate. *Particulate antacids should be avoided because they can cause severe pneumonitis if aspirated.* A disadvantage of antacids is that they increase gastric residual volume.

Cimetidine and *ranitidine* are H_2-receptor antagonists that decrease gastric acid secretion, increase gastric pH, and reduce gastric residual volume.[240–242] These drugs can be given orally, intravenously, or intramuscularly. Cimetidine is the H_2 blocker most frequently administered to children 1 to 3 hours before the induction of anesthesia to reduce gastric residual volume. Cimetidine lasts for approximately 3 to 4 hours, whereas ranitidine provides protection for a longer period of 8 to 9 hours.

Metoclopramide is often administered with cimetidine to increase lower esophageal sphincter tone, relax the pyloric sphincter and the duodenal bulb, and promote gastric emptying by increasing peristalsis of the duodenum and jejunum. The drug effect is apparent 30 to 60 minutes after oral administration and 1 to 2 minutes after intravenous or intramuscular administration.[243] Side effects are related to its effect on the central nervous system through blockade of dopaminergic receptors, thus leading to extrapyramidal symptoms. These medications may also be effective in reducing the risk of pulmonary aspiration of gastric contents, even for patients scheduled for emergency surgical procedures, if administered at least 1 hour before anesthetic induction.

Induction of Anesthesia

Inhalation Induction

The anesthetic induction period can be an extremely stressful period for the anesthesiologist, the child, and the parents,

Table 9–3. Doses of Antacids, H_2-Antagonists, and Gastrointestinal Motility Drugs

Drug	Dose
Antacids	
Bicitra	30 mL
Prokinetic	
Metoclopramide	0.1–0.15 mg/kg
H_2-Antagonists	
Cimetidine	5–10 mg/kg
Ranitidine	2–2.5 mg/kg
Famotidine	0.3–0.4 mg/kg

and for observers in the area. Proper evaluation and preparation of children and their families both psychologically and physiologically is extremely important, to avoid problems that could be prevented through better planning (see Chapters 3 and 4). Failure to properly evaluate the severity of underlying medical problems or to correct metabolic abnormalities can lead to critical events during the induction period. Even though a child may appear "normal" before induction, unexpected problems can occur during induction, such as laryngospasm, bradycardia, or cyanosis. Anesthesiologists who care for children must always be prepared for the unexpected. Because of the ever changing psychological and social needs of children and their parents, it is vital to be very flexible in changing to alternative methods of caring for patients and to alter plans "midstream," depending on the needs and responses of a child. This section focuses on anesthetic induction techniques.

Traditional Mask Inhalation Induction

The most common method of inducing anesthesia in children is inhalation of potent anesthetic agents through a face mask. The technique used depends on a number of factors, including the child's developmental age, understanding and ability to cooperate, and previous experiences, and the interaction of these factors with the patient's underlying medical or surgical conditions. Infants up to 8 to 10 months of age, for example, generally are not fearful of strangers and will easily separate from their parents. Thus this age group does not generally require a premedication and will usually respond to the mask induction of anesthesia by sucking or licking the mask. Toddlers frequently require a premedication to be able to cooperate for the smooth gaseous induction of anesthesia. Cooperative older children generally tolerate an inhalation induction, even though they may dislike the odor of the anesthetic gas. Generally when given a choice between an intravenous or intramuscular induction and an inhalation induction, they will choose an inhalation induction.

The traditional mask induction of anesthesia is accomplished by initially administering either 100% oxygen or a nonhypoxic mixture of nitrous oxide and oxygen. Although modern anesthesia machines do not allow the delivery of hypoxic mixtures, older machines are still available that will allow this to occur. Hypoxic mixtures have no place in pediatric anesthesia; they are potentially hazardous and unnecessary. Following several breaths of oxygen or the nitrous oxide–oxygen mixture, a potent inhalation agent (e.g., halothane) is added, beginning at 0.25%. The inspired concentration of the potent anesthetic is gradually increased 0.5% every three to four breaths until anesthesia is induced. Raising the concentration at this rate generally leads to a smooth induction of anesthesia. Increasing the concentration more rapidly for an agent with a pungent odor, such as halothane, may irritate a patient's airway and cause coughing. Conversely, a slower rate of increase prolongs induction time and makes patients vulnerable to all the problems, such as airway obstruction and vomiting, that could arise during a prolonged excitement period. After anesthesia is induced, the potent inhalation agent concentration is reduced to a maintenance concentration while the intravenous line is secured.

If vital signs become abnormal at any time during the

induction period, the concentration of the potent anesthetic is reduced or it is discontinued and the circuit flushed with 100% oxygen. If the oxygen saturation declines, nitrous oxide is discontinued and 100% oxygen is administered until the oxygen saturation returns to normal while dealing with the cause of the desaturation. Often there is mild to moderate airway obstruction due to collapse of the hypopharyngeal structures or the development of mild laryngospasm. It is recommended that a precordial stethoscope be placed over the larynx at the sternal notch, thus providing immediate input into the early stages of upper airway events. Generally this airway obstruction is readily relieved by gently obtaining a tight mask fit, slightly closing the pop-off valve so as to generate 5 to 10 cm of positive end-expiratory pressure, and simply allowing the distending pressure of the bag to stent open the airway (see Fig. 7–10). In most cases, there is no need to squeeze the bag.

Isoflurane is a more pungent drug than halothane; because of its pungency, inducing anesthesia in unpremedicated patients by slowly increasing the concentration of the drug is more difficult. An isoflurane induction of anesthesia is associated with a several-fold higher incidence of airway problems and is generally not recommended.[244, 245] If isoflurane must be used, increasing the concentration gradually (0.25 to 0.5% increase in concentration every 10 breaths) seems to reduce the propensity to airway irritation.

The induction, recovery, and safety characteristics of sevoflurane compared to halothane with and without nitrous oxide have been evaluated extensively.[246–251] There is little doubt that the gaseous induction of anesthesia is more rapid and that the increase in the inspired sevoflurane concentration can proceed more rapidly than with halothane.[246, 252, 253] Sevoflurane has replaced halothane in many institutions where cost is not a factor, whereas others limit its use to the induction period, changing to halothane or isoflurane for the maintenance of anesthesia. One pharmacodynamic effect is the apparent disparity between loss of consciousness and analgesia. It is very common to observe children respond to attempts at insertion of the intravenous catheter despite having lost consciousness. This may in part relate to the fact that sevoflurane opposes the analgesic properties of nitrous oxide.[254] Another concern is the rare case of electrically generalized but clinically silent seizure activity in both normal children and children with seizure disorders.[248, 255, 256] The clinical importance of this observation is not yet clear.

Induction Using Scented Masks

The odor of the anesthetic may be very objectionable to some children. If patients are instructed to breathe through their mouth instead of their nose, they may find the odor less objectionable. Often offering children the choice of smells provides sufficient distraction to allow a smooth induction of anesthesia. A small amount of a scented liquid, such as bubble gum, strawberry, or grape flavor (Lorann Oils, Lansing, MI), applied to the inside of the face mask may disguise the odor of the inhalation anesthetic. Too much liquid applied to the mask may result in too strong a scent for a child. Patients may select a scent before the induction of anesthesia or during the preanesthetic visit. An alternative to liquid scents is flavored lip balm such as Chapstick (A. H. Robins Co., Richmond, VA). Children can be presented with the various tubes before the induction of anesthesia and allowed to paint the inside of the anesthetic mask with the flavor they wish to breathe while they fall asleep.

Distraction Techniques

Since young children are often very susceptible to suggestions and distraction, a common method for induction is to ask them to "blow up the balloon" (the anesthesia bag) or to try and "blow out the candles." This can be accomplished with the child sitting in the lap of the anesthesiologist or in a parent's lap, or with the child sitting on the operating room table leaning against the chest of the anesthesiologist. Generally allowing the child this degree of freedom without forcing him or her to be supine on the operating room table provides excellent conditions for a smooth induction.

Hypnotic Induction

Another very common method of gaseous induction is to use hypnotic suggestions as a means of distraction. Hypnosis can be successfully used in pediatric patients. The safe use of hypnosis as the sole anesthetic technique requires an understanding of the hypnotic process and formal training. Although an anesthesiologist may not have had training in hypnosis, a competent practitioner can use hypnotic suggestions to help patients even though an actual trance state is not induced. Carefully worded suggestions that are reassuringly spoken can direct a patient's attention to the positive aspects of events. Phrases such as *"you will feel very comfortable and relaxed as you concentrate on your breathing,"* or *"everything will feel warm and tingly"* spoken slowly and rhythmically with meaningful pauses and emphasis on key words, can instill confidence in a child and assist the induction of anesthesia. To a child, the anesthesiologist is not only an adult but an authority figure, further enhancing the aura of the doctor as a hypnotist. In this instance, words are exceedingly powerful tools that can have a profound influence on the mental attitude of patients toward the therapeutic regimen and illness. Often younger children can be "taken for a trip to the zoo." By the anesthesiologist's describing sights and sounds that are familiar and by repeatedly telling the children how good they feel, children become very susceptible to the hypnotic sound of the voice and the repeated imagery suggested. An example of a hypnotic induction is as follows:

"Do you like to go to the zoo?" *"Today let's pretend that you are going to the zoo with mom and dad."* *"It is a beautiful day and the sun is shining and everything feels warm and tingly."* (Start the nitrous oxide and oxygen) *"As we get closer to the zoo you can hear some of the animals and the first animal we will see is the elephant."* *"The elephant has great big floppy ears and a big long trunk and they love to eat hay, but those elephants really stink"* (Turn on the potent inhalation agent to a low concentration) *"but you are having a wonderful time with your family and the sun is shining and everything feels warm and tingly."* *"Now we are going to see the giraffes, and they are very beautiful with big long necks and pretty orange and yellow colors and they love to eat hay also, but they smell even worse than the elephants."* (Increase the concentration of potent agent) *"but it is a beautiful day and the sun is shining and everything*

feels warm and tingly and you are having a wonderful time with your parents." "Now we are going to see the hippos and they are flopping around in the water and you can throw apples at them but they smell even worse than the giraffes" (Increase the concentration of the agent further) *"but it is a beautiful day and the sun is shining and everything feels warm and tingly and you are having a wonderful time with your parents."*

This type of hypnotic suggestion distracts the child so that the smell of anesthetic agent is the smell of the animals and the warm feeling during induction is the sunshine while at the same time suggesting a feeling of love from their parents and a feeling of enjoyment. In older children, one can substitute flying a jet with the mask being the pilot's mask and the smell of agent the smell of aviation fuel. The faster the jet goes, the stronger the fuel smell. One can repeatedly describe the blue sky–white clouds, blue water–white sand, blue water–white sails. Any number of stories can be told with the same result as long as one remembers to repeatedly say things that can be identified by the child and that fit with what the child is experiencing at the time of induction.

Noise in the room should be kept to a minimum during the induction of anesthesia. The anesthesiologist can tell the child a story with a nonthreatening, soothing voice. It is probably wise not to ask patients questions during the induction because they may become upset if they are unable to answer the questions. Some children may object to having a mask placed over their face because they have the feeling of suffocation. They may feel better if the mask is held a few inches away from their face. If a mask is objectionable, removing the mask from the elbow (anesthetic delivery hose) allows the anesthesiologist to cup the hand around the orifice of the elbow to concentrate the flow of gases in the area under the palm of the hand. Holding the elbow between two fingers just above the child's face may be more acceptable. As the child becomes drowsy, the anesthesiologist can move the hand closer to the child's face. Once the child is lightly anesthetized (and hopefully amnesic), the anesthetic mask can be attached to the elbow and gently applied to the child's face. Care should always be taken to direct the flow of gas downward away from the eyes because the sensation of "wind" blowing in their eyes is distracting and can be uncomfortable. Care must also be taken with how gently the mask is applied to the face and to ensure that it fits properly.

Modified Single-Breath Induction

Some children will be very cooperative until they smell the anesthetic agent. This change in attitude can usually be circumvented if the inhalation induction time is shortened. We have had success using a modification of the single-breath halothane or sevoflurane induction technique as an alternative to the traditional method of inducing anesthesia.[183, 248, 253, 257–261] Children as young as 3 years can be anesthetized with this modified technique if they are cooperative. This method of inducing anesthesia is especially useful in children who desire "to go to sleep" with a face mask but who may struggle during a traditional mask induction of anesthesia.

Before going into the induction area, a child is coached through a mock induction; practicing with the anesthesia

mask without the circuit assists the child in understanding what will be required. The success of this technique depends almost entirely on the full coordination of the child's breathing and the application of the face mask. Generally, demonstrating for the child a full vital capacity breath in and holding it is the first step. The next step is making a full exhalation and holding it. This is followed by applying the mask (with a good fit) to the face while the child pauses in full exhalation and then asking him or her to make a full inspiration and then hold it in before resuming normal respirations. An assessment of whether a child is able to follow commands should be made at this time. If the child understands and is cooperative, the induction of anesthesia will be attempted using the modified single-breath induction technique; otherwise, another method should be selected.

Before induction, the face mask is attached to the anesthetic elbow and the anesthetic circuit is filled with maximum concentrations of halothane or sevoflurane in 3 L/min of nitrous oxide and 2 L/min of oxygen by occluding the outflow from the anesthetic elbow. Venting the anesthesia bag several times allows equilibration of the appropriate gas concentration throughout the breathing circuit. The child is then asked to take a deep breath of room air, to blow it all out, and then to hold his or her breath. After removing the occlusion from the outflow of the anesthesia elbow, the anesthesiologist gently places the face mask over the face, making a conscious effort not to grip the child's jaw. Gripping the jaw can frighten an awake child and could lead to a stormy induction. After the mask is securely placed on the patient's face, the child is asked to take a deep breath and then to breathe normally. Once anesthesia is induced, the concentration of the potent inhalation agent is decreased to a concentration that is appropriate to maintain anesthesia.

The induction technique just described usually induces anesthesia in children faster than the traditional inhalation method of having the child inhale increasing concentrations of the potent anesthetic gas.[262] This is true whether the child holds his or her breath or breathes normally after the initial breath of anesthetic gas. If a patient fails to exhale completely or takes a very small breath of room air before breathing the anesthetic gas mixture, anesthesia will still be induced within 2 minutes as long as the next breath, whether it is a deep or a normal breath, is of the maximum concentration of the potent anesthetic gas. Adding nitrous oxide to the inhaled gases decreases induction time with halothane but may not significantly alter the induction time with sevoflurane.[260, 262, 263] Anesthetic induction, as noted by the loss of the eyelash reflex, is induced almost as rapidly as with intravenous thiopental (30 to 45 seconds) and three times faster than with the traditional inhalation induction of anesthesia.[262, 264]

Intravenous Induction

The intravenous method of inducing anesthesia is generally reserved for older children, those who request an intravenous induction, those who have a pre-existing intravenous catheter, and those who need a rapid-sequence induction because of a full stomach. A child is also a candidate for intravenous induction of anesthesia if an intravenous catheter can be inserted without undue trauma.

Intravenous anesthesia began in 1934 with the introduction of thiopental.[265] Despite the release of other ultrashort-acting barbiturates for inducing anesthesia, such as thiamylal and methohexital, thiopental remained the most popular intravenous induction agent. It was not until 1967 that the first nonbarbiturate anesthetic, ketamine, was released. Subsequently, a number of other intravenous anesthetic drugs, such as gamma-hydroxybutyric acid, etomidate, propanidid, and propofol, have become available. Although many of these drugs are still not recommended for children because safety and efficacy studies in children were not performed before their release, many of them are used in the anesthetic care of pediatric patients (Table 9–4) (see Chapter 8 for discussion of drug labeling).

The most frequently used intravenous anesthetic-inducing drug for children is *thiopental*. It is an ultrashort-acting barbiturate that produces sedation within 1 minute after administration. The beta elimination half-life in newborns is twice that of their mothers (15 hours versus 7 hours) so this agent may produce excessively long effects in this population.[266] Children require more thiopental per kilogram of body weight than adults. The recommended inducing dose for healthy unpremedicated children is 5 to 6 mg/kg.[267–269] Neonates, debilitated patients, severely ill patients, and those that have been premedicated require less drug, whereas infants beyond the neonatal period may require more.[269, 270]

Thiamylal is an ultrashort-acting thiobarbiturate that is very similar to thiopental. Like thiopental, a 2.5% solution is recommended for intravenous administration. The recommended anesthetic induction dose is similar to thiopental.

Methohexital is an ultrashort-acting oxybarbiturate that is used intravenously as a 1% solution. Recovery from intravenous anesthesia after this drug is more rapid than after thiopental.[271, 272] Pharmacokinetic studies demonstrate that methohexital is cleared more rapidly than thiopental.[86, 92] The intravenous induction dose for children ranges from 1 to 2.5 mg/kg. Unpremedicated children require an induction dose of 2.0 to 2.5 mg/kg IV.[273] Higher doses cause skeletal muscle hyperactivity. Pain at the injection site is more common after methohexital than after thiopental, and the incidence of pain is directly related to the dose. Intravenous methohexital is associated with hiccoughs and pain.[273]

Propofol is an alkylphenol that is an oil at room temperature. Because it is only slightly soluble in water, it is formulated as a 1% solution in a white soybean oil, egg lecithin, and glycerol emulsion. Propofol is highly lipophilic and protein bound and rapidly distributes and redistributes throughout body compartments. The initial distribution half-life is about 2 minutes, and the elimination half-life is about 30 minutes.[274] Clearance is very high (2.3 ± 0.6 L/min) and exceeds liver blood flow.[274] The dose of propofol for the induction of anesthesia varies with age. In children, the dose ratio for the induction of anesthesia with propofol compared with thiopental is 1:2.5.[275] Healthy children require about 2.5 to 3.5 mg/kg for satisfactory induction of anesthesia.[276, 277] The induction dose of propofol for infants is higher than for older children. In one study, the effective dose in 50% (ED_{50}) for satisfactory induction was 3.0 ± 0.2 mg/kg for infants 1 to 6 months old and 2.4 ± 0.1 mg/kg for children 10 to 16 years old.[278]

There are major advantages to using propofol for the induction of anesthesia. A number of studies have demonstrated a lower incidence of airway-related problems (laryngospasm) and a more rapid emergence.[279–281] Another major advantage, particularly for ambulatory patients, is a lower incidence of nausea and vomiting.[282–286] The major disadvantage of propofol is the pain it produces during injection, especially when administered into small veins.[278] Lidocaine (0.5 to 1.0 mg/kg) administered before or concomitantly with propofol may decrease the incidence of pain. One easy method of reducing this pain is to apply a tourniquet to the extremity with the intravenous line and inject 0.5 to 1.0 mg/kg lidocaine in the running intravenous line, creating a "mini-Bier block." The induction dose of propofol is administered through the running intravenous line, and once the entire dose is in the patient's veins the tourniquet is released, resulting in a relatively pain-free administration. Approximately 15% of patients will experience a decrease in blood pressure and apnea.[275, 277, 278, 287, 288]

In addition to its use as an induction drug, propofol can also be administered intravenously to maintain anesthesia. The availability of this rapid and short-acting intravenous anesthetic has encouraged the use of continuous intravenous infusion techniques as an alternative to standard inhalation anesthetics for maintenance of general anesthesia in pediatric patients undergoing short procedures such as radiation therapy or intrathecal chemotherapy. The drug is especially useful in children who require multiple treatments over the course of a few weeks. Minimal cardiovascular or respiratory depression is observed when the drug is titrated to sedate children for these procedures. A variable-rate infusion pump can provide a stable anesthetic state and allow the anesthesiologist to titrate the dose to a desired effect.

Etomidate is a hypnotic drug that is available as a 2 mg/mL solution. A dose of 0.3 mg/kg induces sleep in adults. Cardiovascular and respiratory depression are rare, but nausea and vomiting are common during recovery, especially when combined with an opioid.[289] The major advantage of etomidate is the marked cardiovascular stability; this is perhaps the best induction agent for patients with known cardiovascular dysfunction, such as children with cardiomyopathy.[290, 291]

Ketamine is another very useful induction agent for patients with cardiovascular instability, especially in hypovolemic states, or patients in whom it is vital to maintain peripheral vascular resistance, such as those with aortic stenosis or other forms of congenital heart disease in whom the balance between pulmonary and systemic blood flow is vital for maintaining cardiovascular homeostasis. It should be noted that ketamine is a myocardial depressant and can result in systemic hypotension in patients who already are maximally responding with endogenous catecholamines.[292] The usual induction dose is 2 mg/kg, which is reduced to 1

Table 9–4. Doses of Commonly Used Intravenous Induction Agents

Drug	Dose (mg/kg)
Thiopental or thiamylal	5–8
Methohexital	1–2.5
Propofol	2.5–3.5
Etomidate	0.3
Ketamine	1–2

mg/kg if there is the possibility of severe hypovolemia. Lower doses of intravenous ketamine (0.25–0.5 mg/kg) have been successfully used for procedural sedation. It should be noted that atropine or another antisialagogue should be administered so as to avoid the copious secretions often produced by ketamine.

Intramuscular Induction

There are occasions when a well-planned induction of anesthesia goes awry and the anesthesiologist is confronted with a child who suddenly loses composure or becomes upset and uncooperative. In these situations, administering drugs intramuscularly may be the least traumatic way to induce anesthesia, especially in a child who strenuously objects to oral, rectal, or intranasal medication or who has poor venous access. In infants and very small children, intramuscular *methohexital* (10 mg/kg of a 5% solution) produces sleep in the majority of patients within several minutes. In older patients, *ketamine* is a useful drug. An initial dose of 6 to 10 mg/kg IM is generally required for anesthesia, whereas a dose of 2 to 3 mg/kg IM produces sedation in the majority of the children.[11] The cardiovascular stimulating properties of the drug are particularly appealing in situations in which hypotension is a potential problem, such as in hypovolemic patients or the cardiovascular patients described earlier. Ketamine can be very unpredictable in infants. Some may require extremely large doses, whereas others are anesthetized after receiving low doses.[293] Ketamine may also be contraindicated in children with airway problems, especially those with an upper respiratory tract infection. The increase in airway secretions following ketamine administration may stimulate laryngospasm.[140] Administering anticholinergic drugs may eliminate this side effect. Although ketamine generally stimulates respiration, severe respiratory depression can occur. The occasional occurrence of hallucinations in children following administration of ketamine is another disadvantage. This can be minimized by administering a benzodiazepine, such as diazepam or midazolam.

Ketamine and methohexital are rapidly absorbed after intramuscular administration. The induction of anesthesia, however, might be delayed when tissue perfusion is poor. Although a speedy induction of anesthesia and easy administration are the appealing characteristics of an intramuscular induction, disadvantages include injection pain and the possibility of sterile abscess formation.

Rectal Induction

Rectal sedation produces a spectrum from drowsiness to general anesthesia. In general, the dose of the rectally administered drug should be higher when the situation calls for anesthesia rather than sedation. Methohexital, thiopental, ketamine, and midazolam have all been utilized by this route of administration. For certain procedures, such as computed tomographic scans, dressing changes, suture removal, and some eye examinations, rectally administered ketamine or methohexital may be all that is needed for the procedure.

Rectal drug administration is ideally suited for an extremely frightened child who rejects a needle or a mask induction of anesthesia but who does not object to rectal thermometers. It is also useful in mentally handicapped patients. Other advantages include ease of drug administration, easy repetition of the dose if sleep does not ensue, and elimination of anxiety produced by separating a child from parents when the child is awake. Disadvantages include failure of inducing anesthesia in a small percentage of patients owing to poor bioavailability of the drug or defecation, as well as delayed recovery from anesthesia after brief procedures due to the variability of absorption of rectal drugs.[101, 294]

Rapid-Sequence Induction

Patients with a full stomach or gastroesophageal reflux should receive oxygen before the induction of anesthesia to ensure adequate oxygenation. In some children who are very frightened by the anesthesia mask, the best that can be done is to "enrich" the environment by using high oxygen flows and holding the mask in close proximity but not touching the face of the child. Intravenous induction agents and muscle relaxants should be rapidly administered followed by the application of cricoid pressure (Sellick maneuver) as the child loses consciousness.[295] Cricoid pressure should be maintained until the endotracheal tube is in place and the cuff is inflated (if a cuffed endotracheal tube is used) to prevent potential aspiration of gastric contents (see Chapters 4 and 7).

Parental Presence During Induction

The presence of the parents during the induction of anesthesia is desirable if a child will be more cooperative and if it will allay their anxieties. The presence of parents during induction is controversial, but at some institutions they are present during the induction of every elective case unless the patient does not want them present. It should be noted that parental presence is for the welfare of the child and not the parent. Since the child is the patient, parental presence at the time of induction is only considered if it will benefit the patient. It is unlikely that parental presence will be of any benefit to the neonate or infant who is not fearful of strangers, nor is it appropriate for parents to attend a rapid sequence induction. Studies suggest that children are more secure when their parents are present, although they may "act out" or express vocal or physical opposition to anesthesia in their presence.[296, 297] Parental presence may decrease the requirement for heavy sedation and minimize anxiety. It can also allay parents' anxiety about the transition to general anesthesia, that is, the parents' concern to make this process as psychologically atraumatic as possible. There are three groups of patients who seem to benefit most from parental presence. They are (1) children who are older than 4 years of age, (2) children with parents who have a low baseline level of anxiety (less anxious), and (3) children who have a low baseline level of anxiety (less anxious).[298] It was further found that oral midazolam premedication was more effective in allaying anxiety than parental presence.[299]

Major arguments against parents' presence during induction are that the parents may interfere with the induction procedure through disruptive behavior or may cause the anesthesiologist discomfort at being watched, especially if a critical incident occurs. Difficulties with parents during induction are uncommon and usually not severe.[300] Rarely, a parent may disrupt the induction; this is often related to anxiety or to distress about the anesthetic or surgical procedure. The education of parents and the selection of those who should be present during induction of anesthesia are critical if induction is to proceed smoothly. Whenever parental presence during induction is contemplated, the anxiety level of the parents should be assessed as part of the routine preoperative evaluation. Parents who are extremely anxious or distressed about the anesthetic procedure should probably not be present during induction because children in this setting are usually more upset if their parents are present than if they are separated from them.[301] Parents must be informed about what to anticipate in terms of the operating room itself (equipment, surgical devices) and in terms of what they may observe during induction (eyes rolling back, laryngeal noises, anesthetic monitor alarms, excitation) and when they will be asked to leave. They must also be instructed about how they can be most helpful to the induction process, such as by comforting their child and reassuring him or her to trust the anesthesiologist, distracting the child, and consoling the child. Personnel should be immediately available to escort parents back to the waiting area at the appropriate time. Someone should also be available to care for a parent who wishes to leave the induction area or who becomes lightheaded or faints. An anesthesiologist's anxiety about parents' presence during induction decreases significantly with experience.[302]

Explaining what parents might see or hear is very important. We generally tell parents the following:

"As you see your child fall asleep today there are several things you might observe that you are not used to seeing. First, when anyone falls asleep, the eyes roll up, but since we are sleeping we do not generally see it. You may see your child do that today and I do not want you to be frightened by that—it is expected and normal. The second thing is that as children go to sleep from the anesthesia medications, the tone of the structures in the neck decreases so that some children will begin to snore or make vibrating noises. Again, I do not want you to be frightened or think that something is wrong. We expect this and it is normal. The third thing you might see is what we call excitement. As the brain begins to go to sleep it can actually get excited first. About 30 to 60 seconds after breathing the anesthesia medications, your child might suddenly look around or suddenly move his or her arms and legs. To you it appears that he is awaking from anesthesia or that he is upset. In reality, this is a good sign because it indicates to us that the child is falling asleep and that about 15 to 30 seconds after that he or she will be completely anesthetized. Also you should know that even though your child appears to be awake to you, in reality he or she will not remember any of that."

This kind of careful preparation, and also pointing out to the parents the various events as they happen, actually gives parents confidence that the anesthesiologist really knows what he or she is talking about and it avoids frightening the parents. Some parents are still frightened by this process and will likely decline the opportunity to participate in the next anesthetic procedure, whereas others are grateful for the information and the warning of what they might observe. In general, the more information you can provide, the happier the parents are.

REFERENCES

1. Sigurdsson GH, Lindahl S, Norden N: Influence of premedication on the sympathetic and endocrine responses and cardiac arrhythmias during halothane anaesthesia in children undergoing adenoidectomy. Br J Anaesth 1983;55:961–968.
2. Vetter TR: The epidemiology and selective identification of children at risk for preoperative anxiety reactions. Anesth Analg 1993;77:96–99.
3. Kain ZN, Mayes LC, O'Connor TZ, et al: Preoperative anxiety in children: Predictors and outcomes. Arch Pediatr Adolesc Med 1996;150:1238–1245.
4. Cassady JF Jr, Wysocki TT, Miller KM, et al: Use of a preanesthetic video for facilitation of parental education and anxiolysis before pediatric ambulatory surgery. Anesth Analg 1999;88:246–250.
5. Karl HW, Pauza KJ, Heyneman N, et al: Preanesthetic preparation of pediatric outpatients: The role of a videotape for parents. J Clin Anesth 1990;2:172–177.
6. Kain ZN, Mayes LC, Wang SM, et al: Postoperative behavioral outcomes in children: Effects of sedative premedication. Anesthesiology 1999;90:758–765.
7. Waters RM; Pain relief for children. Am J Surg 1938;39:470–475.
8. Smalley A: Needle phobia. Paediatr Nurs 1999;11:17–20.
9. Rice LJ: Needle phobia: An anesthesiologist's perspective. J Pediatr 1993;122:S9–S13.
10. Brzustowicz RM, Nelson DA, Betts EK, et al: Efficacy of oral premedication for pediatric outpatient surgery. Anesthesiology 1984;60:475–477.
11. Hannallah RS, Patel RI: Low-dose intramuscular ketamine for anesthesia pre-induction in young children undergoing brief outpatient procedures. Anesthesiology 1989;70:598–600.
12. Kain ZN, Mayes LC, Bell C, et al: Premedication in the United States: A status report. Anesth Analg 1997;84:427–432.
13. Greenblatt DJ, Abernethy DR, Locniskar A, et al: Effect of age, gender, and obesity on midazolam kinetics. Anesthesiology 1984;61:27–35.
14. Feld LH, Negus JB, White PF: Oral midazolam preanesthetic medication in pediatric outpatients. Anesthesiology 1990;73:831–834.
15. Rita L, Seleny FL, Mazurek A, et al: Intramuscular midazolam for pediatric preanesthetic sedation: A double-blind controlled study with morphine. Anesthesiology 1985;63:528–531.
16. Taylor MB, Vine PR, Hatch DJ: Intramuscular midazolam premedication in small children: A comparison with papaveretum and hyoscine. Anaesthesia 1986;41:21–26.
17. Saint-Maurice C, Landais A, Delleur MM, et al: The use of midazolam in diagnostic and short surgical procedures in children. Acta Anaesthesiol Scand Suppl 1990;92:41–47.
18. Saarnivaara L, Lindgren L, Klemola U-M, et al: Comparison of chloral hydrate and midazolam by mouth as premedicants in children undergoing otolaryngological surgery. Br J Anaesth 1988;61:390–396.
19. Wilton NC, Leigh J, Rosen DR, et al: Preanesthetic sedation of preschool children using intranasal midazolam. Anesthesiology 1988;69:972–975.
20. Walbergh EJ, Wills RJ, Eckhert J: Plasma concentrations of midazolam in children following intranasal administration. Anesthesiology 1991;74:233–235.
21. Saint-Maurice C, Meistelman C, Rey E, et al: The pharmacokinetics of rectal midazolam for premedication in children. Anesthesiology 1986;65:536–538.
22. Lindahl SGE: The use of midazolam in premedication. Acta Anaesthesiol Scand 1990;34(Suppl 92):79–83.
23. Riva J, Lejbusiewicz G, Papa M, et al: Oral premedication with midazolam in paediatric anaesthesia: Effects on sedation and gastric contents. Paediatr Anaesth 1997;7:191–196.
24. Gillerman RG, Hinkle AJ, Green HM, et al: Parental presence plus oral midazolam decreases frequency of 5% halothane inductions in children. J Clin Anesth 1996;8:480–485.
25. Suresh S, Cohen IJ, Matuszczak M, et al: Dose ranging, safety, and efficacy of a new oral midazolam syrup in children. Anesthesiology 1998;89:A1313.
26. Palkama VJ, Ahonen J, Neuvonen PJ, et al: Effect of saquinavir on

the pharmacokinetics and pharmacodynamics of oral and intravenous midazolam. Clin Pharmacol Ther 1999;66:33–39.

27. Bailey DG, Malcolm J, Arnold O, et al: Grapefruit juice-drug interactions. Br J Clin Pharmacol 1998;46:101–110.

28. Ameer B, Weintraub RA: Drug interactions with grapefruit juice. Clin Pharmacokinet 1997;33:103–121.

29. Thummel KE, O'Shea D, Paine MF, et al: Oral first-pass elimination of midazolam involves both gastrointestinal and hepatic CYP3A-mediated metabolism. Clin Pharmacol Ther 1996;59:491–502.

30. Olkkola KT, Aranko K, Luurila H, et al: A potentially hazardous interaction between erythromycin and midazolam. Clin Pharmacol Ther 1993;53:298–305.

31. Hiller A, Olkkola KT, Isohanni P, et al: Unconsciousness associated with midazolam and erythromycin. Br J Anaesth 1994;65:826–828.

32. Gorski JC, Hall SD, Jones DR, et al: Regioselective biotransformation of midazolam by members of the human cytochrome P450 3A (CYP3A) subfamily. Biochem Pharmacol 1994;47:1643–1653.

33. Massanari M, Novitsky J, Reinstein LJ: Paradoxical reactions in children associated with midazolam use during endoscopy. Clin Pediatr (Phila) 1997;36:681–684.

34. McGraw T: Oral midazolam and post-operative behaviour in children. Can J Anaesth 1993;40:682–683.

35. Karl HW, Keifer AT, Rosenberger JL, et al: Comparison of the safety and efficacy of intranasal midazolam or sufentanil for preinduction of anesthesia in pediatric patients. Anesthesiology 1992;76:209–215.

36. Fishbein M, Lugo RA, Woodland J, et al: Evaluation of intranasal midazolam in children undergoing esophagogastroduodenoscopy. J Pediatr Gastroenterol Nutr 1997;25:261–266.

37. Zedie N, Amory DW, Wagner BK, et al: Comparison of intranasal midazolam and sufentanil premedication in pediatric outpatients. Clin Pharmacol Ther 1996;59:341–348.

38. Zatta P, Favarato M, Nicolini M: Deposition of aluminum in brain tissues of rats exposed to inhalation of aluminum acetylacetonate. Neuro Report 1993;4:1119–1122.

39. Jackson RT, Tigges J, Arnold W: Subarachnoid space of the CNS, nasal mucosa, and lymphatic system. Arch Otolaryngol 1979;105:180–184.

40. Harkema JR: Comparative aspects of nasal airway anatomy: Relevance to inhalation toxicology. Toxicol Pathol 1991;19:321–336.

41. Malinovsky JM, Cozian A, Lepage JY, et al: Ketamine and midazolam neurotoxicity in the rabbit. Anesthesiology 1991;75:91–97.

42. Committee on Drugs American Academy of Pediatrics: Alternate routes of drug administration: Advantages and disadvantages. Pediatrics 1997;100:143–152.

43. Davis PJ, Tome JA, McGowan FX Jr, et al: Preanesthetic medication with intranasal midazolam for brief pediatric surgical procedures: Effect on recovery and hospital discharge times. Anesthesiology 1995;82:2–5.

44. Weldon BC, Watcha MF, White PF: Oral midazolam in children: effect of time and adjunctive therapy. Anesth Analg 1992;75:51–55.

45. Mitchell V, Grange C, Black A, et al: A comparison of midazolam with trimeprazine as an oral premedicant for children. Anaesthesia 1997;52:416–421.

46. Patel D, Meakin G: Oral midazolam compared with diazepam-droperidol and trimeprazine as premedicants in children. Paediatr Anaesth 1997;7:287–293.

47. Mandelli M, Tognoni G, Garattini S: Clinical pharmacokinetics of diazepam. Clin Pharmacokinet 1978;3:72–91.

48. Hardman JG, Limbird LE, Molinoff PB, et al: In: Gilman AG, Goodman LS, Gilman A, eds: Goodman & Gilman's The Pharmacological Basis of Therapeutics, 9th ed. New York: Macmillan Publishing Co.; 1996:1734.

49. Hillestad L, Hansen T, Melsom H, et al: Diazepam metabolism in normal man. I. Serum concentrations and clinical effects after intravenous, intramuscular, and oral administration. Clin Pharmacol Ther 1974;16:479–484.

50. Hung OR, Dyck JB, Varvel J, et al: Comparative absorption kinetics of intramuscular midazolam and diazepam. Can J Anaesth 1996;43:450–455.

51. Kanto J: Plasma levels of diazepam after oral and intramuscular administration. Br J Anaesth 1974;46:817.

52. Gamble JA, MacKay JS, Dundee JW: Correspondence: Plasma levels of diazepam. Br J Anaesth 1973;45:1085.

53. Mattila MA, Ruoppi MK, Ahlstrom-Bengs E, et al: Diazepam in rectal

54. Sonander H, Arnold E, Nilsson K: Effects of the rectal administration of diazepam: Diazepam concentrations in children undergoing general anaesthesia. Br J Anaesth 1985;57:578–580.

55. van der Walt JH, Jacob R, Murrell D, et al: The perioperative effects of oral premedication in children. Anaesth Intensive Care 1990;18:5–10.

56. Relling MV, Mulhern RK, Dodge RK, et al: Lorazepam pharmacodynamics and pharmacokinetics in children. J Pediatr 1989;114:641–646.

57. Van de Velde A, Schneider I, Camu F: A double-blind comparison of the efficacy of lorazepam FDDF versus placebo for anesthesia premedication in children. Acta Anaesthesiol Belg 1987;38:207–212.

58. Buhrer M, Maitre PO, Hung O, et al: Electroencephalographic effects of benzodiazepines. I. Choosing an electroencephalographic parameter to measure the effect of midazolam on the central nervous system. Clin Pharmacol Ther 1990;48:544–554.

59. Buhrer M, Maitre PO, Crevoisier C, et al: Electroencephalographic effects of benzodiazepines. II. Pharmacodynamic modeling of the electroencephalographic effects of midazolam and diazepam. Clin Pharmacol Ther 1990;48:555–567.

60. Nicolson SC, Kaya KM, Betts EK: The effect of preoperative oral droperidol on the incidence of postoperative emesis after paediatric strabismus surgery. Can J Anaesth 1988;35:364–367.

61. Karlsson E, Larsson LE, Nilsson K: Postanaesthetic nausea in children. Acta Anaesthesiol Scand 1990;34:515–518.

62. Blanc VF, Ruest P, Milot J, et al: Antiemetic prophylaxis with promethazine or droperidol in paediatric outpatient strabismus surgery. Can J Anaesth 1991;38:54–60.

63. Brown RE Jr, James DJ, Weaver RG, et al: Low-dose droperidol versus standard-dose droperidol for prevention of postoperative vomiting after pediatric strabismus surgery. J Clin Anesth 1991;3:306–309.

64. Davis A, Krige S, Moyes D: A double-blind randomized prospective study comparing ondansetron with droperidol in the prevention of emesis following strabismus surgery. Anaesth Intens Care 1995;23:438–443.

65. Lerman J, Eustis S, Smith DR: Effect of droperidol pretreatment on postanesthetic vomiting in children undergoing strabismus surgery. Anesthesiology 1986;65:322–325.

66. Lin DM, Furst SR, Rodarte A: A double-blinded comparison of metoclopramide and droperidol for prevention of emesis following strabismus surgery. Anesthesiology 1992;76:357–361.

67. Grunwald Z, Torjman M, Schieren H, et al: The pharmacokinetics of droperidol in anesthetized children. Anesth Analg 1993;76:1238–1242.

68. Dupre LJ, Stieglitz P: Extrapyramidal syndromes after premedication with droperidol in children. Br J Anaesth 1980;52:831–833.

69. Gaal DG, Rice LJ, Hannallah RS: Droperidol-induced extrapyramidal symptoms in an adolescent following strabismus surgery. Middle East J Anesthesiol 1990;10:527–531.

70. Terndrup TE, Dire DJ, Madden CM, et al: Comparison of intramuscular meperidine and promethazine with and without chlorpromazine: A randomized, prospective, double-blind trial. Ann Emerg Med 1993;22:206–211.

71. Terndrup TE, Cantor RM, Madden CM: Intramuscular meperidine, promethazine, and chlorpromazine: Analysis of use and complications in 487 pediatric emergency department patients. Ann Emerg Med 1989;18:528–533.

72. Saravia ME, Currie WR, Campbell RL: Cardiopulmonary parameters during meperidine, promethazine, and chlorpromazine sedation for pediatric dentistry. Anesth Prog 1987;34:92–96.

73. Taylor G, Houston JB, Shaffer J, et al: Pharmacokinetics of promethazine and its sulphoxide metabolite after intravenous and oral administration to man. Br J Clin Pharmacol 1983;15:287–293.

74. Bloomfield EL, Masaryk TJ, Caplin A, et al: Intravenous sedation for MR imaging of the brain and spine in children: Pentobarbital versus propofol. Radiology 1993;186:93–97.

75. Cook BA, Bass JW, Nomizu S, et al: Sedation of children for technical procedures: Current standard of practice. Clin Pediatr (Phila) 1992;31:137–142.

76. Temme JB, Anderson JC, Matecko S: Sedation of children for CT and MRI scanning. Radiol Technol 1990;61:283–285.

77. Nicolson SC, Betts EK, Jobes DR, et al: Comparison of oral and intramuscular preanesthetic medication for pediatric inpatient surgery. Anesthesiology 1989;71:8–10.

78. Dundee JW, Nair SG, Assaf RA, et al: Pentobarbitone premedication

for anaesthesia: The influence of the preparation and route of administration on its clinical action. Anaesthesia 1976;31:1025–1031.

79. Christensen PA, Balslev T, Hasselstrom L: Comparison of methohexital and pentobarbital for premedication in children. Acta Anaesthesiol Scand 1990;34:478–481.

80. Mark LC, Fox JL, Burstein CL: Preanesthetic hypnosis with rectal pentothal in children. Anesthesiology 1949;10:401–405.

81. Beekman RP, Hoorntje TM, Beek FJ, et al: Sedation for children undergoing magnetic resonance imaging: efficacy and safety of rectal thiopental. Eur J Pediatr 1996;155:820–822.

82. White TJ 3d, Siegle RL, Burckart GJ, et al: Rectal thiopental for sedation of children for computed tomography. J Comput Assist Tomogr 1979;3:286–288.

83. Glasier CM, Stark JE, Brown R, et al: Rectal thiopental sodium for sedation of pediatric patients undergoing MR and other imaging studies. AJNR 995;16:111–114.

84. Liu LMP, Goudsouzian NG, Liu P: Rectal methohexital premedication in children: A dose comparison study. Anesthesiology 1980;53:343–345.

85. Manuli MA, Davies L: Rectal methohexital for sedation of children during imaging procedures. AJR Am J Roentgenol 1993;160:577–580.

86. Hardman JG, Limbird LE, Molinoff PB, et al: In: Gilman AG, Goodman LS, Gilman A, eds: Goodman & Gilman's The Pharmacological Basis of Therapeutics, 9th ed. New York: Macmillan Publishing Co.; 1996:1758.

87. Hudson RJ, Stanski DR, Burch PG: Pharmacokinetics of methohexital and thiopental in surgical patients. Anesthesiology 1983;59:215–219.

88. Jung D, Mayersohn M, Perrier D, et al: Thiopental disposition in lean and obese patients undergoing surgery. Anesthesiology 1982;56:269–274.

89. Breimer DD: Pharmacokinetics of methohexitone following intravenous infusion in humans. Br J Anaesth 1976;48:643–649.

90. Morgan DJ, Blackman GL, Paull JD, et al: Pharmacokinetics and plasma binding of thiopental. I: Studies in surgical patients. Anesthesiology 1981;54:468–473.

91. Audenaert SM, Montgomery CL, Thompson DE, et al: A prospective study of rectal methohexital: Efficacy and side effects in 648 cases. Anesth Analg 1995;81:957–961.

92. Bjorkman S, Gabrielsson J, Quaynor H, et al: Pharmacokinetics of I.V. and rectal methohexitone in children. Br J Anaesth 1987;59:1541–1547.

93. Daniels AL, Coté CJ, Polaner DM: Continuous oxygen saturation monitoring following rectal methohexitone induction in paediatric patients. Can J Anaesth 1992;39:27–30.

94. Griswold JD, Liu LM: Rectal methohexital in children undergoing computerized cranial tomography and magnetic resonance imaging scans. Anesthesiology 1987;67:A 494.

95. Laishley RS, O'Callaghan AC, Lerman J: Effects of dose and concentration of rectal methohexitone for induction of anaesthesia in children. Can Anaesth Soc J 1986;33:427–432.

96. Forbes RB, Vandewalker GE: Comparison of two and ten per cent rectal methohexitone for induction of anaesthesia in children. Can J Anaesth 1988;35:345–349.

97. Forbes RB, Murray DJ, Dull DL, et al: Haemodynamic effects of rectal methohexitone for induction of anaesthesia in children. Can J Anaesth 1989;36:5:526–529.

98. Forbes RB, Murray DJ, Dillman JB, et al: Pharmacokinetics of two per cent rectal methohexitone in children. Can J Anaesth 1989;36:160–164.

99. Khalil SN, Florence FB, Van den Nieuwenhuyzen MCO, et al: Rectal methohexital: Concentration and length of the rectal catheters. Anesth Analg 1990;70:645–649.

100. Goresky GV, Steward DJ: Rectal methohexitone for induction of anaesthesia in children. Can Anaesth Soc J 1979;26:213–215.

101. Liu LM, Gaudreault P, Friedman PA, et al: Methohexital plasma concentrations in children following rectal administration. Anesthesiology 1985;62:567–570.

102. Quaynor H, Corbey M, Bjorkman S: Rectal induction of anaesthesia in children with methohexitone: Patient acceptability and clinical pharmacokinetics. Br J Anaesth 1985;57:573–577.

103. Liu LM, Liu PL, Moss J: Severe histamine-mediated reaction to rectally administered methohexital. Anesthesiology 1984;61:95–97.

104. Rockoff MA, Goudsouzian NG: Seizures induced by methohexital. Anesthesiology 1981;54:333–335.

105. Parikh RK, Moore MR: Proceedings: Anaesthetics in porphyria: intravenous induction agents. Br J Anaesth 1975;47:907.

106. Mayers DJ, Hindmarsh KW, Sankaran K, et al: Chloral hydrate disposition following single-dose administration to critically ill neonates and children. Dev Pharmacol Ther 1991;16:71–77.

107. Greenberg SB, Faerber EN, Aspinall CL: High dose chloral hydrate sedation for children undergoing CT. J Comput Assist Tomogr 1991;15:467–469.

108. Greenberg SB, Faerber EN, Aspinall CL, et al: High-dose chloral hydrate sedation for children undergoing MR imaging: Safety and efficacy in relation to age. AJR 1993;161:639–641.

109. Hubbard AM, Markowitz RI, Kimmel B, et al: Sedation for pediatric patients undergoing CT and MRI. J Comput Assist Tomogr 1992;16:3–6.

110. Anyebuno MA, Rosenfeld CR: Chloral hydrate toxicity in a term infant. Dev Pharmacol Ther 1991;17:116–120.

111. Laptook AR, Rosenfeld CR: Chloral hydrate toxicity in a preterm infant. Pediatr Pharmacol (New York) 1984;4:161–165.

112. American Academy of Pediatrics, Committee on Drugs, Committee on Environmental Health: Use of chloral hydrate for sedation in children. Pediatrics 1993;92:471–473.

113. Salmon AG, Kizer KW, Zeise L, et al: Potential carcinogenicity of chloral hydrate: A review. J Toxicol Clin Toxicol 1995;33:115–121.

114. Westerling D: Rectally administered morphine: Plasma concentrations in children premedicated with morphine in hydrogel and in solution. Acta Anaesthesiol Scand 1985;29:653–656.

115. Gourlay GK, Boas RA: Fatal outcome with use of rectal morphine for postoperative pain control in an infant. Br Med J 1992;304:766–767.

116. Lindahl SG, Olsson AK, Thormson D: Rectal premedication in children: Use of diazepam, morphine, and hyoscine. Anaesthesia 1981;36:376–379.

117. Haagensen RE: Rectal premedication in children: Comparison of diazepam with a mixture of morphine, scopolamine and diazepam. Anaesthesia 1985;40:956–959.

118. Smith BL, Manford ML: Postoperative vomiting after paediatric adenotonsillectomy: A survey of incidence following differing pre- and postoperative drugs. Br J Anaesth 1974;46:373–378.

119. Booker PD, Chapman DH: Premedication in children undergoing day-care surgery. Br J Anaesth 1979;51:1083–1087.

120. Dahlstrom B, Bolme P, Feychting H, et al: Morphine kinetics in children. Clin Pharmacol Ther 1979;26:354–365.

121. Lynn AM, Slattery JT: Morphine pharmacokinetics in early infancy. Anesthesiology 1987;66:136–139.

122. Way WL, Costley EC, Way EI: Respiratory sensitivity of the newborn infant to meperidine and morphine. Clin Pharmacol Ther 1965;6:454–461.

123. Armstrong PJ, Bersten A: Normeperidine toxicity. Anesth Analg 1986;65:536–538.

124. Dsida RM, Wheeler M, Birmingham PK, et al: Premedication of pediatric tonsillectomy patients with oral transmucosal fentanyl citrate. Anesth Analg 1998;86:66–70.

125. Feld LH, Champeau MW, van Steennis CA, et al: Preanesthetic medication in children: A comparison of oral transmucosal fentanyl citrate versus placebo. Anesthesiology 1989;71:374–377.

126. Epstein RH, Mendel HG, Witkowski TA, et al: The safety and efficacy of oral transmucosal fentanyl citrate for preoperative sedation in young children. Anesth Analg 1996;83:1200–1205.

127. Friesen RH, Lockhart CH: Oral transmucosal fentanyl citrate for preanesthetic medication of pediatric day surgery patients with and without droperidol as a prophylactic anti-emetic. Anesthesiology 1992;76:46–51.

128. Schutzman SA, Burg J, Liebelt E, et al: Oral transmucosal fentanyl citrate for premedication of children undergoing laceration repair. Ann Emerg Med 1994;24:1059–1064.

129. Greeley WJ, de Bruijn NP: Changes in sufentanil pharmacokinetics within the neonatal period. Anesth Analg 1988;67:86–90.

130. Henderson JM, Brodsky DA, Fisher DM, et al: Pre-induction of anesthesia in pediatric patients with nasally administered sufentanil. Anesthesiology 1988;68:671–675.

131. Tobias JD, Rasmussen GE: Transnasal butorphanol for postoperative analgesia following paediatric surgery in a Third World country. Paediatr Anaesth 1995;5:63–66.

132. Splinter WM, O'Brien HV, Komocar L: Butorphanol: an opioid for day-care paediatric surgery. Can J Anaesth 1995;42:483–486.

133. Bennie RE, Boehringer LA, Dierdorf SF, et al: Transnasal butorphanol is effective for postoperative pain relief in children undergoing myringotomy. Anesthesiology 1998;89:385–390.

134. Bailey PL, Pace NL, Ashburn MA, et al: Frequent hypoxemia and apnea after sedation with midazolam and fentanyl. Anesthesiology 1990;73:826–830.

135. Yaster M, Nichols DG, Deshpande JK, et al: Midazolam-fentanyl intravenous sedation in children: Case report of respiratory arrest. Pediatrics 1990;86:463–467.

136. Cook DR, Davis PJ: Pediatric anesthesia pharmacology. In: Lake CL, ed. Pediatric Cardiac Anesthesia, 3rd ed. Stamford, Connecticut: Appleton & Lange; 1998:123–164.

137. Lockhart CH, Nelson WL: The relationship of ketamine requirement to age in pediatric patients. Anesthesiology 1974;40:507–508.

138. Krantz EM: Low-dose intramuscular ketamine and hyaluronidase for induction of anaesthesia in non-premedicated children. S Afr Med J 1980;58:161–162.

139. Stevens RW, Hain WR: Tolerance to rectal ketamine in paediatric anaesthesia. Anaesthesia 1981;36:1089–1093.

140. Gingrich BK: Difficulties encountered in a comparative study of orally administered midazolam and ketamine. Anesthesiology 1994;80:1414–1415.

141. Gutstein HB, Johnson KL, Heard MB, et al: Oral ketamine preanesthetic medication in children. Anesthesiology 1992;76:28–33.

142. Alderson PJ, Lerman J: Oral premedication for paediatric ambulatory anaesthesia. A comparison of midazolam and ketamine. Can J Anaesth 1994;41:221–226.

143. Warner DL, Cabaret J, Velling D: Ketamine plus midazolam, a most effective paediatric oral premedicant. Pediatr Anaesth 1995;5:293–295.

144. Rainey L, van der Walt JH: The anaesthetic management of autistic children. Anaesth Intensive Care 1998;26:682–686.

145. Cioaca R, Canavea I: Oral transmucosal ketamine: An effective premedication in children. Paediatr Anaesth 1996;6:361–365.

146. Qureshi FA, Mellis PT, McFadden MA: Efficacy of oral ketamine for providing sedation and analgesia to children requiring laceration repair. Pediatr Emerg Care 1995;11:93–97.

147. Lin SM, Liu K, Tsai SK, et al: Rectal ketamine versus intranasal ketamine as premedicant in children. Ma Tsui Hsueh Tsa Chi 1990;28:177–183.

148. Diaz JH: Intranasal ketamine preinduction of paediatric outpatients. Pediatr Anaesth 1997;7:273–278.

149. Weksler N, Ovadia L, Muati G, et al: Nasal ketamine for paediatric premedication. Can J Anaesth 1993;40:119–121.

150. Malinovsky JM, Lepage JY, Cozian A, et al: Is ketamine or its preservative responsible for neurotoxicity in the rabbit? Anesthesiology 1993;78:109–115.

151. Eisenach JC, De Kock M, Klimscha W: Alpha(2)-adrenergic agonists for regional anesthesia. A clinical review of clonidine (1984–1995). Anesthesiology 1996;85:655–674.

152. Ramesh VJ, Bhardwaj N, Batra YK: Comparative study of oral clonidine and diazepam as premedicants in children. Int J Clin Pharmacol Ther 1997;35:218–221.

153. Nishina K, Mikawa K, Maekawa N, et al: Clonidine decreases the dose of thiamylal required to induce anesthesia in children. Anesth Analg 1994;79:766–768.

154. Mikawa K, Nishina K, Maekawa N, et al: Attenuation of the catecholamine response to tracheal intubation with oral clonidine in children. Can J Anaesth 1995;42:869–874.

155. Nishina K, Mikawa K, Maekawa N, et al: The efficacy of clonidine for reducing perioperative haemodynamic changes and volatile anaesthetic requirements in children. Acta Anaesthesiol Scand 1996;40:746–751.

156. Nishina K, Mikawa K, Shiga M, et al: Oral clonidine premedication reduces minimum alveolar concentration of sevoflurane for tracheal intubation in children. Anesthesiology 1997;87:1324–1327.

157. Lavrich PS, Hermann D, Pang LM, Jonassen AE: Clonidine as a premedicant in children. Anesthesiology 1996;85:A1085.

158. Mikawa K, Nishina K, Maekawa N, et al: Oral clonidine premedication reduces postoperative pain in children. Anesth Analg 1996;82:225–230.

159. Reimer EJ, Dunn GS, Montgomery CJ, et al: The effectiveness of clonidine as an analgesic in paediatric adenotonsillectomy. Can J Anaesth 1998;45:1162–1167.

160. Mikawa K, Nishina K, Maekawa N, et al: Oral clonidine premedication reduces vomiting in children after strabismus surgery. Can J Anaesth 1995;42:977–981.

161. Nishina K, Mikawa K, Maekawa N, et al: Oral clonidine premedication does not affect preoperative gastric fluid pH and volume in children. Anesth Analg 1995;80:1065–1066.

162. Andersen TW, Gravenstein JS: Cardiovascular effects of sedative doses of pentobarbital and hydroxyzine. Anesthesiology 1966;27:272–278.

163. Lauria JI, Markello R, King BD: Circulatory and respiratory effects of hydroxyzine in volunteers and geriatric patients. Anesth Analg 1968;47:378–382.

164. Koseoglu V, Kurekci AE, Sarici U, et al: Comparison of the efficacy and side-effects of ondansetron and metoclopramide-diphenhydramine administered to control nausea and vomiting in children treated with antineoplastic chemotherapy: A prospective randomized study. Eur J Pediatr 1998;157:806–810.

165. Simons KJ, Watson WT, Martin TJ, et al: Diphenhydramine: pharmacokinetics and pharmacodynamics in elderly adults, young adults, and children. J Clin Pharmacol 1990;30:665–671.

166. Mirakhur RK, Jones CJ: Atropine and glycopyrrolate: Changes in cardiac rate and rhythm in conscious and anaesthetized children. Anaesth Intensive Care 1982;10:328–332.

167. Warran P, Radford P, Manford ML: Glycopyrrolate in children. Br J Anaesth 1981;53:1273–1276.

168. Wyant GM, Kao E: Glycopyrrolate methobromide. 1. Effect on salivary secretion. Can Anaesth Soc J 1974;21:230–241.

169. Zimmerman G, Steward DJ: Bradycardia delays the onset of action of intravenous atropine in infants. Anesthesiology 1986;65:320–322.

170. Berghem L, Bergman U, Schildt B, et al: Plasma atropine concentrations determined by radioimmunoassay after single-dose I.V. and I.M. administration. Br J Anaesth 1980;52:597–601.

171. Stratelak PA, White W, Wenzel D: The effect of glycopyrrolate premedication on postoperative sore throat. AANA J 1996;64:545–548.

172. Anderson BJ, Holford NH, Woollard GA, et al: Perioperative pharmacodynamics of acetaminophen analgesia in children. Anesthesiology 1999;90:411–421.

173. Bean-Lijewski JD, Stinson JC: Acetaminophen or ketorolac for post myringotomy pain in children? A prospective, double-blinded comparison. Paediatr Anaesth 1997;7:131–137.

174. Romej M, Voepel-Lewis T, Merkel SI, et al: Effect of preemptive acetaminophen on postoperative pain scores and oral fluid intake in pediatric tonsillectomy patients. AANA J 1996;64:535–540.

175. Korpela R, Korvenoja P, Meretoja OA: Morphine-sparing effect of acetaminophen in pediatric day-case surgery. Anesthesiology 1999;91:442–447.

176. Tobias JD, Lowe S, Hersey S, et al: Analgesia after bilateral myringotomy and placement of pressure equalization tubes in children: Acetaminophen versus acetaminophen with codeine. Anesth Analg 1995;81:496–500.

177. Birmingham PK, Tobin MJ, Henthorn TK, et al: Twenty-four-hour pharmacokinetics of rectal acetaminophen in children: An old drug with new recommendations. Anesthesiology 1997;87:244–252.

178. Birmingham PK, Tobin MJ, Henthorn TK, et al: "Loading" and subsequent dosing of rectal acetaminophen in children: A 24 hour pharmacokinetic study of new dosing recommendations. Anesthesiology 1996;85:A1105.

179. Montgomery CJ, McCormack JP, Reichert CC, et al: Plasma concentrations after high-dose (45 mg.kg-1) rectal acetaminophen in children. Can J Anaesth 1995;42:982–986.

180. Houck CS, Sullivan LJ, Wilder RT, et al: Pharmacokinetics of a higher dose of rectal acetaminophen in children. Anesthesiology 1995;83:A1126.

181. Maunuksela EL, Ryhanen P, Janhunen L: Efficacy of rectal ibuprofen in controlling postoperative pain in children. Can J Anaesth 1992;39:226–230.

182. Harley EH, Dattolo RA: Ibuprofen for tonsillectomy pain in children: Efficacy and complications. Otolaryngol Head Neck Surg 1998;119:492–496.

183. Moghal NE, Hulton SA, Milford DV: Care in the use of ibuprofen as an antipyretic in children. Clin Nephrol 1998;49:293–295.

184. Lesko SM, Mitchell AA: Renal function after short-term ibuprofen use in infants and children. Pediatrics 1997;100:954–957.

185. Davis PJ, Greenberg JA, Gendelman M, et al: Recovery characteristics of sevoflurane and halothane in preschool-aged children undergoing

bilateral myringotomy and pressure equalization tube insertion. Anesth Analg 1999;88:34–38.

186. Rusy LM, Houck CS, Sullivan LJ, et al: A double-blind evaluation of ketorolac tromethamine versus acetaminophen in pediatric tonsillectomy: Analgesia and bleeding. Anesth Analg 1995;80:226–229.

187. Splinter WM, Rhine EJ, Roberts DW, et al: Preoperative ketorolac increases bleeding after tonsillectomy in children. Can J Anaesth 1996;43:560–563.

188. Fitz-James I, Ho J, Pang LM, et al: Effect of ketorolac on perioperative bleeding and analgesia in pediatric tonsillectomy and adenoidectomy patients. Anesth Analg 1995;80:S127.

189. Gunter JB, Varughese AM, Harrington JF, et al: Recovery and complications after tonsillectomy in children: A comparison of ketorolac and morphine. Anesth Analg 1995;81:1136–1141.

190. Splinter WM, Reid CW, Roberts DJ, et al: Reducing pain after inguinal hernia repair in children: Caudal anesthesia versus ketorolac tromethamine. Anesthesiology 1997;87:542–546.

191. Rose JB, Brenn BR, Corddry DH, et al: Preoperative oral ondansetron for pediatric tonsillectomy. Anesth Analg 1996;82:558–562.

192. Splinter WM, Baxter MR, Gould HM, et al: Oral ondansetron decreases vomiting after tonsillectomy in children. Can J Anaesth 1995;42:277–280.

193. Khalil S, Rodarte A, Weldon BC, et al: Intravenous ondansetron in established postoperative emesis in children. S3A–381 Study Group. Anesthesiology 1996;85:270–276.

194. Patel RI, Davis PJ, Orr RJ, et al: Single-dose ondansetron prevents postoperative vomiting in pediatric outpatients. Anesth Analg 1997;85:538–545.

195. Rose JB, Martin TM: Posttonsillectomy vomiting. Ondansetron or metoclopramide during paediatric tonsillectomy: Are two doses better than one? Paediatr Anaesth 1996;6:39–44.

196. Splinter WM, Rhine EJ: Prophylactic antiemetics in children undergoing tonsillectomy: High-dose vs low-dose ondansetron. Paediatr Anaesth 1997;7:125–129.

197. Stene FN, Seay RE, Young LA, et al: Prospective, randomized, double-blind, placebo-controlled comparison of metoclopramide and ondansetron for prevention of posttonsillectomy or adenotonsillectomy emesis. J Clin Anesth 1996;8:540–544.

198. Litman RS, Wu CL, Catanzaro FA: Ondansetron decreases emesis after tonsillectomy in children. Anesth Analg 1994;78:478–481.

199. Rose JB, Martin TM, Corddry DH, et al: Ondansetron reduces the incidence and severity of poststrabismus repair vomiting in children. Anesth Analg 1994;79:486–489.

200. Watcha MF, Bras PJ, Cieslak GD, et al: The dose-response relationship of ondansetron in preventing postoperative emesis in pediatric patients undergoing ambulatory surgery. Anesthesiology 1995;82:47–52.

201. Davis PJ, McGowan FX Jr, Landsman I, et al: Effect of antiemetic therapy on recovery and hospital discharge time: A double-blind assessment of ondansetron, droperidol, and placebo in pediatric patients undergoing ambulatory surgery. Anesthesiology 1995;83:956–960.

202. Furst SR, Rodarte A: Prophylactic antiemetic treatment with ondansetron in children undergoing tonsillectomy. Anesthesiology 1994;81:799–803.

203. Cieslak GD, Watcha MF, Phillips MB, et al: The dose-response relation and cost-effectiveness of granisetron for the prophylaxis of pediatric postoperative emesis. Anesthesiology 1996;85:1076–1085.

204. Fujii Y, Tanaka H, Ito M: Preoperative oral granisetron for the prevention of vomiting after strabismus surgery in children. Ophthalmology 1999;106:1713–1715.

205. Fujii Y, Saitoh Y, Tanaka H, et al: Prophylactic therapy with combined granisetron and dexamethasone for the prevention of post-operative vomiting in children. Eur J Anaesthesiol 1999;16:376–379.

206. Fujii Y, Saitoh Y, Tanaka H, et al: Combination of granisetron and droperidol for the prevention of vomiting after paediatric strabismus surgery. Paediatr Anaesth 1999;9:329–333.

207. Munro HM, D'Errico CC, Lauder GR, et al: Oral granisetron for strabismus surgery in children. Can J Anaesth 1999;46:45–48.

208. Fujii Y, Tanaka H: Granisetron reduces post-operative vomiting in children: A dose-ranging study. Eur J Anaesthesiol 1999;16:62–65.

209. Fujii Y, Toyooka H, Tanaka H: Oral granisetron prevents postoperative vomiting in children. Br J Anaesth 1998;81:390–392.

210. Fujii Y, Saitoh Y, Tanaka H, et al: Comparison of granisetron and droperidol in the prevention of vomiting after strabismus surgery or tonsillectomy in children. Paediatr Anaesth 1998;8:241–244.

211. Carnahan D, Dato K, Hartsuff J: The safety and efficacy of granisetron in postoperative vomiting in pediatric patients undergoing tonsillectomy. AANA J 1997;65:154–159.

212. Fujii Y, Tanaka H, Toyooka H: Granisetron and dexamethasone provide more improved prevention of postoperative emesis than granisetron alone in children. Can J Anaesth 1996;43:1229–1232.

213. Fujii Y, Toyooka H, Tanaka H: Effective dose of granisetron for preventing postoperative emesis in children. Can J Anaesth 1996;43:660–664.

214. Abramowitz MD, Oh TH, Epstein BS, et al: The antiemetic effect of droperidol following outpatient strabismus surgery in children. Anesthesiology 1983;59:579–583.

215. Lawhorn CD, Bower C, Brown RE Jr, et al: Ondansetron decreases postoperative vomiting in pediatric patients undergoing tonsillectomy and adenoidectomy. Int J Pediatr Otorhinolaryngol 1996;36:99–108.

216. Klockgether-Radke A, Neumann S, Neumann P, et al: Ondansetron, droperidol and their combination for the prevention of post-operative vomiting in children. Eur J Anaesthesiol 1997;14:362–367.

217. Kymer PJ, Brown RE Jr, Lawhorn CD, et al: The effects of oral droperidol versus oral metoclopramide versus both oral droperidol and metoclopramide on postoperative vomiting when used as a premedicant for strabismus surgery. J Clin Anesth 1995;7:35–39.

218. Alexander R, Lovell AT, Seingry D, et al: Comparison of ondansetron and droperidol in reducing postoperative nausea and vomiting associated with patient-controlled analgesia. Anaesthesia 1995;50:1086–1088.

219. Fujii Y, Toyooka H, Tanaka H: A granisetron-droperidol combination prevents postoperative vomiting in children. Anesth Analg 1998;87:761–765.

220. April MM, Callan ND, Nowak DM, et al: The effect of intravenous dexamethasone in pediatric adenotonsillectomy. Arch Otolaryngol Head Neck Surg 1996;122:117–120.

221. Pappas AL, Sukhani R, Hotaling AJ, et al: The effect of preoperative dexamethasone on the immediate and delayed postoperative morbidity in children undergoing adenotonsillectomy. Anesth Analg 1998;87:57–61.

222. Splinter WM, Roberts DJ: Dexamethasone decreases vomiting by children after tonsillectomy. Anesth Analg 1996;83:913–916.

223. Splinter WM, Rhine EJ: Low-dose ondansetron with dexamethasone more effectively decreases vomiting after strabismus surgery in children than does high-dose ondansetron. Anesthesiology 1998;88:72–75.

224. Vener DF, Carr AS, Sikich N, et al: Dimenhydrinate decreases vomiting after strabismus surgery in children. Anesth Analg 1996;82:728–731.

225. Hamid SK, Selby IR, Sikich N, et al: Vomiting after adenotonsillectomy in children: A comparison of ondansetron, dimenhydrinate, and placebo. Anesth Analg 1998;86:496–500.

226. Splinter W, Roberts DJ: Prophylaxis for vomiting by children after tonsillectomy: Dexamethasone versus perphenazine. Anesth Analg 1997;85:534–537.

227. Fujii Y, Saitoh Y, Tanaka H, et al: Preoperative oral antiemetics for reducing postoperative vomiting after tonsillectomy in children: Granisetron versus perphenazine. Anesth Analg 1999;88:1298–1301.

228. Maxwell LG, Deshpande JK, Wetzel RC: Preoperative evaluation of children. Pediatr Clin North Am 1994;41:93–110.

229. Dajani AS, Bisno AL, Chung KJ, et al: Prevention of bacterial endocarditis. Recommendations by the American Heart Association. JAMA 1990;264:2919–2922.

230. Mendelson CL: The aspiration of stomach contents into the lungs during obstetric anesthesia. Am J Obstet Gynecol 1946;52:191–205.

231. Roberts RB, Shirley MA: Reducing the risk of acid aspiration during cesarean section. Anesth Analg 1974;53:859–868.

232. Coté CJ, Goudsouzian NG, Liu LM, et al: Assessment of risk factors related to the acid aspiration syndrome in pediatric patients—gastric pH and residual volume. Anesthesiology 1982;56:70–72.

233. Tiret L, Nivoche Y, Hatton F, et al: Complications related to anaesthesia in infants and children: A prospective survey of 40,240 anaesthetics. Br J Anaesth 1988;61:263–269.

234. Warner MA, Warner ME, Weber JG: Clinical significance of pulmonary aspiration during the perioperative period. Anesthesiology 1993;78:56–62.

235. Borland LM, Sereika SM, Woelfel SK, et al: Pulmonary aspiration in pediatric patients during general anesthesia: Incidence and outcome. J Clin Anesth 1998;10:95–102.

236. Coté CJ: NPO after midnight for children: A reappraisal. Anesthesiology 1990;72:589–592.

237. Raidoo DM, Marszalek A, Brock-Utne JG: Acid aspiration in primates (A surprising experimental result). Anaesth Intens Care 1988;16:375–376.

238. Goudsouzian NG, Coté CJ, Liu LM, et al: The dose-response effects of oral cimetidine on gastric pH and volume in children. Anesthesiology 1981;55:53–56.

239. Tryba M, Yildiz F, Kuhn K, et al: Rectal and oral cimetidine for prophylaxis of aspiration pneumonitis in paediatric anaesthesia. Acta Anaesthesiol Scand 1983;27:328–330.

240. Manchikanti L, Marrero TC, Roush JR: Preanesthetic cimetidine and metoclopramide for acid aspiration prophylaxis in elective surgery. Anesthesiology 1984;61:48–54.

241. Morison DH, Dunn GL, Fargas-Babjak AM, et al: A double-blind comparison of cimetidine and ranitidine as prophylaxis against gastric aspiration syndrome. Anesth Analg 1982;61:988–992.

242. Durrant JM, Strunin L: Comparative trial of the effect of ranitidine and cimetidine on gastric secretion in fasting patients at induction of anaesthesia. Can Anaesth Soc J 1982;29:446–451.

243. Howard FA, Sharp DS: Effect of metoclopramide on gastric emptying during labour. Br Med J 1973;1:446–448.

244. Fisher DM, Robinson S, Brett CM, et al: Comparison of enflurane, halothane, and isoflurane for diagnostic and therapeutic procedures in children with malignancies. Anesthesiology 1985;63:647–650.

245. McAteer PM, Carter JA, Cooper GM, et al: Comparison of isoflurane and halothane in outpatient paediatric dental anaesthesia. Br J Anaesth 1986;58:390–393.

246. Piat V, Dubois MC, Johanet S, et al: Induction and recovery characteristics and hemodynamic responses to sevoflurane and halothane in children. Anesth Analg 1994;79:840–844.

247. Black A, Sury MR, Hemington L, et al: A comparison of the induction characteristics of sevoflurane and halothane in children. Anaesthesia 1996;51:539–542.

248. Haga S, Shima T, Momose K, et al: Anesthetic induction of children with high concentrations of sevoflurane. [in Japanese]. Masui 1992;41:1951–1955.

249. Kataria B, Epstein R, Bailey A, et al: A comparison of sevoflurane to halothane in paediatric surgical patients: Results of a multicentre international study. Pediatr Anaesth 1996;6:283–292.

250. Lerman J, Davis PJ, Welborn LG, et al: Induction, recovery, and safety characteristics of sevoflurane in children undergoing ambulatory surgery: A comparison with halothane. Anesthesiology 1996;84:1332–1340.

251. Sarner JB, Levine M, Davis PJ, et al: Clinical characteristics of sevoflurane in children: A comparison with halothane. Anesthesiology 1995;82:38–46.

252. Ariffin SA, Whyte JA, Malins AF, et al: Comparison of induction and recovery between sevoflurane and halothane supplementation of anaesthesia in children undergoing outpatient dental extractions. Br J Anaesth 1997;78:157–159.

253. Baum VC, Yemen TA, Baum LD: Immediate 8% sevoflurane induction in children: A comparison with incremental sevoflurane and incremental halothane. Anesth Analg 1997;85:313–316.

254. Janiszewski DJ, Galinkin JL, Klock PA, et al: The effects of subanesthetic concentrations of sevoflurane and nitrous oxide, alone and in combination, on analgesia, mood, and psychomotor performance in healthy volunteers. Anesth Analg 1999;88:1149–1154.

255. Komatsu H, Taie S, Endo S, et al: Electrical seizures during sevoflurane anesthesia in two pediatric patients with epilepsy. Anesthesiology 1994;81:1535–1537.

256. Osawa M, Shingu K, Murakawa M, et al: Effects of sevoflurane on central nervous system electrical activity in cats. Anesth Analg 1994;79:52–57.

257. Ruffle JM, Snider MT, Rosenberger JL, et al: Rapid induction of halothane anaesthesia in man. Br J Anaesth 1985;57:607–611.

258. Sigston PE, Jenkins AM, Jackson EA, et al: Rapid inhalation induction in children: 8% sevoflurane compared with 5% halothane. Br J Anaesth 1997;78:362–365.

259. Lewis MC, Schauer JC, Gold MI: Single breath induction technique: Comparison of sevoflurane and isoflurane. Anesth Analg 1996;83:890–891.

260. Agnor RC, Sikich N, Lerman J: Single-breath vital capacity rapid inhalation induction in children: 8% sevoflurane versus 5% halothane. Anesthesiology 1998;89:379–384.

261. Ruffle JM, Snider MT: Comparison of rapid and conventional inhalation inductions of halothane oxygen anesthesia in healthy men and women. Anesthesiology 1987;67:584–587.

262. Liu LMP, Miler V, Ryan JF: Comparison of inhalation anesthetic induction methods in children: Traditional vs. modified single breath technique. Anesthesiology 1989;71:A1007.

263. Yurino M, Kimura H: Comparison of induction time and characteristics between sevoflurane and sevoflurane/nitrous oxide. Acta Anaesthesiol Scand 1995;39:356–358.

264. Liu LMP, Ryan JF: Modified single breath induction of anesthesia in children with halothane with and without nitrous oxide. Anesthesiology 1989;71:A1008.

265. Lundy JS: Intravenous anesthesia: Preliminary report of the use of two new thiobarbiturates. Proc Staff Meet Mayo Clin 1935;10:536–543.

266. Gaspari F, Marraro G, Penna GF, et al: Elimination kinetics of thiopentone in mothers and their newborn infants. Eur J Clin Pharmacol 1985;28:321–325.

267. Coté CJ, Goudsouzian NG, Liu LM, et al: The dose response of intravenous thiopental for the induction of general anesthesia in unpremedicated children. Anesthesiology 1981;55:703–705.

268. Brett CM, Fisher DM: Thiopental dose-response relations in unpremedicated infants, children, and adults. Anesth Analg 1987;66:1024–1027.

269. Jonmarker C, Westrin P, Larsson S, et al: Thiopental requirements for induction of anesthesia in children. Anesthesiology 1987;67:104–107.

270. Westrin P, Jonmarker C, Werner O: Thiopental requirements for induction of anesthesia in neonates and in infants one to six months of age. Anesthesiology 1989;71:344–346.

271. Korttila K, Linnoila M, Ertama P, et al: Recovery and simulated driving after intravenous anesthesia with thiopental, methohexital, propanidid, or alphadione. Anesthesiology 1975;43:291–299.

272. Beskow A, Werner O, Westrin P: Faster recovery after anesthesia in infants after intravenous induction with methohexital instead of thiopental. Anesthesiology 1995;83:976–979.

273. Liu LMP, Coté CJ, Goudsouzian NG, et al: Response to intravenous induction doses of methohexital in children. Anesthesiology 1981;55:A330.

274. Servin F, Desmonts JM, Haberer JP, et al.:Pharmacokinetics and protein binding of propofol in patients with cirrhosis. Anesthesiology 1988;69:887–891.

275. Morton NS, Wee M, Christie G, et al:. Propofol for induction of anaesthesia in children: A comparison with thiopentone and halothane inhalational induction. Anaesthesia 1988;43:350–355.

276. Patel DK, Keeling PA, Newman GB, et al: Induction dose of propofol in children. Anaesthesia 1988;43:949–952.

277. Hannallah RS, Baker SB, Casey W, et al: Propofol: Effective dose and induction characteristics in unpremedicated children. Anesthesiology 1991;74:217–219.

278. Westrin P: The induction dose of propofol in infants 1–6 months of age and in children 10–16 years of age. Anesthesiology 1991;74:455–458.

279. Schrum SF, Hannallah RS, Verghese PM, et al: Comparison of propofol and thiopental for rapid anesthesia induction in infants. Anesth Analg 1994;78:482–485.

280. Crawford MW, Lerman J, Sloan MH, et al: Recovery characteristics of propofol anaesthesia, with and without nitrous oxide: A comparison with halothane/nitrous oxide anaesthesia in children. Pediatr Anaesth 1998;8:49–54.

281. Hannallah RS, Britton JT, Schafer PG, et al: Propofol anaesthesia in paediatric ambulatory patients: A comparison with thiopentone and halothane. Can J Anaesth 1994;41:12–18.

282. Barst SM, Markowitz A, Yossefy Y, et al: Propofol reduces the incidence of vomiting after tonsillectomy in children. Pediatr Anaesth 1995;5:249–252.

283. Watcha MF, Simeon RM, White PF, et al: Effect of propofol on the incidence of postoperative vomiting after strabismus surgery in pediatric outpatients. Anesthesiology 1991;75:204–209.

284. Standl T, Wilhelm S, von Knobelsdorff G, et al: Propofol reduces emesis after sufentanil supplemented anaesthesia in paediatric squint surgery. Acta Anaesthesiol Scand 1996;40:729–733.

285. Martin TM, Nicolson SC, Bargas MS: Propofol anesthesia reduces emesis and airway obstruction in pediatric outpatients. Anesth Analg 1993;76:144–148.

286. Habre W, Sims C: Propofol anaesthesia and vomiting after myringoplasty in children. Anaesthesia 1997;52:544–546.

287. Purcell-Jones G, Yates A, Baker JR, et al: Comparison of the induction characteristics of thiopentone and propofol in children. Br J Anaesth 1987;59:1431–1436.

288. Valtonen M, Iisalo E, Kanto J, et al: Comparison between propofol and thiopentone for induction of anaesthesia in children. Anaesthesia 1988;43:696–699.

289. McDowall RH, Scher CS, Barst SM: Total intravenous anesthesia for children undergoing brief diagnostic or therapeutic procedures. J Clin Anesth 1995;7:273–280.

290. Schechter WS, Kim C, Martinez M, et al: Anaesthetic induction in a child with end-stage cardiomyopathy. Can J Anaesth 1995;42:404–408.

291. Donmez A, Kaya H, Haberal A, et al: The effect of etomidate induction on plasma cortisol levels in children undergoing cardiac surgery. J Cardiothorac Vasc Anesth 1998;12:182–185.

292. Christ G, Mundigler G, Merhaut C, et al: Adverse cardiovascular effects of ketamine infusion in patients with catecholamine-dependent heart failure. Anaesth Intens Care 1997;25:255–259.

293. Cook DR: Paediatric anaesthesia: Pharmacological considerations. Drugs 1976;12:212–221.

294. Idvall J, Holasek J, Stenberg P: Rectal ketamine for induction of anaesthesia in children. Anaesthesia 1983;38:60–64.

295. Sellick BA: Cricoid pressure to control regurgitation of stomach contents during induction of anaesthesia. Lancet 1961;2:404–406.

296. Hannallah RS, Rosales JK: Experience with parent's presence during anesthesia induction in children. Can Anaesth Soc J 1983;30:287–290.

297. Schulman JL, Foley JM, Vernon DTA, et al: A study of the effect of the mother's presence during anesthesia induction. Pediatrics 1967;39:111–114.

298. Kain ZN, Mayes LC, Caramico LA, et al: Parental presence during induction of anesthesia. A randomized controlled trial. Anesthesiology 1996;84:1060–1067.

299. Kain ZN, Mayes LC, Wang SM, et al: Parental presence during induction of anesthesia versus sedative premedication: Which intervention is more effective? Anesthesiology 1998;89:1147–1156.

300. Schofield NM, White JB: Interrelations among children, parents, premedication, and anaesthetists in paediatric day stay surgery. Br Med J [Clin Res] 1989;299:1371–1375.

301. Bevan JC, Johnston C, Haig MJ, et al: Preoperative parental anxiety predicts behavioral and emotional responses to induction of anaesthesia in children. Can J Anaesth 1990;37:177–182.

302. Hannallah RS, Abramowitz MD, Oh TH, et al: Residents' attitudes toward parents' presence during anesthesia induction in children: Does experience make a difference? Anesthesiology 1984;60:598–601.

10 Muscle Relaxants in Children

Nishan G. Goudsouzian

Monitoring Neuromuscular Function
    Frequency of Stimulation
Depolarizing Muscle Relaxants
    Succinylcholine
Short-Acting Relaxants
    Mivacurium
    Rapacuronium
Intermediate-Acting Nondepolarizing Relaxants
    Atracurium
    Cisatracurium
    Vecuronium
    Rocuronium
Long-Acting Nondepolarizing Relaxants
    Tubocurarine
    Metocurine
    Pancuronium
    Doxacurium
    Pipecuronium
Antagonism of Muscle Relaxants
Relaxants in Special Situations
    Progressive Muscular Dystrophy
    Myotonia
    Myasthenia Gravis
    Burns

This chapter reviews basic principles in the evaluation of the myoneural junction of children, the pharmacology of muscle relaxants relative to age, and the practice of muscle relaxant use in both healthy and diseased pediatric patients.

Monitoring Neuromuscular Function

The measurement of evoked responses following an electrical stimulus is the standard method for evaluating neuromuscular function. This method allows nearly instantaneous evaluation of muscle activity: either electrically (by electromyogram), or mechanically (by twitch), in an unconscious individual. With the electromyographic techniques, the compound muscle action potential is recorded by surface or needle electrodes applied to any muscle, usually the adductor pollicis brevis, the abductor digiti minimi, or the first dorsal interosseous muscle of the hand. Twitch tension measurements, by contrast, use the force of contraction of the adductor pollicis. This muscle is the only thumb muscle supplied by the ulnar nerve; measurements therefore approach the single-muscle precision of the experimental nerve muscle preparation.[1] The evoked tension of the adductor pollicis in response to stimulation of the ulnar nerve can be recorded by a force displacement transducer (Fig. 10–1). To achieve reproducibility and to ensure full activation of all stimulated nerve and muscle fibers, the stimuli should be supramaximal in intensity, square wave in nature, and no longer than 0.2 msec.

Frequency of Stimulation

Clinically, three types of stimulation are used (Fig. 10–2):

1. Single twitch (0.1 to 0.25 Hz [cycles/sec])
2. Train-of-four (2 Hz for 2 sec)
3. Tetanus (50 Hz, usually for 5 sec)

Single-twitch rates are useful whenever there is an observable control response. By comparing the percentage change of twitch tension before and after administration of the neuromuscular blocking agent, one can obtain a simple mathematic value and predict the degree of paralysis. Single stimuli detect relatively high degrees of neuromuscular blockade. In fact, depression of the twitch response can be observed only if more than three fourths of the postsynaptic receptors are blocked.[2]

The *train-of-four* is a simple quantitative technique used primarily for measurement of nondepolarizing neuromuscular blockade. It consists of four supramaximal stimuli applied to the ulnar nerve at a frequency of 2 cycles/sec. The ratio of the amplitude of the fourth twitch to the first is an indicator of the degree of neuromuscular blockade. The main advantage of the train-of-four over single-twitch response is that it does not require a control. Further, the train-of-four technique can be repeated every 10 seconds, thus allowing rapid changes in neuromuscular blockade to be closely monitored.[1]

The theory of train-of-four is based on the premise that a rate of stimulation of 2 cycles/sec is rapid enough to produce depletion of the immediately available stores of acetylcholine, yet slow enough to prevent transmitter facilitation. Four stimuli were chosen because, during partial nondepolarizing neuromuscular blockade, the fourth response was found to be maximally depressed; thereafter, the twitch height leveled off.[3] In fact, in infants and children, the train-of-four correlates directly with the twitch height and is a more sensitive indicator of neuromuscular blockade than the single twitch recorded every 15 seconds (Fig. 10–3).[4]

Premature infants less than 32 weeks of post-conceptual age have lower train-of-four values (83 ± 2%) than more mature neonates (Fig. 10–4).[5] In infants less than 1 month of age, the height of the fourth evoked response of the train is about 95%.[6] The change to the higher value in the first month of development probably indicates maturation of the myoneural junction. In children anesthetized with halothane, all components of the train-of-four are practically equal in

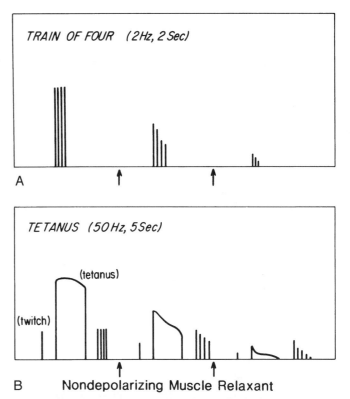

B   Nondepolarizing Muscle Relaxant

Figure 10–2. Idealized recording of the effect of nondepolarizing muscle relaxants on the train-of-four and tetanic stimulation. (A) Note the four equal twitches before the administration of a nondepolarizing muscle relaxant (arrows). After curare, the fourth twitch is less in amplitude than the first (train-of-four). The last sequence indicates greater neuromuscular blockade, because only three of the four twitches are observed. (B) Corresponding single-twitch/tetanus observations at a lower amplification. Note the marked fade and post-tetanic facilitation after the second dose of nondepolarizing muscle relaxant (arrows).

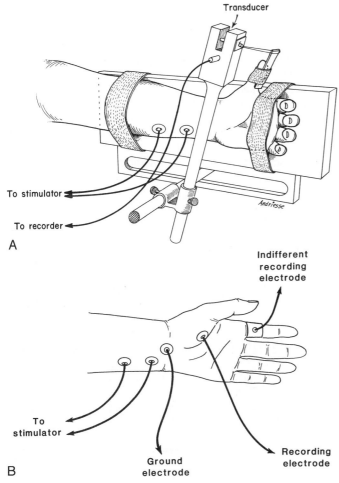

Figure 10–1. (A) The arrangement used for studying evoked tensions in infants and children. (B) The position of electrodes for recording an evoked electromyogram. In a clinical setting and in the absence of recording apparatus, feeling the twitch response is adequate.

size (100%). Adults with a train-of-four value above 75% can usually sustain head-lift for 3 seconds or longer while tidal volume, vital capacity, inspiratory flow, and peak expiratory flow are not significantly altered.[7, 8]

Tetanic stimulation is usually obtained by supramaximally stimulating the nerve for 5 seconds or more. During tetanic stimulation, synthesis of acetylcholine increases; however, this increase is limited. If the duration of stimulation is too long or the frequency of stimulation too high, *fade* occurs—that is, a decrement in the height of tetanus is noted. The usual explanation for the occurrence of fade is that during repetitive stimulation, the acetylcholine output per impulse falls off. Under normal circumstances, the diminution of acetylcholine output does not affect transmission because of the continuing excess of both acetylcholine and receptors at the myoneural junction (safety factor). During partial receptor blockade with a nondepolarizing relaxant, the progressive diminution of acetylcholine output eventually results in a decreased number of stimulated receptors and a consequent decrease in the amplitude of contraction. An alternative notion holds that fade is not simply the consequence of a spontaneously occurring fall in the transmitter action, but is in fact due to a different and separate action of the drug. This line of thought suggests that the

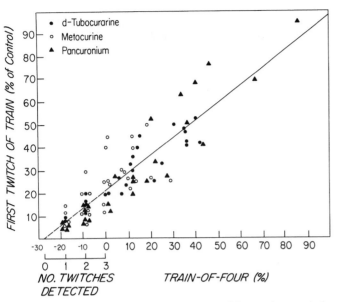

Figure 10-3. Correlation between the train-of-four values and the twitch heights (percent of control). Note that at 20 to 25% of control twitch height, the fourth response of the train-of-four disappears.

relaxant has a prejunctional effect, resulting in a decline of transmitter release.[9]

In infants and children anesthetized with halothane, the percentage of fade during tetanic stimulation for 5 seconds at 20 cycles/sec is 5% and at 50 cycles/sec is 9%.[6] These values are comparable to those for adults.[10] If the duration of stimulation is prolonged, an even greater degree of fade may be noted. In small infants, a more than 50% decrement in the height of tetanus has been observed during 15 seconds of tetanic stimulation; this decrement is more marked in premature infants.[11, 12] Increasing the rate of stimulation from 20 cycles/sec to 50 cycles/sec to 100 cycles/sec increases the degree of fade from 5% to 9% to 17%, respectively, during a 5-second tetanic stimulation.[6] With fast-sweep electromyography, infants less than 12 weeks of age have shown more marked fade than older children and adults; this difference is greater at high frequencies (50 Hz).[13] These findings suggest that small infants can indeed sustain short periods of tetanic stimulation, but their musculature becomes fatigued more quickly than that of older children in response to sustained stimulation.

The integrity of the myoneural junction can also be analyzed by evaluation of *post-tetanic facilitation.* The increased synthesis and release of acetylcholine that occur during tetanic stimulation continue for a short interval after the stimulation has stopped. This increased production normally does not result in facilitation because all the muscle fibers are excited by the stimulus. In the presence of nondepolarizing (competitive) neuromuscular blockade, however, the increased post-tetanic acetylcholine release stimulates a greater number of muscle fibers, producing the characteristic post-tetanic facilitation.[10]

In infants and children, the normal post-tetanic facilitation following tetanus of 5 seconds at 20 cycles/sec is 10%. It increases to 18% when the tetanic stimulation is increased to 50 cycles/sec. When the rate of stimulation reaches the

nonphysiologic range of 100 cycles/sec, post-tetanic exhaustion occurs; that is, the post-tetanic twitch is lower than the pretetanic one, indicating the depletion of acetylcholine reserves.[6]

The *post-tetanic count* has been used to evaluate intense neuromuscular blockade in children.[14, 15] This is a measure obtained by applying a 50-cycle/sec tetanic stimulus to the ulnar nerve for 5 sec, followed by single twitch stimulation at 1 cycle/sec; the number of twitches observed in the posttetanic period is known as the *post-tetanic count* (Fig. 10-5). Because tetanus and post-tetanic responses are indicators of deep neuromuscular blockade, they can usually be elicited during recovery before the appearance of the train-of-four. At very deep levels of blockade, no tetanus or post-tetanic effect can be seen; as the patient recovers, a single posttetanic response eventually manifests itself. The number of post-tetanic counts increases as recovery proceeds until, at post-tetanic counts of six to seven, the first twitch of the train-of-four appears. It has been shown that during recovery, the first post-tetanic response precedes the first response of the train-of-four by 5 to 10 minutes with atracurium or vecuronium and by 20 to 30 minutes with pancuronium or tubocurarine.[14, 15]

The *tetanus to twitch ratio,* which is the ratio of the highest tetanic response to the preceding twitch height, changes with age. In infants younger than 1 month, the ratio is 4:1; in children older than 1 month, it increases to 6:1, indicating maturation of the myoneural junction or the muscle itself.[6] This ratio is lower in patients who have received a muscle relaxant and increases after the reversal of neuromuscular blockade.

As a practical matter, the single twitch or the train-offour is usually the method of choice for monitoring neuromuscular blockade. Slow rates of stimulation (4–6 per minute) are more helpful because the necessary levels of clinical neuromuscular blockade can be identified without first abol-

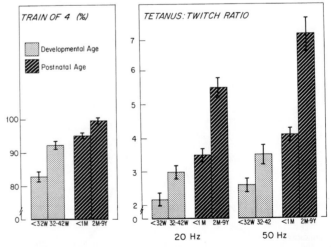

Figure 10-4. The train-of-four values and tetanus:twitch ratios of critically ill infants less than 42 weeks of developmental age in the neonatal intensive care unit and term infants anesthetized with halothane. Note the evidence of maturation of the myoneural junction in the older children, especially during tetanic stimulation at 50 cycles/second. (From Goudsouzian NG, Crone RK, Todres ID: Recovery from pancuronium blockade in the neonatal intensive care unit. Br J Anaesth 1981;53(12):1303–1309.)

Figure 10–5. The recovery pattern of train-of-four and post-tetanic response following a nondepolarizing muscle relaxant. Note that despite deep neuromuscular blockade (absent train-of-four), the post-tetanic response is evident. The less intense the neuromuscular blockade, the greater the number of post-tetanic counts (see text).

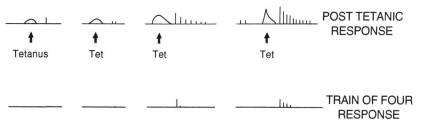

ishing the twitch response. The main drawback of the single-twitch rate of stimulation is the necessity of obtaining a control twitch tension for quantitative assessment of blockade; the train-of-four obviates the need for a control response because the ratio of the fourth twitch to the first is the quantitated parameter.

In a clinical situation in which neuromuscular recording instruments are not available, the number of contractions during train-of-four are counted. This technique depends on the fact that the number of twitches in the train-of-four usually correlates well with the degree of blockade. When the height of the first twitch is about 21% of control, three contractions are usually detected during train-of-four stimulation; at a single twitch height of 14% of control, two contractions are in evidence, and when the single twitch height is about 7%, only one contraction is detected.[16] During procedures in which a child's hand is covered by surgical drapes, palpating the number of contractions provides a satisfactory alternative. The number of contractions during train-of-four stimulation thus yields a practical assessment of neuromuscular blockade. For more profound blockade, the post-tetanic counts can be used intermittently. However, repeated tetanic stimulation is not ideal because it is painful and can lead to post-tetanic exhaustion.

Although twitch monitoring is the standard method of evaluating neuromuscular block, it has been realized that the block at one group of muscles will differ from that at another group. For example, 1.7 times more relaxant is needed to block the diaphragm and the vocal cords than is required to depress the adductor pollicis.[17, 18] The recovery is about 50% faster in these central muscles; however, there is the possibility that patients might cough or react during intubation in the absence of the twitch response. If the twitch response has recovered at the end of the procedure, that is a clear indication that the diaphragm and the vocal cords are in a more advanced stage of recovery. An estimate of the relaxation of central muscles as a predictor for the conditions for intubation can be obtained by monitoring the orbicularis oculi contraction, where relaxation occurs before the adductor of the thumb.[19]

Depolarizing Muscle Relaxants

Succinylcholine

Succinylcholine is the only depolarizing relaxant used in children. Infants have been found to be more resistant than adults to its neuromuscular effects.[20] Early studies demonstrated that the degree of neuromuscular blockade achieved by 1 mg/kg IV in infants is about equal to that produced by 0.5 mg/kg in older children.[21] Determinations of effective doses of succinylcholine during thiopental-opioid anesthesia have shown the effective dose that causes 95% depression of the twitch response (ED_{95}) of neonates, infants, and children to be 0.62, 0.73, and 0.42 mg/kg, respectively.[22] These values are higher than those reported in adults, in whom the ED_{95} is about 0.29 mg/kg.[22] The increase in dose requirement in younger patients is thought to result from the drug's rapid distribution into the infant's large extracellular fluid volume (Tables 10–1 and 10–2).[12] The extracellular volume constitutes 45% of the body weight at birth, 30% at 2 months of age, 20% at 6 years, and 16% to 18% at adulthood.[23] Because the extracellular space and body surface area are related throughout childhood, it is not surprising to find a correlation between neuromuscular response and the dose of succinylcholine for each square meter of body surface area.[12]

As in adults, administration of a continuous infusion of succinylcholine in infants and children results in tachyphylaxis (increased requirement). In addition, phase II block may be produced, as evidenced by a train-of-four less than 50% (blockade similar to that produced by nondepolarizing muscle relaxants). In general, tachyphylaxis develops after the administration of about 3 mg/kg succinylcholine and phase II block develops during tachyphylaxis following 4 mg/kg in children.[24, 25] The exact cause of phase II block is unknown. It is theorized that the receptors may become refractory to the transmitter because of desensitization and that some sodium channels are blocked by the agonist.[26] It should be noted that some infants, unpredictably, are extremely resistant to the neuromuscular effects of a succinylcholine infusion, requiring three to four times the usual dose.[25] As a group, infants have an increased requirement, partly because of the large extracellular fluid volume. If

Table 10–1. Effective Doses of Relaxants in Neonates, Infants, Children, and Adults*

	Dose (μg/kg)			
	Neonates	*Infants*	*Children*	*Adults*
Succinylcholine	620	729	423	290
Mivacurium		65–94	82–110	58–120
Atracurium	120	156–175	170–350	110–280
Vecuronium	47	42–47	56–80	27–56
Rocuronium		255	402	350
Cisatracurium			41	32–50
Metocurine		180	180–340	180–280
Tubocurarine	340	320	320–600	290–510
Pancuronium		55–92	55–81	50–70
Doxacurium		25	27–32	14–19
Pipecuronium	46	33–48	49–79	42–59

*Blank spaces indicate lack of published data at the time of writing this chapter.

Table 10–2. Suggested Standard Intubating Doses of Relaxants in Infants and Children

	Dose mg/kg (μg/kg)	
	Infants	*Children*
Succinylcholine	3 (3000)	1.5–2 (1500–2000)
Mivacurium	0.3 (300)	0.2–0.3 (200–300)
Atracurium	0.5 (500)	0.5 (500)
Vecuronium	0.07–0.1 (70–100)	0.1 (100)
Rocuronium	0.25–0.5 (250–500)	0.6–1.2 (600–1200)
Cisatracurium	0.1 (100)	0.1-0.2 (100–200)
Metocurine		0.3 (300)
Tubocurarine	0.2–0.5 (200–500)	0.3–0.6 (300-600)
Pancuronium	0.1 (100)	0.1 (100)
Doxacurium		0.05 (50)
Pipecuronium	0.07–0.1 (70–100)	0.1 (100)

needed, the residual phase II block in infants and children may be antagonized by the usual doses of atropine and neostigmine.[27]

Succinylcholine is also effective when administered by the intramuscular route; in this instance, complete paralysis is achieved in 3 to 4 minutes. Evidence of relaxation of the respiratory muscles, as manifest by decreased positive pressure required to ventilate by face mask, can be detected before the abolishment of the twitch response. A dose of 2 mg/kg IM does not achieve satisfactory relaxation in all children, whereas the higher dose of 3 mg/kg IM produces a mean twitch depression of 85%; 4 mg/kg produces profound relaxation in all children, but its effects may last up to 20 minutes.[26] In infants less than 6 months of age, a dose of 5 mg/kg is required to achieve profound relaxation.[28] Recovery from the neuromuscular effect of intramuscular succinylcholine is faster in infants than in children. Changes in the heart rate following intramuscular succinylcholine are not pronounced. Consequently, routine intramuscular administration of atropine with intramuscular succinylcholine is not generally indicated.[29]

The short duration of action of succinylcholine is due to its rapid hydrolysis by plasma cholinesterase (pseudocholinesterase), which is synthesized by the liver. Plasma cholinesterase is present in serum as a tetrameric glycoprotein consisting of four identical subunits made of nine sugar chains.[30] The normal function of human plasma cholinesterase is unknown, but it hydrolyzes several compounds that reach the circulation such as heroine, cocaine, procaine, chloroprocaine, succinylcholine, and mivacurium.[31]

The most common cause of decreased plasma cholinesterase activity in children is the presence of the atypical enzyme. This nucleotide-substituted altered esterase can be present in the usual concentration, but it has a markedly diminished hydrolytic activity. Plasma cholinesterase deficiency is an inherited condition that occurs in a mild form (heterozygous) in about 4% of people of European descent. The incidence of more severe forms (homozygous) is about 1 in 2000.[32] In patients with plasma cholinesterase deficiency, prolonged duration of the effect of succinylcholine is expected. In heterozygous patients, the prolongation is only for

a few minutes. Consequently, it might not be noted clinically. Homozygous patients, however, with two atypical genes (two fluoride or two silent) may have prolonged paralysis for several hours.

Side Effects of Succinylcholine

Jaw Stiffness. Succinylcholine administration is occasionally associated with an increase in masseter muscle tone and hence a decrease in the ability to open the mouth. This increase in tone is a transient phenomenon lasting for only a few minutes and occurs despite abolition of the evoked twitch response in the masseter or the peripheral muscles. This increased muscle tone is seen to a much lesser degree in peripheral muscles, but the onset is earlier in the masseter group.[33, 34] The increase in muscle tone is usually mild and can be overcome by manually opening the mouth.[35] On rare occasions, it may be so severe that extreme force will be required to open the mouth, thus interfering with smooth endotracheal intubation. This phenomenon seems to occur more frequently during halothane anesthesia than with thiopental induction.[36] Whether this increased masseter tone is related to the "trismus" encountered in patients with malignant hyperthermia remains a matter of speculation.[37] Prospective studies designed to evaluate masseter tone have failed to demonstrate a patient with a marked increase in masseter tone who went on to develop any evidence of malignant hyperthermia.[34, 38] In several retrospective reports, however, a number of patients had trismus and did develop or have a positive test response for malignant hyperthermia.[39–41] These studies have left clinicians in a bit of quandary about how to proceed when a patient develops trismus. Some have advocated canceling the surgical procedure, treating the patient as susceptible to malignant hyperthermia, and recommending a muscle biopsy.[41, 42] Others advocate continuing the procedure, avoiding further exposure to triggering agents by changing anesthetic technique, carefully observing for early signs of malignant hyperthermia, e.g., increased carbon dioxide (CO_2) production or tachycardia, and if indicated, initiating arterial and central venous blood gas sampling as well as early treatment.[43]

Arrhythmias. Changes in heart rate (usually mild, transient increases) are frequently observed after the administration of succinylcholine. The tachycardia is more pronounced in the presence of sevoflurane than halothane.[44] Of greater concern is the occasional bradycardia.[45] These fluctuations in heart rate appear to be more common in children anesthetized with halothane. Most arrhythmias are transient (mostly two to three beats), predominantly vagal in origin, and usually detected through continuous electrocardiographic recording. Succinylcholine-associated arrhythmias are rarely due to ventricular irritability. Prior intravenous administration of anticholinergic agents (atropine) markedly decreases but does not completely abolish the incidence of these arrhythmias.[45] As in adults, the incidence and severity of these irregularities in heart rate increase after a second dose.[46, 47]

Hyperkalemia. An elevation in serum potassium level occurs after intravenous administration of succinylcholine in normal children, but the change is too small to have a clinically important cardiovascular effect.[48] A life-threatening arrhythmia related to hyperkalemia may occur after intravenous administration of succinylcholine in patients with burn injury, tetanus, paraplegia, encephalitis, crush injuries, or neuromuscular (Duchenne or Becker muscular dystrophy) disease.[49-55] In some of these situations, especially following burn injuries, the muscle tissue develops an increased number of receptors and becomes more permeable so that the entire muscle becomes capable of releasing potassium during depolarization. Thus, the prolonged depolarization caused by succinylcholine may induce a massive efflux of potassium, producing cardiac arrest.[56] In contrast to these situations, spastic quadriparetic children from cerebral palsy respond normally to succinylcholine and do not demonstrate hyperkalemia.[56-58]

Biochemical Changes. An increase in serum creatine kinase concentrations can be detected following succinylcholine in the presence of inhalational agents, especially with halothane.[59] This increase is less pronounced during a thiopental nitrous oxide anesthetic. In patients with neuromuscular disease, this increase in creatine kinase activity is much more pronounced.[60]

Myoglobinemia. Myoglobinemia, another sensitive indicator of muscle injury, occurs in 40% of children who are anesthetized with halothane and receive succinylcholine. Eight percent of patients achieve sufficiently high blood myoglobin levels to cause myoglobinuria (an effect seen in only 3% of adults).[61] Myoglobinuria occurs more frequently after inhalation induction with halogenated agents than after intravenous inductions. It is also seen less frequently in children anesthetized with enflurane than with halothane.[62, 63] It does not occur with intramuscular succinylcholine. Such an increase can be attenuated by the prior administration of small doses of pancuronium or tubocurarine (20 and 50 μg/kg, respectively), oral dantrolene, or thiopental (4 mg/kg).[64-66]

Fasciculations. Fasciculations are usually observed in adolescents and children but rarely in infants; in children 1 to 3 years old, they are described as gross muscle movements.[59, 67] Prior administration of small doses of succinylcholine (100 μg/kg), curare (50 μg/kg), pancuronium (20 μg/kg), fentanyl (1–2 μg/kg), or alfentanil (50 μg/kg) will usually decrease the frequency and intensity of the fasciculations and the consequent rise of intragastric pressure.[59, 65, 67-69] Neither the incidence nor the severity of fasciculations correlate with the occurrence of myoglobinemia, but may be mildly correlated with the increase in serum creatine phosphokinase activity.[60]

Intraocular pressure rises after succinylcholine administration in children whether they fasciculate or not.[70] The exact mechanism of this rise in intraocular pressure is not clear. Initially, it was presumed to be due to tonic contractions of extraocular muscles. However, observations on patients with detached extraocular muscles prior to enucleation showed rises of intraocular pressure similar to the level of intact eyes.[71] The increase in intraocular pressure is probably due to a number of factors, but is chiefly due to the cycloplegic action of succinylcholine with deepening of the anterior chamber and increased outflow resistance. The intraocular pressure usually rises by about 10 mm Hg, peaks in 2 to 3 minutes, and then returns to baseline in 5 to 7 minutes.[70] It is advisable to perform tonometry measurements before succinylcholine administration or wait at least 7 minutes following succinylcholine administration before performing tonometry in children. Although use of succinylcholine free of untoward side effects has been reported in patients with open eye injuries,[72] it is nonetheless prudent to refrain from its use in situations of penetrating ocular wounds unless the eye is not salvageable. High-dose rocuronium (1.2 mg/kg) may be a reasonable alternative for rapid sequence intubation.[73]

Perioperative Dreaming. Children receiving succinylcholine during narcotic-based anesthesia have reported a 19% incidence of dreaming. This dream activity is not associated with awareness and can be curtailed by pretreatment with tubocurarine. Speculation as to the cause of this activity centers on the notion that increased muscle spindle discharge causes cerebral arousal and dream stimulation.[74, 75]

Clinical Uses of Succinylcholine

The use of succinylcholine for routine surgical procedures has declined, primarily because of rare but life-threatening complications such as unexpected malignant hyperthermia or cardiac arrest in patients with undiagnosed muscular dystrophy.[76] On the other hand, succinylcholine does have the most rapid onset and brief duration of action of all muscle relaxants and therefore remains the most desirable for rapid-sequence endotracheal intubation and for the treatment of laryngospasm.[77-79] Since the rapidity of onset is dose related, children can be given 1.5 to 2.0 mg/kg IV to obtain 95% neuromuscular depression in about 40 seconds; the smaller dose of 1.0 mg/kg would achieve the same degree of depression in about 50 seconds.[77, 78] In infants younger than 1 year, a dose of 3 mg/kg IV would be more appropriate because of their large extracellular volume. These doses provide excellent intubating conditions in all patients.[78] To decrease the incidence of arrhythmias, one should precede the intravenous dose of succinylcholine with atropine 0.01 to 0.02 mg/kg IV.

The value of preventing succinylcholine fasciculations and the consequent increase in intragastric pressure is a frequently debated issue.[79] In children younger than 3 years, in whom fasciculations are in the form of gross movements, the consequent rise in intragastric pressure would be insignificant; therefore, pretreatment with nondepolarizing agents is not necessary.[67] In older children, prevention of fasciculations may be considered, although it should be noted that small doses of nondepolarizing relaxants might cause undesirable side effects such as diplopia. One must also recognize that the advantage of abolishing fasciculations in emergency situations is mostly theoretical and that the consequences of a rise in intragastric pressure (regurgitation and aspiration) can be prevented by applying cricoid pressure (Sellick maneuver).[67]

Controversies in Succinylcholine Use

In 1993, the Food and Drug Administration issued a directive against the routine use of succinylcholine in children and adolescents except for emergency airway management. This was based on several case reports of hyperkalemic cardiac arrests, primarily in children with undiagnosed Duchenne muscular dystrophy.[80] The disturbing observation about this complication was the high mortality rate of 55%. Almost all of these cases, however, occurred in male children 8 years of age and younger. Thereafter the Food and Drug Administration and the manufacturer revised the product label (package insert) stating:

> Since it is difficult to identify which patients are at risk, it is recommended that the use of succinylcholine in pediatric patients be reserved for emergency intubation or in instances when immediate securing of the airway is necessary, e.g., laryngospasm, difficult airway, and full stomach, or for intramuscular route when a suitable vein is inaccessible.

Although it is frequently stated that rapid intubation can avoid pulmonary aspiration of gastric contents, no data prove this statement to be true. In cases in which the child has eaten and is at potential risk for an adverse response to succinylcholine, but there is no obvious distention of the abdomen or active regurgitation, a controlled induction with nondepolarizing muscle relaxant with a relatively fast onset, such as rocuronium, may be as safe as succinylcholine. It is reasonable in these situations to administer the induction agent (thiopental or propofol) and follow with a relatively large dose of nondepolarizing muscle relaxant, apply cricoid pressure, ventilate the child with *low* positive pressure (<20 cm water), and perform the tracheal intubation about a minute after the point at which relaxation has taken full effect. The main disadvantage is that the duration of the nondepolarizing relaxant may exceed the duration of the planned procedure. One study has found comparable intubating conditions 30 seconds after administration of succinylcholine (1.5 mg/kg) and rocuronium (1.2 mg/kg) following 5 mg/kg thiopental, thus avoiding the need for ventilation prior to intubation.[73]

There will be still some emergency situations, however, in which a short-acting agent with rapid onset is most desirable, such as in patients undergoing a short procedure who have a full stomach. In these circumstances, succinylcholine is still the most suitable muscle relaxant. A recent survey has noted that one-half of pediatric centers have stopped the routine use of succinylcholine for intubation and limit its use for special indications without an apparent increase in morbidity or mortality.[81]

Concerning the most feared complication of succinylcholine, rhabdomyolysis, there is no specific treatment. Cardiac arrest immediately following administration of succinylcholine is almost always due to hyperkalemia. Since hyperkalemia is the cause of cardiac arrest, a successful outcome depends on immediate counteracting of the cardiac arrhythmogenic effects of hyperkalemia. Hyperventilation in normal situations decreases plasma potassium levels; a 10 mm Hg decrease in $PaCO_2$ causes a 0.5 mEq/L decrease in plasma potassium concentration. Calcium is recommended as an antagonist for the cardiac effects of potassium. The specific dose is unknown and variable for each patient, but 2 to 4 mg/kg of calcium chloride are reasonable initial doses. Further calcium is administered until the arrhythmia is abolished. Modes for treatment of hyperkalemia are glucose (0.5 g/kg) and insulin (0.1 U/kg) over 30 minutes and sodium polystyrene sulfonate (Kayexalate; 1–2 g/kg retention enema). It

should be noted that successful treatment of this complication might require a very prolonged resuscitation.

Short-Acting Relaxants

Mivacurium

Mivacurium chloride is a short-acting nondepolarizing muscle relaxant. It is a *bis*-quaternary benzylisoquinolinium choline-like diester consisting of three stereoisomers, *cis-trans*, *trans-trans*, and *cis-cis*. The important active isomers are the *cis-trans* and *trans-trans*, each with a half-life of about 2 minutes.[82] Similar to succinylcholine, these two active isomers are rapidly hydrolyzed by plasma cholinesterase into pharmacologically inactive monoquaternary compounds.[83]

During halothane anesthesia, the ED_{50} of mivacurium is approximately 50 μg/kg and the ED_{95} is 89–95 μg/kg (Fig. 10–6).[84, 85] The corresponding values during $N_2O:O_2$ opioid anesthesia are slightly higher. Infants (2 months–1 year) tend to have slightly lower effective doses than children. In infants, the ED_{50} is about 45 μg/kg and the ED_{95} varies from 65 to 94 μg/kg.[86, 87]

Usually, 2 to 2.5 times the ED_{95} dose of a muscle relaxant is administered to achieve adequate conditions for tracheal intubation (see Tables 10–1 and 10–2). Consequently, a dose of 200 to 250 μg/kg mivacurium was initially administered to children for tracheal intubation. At this dose, maximum twitch suppression occurred in about 1.5 to 2 minutes; recovery to 5% was 6 to 10 minutes and complete recovery was within 15 to 20 minutes.[84, 85]

Subsequently, it was found that the recommended intubating dose of 250 μg/kg did not provide adequate conditions for intubation in all children. Therefore, higher doses were used.[26, 86] By increasing the dose to 300 μg/kg, the onset time (time to maximum depression) was decreased to 1.3 minutes.[88] A further increase in dose to 400 μg/kg produced

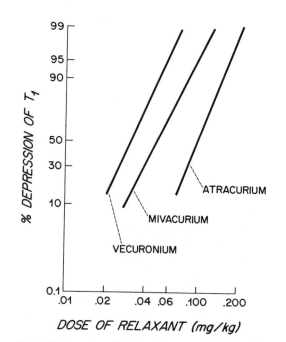

Figure 10–6. Comparative dose response curves for vecuronium, mivacurium, and atracurium.

no significant decrement in onset time, but prolonged the recovery. With propofol and fentanyl, the intubating conditions with 300 μg/kg were classified as good or excellent in all patients. The onset time of 1.5 minutes, even at these higher doses, was still significantly longer than the onset time of 0.7 to 0.9 minutes with succinylcholine.[89, 90]

The recovery times of mivacurium in children are about 30% faster than those observed in adults.[91–93] In comparison with other muscle relaxants, mivacurium's neuromuscular blockade is twice as long as that of succinylcholine, but only 30% to 50% as long as atracurium or vecuronium. Increasing the initial dose of mivacurium prolongs only the immediate time of recovery (to 5%). Subsequent recovery indices (25–75%, 75–95%) are not affected by the initial dose or by the subsequent doses, whether it is given by repeated bolus doses or by continuous infusion.

As with other nondepolarizing muscle relaxants, potentiation of the neuromuscular effects of mivacurium can be observed in the presence of halogenated agents. Since halothane produces the smallest degree of potentiation, the neuromuscular blockade is more marked with isoflurane and sevoflurane.[93]

Since mivacurium is short acting and the recovery is independent of the dose and duration of administration, it is most suitable for continuous administration. In children, the infusion requirements to achieve 95% neuromuscular block during halothane anesthesia are 10 to 12 μg/kg/min and 13 to 16 μg/kg/min during $N_2O:O_2$ opioid anesthesia.[91, 92] These infusion requirements decrease exponentially during isoflurane anesthesia.[93, 94]

Caution is always in order when delivering drugs by infusion in children because of the possibility that the intravenous infusion will stop flowing and a "piggy-back" infusion will accumulate in the main intravenous line; upon clearing the intravenous line, the patient may in effect receive a bolus dose of the drug. This has been reported in an infant when, upon clearing the intravenous line in the recovery room, immediate respiratory arrest occurred.[95]

Since mivacurium is a benzylisoquinolinium compound, it has the potential to cause histamine release from mast cells. Most often this manifests as a generalized flushing and very rarely as mild hypotension. These hypotensive episodes usually last about 5 minutes in unstimulated patients. In the clinical setting, however, tracheal intubation at this period will counteract the hypotensive effect. In children, the cardiovascular effect at doses up to 200 μg/kg occasionally (< 5%) causes hypotension. Increasing the dose of mivacurium from 200 to 300 and 400 μg/kg will increase the incidence of flushing and decreased arterial blood pressure. These hypotensive episodes, even at high doses, are transient and self-limiting.[88]

One rare complication is prolonged neuromuscular blockade in patients with plasma cholinesterase deficiency. In a heterozygous patient with plasma cholinesterase deficiency, a modest increase in duration (15–20 min) can be detected, whereas in homozygous patients there is a considerable delay in recovery. Patients with prolonged block beyond the duration of the surgical procedure are usually treated with sedation and mechanical ventilation. Reversal with anticholinergic agents is indicated when there is evidence of muscle activity.[96]

Rapacuronium (has been withdrawn from the market)

Rapacuronium is an aminosteroid neuromuscular blocking agent. It has a relatively rapid onset similar to rocuronium. Its rapid onset is due to its low potency (ED_{90} 1.15 mg/kg in adults) and hence the higher concentration gradient between plasma and the postsynaptic nicotinic receptor.[97] Clearance of rapacuronium depends largely on hepatic uptake and biliary excretion (similar to vecuronium). Rapacuronium's most important degradation product is the 3-desacetyl metabolite that has neuromuscular blocking properties half as potent as rapacuronium with a slower onset time. The lower clearance of the metabolite will gradually prolong the time course of neuromuscular blockade during maintenance with rapacuronium.[98] Therefore, a single intubating dose of rapacuronium has a duration similar to that of mivacurium, but at larger or repeated doses it will have a duration similar to an intermediate muscle relaxant.

Rapacuronium has minimal cardiovascular effects. However, it appears that a higher than usual (up to 10%) incidence of bronchospasm occurs. Usually the bronchospasm is mild in nature and responds to the administration of an inhalation agent. However, some episodes of bronchospasm have required more aggressive treatment.[99]

Rapacuronium provides good to excellent conditions for intubation at 60 seconds in infants after 1.5 mg/kg and in children after 2 mg/kg. At these doses the twitch response reappears in about 10 minutes.[100] An advantage is that this relaxant can be safely administered intramuscularly in patients without venous access. In infants and children, a deltoid muscle injection of rapacuronium (2.8 and 4.8 mg/kg) is effective in producing neuromuscular relaxation, but these doses do not provide adequate intubating conditions in all patients in less than 3 minutes.[101] A longer period of observation increases the number of patients with satisfactory intubating conditions.

In adults, the duration of action of 1.5 mg/kg of rapacuronium (IV) is similar to 0.25 mg/kg of mivacurium. Recovery of the train-of-four to more than 70% occurs within 30 minutes. At larger doses, however, especially in patients with renal failure, prolongation of effect is observed because of formation and accumulation of the diacetyl active metabolite.[102]

Intermediate-Acting Nondepolarizing Relaxants

Atracurium

Chemically, atracurium is an imidazoline bisquaternary compound that undergoes spontaneous decomposition into inactive metabolites. At physiologic (alkaline) pH, it undergoes nonenzymatic hydrolysis independent of plasma cholinesterase (Hofmann elimination). In blood and other tissue fluids, the quaternary ammonium compound breaks down primarily into laudanosine and a related quaternary acid (methylacrylate).

The studies that have evaluated the effective dose of atracurium in children have found the ED_{50} to be 100 to 160 μg/kg and the ED_{95} from 170 to 280 μg/kg (see Fig. 10–6). The higher values are reported in the presence of $N_2O:O_2$ opioid anesthesia and the lower ones with halothane anesthesia; however, the difference in potency between these two anesthetic techniques is only on the order of 10 to 20% (see Tables 10–1 and 10–2).

The effective dose in infants has varied from 85 to 100 μg/kg for the ED_{50} and 100 to 170 μg/kg for the ED_{95}.[103–111] The studies that have shown infants to be more sensitive to atracurium have also demonstrated that at these smaller doses, the duration of action of the drug is shorter.[105, 107] Although these data may have a certain theoretical importance, the observed differences are clinically unimportant; therefore, the same dose can be used in infants and children.

For intubating purposes, two to three times the ED_{95} (300 to 600 μg/kg) is given to produce rapid and effective blockade in most children and adolescents.[108, 109] Such doses provide satisfactory conditions for intubation within 2 minutes. The period of absence of twitch response after an intubating dose of atracurium usually lasts 15 to 30 minutes. Hence, in clinical situations, an intubating dose should provide complete neuromuscular blockade for such an interval, followed by another 20 minutes of intermediate blockade (twitch height 5 to 25%); complete recovery usually occurs within 40 to 60 minutes. Comparison of data from children and adults demonstrates that children require more atracurium per kilogram body weight and generally recover faster. This difference, however, is relatively small and is masked in most cases by the wide range of individual patient responses.

Since atracurium is degraded spontaneously and its metabolites do not have neuromuscular blocking properties, it can be easily administered by continuous infusion. The infusion requirement to maintain 90 to 99% twitch depression in children is 6 μg/kg/min during isoflurane anesthesia, 7 to 8 μg/kg/min with halothane, and 9 μg/kg/min with a $N_2O:O_2$ opioid technique.[112, 113] It has been noted, however, that required doses of atracurium increase during prolonged infusion (90 hours) in an intensive care setting.[105] This is most probably due to immobilization, which produces resistance to muscle relaxants because of the development of extrajunctional receptors. These patients recover promptly following discontinuation of the atracurium.

No significant differences in the volume of distribution, clearance, or half-lives have been detected between normal infants and children with impaired hepatic function.[114] Plasma laudanosine concentrations tend to be higher in children with hepatic impairment than in children with normal hepatic function.[114] In a two-compartment pharmacokinetic model, it was noted that the volume of distribution at steady state was largest in infants, intermediate in children, and smallest in adults. Clearance of atracurium follows the same trend: fastest in infants, intermediate in children, and slowest in adults.[112] These data explain the minimal differences in the recovery parameters of atracurium between infants, children, and adults.[115]

The *side effects* of atracurium are minimal. At clinical doses of up to 600 μg/kg, the compound does not significantly alter the heart rate or blood pressure in children. Mild cutaneous reactions in the form of flushing of the neck or the face can sometimes be observed.[108] Extremely rare instances of anaphylactoid reactions or bronchospasm have been reported, although it is interesting that these have occurred when atracurium was preceded by thiopental.

Cisatracurium

Cisatracurium is one of the 10 stereoisomers of atracurium (1R-*Cis*, 1′R-*Cis*). In the original atracurium formula, it made up 15% of the mixture. In clinical studies, it was found that cisatracurium is three times more potent than atracurium with a similar duration of action.[116] Similar to other nondepolarizing relaxants, its onset can be accelerated by increasing the dose (see Tables 10–1 and 10–2). This will increase the duration of the action; doubling the dose of the cisatracurium prolongs its effect. This is consistent with its decomposition and metabolism by Hofmann elimination. This suggests that cisatracurium, like atracurium, is a noncumulative agent with recovery occurring during the elimination phase rather than during the distribution phase.

The ED_{95} dose of cisatracurium during halothane anesthesia in children is 41 μg/kg.[117] In comparison, in adults the ED_{95} is about 50 μg/kg during $N_2O:O_2$ opioid anesthesia.[118] Twice the ED_{95} dose has an onset time of 2 to 2.5 minutes with recovery to 25% in 27 to 34 minutes. Cisatracurium has a tendency to have slightly slower onset of action than atracurium consistent with its relative potency; more potent nondepolarizing relaxants have slower onsets than the less potent nondepolarizing relaxants. Twice the ED_{95} dose (80 μg/kg) of cisatracurium leads to complete suppression of the twitch response in 2.5 minutes. The recovery to 25 and 95% of control response occurs in 31 and 53 minutes, respectively.[116–119] The recovery index to 25 to 75% in children is 11 minutes.[117] Its duration and recovery profile is essentially the same as for atracurium and is independent of the dose.

The higher potency of cisatracurium offers some advantages over atracurium. Since a lower amount of relaxant is administered and histamine-related effects can be related to the molar concentration of the drug, its histamine-releasing effects are minimal. At doses up to five times ED_{95} in adults (250 μg/kg), no cutaneous flushing or bronchospasm occurs. In addition, there are no concomitant changes in heart rate, blood pressure, or plasma histamine concentration.[119]

The clearance of cisatracurium is faster in pediatric patients than in adults, with a shorter duration of neuromuscular blockade. In patients with renal failure, the clearance of cisatracurium is reduced by 13%; plasma laudanosine levels were higher but were only about 10% of those reported with atracurium.[120] The duration of action of cisatracurium in renal failure patients is not significantly prolonged.[121]

The safety profile of cisatracurium is manifested in one case report of a 7-month-old infant who unintentionally received 6 mg cisatracurium, a dose of 860 μg/kg that is equivalent to 20 times the ED_{95}. After 100 minutes, this infant showed evidence of recovery of the twitch response and within another 10 minutes four responses on train-of-four were recorded.[122]

Vecuronium

Vecuronium is the monoquaternary analogue of pancuronium in which the methyl group of the position 2 nitrogen atom is absent. The specific advantage of vecuronium is the absence of any adverse cardiovascular effects even in doses several times greater than the usually recommended clinical doses (see Tables 10–1 and 10–2).[123] Vecuronium is primarily metabolized by the liver and excreted in bile.[124]

With vecuronium, the dose requirements according to age groups are much more pronounced (more than 50%), with a biphasic distribution of the dose requirement and duration of action varying with age. Infants less than 1 year of age are significantly more sensitive to the action of vecuronium than older children. As adolescence is reached, the requirement diminishes to that of adults.[125-128] These observations have been made with bolus dose response as well as with infusion techniques.[129] A similar trend is observed in the duration of action, when a fixed dose produces a relatively long-lasting effect in infants, a shorter one in children, and a longer one again in adolescents. This observation has led some investigators to conclude that vecuronium should be considered a long-acting neuromuscular agent in infants less than 1 year of age.[130] The long-acting effect is even more pronounced in neonates. The *pharmacokinetic* explanation is that the plasma concentration required for a certain degree of paralysis is lower in infants than in children but that this effect is partly compensated in the dose requirement by an infant's larger distribution volume. The implication is that a greater amount of the drug needs to be administered to produce a given effect at the neuromuscular junction. The lower plasma concentration in combination with the larger distribution volume leads to a relatively slow decrease in the plasma concentration during recovery, which is expressed as a prolonged mean residence time.[131] Consequently, the dose of vecuronium (especially repeat doses) needs to be more carefully adjusted in very young patients.

Long-Term Administration of Vecuronium. Muscle relaxants are often administered to critically ill patients. Vecuronium has been popular because of the absence of cardiovascular effects and because its metabolites do not seem to have central nervous system effects. However, several adult patients have had residual weakness following the discontinuation of vecuronium.[132, 133] A common feature in these patients was renal failure and high plasma concentration of the metabolite of vecuronium (3-desacetylvecuronium). In contrast to adults, such a response seems to be extremely rare in children. In one study in which the rate of infusion was adjusted by accelerometry, all children recovered within 1 hour. Of note in these pediatric patients, the requirements of neonates and small infants was 45% less than in older children.[134]

Rocuronium

Rocuronium is a monoquaternary steroidal muscle relaxant similar to vecuronium. It has the fastest onset of action of the intermediate-acting nondepolarizing relaxants because of its low potency and higher dose requirements. The clinical duration of action of rocuronium is similar to that of vecuronium.[135] In animals it is primarily eliminated by the liver and the kidney excretes about 10%.

Studies with rocuronium in children during halothane anesthesia show that the ED_{50} and ED_{95} are 179 and 303 μg/kg respectively.[136] During $N_2O:O_2$ opioid anesthesia, it is slightly higher.[137-139] Following the administration of 600 μg/kg rocuronium, 90% and 100% neuromuscular block occurs in 0.8 and 1.3 minutes (see Tables 10–1 and 10–2). At this dose, the heart rate in these children increased by about 15 beats per minute. The mean recovery to 25% of control was about 28 minutes and to 90%, 46 minutes.[139] Based on these data, it can be stated that rocuronium is about one fourth to one third as potent as mivacurium and one tenth as potent as vecuronium.

Infants 2 to 11 months of age have a slightly faster onset following the same dose of 600 μg/kg rocuronium, the times to 90% and 100% twitch depression being 37 and 64 seconds, respectively. The recovery to 25% was 42 minutes, 15 minutes longer than in children.[140] Rocuronium has a fast onset, but it is still not as fast as succinylcholine in adults or children. The exception is in infants, in whom the 60-second neuromuscular depression of rocuronium is similar to that of succinylcholine.[136, 141] When the intubating conditions of rocuronium (600 μg/kg) in children were compared with those of vecuronium (100 μg/kg), atracurium (500 μg/kg), or succinylcholine (1 mg/kg), it was found that tracheal intubation could be performed within 60 seconds in all the children receiving rocuronium or succinylcholine, whereas with vecuronium, 120 seconds were required and with atracurium 180 seconds.[142, 143] The twitch response during intubation was not significantly different between the three nondepolarizing drugs, as all were between 25 and 37%. The fact that intubation could be performed in the absence of complete suppression of the twitch response can be explained by the observation that the peak effects of rocuronium at the laryngeal adductor muscles occur about 40 seconds faster than on the adductor pollicis in humans.[144] The 1-minute intubating conditions can be slightly improved by increasing the dose of rocuronium from 600 to 900 μg/kg.[145] At 600 μg/kg, better intubating conditions can be obtained at 60 seconds than at 50 seconds.[146] At these doses, a slight increase in heart rate (11–18%) with no change in systolic or diastolic pressure is seen. These increases in heart rate are transient and of no clinical importance in a healthy patient.[136, 147] The onset time of rocuronium can be further hastened by increasing the dose to 1.2 mg/kg (three to four times the ED_{95}).[73, 139] Two pediatric studies have demonstrated that 1.2 mg/kg rocuronium provides intubating conditions similar to those provided by 1.5 to 2.0 mg/kg succinylcholine within 30 seconds of administration following 5 mg/kg thiopental.[73, 148] The time to recovery of 25% of twitch response after such a dose is about 40 to 75 minutes.

In a pharmacokinetic study of rocuronium, it was found that infants cleared rocuronium at a slower rate than children (4 vs. 7 mL/kg/min), with the distribution volume being larger in infants. The mean residence time was 56 minutes in infants vs. 26 minutes in children, which explains the prolonged effect of rocuronium in infants compared with children. When these data are compared with data from adults, it can be noted that the larger plasma clearance and lower volume of distribution in children compared with infants and adults results in markedly lower mean residence time and a shorter neuromuscular block.[149] The observation in infants of their need for a lower concentration of rocuronium as compared with children to produce the same degree of neuromuscular block has been previously observed with curare and vecuronium.[150] Plasma clearance of rocuronium decreases with weight in children 4 to 11 years of age. In turn, distribution and elimination half-lives increase with weight and presumably with age, which explains the larger dose requirement and the more rapid recovery in younger compared with older children.[151]

In adult patients with liver disease, the elimination half-life is increased from 76 minutes to 110 minutes. The delayed elimination half-life is secondary to the increased distribution volume in liver disease.[152] During renal failure, the clearance of rocuronium is decreased by 30 to 40%, which results in an increase in duration of action of a single dose by about 10 minutes.[152] Even in patients with hepatic or renal dysfunction, rocuronium still remains a fast-onset drug.[153] The duration of action of this drug can be markedly prolonged in patients with hepatorenal disease when repeated doses are administered.

Intramuscular Rocuronium. In infants and children, it is considered desirable that a nondepolarizing agent be available for producing neuromuscular relaxation in the absence of intravenous access as an alternative to succinylcholine. In one study, it was found that deltoid injection of 1.8 mg/kg (1800 μg/kg) rocuronium in children and 1 mg/kg (1000 μg/kg) in infants can produce satisfactory relaxation to perform endotracheal intubation in 2.5 to 3 minutes.[154] However, a subsequent multicenter study could not confirm these findings. The conditions for intubation were poor in most of these patients in 3.5 to 4 minutes, although neuromuscular depression was obtained in 6 to 8 minutes.[155] The bioavailability of intramuscular rocuronium at these doses is about 80%.[156] It would appear the intramuscular rocuronium is a possible alternative to intramuscular succinylcholine but that the time of onset and the duration of action are much longer than with succinylcholine.

Clinical Implications When Using Short- and Intermediate-Acting Relaxants

Short- and intermediate-acting relaxants have great utility in the pediatric population because of the large number of short surgical procedures performed in children. Because of their short duration of action, these drugs can be given in one intubating dose (atracurium, 500 μg/kg; cisatracurium 200 μg/kg; vecuronium, 100 μg/kg; rocuronium 600 μg/kg) and a light anesthetic level maintained throughout the procedure. If more than 45 minutes have elapsed since the final dose of either drug, one may reasonably assume that neuromuscular function has nearly recovered, and clinical reversal may not be necessary. This assumption must be confirmed by clinical signs or by the twitch monitor.

One of the main disadvantages of nondepolarizing relaxants is the delayed onset. With most of them, complete paralysis does not occur until at least 2 minutes pass. With rocuronium, paralysis tends to occur faster, though this is not consistent in all clinical situations. None of these nondepolarizing drugs compare to succinylcholine, which provides complete paralysis in all patients within 45 seconds.[157] If complete paralysis is required in children, the dose should be increased to four to six times the ED$_{95}$ dose; for example, 0.3 mg/kg for vecuronium, 0.3 mg/kg for cisatracurium, or 1.2 mg/kg for rocuronium. The drawback of these larger doses is the prolonged duration of complete paralysis, which might be longer than 1 hour. Although onset of paralysis is faster with succinylcholine, comparable intubating conditions are provided by 45 seconds with rocuronium (1.2 mg/kg).[73]

It should be noted that complete paralysis at the thumb is not an absolute prerequisite for adequate relaxation to perform tracheal intubation, since equilibration of relaxants between the plasma and laryngeal adductors occurs earlier than in the adductor of the thumb.[158] During recovery, the laryngeal adductors recover earlier because of their faster equilibration and because of their lesser sensitivity to relaxants.

The use of these intermediate-acting neuromuscular blocking drugs has increased markedly in the last decade, whereas the use of long-acting agents has declined. This trend is probably due to the absence of clinically significant side effects and the fact that the shorter duration of action gives an extra measure of security; a child who demonstrates "mild" neuromuscular weakness at the end of surgery is generally able to overcome it within a short interval. This weakness can be observed frequently at the end of a procedure (in the absence of reversal) when a "typical" patient might barely be able to lift an arm; within 2 or 3 minutes, much improvement is usually noted. This recovery from neuromuscular blockade is more predictable with atracurium or cisatracurium because of the many pathways for degradation that these drugs have, both at the tissue level and at the extracellular compartment level.

Nondepolarizing muscle relaxants have minimal or practically no effect on intraocular pressure. In the presence of an open eye injury, a large dose of vecuronium or rocuronium would seem to be an alternative choice when there is the need for rapid intubation.[73, 159]

It is important to realize that atracurium and vecuronium are acidic compounds (pH 3 to 4) and can therefore be easily deactivated in alkaline media. In a slowly running intravenous system in which thiopental (pH 10 to 11) is injected with a muscle relaxant, precipitation and loss of the relaxant's potency might occur. Consequently, if these drugs are to be administered in tandem, clinicians should ensure that the thiopental is washed through the intravenous line before administering the atracurium.[73]

Long-Acting Nondepolarizing Relaxants

Tubocurarine

Early studies based on clinical requirements demonstrated that infants less than 1 month of age are markedly sensitive to the action of curare.[160] A follow-up study (in children anesthetized with halothane and using a twitch monitor) did not observe this sensitivity; instead, marked variation in the response to tubocurarine of infants less than 2 months of age was noted.[4] The dose that caused 95% depression of the twitch (ED$_{95}$) varied between 160 and 640 μg/kg IV in infants younger than 10 days, whereas the range for the ED$_{95}$ in older children was 230 to 460 μg/kg IV. The mean ED$_{95}$ in all infants and children for tubocurarine was 300 μg/kg (see Tables 10–1 and 10–2).

Pharmacokinetic studies have demonstrated that the plasma concentration at which 50% depression of the twitch height occurs is lower in neonates and infants than in children and adults, whereas the steady-state distribution volume is greater in neonates than in infants, children, or adults.[150, 161] The product of the two—the quantity of tubocurarine present at a steady state to produce 50% paralysis—was nearly the same in all age groups. These data indicate that small infants demonstrate neuromuscular blockade at lower plasma concentrations but that the total dose (milligrams per kilogram) does not change because it is counterbalanced by an infant's larger volume of distribution. Clearance of tubocurarine in infants and children is similar to that in young adults. Because of a neonate's larger distribution volume, however, a smaller fraction of the drug is eliminated each minute. This longer elimination half-life may result in a slower rate of recovery from neuromuscular blockade.[150]

Infants demonstrate marked variability in response to all muscle relaxants; the reasons for this are not entirely clear. It may in part be related to a nonhomogeneous group of patients in whom the myoneural junction is at different stages of development. The sensitivity of some individuals can be explained by the immaturity of the junction, whereas relative resistance to the effects of the blocking agents can be due to residual fetal-type receptors that might behave like extrajunctional receptors.[162]

In pediatric practice, the initial dose of tubocurarine has varied between 250 and 800 µg/kg. The lower dose is used in children already intubated and anesthetized with a halogenated agent. This dose produces clinical relaxation lasting for approximately 25 minutes. The larger dose can be used for tracheal intubation, with the clinical effect lasting for more than 1 hour in children.[16]

Side Effects. The histamine-releasing effects of tubocurarine have been frequently observed in adults. In children, only indirect evidence of histamine release has been seen, such as erythema along the injected vein and mild hypotension.[163] This effect is more prominent in adolescents than in children and nearly absent in infants.

Metocurine

Metocurine iodide is a methyl derivative of tubocurarine with a parallel dose-response curve and a potency ratio of 2:1 (Fig. 10–7). It causes less histamine release than tubocurarine and therefore minimal changes in cardiovascu-

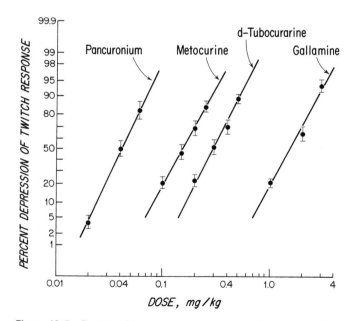

Figure 10–7. Comparative dose-response curves for pancuronium, metocurine, tubocurarine, and gallamine. (From Goudsouzian NG, Martyn JJ, Liu LM, Ali HH: The dose-response effect of long-acting nondepolarizing neuromuscular blocking agents in children. Can Anaesth Soc J 1984;31:246–250.)

lar parameters.[164] In infants and children, a dose of 500 µg/kg provides satisfactory to excellent conditions for intubation (see Tables 10–1 and 10–2). After this dose, the period of tetanic fade and post-tetanic facilitation is about 38 minutes during halothane anesthesia and 19 minutes in the presence of thiopental $N_2O:O_2$ opioid anesthesia. These recovery rates are shorter than those reported in adults.

Pancuronium

Pancuronium bromide is a bisquaternary ammonium steroidal compound with nondepolarizing neuromuscular blocking properties. It is more potent than tubocurarine, metocurine, and gallamine and has a slightly shorter duration of action.[165] Pancuronium has some advantages over tubocurarine in that it induces tachycardia (increased cardiac output in infants) and has no histamine-releasing properties. As a result, the systolic blood pressure tends to rise after its administration.[163]

Pancuronium at a dose of 100 µg/kg IV offers satisfactory conditions for tracheal intubation in 70 to 90% of infants and children within 150 seconds of administration. Increasing the initial dose to 150 µg/kg provides satisfactory intubating conditions in all children within 80 seconds (see Tables 10–1 and 10–2).[77, 166]

Pancuronium is frequently advocated for various cardiac surgical and other high-risk procedures in infants. The anesthetic technique of high-dose fentanyl (50 to 75 µg/kg) or sufentanil (5 to 10 µg/kg) with air-O_2-pancuronium is well tolerated by infants. The vagolytic effect (tachycardia) of pancuronium counteracts the vagotonic effect (bradycardia) of fentanyl and sufentanil, and its relaxant properties counteract narcotic-induced chest wall and glottic rigidity.[167] In the postoperative period, pancuronium, by abolishing voluntary movement, has the advantage of decreasing O_2 consumption in mechanically ventilated patients.[168]

Pancuronium has been used to facilitate ventilation in premature infants in *neonatal intensive care units*.[169] Because pancuronium increases the heart rate, blood pressure, and plasma epinephrine and norepinephrine levels in neonates, there is some concern that it may be a factor in causing cerebral hemorrhage.[170] With this concern in mind, the best approach is to administer pancuronium with either general anesthesia or with adequate sedation to blunt adverse cardiovascular responses. Vecuronium may offer an advantage over pancuronium because it does not significantly increase the blood pressure. In sick neonates, cerebral blood flow is directly related to blood pressure.[171–175] In patients at risk, it should be noted that nasotracheal intubation or intratracheal suctioning in the presence of pancuronium causes smaller changes in intracranial pressure than such activity in patients not receiving the drug.[175, 176] By abolishing fluctuations in cerebral blood flow through the use of muscle relaxants, one may theoretically reduce the incidence and severity of intraventricular hemorrhages.

Doxacurium

Doxacurium is a long-acting bisquaternary benzylisoquinolinium relaxant. It has practically no side effects at doses up to three times the ED_{95}. The ED_{95} for doxacurium in children is 30 µg/kg,[177, 178] making it the most potent neuromuscular blocking agent available and twice as potent as vecuronium or pipecuronium (see Tables 10–1 and 10–2). As with other muscle relaxants, its effect is potentiated by halothane and isoflurane.[179] Infants require smaller doses than children.[180] Its duration of action is similar to that of any of the long-acting relaxants. Similar to other relaxants, the effective dose of doxacurium is higher in children than in adults and the duration of action of an effective dose in children is shorter than that reported for adults. In one study, doxacurium was administered by titrated infusion for 5 to 12 days in a group of pediatric patients following laryngotracheal reconstruction. Although these patients recovered satisfactorily upon discontinuation of the relaxant, about 40% had residual weakness and decreased coordination for several days to weeks postextubation.[181]

Pipecuronium

Pipecuronium is a steroidal nondepolarizing relaxant with a duration of action similar to that of doxacurium. The ED_{95} of pipecuronium in children during fentanyl $N_2O{:}O_2$ anesthesia is about 80 µg/kg versus 60 µg/kg in adults. The requirements of infants are less than those of children, whose dosage is similar to that of adults (see Tables 10–1 and 10–2). Isoflurane markedly potentiates the action of pipecuronium, whereas halothane has a minimal effect.[182–184] Again, children tend to recover faster from its effects than adults. Infants require lesser amounts of pipecuronium and recover faster than children.

Antagonism of Muscle Relaxants

In children and especially in infants, the O_2 consumption for each kilogram of body weight is higher than in adults. Therefore, a slight diminution in respiratory muscle power may lead to hypoxemia and CO_2 retention. Consequently, it is very important that neuromuscular function return to normal at the end of the surgical procedure.

In this respect, neonates are more vulnerable than adults for the following reasons: (1) immaturity of the neuromuscular system, as evidenced by the lower values of train-of-four, post-tetanic facilitation, tetanus:twitch ratios, and the marked fade during prolonged tetanic stimulation; (2) longer elimination half-life of relaxants; (3) the presence of a greater number of fast muscles in the ventilatory musculature (these types of fibers being more liable to fatigue than slow muscles)[185]; and (4) the closing volume of a neonate, which is within the tidal volume; that is, airway closure occurs at the end of expiration.[186] If respiration is mildly impaired as a result of residual muscle paralysis, more alveoli will collapse. The result may be dangerous hypoxemia and acidosis, which might potentiate and prolong the action of the muscle relaxant, thus creating a vicious cycle.

When monitoring pediatric patients, one should keep in mind that higher doses of muscle relaxants are required to block the diaphragm than the adductor pollicis; train-of-four monitoring of the adductor pollicis overestimates the degree of neuromuscular blockade in the diaphragm.[18] Therefore, if the train-of-four of the adductor is near normal, it can be reasonably assumed that the diaphragm is fully recovered.

Clinical evaluation of the adequacy of antagonism in infants and children is more difficult than in adults. Neither grip strength nor voluntary head lifting can be expected from small children. Rather, it is important when working with infants to observe the clinical conditions preoperatively (muscle tone, depth of respiration, vigor of crying) and then to aim for a return to those levels in the post-reversal period. An exception to this rule is a child who will be ventilated postoperatively. In this instance, antagonism of muscle relaxation may not be indicated.

Useful clinical signs of antagonism are the ability to flex the arm and lift the legs and the return of abdominal muscle tone.[187] Inspiratory force may be measured; a negative force less than -25 cm H_2O is an indicator of adequate reversal.[188] A crying vital capacity of more than 15 mL/kg is considered an adequate sign of recovery of respiratory reserve. The train-of-four is a valuable aid; it can even be used in the smallest infants, in whom the force of contraction can easily be felt (four equal contractions, indicating adequate antagonism). Alternatively, tetanic stimulation can be used and the post-tetanic count evaluated. The post-tetanic twitch response can be detected before the return of single twitches or train-of-four responses.

The dose requirement of reversal agents in children is different than that in adults; the requirement of *neostigmine* is lower in children.[189] In most situations (as long as the twitch response is present), 20 µg/kg neostigmine preceded by 10 µg/kg atropine or 5 µg/kg glycopyrrolate is satisfactory. Infants and neonates may require higher doses of atropine; my minimal dose of atropine is 0.1 mg. If needed, this dose can be repeated. *Edrophonium* has the theoretic advantage of an onset of action 2 to 3 minutes faster than that of neostigmine. Whether this difference is of any clinical importance is a matter of opinion. The dose required for children is higher than for adults; at least 0.3 mg/kg is needed, but 0.5 to 1.0 mg/kg is most often used.[190, 191] A minor advantage of edrophonium is that less atropine (10 µg/kg) is needed to antagonize bradycardia. Because heart rate changes seem to occur earlier with this agent, its administration should be delayed until the vagolytic effect (tachycardia) of the atropine has occurred. Alternatively, glycopyrrolate can be given before the edrophonium at a dose of 10 µg/kg to block edrophonium's vagal effects.[191] It should be realized, however, that besides the type and the dose of the reversal agent, the degree of blockade before the reversal is extremely important; the less blockade, the faster the antagonism.[192–194]

The question arises about whether the neuromuscular effects of all the various nondepolarizing muscle relaxants should be reversed in all cases, even if a lengthy interval has elapsed since the administration of the last dose. Routine reversal was almost essential a decade ago because the techniques for evaluating the effects of the relaxants were in their infancy and all muscle relaxants were long acting. With the advent of reliable neuromuscular monitors and their use in conjunction with clinical observations and measurements of respiratory adequacy, one can be more confident that reversal will not always be required. This is especially true of the recently developed short- and intermediate-acting relaxants, particularly mivacurium, atracurium, or cisatracurium, which are hydrolyzed in plasma. Children have the additional advantage of recovering faster than adults from residual neuromuscular block.[193, 194] In infants (though not in children), the excretion of vecuronium might be delayed, necessitating the prophylactic use of reversing agents. If any doubts remain about a particular patient's condition, clinicians should always err on the side of reversal.

The classical teaching has been that reversal should not be attempted until the twitch response has returned to a reasonable level (about 25%). Recent studies, however, have demonstrated that early reversal with neostigmine 5 minutes after the administration of rocuronium or vecuronium is possible.[195] However, there was no marked difference in recovery of the train-of-four to 70% whether the reversal was given 5 minutes after the relaxant or when the twitch response had recovered to 25%. With a single dose of rapacuronium, earlier reversal (2 min) or so-called rescue reversal is also possible.[196]

Hypothermia potentiates the action of most of the nondepolarizing muscle relaxants and delays their excretion.[197] This effect can create a special problem at the end of a surgical procedure. Shivering in children increases O_2 consumption and augments the load on the respiratory system, whereas small infants increase their oxygen consumption through brown fat metabolism. If the respiratory muscles are unable to match this increased load, hypoxemia and CO_2 retention occur, leading to acidosis, which again potentiates the action of the relaxant. To avoid the extra cardiorespiratory load in a postsurgical patient, it is reasonable to warm the infant if his or her temperature has fallen below 35°C. Once the core temperature is safely above this level, reversal may be attempted if appropriate.

All *antibiotics* theoretically have neuromuscular depressing properties when administered in association with relaxants.[198] Aminoglycoside derivatives such as gentamicin, tobramycin, and neomycin have the greatest effect. In general, a single clinical dose of antibiotic does not have any appreciable neuromuscular blocking effect.[199] This factor alone does not rule out the possibility that large concentrations of antibiotics, especially in the presence of other potentiating factors, may indeed contribute to neuromuscular paralysis. The clinical importance of this factor with regard to inadequate or difficult reversal has decreased since the introduction of intermediate-acting neuromuscular blocking agents.

Relaxants in Special Situations

In certain diseases, the response of a patient to a given anesthetic or relaxant may be different from what is expected; even a minor or seemingly insignificant side effect can be catastrophic. Of the many drug combinations possible, that of succinylcholine and halothane seems to be most likely to trigger malignant hyperthermia[200] (see Chapter 27). The use of depolarizing neuromuscular blocking agents in combination with halogenated agents should be avoided in patients at risk for this syndrome.[201] The safest general anesthetic technique is the use of an opioid:N_2O:O_2 combination with a nondepolarizing relaxant. Nondepolarizing agents devoid of cardiovascular side effects may offer an advantage in not masking tachycardia, one of the early signs of malignant hyperthermia.[202]

Progressive Muscular Dystrophy

The Duchenne form is the most common and one of the most severe types of the muscular dystrophies in children.[203, 204] It is estimated that it occurs in 1 in 3300 male births. It is due to mutation of an X-linked recessive gene that results in abnormalities of dystrophin.[205] The Duchenne dystrophy gene has been isolated and its locus defined in the short arm of the X chromosome, position 21.[206] Affected persons are almost always males who present with proximal muscle weakness before the age of 5 years; they are likely to be brought to a pediatrician because of a waddling, clumsy gait and frequent falls. The disease initially affects the proximal muscles of the pelvis and the shoulders; the latter enlarge from fatty infiltration and become extremely weak (pseudohypertrophy). A characteristic movement of affected children is using the hands to grasp the ankles, shins, knees, and thighs to help stand when arising from the floor (Gower sign). The weakness eventually progresses to all the muscles of the body; young victims lose their ability to ambulate and develop contractures. Unfortunately, this disease is progressive, with death occurring 5 to 20 years after its onset. The female carriers of the gene do not have peripheral muscular anomalies but can show evidence of cardiomyopathy.[207] Some progress has been made in the management of these cases using prolonged treatment with prednisone.[208]

The probable cause of Duchenne muscular dystrophy is the virtual absence of the intracellular protein dystrophin.[205] In the milder forms of muscular dystrophy such as facioscapulohumeral, limb-girdle, and Becker dystrophies, lower than normal levels of dystrophin or abnormal dystrophins are present. The absence of dystrophin weakens the attachment of intracellular calcium to the extracellular basal lamina and hence the stability of the myofibrillar membrane during contraction.[206] Initially, an association was suggested with Duchenne's muscular dystrophy and malignant hyperthermia. It has been concluded, however, that the absence of dystrophin per se is not the primary cause of malignant hyperthermia crisis.[209–211]

Affected patients with Duchenne dystrophy frequently have myocardial involvement (70%), which is symptomatic in only a small proportion of cases (10%). Myocardial damage starts from an asymptomatic stage that is only recognized by the electrocardiogram to a preclinical period of myocardial hypertrophy (chaotic hypertrophy) localized at the septum, leading to conduction defects such as heart block or arrhythmias. This is followed by the development of a cardiomyopathy characterized by poor contraction of the ventricles, cardiac dilatation, and reduced ejection fraction.[207] The electrocardiogram typically demonstrates tall R waves in the right precordial leads and deep Q waves in the lateral precordial or limb leads. Echocardiographic imaging demonstrates wall motion abnormalities and fibrosis in the lateral and posterobasal walls of the left ventricle. Previously undetected cardiac involvement may appear during anesthesia as tachycardia (shortened PR interval), ventricular fibrillation, and even cardiac arrest.[210] Cardiac arrest in an undiagnosed case in an infant prompted anesthesiologists to question the routine use of succinylcholine in infants and children in 1987.[76] Since that time, most anesthesiologists have altered their practice away from the routine use of succinylcholine in children. During this time, the Food and Drug Administration issued a warning against the routine use of succinylcholine in infants and children[80] and recommended the use of nondepolarizing relaxants for routine intubation. Besides the skeletal muscle weaknesses, myopathic patients have blunted pharyngeal reflexes, difficulty in swallowing, and pronounced gastric hypomotility. These factors make them prone to aspiration pneumonitis.[212]

Patients with diagnosed muscular dystrophy commonly present for two surgical procedures. One is for muscle biopsy to establish the diagnosis, and the other is for correction of contractures or kyphoscoliosis. In patients with Duchenne muscular dystrophy, succinylcholine causes rhabdomyolysis as evidenced by myoglobinuria, increased levels of creatine phosphokinase, hyperkalemia, and occasionally metabolic acidosis.[213] During the anesthetic course in these patients, a moderate rise in body temperature is often observed. Complications most often occur when halothane is combined with succinylcholine. The incidence of complications is much less with local than with general anesthesia. It is reasonable if possible to perform most biopsies with local anesthesia with sedation and reserve general anesthesia ($N_2O:O_2$:opioid:relaxant) for the more involved procedures.[210, 213]

If needed, nondepolarizing agents can be safely administered to these patients.[214–216] The dose requirement of atracurium, for instance, is similar to that in normal patients, but the effects may last longer.[214] The same effect has been reported from mivacurium when a slight prolongation and moderately decreased infusion requirements were observed.[215] Also of clinical importance is the fact that such patients have weakness of the respiratory muscles that may lead to respiratory failure. Consequently, adequacy of reversal should be thoroughly evaluated before extubation is attempted. If there is any doubt, patients should remain intubated until their strength returns.

Myotonia

Myotonic dystrophy (myotonia dystrophica) is an autosomal dominant disease that results from abnormal muscle calcium metabolism.[217] Because the cellular adenosine triphosphate system fails to return the calcium ions to the sarcoplasmic reticulum, they remain available to produce sustained muscle contracture. Because of this intracellular calcium defect, muscle contractions are not prevented by relaxants or regional anesthesia; infiltration of the affected muscles with local anesthetic is necessary to induce relaxation. Myotonic patients have an expressionless face because of facial weakness; they also have frontal baldness, ptosis, dysarthria, and wasting of the sternocleidomastoid muscles. Cardiac involvement consists mainly in conduction system abnormalities, mitral valve prolapse, and wall motion anomalies; however, alterations in myocardial relaxation (in contrast to skeletal muscles) are minor.[216] Progressive distal muscle weakness occurs with additional muscle wasting. A characteristic feature of these patients is their inability to relax the hand muscles on stimulation (hence the term *myotonia*).

Though myotonia dystrophica is a disease of adults, its other variants do occur in infants and children. These include myotonia congenita (Thomsen disease), characterized by general myotonia and hypertrophy of voluntary muscles, and paramyotonia, in which the syndrome appears only on exposure to cold. Another subvariant is congenital dystrophia myotonica, which presents in the neonatal period as generalized hypotonia and facial diplegia.[217] Affected neonates have difficulty in breathing as well as swallowing and are usually mentally subnormal. Such babies slowly improve during the first decade of life but then develop the adult form of the disease.

Myotonic patients are known to be extremely sensitive to thiopental and opioids. Therefore, the dose of these drugs should be carefully titrated. In such patients, succinylcholine may exacerbate myotonia, causing respiratory and jaw muscle rigidity, leading to hypoxemia and the inability to open the mouth adequately. An increased myotonic response has occasionally been observed following neostigmine, presumably from the stimulating effect of acetylcholine.

One should avoid succinylcholine in myotonic patients and substitute a nondepolarizing agent. Atracurium or cisatracurium seem to be the most favored because of their predictable rapid recovery rate; this feature obviates the need for reversal agents in most clinical situations.[218, 219] As expected, these dystrophic patients (especially infants) have respiratory muscle weakness. Consequently, their respiratory parameters should be carefully monitored even after adequate reversal.

Myasthenia Gravis

Myasthenia gravis is a disorder of neuromuscular function due to reduction of available acetylcholine receptors at the neuromuscular junction. It is caused by an autoimmune process that induces the development of highly specific antibodies to these receptors.[220, 221] When the density of postsynaptic receptors is reduced to 20 to 30% of baseline, the safety margin for neuromuscular transmission is lost and the patient develops signs of weakness and fatigue on exertion. In myasthenic patients, the muscle weakness is typically worse after effort and improves with rest. It is characteristically distributed in the following order: extraocular, bulbar, neck, limb-girdle, distal limb, and trunk muscles.

Two thirds of myasthenic patients are women with a peak age of onset between 20 and 30 years. About 15% of infants born to mothers with myasthenia develop signs of transient *neonatal myasthenia* due to transplacental transfer of antibodies.[222] The symptoms appear within 72 hours of birth and persist for several days; rarely do they persist for more than 3 months. The course of transient neonatal myasthenia seems to be different from the extremely rare *congenital myasthenia*, which has a prolonged course.

Because the extent and course of neonatal myasthenia is variable, with gradual improvement, treatment is tailored to the situation. All babies born to myasthenic mothers should be closely observed for signs of weakness. The critical period is during feeding. If needed, the clinical response to a relatively large but frequently used dose of reversal agents (atropine 20 μg/kg followed by neostigmine 40 to 60 μg/kg) can be tested. If improvement is noted, pyridostigmine (5 mg/kg) can be given orally before each feeding. If the symptoms are severe, however, and the baby is developing respiratory failure, endotracheal intubation and ventilation should be carried out and the dose of pyridostigmine titrated.

Burns

Since the early reports of cardiac arrest in burned patients receiving succinylcholine, extensive investigations have sought to define and understand the effect of muscle relaxants in these individuals.[223] Succinylcholine causes hyperkalemia, which predisposes to cardiac arrest. The more extensive the burn is, the more likely and the greater the hyperkalemic response. Although most cases of cardiac arrest have occurred 20 to 50 days after the burn injury, abnormal elevations of plasma potassium levels following administration of succinylcholine can occur within a few days of the burn. Hyperkalemia probably results from the development of new acetylcholine receptors along the surface of the muscle membrane in the postburn phase.[224] Such receptors are thought to be extremely sensitive to the usual doses of agonists, such as acetylcholine or succinylcholine; instead of the discrete potassium movement at the end plate, more general leakage occurs along the entire muscle membrane.

The requirement for nondepolarizing relaxants tends to be increased for burned patients (except with mivacurium).[225, 226] In fact, such patients may require two to three times the usual intravenous dose to produce the desired clinical effect (see Chapter 23). This resistance peaks about 2 weeks after the burn, persists for many months in patients with major burns, and decreases gradually with healing; it correlates with both the magnitude of the burn and the period of healing. This resistance can be partially explained by the increased drug binding as a result of increased plasma alpha 1-acid glycoprotein levels found in the presence of a burn and an increase in extrajunctional receptors.

Although no cases of cardiac arrest have been reported in the first few days after a large burn injury, the use of succinylcholine at that time should be avoided because of the ever-present possibility of hyperkalemia. Patients can usually be adequately managed with a nondepolarizing relaxant, although in most cases they require up to three times the usual dose. The relaxant effect can, however, be antagonized by the usual doses of the anticholinesterases.

REFERENCES

1. Ali HH, Savarese JJ: Monitoring of neuromuscular function. Anesthesiology 1976;45:216–249.
2. Waud BE, Waud DR: The relation between the response to "train-of-four" stimulation and receptor occlusion during competitive neuromuscular block. Anesthesiology 1972;37:413–416.
3. Ali HH, Utting JE, Gray TC: Quantitative assessment of residual antidepolarizing block. II. Br J Anaesth 1971;43:478–485.
4. Goudsouzian NG, Donlon JV, Savarese JJ, et al: Re-evaluation of dosage and duration of action of d-tubocurarine in the pediatric age group. Anesthesiology 1975;43:416–425.
5. Goudsouzian NG, Crone RK, Todres ID: Recovery from pancuronium blockade in the neonatal intensive care unit. Br J Anaesth 1981;53:1303–1309.
6. Goudsouzian NG: Maturation of neuromuscular transmission in the infant. Br J Anaesth 1980;52:205–214.
7. Ali HH, Wilson RS, Savarese JJ, et al: The effect of tubocurarine on indirectly elicited train-of-four muscle response and respiratory measurements in humans. Br J Anaesth 1975;47:570–574.
8. Engbaek J, Ostergaard D, Viby-Mogensen J, et al: Clinical recovery and train-of-four ratio measured mechanically and electromyographically following atracurium. Anesthesiology 1989;71:391–395.
9. Bowman WC: Pharmacology of Neuromuscular Function, 2nd ed. London: Butterworth & Co., 1990.
10. Stanec A, Heyduk J, Stanec G, et al: Tetanic fade and post-tetanic tension in the absence of neuromuscular blocking agents in anesthetized man. Anesth Analg 1978;57:102–107.
11. Churchill-Davidson HC, Wise RP: The response of the newborn infant to muscle relaxants. Can Anaesth Soc J 1964;11:1–6.
12. Koenigsberger MR, Patten B, Lovelace RE: Studies of neuromuscular function in the newborn: I. A comparison of myoneural function in the full-term and the premature infant. Neuropaediatrie 1973;4:350–361.
13. Crumrine RS, Yodlowski EH: Assessment of neuromuscular function in infants. Anesthesiology 1981;54:29–32.
14. Gwinnutt CL, Meakin G: Use of the post-tetanic count to monitor recovery from intense neuromuscular blockade in children. Br J Anaesth 1988;61:547–550.
15. Ridley SA, Braude N: Post-tetanic count and intense neuromuscular blockade with vecuronium in children. Br J Anaesth 1988;61:551–556.
16. Goudsouzian NG, Liu LM, Coté CJ: Comparison of equipotent doses of non-depolarizing muscle relaxants in children. Anesth Analg 1981;60:862–866.
17. Donati F, Meistelman C, Plaud B: Vecuronium neuromuscular blockade at the adductor muscles of the larynx and adductor pollicis. Anesthesiology 1991;74:833–837.
18. Laycock JR, Baxter MK, Bevan JC, et al: The potency of pancuronium at the adductor pollicis and diaphragm in infants and children. Anesthesiology 1988;68:908–911.
19. Plaud B, Laffon M, Ecoffey C, et al: Monitoring orbicularis oculi predicts good intubating conditions after vecuronium in children. Can J Anaesth 1997;44:712–716.
20. Stead AL: The response of the newborn infant to muscle relaxants. Br J Anaesth 1955;27:124–130.
21. Cook DR, Fisher CG: Neuromuscular blocking effects of succinylcholine in infants and children. Anesthesiology 1975;42:662–665.
22. Meakin G, McKiernan EP, Morris P, et al: Dose-response curves for suxamethonium in neonates, infants and children. Br J Anaesth 1989;62:655–658.
23. Widdowson EM: Changes in body proportions and composition during growth. In: Davis JA, Dobbing J (eds): Scientific Foundations of Paediatrics, pp 153–163. Philadelphia: W.B. Saunders; 1974.
24. DeCook TH, Goudsouzian NG: Tachyphylaxis and phase II block development during infusion of succinylcholine in children. Anesth Analg 1980;59:639–643.
25. Goudsouzian NG, Liu LM: The neuromuscular response of infants to a continuous infusion of succinylcholine. Anesthesiology 1984;60:97–101.
26. Gronert BJ, Brandom BW: Neuromuscular blocking drugs in infants and children. Pediatr Clin North Am 1994;41:73–91.
27. Bevan JC, Donati F, Bevan DR: Prolonged infusion of suxamethonium in infants and children. Br J Anaesth 1986;58:839–843.
28. Liu LM, DeCook TH, Goudsouzian NG, et al: Dose response to intramuscular succinylcholine in children. Anesthesiology 1981;55:599–602.
29. Hannallah RS, Oh TH, McGill WA, et al: Changes in heart rate and rhythm after intramuscular succinylcholine with or without atropine in anesthetized children. Anesth Analg 1986;65:1329–1332.
30. Davis L, Britten JJ, Morgan M: Cholinesterase: Its significance in anaesthetic practice. Anaesthesia 1997;52:244–260.
31. Hoffman RS, Morasco R, Goldfrank LR: Administration of purified human plasma cholinesterase protects against cocaine toxicity in mice. J Toxicol Clin Toxicol 1996;34:259–266.
32. Whittaker M: Plasma cholinesterase variants and the anaesthetist. Anaesthesia 1980;35:174–197.
33. van der Spek AF, Fang WB, Ashton-Miller JA, et al: Increased masticatory muscle stiffness during limb muscle flaccidity associated with succinylcholine administration. Anesthesiology 1988;69:11–16.
34. Plumley MH, Bevan JC, Saddler JM, et al: Dose-related effects of succinylcholine on the adductor pollicis and masseter muscles in children. Can J Anaesth 1990;37:15–20.
35. Hannallah RS, Kaplan RF: Jaw relaxation after a halothane/succinylcholine sequence in children. Anesthesiology 1994;81:99–103.
36. Lazzell VA, Carr AS, Lerman J, et al: The incidence of masseter muscle rigidity after succinylcholine in infants and children. Can J Anaesth 1994;41:475–479.
37. Schwartz L, Rockoff MA, Koka BV: Masseter spasm with anesthesia: incidence and implications. Anesthesiology 1984;61:772–775.
38. Saddler JM, Bevan JC, Plumley MH, et al: Jaw muscle tension after succinylcholine in children undergoing strabismus surgery. Can J Anaesth 1990;37:21–25.
39. Ellis FR, Halsall PJ: Suxamethonium spasm: A differential diagnostic conundrum. Br J Anaesth 1984;56:381–384.
40. Donlon JV, Newfield P, Sreter F, et al: Implications of masseter spasm after succinylcholine. Anesthesiology 1978;49:298–301.

41. O'Flynn RP, Shutack JG, Rosenberg H, et al: Masseter muscle rigidity and malignant hyperthermia susceptibility in pediatric patients: An update on management and diagnosis. Anesthesiology 1994;80:1228–1233.

42. Rosenberg H: Trismus is not trivial. Anesthesiology 1987;67:453–455.

43. Berry FA, Lynch C 3d: Succinylcholine and trismus. Anesthesiology 1989;70:161–163.

44. Rieger A, Hass I, Striebel HW, et al: Marked increases in heart rate associated with sevoflurane but not with halothane following suxamethonium administration in children. Eur J Anaesthesiol 1996;13:616–621.

45. Goudsouzian NG: Turbe del ritmo cardiaco durante intubazione tracheale nei bambini. Acta Anesthesiol Italica 1981;32:293–299.

46. Blanc VF: Atropine and succinylcholine: Beliefs and controversies in paediatric anaesthesia. Can J Anaesth 1995;42:1–7.

47. Mazze RI, Dunbar RW: Intralingual succinylcholine administration in children: An alternative to intravenous and intramuscular routes? Anesth Analg 1968;47:605–615.

48. Keneally JP, Bush GH: Changes in serum potassium after suxamethonium in children. Anaesth Intensive Care 1974;2:147–150.

49. McCaughty TJ: Hazards of anaesthesia for the burned child. Can Anaesth Soc J 1962;9:220–233.

50. Cooperman LH: Succinylcholine-induced hyperkalemia in neuromuscular disease. JAMA 1970;213:1867–1871.

51. Roth F, Wuthrich H: The clinical importance of hyperkalaemia following suxamethonium administration. Br J Anaesth 1969;41:311–316.

52. Smith RB, Grenvik A: Cardiac arrest following succinylcholine in patients with central nervous system injuries. Anesthesiology 1970;33:558–560.

53. Mazze RI, Escue HM, Houston JB: Hyperkalemia and cardiovascular collapse following administration of succinylcholine to the traumatized patient. Anesthesiology 1969;31:540–547.

54. Larach MG, Rosenberg H, Gronert GA, et al: Hyperkalemic cardiac arrest during anesthesia in infants and children with occult myopathies. Clin Pediatr (Phila) 1997;36:9–16.

55. Pedrozzi NE, Ramelli GP, Tomasetti R, et al: Rhabdomyolysis and anesthesia: A report of two cases and review of the literature. Pediatr Neurol 1996;15:254–257.

56. Gronert GA, Theye RA: Pathophysiology of hyperkalemia induced by succinylcholine. Anesthesiology 1975;43:89–99.

57. Theroux MC, Brandom BW, Zagnoev M, et al: Dose response of succinylcholine at the adductor pollicis of children with cerebral palsy during propofol and nitrous oxide anesthesia. Anesth Analg 1994;79:761–765.

58. Dierdorf SF, McNiece WL, Rao CC, et al: Effect of succinylcholine on plasma potassium in children with cerebral palsy. Anesthesiology 1985;62:88–90.

59. Cozanitis DA, Erkola O, Klemola UM, et al: Precurarisation in infants and children less than three years of age. Can J Anaesth 1987;34:17–20.

60. Karhunen U: Serum creatine kinase levels after succinylcholine in children with "muscle, eye and brain disease." Can J Anaesth 1988;35:90–92.

61. Ryan JF, Kagen LJ, Hyman AI: Myoglobinemia after a single dose of succinylcholine. N Engl J Med 1971;285:824–827.

62. Laurence AS: Serum myoglobin release following suxamethonium administration to children. Eur J Anaesthesiol 1988;5:31–38.

63. Shono S, Higa K, Watanabe R, et al: Myoglobinuria following anesthesia with enflurane and succinylcholine in an asthmatic child on theophylline. [in Japanese]. Masui 1996;45:91–95.

64. Blanc VF, Vaillancourt G, Brisson G: Succinylcholine, fasciculations and myoglobinaemia. Can Anaesth Soc J 1986;33:178–184.

65. Asari H, Inoue K, Maruta H, et al: The inhibitory effect of intravenous d-tubocurarine and oral dantrolene on halothane-succinylcholine-induced myoglobinemia in children. Anesthesiology 1984;61:332–333.

66. Noguchi I, Suzuki G, Amemiya Y: Effects of different doses of thiopentone on the increase in serum myoglobin induced by suxamethonium in children. Br J Anaesth 1993;71:291–293.

67. Salem MR, Wong AY, Lin YH: The effect of suxamethonium on the intragastric pressure in infants and children. Br J Anaesth 1972;44:166–170.

68. Lindgren L, Saarnivaara L: Increase in intragastric pressure during suxamethonium-induced muscle fasciculations in children: Inhibition by alfentanil. Br J Anaesth 1988;60:176–179.

69. Lindgren L, Saarnivaara L: Effect of competitive myoneural blockade and fentanyl on muscle fasciculation caused by suxamethonium in children. Br J Anaesth 1983;55:747–751.

70. Craythorne NWB, Rottenstein HS, Dripps RD: The effect of succinylcholine on intraocular pressure in adults, infants, and children during general anesthesia. Anesthesiology 1960;21:59–63.

71. Kelly RE, Dinner M, Turner LS, et al: Succinylcholine increases intraocular pressure in the human eye with the extraocular muscles detached. Anesthesiology 1993;79:948–952.

72. Libonati MM, Leahy JJ, Ellison N: The use of succinylcholine in open eye surgery. Anesthesiology 1985;62:637–640.

73. Mazurek AJ, Rae B, Hann S, et al: Rocuronium versus succinylcholine: Are they equally effective during rapid-sequence induction of anesthesia? Anesth Analg 1998;87:1259–1262.

74. Hobbs AJ, Bush GH, Downham DY: Peri-operative dreaming and awareness in children. Anaesthesia 1988;43:560–562.

75. O'Sullivan EP, Childs D, Bush GH: Peri-operative dreaming in paediatric patients who receive suxamethonium. Anaesthesia 1988;43:104–106.

76. Delphin E, Jackson D, Rothstein P: Use of succinylcholine during elective pediatric anesthesia should be reevaluated. Anesth Analg 1987;66:1190–1192.

77. Cunliffe M, Lucero VM, McLeod ME, et al: Neuromuscular blockade for rapid tracheal intubation in children: Comparison of succinylcholine and pancuronium. Can Anaesth Soc J 1986;33:760–764.

78. Meakin G, Walker RW, Dearlove OR: Myotonic and neuromuscular blocking effects of increased doses of suxamethonium in infants and children. Br J Anaesth 1990;65:816–818.

79. Robinson AL, Jerwood DC, Stokes MA: Routine suxamethonium in children: A regional survey of current usage. Anaesthesia 1996;51:874–878.

80. Goudsouzian NG: Recent changes in the package insert for succinylcholine chloride: Should this drug be contraindicated for routine use in children and adolescents? (Summary of the discussions of the anesthetic and life support drug advisory meeting of the Food and Drug Administration, FDA building, Rockville, MD, June 9, 1994). Anesth Analg 1995;80:207–208.

81. O'Flynn RP, Shutack JG, Rosenberg H: Succinylcholine in pediatric centers before and after 1992. Am J Anesth 1992;26:200–203.

82. Lien CA, Schmith VD, Embree PB, et al: The pharmacokinetics and pharmacodynamics of the stereoisomers of mivacurium in patients receiving nitrous oxide/opioid/barbiturate anesthesia. Anesthesiology 1994;80:1296–1302.

83. Cook DR, Stiller RL, Weakly JN, et al: In vitro metabolism of mivacurium chloride (BW B1090U) and succinylcholine. Anesth Analg 1989;68:452–456.

84. Goudsouzian NG, Alifimoff JK, Eberly C, et al: Neuromuscular and cardiovascular effects of mivacurium in children. Anesthesiology 1989;70:237–242.

85. Sarner JB, Brandom BW, Woelfel SK, et al: Clinical pharmacology of mivacurium chloride (BW B1090U) in children during nitrous oxide-halothane and nitrous oxide-narcotic anesthesia. Anesth Analg 1989;68:116–121.

86. Goudsouzian NG, Denman W, Schwartz A, et al: Pharmacodynamic and hemodynamic effects of mivacurium in infants anesthetized with halothane and nitrous oxide. Anesthesiology 1993;79:919–925.

87. Woelfel SK, Brandom BW, McGowan FX Jr, et al: Clinical pharmacology of mivacurium in pediatric patients less than two years old during nitrous oxide-halothane anesthesia. Anesth Analg 1993;77:713–720.

88. Shorten GD, Crawford MW, St. Louis P: The neuromuscular effects of mivacurium chloride during propofol anesthesia in children. Anesth Analg 1996;82:1170–1175.

89. Cook DR, Gronert BJ, Woelfel SK: Comparison of the neuromuscular effects of mivacurium and suxamethonium in infants and children. Acta Anaesthesiol Scand Suppl 1995;106:35–40.

90. Mangat PS, Evans DEN, Harmer M, et al: A comparison between mivacurium and suxamethonium in children. Anaesthesia 1993;48:866–869.

91. Kaplan RF, Garcia M, Hannallah RS: Mivacurium-induced neuromuscular blockade during sevoflurane and halothane anaesthesia in children. Can J Anaesth 1995;42:16–20.

92. Alifimoff JK, Goudsouzian NG: Continuous infusion of mivacurium in children. Br J Anaesth 1989;63:520–524.

93. Meretoja OA, Wirtavuori K, Taivainen T, et al: Time course of potentiation of mivacurium by halothane and isoflurane in children. Br J Anaesth 1996;76:235–238.

94. Jalkanen L, Meretoja OA: The influence of the duration of isoflurane anaesthesia on neuromuscular effects of mivacurium. Acta Anaesthesiol Scand 1997;41:248–251.

95. Litman RS, Younan MM, Patt RB, et al: Postoperative recurrent paralysis in an infant after mivacurium infusion. Can J Anaesth 1994;41:758–759.

96. Goudsouzian NG, d'Hollander AA, Viby-Mogensen J: Prolonged neuromuscular block from mivacurium in two patients with cholinesterase deficiency. Anesth Analg 1993;77:183–185.

97. Goulden MR, Hunter JM: Rapacuronium (Org 9487): Do we have a replacement for succinylcholine? Br J Anaesth 1999;82:489–492.

98. Schiere S, Proost JH, Schuringa M, et al: Pharmacokinetics and pharmacokinetic-dynamic relationship between rapacuronium (Org 9487) and its 3-desacetyl metabolite (Org 9488). Anesth Analg 1999;88:640–647.

99. Sparr HJ, Mellinghoff H, Blobner M, et al: Comparison of intubating conditions after rapacuronium (Org 9487) and succinylcholine following rapid sequence induction in adult patients. Br J Anaesth 1999;82:537–541.

100. Meakin GH, Meretoja OA, Motsch J, et al: A dose-ranging study of rapacuronium in pediatric patients. Anesthesiology 2000;92:1002–1009.

101. Reynolds LM, Infosino A, Brown R, et al: Intramuscular rapacuronium in infants and children. Anesthesiology 1999;91:1285–1292.

102. Szenohradszky J, Caldwell JE, Wright PM, et al: Influence of renal failure on the pharmacokinetics and neuromuscular effects of a single dose of rapacuronium bromide. Anesthesiology 1999;90:24–35.

103. Goudsouzian NG: Atracurium in infants and children. Br J Anaesth 1986;58(Suppl 1):23S–28S.

104. Brandom BW, Woelfel SK, Cook DR, et al: Clinical pharmacology of atracurium in infants. Anesth Analg 1984;63:309–312.

105. Kushimo OT, Darowski MJ, Morris P, et al: Dose requirements of atracurium in paediatric intensive care patients. Br J Anaesth 1991;67:781–783.

106. Goudsouzian N, Liu LM, Gionfriddo M, et al: Neuromuscular effects of atracurium in infants and children. Anesthesiology 1985;62:75–79.

107. Meakin G, Shaw EA, Baker RD, et al: Comparison of atracurium-induced neuromuscular blockade in neonates, infants and children. Br J Anaesth 1988;60:171–175.

108. Goudsouzian NG, Liu LM, Coté CJ, et al: Safety and efficacy of atracurium in adolescents and children anesthetized with halothane. Anesthesiology 1983;59:459–462.

109. Goudsouzian NG, Young ET, Moss J, et al: Histamine release during the administration of atracurium or vecuronium in children. Br J Anaesth 1986;58:1229–1233.

110. Charlton AJ, Harper NJN, Wilson AC, et al: Atracurium in the neonate: Dose-response with halothane. Paediatr Anaesth 1994;4:17–20.

111. Meretoja OA, Kalli I: Spontaneous recovery of neuromuscular function after atracurium in pediatric patients. Anesth Analg 1986;65:1042–1046.

112. Goudsouzian N, Martyn J, Rudd GD, et al: Continuous infusion of atracurium in children. Anesthesiology 1986;64:171–174.

113. Brandom BW, Cook DR, Woelfel SK, et al: Atracurium infusion requirements in children during halothane, isoflurane, and narcotic anesthesia. Anesth Analg 1985;64:471–476.

114. Brandom BW, Stiller RL, Cook DR, et al: Pharmacokinetics of atracurium in anaesthetized infants and children. Br J Anaesth 1986;58:1210–1213.

115. Fisher DM, Canfell PC, Spellman MJ, et al: Pharmacokinetics and pharmacodynamics of atracurium in infants and children. Anesthesiology 1990;73:33–37.

116. Belmont MR, Lien CA, Quessy S, et al: The clinical neuromuscular pharmacology of 51W89 in patients receiving nitrous oxide/opioid/barbiturate anesthesia. Anesthesiology 1995;82:1139–1145.

117. Meretoja OA, Taivainen T, Wirtavuori K: Pharmacodynamic effects of 51W89, an isomer of atracurium, in children during halothane anaesthesia. Br J Anaesth 1995;74:6–11.

118. Lepage JY, Malinovsky JM, Malinge M, et al: Pharmacodynamic dose-response and safety study of cisatracurium (51W89) in adult surgical patients during N_2O-O_2-opioid anesthesia. Anesth Analg 1996;83:823–829.

119. Lien CA, Belmont MR, Abalos A, et al: The cardiovascular effects and histamine-releasing properties of 51W89 in patients receiving nitrous oxide/opioid/barbiturate anesthesia. Anesthesiology 1995;82:1131–1138.

120. Eastwood NB, Boyd AH, Parker CJ, et al: Pharmacokinetics of 1R-cis 1'R-cis atracurium besylate (51W89) and plasma laudanosine concentrations in health and chronic renal failure. Br J Anaesth 1995;75:431–435.

121. Boyd AH, Eastwood NB, Parker CJ, et al: Pharmacodynamics of the 1R cis-1'R cis isomer of atracurium (51W89) in health and chronic renal failure. Br J Anaesth 1995;74:400–404.

122. Brandom BW, Westman HR: Effects of 0.86 mg/kg cisatracurium in an infant. Anesthesiology 1996;85:688–689.

123. Tullock WC, Diana P, Cook DR, et al: Neuromuscular and cardiovascular effects of high-dose vecuronium. Anesth Analg 1990;70:86–90.

124. Bencini AF, Scaf AH, Sohn YJ, et al: Hepatobiliary disposition of vecuronium bromide in man. Br J Anaesth 1986;58:988–995.

125. Goudsouzian NG, Martyn JJ, Liu LM, et al: Safety and efficacy of vecuronium in adolescents and children. Anesth Analg 1983;62:1083–1088.

126. Fisher DM, Miller RD: Neuromuscular effects of vecuronium (ORG NC45) in infants and children during N_2O halothane anesthesia. Anesthesiology 1983;58:519–523.

127. Motsch J, Hutschenreuter K, Ismaily AJ, et al: Vecuronium in infants and children: clinical and neuromuscular effects. [in German]. Anaesthesist 1985;34:382–387.

128. Meretoja OA, Wirtavuori K, Neuvonen PJ: Age-dependence of the dose-response curve of vecuronium in pediatric patients during balanced anesthesia. Anesth Analg 1988;67:21–26.

129. Meretoja OA: Vecuronium infusion requirements in pediatric patients during fentanyl-N_2O-O_2 anesthesia. Anesth Analg 1989;68:20–24.

130. Meretoja OA: Is vecuronium a long-acting neuromuscular blocking agent in neonates and infants? Br J Anaesth 1989;62:184–187.

131. Fisher DM, Castagnoli K, Miller RD: Vecuronium kinetics and dynamics in anesthetized infants and children. Clin Pharmacol Ther 1985;37:402–406.

132. Kupfer Y, Namba T, Kaldawi E, et al: Prolonged weakness after long-term infusion of vecuronium bromide. Ann Intern Med 1992;117:484–486.

133. Segredo V, Caldwell JE, Matthay MA, et al: Persistent paralysis in critically ill patients after long-term administration of vecuronium. N Engl J Med 1992;327:524–528.

134. Hodges UM: Vecuronium infusion requirements in paediatric patients in intensive care units: The use of acceleromyography. Br J Anaesth 1996;76:23–28.

135. Wierda JM, Hommes FD, Nap HJ, et al: Time course of action and intubating conditions following vecuronium, rocuronium and mivacurium. Anaesthesia 1995;50:393–396.

136. Woelfel SK, Brandom BW, Cook DR, et al: Effects of bolus administration of ORG-9426 in children during nitrous oxide-halothane anesthesia. Anesthesiology 1992;76:939–942.

137. Taivainen T, Meretoja OA, Erkola O, et al: Rocuronium in infants, children and adults during balanced anaesthesia. Pediatr Anaesth 1996;6:271–275.

138. Hopkinson JM, Meakin G, McCluskey A, et al: Dose-response relationship and effective time to satisfactory intubation conditions after rocuronium in children. Anaesthesia 1997;52:428–432.

139. Woolf RL, Crawford MW, Choo SM: Dose-response of rocuronium bromide in children anesthetized with propofol: A comparison with succinylcholine. Anesthesiology 1997;87:1368–1372.

140. Vuksanaj D, Skjonsby B, Dunbar BS: Neuromuscular effects of rocuronium in children during halothane anaesthesia. Pediatr Anaesth 1996;6:277–281.

141. Woelfel SK, Brandom BW, McGowan FX, et al: Neuromuscular effects of 600 μg•kg^{-1} of rocuronium in infants during nitrous oxide-halothane anaesthesia. Paediatr Anaesth 1994;4:173–177.

142. Stoddart PA, Mather SJ: Onset of neuromuscular blockade and intubating conditions one minute after the administration of rocuronium in children. Paediatr Anaesth 1998;8:37–40.

143. Scheiber G, Ribeiro FC, Marichal A, et al: Intubating conditions and onset of action after rocuronium, vecuronium, and atracurium in young children. Anesth Analg 1996;83:320–324.

144. Debaene B, Lieutaud T, Billard V, et al: ORG 9487 neuromuscular block at the adductor pollicis and the laryngeal adductor muscles in humans. Anesthesiology 1997;86:1300–1305.

145. Fuchs-Buder T, Tassonyi E: Intubating conditions and time course of rocuronium-induced neuromuscular block in children. Br J Anaesth 1996;77:335–338.

146. McDonald PF, Sainsbury DA, Laing RJ: Evaluation of the onset time

and intubation conditions of rocuronium bromide in children. Anaesth Intensive Care 1997;25:260–261.

147. Motsch J, Leuwer M, Bottiger BW, et al: Dose-response, time-course of action and recovery of rocuronium bromide in children during halothane anaesthesia. Eur J Anaesthesiol Suppl 1995;11:73–78.

148. Schultz J, Crawford M: Intubating conditions 30 seconds after rocuronium or succinylcholine in children. Anesth Analg 1998; 86:S417.

149. Wierda JM, Meretoja OA, Taivainen T, et al: Pharmacokinetics and pharmacokinetic-dynamic modelling of rocuronium in infants and children. Br J Anaesth 1997;78:690–695.

150. Fisher DM, O'Keefe C, Stanski DR, et al: Pharmacokinetics and pharmacodynamics of d-tubocurarine in infants, children, and adults. Anesthesiology 1982;57:203–208.

151. Vuksanaj D, Fisher DM: Pharmacokinetics of rocuronium in children aged 4–11 years. Anesthesiology 1995;82:1104–1110.

152. Magorian T, Wood P, Caldwell J, et al: The pharmacokinetics and neuromuscular effects of rocuronium bromide in patients with liver disease. Anesth Analg 1995;80:754–759.

153. Szenohradszky J, Fisher DM, Segredo V, et al: Pharmacokinetics of rocuronium bromide (ORG 9426) in patients with normal renal function or patients undergoing cadaver renal transplantation. Anesthesiology 1992;77:899–904.

154. Reynolds LM, Lau M, Brown R, et al: Intramuscular rocuronium in infants and children: Dose-ranging and tracheal intubating conditions. Anesthesiology 1996;85:231–239.

155. Kaplan RF, Uejima T, Lobel G, et al: Intramuscular rocuronium in infants and children: A multicenter study to evaluate tracheal intubating conditions, onset, and duration of action. Anesthesiology 1997;91:633–638.

156. Reynolds LM, Lau M, Brown R, et al: Bioavailability of intramuscular rocuronium in infants and children. Anesthesiology 1997;87:1096–1105.

157. Churchill-Davidson HC, Wise RP: Neuromuscular transmission in the newborn infant. Anesthesiology 1963;24:271–278.

158. Wright PM, Caldwell JE, Miller RD: Onset and duration of rocuronium and succinylcholine at the adductor pollicis and laryngeal adductor muscles in anesthetized humans. Anesthesiology 1994;81:1110–1115.

159. Vinik HR: Intraocular pressure (IOP) changes during rapid sequence induction with succinylcholine or rocuronium. Anesth Analg 1995;80:S530.

160. Bush GH, Stead AL: The use of d-tubocurarine in neonatal anaesthesia. Br J Anaesth 1962;34:721–728.

161. Matteo RS, Lieberman IG, Salanitre E, et al: Distribution, elimination, and action of d-tubocurarine in neonates, infants, children, and adults. Anesth Analg 1984;63:799–804.

162. Goudsouzian NG, Standaert FG: The infant and the myoneural junction. Anesth Analg 1986;65:1208–1217.

163. Nightingale DA, Bush GH: A clinical comparison between tubocurarine and pancuronium in children. Br J Anaesth 1973;45:63–70.

164. Goudsouzian NG, Liu LM, Savarese JJ: Metocurine in infants and children: Neuromuscular and clinical effects. Anesthesiology 1978;49:266–269.

165. Goudsouzian NG, Ryan JF, Savarese JJ: The neuromuscular effects of pancuronium in infants and children. Anesthesiology 1974;41:95–98.

166. Yamamoto T, Baba H, Shiratsuchi T: Clinical experience with pancuronium bromide in infants and children. Anesth Analg 1972;51:919–924.

167. Robinson S, Gregory GA: Fentanyl-air-oxygen anesthesia for ligation of patent ductus arteriosus in preterm infants. Anesth Analg 1981;60:331–334.

168. Palmisano BW, Fisher DM, Willis M, et al: The effect of paralysis on oxygen consumption in normoxic children after cardiac surgery. Anesthesiology 1984;61:518–522.

169. Greenough A, Wood S, Morley CJ, et al: Pancuronium prevents pneumothoraces in ventilated premature babies who actively expire against positive pressure inflation. Lancet 1984;1:1–3.

170. Cabal LA, Siassi B, Artal R, et al: Cardiovascular and catecholamine changes after administration of pancuronium in distressed neonates. Pediatrics 1985;75:284–287.

171. Kelly MA, Finer NN: Nasotracheal intubation in the neonate: Physiologic responses and effects of atropine and pancuronium. J Pediatr 1984;105:303–309.

172. Ment LR: Prevention of neonatal intraventricular hemorrhage. N Engl J Med 1985;312:1385–1387.

173. Perlman JM, Goodman S, Kreusser KL, et al: Reduction in intraventricular hemorrhage by elimination of fluctuating cerebral blood-flow velocity in preterm infants with respiratory distress syndrome. N Engl J Med 1985;312:1353–1357.

174. Kuban KC, Skouteli H, Cherer A, et al: Hemorrhage, phenobarbital, and fluctuating cerebral blood flow velocity in the neonate. Pediatrics 1988;82:548–553.

175. Stow PJ, McLeod ME, Burrows FA, et al: Anterior fontanelle pressure responses to tracheal intubation in the awake and anaesthetized infant. Br J Anaesth 1988;60:167–170.

176. Friesen RH, Honda AT, Thieme RE: Perianesthetic intracranial hemorrhage in preterm neonates. Anesthesiology 1987;67:814–816.

177. Goudsouzian NG, Alifimoff JK, Liu LM, et al: Neuromuscular and cardiovascular effects of doxacurium in children anaesthetized with halothane. Br J Anaesth 1989;62:263–268.

178. Sarner JB, Brandom BW, Cook DR, et al: Clinical pharmacology of doxacurium chloride (BW A938U) in children. Anesth Analg 1988;67:303–306.

179. Kern C, Tassonyi E, Rouge JC, et al: Doxacurium pharmacodynamics in children during volatile and opioid-based anaesthesia. Anaesthesia 1996;51:361–364.

180. Taivainen TR, Meretoja OA: Potency of doxacurium in infants, children, and adolescents during N_2O-O_2-alfentanil anesthesia. J Clin Anesth 1996;8:225–228.

181. Brandom BW, Yellon RF, Lloyd ME, et al: Recovery from doxacurium infusion administered to produce immobility for more than four days in pediatric patients in the intensive care unit. Anesth Analg 1997;84:307–314.

182. Pittet JF, Tassonyi E, Morel DR, et al: Pipecuronium-induced neuromuscular blockade during nitrous oxide, fentanyl, isoflurane, and halothane anesthesia in adults and children. Anesthesiology 1989;71:210–213.

183. Pittet JF, Tassonyi E, Morel DR, et al: Neuromuscular effect of pipecuronium bromide in infants and children during nitrous oxide-alfentanil anesthesia. Anesthesiology 1990;72:432–435.

184. Meretoja OA, Erkola O: Pipecuronium revisited: dose-response and maintenance requirement in infants, children, and adults. J Clin Anesth 1997;9:125–129.

185. Keens TG, Bryan AC, Levison H, et al: Developmental pattern of muscle fiber types in human ventilatory muscles. J Appl Physiol Resp 1978;44:909–913.

186. Mansell A, Bryan C, Levison H: Airway closure in children. J Appl Physiol 1972;33:711–714.

187. Mason LJ, Betts EK: Leg lift and maximum inspiratory force, clinical signs of neuromuscular blockade reversal in neonates and infants. Anesthesiology 1980;52:441–442.

188. Shimada Y, Yoshiya I, Tanaka K, et al: Crying vital capacity and maximal inspiratory pressure as clinical indicators of readiness for weaning of infants less than a year of age. Anesthesiology 1979;51:456–459.

189. Fisher DM, Cronnelly R, Miller RD, et al: The neuromuscular pharmacology of neostigmine in infants and children. Anesthesiology 1983;59:220–225.

190. Fisher DM, Cronnelly R, Sharma M, et al: Clinical pharmacology of edrophonium in infants and children. Anesthesiology 1984;61:428–433.

191. Meakin G, Sweet PT, Bevan JC, et al: Neostigmine and edrophonium as antagonists of pancuronium in infants and children. Anesthesiology 1983;59:316–321.

192. Goldhill DR, Pyne A, Jones CJ: Antagonism of neuromuscular blockade: The cardiovascular effects in children of the combination of edrophonium and glycopyrronium. Anaesthesia 1988;43:930–934.

193. Bevan JC, Tousignant C, Stephenson C, et al: Dose responses for neostigmine and edrophonium as antagonists of mivacurium in adults and children. Anesthesiology 1996;84:354–361.

194. Bevan DR, Kahwaji R, Ansermino JM, et al: Residual block after mivacurium with or without edrophonium reversal in adults and children. Anesthesiology 1996;84:362–367.

195. Bevan JC, Collins L, Fowler C, et al: Early and late reversal of rocuronium and vecuronium with neostigmine in adults and children. Anesth Analg 1999;89:333–339.

196. Bevan DR, Purdy FR, Donati F, Lichtor JL: "Rescue" reversal of ORG 9487 blockade. Anesth Analg 1998;86:S428.

197. Heier T, Caldwell JE, Sessler DI, et al: Mild intraoperative hypothermia increases duration of action and recovery time of vecuronium. Anesth Analg 1999;70:S153.

198. Sokoll MD, Gergis SD: Antibiotics and neuromuscular function. Anesthesiology 1981;55:148–159.
199. Lippmann M, Yang E, Au E, et al: Neuromuscular blocking effects of tobramycin, gentamicin, and cefazolin. Anesth Analg 1982;61:767–770.
200. Mader N, Gilly H, Bittner RE: Dystrophin-deficient mdx muscle is not prone to MH susceptibility: An in vitro study. Br J Anaesth 1997;79:125–127.
201. Wedel DJ: Malignant hyperthermia and neuromuscular disease. Neuromuscul Disord 1992;2:157–164.
202. Michel PA, Fronefield HP: Use of atracurium in a patient susceptible to malignant hyperthermia. Anesthesiology 1985;62:213.
203. Smith CL, Bush GH: Anaesthesia and progressive muscular dystrophy. Br J Anaesth 1985;57:1113–1118.
204. Morris P: Duchenne muscular dystrophy: A challenge for the anaesthetist. Pediatr Anaesth 1997;7:1–4.
205. Hoffman EP, Fischbeck KH, Brown RH, et al: Characterization of dystrophin in muscle-biopsy specimens from patients with Duchenne's or Becker's muscular dystrophy. N Engl J Med 1988;318:1363–1368.
206. Duggan DJ, Gorospe JR, Fanin M, et al: Mutations in the sarcoglycan genes in patients with myopathy. N Engl J Med 1997;336:618–624.
207. Politano L, Nigro V, Nigro G, et al: Development of cardiomyopathy in female carriers of Duchenne and Becker muscular dystrophies. JAMA 1996;275:1335–1338.
208. Brown RH Jr: Prednisone therapy for Duchenne's muscular dystrophy. N Engl J Med 1989;320:1621–1623.
209. Rosenberg H, Heiman-Patterson T: Duchenne's muscular dystrophy and malignant hyperthermia: another warning. Anesthesiology 1983;59:362.
210. Sethna NF, Rockoff MA, Worthen HM, et al: Anesthesia-related complications in children with Duchenne muscular dystrophy. Anesthesiology 1988;68:462–465.
211. Ackerman MJ, Clapham DE: Ion channels: Basic science and clinical disease. N Engl J Med 1997;336:1575–1586.
212. Barohn RJ, Levine EJ, Olson JO, et al: Gastric hypomotility in Duchenne's muscular dystrophy. N Engl J Med 1988;319:15–18.
213. Iaizzo PA, Lehmann-Horn F: Anesthetic complications in muscle disorders. Anesthesiology 1995;82:1093–1096.
214. Buzello W, Huttarsch H: Muscle relaxation in patients with Duchenne's muscular dystrophy: Use of vecuronium in two patients. Br J Anaesth 1988;60:228–231.
215. Tobias JD, Atwood R: Mivacurium in children with Duchenne muscular dystrophy. Paediatr Anaesth 1994;4:57–60.
216. Tokgozoglu LS, Ashizawa T, Pacifico A, et al: Cardiac involvement in a large kindred with myotonic dystrophy: Quantitative assessment and relation to size of CTG repeat expansion. JAMA 1995;274:813–819.
217. Bray RJ, Inkster JS: Anaesthesia in babies with congenital dystrophia myotonica. Anaesthesia 1984;39:1007–1011.
218. Nightingale P, Healy TE, McGuinness K: Dystrophia myotonica and atracurium: A case report. Br J Anaesth 1985;57:1131–1135.
219. Stirt JA, Stone DJ, Weinberg G, et al: Atracurium in a child with myotonic dystrophy. Anesth Analg 1985;64:369–370.
220. Oosterhuis HJ: Myasthenia gravis: A survey. Clin Neurol Neurosurg 1981;83:105–135.
221. Scadding GK, Havard CW: Pathogenesis and treatment of myasthenia gravis. Br Med J (Clin Res Ed) 1981;283:1008–1012.
222. Wise GA, McQuillen MP: Transient neonatal myasthenia: Clinical and electromyographic studies. Arch Neurol 1970;22:556–565.
223. Martyn J, Goldhill DR, Goudsouzian NG: Clinical pharmacology of muscle relaxants in patients with burns. J Clin Pharmacol 1986;26:680–685.
224. Kim C, Fuke N, Martyn JA: Burn injury to rat increases nicotinic acetylcholine receptors in the diaphragm. Anesthesiology 1988;68:401–406.
225. Martyn JA, Goudsouzian NG, Matteo RS, et al: Metocurine requirements and plasma concentrations in burned paediatric patients. Br J Anaesth 1983;55:263–268.
226. Mills AK, Martyn JA: Evaluation of atracurium neuromuscular blockade in paediatric patients with burn injury. Br J Anaesth 1988;60:450–455.

11 Pediatric Fluid Management

Michael L. McManus

Regulatory Mechanisms: Fluid Volume, Osmolality, and Arterial Pressure

Maturation of Fluid Compartments and Homeostatic Mechanisms

    Body Water and Electrolyte Distribution

    Circulating Blood Volume

    Maturation of Homeostatic Mechanisms

Fluid and Electrolyte Requirements

Neonatal Fluid Management

Intraoperative Fluid Management

    Intravenous Access and Fluid Administration Devices

    Choice and Composition of Intravenous Fluids

    Fasting Recommendations and Deficit Replacement

    Assessment of Intravascular Volume

    Ongoing Losses and Third-Spacing

Postoperative Fluid Management

    General Approach

    Postoperative Physiology and Hyponatremia

    Postoperative Pulmonary Edema

Pathophysiologic States and Their Management

    Fluid Overload and Edema

    Dehydration States

    Hypernatremia and Hyponatremia

    Disorders of Potassium Homeostasis

    Syndrome of Inappropriate Antidiuretic Hormone Secretion

    Diabetes Insipidus

Electrolyte disturbances are common in children because of their small size, large surface area to volume ratio, and

The author acknowledges the contribution of Letty M.P. Liu to the previous edition of this chapter.

immature homeostatic mechanisms. As a result, fluid management can be challenging. On the ward, in the operating room, or in the intensive care unit, additional difficulties may result when fluid management is not tailored to the individual or when therapeutic decisions are based on extrapolations from adult data. To better understand the former and to limit the latter, this chapter reviews the basic mechanisms underlying fluid and electrolyte regulation, the developmental anatomy and physiology of fluid compartments, and the management of selected pediatric disease states relevant to anesthesia and critical care.

Regulatory Mechanisms: Fluid Volume, Osmolality, and Arterial Pressure

Water is in thermodynamic equilibrium across cell membranes and moves only in response to the movement of solute (Fig. 11–1). Movement of water is described by the Starling equation:

$$Q_f = K_f ((P_c - P_i) - \sigma (\pi_c - \pi_i))$$

where Q_f is fluid flow, K_f is membrane fluid filtration coefficient, P_i, P_o, π_c, and π_i are hydrostatic and osmotic pressures on either side of the membrane, and σ is the reflection coefficient for the solute and membrane of interest. The reflection coefficient gives a measure of a solute's permeability and, therefore, its contribution to osmotic force after equilibration. Across the blood-brain barrier, for example, σ for sodium approaches 1.0,[1] whereas in muscle and other cell membranes, σ is on the order of 0.15 to 0.3.[2] Thus, when isotonic sodium–containing solutions are given intravenously, usually only 15 to 30% of administered salt and water remains in the intravascular space while the remainder contributes to accumulating interstitial edema.[3, 4] In contrast, hypertonic solutions permit greater expansion of circulating blood volume with lower fluid loads and less edema.[5–7]

Both the amount and concentration of solute are tightly regulated to maintain the volumes of intravascular and intracellular compartments. Since sodium is the primary extracellular solute, this ion is the focus of homeostatic mechanisms concerned with maintenance of intravascular volume. With

$$Q_f = K_f [(P_c - P_i) - \sigma (\pi_c - \pi_i)]$$

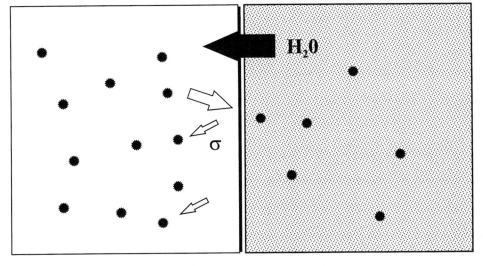

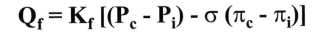

Figure 11–1. Movement of water from the intracellular to extracellular compartments is described by the Starling equation.

osmolality held constant, water movement tends to follow sodium movement. As a result, total body sodium (although not necessarily serum Na$^+$) and total body water generally parallel one another. Since sodium "leak" across membranes limits its contribution to the support of intravascular volume, this compartment is also critically dependent on large, impermeable molecules such as protein. In contrast to sodium, albumin molecules, for example, follow Starling equilibrium with a reflection coefficient above 0.8.[8] Soluble proteins create the so-called colloid oncotic pressure, approximately 80% of which is contributed by albumin.

Although the presence of albumin supports intravascular volume, protein leak into the interstitium may limit its effectiveness. It has been observed, for example, that the reflection coefficient for albumin is decreased by as much as one third following mechanical trauma[9] and that, because of ongoing leakage, slow continuous infusion is superior to bolus administration for raising serum albumin levels in critically ill individuals.[10]

Potassium is the primary intracellular solute, with approximately one third of cellular energy metabolism devoted to Na$^+$/K$^+$ exchange. Sodium continuously leaks into the cell along its concentration gradient yet is rapidly extruded in exchange for potassium. As the cell is exposed to varying osmolarity, water movement occurs, causing cell swelling or shrinkage. Since stable cell volume is critical for survival, complex regulatory mechanisms have evolved to ensure this.[11, 12] The processes by which swollen cells return to normal are collectively termed *regulatory volume decrease*, and those returning a shrunken cell are termed *regulatory volume increase* (Fig. 11–2). With sudden, brief changes in osmolality, regulatory volume increase, or regulatory volume decrease processes are activated after small (1–2%) changes in cell volume, returning cell volume to normal primarily through transport of electrolytes. If anisosmotic conditions persist, chronic compensation occurs through accumulation or loss of small organic molecules termed *osmolytes*, (e.g., polyols, sorbitol, myo-inositol), amino acids and their derivatives (e.g., taurine, alanine, proline), and methylamines (e.g., betaine and glycerylphosphorylcholine).

Like intracellular volume, circulating blood volume is also tightly controlled. Increases in intravascular volume result from increases in sodium and water retention, while decreases in intravascular volume result from increases in excretion of sodium and water. As noted earlier, serum osmolality must be maintained within a very narrow range if serum sodium is to be an effective focus of intravascular volume control. Thus, serum osmolality is generally maintained between 280 to 300 mOsm/L and osmolality changes of as little as 1% begin to elicit regulatory mechanisms.

Serum osmolality is primarily regulated by antidiuretic hormone (ADH), thirst, and renal concentrating ability. Because the indirect aim of osmolar control is actually volume control, these same osmoregulatory mechanisms are also influenced by factors such as blood pressure, cardiac output, and vascular capacitance.[13, 14] In pathologic conditions such as ascites or hemorrhage, intravascular volume preservation takes precedence over osmolality, and osmoregulatory mechanisms operate to restore intravascular volume even at the expense of disrupting physiologic solute balance.

For example, ADH (or *arginine vasopressin*) is released from neurons of the supraoptic and paraventricular nuclei in response to osmolar fluctuations in cell size. Solutes that readily permeate cell membranes, such as urea, raise serum osmolality without eliciting ADH release. Infusion of solutes with high actual or effective σ's at the cell membrane (such as sodium and mannitol) elicits a robust ADH release. ADH release begins when serum osmolality reaches a threshold of approximately 280 mOsm. Rapid increases in osmolality lead to more vigorous release of ADH than do slow increases. Hypovolemia and hypotension diminish the threshold for ADH release and increase the "gain" of the system by exaggerating the rate of rise of serum ADH levels (Fig. 11–3). Thus, in a volume-depleted or hypotensive patient, brisk ADH release may be seen with plasma osmolalities as low as 260 to 270 mOsm. It has been hypothesized that different populations of vasopressin-secreting cells are responsive to osmotic and baroreceptor-mediated information.

Intravascular fluid volume, salt and water intake, electrolyte balance, and cardiovascular status are joined at many

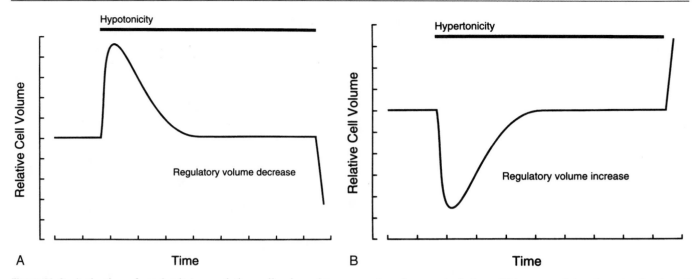

Figure 11–2. Activation of mechanisms regulating cell volume in response to volume perturbations. Volume-regulatory losses and gains of solutes are termed regulatory volume decrease (A) and regulatory volume increase (B), respectively. The course of these decreases and increases varies with the type of cell and experimental conditions. Typically, however, a regulatory volume increase mediated by the uptake of electrolytes and a regulatory volume decrease mediated by the loss of electrolytes and organic osmolytes occur over a period of minutes. When cells that have undergone a regulatory volume decrease (A) or increase (B) are returned to normotonic conditions, they swell above or shrink below their resting volume. This is due to volume-regulatory accumulation or loss of solutes, which effectively makes the cytoplasm hypertonic or hypotonic, respectively, as compared with normotonic extracellular fluid. (From McManus ML, Churchwell KB, Strange K: Regulation of cell volume in health and disease. N Engl J Med 1995;333:1260–1266. © Massachusetts Medical Society.)

levels.[15] For example, as vascular fullness increases and systemic blood pressure rises, ADH release ceases and both *pressure diuresis* and *natriuresis* occur.[16] The resulting relationship of urinary output versus arterial pressure is termed the *renal function curve* and its intersection with salt and water intake determines the *equilibrium point* at which arterial blood pressure ultimately rests (Fig. 11–4). Equilibrium (chronic) blood pressure is only influenced by shifts of the renal function or fluid intake curves. Transient changes in arterial pressure secondary to peripheral resistance changes are always resolved by opposing changes in total body salt and water.

In response to falling arterial pressure, the renin-angiotensin system is mobilized. With decreased renal perfusion, juxtaglomerular cells release renin, which, in turn, converts renin substrate *(angiotensinogen)* to angiotensin I. Angiotensin I is then rapidly converted to angiotensin II by angiotensin-converting enzyme present in lung endothelium. Angiotensin II supports arterial pressure in three ways: (1) direct vasoconstriction, (2) increased salt and water retention (via renal vasoconstriction and decreased glomerular filtration), and (3) stimulation of aldosterone secretion (Fig. 11–5).

Antidiuretic hormone, pressure diuresis, and the renin-angiotensin system permit wide ranges in salt and water intake without large fluctuations in blood pressure or volume status. All serve to support the systemic circulation when threatened and complement the more immediate activity of the sympathetic nervous system. In addition to high pressure sensors, such as aortic baroreceptors, intravascular volume information is provided by low pressure thoracic sensors. For this reason, effective increases or decreases in intrathoracic blood volume may mimic changes in whole-body volume status and produce natriuresis, diuresis, or fluid retention. Intravascular volume may also be sensed as the stretch

of atrial muscle fibers leading to release of atrial natriuretic peptide.[17] Although its complete physiologic role is uncertain, atrial natriuretic peptide may serve to "fine-tune" volume status by causing modest vasodilation, gently increasing glomerular filtration rate (GFR), and decreasing reabsorption of sodium. The combination of complex autoregulatory mechanisms with complementary actions operating on varying time scales, all responding to different, yet interrelated, effector stimuli yields an elegant system by which the mature individual may maintain circulation amidst a variety of challenges. In this context, it is interesting to observe that successful heart transplant recipients, despite general cardiovascular stability, typically manifest fundamental derangements in body fluid homeostasis.[18]

Maturation of Fluid Compartments and Homeostatic Mechanisms

Body Water and Electrolyte Distribution

Much of our understanding of the development of body water compartments is derived from deuterium oxide dilution studies performed in the 1950s.[19] In a series of 21 newborn infants, total body water (TBW) was measured as 78 ± ~5% body weight. Subsequent measurements in fewer subjects showed TBW to decrease to approximately 60% in the second 6 months of life with most of the loss being extracellular. A smaller decrease (to ~57%) is observed late in childhood (Fig. 11–6). When TBW is expressed in terms of surface area rather than weight, it is seen to fall briefly in the first month of life and then to increase steadily to adulthood. This "increase" reflects growth and the steady decrease of surface area to volume ratio. After 3 months of life, extracellular water and plasma volume, expressed as

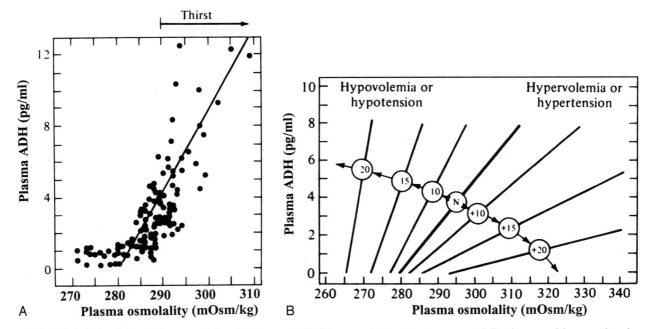

Figure 11–3. (A) Relationship of plasma antidiuretic hormone (ADH) concentration to plasma osmolality in normal humans in whom the plasma osmolality was changed by varying the state of hydration. Notice that the osmotic threshold for thirst is a few mOsm/kg higher than that for ADH. (Adapted from Robertson GL, Aycinena P, Zerbe RL: Neurogenic disorders of osmoregulation. Am J Med 1982;72:339.) (B) The influence of hemodynamic status on the osmoregulation of ADH in otherwise healthy humans. The numbers in the center circles refer to the percentage change in volume or pressure; N refers to the normovolemic normotensive subject. Notice that the hemodynamic status affects both the slope of the relationship between the plasma ADH and osmolality and the osmotic threshold for ADH release. (From Rose DB: Clinical Physiology of Acid-Base and Electrolyte Disorders, 4th ed. New York: McGraw-Hill;1994:159, 163.)

functions of surface area and ideal body weight, remain constant. Using these data, formulas such as TBW = 0.135 × $W^{0.666}$ × $H^{0.535}$ (S.D. = 8.7%) and TBW = 0.843 × $W^{0.891}$ (S.D. = 9.2%) have been generated and nomograms constructed (W = weight, H = height).

The importance of the extracellular compartment, its rela-

tionship to the intracellular space, and much of the chemical anatomy of both was first described by Gamble in educational monographs issued during the first part of the twentieth century (Fig. 11–7).[20, 21] The chemical compositions of mature body fluid compartments are provided in Table 11–1.

Circulating Blood Volume

Circulating blood volume in infants and children has been studied extensively using a variety of methods. Using the 121-iodinated human serum albumin technique, the blood volume of newborns was found to be 82 ± 9 mL/kg, although substantial variability may result from the degree of placental-fetal transfusion.[22] In low birth weight, premature, or critically ill infants, values as high as 100 mL/kg have been measured.[23] Blood volume then rises slightly during the first few months of life, peaking at 2 months of age (~86 mL/kg), returning to near 80 mL/kg in the second year of life, and then stabilizing between 75 and 80 mL/kg until adolescence. In general, the blood volume to weight ratio decreases with growth. The most accurate basis for prediction of blood volume is lean body mass, the consideration of which removes any male to female variation even into adulthood.[24] An estimate of the circulating blood volume is presented in Table 11–2.

Maturation of Homeostatic Mechanisms

Renal development begins at around 5 weeks of gestation and continues in a centrifugal pattern until the full complement of nephrons is in place by around the 38th week. In the outermost regions of the renal cortex, postnatal nephron

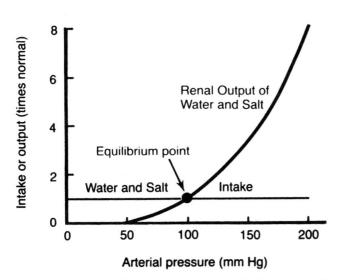

Figure 11–4. Analysis of arterial pressure regulation by equating the renal output curve with the salt and water intake curve. The equilibrium point describes the level to which the arterial pressure will be regulated. (That portion of the salt and water intake that is lost from the body through nonrenal routes is ignored in this figure.) (From Guyton AC, Hall JC, eds: Textbook of Medical Physiology. Philadelphia: WB Saunders;1996:221–237.)

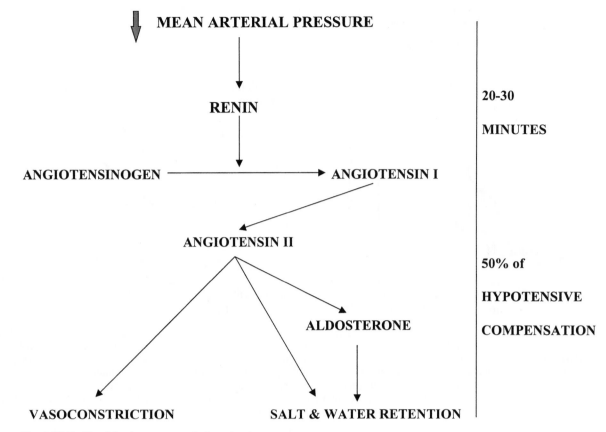

Figure 11–5. Physiologic responses to hypotension.

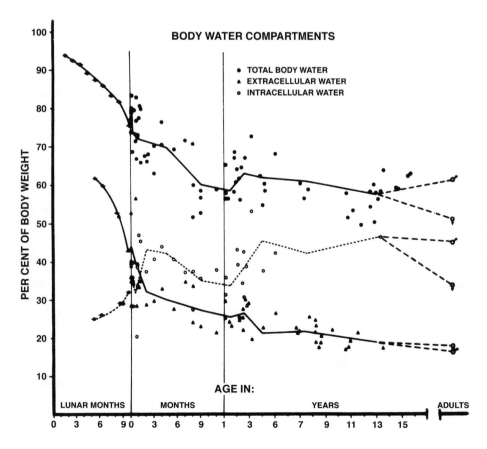

Figure 11–6. Total body water (solid circles), extracellular water (triangles), and intracellular water (open circles) as percentages of body weight in infants and children, compared with corresponding values for the fetus and adults. (From Friis-Hansen B: Body water compartments in children: Changes during growth and related changes in body composition. Pediatrics 1961;28:169–181.)

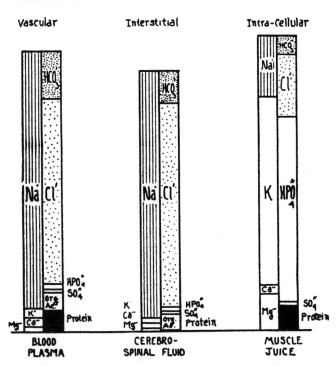

Figure 11–7. Acid-base composition of body fluids. These diagrams are constructed from average values for the individual factors expressed in terms of acid-base equivalence—that is, as cubic centimeters of one-tenth normal solutions per hundred cubic centimeters of fluid. The base factors are superimposed in the left-hand column and the acid factors in the right-hand column of each diagram. They represent, as is actually the case, a structure composed not of salt but of individually sustained concentrations of ions. The exact acid-base equivalence indicated by the equal height of the two columns is obtained by adjustability of the bicarbonate ion concentration (HCO_3^-) to any change elsewhere in the structure. (From McIver MA, Gamble JL: Body fluid changes due to upper intestinal obstruction. JAMA 1928;92:1589–1592. Copyright 1928, American Medical Association.)

Table 11–1. Composition of Body Fluid Compartments

	Extracellular Fluid	Intracellular Fluid
Osmolality (mOsm)	290–310	290–310
Cations (mEq/L)	155	155
Na^+	138–142	10
K^+	4.0–4.5	110
Ca^{++}	4.5–5.0	—
Mg^{++}	3	40
Anions (mEq/L)	155	155
Cl^-	103	—
HCO_3^-	27	—
HPO_4^{--}	—	10
SO_4^{--}	—	110
PO_4^{--}	3	—
Organic acids	6	—
Protein	16	40

half that of the adult (700–800 mEq/L vs. 1300–1400 mEq/L). In part, this also relates to low circulating ADH levels and decreased renal responsiveness to ADH. Although overall ADH production is not impaired, excessive secretion may occur in some disease states. Limited urine concentrating ability necessitates large urine volumes for elimination of large solute loads.

In the first year of life, renal plasma flow and GFR are approximately half the adult values of 350 and 70 mL/min/m², respectively.[25] Consequently, serum creatinine is elevated in term and preterm infants yet normalizes in the second month of life. Fractional excretion of sodium (FE_{Na}) is markedly elevated in prematures, falls somewhat by term, and stabilizes at adult levels by the second month of life. Although the adult kidney may easily achieve Fe_{Na} values as low as 0.5%, the 34-week infant is limited to no less than 2%.

These maturational features make it very difficult for the preterm or young infant to handle fluctuations in fluid and solute loads. Both sodium conservation and regulation of extracellular fluid volume are impaired relative to the older child and adult. Limited GFR makes excretion of a fluid challenge difficult. Excessive urinary sodium loss leads to increased maintenance requirements. Hyponatremia is common. Conversely, diminished concentrating ability increases free water losses during excretion of a solute load while high surface area to volume ratios produce increased evaporative water loss. Consequently, fluid requirements are relatively high and dehydration is common. Errors in medical management are poorly tolerated. Fortunately, the most se-

differentiation may continue for several weeks to months. In the early stages of gestation, renal blood flow is approximately one fifth of normal. Initially this is related to structural immaturity and later it is due to elevated renovascular resistance. By 38 weeks, renal blood flow is approximately one third of normal. High renovascular resistance protects the developing nephron from both pressure and volume overload. Resulting renal contribution to metabolic homeostasis in utero is limited.

As with the pulmonary bed, vascular resistance in the kidney falls after birth, leading to abrupt rises in renal blood flow and GFR. In utero, despite lower GFR, urine output is brisk owing to poor reabsorption of salt and water. Plasma renin activity is high in utero, falls immediately after birth, and then rises again as excess extracellular water is mobilized and excreted. Aldosterone levels are elevated in cord blood and remain so for the first 3 days of life. Elevated aldosterone may be necessary for sodium retention during periods of high anabolism early in life.

Intrarenal gradients of NaCl and urea are less steep in the immature kidney, and full nephron length has yet to be achieved. Consequently, urine concentrating ability is limited in newborns, with maximum urine osmolality being about

Table 11–2. Estimate of Circulating Blood Volume

Age	Estimated Blood Volume (mL/kg)
Preterm infant	100
Full-term newborn	90
Infant	80
School age	75
Adults	70

vere impairment exists in preterm infants and the majority of homeostatic mechanisms are fully developed after the first year of life.

Fluid and Electrolyte Requirements

Holliday has summarized the evolution of contemporary hydration therapy.[20] In 1832, Latta first reported the use of intravenous fluids in the resuscitation of patients dehydrated by cholera.[26] In 1918, growing information on the subject permitted Blackfan and Maxcy to successfully treat nine infants by intraperitoneal injection.[27] In 1923, Gamble detailed the anatomy of fluid and electrolyte compartments, introducing the use of milliequivalents to clinical practice.[21] This paved the way for the development of the "deficit therapy" regimen of Darrow.[28]

In subsequent decades, various recipes for replacement of extracellular and intracellular fluid losses were suggested. For the most part, these failed because of excessive potassium and insufficient sodium content. Hyponatremia was common. When repletion of extracellular losses became the focus, rapid restoration of extracellular fluid using solutions high in sodium became commonplace. This, along with oral rehydration, is the preferred method of treatment today.

The concept of "maintenance fluids" is a complex one. While water and salt are required to sustain life, it is fair to say that for an individual patient at any particular time the precise amounts necessary are unknown (and perhaps unknowable). In the context of individual variability, complex homeostatic mechanisms, and changing requirements, the "dose" of salt and water required for "maintenance" cannot be calculated precisely. Instead, fluids and electrolytes, like anesthetics, are titrated to effect with general guideposts provided by clinical assessment, basic physio-

logic principles, and limited published data. The term "maintenance fluids" is often more limiting than helpful and in all cases is less precise than other terms familiar to anesthesiologists such as minimum alveolar concentration (MAC) or effective dose 50% (ED_{50}).

Calculations for a first approximation of "the maintenance need for water in parenteral fluid therapy" were provided by Holliday and Seger in 1957.[29] Integrating the relevant known physiology to date, these authors observed that, "insensible loss of water and urinary water loss roughly parallel energy metabolism and do not parallel weight." However, since water utilization parallels energy metabolism, energy metabolism follows surface area, and surface area follows weight, it should be possible to "estimate" water requirement (in a nonlinear fashion) from weight alone. The authors then proceeded under a series of assumptions to extrapolate from limited data to a "relationship between weight and energy expenditure that might easily be remembered."

Assuming energy requirements of "hospitalized patients" to be "roughly midway between basal and normal levels," a curve of caloric requirement versus weight was constructed. Such a curve could be seen as composed of three linear sections: 0–10 kg, 10–20 kg, and 20–70 kg (Fig. 11–8). Viewed in this manner, the authors reasoned that "fortuitously, the average needs for water, expressed in milliliters, equals energy expenditure in calories": 100 mL/kg/d for weights to 10 kg, an additional 50 mL/kg/d each kilogram from 11 to 20 kg, and 20 mL/kg/d more for each kilogram beyond 20 kg. In anesthetic practice, this has been further simplified to yield the following estimated hourly fluid requirements: 4 mL/kg for first 10 kg of weight plus 2 mL/kg for the next 10 kg plus 1 mL/kg for each kilogram thereafter (Table 11–3).

Estimation of pediatric electrolyte needs was difficult and

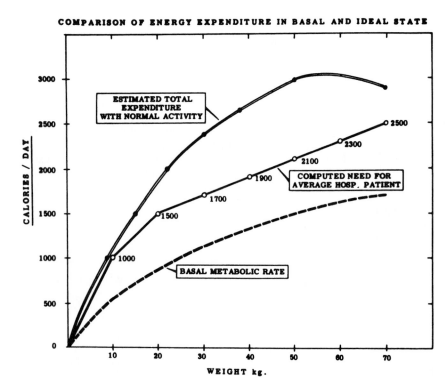

COMPARISON OF ENERGY EXPENDITURE IN BASAL AND IDEAL STATE

Figure 11–8. The upper and lower lines were plotted from data from the study by Talbot.[107] Weights at the 50th percentile level were selected for converting calories at various ages to calories related to weight. The computed line was derived from the following equations:

1. 0–10 kg: 100 kcal/kg.
2. 10–20 kg: 1000 kcal + 50 kcal/kg for each kg over 10 kg.
3. 20 kg and up: 1500 kcal + 20 kcal/kg for each kg over 20 kg.

(From Holliday MA, Segar WE: The maintenance need for water in parenteral fluid therapy. Pediatrics 1957;19:823–832.)

Table 11-3. Relationship Between Weight and Hourly or Daily Maintenance Fluid Requirements of Patients

	Maintenance Fluid Requirements	
Weight (kg)	*Hour*	*Day*
<10	4 mL/kg	100 mL/kg
10–20	40 mL + 2 mL/kg for every kg >10 kg	1000 mL + 50 mL/kg for every kg >10
>20	60 mL + 1 mL/kg for every kg >20 kg	1500 mL + 20 mL/kg for every kg >20

required use of less precise data. Assuming that human milk contained the minimal electrolyte requirement for infants and coupling this observation with Darrow's work,[30] Holliday and Seger concluded that "maintenance requirements for sodium, chloride, and potassium were 3.0, 2.0, and 2.0 mEq/100 cal/d, respectively."

The simplicity and elegance of the Holliday and Seger formula have made it a great service to all physicians as the starting point for fluid management in healthy children. In the operating room, the formula is particularly useful in estimating deficits after a period of NPO status. Clearly, however, its blind application to all situations is unwarranted and its uncritical use was unintended. As the authors cautioned, "understanding of the limitations and of exceptions to the system are required. Even more essential is the clinical judgment to modify the system as circumstances dictate."

General water losses for infants and children are summarized in Table 11–4.

Neonatal Fluid Management

In the first few days of life, isotonic losses of salt and water cause the normal newborn to lose 5 to 15% of its body weight. Although GFR rises rapidly, urine output is initially low and renal losses are modest. Day 1 fluid requirements of the wrapped newborn, therefore, are relatively low. Over the first few days of life, losses and requirements increase. In the poorly feeding infant, progression to hypernatremia and dehydration are common. When intake is appropriate, the term infant will regain body weight in the first week of life.

Three distinct phases of fluid and electrolyte homeostasis

Table 11-4. Normal Water Losses for Infants and Children

Cause of Loss	Volume of Loss (mL/100 kcal)
Output	
Urine	70
Insensible loss	
Skin	30
Respiratory tract	15
"Hidden intake" (from burning 100 calories)	15
Total	100

have been described in low[31] and very low birth weight[32] infants. In the first day of life, there is minimal urine output and body weight is stable despite low fluid intake. In the second phase, days 2 and 3 of life, diuresis occurs irrespective of the amount of fluid administered. By the fourth and fifth days of life, urine output begins to vary with changes in fluid intake and state of health.

Prematurity increases neonatal fluid requirements significantly. Fluid requirements are therefore estimated and then titrated to the infant's changing weight, urine output, and serum sodium. Sodium levels are routinely measured every 6 to 8 hours until equilibrium is established around 150 mEq/L.

No less important is glucose homeostasis. In the ninth month of gestation, the fetus begins to form glycogen stores at a rate of over 100 kcal/d. Thus, in the unstressed, term infant, hepatic glycogen stores are 5% by weight. Immediately after birth, glycogenolysis depletes most of these stores within the first 24 to 48 hours. Gluconeogenesis must then proceed to yield glucose at a rate of around 4 mg/kg/min.

At birth, fetal serum glucose is 60 to 70% of maternal levels. Levels may fall in the first hours of life before recovering, but should be kept above 45 mg/100 mL to avoid neurologic injury. Symptoms of hypoglycemia may include jitteriness, lethargy, temperature instability, and convulsions. Ten percent dextrose in water ($D_{10}W$) may be given as a bolus of 2 to 4 mL/kg followed by a continuous infusion providing 4 to 6 mg/kg/min. The serum glucose level is then followed every 30 minutes and the infusion titrated upward as necessary. It is important that the amount of glucose being provided is calculated in mg/kg/min to avoid errors during fluid changes and to facilitate the diagnosis of persistent hypoglycemia.

Typical *Day 1* infant fluid orders call for 70 to 80 mL/kg of $D_{10}W$. Since $D_{10}W$ contains 10 g glucose/100 mL, this provides

$$10 \text{ g}/100 \text{ mL} \times 70\text{–}80 \text{ mL/kg/d}$$
$$= 7\text{–}8 \text{ g/kg/d}$$
$$= 0.333 \text{ g/kg/h}$$
$$= \text{approximately } 5 \text{ mg/kg/min.}$$

On *Day 2*, fluids are routinely increased to at least 100 mL/kg/d and sodium added at 2 to 3 mEq/100 mL. When urine output is established, potassium is added at 1 to 2 mEq/100 mL. The final solution, containing 30 mEq Na^+ and 10 to 20 mEq K^+/L, approximates the 0.2 normal saline (NS) "maintenance" solution commonly used in older children.

In the neonatal intensive care unit, fluid management focuses on provision of adequate nutrition, maintenance of electrolyte balance, and limitation of fluid overload. The last factor is of particular concern because plasma oncotic pressure is lowered in premature infants and the whole-body protein reflection coefficient is below adult values.[33] Very low birth weight infants are at particular risk for fluid and electrolyte imbalances.[34] Even modest fluid overload, therefore, may exacerbate pulmonary edema, prolong ductal patency, and more readily produce congestive heart failure. This perspective typically accompanies the infant to the operating room, where the primary considerations are routinely quite the opposite: restoration of circulating blood volume after third-space accumulation, maintenance of intra-vascular volume amidst ongoing blood loss, replacement of potentially massive evaporative losses, and maintenance of blood pressure despite anesthetic-induced vasodilatation and increased venous capacitance. During surgery, these concerns must take precedence, yet unnecessary administration of fluid is best avoided.

Intraoperative Fluid Management

Intravenous Access and Fluid Administration Devices

In pediatrics, the first step toward intraoperative fluid management is often the most challenging—that is, gaining intravenous access. In general, simple procedures in healthy patients are successfully approached using a single peripheral intravenous line. Although preferences vary among anesthesiologists, line placement is most easily accomplished after induction of anesthesia. Routinely in very young children, anesthesia is induced by inhalation and a catheter is inserted by an assistant into any available hand or foot vein. In older children, or when intravenous access is desirable prior to induction, catheter placement may be facilitated by the use of topical anesthesia (e.g., EMLA cream, amethocaine, lidocaine infiltration) or sedation or both.

Larger procedures in sicker patients usually require placement of at least two wide-bore catheters. In pediatrics, however, "wide-bore" is a relative term, with 22-gauge catheters typically providing sufficient access in infants. Preferred sites for larger catheters include antecubital and saphenous veins. In cases in which access to the central circulation is required (as for pressure monitoring, infusion of vasoactive medications, or prolonged access), longer catheters may be placed via the femoral, subclavian, or internal jugular veins (the latter usually via a high, anterior approach).[35] Although secure access may also be obtained via the external jugular vein, it is often difficult to negotiate the J-wire or catheter tip into the central circulation.[36]

In selecting the appropriate intravenous catheter, it is useful to consider the relative effects of catheter length and diameter on solution flow rates. Longer catheters produce increased flow resistance and are therefore inferior to shorter catheters when rapid infusion is required. In vitro, catheters designed for peripheral venous insertion showed an 18 to 164% greater flow rate when compared with the same-gauge catheters designed for central venous use. Under pressure, as might be employed during emergent volume resuscitation, rates differed up to 17-fold.[37] While this seems to suggest that short peripheral catheters should be preferred, in vivo data are more complex. In animal models, it seems that overall catheter flow rates are below in vitro rates, and that central access presents somewhat less resistance to flow than peripheral access.[38] Finally, when weighing the risks and benefits of central versus peripheral access, it is also interesting to consider that central administration of resuscitation medications may provide little practical advantage over peripheral administration.[39]

Intraosseous catheters are now commonly used in the initial resuscitation of critically ill or injured children.[40, 41] Flow rates via these lines seem to be less dependent on catheter diameter than on resistance in the marrow compartment.[42] In the operating room, the intraosseous route has been used for both induction and maintenance of anesthesia.[43–45] However, onset of drug effect is less predictable than with the intravenous route and intraosseous lines are easily dislodged. Potential complications include compartment syndrome[46–48] and, very rarely, damage to the growth plate.[41, 49] Thus, such lines are probably best considered an emergency or last-resort option (see Figs. 32–4 and 16–3).[44]

To prevent accidental volume overload, the amount of intravenous fluid available to a child at any one time should not exceed the child's calculated hourly requirement. Particularly in infants, a volumetric chamber should be used to limit the amount of fluid available for infusion. Similarly, a micro-drip infusion set limits the rate of fluid administration and permits much greater control. Although a fluid infusion pump provides the most precise mode of regulating the rate of fluid administration (and is therefore very useful in providing supplemental fluids or medications), such devices are impractical on primary access lines, since they hinder the ability to administer drugs or fluids rapidly.

In babies, when rapid infusion of resuscitation solutions or blood products is anticipated, many practitioners find it helpful to include a stopcock manifold in-line. Additional fluids may then be drawn up into 60 mL syringes and warmed separately. During periods of sudden blood loss, stored syringes may then be inserted into the manifold and a known volume rapidly infused.

Finally, in prolonged surgeries, or when volume replacement is great, it is imperative that all intravenous infusions be adequately warmed. Also, in younger patients in whom patency of the foramen ovale is a concern, an in-line "bubble" filter is desirable.

Choice and Composition of Intravenous Fluids

In the early 1960s,[50] simultaneous measurements of plasma and extracellular fluid volumes demonstrated that, during surgery, plasma volume is supported at the expense of the extravascular space. At the same time, isotonic fluid is, to varying extents, redistributed from the extracellular and intravascular spaces to a third, nonfunctional space. Because of their differing fluid composition and renal function, it was at first unclear that these findings could be extended to infancy. Thus, fluid restriction remained the standard of care until careful studies specifically demonstrated that fluid and electrolyte requirements are often extremely large in neonates undergoing major surgical procedures.[51–53]

Although hypotonic fluids are selected for maintenance hydration throughout the hospital (according to the reasoning outlined previously), isotonic solutions are preferred intraoperatively for several reasons. First, most ongoing volume losses are isotonic, consisting of shed blood and interstitial fluids. Second, large volumes of hypotonic solutions may rapidly diminish serum osmolality, producing electrolyte instability and undesirable fluid shifts. Indeed, even large volumes of "isotonic" fluids have been shown to significantly decrease serum osmolality in adult volunteers.[54] Third, as discussed earlier, the plasma volume expansion necessary in response to diminished vascular tone under anesthesia is difficult to achieve even with isotonic fluids. Finally, increases in ADH and other elements of intraoperative physiol-

Table 11-5. Composition of Extracellular Fluid and Common Intravenous Solutions

	Cations (mEq/L)					Anions (mEq/L)		
	Na^+	K^+	Ca^{++}	Mg^{++}	NH_4^+	Cl^-	HCO_3^-	HPO_4^-
Extracellular fluid	142	4	5	3	0.3	103	27	3
Lactated Ringer solution	130	4	3			109	28	
0.45 NaCl	77					77		
0.9% NaCl (normal saline)	154					154		
3% NaCl	590					590		

ogy result in free water retention in excess of sodium if inadequate amounts of the latter are provided.

The compositions of commonly used intravenous solutions are presented in Table 11–5. Assuming normal plasma osmolality of 275 to 290 mOsm/L, it is noteworthy that 0.9 NS is slightly hypertonic to plasma and that lactated Ringer solution is isotonic, though perhaps slightly hyponatremic. For dextrose-containing solutions, added osmolality is rapidly dissipated as sugar is metabolized. Thus, administration of 5% dextrose in water is ultimately equivalent to administration of free water.

The routine intraoperative use of glucose-containing solutions has been a subject of debate. As a rule, operative stress evokes physiologic responses that increase serum glucose. In practice, therefore, hypoglycemia is seldom a problem in healthy children when glucose is omitted from operative fluids.[55, 56] Indeed, the risk should be particularly small if the period of fasting is limited to less than 10 hours.[56] At the same time, rapid administration of dextrose solutions may certainly produce acute hyperglycemia and hyperosmolality.[55, 56] Thus glucose-containing solutions should not be used to replace fluid deficits, third-space losses, or blood losses. Some populations, such as debilitated infants[57] or those undergoing cardiac surgery, have been shown, however, to be at risk for intraoperative hypoglycemia.[58, 59] Thus, intraoperative glucose monitoring may be useful in small or debilitated patients.

When necessary, glucose-containing solutions are best administered as a separate "piggyback" infusion using an infusion pump or other rate- or volume-limiting device so as to avoid accidental bolus administration. Patients receiving parenteral nutrition preoperatively should continue receiving those infusions separately, and a corresponding volume should be deducted from isotonic operative fluids. Because of hyperglycemic responses to the stress of surgery, some practitioners routinely decrease hyperalimentation infusion rates by one third to one half.

Fasting Recommendations and Deficit Replacement

Fasting recommendations have evolved significantly over the past decade. The goal of fasting is to minimize the volume of gastric contents and thereby lessen the risk of vomiting and aspiration during induction of anesthesia. In pediatric as compared with adult anesthesia, this is of particular concern since induction is more often accomplished via inhalation and the period of vulnerability to aspiration is longer than with an intravenous induction of anesthesia.

At issue are (1) the effectiveness of fasting in lowering a child's gastric volume and (2) the benefits of this when weighed against the added discomfort and risk of dehydration. It seems unlikely, for example, that a hungry, thirsty, and agitated child who has been NPO since bedtime the prior evening is at an overall decreased anesthetic risk when compared with the child who has been permitted clear liquids 2 to 3 hours before surgery. Nonetheless, until recently, long periods of NPO status were the preoperative rule. Fortunately, numerous studies of gastric volume and pH have convincingly demonstrated that clear liquids are rapidly emptied from the stomach and the stimulated peristalsis actually serves to decrease gastric volume and acidity. Taking this together with the benefits of improved hydration and mental status, it is clear that prolonged NPO status is unwarranted. The specific NPO guidelines currently in use in many institutions are included in Table 11–6.

With shorter NPO periods, replacement of the fasting deficit becomes less critical. Typically, in calculating maintenance requirements and deficits, anesthesiologists have reduced the work of Holliday and Seger to the following shorthand:

Hourly maintenance fluid rate =
  4 mL/kg/h for the first 10 kg = 40 mL/h
  +2 mL/kg/h for the second 10 kg (11–20 kg) = 20 mL/h
  +1 mL/kg/h for each kilogram > 20 kg thereafter

Thus, fluid requirements for a 30 kg child would be 40 + 20 + 10 = 70 mL/kg/h. The estimated deficit is calculated as the above hourly requirement multiplied by the number of NPO hours. Such calculations provide a margin for error, as they tend to overestimate true requirements. Physiologic conservation of water with increasing dehydration is neglected. Thus, complete replacement of the calculated deficit is frequently unnecessary. Conversely, as discussed earlier, factors such as fever, prematurity, and renal concentrating ability may significantly increase real fluid requirements above these estimates.

Table 11-6. Fasting (NPO) Guidelines for Children and Adults

	Fasting Time (Hours)	
Age	*Solids*	*Clear Liquids*
<6 months	4	2
6–36 months	6	3
>36 months	8	3

In practice, there is considerable variability in the speed and extent to which estimated deficits are replaced. As a general principle, however, deficits are usually replaced by 50% in the first hour and the remainder over the subsequent 2 hours.

Assessment of Intravascular Volume

In the operating room while the patient is under anesthesia, many clinical clues to volume status are lost or confounded by operative events. For example, though a fairly reliable indicator of volume status in the quietly resting preoperative child, tachycardia may result from any number of factors beyond volume status during surgery. It is the challenge of the anesthesiologist to view the entire clinical picture, consider the possibilities, integrate them into a hypothesis and then test the hypothesis.

Assessment of intravascular volume begins with knowledge of age-related norms for heart rate and blood pressure (see Tables 2–9 and 2–10). Is the heart rate persistently high or does it vary with surgical stimulation? Is the pulse pressure narrow or, more ominously, is the blood pressure low for age? Does it vary with positive pressure breaths? Are the extremities warm? Is capillary refill brisk? What is the urine output? Are these variables changing? What is the rate of the change? When hypovolemia is suspected, observing the response to a 10 to 20 mL/kg bolus of isotonic crystalloid or colloid may test the hypothesis.

Measurement and continuous monitoring of central venous pressure are often helpful in assessing the status of circulating volume (see Figs. 32–1, 32–2, and 32–3). In addition to traditional central lines introduced from above into the superior vena cava or left atrium, there are animal[60] and limited clinical[61] data suggesting that femoral lines terminating in the abdominal vena cava may also be useful. In one study of 20 infants and children, comparison of right atrial and inferior vena caval pressures found close agreement with average end-expiratory pressure differences of less than 1 mm Hg.[61] Assessment of changes in the contour of the arterial waveform may also be helpful in assessing volume status and the response to volume administration (see Fig. 12–7).

Ongoing Losses and Third-Spacing

During all surgical procedures, fluid loss from the vascular space is primarily the result of three simultaneous physiologic processes. First, whole blood is shed at various rates and must be replaced. Second, capillary leak and surgical trauma result in extravasation of isotonic, protein-containing fluid into nonfunctional compartments (the so-called "third space"). Third, anesthetic-induced relaxation of sympathetic tone produces vasodilatation and relative hypovolemia (a "virtual" loss). In very small patients, a fourth source of losses must also be carefully considered: direct evaporation. These ongoing losses are often difficult to quantitate (or even estimate). Nonetheless, the small circulating blood volume of an infant (e.g., for a 5 kg infant = 80 mL/kg × 5 kg = 400 mL) leaves little room for error. Faced with uncertainty, the prudent response is constant vigilance and reliance on general principles.

As a rule, just as in adults, shed blood is replaced 1 mL for 1 mL of blood loss with colloid (5% albumin or blood) or 3 mL for 1 mL of blood loss with isotonic crystalloid, such as lactated Ringer solution. Isotonic crystalloid is also used to replenish third-space losses. Surgical procedures involving only mild tissue trauma may entail third space losses of 3 to 4 mL/kg/h. More extensive surgical procedures involving moderate trauma may require replacement equivalent to 5 to 7 mL/kg/h to adequately support intravascular volume. In small infants undergoing very large abdominal procedures, the losses may approach 10 mL/kg/h or more.[51, 53] These "losses" are to the vascular compartment and include both evaporation and redistribution of fluid. The latter must be most carefully considered, since, for reasons outlined previously, such redistribution is exacerbated by continued fluid administration.

Although necessary intraoperatively, third-space accumulation represents whole body salt and water overload that will need to be mobilized postoperatively. The price of unchecked fluid administration is generalized anasarca, pulmonary edema, bowel swelling, and laryngotracheal edema. In the relatively healthy child, this relative fluid overload is well tolerated, with most excess fluid excreted over the first 2 postoperative days. In children with impaired pulmonary, cardiac, or renal function, however, such fluid excess may result in clinically important postoperative morbidity.

Postoperative Fluid Management

General Approach

Well-planned postoperative fluid management complements the intraoperative plan and accounts for evolving physiology as the child recovers. Replacement of fluid deficits is completed. Ongoing losses are replaced. The patient is repeatedly reassessed and intake adjusted until normal fluid and electrolyte homeostasis has returned. To aid in decision-making, trends in vital signs are identified, all sources of fluid intake and output are quantitated, urine specific gravity is followed, daily weights are obtained, and serum electrolytes are measured.

In simple outpatient surgeries, discharge is possible when fluid deficits are replaced. In complex patients, replacement fluids may require hourly readjustment that is based on the prior hour's intake and output. Rather than reacting to single pieces of data, such as low urine output, overall patterns must be discerned. High urine output and low urine specific gravity may indicate overhydration or diabetes insipidus. Oliguria may suggest hypovolemia when accompanied by high urine specific gravity and clinical signs of dehydration or low cardiac output when accompanied by signs of poor perfusion. In the well-hydrated patient, oliguria may represent renal failure if the urine specific gravity is normal (or dilute) but syndrome of inappropriate antidiuretic hormone secretion (SIADH) if the urine is concentrated. A careful physical examination is necessary; in many cases, certainty in diagnosis requires simultaneous measurement of serum and urine electrolytes.

Frequently, losses via surgical or gastric drains may be large in both real and relative terms. For example, a neonate with a nasogastric tube may lose more than 100 mL/kg/d (normally 20–40 mL/kg/d) in gastric fluid. Therefore, in determining the volume and composition of replacement fluids, it is sometimes helpful to consider the electrolyte content of various losses (Table 11–7).

Postoperative Physiology and Hyponatremia

For a variety of reasons, postoperative patients retain salt and water. Contributing factors include neuroendocrine activation by stress, continued capillary leak with third-space accumulation, and hypovolemic stimulation of ADH or renin secretion. As outlined earlier, intravascular volume depletion is a potent nonosmotic signal for fluid retention and may override osmotic signals under a variety of clinical circumstances.

At the same time, ongoing fluid and electrolyte losses following surgery may be large. Chest tubes, nasogastric suction, weeping incisions, and even continued slow bleeding can account for significant losses in adults and even greater losses, proportionately, in children. Postoperative patients are often entirely dependent on intravenous fluids for replacement of these and other losses.

Thus, unless isotonic, sodium-containing fluids are provided, postoperative patients are universally at risk for developing hyponatremia. In a retrospective review of 24,412 surgical admissions to a large children's hospital, the incidence of significant postoperative hyponatremia was found to be 0.34% and mortality in these previously healthy patients was high (8.4%).[62] This measured incidence, 340 cases and 29 deaths per 100,000, would suggest 7448 cases of postoperative hyponatremia and 626 associated deaths per year in the United States alone.

In reviewing the etiology of hyponatremia, two factors stand out: extensive extrarenal loss of electrolyte-containing fluid and intravenous replacement with hypotonic fluids.[62] In addition, delay in recognition often plays a major role in associated morbidity. The solution seems a simple one: (1) administration of hypotonic fluids without a specific indication should be minimized postoperatively, (2) ongoing losses should be replaced in a timely fashion, and (3) serum electrolytes should be measured in patients exhibiting potential symptoms of hyponatremia (see subsequent discussion).

Postoperative Pulmonary Edema

Patients receiving large volumes of fluid intraoperatively are at risk for developing pulmonary edema as third-space fluids are mobilized. Usually, fluid mobilization begins to occur on the second postoperative day and continues through day 3 or 4. Although this is less common in children than in the elderly, it occurs occasionally in children with burn injuries[63] or pediatric patients receiving large amounts of fluid during resuscitation from trauma or sepsis. In one review,[64] 13 patients (11 adults and 2 children) were identified who developed postoperative pulmonary edema. All began to exhibit symptoms within 36 hours following surgery and all received perioperative fluids in excess of 67 mL/kg.

Pathophysiologic States and Their Management

Fluid Overload and Edema

Edema is essentially a "sodium disease" representing sodium and water overload, with excessive fluid residing in the extracellular space. Although intracellular volume changes can sometimes be substantial, prolonged cell swelling represents failure of essential volume regulatory functions and is likely a preterminal event. In fluid overload states, plasma volume is generally elevated unless the balance of Starling forces is disturbed, as in nephrotic syndrome or lymphatic obstruction. Edema formation is opposed by (1) low compliance of the interstitial compartment, (2) increased lymphatic flow, (3) osmotic washout of interstitial proteins, and (4) impedance and elasticity of the proteoglycan gel. The differential diagnosis of fluid overload and edema formation is presented in Table 11–8. Principles of therapy for fluid overload states include the following:

- Fluid restriction
- Salt restriction
- Diuresis, dialysis
- Salt-poor albumin for diminished plasma volume

Dehydration States

For reasons outlined earlier, dehydration states are common in children. The extent of dehydration is best assessed by weight, as clinical signs such as tachycardia, capillary refill, and skin elasticity,[65] although often reliable, may be influenced by factors other than hydration status. Capillary refill time of 1.5 to 3.0 seconds, for example, suggests a fluid

Table 11–7. Composition of Body Fluids

Source	Na+ (mEq/L)	K+ (mEq/L)	Cl− (mEq/L)	HCO₃− (mEq/L)	pH	Osmolality (mOsm/L)
Gastric	50	10–15	150	0	1	300
Pancreas	140	5	50–100	100	9	300
Bile	130	5	100	40	8	300
Ileostomy	130	15–20	120	25–30	8	300
Diarrhea	50	35	40	50	Alkaline	
Sweat	50	5	55	0		
Blood	140	4–5	100	25	7.4	285–295
Urine	0–100*	20–100*	70–100*	0	4.5–8.5*	50–1400*

*Varies considerably with fluid intake.
From Herrin J: Fluid and electrolytes. In: Graef JW, ed: Manual of Pediatric Therapeutics, 6th ed. Philadelphia: Lippincott-Raven; 1997:63–75.

Table 11–8. Differential Diagnosis of Fluid Overload and Edema Formation

Condition	Differential
Imbalance of intake and output	Salt poisoning
	Formula dilution errors
	Intravenous infusion errors
	Drugs given as sodium salts
Steroid excess with normal sodium intake	Congenital adrenal hyperplasia
	Exogenous steroids
Perceived decreases in effective plasma volume	$\downarrow$ MAP $\rightarrow$ baroreceptors $\rightarrow$ $\uparrow$ sympathetic tone, ADH, renin, aldosterone
	Vasodilators
	Congestive heart failure
	Cirrhosis
	Nephrotic syndrome
Impaired sodium excretion	Chronic renal failure
	Acute glomerular disease ($\downarrow$ GFR with normal tubular function)
	Nonsteroidal anti-inflammatory drugs ($\downarrow$ PGE_2 and RBF)
Water excess	SIADH
	Hypotonic infusion
	Stress ($\uparrow$ ADH)

ADH, antidiuretic hormone; GFR, glomerular filtration rate; PGE_2, prostaglandin E_2; RBF, renal blood flow; SIADH, syndrome of inappropriate antidiuretic hormone secretion.

deficit of between 50 and 100 mL/kg, yet this sign is extremely dependent on ambient temperature.[66] Similarly, poor skin elasticity reflects significant volume loss, yet elasticity may be well preserved in patients with hypernatremic dehydration.[65] Clinical signs associated with varying levels of dehydration are presented in Table 11–9.

As a first approximation, correction of most dehydration states in older children is most readily achieved with administration of a simple bolus of 0.9 or 0.45 NS. In mild-to-moderate acute dehydration states, 0.33 NS in 20 mL/kg boluses has also been applied with good results.[67] When caring for infants or children with unusual, prolonged, or severe dehydration, however, management must be more precise. Kallen has proposed a framework for approaching the dehydrated child which, though intended for the pediatrician, may also be used by the anesthesiologist when facing a complex condition.[68] This approach uses a five-point assessment that calls attention to the following questions:

1. Does a volume deficit exist and, if so, how great is it?
As noted previously, assessment of this is best made by weight, yet ballpark estimates of 3% (mild), 6% (moderate), and 9% (severe) may be made in older children based on

clinical signs (see Table 11–9). Infants must be managed by weight only.

2. Does an osmolar disturbance exist? Is it acute or chronic?
Identification of osmolar imbalance is made through measurement of serum sodium. The majority of clinically encountered dehydration states ($\sim$80%) are isotonic (Na^+ = 130–150 mEq/L). These patients have experienced isotonic losses and are easily managed by almost any strategy.

Approximately 15% of dehydrated patients present with hypertonic dehydration (Na^+ > 150 mEq/L). These patients are at greatest risk and have usually experienced the greatest fluid losses for a given set of clinical signs.[69] If the condition is chronic, they may require extensive, slow rehydration over much longer periods.[70]

Five percent of patients may present with hypotonic dehydration and serum sodium levels below 130 mEq/L. For a given fluid deficit, these individuals are often more symptomatic than others and their requirement for sodium replacement is greatest. Surprisingly, rapid improvement in clinical condition often results from the first fluid bolus.

In general, chronic dehydration states must be repaired slowly and acute dehydration states (< 24 hours) may be

Table 11–9. Clinical Signs and Symptoms for Estimation of Severity of Dehydration

Clinical Signs	Degree of Dehydration		
	Mild	*Moderate*	*Severe*
Weight loss (%)	5	10	15
Behavior	Normal	Irritable	Hyperirritable to lethargic
Thirst	Slight	Moderate	Intense
Mucous membranes	May be normal	Dry	Parched
Tears	Present	$\pm$	Absent
Anterior fontanelle	Flat	$\pm$	Sunken
Skin turgor	Normal	$\pm$	Increased

Modified from Herrin J: Fluid and electrolytes. In: Graef J, ed: Manual of Pediatric Therapeutics, 6th ed. Philadelphia: Lippincott-Raven; 1997:63–75.

corrected more rapidly. This is because cell volume equilibration occurs acutely through gain or loss of electrolytes (which may be moved rapidly) and chronically through gain or loss of osmolytes (which are moved more slowly).[11] Re-equilibration of brain cell volume during correction of hypertonicity is often very slow, mandating patience in repair of chronic fluid deficits. Similarly, rapid repair of hyponatremic disturbances can be hazardous,[62] even when seemingly "safe" isotonic solutions are employed.[71]

3. Does an acid-base abnormality exist?

Quantitation of the patient's acid-base status gives useful, though limited, information as to the severity of dehydration. When evaluating acid-base status, it is important to recall that bicarbonate reabsorption and urine acidification are limited in premature and young infants, leaving even the normal infant in a state of mild metabolic acidosis (pH, 7.3; TCO_2 20–21 mEq/L [normal 22–26 mEq/L]). While slow spontaneous correction of acid-base status is typically observed upon rehydration, rapid fluid boluses in poorly perfused individuals may result in a transient "reperfusion acidosis" as returning circulation washes the products of anaerobic metabolism out of the tissues. In this setting, or when renal insufficiency exists, blood buffering capacity is such that patients with serum bicarbonate concentrations below 8 mEq/L or pH less than 7.2 may benefit from administration of supplemental base (sodium bicarbonate) (Fig. 11–9).[68]

Rapid bedside evaluation of acid-base status utilizes the following general relationships: a pH decrease of 0.1 units accompanies a base excess of approximately 6 mEq/L or an increase in P_{CO_2} of 10 to 12 mm Hg. The total replacement base required is then determined by the following equation:

$$\text{Dose (mEq)} = 0.3 \times \text{Wt (kg)} \times \text{BE (mEq/L)}$$

Clinically, a smaller sodium bicarbonate dose (1–2 mEq/kg) is given initially, the response verified by blood gas analysis, and the remaining doses titrated to effect.

4. Is renal function impaired?

Initial evaluation includes information as to last urine void and recent urine output, measurement of urine specific gravity, and serum levels of blood urea nitrogen and creatinine. If uncertainty persists, measurement of serum and urine electrolytes for comparison and calculation of the FE_{Na} is indicated:

$$FE_{(Na)} = \frac{U_{(Na)}/P_{(Na)}}{U_{(Cr)}/P_{(Cr)}} \times 100$$

U = urine
P = plasma
Na = sodium
Cr = creatinine

FE_{Na} values less than 1% imply prerenal conditions causing renal dysfunction, whereas FE_{Na} values greater than 2 to 3% suggest renal insufficiency. In prematurity, however, values as high as 9% may be seen in otherwise normal infants.

5. What is the state of potassium balance?

Potassium homeostasis is critical to life, and serum potassium levels are generally maintained within a very narrow range. Nonetheless, serum potassium levels do not reflect whole body stores and substantial potassium depletion may exist in the presence of modest changes in serum potassium

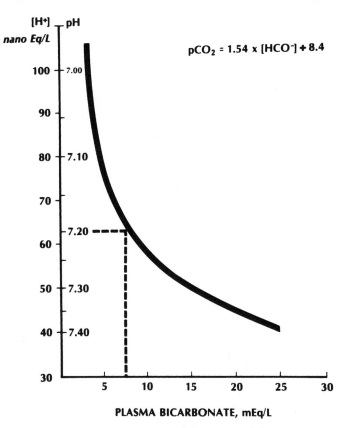

$$pCO_2 = 1.54 \times [HCO_3^-] + 8.4$$

Figure 11–9. This figure, based on data from children with metabolic acidosis,[108] depicts the displacement of pH as serum bicarbonate declines. The zone of rapid pH displacement (pH less than 7.20) has a slope that is several times greater than the zone of gradual pH displacement (pH 7.20 or higher). As the pH moves through the zone of rapid pH displacement, a further decline of serum bicarbonate, of as little as 1 or 2 mEq/L, produces a highly leveraged further decrease of pH. (From Kallen RJ: The management of diarrheal dehydration in infants using parenteral fluids. Pediatr Clin North Am 1990;37:265–286.)

concentration ($\{K^+\}_{serum}$). Gastrointestinal losses or metabolic acidosis is usually accompanied by a potassium deficit, whereas other dehydration states are not. Rapid fluid boluses or pH correction, or both, may acutely reduce $\{K^+\}_{serum}$,[72] and refractory hypokalemia may occur in patients deficient in magnesium.[73] In all cases, adequate renal function should be present before administration of potassium and complete repletion should be accomplished over 48 to 72 hours.

Once the nature and severity of dehydration have been determined, the clinician may proceed using any one of a variety of correction strategies. In one approach, moderate to severe dehydration deficits may be estimated, as in Table 11–9. Fluid and electrolyte repair may then proceed according to a three-phase approach wherein circulating plasma volume, perfusion, and urine output are restored rapidly using isotonic crystalloid or colloid solution and remaining deficits are corrected over 24 hours as outlined[74]:

- *Emergency Phase:* 20–30 mL/kg isotonic crystalloid/colloid bolus
- *Repletion Phase 1:* 25–50 mL/kg (or half of deficit) over 6 to 8 hours. Anions: Cl^- 75%, acetate 25%
- *Repletion Phase 2:* remainder of deficit over 24 hours

(isotonic) or 48 hours (hypertonic). Include calcium replacement as necessary

Hypernatremia and Hyponatremia

As previously detailed, disorders of sodium equilibrium are primarily marked by disturbances of fluid balance and are repaired according to the principles outlined earlier. Serious hypernatremia or hyponatremia is accompanied by neurologic symptoms whose severity is determined by the degree and rate of change of serum sodium concentration ($\{Na^+\}_{serum}$).

Hypernatremia

Unlike in adults, *acute hypernatremia* is common in children. A mortality rate of greater than 40% for acute and 10% for chronic has been quoted for hypernatremia (serum sodium > 160 mEq/L). Mortality and permanent neurologic injury are even more common in infants. Depending on degree and duration, neurologic findings include irritability and coma. Seizures may be a presenting symptom, yet are more commonly encountered after the start of therapy. Patients with acute conditions are usually symptomatic, whereas those with chronic conditions (acclimated individuals) may be asymptomatic. General principles for treatment of hypernatremia are as follows:

- In the setting of circulatory collapse, colloid or NS bolus should be administered. Though debatable, colloid bolus provides the theoretical benefit of sustained hemodynamic support with lower fluid load. Saline, in contrast, rapidly re-equilibrates, necessitating repeated boluses while adding to the total salt burden.
- On the basis of the principles outlined above, fluid deficit should be assessed as accurately as possible and repaired over 48 hours. Free water excess will be required. Continued reassessment of serum sodium and osmolality should be made, aiming for correction of no more than 1 to 2 mOsm/L/h. Because of possible associated hypoglycemia, some solutions should be glucose-containing and serum glucose levels should be monitored.
- Vigilance for seizures, apnea, and cardiovascular compromise should be maintained, since such complicating factors can be the primary determinates of successful outcome.

Hyponatremia

Hyponatremia is also common in infants and children. Increasing prevalence due to erroneous formula dilution has intermittently been reported.[75, 76] In the practice of anesthesiology, mild hyponatremia is a common postoperative condition following surgery of any severity[77]; in neurosurgical patients, hyponatremia may represent cerebral salt wasting or inappropriate secretion of antidiuretic hormone.[78] In general, symptomatic patients are acutely hyponatremic and asymptomatic individuals are chronically hyponatremic.[79] Following surgery, acutely hyponatremic patients may present with nonspecific symptoms that are often erroneously attributed to other causes. Early central nervous system symptoms include headache, nausea, weakness, and anorexia. Advanc-

ing symptoms include mental status changes, confusion, irritability, progressive obtundation, and seizures. Respiratory arrest (or irregularity) is a common manifestation of advanced hyponatremia.

When approaching the correction of hyponatremia, symptomatic patients must be considered a medical emergency while asymptomatic patients do not require rapid intervention. Correction of chronic hyponatremia must be slow and limited to no more than 0.5 mEq/L/h so as to avoid neurologic complications.[80] The best treatment for acute hyponatremia is early recognition and intervention. Because hypoxia will exacerbate neurologic injury, simple ABCs are attended to first and the airway is secured in the child with seizures or respiratory irregularity. Hyponatremic seizures may be quieted by relatively modest (3–6 mEq/L) increases of serum sodium.[81] In several series[76, 82, 83] such limited, rapid correction of symptomatic hyponatremia with hypertonic saline (514 mEq/L NaCl) was found to be well tolerated. It should be emphasized, however, that complete correction is unnecessary and unwise.[84] Initial therapy is aimed at raising serum sodium no more than is necessary to stop seizure activity (usually 3–5 mEq/L). Further correction is carried out over several days. Hypertonic saline may be used for correction until the serum sodium increases to greater than 120 mEq/L. Total sodium deficit is estimated as follows:

$$\text{Sodium change (mEq/L)} \times \text{fraction TBW (L/kg)} \times \text{weight (kg)} = \text{mEq sodium}$$

$$(\text{Desired } [Na^+]_{serum} - \text{Observed } [Na^+]_{serum}) \times 0.6^* \times \text{weight (kg)} = \text{mEq sodium required}$$

*As discussed earlier, TBW may range from 75% in infancy to 60% or lower in older children.

In the 25 kg child with a serum sodium of 110 mEq/L, to correct to 125 mEq/L using hypertonic saline (514 mEq/L), infuse

$$(125 \text{ mEq/L} - 110 \text{ mEq/L}) \times 0.6 \times 25 = 225 \text{ mEq total}$$
$$or$$
$$225 \text{ mEq}/514 \text{ mEq/L} = 0.44 \text{ L over 48 hours} \cong 9 \text{ mL/h}$$

Because such calculations involve estimates, frequent measurement of serum sodium values is necessary during correction. As with hypernatremia, much of the morbidity and mortality associated with hyponatremia relates to complicating factors such as seizures and hypoxia that may occur during therapy. Thus, patients undergoing therapy should be cared for in a monitored setting. When overzealous correction has occurred (seizures), there may be value in acutely re-lowering $\{Na^+\}_{serum}$ using hypotonic fluids,[79] although such therapy is not without its own hazards.

General principles for treatment of hyponatremia are as follows:

- Asymptomatic hyponatremia in and of itself need not be rapidly corrected. Associated cardiovascular compromise due to volume depletion may be addressed by colloid bolus or administration of isotonic saline (1 L/m²/d). Provision of sodium is accompanied by free water restriction.
- Symptomatic hyponatremia is a medical emergency and

may sometimes reflect irreversible neurologic injury. Correction should be rapid, yet limited, as discussed previously. A dose of 3 mL/kg of 3% saline (514 mEq/L) may be administered over 20 to 30 minutes to halt seizures.

■ Subsequent correction is accomplished through calculation of sodium deficit and provision of sodium so as to slowly correct at a rate not to exceed 0.5 mEq/L/h or 25 mEq/L (total) in 24 to 48 hours.

■ If attendant fluid load is excessive or if oliguria is present, diuretics may be useful.

Disorders of Potassium Homeostasis

Hyperkalemia

Hyperkalemia is occasionally the presenting finding in conditions such as congenital adrenal hyperplasia. More commonly, it results from acute renal insufficiency, massive tissue injury, acidosis, or iatrogenic mishaps. In the operating room, acute hyperkalemia accompanies malignant hyperthermia, the use of succinylcholine in patients with undiagnosed muscular dystrophies, and occasionally during rapid transfusion of red blood cells or whole blood.[85] While neurologic status is the main concern for patients with abnormal serum sodium levels, cardiac status (rate and rhythm) determines the care of patients with hyperkalemia. In hyperkalemia, peaked T waves are followed by lengthening of the PR interval and widening of the QRS until P-waves are lost and the QRS merges with its T wave to produce a sinusoidal pattern (Fig. 11–10). Successful treatment traditionally utilizes the following approach:

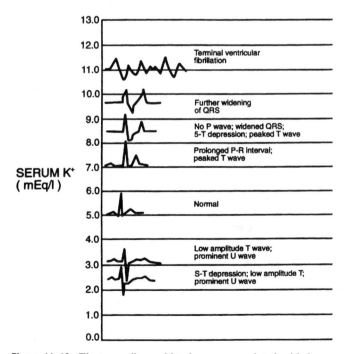

SERUM K⁺ (mEq/l)

Serum K⁺ value	Description
~11.0	Terminal ventricular fibrillation
~9.75	Further widening of QRS
~9.0	No P wave; widened QRS; S-T depression; peaked T wave
~7.75	Prolonged P-R interval; peaked T wave
~5.5	Normal
~3.0	Low amplitude T wave; prominent U wave
~2.5	S-T depression; low amplitude T; prominent U wave

Figure 11–10. Electrocardiographic changes associated with hyperkalemia. (From Williams GS, Klenk EL, Winters RW: Acute renal failure in pediatrics. In: Winters RW, ed: The Body Fluids in Pediatrics: Medical, Surgical, and Neonatal Disorders of Acid-Base Status, Hydration, and Oxygenation. Boston: Little, Brown and Company; 1973:523–557.)

■ Emergent therapy is first directed toward antagonism of potassium's cardiac effects by administration of calcium (calcium chloride 0.1 to 0.3 mL/kg of a 10% solution or calcium gluconate 0.3 to 1.0 mL/kg of a 10% solution over 3 to 5 min).

■ Serum potassium is then reduced by returning potassium to the intracellular space by reversal of acidosis through administration of sodium bicarbonate (1–2 mEq/kg) and mild to moderate hyperventilation.

■ To maintain potassium in the intracellular space, glucose and insulin are administered by infusion (0.5–1 g/kg glucose with 0.1 U/kg insulin over 30–60 minutes).

■ After stabilization, attention is directed toward removal of the whole-body potassium burden (kayexalate, dialysis) and correction of the underlying cause.

The knowledge that beta-adrenergic stimulation modulates the translocation of potassium into the intracellular space[86, 87] has prompted the consideration of beta-agonists in the treatment of acute hyperkalemia.[88–91] In children, a single infusion of salbutamol (5 μg/kg over 15 min) has been shown to effectively lower serum potassium concentrations within 30 minutes. The rapidity, efficacy, and safety observed with this therapy in a study of 15 children led its authors to conclude that salbutamol is a reasonable first choice treatment for hyperkalemia.[88] In addition to intravenous therapy, both salbutamol[92] and albuterol[91] have been found to be effective when given by inhalation.

This route has the significant advantages of being readily available in emergency departments and not requiring intravenous access. However, the observation that a paradoxical exacerbation of hyperkalemia sometimes occurs upon initiation of treatment,[92] together with concerns regarding the possibility of associated arrhythmias,[93] suggests that more experience is required before such therapy can be considered the standard of care. Certainly inhalation of albuterol during such an event in the operating room may help speed the reduction in serum potassium while instituting other methods of treatment.

Hypokalemia

Hypokalemia is most common in children as a complication of diarrhea or persistent vomiting associated with gastroenteritis. In the operating room or intensive care unit, hypokalemia may also accompany a wide variety of other conditions, including diabetes, hyperaldosteronism, pyloric stenosis, starvation, renal tubular disease, chronic steroid or diuretic use, and beta-agonist therapy. Severe hypokalemia is accompanied by electrocardiographic changes including QT prolongation, diminution of the T-wave, and appearance of U-waves (see Fig. 11–10).

As noted previously, serum potassium levels do not accurately reflect total potassium homeostasis, and low serum levels may or may not be associated with significant total body potassium depletion. The precise point to begin replacement therapy, therefore, is controversial, and total replacement requirements are impossible to calculate. In general practice, serum potassium values ($\{K^+\}_{serum}$) between 2.0 and 2.5 mEq/L are corrected prior to surgery on the assumption that further decreases may predispose the child to arrhythmias and hemodynamic instability.

Potassium replacement is best accomplished orally over an extended period while the underlying cause is evaluated and treated. When intravenous correction is required, concentrations up to 40 mEq/L may be given slowly (not to exceed 1 mEq/kg/h) in a monitored setting. Because such solutions often cause phlebitis, large-bore or central catheters are preferred. In the setting of hypochloremic hypokalemia, chloride deficits must first be replaced, usually via administration of normal saline.

Syndrome of Inappropriate Antidiuretic Hormone (SIADH) Secretion

The many factors capable of stimulating ADH release make the syndrome of inappropriate ADH release common. As detailed earlier, intravascular depletion is the most potent stimulus for vasopressin release, yet the term "inappropriate" generally refers to control of osmolality. Pain, surgical stress, critical illness, sepsis, pulmonary disease, central nervous system injury, and a variety of drugs may all stimulate ADH release above and beyond that necessary to maintain osmolar balance.

The SIADH is common in children yet often overlooked. Minor head trauma, for example, may elicit spikes in ADH levels, though infrequently to the point of producing serious hyponatremia and seizures.[94] Urine output in postoperative spinal fusion patients is often reduced by elevated ADH levels and routinely returns within 24 hours without specific therapy.[95] Infants with bronchiolitis and hyperinflated lungs frequently possess markedly elevated plasma ADH levels and exhibit fluid retention, weight gain, urinary concentration, and plasma hypo-osmolality until their illness begins to resolve.[96] Hyponatremia to the point of seizures, however, is only occasionally observed. Overall, elevated ADH levels are probably more common than generally appreciated in the intensive care unit and operating room. The challenge, therefore, is to maintain vigilance and to intervene when potentially dangerous conditions present themselves.

The diagnosis of SIADH rests on the identification of impaired urinary dilution in the setting of plasma hypo-osmolality. Hyponatremia ($Na^+ < 135$ mEq/L), serum osmolality less than 280 mOsm/L, and urine osmolality greater than 100 mOsm/L in the absence of volume depletion, cardiac failure, nephropathy, adrenal insufficiency, or cirrhosis is generally considered sufficient for diagnosis. Therapeutic principles are similar to those of hyponatremia and rest upon the following:

- Free water restriction
- Repletion of sodium deficits (if present)
- Countering of vasopressin effects with judicious use of diuretics

Diabetes Insipidus

In the operating room and the intensive care unit, diabetes insipidus is most commonly associated with the care of neurosurgical patients.[97–99] Diabetes insipidus also results from neuroendocrine failure in brain death, and management may be necessary if organ donation is requested.[100, 101] Diabetes insipidus results from decreased secretion of, or renal insensitivity to, vasopressin. Manifestations include massive polyuria, volume contraction, dehydration, and plasma hyperosmolality. Dilute polyuria (<250 mOsm, > 2 mL/kg/h) in the presence of hypernatremia ($Na^+ > 145$ mEq/L) with hyperosmolality (> 300 mOsm/L) is the hallmark. In central diabetes insipidus, administration of desmopressin produces urine concentration, yet water deprivation does not. Postoperative diabetes insipidus may initially be difficult to distinguish from mobilization of operative fluids.

Children with craniopharyngiomas or a similarly situated pathologic lesion, may not initially manifest vasopressin deficiency yet become symptomatic preoperatively after steroid administration or intraoperatively upon surgical manipulation. Postoperative diabetes insipidus typically begins the evening following surgery and may resolve in 3 to 5 days if osmoregulatory structures have not been permanently injured. An often-confusing triphasic response may also occur wherein postoperative diabetes insipidus appears to resolve, fluid status normalizes, or SIADH appears, and then vasopressin secretion ceases and diabetes insipidus returns. It is hypothesized that this pattern reflects nonspecific vasopressin release from a degenerating pituitary gland.

Management of diabetes insipidus in the conscious patient with intact thirst mechanism is relatively straightforward. Desmopressin may be administered intranasally on a daily basis and fluid intake monitored closely. Management through fluid restriction and volume contraction alone is also possible if the volume of urine presented to the distal collecting tubules (and subject to the actions of vasopressin) is sufficiently limited.

Management of the unconscious surgical patient is more challenging. Preoperatively, in the patient with pre-existing diabetes insipidus, desmopressin may be either withheld several days before surgery (with additional fluids provided intravenously) or continued until the evening before surgery. Intraoperatively, osmotic diuresis with mannitol is avoided and urine output monitored closely. If urine output abruptly rises and simultaneously obtained urine and serum osmolalities suggest diabetes insipidus, vasopressin administration should begin. Although some authors suggest intranasal or intramuscular administration of desmopressin, in the unconscious patient we prefer the control of continuous intravenous vasopressin infusion starting at 0.5 mU/kg/h and titrated upward to effect (1–10 mU/kg/h). A novel and simple strategy has also been suggested wherein vasopressin is added directly to crystalloid replacement fluids, which are then titrated to match urine output.[102]

REFERENCES

1. Fenstermacher JD, Johnson JA: Filtration and reflection coefficients of the rabbit blood-brain barrier. Am J Physiol 1966;211:341–346.
2. Perl W, Chowdhury P, Chinard FP: Reflection coefficients of dog lung endothelium to small hydrophilic solutes. Am J Physiol 1975;228:797–809.
3. Lamke LO, Liljedahl SO: Plasma volume changes after infusion of various plasma expanders. Resuscitation 1976;5:93–102.
4. Moon PF, Hollyfield-Gilbert MA, Myers TL, et al: Effects of isotonic crystalloid resuscitation on fluid compartments in hemorrhaged rats. Shock 1994;2:355–361.
5. Svensen C, Hahn RG: Volume kinetics of Ringer solution, dextran 70, and hypertonic saline in male volunteers. Anesthesiology 1997;87:204–212.
6. Christ F, Niklas M, Kreimeier U, et al: Hyperosmotic-hyperoncotic solutions during abdominal aortic aneurysm (AAA) resection. Acta Anaesthesiol Scand 1997;41:62–70.

7. Younes RN, Aun F, Accioly CQ, et al: Hypertonic solutions in the treatment of hypovolemic shock: a prospective, randomized study in patients admitted to the emergency room. Surgery 1992;111:380–385.

8. Richardson PD, Granger DN, Mailman D, et al: Permeability characteristics of colonic capillaries. Am J Physiol 1980;239:G300–G305.

9. Kongstad L, Moller AD, Grande PO: Reflection coefficient for albumin and capillary fluid permeability in cat calf muscle after traumatic injury. Acta Physiol Scand 1999;165:369–377.

10. Greissman A, Silver P, Nimkoff L, et al: Albumin bolus administration versus continuous infusion in critically ill hypoalbuminemic pediatric patients. Intensive Care Med 1996;22:495–499.

11. McManus ML, Churchwell KB, Strange K: Regulation of cell volume in health and disease. N Engl J Med 1995;333:1260–1266.

12. Chamberlin ME, Strange K: Anisosmotic cell volume regulation: A comparative view. Am J Physiol 1989;257:C159–C173.

13. Schrier RW, Abraham WT: Hormones and hemodynamics in heart failure. N Engl J Med 1999;341:577–585.

14. Abraham WT, Schrier RW: Body fluid volume regulation in health and disease. Adv Intern Med 1994;39:23–47.

15. Fitzsimons JT: Angiotensin, thirst, and sodium appetite. Physiol Rev 1998;78:583–686.

16. Navar LG: The kidney in blood pressure regulation and development of hypertension. Med Clin North Am 1997;81:1165–1198.

17. Levin ER, Gardner DG, Samson WK: Natriuretic peptides. N Engl J Med 1998;339:321–328.

18. Braith RW, Mills RM Jr, Wilcox CS, et al: Breakdown of blood pressure and body fluid homeostasis in heart transplant recipients. J Am Coll Cardiol 1996;27:375–383.

19. Friis-Hansen B: Body water compartments in children: Changes during growth and related changes in body composition. Pediatrics 1961;28:169–181.

20. Holliday M: The evolution of therapy for dehydration: Should deficit therapy still be taught? Pediatrics 1996;98:171–177.

21. Gamble J, Ross G, Tisdall F: The metabolism of fixed base in fasting. J Biol Chem 1923;57:633–695.

22. Linderkamp O, Versmold HT, Riegel KP, et al: Estimation and prediction of blood volume in infants and children. Eur J Pediatr 1977;125:227–234.

23. Cassady G: Plasma volume studies in low birth weight infants. Pediatrics 1966;38:1020–1027.

24. Feldschuh J, Enson Y: Prediction of the normal blood volume: Relation of blood volume to body habitus. Circulation 1977;56:605–612.

25. Herrin J: Fluid and electrolytes. In: Graef JW, ed: Manual of Pediatric Therapeutics, 6th ed. Philadelphia: Lippincott-Raven; 1997:63–75.

26. Latta T: Central Board of Health, London: Relative to the treatment of cholera by the copious injection of aqueous and saline fluids into the vein. Lancet 1831;2:274–277.

27. Blackfan K, Maxcy K: Intraperitoneal injection of saline solution. Am J Dis Child 1918;15:19–28.

28. Darrow D: Therapeutic measures promoting recovery from the physiologic disturbances of infantile diarrhea. Pediatrics 1952;9:519–533.

29. Holliday MA, Segar WE: The maintenance need for water in parenteral fluid therapy. Pediatrics 1957;19:823–832.

30. Darrow D, Council on Food and Nutrition: Fluid therapy; relation to tissue composition and expenditure of water and electrolyte. JAMA 1950;143:365.

31. Lorenz JM, Kleinman LI, Kotagal UR, et al: Water balance in very low-birth-weight infants: Relationship to water and sodium intake and effect on outcome. J Pediatr 1982;101:423–432.

32. Lorenz JM, Kleinman LI, Ahmed G, et al: Phases of fluid and electrolyte homeostasis in the extremely low birth weight infant. Pediatrics 1995;96:484–489.

33. Gold PS, Brace RA: Fetal whole-body permeability: Surface area product and reflection coefficient for plasma proteins. Microvasc Res 1988;36:262–274.

34. Takahashi N, Hoshi J, Nishida H: Water balance, electrolytes and acid-base balance in extremely premature infants. Acta Paediatr Jpn 1994;36:250–255.

35. Coté CJ, Jobes DR, Schwartz AJ, et al: Two approaches to cannulation of a child's internal jugular vein. Anesthesiology 1979;50:371–373.

36. Nicolson SC, Sweeney MF, Moore RA, et al: Comparison of internal and external jugular cannulation of the central circulation in the pediatric patient. Crit Care Med 1985;13:747–749.

37. Hodge D 3d, Fleisher G: Pediatric catheter flow rates. Am J Emerg Med 1985;3:403–407.

38. Hodge D 3d, Delgado-Paredes C, Fleisher G: Central and peripheral catheter flow rates in "pediatric" dogs. Ann Emerg Med 1986;15:1151–1154.

39. Fleisher G, Caputo G, Baskin M: Comparison of external jugular and peripheral venous administration of sodium bicarbonate in puppies. Crit Care Med 1989;17:251–254.

40. Rosetti VA, Thompson BM, Miller J, et al: Intraosseous infusion: An alternative route of pediatric intravascular access. Ann Emerg Med 1985;14:885–888.

41. Fiser DH: Intraosseous infusion. N Engl J Med 1990;322:1579–1581.

42. Hodge D 3d, Delgado-Paredes C, Fleisher G: Intraosseous infusion flow rates in hypovolemic "pediatric" dogs. Ann Emerg Med 1987;16:305–307.

43. Selby IR, James MR: The intraosseous route for induction of anaesthesia. Anaesthesia 1993;48:982–984.

44. Schwartz RE, Pasquariello CA, Stayer SA: Elective use in pediatric anesthesia of intraosseous infusion: Proceed only with extreme caution. Anesth Analg 1993;76:918–919.

45. Stewart FC, Kain ZN: Intraosseous infusion: elective use in pediatric anesthesia. Anesth Analg 1992;75:626–629.

46. Moscati R, Moore GP: Compartment syndrome with resultant amputation following intraosseous infusion. Am J Emerg Med 1990;8:470–471.

47. Galpin RD, Kronick JB, Willis RB, et al: Bilateral lower extremity compartment syndromes secondary to intraosseous fluid resuscitation. J Pediatr Orthop 1991;11:773–776.

48. Ribeiro JA, Price CT, Knapp DR Jr: Compartment syndrome of the lower extremity after intraosseous infusion of fluid: A report of two cases. J Bone Joint Surg Am 1993;75:430–433.

49. Fiser RT, Walker WM, Seibert JJ, et al: Tibial length following intraosseous infusion: A prospective, radiographic analysis. Pediatr Emerg Care 1997;13:186–188.

50. Shires T, Williams J, Brown F: Acute change in extracellular fluids associated with major surgical procedures. Ann Surg 1961;154:803–810.

51. Bennett EJ, Daughety MJ, Jenkins MT: Fluid requirements for neonatal anesthesia and operation. Anesthesiology 1970;32:343–350.

52. Philippart AI, Canty TG, Filler RM: Acute fluid volume requirements in infants with anterior abdominal wall defects. J Pediatr Surg 1972;7:553–558.

53. Mollitt DL, Ballantine TV, Grosfeld JL, et al: A critical assessment of fluid requirements in gastroschisis. J Pediatr Surg 1978;13:217–219.

54. Williams EL, Hildebrand KL, McCormick SA, et al: The effect of intravenous lactated Ringer's solution versus 0.9% sodium chloride solution on serum osmolality in human volunteers. Anesth Analg 1999;88:999–1003.

55. Mikawa K, Maekawa N, Goto R, et al: Effects of exogenous intravenous glucose on plasma glucose and lipid homeostasis in anesthetized children. Anesthesiology 1991;74:1017–1022.

56. Welborn LG, McGill WA, Hannallah RS, et al: Perioperative blood glucose concentrations in pediatric outpatients. Anesthesiology 1986;65:543–547.

57. Mercer S, Bass J: Hypoglycemia associated with pediatric surgical procedures. Can J Surg 1983;26:246–249.

58. Aouifi A, Neidecker J, Vedrinne C, et al: Glucose versus lactated Ringer's solution during pediatric cardiac surgery. J Cardiothorac Vasc Anesth 1997;11:411–414.

59. Nicolson SC, Jobes DR, Zucker HA, et al: The effect of administering or withholding dextrose in pre-bypass intravenous fluids on intraoperative blood glucose concentrations in infants undergoing hypothermic circulatory arrest. J Cardiothorac Vasc Anesth 1992;6:316–318.

60. Berg RA, Lloyd TR, Donnerstein RL. Accuracy of central venous pressure monitoring in the intraabdominal inferior vena cava: a canine study. J Pediatr 1992;120:67–71.

61. Lloyd TR, Donnerstein RL, Berg RA. Accuracy of central venous pressure measurement from the abdominal inferior vena cava. Pediatrics 1992;89:506–508.

62. Arieff AI, Ayus JC, Fraser CL. Hyponatraemia and death or permanent brain damage in healthy children. BMJ 1992;304:1218–1222.

63. Zak AL, Harrington DT, Barillo DJ, et al. Acute respiratory failure that complicates the resuscitation of pediatric patients with scald injuries. J Burn Care Rehabil 1999;20:391–399.

64. Arieff AI. Fatal postoperative pulmonary edema: pathogenesis and literature review. Chest 1999;115:1371–1377.

65. Laron Z: Skin turgor as a quantitative index of dehydration in children. Pediatrics 1957;19:816–821.

66. Saavedra JM, Harris GD, Li S, et al: Capillary refilling (skin turgor) in the assessment of dehydration. Am J Dis Child 1991;145:296–298.

67. Moineau G, Newman J: Rapid intravenous rehydration in the pediatric emergency department. Pediatr Emerg Care 1990;6:186–188.

68. Kallen RJ: The management of diarrheal dehydration in infants using parenteral fluids. Pediatr Clin North Am 1990;37:265–286.

69. Conley SB: Hypernatremia. Pediatr Clin North Am 1990;37:365–372.

70. Lee JH, Arcinue E, Ross BD: Brief report: Organic osmolytes in the brain of an infant with hypernatremia. N Engl J Med 1994;331:439–442.

71. Ellis SJ: Extrapontine myelinolysis after correction of chronic hyponatraemia with isotonic saline. Br J Clin Pract 1995;49:49–50.

72. Malone DR, McNamara RM, Malone RS, et al: Hypokalemia complicating emergency fluid resuscitation in children. Pediatr Emerg Care 1990;6:13–16.

73. Whang R, Flink EB, Dyckner T, et al: Magnesium depletion as a cause of refractory potassium repletion. Arch Intern Med 1985;145:1686–1689.

74. Finberg L: Hypernatremic (hypertonic) dehydration in infants. N Engl J Med 1973;289:196–198.

75. Vanapruks V, Prapaitrakul K: Water intoxication and hyponatraemic convulsions in neonates. Arch Dis Child 1989;64:734–735.

76. Keating JP, Schears GJ, Dodge PR: Oral water intoxication in infants: An American epidemic. Am J Dis Child 1991;145:985–990.

77. Guy AJ, Michaels JA, Flear CT: Changes in the plasma sodium concentration after minor, moderate and major surgery. Br J Surg 1987;74:1027–1030.

78. Sivakumar V, Rajshekhar V, Chandy MJ: Management of neurosurgical patients with hyponatremia and natriuresis. Neurosurgery 1994;34:269–274.

79. Soupart A, Ngassa M, Decaux G: Therapeutic relowering of the serum sodium in a patient after excessive correction of hyponatremia. Clin Nephrol 1999;51:383–386.

80. Gross P, Reimann D, Neidel J, et al: The treatment of severe hyponatremia. Kidney Int Suppl 1998;64:S6–S11.

81. Gruskin AB, Sarnaik A: Hyponatremia: Pathophysiology and treatment, a pediatric perspective. Pediatr Nephrol 1992;6:280–286.

82. Sharf RE: Seizure from hyponatremia in infants: Early recognition and treatment. Arch Fam Med 1993;2:647–652.

83. Sarnaik AP, Meert K, Hackbarth R, et al: Management of hyponatremic seizures in children with hypertonic saline: A safe and effective strategy. Crit Care Med 1991;19:758–762.

84. Ayus JC, Krothapalli RK, Arieff AI: Changing concepts in treatment of severe symptomatic hyponatremia: Rapid correction and possible relation to central pontine myelinolysis. Am J Med 1985;78:897–902.

85. Larach MG, Rosenberg H, Gronert GA, et al: Hyperkalemic cardiac arrest during anesthesia in infants and children with occult myopathies. Clin Pediatr (Phila) 1997;36:9–16.

86. Rosa RM, Silva P, Young JB, et al: Adrenergic modulation of extrarenal potassium disposal. N Engl J Med 1980;302:431–434.

87. Williams ME, Gervino EV, Rosa RM, et al: Catecholamine modulation of rapid potassium shifts during exercise. N Engl J Med 1985;312:823–827.

88. Kemper MJ, Harps E, Hellwege HH, et al: Effective treatment of acute hyperkalaemia in childhood by short-term infusion of salbutamol. Eur J Pediatr 1996;155:495–497.

89. Kim HJ: Acute therapy for hyperkalemia with the combined regimen of bicarbonate and beta(2)-adrenergic agonist (salbutamol) in chronic renal failure patients. J Korean Med Sci 1997;12:111–116.

90. Hanna MG, Stewart J, Schapira AH, et al: Salbutamol treatment in a patient with hyperkalaemic periodic paralysis due to a mutation in the skeletal muscle sodium channel gene (SCN4A). J Neurol Neurosurg Psychiatry 1998;65:248–250.

91. Greenberg A: Hyperkalemia: Treatment options. Semin Nephrol 1998;18:46–57.

92. Mandelberg A, Krupnik Z, Houri S, et al: Salbutamol metered-dose inhaler with spacer for hyperkalemia: How fast? How safe? Chest 1999;115:617–622.

93. Semmekrot BA, Monnens LA: A warning for the treatment of hyperkalaemia with salbutamol. Eur J Pediatr 1997;156:420.

94. Padilla G, Leake JA, Castro R, et al: Vasopressin levels and pediatric head trauma. Pediatrics 1989;83:700–705.

95. Burrows FA, Shutack JG, Crone RK: Inappropriate secretion of antidiuretic hormone in a postsurgical pediatric population. Crit Care Med 1983;11:527–531.

96. Gozal D, Colin AA, Jaffe M, et al: Water, electrolyte, and endocrine homeostasis in infants with bronchiolitis. Pediatr Res 1990;27:204–209.

97. Balestrieri FJ, Chernow B, Rainey TG: Postcraniotomy diabetes insipidus. Who's at risk? Crit Care Med 1982;10:108–110.

98. Baskin DS, Wilson CB: Surgical management of craniopharyngiomas: A review of 74 cases. J Neurosurg 1986;65:22–27.

99. Honegger J, Buchfelder M, Fahlbusch R: Surgical treatment of craniopharyngiomas: Endocrinological results. J Neurosurg 1999;90:251–257.

100. Staworn D, Lewison L, Marks J, et al: Brain death in pediatric intensive care unit patients: Incidence, primary diagnosis, and the clinical occurrence of Turner's triad. Crit Care Med 1994;22:1301–1305.

101. Kissoon N, Frewen TC, Bloch M, et al: Pediatric organ donor maintenance: Pathophysiologic derangements and nursing requirements. Pediatrics 1989;84:688–693.

102. Ralston C, Butt W: Continuous vasopressin replacement in diabetes insipidus. Arch Dis Child 1990;65:896–897.

103. Robertson GL, Aycinena P, Zerbe RL: Neurogenic disorders of osmoregulation. Am J Med 1982;72:339–353.

104. Rose BD: Clinical Physiology of Acid-Base and Electrolyte Disorders, 4th ed. New York: McGraw-Hill; 1994.

105. Guyton AC, Hall JC, eds: Dominant role of the kidneys in long-term regulation of arterial pressure and in hypertension: The integrated system for pressure control. In: Textbook of Medical Physiology, 9th ed. Philadelphia: WB Saunders; 1996:221–237.

106. McIver MA, Gamble JL: Body fluid changes due to upper intestinal obstruction. JAMA 1928;91:1589–1592.

107. Talbot FB: Basal metabolism in children. Brennemann's Practice of Pediatrics. Hagerstown: Prior; 1949.

108. Albert MS, Dell RB, Winters RW: Quantitative displacement of acid-base equilibrium in metabolic acidosis. Ann Intern Med 1967;66:312–322.

109. Link D: Fluids, electrolytes, acid-base disturbances, and diuretics. In: Todres ID, Fugate JH, eds: Critical Care of Infants and Children. Boston: Little, Brown and Company; 1996:410–435.

12

Strategies for Blood Product Management and Transfusion Reduction

Charles J. Coté *and* Richard M. Dsida

Blood Volume

Blood Products and Adjuvants

    Whole Blood and Other Products Containing Red Blood Cells

    Fresh Frozen Plasma

    Platelets

    Cryoprecipitate

    Factor Concentrates

    Desmopressin (DDAVP)

Massive Blood Transfusion

    Coagulopathy

    Hyperkalemia

    Hypocalcemia

    Disseminated Intravascular Coagulopathy

    Acid-Base Balance

    Hypothermia

    Oxygen-Hemoglobin Dissociation

    Pulmonary Effects

    Miscellaneous Complications

    Monitoring During Massive Blood Transfusion

    Infectious Disease Considerations for Anesthesiologists

Methods to Reduce Exposure to Blood Products

    Eyrthropoietin

    Pre-donation

    Directed Donation

    Autotransfusion (Intraoperative Blood Scavenging)

    Controlled Hypotension

    Hemodilution

Despite advances in pediatric surgery, the number of infants and children sustaining major operative blood loss remains high. Little information has been gathered about when to expect coagulation defects in the pediatric age group. Advances in blood banking, use of component therapy, use of blood salvage techniques, preoperative autodonation, and directed donor blood have altered the problems associated with blood replacement. Most studies of massive blood transfusion have involved adult patients whose blood replacement has been with either whole blood or modified whole blood. The majority of recommendations regarding the use of fresh frozen plasma (FFP) and platelets are based on these studies and not on large series of patients whose blood replacement has been made exclusively with component therapy.

Perhaps nothing has changed the use of blood products by surgeons and anesthesiologists more than the threat of the acquired immunodeficiency syndrome (AIDS).[1-3] Although infection with human immunodeficiency virus (HIV) is by no means the most common disease associated with blood transfusion, it has been the most publicized in the lay press and the most feared in the public mind. An estimated 30 million people worldwide are currently infected with HIV; the incidence varies from country to country.[4] All blood products are capable of transmitting HIV, with infection ultimately resulting in AIDS in most individuals.[5] A number of other diseases may be transmitted with blood products, including human T-cell leukemia/lymphoma virus I and II, hepatitis B, hepatitis C, hepatitis D, hepatitis A, hepatitis E, hepatitis G, Parvo B19, cytomegalovirus, human herpes viruses 6 and 8, syphilis, parasites (malaria, Chagas disease, babesiosis), toxoplasmosis, and bacterial infections.[4] Table 12–1 defines the current screening processes used in the United States.[6] It is estimated that the risk of transfusion-associated disease from blood products that have been screened as negative is approximately 1 in 66,000 units of blood for hepatitis B, less than 1 in 100,000 units for

Table 12–1. Current Blood Screening Tests Used on Donated Blood in the United States

Hepatitis B surface antigen (HBsAg)
Hepatitis B core antigen (anti-HBc)
Hepatitis C virus antibody (anti-HCV)
HIV-1 antibody (anti-HIV-1)
HIV-2 antibody (anti-HIV-2)
HIV p24 antigen
HTLV-1 antibody (anti-HTLV-1)
HTLV-II antibody (anti-HTLV-II)
Serologic test for syphilis

HIV, human immunodeficiency virus; HTLV, human T-cell lymphoma virus.

hepatitis C, and 1 in 825,000 units for HIV. The reason for missed screening tests is the period of incubation between the time of disease transmission to the donor and the development of detectable antibodies or antigens.[4-14] This "window" of negative response may last for a period of weeks to several years.[5, 12, 15, 16] The incidence of donated blood that tests negative but is infected may have some geographic variation that is somewhat dependent on the local pool of donors.[17]

Despite these efforts at cleansing the donor pool, it is still vital that there be clear medical justification for every blood transfusion.[15, 18] The benefits of each transfusion must be weighed against the potential infectious, immunologic, and metabolic risks.[19] It is in the patient's best interest to minimize the number of transfusions administered and in the anesthesiologist's best interest to document the reason for each transfusion. It is not good medical practice to administer a transfusion when it is of questionable benefit.

Blood Volume

An estimation of circulating blood volume should be made before induction of anesthesia. The blood volume of a premature infant (90 to 100 mL/kg) constitutes a greater portion of body weight than that of a full-term newborn (80 to 90 mL/kg), an infant 3 months to 1 year old (70 to 80 mL/kg), or an older child (70 mL/kg). Consideration must also be given to body habitus. In an obese child, the blood volume would be 60 to 65 mL/kg. From the estimated blood volume (EBV), the initial hemoglobin or hematocrit, and the minimum acceptable hematocrit, an estimation can be made of the maximum allowable blood loss (MABL) before red blood cell (RBC) transfusion would be indicated.

The minimum acceptable hematocrit varies according to an individual patient's need. The balance between oxygen supply and demand depends on a number of factors, including the oxygen content of blood, cardiac output and its regional distribution, and metabolic needs. With these concepts in mind, it is obvious that a child with severe pulmonary disease or cyanotic congenital heart disease probably requires a higher hematocrit than does a healthy child. Premature infants may require a higher hematocrit (40%) to prevent apnea. The decision to transfuse such infants should be made in conjunction with a neonatologist.[20] A healthy child readily tolerates a hematocrit well below 30%. It is our practice not to transfuse otherwise healthy children until

their hematocrit has fallen to the 20 to 25% range if there is little potential for postoperative bleeding. In this circumstance, it is essential that the circulating blood volume be maintained. Observing the operative field (to estimate blood loss) and monitoring the vital signs, hematocrit, urine output, and central venous pressure can help assess the adequacy of volume replacement. Although the hematocrit does not equilibrate instantaneously, it is a useful piece of information. If a procedure is expected to result in significant blood loss or fluid shifts, the anesthesiologist should strongly consider the use of a urine catheter and central venous line. Patient size or age should not be a deterrent to the use of central venous lines (Table 12–2).

Methods for estimating the MABL include (1) an approximation of circulating RBC mass, (2) a modified logarithmic equation, and (3) a simple proportion.[21-23] Any of the three techniques is acceptable, since the numbers calculated by each do not differ clinically. The most straightforward method is to estimate the MABL by simple proportion.[21] For purposes of discussion, we will use a hematocrit of 25% as the minimum acceptable hematocrit.

$$MABL = \frac{EBV \times (\text{patient's Hct} - \text{minimum accepted Hct})}{\text{Patient's Hct}}$$

For example, a 10 kg child would have an EBV of 10 (kg) $\times$ 70 (mL/kg), equaling 700 mL. If the patient's hematocrit were 42, the MABL would be:

$$MABL = \frac{700 \times (42 - 25)}{42}$$
$$= \frac{700 \times 17}{42}$$
$$= 285 \text{ mL}$$

It is critical to understand that these calculations for MABL provide only an estimate. The actual hematocrit will vary with the rapidity of blood loss and the rate of concurrent crystalloid replacement.

Initial therapy is directed at replacing fluid deficits and providing maintenance requirements (see Chapter 11). Additional fluid administration is directed at replacing blood loss and third-space losses. Each milliliter of blood lost should be replaced by 2 to 3 mL of isotonic crystalloid or 1 mL of 5% albumin.[24, 25] The latter type of replacement is expensive, and there is no clear evidence that colloid is superior to crystalloid.

In the previous example of a 10 kg child with a 700 mL blood volume and 285/mL MABL, replacement of blood loss up to that point could be made in two ways: either 570 to 855 mL of isotonic crystalloid (2 to 3 mL per milliliter of blood loss) or 285 mL of 5% albumin. If blood loss exceeds the MABL or if the hematocrit decreases to 20 to 25% (particularly if additional blood loss is expected) during surgery or in the recovery period, transfusion with packed red blood cells (PRBCs) or whole blood should be started. If postoperative bleeding is likely to occur, such as in posterior spinal fusion or open heart operations, then it is reasonable to transfuse to a level greater than the minimum acceptable hematocrit. This is especially true if a higher hematocrit can be provided without exposure to additional units of

Table 12–2. Estimated Predicted Blood Loss and Recommended Monitoring and Equipment

Predicted Blood Loss	Recommended Monitors/Equipment
<0.5 blood volumes	Routine monitoring
0.5–1.0 blood volumes	Routine monitoring + urine catheter
≥1.0 blood volumes	Routine monitoring + urine catheter + CVP line + arterial line
≥1.0 blood volumes with potential for rapid blood loss	Routine monitoring + urine catheter + CVP line + arterial line + large bore IV line + rapid infusion device
Severe head injury	Routine monitoring + urine catheter + CVP line + arterial line + large bore IV line
Major trauma with unknown severity	Routine monitoring + urine catheter + CVP line + arterial line + large bore IV line + rapid infusion device

CVP, central venous prassure; IV, intravenous.

blood (completion of units already begun). *If 1 unit of blood has been started, it is reasonable to give the patient an additional 5 to 10% rather than risk the exposure to a second unit postoperatively.* It is our practice to administer as much of the unit as will be safely tolerated by a patient rather than expose the patient to another unit of blood postoperatively.

There seems to be little danger in replacing up to the MABL entirely with crystalloid, provided that the patient is healthy and that postoperative oozing will not exceed the MABL. If replacement of lost RBCs is necessary, it is simple to calculate the volume of PRBCs needed to return the hemoglobin to an acceptable value. For example if a 10 kg child's hematocrit has fallen to 23% and one anticipates continued blood loss either intraoperatively or postoperatively, the following calculations would be made to increase the hematocrit to 35%:

$$\text{Volume of PRBCs} = \frac{(\text{Desired Hct} - \text{Present Hct}) \times \text{Estimated Blood Volume (70 mL/kg} \times 10 \text{ kg)}}{\text{Hematocrit of PRBCs}}$$

$$= \frac{(35-23) \times (70 \times 10)}{60}$$

$$= 140 \text{ mL PRBCs}$$

Because this volume is less than 1 unit, it may be reasonable to transfuse the patient up to a hematocrit of 40 (200 mL PRBCs) to allow an additional margin of safety for postoperative blood loss.

Blood Products and Adjuvants

With the recognition that certain disease states, such as von Willebrand's disease, hemophilia, other clotting factor deficiencies, and thrombocytopenia, call for specific fractions of a unit of blood, component therapy has replaced whole blood transfusion in the majority of cases. In addition, many blood banks separate units of blood into "pediatric" units, so that multiple RBC transfusions can be administered to an infant from a single adult unit. Table 12–3 presents a summary of blood transfusion compatibilities with a variety of blood products.

Whole Blood and Other Products Containing Red Blood Cells

Blood products containing RBCs are indicated for the treatment of symptomatic deficits of oxygen-carrying capacity.[26]

Table 12–3. Compatibilities of Various Blood Products

Recipient	Acceptable Donor			
	Whole Blood	*Packed Red Blood Cells**	*Fresh Frozen Plasma*	*Platelets†*
AB+	AB+, AB−	AB+, AB−, A+, A−, B+, B−, O−, O+	AB	AB+, AB− (A+, A−, B+, B−, O+, O− if hyperconcentrated)
AB−	AB−	AB−, A−, B−, O−	AB	AB− (A−, B−, O− if hyperconcentrated)
A+	A+, A−	A+, A−, O−, O+	A, AB	A+, A−, AB+, AB− (B+, B−, O+, O− if hyperconcentrated)
A−	A−	A−, O−	A, AB	A−, AB− (B−, O− if hyperconcentrated)
B+	B+, B−	B+, B−, O−, O+	B, AB	B+, B−, AB+, AB− (A+, A−, O+, O− if hyperconcentrated)
B−	B−	B−, O−	B, AB	B−, AB− (A−, O− if hyperconcentrated)
O+	O+, O−	O−, O+	O, A, B, AB	O+, O−, A+, A−, B+, B−, AB+, AB−
O−	O−	O−	O, A, B, AB	O−, A−, B−, AB−

*Rh− patients, particularly females, should not receive Rh+ red blood cells unless in emergency to avoid Rh sensitization.
†Platelets have a minute amount of red blood cells that might potentially cause Rh sensitization in Rh− patients. If giving Rh+ platelets is necessary, Rh immune globulin should be considered (Rh+ patients can always receive any Rh− products).
We wish to thank the Blood Bank of Children's Memorial Hospital.

RBCs may be transfused in several forms: fresh whole blood, citrated whole blood, citrated PRBCs, or frozen PRBCs (Table 12–4). Ease of administration and availability greatly favors citrated PRBCs, the preferred means of red cell transfusion in clinical practice. Frozen PRBCs offer theoretical advantages in that they pose less chance for transmission of viral disease, cause less HLA and blood group sensitization, offer better preservation of 2,3-diphosphoglycerate (2,3-DPG), and cause no elevation of potassium or citrate. However, for a variety of reasons, especially cost, frozen PRBCs are not generally available.

Although some benefits may exist with transfusion of whole blood in children, its availability limits its utility on a widespread basis.[27] Directed donor blood is the most common source of whole blood for children. Donor whole blood must be ABO-identical to the recipient. PRBCs must be ABO-compatible, but because of the reduced plasma volume contained therein, it need not be ABO-identical. Whole blood units typically contain a volume of 450 to 500 mL with a hematocrit of 35% to 38%; PRBCs contain approximately 350 mL with a hematocrit of 55% to 65%. Directed donor blood products from first- or second-degree relatives should be irradiated to prevent the possibility of transfusion-associated graft-versus-host disease.[28]

Fresh Frozen Plasma

Fresh frozen plasma (FFP) represents the fluid portion of whole blood that is separated and frozen within 8 hours of collection. It contains all clotting factors at normal concentrations when administered within 6 hours of thawing. The volume of 1 unit varies from 180 to 300 mL and represents approximately 7 to 10% of the coagulation factor activity in a 70 kg patient. After 6 hours, the levels of labile factors V and VIII begin to diminish.[29] FFP does not provide functional platelets and usually requires 30 to 45 minutes to thaw and crossmatch. FFP should be ABO-compatible with recipient red cells. If the recipient's blood type is not known, plasma from a donor with blood type AB may be administered. FFP contains proportionally more citrate than whole blood. Its use may be associated with citrate toxicity, particularly with rapid administration (see later).

Fresh frozen plasma is frequently administered without clear hematologic indication. The major surgical indication for FFP is coagulopathy associated with massive blood transfusion. Other indications include the emergency reversal of warfarin and the presence of a specific coagulation abnormality, congenital or acquired, in which a factor concentrate is either not available or insufficient to correct. Relatively strict guidelines are worth emphasis, because there is evidence that should a unit of FFP be capable of transmitting HIV, then there is a greater likelihood that the recipient will develop the disease with FFP than with PRBCs, presumably because of greater viral exposure.[30]

Platelets

Platelets are essential to hemostasis associated with the vascular injury of surgery and thus are necessary for the control of surgical bleeding. Two major categories of patients may require platelet transfusion therapy: (1) those whose platelet count or function, or both, has fallen gradually, secondary to disease or therapeutic intervention, and (2) those whose platelet count has decreased rapidly because of massive blood loss and subsequent transfusion (dilutional thrombocytopenia). Many medications, such as aspirin and ketorolac, cause abnormal platelet function, which may interfere with surgical hemostasis.[31–33]

A patient whose platelet count has fallen gradually to the 10,000 to 20,000/mm³ range does not usually require additional platelets unless there are overt signs of clinical bleeding or a surgical procedure is imminent.[34–37] A patient whose platelet count has rapidly decreased secondary to massive transfusion may require a significantly higher platelet count for hemostasis (50,000 to 75,000/mm³).[35, 38, 39]

There is no clear-cut threshold regarding platelet count and clinical bleeding in the perioperative period; each patient must be individually assessed by the constant observation of the surgical field for evidence of abnormal bleeding.[40] If the thrombocytopenia relates to drug therapy, fewer platelets

Table 12–4. Differences in Composition of Major Blood Products

	Normal Whole Blood (In Vivo)	Citrated Whole Blood (2 wk old) ACD/CPD	Citrated PRBCs*	Frozen PRBCs	Fresh Frozen Plasma
Ph	7.4	6.6–6.9	6.6–6.9	6.6–7.2	6.6–6.9
Pco₂	35–45	180–210	180–210	0–10	180–210
Base deficit (mEq/L)	0	9–15	9–15	?	9–15
Potassium† (mEq/L)	3.5–5.0	18–26	18–26	1–2	4–8
Citrate	None	2 +	1 +	None	4 +
Factors V and VIII	Normal	20–50%	20–50%	None	85–100%
Fibrinogen	Normal	Normal	Normal	None	Normal
Platelets	240,000–400,000	None	None	None	None
2,3-DPG	Normal	3% of normal	3% of normal	Nearly normal	—
Hematocrit	35–45	35–45	60–70	50–95	—
Temperature (°C)	37	4–6	4–6	4–6	Cold

*Citrated whole blood and citrated PRBCs have the same chemical composition, but citrated PRBCs have considerably less plasma volume.
†Potassium values may increase up to 50–60 mEq/L depending on how long the blood is stored or the length of time after thawing.[124, 126–131, 133, 433, 434]
ACD/CPD, acid-citrate-dextrose/citrate-phosphate-dextrose; 2,3-DPG, 2,3-diphosphoglycerate; Pco₂, carbon dioxide tension; PRBCs, packed red blood cells.
Modified from Miller RD: Transfusion therapy and associated problems. Refresher Courses in Anesthesiology 1973;1:101.

will be required than if the thrombocytopenia is secondary to an immunologic abnormality. Similarly, a patient with ongoing consumption of platelets, as in disseminated intravascular coagulopathy (DIC), has much higher platelet requirements than a patient with dilutional thrombocytopenia, owing to massive blood replacement. Some patients who have suffered massive trauma and had multiple transfusions may develop a thrombocytopathy in which platelets are present in adequate numbers but their function is impaired.[41] The most expeditious way to assess platelet function preoperatively is to measure the bleeding time.[36, 42–44] This is rarely an option in the operating room, so other means (clinical observation, thromboelastography) become necessary.[45–48]

A patient occasionally presents for surgery with a prolonged bleeding time, and the hematologist recommends a platelet transfusion before the operation. If the patient has a normal platelet count and the prolonged bleeding time can be ascribed to platelet dysfunction (thrombocytopathy), then it is our practice to have the platelets available in the operating room but to withhold transfusion until the patient demonstrates pathologic bleeding. Such patients frequently do not require platelet transfusion. Conversely, if bleeding poses a threat to the patient's life or the success of the operation, as in neurosurgery or middle ear surgery, then it is reasonable to administer platelets immediately before the surgical procedure or, if possible, to postpone the surgery until the bleeding time has returned to normal.[36] Transfusion with platelets obtained from a single donor (apheresis) reduces the total donor pool exposure.

One standard unit of platelets represents the platelets separated from a unit of whole blood that are then suspended in a small volume of plasma from that unit. Platelets must be stored at 20° to 24°C with gentle continuous agitation for a maximum of 5 days. Platelets obtained by apheresis represent a greater number of platelets per unit and are equivalent to approximately 6 to 8 units of individual donor platelets.[49]

One standard unit of single donor platelets would be expected to increase the platelet count of a 70 kg adult by 5000 to 10,000/mm^3 and increase the count in an 18 kg child by 20,000/mm^3.[50, 51] A common dose for pediatric patients is 0.1 to 0.3 U/kg of body weight; this usually produces an increment of 20,000 to 70,000/mm^3. If one is dealing with dilutional thrombocytopenia with ongoing losses, a larger transfusion of platelets (0.3 U/kg or more) may be required to boost the platelet count above 50,000/mm^3. The use of platelet apheresis has the potential to markedly reduce the exposure to different donors and therefore the risk of disease transmission.[52] In addition, there are some data suggesting that a greater initial increment of platelets reduces the need for additional platelets.[53, 54] Anesthesiologists should anticipate the need for platelets so that excessive surgical bleeding does not occur during the wait for platelets to be prepared by the blood bank. The decision to administer platelets must not be made lightly. The more frequently platelets are administered, the greater will be the antibody production, which may lead to a shortened half-life for future transfused platelets.[50, 51] Additionally, platelet transfusions may result in the exposure to multiple donors and therefore increase the risk of viral disease transmission. When the use of multiple platelet units is expected, single donor apheresis platelet concentrates should be sought and utilized if available.

Several additional points should be considered: (1) Not all hospitals have platelets readily available. Unless the need is anticipated before surgery, platelets may not be available when required. (2) For patients who are thrombocytopenic before surgery, it is recommended that platelets be infused just before the surgical procedure to ensure the highest levels during the time of peak demand. (3) Platelets should be filtered only by the large-pore filters ($\geq$ 150 μm); micropore filters may adsorb large numbers of platelets and therefore diminish the effectiveness of a platelet transfusion.[55] (4) Platelets are suspended in plasma, which may help to replenish diminished coagulation factors and decrease the need for FFP.[56] Four to five units of platelets provide clotting factors equivalent to 1 unit of FFP. (5) Platelets should not be refrigerated once released from the blood bank and prior to administration. They should be gently agitated to decrease clumping.

Cryoprecipitate

Cryoprecipitate is a concentrated plasma protein fraction that contains 20 to 50% of the factor VIII of plasma.[57, 58] It also contains von Willebrand factor (vWF), fibrinogen, and factor XIII. It is indicated for the treatment of von Willebrand disease unresponsive to desmopressin (DDAVP), hemophilia A when factor VIII concentrates are unavailable (rare), factor XIII deficiency, and hypofibrinogenemia.

In patients who have von Willebrand disease and are resistant to DDAVP, we withhold infusion of cryoprecipitate until surgery has begun to reduce unnecessary transfusions, unless surgery is performed in an area where bleeding is potentially life threatening. These patients often do not demonstrate pathologic bleeding despite a prolonged bleeding time or other hematologic abnormality.

Factor Concentrates

The most commonly administered factor concentrate is factor VIII, utilized in the treatment of hemophilia A. Patients with hemophilia have many problems related to their disease, including splenomegaly, abnormal liver function, joint disease related to hemarthrosis, the possibility of the hepatitis or the HIV carrier state, or fully manifested AIDS.[59–61] Careful planning of any surgical procedure must entail close communication with the patient's hematologist to ensure optimal therapy while reducing unnecessary transfusions. This is particularly important if one is considering the use of pooled concentrates, which may contain the blood products from 2500 to 25,000 donors.[58, 59, 62]

The treatment of patients with hemophilia has undergone radical changes during recent years.[58, 62] At one point, it was estimated that approximately 70% of patients with hemophilia were infected with HIV, and a massive effort was made to remove viral contamination from the donor pool. Additionally, increasing evidence suggests that extraneous proteins and living or killed virus material are suppressive to the immunologic system, making the hemophilia recipient even more susceptible to HIV activation—that is, converting from HIV carrier to active AIDS.[57, 58, 62]

Many methods to kill live virus have been developed to improve the safety of transfused blood products; these include at least eight variations of heat treatment, viral detergent cleansing, and affinity chromatography. Although these steps are positive and necessary, the greater purity has resulted in markedly higher costs and shortages.[57, 59] Genetically engineered factor VIII and factor IX provide hope for the future by eliminating all of these steps and safely controlling the disease.[63–66] In addition, there is some evidence suggesting a better response and a reduced level of factor inhibitors in patients who receive recombinant therapy compared with standard purified factor therapy.[67, 68] Some patients with mild hemophilia may respond to DDAVP therapy.[69, 70]

In patients with hemophilia, replacement is aimed at increasing the deficient factors, which are determined by measuring their content in a patient's plasma and knowing the concentrations in cryoprecipitate, factor concentrate, or recombinant replacement. The activity of 1 mL of normal plasma is defined as 1 unit. Each unit of factor VIII per kilogram results in an increase of factor VIII of approximately 2%, whereas the in vivo response to factor IX is less and ranges from 0.5 to 1.0% for each unit per kilogram. Consultation with a patient's hematologist is essential, especially in the presence of complicating factors such as factor VIII or factor IX inhibitors, which would greatly increase the factor replacement requirements.

In the past, patients with hemophilia B (Christmas disease), factor IX deficiency, were generally treated with commercially available concentrates that contain prothrombin and factors VII, IX, and X. These concentrates pose a significant risk of hepatitis and HIV, so judicious use must be planned. For minor surgical procedures, an attempt is often made to manage the bleeding with single-donor FFP rather than the commercially available pooled concentrates, which pose a much higher risk than single donor products. Clinical trials using recombinant human factor IX in animals and human studies of patients using highly purified factor IX (preparations devoid of factors VII, X, and prothrombin) are very promising.[71–76]

Desmopressin (DDAVP)

Desmopressin, or DDAVP (1-deamino-8-D-arginine vasopressin), a synthetic analogue of vasopressin, can increase factor VIII:C and factor VIII:vWF.[70, 77–81] A dose of 0.3 μg/kg (IV or SC) increases factor VIII:C and VIII:vWF two- to threefold within 30 to 60 minutes, with a half-life for factors VIII:C and VIII:vWF of 3 to 6 hours.[78] Intranasal DDAVP is also effective but less rapid. It is important to be aware that not all patients are "responders" and that such therapy may be suitable for minor but not for major surgical procedures.[82, 83]

DDAVP has also been used to treat the coagulopathy associated with uremia and cirrhosis.[84] It may also have a role in patients undergoing elective surgical procedures with the high potential for blood loss, such as cardiac surgery and spine fusion.[70, 85–88] Although these studies demonstrated a benefit in patients without a pre-existing coagulopathy, other studies show none, despite increases in factors VIII:C and VIII:vWF.[89–91] Because of the potential for hyponatremia secondary to water retention, particularly in small children, and other problems such as tachyphylaxis, stimulation of fibrinolysis, mild hypotension, and tachycardia, therapy

should be reserved for those with a high likelihood of clinical effect.[70]

Massive Blood Transfusion

Massive blood transfusion may be defined as replacing a patient's entire blood volume one or more times. As previously emphasized, when dealing with children, the anesthesiologist must think in terms of percent of blood volume lost rather than units of blood lost. In addition, it is important to appreciate the composition of each blood component to anticipate problems and at what stage of transfusion these problems might occur (see Table 12–4). The use of large quantities of blood components may seriously affect coagulation, potassium and calcium concentrations, acid-base balance, body temperature, oxygen-hemoglobin dissociation, and hematocrit.

Coagulopathy

The coagulopathy of massive blood transfusion is primarily related to dilution of either clotting factors or platelets. The point at which clotting factor deficiency sufficient to produce coagulopathy occurs is dependent on the volume of blood lost, the type of blood component transfused (PRBCs vs whole blood), and the presence or absence of DIC.[38, 92–104] Coagulopathy is also related to severity of hypothermia, thus indicating the importance of maintaining body temperature through the use of efficient blood warming devices.[105–107] Coagulopathy in the trauma patient is also related to the severity of metabolic acidosis at the time of presentation to the hospital.[108] Dilutional thrombocytopenia sufficient to cause clinical bleeding depends on the starting platelet count, the volume of blood lost, and the presence or absence of DIC. Excluding the use of fresh whole blood, which is exceedingly rare, the platelet count is not affected by the type of blood product transfused, since no other red cell product contains viable platelets.

Factor Deficiency

There are minimal published data regarding the effects of massive blood transfusion in children. As clinicians, we are dependent on clinical experience and extrapolation from investigations using adult patients. A study of trauma patients during the Vietnam War found that the onset of clinical bleeding occurred after about 15 units of *whole blood* had been transfused. The incidence of coagulopathy was unrelated to abnormal prothrombin time (PT) or partial thromboplastin time (PTT) but was highly correlated with a platelet count of less than 65,000/mm³.[38] In an average-sized adult male who weighs 70 kg, the estimated blood volume is approximately 5 L (70 mL/kg × 70 kg = 4900 mL), or approximately 10 units of whole blood. To relate the data given in Figure 12–1 to children, one should assume each 10 units of whole blood in a normal-sized adult male to be equivalent to one blood volume. One would thus anticipate that some children would develop coagulopathy after 1.5 blood volumes lost, but the majority of children would develop clinical bleeding after 2.0 to 2.5 blood volumes lost. *This applies only if replacement is with citrated whole blood*

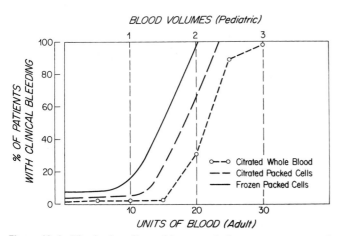

BLOOD VOLUMES (Pediatric)

Figure 12–1. The broken line with open circles represents a study of the use of citrated whole blood in adults; bleeding in most cases was secondary to dilutional thrombocytopenia. Other lines represent postulated points of dilutional clotting factor deficiency if solely citrated packed cells or frozen cells are transfused. Note that because no clotting factors are present in frozen blood, dilutional clotting factor deficiency would likely occur earliest with exclusively frozen red blood cell transfusions. (Modified from Miller RD: Transfusion therapy and associated problems. ASA Refresher Courses in Anesthesiology 1973;1:107.)

or modified whole blood, which still contains moderate quantities of clotting factors. The coagulopathy would be due to thrombocytopenia, not clotting factor deficiency. Other studies of massive blood loss with whole blood replacement appear to support this conclusion.[38, 92–99]

Laboratory assessment of developing coagulopathy can play an important part in transfusion decisions; however, availability of results in a timely fashion can limit their utility. The PT measures the adequacy of factors VII, X, V, prothrombin, and fibrinogen (the extrinsic system).[38] The PTT assesses the adequacy of factors XII, XI, IX, VIII, X, V, prothrombin, and fibrinogen (intrinsic system).[109] Banked citrated whole blood has all blood components but a reduced concentration of factors V and VIII (20 to 50% of normal [see Table 12–4]). For coagulopathy secondary to a clotting factor deficiency to develop, factor VIII must decrease to less than 30% of normal, and factor V to less than 20% of normal.[92] For this to occur, at least three blood volumes must be exchanged with citrated *whole blood.* The first coagulation test result to be altered is the PTT, because factor VIII would be diluted to less than 30%.

If replacement is being made with citrated PRBCs, as is current practice with modern blood banking techniques, then minimal plasma is administered, because 70 to 80% of the plasma has been separated into the FFP fraction. Massive replacement with PRBCs results in dilution of factors V and VIII, as well as all other clotting factors including fibrinogen.[97, 99, 100, 110] Clotting factor deficiency is unlikely when replacement is made with whole blood but is very likely with massive PRBC transfusion (see Fig. 12–1). Data suggest that prolongation of the PT or PTT occurs at higher clotting factor values in patients with multiple clotting factor deficiencies, as during massive blood replacement with component therapy, than with isolated individual clotting factor deficiency, as in congenital coagulopathies or massive trans-

fusion with *whole* blood (isolated factor V and VIII deficiency).[99, 100] One study of adult patients transfused exclusively with PRBCs and crystalloid demonstrated a clear relationship between dilution of multiple clotting factors and the volume of blood transfused; moderate prolongations of the PT and PTT exist without overt signs of clinical bleeding.[99] The indication for FFP should be onset of clinical coagulopathy or a documented deficiency of fibrinogen (< 75 mg/100 mL). No published studies have examined massive blood replacement in the pediatric population using exclusively component therapy.

Our experience with 26 children 12 ± 4 years, weight 41.9 ± 15.8 kg (22 Harrington Rod procedures, 3 tumor excisions, 1 Whipple procedure) who did not receive FFP or whole blood during surgical procedures involving blood loss of 0.5 to 1.0 blood volumes found that none of the children demonstrated clinical signs of coagulopathy. Slight prolongations of the PT or PTT occurred when blood loss was 1 blood volume or less (Table 12–5). Two children lost 1.5 blood volumes, and one lost 2.0 blood volumes; all had prolongations of the PT, and two had prolongations of the PTT (>1.5 × control). The only patient who had signs of coagulopathy was the child who lost 2 blood volumes, and the coagulopathy could also have been ascribed to simultaneous dilutional thrombocytopenia.[111, 112]

Few data are available to clearly define how much of a change in the PT or PTT correlates with clinical coagulopathy. However, the consensus panel of the National Institutes of Health and others suggest that greater than 1.5 times normal should be considered in the pathologic range.[40, 94, 98, 113–117] Our studies suggest that clinically important prolongations of the PT and PTT to greater than 1.5 times normal occur when blood loss equals or exceeds 1.5 blood volumes and replacement has been made exclusively with either citrated or frozen PRBCs and crystalloid or 5% albumin.[111, 112] Our clinical practice is to transfuse FFP in a volume of at least 25 to 33% for each blood volume lost after blood losses exceed specific volumes and replacement has been made exclusively with one type of blood product (Table 12–6). The indications for and timing of FFP transfusion therefore depend on which blood product has been transfused, the volume of that transfusion as it relates to a

Table 12–5. Changes in Prothrombin and Partial Thromboplastin Times During Massive Blood Transfusions in Children Receiving Either Packed Red Blood Cells and 5% Albumin or Packed Red Blood Cells and Crystalloid

	Prothrombin Time			
Blood Volumes Lost	Baseline	0.5	0.75	1.0
N	26	16	12	10
Mean ± SD	10.9 ± 0.96	12.5 ± 0.77	13.2 ± 0.76	13.6 ± 0.98
Range	9.3–12.0	11.4–14.0	11.4–14.2	11.9–15.8
	Partial Thromboplastin Time			
Mean ± SD	31.8 ± 4.4	38.0 ± 4.9	40 ± 5.4	45.1 ± 13.1
Range	25–45.9	28.1 – 59.6	33–51.5	25.6–60

Table 12–6. Minimal Fresh Frozen Plasma (FFP) Recommendations According to the Type of Blood Product Transfused and the Volume of Blood Lost

Type of Blood Replaced	Junction at Which FFP Is Indicated	Volume FFP to Be Transfused
Citrated whole blood	2.0–3.0 blood volumes and each blood volume thereafter	25–33% of each blood volume lost
Citrated PRBCs	1–2 blood volumes and each blood volume thereafter	25–33% of each blood volume lost
Frozen PRBCs	0.75–1.50 blood volumes and each blood volume thereafter	25–33% of each blood volume lost

PRBCs, packed red blood cells.

patient's blood volume, and whether blood loss will continue either intraoperatively or postoperatively.

Thrombocytopenia (Dilutional)

A platelet count gives the number of circulating platelets (normal = 150,000 to 350,000/mm³), but the only uncomplicated laboratory test that is helpful in determining whether platelet function is normal is the bleeding time, and even this is controversial.[42–44, 118] For a patient with acute blood loss, a platelet count in excess of 50,000 to 75,000/mm³ is adequate to maintain hemostasis, whereas for a patient with a chronic platelet deficiency, the platelet count may be sufficient when greater than 10,000 to 15,000/mm³.[37, 119, 120] The reason for this difference is unknown.[38, 39, 41, 94–96, 117, 120]

Studies of adult and pediatric patients with acute dilutional thrombocytopenia found a high correlation of clinical bleeding with a platelet count of 65,000/mm³ or less.[36, 38, 92–100, 118] Figure 12–2 represents the calculated reduction in platelet count compared with the observed decline in platelet count in both adult and pediatric patients. The observed decrement is probably different from the calculated reduction because of increased platelet release from the bone marrow, lungs, and lymphatic tissue. The important point is that the platelet count usually did not decline to dangerous levels until 20 to 25 units of whole blood in adults or 2 blood volumes in children were lost.[39, 98, 120] Our observations of pediatric patients who lost 1 to 5 blood volumes correlate well with the studies of adults. Clinical bleeding did not occur in children whose platelet count remained above 50,000/mm³, despite blood losses as great as 5 blood volumes (Fig. 12–3A).[39] The starting platelet count was very important. For example, if a patient began surgery with 600,000/mm³ of platelets, dilutional thrombocytopenia did not occur until 4 or more blood volumes were lost. If the starting platelet count was approximately 100,000/mm³, however, then dilutional thrombocytopenia occurred after 1 blood volume was lost (Fig. 12–3B). Prophylactic transfusion of platelets is generally not indicated without documented evidence of dilutional thrombocytopenia, visible microvascular bleeding, and ongoing blood loss.[39, 40, 121] Some data suggest that platelets may not function normally (thrombocytopathy) after massive trauma, in patients with severe

liver disease, or in the presence of hypothermia.[42, 107, 122, 123] This did not occur in the pediatric patients we studied, whose temperature remained within the normal range.[39, 41, 92]

It is therefore important to perform basic clotting studies, especially a platelet count, before elective surgery when major blood loss can be anticipated, so that adequate blood is available. If coagulopathy appears earlier than expected, that is, before 1 blood volume loss, one should search for other causes of bleeding, such as increased arterial or venous pressure in the surgical field or possibly DIC.

In summary, the coagulopathy associated with massive blood transfusion using *whole blood* is usually secondary to dilutional thrombocytopenia, not clotting factor deficiency. When blood loss of 3 blood volumes or more occurs, dilution of labile clotting factors V and VIII may result. However, other factors such as thrombocytopathy must also be considered during such situations. In addition, with the increased use of component therapy, there is a greater tendency for dilution of all clotting factors and platelets. Thus, when any form of PRBCs is transfused in large quantity, the use of FFP must be considered early, that is, FFP should be thawed and ready to administer after loss of 1 blood volume, with anticipated need occurring after loss of approximately 1.5 blood volumes.

Hyperkalemia

Hyperkalemia is primarily a problem when whole blood is administered rapidly; whole blood may have a plasma potassium level as high as 26 mEq/L, the degree of potassium elevation being related to the shelf age.[92, 93] Hyperka-

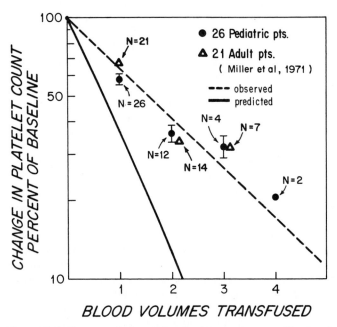

Figure 12–2. Percent of change in platelet count versus blood volumes transfused in adults and children.[39, 120] The broken line represents observed values, whereas the solid line represents calculated values. This difference suggests mobilization of platelets during massive transfusion. (From Coté CJ, Liu LMP, Szyfelbein SK, et al: Changes in serial platelet counts following massive blood transfusions in pediatric patients. Anesthesiology 1985;62:197–201.)

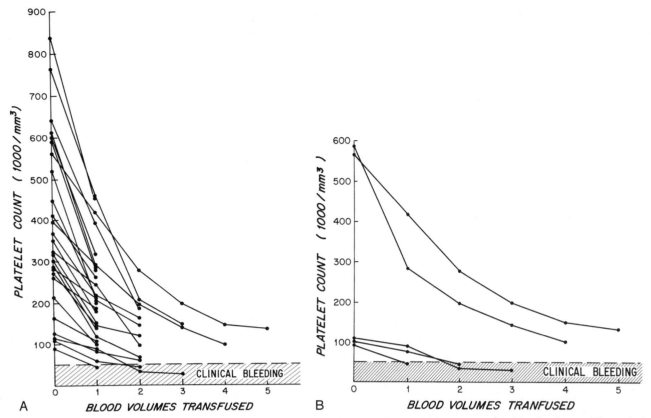

Figure 12–3. (A) Serial changes in platelet counts are plotted for 26 pediatric patients who lost one to five blood volumes. The majority of these patients suffered from severe thermal injuries, and many had relatively high platelet counts at baseline. Clinically evident signs of coagulopathy appeared when the platelet count fell below 50,000/mm³. (B) This illustration abstracts the platelet counts of five patients from the group represented in part A. The baseline platelet count is invaluable in estimating potential platelet needs in relation to blood volumes transfused. A low initial count suggests the potential need for early exogenous platelet transfusion, whereas a high initial platelet count indicates that exogenous platelets may not be required until several blood volumes have been lost. Note that the three patients who developed a coagulopathy began surgery with a relatively low platelet count, whereas the two patients with a very high platelet count did not require platelet transfusion despite the loss of four and five blood volumes. (From Coté CJ, Liu LMP, Szyfelbein SK, et al: Changes in serial platelet counts following massive blood transfusions in pediatric patients. Anesthesiology 1985;62:197–201.)

lemia reflects leakage of intracellular potassium into the extracellular space and has occurred in adults who receive more than 120 mL/min of citrated whole blood and in children undergoing massive blood transfusion.[124–126] Relating this amount to a patient's weight:

$$120 \text{ mL} = 1/4 \text{ adult unit of whole blood/min}$$
$$= 1/40 \text{ blood volume/min}$$
$$= 1.5 \text{ to } 2.0 \text{ mL/kg/min.}$$

The need to relate the size of the patient to the speed of blood replacement rarely occurs clinically in adults but is important to consider in an infant or small child. Table 12–4 clearly shows that hyperkalemia would be a problem with old whole blood and would not usually occur with citrated PRBCs because of the small plasma volume. Although citrated PRBCs have significant intracellular loss of potassium, resulting in a supernatant potassium concentration in excess of 60 mEq/L after 14 days of storage, clinically important hyperkalemia following *routine* transfusion has not been reported.[127–129] A study of serum potassium in neonates following exchange transfusion with PRBCs has documented a decrease in serum potassium values despite the high potas-

sium content in the supernatant measured before administration.[130] A retrospective study of children undergoing massive intraoperative transfusion with PRBCs documented transient, but not life-threatening, hyperkalemia.[126] It appears that despite very high supernatant potassium values, clinically important hyperkalemia does not usually occur when citrated PRBCs are administered. This may be because of the combination of rapid absorption of potassium into the potassium-depleted cells following transfusion, dilution with crystalloid or albumin during administration, dilution by the patient's blood, or slow administration due to the high viscosity when not diluted.

With the use of autologous predonated blood and with directed donor blood, the availability of whole blood has increased; it is advisable to transfuse whole blood to children with caution, because hyperkalemia may occur. We observed a 15-year-old 40 kg child (EBV 2800 mL) who donated his own blood before spinal instrumentation, whose intraoperative potassium level rose from 3.5 to 6.3 mEq/L following transfusion of 2 units of whole blood (900 mL). This child did not require treatment; however, the remaining 3 units of whole blood were returned to the blood bank and converted to PRBCs. In this situation, it would be advisable to pack the oldest blood and retain the freshest as whole blood. These concerns about hyperkalemia are more important in young pediatric patients, in whom a unit of blood product constitutes a relatively large proportion of the circulating blood volume and to whom the blood is rapidly administered.

When the rate of infusion of citrated whole blood exceeds 1.5 to 2.0 mL/kg/min, the electrocardiogram must be closely monitored. Should ventricular arrhythmias occur with peaked T waves, appropriate treatment for hyperkalemia is instituted pending measurement of the serum potassium level (calcium chloride or calcium gluconate, hyperventilation, sodium bicarbonate, glucose and insulin, Kayexalate). One death has been reported following neonatal exchange transfusion with whole blood that was less than 48 hours old. A study of the fresh whole blood used for exchange transfusion at that institution revealed 30% of units to have a potassium level greater than 9 mEq/L and 21% to have a potassium level greater than 11 mEq/L.[131] This complication occurred with relatively fresh blood. It would be advantageous to administer citrated PRBCs or washed PRBCs that are less than 5 days old to avoid hyperkalemia in neonates requiring massive blood transfusion. *If whole blood is to be used in a neonate, it is advised that the potassium level be measured before administration.* Another potential source of hyperkalemia is blood that has been irradiated to reduce the potential for graft-versus-host disease. Units of red blood cells that have been irradiated have a higher potassium value than nonirradiated PRBCs, especially if they have been stored for greater than 1 week after irradiation.[132] Cardiac arrest and death of an adult patient with the use of a rapid transfusion device has been reported. This patient received adenosine/dextrose/saline-preserved PRBCs with a supernatant potassium concentration of approximately 24 to 34 mEq/L at a rate of 6.4 mL/kg/min.[133] Such high rates of transfusion are possible in infants and children even without such devices.[126, 134, 135] If the potential for such a rapid transfusion can be anticipated, washing the cells just before infusion may reduce the potential for transfusion-related hyperkalemia.[133]

Hypocalcemia

Hypocalcemia may occur with massive blood transfusion of whole blood due to the binding of ionized calcium (Ca^{++}) with sodium citrate.[136–139] Clinically, it is rare for hypocalcemia to occur unless the rate of transfusion is very rapid; in adults, this rate must be 1 unit of whole blood over 3 to 4 minutes.[136] In adult cardiac surgical patients who received citrated whole blood at 1.5 mL/kg/min, there was no improvement in the ventricular function curve, that is, no increase in cardiac output and a decrease in Ca^{++} occurred. When a similar volume of heparinized blood was administered at the same rate, there was an increase in cardiac output and no change in Ca^{++}, that is, there was a normal Frank-Starling response to volume loading.[140] These findings correlate well with earlier studies; one would expect ionized hypocalcemia of clinical importance (decreased cardiac contractility) to occur when the rate of infusion of citrated whole blood exceeds 1.5 to 2.0 mL/kg/min.[136, 140] The problem of ionized hypocalcemia following large volumes of *citrated PRBCs* has not been examined, but it is unlikely that clinically significant hypocalcemia would result.

The rates of infusion of citrated whole blood that produce hypocalcemia and hyperkalemia are nearly identical. Although the cardiac electrophysiologic effects produced by hypocalcemia and hyperkalemia are opposite, the treatment for both is administration of exogenous calcium. It is important to observe the electrocardiogram for abnormalities, especially widening of the QRS complex, prolonged QT interval, and flattening or peaking of the T wave.[92, 141] Studies of laboratory animals and children with extensive thermal injuries demonstrated that both calcium chloride and calcium gluconate dissociate at a similar rate, that is, hepatic metabolism of the gluconate moiety is not necessary (Fig. 12–4A, B).[142] Other studies during the anhepatic phase of liver transplantation also found equal ionization of calcium chloride and calcium gluconate, clearly proving that hepatic metabolism is not required to release calcium from gluconate.[143] Therefore, either calcium chloride or calcium gluconate may be used to treat acute ionized hypocalcemia. Note that calcium gluconate contains one third the ionizable calcium of calcium chloride and therefore should be administered at a threefold higher dose (milligrams per kilogram) than calcium chloride. Frequent small boluses are as effective as single large boluses and result in smaller fluctuations in plasma Ca^{++} values.[142] Ideally, both forms of calcium should be slowly administered through a large peripheral or central vein, because both are highly sclerosing.

Fresh frozen plasma contains relatively more citrate than whole blood, and thus, milliliter for milliliter, FFP is potentially more hazardous than citrated whole blood. Caution is urged whenever FFP is rapidly infused, especially if the patient already has a low Ca^{++} level. Figure 12–5A presents the changes in Ca^{++} that occurred in children who had extensive thermal injury and received rapid FFP infusions of 1.0 to 2.5 mL/kg/min for 5 minutes. The maximal change in Ca^{++} occurred between the fourth and fifth minute; there was no difference between the three highest rates of FFP infusion.[144] If exogenous calcium is administered *during* rapid FFP transfusion, dangerous ionized hypocalcemia can be avoided (Fig. 12–5B). We also studied six children who received FFP at a rate of 2 mL/kg/min for 10 minutes (equivalent to an average-sized adult receiving 1400 mL FFP over 10 minutes). We found highly significant reductions in Ca^{++}, but no consistent adverse cardiovascular events.[144] A laboratory study examining the effects of citrate-induced ionized hypocalcemia and halothane anesthesia in a dog model found significantly greater cardiovascular depression with the higher level of expired halothane.[145] These findings are consistent with the combined myocardial depression caused by ionized hypocalcemia and the myocardial depressant effects of calcium channel blockade caused by the halothane.[146, 147]

The adverse cardiac effects of citrate-induced hypocalcemia may be increased if FFP is rapidly administered through a central venous catheter. Therefore, FFP may be more safely administered through a peripheral intravenous site. Calcium administration should be carried out *during* rapid transfusion of FFP (more than 1 mL/kg/min) to minimize this transient but dangerous citrate toxicity, especially in the presence of anesthesia with potent anesthetic agents.[145–147] Our clinical impression is that neonates and small infants are particularly susceptible to the development of citrate toxicity because it is easier to administer a rela-

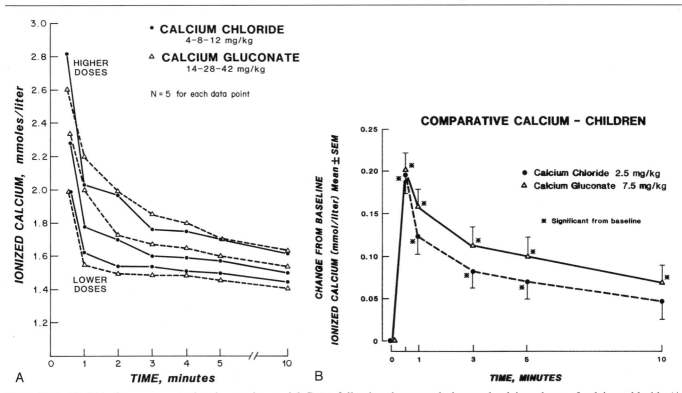

Figure 12–4. (A) This figure presents the changes in arterial Ca^{++} following three equal elemental calcium doses of calcium chloride (4, 8, 12 mg/kg) or calcium gluconate (14, 28, 42 mg/kg) in dogs. The rate of change in Ca^{++} was identical for each form of calcium at each dose. There was no significant difference between the highest and lowest doses after 2 minutes, suggesting that frequent low doses are equally effective and perhaps safer than large boluses of exogenous calcium. (B) Changes in arterial ionized calcium in children who received equal elemental doses of calcium chloride and calcium gluconate. Note that at 30 seconds, both forms of calcium have dissociated equally; these data indicate that hepatic metabolism of the gluconate moiety is not required to liberate ionized calcium from calcium gluconate. (From Coté CJ, Drop LJ, Daniels AL, et al: Calcium chloride versus calcium gluconate: Comparison of ionization and cardiovascular effects in children and dogs. Anesthesiology 1987; 66:465–470.)

tively large quantity of FFP over a brief period of time and because the elimination of citrate (first-pass effect through the liver) may be compromised in these patients. In addition to thermally injured patients, patients undergoing liver transplantation and cardiac surgery are also likely to require FFP and develop hypocalcemia.[148, 149] Liver transplantation patients in particular are susceptible to ionized hypocalcemia during the anhepatic phase and during the preanhepatic phase of surgery because of impaired hepatic metabolism, impaired hepatic blood flow, and the inability to metabolize citrate.[150–153] An intravenous preparation of calcium should always be available whenever major blood loss is anticipated.

Disseminated Intravascular Coagulopathy

Disseminated intravascular coagulopathy is frequently associated with shock. When dealing with massive blood loss, it is crucial that DIC be differentiated from dilutional coagulopathy. Making the distinction may be difficult, because both are associated with pathologic oozing of blood in the surgical field and each may result in prolongation of the PT and PTT, as well as thrombocytopenia. With massive replacement using whole blood or PRBCs and *adequate* FFP, the fibrinogen level should remain normal; with DIC, it may be decreased. However, it is important to appreciate that replacement with PRBCs, albumin, and crystalloid also leads to a reduction in fibrinogen. The most helpful test for DIC is to document a

significant increase in fibrin split products.[154–158] If pathologic oozing in the surgical field is observed and 1 blood volume or less has been lost in a patient who had a normal platelet count as well as normal PT and PTT, it should be suspected that the patient has developed a coagulopathy. The most effective treatment for DIC is to eliminate the cause, for example, by correcting shock, acidosis, or sepsis; heparin therapy remains controversial.[154, 158]

Acid-Base Balance

Massive transfusion is usually needed in two situations:

1. Severe trauma with shock
2. Major surgery in which the intravascular volume is maintained.

In the first situation, severe metabolic acidosis may result because of low cardiac output and diminished oxygen delivery. In this circumstance, correction of the acidosis with sodium bicarbonate may be a necessary part of the resuscitation, along with blood volume replacement. In this situation, impaired coagulation may occur because of the acidosis.[105] In the operating room, intravascular volume is usually maintained and replacement of the blood loss is more controlled. Even with repeated massive blood loss, metabolic acidosis is not usually a problem, provided severe hypovolemia is avoided.[159–161] *Sodium bicarbonate therapy must therefore be*

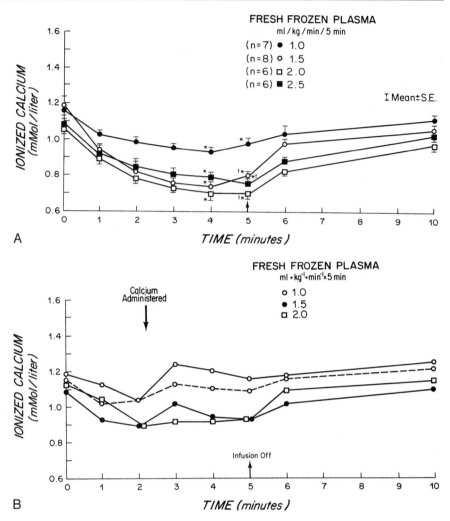

Figure 12–5. (A) Changes in arterial Ca^{++} in children with severe thermal injuries during fresh frozen plasma infusions of 1.0 to 2.5 mL/kg/min for 5 minutes administered by an infusion pump. Note the dangerous though transient fall in Ca^{++}, with the nadir occurring between the fourth and fifth minute. Ionized hypocalcemia occurs whenever the infusion rate equals or exceeds 1 mL/kg/min. (B) This figure demonstrates the change in Ca^{++} in four thermally injured patients who received calcium chloride (arrow) after 2 minutes of fresh frozen plasma infusion. Note that there were no sharp increases or decreases in Ca^{++}. (From the International Anesthesia Research Society: Anesthesia and Analgesia 1988;67:152–160.)

governed by actual measurement of acid-base status, because metabolic acidosis does not occur with massive transfusion unless accompanied by severe hypovolemia, low cardiac output, or hypoxemia. To the contrary, with uncomplicated massive blood transfusion, the patient may develop a moderate to severe *metabolic alkalosis* due to the metabolism of citrate.[137, 149, 162] Routine administration of alkali may have deleterious effects on oxygen-hemoglobin dissociation (see later).

Hypothermia

Hypothermia is a significant problem associated with major blood loss and its replacement. Hypothermia causes an increase in oxygen consumption, a leftward shift of the oxygen-hemoglobin dissociation curve, and a potential for refractory ventricular tachycardia.[92, 163, 164] In addition, hypothermia can have profound effects on platelet function and the coagulation cascade.[105–107] As shown in Table 12–4, all banked blood products except platelets and freshly thawed FFP have a temperature of 4° to 6°C and therefore must be warmed before infusion. Prolonged warming or overheating (greater than 42°C) may result in RBC hemolysis. Warming blood and all other intravenous infusions with a high capacity blood warmer, using hot air warming blankets and radiant warmers, placing plastic wrap around ex-

tremities, inserting a heated humidifier in the anesthesia circuit, covering the patient's head, and maintaining a warm operating room all help maintain body heat (see Chapter 27). Rapid transfusion devices markedly improve both the rapidity of transfusion and the thermokinetics involved.[165–170] Such devices can be important in the management of trauma, liver transplantation, reconstruction, cardiac, or oncologic surgical cases, when patients may require rapid, massive blood transfusion.

Oxygen-Hemoglobin Dissociation

Oxygen binding to hemoglobin is primarily dependent on temperature, acid-base status, and 2,3-DPG. Figure 12–6 illustrates these effects on the oxygen-hemoglobin dissociation curve. Citrate is rapidly metabolized to bicarbonate and thus causes metabolic alkalosis within hours of massive transfusion.[131, 149] If exogenous bicarbonate therapy is superimposed on this endogenous metabolic alkalosis, a significant effect on the dissociation of oxygen and hemoglobin could result. It is important to determine the acid-base status *before* administering sodium bicarbonate to avoid intensifying the left shift caused by hypothermia and metabolized citrate. Citrated whole blood and FFP therefore have the greatest effect on the oxygen-hemoglobin dissociation curve because of the large volume of citrate contained in these

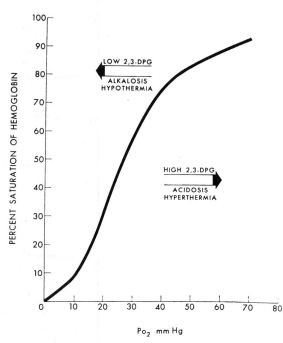

Figure 12–6. Oxygen-hemoglobin dissociation curve with alterations that can shift the curve to the right or left. A leftward shift indicates a low P_{50} or increased affinity of hemoglobin for oxygen; thus, less oxygen is released to tissues. (From Miller RD: Transfusion therapy and associated problems. ASA Refresher Courses in Anesthesiology 1973;1:102.)

blood products. Citrated PRBCs have little citrate and therefore minimal effects.

Oxygen binding to hemoglobin is affected by 2,3-DPG; a low 2,3-DPG level results in less oxygen delivery to tissue secondary to increased affinity of oxygen for hemoglobin.[164, 171] Citrated whole blood and PRBCs rapidly lose 2,3-DPG, but frozen blood maintains it at nearly normal levels (Tables 12–4 and 12–7).

Each type of blood component has slightly different effects on the oxygen-hemoglobin dissociation curve; the point at which these factors are clinically important has yet to be fully evaluated in pediatric patients. Frozen blood would

Table 12–7. The Effect of Stored Blood Products on the Oxygen-Hemoglobin Dissociation Curve

	Temperature	2,3-Diphospho-glycerate	Acid Load
Fresh Frozen Plasma	←	0	→
			→
Citrated Whole Blood	←	←	→
	←	←	→
	←	←	
Citrated Packed Cells	←	←	→
	←	←	
Frozen Packed Cells	←	0	→
	←		

←, Left shift; →, right shift; 0, none present. Multiple arrows indicate greater effect.

appear to have significant advantages, because 2,3-DPG levels are preserved and it is citrate free (see Table 12–4). For most patients, any shift in the oxygen-hemoglobin dissociation curve is readily corrected by compensatory mechanisms, such as increased cardiac output or vasodilation. However, when a vascular bed is compromised (e.g., cardiac and cerebral), then severe shifts in the oxygen-hemoglobin dissociation curve may result in tissue hypoxemia.[172, 173]

Pulmonary Effects

Laboratory evidence suggests that embolism of fibrinous debris contained in blood products may be detrimental to pulmonary function; however, this has not been confirmed clinically.[174, 175] Large quantities of fibrinous material are removed by micropore filtration.[176, 177] If large transfusions are expected, a micropore filter should be used with all blood products except platelets.[13]

Miscellaneous Complications

Many other problems associated with massive transfusion are related to volume as well as rate of administration. Transmission of malaria and viral diseases such as many forms of hepatitis, HIV, cytomegalovirus, and Epstein-Barr virus may occur, although more rigorous donor screening and intensive blood testing have decreased the incidence of these complications (see earlier discussion).

Monitoring During Massive Blood Transfusion

If massive blood loss can be anticipated before surgery, then adequate monitoring should be instituted *before* surgery begins so that all baseline information may be gathered. If a patient arrives in the operating room in shock, such as a trauma patient, one must be careful to distinguish hypovolemia from other causes of shock, such as tension pneumothorax or cardiac tamponade (see Chapters 15 and 16). Invasive monitoring inserted during resuscitation helps with the differentiation. Our philosophy is one of aggressive invasive monitoring to provide maximal data for evaluation and management of a critically hypovolemic child.

1. Routine monitoring includes electrocardiogram, blood pressure cuff, stethoscope, temperature, pulse oximetry, and expired carbon dioxide. The use of a pulse oximeter placed on the tongue may be particularly valuable in special circumstances when a patient is vasoconstricted, hypothermic, or without peripheral pulses.[178, 179] Hypovolemia may occasionally manifest with pulsus paradoxus identified by the peripheral pulse oximeter.[180]
2. A urinary catheter allows accurate quantitation of urine output and assessment of organ perfusion and intravascular volume status.
3. An arterial catheter enables continuous blood pressure monitoring and measurements of arterial blood gas, hematocrit, glucose, calcium, and potassium. The adequacy of the circulating blood volume may be inferred from the shape of the arterial waveform, presence of the dicrotic notch, and absence of exaggerated respiratory variation (Fig. 12–7).
4. A central venous pressure (CVP) line may provide useful

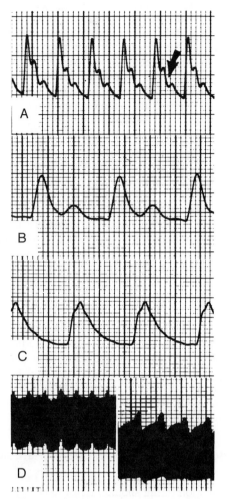

Figure 12–7. Changes in the contour of an arterial tracing with hypovolemia. In the normal tracing (A), note the sharp upswing of arterial pulse wave and position of the dicrotic notch. A slightly slower recording speed was used for A than for B and C. In B, there is movement of the dicrotic notch and widening of the pulse wave. In C, we see further widening of the pulse wave and loss of the dicrotic notch. An exaggerated ("picket-fence") respiratory variation of pulse wave is shown in D (right tracing compared with left). *Caution:* Factors other than hypovolemia—such as hypothermia, deep anesthesia, vasodilator therapy, or damped tracing (clot, air bubble)—may produce artifactual changes in the shape of the arterial waveform.

information, and its ease and safety of insertion have been demonstrated for children of all sizes.[181] It is our clinical impression that in healthy, anesthetized, supine patients, a very small change in CVP (2–3 mm Hg) may represent a change of as much as 10 to 15% of a patient's blood volume. In most pediatric patients, right-sided pressures correlate well with left-sided pressures; the CVP is generally an accurate indicator of cardiac filling pressures of both ventricles. A CVP also provides access for blood sampling as well as a reliable site for intravenous administration of medications, fluid, and blood.

5. A pulmonary artery flow-directed catheter provides more direct measurement of left-sided cardiac filling pressures and is a useful monitor in any patient in whom pulmonary or cardiac pathology might lead to confusion in interpretation of CVP.[182]

Monitors and the data they generate are helpful, but one must not rely on "numbers." *It serves no purpose to have sophisticated monitoring if the data provided cannot be interpreted and related to clinical events. The final monitor is ultimately the anesthesiologist's attention and judgment.*

Thromboelastography provides a standardized means of quantitating the rapidity and quality of clot formation as well as a means for identifying fibrinolysis.[183, 184] This device was first used primarily during massive blood transfusion situations related to liver transplantation and now is used in a number of areas, particularly cardiac surgery.[45–47, 183–186] Some studies have found that thromboelastography screening was not useful in predicting post-cardiac surgical bleeding and was associated with a high percentage of false-positive results.[187, 188] Use of heparinase helps improve the accuracy of the results by eliminating the effects of heparin, but this then requires two machines to simultaneously sample blood (with and without heparinase) to have results within a useful period of time.[189] This monitor may also be used to guide the effectiveness of antifibrinolytic therapy.[190] The role of thromboelastography in the care of pediatric cardiac surgical patients, liver transplant patients, and patients who have had massive blood loss with ongoing coagulopathy is yet to be clearly proven.

Infectious Disease Considerations for Anesthesiologists

It is important for anesthesiologists to use basic precautions to minimize their risk when administering blood products and being exposed to body fluids. There is no doubt that blood and body fluids, even in infants, are capable of transmitting HIV through parenteral exposure (cuts, needle stick), mucous membrane contact, or exposure to non-intact skin.[1, 191–202] Accidental needle sticks seem to be the most common means of exposure in the operating room for anesthesiologists; a needleless system, the use of stop cocks, or never attempting to recap used needles help reduce the incidence of this problem.[203–205] The incidence of HIV seroconversion following needle puncture is estimated to be 0.3 to 0.5% (1 in 200–300).[1, 191, 197–200, 206] Anesthesiologists must use universal blood and body fluid precautions (gloves, goggles) and should minimize the use of needles and especially the practice of recapping needles.[201] The management of infants may be less than optimal with the use of three-way stopcocks because of the fluid required to flush the system and the ease of introducing air into the intravenous line. In these patients, single-use needles without recapping or needleless systems are recommended. *Should an exposure occur from a known HIV-positive patient or puncture from a needle of unknown origin, then consultation with a specialist should occur immediately so as to determine the need for prophylactic medical therapy.*[207, 208]

Methods to Reduce Patient Exposure to Blood Products

Erythropoietin

The development of recombinant erythropoietin to promote red blood cell production provides a tool for physicians to use in reducing the need for transfusions. This therapy has proved useful in a wide variety of patient populations, including preterm infants, children on chemotherapy, children with renal failure, and children undergoing major reconstructive and cardiac surgery. Coordination with hematology, blood banking, and the primary patient care team are required to take full advantage of this form of therapy.[209-217]

Pre-donation

Modern blood banking procedures and the motivation to avoid homologous blood transfusions have made presurgical autologous blood donation more acceptable and, despite the cost, a new source of blood that can reduce exposure to exogenous blood.[14, 218-228] New blood preservatives have increased the shelf life to 35 days with the hope in the future for an even longer shelf life.[229-231] Erythropoietin has been used to stimulate RBC production and allow older pediatric patients to predeposit several units of blood before elective major surgical procedures as well as to increase red cell mass in children on chemotherapy or with renal failure.[213, 232-236] The advantages to patients are obvious; surgeons and blood banks should encourage pre-donation. Blood banks are generally receptive to presurgical donation and the processing costs are lower.[237] If the blood is not used during that donor's hospitalization, then the blood either is added to the general donor pool (after appropriate screening) or discarded.

Directed Donation

Directed blood donation is another method of reducing exposure of children to sources of blood other than the family. Parents or other blood relatives may donate blood with the theory that this donor pool might be "safer" than the general pool of donors. This assumes that family members are honest about high-risk behavior such as drug abuse and unprotected sexual activity that places them at risk for HIV infection that could possibly not be detected by screening tests. Another concern is the possibility of graft-versus-host disease. Blood from first-degree relatives is irradiated to prevent this possibility.[28, 238, 239]

Autotransfusion (Intraoperative Blood Scavenging)

Blood scavenging techniques have been applied to major vascular, cardiac, and multiple trauma situations for many years.[14, 240-249] Currently used techniques enable the patient to receive primarily RBCs suspended in saline.[240, 247] Cellular debris, excess citrate or heparin, free hemoglobin, and clotted blood are almost completely removed. Thus the blood returned to the patient is very similar to frozen PRBCs; it is usually of high hematocrit value, and nearly free of clotting factors. Autotransfusion poses no risk of hepatitis, HIV transmission, or transfusion reaction.[247, 248, 250]

Intraoperative blood salvage is underused in pediatric patients.[225, 226, 243, 244, 247-249] At present, the equipment available is primarily designed for adults, limiting its use to larger pediatric patients. We have found it a useful adjunct in minimizing homologous blood transfusions in scoliosis surgery. Additionally, if a patient has been able to donate blood before elective surgery, it may prevent the need for homologous blood entirely.[243, 244] At present, the equipment is expensive; however, if at least 3 units of blood are reinfused, there is a net monetary saving to the patient. Certainly the avoidance of homologous blood transfusions is a desirable goal, and the development of pediatric-sized equipment should make this technique more widely used and more cost-effective even in smaller children.[251]

The indications for intraoperative blood salvage include (1) major vascular or reconstructive procedures in which there is potential for massive blood loss; (2) patients with very rare blood types; and (3) multiple trauma without fecal contamination. The major contraindications are surgery on malignant lesions, contamination secondary to bowel trauma or abscess, and sickle cell disease.[252, 253]

Controlled Hypotension

Controlled hypotension, the intentional reduction of systemic perfusion pressure, has been used for many years to reduce intraoperative blood loss or to provide a relatively "bloodless" operating field.[254-264] Hypotensive anesthesia may be accomplished with a number of techniques, including continuous infusion of vasodilators, beta-adrenergic blockade, deep inhalation anesthesia, infusion of calcium channel blockers (vasodilation), or administration of adenosine. Controlled hypotension is generally reserved for older children and teenagers undergoing major reconstructive or orthopedic surgery. The choice of technique and the degree of induced hypotension depend on the surgical procedure. For procedures in which a dry surgical field is the end point with little potential for rapid blood loss, a technique that may take a period of time to recover from is acceptable, such as deep inhalational agent, beta blockade, or calcium channel blockade. If, however, the surgical procedure carries the possibility of rapid or massive blood loss, then a technique that is rapidly reversed, such as nitroprusside, nitroglycerin, adenosine, or prostaglandin E_1, is likely safer. It should be noted that there is limited published information on the use of adenosine, prostaglandin E_1, or calcium channel blockade in pediatric patients. These techniques, although purported to have advantages, should be used with caution in children until there is a greater published experience.

Physiology

Central Nervous System

All potent anesthetic agents decrease the cerebral metabolic rate of oxygen consumption ($CMRO_2$) and increase cerebral blood flow. Isoflurane appears to offer the greatest advantage because it causes the greatest depression of $CMRO_2$, and it has been used as the sole hypotensive agent.[265-271] The degree of decreased metabolic demand is unpredictable and cannot be depended on for cerebral protection during controlled hypotension. Sevoflurane has also been used to help facilitate controlled hypotension in conjunction with beta blockade or other vasodilating agent.[272-274]

One of the most important considerations of any hypotensive technique is the effect that it will have on cerebral blood flow (CBF). Studies of adults demonstrate that little change occurs in cerebral metabolism when mean arterial pressure (MAP) is maintained above 55 mm Hg.[265] There are no comparable data for pediatric patients; however, experience with children during cardiac bypass suggests that children tolerate pressures below this level on an age-related basis—that is, neonates tolerate a lower MAP than small children, who in turn tolerate a lower MAP better than adults. It appears that CBF is maintained in adults during isoflurane-induced hypotension.[267] Brain ischemia has been documented when a MAP of 55 mm Hg is combined with hypocarbia; however, no similar pediatric studies have been carried out.[270, 271] Animal data suggest that direct vasodilating agents may reduce cerebral blood vessel responsiveness to carbon dioxide.[275] Maintenance of normal arterial carbon dioxide tension ($PaCO_2$) is vitally important to ensure adequate CBF during induced hypotension; the relationship of CBF to $PaCO_2$ is described in greater detail in Chapter 22. To optimize CBF, we generally maintain the MAP at 55 mm Hg and the $PaCO_2$ at 35 to 45 mm Hg.

During induced hypotension, CBF may decrease from baseline with trimethaphan, nitroglycerin, and nitroprusside; the extent of altered CBF varies with each agent and the degree of induced hypotension.[276–278] Studies attempting to find the ideal vasodilator agent have demonstrated significant differences in cerebral metabolites and regional distribution of CBF between trimethaphan, sodium nitroprusside, and nitroglycerin. Trimethaphan, which has generally fallen out of use, produces a profound reduction in CBF, with possible redistribution away from cortical areas.[271, 277–281] Calcium channel blocker–induced vasodilation increases regional cerebral blood flow despite induced hypotension.[282] This increase in CBF lasts approximately 1 hour after drug cessation. It would appear that use of this drug category would not be a good choice for control of blood pressure in patients with increased intracranial pressure. On the other hand, beta-adrenergic blockade does not appear to affect cerebral blood flow even in the presence of halothane anesthesia.[283–285]

Sodium nitroprusside and nitroglycerin appear to maintain a more homogeneous distribution of CBF and better cerebral perfusion for any given MAP than does trimethaphan and thus may be safer.[271, 278, 279] The use of vasodilating agents in the presence of increased intracranial pressure is controversial; all vasodilators and inhalation agents have been found to increase intracranial pressure under these conditions.[265, 276, 277, 286] Both increased flow and increased capacitance of the cerebral blood vessels have been implicated. The key to safe administration of vasodilators in this circumstance is careful monitoring of cerebral perfusion pressure. Cerebral perfusion pressure is the MAP minus the intracranial pressure; cerebral perfusion pressure should be maintained above 50 mm Hg. Hypotensive techniques must be used with great caution in the presence of elevated intracranial pressure, with the risk-benefit ratio carefully evaluated.

Hypotensive anesthesia may also affect spinal cord blood flow.[287] Studies of animals suggest that regulation of spinal cord blood flow is similar to regulation of CBF; factors that increase or decrease CBF have the same effect on spinal cord blood flow.[287, 288] Studies of animals also suggest that there is little compromise and possibly an increase in spinal cord blood flow with sodium nitroprusside- or nitroglycerin-induced hypotension, assuming that MAP does not decline below 50 mm Hg.[281, 289, 290] Potent inhalation agents tend to increase spinal cord blood flow and may offer some advantage during spinal cord instrumentation.[291, 292] However, this potentially protective effect may be reduced because of the need to limit inhalation anesthetic concentrations to allow monitoring of evoked potentials. One limited clinical study of only 14 patients found no change in evoked spinal cord potential and spinal cord blood flow during prostaglandin E_1–induced hypotension.[293] Trimethaphan has been demonstrated to *reduce* spinal cord blood flow in animal models and this is exacerbated with spinal distraction. *These studies suggest that trimethaphan should not be used for hypotensive anesthesia during scoliosis surgery.*[262, 281, 289, 290, 294–296] Controlled hypotension has been safely used for reduction of blood loss during posterior spinal fusion; blood loss seems to be reduced to a greater extent in children than in adults.[261, 262, 264, 297, 298] However, with anterior spinal fusion, if there is any danger of disruption of spinal cord blood flow due to aortic dissection, hypotensive anesthesia may be contraindicated. Neuropsychiatric testing during and after hypotensive anesthesia indicates that effects on memory and electroencephalographic findings are no different than in normotensive control subjects.[299]

Myocardium

Coronary blood flow autoregulates with metabolic demand and is dependent on diastolic filling pressure. All vasodilators appear to improve left ventricular function by reducing afterload.[300–302] For children who have a normal coronary circulation, trimethaphan, nitroprusside, and nitroglycerin appear to be equally well tolerated. Trimethaphan appears to have a less predictable response because its major effect is on sympathetic tone, which is quite variable from one patient to another, especially children.[280, 281, 303] Cardiac work is decreased because of reduced afterload. Coronary blood flow is generally matched to cardiac metabolic demands but may be reduced precipitously because of the sharp decline in diastolic pressure; this reduction is potentially dangerous in patients with a compromised coronary circulation.[280, 302] Sodium nitroprusside improves cardiovascular hemodynamics by rapidly reducing afterload, reducing myocardial oxygen consumption, and maintaining coronary blood flow.[302–304] Coronary flow may be increased compared with cardiac metabolic demand with nitroprusside.[280, 281] Nitroprusside tends to cause tachycardia, especially in children. Central toxicity (poisoning of the cytochrome oxidase system) appears to precede direct cardiac toxicity.[305] Nitroglycerin is a more potent coronary artery dilator than sodium nitroprusside and increases myocardial blood flow.[280, 306, 307] From a cardiac standpoint, nitroglycerin or nitroprusside may offer advantages over trimethaphan.

Hypotensive anesthesia may also be induced by direct myocardial depression with potent inhalation agents either alone or in combination with beta-adrenergic blockade.[267, 272, 308] Since this technique relies on depression of myocardial function, there is less ability to rapidly reverse the effects of the drugs depressing the heart. It is our belief that vasodilating agents provide a more precise control of blood pressure without depressing the heart. For patients undergoing procedures that have the potential for rapid blood loss, a vasodilating technique that rapidly reverses upon stopping the infusion may be advantageous. If the procedure is not one associated with rapid blood loss, then techniques that take longer to reverse may be a reasonable alternative. Cardiac arrest can occur with the administration of beta-blockers to children.[309] Beta-adrenergic blockade has been shown to decrease the requirements of the vasodilator.[310] It is imperative, if beta blockade is to be used, that clinicians clearly understand the differences in half-lives between agents and the best means for reversing their effect. Esmolol is very short acting with a half-life in children of approximately 3 minutes.[311] Nonanesthetized children have a greater requirement per kilogram body weight than adults.[312] In nonanesthetized children, a loading dose of 500 μg/kg/min is then followed by a maintenance rate of 25 to 200 μg/kg/min. Since there is minimal published experience in children under anesthesia, a lower starting dose (50–100 μg/kg/min) and titration of dose every 3 to 5 minutes (increase by 12.5–25 μg/kg/min) would seem indicated. Labetalol[308, 313–315] and propranolol[316, 317] have also been used to help induce hypotensive anesthesia. The half-lives, onset of effect, and time to peak effect of these medications are much longer and therefore the effects are less controllable. Acute beta-blocker toxicity can be reversed with high-dose intravenous glucagon (50 μg/kg followed by an infusion of 0.3–3.0 μg/kg/min). *Note that this dose is extrapolated from adult data.*[318, 319]

Renal System

Renal blood flow autoregulates between a MAP of 80 and 180 mm Hg; however, general anesthesia has profound effects on autoregulation, depending on the anesthetic agent used.[320] Renal blood flow may be diminished by trimethaphan, with resultant increase in renal vascular resistance.[302] Sodium nitroprusside maintains and perhaps increases renal blood flow during induced hypotension, compared with trimethaphan.[301, 302, 321] A transient reduction in creatinine clearance and sodium reabsorption occurs with both drugs.[321–323] Nitroglycerin maintains renal blood flow.[280, 281] Measuring urinary output is a simple method of monitoring the adequacy of intraoperative renal perfusion and function. One study of adults compared isoflurane-induced with sevoflurane-induced hypotension; following 2 hours of hypotension, there was a temporarily reversible abnormality in renal function as indicated by a rise in N-acetyl-beta-D-glucosaminidase.[324] The clinical importance of this is unknown.

Adenosine-induced hypotension has been shown to compromise renal function by increasing renovascular resistance and renal blood flow to a greater extent than nitroprusside.[325] This may explain in part why this drug has not had widespread use. Calcium channel blockers have also been used to induce controlled hypotension: renal blood flow is increased and renal function preserved.[263, 264, 326, 327] Beta blockade seems to have a mixed effect on renal function. Lowering MAP decreases renal blood flow, but overall there appears to be minimal impairment of renal function by any of the beta blockers commonly used to facilitate controlled hypotension; renal function returns to normal after the period of controlled hypotension.[313, 328–331]

Pulmonary System

An increase in physiologic dead space and intrapulmonary shunting during induced hypotension has been reported in adults and children.[258, 260, 332–334] This does not seem to be a clinically important problem in children, possibly because of less gravitational pooling of blood in the lungs; however, it is important to measure arterial blood gases and expired CO_2 and to monitor oxygen saturation to assess this possibility.[258, 260] Pulmonary blood flow is usually diminished by all vasodilators because of redistribution of blood into the peripheral circulation. An increasing difference between end-expired carbon dioxide values and measured arterial blood gas values would suggest the development of shunting and increased physiologic dead space.

Hepatic System

Catecholamines, Pa_{CO_2}, circulating blood volume, and anesthetic agents influence the portal circulation.[335] The liver is oxygenated by the arterial circulation but receives most of its blood flow through the portal circulation; changes in portal blood flow may have profound effects on total hepatic blood flow. In dogs, reduction of both hepatic arterial and portal blood flow occurred during sodium nitroprusside-induced hypotension, but hepatic oxygenation was preserved by increases in arterial flow during periods of insufficient portal vein flow.[336, 337] Studies of animals suggest that hepatic blood flow is generally maintained with nitroglycerin or nitroprusside but may be reduced with trimethaphan.[280, 281] A prospective study of adults using either deep halothane anesthesia or nitroprusside-induced hypotension detected no postoperative abnormalities in hepatic function for either group.[338] It appears that adequate hepatic oxygenation is maintained during induced hypotensive anesthesia, provided the Pa_{CO_2} is within the normal range and an adequate circulating blood volume is maintained.[339] A study of animals suggests that nitroglycerin has less effect on the hepatic microcirculation than nitroprusside.[340] Beta blockade seems to have minimal effect on splanchnic blood flow.[341–343] Hepatic clearance of drugs secondary to altered perfusion does not appear to be an issue with propranolol; rather, the reported decreased clearance of lidocaine and other medications is likely due to propranolol's direct effects on enzyme inhibition.[344] It appears that the potent anesthetic agents have a greater effect on hepatic drug metabolism than beta-adrenergic blockade.[344] Nicardipine has been shown to decrease hepatic blood flow by 50% during induced hypotension using a rabbit model.[345]

Another study in humans found less impairment of hepatic drug excretion with nicardipine and halothane compared with nitroglycerin and halothane.[346] In unanesthetized humans, it appears that therapeutic doses of nicardipine have no adverse effects on hepatic blood flow. These studies suggest that there would be some decrease in hepatic blood flow during nicardipine-induced hypotension, particularly if combined with potent inhalation agent. The clinical importance of this is unclear, but one could expect that there might be some impairment of drug clearance during the period of induced hypotension.

Skin and Muscle

Blood flow redistribution to skin and muscle may be an undesirable side effect of hypotensive anesthesia, especially during a reconstructive plastic surgical procedure. Data gathered from studies of animals document this effect with trimethaphan but not with sodium nitroprusside.[280, 302] All commonly used vasodilating hypotensive agents diminish muscle blood flow.[281] It appears that beta-adrenergic blockade reduces skin blood flow but that nicardipine increases skin blood flow.[282, 347-349] There may also be differences in skin blood flow with potent inhalation agents combined with nicardipine; in humans, skin blood flow tended to increase in patients anesthetized with sevoflurane compared with patients anesthetized with isoflurane.[350]

Pharmacology

Trimethaphan (Arfonad)

Trimethaphan is a ganglionic blocking drug that also has direct vasodilator properties. Its advantages are a rapid onset of action (several minutes) and, because its duration of action is brief (several minutes), it can be conveniently titrated by intravenous infusion. Disadvantages include tachycardia, tachyphylaxis, histamine release, inhibition of pseudocholinesterase hydrolysis of succinylcholine, potentiation of nondepolarizing neuromuscular blockade, alteration of cerebral and spinal cord blood flow distribution, possible decreases in coronary, renal, and hepatic blood flow, and redistribution of blood flow to skin and muscle.[280, 281, 289, 290, 294-296, 302, 351-353] In children, resistance to hypotension may occur secondary to reflex tachycardia.[351] Trimethaphan may be contraindicated in asthmatic patients because of its histamine-releasing properties. In high doses, this medication produces markedly dilated pupils, which could be confused as a sign of an intracerebral catastrophe. The usual starting dosage is 25 to 100 μg/kg/min, which may be gradually increased as clinically indicated. It would appear that this agent's disadvantages far outweigh its advantages for most circumstances, except perhaps for very minimal reductions in MAP.

Sodium Nitroprusside

Sodium nitroprusside has a very rapid onset of action (seconds), brief duration of action (1–2 minutes), and minimal side effects when used in the recommended dose range.[354] This agent is extremely potent and is *most safely administered by an infusion pump through a separate intravenous site.* Its principal mechanism of action is direct vascular smooth-muscle relaxation, primarily causing arteriolar dilation, as well as some venodilation.

DOSAGE. It is recommended to commence sodium nitroprusside infusion at 0.5 to 1.0 μg/kg/min and gradually increase the dose as needed.[355, 356] A satisfactory reduction of systemic perfusion pressure can usually be obtained well below the recommended maximum of 10 μg/kg/min.

TOXICITY. Cyanide toxicity is characterized by the unexplained development of metabolic acidosis, elevated blood lactate levels, and an elevated mixed venous oxygen content.[356, 357] The nitroprusside radical interacts with the sulfhydryl groups of erythrocytes, causing the release of cyanide. Nitroprusside contains five cyanide molecules, and as the cyanide is released, it is converted to nontoxic thiocyanate by the rhodanase enzyme system in the liver and is then excreted by the kidneys.[357] If the amount of cyanide released overwhelms the capacity of the rhodanase system, cyanide toxicity (binding to the cytochrome electron transport system) results; this in turn produces a change to anaerobic metabolism, metabolic acidosis, a rise in mixed venous oxygen content, and eventually death.[305, 356, 358-361] Several pediatric anesthetic-related deaths have resulted from both cyanide toxicity and its treatment.[358-360] Three responses to sodium nitroprusside infusion may herald impending cyanide toxicity:

1. Greater than 10 μg/kg/min required for response
2. Tachyphylaxis developing within 30 to 60 minutes
3. Immediate resistance to the drug.[357]

If any of these occur, sodium nitroprusside should be discontinued and the patient investigated for possible cyanide toxicity. Treatment of cyanide poisoning is directed at reversal of the binding of cyanide to the cytochrome enzymes. This can be accomplished by producing methemoglobinemia with amyl nitrite. Methemoglobin has a greater affinity for cyanide than it does for the cytochrome system; thus, the reaction is forced in the direction of forming cyanomethemoglobin. The breakdown of cyanomethemoglobin is promoted by administering thiosulfate, which reacts with the cyanide to form nontoxic thiocyanate, which is then excreted by the kidneys. Hydroxocobalamin may prevent toxicity by formation of cyanocobalamin.[362] It is important to emphasize, however, that this treatment is not without hazard. As Posner states, "Overzealous treatment may merely convert a cytotoxic hypoxia to an anemic hypoxia."[362] In addition, prophylactic infusion of sodium thiosulfate may be helpful in reducing toxicity by promoting the production of thiocyanate.[362-367] The first step in treatment of toxicity is the *intermittent* administration of amyl nitrite (by inhalation), until sodium nitrite can be administered intravenously. The second step is sodium nitrite given as a 3% solution (300 mg/mL, 0.2 mL/kg, not to exceed 10 mL [3 g]). Immediately afterward, sodium thiosulfate in a dose of 175 mg/kg, not to exceed 12.5 g, should be administered. One hundred percent oxygen should be delivered continuously. A cyanide antidote (Taylor Pharmaceuticals, Decatur, IL 62522) is available.

Sodium nitroprusside is a safe medication, provided that doses remain well within the guidelines that have been established by various investigators.[364-366] *For children, this is a maximum of 50 μg/kg/min for 30 minutes and about 8 to 10 μg/kg/min for 3 hours*, with frequent blood gas analysis.[356, 366]

Nitroglycerin

Nitroglycerin has been used to induce controlled hypotension; one report suggests that sodium nitroprusside produces more predictable hypotension when used as an adjunct to nitrous oxide:narcotic anesthesia.[260] The main advantages of nitroglycerin are its relatively rapid onset of action (several minutes), lack of tachyphylaxis and toxicity, and brief duration of action (several minutes).

DOSAGE. The infusion should be started at a rate of 1 μg/kg/min and the dose increased until the desired response is obtained. Resistance to the hypotensive effects of nitroglycerin may occur in children; however, in view of the reduced potential for toxicity when compared with nitroprusside, nitroglycerin appears to be a reasonable alternative.

TOXICITY. Nitroglycerin is relatively free of toxic side effects in the usual doses applied during hypotensive anesthesia.[260, 300, 368, 369] No toxicities or deaths have been reported with nitroglycerin when used for hypotensive anesthesia.[260, 300, 368–370] Several reports have described nitroglycerin-induced methemoglobinemia; a study of patients undergoing anesthetic procedures using controlled hypotension did not find a relation between the development of methemoglobin and the dose of nitroglycerin.[371, 372] Pulse oximetry may be of value in making the initial diagnosis (decreased saturation). Should this occur, however, accurate saturation determinations will not be possible because of the interference in light absorbance caused by methemoglobin at both ends of the absorbance spectrum used by pulse oximeters.[373, 374] The use of other adjuncts (potent inhalation agents, other vasodilators, or beta-adrenergic blockade) reduces the total dose of nitroglycerin administered and provides greater control of the blood pressure.

General Concepts of Hypotensive Anesthesia

Before using controlled hypotension, it is important to understand the rationale for using this technique.[375] If it is used to reduce surgical blood loss, the preparation and monitoring of a patient are different from those of a procedure in which the main objective for lowering the perfusion pressure is to improve operating conditions, as in microsurgical techniques. In the former case, direct assessment of circulating blood pressure and volume with an arterial line and central venous or flow-directed pulmonary artery catheter is important, whereas in the latter case, only a direct means of measuring blood pressure (arterial line) is needed.

Premedication

Premedication of a patient scheduled for hypotensive anesthesia may include a drug with vasodilating properties such as morphine, chlorpromazine, or droperidol. These drugs help reduce anxiety as well as facilitate the hypotensive technique.

Anesthetic Management

All inhalation agents, by directly depressing cardiac output, have been used with various degrees of success as a single drug to produce controlled hypotension. Isoflurane may be the most advantageous because of its effects on $CMRO_2$; however, profound cardiovascular depression may be difficult to control and certainly is not readily reversible.[267–269] Sevoflurane or desflurane may provide slightly better control of blood pressure if combined with beta-adrenergic blockade.[272, 376] We do not advocate hypotensive anesthesia using potent inhalation agents as the sole hypotensive agents because the cardiovascular depression is not rapidly reversed if a problem arises with relative anesthetic overdose. However, low to moderate concentrations of potent inhalation agents used with other medications reduce the amounts of vasodilator or beta blocker necessary to reduce blood pressure and thereby may reduce the potential for toxicity.[377]

The availability of short-acting beta-adrenergic-blocking agents offers an alternative method for decreasing MAP by directly depressing cardiac output. Beta-adrenergic blockade removes a valuable guide to the depth of anesthesia and volume status. Because children approximately 2 years of age and younger have heart rate–dependent cardiac output (see Chapter 17), beta-adrenergic blockade is not recommended in this age group. Low-dose, short-acting beta-adrenergic blockade may be a reasonable supplement to hypotensive anesthesia with potent inhalation agents as a means of reducing the inspired anesthetic agent requirement or as a supplement to reduce vasodilator requirements.[378] Short-acting beta blockers such as esmolol may be the best compromise, because, with a half-life of approximately 3 minutes, it may be administered as an infusion and adjusted up or down as needed. Even with this type of control, serious adverse events as a result of beta blockade have been reported.[309] Nicardipine also offers a reasonable alternative because its action is primarily peripheral vasodilation rather than myocardial depression.[264, 264, 327, 379–381] The main disadvantage is the 20 minutes it takes for the hypotensive effects to subside once the infusion is stopped.[264] Several studies, mostly by the same author, suggest a starting dose of 5 to 10 μg/kg/min that is rapidly reduced to 1 to 2 μg/kg/min as indicated to maintain the blood pressure in the desired range.[263, 264]

The best method for administration of vasodilating agents or ultra-short-acting beta blocking agents is by continuous infusion pumps; one pump maintains a continuous and constant flow through the intravenous catheter and another infuses the hypotensive agent, allowing easy titration. *It is particularly important to use a separate intravenous site to minimize accidental bolus infusion of the vasodilator during changes in fluid requirements or during the administration of other medications; this method provides a measure of safety.* The vasodilator or ultra-short-acting beta-blocker should be administered as close to the vein as possible to eliminate dead space and the possibility of accidental bolus administration.

Monitoring

The following baseline parameters should be carefully monitored: oxygen saturation and expired carbon dioxide, electrocardiogram, temperature, hematocrit, blood glucose, arterial blood gases and acid-base status, MAP, and CVP or pulmonary artery occlusion pressure. Arterial pressure is usually measured using the radial artery; a report of spurious arterial pressure measurements when using the dorsalis pedis artery in adults suggests that this artery should be used with caution.[382]

When the desired MAP has been attained, a new baseline CVP or pulmonary artery occlusion pressure should be measured and maintained at this, or slightly higher than the new, lower level throughout the procedure. *To use any hypotensive technique safely, it is mandatory that the patient remain normovolemic at all times; this means strict correction of a change of even 1 or 2 mm Hg in CVP or PAOP.* A small change in cardiac filling pressures in a healthy, supine, anesthetized pediatric patient may represent a significant reduction in circulating blood volume. A pulmonary artery catheter is rarely indicated in children with normal cardiovascular and pulmonary function because right-sided filling pressures parallel left-sided filling pressures.

A useful indicator of intravascular volume status is urine

output. Even during hypotensive anesthesia, the kidneys should produce 0.5 to 1.0 mL/kg of urine per hour. The failure to detect urine output frequently is due to obstruction or kinking of the urinary catheter. If the catheter is patent, then an intravenous fluid challenge should be considered. Urine output is one of the best indicators of organ perfusion and function; for this reason, it is perhaps the most useful monitor during hypotensive anesthesia.

Constant monitoring of oxygen saturation and expired carbon dioxide is extremely important for the early warning of adverse anesthetic events.[383–385] A large difference between arterial and expired carbon dioxide values may indicate the development of a pulmonary shunt or air embolization. A rise in mixed venous oxygen content may signal development of cyanide toxicity. Pulse oximetry is generally unaffected by controlled hypotensive anesthesia; however, the oximeter probe can be placed on the tongue or ear lobe should an unsatisfactory recording develop.[178, 179]

Once hypotension has been induced and the surgical field is bloodless, the MAP should be slowly raised until increased bleeding is noted; then the MAP can be again reduced by approximately 5 mm Hg to achieve optimal conditions. With this method, it is sometimes necessary to reduce the MAP only 10 to 20% from baseline to achieve satisfactory hemostasis with hypotensive anesthesia.

Position

It is most desirable to make the operative field the highest point of the patient's body to take advantage of gravitational forces to help reduce blood pressure and the potential for air embolization.[386–388] When positioning a patient, the clinician must also take care to minimize any possible impedance to venous drainage that might contribute to blood loss. For example, abdominal pressure from a misplaced roll of sheets can markedly increase venous pressure during posterior spine instrumentation and completely offset any beneficial effects from reduced arterial pressure.[262, 375, 386, 388, 389] If the head is the surgical site, then the arterial transducer must be calibrated at head level rather than heart level to ensure adequate cerebral perfusion pressure.[389]

Laboratory Parameters

Adequate levels of hemoglobin must be maintained to have sufficient oxygen-carrying capacity. Studies have indicated that at normal blood pressures, a hemoglobin value of 5 g/100 mL is well tolerated in laboratory animals, but ischemia may occur with a lower hemoglobin value.[390] There is some evidence to suggest that the combination of hemodilution and hypotensive anesthesia may result in inadequate oxygenation of some vascular beds (renal, enteric mucosa).[391, 392] *Although no similar studies have been conducted in children, for additional safety we maintain the hemoglobin level at approximately 10 g/100 mL or higher during controlled hypotensive anesthesia.* This would seem to be particularly important for children undergoing spinal instrumentation in which traction on the spinal cord may alter spinal cord blood flow.

Arterial blood gases must be carefully evaluated on a 30- to 60-minute basis to diagnose changes in oxygenation, ventilation, or perfusion, or the development of drug toxicity

(nitroprusside). It is exceedingly important that adequate arterial oxygen pressure be maintained at all times. In addition, examination of the $PaCO_2$ is mandatory during any hypotensive anesthetic technique, because cerebral perfusion is directly related to $PaCO_2$.[393, 394] For this reason, normocarbia should be maintained; *the combination of hypocarbia and hypotension should be avoided.* Controlled ventilation is desirable because it maintains a constant $PaCO_2$. The metabolic components of acid-base equilibrium must also be carefully monitored; the development of acidosis reflects inadequate oxygen delivery or toxicity from the hypotensive agent (e.g., sodium nitroprusside).[354]

Although we do not advocate the routine use of beta-adrenergic blockade, blood glucose values should be measured serially if these drugs are part of the chosen hypotensive technique. Beta-adrenergic blockade inhibits glycogenolysis and may cause severe unsuspected hypoglycemia in children.[258, 395] A further consideration is the rate at which hypotensive anesthesia is reversed; data suggest that less profound rebound hyperemia and hypertension occur if blood pressure is allowed to return to normal gradually.[258, 396]

Contraindications

The risks of hypotensive anesthesia are significant. The risk-to-benefit ratio must always be considered on an individual patient basis, particularly with neurosurgical patients and those undergoing spinal instrumentation. Any systemic disease compromising function of a major organ is a relative contraindication to the use of controlled hypotension. The majority of complications reported, however, relate to the inexperience of the practitioner, inappropriate patient selection, unfamiliarity with the drugs involved, or inattention to details such as blood volume status, pH, $PaCO_2$, and blood glucose.[258, 358, 359, 375, 386, 397, 398] If a patient is healthy and meticulous attention is paid to all the parameters previously detailed, the benefits of improved surgical technique, shorter surgical time, and decreased need for blood transfusion usually outweigh the potential risks. We caution that this technique should be attempted only after a clear understanding is attained of its physiology and pharmacology and after experience is gained by working with colleagues intimately familiar with controlled hypotensive anesthesia.

Hemodilution

Intentional *isovolemic* hemodilution is a useful adjunct to an anesthesiologist's strategy to reduce blood transfusions.[14, 390, 399, 400] Two basic methods can be applied: (1) Allow the surgical blood loss to continue to the point at which the patient's hematocrit is in the high "teens" and *maintain at that hematocrit value* until near the end of the procedure; at that point, the hematocrit can be raised to the desired value through transfusion of PRBCs. This technique allows surgical bleeding to occur at a reduced hematocrit value, resulting in less loss of RBC mass (300 mL of blood loss at a hematocrit of 40% is twice as much RBC mass as 300 mL of blood loss at a hematocrit of 20%). (2) Blood can be removed from a patient at the beginning of the operation and returned at the end. The latter technique is preferable because it reserves a quantity of the patient's own fresh whole blood, which can be returned at the end of the surgical procedure; for a Jehovah's Witness, this technique often conforms to religious guidelines (if continuity is maintained with the patient's blood).[390, 401–406] There is at least one report of acute hypervolemic hemodilution in adults that was apparently well tolerated by patients free of cardiac disease[407]; we cannot support this technique in children without further study.

Physiology

Blood Viscosity

One of the major effects of hemodilution is a marked reduction in blood viscosity, primarily as a result of the reduction in red blood cell mass but also partly because of dilution of the plasma.[408] The reduced viscosity improves blood flow through capillary beds.[390, 409–411]

Cardiac Output

Venous return is increased with isovolemic hemodilution, and cardiac output is increased, apparently related to increased stroke volume.[412–414] However, in our experience it is not unusual to observe little or no increase in cardiac output in children undergoing hemodilution under anesthesia.

Tissue Oxygenation

The delivery of oxygen to tissues during acute anemia may be maintained by several compensatory mechanisms: increased blood flow, increased oxygen extraction, increased utilization of dissolved oxygen, and changes in the oxygen-hemoglobin dissociation curve.[409–420] During acute normovolemic hemodilution, there is an improvement in blood flow distribution with a lowered hematocrit. This improved blood rheology is the major compensatory mechanism maintaining oxygen delivery. Increased oxygen extraction occurs only in the presence of inadequate circulating blood volume or when the hematocrit decreases below 20%; if the hematocrit declines below 15%, myocardial ischemia may develop, as demonstrated by impaired subendocardial perfusion.[416, 418, 421] It is at this extreme level of anemia that dissolved oxygen begins to assume a more important role. There are a number of reports of extreme hemodilution with successful outcome (hemoglobin as low as 2 g/100 mL) without the production of lactic acid.[422, 423]

Control of the patient's metabolic rate is very important during extreme hemodilution. Therefore, inducing a slight degree of hypothermia (33–34°C), controlled ventilation to maintain a constant carbon dioxide value, and a high inspired oxygen tension (and therefore a high dissolved oxygen value) have allowed the survival of patients with hematocrits as low as 4%.[423] These extreme levels of hemodilution cannot be recommended as an elective effort to reduce blood transfusions. However, these reports[422, 423] do indicate how well healthy patients tolerate such low oxygen carrying capacity, provided that they are under the effects of anesthesia, they are normovolemic, they are slightly hypothermic, and they are on 100% oxygen.

A right shift in the oxygen-hemoglobin dissociation curve secondary to increased erythrocyte 2,3-DPG improves oxygen release to tissues. This compensatory mechanism occurs primarily during chronic anemia and becomes important when the hematocrit falls below 20%; this compensatory mechanism is less important during the development of acute anemia.[390, 401, 402, 416] Patients who underwent isovolemic hemodilution and received their own fresh blood back at the end of surgery had a higher P_{50} than patients receiving hemodilution and replacement with banked blood.[424] It is our practice never to allow the hematocrit to fall below 15%, and we prefer to maintain it closer to 20%.

Lung Water

Pulmonary interstitial water increases with hemodilution; this amount is quantitatively greater with crystalloid than colloid replacement. There is no clinical difference as measured by arterial blood gases.[425–427] There appears to be no clinical advantage of colloid over crystalloid hemodilution, and the cost of the latter is much less.

Effects on Muscle Relaxants

Several studies have demonstrated a prolonged duration of action and an increased potency of many muscle relaxants (succinylcholine, pancuronium, curare, rocuronium, and vecuronium).[428–432] It is unclear why the potency of muscle relaxants is increased. These effects may relate to a number of factors, including alterations in protein binding, volume of distribution, alterations in distribution of blood flow to organs that metabolize or excrete these medications, and acute changes in electrolytes, ionized calcium, and blood flow to tissues.[428]

Technique

We allow blood to run directly from an arterial line into sterile acid-citrate-dextrose or citrate-phosphate-dextrose blood collection bags. The bag is placed on a scale below the level of the patient so as to accurately measure the amount of blood withdrawn. The bag is frequently but gently agitated to ensure even distribution of the anticoagulant. Each unit is weighed before any blood is transferred so as to determine precisely the volume that has been removed. This volume should be calculated preoperatively, and it usually amounts to 30 to 40% of the estimated blood volume of the child. The blood removed most often reduces the hematocrit to the 20 to 25% range. Care must be taken to replace the blood removed with either 5% albumin, milliliter for milliliter, or 2 to 3 mL of lactated Ringer solution for each milliliter of blood removed. Sometimes an even greater volume of replacement fluids is needed.[400] It is preferable to hemodilute before the surgical incision, although this can also be done during the initial phases of surgery. The major concern is to maintain a normal circulating blood volume, provide adequate oxygen-carrying capacity, minimize exposure to homologous blood products, and ensure hemostasis. It is therefore important to make an educated guess about how much blood loss is anticipated so that the autologous blood can be reinfused in place of homologous blood. Once surgical blood loss has ceased or if apparent coagulopathy secondary to dilution of clotting factors or platelets has developed, the autologous blood may be reinfused. It may be administered one unit at a time or saved and reinfused at the end of the procedure.

To apply this technique most effectively, the anesthesiologist must be familiar with the differences in composition of the various blood components used (see Table 12–4). If exclusively whole blood is used for replacement, coagulopathy most commonly occurs secondary to thrombocytopenia and does not usually develop until 2 to 3 blood volumes have been lost. If exclusively PRBCs are used, coagulopathy secondary to dilution of clotting factors develops first, probably after 1 to 1.5 blood volumes have been lost. Blood removed at the beginning of the procedure acts as a ready source of fresh plasma and platelets. It is important to remember that a small-pore filter (20 μm) traps many of the platelets that a large-pore filter (≥ 150 μm) allows to pass. The time at which a patient's blood is best reinfused must be determined according to the type of blood replaced, the volume lost, and the total clinical picture.

Indications

Hemodilution may be indicated in any procedure in which blood loss is expected to exceed half the patient's blood volume.

Contraindications

Hemodilution is contraindicated in patients with sickle cell disease, septicemia, or compromised function of any major organ that may be significantly affected by changes in perfusion and oxygenation. *We do not recommend combining extreme hemodilution (hematocrit < 25%) with controlled hypotensive anesthesia.*

Complications

The major complications of hemodilution relate to blood volume status, hemoglobin content, and coagulopathy. Anesthesiologists must pay meticulous attention to blood volume replacement. As long as normovolemia is maintained and the hematocrit kept above 15% (preferably around 20%), problems with organ perfusion or oxygenation should not occur.

Advantages

Hemodilution provides a ready source of fresh whole blood rich in platelets and clotting factors. It poses no problems such as hepatitis, infection with human immunodeficiency virus, or inexact crossmatch and yields a net saving in loss of red blood cell mass, because the surgical losses occur at a hematocrit of 15 to 20% compared with 30 to 45%.

REFERENCES

1. Berkelman RL, Heyward WL, Stehr-Green JK, et al.: Epidemiology of human immunodeficiency virus infection and acquired immunodeficiency syndrome. Am J Med 1989;86:761–770.
2. Novello AC, Wise PH, Willoughby A, et al.: Final report of the United States Department of Health and Human Services Secretary's Work Group on pediatric human immunodeficiency virus infection and disease: Content and implications. Pediatrics 1989;84:547–555.
3. Surgenor DM: The patient's blood is the safest blood. N Engl J Med 1987;316:542–544.
4. Moor AC, Dubbelman TM, VanSteveninck J, et al.: Transfusion-transmitted diseases: Risks, prevention and perspectives. Eur J Haematol 1999;62:1–18.
5. Ward JW, Holmberg SD, Allen JR, et al.: Transmission of human immunodeficiency virus (HIV) by blood transfusions screened as negative for HIV antibody. N Engl J Med 1988;318:473–478.
6. American Association of Blood Banks: Facts about Blood and Blood Banking. 1999. www.aabb.org
7. Lackritz EM, Satten GA, Aberle-Grasse J, et al.: Estimated risk of transmission of the human immunodeficiency virus by screened blood in the United States. N Engl J Med 1995;333:1721–1725.
8. Korelitz JJ, Busch MP, Kleinman SH, et al.: A method for estimating hepatitis B virus incidence rates in volunteer blood donors. National Heart, Lung, and Blood Institute Retrovirus Epidemiology Donor Study. Transfusion 1997;37:634–640.
9. Schreiber GB, Busch MP, Kleinman SH, et al.: The risk of transfusion-transmitted viral infections. The Retrovirus Epidemiology Donor Study. N Engl J Med 1996;334:1685–1690.
10. Kleinman S, Busch MP, Hall L, et al.: False-positive HIV-1 test results in a low-risk screening setting of voluntary blood donation. Retrovirus Epidemiology Donor Study. JAMA 1998;280:1080–1085.
11. Kleinman S, Busch MP, Korelitz JJ, et al.: The incidence/window period model and its use to assess the risk of transfusion-transmitted human immunodeficiency virus and hepatitis C virus infection. Transfus Med Rev 1997;11:155–172.
12. Cumming PD, Wallace EL, Schorr JB, et al.: Exposure of patients to human immunodeficiency virus through the transfusion of blood components that test antibody-negative. N Engl J Med 1989; 321:941–946.
13. Goodnough LT, Brecher ME, Kanter MH, et al.: Transfusion medicine. First of two parts: Blood transfusion. N Engl J Med 1999;340:438–447.
14. Goodnough LT, Brecher ME, Kanter MH, et al.: Transfusion medicine. Second of two parts: Blood conservation. N Engl J Med 1999; 340:525–533.
15. Imagawa DT, Lee MH, Wolinsky SM, et al.: Human immunodeficiency virus type 1 infection in homosexual men who remain seronegative for prolonged periods. N Engl J Med 1989;320:1458–1462.
16. Haseltine WA: Silent HIV infections. N Engl J Med 1989;320:1487–1489.
17. Prati D, Capelli C, Rebulla P, et al: The current risk of retroviral infections transmitted by transfusion in patients who have undergone multiple transfusions. Cooleycare Cooperative Group. Arch Intern Med 1998;158:1566–1569.
18. Schwartz JS, Kinosian BP, Pierskalla WP, et al.: Strategies for screening blood for human immunodeficiency virus antibody: Use of a decision support system. JAMA 1990;264:1704–1710.
19. Crosby ET: Perioperative haemotherapy: II. Risks and complications of blood transfusion. Can J Anaesth 1992;39:822–837.
20. Joshi A, Gerhardt T, Shandloff P, et al.: Blood transfusion effect on the respiratory pattern of preterm infants. Pediatrics 1987;80:79–84.
21. Kallos T, Smith TC: Replacement for intraoperative blood loss. Anesthesiology 1974;41:293–295.
22. Furman EB, Roman DG, Lemmer LA, et al.: Specific therapy in water, electrolyte and blood-volume replacement during pediatric surgery. Anesthesiology 1975;42:187–193.
23. Bourke DL, Smith TC: Estimating allowable hemodilution. Anesthesiology 1974;41:609–612.
24. Shires T, Williams J, Brown F: Acute change in extracellular fluids associated with major surgical procedures. Ann Surg 1961;154:803–810.
25. Shires T, Coln D, Carrico J, et al: Fluid therapy in hemorrhagic shock. Arch Surg 1964;88:688–693.
26. Consensus statement on red cell transfusion. Proceedings of a Consensus Conference Held by the Royal College of Physicians of Edinburgh, May 9–10, 1994. Br J Anaesth 1994;73:857–859.
27. Manno CS, Hedberg KW, Kim HC, et al: Comparison of the hemostatic effects of fresh whole blood, stored whole blood, and components after open heart surgery in children. Blood 1991;77:930–936.
28. Manno CS: What's new in transfusion medicine? Pediatr Clin North Am 1996;43:793–808.
29. Moss GS, Gould SA: Plasma expanders: An update. Am J Surg 1988;155:425–434.

30. Blumberg N, Heal JM: Evidence for plasma-mediated immunomodulation: Transfusions of plasma-rich blood components are associated with a greater risk of acquired immunodeficiency syndrome than transfusions of red blood cells alone. Transplant Proc 1988;20:1138–1142.

31. Weiss HJ: Antiplatelet drugs: A new pharmacologic approach to the prevention of thrombosis. Am Heart J 1976;92:86–102.

32. Schafer AI: Effects of nonsteroidal anti-inflammatory therapy on platelets. Am J Med 1999;106:25S–36S.

33. Schror K: Antiplatelet drugs: A comparative review. Drugs 1995;50:7–28.

34. George JN, Shattil SJ: The clinical importance of acquired abnormalities of platelet function. N Engl J Med 1991;324:27–39.

35. Pisciotto PT, Benson K, Hume H, et al: Prophylactic versus therapeutic platelet transfusion practices in hematology and/or oncology patients. Transfusion 1995;35:498–502.

36. Menitove JE, Aster RH: Transfusion of platelets and plasma products. Clin Haematol 1983;12:239–266.

37. Wandt H, Frank M, Ehninger G, et al: Safety and cost effectiveness of a 10 x 10(9)/L trigger for prophylactic platelet transfusions compared with the traditional 20 x 10(9)/L trigger: A prospective comparative trial in 105 patients with acute myeloid leukemia. Blood 1998;91:3601–3606.

38. Miller RD, Robbins TO, Tong MJ, et al: Coagulation defects associated with massive blood transfusions. Ann Surg 1971;174:794–801.

39. Coté CJ, Liu LM, Szyfelbein SK, et al: Changes in serial platelet counts following massive blood transfusion in pediatric patients. Anesthesiology 1985;62:197–201.

40. Practice Guidelines for blood component therapy: A report by the American Society of Anesthesiologists Task Force on Blood Component Therapy. Anesthesiology 1996;84:732–747.

41. Harrigan C, Lucas CE, Ledgerwood AM, et al: Serial changes in primary hemostasis after massive transfusion. Surgery 1985;98:836–844.

42. Sutor AH: The bleeding time in pediatrics. Semin Thromb Hemost 1998;24:531–543.

43. Levine PL: Editorial. Platelet-function tests: Predictive value. N Engl J Med 1975;292:1346–1347.

44. Harker LA, Slichter SJ: The bleeding time as a screening test for evaluation of platelet function. N Engl J Med 1972;287:155–159.

45. Spiess BD: Thromboelastography and cardiopulmonary bypass. Semin Thromb Hemost 1995;21:27–33.

46. Chandler WL: The thromboelastography and the thromboelastograph technique. Semin Thromb Hemost 1995;21:1–6.

47. Essell JH, Martin TJ, Salinas J, et al: Comparison of thromboelastography to bleeding time and standard coagulation tests in patients after cardiopulmonary bypass. J Cardiothorac Vasc Anesth 1993;7:410–415.

48. Kang Y: Thromboelastography in liver transplantation. Semin Thromb Hemost 1995;21(Suppl 4):34–44.

49. Kirkley SA, Blumberg N: Use of single donor platelets. Blood Rev 1994;8:142–147.

50. Herman JH, Kamel HT: Platelet transfusion: Current techniques, remaining problems, and future prospects. Am J Pediatr Hematol Oncol 1987;9:272–286.

51. McCullough J, Steeper TA, Connelly DP, et al: Platelet utilization in a university hospital. JAMA 1988;259:2414–2418.

52. Rosenberg EM, Chambers LA, Gunter JM, et al: A program to limit donor exposures to neonates undergoing extracorporeal membrane oxygenation. Pediatrics 1994;94:341–346.

53. Strauss RG: Clinical perspectives of platelet transfusions: Defining the optimal dose. J Clin Apheresis 1995;10:124–127.

54. Norol F, Bierling P, Roudot-Thoraval F, et al: Platelet transfusion: A dose-response study. Blood 1998;92:1448–1453.

55. Marshall BE, Wurzel HA, Neufeld GR, et al: Effects of Fenwal 4C2423 transfusion microfilter on microaggregates and other constituents of stored blood. Transfusion 1978;18:38–45.

56. Miller BE, Mochizuki T, Levy JH, et al: Predicting and treating coagulopathies after cardiopulmonary bypass in children. Anesth Analg 1997;85:1196–1202.

57. Brettler DB, Levine PH: Factor concentrates for treatment of hemophilia: Which one to choose? Blood 1989;73:2067–2073.

58. Pierce GF, Lusher JM, Brownstein AP, et al: The use of purified clotting factor concentrates in hemophilia: Influence of viral safety, cost, and supply on therapy. JAMA 1989;261:3434–3438.

59. Levine PH: HIV infection in hemophilia. J Clin Apheresis 1993;8:120–125.

60. Eyster ME, Rabkin CS, Hilgartner MW, et al: Human immunodeficiency virus-related conditions in children and adults with hemophilia: rates, relationship to CD4 counts, and predictive value. Blood 1993;81:828–834.

61. Rosenberg PS, Goedert JJ: Estimating the cumulative incidence of HIV infection among persons with haemophilia in the United States of America. Stat Med 1998;17:155–168.

62. Kasper CK, Dietrich SL: Comprehensive management of haemophilia. Clin Haematol 1985;14:489–512.

63. Levine PH: Factor VIII:C purified from plasma via monoclonal antibodies: Human studies. Semin Hematol 1988;25(Suppl 1):38–41.

64. White GC 2d, McMillan CW, Kingdon HS, et al: Use of recombinant antihemophilic factor in the treatment of two patients with classic hemophilia. N Engl J Med 1989;320:166–170.

65. Shapiro AD: American experience with home use of NovoSeven: Recombinant factor VIIa in hemophiliacs with inhibitors. Haemostasis 1996;26:143–149.

66. Lusher JM: Recombinant factor VIIa (NovoSeven) in the treatment of internal bleeding in patients with factor VIII and IX inhibitors. Haemostasis 1996;26:24–30.

67. Kelly KM, Butler RB, Farace L, et al: Superior in vivo response of recombinant factor VIII concentrate in children with hemophilia A. J Pediatr 1997;130:537–540.

68. Lusher JM, Arkin S, Abildgaard CF, et al: Recombinant factor VIII for the treatment of previously untreated patients with hemophilia A: Safety, efficacy, and development of inhibitors. Kogenate Previously Untreated Patient Study Group. N Engl J Med 1993;328:453–459.

69. Rodeghiero F, Castaman G, Mannucci PM: Prospective multicenter study on subcutaneous concentrated desmopressin for home treatment of patients with von Willebrand disease and mild or moderate hemophilia A. Thromb Haemost 1996;76:692–696.

70. Sutor AH: Desmopressin (DDAVP) in bleeding disorders of childhood. Semin Thromb Hemost 1998;24:555–566.

71. Brinkhous KM, Sigman JL, Read MS, et al: Recombinant human factor IX: Replacement therapy, prophylaxis, and pharmacokinetics in canine hemophilia B. Blood 1996;88:2603–2610.

72. Roberts HR, Eberst ME: Current management of hemophilia B. Hematol Oncol Clin North Am 1993;7:1269–1280.

73. Kurachi K, Furukawa M, Yao SN, et al: Biology of factor IX. Hematol Oncol Clin North Am 1992;6:991–997.

74. Schaub R, Garzone P, Bouchard P, et al: Preclinical studies of recombinant factor IX. Semin Hematol 1998;35:28–32.

75. White G, Shapiro A, Ragni M, et al: Clinical evaluation of recombinant factor IX. Semin Hematol 1998;35:33–38.

76. White GC, Beebe A, Nielsen B: Recombinant factor IX. Thromb Haemost 1997;78:261–265.

77. Mannucci PM: Desmopressin: A nontransfusional form of treatment for congenital and acquired bleeding disorders. Blood 1988;72:1449–1455.

78. Richardson DW, Robinson AG: Desmopressin. Ann Intern Med 1985;103:228–239.

79. Salva KM, Kim HC, Nahum K, et al: DDAVP in the treatment of bleeding disorders. Pharmacotherapy 1988;8:94–99.

80. Naranja RJ Jr, Chan PS, High K, et al: Treatment considerations in patients with compartment syndrome and an inherited bleeding disorder. Orthopedics 1997;20:706–709.

81. Lethagen S: Desmopressin (DDAVP) and hemostasis. Ann Hematol 1994;69:173–180.

82. Deitcher SR, Tuller J, Johnson JA: Intranasal DDAVP induced increases in plasma von Willebrand factor alter the pharmacokinetics of high-purity factor VIII concentrates in severe haemophilia A patients. Haemophilia 1999;5:88–95.

83. Berntorp E: The treatment of haemophilia, including prophylaxis, constant infusion and DDAVP. Baillieres Clin Haematol 1996;9:259–271.

84. Zachee P, Vermylen J, Boogaerts MA: Hematologic aspects of end-stage renal failure. Ann Hematol 1994;69:33–40.

85. Salzman EW, Weinstein MJ, Reilly D, et al: Adventures in hemostasis: Desmopressin in cardiac surgery. Arch Surg 1993;128:212–217.

86. Salzman EW, Weinstein MJ, Weintraub RM, et al: Treatment with desmopressin acetate to reduce blood loss after cardiac surgery: A double-blind randomized trial. N Engl J Med 1986;314:1402–1406.

87. Kobrinsky NL, Letts RM, Patel LR, et al: 1-Desamino-8-D-arginine vasopressin (desmopressin) decreases operative blood loss in patients having Harrington rod spinal fusion surgery: A randomized, double-blinded, controlled trial. Ann Intern Med 1987;107:446–450.

88. Spiess BD: Cardiac anesthesia risk management. Hemorrhage, coagulation, and transfusion: a risk-benefit analysis. J Cardiothorac Vasc Anesth 1994;8:19–22.

89. Hackmann T, Naiman SC: Con: Desmopressin is not of value in the treatment of post-cardiopulmonary bypass bleeding. J Cardiothorac Vasc Anesth 1991;5:290–293.

90. Brown MR, Swygert TH, Whitten CW, et al: Desmopressin acetate following cardiopulmonary bypass: Evaluation of coagulation parameters. J Cardiothorac Anesth 1989;3:726–729.

91. Theroux MC, Corddry DH, Tietz AE, et al: A study of desmopressin and blood loss during spinal fusion for neuromuscular scoliosis: A randomized, controlled, double-blinded study. Anesthesiology 1997;87:260–267.

92. Miller RD: Complications of massive blood transfusions. Anesthesiology 1973;39:82–93.

93. Collins JA: Problems associated with the massive transfusion of stored blood. Surgery 1974;75:274–295.

94. Counts RB, Haisch C, Simon TL, et al: Hemostasis in massively transfused trauma patients. Ann Surg 1979;190:91–99.

95. Noe DA, Graham SM, Luff R, et al: Platelet counts during rapid massive transfusion. Transfusion 1982;22:392–395.

96. Phillips TF, Soulier G, Wilson RF: Outcome of massive transfusion exceeding two blood volumes in trauma and emergency surgery. J Trauma 1987;27:903–910.

97. Hewson JR, Neame PB, Kumar N, et al: Coagulopathy related to dilution and hypotension during massive transfusion. Crit Care Med 1985;13:387–391.

98. Collins JA: Recent developments in the area of massive transfusion. World J Surg 1987;11:75–81.

99. Murray DJ, Olson J, Strauss R, et al: Coagulation changes during packed red cell replacement of major blood loss. Anesthesiology 1988;69:839–845.

100. Ciavarella D, Reed RL, Counts RB, et al: Clotting factor levels and the risk of diffuse microvascular bleeding in the massively transfused patient. Br J Haematol 1987;67:365–368.

101. Harvey MP, Greenfield TP, Sugrue ME, et al: Massive blood transfusion in a tertiary referral hospital: Clinical outcomes and haemostatic complications. Med J Aust 1995;163:356–359.

102. Donaldson MD, Seaman MJ, Park GR: Massive blood transfusion. Br J Anaesth 1992;69:621–630.

103. Irving GA: Perioperative blood and blood component therapy. Can J Anaesth 1992;39:1105–1115.

104. Crosby ET: Perioperative haemotherapy: I. Indications for blood component transfusion. Can J Anaesth 1992;39:695–707.

105. Cosgriff N, Moore EE, Sauaia A, et al: Predicting life-threatening coagulopathy in the massively transfused trauma patient: Hypothermia and acidoses revisited. J Trauma 1997;42:857–861.

106. Rohrer MJ, Natale AM: Effect of hypothermia on the coagulation cascade. Crit Care Med 1992;20:1402–1405.

107. Valeri CR, Feingold H, Cassidy G, et al: Hypothermia-induced reversible platelet dysfunction. Ann Surg 1987;205:175–181.

108. Davis JW, Parks SN, Kaups KL, et al: Admission base deficit predicts transfusion requirements and risk of complications. J Trauma 1996;41:769–774.

109. Triplett DA: The extrinsic system. Clin Lab Med 1984;4:221–244.

110. Murray DJ, Pennell BJ, Weinstein SL, et al: Packed red cells in acute blood loss: Dilutional coagulopathy as a cause of surgical bleeding. Anesth Analg 1995;80:336–342.

111. Coté CJ: Blood, colloid, and crystalloid therapy. Anesth Clin North Am 1991;9:865–884.

112. Coté CJ: Changes in prothrombin and partial thromboplastin times during massive blood loss in children undergoing Harrington rod instrumentation. [abstract] Section on Anesthesiology, American Academy of Pediatrics. 1988.

113. Fresh-Frozen Plasma, Cryoprecipitate, and Platelets Administration Practice Guidelines Development Task Force of the College of American Pathologists: Practice parameter for the use of fresh-frozen plasma, cryoprecipitate, and platelets. JAMA 1994;271:777–781.

114. Oberman HA: Inappropriate use of fresh-frozen plasma. JAMA 1985;253:556–557.

115. Consensus conference. Fresh-frozen plasma. Indications and risks. JAMA 1985;253:551–553.

116. Braunstein AH, Oberman HA: Transfusion of plasma components. Transfusion 1984;24:281–286.

117. Blumberg N, Laczin J, McMican A, et al: A critical survey of fresh-frozen plasma use. Transfusion 1986;26:511–513.

118. Barrer MJ, Ellison N: Platelet function. Anesthesiology 1977;46:202–211.

119. Rebulla P, Finazzi G, Marangoni F, et al: The threshold for prophylactic platelet transfusions in adults with acute myeloid leukemia. Gruppo Italiano Malattie Ematologiche Maligne dell'Adulto. N Engl J Med 1997;337:1870–1875.

120. Lim RC Jr, Olcott C 4th, Robinson AJ, et al: Platelet response and coagulation changes following massive blood replacement. J Trauma 1973;13:577–582.

121. Reed RL 2d, Ciavarella D, Heimbach DM, et al: Prophylactic platelet administration during massive transfusion: A prospective, randomized, double-blind clinical study. Ann Surg 1986;203:40–48.

122. Mammen EF: Coagulopathies of liver disease. Clin Lab Med 1994;14:769–780.

123. Mammen EF: Coagulation defects in liver disease. Med Clin North Am 1994;78:545–554.

124. Marshall M: Potassium intoxication from blood and plasma transfusions. Anaesthesia 1962;17:145–148.

125. Brown KA, Bissonnette B, MacDonald M, et al: Hyperkalaemia during massive blood transfusion in paediatric craniofacial surgery. Can J Anaesth 1990;37:401–408.

126. Brown KA, Bissonnette B, McIntyre B: Hyperkalaemia during rapid blood transfusion and hypovolaemic cardiac arrest in children. Can J Anaesth 1990;37:747–754.

127. Moroff G, Morse EE, Katz AJ, et al: Survival and biochemical characteristics of stored red cells preserved with citrate-phosphate-dextrose-adenine-one and two and prepared from whole blood maintained at 20 to 24 degrees C for eight hours following phlebotomy. Transfusion 1984;24:115–119.

128. Moroff G, Dende D: Characterization of biochemical changes occurring during storage of red cells. Comparative studies with CPD and CPDA-1 anticoagulant-preservative solutions. Transfusion 1983;23:484–489.

129. Wolfe LC: Oxidative injuries to the red cell membrane during conventional blood preservation. Semin Hematol 1989;26:307–312.

130. Batton DG, Maisels MJ, Shulman G: Serum potassium changes following packed red cell transfusions in newborn infants. Transfusion 1983;23:163–164.

131. Scanlon JW, Krakaur R: Hyperkalemia following exchange transfusion. J Pediatr 1980;96:108–110.

132. Fukuoka Y, Ishiyama T, Oguchi T, et al: Hyperkalemia after irradiated blood transfusion. [in Japanese] Masui 1999;48:192–194.

133. Jameson LC, Popic PM, Harms BA: Hyperkalemic death during use of a high-capacity fluid warmer for massive transfusion. Anesthesiology 1990;73:1050–1052.

134. de la Roche MR, Gauthier L: Rapid transfusion of packed red blood cells: Effects of dilution, pressure, and catheter size. Ann Emerg Med 1993;22:1551–1555.

135. Gibbs N, Murphy T, Campbell R: Maximum transfusion rates in neonates and infants. Anaesth Intensive Care 1986;14:347–349.

136. Bunker JP: Metabolic effects of blood transfusion. Anesthesiology 1966;27:446–455.

137. Dzik WH, Kirkley SA: Citrate toxicity during massive blood transfusion. Transfus Med Rev 1988;2:76–94.

138. Olinger GN, Hottenrott C, Mulder DG, et al: Acute clinical hypocalcemic myocardial depression during rapid blood transfusion and postoperative hemodialysis: A preventable complication. J Thorac Cardiovasc Surg 1976;72:503–511.

139. Vagianos C, Steen S, Masson P, et al: Reversal of lethal citrate intoxication by intravenous infusion of calcium: An experimental study in pigs. Acta Chir Scand 1990;156:671–675.

140. Stulz PM, Scheidegger D, Drop LJ, et al: Ventricular pump performance during hypocalcemia: Clinical and experimental studies. J Thorac Cardiovasc Surg 1979;78:185–194.

141. Scheidegger D, Drop LJ: The relationship between duration of Q-T interval and plasma ionized calcium concentration: Experiments with acute, steady-state $[Ca++]$ changes in the dog. Anesthesiology 1979;51:143–148.

142. Coté CJ, Drop LJ, Daniels AL, et al: Calcium chloride versus calcium gluconate: Comparison of ionization and cardiovascular effects in children and dogs. Anesthesiology 1987;66:465–470.

143. Martin TJ, Kang Y, Robertson KM, et al: Ionization and hemodynamic effects of calcium chloride and calcium gluconate in the absence of hepatic function. Anesthesiology 1990;73:62–65.

144. Coté CJ, Drop LJ, Hoaglin DC, et al: Ionized hypocalcemia after fresh

frozen plasma administration to thermally injured children: Effects of infusion rate, duration, and treatment with calcium chloride. Anesth Analg 1988;67:152–160.

145. Coté CJ: Depth of halothane anesthesia potentiates citrate-induced ionized hypocalcemia and adverse cardiovascular events in dogs. Anesthesiology 1987;67:676–680.

146. Komai H, Rusy BF: Contribution of the known subcellular effects of anesthetics to their negative inotropic effect in intact myocardium. Adv Exp Med Biol 1991;301:115–123.

147. Rusy BF, Komai H: Anesthetic depression of myocardial contractility: A review of possible mechanisms. Anesthesiology 1987;67:745–766.

148. Marquez J, Martin D, Virji MA, et al: Cardiovascular depression secondary to ionic hypocalcemia during hepatic transplantation in humans. Anesthesiology 1986;65:457–461.

149. Driscoll DF, Bistrian BR, Jenkins RL, et al: Development of metabolic alkalosis after massive transfusion during orthotopic liver transplantation. Crit Care Med 1987;15:905–908.

150. Borland LM, Roule M, Cook DR: Anesthesia for pediatric orthotopic liver transplantation. Anesth Analg 1985;64:117–124.

151. Borland LM, Martin DJ: Anesthesia considerations for orthotopic liver transplantation. Contemp Anesth Pract 1987;10:157–182.

152. Carmichael FJ, Lindop MJ, Farman JV: Anesthesia for hepatic transplantation: Cardiovascular and metabolic alterations and their management. Anesth Analg 1985;64:108–116.

153. Davis PJ, Cook DR: Anesthetic problems in pediatric liver transplantation. Transplant Proc 1989;21:3493–3496.

154. Rocha E, Paramo JA, Montes R, et al: Acute generalized, widespread bleeding. Diagnosis and management. Haematologica 1998;83:1024–1037.

155. Ellison N: Diagnosis and management of bleeding disorders. Anesthesiology 1977;47:171–180.

156. Giddings JC, Peake IR: Laboratory support in the diagnosis of coagulation disorders. Clin Haematol 1985;14:571–595.

157. Prentice CR: Acquired coagulation disorders. Clin Haematol 1985;14:413–442.

158. Risberg B, Andreasson S, Eriksson E: Disseminated intravascular coagulation. Acta Anaesthesiol Scand Suppl 1991;95:60–71.

159. Miller RD, Tong MJ, Robbins TO: Effects of massive transfusion of blood on acid-base balance. JAMA 1971;216:1762–1765.

160. Collins JA, Simmons RL, James PM, et al: Acid-base status of seriously wounded combat casualties. II. Resuscitation with stored blood. Ann Surg 1971;173:6–18.

161. Collins JA, Simmons RL, James PM, et al: The acid-base status of seriously wounded combat casualties. I. Before treatment. Ann Surg 1970;171:595–608.

162. Kahn RC, Jascott D, Carlon GC, et al: Massive blood replacement: Correlation of ionized calcium, citrate, and hydrogen ion concentration. Anesth Analg 1979;58:274–278.

163. Boyan CP: Cold or warmed blood for massive transfusions. Ann Surg 1964;160:282–286.

164. Wagner PD: The oxyhemogolobin dissociation curve and pulmonary gas exchange. Semin Hematol 1974;11:405–421.

165. Presson RG Jr, Bezruczko AP, Hillier SC, et al: Evaluation of a new fluid warmer effective at low to moderate flow rates. Anesthesiology 1993;78:974–980.

166. Presson RG Jr, Hillier SC: Perioperative fluid and transfusion management. Semin Pediatr Surg 1992;1:22–31.

167. Presson RG Jr, Haselby KA, Bezruczko AP, et al: Evaluation of a new high-efficiency blood warmer for children. Anesthesiology 1990;73:173–176.

168. Arndt M, Hofmockel R, Benad G: Level 1: A new blood warming device. [in German]. Anaesthesiol Reanim 1994;19:78–79.

169. Browne DA, de Boeck R, Morgan M: An evaluation of the Level 1 blood warmer series. Anaesthesia 1990;45:960–963.

170. Smallman JM, Morgan M: Evaluation of the Level 1 Hotline blood warmer. Anaesthesia 1992;47:869–871.

171. Bunn HF, Jandl JH: Control of hemoglobin function within the red cell. N Engl J Med 1970;282:1414–1421.

172. Sheldon GF: Diphosphoglycerate in massive transfusion and erythropoiesis. Crit Care Med 1979;7:407–411.

173. Woodson RD: Physiological significance of oxygen dissociation curve shifts. Crit Care Med 1979;7:368–373.

174. McNamara JJ, Burran EL, Stremple JF, et al: Coagulopathy after major combat injury: Occurrence, management, and pathophysiology. Ann Surg 1972;176:243–246.

175. Connell RS, Swank RL: Pulmonary microembolism after blood transfusion: An electron microscopic study. Ann Surg 1973;177:40–50.

176. Cullen DJ, Ferrara L: Comparative evaluation of blood filters: A study in vitro. Anesthesiology 1974;41:568–575.

177. Marshall BE, Wurzel HA, Ewing BC, et al: An evaluation of the Bentley PFF-100 transfusion filter. Can Anaesth Soc J 1978;25:204–210.

178. Coté CJ, Daniels AL, Connolly M, et al: Tongue oximetry in children with extensive thermal injury: Comparison with peripheral oximetry. Can J Anaesth 1992;39:454–457.

179. Jobes DR, Nicolson SC: Monitoring of arterial hemoglobin oxygen saturation using a tongue sensor. Anesth Analg 1988;67:186–188.

180. Partridge BL: Use of pulse oximetry as a noninvasive indicator of intravascular volume status. J Clin Monit 1987;3:263–268.

181. Coté CJ, Jobes DR, Schwartz AJ, et al: Two approaches to cannulation of a child's internal jugular vein. Anesthesiology 1979;50:371–373.

182. Todres ID, Crone RK, Rogers MC, et al: Swan-Ganz catheterization in the critically ill newborn. Crit Care Med 1979;7:330–334.

183. Williams GD, Bratton SL, Nielsen NJ, et al: Fibrinolysis in pediatric patients undergoing cardiopulmonary bypass. J Cardiothorac Vasc Anesth 1998;12:633–638.

184. Shore-Lesserson L, Manspeizer HE, DePerio M, et al: Thromboelastography-guided transfusion algorithm reduces transfusions in complex cardiac surgery. Anesth Analg 1999;88:312–319.

185. Stammers AH, Bruda NL, Gonano C, et al: Point-of-care coagulation monitoring: Applications of the thromboelastography. Anaesthesia 1998;53:58–59.

186. Gillies BS: Thromboelastography and liver transplantation. Semin Thromb Hemost 1995;21:45–49.

187. Wang JS, Lin CY, Hung WT, et al: Thromboelastogram fails to predict postoperative hemorrhage in cardiac patients. Ann Thorac Surg 1992;53:435–439.

188. Dorman BH, Spinale FG, Bailey MK, et al: Identification of patients at risk for excessive blood loss during coronary artery bypass surgery: Thromboelastography versus coagulation screen. Anesth Analg 1993;76:694–700.

189. Pivalizza EG, Abramson DC, King FS Jr: Thromboelastography with heparinase in orthotopic liver transplantation. J Cardiothorac Vasc Anesth 1998;12:305–308.

190. Slaughter TF, Greenberg CS: Antifibrinolytic drugs and perioperative hemostasis. Am J Hematol 1997;56:32–36.

191. Ippolito G, Puro V, Heptonstall J, et al: Occupational human immunodeficiency virus infection in health care workers: Worldwide cases through September 1997. Clin Infect Dis 1999;28:365–383.

192. Rodriguez-Merchan EC: Intraoperative transmission of blood-borne disease in haemophilia. Haemophilia 1998;4:75–78.

193. Bell DM: Occupational risk of human immunodeficiency virus infection in healthcare workers: An overview. Am J Med 1997;102:9–15.

194. Sistrom MG, Coyner BJ, Gwaltney JM Jr, et al: Frequency of percutaneous injuries requiring postexposure prophylaxis for occupational exposure to human immunodeficiency virus. Infect Control Hosp Epidemiol 1998;19:504–506.

195. Cuny E, Carpenter WM: Occupational exposure to blood and body fluids: New postexposure prophylaxis recommendations. United States Occupational Safety and Health Administration. J Calif Dent Assoc 1998;26:261–267.

196. Local Collaborators, PHLS AIDS and STD Centre, Scottish Centre for Infection and Environmental Health: Occupational acquisition of HIV infection among health care workers in the United Kingdom: Data to June 1997. Commun Dis Public Health 1998;1:103–107.

197. Jagger J, Hunt EH, Pearson RD: Estimated cost of needlestick injuries for six major needled devices. Infect Control Hosp Epidemiol 1990;11:584–588.

198. Jagger J, Hunt EH, Pearson RD: Sharp object injuries in the hospital: Causes and strategies for prevention. Am J Infect Control 1990;18:227–231.

199. Jagger J, Hunt EH, Brand-Elnaggar J, et al: Rates of needle-stick injury caused by various devices in a university hospital. N Engl J Med 1988;319:284–288.

200. Marcus R: Surveillance of health care workers exposed to blood from patients infected with the human immunodeficiency virus. N Engl J Med 1988;319:1118–1123.

201. Greene ER Jr: Acquired immunodeficiency syndrome: An overview for anesthesiologists. Anesth Analg 1986;65:1054–1058.

202. Falloon J, Eddy J, Wiener L, et al: Human immunodeficiency virus infection in children. J Pediatr 1989;114:1–30.

203. Tomkins DP, van der Walt JH: Needleless and sharp-free anaesthesia. Anaesth Intensive Care 1996;24:164–168.
204. O'Neill TM, Abbott AV, Radecki SE: Risk of needlesticks and occupational exposures among residents and medical students. Arch Intern Med 1992;152:1451–1456.
205. Melzer SM, Vermund SH, Shelov SP: Needle injuries among pediatric housestaff physicians in New York City. Pediatrics 1989;84:211–214.
206. Cheung RJ, DiMarino AJ Jr: Risk to the health care worker of HIV infection and how to minimize it. Gastrointest Endosc Clin N Am 1998;8:769–782.
207. Lurie P, Miller S, Hecht F, et al: Postexposure prophylaxis after nonoccupational HIV exposure: Clinical, ethical, and policy considerations. JAMA 1998;280:1769–1773.
208. Danila RN: Recommendations for chemoprophylaxis after occupational exposure to human immunodeficiency virus: A public health agency perspective. Am J Med 1997;102:98–101.
209. MacMillan ML, Freedman MH: Recombinant human erythropoietin in children with cancer. J Pediatr Hematol Oncol 1998;20:187–189.
210. Varan A, Buyukpamukcu M, Kutluk T, et al: Recombinant human erythropoietin treatment for chemotherapy-related anemia in children. Pediatrics 1999;103:E16.
211. Burke JR: Low-dose subcutaneous recombinant erythropoietin in children with chronic renal failure. Australian and New Zealand Paediatric Nephrology Association. Pediatr Nephrol 1995;9:558–561.
212. Shimpo H, Mizumoto T, Onoda K, et al: Erythropoietin in pediatric cardiac surgery: Clinical efficacy and effective dose. Chest 1997;111:1565–1570.
213. Vitale MG, Stazzone EJ, Gelijns AC, et al: The effectiveness of preoperative erythropoietin in averting allogenic blood transfusion among children undergoing scoliosis surgery. J Pediatr Orthop B 1998;7:203–209.
214. Smith SN, Milov DE: Use of erythropoietin in Jehovah's Witness children following acute gastrointestinal blood loss. J Fla Med Assoc 1993;80:103–105.
215. Scharer K, Klare B, Braun A, et al: Treatment of renal anemia by subcutaneous erythropoietin in children with preterminal chronic renal failure. Acta Paediatr 1993;82:953–958.
216. Goodnough LT, Verbrugge D, Marcus RE, et al: The effect of patient size and dose of recombinant human erythropoietin therapy on red blood cell volume expansion in autologous blood donors for elective orthopedic operation. J Am Coll Surg 1994;179:171–176.
217. Damme-Lombaerts R, Broyer M, Businger J, et al: A study of recombinant human erythropoietin in the treatment of anaemia of chronic renal failure in children on haemodialysis. Pediatr Nephrol 1994;8:338–342.
218. Anand N, Idio FG Jr, Remer S, et al: The effects of perioperative blood salvage and autologous blood donation on transfusion requirements in scoliosis surgery. J Spinal Disord 1998;11:532–534.
219. Kruskall MS, Glazer EE, Leonard SS, et al: Utilization and effectiveness of a hospital autologous preoperative blood donor program. Transfusion 1986;26:335–340.
220. Ferguson KJ, Strauss RG, Toy PT: Physician recommendation as the key factor in patients' decisions to participate in preoperative autologous blood donation programs: Preoperative Autologous Blood Donation Study Group. Am J Surg 1994;168:2–5.
221. McVay PA, Andrews A, Kaplan EB, et al: Donation reactions among autologous donors. Transfusion 1990;30:249–252.
222. Toy PT, Strauss RG, Stehling LC, et al: Predeposited autologous blood for elective surgery: A national multicenter study. N Engl J Med 1987;316:517–520.
223. Novak RW: Autologous blood transfusion in a pediatric population: Safety and efficacy. Clin Pediatr (Phila) 1988;27:184–187.
224. Luban NL, DePalma L: Transfusion-associated graft-versus-host disease in the neonate-expanding the spectrum of disease. Transfusion 1996;36:101–103.
225. DePalma L, Luban NL: Autologous blood transfusion in pediatrics. Pediatrics 1990;85:125–128.
226. DePalma L, Luban NL: Blood component therapy in the perinatal period: Guidelines and recommendations. Semin Perinatol 1990;14:403–415.
227. Stehling L: Autologous transfusion. Int Anesthesiol Clin 1990;28:190–196.
228. Stehling L: Predeposit autologous blood donation. Acta Anaesthesiol Scand Suppl 1988;89:58–62.
229. Greenwalt TJ, Dumaswala UJ, Dhingra N, et al: Studies in red blood cell preservation. 7. In vivo and in vitro studies with a modified phosphate-ammonium additive solution. Vox Sang 1993;65:87–94.
230. Moore GL: Additive solutions for better blood preservation. Crit Rev Clin Lab Sci 1987;25:211–229.
231. Knight JA, Searles DA, Clayton FC: The effect of desferrioxamine on stored erythrocytes: Lipid peroxidation, deformability, and morphology. Ann Clin Lab Sci 1996;26:283–290.
232. Laupacis A, Fergusson D: Erythropoietin to minimize perioperative blood transfusion: A systematic review of randomized trials. The International Study of Peri-operative Transfusion (ISPOT) Investigators. Transfus Med 1998;8:309–317.
233. Jabs K, Harmon WE: Recombinant human erythropoietin therapy in children on dialysis. Adv Ren Replace Ther 1996;3:24–36.
234. Csaki C, Ferencz T, Schuler D, et al: Recombinant human erythropoietin in the prevention of chemotherapy-induced anaemia in children with malignant solid tumours. Eur J Cancer 1998;34:364–367.
235. Eschbach JW, Kelly MR, Haley NR, et al: Treatment of the anemia of progressive renal failure with recombinant human erythropoietin. N Engl J Med 1989;321:158–163.
236. Rhondeau SM, Christensen RD, Ross MP, et al: Responsiveness to recombinant human erythropoietin of marrow erythroid progenitors from infants with the "anemia of prematurity." J Pediatr 1988;112:935–940.
237. Roberts WA, Kirkley SA, Newby M: A cost comparison of allogeneic and preoperatively or intraoperatively donated autologous blood. Anesth Analg 1996;83:129–133.
238. BCSH Blood Transfusion Task Force: Guidelines on gamma irradiation of blood components for the prevention of transfusion-associated graft-versus-host disease. Transfus Med 1996;6:261–271.
239. Przepiorka D, LeParc GF, Stovall MA, et al: Use of irradiated blood components: Practice parameter. Am J Clin Pathol 1996;106:6–11.
240. Blais RE, Hadjipavlou AG, Shulman G: Efficacy of autotransfusion in spine surgery: Comparison of autotransfusion alone and with hemodilution and apheresis. Spine 1996;21:2795–2800.
241. Due TL, Johnson JM, Wood M, et al: Intraoperative autotransfusion in the management of massive hemorrhage. Am J Surg 1975;130:652–658.
242. Lennon RL, Hosking MP, Gray JR, et al: The effects of intraoperative blood salvage and induced hypotension on transfusion requirements during spinal surgical procedures. Mayo Clin Proc 1987;62:1090–1094.
243. Glover JL, Smith R, Yaw PB, et al: Autotransfusion of blood contaminated by intestinal contents. JACEP 1978;7:142–144.
244. Glover JL, Smith R, Yaw P, et al: Intraoperative autotransfusion: An underutilized technique. Surgery 1976;80:474–479.
245. Stillman RM, Wrezlewicz WW, Stanczewski B, et al: The haematological hazards of autotransfusion. Br J Surg 1976;63:651–654.
246. Mattox KL: Comparison of techniques of autotransfusion. Surgery 1978;84:700–702.
247. Csencsitz TA, Flynn JC: Intraoperative blood salvage in spinal deformity surgery in children. J Fla Med Assoc 1979;66:39–41.
248. McShane AJ, Power C, Jackson JF, et al: Autotransfusion: quality of blood prepared with a red cell processing device. Br J Anaesth 1987;59:1035–1039.
249. Solem JO, Vagianos C: Peroperative blood salvage. Acta Anaesthesiol Scand Suppl 1988;89:71–75.
250. Tawes RL Jr, Duvall TB: Is the "salvaged-cell syndrome" myth or reality? Am J Surg 1996;172:172–174.
251. Booke M, Hagemann O, Van Aken H, et al: Intraoperative autotransfusion in small children: An in vitro investigation to study its feasibility. Anesth Analg 1999;88:763–765.
252. Hansen E, Wolff N, Knuechel R, et al: Tumor cells in blood shed from the surgical field. Arch Surg 1995;130:387–393.
253. Mercuriali F, Inghilleri G, Biffi E, et al: Autotransfusion program: Integrated use of different techniques. Int J Artif Organs 1993;16:233–240.
254. Leigh JM: The history of controlled hypotension. Br J Anaesth 1975;47:745–749.
255. Salem MR, Toyama T, Wong AY, et al: Haemodynamic responses to induced arterial hypotension in children. Br J Anaesth 1978;50:489–494.
256. Diaz JH, Lockhart CH: Hypotensive anaesthesia for craniectomy in infancy. Br J Anaesth 1979;51:233–235.
257. McNeill TW, DeWald RL, Kuo KN, et al: Controlled hypotensive anesthesia in scoliosis surgery. J Bone Joint Surg Am 1974;56:1167–1172.

258. Salem MR, Wong AY, Bennett EJ, et al: Deliberate hypotension in infants and children. Anesth Analg 1974;53:975–981.

259. Viguera MG, Terry RN: Induced hypotension for extensive surgery in an infant. Anesthesiology 1966;27:701–702.

260. Yaster M, Simmons RS, Tolo VT, et al: A comparison of nitroglycerin and nitroprusside for inducing hypotension in children: A double-blind study. Anesthesiology 1986;65:175–179.

261. Mandel RJ, Brown MD, McCollough NC, III, et al: Hypotensive anesthesia and autotransfusion in spinal surgery. Clin Orthop 1981;154:27–33.

262. Phillips WA, Hensinger RN: Control of blood loss during scoliosis surgery. Clin Orthop 1988;229:88–93.

263. Tobias JD: Nicardipine for controlled hypotension during orthognathic surgery. Plast Reconstr Surg 1997;99:1539–1543.

264. Tobias JD, Hersey S, Mencio GA, et al: Nicardipine for controlled hypotension during spinal surgery. J Pediatr Orthop 1996;16:370–373.

265. Smith AL, Wollman H: Cerebral blood flow and metabolism: Effects of anesthetic drugs and techniques. Anesthesiology 1972;36:378–400.

266. Newberg LA, Milde JH, Michenfelder JD: The cerebral metabolic effects of isoflurane at and above concentrations that suppress cortical electrical activity. Anesthesiology 1983;59:23–28.

267. Madsen JB, Cold GE, Hansen ES, et al: Cerebral blood flow and metabolism during isoflurane-induced hypotension in patients subjected to surgery for cerebral aneurysms. Br J Anaesth 1987;59:1204–1207.

268. Seyde WC, Longnecker DE: Cerebral oxygen tension in rats during deliberate hypotension with sodium nitroprusside, 2-chloroadenosine, or deep isoflurane anesthesia. Anesthesiology 1986;64:480–485.

269. Newman B, Gelb AW, Lam AM: The effect of isoflurane-induced hypotension on cerebral blood flow and cerebral metabolic rate for oxygen in humans. Anesthesiology 1986;64:307–310.

270. Harp JR, Wollman H: Cerebral metabolic effects of hyperventilation and deliberate hypotension. Br J Anaesth 1973;45:256–262.

271. McDowall DG: Induced hypotension and brain ischaemia. Br J Anaesth 1985;57:110–119.

272. Tobias JD: Sevoflurane for controlled hypotension during spinal surgery: Preliminary experience in five adolescents. Paediatr Anaesth 1998;8:167–170.

273. Fukusaki M, Miyako M, Hara T, et al: Effects of controlled hypotension with sevoflurane anaesthesia on hepatic function of surgical patients. Eur J Anaesthesiol 1999;16:111–116.

274. Yukioka H, Asada K, Fujimori M, et al: Prostaglandin E₁ as a hypotensive drug during general anesthesia for total hip replacement. J Clin Anesth 1993;5:310–314.

275. Artru AA: Cerebral metabolism and EEG during combination of hypocapnia and isoflurane-induced hypotension in dogs. Anesthesiology 1986;65:602–608.

276. Turner JM, Powell D, Gibson RM, et al: Intracranial pressure changes in neurosurgical patients during hypotension induced with sodium nitroprusside or trimetaphan. Br J Anaesth 1977;49:419–425.

277. Stoyka WW, Schutz H: The cerebral response to sodium nitroprusside and trimethaphan controlled hypotension. Can Anaesth Soc J 1975;22:275–283.

278. Michenfelder JD, Theye RA: Canine systemic and cerebral effects of hypotension induced by hemorrhage, trimethaphan, halothane, or nitroprusside. Anesthesiology 1977;46:188–195.

279. Maekawa T, McDowall DG, Okuda Y: Brain-surface oxygen tension and cerebral cortical blood flow during hemorrhagic and drug-induced hypotension in the cat. Anesthesiology 1979;51:313–320.

280. Sivarajan M, Amory DW, McKenzie SM: Regional blood flows during induced hypotension produced by nitroprusside or trimethaphan in the rhesus monkey. Anesth Analg 1985;64:759–766.

281. Norlen K: Central and regional haemodynamics during controlled hypotension produced by adenosine, sodium nitroprusside and nitroglycerin: Studies in the pig. Br J Anaesth 1988;61:186–193.

282. Takakura S, Satoh Y, Satoh H, et al: Effects of nilvadipine on regional cerebral blood flow and skin blood flow in anesthetized cats. Arch Int Pharmacodyn Ther 1992;319:38–48.

283. James IM, Yogendran L, McLaughlin K, et al: Blood pressure lowering and cerebral blood flow: A comparison of the effects of carvedilol and propranolol on the cerebral circulation in hypertensive patients. J Cardiovasc Pharmacol 1992;19:S40–S43.

284. Madsen PL, Vorstrup S, Schmidt JF, et al: Effect of acute and prolonged treatment with propranolol on cerebral blood flow and cerebral oxygen metabolism in healthy volunteers. Eur J Clin Pharmacol 1990;39:295–297.

285. Nikki PH, Nemoto EM, Bleyaert AL, et al: Absence of beta-adrenergic receptor involvement in cerebrovascular dilation by halothane in monkeys. Anesth Analg 1987;66:39–46.

286. Rogers MC, Hamburger C, Owen K, et al: Intracranial pressure in the cat during nitroglycerin-induced hypotension. Anesthesiology 1979;51:227–229.

287. Hickey R, Albin MS, Bunegin L, et al: Autoregulation of spinal cord blood flow: Is the cord a microcosm of the brain? Stroke 1986;17:1183–1189.

288. Grundy BL, Nash CL Jr, Brown RH: Deliberate hypotension for spinal fusion: Prospective randomized study with evoked potential monitoring. Can Anaesth Soc J 1982;29:452–462.

289. Spargo PM, Tait AR, Knight PR, et al: Effect of nitroglycerine-induced hypotension on canine spinal cord blood flow. Br J Anaesth 1987;59:640–647.

290. Jacobs HK, Lieponis JV, Bunch WH, et al: The influence of halothane and nitroprusside on canine spinal cord hemodynamics. Spine 1982;7:35–40.

291. Salzman SK, Lee WA, Sabato S, et al: Halothane anesthesia is neuroprotective in experimental spinal cord injury: early hemodynamic mechanisms of action. Res Commun Chem Pathol Pharmacol 1993;80:59–81.

292. Hoffman WE, Edelman G, Kochs E, et al: Cerebral autoregulation in awake versus isoflurane-anesthetized rats. Anesth Analg 1991;73:753–757.

293. Kien ND, White DA, Reitan JA, et al: Cardiovascular function during controlled hypotension induced by adenosine triphosphate or sodium nitroprusside in the anesthetized dog. Anesth Analg 1987;66:103–110.

294. Wilton NC, Tait AR, Kling TF Jr, et al: The effect of trimethaphan-induced hypotension on canine spinal cord blood flow: Measurement at different cord levels using radiolabelled microspheres. Spine 1988;13:490–493.

295. Kling TF Jr, Wilton N, Hensinger RN, et al: The influence of trimethaphan (Arfonad)-induced hypotension with and without spine distraction on canine spinal cord blood flow. Spine 1986;11:219–224.

296. Kling TF Jr, Fergusson NV, Leach AB, et al: The influence of induced hypotension and spine distraction on canine spinal cord blood flow. Spine 1985;10:878–883.

297. Patel NJ, Patel BS, Paskin S, et al: Induced moderate hypotensive anesthesia for spinal fusion and Harrington-rod instrumentation. J Bone Joint Surg Am 1985;67:1384–1387.

298. Lawhon SM, Kahn A 3d, Crawford AH, et al: Controlled hypotensive anesthesia during spinal surgery: A retrospective study. Spine 1984;9:450–453.

299. Townes BD, Dikmen SS, Bledsoe SW, et al: Neuropsychological changes in a young, healthy population after controlled hypotensive anesthesia. Anesth Analg 1986;65:955–959.

300. Fahmy NR: Nitroglycerin as a hypotensive drug during general anesthesia. Anesthesiology 1978;49:17–20.

301. Page IH, Corcoran AC, Dustan HP, et al: Cardiovascular actions of sodium nitroprusside in animals and hypertensive patients. Circulation 1955;11:188–198.

302. Wang HH, Liu LM, Katz RL: A comparison of the cardiovascular effects of sodium nitroprusside and trimethaphan. Anesthesiology 1977;46:40–48.

303. Miletich DJ, Ivankovich AD: Cardiovascular effects of ganglionic blocking drugs. Int Anesthesiol Clin 1978;16:151–170.

304. Chatterjee K, Parmley WW, Ganz W, et al: Hemodynamic and metabolic responses to vasodilator therapy in acute myocardial infarction. Circulation 1973;48:1183–1193.

305. Tinker JH, Michenfelder JD: Cardiac cyanide toxicity induced by nitroprusside in the dog: potential for reversal. Anesthesiology 1978;49:109–116.

306. Goldstein RE, Michaelis LL, Morrow AG, et al: Coronary collateral function in patients without occlusive coronary artery disease. Circulation 1975;51:118–125.

307. Chiariello M, Gold HK, Leinbach RC, et al: Comparison between the effects of nitroprusside and nitroglycerin on ischemic injury during acute myocardial infarction. Circulation 1976;54:766–773.

308. Lam AM: The choice of controlled hypotension during repair of intracranial aneurysms: Techniques and complications. Agressologie 1990;31:357–359.

309. Litman RS, Zerngast BA: Cardiac arrest after esmolol administration: A review of acute beta-blocker toxicity. J Am Osteopath Assoc 1996;96:616–618.

310. Shah N, Del Valle O, Edmondson R, et al: Esmolol infusion during nitroprusside-induced hypotension: Impact on hemodynamics, ventricular performance, and venous admixture. J Cardiothorac Vasc Anesth 1992;6:196–200.

311. Cuneo BF, Zales VR, Blahunka PC, et al: Pharmacodynamics and pharmacokinetics of esmolol, a short-acting beta-blocking agent, in children. Pediatr Cardiol 1994;15:296–301.

312. Wiest DB, Trippel DL, Gillette PC, et al: Pharmacokinetics of esmolol in children. Clin Pharmacol Ther 1991;49:618–623.

313. De Hert S, Boeckx E, Vercauteren M, et al: Safety of labetalol–induced controlled hypotension during middle ear microsurgery. Acta Otorhinolaryngol Belg 1989;43:157–162.

314. Jones SE: Coarctation in children: Controlled hypotension using labetalol and halothane. Anaesthesia 1979;34:1052–1055.

315. Gurevich B, Artru AA, Geva D, et al: Labetalol-induced hypotension decreases blood loss during uncontrolled hemorrhage. Resuscitation 1998;38:25–32.

316. Marshall WK, Bedford RF, Arnold WP, et al: Effects of propranolol on the cardiovascular and renin-angiotensin systems during hypotension produced by sodium nitroprusside in humans. Anesthesiology 1981;55:277–280.

317. Hellewell J, Potts MW: Propranolol during controlled hypotension. Br J Anaesth 1966;38:794–801.

318. Critchley JA, Ungar A: The management of acute poisoning due to beta-adrenoceptor antagonists. Med Toxicol Adverse Drug Exp 1989;4:32–45.

319. Peterson CD, Leeder JS, Sterner S: Glucagon therapy for beta-blocker overdose. Drug Intell Clin Pharm 1984;18:394–398.

320. Larson CP Jr, Mazze RI, Cooperman LH, et al: Effects of anesthetics on cerebral, renal, and splanchnic circulations: Recent developments. Anesthesiology 1974;41:169–181.

321. Leighton KM, Bruce C, MacLeod BA: Sodium nitroprusside-induced hypotension and renal blood flow. Can Anaesth Soc J 1977;24:637–640.

322. Behnia R, Siqueira EB, Brunner EA: Sodium nitroprusside-induced hypotension: Effect on renal function. Anesth Analg 1978;57:521–526.

323. Behnia R, Martin A, Koushanpour E, et al: Trimethaphan-induced hypotension: Effect on renal function. Can Anaesth Soc J 1982;29:581–586.

324. Hara T, Fukusaki M, Nakamura T, et al: Renal function in patients during and after hypotensive anesthesia with sevoflurane. J Clin Anesth 1998;10:539–545.

325. Zall S, Eden E, Winso I, et al: Controlled hypotension with adenosine or sodium nitroprusside during cerebral aneurysm surgery: Effects on renal hemodynamics, excretory function, and renin release. Anesth Analg 1990;71:631–636.

326. Smith SA, Rafiqi EI, Gardener EG, et al: Renal effects of nicardipine in essential hypertension: Differences between acute and chronic therapy. J Hypertens 1987;5:693–697.

327. Testa LD, Tobias JD: Pharmacologic drugs for controlled hypotension. J Clin Anesth 1995;7:326–337.

328. Nitenberg A, Chemla D, Blanchet F, et al: Beta blockers induce different intrarenal effects in humans: Demonstration by selective infusion of tertatolol and propranolol. J Clin Pharmacol 1990;30:930–937.

329. Toivonen J, Kaukinen S, Oikkonen M, et al: Effects of deliberate hypotension induced by labetalol on renal function. Eur J Anaesthesiol 1991;8:13–20.

330. Wallin JD: Adrenoreceptors and renal function. J Clin Hypertens 1985;1:171–178.

331. Epstein M, Oster JR: Beta blockers and renal function: A reappraisal. J Clin Hypertens 1985;1:85–99.

332. Askrog VF, Pender JW, Eckenhoff JE: Changes in physiological dead space during deliberate hypotension. Anesthesiology 1964;25:744–751.

333. Casthely PA, Lear S, Cottrell JE, et al: Intrapulmonary shunting during induced hypotension. Anesth Analg 1982;61:231–235.

334. Eckenhoff JE, Enderby GEH, Larson A, et al: Pulmonary gas exchange during deliberate hypotension. Br J Anaesth 1963;35:750–759.

335. Strunin L: Organ perfusion during controlled hypotension. Br J Anaesth 1975;47:793–798.

336. Gelman S, Ernst EA: Hepatic circulation during sodium nitroprusside infusion in the carbon tetrachloride–treated dog. Ala J Med Sci 1982;19:371–374.

337. Gelman S, Ernst EA: Hepatic circulation during sodium nitroprusside infusion in the dog. Anesthesiology 1978;49:182–187.

338. Thompson GE, Miller RD, Stevens WC, et al: Hypotensive anesthesia for total hip arthroplasty: A study of blood loss and organ function (brain, heart, liver, and kidney). Anesthesiology 1978;48:91–96.

339. Chauvin M, Bonnet F, Montembault C, et al: Hepatic plasma flow during sodium nitroprusside–induced hypotension in humans. Anesthesiology 1985;63:287–293.

340. Endrich B, Franke N, Peter K, et al: Induced hypotension: action of sodium nitroprusside and nitroglycerin on the microcirculation: A micropuncture investigation. Anesthesiology 1987;66:605–613.

341. Sweeney MO, Cinquegrani M, Liang CS: Effects of oral labetalol on forearm and hepatic circulations in normotensive humans. J Lab Clin Med 1987;109:589–594.

342. Zoller WG, Wagner DR, Zentner J: Effect of propranolol on portal vein hemodynamics: Assessment by duplex sonography and indocyanine green clearance in healthy volunteers. Clin Invest 1993;71:654–658.

343. Soons PA, De Boer A, Cohen AF, et al: Assessment of hepatic blood flow in healthy subjects by continuous infusion of indocyanine green. Br J Clin Pharmacol 1991;32:697–704.

344. Bax ND, Tucker GT, Lennard MS, et al: The impairment of lignocaine clearance by propranolol: Major contribution from enzyme inhibition. Br J Clin Pharmacol 1985;19:597–603.

345. Kito K, Arai T, Mori K, et al: Hepatic blood flow and energy metabolism during hypotension induced by prostaglandin E_1 and nicardipine in rabbits: An in vivo magnetic resonance spectroscopic study. Anesth Analg 1993;77:606–612.

346. Aono J, Ueda W, Hirakawa M: Effect of nitroglycerin and nicardipine on ICG excretion during halothane anesthesia. [in Japanese] Masui 1991;40:406–409.

347. Hyer SL, Taylor D, Barham J, et al: The effects of propranolol and metoprolol on skin blood flow in diabetic patients. Br J Clin Pharmacol 1987;23:769–771.

348. McSorley PD, Warren DJ: Effects of propranolol and metoprolol on the peripheral circulation. Br Med J 1978;2:1598–1600.

349. Mashimo T, Pak M, Choe H, et al: Effects of vasodilators guanethidine, nicardipine, nitroglycerin, and prostaglandin E_1 on primary afferent nociceptors in humans. J Clin Pharmacol 1997;37:330–335.

350. Kobori M, Negishi H, Hosoyamada A: Effects of nicardipine on hemodynamics and skin blood flow: Comparison between N_2O-sevoflurane and N_2O-isoflurane anesthesia. [in Japanese] Masui 1993;42:1435–1439.

351. Salem MR: Therapeutic uses of ganglionic blocking drugs. Int Anesthesiol Clin 1978;16:171–200.

352. Klowden AJ, Ivankovich AD, Miletich DJ: Ganglionic blocking drugs: General considerations and metabolism. Int Anesthesiol Clin 1978;16:113–150.

353. Sklar GS, Lanks KW: Effects of trimethaphan and sodium nitroprusside on hydrolysis of succinylcholine in vitro. Anesthesiology 1977;47:31–33.

354. Tinker JH, Michenfelder JD: Sodium nitroprusside: Pharmacology, toxicology and therapeutics. Anesthesiology 1976;45:340–354.

355. Wildsmith JA, Marshall RL, Jenkinson JL, et al: Haemodynamic effects of sodium nitroprusside during nitrous oxide-halothane anaesthesia. Br J Anaesth 1973;45:71–74.

356. Bennett NR, Abbott TR: The use of sodium nitroprusside in children. Anaesthesia 1977;32:456–463.

357. Ivankovich AD, Miletich DJ, Tinker JH: Sodium nitroprusside: Metabolism and general considerations. Int Anesthesiol Clin 1978;16:1–29.

358. Davies DW, Kadar D, Steward DJ, et al: A sudden death associated with the use of sodium nitroprusside for induction of hypotension during anaesthesia. Can Anaesth Soc J 1975;22:547–552.

359. Pershau RA, Modell JH, Bright RW, et al: Suspected sodium nitroprusside-induced cyanide intoxication. Anesth Analg 1977;56:533–537.

360. Berlin CM Jr: The treatment of cyanide poisoning in children. Pediatrics 1970;46:793–796.

361. Palmer RF, Lasseter KC: Drug therapy. Sodium nitroprusside. N Engl J Med 1975;292:294–297.

362. Posner MA, Tobey RE, McElroy H: Hydroxocobalamin therapy of cyanide intoxication in guinea pigs. Anesthesiology 1976;44:157–160.

363. Vesey CJ, Cole PV, Simpson PJ: Cyanide and thiocyanate concentrations following sodium nitroprusside infusion in man. Br J Anaesth 1976;48:651–660.

364. Michenfelder JD, Tinker JH: Cyanide toxicity and thiosulfate protec-

tion during chronic administration of sodium nitroprusside in the dog: Correlation with a human case. Anesthesiology 1977;47:441–448.

365. Michenfelder JD: Cyanide release from sodium nitroprusside in the dog. Anesthesiology 1977;46:196–201.

366. Aitken D, West D, Smith F, et al: Cyanide toxicity following nitroprusside induced hypotension. Can Anaesth Soc J 1977;24:651–660.

367. Ivankovich AD, Braverman B, Shulman M, et al: Prevention of nitroprusside toxicity with thiosulfate in dogs. Anesth Analg 1982;61:120–126.

368. Mason DT, Zelis R, Amsterdam EA: Actions of the nitrites on the peripheral circulation and myocardial oxygen consumption: Significance in the relief of angina pectoris. Chest 1971;59:296–305.

369. Guggiari M, Dagreou F, Lienhart A, et al: Use of nitroglycerine to produce controlled decreases in mean arterial pressure to less than 50 mm Hg. Br J Anaesth 1985;57:142–147.

370. Pasch T, Hoppelshauser G: Methaemoglobin levels during nitroglycerin infusion for the intraoperative induction of controlled hypotension. Arzneimittelforschung 1983;33:879–882.

371. Kaplan KJ, Taber M, Teagarden JR, et al: Association of methemoglobinemia and intravenous nitroglycerin administration. Am J Cardiol 1985;55:181–183.

372. Zurick AM, Wagner RH, Starr NJ, et al: Intravenous nitroglycerin, methemoglobinemia, and respiratory distress in a postoperative cardiac surgical patient. Anesthesiology 1984;61:464–466.

373. Eisenkraft JB: Pulse oximeter desaturation due to methemoglobinemia. Anesthesiology 1988;68:279–282.

374. Barker SJ, Tremper KK, Hyatt J: Effects of methemoglobinemia on pulse oximetry and mixed venous oximetry. Anesthesiology 1989;70:112–117.

375. Sollevi A: Hypotensive anesthesia and blood loss. Acta Anaesthesiol Scand Suppl 1988;89:39–43.

376. Crawford MW, Carmichael FJ, Orrego H, et al: Systemic hemodynamics and organ blood flow during adenosine-induced hypotension: Effects of halothane and sevoflurane anaesthesia. Can J Anaesth 1990;37:S19.

377. Bedford RF: Increasing halothane concentrations reduce nitroprusside dose requirement. Anesth Analg 1978;57:457–462.

378. Ornstein E, Matteo RS, Weinstein JA, et al: A controlled trial of esmolol for the induction of deliberate hypotension. J Clin Anesth 1988;1:31–35.

379. Hersey SL, O'Dell NE, Lowe S, et al: Nicardipine versus nitroprusside for controlled hypotension during spinal surgery in adolescents. Anesth Analg 1997;84:1239–1244.

380. Tobias JD: Nicardipine: Applications in anesthesia practice. J Clin Anesth 1995;7:525–533.

381. Tobias JD, Lowe S, Deshpande JK: Nicardipine: Perioperative applications in children. Paediatr Anaesth 1995;5:171–176.

382. Abou-Madi M, Lenis S, Archer D, et al: Comparison of direct blood pressure measurements at the radial and dorsalis pedis arteries during sodium nitroprusside- and isoflurane-induced hypotension. Anesthesiology 1986;65:692–695.

383. Coté CJ, Goldstein EA, Coté MA, et al: A single-blind study of pulse oximetry in children. Anesthesiology 1988;68:184–188.

384. Coté CJ, Rolf N, Liu LM, et al: A single-blind study of combined pulse oximetry and capnography in children. Anesthesiology 1991;74:980–987.

385. Coté CJ, Liu LM, Szyfelbein SK, et al: Intraoperative events diagnosed by expired carbon dioxide monitoring in children. Can Anaesth Soc J 1986;33:315–320.

386. Edwards MW Jr, Flemming DC: Deliberate hypotension. Surg Clin North Am 1975;55:947–957.

387. Adams AP: Techniques of vascular control for deliberate hypotension during anaesthesia. Br J Anaesth 1975;47:777–792.

388. Lee TC, Yang LC, Chen HJ: Effect of patient position and hypotensive anesthesia on inferior vena caval pressure. Spine 1998;23:941–947.

389. Stoelting RK, Viegas O, Campbell RL: Sodium nitroprusside-produced hypotension during anesthesia and operation in the head-up position. Anesth Analg 1977;56:391–394.

390. Kreimeier U, Messmer K: Hemodilution in clinical surgery: State of the art 1996. World J Surg 1996;20:1208–1217.

391. Fukusaki M, Hara T, Maekawa T, et al: Effect of controlled hypotension combined with hemodilution on gastric intramural pH. J Clin Anesth 1998;10:222–227.

392. Fukusaki M, Matsumoto M, Yamaguchi K, et al: Effects of hemodilution during controlled hypotension of hepatic, renal, and pancreatic function in humans. J Clin Anesth 1996;8:545–550.

393. Kety SS, Schmidt CF: The effects of active and passive hyperventilation on cerebral blood flow, cerebral oxygen consumption, cardiac output, and blood pressure in normal young men. J Clin Invest 1946;25:107–119.

394. Kety SS, Schmidt CF: The effects of altered arterial tensions of carbon dioxide and oxygen on cerebral blood flow and cerebral oxygen consumption in normal young men. J Clin Invest 1948;27:484–492.

395. Merin RG: Anesthetic management problems posed by therapeutic advances: 3. Beta-adrenergic blocking drugs. Anesth Analg 1972;51:617–624.

396. Karlin A, Hartung J, Cottrell JE: Rate of induction of hypotension with trimetaphan modifies the intracranial pressure response in cats. Br J Anaesth 1988;60:161–166.

397. Eckenhoff JE: Deliberate hypotension. Anesthesiology 1978;48:87-88.

398. Lindop MJ: Complications and morbidity of controlled hypotension. Br J Anaesth 1975;47:799–803.

399. Hur SR, Huizenga BA, Major M: Acute normovolemic hemodilution combined with hypotensive anesthesia and other techniques to avoid homologous transfusion in spinal fusion surgery. Spine 1992;17:867–873.

400. Payen JF, Vuillez JP, Geoffray B, et al: Effects of preoperative intentional hemodilution on the extravasation rate of albumin and fluid. Crit Care Med 1997;25:243–248.

401. Messmer K: Hemodilution. Surg Clin North Am 1975;55:659–678.

402. Messmer K, Kreimeier U, Intaglietta M: Present state of intentional hemodilution. Eur Surg Res 1986;18:254–263.

403. Schaller RT Jr, Schaller J, Morgan A, et al: Hemodilution anesthesia: A valuable aid to major cancer surgery in children. Am J Surg 1983;146:79–84.

404. Adzick NS, deLorimier AA, Harrison MR, et al: Major childhood tumor resection using normovolemic hemodilution anesthesia and hetastarch. J Pediatr Surg 1985;20:372–375.

405. Martin E, Hansen E, Peter K: Acute limited normovolemic hemodilution: A method for avoiding homologous transfusion. World J Surg 1987;11:53–59.

406. Van Hemelen G, Avery CM, Venn PJ, et al: Management of Jehovah's Witness patients undergoing major head and neck surgery. Head Neck 1999;21:80–84.

407. van Daele ME, Trouwborst A, van Woerkens LC, et al: Transesophageal echocardiographic monitoring of preoperative acute hypervolemic hemodilution. Anesthesiology 1994;81:602–609.

408. Murray JF, Escobar E, Rapaport E:. Effects of blood viscosity on hemodynamic responses in acute normovolemic anemia. Am J Physiol 1969;216:638–642.

409. Schmid-Schonbein H: Blood rheology and physiology of microcirculation. Ric Clin Lab 1981;11(Suppl 1):13–33.

410. Schmid-Schonbein H: Microrheology of erythrocytes, blood viscosity, and the distribution of blood flow in the microcirculation. Int Rev Physiol 1976;9:1–62.

411. Schmid-Schonbein H: Blood rheology and the distribution of blood flow within the nutrient capillaries. Bibl Haematol 1975;41:1–15.

412. Guyton AC, Richardson TQ: Effect of hematocrit on venous return. Circ Res 1961;9:157–164.

413. Messmer K, Sunder-Plassmann L, Kloevekorn WP, et al: Circulatory significance of hemodilution: Rheological changes and limitations. Adv Microcirc 1972;4:1–2.

414. Hagl S, Bornikoel K, Mayr N, et al: Cardiac performance during limited hemodilution. Bibl Haematol 1975;41:152–172.

415. Neuhof H, Wolf H: Oxygen uptake during hemodilution. Bibl Haematol 1975;41:66–75.

416. Sunder-Plassmann L, Kessler M, Jesch F, et al: Acute normovolemic hemodilution: Changes in tissue oxygen supply and hemoglobin-oxygen affinity. Bibl Haematol 1975;41:44–53.

417. Kessler M, Messmer K: Tissue oxygenation during hemodilution. Bibl Haematol 1975;41:16–33.

418. Buckberg G, Brazier J: Coronary blood flow and cardiac function during hemodilution. Bibl Haematol 1975;41:173–189.

419. Messmer K: Hemodilution: Possibilities and safety aspects. Acta Anaesthesiol Scand Suppl 1988;89:49–53.

420. Lisander B: Preoperative haemodilution. Acta Anaesthesiol Scand Suppl 1988;89:63–70.

421. Crystal GJ, Rooney MW, Salem MR: Myocardial blood flow and oxygen consumption during isovolemic hemodilution alone and in combination with adenosine-induced controlled hypotension. Anesth Analg 1988;67:539–547.

422. Fontana JL, Welborn L, Mongan PD, et al: Oxygen consumption and cardiovascular function in children during profound intraoperative normovolemic hemodilution. Anesth Analg 1995;80:219–225.

423. Lichtenstein A, Eckhart WF, Swanson KJ, et al: Unplanned intraoperative and postoperative hemodilution: Oxygen transport and consumption during severe anemia. Anesthesiology 1988;69:119–122.

424. Parris WC, Kambam JR, Blanks S, et al: The effect of intentional hemodilution on P_{50}. J Cardiovasc Surg (Torino) 1988;29:560–562.

425. Cooper JD, Maeda M, Lowenstein E: Lung water accumulation with acute hemodilution in dogs. J Thorac Cardiovasc Surg 1975;69:957–965.

426. Laks H, O'Connor NE, Anderson W, et al: Crystalloid versus colloid hemodilution in man. Surg Gynecol Obstet 1976;142:506–512.

427. Lowenstein E, Cooper JD, Erdman AJ, et al: Lung and heart water accumulation associated with hemodilution. Bibl Haematol 1975;41:190–202.

428. Schuh FT: Influence off haemodilution on the potency of neuromuscular blocking drugs. Br J Anaesth 1981;53:263–265.

429. Schuh FT: Haemodilution and duration of action of muscle relaxants. [in German] Anaesthesist 1981;30:44–45.

430. Xue FS, Liu JH, Liao X, et al: The influence of acute normovolemic hemodilution on the dose-response and time course of action of vecuronium. Anesth Analg 1998;86:861–866.

431. Xue FS, Liao X, Tong SY, et al: Pharmacokinetics of vecuronium during acute isovolaemic haemodilution. Br J Anaesth 1997;79:612–616.

432. Xue FS, Liao X, Tong SY, et al: Influence of acute normovolaemic haemodilution on the relation between the dose and response of rocuronium bromide. Eur J Anaesthesiol 1998;15:21–26.

433. Wolfe LC: The membrane and the lesions of storage in preserved red cells. Transfusion 1985;25:185–203.

434. Rao TL, Mathru M, Salem MR, et al: Serum potassium levels following transfusion of frozen erythrocytes. Anesthesiology 1980;52:170–172.

Charles L. Schleien *and* I. David Todres

Historical Background

Epidemiology and Outcome of Cardiopulmonary Arrest

Management

   Airway

   Ventilation

   Laryngeal Mask Airway

Perioperative Cardiac Arrest

   Mechanisms of Blood Flow

   Newer Cardiopulmonary Resuscitation Techniques

   Pharmacology

Ventricular Fibrillation

   Electric Countershock

   Clinical Aspects of Pediatric Defibrillation

   Pharmacotherapy of Life-Threatening Arrhythmias

Supraventricular Tachycardia

Pulseless Electrical Activity

Cardiopulmonary arrest results in total cessation of oxygen delivery to vital organs of the body. Efforts at resuscitation may lead to resumption of heart and lung function but if carried out too late or ineffectively may result in profound cerebral injury. The primary goal of cardiopulmonary resuscitation (CPR) is to utilize the most effective methods to maintain adequate myocardial and cerebral perfusion. Thus, proponents of CPR should embrace the concept of cerebral resuscitation.

Historical Background

A biblical reference (2 Kings 4:34–35) suggests the first documented successful mouth-to-mouth resuscitation when Elisha the prophet resuscitated a child: *"And he went up,*

and lay upon the child, and put his mouth upon his mouth, and his eyes upon his eyes, and his hands upon his hands; and he stretched himself upon the child; and the child waxed warm."

Newborn infants were successfully resuscitated with mouth-to-mouth resuscitation in the early part of the 19th century, but this technique was abandoned because of the fear of contracting a contagious disease from a technique that was also considered aesthetically unclean. In 1814, a description in poetical form of the Rules of the Humane Society for recovering drowned persons included the following description of mouth-to-mouth resuscitation.[1]

Let one the mouth, and either nostril close
While through the other the bellows gently blows.
Thus the pure air with steady force convey,
To put the flaccid lungs again in play.
Should bellows not be found, or found too late,
Let some kind soul with willing mouth inflate;
Then downward, though but lightly, press the chest.
And let the inflated air be upward prest.

Following reports by Elam, Gordon, and Safar demonstrating the effectiveness of mouth-to-mouth resuscitation,[2–4] in 1958 the National Academy of Sciences National Research Council recommended mouth-to-mouth resuscitation as the preferred technique for all individuals requiring emergency artificial ventilation. Maximum backward tilt of the head was shown by radiography and cinefluoroscopy to be the most important step for opening the air passages and proved to be the quickest and easiest maneuver to apply.[5] This became the preferred method for mouth-to-mouth resuscitation.[6, 7] External cardiac massage was successfully conducted over 100 years ago in two children (ages 8 and 13 years) following circulatory arrest precipitated by chloroform anesthesia.[8] In 1904, Crile described the effectiveness of external cardiac compressions in maintaining the circulation of dogs.[9] External cardiac compressions as a resuscitation technique was revived in 1960, when Kouwenhoven et al.[10] demonstrated the effectiveness of external cardiac compressions and this method became the standard form of cardiac support, combined with artificial respiration. In their paper, external cardiac massage was successful in 20 patients (including pediatric patients) with a 70% survival rate. Their

The authors acknowledge the contribution to the previous version of this chapter by James K. Alifimoff.

paper stated, "Anyone, anywhere can now initiate cardiac resuscitative procedures. All that is needed is two hands."[10] Prior to this study, internal cardiac compressions was the accepted technique; its effectiveness demonstrated by experience in cardiac bypass surgery. In 1947, Beck successfully internally defibrillated the human heart and in 1956, Zoll performed the first successful external defibrillation of a human heart.[11, 12]

Epidemiology and Outcome of Cardiopulmonary Arrest

Cardiopulmonary arrest is most common in the child less than 2 years of age, with the majority of arrests occurring in infants under 5 months of age. Leading causes in out-of-hospital cardiac arrest are sudden infant death syndrome, trauma (motor vehicle, abuse), near-drowning, and upper airway obstruction (foreign body, smoke inhalation). Most common in-hospital arrests are due to respiratory infections and disorders, congenital diseases, overwhelming sepsis, and hypoxemic encephalopathy.

It is uncommon for cardiopulmonary arrest to be caused by a primary cardiac event in children. Cardiopulmonary arrest most commonly arises as a result of respiratory dysfunction leading to bradyarrhythmia secondary to hypoxemia, hypercarbia, and acidosis, followed by asystolic arrest. This is in contrast to the adult, in whom cardiac arrest follows a primary cardiac insult such as myocardial infarction or arrhythmia. Survival rates are unfortunately dismal, in a range of 3 to 17%, with the majority of patients left with significant neurologic impairment.[13–26] This is probably the outcome of prolonged hypoxemia prior to total cardiac arrest, hence the need to intervene before cardiopulmonary failure proceeds to cardiac arrest. Outcomes are more favorable with respiratory arrest alone.

Patients who do not experience a return of spontaneous circulation at the site of the event (prehospital care) were found to be unlikely to survive. One in three patients who arrived in the emergency room in full cardiopulmonary arrest survived, and that cohort was neurologically devastated. Most patients with good neurologic survival following resuscitation outside of the hospital venue have experienced return of spontaneous circulation before hospital arrival (with the possible exception of hypothermic patients).[23]

In a multicenter pediatric trial examining the efficacy of high-dose epinephrine, of 213 patients, 3 patients who presented to the emergency department in full arrest survived with good neurologic outcomes.[27] Of concern is a report of pediatric patients in cardiopulmonary arrest being significantly less likely to receive advanced life support intervention than adult cases.[28] Only 55% of children compared with 93% of adults were intubated. Thirty-eight percent of pediatric patients versus 83% of adults had vascular access. Also, 40% of pediatric patients did not receive epinephrine compared with 7% of adults.

Improved survival rates using high-dose epinephrine has been observed with resuscitation efforts lasting less than 20 minutes and requiring fewer than two doses of epinephrine.[26, 29] More favorable outcomes were also associated with witnessed cardiac arrest, bystander CPR, and emergency service system arrival in less than 10 minutes.[29] Patients presenting with ventricular fibrillation had improved survival rates compared with those presenting with asystole or pulseless electrical activity. It has been demonstrated that Pediatric Advanced Life Support training of emergency personnel in the operating room led to an increase in intubation rate from 48% to 90% in children younger than 18 months, and vascular access increased from 18% to 64%.[30]

The nonstandardization of the nature of the cardiac arrest and the location of the patient have compounded evaluating outcomes. The development of the Utstein style for uniform reporting of data from out-of-hospital cardiac arrest, which was adapted to pediatrics in 1995, will allow this form of reporting template to make studies comparable and assist in recommended evidence-based guidelines for cardiopulmonary resuscitation.[31]

Management

The diagnosis of cardiopulmonary arrest rests on the absence of a *major* pulse (carotid, femoral, brachial) by palpation. In addition, there will be unconsciousness (recognized through verbal and physical stimulation) and absence of respirations (looking and listening). Management proceeds along the following lines, recognizing that tasks may be accomplished simultaneously and that *prioritizing tasks is essential.*

Airway

A *clear* airway is a primary requirement for effective CPR. In children, respiratory arrest usually precedes cardiac arrest. Thus, urgent reaction to the child experiencing respiratory difficulty is essential. Proper head positioning (extension) and securing of the airway to provide oxygen and ventilation may be all that is necessary to save the child's life. Anterior thrust of the mandible may be necessary to obtain a clear airway should chin lift alone prove inadequate.[32–35] In the child undergoing CPR, airway patency is compromised by posterior displacement of the tongue, the epiglottis, and the soft palate toward the posterior pharyngeal wall. Traditional teaching cautioned against excessive extension of the head of infants to "open the airway." It was thought that this resulted in a "tethering" of the trachea with reduction of its caliber. A recent study has refuted this traditional thinking.[36] However, supraglottic obstruction with extreme head extension has not been systematically examined.

Of special concern is the patient who has sustained possible cervical vertebrae or spinal cord injury. In this situation, stabilizing the neck is critical. Positioning on a standard backboard may result in flexion of the young child's neck. For the head to remain in the neutral position—a position which corresponds approximately to an alignment of the external auditory meatus with the shoulders—the child should be supported on a backboard that has a recess for the occiput to lower the head or on a double mattress to raise the chest and shoulders.[37]

Endotracheal intubation provides the most secure way to establish airway control. The child's airway can be managed effectively prior to tracheal intubation with proper head positioning and jaw thrust, and with bag and mask ventilation. In this situation, care should be taken to avoid inflating the stomach with excessive tidal volumes. Abdominal distension can significantly compromise oxygenation; therefore, the child should always be uncovered and the stomach vented in case excessive gastric inflation has occurred. Bag and mask ventilation with 100% oxygen should precede any attempt at tracheal intubation.

The laryngeal mask airway (LMA) may help to secure an effective airway should tracheal intubation fail. Studies have shown that more effective tidal volumes are achieved with the LMA than with conventional face mask techniques.[38-40]

Ventilation

If there is no chest movement, there is no ventilation. It is imperative to exclude upper airway obstruction as the cause of failure to effectively ventilate the child.

Mouth-to-Mouth and Mouth-to-Mask Ventilation

Mouth-to-mouth and mouth-to-mask are effective basic life-support methods to achieve adequate ventilation.[41] Mouth-to-mask is more acceptable because of its aesthetic appeal and concerns for the spread of infectious diseases. In addition, the mask may allow for the provision of supplemental oxygen.

Bag-Valve-Mask Devices

Bag-valve mask devices (BVMs), when effectively used, will provide adequate ventilation for the child. The self-inflating bag is the most commonly utilized and is available in sizes ranging from 250 mL to 2 L. It should be noted that the small-volume self-inflating devices may deliver inadequate tidal volumes to the infant with poorly compliant lungs or high airway resistance. The child-size and adult-size self-inflating bags will function effectively for the entire range of infants and children. To optimize oxygenation, the self-inflating devices should have an oxygen reservoir attached. It is necessary to have a flow of oxygen of 15 L/min to achieve the best oxygen delivery through the system. Even then, effective FIO_2 may not exceed 90%.

An alternate device for ventilating children is the "anesthesia bag." This is a very effective device but requires skill and practice for its optimal functioning.[42, 43] Self-inflating bags function independently of a gas-flow delivery system. In comparison, the anesthesia bag device is gas-flow dependent and is therefore ineffective in the absence of a gas-flow system or incomplete mask fit.

To prevent overinflation of the lungs with its attendant risks of air-leaks and life-threatening tension pneumothorax, some BVM devices are fitted with pop-off valves set at 30 to 35 cm H_2O pressure.[44] The rationale for this preset pop-off pressure level is based on a single experimental study of excised newborn lungs—a condition that is not relevant to the clinical state.[45] It is important to appreciate that in situations with decreased lung compliance or increased airway resistance, effective ventilation may necessitate exceeding pressures greater than 30 cm H_2O. Activation of the pop-off valve also causes reduced delivery of oxygen and thus limits the reliability of the device to deliver maximal oxygen concentrations. Therefore, when inspiratory pressures greater than the pop-off pressure are required, the pop-off valve should be deactivated.

Mask fit is crucial to ensuring effective ventilation. An air-leak under the mask will cause underventilation, particularly in patients with poor lung compliance or high airway resistance. In most situations, a single operator can maintain a good face mask seal with one hand while delivering the breaths with the other. However, when it is difficult to secure an air-tight face mask fit, the operator should employ both hands on the face-mask and have a second individual provide effective ventilation squeezing the bag (see Fig. 7–22).[46, 47] For individuals with "smaller hands," the open palm method of squeezing the bag against one's body will effectively deliver an adequate tidal volume.[48] Attempts to control the airway and effectively ventilate the child from positions other than behind the patient's head are often suboptimal in achieving adequate head extension and chin lift to open the airway.

Cricoid pressure (Sellick maneuver) is performed by a second person during BVM ventilations to reduce the risk of gastric distension and regurgitation with its potential for pulmonary aspiration. It is recommended that orogastric or nasogastric tubes be left in place during the maneuver of cricoid pressure, as their presence enhances the effect.[49, 50] The technique of cricoid pressure is carried out in variable ways. Complete airway obstruction may occur with excessive pressure or if applied in a caudal direction.[51] Cricoid pressure may be applied with one hand or bimanually with a hand supporting the posterior cervical spine.[52] The latter technique should be carried out in any patient with a suspected cervical injury.[53] When an LMA is employed, cricoid pressure may affect the proper positioning of the device.[54-57]

In the infant and young child, the airway is structurally less stable than in the adult. Obstruction of the airway causes marked increase in negative pressure on inspiration producing significant dynamic collapse of the airway at the thoracic inlet, further aggravating the airway obstruction (see Fig. 7–10). Positive pressure ventilation with the BVM device will stent the airway open and help provide effective ventilation for the child (see Fig. 15–1).

Guidelines for CPR have recommended employing a manometer to monitor airway pressures as tidal volumes are delivered. It should be noted, however, that effective ventilation is *best judged by visualizing chest excursions and listening to the quality of breath sounds* rather than setting a preset pressure not to be exceeded as a guide to the adequacy of ventilation. The recommended rate of ventilation is 20 breaths per minute. When cardiac arrest has supervened, these breaths need to be synchronized with cardiac compressions to ensure effective ventilation at all times. In clinical situations such as raised intracranial pressure, increased ventilation rates may be necessary.

With bag-valve mask devices, there is a significant risk of gastric inflation followed by pulmonary aspiration. In one study, there was a 28% incidence of pulmonary aspiration in a series of failed resuscitations.[58] For this reason, inflation pressures limited to 20 cm H_2O have been recommended by some.[59] Tidal volumes of 400 to 500 mL (i.e., 5–6 mL/kg) have corresponded to perceived adequate chest movement and are recommended.[60, 61]

Ventilation/compression sequences originally were based on normal cardiopulmonary function. In cardiopulmonary arrest, frequency of ventilation and tidal volume is less relevant, as delivery of CO_2 to the lungs is low. Of paramount importance in cardiac arrest is oxygenation.[62, 63]

Tracheal Intubation

Tracheal intubation ensures optimal control of the airway for effective ventilation. However, one should recognize that BVM ventilation is generally effective in providing adequate ventilation, making tracheal intubation an elective procedure. Multiple attempts at intubation by the inexperienced operator may seriously compromise the child's ability to recover. Ventilation via a tracheal tube will ensure that all the delivered gas is directed into the lungs, avoiding gastric inflation that may occur with BVM ventilation. Also, tracheal intubation protects the lungs from aspiration of gastric contents and provides for suctioning secretions, blood, or gastric contents that may have contributed to airway obstruction.

Tracheal intubation must be performed expeditiously and skillfully. Proper positioning of the child is important (see Fig. 7–14). Appropriate equipment and drugs must be at hand. Endotracheal tube size is usually estimated using the child's age as standard formulae (see Table 7–2). It appears that the child's height reliably predicts the appropriate endotracheal tube size.[64] Following intubation, the endotracheal tube is securely fixed in place and the head of the child stabilized in the neutral position, as flexion or extension of the head may displace the endotracheal tube into a mainstem bronchus or up into the pharynx, respectively, with potentially catastrophic consequences.[65, 66] *Any deterioration in the child's condition following tracheal intubation necessitates immediate attention to the patency and position of the endotracheal tube.* The endotracheal tube may have passed accidentally into the esophagus or down a mainstem bronchus or it may be plugged with mucus, blood, or vomitus. Measuring oxygen saturation is a valuable rapid indicator of any deleterious change in the child's condition; a persistent 5% decrease in oxygen saturation may indicate partial endobronchial intubation.[67] It should also be appreciated that in the child who is poorly perfused, peripheral vasoconstriction limits ability of the device to accurately record oxygen saturations. It is hoped that the next generation of pulse oximeters will overcome interference caused by motion and low flow states and therefore provide more meaningful information during adverse cardiovascular events.

Aids to tracheal intubation include bougies, stylets, light wands, LMAs, and fiberoptic technology (Bullard laryngoscope and fiberoptic laryngoscope). With the gum elastic bougie, successful tracheal intubation was enhanced in patients with suspected cervical spine injuries in whom manual in-line stabilization was carried out (see also Chapter 7 and Figs. 16–1 and 16–2).[68]

The measurement of end-tidal carbon dioxide ($ETCO_2$) is a valuable method of confirming the correct position of the endotracheal tube, namely in the trachea as opposed to outside the trachea. A disposable colorimetric $ETCO_2$ is useful in verifying endotracheal tube placement in children when in-line capnography is not available (see Fig. 16–4).[69] It is important to appreciate that $ETCO_2$ measurements are only evident when there is effective pulmonary circulation, either spontaneously or with adequate cardiac compressions.

Transtracheal catheter ventilation may be a life-saving maneuver when all other methods to secure an airway and oxygenate the child have failed. This method has proved effective in adults. In young children, however, it is particularly difficult to perform due to the relatively small and not easily identifiable cricothyroid membrane. Experimentally in animals (dogs weighing 21–30 pounds) the procedure has been demonstrated to effectively oxygenate the animal while resulting in tolerable hypercarbia.[70] In spontaneously breathing animals with near total airway obstruction, the simple delivery of oxygen via a transtracheal catheter may be all that is required for oxygenation (Fig. 13–1). In animals without respiratory efforts, some degree of ventilation is achieved (Fig. 13–2). Marked hypercarbia (>150 mm Hg) is well tolerated, provided oxygenation is adequate (see Fig. 7–23).[71]

Laryngeal Mask Airway

Ventilation may be more effective with an LMA than with a bag-mask device.[40, 72] The LMA can be inserted with the neck in the neutral position, thus avoiding extension or flexion that may be hazardous if there is an underlying cervical injury. Effective positive pressure ventilation may be carried out via the LMA provided airway pressures do not exceed 20 to 25 cm H_2O. Underventilation will occur in patients with poorly compliant lungs or whose airway resistance is significantly increased.

One concern with the use of the LMA is the potential for pulmonary aspiration.[73, 74] However, this occurs infrequently and has been reported in a recent study of cardiac arrests to have an incidence of about 2%.[75] Cricoid pressure may cause upward displacement of the LMA and impair ventilation.[55]

Perioperative Cardiac Arrest

The incidence, causes, and risk factors associated with perioperative cardiac arrest have been evaluated by the Pediatric Perioperative Cardiac Arrest registry and reported by Geiduschek.[76] In an earlier analysis (1994–1996), cardiac arrest or death in the perioperative period (pre-induction, induction, maintenance, or recovery from anesthesia) occurred at a rate of 2.8 per 10,000 anesthetic procedures. Twenty-one percent of cardiac arrests occurred during induction and 67% during maintenance. Death occurred in 47% of cases within 24 days following cardiac arrest. Four percent of survivors suffered permanent injuries. With regard to risk factors, 25% of arrests occurred in infants less than 1 month of age, with a mortality rate greater than in all other age groups. American Society of Anesthesiologists (ASA) physical status was also higher in this age group. A significant number of infants failed to be weaned from cardiopulmonary bypass following repair of a congenital heart defect. It is noteworthy that only 8% of cases were respiratory in origin, of which the majority were related to airway obstruction. This relatively low incidence of airway-associated events may be related to the introduction of oxygen saturation and $ETCO_2$ as standard monitoring practices. Of the cardiovascular causes, hemorrhage was responsible for the largest number of cardiac arrests. Overdose of inhalation anesthetic was also a significant factor, but all patients were successfully resuscitated.

Cardiac arrest in the operating room should have the greatest potential for a successful outcome (successful res-

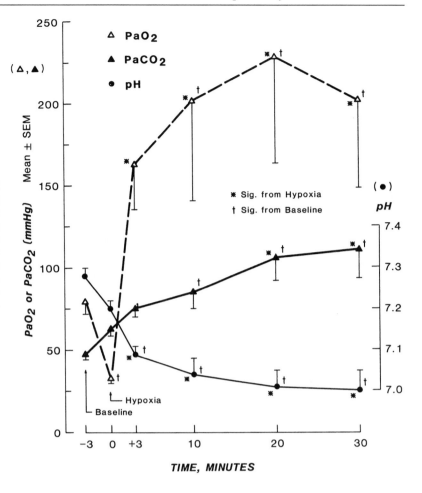

Figure 13–1. Changes in arterial blood gases and pH are plotted over time for six dogs with spontaneous ventilation; baseline in room air is time −3; 2 to 3 minutes of hypoxemia as a result of airway obstruction is time 0. Marked, sustained increases in PaO_2 follow cricothyroid membrane puncture with delivery of only 1.0 L/min oxygen. (From Coté CJ, Eavey RD, Todres ID, et al: Cricothyroid membrane puncture: Oxygenation and ventilation in a dog model using an intravenous catheter. Crit Care Med 16:615–619, © by Williams & Wilkins, 1988.)

cue) because it is a witnessed arrest with virtually instantaneous availability of skilled personnel, monitoring equipment, resuscitative equipment, and drugs. Whenever a cardiac arrest occurs in the operating room, one must consider the circumstance to rapidly determine the cause. Use of all the available monitors will also help to make the diagnosis and to guide the adequacy of resuscitative efforts. A precordial stethoscope will immediately inform the anesthesiologist of muffled heart tones consistent with a low cardiac output (e.g., anesthetic overdose). This is particularly important during anesthetic induction and also why extraneous room noises should be minimized during this critical phase of the anesthetic process. Since the majority of children who suffer cardiac arrest are high-risk patients with cardiovascular anomalies and who suffer the arrest as a consequence of surgical interventions, an arterial line is often in place. In this situation, the quality and area under the curve of cardiac output generated by chest compressions can be readily monitored as can the effectiveness of changing the depth and ratio of compression to relaxation. In cases in which an arterial line is not in place, the audible pulse of the plethysmograph from a pulse oximeter at the same rate as chest compressions may be a reflection of adequacy of perfusion. Likewise, the capnograph is useful in determining cardiac output and pulmonary blood flow. Again, changes in the depth and ratio of compression to relaxation of the sternum may yield improved expired carbon dioxide levels, indicating improved pulmonary blood flow. Restoration of

the circulation with epinephrine and ensuring adequate circulating blood volume will also manifest as improved carbon dioxide elimination.

The circumstances of the arrest may also provide a clue as to the cause, such as hyperkalemia following succinylcholine or rapid blood transfusion, hypocalcemia during a rapid infusion of fresh frozen plasma, or a sudden fall in end-expired carbon dioxide indicating an air embolism. Thus the sequence of drugs used in operating room resuscitation may be slightly different than those currently recommended for cardiopulmonary resuscitation outside of the operating room; for example, calcium would certainly be immediately indicated to correct ionized hypocalcemia (citrate toxicity) or to oppose the cardiac electrophysiologic effects of hyperkalemia. A bradyarrhythmia must always first be assumed to be due to hypoxemia, second due to anesthetic overdose (real or relative), and third, possibly related to a vagal reflex due to surgical manipulations. Oxygen 100% and assurance of the adequacy of ventilation is always the first drug of choice regardless of the cause of the bradycardia. Since cardiac output is rate dependent, especially in neonates and toddlers, atropine and epinephrine are indicated. In reflex-induced bradycardia, atropine may be the first drug of choice, but in extreme cases of bradycardia whatever the mechanism, epinephrine is the drug of choice. Hypotension and a low cardiac output state must be rapidly corrected by appropriate administration of drugs and adequate chest compressions to circulate drugs so that they can have the

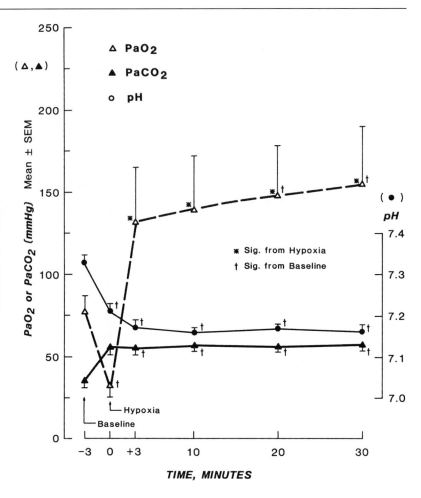

Figure 13–2. Changes in arterial blood gases and pH are plotted over time for five animals who were not making spontaneous ventilatory efforts. Both oxygenation and ventilation were achieved with a self-inflating bag attached to the intravenous catheter, which had been introduced through the cricothyroid membrane. (From Coté CJ, Eavey RD, Todres ID, et al: Cricothyroid membrane puncture: Oxygenation and ventilation in a dog model using an intravenous catheter. Crit Care Med 16:615–619, © by Williams & Wilkins, 1988.)

needed clinical effect. Once there is need for chest compressions, then the standard American Heart Association recommendations for cardiopulmonary resuscitation generally apply and this includes the frequent administration of epinephrine. Figure 13–3 presents a proposed algorithm for the differential diagnosis and treatment of the more common causes of acute operating room–associated cardiac dysfunction.

Mechanisms of Blood Flow

Cardiac Pump Mechanism

By the cardiac pump mechanism of blood flow, cardiac output is generated during closed-chest compressions by the heart being squeezed between the sternum and the vertebral column (Fig. 13–4). This mechanism of flow implies that ventricular compression results in closure of the atrioventricular valves and that the ejection of blood reduces ventricular volume. In between compressions, ventricular pressure falls below atrial pressure, allowing the atrioventricular valves to open and the ventricles to fill. This sequence of events resembles the normal cardiac cycle and definitely occurs during cardiac compression when open-chest CPR is used.[77]

Despite the abundant evidence supporting the thoracic pump mechanism (see subsequent discussion), other specific clinical situations have been identified in which the cardiac pump mechanism appears to predominate during closed-chest CPR. Increasing the applied force during chest compressions increases the likelihood of direct cardiac compression.[78] A smaller chest size may allow for more direct cardiac compression. Adult dogs with small chests have better hemodynamics during closed-chest CPR than dogs with large chests.[79] Since the infant's chest is smaller and more compliant than the adult's, direct compression of the heart during CPR is more likely to occur (Fig. 13–5). Blood flow during closed-chest CPR in a piglet model of cardiac arrest is higher than what is achieved in adult models.[80] Unlike in adult animals, increasing intrathoracic pressure by simultaneous compressions and ventilation (SCV-CPR), thus increasing the thoracic pump contribution to blood flow, does not augment vascular pressure or regional organ blood flow during CPR in piglets.[81] The failure of SCV-CPR to increase blood flow in the infant implies that direct compression occurs with conventional CPR, and that additional intrathoracic pressure is of no benefit.

Thoracic Pump Mechanism

Several observations of the hemodynamics during CPR do not support the cardiac pump mechanism of blood flow. Closed-chest CPR produces similar elevations in arterial and venous intravascular pressures due to a generalized increase in intrathoracic pressure.[82] In 1976, Criley made the dramatic observation that several patients who developed ventricular fibrillation during cardiac catheterization produced enough blood flow to maintain consciousness by repetitive

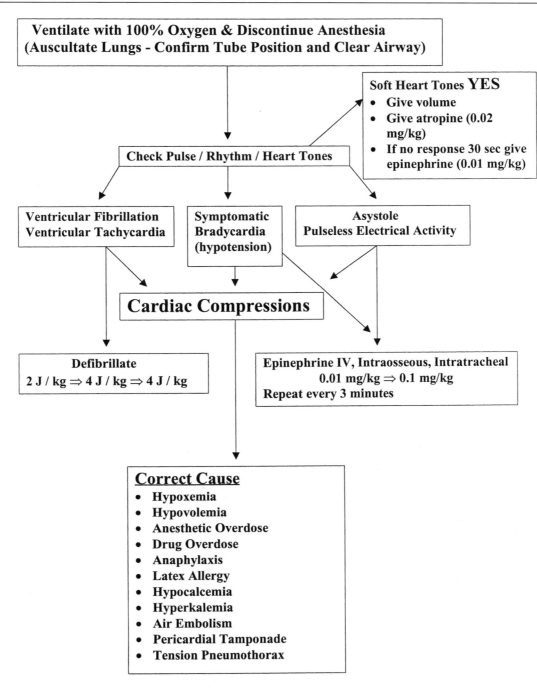

Figure 13–3. Algorithm for diagnosis and treatment of acute cardiac dysfunction in the operating room.

coughing.[83] The production of blood flow by increasing thoracic pressure without direct cardiac compression describes the thoracic pump mechanism (Fig. 13–6).

Chest compression during CPR generates almost equal pressures in the left ventricle, aorta, right atrium, pulmonary artery, and esophagus.[84] Since all intrathoracic vascular pressures are equal, the suprathoracic arterial pressures must be higher than the suprathoracic venous pressures for blood to flow. Venous valves prevent the transmission of intrathoracic pressure to the suprathoracic veins. The presence of these jugular venous valves has been demonstrated in animals[84] and humans[85–87] undergoing CPR. This unequal transmission of intrathoracic pressure to the suprathoracic vasculature

establishes the gradient necessary for blood to flow forward (see Fig. 13–6).

During normal cardiac function, the lowest pressure in the vascular circuit occurs on the atrial side of the atrioventricular valves. This low-pressure compartment is the downstream pressure for the systemic circulation that allows venous return to the heart. Angiographic studies show that blood passes from the vena cavae through the right heart into the pulmonary artery and from the pulmonary veins through the left heart into the aorta during a single chest compression.[86, 88] Echocardiographic studies show that, unlike normal cardiac activity or during open-chest CPR, during closed-chest CPR in both dogs[86] and humans[89, 90] the

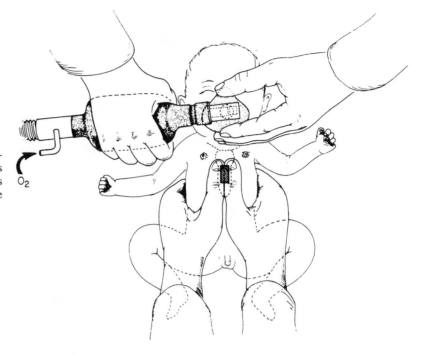

Figure 13–4. Chest-encircling method for cardiac compressions in a neonate: Thumbs are placed one finger's breadth below the nipple line. (Modified from Todres ID, Rogers MC: Methods of external cardiac massage in the newborn infant. J Pediatr 1975; 86:781–782.)

CARDIAC PUMP

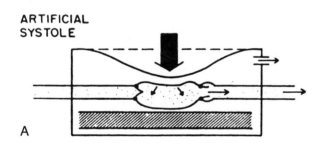

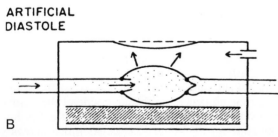

Figure 13–5. Schematic representations of the mechanism of blood flow during external cardiac compressions. (A) The cardiac pump mechanism by which the heart is directly squeezed between the sternum and vertebral column, representing artificial systole. (B) Artificial diastole occurs with relaxation of the compressions. (From Babbs CF: New versus old theories of blood flow during CPR. Crit Care Med 8:191–195, © by Williams & Wilkins, 1980.)

THORACIC PUMP

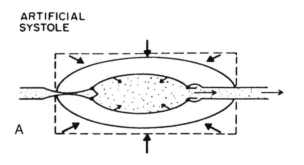

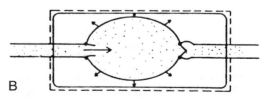

Figure 13–6. Schematic representation of the mechanism of blood flow during external cardiac compression. (A) The thoracic pump mechanism by which blood flow occurs through a general increase in intrathoracic pressure with external compressions (i.e., the heart is a passive conduit). (B) Artificial diastole occurs with release of external compressions. (From Babbs CF: New versus old theories of blood flow during CPR. Crit Care Med 8:191–195, © by Williams & Wilkins, 1980.)

atrioventricular valves are open during blood ejection and aortic diameter decreases rather than increases during blood ejection.[86, 90] These findings during closed-chest CPR support the thoracic pump theory and demonstrate that the heart is a passive conduit for blood flow.

Rate and Duty Cycle

The recommended rate of chest compressions for all patients is 80 to 100 per minute (Table 13–1).[91] This rate represents a compromise between advocates of the thoracic pump and cardiac pump mechanism of blood flow. Duty cycle is defined as the ratio of the duration of the compression phase to the entire compression-relaxation cycle expressed as a percent. For example, at a rate of 30 compressions per minute, a 1.2 second compression time produces a 60% duty cycle. If blood flow is generated by direct cardiac compression, then the stroke volume is determined primarily by the force of compression. Prolonging the compression (increasing the duty cycle) beyond the time necessary for full ventricular ejection should have no additional effect on stroke volume. Increasing the rate of compressions should increase cardiac output, since a fixed, relatively small volume of blood is ejected with each cardiac compression. In contrast, if blood flow is produced by the thoracic pump mechanism, the volume of blood to be ejected comes from a large reservoir of blood contained within the capacitance vessels in the chest. With the thoracic pump mechanism, flow is enhanced by increasing either the force of compression or the duty cycle, but is not affected by changes in compression rate over a wide range of rates.[85]

Mathematical models of the cardiovascular system have confirmed that both the applied force and the compression duration determine blood flow with the thoracic pump mechanism.[92] It appears from experimental animal data that both the thoracic pump and cardiac pump mechanisms can effectively generate blood flow during closed-chest CPR. Differences between various studies may be attributed to differences in animal models or compression techniques. Important differences in animal models include chest wall geometry, compliance and elastic recoil, compliance of the diaphragm, and intra-abdominal pressure. Differences in technique include the magnitude of sternal displacement, compression force, momentum of chest compression, compression rate, and duty cycle. Experimental and clinical data support both mechanisms of blood flow during CPR in human infants.

Results of several studies in dogs have demonstrated a

benefit of a compression rate of 120 per minute compared with slower rates during conventional CPR.[93–96] Studies in piglets,[97] puppies,[98] and humans[85, 98] found no differences between various rates of compression during conventional CPR. In a study of piglet CPR, duty cycle was the major determinant of cerebral perfusion pressure. The duty cycle at which venous return became limited varied with age. A longer duty cycle was more effective in younger piglets.[97]

The discrepancy between the importance of rate and duty cycle in various models by different investigators generates confusion. However, a rate of compression during conventional CPR of 100 per minute satisfies both those who prefer the faster rates and those who support a longer duty cycle. This is true because it is easier to produce a longer duty cycle when compressions are administered at a faster rate.[93, 99]

Chest Geometry

Chest geometry plays an important role in the ability of extrathoracic compressions to generate intrathoracic pressure. Shape, compliance, and deformability, which change greatly with age, are the characteristics of the chest that have the greatest impact during CPR. The change in cross-sectional area of the chest during anterior to posterior delivered compressions is related to its shape[100] and explains some of the findings in animal studies. The rounder, flatter chests of small dogs, pigs, and humans may require less chest displacement than the keel-shaped chests of adult dogs to generate thoracic ejection of blood. This has been demonstrated in small dogs with round chests compared to adult dogs with keel-shaped chests.[79]

As humans age, the cartilage of the rib cage calcifies and chest wall compliance decreases. Older patients may require greater compression force to generate the same sternal displacement. A 3-month-old piglet requires a much greater compression force for anteroposterior displacement than its 1-month-old counterpart.[100] Direct cardiac compression is more likely to occur in the more compliant chest of younger animals and infants. Cerebral and myocardial blood flow during closed-chest conventional CPR was much higher in infant piglets than in adults.[80] This finding supports the cardiac pump mechanism of blood flow in infants, because the level of organ blood flow achieved during closed-chest CPR in piglets approaches what is achieved during open-chest cardiac massage in adults.

Marked deformation of the chest can occur during prolonged CPR and may alter the effectiveness of CPR.[92] Over time, the chest assumes a flatter shape, producing a larger percent decrease in cross-sectional area at the same absolute chest displacement. Progressive deformation may be beneficial if it leads to more direct cardiac compression. Unfortunately, too much deformation may decrease the recoil of the chest wall during the relaxation phase, leading to decreased cardiac filling. A progressive decrease in the effectiveness of chest compressions to produce blood flow is seen in piglets receiving conventional CPR.[80] The permanent deformation of the chest in this model approaches 30% of the original anteroposterior diameter. Attempting to limit deformation by increasing intrathoracic pressure from within during CPR with SCV-CPR was ineffective.[81] Using a thoracic vest to limit deformation when performing CPR greatly

Table 13–1. Guidelines for Chest Compression and Ventilatory Rates During Cardiopulmonary Resuscitation

Age	Chest Compressions (min)	Ventilatory Rates (min)	Ratio
Neonate	120	40	3:1
Infant	100	20	5:1
Child and adolescent	80	16	5:1

Data from The American Heart Association: American Academy of Pediatrics, Pediatric Advanced Life Support. Dallas, Texas, 1997.

decreased the permanent chest deformation (3 vs. 30%), but did not attenuate the deterioration of vital organ blood flow with time.[101]

The characteristics of chest geometry of animals may relate to humans. Body weight, surface area, chest circumference, and diameter did not correlate with the magnitude of aortic pressure produced during CPR in a study of nine adults already declared dead.[102] The higher intravascular pressures and organ blood flow during CPR in infants compared with adults may be due to more effective transmission of the force of chest compression because of the higher compliance and greater deformability of the infant chest.

Newer Cardiopulmonary Resuscitation Techniques

Active Compression-Decompression

Active compression-decompression CPR utilizes a negative pressure "pull" on the thorax during the release phase of chest compression using a hand-held suction device.[103] This technique has been shown to improve vascular pressures and minute ventilation[104] during CPR in animals and humans.[104–108] The mechanism of benefit of this technique is attributed to enhancement of venous return by the negative intrathoracic pressure generated during the decompression phase. However, its benefit may actually result from the greater chest expansion and filling with air between compressions. Thus, when this technique was used with impedance to inspiratory gas exchange, vascular pressures and flow increased further.[109] Its effectiveness in adults shows promise, with increased survival and a trend toward neurologic improvement in pre-hospital victims.[103, 110, 111] However, two recent, larger trials did not demonstrate improved survival in in-hospital or pre-hospital victims of cardiac arrest, nor demonstrate any subgroup that appeared to benefit from active compression-decompression CPR.[112–114] The complication rate, including fatal rib and sternal fractures, may be higher with this technique.[115]

Simultaneous Compression and Ventilation

Simultaneous compression-ventilation CPR is a technique designed to increase blood flow during conventional CPR by increasing the thoracic pump mechanism contribution to blood flow. Delivering a breath simultaneously with every compression (instead of after every fifth compression) increases intrathoracic pressure and augments cardiac output produced by closed-chest CPR.

Experimental studies have shown that SCV-CPR increases cardiac output when compared with conventional CPR alone.[79, 116] However, in infant piglets and small dogs, SCV-CPR offered no advantage over conventional CPR.[79, 81] In these small animals, the compliance and geometry of the chest may allow more direct cardiac compression. Thus, higher intrathoracic pressure may be achieved with conventional CPR alone.[80] In human studies, coronary perfusion pressure was either only minimally increased or decreased with SCV-CPR compared with conventional CPR.[117] Survival was significantly worse in pre-hospital victims of cardiac arrest who received SCV-CPR compared to conventional CPR.[118] No study has shown an increased survival with this technique of CPR.

Vest Technique

Vest CPR employs an inflatable bladder resembling a blood pressure cuff wrapped circumferentially around the chest that is inflated phasically to increase intrathoracic pressure. Chest dimensions are changed minimally and so direct cardiac compression is unlikely. In addition, the even distribution of the force of compression over the entire chest wall decreases the likelihood of trauma to the skeletal chest wall and its thoracic contents.

Improvement of cerebral and myocardial blood flows and survival with vest CPR as compared with conventional CPR was seen in dogs, but not in piglets in spite of decreasing permanent chest deformation.[101, 119–121] In a human study, vest CPR increased aortic systolic pressure but had little effect on diastolic pressure when compared with conventional CPR.[102] Despite its late application, vest CPR improved the hemodynamics and the rate of return to spontaneous circulation in adult patients in another study.[122] The vest has also been used as an external cardiac assist device in nonarrested dogs with heart failure.[123] Clinically, the use of vest CPR depends on sophisticated equipment; thus, this technique remains experimental at this time.

Abdominal Binding

Abdominal binders and military antishock trousers have been used to augment closed-chest CPR. Both methods apply continuous compression circumferentially below the diaphragm. Three mechanisms have been proposed for the augmentation of blood flow during CPR by these binders. First, binding the abdomen decreases the compliance of the diaphragm and raises intrathoracic pressure. Second, blood may be moved out of the intrathoracic structures to increase circulating blood volume. Third, applying pressure to the subdiaphragmatic vasculature and increasing its resistance may increase suprathoracic blood flow. This method has resulted in increased aortic pressure and carotid blood flow in both animals and humans.[116, 124, 125] Unfortunately, as aortic pressure increases, the downstream component of coronary perfusion pressure, namely, right atrial pressure, increases to an even greater extent, resulting in a decrease in coronary perfusion pressure and myocardial blood flow.[124] These techniques also lower the cerebral perfusion pressure by increasing intracranial pressure, the downstream component of cerebral perfusion pressure.[126] Clinical studies have failed to show an increased survival when an abdominal binder or military anti-shock trousers was used to augment CPR.[127, 128]

Abdominal Compression

Interposed abdominal compression CPR (IAC-CPR) represents the delivery of an abdominal compression during the relaxation phase of chest compression. IAC-CPR may augment conventional CPR in several ways. First IAC-CPR may return venous blood to the chest during chest relaxation.[129, 130] Second, IAC-CPR increases intrathoracic pressure and augments the duty cycle of chest compression.[131] Third, IAC-CPR may compress the aorta and return blood retrograde to the carotid or coronary arteries.[130]

In animal experiments, cardiac output and cerebral and coronary blood flow were improved when IAC-CPR was compared with conventional CPR[129, 131, 132] but not in an infant model.[133] Human studies also demonstrated an increase in aortic pressure and coronary perfusion pressure during IAC-CPR compared with conventional CPR.[85, 134, 135] Clinically, IAC-CPR requires additional manpower and equipment and remains experimental until additional outcome studies prove its superiority over conventional techniques of CPR.

Open Chest Technique

The use of open-chest cardiac massage has generally been replaced by closed-chest CPR.[10] Compared with closed-chest CPR, open-chest CPR generates higher cardiac output and vital organ blood flow. During open-chest CPR, there is less elevation of intrathoracic, right atrial, and intracranial pressure, resulting in higher coronary and cerebral perfusion pressure and higher myocardial and cerebral blood flow.[77, 136, 137]

Open-chest CPR is obviously not a technique that can be applied by most health care personnel. It can be used in the operating room, intensive care unit, or emergency department equipped with the necessary surgical and technical equipment and personnel. Open-chest CPR is indicated for cardiac arrest secondary to cardiac tamponade, hypothermia, critical aortic stenosis, and ruptured aortic aneurysm. Other indications include cardiac arrest secondary to penetrating or crushed chest wall abnormalities that make closed-chest CPR impossible or ineffective.[91] Open-chest CPR is also indicated for selected patients when closed-chest CPR has failed, although exactly which patients should receive this method of resuscitation under this condition is controversial. When initiated early following failure of closed-chest CPR, open-chest CPR may improve outcome.[138–140] When performed after 15 minutes of closed-chest CPR, open chest CPR significantly improves coronary perfusion pressure and the rate of successful resuscitation.[141]

Cardiopulmonary Bypass

Cardiopulmonary bypass (CPB) represents one of the most effective ways to restore circulation after cardiac arrest. Animal studies show that CPB improves survival and neurologic recovery and preserves the myocardium better than conventional CPR.[142] In dogs, CPB resulted in better neurologic outcome than with conventional CPR after a 4-minute ischemic period, but neurologic outcome was dismal in both groups when the ischemic period lasted 12 minutes.[142] Ninety percent of dogs survived 24 hours after 15 to 20 minutes of cardiac arrest, but only 10% survived when the arrest time was prolonged to 30 minutes when CPB was used for stabilization during defibrillation.[143] CPB decreased myocardial infarct size in a model involving coronary artery occlusion when compared with conventional CPR.[144] In all animal models, CPB improves the success of resuscitation when compared to conventional CPR.

Human experience with CPB for cardiac arrest outside the operating room is limited.[145, 146] Following limited but positive experiences with CPB for "refractory" cardiac arrest,[145, 146] more recent, larger studies have been performed in humans. In the first of these studies, only 7 of 29 patients with cardiac arrest placed on CPB were weaned from bypass

and only one of those seven patients survived to hospital discharge.[147] In the second of these studies, of the 36 patients with cardiac arrest placed on CPB, 18 patients were weaned from bypass and six survived to hospital discharge.[148] In another, 6 of 10 patients were weaned from CPB after failing conventional CPR; however, none survived to hospital discharge.[149] An additional study had none out of six patients survive emergency cardiac resuscitation with CPB.[150] Other clinical situations where CPB may be rapidly and successfully instituted include resuscitation after cardiac surgery,[151] resuscitation from severe hypothermia,[152, 153] treatment for acute pulmonary embolectomy,[154] and after penetrating cardiac trauma.[155] Successful emergency CPB has been used in pediatric patients who suffer refractory cardiac arrest in the cardiac catheterization laboratory and to treat refractory hyperkalemia.[156, 157]

Cardiopulmonary bypass requires a great deal of technical support and sophistication. It can be implemented quickly in systems set up to do so.[145, 148, 153] Despite rapid availability and restoration of circulation, the lack of effective resuscitation prior to institution of CPB limits the ability to preserve neurologic or cardiac function. Because of these limitations, CPB is not recommended for patients who suffer out-of-hospital cardiac arrest or undergo more than 30 minutes of conventional CPR in any setting.[148]

Monitoring During Cardiopulmonary Resuscitation

Monitoring and assessment of the patient during CPR is similar to other clinical situations. A basic clinical examination including inspection, palpation, and auscultation of the patient is performed. The chest is carefully observed for adequacy of chest expansion with artificial ventilation and for equal and normal breath sounds. In addition, one should constantly re-evaluate the depth of compression and the position of the rescuer's hands in performing chest compressions. Palpation is essential in establishing pulselessness, in assessing the adequacy of blood flow during chest compressions, and in locating landmarks. Simply palpating the peripheral pulses may not allow for an accurate assessment of blood flow during CPR, especially during intense vasoconstriction following the use of epinephrine.

Adequacy of vital organ blood flow or function may not be well assessed by the clinical examination. The use of an indwelling arterial catheter, when available, is a valuable monitor in assessing the arterial blood pressure. The effects of volume expansion and drugs on arterial blood pressure are critical. Aortic diastolic pressure relates directly to adequacy of coronary perfusion during CPR.[158, 159] In addition, an arterial line allows for frequent blood sampling, particularly for measurement of arterial pH and blood gases. The state of oxygen delivery can also be determined by transcutaneous monitoring of PO_2 or by pulse oximetry. Pulse oximetry can be used during CPR to determine the oxygen saturation and the level of cardiac output, as reflected in the plethysmograph.[160–162]

The electrocardiogram (ECG) is an integral part of monitoring the patient during CPR. The ECG can reflect the adequacy of myocardial blood flow, reveal metabolic imbalances, and show electrical disturbances (see Fig. 11–10).

The neurologic examination should not be utilized as a predictor of outcome.[163] Use of the electroencephalogram has been shown to be a poor predictor of survival during CPR.[164–166] Somatosensory evoked potentials have been used as a monitor of adequacy of cerebral blood flow and function during and after CPR in animals.[167, 168] Clinical studies have indicated that the bilateral absence of cortical somatosensory evoked potentials portends a poor neurologic outcome.[169]

Temperature should be monitored routinely during CPR as it may vary widely during the resuscitation or at presentation to the hospital. The resuscitation of the patient with hypothermia as the cause of cardiac arrest must be continued until the patient's core temperature has risen above 35°C. Use of a glass bulb thermometer allows measurement of temperature to very low levels. Repeated measurements of core body temperature should be made at several sites (rectal, bladder, esophageal, axillary, and tympanic membrane) if possible to avoid misleading temperature readings from a single site, which might be affected by alterations in regional blood flow during CPR. Temperature can affect the success of resuscitation, the short-term neurologic status and eventual neurologic outcome. External rewarming should be done carefully to avoid overheating the patient once spontaneous circulation has been restored. Conversely, the therapeutic use of hypothermia may be applied eventually to improve outcome from resuscitation.

Vascular Access and Fluid Administration

One of the key aspects of successful CPR is the early establishment of an intravascular line for the administration of fluids and medications. If an intravenous line cannot be established rapidly, then one of the other alternatives, the intraosseous or endotracheal route, must be used.

Intravenous Access

During CPR, the rapid establishment of intravenous access is critical. Central venous access is always the preferable route for fluid and drug administration but should not be the first site for attempting to gain venous access. In children less than 5 years old, a brief attempt should be made to start a peripheral intravenous line when cardiac arrest has occurred. If access is not achieved quickly, then an intraosseous needle should be placed for vascular access (see Fig. 32–4).[170] A large peripheral vein such as the antecubital vein can be used. Attempts at either the jugular or subclavian vein frequently interfere with bag-mask ventilation during CPR. When additional skilled help is available and after tracheal intubation, then central venous cannulation can be attempted. Peripheral venous access generally is easier in the older child than in the younger patient. If peripheral intravenous placement fails, then a saphenous venous cutdown or other central venous line should be placed. There may be a significant delay in the circulation time of drugs administered from a peripheral site compared with a central site during CPR.[171, 172]

Intraosseous Access

The intraosseous route of fluid and medication administration, described originally in 1934,[173] is an important adjunct to the arrest protocol. All medications used during CPR and fluids, including whole blood, can be given by the intraos-seous route. This technique should be considered a temporary measure during emergencies when other vascular sites are not available. In the young child, this route should be utilized after approximately 90 seconds of attempting peripheral venous access. The placement of an intraosseous needle in the older child or adult, although possible, is difficult due to the thick bony cortex.[174]

The technique of placing an intraosseous line is straight-forward. A specialized intraosseous needle or, if not available, a standard 16- or 18-gauge needle, spinal needle with stylet, or bone marrow needle (see Fig. 16–3) is inserted into the anterior surface of the tibia, 1 to 3 cm below the tibial tuberosity. The needle is directed in a 90° angle to the medial surface of the tibia or slightly inferior to avoid the epiphyseal plate (see Fig. 32–4). When the needle passes through the cortex into the marrow, there is loss of resistance. The infusion is successful if the needle is in the marrow cavity, as evidenced by the needle standing upright without support. It loses the upright position if it has slipped into the subcutaneous tissue. At times bone marrow can be aspirated into a syringe connected to the needle. Free flow of the drug or fluid infusion without significant subcutaneous infiltration should also be demonstrated.[175] The technique has a low complication rate[176]; possible complications include osteomyelitis, fat and bone marrow embolism, and compartment syndrome.[177, 178] Succinylcholine has been administered by this route.[179]

Endotracheal Access

When intravenous access is difficult, medications including lidocaine, atropine, naloxone, and epinephrine can be given through the endotracheal tube. The use of ionized medications such as sodium bicarbonate or calcium chloride is not recommended by this route. The rate of absorption and physiologic effects of lidocaine, epinephrine, and atropine administered via the endotracheal route compare favorably to the intravenous route in most studies.[180–182] The peak level of epinephrine or lidocaine administered via the endotracheal route may be lower compared with the intraosseous route. There is inconsistency in obtaining therapeutic levels of lidocaine when administration is by the endotracheal route to humans during CPR.[183] The peak drug concentration of epinephrine was one tenth following endotracheal administration compared with intravenous administration in anesthetized dogs. The endotracheal dose of epinephrine producing a 50% success of resuscitation was 130 μg/kg.[184] Thus, the effective dose of epinephrine by the endotracheal route may be much larger than currently recommended. The recommended dose of endotracheal epinephrine is 10 times the intravenous or intraosseous dose: 0.1 mg/kg for bradycardia or pulseless arrest.

The volume and the diluent in which the medications are administered through an endotracheal tube may be important. When large volumes of fluid are used, pulmonary surfactant may be altered or destroyed, resulting in atelectasis. The total volume of fluid delivered into the trachea should not exceed 10 mL in the adult or 5 mL in the infant.[185] Normal saline may be the least detrimental on lung mechanics[185] and may be important for the absorption of medication from the bronchial tree.[186] Absorption into the systemic circulation may also be enhanced by deep intrapulmonary administration. This distal placement of drug can be performed by passing a Swan-Ganz catheter or suction catheter to a wedged position deep into the bronchial tree.[187] The current recommendation is to dilute drugs given by this route into 1 to 2 mL of normal or half-normal saline. The risk associated with the endotracheal route of drug administration is the formation of an intrapulmonary depot of drug, which may prolong the drugs' effect. This could theoretically result in post-resuscitation hypertension or the recurrence of fibrillation after normal circulation is restored.

Transcutaneous Cardiac Pacing

Transcutaneous cardiac pacing (TCP) is an external noninvasive method of pacing the ventricles for a relatively short period of time. In the absence of in situ pacing wires or an indwelling transvenous or esophageal pacing catheter, TCP is the preferred method for temporary electrical cardiac pacing. The 1992 American Heart Association's advanced cardiac life support (ACLS) guidelines recommend the early use of an external pacemaker in patients with symptomatic bradycardia or asystole.[91]

Since Zoll established TCP in 1952 as a clinically useful method of pacing adult patients during ventricular standstill (Stokes-Adams attacks) and bradycardia-associated hypotension,[188] a number of reports have supported its use for bradycardic or asystolic in-hospital and pre-hospital arrests.[189-192] Emergency cardiac pacing was successful in resuscitation only when it was initiated soon after the onset of the cardiac arrest.

To date there have been no studies of the efficacy of TCP in pediatric resuscitation. Beland et al.[193] showed that effective TCP could be achieved in hemodynamically stable children during induction of anesthesia for heart surgery. They were successful in 53 of 56 pacing trials and these patients suffered no complications.

Transcutaneous cardiac pacing is indicated for patients whose primary problem is impulse formation or conduction, with preserved myocardial function. TCP is most effective in patients with sinus bradycardia or high-grade atrioventricular (AV) block with slow ventricular response that also have a stroke volume sufficient to generate a pulse. TCP is not indicated for patients in prolonged arrest, since in this situation it usually results in electrical but not mechanical cardiac capture and its use may delay or interfere with other resuscitative efforts.

To set up pacing, one electrode is placed anteriorly at the left sternal border and the other posteriorly just below the left scapula. Smaller electrodes are available for infants and children; adult-size electrodes can be used in children over 15 kg.[193] ECG leads should be connected to the pacemaker, the demand or asynchronous mode selected, and an age-appropriate heart rate used. The stimulus output should be set at zero when the pacemaker is turned on and then increased gradually until electrical capture is seen on the monitor. The output required for a hemodynamically unstable rhythm is higher than that for a stable rhythm in children in whom the mean stimulus required for capture was between 52 and 65 mA. After electrical capture is achieved, one must ascertain whether an effective arterial pulse is generated. If pulses are not adequate, other resuscitative efforts should be employed.

The most serious complication of TCP is the induction of a ventricular arrhythmia.[194] Fortunately, this is rare and may be prevented by pacing only in the demand mode. Mild transient erythema beneath the electrodes is common. Skeletal muscle contraction can be minimized by using large electrodes, a 40 msec pulse duration and the smallest stimulus required for capture. Sedatives or analgesics may be necessary in the awake patient. If defibrillation or cardioversion is necessary, one must allow a distance of 2 to 3 cm between the electrode and paddles to prevent arcing of the current.

Pharmacology

Adrenergic Agonists

In 1963, only 3 years after the original description of closed-chest CPR, Redding and Pearson[195] described the use of adrenergic agonists for resuscitation. They subsequently showed that early administration of epinephrine in a canine model of cardiac arrest improved the success rate of CPR. They also demonstrated that the increase in aortic diastolic pressure by the administration of α-adrenergic agonists was responsible for the improved success of resuscitation. They theorized that vasopressors such as epinephrine were of value because the drug increased peripheral vascular tone and not by any direct effect on the heart.

The relative importance of α- and β-adrenergic agonist actions during resuscitation has been investigated.[196] Only 27% of dogs that received a pure β-adrenergic receptor agonist along with an α-adrenergic antagonist were resuscitated successfully, compared with all of the dogs that received a pure α-adrenergic agonist and a β-adrenergic antagonist. Other investigators have demonstrated that the α-adrenergic effects of epinephrine result in intense vasoconstriction of the resistance vessels of all organs of the body, except those supplying the heart and brain.[197] Because of the widespread vasoconstriction in non-vital organs, adequate perfusion pressure and thus blood flow to the heart and brain can be achieved despite the fact that cardiac output is very low during CPR.[80, 197, 198]

The increase in aortic diastolic pressure associated with epinephrine administration during CPR is critical for maintaining coronary blood flow and enhancing the success of resuscitation. Even though the contractile state of the myocardium is increased by the use of β-adrenergic agonists in the spontaneously beating heart during CPR, β-adrenergic agonists may actually decrease myocardial blood flow by increasing intramyocardial wall pressure and vascular resistance.[199] This could redistribute intramyocardial blood flow away from the subendocardium, increasing the likelihood of ischemic injury to this region.[200] By its inotropic and chronotropic effects, β-adrenergic stimulation increases myocardial oxygen demand, which, when superimposed on low coronary blood flow, increases the risk of ischemic injury. This combination of increased oxygen demand by β-adrenergic agonists and decreased oxygen supply may cause damage to an already ischemic heart.[201]

Any medication that causes vasoconstriction of systemic arterioles can be used successfully to increase aortic diastolic pressure and resuscitate the heart. For example, α-adrenergic agonists can be used in place of epinephrine during CPR.

Phenylephrine and methoxamine, two pure α-adrenergic agonists, have been used in animal models of CPR with success equal to that of epinephrine. Their use results in a higher oxygen supply to demand ratio in the ischemic heart and at least a theoretical advantage over the combined α- and β-adrenergic agonist effects of epinephrine. These agonists, as well as other classes of vasopressors such as vasopressin, have been used successfully for resuscitation.[167, 195, 196, 202, 203] These drugs maintain blood flow to the heart during CPR as well as epinephrine. In an animal model of ventricular fibrillation cardiac arrest, a resuscitation rate of 75% was reported for both epinephrine-treated and phenylephrine-treated groups. In this study, the ratio of endocardial to epicardial blood flow was lower in the epinephrine-treated group, suggesting the presence of subendocardial ischemia. However, studies of this kind are difficult to interpret because of the inability to measure the degree of α-receptor activation by the different vasopressors. The higher subendocardial blood flow in the phenylephrine group may have been due to less α-receptor activation.[204–206] Moreover, the merits of using a pure α-adrenergic agonist during CPR have been questioned by some investigators. While the inotropic and chronotropic effects of β-adrenergic agonists may have deleterious hemodynamic effects during CPR for ventricular fibrillation, increases in both heart rate and contractility will increase cardiac output when spontaneous coordinated ventricular contractions are achieved.

Cerebral blood flow during CPR, like coronary blood flow, depends on peripheral vasoconstriction and is also enhanced by the use of α-adrenergic agonists. This action produces selective vasoconstriction of non-cerebral peripheral vessels to areas of the head and scalp without causing cerebral vasoconstriction.[80, 187, 197] As with myocardial blood flow, pure α agents are as effective as epinephrine in generating and sustaining cerebral blood flow during CPR in adult[167] and in infant[207] animal models. No difference in neurologic deficits 24 hours after cardiac arrest was found between animals receiving either epinephrine or phenylephrine during CPR.[208]

Adrenergic agonists may vasoconstrict or dilate cerebral vessels depending on the balance between α and β-adrenergic receptors if they cross the blood-brain barrier.[209] Epinephrine and phenylephrine had similar effects on cerebral blood flow and metabolism, maintaining normal cerebral oxygen uptake for 20 minutes of CPR in dogs. This implies that cerebral blood flow was high enough to maintain adequate cerebral metabolism and that β-receptor stimulation did not increase cerebral oxygen uptake, despite the fact that the combined effects of brain ischemia and CPR can increase the permeability of the blood-brain barrier to drugs used during CPR or when enzymatic barriers to vasopressors, such as by monoamine oxidase, are overwhelmed during tissue hypoxia.[210, 211] Mechanical disruption of the barrier could occur during chest compressions due to hyperemia by large fluctuations in cerebral venous and arterial pressures.[212] In addition, mechanical disruption could be due to hyperemia, the large increase in cerebral blood flow that occurs during the early reperfusion period when the cerebral vascular bed is maximally dilated following resuscitation, particularly if systemic hypertension occurs.[213] We found no blood-brain barrier permeability changes during CPR, immediately after or 4 hours after resuscitation in adult dogs.[213] However,

in piglets following 8 minutes of cardiac arrest and 6 minutes of CPR, the blood-brain barrier was permeable to a small neutral amino acid (α-aminoisobutyric acid) 4 hours after cardiac arrest.[214] We also found that this increase in permeability could be prevented by pre-arrest administration of conjugated superoxide dismutase and catalase,[215] indicating a role for oxygen free radicals in the pathogenesis of this injury to the blood-brain barrier.

Using the same infant piglet model, we later found that these endothelial membrane changes were frequently associated with the presence of intravascular polymorphonuclear and monocytic leukocytes.[216] Whether leukocytes cause disruption of the blood-brain barrier by release of toxic substances such as oxygen free radicals or proteases, or they appear in the post-ischemic microvessels as an epiphenomenon of a more important derangement is presently unknown.

High-Dose Epinephrine

The epinephrine dosage recommended for cardiac arrest remains controversial because of conflicting reports between anecdotes suggesting increased survival when higher doses were administered after cardiac arrest in children.[91] Several larger clinical studies in adults did not demonstrate any beneficial effects of higher doses of epinephrine on short- or long-term survival. The physiologic responses of animals and humans to higher doses of epinephrine have been studied. Cerebral blood flow increased in response to administration of larger doses of epinephrine.[208, 217, 218]

In animals, high-dose epinephrine increases myocardial and sub-myocardial blood flow, improves oxygen delivery relative to oxygen consumption, and is associated with less depletion of myocardial adenosine triphosphate (ATP) stores and more rapid repletion of phosphocreatine.[219–224] In neonatal lambs following asphyxia-induced bradycardia, high-dose epinephrine resulted in higher heart rate but a lower stroke volume and cardiac output.[225] Contrary results, with increased myocardial oxygen consumption and decreased myocardial blood flow, have been demonstrated during CPR following ventricular fibrillation cardiac arrest.[200, 226, 227] In a piglet model, high-dose epinephrine produced lower myocardial blood flow than achieved with lower doses of epinephrine.[217]

Studies in humans have also been contradictory regarding survival of patients who were given high-dose epinephrine. In out-of-hospital cardiac arrest patients, high-dose epinephrine produced higher aortic diastolic pressure during CPR and increased the rate of return of spontaneous circulation compared with standard doses of epinephrine. A dose-dependent increase in aortic blood pressure by epinephrine has been demonstrated in patients who failed to respond to prolonged resuscitative efforts.[228, 229] One group showed that high-dose epinephrine increased aortic diastolic pressure and improved the rate of successful resuscitation in patients who failed ACLS protocols.[230] That group also reported seven pediatric patients treated successfully with 200 μg/kg of epinephrine.[231] Other centers have claimed that higher than standard doses of epinephrine during CPR in children improves the hemodynamics and increases the success of CPR; however, none has provided any valid data that suggest that high-dose epinephrine improves survival beyond the immediate post-resuscitation period.[230, 232–234]

Three large multicenter studies were published that subsequently dampened the enthusiasm for the use of high-dose epinephrine. One group studied 650 adult patients after cardiac arrests who were randomly assigned to receive either standard- or high-dose (7 mg) epinephrine protocol. No differences were observed between the groups in survival (23% versus 18% 1-hour survival), rate of hospital discharge (5% versus 3%), or neurologic outcome.[235] Another group reported their experience with 1280 adult patients who received either standard-dose (0.02 mg/kg) or high-dose (0.2 mg/kg) epinephrine after cardiac arrest. Again, there were no differences in the rate of return to spontaneous circulation, short-term survival, survival to hospital discharge, or neurologic outcome between these two groups of patients.[236] In another study of 816 adults, a higher rate of return of spontaneous circulation was found in the high-dose epinephrine group. However, there were no differences in the rates of hospital discharge or ultimate survival of these patients.[237]

High doses of epinephrine may account for some of the adverse effects that may occur after resuscitation.[238] Epinephrine could worsen myocardial ischemic injury secondary to increased oxygen demand and result in tachyarrhythmias, hypertension, pulmonary edema, and increased shunting due to ventilation/perfusion ($\dot{V}/\dot{Q}$) mismatch resulting in hypoxemia and cardiac arrest.[175, 197, 214, 239] Use of a β-adrenergic antagonist after return of spontaneous circulation has been suggested to attenuate the adverse effects of epinephrine.[168, 240, 241] Epinephrine causes hypoxemia and an increase in alveolar dead space ventilation by redistributing pulmonary blood flow.[242, 243] In one study, high doses of epinephrine (greater than 15 mg) given to adults during CPR resulted in a lower cardiac index, systemic oxygen consumption, and oxygen delivery immediately after resuscitation.[225] Prolonged peripheral vasoconstriction by excessive doses of epinephrine may delay or impair reperfusion of systemic organs, particularly the kidneys and gastrointestinal tract.

Given the conflicting results and bias by some investigators to their own and to other published anecdotal experiences, the recommendations for epinephrine dosing were modified in 1992 in the American Heart Association's Standards and Guidelines for CPR and Emergency Cardiac Care.[91] To treat a pulseless arrest in children, the first intravenous or intraosseous dose remains 0.01 mg/kg. All endotracheal doses are 10 times this dose, or 0.1 mg/kg. The second dose by any route is 0.1 mg/kg administered every 3 to 5 minutes during arrest. In adults, the guidelines do not specifically recommend or discourage the use of high-dose epinephrine. Possible regimens include an intermediate dose of 2 to 5 mg, escalating doses from 1, to 3, to 5 mg, and a high dose of 0.1 mg/kg.

Atropine

Atropine, a parasympatholytic agent, acts by blocking cholinergic stimulation of the muscarinic receptors of the heart.[244] This usually results in an increase in the sinus rate and shortening of the atrioventricular node conduction time.[245] Atropine may also activate latent ectopic pacemakers. Atropine has little effect on systemic vascular resistance, myocardial perfusion pressure, or contractility.[246]

Atropine is indicated for the treatment of asystole, pulseless electrical activity, bradycardia associated with hypotension,[247] second- and third-degree heart block, and slow idioventricular rhythms.[244] In children who present in cardiac arrest, sinus bradycardia and asystole are the most common initial rhythms, which makes atropine useful as a first-line drug. Atropine is particularly effective in clinical conditions associated with excessive parasympathetic tone.

The recommended dose of atropine is 0.02 mg/kg, with a minimum dose of 0.15 mg and a maximum dose of 2.0 mg. Smaller doses than 0.15 mg even in small infants may result paradoxically in bradycardia due to a central stimulatory effect on the medullary vagal nuclei by a dose that is too low to provide anticholinergic effects on the heart.[248] Atropine may be given by any route, including intravenous, intraosseous, endotracheal, intramuscular, and subcutaneous. Its onset of action occurs within 30 seconds and its peak effect occurs between 1 and 2 minutes after an intravenous dose. The recommended adult dose is 0.5 mg every 5 minutes until the desired heart rate is obtained, up to a maximum of 2.0 mg. For asystole, 1.0 mg IV is given and repeated every 5 minutes if asystole persists. Full vagal blockade is usually obtained in adults with a dose of 2.0 mg.

Because of its parasympatholytic effects, atropine should not be used in patients in whom tachycardia is undesirable. In patients after myocardial infarction or ischemia with persistent bradycardia, atropine should be used in the lowest dose possible to increase heart rate. This will limit tachycardia, a potent contributor to increased myocardial oxygen consumption, which could lead to ventricular fibrillation. In addition, atropine should not be used in patients with pulmonary or systemic outflow tract obstruction or idiopathic hypertrophic subaortic stenosis, as tachycardia decreases ventricular filling and lowers cardiac output in this setting.

Sodium Bicarbonate

The administration of sodium bicarbonate results in an acid-base reaction in which bicarbonate combines with hydrogen to form carbonic acid, which dissociates into water and carbon dioxide. Because of the generation of carbon dioxide, adequate alveolar ventilation must be present to achieve the normal buffering action of bicarbonate. The use of sodium bicarbonate during CPR remains controversial because of its potential side effects and the lack of evidence showing any benefit from its use during CPR.[249–251]

Sodium bicarbonate is indicated for correction of significant metabolic acidosis, especially when there are signs of cardiovascular compromise. Acidosis itself may have a number of negative effects on the circulation including depression of myocardial function by prolonging diastolic depolarization, depressing spontaneous cardiac activity, decreasing the electrical threshold for ventricular fibrillation, decreasing the inotropic state of the myocardium, and reducing the cardiac response to catecholamines.[252] Acidosis also vasodilates systemic vessels and attenuates the vasoconstrictive response of peripheral vessels to catecholamines,[253] which is the opposite of the desired vascular effect during CPR. In patients with a reactive pulmonary vascular bed, acidosis causes pulmonary hypertension. Rudolph et al.[254] observed a twofold increase in pulmonary vascular resistance in calves when pH was lowered from 7.40 to 7.20 under normoxic conditions. Therefore, correction of even mild acidosis may be helpful in resuscitating patients who have the potential for increased right-to-left shunting through a cardiac septal defect, patent ductus arteriosus, or an aortic to pulmonary shunt during periods of elevated pulmonary vascular resistance.

Multiple side effects of bicarbonate administration include metabolic alkalosis, hypercapnia, hypernatremia, and hyperosmolality.[255] All of these side effects are associated with a high mortality rate. Alkalosis causes a leftward shift of the oxyhemoglobin dissociation curve and so impairs release of oxygen from hemoglobin to tissues, at a time when oxygen delivery may already be low.[256] Alkalosis can also result in hypokalemia by enhancing potassium influx into cells and ionic hypocalcemia by increasing protein binding of ionized calcium. Hypernatremia and hyperosmolality may decrease tissue perfusion by increasing interstitial edema in microvascular beds. The marked hypercapnic acidosis that occurs during CPR on the venous side of the circulation, including the coronary sinus, may be worsened by the administration of bicarbonate.[257] Myocardial acidosis during cardiac arrest is associated with decreased myocardial contractility.[252] Paradoxical intracellular acidosis after bicarbonate administration is possible due to the rapid entry of carbon dioxide into cells with a slow egress of hydrogen ions out of cells; however, in neonatal rabbits recovering from hypoxic acidosis, bicarbonate administration increased both arterial pH and intracellular brain pH as measured by nuclear magnetic resonance spectroscopy.[258] Likewise, intracellular brain ATP concentration did not change during severe intracellular acidosis in the brain produced by extreme hypercapnia in rats.[259] The rats who maintained ATP concentration, even in the face of severe brain acidosis, had no functional or histologic differences from normal control subjects.

In another study using nuclear magnetic resonance spectroscopy of the brain in dogs during cardiac arrest and CPR, intracellular brain pH decreased to 6.29, with total depletion of brain ATP after 6 minutes of cardiac arrest; however, following effective CPR, ATP levels rose to 86% of prearrest levels and to normal by 35 minutes of CPR despite ongoing peripheral arterial acidosis.[260] Cerebral pH decreased in parallel with blood pH when CPR was started immediately after arrest. Bicarbonate administration ameliorated and did not worsen the cerebral acidosis, indicating that the blood-brain pH gradient is maintained during CPR.[261]

When Pa_{CO_2} and pH are known, the dose of bicarbonate to correct the pH to 7.40 is calculated using the following formula: $0.3 \times$ weight (kg) $\times$ base deficit = mEq sodium bicarbonate. Because of its possible side effects and the large venous to arterial carbon dioxide gradient that develops during CPR, we recommend giving half the dose based on a volume distribution of 0.6. If blood gases are not available, the initial dose is 1 mEq/kg followed by 0.5 mEq/kg every 10 minutes of ongoing arrest.[262] Alveolar ventilation must be maintained because of the generation of carbon dioxide, and can be assessed only by serial measurements of arterial blood gases and pH. Because of the potential side effects of bicarbonate, the indications for its use are limited to cardiac arrest associated with hyperkalemia, patients with preexisting metabolic acidosis, and after approximately 10 minutes of CPR.

The $ETCO_2$ monitor is very useful during CPR because it provides important information regarding both pulmonary and cardiac function. $ETCO_2$ is measured instantaneously in the exhaled gas of every breath. In the absence of lung disease, $ETCO_2$ correlates closely with Pa_{CO_2}, provided that pulmonary blood flow is at least 20 to 25% of normal. As a respiratory monitor, $ETCO_2$ analyzers accurately distinguish a tracheal ($ETCO_2 > 10$ mm Hg) from an esophageal ($ETCO_2 < 5$ mm Hg) intubation in infants and children.[69] Because measurements are made with every breath, dislodgement of the endotracheal tube from the trachea can be identified immediately (see Fig. 16–3). When cardiac output is extremely low, as occurs during ineffective CPR, delivery of carbon dioxide to the lungs is so limited that the total amount exchanged across the alveolar-capillary membrane is markedly reduced. In this situation, the measured $ETCO_2$ is very low even when the Pa_{CO_2} is elevated because of an absolute low CO_2 volume. As the cardiac output increases, the $ETCO_2$ increases and the difference between end-tidal and arterial CO_2 becomes smaller.[263, 264] $ETCO_2$ has been correlated with coronary perfusion pressure,[264] the critical parameter for resuscitation of the heart. However, a low $ETCO_2$ may occur in the presence of adequate cardiac output during CPR after epinephrine owing to its ability to increase intrapulmonary shunting.[242] In this case, a low $ETCO_2$ would underestimate cardiac output. Other causes of a low $ETCO_2$ include airway obstruction, tension pneumothorax, pericardial tamponade, pulmonary embolism, hypothermia, and severe hypocapnia (which occurs commonly with overaggressive hand ventilation). Esophageal intubation would be indicated by the virtual absence of carbon dioxide detection.

Other Alkalinizing Agents

Other alkalinizing agents have been used experimentally in animals and humans. None, however, have demonstrated any real advantages over sodium bicarbonate. Carbicarb, a solution of equimolar amounts of sodium bicarbonate and sodium carbonate, corrects metabolic acidosis without many of the side effects of sodium bicarbonate.[265] The buffering action of sodium carbonate is by consumption of carbon dioxide with generation of bicarbonate ion. During CPR, Carbicarb administration resulted in a greater increase in arterial pH, and a smaller increase in Pa_{CO_2}, lactate, and serum osmolality in animals.[265, 266] However, Carbicarb was not superior to sodium bicarbonate when used for hypovolemic shock in rats.[267]

Dichloroacetate increases the activity of pyruvate dehydrogenase, which facilitates the conversion of lactate to pyruvate.[268] When administered to patients with lactic acidosis, dichloroacetate decreased lactate concentration by one half and increased bicarbonate concentration and pH.[269] In other studies, dichloroacetate improved cardiac output, possibly by increasing myocardial metabolism of lactate and carbohydrate.[270, 271] In a multicenter trial of patients with lactic acidosis, dichloroacetate did not improve outcome when compared with sodium bicarbonate.[272]

Tromethamine (tris-hydroxymethyl-aminomethane) is an organic amine that attracts and combines with hydrogen ion, causing CO_2 and H_2O to combine to form bicarbonate and hydrogen ion. A dose of 3 mL/kg should raise the bicarbonate concentration by 3 mEq/L. Side effects of tromethamine include hyperkalemia, hypoglycemia, and acute hypocarbia resulting in apnea. In addition, peripheral vasodilation may occur after administration of tromethamine during CPR, an undesirable effect. Tromethamine is contraindicated in patients with renal failure.[273, 274]

Calcium

Calcium administration during CPR is restricted to the treatment of hypocalcemia, hyperkalemia, hypermagnesemia, and calcium channel blocker overdose. These restrictions are based on the possibility that exogenously administered calcium may worsen ischemia-reperfusion injury. Intracellular calcium overload occurs during cerebral ischemia by the influx of calcium through voltage-dependent and agonist-dependent (e.g., NMDA) calcium channels. Calcium plays an important role in the process of cell death in many organs,[275, 276] possibly by activation of intracellular enzymes such as nitric oxide synthase, phospholipase A and C, and others.[277] Calcium channel blockers have been found to improve blood flow and function after ischemia to the heart,[278] kidney[279] and brain.[280] Calcium channel blockers also raise the threshold of the ischemic heart to ventricular fibrillation.[281] For these reasons, it appears that the recommended restrictions for the use of calcium during CPR are well founded.

No studies have shown that the elevation of plasma calcium concentration, which occurs after its administration, worsens outcome from cardiac arrest. Since the normal ratio of extracellular to intracellular calcium is on the order of 1000:1 to 10,000:1, it seems unlikely that the rate of influx of calcium into cells would be influenced by a relatively small increase in its extracellular concentration.

The calcium ion is essential in myocardial excitation-contraction coupling, in increasing ventricular contractility, and in enhancing ventricular automaticity during asystole. Ionized hypocalcemia is associated with decreased ventricular performance, and peripheral blunting of the hemodynamic response to catecholamines.[282, 283] In addition, severe ionized hypocalcemia has been documented in adults suffering from out-of-hospital cardiac arrest (mean Ca^{++} 0.67 mmol/L),[284] during sepsis,[285] and in animals during prolonged CPR.[286] Thus, patients at risk for ionized hypocalcemia should be identified and treated as expeditiously as possible (see Chapter 12). Both total and ionized hypocalcemia may occur in patients with either chronic or acute disease. Total body calcium depletion leading to total serum hypocalcemia occurs in patients with hypoparathyroidism, Di George syndrome, renal failure, pancreatitis and long term use of loop diuretics. Ionized hypocalcemia also occurs after massive or rapid transfusion of blood products because of citrate and other preservatives in stored blood products that bind calcium. The magnitude of hypocalcemia in this setting depends on the rate of blood administration, the total dose, and the hepatic and renal function of the patient (see Chapter 12). Administration of fresh frozen plasma at a rate greater than 1 mL/kg/min causes a significant decrease in ionized calcium concentration in anesthetized children.[287]

The pediatric dose of calcium chloride for resuscitation is 20 mg/kg. The adult dose is 200 mg (2 mL of the 10% solution). Calcium gluconate is as effective as calcium chloride in raising ionized calcium concentration during CPR.[288, 289] Calcium gluconate is given at a dose of 30 to 100 mg/kg, with a maximum dose of 2 g in pediatric patients. Calcium should be given slowly through a large-bore, free-flowing intravenous line, preferably a central venous line. Severe tissue necrosis occurs when calcium infiltrates into subcutaneous tissue. When administered too rapidly, calcium may cause bradycardia, heart block, or ventricular standstill.

Glucose

The administration of glucose during CPR should be restricted to patients with documented hypoglycemia because of the possible detrimental effects of hyperglycemia on the brain during or following ischemia. Infant monkeys that received glucose before cardiac arrest were more likely to develop seizures, prolonged coma, and brain death with cerebral necrosis than those that received saline.[290] The neurologic recovery of hyperglycemic rats was worse than that of normoglycemic controls after 10 minutes of global brain ischemia.[291] The mechanism by which hyperglycemia exacerbates ischemic neurologic injury may be due to an increased production of lactic acid in the brain by anaerobic metabolism. During ischemia under normoglycemic conditions, brain lactate concentration reaches a plateau. In a hyperglycemic milieu, however, brain lactate concentration continues to rise for the duration of the ischemic period.[292] The severity of intracellular acidosis during ischemia is directly proportional to the preischemic glucose concentration.[293] The negative effect of hyperglycemia during brain ischemia is predicated on at least a small amount of blood flow to brain tissue. In one study, collaterally perfused but not end-arterial brain tissue had greater neuronal damage during hyperglycemic focal ischemia.[294]

Clinical studies have shown a direct correlation between the initial postcardiac arrest serum glucose concentration and poor neurologic outcome.[295–297] A higher glucose concentration may just be an endogenous response to severe stress and thus a marker and not the cause of more severe brain injury.[298] In piglets, postischemic administration of glucose did not worsen neurologic outcome after global hypoxia-ischemia.[299] However, given the likelihood of additional ischemic and hypoxic events in the post-resuscitation period, it seems prudent to maintain serum glucose in the normal range. The administration of insulin to hyperglycemic rats after global brain ischemia improved neurologic outcome.[300] The effect of insulin may be independent of its ability to lower blood glucose, since these investigators later showed that normoglycemic insulin-treated rats had a better outcome than normoglycemic placebo-treated control subjects.[301] Additional studies need to be done to determine if the benefit from tight control of serum glucose following cardiac arrest or the use of insulin outweighs the risk of iatrogenic hypoglycemia.

Some groups of patients, including premature infants and debilitated patients with low endogenous glycogen stores, are more prone to developing hypoglycemia during and after a physiologic stress such as surgery.[302] Bedside monitoring of serum glucose is critical during and following a cardiac arrest and allows for intervention before the critical point of low substrate delivery has been reached. The dose of glucose needed to correct hypoglycemia is 0.5 to 1.0 g/kg given as 10% dextrose in infants. The osmolarity of 50% dextrose is approximately 2700 mOsm/L and has been associated with intraventricular hemorrhage in neonates and infants: therefore, the more dilute concentration is recommended in neonates.

Ventricular Fibrillation

Ventricular fibrillation is a sustained burst of multiple, uncoordinated regional ventricular depolarizations and contractions, associated with both absent cardiac output and myocardial blood flow. The rhythm is maintained by re-entrant impulses generated within the ventricles with multiple, shifting circuits. Physiologic conditions that lower the threshold for ventricular fibrillation include hypoxemia, respiratory or metabolic acidosis, myocardial ischemia, hypothermia, and electrolyte disturbances including Na^+, K^+, Ca^{++}, and Mg^{++}.

Ventricular fibrillation and ventricular tachycardia are relatively uncommon rhythms during cardiac arrest in children. Examination of the terminal electrocardiograms in 100 inhospital pediatric arrest patients found that the initial electrical disturbance was a bradyarrhythmia that progressed to asystole, without any evidence for ventricular ectopy in over 90% of cases. However, with increasing numbers of children with congenital heart disease, particularly those with a history of cardiac surgery, and an increasing incidence of toxic ingestions, ventricular fibrillation is increasing as the cause of cardiac arrest in children. A recent study showed ventricular fibrillation as the initial rhythm in 19% of children presenting with cardiac arrest.[24] The cause of ventricular fibrillation was due to medical illnesses, toxic overdose, drowning, trauma, and congenital heart defects.

Electric Countershock

Electric countershock is the treatment of choice for ventricular fibrillation and ventricular tachycardia when a pulse is not present or when the patient is comatose due to the arrhythmia. Drug treatment by itself cannot be relied on to terminate ventricular fibrillation in these instances. Antiarrhythmic agents such as lidocaine are known cardiac depressants and may transform ventricular fibrillation into intractable asystole.[303] High-voltage electric shock, when properly applied, sends more than 2 A through the heart. Ventricular fibrillation is terminated by simultaneously depolarizing and causing a sustained contraction of the entire myocardium, which allows return of spontaneous, coordinated cardiac contractions, assuming the myocardium is well oxygenated and the acid-base status is normal. Modern day defibrillators deliver only direct current shocks using a dampened sine wave form, although some use a trapezoidal wave form.

Higher energy levels cause a greater amount of myocardial damage,[304, 305] and increase the incidence of post-defibrillation arrhythmias.[306] With prolonged depolarization of the myocardial cell membrane, stimulus intensity increases and provides an ideal setting for these re-entrant arrhythmias.[307]

In the majority of adult cases, energy levels of 100 to 200 J are successful when shocks are delivered with minimal delay.[308, 309] There were no differences in heart weight or energy per gram of heart weight to defibrillate in patients who ultimately had an autopsy.[310] The goal of defibrillation is to deliver a minimum of electrical energy to a critical mass of ventricular muscle, while avoiding high current that could further damage the heart.

A dose of 2 J/kg is used initially in children. This dose is based on 71 defibrillatory attempts in 27 children. Fifty-seven shocks were within 10 J above or below an energy dose of 2 J/kg of body weight. Ninety-one percent of these shocks were effective.[311]

One study found that a critical amount of myocardial tissue must be depolarized to terminate ventricular fibrillation.[312] However, depolarization of every myocardial cell is not necessary to terminate fibrillation of the heart. Electric shocks terminate ventricular fibrillation most often when the shocks are delivered between electrodes located at the apex of the right ventricle and the posterior base of the left ventricle, and least often when the shock is delivered between two right ventricular electrodes.

Several clinical factors affect the efficacy of ventricular defibrillation in humans. The most reliable predictor of success of defibrillation is the duration of fibrillation prior to the first countershock.[310] The success of defibrillation decreases with an increased duration of fibrillation. Defibrillatory attempts were successful in patients who were shocked before 8 minutes elapsed after the onset of ventricular fibrillation, whereas attempts were unsuccessful in patients shocked with a mean of 17 minutes after the onset of fibrillation.[310] Acidosis and hypoxia also decrease the success of defibrillation.[310] Patients with terminal illness are more resistant to successful defibrillation,[313] as are those who fibrillate later in the course of their myocardial infarction.

Clinical Aspects of Pediatric Defibrillation

For the first defibrillatory attempt, 200 to 300 J delivered energy should be administered to adults and 2 J/kg to children. If this attempt is unsuccessful, a second and third attempt is made immediately, using the same energy dose in adults and 4 J/kg in children. If these attempts are unsuccessful, then basic life support is continued, epinephrine is administered, and sodium bicarbonate is given if metabolic acidosis is documented or if the duration of cardiac arrest warrants its administration. A fourth defibrillatory attempt is then made at a setting that does not exceed 360 J of delivered energy in adults or 4 J/kg in children. If ventricular fibrillation recurs frequently, lidocaine, bretylium, amiodarone, or procainamide may be used. It is not necessary to increase the energy dose on each successive shock during defibrillation. On the contrary, the threshold for ventricular fibrillation often increases after CPR and resuscitation drugs are administered.

Correct paddle size and position are critical to the success of defibrillation. Three paddle sizes are used to defibrillate externally: 13 cm in diameter for adults, 8 cm for older children, and 4.5 cm for infants. The largest paddle size appropriate for the patient should be used because a larger size reduces the density of current flow, which in turns reduces myocardial damage. If the entire paddle does not rest firmly on the chest wall, a current of high density will be delivered to a small contact point. The paddles should be positioned on the chest wall so that a majority of myocardium lies directly between them. One paddle is placed to the right of the upper sternum below the clavicle, the other positioned just below and to the left of the left nipple. For patients with dextrocardia, the position of the paddles should be a mirror image. An alternative approach is to place one paddle anteriorly over the left precordium and the other paddle posteriorly between the scapulae.

The interface between the paddle and chest wall can be electrode cream, paste, saline, soap, or moist gauze pads. The electrode cream produces lower impedance than the paste. Electric current follows the path of least resistance, so care should be taken that the substance from one paddle does not touch that of the other paddle. *This is especially important in infants, in whom the distance between paddles is short. If the gel is continuous between paddles, a short circuit is created, and an insufficient amount of current will cross the heart.*

If the duration of ventricular fibrillation is less than 2 minutes, then a defibrillatory attempt should be administered as soon as possible. If ventricular fibrillation has been present for longer than 2 minutes or for an undetermined period of time, then basic life support should be initiated for at least 2 minutes before attempting defibrillation in order to improve myocardial oxygenation and acid-base status.[314]

Open-Chest Defibrillation

If the chest is already opened, ventricular fibrillation should be treated with open-chest defibrillation, using internal paddles applied directly to the heart. These should have a diameter of 6 cm for adults, 4 cm for children, and 2 cm for infants. Handles should be insulated. Saline-soaked pads or gauzes should be placed between the paddles and the heart. One electrode is placed behind the left ventricle and the other over the right ventricle on the anterior surface of the heart. The dosage used should begin at 5 J in infants and 20 J in adults.

Automated External Defibrillation

With increasing awareness that time to defibrillation is key in the success of resuscitation, automated external defibrillation (AED) is now standard therapy in out-of-hospital resuscitation of adults.[315] Low-energy (150 J), impedance-adjusted shocks for adults appear to be clinically effective and safe.[316] Engineering issues continue to allow for improvements in the AED units and include size and weight, expense, ease of public use, waveform, and energy dose.[317]

The use of AEDs has generally been limited to adults because of the lower incidence of ventricular fibrillation in children and because the delivered energy dose of 100 to 200 J is higher than the standard dose for most children. However, with recognition that ventricular fibrillation occurs more frequently in children than previously thought,[24, 318] the use of AED in emergency situations would be beneficial. A published, retrospective review of 18 adolescents and children (5–15 years), receiving AED by emergency medical crews, showed accurate rhythm detection and shock delivery.[319] AEDs are potentially effective for all children. Its widespread usage remains a public health issue.

Pharmacotherapy of Life-Threatening Arrhythmias

Even though rapid electric defibrillation and cardioversion remain the mainstay of therapy for life-threatening ventricu-lar arrhythmias, medications such as lidocaine remain important adjuncts for therapy. The role for other agents such as amiodarone, sotalol, and others is becoming increasingly important.

Lidocaine

Lidocaine is a class IB anti-arrhythmic. The chemical structure of lidocaine is an aromatic group 2-6 xylidine coupled to diethylglycine via an amide bond. It is a weak base with a pKa of 7.85. Lidocaine decreases automaticity of pacemaker tissue that prevents or terminates ventricular arrhythmias due to accelerated ectopic foci. Lidocaine abolishes re-entrant ventricular arrhythmias by decreasing the action potential duration and the conduction time of Purkinje fibers, and increases the effective refractory period of Purkinje fibers, reducing the nonuniformity of contraction. Because the microcirculation of ischemic myocardium may differ greatly from that of normal tissue, and since ventricular arrhythmias are thought to originate from ischemic areas of myocardium, lidocaine concentration as well as oxygen content may be much lower in ischemic zones than seen in vitro.[320]

Lidocaine has been shown to be effective in terminating ventricular premature beats (VPB) and ventricular tachycardia in humans during general surgery, before or after cardiac surgery, during cardiac catheterization, after an acute myocardial infarction, and in patients with digitalis intoxication. Treatment of VPBs after myocardial infarction is indicated if they occur at a rate of more than 5 per minute of unifocal origin, on a normal T-wave, with multifocal VPBs or with ventricular tachycardia. The drug is indicated after cardioversion from ventricular fibrillation especially with recurrent ventricular fibrillation or tachycardia. Lidocaine has no effect on atrioventricular nodal conduction time, so it is ineffective in the treatment of atrial or atrioventricular junctional arrhythmias.

In dogs, when lidocaine is given by a rapid intravenous bolus, there is a transient decrease in stroke work, blood pressure, systemic vascular resistance,[321] left ventricular contractility,[322] as well as a slight increase in the heart rate. In healthy adults, no change in heart rate or blood pressure occurs with lidocaine administration. In patients with more severe cardiac disease, there is only a slight or no decrease in ventricular function when a lidocaine bolus is administered intravenously. In patients with more severe cardiac disease, especially in those with acute myocardial infarction, excessive doses of lidocaine given by rapid infusion may lead to a decrease in cardiac function. Therefore, slow intravenous administration, no greater than 50 to 100 mg/min in adults or 1 mg/kg/min in children, is recommended.[320]

Lidocaine is metabolized mainly in the liver by the microsomal enzyme system.[320] Its major degradative pathway is by oxidative N-de-ethylation, followed by hydrolysis to 2-6 xylidine. Its minor degradative pathway is by hydroxylation of its aromatic nitrogen. Normally up to 10% of the dose is excreted unchanged in the urine, but this fraction is increased when the urine is acidic. There is neither biliary excretion nor intestinal absorption in humans. In patients with normal liver function, the hepatic extraction ratio for lidocaine is approximately 70%.

To achieve and maintain therapeutic levels of the drug, a

bolus dose of lidocaine should be given at the same time that a constant infusion is initiated. Without an initial bolus, approximately five half-lives are required to approach plateau concentration of any infused drug.[320] With a half-life of approximately 90 minutes, a 7½ hour infusion of lidocaine would be required to reach a plateau concentration. Ventricular arrhythmias often return within 15 to 20 minutes after an intravenous bolus as a result of rapid clearance from the central compartment.

Lidocaine toxicity occurs when the serum concentration exceeds 7 to 8 μg/mL and occurs most commonly in patients with severe hepatic disease or severe congestive heart failure. Lidocaine clearance decreases during low cardiac output states because of the concomitant fall of hepatic blood flow. During CPR, lidocaine clearance is decreased because of the inherent decrease in cardiac output. In dogs, with use of conventional CPR to attain a blood pressure of 20% of control, a bolus of lidocaine of 2 mg/kg IV resulted in very elevated blood and tissue concentrations, as compared with control animals. Distribution of the drug, as measured by tissue extraction, was complete in 20 minutes. Also, lidocaine clearance and distribution may be altered due to changes in protein binding and metabolism during CPR.[323] In humans, high peak blood and tissue concentrations of lidocaine are observed during CPR, with a delay in the time to the peak concentration of the drug.[324]

In patients with normal cardiac and hepatic function, an initial intravenous bolus of 1.5 to 2 mg/kg of lidocaine is given followed by a constant intravenous infusion at a rate of 55 μg/kg/minute. If the arrhythmia recurs, a second intravenous bolus at the same dose can be given.[325] The eventual steady state plasma concentration of the drug is not affected by this dose. Patients with a moderate decrease in cardiac output or those suffering an acute myocardial infarction should receive only 1 to 1.5 mg/kg IV bolus, with an infusion rate of 30 μg/kg/min. In patients with severe diminution of cardiac output, a bolus of no greater than 0.75 mg/kg, followed by an infusion at the rate of 10 to 20 μg/kg/min, is administered. In patients with hepatic disease, dosages should be decreased by 50% of normal. Patients with chronic renal disease on hemodialysis have normal lidocaine pharmacokinetics; however, toxic metabolites may accumulate in patients receiving infusions over a long period of time. In patients with hypoproteinemia, the dose of lidocaine should also be lowered, due to the increase in free fraction of drug. Measurement of steady-state lidocaine concentration is useful in achieving the therapeutic effects of lidocaine while avoiding side effects.

Drug interactions with lidocaine are common. Phenobarbital increases lidocaine metabolism, so higher doses of lidocaine are needed. Isoniazid and chloramphenicol decrease lidocaine metabolism, so lower doses should be used with those drugs. Propranolol increases the serum concentration by decreasing cardiac output, while positive inotropics have the opposite effect.

Toxic effects of lidocaine are seen when the serum concentration of free drug exceeds 7 μg/mL and usually involve the central nervous system. These symptoms include seizures, psychosis, drowsiness, paresthesias, disorientation, agitation, tinnitus, muscle spasms, and respiratory arrest. The treatment of choice for lidocaine-induced seizures is a benzodiazepine such as midazolam or lorazepam or a barbiturate such as phenobarbital. Barbiturates may be the better choice since they also increase the hepatic metabolism of lidocaine. True allergic reactions to lidocaine are extremely rare. Cardiovascular side effects, as discussed above, are usually seen when large intravenous boluses are given rapidly to patients with severe myocardial dysfunction. Conversion of second-degree heart block to complete heart block has been described,[326] as well as severe sinus bradycardia.

Bretylium

Bretylium, a class III anti-arrhythmic, is a bromobenzyl quaternary ammonia compound and is not structurally related to lidocaine. The half-life of bretylium gradually increases over time, with a mean elimination half-life of 9.8 hours.[327] The drug is 80% excreted unchanged in the urine over the first 24 hours. An additional 10% of the drug is excreted in the urine over the next 72 hours.[328]

The mechanism of action of bretylium appears to be by adrenergic stimulation. There is an initial release of norepinephrine from adrenergic nerve endings, with subsequent inhibition of release of norepinephrine.[329] The drug also blocks the reuptake of norepinephrine and epinephrine into these adrenergic nerve endings, thereby potentiating the action of these agonists.

Bretylium appears to have direct cardiac effects, which are not abolished by β-adrenergic blockade,[330] nor prevented by pretreatment with reserpine or denervation of the heart.[331] Bretylium increases the action potential duration of cardiac muscle and the effective refractory period of Purkinje and ventricular muscle fibers. In dogs, bretylium decreases the disparity in action potential duration between normal and infarcted areas of the heart, probably the explanation for its antiarrhythmic actions.[331] Bretylium also increases the electrical threshold for ventricular fibrillation in normal and infarcted hearts. Bretylium has been noted to defibrillate a heart without electric countershock.[332, 333] It may be more effective in raising the ventricular fibrillatory threshold than lidocaine, phenytoin, procainamide, propranolol, or quinidine.

Bretylium may suppress a ventricular arrhythmia when other antiarrhythmics have not, including ventricular fibrillation resistant to electric countershock.[334] The drug is indicated for the treatment of ventricular fibrillation and ventricular tachycardia that have failed to respond to electric cardioversion and the first-line antiarrhythmic agents, lidocaine or procainamide. The drug is not used to suppress asymptomatic VPBs, nor to treat atrial arrhythmias. When lidocaine and bretylium were compared as the initial treatment for 146 patients suffering from out-of-hospital ventricular fibrillation, there was no difference in resuscitation rate or the rate of hospital discharge.[335]

The dose of bretylium is 5 to 10 mg/kg given by rapid intravenous bolus. When the drug is given less urgently for refractory ventricular tachycardia, 500 mg is diluted in 50 mL of fluid and *the appropriate dose (mg/kg)*, given over 10 minutes. This decreases the severity of orthostatic hypotension in the awake patient. Its onset of action in suppressing ventricular fibrillation is usually within minutes. After an intramuscular injection, the drug is not effective for 20 to 60 minutes. Its duration of action is 6 to 12 hours.[334, 335]

After an intravenous bolus of bretylium is given, an

electric countershock should be administered. If the arrhythmia persists, the drug can be repeated every 15 to 30 minutes, up to a total dose of 30 mg/kg. If the arrhythmia is eradicated, a maintenance dose, the same as the initial dose, is then given every 6 to 8 hours. If ventricular tachycardia is being treated, the second dose should be repeated in 1 to 2 hours and then every 6 to 8 hours for maintenance. The drug can also be given by constant infusion at 1 to 2 mg/min in adults.

After a dose of bretylium, an initial increase in blood pressure due to norepinephrine release is usually seen, along with a slight increase in heart rate, cardiac output, and frequency of VPBs.[329] Subsequently, over half of the patients show a mild decrease in blood pressure due to its adrenergic-blocking effects.[334] If hypotension is severe, fluids and vasopressors should be given. After a patient has received bretylium, he or she may have an exaggerated response to dopamine, norepinephrine, and epinephrine because of the impaired reuptake of these drugs. Patients on maintenance doses become tolerant to its hypotensive effect within a few days. With a rapid infusion of the drug, nausea and vomiting are common. Parotid swelling and pain have been seen following oral bretylium administration.[334]

Newer Antiarrhythmics

There is increasing evidence for the effectiveness of class III anti-arrhythmic agents to treat ventricular tachyarrhythmias. These include sotalol and amiodarone.

Sotalol

Sotalol both has β-adrenergic blocking activity (class II activity) and prolongs action potential duration (class III activity). It is a racemic compound consisting of equal concentrations of the l- and d-isomers. l-sotalol possesses the majority of the β-blocking activity. The mechanism of its class III effects, prolonging the action potential duration, is by inhibiting the rapid component of the outward potassium current.[336]

Sotalol has been shown to be an effective anti-arrhythmic and defibrillating agent in animal models of myocardial ischemia and infarction.[337] A number of trials show the efficacy of short-term and long-term use of sotalol in adult patients with sustained ventricular tachycardia or ventricular fibrillation.[338, 339] However, it is not known whether sotalol is more effective than conventional β-blockers, amiodarone, or implantable cardioverter-defibrillators alone.[340]

Following an oral dose, sotalol has greater than 90% absorption, almost 100% bioavailability, has no hepatic metabolism, and is excreted unchanged by the kidneys[341]; dosage therefore needs to be adjusted in patients with renal failure. The mean elimination half-life is 10 to 20 hours. The usual starting oral dosage in children is 2 mg/kg in two daily doses. Because its plasma protein binding is poor, it has limited drug interactions. Its side effects include proarrhythmias, which occur in 4% of adult patients, with half those having torsades de pointes[342]; however, this side effect is seen less frequently in children.[343] The drug seems to be well tolerated in children with impaired left ventricular function. In children, the best documented use is for various forms of supraventricular tachycardia, with a success rate of

90%.[344, 345] Few children have been treated for ventricular arrhythmias.

Amiodarone

Amiodarone, another class III anti-arrhythmic, is also being used more frequently for ventricular tachyarrhythmias. The predominant activity associated with long-term therapy is an increase in the action potential duration. Amiodarone is a lipophilic drug. It is hepatically metabolized and is highly bound to protein. It is excreted mainly in the bile; renal excretion is minimal.

Clinically it is used to treat both ventricular[346] and supraventricular[347] tachycardia in adult patients. It has been used in children with supraventricular tachycardia and ventricular tachycardia at a loading dose of 5 mg/kg followed by a maintenance dose of 7 to 20 mg/kg/day. Hypotension is the most common adverse reaction, occurring in approximately 15% of patients, due to both its vasodilating and negative inotropic effects. The drug may also cause bradycardia and heart failure, although its proarrhythmic effects appear less often than with other class III agents. Pulmonary fibrosis, probably the best known side effect of long-term oral amiodarone therapy, occurs in only 0.1% of patients.[348] Hepatotoxicity, another important concern with oral therapy, also appears less often after intravenous therapy. Drug interactions include an increase in serum lidocaine and cyclosporine levels. In addition, there are additive pharmacologic effects with β-blockers and calcium-channel blockers.

Supraventricular Tachycardia

Supraventricular tachycardia (SVT), a common arrhythmia in infants and children, may be associated with severe circulatory compromise or even cardiac arrest. Therapy for this arrhythmia should be based on the child's hemodynamic status. SVT associated with poor circulation, including poor peripheral perfusion, hypotension, or a depressed level of consciousness, should be immediately treated with synchronized cardioversion beginning at a dose of 0.5 J/kg. If intravenous access is available, adenosine can be used as cardioversion is being prepared; however, cardioversion should not be delayed while intravenous access is being obtained.

Adenosine is the medical treatment of choice for SVT.[349, 350] The underlying mechanism in children is usually a re-entry circuit involving the atrioventricular node. Adenosine is an endogenous nucleoside that causes a temporary block in the atrioventricular node and interrupts this re-entry circuit. It is rapidly and highly effective with minimal side effects.[351] It has been used in a variety of settings, including during general anesthesia, open heart surgery, and in the intensive care unit.[352–354] There is now considerable experience in treating adult patients with SVT by emergency services personnel in the pre-hospital setting.[355, 356] The initial dose is 0.1 mg/kg given as a rapid IV bolus. Central venous administration is preferable since the drug is rapidly metabolized by red blood cell adenosine deaminase and so has a half-life of only 10 seconds; higher doses may be necessary when the drug is given peripherally.[349] If there is no interruption in the re-entry circuit, successive doses should be doubled up to a maximum single dose of 12 mg until the arrhythmia is broken. In neonates, a smaller initial dose of 0.05 mg/kg is given and increased by 0.05 mg/kg/dose until termination of the arrhythmia up to a maximum dose of 0.25 mg/kg.[357] When SVT appears without any circulatory compromise, conversion of the arrhythmia may first be attempted with a vagal maneuver such as ice water to the face. If ineffective, then adenosine should be utilized.

All other medications to treat SVT have a higher incidence of side effects. Digoxin is often ineffective and causes frequent arrhythmias. Verapamil should be avoided in infants because of its association with congestive heart failure and cardiac arrest due to its negative inotropic effects.[358] Flecainide is effective in treating SVT but has many cardiac and non-cardiac side effects.[359] Its role for hemodynamically unstable SVT still needs to be established. Other therapies include β-adrenergic blockers, edrophonium, and α-agonists. If SVT persists despite medical therapy and the patient progresses to circulatory instability, electrical cardioversion should proceed immediately.

Pulseless Electrical Activity

Pulseless electrical activity (PEA), formerly known as electromechanical dissociation is defined as organized ECG activity, excluding ventricular tachycardia and fibrillation, without clinical evidence of a palpable pulse or myocardial contractions. It may occur spontaneously following cardiac arrest or as an intervening rhythm associated with treatment for cardiac arrest. The etiology of PEA is divided into primary (cardiac) and secondary (non-cardiac) causes. Primary PEA, associated with cardiac arrest, is due to depletion of myocardial energy stores and, as such, responds poorly to therapy. Drugs used for primary PEA include epinephrine, atropine, calcium, and sodium bicarbonate. The causes of secondary PEA include hypovolemia, tension pneumothorax, pericardial tamponade, pulmonary embolism, and sympathetic nervous system failure.[360] In secondary PEA, intervention is directed at the underlying disorder and usually results in a successful resuscitation. In contrast, patients with primary PEA are difficult to resuscitate. When the cause of PEA is unknown and the patient does not respond to medications, one should consider giving a fluid bolus and inserting needles into the pleural space to rule out pneumothorax and into the pericardial space to rule out an effusion tamponade. In a study of 503 adults with PEA, patients who were successfully resuscitated more commonly had normal QRS and QT intervals, tachycardia, presence of P waves, and return of P waves after pharmacologic intervention, compared with those not resuscitated from PEA.[361] Resuscitation of patients with PEA, but not survival was improved with the use of cardiopulmonary bypass and epinephrine.[362]

REFERENCES

1. Scherlis L: Poetical version of the Rules of the Humane Society for recovering drowned persons. Crit Care Med 1981;9:430–431.
2. Elam JO, Brown ES, Elder JD Jr: Artificial respiration by mouth-to-mask method. N Engl J Med 1954;250:749–754.
3. Gordon AS, Frye CW, Gittelson L, et al: Mouth-to-mouth versus manual artificial respiration for children and adults. JAMA 1958;167:320–328.
4. Safar P: Ventilatory efficiency of mouth-to-mouth respiration. JAMA 1958;167:335–341.
5. Ruben HM, Elam JO, Ruben AM, et al: Investigations of upper airway problems in resuscitation: Studies of pharyngeal x-rays and performance by laymen. Anesthesiology 1961;22:271–279.
6. Elam JO, Greene DG, Schneider MA, et al: Head-tilt method of oral resuscitation. JAMA 1960;172:812–815.
7. Elam JO, Greene DG: Mission accomplished: Successful mouth-to-mouth resuscitation. Anesth Analg 1961;40:578–580.
8. Pearson JW: Historical and Experimental Approaches to Modern Resuscitation. Springfield IL: Thomas; 1965.
9. Crile GW: The resuscitation of the apparently dead and a demonstration of the pneumatic rubber suit as a means of controlling blood pressure. Trans South Surg Gynecol Assoc 1904;16:362.
10. Kouwenhoven WB, Jude JR, Knickerbocker GG: Closed-chest cardiac massage. JAMA 1960;173:1064–1067.
11. Beck CS, Pritchard WH, Feil HS: Ventricular fibrillation of long duration abolished by electric shock. JAMA 1947;135:985–986.
12. Zoll PM, Linenthal AJ, Norman LR, et al: Treatment of unexpected cardiac arrest by external electric stimulation of the heart. N Engl J Med 1956;254:541–546.
13. Friesen RM, Duncan P, Tweed WA, et al: Appraisal of pediatric cardiopulmonary resuscitation. Can Med Assoc J 1982;126:1055–1058.
14. Eisenberg M, Bergner L, Hallstrom A: Epidemiology of cardiac arrest and resuscitation in children. Ann Emerg Med 1983;12:672–674.
15. Torphy DE, Minter MG, Thompson BM: Cardiorespiratory arrest and resuscitation of children. Am J Dis Child 1984;138:1099–1102.
16. O'Rourke PP: Outcome of children who are apneic and pulseless in the emergency room. Crit Care Med 1986;14:466–468.
17. Zaritsky A, Nadkarni V, Getson P, et al: CPR in children. Ann Emerg Med 1987;16:1107–1111.
18. Losek JD, Hennes H, Glaeser PW, et al: Prehospital countershock treatment of pediatric asystole. Am J Emerg Med 1989;7:571–575.
19. Quan L, Wentz KR, Gore EJ, et al: Outcome and predictors of outcome in pediatric submersion victims receiving prehospital care in King County, Washington. Pediatrics 1990;86:586–593.
20. Quan L, Kinder D: Pediatric submersions: Prehospital predictors of outcome. Pediatrics 1992;90:909–913.
21. Innes PA, Summers CA, Boyd IM, et al: Audit of paediatric cardiopulmonary resuscitation. Arch Dis Child 1993;68:487–491.
22. Dieckmann RA, Vardis R: High-dose epinephrine in pediatric out-of-hospital cardiopulmonary arrest. Pediatrics 1995;95:901–913.
23. Hickey RW, Cohen DM, Strausbaugh S, et al: Pediatric patients requiring CPR in the prehospital setting. Ann Emerg Med 1995;25:495–501.
24. Mogayzel C, Quan L, Graves JR, et al: Out-of-hospital ventricular fibrillation in children and adolescents: Causes and outcomes. Ann Emerg Med 1995;25:484–491.
25. Ronco R, King W, Donley DK, et al: Outcome and cost at a children's hospital following resuscitation for out-of-hospital cardiopulmonary arrest. Arch Pediatr Adolesc Med 1995;149:210–214.
26. Schindler MB, Bohn D, Cox PN, et al: Outcome of out-of-hospital cardiac or respiratory arrest in children. N Engl J Med 1996;335:1473–1479.
27. Patterson M, Boenning D, Klein B, et al: High dose epinephrine in pediatric cardiopulmonary arrest. Pediatr Res 1998;43:69.
28. Kumar VR, Bachman DT, Kiskaddon RT: Children and adults in cardiopulmonary arrest: Are advanced life support guidelines followed in the prehospital setting? Ann Emerg Med 1997;29:743–747.
29. Kuisma M, Suominen P, Korpela R: Paediatric out-of-hospital cardiac arrests: Epidemiology and outcome. Resuscitation 1995;30:141–150.
30. Losek JD, Szewczuga D, Glaeser PW: Improved prehospital pediatric ALS care after an EMT-paramedic clinical training course. Am J Emerg Med 1994;12:429–432.
31. Cummins RO, Chamberlain D, Hazinski MF, et al: Recommended guidelines for reviewing, reporting, and conducting research on in-hospital resuscitation: The in-hospital 'Utstein style'. American Heart Association. Circulation 1997;95:2213–2239.
32. Morikawa S, Safar P, DeCarlo J: Influence of the head-jaw position upon upper airway patency. Anesthesiology 1961;22:265–279.
33. Boidin MP: Airway patency in the unconscious patient. Br J Anaesth 1985;57:306–310.
34. Rodenstein DO, Stanescu DC: The soft palate and breathing. Am Rev Respir Dis 1986;134:311–325.

35. Nandi PR, Charlesworth CH, Taylor SJ, et al: Effect of general anaesthesia on the pharynx. Br J Anaesth 1991;66:157–162.

36. Wheeler M, Roth AG, Dunham ME, et al: A bronchoscopic, computer-assisted examination of the changes in dimension of the infant tracheal lumen with changes in head position: Implications for emergency airway management. Anesthesiology 1998;88:1183–1187.

37. Herzenberg JE, Hensinger RN, Dedrick DK, et al: Emergency transport and positioning of young children who have an injury of the cervical spine: The standard backboard may be hazardous. J Bone Joint Surg Am 1989;71:15–22.

38. Brain AI: The laryngeal mask: A new concept in airway management. Br J Anaesth 1983;55:801–805.

39. Brain AI: The laryngeal mask airway: A possible new solution to airway problems in the emergency situation. Arch Emerg Med 1984;1:229–232.

40. Martin PD, Cyna AM, Hunter WA, et al: Training nursing staff in airway management for resuscitation: A clinical comparison of the facemask and laryngeal mask. Anaesthesia 1993;48:33–37.

41. Nickalls RW, Thomson CW: Mouth to mask respiration. Br Med J (Clin Res Ed) 1986;292:1350.

42. Terndrup TE, Kanter RK, Cherry RA: A comparison of infant ventilation methods performed by prehospital personnel. Ann Emerg Med 1989;18:607–611.

43. Kanter RK: Evaluation of mask-bag ventilation in resuscitation of infants. Am J Dis Child 1987;141:761–763.

44. Hirschman AM, Kravath RE: Venting vs ventilating: A danger of manual resuscitation bags. Chest 1982;82:369–370.

45. Rosen M, Laurence KM: Expansion pressures and rupture pressures in the newborn lung. Lancet 1965;2:721–722.

46. Jesudian MC, Harrison RR, Keenan RL, et al: Bag-valve-mask ventilation. Two rescuers are better than one: preliminary report. Crit Care Med 1985;13:122–123.

47. Hess D, Goff G: The effects of two-hand versus one-hand ventilation on volumes delivered during bag-valve ventilation at various resistances and compliances. Resp Care 1987;32:268–273.

48. Thomas AN, Dang PT, Hyatt J, et al: A new technique for two-hand bag valve mask ventilation. Br J Anaesth 1992;69:397–398.

49. Salem MR, Joseph NJ, Heyman HJ, et al: Cricoid compression is effective in obliterating the esophageal lumen in the presence of a nasogastric tube. Anesthesiology 1985;63:443–446.

50. Vanner RG, Pryle BJ: Regurgitation and oesophageal rupture with cricoid pressure: A cadaver study. Anaesthesia 1992;47:732–735.

51. Allman KG: The effect of cricoid pressure application on airway patency. J Clin Anesth 1995;7:197–199.

52. Moynihan RJ, Brock-Utne JG, Archer JH, et al: The effect of cricoid pressure on preventing gastric insufflation in infants and children. Anesthesiology 1993;78:652–656.

53. Gabbott DA: The effect of single-handed cricoid pressure on neck movement after applying manual in-line stabilisation. Anaesthesia 1997;52:586–588.

54. Ansermino JM, Blogg CE: Cricoid pressure may prevent insertion of the laryngeal mask airway. Br J Anaesth 1992;69:465–467.

55. Aoyama K, Takenaka I, Sata T, et al: Cricoid pressure impedes positioning and ventilation through the laryngeal mask airway. Can J Anaesth 1996;43:1035–1040.

56. Asai T, Barclay K, McBeth C, et al: Cricoid pressure applied after placement of the laryngeal mask prevents gastric insufflation but inhibits ventilation. Br J Anaesth 1996;76:772–776.

57. Brimacombe JR, Berry A: Mechanical airway obstruction after cricoid pressure with the laryngeal mask airway. Anesth Analg 1994;78:604–605.

58. Lawes EG, Baskett PJ: Pulmonary aspiration during unsuccessful cardiopulmonary resuscitation. Intens Care Med 1987;13:379–382.

59. Weiler N, Heinrichs W, Dick W: Assessment of pulmonary mechanics and gastric inflation during mask ventilation. Prehosp Disas Med 1995;10:101–105.

60. Baskett P, Nolan J, Parr M: Tidal volumes which are perceived to be adequate for resuscitation. Resuscitation 1996;31:231–234.

61. Airway and Ventilation Management Working Group of the European Resuscitation Council: Guidelines for the basic management of the airway and ventilation during resuscitation. Resuscitation 1996; 31:187–200.

62. Gabbott DA, Baskett PJ: Management of the airway and ventilation during resuscitation. Br J Anaesth 1997;79:159–171.

63. Zideman DA: Resuscitation. Br J Anaesth 1999;83:157–168.

64. Luten RC, Wears RL, Broselow J, et al: Length-based endotracheal tube and emergency equipment in pediatrics. Ann Emerg Med 1992;21:900–904.

65. Todres ID, deBros F, Kramer SS, et al: Endotracheal tube displacement in the newborn infant. J Pediatr 1976;89:126–127.

66. Donn SM, Kuhns LR: Mechanism of endotracheal tube movement with change of head position in the neonate. Pediatr Radiol 1980;9:37–40.

67. Rolf N, Coté CJ: Diagnosis of clinically unrecognized endobronchial intubation in paediatric anaesthesia: Which is more sensitive, pulse oximetry or capnography? Paediatr Anaesth 1992;2:31–35.

68. Nolan JP, Wilson ME: Orotracheal intubation in patients with potential cervical spine injuries: An indication for the gum elastic bougie. Anaesthesia 1993;48:630–633.

69. Bhende MS, Thompson AE, Cook DR, et al: Validity of a disposable end-tidal CO2 detector in verifying endotracheal tube placement in infants and children. Ann Emerg Med 1992;21:142–145.

70. Coté CJ, Eavey RD, Todres ID, et al: Cricothyroid membrane puncture: Oxygenation and ventilation in a dog model using an intravenous catheter. Critical Care Medicine 1988;16:615–619.

71. Goldstein B, Shannon DC, Todres ID: Supercarbia in children: clinical course and outcome. Crit Care Med 1990;18:166–168.

72. Alexander R, Hodgson P, Lomax D, et al: A comparison of the laryngeal mask airway and Guedel airway, bag and facemask for manual ventilation following formal training. Anaesthesia 1993; 48:231–234.

73. Stone BJ, Chantler PJ, Baskett PJ: The incidence of regurgitation during cardiopulmonary resuscitation: A comparison between the bag valve mask and laryngeal mask airway. Resuscitation 1998;38:3–6.

74. Samarkandi AH, Seraj MA, el Dawlatly A, et al: The role of laryngeal mask airway in cardiopulmonary resuscitation. Resuscitation 1994;28:103–106.

75. Kokkinis K: The use of the laryngeal mask airway in CPR. Resuscitation 1994;27:9–12.

76. Geiduschek JM: Registry offers insight on preventing cardiac arrests in children. Am Soc Anesth (newsletter) 1998;62:6–18.

77. DelGurecio LRM, Feins NR, Cohn JD, et al: Comparison of blood flow during external and internal cardiac message in man. Circulation 1965;3 (Suppl1): I171.

78. Feneley MP, Maier GW, Gaynor JW, et al: Sequence of mitral valve motion and transmitral blood flow during manual cardiopulmonary resuscitation in dogs. Circulation 1987;76:363–375.

79. Babbs CF, Tacker WA, Paris RL, et al: CPR with simultaneous compression and ventilation at high airway pressure in 4 animal models. Crit Care Med 1982;10:501–504.

80. Schleien CL, Dean JM, Koehler RC, et al: Effect of epinephrine on cerebral and myocardial perfusion in an infant animal preparation of cardiopulmonary resuscitation. Circulation 1986;73:809–817.

81. Berkowitz ID, Chantarojanasiri T, Koehler RC, et al: Blood flow during cardiopulmonary resuscitation with simultaneous compression and ventilation in infant pigs. Pediatr Res 1989;26:558–564.

82. Weale FE, Lond MS, Rothwell-Jackson RL: The efficacy of cardiac message. Lancet 1962;1:990.

83. Criley JM, Blaufuss AH, Kissel GL: Cough-induced cardiac compression: Self-administered from of cardiopulmonary resuscitation. JAMA 1976;236:1246–1250.

84. Rudikoff MT, Maughan WL, Effron M, et al: Mechanisms of blood flow during cardiopulmonary resuscitation. Circulation 1980;61:345–352.

85. Chandra NC, Tsitlik JE, Halperin HR, et al: Observations of hemodynamics during human cardiopulmonary resuscitation. Crit Care Med 1990;18:929–934.

86. Niemann JT, Rosborough JP, Hausknecht M, et al: Pressure-synchronized cineangiography during experimental cardiopulmonary resuscitation. Circulation 1981;64:985–991.

87. Paradis NA, Martin GB, Goetting MG, et al: Simultaneous aortic, jugular bulb, and right atrial pressures during cardiopulmonary resuscitation in humans: Insights into mechanisms. Circulation 1989; 80:361–368.

88. Cohen JM, Chandra N, Alderson PO, et al: Timing of pulmonary and systemic blood flow during intermittent high intrathoracic pressure cardiopulmonary resuscitation in the dog. Am J Cardiol 1982; 49:1883–1889.

89. Rich S, Wix HL, Shapiro EP: Clinical assessment of heart chamber size and valve motion during cardiopulmonary resuscitation by two-dimensional echocardiography. Am Heart J 1981;102:368–373.

90. Werner JA, Greene HL, Janko CL, et al: Visualization of cardiac valve motion in man during external chest compression using two-dimensional echocardiography: Implications regarding the mechanism of blood flow. Circulation 1981;63:1417–1421.

91. Emergency Cardiac Care Committee and Subcommittees, American Heart Association: Guidelines for cardiopulmonary resuscitation and emergency cardiac care. Part VI. Pediatric advanced life support. JAMA 1992;268:2262–2275.

92. Halperin HR, Tsitlik JE, Beyar R, et al: Intrathoracic pressure fluctuations move blood during CPR: Comparison of hemodynamic data with predictions from a mathematical model. Ann Biomed Eng 1987;15:385–403.

93. Maier GW, Tyson GSJ, Olsen CO, et al: The physiology of external cardiac massage: High-impulse cardiopulmonary resuscitation. Circulation 1984;70:86–101.

94. Fitzgerald KR, Babbs CF, Frissora HA, et al: Cardiac output during cardiopulmonary resuscitation at various compression rates and durations. Am J Physiol 1981;241:H442–H448.

95. Feneley MP, Maier GW, Kern KB, et al: Influence of compression rate on initial success of resuscitation and 24 hour survival after prolonged manual cardiopulmonary resuscitation in dogs. Circulation 1988;77:240–250.

96. Sanders AB, Kern KB, Fonken S, et al: The role of bicarbonate and fluid loading in improving resuscitation from prolonged cardiac arrest with rapid manual chest compression CPR. Ann Emerg Med 1990;19:1–7.

97. Dean JM, Koehler RC, Schleien CL, et al: Age-related effects of compression rate and duration in cardiopulmonary resuscitation. J Appl Physiol 1990;68:554–560.

98. Fleisher G, Delgado-Paredes C, Heyman S: Slow versus rapid closed-chest cardiac compression during cardiopulmonary resuscitation in puppies. Crit Care Med 1987;15:939–943.

99. Ornato JP, Gonzalez ER, Garnett AR, et al: Effect of cardiopulmonary resuscitation compression rate on end-tidal carbon dioxide concentration and arterial pressure in man. Crit Care Med 1988;16:241–245.

100. Dean JM, Koehler RC, Schleien CL, et al: Age-related changes in chest geometry during cardiopulmonary resuscitation. J Appl Physiol 1987;62:2212–2219.

101. Shaffner DH, Schleien CL, Koehler RC, et al: Effect of vest cardiopulmonary resuscitation on cerebral and coronary perfusion in an infant porcine model. Crit Care Med 1994;22:1817–1826.

102. Swenson RD, Weaver WD, Niskanen RA, et al: Hemodynamics in humans during conventional and experimental methods of cardiopulmonary resuscitation. Circulation 1988;78:630–639.

103. Lurie KG, Shultz JJ, Callaham ML, et al: Evaluation of active compression-decompression CPR in victims of out-of-hospital cardiac arrest. JAMA 1994;271:1405–1411.

104. Tucker KJ, Khan JH, Savitt MA: Active compression-decompression resuscitation: Effects on pulmonary ventilation. Resuscitation 1993;26:125–131.

105. Cohen TJ, Tucker KJ, Lurie KG, et al: Active compression-decompression: A new method of cardiopulmonary resuscitation. Cardiopulmonary Resuscitation Working Group. JAMA 1992;267:2916–2923.

106. Lindner KH, Pfenninger EG, Lurie KG, et al: Effects of active compression-decompression resuscitation on myocardial and cerebral blood flow in pigs. Circulation 1993;88:1254–1263.

107. Cohen TJ, Tucker KJ, Redberg RF, et al: Active compression-decompression resuscitation: A novel method of cardiopulmonary resuscitation. Am Heart J 1992;124:1145–1150.

108. Shultz JJ, Coffeen P, Sweeney M, et al: Evaluation of standard and active compression-decompression CPR in an acute human model of ventricular fibrillation. Circulation 1994;89:684–693.

109. Lurie KG, Coffeen P, Shultz J, et al: Improving active compression-decompression cardiopulmonary resuscitation with an inspiratory impedance valve. Circulation 1995;91:1629–1632.

110. Cohen TJ, Goldner BG, Maccaro PC, et al: A comparison of active compression-decompression cardiopulmonary resuscitation with standard cardiopulmonary resuscitation for cardiac arrests occurring in the hospital. N Engl J Med 1993;329:1918–1921.

111. Plaisance P, Adnet F, Vicaut E, et al: Benefit of active compression-decompression cardiopulmonary resuscitation as a prehospital advanced cardiac life support: A randomized multicenter study. Circulation 1997;95:955–961.

112. Stiell IG, Hebert PC, Wells GA, et al: The Ontario trial of active compression-decompression cardiopulmonary resuscitation for in-hospital and prehospital cardiac arrest. JAMA 1996;275:1417–1423.

113. Schwab TM, Callaham ML, Madsen CD, et al: A randomized clinical trial of active compression-decompression CPR vs standard CPR in out-of-hospital cardiac arrest in two cities. JAMA 1995;273:1261–1268.

114. Mauer D, Schneider T, Dick W, et al: Active compression-decompression resuscitation: A prospective, randomized study in a two-tiered EMS system with physicians in the field. Resuscitation 1996;33:125–134.

115. Rabl W, Baubin M, Broinger G, et al: Serious complications from active compression-decompression cardiopulmonary resuscitation. Int J Legal Med 1996;109:84–89.

116. Koehler RC, Chandra N, Guerci AD, et al: Augmentation of cerebral perfusion by simultaneous chest compression and lung inflation with abdominal binding after cardiac arrest in dogs. Circulation 1983;67:266–275.

117. Babbs CF, Fitzgerald KR, Voorhees WD, et al: High-pressure ventilation during CPR with 95% O$_2$:5% CO$_2$. Crit Care Med 1982;10:505–508.

118. Krischer JP, Fine EG, Weisfeldt ML, et al: Comparison of prehospital conventional and simultaneous compression-ventilation cardiopulmonary resuscitation. Crit Care Med 1989;17:1263–1269.

119. Luce JM, Ross BK, O'Quin RJ, et al: Regional blood flow during cardiopulmonary resuscitation in dogs using simultaneous and nonsimultaneous compression and ventilation. Circulation 1983;67:258–265.

120. Halperin HR, Guerci AD, Chandra N, et al: Vest inflation without simultaneous ventilation during cardiac arrest in dogs: Improved survival from prolonged cardiopulmonary resuscitation. Circulation 1986;74:1407–1415.

121. Criley JM, Niemann JT, Rosborough JP, et al: Modifications of cardiopulmonary resuscitation based on the cough. Circulation 1986;74:IV 42–50.

122. Halperin HR, Tsitlik JE, Gelfand M, et al: A preliminary study of cardiopulmonary resuscitation by circumferential compression of the chest with use of a pneumatic vest. N Engl J Med 1993;329:762–768.

123. Beyar R, Halperin HR, Tsitlik JE, et al: Circulatory assistance by intrathoracic pressure variations: Optimization and mechanisms studied by a mathematical model in relation to experimental data. Circ Res 1989;64:703–720.

124. Niemann JT, Rosborough JP, Ung S, et al: Hemodynamic effects of continuous abdominal binding during cardiac arrest and resuscitation. Am J Cardiol 1984;53:269–274.

125. Chandra N, Snyder LD, Weisfeldt ML: Abdominal binding during cardiopulmonary resuscitation in man. JAMA 1981;246:351–353.

126. Guerci AD, Shi AY, Levin H, et al: Transmission of intrathoracic pressure to the intracranial space during cardiopulmonary resuscitation in dogs. Circ Res 1985;56:20–30.

127. Sanders AB, Ewy GA, Alferness CA, et al: Failure of one method of simultaneous chest compression, ventilation, and abdominal binding during CPR. Crit Care Med 1982;10:509–513.

128. Mahoney BD, Mirick MJ: Efficacy of pneumatic trousers in refractory prehospital cardiopulmonary arrest. Ann Emerg Med 1983;12:8–12.

129. Ralston SH, Babbs CF, Niebauer MJ: Cardiopulmonary resuscitation with interposed abdominal compression in dogs. Anesth Analg 1982;61:645–651.

130. Hoekstra OS, van Lambalgen AA, Groeneveld AB, et al: Abdominal compressions increase vital organ perfusion during CPR in dogs: Relation with efficacy of thoracic compressions. Ann Emerg Med 1995;25:375–385.

131. Einagle V, Bertrand F, Wise RA, et al: Interposed abdominal compressions and carotid blood flow during cardiopulmonary resuscitation: Support for a thoracoabdominal unit. Chest 1988;93:1206–1212.

132. Voorhees WD, Niebauer MJ, Babbs CF: Improved oxygen delivery during cardiopulmonary resuscitation with interposed abdominal compressions. Ann Emerg Med 1983;12:128–135.

133. Eberle B, Schleien CL, Shaffner DH, et al: Effects of three models of abdominal compression on vital organ blood flow in a piglet CPR model. Anesthesiology 1990;73:A300.

134. Berryman CR, Phillips G: Interposed abdominal compression-CPR in human subjects. Ann Emerg Med 1984;13:226–229.

135. Howard M, Carrubba C, Foss F, et al: Interposed abdominal compression-CPR: Its effects on parameters of coronary perfusion in human subjects. Ann Emerg Med 1987;16:253–259.

136. Bircher N, Safar P, Stewart R: A comparison of standard, "MAST"-augmented, and open-chest CPR in dogs. A preliminary investigation. Crit Care Med 1980;8:147–152.

137. Weiser FM, Adler LN, Kuhn LA: Hemodynamic effects of closed and open-chest cardiac resuscitation in normal dogs and those with acute myocardial infarction. Am J Cardiol 1962;10:555.

138. Kern KB, Sanders AB, Ewy GA: Open-chest cardiac massage after closed-chest compression in a canine model: When to intervene. Resuscitation 1987;15:51–57.

139. Sanders AB, Kern KB, Atlas M, et al: Importance of the duration of inadequate coronary perfusion pressure on resuscitation from cardiac arrest. J Am Coll Cardiol 1985;6:113–118.

140. Hachimi-Idrissi S, Leeman J, Hubloue Y, et al: Open chest cardiopulmonary resuscitation in out-of-hospital cardiac arrest. Resuscitation 1997;35:151–156.

141. Sanders AB, Kern KB, Ewy GA, et al: Improved resuscitation from cardiac arrest with open-chest massage. Ann Emerg Med 1984; 13:672–675.

142. Levine R, Gorayeb M, Safar P, et al: Cardiopulmonary bypass after cardiac arrest and prolonged closed-chest CPR in dogs. Ann Emerg Med 1987;16:620–627.

143. Reich H, Angelos M, Safar P, et al: Cardiac resuscitability with cardiopulmonary bypass after increasing ventricular fibrillation times in dogs. Ann Emerg Med 1990;19:887–890.

144. Angelos MG, Gaddis M, Gaddis G, et al: Cardiopulmonary bypass in a model of acute myocardial infarction and cardiac arrest. Ann Emerg Med 1990;19:874–880.

145. Phillips SJ, Ballentine B, Slonine D, et al: Percutaneous initiation of cardiopulmonary bypass. Ann Thorac Surg 1983;36:223–225.

146. Mattox KL, Beall AC Jr: Resuscitation of the moribund patient using portable cardiopulmonary bypass. Ann Thorac Surg 1976;22:436–442.

147. Reichman RT, Joyo CI, Dembitsky WP, et al: Improved patient survival after cardiac arrest using a cardiopulmonary support system. Ann Thorac Surg 1990;49:101–104.

148. Hartz R, LoCicero J III, Sanders JH Jr, et al: Clinical experience with portable cardiopulmonary bypass in cardiac arrest patients. Ann Thorac Surg 1990;50:437–441.

149. Martin GB, Rivers EP, Paradis NA, et al: Emergency department cardiopulmonary bypass in the treatment of human cardiac arrest. Chest 1998;113:743–751.

150. Magovern GJ Jr, Simpson KA: Extracorporeal membrane oxygenation for adult cardiac support: The Alleghenny experience. Ann Thorac Surg 1999;68:655–661.

151. Feng WC, Bert AA, Browning RA, et al: Open cardiac massage and periresuscitative cardiopulmonary bypass for cardiac arrest following cardiac surgery. J Cardiovasc Surg (Torino) 1995;36:319–321.

152. Mair P, Schwarz B, Kornberger E, et al: Case 5–1997. Successful resuscitation of a patient with severe accidental hypothermia and prolonged cardiocirculatory arrest using cardiopulmonary bypass. J Cardiothorac Vasc Anesth 1997;11:901–904.

153. Jones AI, Swann IJ: Prolonged resuscitation in accidental hypothermia: Use of mechanical cardio-pulmonary resuscitation and partial cardio-pulmonary bypass. Eur J Emerg Med 1994;1:34–36.

154. Ohteki H, Norita H, Sakai M, et al: Emergency pulmonary embolectomy with percutaneous cardiopulmonary bypass. Ann Thorac Surg 1997;63:1584–1586.

155. Karmy-Jones R, van Wijngaarden MH, Talwar MK, et al: Cardiopulmonary bypass for resuscitation after penetrating cardiac trauma. Ann Thorac Surg 1996;61:1244–1245.

156. Cochran JB, Tecklenburg FW, Lau YR, et al: Emergency cardiopulmonary bypass for cardiac arrest refractory to pediatric advanced life support. Pediatr Emerg Care 1999;15:30–32.

157. Lee G, Antognini JF, Gronert GA: Complete recovery after prolonged resuscitation and cardiopulmonary bypass for hyperkalemic cardiac arrest. Anesth Analg 1994;79:172–174.

158. Voorhees WD III, Ralston SH, Kougias C, et al: Fluid loading with whole blood or Ringer's lactate solution during CPR in dogs. Resuscitation 1987;15:113–123.

159. Tomaszewski CA, Meador SA: Theoretical effects of fluid infusions during cardiopulmonary resuscitation as demonstrated in a computer model of the circulation. Resuscitation 1987;15:97–112.

160. Maxwell LG, Harris AP, Sendak MJ, et al: Monitoring the resuscitation of preterm infants in the delivery room using pulse oximetry. Clin Pediatr (Phila) 1987;26:18–20.

161. Stratmann B, Richter J, Muhr G: Experiences with the pulse oximeter during preclinical cardiopulmonary resuscitation [German]. Unfallchirurg 1997;100:465–468.

162. Spittal MJ: Evaluation of pulse oximetry during cardiopulmonary resuscitation. Anaesthesia 1993;48:701–703.

163. Jorgensen EO, Malchow-Moller AM: Cerebral prognostic signs during cardiopulmonary resuscitation. Resuscitation 1978;6:217–225.

164. Morillo LE, Tulloch JW, Gumnit RJ, et al: Compressed spectral array patterns following cardiopulmonary arrest: A preliminary report. Arch Neurol 1983;40:287–289.

165. Moss J, Rockoff M: EEG monitoring during cardiac arrest and resuscitation. JAMA 1980;244:2750–2751.

166. Young WL, Ornstein E: Compressed spectral array EEG monitoring during cardiac arrest and resuscitation. Anesthesiology 1985;62:535–538.

167. Schleien CL, Koehler RC, Gervais H, et al: Organ blood flow and somatosensory-evoked potentials during and after cardiopulmonary resuscitation with epinephrine or phenylephrine. Circulation 1989; 79:1332–1342.

168. Gervais HW, Schleien CL, Koehler RC, et al: Effect of adrenergic drugs on cerebral blood flow, metabolism, and evoked potentials after delayed cardiopulmonary resuscitation in dogs. Stroke 1991;22:1554–1561.

169. Goodwin SR, Friedman WA, Bellefleur M: Is it time to use evoked potentials to predict outcome in comatose children and adults? Crit Care Med 1991;19:518–524.

170. Schleien CL: Cardiopulmonary resuscitation. In: Nichols DG, Yaster M, Lappe DG, et al, eds: Golden Hour: The Handbook of Advanced Pediatric Life Support. St. Louis: Mosby Year Book; 1996:105–136.

171. Hedges JR, Barsan WB, Doan LA, et al: Central versus peripheral intravenous routes in cardiopulmonary resuscitation. Am J Emerg Med 1984;2:385–390.

172. Kuhn GJ, White BC, Swetnam RE, et al: Peripheral vs central circulation times during CPR: A pilot study. Ann Emerg Med 1981;10:417–419.

173. Josefson LM: A new method of treatment-intraosseal injections. Acta Med Scand 1934;81:550.

174. Waisman M, Waisman D: Bone marrow infusion in adults. J Trauma 1997;42:288–293.

175. Berg RA: Emergency infusion of catecholamines into bone marrow. Am J Dis Child 1984;138:810–811.

176. Meola F: Bone marrow infusions as routine procedure in children. J Pediatr 1944;25:13–16.

177. Heinild S, Sondergaard T, Tudvad F: Bone marrow infusion in childhood: Experiences from a thousand infusions. J Pediatr 1947;30:400–412.

178. Orlowski JP, Julius CJ, Petras RE, et al: The safety of intraosseous infusions: Risks of fat and bone marrow emboli to the lungs. Ann Emerg Med 1989;18:1062–1067.

179. Tobias JD, Nichols DG: Intraosseous succinylcholine for orotracheal intubation. Pediatr Emerg Care 1990;6:108–109.

180. Hornchen U, Schuttler J, Stoeckel H, et al: Endobronchial instillation of epinephrine during cardiopulmonary resuscitation. Crit Care Med 1987;15:1037–1039.

181. Roberts JR, Greenburg MI, Knaub M, et al: Comparison of the pharmacological effects of epinephrine administered by the intravenous and endotracheal routes. JACEP 1978;7:260–264.

182. Roberts JR, Greenberg MI, Knaub MA, et al: Blood levels following intravenous and endotracheal epinephrine administration. JACEP 1979;8:53–56.

183. McDonald JL: Serum lidocaine levels during cardiopulmonary resuscitation after intravenous and endotracheal administration. Crit Care Med 1985;13:914–915.

184. Ralston SH, Tacker WA, Showen L, et al: Endotracheal versus intravenous epinephrine during electromechanical dissociation with CPR in dogs. Ann Emerg Med 1985;14:1044–1048.

185. Greenberg MI, Roberts JR, Baskin SI: Use of endotracheally administered epinephrine in a pediatric patient. Am J Dis Child 1981;135:767–768.

186. Redding JS, Asuncion JS, Pearson JW: Effective routes of drug administration during cardiac arrest. Anesth Analg 1967;46:253–258.

187. Ralston SH, Voorhees WD, Babbs CF: Intrapulmonary epinephrine during prolonged cardiopulmonary resuscitation: Improved regional blood flow and resuscitation in dogs. Ann Emerg Med 1984;13:79–86.

188. Zoll PM: Resuscitation of the heart in ventricular standstill by external electrical stimulation. N Engl J Med 1952;247:768–771.

189. Zoll PM, Zoll RH, Falk RH, et al: External noninvasive temporary cardiac pacing: Clinical trials. Circulation 1985;71:937–944.

190. Barthell E, Troiano P, Olson D, et al: Prehospital external cardiac pacing: A prospective, controlled clinical trial. Ann Emerg Med 1988;17:1221–1226.

191. Hedges JR, Syverud SA, Dalsey WC, et al: Prehospital trial of emergency transcutaneous cardiac pacing. Circulation 1987;76:1337–1343.

192. Hedges JR, Feero S, Shultz B, et al: Prehospital transcutaneous cardiac pacing for symptomatic bradycardia. Pacing Clin Electrophysiol 1991;14:1473–1478.

193. Beland MJ, Hesslein PS, Finlay CD, et al: Noninvasive transcutaneous cardiac pacing in children. Pacing Clin Electrophysiol 1987;10:1262–1270.

194. Beland MJ, Hesslein PS, Rowe RD: Ventricular tachycardia related to transcutaneous pacing. Ann Emerg Med 1988;17:279–281.

195. Redding JS, Pearson JW: Evaluation of drugs for resuscitation. Anesthesiology 1963;24:203.

196. Yakaitis RW, Otto CW, Blitt CD: Relative importance of alpha and beta adrenergic receptors during resuscitation. Crit Care Med 1979;7:293–296.

197. Michael JR, Guerci AD, Koehler RC, et al: Mechanisms by which epinephrine augments cerebral and myocardial perfusion during cardiopulmonary resuscitation in dogs. Circulation 1984;69:822–835.

198. Koehler RC, Michael JR: Cardiopulmonary resuscitation, brain blood flow, and neurologic recovery. Crit Care Clin 1985;1:205–222.

199. Downey JM, Chagrasulis RW, Hemphill V: Quantitative study of intramyocardial compression in the fibrillating heart. Am J Physiol 1979;237:H191–H196.

200. Livesay JJ, Follette DM, Fey KH, et al: Optimizing myocardial supply/demand balance with alpha-adrenergic drugs during cardiopulmonary resuscitation. J Thorac Cardiovasc Surg 1978;76:244–251.

201. Ditchey RV, Goto Y, Lindenfeld J: Myocardial oxygen requirements during experimental cardiopulmonary resuscitation. Cardiovasc Res 1992;26:791–797.

202. Pearson JW, Redding JS: Influence of peripheral vascular tone on resuscitation. Anesth Analg 1965;44:746–750.

203. Lindner KH, Prengel AW, Pfenninger EG, et al: Vasopressin improves vital organ blood flow during closed-chest cardiopulmonary resuscitation in pigs. Circulation 1995;91:215–221.

204. Brown CG, Werman HA, Davis EA, et al: The effect of high-dose phenylephrine versus epinephrine on regional cerebral blood flow during CPR. Ann Emerg Med 1987;16:743–748.

205. Brown CG, Davis EA, Werman HA, et al: Methoxamine versus epinephrine on regional cerebral blood flow during cardiopulmonary resuscitation. Crit Care Med 1987;15:682–686.

206. Holmes HR, Babbs CF, Voorhees WD, et al: Influence of adrenergic drugs upon vital organ perfusion during CPR. Crit Care Med 1980;8:137–140.

207. Schleien CL, Koehler RC, Berkowitz ID, et al: Effect of phenylephrine on cerebral and myocardial perfusion during cardiopulmonary resuscitation in infant piglets. Anesthesiology 1986;65:A76–A76.

208. Brillman JA, Sanders AB, Otto CW, et al: Outcome of resuscitation from fibrillatory arrest using epinephrine and phenylephrine in dogs. Crit Care Med 1985;13:912–913.

209. Winquist RJ, Webb RC, Bohr DF: Relaxation to transmural nerve stimulation and exogenously added norepinephrine in porcine cerebral vessels: A study utilizing cerebrovascular intrinsic tone. Circ Res 1982;51:769–776.

210. Edvinsson L, Hardebo JE, MacKenzie ET, et al: Effect of exogenous noradrenaline on local cerebral blood flow after osmotic opening of the blood-brain barrier in the rat. J Physiol (Lond) 1978;274:149–156.

211. Lasbennes F, Sercombe R, Seylaz J: Monoamine oxidase activity in brain microvessels determined using natural and artificial substrates: relevance to the blood-brain barrier. J Cereb Blood Flow Metab 1983;3:521–528.

212. Arai T, Watanabe T, Nagaro T, et al: Blood-brain barrier impairment after cardiac resuscitation. Crit Care Med 1981;9:444–448.

213. Schleien CL, Koehler RC, Shaffner DH, et al: Blood-brain barrier integrity during cardiopulmonary resuscitation in dogs. Stroke 1990;21:1185–1191.

214. Schleien CL, Koehler RC, Shaffner DH, et al: Blood-brain barrier disruption after cardiopulmonary resuscitation in immature swine. Stroke 1991;22:477–483.

215. Schleien CL, Eberle B, Shaffner DH, et al: Reduced blood-brain barrier permeability after cardiac arrest by conjugated superoxide dismutase and catalase in piglets. Stroke 1994;25:1830–1834.

216. Caceres MJ, Schleien CL, Kuluz JW, et al: Early endothelial damage and leukocyte accumulation in piglet brains following cardiac arrest. Acta Neuropathol (Berl) 1995;90:582–591.

217. Berkowitz ID, Gervais H, Schleien CL, et al: Epinephrine dosage effects on cerebral and myocardial blood flow in an infant swine model of cardiopulmonary resuscitation. Anesthesiology 1991;75:1041–1050.

218. Brown CG, Werman HA, Davis EA, et al: Comparative effect of graded doses of epinephrine on regional brain blood flow during CPR in a swine model. Ann Emerg Med 1986;15:1138–1144.

219. Brown CG, Werman HA, Davis EA, et al: The effects of graded doses of epinephrine on regional myocardial blood flow during cardiopulmonary resuscitation in swine. Circulation 1987;75:491–497.

220. Brown CG, Taylor RB, Werman HA, et al: Myocardial oxygen delivery/consumption during cardiopulmonary resuscitation: A comparison of epinephrine and phenylephrine. Ann Emerg Med 1988;17:302–308.

221. Brown CG, Taylor RB, Werman HA, et al: Effect of standard doses of epinephrine on myocardial oxygen delivery and utilization during cardiopulmonary resuscitation. Crit Care Med 1988;16:536–539.

222. Chase PB, Kern KB, Sanders AB, et al: Effects of graded doses of epinephrine on both noninvasive and invasive measures of myocardial perfusion and blood flow during cardiopulmonary resuscitation. Crit Care Med 1993;21:413–419.

223. Jackson RE, Joyce K, Danosi SF, et al: Blood flow in the cerebral cortex during cardiac resuscitation in dogs. Ann Emerg Med 1984;13:657–659.

224. Hoekstra JW, Griffith R, Kelley R, et al: Effect of standard-dose versus high-dose epinephrine on myocardial high-energy phosphates during ventricular fibrillation and closed-chest CPR. Ann Emerg Med 1993;22:1385–1391.

225. Burchfield DJ, Preziosi MP, Lucas VW, et al: Effects of graded doses of epinephrine during asphxia-induced bradycardia in newborn lambs. Resuscitation 1993;25:235–244.

226. Berg RA, Otto CW, Kern KB, et al: High-dose epinephrine results in greater early mortality after resuscitation from prolonged cardiac arrest in pigs: a prospective, randomized study. Crit Care Med 1994;22:282–290.

227. Ditchey RV, Lindenfeld J: Failure of epinephrine to improve the balance between myocardial oxygen supply and demand during closed-chest resuscitation in dogs. Circulation 1988;78:382–389.

228. Gonzalez ER, Ornato JP, Levine RL: Vasopressor effect of epinephrine with and without dopamine during cardiopulmonary resuscitation. Drug Intell Clin Pharm 1988;22:868–872.

229. Gonzalez ER, Ornato JP, Garnett AR, et al: Dose-dependent vasopressor response to epinephrine during CPR in human beings. Ann Emerg Med 1989;18:920–926.

230. Paradis NA, Martin GB, Rivers EP, et al: Coronary perfusion pressure and the return of spontaneous circulation in human cardiopulmonary resuscitation. JAMA 1990;263:1106–1113.

231. Goetting MG, Paradis NA: High dose epinephrine in refractory pediatric cardiac arrest. Crit Care Med 1989;17:1258–1262.

232. Polin K, Leikin JB: High-dose epinephrine in cardiopulmonary resuscitation. JAMA 1993;269:1383–1384.

233. Cipolotti G, Paccagnella A, Simini G: Successful cardiopulmonary resuscitation using high doses of epinephrine. Int J Cardiol 1991;33:430–431.

234. Martin D, Werman HA, Brown CG: Four case studies: high-dose epinephrine in cardiac arrest. Ann Emerg Med 1990;19:322–326.

235. Stiell IG, Hebert PC, Weitzman BN, et al: High-dose epinephrine in adult cardiac arrest. N Engl J Med 1992;327:1045–1050.

236. Brown CG, Martin DR, Pepe PE, et al: A comparison of standard-dose and high-dose epinephrine in cardiac arrest outside the hospital. The Multicenter High-Dose Epinephrine Study Group. N Engl J Med 1992;327:1051–1055.

237. Callaham M, Madsen CD, Barton CW, et al: A randomized clinical trial of high-dose epinephrine and norepinephrine vs standard-dose epinephrine in prehospital cardiac arrest. JAMA 1992;268:2667–2672.

238. Rivers EP, Wortsman J, Rady MY, et al: The effect of the total cumulative epinephrine dose administered during human CPR on hemodynamic, oxygen transport, and utilization variables in the post-resuscitation period. Chest 1994;106:1499–1507.

239. Angelos MG, Ward KR, Beckley PD: Norepinephrine-induced hypertension following cardiac arrest: Effects on myocardial oxygen use in a swine model. Ann Emerg Med 1994;24:907–914.

240. Ditchey RV, Slinker BK: Phenylephrine plus propranolol improves the balance between myocardial oxygen supply and demand during experimental cardiopulmonary resuscitation. Am Heart J 1994;127:324–330.

241. Ditchey RV, Rubio-Perez A, Slinker BK: Beta-adrenergic blockade

reduces myocardial injury during experimental cardiopulmonary resuscitation. J Am Coll Cardiol 1994;24:804–812.

242. Tang W, Weil MH, Gazmuri RJ, et al: Pulmonary ventilation/perfusion defects induced by epinephrine during cardiopulmonary resuscitation. Circulation 1991;84:2101–2107.

243. von Planta I, Wagner O, von Planta M, et al: Coronary perfusion pressure, end-tidal CO2 and adrenergic agents in haemodynamic stable rats. Resuscitation 1993;25:203–217.

244. Dhingra RC, Amat YL, Wyndham C, et al: Electrophysiologic effects of atropine on human sinus node and atrium. Am J Cardiol 1976;38:429–434.

245. Gillette PC, Garson A: Pediatric Cardiac Dysrhythmias. New York: Grune and Stratton; 1981.

246. Brown JH: Atropine, scopolamine, and related antimuscarinic drugs. In: Gilman AG, Rall TW, Nies AS, et al, eds: Goodman & Gilman's The Pharmacological Basis of Therapeutics. Elmsford, NY: Pergamon Press; 1990:150–165.

247. Goldberg AH: Cardiopulmonary arrest. N Engl J Med 1974;290:381–385.

248. Kottmeier CA, Gravenstein JS: The parasympathomimetic activity of atropine and atropine methylbromide. Anesthesiology 1968;29:1125–1133.

249. Stacpoole PW: Lactic acidosis: The case against bicarbonate therapy. Ann Intern Med 1986;105:276–279.

250. Guerci AD, Chandra N, Johnson E, et al: Failure of sodium bicarbonate to improve resuscitation from ventricular fibrillation in dogs. Circulation 1986;74:IV75–79.

251. Graf H, Leach W, Arieff AI: Evidence for a detrimental effect of bicarbonate therapy in hypoxic lactic acidosis. Science 1985;227:754–756.

252. Pannier JL, Leusen I: Contraction characteristics of papillary muscle during changes in acid-base composition of the bathing-fluid. Arch Int Physiol Biochim 1968;76:624–634.

253. Wood WB, Manley ES Jr, Woodbury RA: The effects of CO_2 induced respiratory acidosis on the depressor and pressor components of the dog's blood pressure to epinephrine. J Pharmacol Exp Ther 1963;139:238.

254. Rudolph AM, Yuan S: Response of the pulmonary vasculature to hypoxia and H+ ion concentration changes. J Clin Invest 1966;45:399–411.

255. Mattar JA, Weil MH, Shubin H, et al: Cardiac arrest in the critically ill. II. Hyperosmolal states following cardiac arrest. Am J Med 1974;56:162–168.

256. Bishop RL, Weisfeldt ML: Sodium bicarbonate administration during cardiac arrest. Effect on arterial pH, Pco_2, and osmolality. JAMA 1976;235:506–509.

257. Grundler W, Weil MH, Rackow EC: Arteriovenous carbon dioxide and pH gradients during cardiac arrest. Circulation 1986;74:1071–1074.

258. Sessler D, Mills P, Gregory G, et al: Effects of bicarbonate on arterial and brain intracellular pH in neonatal rabbits recovering from hypoxic lactic acidosis. J Pediatr 1987;111:617–623.

259. Cohen Y, Chang LH, Litt L, et al: Stability of brain intracellular lactate and 31P-metabolite levels at reduced intracellular pH during prolonged hypercapnia in rats. J Cereb Blood Flow Metab 1990;10:277–284.

260. Eleff SM, Schleien CL, Koehler RC, et al: Brain bioenergetics during cardiopulmonary resuscitation in dogs. Anesthesiology 1992;76:77–84.

261. Eleff SM, Sugimoto H, Shaffner DH, et al: Acidemia and brain pH during prolonged cardiopulmonary resuscitation in dogs. Stroke 1995;26:1028–1034.

262. Martinez LR, Holland S, Fitzgerald J, et al: pH homeostasis during cardiopulmonary resuscitation in critically ill patients. Resuscitation 1979;7:109–117.

263. Gudipati CV, Weil MH, Bisera J, et al: Expired carbon dioxide: A noninvasive monitor of cardiopulmonary resuscitation. Circulation 1988;77:234–239.

264. Sanders AB, Kern KB, Otto CW, et al: End-tidal carbon dioxide monitoring during cardiopulmonary resuscitation: A prognostic indicator for survival. JAMA 1989;262:1347–1351.

265. Gazmuri RJ, von Planta M, Weil MH, et al: Cardiac effects of carbon dioxide-consuming and carbon dioxide-generating buffers during cardiopulmonary resuscitation. J Am Coll Cardiol 1990;15:482–490.

266. Bersin RM, Arieff AI: Improved hemodynamic function during hypoxia with Carbicarb, a new agent for the management of acidosis. Circulation 1988;77:227–233.

267. Beech JS, Nolan KM, Iles RA, et al: The effects of sodium bicarbonate and a mixture of sodium bicarbonate and carbonate ("Carbicarb") on skeletal muscle pH and hemodynamic status in rats with hypovolemic shock. Metabolism 1994;43:518–522.

268. Stacpoole PW: The pharmacology of dichloroacetate. Metabolism 1989;38:1124–1144.

269. Stacpoole PW, Lorenz AC, Thomas RG, et al: Dichloroacetate in the treatment of lactic acidosis. Ann Intern Med 1988;108:58–63.

270. Wargovich TJ, MacDonald RG, Hill JA, et al: Myocardial metabolic and hemodynamic effects of dichloroacetate in coronary artery disease. Am J Cardiol 1988;61:65–70.

271. Stacpoole PW, Gonzalez MG, Vlasak J, et al: Dichloroacetate derivatives. Metabolic effects and pharmacodynamics in normal rats. Life Sci 1987;41:2167–2176.

272. Stacpoole PW, Wright EC, Baumgartner TG, et al: A controlled clinical trial of dichloroacetate for treatment of lactic acidosis in adults. The Dichloroacetate-Lactic Acidosis Study Group. N Engl J Med 1992;327:1564–1569.

273. Bjerneroth G: Alkaline buffers for correction of metabolic acidosis during cardiopulmonary resuscitation with focus on Tribonat: A review. Resuscitation 1998;37:161–171.

274. Brown C, Wiklund L, Bar-Joseph G, et al: Future directions for resuscitation research. IV. Innovative advanced life support pharmacology. Resuscitation 1996;33:163–177.

275. Katz AM, Reuter H: Cellular calcium and cardiac cell death. Am J Cardiol 1979;44:188–190.

276. White BC, Winegar CD, Wilson RF, et al: Possible role of calcium blockers in cerebral resuscitation: A review of the literature and synthesis for future studies. Crit Care Med 1983;11:202–207.

277. Morley P, Hogan MJ, Hakim AM: Calcium-mediated mechanisms of ischemic injury and protection. Brain Pathol 1994;4:37–47.

278. Clark RE, Christlieb IY, Henry PD, et al: Nifedipine: A myocardial protective agent. Am J Cardiol 1979;44:825–831.

279. Burke TJ, Arnold PE, Gordon JA, et al: Protective effect of intrarenal calcium membrane blockers before or after renal ischemia: Functional, morphological, and mitochondrial studies. J Clin Invest 1984;74:1830–1841.

280. Holthoff V, Beil C, Hartmann-Klosterkotter U, et al: Effect of nimodipine on glucose metabolism in the course of ischemic stroke. Stroke 1990;21:95–97.

281. Resnekov L: Calcium antagonist drugs: Myocardial preservation and reduced vulnerability to ventricular fibrillation during CPR. Crit Care Med 1981;9:360–361.

282. Bristow MR, Schwartz HD, Binetti G, et al: Ionized calcium and the heart: Elucidation of in vivo concentration-response relationships in the open-chest dog. Circ Res 1977;41:565–574.

283. Urban P, Scheidegger D, Buchmann B, et al: The hemodynamic effects of heparin and their relation to ionized calcium levels. J Thorac Cardiovasc Surg 1986;91:303–306.

284. Urban P, Scheidegger D, Buchmann B, et al: Cardiac arrest and blood ionized calcium levels. Ann Intern Med 1988;109:110–113.

285. Burchard KW, Simms HH, Robinson A, et al: Hypocalcemia during sepsis: Relationship to resuscitation and hemodynamics. Arch Surg 1992;127:265–272.

286. Cairns CB, Niemann JT, Pelikan PC, et al: Ionized hypocalcemia during prolonged cardiac arrest and closed-chest CPR in a canine model. Ann Emerg Med 1991;20:1178–1182.

287. Coté CJ, Drop LJ, Hoaglin DC, et al: Ionized hypocalcemia after fresh frozen plasma administration to thermally injured children: Effects of infusion rate, duration, and treatment with calcium chloride. Anesth Analg 1988;67:152–160.

288. Heining MP, Band DM, Linton RA: Choice of calcium salt: A comparison of the effects of calcium chloride and gluconate on plasma ionized calcium. Anaesthesia 1984;39:1079–1082.

289. Coté CJ, Drop LJ, Daniels AL, et al: Calcium chloride versus calcium gluconate: Comparison of ionization and cardiovascular effects in children and dogs. Anesthesiology 1987;66:465–470.

290. Myers R: Lactic acid accumulation as a cause of brain edema and cerebral necrosis resulting from oxygen deprivation. In: Korbin R, Gilleminault C, eds: Advances in Perinatal Neurology. New York: Spectrum; 1979.

291. Siemkowicz E, Hansen AJ: Clinical restitution following cerebral ischemia in hypo-, normo- and hyperglycemic rats. Acta Neurol Scand 1978;58:1–8.

292. Siesjo BK: Cerebral circulation and metabolism. J Neurosurg 1984;60:883–908.

293. Chopp M, Welch KM, Tidwell CD, et al: Global cerebral ischemia and intracellular pH during hyperglycemia and hypoglycemia in cats. Stroke 1988;19:1383–1387.

294. Prado R, Ginsberg MD, Dietrich WD, et al: Hyperglycemia increases infarct size in collaterally perfused but not end-arterial vascular territories. J Cereb Blood Flow Metab 1988;8:186–192.

295. Pulsinelli WA, Levy DE, Sigsbee B, et al: Increased damage after ischemic stroke in patients with hyperglycemia with or without established diabetes mellitus. Am J Med 1983;74:540–544.

296. Longstreth WT Jr, Inui TS: High blood glucose level on hospital admission and poor neurological recovery after cardiac arrest. Ann Neurol 1984;15:59–63.

297. Ashwal S, Schneider S, Tomasi L, et al: Prognostic implications of hyperglycemia and reduced cerebral blood flow in childhood near-drowning. Neurology 1990;40:820–823.

298. Longstreth WT Jr, Diehr P, Cobb LA, et al: Neurologic outcome and blood glucose levels during out-of-hospital cardiopulmonary resuscitation. Neurology 1986;36:1186–1191.

299. LeBlanc MH, Huang M, Patel D, et al: Glucose given after hypoxic ischemia does not affect brain injury in piglets. Stroke 1994;25:1443–1447.

300. Voll CL, Auer RN: The effect of postischemic blood glucose levels on ischemic brain damage in the rat. Ann Neurol 1988;24:638–646.

301. Voll CL, Auer RN: Insulin attenuates ischemic brain damage independent of its hypoglycemic effect. J Cereb Blood Flow Metab 1991;11:1006–1014.

302. Auer RN: Progress review: Hypoglycemic brain damage. Stroke 1986;17:699–708.

303. Zoll PM, Linenthal AJ, Gibson W, et al: Termination of ventricular fibrillation in man by externally applied electric countershock. N Engl J Med 1956;254:727–732.

304. Dahl CF, Ewy GA, Warner ED, et al: Myocardial necrosis from direct current countershock: Effect of paddle electrode size and time interval between discharges. Circulation 1974;50:956–961.

305. DiCola VC, Freedman GS, Downing SE, et al: Myocardial uptake of technetium-99m stannous pyrophosphate following direct current transthoracic countershock. Circulation 1976;54:980–986.

306. Peleska B: Cardiac arrhythmias following condenser discharges and their dependence upon strength of current and phase of cardiac cycle. Circ Res 1963;13:21.

307. Jones JL, Lepeschkin E, Jones RE, et al: Response of cultured myocardial cells to countershock-type electric field stimulation. Am J Physiol 1978;235:H214–H222.

308. Weaver WD, Cobb LA, Copass MK, et al: Ventricular defibrillation: A comparative trial using 175-J and 320-J shocks. N Engl J Med 1982;307:1101–1106.

309. Campbell NP, Webb SW, Adgey AA, et al: Transthoracic ventricular defibrillation in adults. Br Med J 1977;2:1379–1381.

310. Kerber RE, Sarnat W: Factors influencing the success of ventricular defibrillation in man. Circulation 1979;60:226–230.

311. Gutgesell HP, Tacker WA, Geddes LA, et al: Energy dose for ventricular defibrillation of children. Pediatrics 1976;58:898–901.

312. Zipes DP, Fischer J, King RM, et al: Termination of ventricular fibrillation in dogs by depolarizing a critical amount of myocardium. Am J Cardiol 1975;36:37–44.

313. Gascho JA, Crampton RS, Cherwek ML, et al: Determinants of ventricular defibrillation in adults. Circulation 1979;60:231–240.

314. Niemann JT, Cairns CB, Sharma J, et al: Treatment of prolonged ventricular fibrillation. Immediate countershock versus high-dose epinephrine and CPR preceding countershock. Circulation 1992;85:281–287.

315. Weaver WD, Hill D, Fahrenbruch CE, et al: Use of the automatic external defibrillator in the management of out-of-hospital cardiac arrest. N Engl J Med 1988;319:661–666.

316. Cummins RO, Hazinski MF, Kerber RE, et al: Low-energy biphasic waveform defibrillation: Evidence-based review applied to emergency cardiovascular care guidelines: a statement for healthcare professionals from the American Heart Association Committee on Emergency Cardiovascular Care and the Subcommittees on Basic Life Support, Advanced Cardiac Life Support, and Pediatric Resuscitation. Circulation 1998;97:1654–1667.

317. Niskanen RA: Automated external defibrillators: Experiences with their use and options for their further development. New Horiz 1997;5:137–144.

318. Safranek DJ, Eisenberg MS, Larsen MP: The epidemiology of cardiac arrest in young adults. Ann Emerg Med 1992;21:1102–1106.

319. Atkins DL, Hartley LL, York DK: Accurate recognition and effective treatment of ventricular fibrillation by automated external defibrillators in adolescents. Pediatrics 1998;101:393–397.

320. Collinsworth KA, Kalman SM, Harrison DC: The clinical pharmacology of lidocaine as an antiarrhythmic drug. Circulation 1974;50:1217–1230.

321. Constantino RT, Crockett SE, Vasko JS: Cardiovascular effects of lidocaine. Ann Thorac Surg 1969;8:425–436.

322. Austen WG, Moran JM: Cardiac and peripheral vascular effects of lidocaine and procainamide. Am J Cardiol 1965;16:701–707.

323. Chow MS, Ronfeld RA, Hamilton RA, et al: Effect of external cardiopulmonary resuscitation on lidocaine pharmacokinetics in dogs. J Pharmacol Exp Ther 1983;224:531–537.

324. Chow MS, Ronfeld RA, Ruffett D, et al: Lidocaine pharmacokinetics during cardiac arrest and external cardiopulmonary resuscitation. Am Heart J 1981;102:799–801.

325. Greenblatt DJ, Gross PL, Bolognini V: Pharmacotherapy of cardiopulmonary arrest. Am J Hosp Pharm 1976;33:579–583.

326. Lichstein E, Chadda KD, Gupta PK: Atrioventricular block with lidocaine therapy. Am J Cardiol 1973;31:277–281.

327. Romhilt DW, Bloomfield SS, Lipicky RJ, et al: Evaluation of bretylium tosylate for the treatment of premature ventricular contractions. Circulation 1972;45:800–807.

328. Kuntzman R, Tsai I, Chang R, et al: Disposition of bretylium in man and rat: A sensitive chemical method for its estimation in plasma and urine. Clin Pharmacol Ther 1970;11:829–837.

329. Markis JE, Koch-Weser J: Characteristics and mechanism of inotropic and chronotropic actions of bretylium tosylate. J Pharmacol Exp Ther 1971;178:94–102.

330. Bigger JT Jr, Jaffe CC: The effect of bretylium tosylate on the electrophysiologic properties of ventricular muscle and Purkinje fibers. Am J Cardiol 1971;27:82–92.

331. Chatterjee K, Mandel WJ, Vyden JK, et al: Cardiovascular effects of bretylium tosylate in acute myocardial infarction. JAMA 1973; 223:757–760.

332. Bacaner MB, Benditt DG: Antiarrhythmic, antifibrillatory, and hemodynamic actions of bethanidine sulfate: An orally effective analog of bretylium for suppression of ventricular tachyarrhythmias. Am J Cardiol 1982;50:728–734.

333. Bacaner MB: Treatment of ventricular fibrillation and other acute arrhythmias with bretylium tosylate. Am J Cardiol 1968;21:530–543.

334. Koch-Weser J: Drug therapy: bretylium. N Engl J Med 1979;300:473–477.

335. Haynes RE, Chinn TL, Copass MK, et al: Comparison of bretylium tosylate and lidocaine in management of out of hospital ventricular fibrillation: A randomized clinical trial. Am J Cardiol 1981;48:353–356.

336. Sanguinetti MC, Jurkiewicz NK: Two components of cardiac delayed rectifier K^+ current. Differential sensitivity to block by class III antiarrhythmic agents. J Gen Physiol 1990;96:195–215.

337. Kwan YW, Solca AM, Gwilt M, et al: Comparative antifibrillatory effects of d- and dl-sotalol in normal and ischaemic ventricular muscle of the cat. J Cardiovasc Pharmacol 1990;15:233–238.

338. Singh BN, Kehoe R, Woosley RL, et al: Multicenter trial of sotalol compared with procainamide in the suppression of inducible ventricular tachycardia: a double-blind, randomized parallel evaluation. Sotalol Multicenter Study Group. Am Heart J 1995;129:87–97.

339. Kehoe RF, MacNeil DJ, Zheutlin TA, et al: Safety and efficacy of oral sotalol for sustained ventricular tachyarrhythmias refractory to other antiarrhythmic agents. Am J Cardiol 1993;72:56A–66A.

340. O'Callaghan PA, McGovern BA: Evolving role of sotalol in the management of ventricular tachyarrhythmias. Am J Cardiol 1996;78:54–60.

341. Cobbe SM, Hoffman E, Ritzenhoff A, et al: Action of sotalol on potential reentrant pathways and ventricular tachyarrhythmias in conscious dogs in the late postmyocardial infarction phase. Circulation 1983;68:865–871.

342. Soyka LF, Wirtz C, Spangenberg RB: Clinical safety profile of sotalol in patients with arrhythmias. Am J Cardiol 1990;65:74A–81A.

343. Pfammatter JP, Paul T: New antiarrhythmic drug in pediatric use: Sotalol. Pediatr Cardiol 1997;18:28–34.

344. Maragnes P, Tipple M, Fournier A: Effectiveness of oral sotalol for treatment of pediatric arrhythmias. Am J Cardiol 1992;69:751–754.

345. Pfammatter JP, Paul T, Lehmann C, et al: Efficacy and proarrhythmia of oral sotalol in pediatric patients. J Am Coll Cardiol 1995;26:1002–1007.

346. Morady F, Scheinman MM, Shen E, et al: Intravenous amiodarone in the acute treatment of recurrent symptomatic ventricular tachycardia. Am J Cardiol 1983;51:156–159.

347. McAlister HF, Luke RA, Whitlock RM, et al: Intravenous amiodarone bolus versus oral quinidine for atrial flutter and fibrillation after cardiac operations. J Thorac Cardiovasc Surg 1990;99:911–918.

348. Lapinsky SE, Mullen JB, Balter MS: Rapid pulmonary phospholipid accumulation induced by intravenous amiodarone. Can J Cardiol 1993;9:322–324.

349. Ng GA, Martin W, Rankin AC: Imaging of adenosine bolus transit following intravenous administration: Insights into antiarrhythmic efficacy. Heart 1999;82:163–169.

350. Rankin AC, Brooks R, Ruskin JN, et al: Adenosine and the treatment of supraventricular tachycardia. Am J Med 1992;92:655–664.

351. Ralston MA, Knilans TK, Hannon DW, et al: Use of adenosine for diagnosis and treatment of tachyarrhythmias in pediatric patients. J Pediatr 1994;124:139–143.

352. Litman RS, Keon TP, Campbell FW: Termination of supraventricular tachycardia with adenosine in a healthy child undergoing anesthesia. Anesth Analg 1991;73:665–667.

353. Stemp LI, Roy WL: Adenosine for the cardioversion of supraventricular tachycardia during general anesthesia and open heart surgery. Anesthesiology 1992;76:849–852.

354. Dimich I, Singh PP, Herschman Z, et al: Role of adenosine in the diagnosis and treatment of postoperative supraventricular tachyarrhythmias. J Clin Anesth 1993;5:325–328.

355. Lozano M Jr, McIntosh BA, Giordano LM: Effect of adenosine on the management of supraventricular tachycardia by urban paramedics. Ann Emerg Med 1995;26:691–696.

356. Furlong R, Gerhardt RT, Farber P, et al: Intravenous adenosine as first-line prehospital management of narrow-complex tachycardias by EMS personnel without direct physician control. Am J Emerg Med 1995;13:383–388.

357. Green AP, Giattina KH: Adenosine administration for neonatal SVT. Neonatal Netw 1993;12:15–18.

358. Epstein ML, Kiel EA, Victorica BE: Cardiac decompensation following verapamil therapy in infants with supraventricular tachycardia. Pediatrics 1985;75:737–740.

359. Hopson JR, Buxton AE, Rinkenberger RL, et al: Safety and utility of flecainide acetate in the routine care of patients with supraventricular tachyarrhythmias: Results of a multicenter trial. The Flecainide Supraventricular Tachycardia Study Group. Am J Cardiol 1996;77:72A–82A.

360. Chin DT, Vincent R, Bagg RL: Adrenaline-responsive electromechanical dissociation. Resuscitation 1994;27:215–219.

361. Vanags B, Thakur RK, Stueven HA, et al: Interventions in the therapy of electromechanical dissociation. Resuscitation 1989;17:163–171.

362. DeBehnke DJ, Angelos MG, Leasure JE: Use of cardiopulmonary bypass, high-dose epinephrine, and standard-dose epinephrine in resuscitation from post-countershock electromechanical dissociation. Ann Emerg Med 1992;21:1051–1057.

363. Todres ID, Rogers MC: Methods of external cardiac massage in the newborn infant. J Pediatr 1975;86:781–782.

364. Babbs CF: New versus old theories of blood flow during CPR. Crit Care Med 1980;8:191–195.

365. American Heart Association, American Academy of Pediatrics: Pediatric Advanced Life Support. Dallas, Texas, 1997.

14 Neonatal Emergencies

Jesse D. Roberts Jr., Jonathan H. Cronin, *and* I. David Todres

Neonatal Physiology Related to Anesthesia
    Cardiopulmonary Function
    Temperature Regulation
    Renal and Metabolic Function
    Gastrointestinal and Hepatic Function
    Neurologic Development
Preparation for Surgery
    Operating Room
    Family
Emergency Surgery
    Respiratory Problems
    Gastrointestinal Problems

Advances in perinatal care have greatly reduced the morbidity and mortality of premature and critically ill newborns. Anesthesiologists have contributed to improving neonatal outcome by integrating knowledge of developmental biology and pharmacology and applying these principles in the care of newborns undergoing surgical procedures. The goals of this chapter are to describe critical developmental processes in newborns and how they may affect the anesthetic management of neonatal emergencies.

Neonatal Physiology Related to Anesthesia

Cardiopulmonary Function

Oxygen Consumption

The cardiopulmonary system is driven by the need to deliver adequate oxygen for a newborn's high metabolic rate. The oxygen consumption of an average newborn is 5 to 8 mL/kg/min, whereas that of an adult is 2 to 3 mL/kg/min (Table 14–1). Although ventilatory gas exchange in adults is nearly 10-fold greater than in newborns, the tidal volume relative to body weight for both is approximately equal (6 mL/kg). Tissue oxygen delivery and CO_2 elimination are facilitated in newborns by increasing the respiratory rate; alveolar ventilation in the perinatal period is approximately 130 mL/kg/min, compared with 60 mL/kg/min in adulthood. In a newborn, the thoracic gas volume on a weight basis is similar to that in an adult. The high rate of oxygen consumption,

however, contributes to the rapid oxygen desaturation of a neonate during periods of hypoventilation.

Pulmonary Gas Exchange

Responsiveness of the chemoreceptors to both hypercarbia and hypoxia develops with advancing conceptual age.[1] Decreased oxygen delivery follows periods of apnea associated with hypoxemia and bradycardia. Conceptually, apnea is differentiated in terms of its etiology: (1) *central apnea*, due to immaturity or depression of the respiratory drive; (2) *obstructive apnea*, due to an infant's inability to maintain a patent airway; and (3) *mixed apnea*, a combination of both central and obstructive apnea.[2]

Apnea of central origin may be secondary to poor organization or integration of afferent proprioceptive input from the diaphragm, intercostal receptors, and chemoreceptors. The prevalence of this form of apnea is related to the degree of prematurity and is exacerbated by disturbances such as hypothermia, hypoglycemia, hypocalcemia, and sepsis. Central apnea due to immaturity of the respiratory drive center is often treated with xanthine derivatives such as caffeine and theophylline (Table 14–2).[3–6] Central respiratory depression due to narcotics is reversed with naloxone. Blood transfusions of preterm infants with a hematocrit less than 27% may reduce the incidence of apnea[7, 8]; however, data suggest a poor correlation between anemia and the incidence of apnea and bradycardia spells.[9]

Apnea of an obstructive or mixed origin is responsible for the majority of apneic episodes in preterm infants.[10–12] Apnea may be due to incomplete maturation and poor coordination of upper airway musculature. These forms of apnea often respond to changes in head position, insertion of an oral or nasal airway, or placement of the infant in the prone position. Application of continuous positive airway pressure may occasionally be beneficial.[13]

Recurrent postoperative apnea has been described in newborns with a history of prematurity, apnea, or chronic lung disease.[14] Postoperative apnea is a common morbidity associated with anesthesia in former premature infants.[15] Almost 20% of such patients can be expected to have postoperative apnea. Apnea may result from prolonged action of anesthetic agents, a shift of the carbon dioxide (CO_2) response curve, immaturity of respiratory control, or fatigue of respiratory muscles.[16] Early recommendations were that operative procedures be carried out with planned postoperative admission to an environment that provides continuous cardiopulmonary

Table 14–1. Lung Function in Human Infants and Adults

Parameter	Infants	Adults	Infant/Adult Ratio
Oxygen consumption (mL/kg/min)	5–8	2–3	2
Respiratory rate (breaths/min)	40–60	12	3–5
Tidal volume (mL/kg/min)	6–8	7	1.0
Total lung capacity (mL/kg)	53	85	0.6
Airway diameter (mm)			
Trachea	5	14–16	0.3
Bronchus	4	11–14	0.3
Bronchiole	0.1	0.2	0.5

Data from Polgar G, Weng TR: The functional development of the respiratory system: From the period of gestation to adulthood. Am Rev Respir Dis 1979;120:625–695.

monitoring for patients less than 46 weeks of post-conceptual age.[17] Kurth et al.[18] extended these recommendations to include hospitalization of infants less than 60 weeks of post-conceptual age with monitoring for at least 12 apnea-free hours after surgery. Several studies suggest that regional anesthesia techniques may reduce postoperative apnea; however, apnea may still occur and the incidence may even be increased when a regional technique is supplemented with sedatives such as midazolam or ketamine.[19–22] An analysis of several hundred former preterm infants studied prospectively from four centers over 6 years revealed the following[23]:

1. The incidence of postoperative apnea is inversely related independently to both post-conceptual age and gestational age—that is. the younger a child was born and the earlier after birth that the child is operated upon, the higher the incidence of apnea.
2. Children with a history of only prematurity are still susceptible to the development of postoperative apnea.
3. Children with anemia (Hct < 30%) are particularly vulnerable, even up to 60 weeks of post-conceptual age and possibly beyond.[23, 24]
4. Infants 55 weeks of post-conceptual age and younger are at greatest risk; that is, the statistical risk does not fall below 1% until approximately 55 weeks of post-conceptual age (see Chapter 4).

Table 14–2. Primary Categories of Apnea in Infants

Etiology	Treatment
Central	Increase oxygen delivery
	Increase fraction of inspired oxygen
	Increase hematocrit (?)
	Xanthine derivatives
	Theophylline
	Caffeine
Obstructive	Neck extension
	Prone/lateral position
	Oral airway
	Nasal continuous positive airway pressure

5. Even full-term infants have been observed to suffer postoperative apnea, although this is exceedingly rare.[25–28]

Although neonates prefer to breathe through their nose, they are not all obligate nasal breathers. Some infants cannot overcome nasal airway obstruction by changing to mouth breathing; this ability to mouth-breathe is inversely related to gestational age.[29, 30] Therefore, in a newborn, airway obstruction caused by choanal stenosis, choanal atresia, or nasal edema (e.g., associated with a nasogastric tube) may lead to cyanosis and apnea. Obstruction due to nasal edema may be relieved by instillation of phenylephrine nose drops. The work of breathing consists of compliance and resistive components. Although the total respiratory compliance (chest wall and lungs) is 20- to 40-fold greater in the adult than in the newborn, compliance relative to tidal volume is nearly the same. Resistive work, however, is nearly six times greater in the newborn. Resistive work is also increased by breathing through an endotracheal tube because the resistance is inversely proportional to the fourth power of the radius and directly proportional to the length of the endotracheal tube. Resistance and compliance work is increased when a neonate breathes spontaneously through a circle system because of the inspiratory force required to open one-way valves. It is for these reasons that in the past a valveless ventilatory circuit (i.e., no one-way valves) such as a Mapleson D system was recommended. Studies suggest, however, that a circle system may be used, provided that the problems associated with this circuit are appreciated (i.e., an infant requires assisted ventilation and adequate inflation pressures to reduce the work of breathing and assure adequate ventilation) (see Chapter 31).[31–34]

Bronchopulmonary dysplasia (BPD) or chronic lung disease in infants has been newly defined in such children as those having a need for supplemental oxygen and abnormal chest radiograph findings at 36 weeks of post-conceptual age.[35] The old definition of requiring supplemental oxygen at 28 days of age became obsolete when it became evident that many very low birth weight infants needing supplemental oxygen at 28 days outgrew this at a post-conceptual age of 36 weeks. This condition is most often seen in premature infants who are subjected to prolonged ventilation with both high inspiratory pressures and oxygen concentrations. Other aggravating factors for developing BPD include persistence of a patent ductus arteriosus (PDA) and air leaks. Patients with BPD have abnormalities in lung compliance and airway resistance and hence prolonged pulmonary time constants. These abnormalities may be present for years after the initial injury[36, 37] and are manifested by abnormal pulmonary function tests and chest radiographic findings (small radiolucent cysts and hyperexpanded lungs), hypercarbia, chronic hypoxemia, and reactive airway disease.[38–43]

The treatment of chronic lung disease in infants often requires ventilatory and medical therapies.[44] Air trapping during assisted ventilation may be reduced by using a prolonged expiratory time. Bronchodilators such as aminophylline, albuterol, or ipramodium may be beneficial in reducing airway resistance. Infants with BPD are often treated with diuretics; as a result of chronic furosemide treatment, metabolic abnormalities may exist. Hypercalciuria may occur from the action of furosemide on the ascending loop of Henle, leading to secondary hyperparathyroidism and nephrocalcinosis in some infants. Hydrochlorothiazide and spironolactone produce less severe metabolic abnormalities. High-dose steroids, especially dexamethasone, have been shown to provide some relief for infants with BPD.[45, 46] However, dexamethasone treatment may result in a hypertrophic cardiomyopathy in some children.[47, 48] Therefore, these children require a very careful history, particularly focused on both pulmonary and cardiovascular systems. Some children may require echocardiographic evaluation.

Surfactant production by type II alveolar pneumocytes occurs predominantly after 32 weeks of gestation. Infants born prematurely may develop respiratory distress syndrome (RDS; also referred to as *hyaline membrane disease*) because of surfactant deficiency. Infants of mothers with gestational diabetes may develop RDS even when born near term. RDS is characterized by grunting respirations, nasal flaring, and chest retractions, developing soon after birth. Radiographic examination demonstrates significant loss of lung volume due to widespread atelectasis. The resultant intrapulmonary shunting of blood reduces oxygen delivery to the tissues. Exogenous surfactant treatment at the time of premature birth or subsequent to the development of RDS may reduce intrapulmonary shunting and thus correct hypoxemia.[49-53] In addition, the incidence and severity of RDS may be decreased altogether by the now routine use of glucocorticoids given to mothers who are threatening to deliver a preterm infant. It should be noted that exogenous surfactant therapy does not prevent the development of BPD.[54]

The relatively large abdomen in a newborn displaces the diaphragm cephalad, placing the lungs' closing capacity within the expiratory reserve volume. With increases in intra-abdominal pressure due to gastric distention, as with overzealous assisted ventilation with a face mask, placement of bowel in the abdomen with repair of gastroschisis or omphalocele, or surgical retraction or manipulation, the closing capacity may occur within the infant's tidal volume. Atelectasis and intrapulmonary shunting may ensue, requiring controlled ventilation with positive end-expiratory pressure.

Oxygen Uptake and Circulation

Uptake of oxygen at the alveolar surface is facilitated by the higher hemoglobin concentration in a newborn and the increased amount of fetal hemoglobin. Fetal hemoglobin has a lower affinity for 2,3-diphosphoglycerate and hence a higher affinity for oxygen. This greater affinity, however, can reduce oxygen release from hemoglobin in the tissue. Red blood cells containing fetal hemoglobin have an average half-life of 100 days, compared with 120 days for those containing adult hemoglobin. The consequences are a rapid turnover of red blood cells, elevation of erythropoietin, and increased reticulocyte production.

Oxygen delivery in newborns is facilitated by a cardiac output that is greater than what is observed in adults. The relationships between preload, myocardial contractility, afterload, and heart rate determine cardiac output. Passive myocardial fiber tension along portions of the length-tension curve is reflective of myocardial compliance, which is significantly lower in the perinatal period.[55] Active myocardial tension, reflecting contractility, is also significantly lower during the neonatal period.[55] At lower end-diastolic volumes,

mild elevations in preload are associated with increased cardiac output. As a result of poor ventricular compliance at high end-diastolic volumes, however, this positive effect is soon overcome, and cardiac output becomes more dependent on heart rate (see Chapter 17).[56-58] The heart rate of a neonate is approximately 120 beats/min; it increases to 160 beats/min by 1 month of age.[59] Parasympathetic control of heart rate in lambs, and probably humans, is developed earlier in gestation and to a greater extent than beta-adrenergic control.[60, 61] For this reason, newborns may not respond to hypovolemia or an inadequate depth of anesthesia with tachycardia. The vagotonic response caused by succinylcholine or its metabolites (succinylmonocholine) and synthetic opioids may lead to bradycardia that can be offset by the vagolytic effects of pancuronium or atropine.[62, 63]

Preterm infants may have persistence of a fetal circulatory pattern. In utero, the lungs are not required for gas exchange; the placenta performs this function. Thus the fetal circulatory pattern consists of atria and ventricles working as units in parallel, with as little as 10% of the fetal right ventricular output circulating through the lungs.[64] Most of the blood return from the lower extremities and a portion of the umbilical venous blood supply passes into the pulmonary arteries and subsequently through the PDA into the systemic circulation (see Chapter 17). The superior vena caval blood supply circulates through the patent foramen ovale (PFO) into the left atria and subsequently into the systemic circulation. With expansion of the lungs during the first breath, pulmonary vascular resistance decreases and blood flow to the lungs increases, matching perfusion with new ventilation.[64, 65] Any factor that increases pulmonary vascular resistance, such as hypoxia, hypercarbia, or acidosis, may result in a return to the fetal-type circulatory pattern with shunting at the PFO or PDA. This right-to-left shunting explains in part why some infants remain hypoxemic despite ventilation with 100% oxygen.

The ductus arteriosus may remain patent in newborns, especially in premature infants.[66] Bounding peripheral pulses, a harsh systolic ejection murmur at the left sternal border, widened pulse-pressure difference, and differential upper and lower extremity oxygen saturations suggest the presence of a PDA. The presence of a PDA and a right-to-left shunting of blood may contribute to ventilation/perfusion mismatch as deoxygenated blood is shunted from the pulmonary arteries to the systemic circulation through the PDA; left-to-right shunting of blood may cause later pulmonary artery remodeling and hypertension. Infants with a PDA often require increased ventilatory support.

A PDA may be treated with indomethacin administration, coil occlusion, or surgical ligation.[67-69] Treatment with indomethacin is associated with renal or platelet dysfunction. Although experience has suggested that infants who have received high volumes of intravascular fluid have a higher incidence of PDA,[70] the mechanism behind this is unknown, and the relationship may not be causal. In fact, if the PDA is associated with ventricular dysfunction and poor organ perfusion, it is *imperative* to improve cardiac output with dopamine infusions and occasionally to increase ventricular filling pressures with carefully titrated fluid administration.

In newborns, increased pulmonary vascular resistance causes intracardiac shunting of desaturated blood through the PFO and PDA and thereby causes severe systemic hypoxemia. Although the etiology of *persistent pulmonary hypertension of the newborn* (PPHN) is incompletely understood, it is associated with increased muscularization of pulmonary arterial vessels[71] and sepsis and aspiration syndromes.[72] PPHN is suspected in severely hypoxic newborns who do not have a significant increase in postductal oxygen saturation when they breathe at FIO_2 1.0. A difference in pre-ductal and post-ductal oxygen saturations supports the diagnosis, since it reflects the extrapulmonary shunting of blood via the PDA. PPHN is diagnosed when pulmonary hypertension and no other structural heart lesions are observed by cardiac ultrasonography.

Treatment of PPHN is directed at decreasing pulmonary vascular resistance and the extrapulmonary shunting of deoxygenated blood. In cases of pneumonia and aspiration syndromes, in which intrapulmonary shunt complicates PPHN, mechanical ventilation and exogenous surfactant are often used to recruit alveoli. To treat the pulmonary vasoconstriction that is pathognomonic of PPHN, hyperoxia and alkalosis therapies are utilized. Although oxygen is a potent vasodilator, maximum dilatation is induced by very low levels of oxygen. For this reason, increasing the FIO_2 often does not improve gas exchange in PPHN. Through means that are incompletely understood, alkalosis causes pulmonary vasodilatation. In many patients, alkalosis induced by hyperventilation, the infusion of base, or both decreases pulmonary vascular resistance and increases oxygen levels in PPHN. Generally, the vasodilatation will be observed when the arterial pH is 7.55 or greater. Intravenous vasodilator drugs cause inconsistent vasodilatation in patients with pulmonary hypertension.[73] Unfortunately, since these agents dilate the systemic as well as the pulmonary vasculature, they often cause severe hypotension.

Inhaled nitric oxide gas (NO) selectively decreases pulmonary vascular resistance and increases systemic oxygen levels in patients with PPHN. NO is a gas that is synthesized by endothelial cells from L-arginine and oxygen and diffuses into subjacent smooth muscle cells where it increases cGMP levels and causes vascular relaxation (Fig. 14–1). It was discovered that inhaling low levels of NO causes selective pulmonary vasodilatation, decreased right-to-left shunting of blood, and increased systemic oxygen levels in newborn animals and babies with pulmonary hypertension.[74–76] Acutely breathing up to 80 ppm NO rapidly and selectively decreases pulmonary vascular resistance and increases systemic oxygen levels by decreasing extrapulmonary shunting of deoxygenated blood. Although methemoglobin is produced during the metabolism of NO, no important increases in methemoglobin were observed in babies breathing low levels of NO gas. Recent large multicenter studies suggest that inhaled NO therapy decreases the requirement for extracorporeal membrane oxygenation (ECMO). Although ECMO is lifesaving for several severely hypoxemic newborns,[77–79] it is expensive and invasive, sometimes causes important complications, and is not available at most hospitals.

Studies also suggest that chronic NO inhalation protects the newborn lung from injury.[80] NO has been observed to decrease proliferation and increase programmed cell death (apoptosis) in culture. Inhaled NO has been observed to decrease pulmonary artery neomuscularization in animals with lungs injured by breathing gases with low levels of

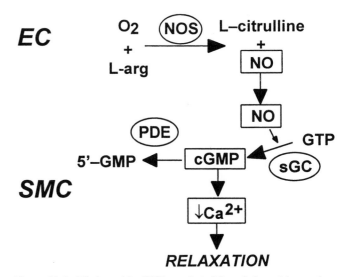

Figure 14–1. Nitric oxide (NO) produced by nitric oxide synthase (NOS) in endothelial cells (EC) diffuses into subjacent smooth muscle cells (SMC), interacts with soluble guanylate cyclase (sGC), and increases the concentration of cGMP to cause vascular relaxation. The effect of NO is decreased by metabolism of cGMP by specific phosphodiesterases (PDE).

oxygen. Although inhaled NO may decrease lung artery remodeling by preventing hypoxic pulmonary vasoconstriction, recent studies suggest that it prevents abnormal pulmonary artery remodeling in injured lungs without hypertension.[81] Although the protective mechanism of inhaled NO is not known, it has been observed to decrease smooth muscle cell proliferation in vitro,[82] possibly by altering the progression of the cell cycle.[83–85] New experiments are underway to test whether chronically inhaled NO prevents lung disease, such as bronchopulmonary dysplasia, in newborn infants exposed to high levels of oxygen and ventilator support.

Temperature Regulation

The neonatal body habitus favors heat loss. The large surface area of the head relative to the body of newborns increases heat dissipation. A head cover may significantly reduce temperature loss.[86, 87] Newborns do not shiver or sweat effectively to maintain body temperature and rely primarily on brown fat metabolism to maintain body heat. Brown fat cells begin to differentiate at 26 to 30 weeks of gestation and hence are absent as a substrate buffer in extremely premature infants.[88] Warming the operating room to 30°C (85°F) and using radiant warming units and forced air heating pads help maintain the neonate's temperature in the neutral thermal range.[89–91] Warming intravenous and irrigation fluids before use may also be beneficial (see Chapter 27).

Renal and Metabolic Function

Renal Function

The placenta acts as an excretory organ of a fetus. A neonate's kidneys are not fully developed until late in gestation, and development is closely related to conceptual age.[92, 93] At birth, the glomerular filtration rate is 15 to 30% of normal adult levels. The glomerular filtration rate reaches adult values at approximately 1 year of age. The kidneys' tubular and hence sodium-retaining ability does not develop until about the 32nd week of gestation.[93, 94] The renal excretion of medications such as penicillin, gentamicin, and neuromuscular blocking agents such as pancuronium may be prolonged, resulting in increased duration of action or the development of excessive blood concentrations. This effect is particularly important when administering medications to an extremely premature infant (see Chapter 8).

The total body water of newborns is higher than in infants, children, or adults. In the preterm infant, 75 to 85% of body weight is water; the lower the gestational age, the higher the percentage of water. In a term infant, 70% of body weight is water.[95] By 6 to 12 months of age, 50 to 60% of body weight is water. Differences between the total body water, renal maturity, and serum protein concentrations in a neonate affect the volume of distribution of most medications. The initial doses of some medications may be greater on a weight basis than for adults to achieve the desired blood concentration; however, immature renal function may necessitate increasing the interval between doses (see Chapter 8).

Fluid Management

The basic principles of fluid maintenance in neonates are similar to those in older children and adults. The highly variable body fluid composition, degree of renal maturity,[96] neuroendocrine control of intravascular fluid status, and insensible fluid loss with age[97] make precise estimates of fluid requirements in neonates very difficult (see Chapter 11). Urine volume and thus measurement of urine concentration may be difficult to ascertain intraoperatively and may not always correlate with volume status. Blood pressure and heart rate may not correlate with intravascular volume status in preterm infants, and anesthetics may mask any subtle changes that might occur. Increased insensible fluid loss, which often occurs in the operating room environment, requires judicious titration of intravenous fluids. Congenital abnormalities, such as gastroschisis and omphalocele, may markedly increase insensible fluid loss through exposure of large mucosal surfaces. The use of humidified gas mixtures reduces insensible fluid loss through the respiratory tract.

Methods of Intravenous Access and Monitoring

Infants who are dehydrated after a prolonged period of fasting or vomiting or who have increased insensible fluid loss may require special procedures for intravenous access. With severe hypovolemia, scalp and peripheral veins may be difficult to cannulate. Many of the superficial veins may be thrombosed from prior use. Fiberoptic light sources may help visualize deeper veins and peripheral arteries. Femoral and axillary veins may be used for delivery of fluids and medications.[98–101] Knowledge of the femoral artery and vein anatomy decreases the incidence of accidental puncture of the femoral head joint and possible septic arthritis.[102] The external or internal jugular veins also provide suitable alternative sites for venous cannulation.

In newborns, fluids and many medications may be infused through the umbilical vessels. The tip of umbilical arterial lines should be placed either in a "low" position, just above

the bifurcation of the femoral arteries (L3-4), or in a "high" position, in the descending aorta above the diaphragm (T6-9). The catheter tip of the umbilical artery catheter should not be left in the descending aorta in the area of the renal or mesenteric arteries (L1-2) because renal or mesenteric artery thrombosis might result (see Fig. 32–9). Aortic thrombosis occurs in approximately 1% of umbilical artery catheterizations, although radiologically detectable thrombi can be detected in 20 to 95% of patients.[103–105] Infants with renal artery thrombosis may present with hypertension, oliguria, hematuria, and elevated blood creatinine levels. The tip of an umbilical venous catheter should rest in the inferior vena cava above the level of the ductus venosus and hepatic veins so that hypertonic solutions are not directly infused into the liver parenchyma, which could result in portal cirrhosis. Aspiration of arterial oxygenated blood suggests that the catheter has entered the left atrium through the foramen ovale.

Some drugs may be effectively delivered through the endotracheal tube. Rapid uptake and minimal effects on gas exchange or the pulmonary parenchyma occur with epinephrine, atropine, lidocaine, and naloxone. Medications administered through an endotracheal tube are generally administered in the usual dose but diluted in a lower concentration (larger volume) to allow dispersion of the drug over a large mucosal surface and therefore rapid absorption. However, administration of large volumes of solutions via the endotracheal tube can cause adverse effects. Complications associated with the endotracheal administration of exogenous surfactant include occasional transient hypoxia and bradycardia, most likely secondary to the relatively large volume of fluid (4–6 mL/kg) associated with the proper dose of surfactant.

Intraosseous cannulation of the tibia with a special intraosseous infusion needle or a styletted spinal needle provides a rapid route for emergency fluid and drug administration and can be life-saving (see Fig. 32–4).

Glucose Homeostasis

The placenta allows the delivery of substrate from the maternal circulation to the fetus; significant glycogen and fat stores do not develop until late in gestation. A number of conditions may lead to hypoglycemia in a newborn. Premature and small-for-gestational-age infants have high glucose requirements; they require glucose infusion rates of 8 to 10 mg/kg/min. In full-term infants, a glucose infusion rate of 5 to 8 mg/kg/min is required to prevent hypoglycemia. Full-term infants who have been excessively fasted and are small for gestational age infants, and infants of diabetic mothers are particularly prone to develop hypoglycemia. Signs and symptoms of hypoglycemia include respiratory distress, apnea, cyanosis, seizures, tremors, high-pitched cry, irritability, limpness, lethargy, eye rolling, poor feeding, temperature instability, and sweating.[106, 107] In infants less than 24 hours old, a plasma glucose concentration of less than 40 mg/dL is cause for concern and should be treated (see Chapter 2).[108] After 24 hours of life, plasma glucose values less than 45 mg/dL should be considered abnormally low. Although hypertonic glucose administration has been used to treat hypoglycemia in neonates, past studies have revealed that administration of hypertonic sodium bicarbonate solutions is associated with an increased incidence of intraventricular hemorrhage in preterm infants.[109] For this reason, it would be prudent to avoid bolus administration of hypertonic glucose to prevent both sudden changes in blood tonicity and hyperglycemia. A bolus of 3 to 4 mL/kg of $D_{10}W$ (0.3 to 0.4 g/kg of glucose) with an increase in the basal glucose infusion may lead to a higher steady-state glucose level. It is extremely important to reassess the blood glucose concentration frequently to determine the effects of the intervention.

Infants undergoing surgical procedures often require less glucose supplementation.[110] This reduced need may be attributed to hormonal responses that decrease glucose uptake as a result of catecholamine release in excess of insulin activity, as well as to reduced metabolic demand due to the effects of the anesthetic agents.[111-113] It is therefore reasonable to administer glucose-containing solutions using a constant-infusion device to avoid large fluctuations in blood glucose values and to monitor blood glucose values. All other fluids replaced (third-space losses, blood loss, deficits) should be glucose-free to avoid hyperglycemia.[110] Since infants treated with high levels of glucose via total parental nutrition may develop severe hypoglycemia if the infusion level is abruptly changed, it is prudent to continue these infusions during surgery and to check the serum glucose levels.

Calcium Homeostasis

Calcium exists in the serum in three fractions: (1) protein bound; (2) chelated to bicarbonate, phosphate, and citrate; and (3) free or ionized calcium (Ca^{++}). The ionized fraction is the physiologically active component. The serum calcium concentration is mainly regulated by the action of parathyroid hormone (PTH) and vitamin D metabolites. PTH acts directly in the bone and kidneys and indirectly through calciferol in the gut.[114]

Ionized hypocalcemia has been reported in 42% of neonatal patients in intensive care.[115] Causes of hypocalcemia include (1) PTH insufficiency and peripheral resistance to PTH, (2) inadequate calcium supplementation, and (3) altered distribution of calcium by transfusion with citrated blood products (see Chapter 12), bicarbonate administration, or diuretics (furosemide), causing renal excretion of ionized calcium.

Hypocalcemia may be asymptomatic, but even when symptomatic, the clinical manifestations are nonspecific, such as seizures and tremors. Thus the diagnosis rests on the determination of total calcium and ionized calcium. In critically ill children, total calcium concentrations do not accurately reflect the ionized calcium concentrations; therefore, the diagnosis of hypocalcemia in these infants should be determined by direct measurement of ionized calcium with an ion-specific electrode.[116] Neonatal hypocalcemia may be defined as a serum ionized calcium level less than 1 mmol/L in full-term infants and less than 0.75 mmol/L in preterm infants. Persistent hypocalcemia necessitates determination of magnesium, phosphorus, PTH, and vitamin D levels.

Treatment of hypocalcemia is not effective in the presence of associated hypomagnesemia. In this situation, administration of supplemental magnesium and treatment of the underlying cause are necessary.[115] Acute symptomatic hypocalcemia is treated with 100 mg/kg calcium gluconate (10%) by slow intravenous infusion (5 min). Maintenance calcium is administered at 100 to 200 mg/kg/day elemental calcium and the clinical response and serum ionized calcium levels are monitored.

Gastrointestinal and Hepatic Function

The fetal gut is not functionally developed until late in gestation. In full-term infants, maturation of esophageal function occurs at term and in the first postnatal weeks. Gastric emptying is prolonged, and lower esophageal sphincters are incompetent; reflux of stomach contents is common. Early feeding of hypertonic formulas in premature infants increases intestinal energy demands and is associated with bowel ischemia and necrotizing enterocolitis.[117] On the other hand, the early use of hypocaloric or trophic feeds has been shown to improve subsequent feeding intolerance, indirect hyperbilirubinemia, cholestatic jaundice, and metabolic bone disease in premature infants.[118, 119]

Following birth, elevated levels of unbound serum bilirubin carry the risk of kernicterus, particularly in infants who are premature, hypoxemic, and acidotic and have low serum protein levels.[120] Highly protein-bound agents such as furosemide, sulfonamides, and benzyl alcohol (found as a preservative in many drugs such as diazepam) may displace bilirubin and increase the possibility of kernicterus (see Chapter 8).[121] Hepatic metabolism is immature in neonates and particularly in preterm infants. Drug metabolism may be prolonged as a result of both immaturity of enzymatic processes and low hepatic perfusion (less drug delivered to the liver). Any factor that further compromises hepatic blood flow, such as increased intra-abdominal pressure, may have profound adverse effects on hepatic drug metabolism.[122] Therefore, careful titration of all hepatically metabolized drugs (e.g., narcotics, barbiturates, benzodiazepines, muscle relaxants) is required to optimize therapeutic effects and prevent toxicity.

Neurologic Development

The central nervous system is incompletely developed at birth. Pain pathways, however, are integrated with somatic, neuroendocrine, and autonomic changes early in gestation. The hormonal responses to pain and stress may be exaggerated in newborns,[111, 112] although the clinical importance of this has not been defined. The potential lack of autoregulation of cerebral blood flow and an infant's fragile cerebral blood vessels may be important factors in the development of intraventricular hemorrhage.[123, 124] Although an association has been noted between the incidence of intraventricular hemorrhage and fluctuations in blood pressure,[125, 126] it is difficult to confirm any causal relationship. This association may be a concern during "awake" laryngoscopy and intubation; however, one study reported no significant change in blood pressure or heart rate in neonates even after awake intubation.[127] In addition, another study questions the lack of autoregulation of cerebral blood flow in premature infants. Using near infrared spectroscopy, investigators found that preterm infants could maintain adequate cerebral perfusion at a mean arterial blood pressure in the range of 23 to 39 mm Hg.[128]

In neonates, the spinal cord extends to a lower segment of the spine than in older children and adults. The volume of cerebrospinal fluid and the spinal surface area are proportionally larger in newborns, whereas the amount of myelination is less than in older children and adults (see Fig. 28–4).[129, 130] These factors may account in part for the increased amount of local anesthetics (mg/kg) required for a successful spinal anesthetic in infants.

Hyperoxia has been associated with retinopathy of prematurity (ROP).[131, 132] Although two case reports of ROP associated with anesthesia in preterm infants implicated hyperoxia as a primary etiologic factor, the etiology of ROP appears to be multifactorial.[133–142] ROP has been reported in full-term infants, in preterm infants never exposed to greater than ambient oxygen unilaterally, and even in infants with congenital cyanotic heart disease.[131] The arterial oxygen tension associated with ROP is unclear. ROP begins as retinal vascular narrowing and obliteration followed by increased vascularity (neovascularization), hemorrhage, and, in the most severe cases, retinal detachment and blindness. Many factors other than hyperoxia are likely more important in the development of ROP (see Chapters 8 and 21).[143]

Preparation for Surgery

Operating Room

Conditions that require emergency surgery in neonates are often accompanied by a multitude of medical problems, and as a consequence management and monitoring considerations can be complex. Routine standard monitoring equipment includes an electrocardiograph, chest or esophageal stethoscope, blood pressure monitor, temperature probe, pulse oximeter, and a CO_2 analyzer. Rapid decreases in arterial oxygen content in neonates after brief periods of ventilatory compromise, coupled with the possible risk of ROP due to hyperoxia, dictate the need for continuous oxygen saturation monitoring. A pulse oximeter probe placed in a preductal position (right hand) can be compared with one placed in a postductal position (foot or left hand) to determine the severity of extrapulmonary (e.g. ductus) shunting. Pulse oximetry may prove to be particularly useful for infants in whom the risk of intra-arterial monitoring cannot be justified.[144] This device can diagnose hypoxemia but not hyperoxia; however, maintaining the oxygen saturation at 93 to 95% (preductal) places most infants on the steep portion of the oxygen hemoglobin dissociation curve and avoids severe hyperoxia.[145] The transcutaneous oxygen analyzer has several drawbacks for intraoperative use, including incompatibility with potent inhalation agents unless a special membrane is used.[146]

An accurate measure of expired CO_2 levels (capnograph), despite the use of a non-rebreathing circuit, may be obtained by using special endotracheal tubes with a sample port located at the tip or with a needle introduced through the side wall of the endotracheal tube 2 to 3 cm distal to the tube's 15 mm connector (see Chapter 31).[147, 148] Using a circle system may allow reasonably accurate measurement of expired CO_2 values. However, regardless of the circuit configuration, the value obtained by the capnograph may not accurately reflect $Paco_2$ in the presence of congenital heart disease or significant intrapulmonary shunting.[149]

In neonates, changes in blood pressure, heart rate, and the intensity of heart sounds are excellent indicators of cardiac function, intravascular volume status, and depth of anesthesia. Under most circumstances, the addition of a urinary catheter to quantify urine output is sufficient to monitor fluid balance in prolonged cases. In cases in which major blood or fluid losses are expected or the physiology is complicated by the presence of cardiac disease, central venous catheters or occasionally pulmonary artery catheters are warranted. Any neonate with significant underlying cardiovascular instability should have an intra-arterial catheter placed for heartbeat-to-heartbeat monitoring of blood pressure and to provide the means to measure arterial blood gases and serum chemistry. Many neonates arrive in the operating room from the intensive care unit with an umbilical artery line in place.

Infrahepatic umbilical venous lines may not be reliable under operative conditions because they may become wedged in the liver. In this position, infusion of hypertonic solutions may lead to parenchymal necrosis and ultimately fibrosis.[150, 151]

Non-rebreathing (open) circuits are simple and effective for delivering anesthetic agents to infants weighing less than 10 kg. The system must have provisions for a humidifier to warm and hydrate the cold, dry anesthetic gases. There is, however, a trend away from the use of non-rebreathing circuits to save money and reduce air pollution.[31–34] With the increasing need for cost savings, there appears to be no significant disadvantage to using circle systems that allow the use of low fresh gas flows. This substitution should be made only if the provider has a clear understanding of the marked increase in compression volume/compliance volume losses compared with non-rebreathing circuits (see Chapter 31).[31, 32–34] The anesthesia machine should also provide compressed air in addition to oxygen and nitrous oxide. The use of air allows regulation of inspired oxygen in cases in which nitrous oxide is contraindicated and hyperoxic levels must be avoided. Table 14–3 lists basic equipment for conducting emergency anesthesia on a newborn.

Family

Close interaction between operating room staff, parents, and nursery staff promotes effective communication of medical concerns and continued emotional support for parents. The birth of a premature infant or illness in a full-term infant does not allow time for preparation of the family or acceptance of the situation by the family because of the suddenness of the event. With the institution of aggressive medical and surgical interventions, parents are often excluded from the care of their infant and develop feelings of isolation and lack of control. The development of rapport between parents of critically ill infants and medical/nursing staff is essential to ensure adequate psychological support during this intensely anxiety-provoking event.

Emergency Surgery

Respiratory Problems

Lesions of the respiratory system can be categorized into those that involve the large airways or the lung parenchyma.

Table 14-3. Suggested Equipment for Emergency Neonatal Anesthesia

Airway Equipment	Environment	Agents	Intravenous Fluids
Suction catheters	Room temperature	Gases	Lactated Ringer
Oral airways	(27–29°C [80–85°F])	Air/oxygen/nitrous oxide	$D_{10}W$
Face masks	Warming blanket†	Volatile anesthetics	Normal saline
Breathing circuit	Circuit humidifier	Drugs	5% albumin
Miller 0, 1 blades* and handle	IV fluid warmer	IV anesthetics	
Uncuffed endotracheal	Warning lights	Thiopental	
tubes–2.5, 3.0, 3.5, 4.0		Ketamine	
Stylet		Propofol	
		Muscle relaxants	
		Succinylcholine	
		Atracurium	
		Rocuronium	
		Pancuronium	
		Narcotics	
		Fentanyl	
		Morphine	
		Local anesthetics	
		Lidocaine 1.0%	
		Tetracaine 1.0%	
		Bupivacaine 0.25%	
		Emergency drugs	
		Atropine	
		Epinephrine (1:10,000)	
		Dopamine	
		Calcium	
		Bicarbonate	
		Isoproterenol	

*Blades modified to deliver oxygen (e.g., oxyscope) are particularly helpful in avoiding desaturation during awake intubation or intubation of spontaneously breathing infants.
†Forced air warming blankets are the most effective.

Abnormalities of the Airway

CHOANAL ATRESIA AND CHOANAL STENOSIS. Not all neonates are able to change to oral breathing when nasal obstruction occurs.[29, 30] Choanal atresia can present as cyanosis at rest that resolves with crying or placement of an oral airway. Choanal atresia and stenosis result from the failure of the bone or membranous portion of the nasopharynx to undergo regression during development. The incidence is approximately 1 in 8000 births. Unilateral lesions are seldom symptomatic and may escape early detection. Bilateral lesions often lead to distress but occasionally may be asymptomatic.[152] These lesions are generally not associated with other craniofacial anomalies. Choanal atresia may be found as part of a constellation of congenital anomalies, the *CHARGE* association: *C*oloboma, *H*eart disease (tetralogy of Fallot, PDA, double-outlet right ventricle with atrioventricular canal, ventricular septal defect, atrial septal defect, right-sided aortic arch), *A*tresia choanae, *R*etarded growth (including other central nervous system anomalies), *G*enital anomalies (hypogonadism), and *E*ar anomalies.[153, 154] These patients may develop airway obstruction during anesthetic induction. Early placement of an oral airway, facilitated by preinduction topical application of viscous lidocaine to the tongue, aids in airway management.

Functional choanal obstruction may result from traumatic nasal suctioning. Obstructive symptoms are often ameliorated by treatment with cool mist therapy or vasoconstrictors such as phenylephrine. The upper airway may also be stented open by nasal placement of a shortened endotracheal tube. Such treatment, however, is only temporary; prolonged use of a nasal airway may increase edema and obstruction.

LARYNGEAL AND UPPER TRACHEAL OBSTRUCTION. Obstruction at the level of the larynx or upper trachea may be due to laryngeal and tracheal webs or subglottic lesions. Subglottic lesions may be due to congenital stenosis, hemangioma, web, or vascular ring. Anesthetic management of obstructive lesions in older children and adults usually includes an inhalation induction while maintaining spontaneous respirations. This method may be difficult in neonates for the following reasons: (1) The combined effects of inhalation anesthetic agents and immature ventilatory drive regulation may predispose to hypoventilation. (2) Hypoventilation leads to elevated alveolar CO_2, which displaces alveolar oxygen. (3) Anesthetic agents decrease intercostal muscle function, resulting in decreased functional residual capacity.[155, 156] The hypoventilation and reduced functional residual capacity combined with a high oxygen consumption predispose infants to desaturation during anesthetic induction while the patient maintains spontaneous ventilation.

WEBS. Laryngeal or tracheal webs generally produce incomplete fibrous membranes, leading to obstruction of the airway with acute respiratory distress or stridor occurring shortly after birth (Fig. 14–2).[157] Complete airway obstruction occasionally results in an emergency in the delivery room. An endotracheal tube may stent open an incomplete lesion. If intubation is not possible, an intravenous catheter passed through the cricothyroid membrane may allow oxygenation and be life saving (see Fig. 7–23).[158] A tracheostomy is then established.

CONGENITAL SUBGLOTTIC STENOSIS. The severity of the symptoms resulting from congenital subglottic stenosis is dependent on the degree of airway occlusion. Treatment depends on the location and length of stenosis. For severe narrowing, a tracheostomy is placed and a series of dilatations attempted.[159] Tracheal dilatations may cause airway disruption, pneumomediastinum, and pneumothorax. Anesthesia induction is performed with an inhalation technique with a face mask and appropriate ventilatory assistance. If a tracheostomy is considered, a small-diameter endotracheal tube may be placed to facilitate ventilation until a tracheostomy is performed. If an endotracheal tube is inserted, it should be of smaller diameter so that it passes beyond the level of obstruction. As resistance increases inversely with the airway radius to the fourth power, ventilatory assistance is required to overcome this significant increase in the work of breathing. The longer time constants due to the increased airway resistance then require a longer expiratory time to avoid gas trapping.

SUBGLOTTIC HEMANGIOMA. Subglottic hemangioma may produce respiratory distress during the first few weeks of life as it rapidly increases in size (Fig. 14–3). The presence of other hemangiomas on an infant's body, especially on the face, is a clue that a subglottic hemangioma may be the source of the respiratory distress.[160] These infants often present with symptoms of upper airway obstruction, which may be life-threatening when additional exacerbating factors such as upper respiratory tract infections or other causes of inspissated mucus result in further airway compromise.[161] Any infant who is less than 3 months of age and presents with symptoms of "croup" must be considered to have causes other than infection as a source of the airway obstruction. If endotracheal intubation is required, it should be carried out as gently as possible because bleeding may occur secondary to trauma from the intubation procedure.

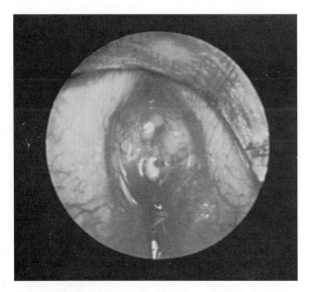

Figure 14–2. Laryngeal web. (Courtesy of Dr. S. Kim.)

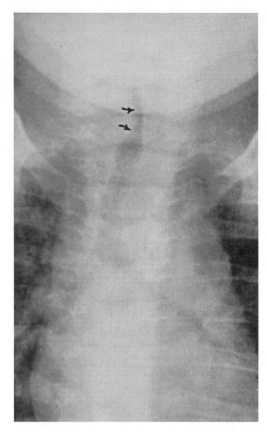

Figure 14–3. Anteroposterior chest film in a patient with a subglottic hemangioma shows marked tracheal narrowing (arrows). Note the asymmetric narrowing; in infectious croup, the subglottic narrowing is concentric. (Courtesy of Dr. P. Donahoe.)

ESOPHAGEAL ATRESIA AND TRACHEOESOPHAGEAL FISTULA. Esophageal atresia and tracheoesophageal fistula (TEF) are often associated with other congenital abnormalities, in particular the VATER association (*V*ertebral abnormalities, imperforate *A*nus, *T*racheo*E*sophageal fistula, *R*adial aplasia, and *R*enal abnormalities),[162] or the more recently described VACTERL association which includes *C*ongenital heart disease and *L*imb abnormalities in addition to those mentioned for the VATER association.[163] The specific cause of these associations is not known. In 90% of cases, esophageal atresia is associated with TEF. Esophageal atresia may be an isolated occurrence.

Affected neonates usually present with excessive oral secretions, regurgitation of the first feeding, and occasionally respiratory distress exacerbated by feedings; recurrent pneumonia is associated with an H-type TEF and is usually diagnosed later in life. The diagnosis is confirmed by the inability to pass a moderately rigid orogastric tube into the stomach or the demonstration of a blind esophageal pouch by air contrast or radiopaque dye and radiographic studies. The presence of bowel gas suggests a TEF; on occasion, the abdominal distention may be severe enough to cause atelectasis and impede ventilation. In the most common form of TEF, the esophagus ends in a blind proximal pouch with the distal end of the esophagus connected to the trachea (usually posteriorly) just above the carina. In the less common form of isolated TEF without esophageal atresia, radiologic studies may be inconclusive (Fig. 14–4A, B).

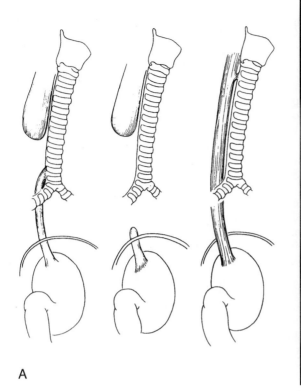

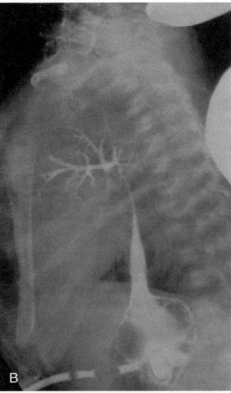

Figure 14–4. (A) The three most common forms of esophageal atresia are presented. The most common form (approximately 85%) consists of a dilated proximal esophageal pouch and a fistula between the distal trachea and esophagus (left). The second most common form consists of esophageal atresia alone (middle). Patients with tracheo-esophageal fistula alone (right) often present with pneumonia as the initial manifestation. (From Coran AG, Behrendt DM, Weintraub WH, Lee DC: Surgery of the Neonate. Boston: Little, Brown, 1978.) (B) Lateral chest film of radiocontrast material refluxing into the esophagus and bronchial tree in a patient with a tracheo-esophageal fistula and esophageal atresia.

Patients with TEF should be maintained prone or in a lateral position on an incline of 30 degrees with the head up to decrease the risk of pulmonary aspiration. A sump suction catheter placed in the upper esophageal pouch preoperatively and connected to constant suction decreases the accumulation of saliva and reduces the potential for aspiration. Patients with esophageal atresia and TEF may have a staged repair of their lesions. A gastrostomy tube to vent the stomach and a central line for parenteral nutrition may be placed with the patient under sedation with local anesthesia or general anesthesia. The procedures will permit the patient to receive long-term nutrition so that growth can occur and an esophageal anastomosis can be performed when the patient is older and the distance between the esophageal pouch and stomach decreases.

To establish an airway for general anesthesia, patients may undergo awake intubation or, if they are medically stable, intubation with intravenous sedation. To properly position the endotracheal tube, an intentional right mainstem endobronchial intubation is performed; subsequently, the practitioner slowly withdraws the endotracheal tube while auscultating the left thorax until breath sounds are heard. At this position, the tip of the endotracheal tube is just above the carina and usually below the fistula. When the endotracheal tube is secured in this location, less gastric insufflation may occur through the fistula. A gastrostomy is occasionally performed with the patient under local anesthesia with seda-

tion to avoid gastric rupture if positive-pressure ventilation is required. With the gastric vent in place, a patient may undergo an inhalation induction even if positive-pressure ventilation is necessary. The endotracheal tube is still secured in a position with the tip distal to the fistula. *The endotracheal tube should be carefully secured; if the endotracheal tube is withdrawn to the position of the fistula opening, adequate pulmonary ventilation cannot be guaranteed.* A stethoscope placed over the left chest may be helpful in detecting accidental displacement of the endotracheal tube into the right mainstem bronchus. An arterial line allows monitoring of blood gas values during the procedure. Pulse oximetry is particularly helpful in detecting partial displacement of the endotracheal tube. Premature infants with poorly compliant lungs occasionally require positive-pressure ventilation. Preferential ventilation through the fistula (the path of least resistance) may result in inadequate pulmonary ventilation because the air leak through the fistula and out the stomach through the gastrostomy is excessive. In this instance, a Fogarty catheter passed retrograde through the gastrostomy can be used to occlude the esophagus from below. This approach offers the advantage of avoiding bronchoscopy to pass a Fogarty catheter into the fistula through the trachea in an infant with pulmonary compromise.[164]

Following correction of the defect, absorptive atelectasis in pulmonary segments may require ventilation with long inspiratory times to re-expand alveoli. This measure is generally a transient necessity. Early extubation after surgery is desirable because it prevents prolonged pressure of the endotracheal tube on the suture line.

Diseases of the Lung Parenchyma

GENERAL PRINCIPLES. Parenchymal lesions may be congenital or acquired. Lesions may include lung hypoplasia if interruption of parenchymal growth occurs early in gestation. Pulmonary cysts may be clinically insignificant until inflation with nitrous oxide or excessive positive-pressure ventilation leads to gas trapping followed by atelectasis of adjacent areas by compression. Shift of mediastinal contents due to marked cyst distention may compromise cardiovascular function.

The small diameter of a neonate's airway makes double-lumen endotracheal tubes impractical. Nevertheless, selective bronchial intubations may be successful, especially on the right. Fiberoptic bronchoscopes and guide wires aid in the placement of left-sided endotracheal tubes. Bronchial blocking with Fogarty catheters or the intrathoracic use of a clamp by the surgeons may allow selective ventilation of the lung.[165, 166]

Avoiding elevations of pulmonary artery pressure by preventing hypoxemia, hypercarbia, acidosis, hypothermia, and surgical stress without analgesia is an essential aspect of managing neonates with compromised pulmonary systems.

Specific Lesions

CONGENITAL DIAPHRAGMATIC HERNIA. Congenital diaphragmatic hernia (CDH) occurs in 1 to 2 of 5000 live births. It represents the failure of complete closure of the pleural and peritoneal canal with subsequent herniation of abdominal organs into the thorax at about the eighth week of gestation. Herniation of abdominal contents into the thorax inhibits normal lung growth, especially during the lungs' pseudoglandular phase, when division of airways and subsequent formation of pulmonary arteries occur. The effects of compression on the lung are ipsilateral lung hypoplasia, decreased lung weight, decreased numbers of bronchi and alveoli, and diminished cross-sectional area of pulmonary arterial branches.[167] The hypoplasia may be bilateral even though herniation has been unilateral. The degree of hypoplasia and the associated morbidity and mortality are related to the time during gestation when herniation occurred.[168] Approximately 90% of herniations occur through the foramen of Bochdalek. Herniation may also occur through the substernal sinus (foramen of Morgagni). Less than 1% of cases have bilateral hernias.

Cardiovascular abnormalities occur in approximately 23% of patients with CDH.[169] Aside from congenital heart lesions that may cause right-to-left shunting of blood, the increase in intrathoracic components during herniation may lead to obstruction of the inferior vena cava and decreased preload and hence decreased cardiac output.[167, 170–172]

The majority of infants with CDH present with signs and symptoms related to lung hypoplasia. Severe respiratory distress is associated with tachypnea and cyanosis. The abdomen may be scaphoid, and transillumination of the thorax on the affected side may be decreased. The mediastinal contents are shifted as a result of the pressure of the herniated viscera in the thorax (Fig. 14–5). Approximately 5% of patients with CDH, however, present with little respiratory distress but with symptoms of bowel obstruction.

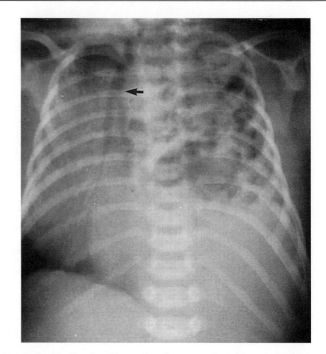

Figure 14–5. Chest radiograph of a neonate with a left diaphragmatic hernia. Note shifting of trachea and bronchi into the right chest (arrow).

For those infants with respiratory failure, initial management is directed at improving ventilation and oxygenation. Airway control is a priority. Mask ventilation should be avoided to reduce the potential for insufflation of the stomach and intestine; visceral distention increases the mass effect in the thorax. However, should conditions warrant (cardiorespiratory collapse), assisted ventilation should be gently instituted until the airway is secured. Awake intubation of these patients is recommended. If the patient is stable, analgesics may be administered to reduce potential increased catecholamine release during instrumentation of the airway.

After the airway is secured with an endotracheal tube, a nasogastric tube should be inserted to evacuate the stomach of gas and fluids. Placing the affected side down before correction may decrease the weight effect of the herniated viscera on the mediastinum and heart. Rapid low-tidal-volume ventilation is advocated to avoid barotrauma and the potential for pneumothorax; alkalosis (respiratory or metabolic) increases pulmonary blood flow.[173–175] Afflicted infants may be treated with sodium bicarbonate infusions in the neonatal intensive care unit to combat the metabolic acidosis resulting from tissue hypoxemia. Although agents such as tromethamine may acutely increase serum pH by chelating hydronium ions without the liberation of CO_2, the ultimate reduction of acid depends on renal excretion. Narcotic infusions (fentanyl or morphine) have been recommended to decrease the release of catecholamines, which may increase pulmonary vascular resistance.[176] The benefit of pharmacologic vasodilator therapy (tolazoline, isoproterenol, prostaglandin E_1, nitroprusside, nitroglycerin) remains controversial. These vasodilators have occasionally been beneficial in reducing pulmonary vascular resistance, but because they are not specific pulmonary vasodilators, systemic hypotension usually results.[174, 177] As a result of the systemic hypotension, vigorous volume replacement is required; it eventually may lead to volume overload and pulmonary edema. In recent years, inhaled NO has been used on an experimental basis to reverse the pulmonary hypertension often seen in patients with congenital diaphragmatic hernia. The potential advantage of inhaled NO over other pharmacologic agents is that it is a specific vasodilator for the pulmonary vascular bed. Unfortunately, inhaled NO has not been found to be as efficacious in this patient population as was once hoped. In the largest study to date evaluating inhaled NO on infants with CDH, inhaled NO demonstrated some short-term improvements in oxygenation, but its use did not reduce the need for ECMO or decrease deaths.[178] Therefore, inhaled NO may be beneficial in the initial stabilization of CDH patients, but it does not appear to significantly reverse pulmonary hypertension and improve oxygenation.

The survival of patients with CDH depends on the degree of pulmonary hypoplasia and associated congenital heart disease. A retrospective investigation before the era of ECMO reported that the mortality of infants with CDH and cardiovascular abnormalities was 73%, versus 27% in infants without cardiac abnormalities.[169] The mortality of infants with CDH has been correlated with the presenting blood gas data. Infants with an initial postsurgical correction alveolar-arterial oxygen difference (A-aDo$_2$) of less than 400 mm Hg usually survived. Infants with a gradient of 400 to 500 mm Hg had intermediate chances of survival and those with an A-aDo$_2$ of greater than 500 mm Hg were unlikely to survive.[179] Hypercarbia (occurring both immediately before and within 2 hours of surgical correction) that is unresponsive to vigorous hyperventilation is associated with a mortality of 90%.[180]

Although ECMO has increased the survival of infants with CDH, morbidity occurs secondary to the effects of anticoagulation and intracranial bleeding.[181-188] These complications may be decreased with the development of smaller, more efficient membranes, reducing the amount of anticoagulant required, reanastomosis of the carotid artery following decannulation, and the use of venovenous ECMO.

The traditional approach to CDH has been emergency surgical correction. However, despite adequate oxygenation immediately after surgery (the so-called honeymoon phase), many of these infants have deteriorated as a result of unrelieved pulmonary hypertension, intrapulmonary shunting of blood, and hypoxemia. Mortality has improved little during the past several decades despite the use of all modern intensive care modalities. Consequently, the approach to CDH has been reassessed. Current practice is to delay surgical correction until the severity of the pulmonary compromise is assessed and the infant has been stable for several days, as with ECMO. The reason for this new approach is that many variables such as loss of body heat, loss of the airway (hypoxemia), hypoventilation (hypercarbia), or the stress of surgery may cause a sudden increase in pulmonary vascular resistance. Such events may result in a nonreversible fetal-type circulation with shunting at the PDA or PFO or both. Stabilization without immediate surgical correction may provide a greater salvage rate.[189-191]

Surgical correction of CDH usually involves a transabdominal approach with closure of the diaphragmatic defect either primarily or with a synthetic patch. A chest tube is placed on the ipsilateral side; some surgeons place another chest tube on the contralateral side because a contralateral tension pneumothorax occasionally occurs. Postoperative decompensation may be due to tension pneumothorax,[192] absorption of intrathoracic gas and mediastinal shift, or pulmonary vascular vasoconstriction with severe right-to-left shunting and hypoxemia.

Congenital Bronchogenic and Pulmonary Cysts. Congenital bronchogenic and pulmonary cysts represent arrests of embryologic pulmonary tissue during fetal lung development.[193] These cysts may be centrally located within the mediastinum and may produce obstruction by a mass effect.[194, 195] They may also be located at the carina and cause obstruction or distal gas trapping by a ball-valve effect. Those located in the hilum, in the paratracheal region, or in the lung parenchyma may lead to chronic respiratory illness from infection and abscess formation.[195, 196] Congenital cysts are occasionally diagnosed only after rupture of the cyst produces hemorrhage and bronchopulmonary fistula formation.[193, 196]

Anesthetic management is directed at minimizing further enlargement of the cyst because a communication may exist with the airway. Awake intubation or intubation with an inhalation induction, followed by maintenance of spontaneous ventilation if possible until the thorax is opened, may reduce the potential for sudden enlargement of the cyst. If assisted ventilation is required, low peak inspiratory pressures should be used. Should the cyst be fluid filled or infected, selective bronchial blocking may be helpful in protecting the unaffected lung.[165, 166] Nitrous oxide and positive-pressure ventilation without adequate expiratory time should be avoided to decrease the potential for cyst enlargement. If these attempts are not successful and cyst enlargement occurs to the point of occluding the airway or causing cardiovascular compromise, then needle aspiration with reduction of cyst size and hence facilitation of oxygenation and ventilation should be attempted. If this method is unsuccessful, emergency thoracostomy may be life saving.

Congenital Lobar Emphysema. Congenital lobar emphysema most commonly affects the left upper lobe but may involve the entire lung (Fig. 14–6).[197, 198] Congenital heart disease coexists in approximately 15% of patients.[199] Patients usually present with progressive respiratory failure, unilateral thoracic hyperexpansion, atelectasis of the contralateral lung, and possibly mediastinal shift with cardiovascular compromise.[200] The anesthetic care is focused on minimizing expansion of the emphysema and is similar to that for patients with pulmonary cysts.

Gastrointestinal Problems

General Principles

The types of emergency surgical conditions that present to an anesthesiologist can be categorized as (1) lesions that are obstructive, (2) those that represent a compromise in intestinal blood supply, and (3) a combination of these two.

Obstructive lesions may be congenital or acquired. Congenital obstruction of the gastrointestinal tract may be suggested by an abnormal increase in maternal weight, polyhydramnios, fetal size greater than normal for gestational age, and fetal abdominal distention detected by ultrasonography. Babies with acquired lesions may present soon after birth

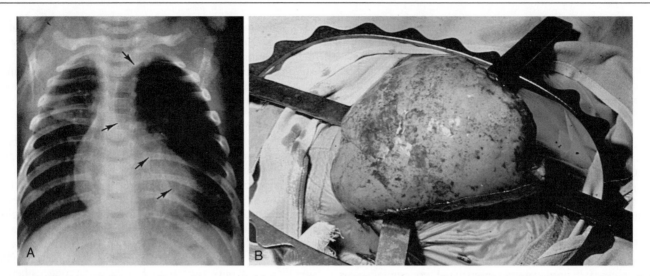

Figure 14–6. Radiograph from a patient with congenital lobar emphysema (A) demonstrates hyperinflation of the left lung with herniation across the midline (arrows) and mediastinal shift. Intraoperative photograph (B) shows the emphysematous lobe bulging through the thoracotomy incision. (From Coté CJ: The anesthetic management of congenital lobar emphysema. Anesthesiology 1978; 49:296–298.)

with vomiting, abdominal distention, and late passage of meconium. Associated findings may include aspiration pneumonia, dehydration, hypovolemia, and metabolic abnormalities. These lesions require emergent care only if life-threatening compromise of organ blood flow occurs. Otherwise, a priority is to re-establish euvolemia and a metabolically stable state before surgery.

Patients with obstructive lesions usually undergo general endotracheal anesthesia. Induction of general anesthesia may follow awake intubation if difficulty is anticipated with intubation or if active vomiting occurs; a rapid-sequence induction may be used if no airway anomaly is apparent. A rapid-sequence intubation may proceed in a manner similar to that for children and adults. Desaturation following apnea is more rapid, however, because the oxygen consumption of a newborn is twice that of an adult. If surgery is an emergency and the intravascular volume status of the patient is tenuous, ketamine may be used for induction in place of a short-acting barbiturate or propofol. A stylet within the endotracheal tube may be used to facilitate placement; however, a stylet may cause injury to the airway if improperly used. After intubation, general anesthesia with either an inhalation or narcotic technique and neuromuscular blockade, while avoiding nitrous oxide, may be used. Air should be blended with oxygen to decrease the inspired oxygen concentration to safe levels. These patients may have poor renal perfusion; therefore, pancuronium bromide and many antibiotics may have prolonged action. In addition, if hepatic blood flow is compromised, metabolism of narcotics and muscle relaxants may be delayed.[122, 201]

Infants with lesions that compromise bowel blood flow, leading to ischemia, are extremely ill. These infants may present with a tender and distended abdomen, bloody stools, vomiting, hypotension, metabolic abnormalities, anemia, leukopenia, and thrombocytopenia. Abdominal radiographic examination may reveal distended intestinal loops, decreased bowel gas, and perforation. These patients are not appropriate candidates for regional anesthesia techniques.

Emergency surgery is required and directed at removing necrotic tissue, closing perforations, and re-establishing normal perfusion to the intestine. Blood and blood products should be immediately available, including un-crossmatched blood if crossmatched blood is not available, fresh frozen plasma, and platelets. Before anesthetic induction, adequate venous access should be ensured because these patients require increased amounts of intraoperative fluids and rapid transfusion of blood products. The umbilical arterial line may be replaced with a peripheral arterial line if it is in a position that may obstruct mesenteric blood flow. The patient's volume status should be optimized by volume administration and dopamine infused to increase blood flow to the gut. If poor peripheral perfusion occurs secondary to a PDA, volume administration should be carefully titrated. In this instance, sympathomimetics may improve cardiac output and organ perfusion.

Specific Lesions

HYPERTROPHIC PYLORIC STENOSIS. Pyloric stenosis usually manifests within the second to sixth week of life with nonbilious vomiting. This lesion occurs more frequently in males; the incidence is approximately 1:500 live births (Fig. 14–7).[202] Pyloric stenosis represents hypertrophy of the muscular layer of the pylorus and can often be palpated as an olive-shaped mass between the midline and right upper quadrant. The lesion may be delineated by ultrasonography[203] or barium swallow.

The renal response to vomiting is twofold: Serum pH initially is defended by excretion of alkaline urine with sodium and potassium loss; with depletion of these electrolytes, the kidneys secrete acidic urine (paradoxic acidosis), further increasing the metabolic alkalosis. Hypocalcemia may be associated with the hyponatremia. With further fluid loss, prerenal azotemia may portend hypovolemic shock and metabolic acidosis. Hemoconcentration may result in polycythemia. This lesion does not mandate an emergency surgical procedure; therefore, intravascular volume and metabolic stabilization and correction are a priority. With protracted vomiting, these patients may be hypokalemic, hypochloremic, and alkalotic.[204]

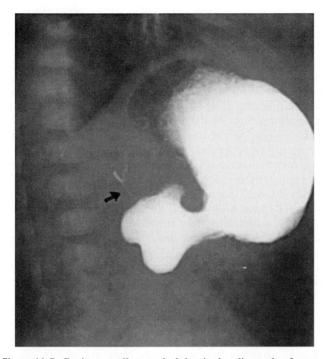

Figure 14–7. Barium swallow and abdominal radiograph of a patient with pyloric stenosis demonstrates a high degree of obstruction of the gastric outflow tract with a "wisp" of barium escaping through the pylorus (arrow).

Suctioning an in situ orogastric or nasogastric tube seldom empties the stomach. A freshly inserted wide-bore orogastric tube almost always removes additional residual gastric contents; this step is especially important for infants who have had a barium contrast radiographic study. One study has shown a nearly complete emptying of the gastric contents if the patient's stomach is suctioned in the right and left lateral as well as the supine positions.[205] Therefore, immediately before induction, the stomach is aspirated using a large-bore orogastric tube as described. These patients should not have a gaseous anesthetic induction because vomiting during induction might result in serious pulmonary aspiration. A rapid-sequence induction is preferred, or awake intubation is carried out before induction of anesthesia, if the intubation is anticipated to be difficult. Inhalation or balanced anesthesia may then be used for maintenance. Patients should be extubated once fully awake and vigorous. Feedings are usually begun soon after surgery, and the postoperative course is generally uncomplicated. Local infiltration of the incision site with a long-acting local anesthetic generally provides complete analgesia. Some centers place these patients on apnea monitors for the first 12 hours after surgery, since there have been several cases of apnea reported.[206]

DUODENAL AND ILEAL OBSTRUCTION. Congenital duodenal and ileal obstructions (atresia, stenosis, annular pancreas, meconium ileus) are often associated with other anomalies. For example, 20 to 30% of patients with duodenal atresia have trisomy 21, and these patients in turn may have cardiac lesions such as atrial septal defect, ventricular septal defect, or atrioventricular canal. Neonates with intestinal atresia are frequently premature or may have other associated anomalies

such as malrotation of the gut, volvulus, and abdominal wall defects.[207] Meconium ileus occurs in 10 to 15% of newborns with cystic fibrosis. It may present either as terminal ileal obstruction by viscid meconium or as bowel atresia. Hyperosmolar enemas are frequently administered to these infants in an effort to clear the viscid meconium plugs; these enemas may result in serious shifts in intravascular volume, leading to hypovolemia requiring aggressive treatment before anesthetic induction.

Duodenal atresia is associated with bilious vomiting beginning within the first 24 to 48 hours after birth. Radiographs of the abdomen demonstrate the pathognomonic double-bubble sign formed by air contrast of the dilated stomach and proximal duodenum; the remaining bowel is devoid of air (Fig. 14–8). With jejunoileal atresia, air-fluid levels are observed throughout the abdomen. With distal ileal obstruction, a barium enema may demonstrate a microcolon. The typical radiographic presentation of meconium ileus is a soap-bubble mass in the right lower abdomen and absence of air-fluid levels.

Initial stabilization of patients with these lesions is directed at fluid and metabolic resuscitation. Anesthetic management proceeds after suctioning of contrast agent and other stomach contents. Awake intubation is generally advocated in volume-depleted or actively vomiting patients; rapid-sequence induction may be used in hemodynamically stable patients with normal airway anatomy. Nitrous oxide should be avoided to minimize intestinal distention. Muscle relaxation is generally necessary to facilitate abdominal ex-

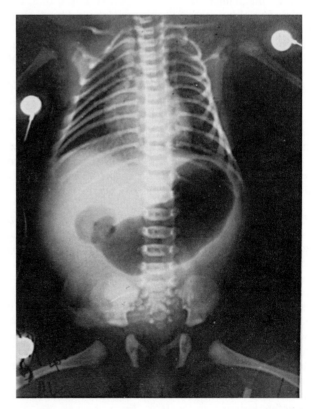

Figure 14–8. Abdominal radiograph of a neonate with congenital duodenal atresia demonstrating a classic double-bubble sign. Note that the remainder of the bowel is devoid of air, indicating complete obstruction.

ploration; use of a neuromuscular blocking agent also decreases or avoids the need for high concentrations of potent inhalation agents, which are poorly tolerated by hypovolemic neonates.

INFANTILE HERNIA. Infantile hernia usually presents within the first 6 months after birth. Although the potential for incarceration through the inguinal canal is present in more than 90% of newborns, it occurs in only 3 to 5% of full-term infants and 30% of preterm infants.[208] With incarceration or strangulation of bowel or gonads, emergency correction is indicated. Incarcerated hernias with or without strangulation should be treated similarly to bowel obstruction. A rapid-sequence or awake intubation should be used for general anesthesia. An inhalation technique without nitrous oxide or a narcotic technique may be used after intubation.

Elective repair of a nonincarcerated hernia can be carried out with either general or regional anesthesia when there is no acute bowel obstruction, such as in a reduced inguinal hernia.[209–212] An intravenous line should be placed before anesthetic induction if there is any concern about the volume status of a patient. Because blood pressure instability is unusual in infants undergoing spinal anesthesia,[213] placement of an intravenous line in the lower extremity may follow the onset of sensory block. Similarly, blood pressure monitoring may be accomplished by using a blood pressure cuff placed on the lower (anesthetized) extremity. Swaddling and a pacifier often are all that is required for sedation.

Spinal anesthesia may be administered through a 1½-inch 22-gauge spinal needle. Once the block is placed, the patient should be maintained in a supine position. Leg lifting, especially during placement of the electrocautery grounding pad, should be avoided because it has been associated with a high spinal blockade (see Figs. 28–5A, B and 28–6).[214] Apnea or sudden cessation of crying may be the presenting sign of a high spinal blockade in a neonate.

Because hernia repair is a common operation in former preterm infants, this population of patients is at greatest risk for postoperative life-threatening apnea.[15–18, 23] Outpatient repair of inguinal hernia in former preterm infants may be contraindicated even in apparently healthy infants 55 weeks of postconceptual age or less.[23] Because apnea may occur after even regional anesthesia, provision for postoperative monitoring must be instituted for all patients at risk.[21]

IMPERFORATE ANUS. Imperforate anus is generally recognized at the initial physical examination or by failure to pass meconium within the first 48 hours of life. Patients with imperforate anus are likely to have associated anomalies of the urogenital sinus as well as those associated with the entire spectrum of the VACTERL syndrome.[163] Some of these patients require a decompressive colostomy before definitive surgery. Before anesthetic induction, it may be prudent to perform echocardiography to rule out associated congenital heart disease. Pre-ductal and post-ductal oxygen saturation determinations may be of value. If these patients exhibit signs of bowel obstruction, they should undergo anesthesia in a manner similar to that in other infants with obstructive lesions.

NECROTIZING ENTEROCOLITIS. Necrotizing enterocolitis is not an anomaly but an illness found predominantly in premature infants.[215] The incidence is 5 to 15% in infants of less than 1500 g birth weight, and the mortality rate is 10 to 30%.[216] Morbidity associated with necrotizing enterocolitis includes short-bowel syndrome, sepsis, and adhesions associated with bowel obstruction. Associated conditions include birth asphyxia, hypotension, RDS, PDA, recurrent apnea, intestinal ischemia, umbilical vessel cannulation, systemic infections, and early feedings.[103, 217–219]

Early signs of necrotizing enterocolitis include temperature instability, poor feeding with gastric residuals or vomiting, malabsorption of feedings (positive stool-reducing substances), lethargy, hyperglycemia, and heme-positive or frankly bloody stools. Affected infants may appear very toxic and have a distended and tender abdomen. Radiographic examination may initially suggest an ileus with edematous bowel and later demonstrate gas in the intestinal wall (pneumatosis intestinalis) and in the biliary tract (Fig. 14–9). When perforation has occurred, free air within the abdominal cavity can be appreciated by radiologic examination of the abdomen.

Patients generally have metabolic and hematologic abnormalities including hyperglycemia, thrombocytopenia, coagulopathy, and anemia. Hypotension, metabolic acidosis, and prerenal azotemia are other significant findings in severe cases. Initial treatment includes discontinuation of enteral feedings and decompression of the abdomen by means of low-pressure intermittent nasogastric or orogastric suctioning. Wide-spectrum antibiotics are administered, although no specific bacteria are associated with necrotizing enterocolitis. Dopamine infusions may be required to increase the cardiac output and improve intestinal perfusion. A high umbilical arterial line is replaced with a peripheral arterial line so that mesenteric blood flow is not compromised. Indications for surgery can vary from surgeon to surgeon but may include abdominal viscus perforation resulting in free air, persistence of a bowel loop on serial abdominal radiographs, or persistent metabolic acidosis with hyperkalemia indicating the presence of necrotic tissue.[220]

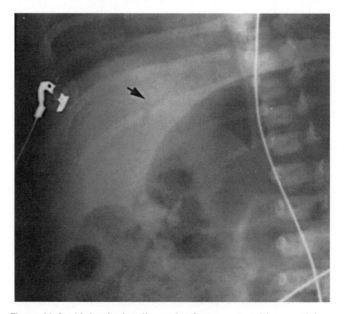

Figure 14–9. Abdominal radiograph of a neonate with necrotizing enterocolitis demonstrating gas in the biliary tract (arrow).

Table 14–4. Comparison of Omphalocele and Gastroschisis

	Omphalocele	Gastroschisis
Etiology	Failure of gut migration from yolk sac into abdomen	Occlusion of omphalomesenteric artery
Location	Within umbilical cord	Periumbilical
Associated Lesions	Beckwith-Wiedemann syndrome (macroglossia, gigantism, hypoglycemia, hyperviscosity) Congenital heart disease Exstrophy of bladder	Exposed gut inflammation, edema, dilation and foreshortened

Adequate preparation before surgery is important. Blood, fresh frozen plasma, and platelets will likely be required. Dopamine infusions may be necessary to improve renal and intestinal perfusion as well as cardiac output. Patients often are already intubated; otherwise, rapid-sequence or awake intubation is indicated. Because these patients are septic and volume depleted, potent inhalation agents are poorly tolerated and are generally avoided. A narcotic and muscle relaxant technique, avoiding nitrous oxide, is preferred. These infants usually have massive volume requirements; it is common for one or more blood volumes of 5% albumin to be required as a result of massive third-space losses. In addition, a severe coagulopathy may result in sudden, catastrophic generalized hemorrhage. Platelet transfusion is often needed prior to surgical incision.

OMPHALOCELE AND GASTROSCHISIS. Patients with omphalocele and gastroschisis have defects in the abdominal wall and may present with impaired blood supply to the herniated organs, intestinal obstruction, and major intravascular fluid deficits. The differences between omphalocele and gastroschisis are summarized in Table 14–4.

Omphalocele represents a failure of the gut to migrate from the yolk sac into the abdomen during gestation (Fig. 14–10A).[221, 222] It occurs in 1 in 6000 births.[223] Infants with omphalocele may have associated genetic, cardiac, urologic (exstrophy of the bladder), and metabolic abnormalities (Beckwith-Wiedemann syndrome, visceromegaly, hypoglycemia, polycythemia).[224] The herniated viscera are covered with a membranous sac; the bowel is morphologically and usually functionally normal.

Gastroschisis develops as a result of occlusion of the omphalomesenteric artery during gestation.[222, 225] It is usually not associated with other congenital anomalies, and its incidence is 1 in 15,000 births. The herniated viscera and intestines are exposed to air after delivery, resulting in inflammation, edema, and dilated, foreshortened, and functionally abnormal bowel (Fig. 14–10B).[226, 227]

Management of these lesions from birth until surgery is directed at reduction of fluid loss from exposed visceral surfaces by covering the mucosal surfaces with sterile, sa-

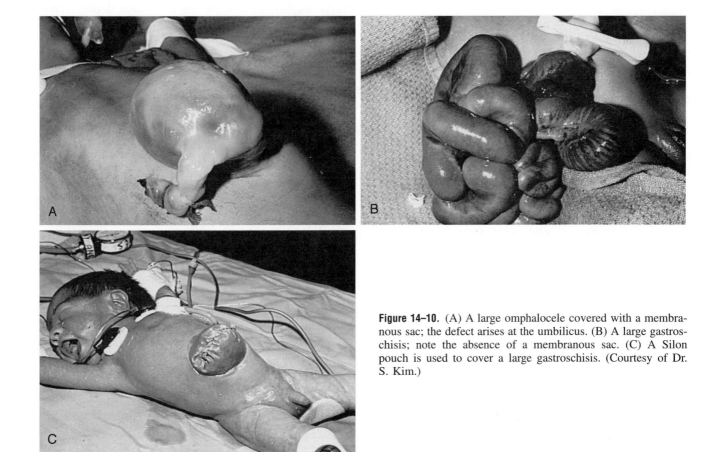

Figure 14–10. (A) A large omphalocele covered with a membranous sac; the defect arises at the umbilicus. (B) A large gastroschisis; note the absence of a membranous sac. (C) A Silon pouch is used to cover a large gastroschisis. (Courtesy of Dr. S. Kim.)

line-soaked dressings. A plastic wrap further decreases evaporative volume losses and the tendency to develop hypothermia. These anomalies represent a wide spectrum of pathology and require individualized assessment of intravascular volume status and fluid replacement. When these infants arrive in the intensive care unit, fluid resuscitation is instituted; patients with gastroschisis require multiple boluses of 20 mL/kg lactated Ringer solution and 5% albumin to replace evaporative and third-space losses.[228]

Anesthetic management is directed at continued volume resuscitation and measures to prevent hypothermia. Aspiration of stomach contents should be performed. Rapid-sequence induction or awake intubation is carried out. Muscle relaxation facilitates reduction of the eviscerated organs and bowel; however, abdominal closure may be associated with markedly increased intra-abdominal pressure. The effects of increased intra-abdominal pressure are twofold: (1) decreased organ perfusion and (2) decreased ventilatory reserve. The increase in intra-abdominal pressure may lead to decreased intestinal, renal, and hepatic perfusion and secondarily impaired organ function. This may lead to markedly altered drug metabolism and prolonged drug effect. The bowel may become edematous, and urine output may be reduced as a result of renal congestion. Venous return from the lower body may also be reduced, resulting in lower extremity congestion and cyanosis. Blood pressure and pulse oximetry determinations from a lower extremity may be different from those in the upper extremity. Significantly decreased diaphragmatic function and bilateral lower lobe atelectasis may occur, leading to respiratory failure.[229] Transduction of intragastric or bladder pressures may be a diagnostic adjunct.[230]

If complete reduction is not possible, a staged reduction is then carried out. The intestine is covered with a prosthetic Silon pouch, and the size of the pouch is subsequently reduced in stages either in the operating room or in the intensive care unit, thus allowing the abdominal cavity to gradually accommodate the increased mass without severely compromising ventilation or organ perfusion (Fig. 14–10C).[231, 232]

MALROTATION AND MIDGUT VOLVULUS. Malrotation and midgut volvulus result from abnormal migration or incomplete rotation of the intestines from the yolk sac back into the abdomen.[233] Rotation of the intestine around the mesentery may produce the abnormal location of the ileocecal valve in the right upper quadrant and kinking or compression of its vascular supply. If the malrotation occurs during development, atretic segments of bowel are formed. If the kinking or compression occurs after the bowel is normally developed, bowel necrosis occurs.

These patients present with a tender, distended abdomen and increasing abdominal girth; bloody stools are an ominous sign. These infants may have hypotension, hypovolemia, and electrolyte abnormalities. Because delay in surgery may result in necrosis of the entire small intestine, fluid and electrolyte resuscitation begins preoperatively and continues during surgery. This is a true neonatal emergency and surgery should proceed as reasonably as possible. Blood and blood products should be available in the operating room. Note that the hematocrit may be falsely elevated secondary to marked intravascular volume depletion. The indications for intra-arterial monitoring depend on the severity of the infant's illness. Central venous pressure monitoring may improve assessment of intravascular volume status and replacement and postoperative fluid management; however, if there is adequate peripheral venous access, the operation should not be delayed to insert the central venous pressure line.

HIRSCHSPRUNG DISEASE AND LARGE-BOWEL OBSTRUCTION. Hirschsprung disease is the most common cause of neonatal colon obstruction and consists of the absence of parasympathetic ganglion cells (Auerbach and Meissner plexus) in the large intestine.[234, 235] This deficiency creates a nonperistaltic segment of variable length, a tonically contracted anorectal sphincter, and delayed passage of meconium. Functional obstruction occurs at the level of the affected segment. The bowel may occasionally become distended to the point where its blood supply is compromised; perforation may occur, with resultant peritonitis. If the condition is not recognized and is left untreated, enteric bacteria may invade the bowel wall and subsequently enter the bloodstream, producing the toxic megacolon syndrome. Infants thus affected present with a distended, tender abdomen and hypotension and require massive volume replacement as well as vasopressor support.

The majority of these cases are diagnosed early because of bowel distention and failure to pass meconium. Bowel obstruction may be intermittent. Initial management is directed at stabilizing the patient's fluid status. For infants with mild to moderate lower intestinal obstruction, induction may be carried out with either rapid-sequence induction or awake intubation. If a patient is volume depleted, potent inhalation agents are poorly tolerated. Nitrous oxide should be avoided to prevent increasing bowel distention.

REFERENCES

1. Frantz ID, Adler SM, Thach BT, et al: Maturational effects on respiratory responses to carbon dioxide in premature infants. J Appl Physiol 1976;41:41–45.
2. Martin RJ, Miller MJ, Carlo WA: Pathogenesis of apnea in preterm infants. J Pediatr 1986;109:733–741.
3. Kuzemko JA, Paala J: Apnoeic attacks in the newborn treated with aminophylline. Arch Dis Child 1973;48:404–406.
4. Shannon DC, Gotay F, Stein IM, et al: Prevention of apnea and bradycardia in low-birthweight infants. Pediatrics 1975;55:589–594.
5. Muttitt SC, Tierney AJ, Finer NN: The dose response of theophylline in the treatment of apnea of prematurity. J Pediatr 1988;112:115–121.
6. Brouard C, Moriette G, Murat I, et al: Comparative efficacy of theophylline and caffeine in the treatment of idiopathic apnea in premature infants. Am J Dis Child 1985;139:698–700.
7. Joshi A, Gerhardt T, Shandloff P, et al.: Blood transfusion effect on the respiratory pattern of preterm infants. Pediatrics 1987;80:79–84.
8. DeMaio JG, Harris MC, Deuber C, et al: Effect of blood transfusion on apnea frequency in growing premature infants. J Pediatr 1989;114:1039–1041.
9. Keyes WG, Donohue PK, Spivak JL, et al: Assessing the need for transfusion of premature infants and role of hematocrit, clinical signs, and erythropoietin level. Pediatrics 1989;84:412–417.
10. Dransfield DA, Fox WW: High incidence of apnea with airway obstruction in recovering premature infants. Pediatr Res 1980;14:595.
11. Thach BT, Brouillette RT, Abu-Osba YK, Wilson SL, Mathew OP: Prevalence of mixed and obstructive apneic spells in preterm infants. Pediatr Res 1080;14:637.
12. Milner AD, Boon AW, Saunders RA, et al: Upper airways obstruction and apnoea in preterm babies. Arch Dis Child 1980;55:22–25.
13. Miller MJ, Carlo WA, Martin RJ: Continuous positive airway pressure

selectively reduces obstructive apnea in preterm infants. J Pediatr 1985;106:91–94.

14. Eichenwald EC, Aina A, Stark AR: Apnea frequently persists beyond term gestation in infants delivered at 24 to 28 weeks. Pediatrics 1997;100:354–359.

15. Steward DJ: Preterm infants are more prone to complications following minor surgery than are term infants. Anesthesiology 1982;56:304–306.

16. Gregory GA, Steward DJ: Life-threatening perioperative apnea in the ex-"premie." Anesthesiology 1983;59:495–498.

17. Liu LM, Coté CJ, Goudsouzian NG, et al: Life-threatening apnea in infants recovering from anesthesia. Anesthesiology 1983;59:506–510.

18. Kurth CD, Spitzer AR, Broennle AM, et al: Postoperative apnea in preterm infants. Anesthesiology 1987;66:483–488.

19. Spear RM, Deshpande JK, Maxwell LG: Caudal anesthesia in the awake, high-risk infant. Anesthesiology 1988;69:407–409.

20. Welborn LG, Rice LJ, Hannallah RS, et al: Postoperative apnea in former preterm infants: prospective comparison of spinal and general anesthesia. Anesthesiology 1990;72:838–842.

21. Cox RG, Goresky GV: Life-threatening apnea following spinal anesthesia in former premature infants. Anesthesiology 1990;73:345–347.

22. Krane EJ, Haberkern CM, Jacobson LE: Postoperative apnea, bradycardia, and oxygen desaturation in formerly premature infants: Prospective comparison of spinal and general anesthesia. Anesth Analg 1995;80:7–13.

23. Coté CJ, Zaslavsky A, Downes JJ, et al: Postoperative apnea in former preterm infants after inguinal herniorrhaphy: A combined analysis. Anesthesiology 1995;82:809–822.

24. Welborn LG, Hannallah RS, Luban NLC, et al. Anemia and postoperative apnea in former preterm infants. Anesthesiology 1991;74:1003–1006.

25. Grylack LJ, Williams AD: Apparent life-threatening events in presumed healthy neonates during the first three days of life. Pediatrics 1996;97:349–351.

26. Coté CJ, Kelly DH: Postoperative apnea in a full-term infant with a demonstrable respiratory pattern abnormality. Anesthesiology 1990;72:559–561.

27. Tetzlaff JE, Annand DW, Pudimat MA, et al: Postoperative apnea in a full-term infant. Anesthesiology 1988;69:426–428.

28. Noseworthy J, Duran C, Khine HH: Postoperative apnea in a full-term infant. Anesthesiology 1989;70:879–880.

29. Rodenstein DO, Perlmutter N, Stanescu DC: Infants are not obligatory nasal breathers. Am Rev Respir Dis 1985;131:343–347.

30. Miller MJ, Carlo WA, Strohl KP, et al: Effect of maturation on oral breathing in sleeping premature infants. J Pediatr 1986;109:515–519.

31. Badgwell JM, Swan J, Foster AC: Volume-controlled ventilation is made possible in infants by using compliant breathing circuits with large compression volume. Anesth Analg 1996;82:719–723.

32. Stevenson GW, Tobin M, Horn B, et al: An adult system versus a Bain system: Comparative ability to deliver minute ventilation to an infant lung model with pressure-limited ventilation. Anesth Analg 1999;88:527–530.

33. Tobin MJ, Stevenson GW, Horn BJ, et al: A comparison of three modes of ventilation with the use of an adult circle system in an infant lung model. Anesth Analg 1998;87:766–771.

34. Stevenson GW, Tobin MJ, Horn BJ, et al: The effect of circuit compliance on delivered ventilation with use of an adult circle system for time cycled volume controlled ventilation using an infant lung model. Paediatr Anaesth 1998;8:139–144.

35. Cordero L, Coley BD, Miller RL, et al: Bacterial and ureaplasma colonization of the airway: radiologic findings in infants with bronchopulmonary dysplasia. J Perinatol 1997;17:428–433.

36. Nickerson BG: Bronchopulmonary dysplasia. Chronic pulmonary disease following neonatal respiratory failure. Chest 1985;87:528–535.

37. Jacob SV, Coates AL, Lands LC, et al: Long-term pulmonary sequelae of severe bronchopulmonary dysplasia. J Pediatr 1998;133:193–200.

38. Baraldi E, Filippone M, Trevisanuto D, et al: Pulmonary function until two years of life in infants with bronchopulmonary dysplasia. Am J Respir Crit Care Med 1997;155:149–155.

39. Calder NA, Williams BA, Smyth J, et al: Absence of ventilatory responses to alternating breaths of mild hypoxia and air in infants who had bronchopulmonary dysplasia: Implications for the risk of sudden infant death. Pediatr Res 1994;35:677–681.

40. Cano A, Payo F: Lung function and airway responsiveness in children and adolescents after hyaline membrane disease: A matched cohort study. Eur Respir J 1997;10:880–885.

41. Carey BE, Trotter C: Bronchopulmonary dysplasia. Neonatal Netw 1996;15:73–77.

42. Chernick V: Long-term pulmonary function studies in children with bronchopulmonary dysplasia: An ever-changing saga. J Pediatr 1998;133:171–172.

43. Giacoia GP, Venkataraman PS, West-Wilson KI, et al: Follow-up of school-age children with bronchopulmonary dysplasia. J Pediatr 1997;130:400–408.

44. Rush MG, Hazinski TA: Current therapy of bronchopulmonary dysplasia. Clin Perinatol 1992;19:563–590.

45. Kari MA, Heinonen K, Ikonen RS, et al: Dexamethasone treatment in preterm infants at risk for bronchopulmonary dysplasia. Arch Dis Child 1993;68:566–569.

46. Rastogi A, Akintorin SM, Bez ML, et al: A controlled trial of dexamethasone to prevent bronchopulmonary dysplasia in surfactant-treated infants. Pediatrics 1996;98:204–210.

47. Brand PL, van Lingen RA, Brus F, et al: Hypertrophic obstructive cardiomyopathy as a side effect of dexamethasone treatment for bronchopulmonary dysplasia. Acta Paediatr 1993;82:614–617.

48. Haney I, Lachance C, van Doesburg NH, et al: Reversible steroid-induced hypertrophic cardiomyopathy with left ventricular outflow tract obstruction in two newborns. Am J Perinatol 1995;12:271–274.

49. Fujiwara T, Maeta H, Chida S, et al: Artificial surfactant therapy in hyaline-membrane disease. Lancet 1980;1:55–59.

50. Hallman M, Merritt TA, Jarvenpaa AL, et al: Exogenous human surfactant for treatment of severe respiratory distress syndrome: A randomized prospective clinical trial. J Pediatr 1985;106:963–969.

51. Gitlin JD, Soll RF, Parad RB, et al: Randomized controlled trial of exogenous surfactant for the treatment of hyaline membrane disease. Pediatrics 1987;79:31–37.

52. Lang MJ, Hall RT, Reddy NS, et al: A controlled trial of human surfactant replacement therapy for severe respiratory distress syndrome in very low birth weight infants. J Pediatr 1990;116:295–300.

53. Soll RF, Hoekstra RE, Fangman JJ, et al: Multicenter trial of single-dose modified bovine surfactant extract (Survanta) for prevention of respiratory distress syndrome. Ross Collaborative Surfactant Prevention Study Group. Pediatrics 1990;85:1092–1102.

54. Pelkonen AS, Hakulinen AL, Turpeinen M, et al: Effect of neonatal surfactant therapy on lung function at school age in children born very preterm. Pediatr Pulmonol 1998;25:182–190.

55. Friedman WF: The intrinsic physiologic properties of the developing heart. In: Friedman WF, Lesch M, Sonnenblick EH, eds. Neonatal Heart Disease. Philadelphia: Grune & Stratton; 1973:21–49.

56. Heymann MA, Rudolph AM: Effects on increasing preload on right ventricular output in fetal lambs in utero. Circulation 1973;48:37.

57. Kirkpatrick SE, Pitlick PT, Naliboff J, et al: Frank-Starling relationship as an important determinant of fetal cardiac output. Am J Physiol 1976;231:495–500.

58. Brinkman CR, Johnson GH, Assali NS: Hemodynamic effects of bradycardia in the fetal lamb. Am J Physiol 1972;223:1465–1469.

59. Southall DP, Richards JM, Johnstone PGB, et al: Study of cardiac rhythm in healthy newborn infants. Br Heart J 1979;41:382.

60. Walker AM, Cannata J, Dowling MH, et al: Sympathetic and parasympathetic control of heart rate in unanaesthetized fetal and newborn lambs. Biol Neonate 1978;33:135–143.

61. Vapaavouri EK, Shinebourne EA, Williams RL, et al: Development of cardiovascular responses to autonomic blockade in intact fetal and neonatal lambs. Biol Neonate 1973;22:177–188.

62. Leigh MD, McCoy DD, Belton MK, et al: Bradycardia following intravenous administration of succinylcholine chloride to infants and children. Anesthesiology 1957;18:698–702.

63. Starr NJ, Sethna DH, Estafanous FG: Bradycardia and asystole following the rapid administration of sufentanil with vecuronium. Anesthesiology 1986;64:521–523.

64. Dawes GS, Mott JC, Widdicombe JG: The foetal circulation in the lamb. J Physiol 1954;126:563–587.

65. Lauer RM, Evans JA, Aoki H, et al: Factors controlling pulmonary vascular resistance in fetal lambs. J Pediatr 1965;67:568–577.

66. Siassi B, Blanco C, Cabal LA, et al: Incidence and clinical features of patent ductus arteriosus in low-birthweight infants: A prospective analysis of 150 consecutively born infants. Pediatrics 1976;57:347–351.

67. Gersony WM, Peckham GJ, Ellison RC, et al: Effects of indomethacin in premature infants with patent ductus arteriosus: Results of a national collaborative study. J Pediatr 1983;102:895–906.

68. Hammerman C, Aramburo MJ: Prolonged indomethacin therapy for the prevention of recurrences of patent ductus arteriosus. J Pediatr 1990;117:771–776.

69. Wessel DL, Keane JF, Parness I, et al: Outpatient closure of the patent ductus arteriosus. Circulation 1988;77:1068–1071.

70. Bell EF, Warburton D, Stonestreet BS, et al: Effect of fluid administration on the development of symptomatic patent ductus arteriosus and congestive heart failure in premature infants. N Engl J Med 1980;302:598–604.

71. Haworth SG, Reid L: Persistent fetal circulation: Newly recognized structural features. J Pediatr 1976;88:614–620.

72. Roberts JD Jr, Shaul PW: Advances in the treatment of persistent pulmonary hypertension of the newborn. Pediatr Clin North Am 1993;40:983–1004.

73. Drummond WH, Gregory GA, Heymann MA, et al: The independent effects of hyperventilation, tolazoline, and dopamine on infants with persistent pulmonary hypertension. J Pediatr 1981;98:603–611.

74. Roberts JD Jr, Fineman JR, Morin FC 3d, et al: Inhaled nitric oxide and persistent pulmonary hypertension of the newborn. The Inhaled Nitric Oxide Study Group. N Engl J Med 1997;336:605–610.

75. Davidson D, Barefield ES, Kattwinkel J, et al: Inhaled nitric oxide for the early treatment of persistent pulmonary hypertension of the term newborn: A randomized, double-masked, placebo-controlled, dose-response, multicenter study. The I-NO/PPHN Study Group. Pediatrics 1998;101:325–334.

76. Kinsella JP, Truog WE, Walsh WF, et al: Randomized, multicenter trial of inhaled nitric oxide and high-frequency oscillatory ventilation in severe, persistent pulmonary hypertension of the newborn. J Pediatr 1997;131:55–62.

77. O'Rourke PP, Crone RK, Vacanti JP, et al: Extracorporeal membrane oxygenation and conventional medical therapy in neonates with persistent pulmonary hypertension of the newborn: A prospective randomized study. Pediatrics 1989;84:957–963.

78. Fugate JH, Ryan DP: Extracorporeal membrane oxygenation. Prob Anesth 1989;3:271–287.

79. Dworetz AR, Moya FR, Sabo B, et al: Survival of infants with persistent pulmonary hypertension without extracorporeal membrane oxygenation. Pediatrics 1989;84:1–6.

80. Roberts JD Jr, Roberts CT, Jones RC, et al: Continuous nitric oxide inhalation reduces pulmonary arterial structural changes, right ventricular hypertrophy, and growth retardation in the hypoxic newborn rat. Circ Res 1995;76:215–222.

81. Roberts JD Jr, Chiche J-D, Weimann J, Steudel W, Zapol WM, Bloch KD: Inhaled nitric oxide gas (NO) prevents pulmonary artery neovascularization in rat pups without pulmonary hypertension. Circulation 1999;98:1–341.

82. Garg UC, Hassid A: Nitric oxide-generating vasodilators and 8-bromo-cyclic guanosine monophosphate inhibit mitogenesis and proliferation of cultured rat vascular smooth muscle cells. J Clin Invest 1989;83:1774–1777.

83. Sarkar R, Gordon D, Stanley JC, et al: Cell cycle effects of nitric oxide on vascular smooth muscle cells. Am J Physiol 1997;272: H1810–1818.

84. Ishida A, Sasaguri T, Kosaka C, et al: Induction of the cyclin-dependent kinase inhibitor p21(Sdi1/Cip1/Waf1) by nitric oxide-generating vasodilator in vascular smooth muscle cells. J Biol Chem 1997;272:10050–10057.

85. Guo K, Andres V, Walsh K: Nitric oxide-induced downregulation of Cdk2 activity and cyclin A gene transcription in vascular smooth muscle cells. Circulation 1998;97:2066–2072.

86. Marks KH, Devenyi AG, Bello ME, et al: Thermal head wrap for infants. J Pediatr 1985;107:956–959.

87. Stothers JK: Head insulation and heat loss in the newborn. Arch Dis Child 1981;56:530–534.

88. Schiff D, Stern L, Leduc J: Chemical thermogenesis in newborn infants: Catecholamine excretion and the plasma non-esterified fatty acid response to cold exposure. Pediatrics 1966;37:577–582.

89. Goudsouzian NG, Morris RH, Ryan JF: The effects of a warming blanket on the maintenance of body temperatures in anesthetized infants and children. Anesthesiology 1973;39:351–353.

90. Hey E: Thermal neutrality. Br Med Bull 1975;31:69–74.

91. Murat I, Berniere J, Constant I: Evaluation of the efficacy of a forced-air warmer (Bair Hugger) during spinal surgery in children. J Clin Anesth 1994;6:425–429.

92. Arant BSJ: Developmental patterns of renal functional maturation compared in the human neonate. J Pediatr 1978;92:705–712.

93. Siegel SR, Oh W: Renal function as a marker of human fetal maturation. Acta Paediatr Scand 1976;65:481–485.

94. Ross B, Cowett RM, Oh W: Renal functions of low birth weight infants during the first two months of life. Pediatr Res 1977;11:1162–1164.

95. Hill LL: Body composition, normal electrolyte concentrations, and the maintenance of normal volume, tonicity, and acid-base metabolism. Pediatr Clin North Am 1990;37:241–256.

96. Siegel SR, Fisher DA, Oh W: Serum aldosterone concentrations related to sodium balance in the newborn infant. Pediatrics 1974;53:410–413.

97. Fanaroff AA, Wald M, Gruber HS, et al: Insensible water loss in low birth weight infants. Pediatrics 1972;50:236–245.

98. Abdulla F, Dietrich KA, Pramanik AK: Percutaneous femoral venous catheterization in preterm neonates. J Pediatr 1990;117:788–791.

99. Kanter RK, Gorton JM, Palmieri K, et al: Anatomy of femoral vessels in infants and guidelines for venous catheterization. Pediatrics 1989;83:1020–1022.

100. Dolcourt JL, Bose CL: Percutaneous insertion of silastic central venous catheters in newborn infants. Pediatrics 1982;70:484–486.

101. Metz RI, Lucking SE, Chaten FC, et al: Percutaneous catheterization of the axillary vein in infants and children. Pediatrics 1990;85:531–533.

102. Asnes RS, Arendar GM: Septic arthritis of the hip: a complication of femoral venipuncture. Pediatrics 1966;38:837–841.

103. O'Neill JAJ, Neblett WW, Born ML: Management of major thromboembolic complications of umbilical artery catheters. J Pediatr Surg 1981;16:972–978.

104. Neal WA, Reynolds JW, Jarvis CW, et al: Umbilical artery catheterization: Demonstration of arterial thrombosis by aortography. Pediatrics 1972;50:6–13.

105. Goetzman BW, Stadalnik RC, Bogren HG, et al: Thrombotic complications of umbilical artery catheters: A clinical and radiographic study. Pediatrics 1975;56:374–379.

106. Fluge G: Clinical aspects of neonatal hypoglycaemia. Acta Paediatr Scand 1974;63:826–832.

107. Pildes R, Forbes AE, O'Connor SM, et al: The incidence of neonatal hypoglycemia: A completed survey. J Pediatr 1967;70:76–80.

108. Srinivasan G, Pildes RS, Cattamanchi G, et al: Plasma glucose values in normal neonates: A new look. J Pediatr 1986;109:114–117.

109. Papile LA, Burstein J, Burstein R, et al: Relationship of intravenous sodium bicarbonate infusions and cerebral intraventricular hemorrhage. J Pediatr 1978;93:834–836.

110. Srinivasan G, Jain R, Pildes RS, et al: Glucose homeostasis during anesthesia and surgery in infants. J Pediatr Surg 1986;21:718–721.

111. Anand KJ, Brown MJ, Bloom SR, et al: Studies on the hormonal regulation of fuel metabolism in the human newborn infant undergoing anaesthesia and surgery. Horm Res 1985;22:115–128.

112. Anand KJS, Hickey PR: Pain and its effects in the human neonate and fetus. N Engl J Med 1987;317:1321–1329.

113. Anand KJ, Hansen DD, Hickey PR: Hormonal-metabolic stress responses in neonates undergoing cardiac surgery. Anesthesiology 1990;73:661–670.

114. Lynch RE: Ionized calcium: Pediatric perspective. Pediatr Clin North Am 1990;37:373–389.

115. Munoz R, Khilnani P, Ziegler J, et al: Ultrafilterable hypomagnesemia in neonates admitted to the neonatal intensive care unit. Crit Care Med 1994;22:815–820.

116. Cardenas-Rivero N, Chernow B, Stoiko MA, et al: Hypocalcemia in critically ill children. J Pediatr 1989;114:946–951.

117. Kosloske AM: A unifying hypothesis for pathogenesis and prevention of necrotizing enterocolitis. J Pediatr 1990;117:S68–S74.

118. Dunn L, Hulman S, Weiner J, et al.: Beneficial effects of early hypocaloric enteral feeding on neonatal gastrointestinal function: Preliminary report of a randomized trial. J Pediatr 1988;112:622–629.

119. Slagle TA, Gross SJ: Effect of early low-volume enteral substrate on subsequent feeding tolerance in very low birth weight infants. J Pediatr 1988;113:526–531.

120. Gartner LM, Snyder RN, Chabon RS, et al: Kernicterus: high incidence in premature infants with low serum bilirubin concentrations. Pediatrics 1970;45:906–917.

121. Lovejoy FHJ: Fatal benzyl alcohol poisoning in neonatal intensive care units: A new concern for pediatricians. Am J Dis Child 1982;136:974–975.

122. Koehntop DE, Rodman JH, Brundage DM, et al: Pharmacokinetics of fentanyl in neonates. Anesth Analg 1986;65:227–232.

123. Papile LA, Burstein J, Burstein R, et al: Incidence and evolution of subependymal and intraventricular hemorrhage: A study of infants with birth weights less than 1,500 gm. J Pediatr 1978;92:529–534.

124. Lou HC, Lassen NA, Friis-Hansen B: Impaired autoregulation of cerebral blood flow in the distressed newborn infant. J Pediatr 1979;94:118–121.

125. Bada HS, Korones SB, Perry EH, et al: Mean arterial blood pressure changes in premature infants and those at risk for intraventricular hemorrhage. J Pediatr 1990;117:607–614.

126. Miall-Allen VM, de Vries LS, Dubowitz LM, et al: Blood pressure fluctuation and intraventricular hemorrhage in the preterm infant of less than 31 weeks' gestation. Pediatrics 1989;83:657–661.

127. Charlton AJ, Greenhough SG: Blood pressure response of neonates to tracheal intubation. Anaesthesia 1988;43:744–746.

128. Tyszczuk L, Meek J, Elwell C, et al: Cerebral blood flow is independent of mean arterial blood pressure in preterm infants undergoing intensive care. Pediatrics 1998;102:337–341.

129. Bridenbaugh PO, Greene NM: Spinal (subarachnoid) neural blockade. In: Cousins MJ, Bridenbaugh PO, eds. Neural Blockade in Clinical Anesthesia and Management of Pain. 2nd ed. Philadelphia: J.B. Lippincott Company; 1988:213–252.

130. Lups S, Haan AMFH, Bailey P: The Cerebrospinal Fluid. Amsterdam: Elsevier Publishing Company; 1954.

131. Lucey JF, Dangman B: A reexamination of the role of oxygen in retrolental fibroplasia. Pediatrics 1984;73:82–96.

132. Purohit DM, Ellison RC, Zierler S, et al: Risk factors for retrolental fibroplasia: Experience with 3,025 premature infants. National Collaborative Study on Patent Ductus Arteriosus in Premature Infants. Pediatrics 1985;76:339–344.

133. Betts EK, Downes JJ, Schaffer DB, et al: Retrolental fibroplasia and oxygen administration during general anesthesia. Anesthesiology 1977;47:518–520.

134. Merritt JC, Sprague DH, Merritt WE, et al: Retrolental fibroplasia: A multifactorial disease. Anesth Analg 1981;60:109–111.

135. Bardin C, Zelkowitz P, Papageorgiou A: Outcome of small-for-gestational age and appropriate-for-gestational age infants born before 27 weeks of gestation. Pediatrics 1997;100:E4.

136. Bossi E, Koerner F: Retinopathy of prematurity. Intensive Care Med 1995;21:241–246.

137. Dobson V, Quinn GE: Retinopathy of prematurity. Optom Clin 1996;5:105–124.

138. Hesse L, Eberl W, Schlaud M, et al: Blood transfusion: Iron load and retinopathy of prematurity. Eur J Pediatr 1997;156:465–470.

139. Holmes JM, Duffner LA, Kappil JC: The effect of raised inspired carbon dioxide on developing rat retinal vasculature exposed to elevated oxygen. Curr Eye Res 1994;13:779–782.

140. Holmes JM, Zhang S, Leske DA, et al: Carbon dioxide-induced retinopathy in the neonatal rat. Curr Eye Res 1998;17:608–616.

141. Inder TE, Clemett RS, Austin NC, et al: High iron status in very low birth weight infants is associated with an increased risk of retinopathy of prematurity. J Pediatr 1997;131:541–544.

142. Keith CG, Doyle LW: Retinopathy of prematurity in extremely low birth weight infants. Pediatrics 1995;95:42–45.

143. Flynn JT: Oxygen and retrolental fibroplasia: Update and challenge. Anesthesiology 1984;60:397–399.

144. Coté CJ, Rolf N, Liu LM, et al: A single-blind study of combined pulse oximetry and capnography in children. Anesthesiology 1991;74:980–987.

145. Bucher HU, Fanconi S, Baeckert P, et al: Hyperoxemia in newborn infants: Detection by pulse oximetry. Pediatrics 1989;84:226–230.

146. Sugioka K, Woodley C: The use of transcutaneous oxygen electrodes in the presence of anaesthetic agents. Can Anaesth Soc J 1981;28:498.

147. Badgwell JM, McLeod ME, Lerman J, et al. End-tidal PCO_2 measurements sampled at the distal and proximal ends of the endotracheal tube in infants and children. Anesth Analg 1987;66:959–964.

148. Rich GF, Sullivan MP, Adams JM: Is distal sampling of end-tidal CO_2 necessary in small subjects? Anesthesiology 1990;73:265–268.

149. Burrows FA: Physiologic dead space, venous admixture, and the arterial to end-tidal carbon dioxide difference in infants and children undergoing cardiac surgery. Anesthesiology 1989;70:219–225.

150. Erkan V, Blankenship W, Stahlman MT: The complications of chronic umbilical vessel catheterization. Pediatr Res 1968;2:317.

151. Brans YW, Ceballos R, Cassady G: Umbilical catheters and hepatic abscesses. Pediatrics 1974;53:264–266.

152. Beligere N, Caldarelli D, Pruzansky S: Bilateral congenital choanal

153. Hall BD: Choanal atresia and associated multiple anomalies. J Pediatr 1979;95:395–398.

154. Ferguson JL, Neel HB: Choanal atresia: Treatment trends in 47 patients over 33 years. Ann Otol Rhinol Laryngol 1989;98:110–112.

155. Motoyama EK, Brinkmeyer SD, Mutich RL, Walczak SA: Reduced FRC in anesthetized infants: Effect of low PEEP. Anesthesiology 1982;57:A418.

156. Tusiewicz K, Bryan AC, Froese AB: Contributions of changing rib cage: Diaphragm interactions to the ventilatory depression of halothane anesthesia. Anesthesiology 1977;47:327–337.

157. Holinger PH, Brown WT: Congenital webs, cysts, laryngoceles and other anomalies of the larynx. Ann Otol Rhinol Laryngol 1967;76:744–752.

158. Coté CJ, Eavey RD, Todres ID, et al: Cricothyroid membrane puncture: Oxygenation and ventilation in a dog model using an intravenous catheter. Crit Care Med 1988;16:615–619.

159. Othersen HBJ: The technique of intraluminal stenting and steroid administration in the treatment of tracheal stenosis in children. J Pediatr Surg 1974;9:683–690.

160. Lampe I, Latourette HB: Management of hemangiomas in infants. Pediatr Clin North Am 1959;6:511–528.

161. Leikensohn JR, Benton C, Cotton R: Subglottic hemangioma. J Otolaryngol 1976;5:487–492.

162. Barry JE, Auldist AW: The Vater association; one end of a spectrum of anomalies. Am J Dis Child 1974;128:769–771.

163. Rittler M, Paz JE, Castilla EE: VACTERL association, epidemiologic definition and delineation. Am J Med Gen 1996;63:529–536.

164. Karl HW: Control of life-threatening air leak after gastrostomy in an infant with respiratory distress syndrome and tracheoesophageal fistula. Anesthesiology 1985;62:670–672.

165. Hogg CE, Lorhan PH: Pediatric bronchial blocking. Anesthesiology 1970;33:560–562.

166. Rao CC, Krishna G, Grosfeld JL, et al: One-lung pediatric anesthesia. Anesth Analg 1981;60:450–452.

167. Kitagawa M, Hislop A, Boyden EA, et al: Lung hypoplasia in congenital diaphragmatic hernia: A quantitative study of airway, artery, and alveolar development. Br J Surg 1971;58:342–346.

168. Nguyen L, Guttman FM, De Chadarevian JP, et al: The mortality of congenital diaphragmatic hernia: Is total pulmonary mass inadequate, no matter what? Ann Surg 1983;198:766–770.

169. Greenwood RD, Rosenthal A, Nadas AS: Cardiovascular abnormalities associated with congenital diaphragmatic hernia. Pediatrics 1976;57:92–97.

170. Reale FR, Esterly JR: Pulmonary hypoplasia: A morphometric study of the lungs of infants with diaphragmatic hernia, anencephaly, and renal malformations. Pediatrics 1973;51:91–96.

171. Naeye RL, Shochat SJ, Whitman V, et al: Unsuspected pulmonary vascular abnormalities associated with diaphragmatic hernia. Pediatrics 1976;58:902–906.

172. Levin DL: Morphologic analysis of the pulmonary vascular bed in congenital left-sided diaphragmatic hernia. J Pediatr 1978;92:805–809.

173. Rudolph AM, Yuan S: Response of the pulmonary vasculature to hypoxia and H^+ ion concentration changes. J Clin Invest 1966;45:399–411.

174. Tiefenbrunn LJ, Riemenschneider TA: Persistent pulmonary hypertension of the newborn. Am Heart J 1986;111:564–572.

175. Schreiber MD, Heymann MA, Soifer SJ: Increased arterial pH, not decreased $PaCO_2$, attenuates hypoxia-induced pulmonary vasoconstriction in newborn lambs. Pediatr Res 1986;20:113–117.

176. Vacanti JP, Crone RK, Murphy JD, et al: The pulmonary hemodynamic response to perioperative anesthesia in the treatment of high-risk infants with congenital diaphragmatic hernia. J Pediatr Surg 1984;19:672–679.

177. Peckham GJ, Fox WW: Physiologic factors affecting pulmonary artery pressure in infants with persistent pulmonary hypertension. J Pediatr 1978;93:1005–1010.

178. The Neonatal Inhaled Nitric Oxide Study Group (NINOS): Inhaled nitric oxide and hypoxic respiratory failure in infants with congenital diaphragmatic hernia. Pediatrics 1997;99:838–845.

179. Harrington J, Raphaely RC, Downes JJ: Relationship of alveolar-arterial oxygen tension difference in diaphragmatic hernia of the newborn. Anesthesiology 1982;56:473–476.

180. Bohn DJ, James I, Filler RM, et al: The relationship between $PaCO_2$

atresia and absence of respiratory distress. Cleft Palate J 1976;13:342–349.

and ventilation parameters in predicting survival in congenital diaphragmatic hernia. J Pediatr Surg 1984;19:666–671.

181. Nagaya M, Tsuda M, Murahashi O, et al: Management of congenital diaphragmatic hernia by extracorporeal membrane oxygenation (ECMO). Eur J Pediatr Surg 1991;1:10–14.

182. Bartlett RH, Roloff DW, Cornell RG, et al: Extracorporeal circulation in neonatal respiratory failure: A prospective randomized study. Pediatrics 1985;76:479–487.

183. Donn SM: Neonatal extracorporeal membrane oxygenation. Pediatrics 1988;82:276–277.

184. Andrews AF, Roloff DW, Bartlett RH: Use of extracorporeal membrane oxygenators in persistent pulmonary hypertension of the newborn. Clin Perinatol 1984;11:729–735.

185. Taylor GA, Short BL, Fitz CR: Imaging of cerebrovascular injury in infants treated with extracorporeal membrane oxygenation. J Pediatr 1989;114:635–639.

186. Krummel TM, Greenfield LJ, Kirkpatrick BV, et al: The early evaluation of survivors after extracorporeal membrane oxygenation for neonatal pulmonary failure. J Pediatr Surg 1984;19:585–590.

187. Schumacher RE, Barks JD, Johnston MV, et al: Right-sided brain lesions in infants following extracorporeal membrane oxygenation. Pediatrics 1988;82:155–161.

188. Glass P, Miller M, Short B: Morbidity for survivors of extracorporeal membrane oxygenation: Neurodevelopmental outcome at 1 year of age. Pediatrics 1989;83:72–78.

189. Breaux CWJ, Rouse TM, Cain WS, et al: Improvement in survival of patients with congenital diaphragmatic hernia utilizing a strategy of delayed repair after medical and/or extracorporeal membrane oxygenation stabilization. J Pediatr Surg 1991;26:333–336.

190. Weber TR, Kountzman B, Dillon PA, et al: Improved survival in congenital diaphragmatic hernia with evolving therapeutic strategies. Arch Surg 1998;133:498–502.

191. Clark RH, Hardin WD Jr, Hirschl RB, et al: Current surgical management of congenital diaphragmatic hernia: A report from the Congenital Diaphragmatic Hernia Study Group. J Pediatr Surg 1998;33:1004–1009.

192. Hansen J, James S, Burrington J, et al: The decreasing incidence of pneumothorax and improving survival of infants with congenital diaphragmatic hernia. J Pediatr Surg 1984;19:385–388.

193. Kirwan WO, Walbaum PR, McCormack RJ: Cystic intrathoracic derivatives of the foregut and their complications. Thorax 1973;28:424–428.

194. Eraklis AJ, Griscom NT, McGovern JB: Bronchogenic cysts of the mediastinum in infancy. N Engl J Med 1969;281:1150–1155.

195. Buntain WL, Isaacs HJ, Payne VCJ, et al: Lobar emphysema, cystic adenomaloid malformation, pulmonary sequestration, and bronchogenic cyst in infancy and childhood: A clinical group. J Pediatr Surg 1974;9:85–93.

196. Crawford TJ, Cahill JL: The surgical treatment of pulmonary cystic disorders in infancy and childhood. J Pediatr Surg 1971;6:251–255.

197. Murray GF: Congenital lobar emphysema. Surg Gynecol Obstet 1967;124:611–625.

198. Hendren WH, McKee DM: Lobar emphysema of infancy. J Pediatr Surg 1966;1:24–39.

199. Pierce WS, DeParedes CG, Friedman S, et al: Concomitant congenital heart disease and lobar emphysema in infants: Incidence, diagnosis, and operative management. Ann Surg 1970;172:951–956.

200. Coté CJ: The anesthetic management of congenital lobar emphysema. Anesthesiology 1978;49:296–298.

201. Meretoja OA: Is vecuronium a long-acting neuromuscular blocking agent in neonates and infants? Br J Anaesth 1989;62:184–187.

202. Guzzetta PC, Randolph JG, Anderson KD, et al: Surgery of the neonate. In: Avery GB, ed. Neonatology: Pathophysiology and Management of the Newborn. Philadelphia: J.B. Lippincott; 1987:944–984.

203. Tunell WP, Wilson DA: Pyloric stenosis: diagnosis by real time sonography, the pyloric muscle length method. J Pediatr Surg 1984;19:795–799.

204. Touloukian RJ, Higgins E: The spectrum of serum electrolytes in hypertrophic pyloric stenosis. J Pediatr Surg 1983;18:394–397.

205. Cook-Sather SD, Liacouras CA, Previte JP, et al: Gastric fluid measurement by blind aspiration in paediatric patients: A gastroscopic evaluation. Can J Anaesth 1997;44:168–172.

206. Andropoulos DB, Heard MB, Johnson KL, et al: Postanesthetic apnea in full-term infants after pyloromyotomy. Anesthesiology 1994;80:216–219.

207. Bishop HC: Small bowel obstructions in the newborn. Surg Clin North Am 1976;56:329–348.

208. Boocock GR, Todd PJ: Inguinal hernias are common in preterm infants. Arch Dis Child 1985;60:669–670.

209. Abajian JC, Mellish RWP, Browne AF, et al: Spinal anesthesia for surgery in the high risk infant. Anesth Analg 1984;63:359–362.

210. Harnik EV, Hoy GR, Potolicchio S, et al: Spinal anesthesia in premature infants recovering from respiratory distress syndrome. Anesthesiology 1986;64:95–99.

211. Mahe V, Ecoffey C: Spinal anesthesia with isobaric bupivacaine in infants. Anesthesiology 1988;68:601–603.

212. Gallagher TM, Crean PM: Spinal anaesthesia for infants born prematurely. Anaesthesia 1989;44:434–436.

213. Dohi S, Naito H, Takahashi T: Age-related changes in blood pressure and duration of motor block in spinal anesthesia. Anesthesiology 1979;50:319–323.

214. Wright TE, Orr RJ, Haberkern CM, et al: Complications during spinal anesthesia in infants: High spinal blockade. Anesthesiology 1990;73:1290–1292.

215. Kliegman RM, Fanaroff AA: Neonatal necrotizing enterocolitis: A nine-year experience. Am J Dis Child 1981;135:603–607.

216. Holman RC, Stehr-Green JK, Zelasky MT: Necrotizing enterocolitis mortality in the United States, 1979–85. Am J Public Health 1989;79:987–989.

217. Kliegman RM, Fanaroff AA: Necrotizing enterocolitis. N Engl J Med 1984;310:1093–1103.

218. Kosloske AM: Pathogenesis and prevention of necrotizing enterocolitis: A hypothesis based on personal observation and a review of the literature. Pediatrics 1984;74:1086–1092.

219. Frantz ID, L'Heureux P, Engel RR, et al: Necrotizing enterocolitis. J Pediatr 1975;86:259–263.

220. Ricketts RR: Surgical treatment of necrotizing enterocolitis and the short bowel syndrome. Clin Perinatol 1994;21:365–387.

221. deVries PA: The pathogenesis of gastroschisis and omphalocele. J Pediatr Surg 1980;15:245–251.

222. Thomas DF, Atwell JD: The embryology and surgical management of gastroschisis. Br J Surg 1976;63:893–897.

223. Kim SH: Omphalocele. Surg Clin North Am 1976;56:361–371.

224. Combs JT, Grunt JA, Brandt IK: New syndrome of neonatal hypoglycemia. Association with visceromegaly, macroglossia, microcephaly and abnormal umbilicus. N Engl J Med 1966;275:236–243.

225. Hoyme HE, Higginbottom MC, Jones KL: The vascular pathogenesis of gastroschisis: Intrauterine interruption of the omphalomesenteric artery. J Pediatr 1981;98:228–231.

226. King DR, Savrin R, Boles ETJ: Gastroschisis update. J Pediatr Surg 1980;15:553–557.

227. Moore TC: Gastroschisis and omphalocele: clinical differences. Surgery 1977;82:561–568.

228. Philippart AI, Canty TG, Filler RM: Acute fluid volume requirements in infants with anterior abdominal wall defects. J Pediatr Surg 1972;7:553–558.

229. Ein SH, Rubin SZ: Gastroschisis: Primary closure or Silon pouch. J Pediatr Surg 1980;15:549–552.

230. Yaster M, Buck JR, Dudgeon DL, et al: Hemodynamic effects of primary closure of omphalocele/gastroschisis in human newborns. Anesthesiology 1988;69:84–88.

231. Schuster SR: A new method for the staged repair of large omphaloceles. Surg Gynecol Obstet 1967;125:837–850.

232. Schwartz MZ, Tyson KR, Milliorn K, et al: Staged reduction using a Silastic sac is the treatment of choice for large congenital abdominal wall defects. J Pediatr Surg 1983;18:713–719.

233. Andrassy RJ, Mahour GH: Malrotation of the midgut in infants and children: A 25-year review. Arch Surg 1981;116:158–160.

234. Martin LW, Torres AM: Hirschsprung's disease. Surg Clin North Am 1985;65:1171–1180.

235. Kapur RP: Hirschsprung disease and other enteric dysganglionoses. Crit Rev Clin Lab Sci 1999;36:225–273.

Pediatric Emergencies

Stephen Campo, William T. Denman, *and* I. David Todres

Anesthesia for Emergency Pediatric Surgery
   History and Physical Examination
   Resuscitation
   Airway Control
   Full Stomach
   Hypovolemia and Intravascular Expansion
   Premedication
   Pain Management in Emergency Pediatric Surgery
   Anxiety and Fear in Patients and Parents
Special Problems
   Airway
   Circulation
   Status Epilepticus
   Poisoning
   Trauma

Anesthesiologists are involved in pediatric emergencies through the administration of anesthesia for emergency surgery and through their roles as consultants for airway management, resuscitation, and intensive care. The basic approach to cardiopulmonary resuscitation is described in Chapter 13. This chapter outlines the approach to anesthetic management for emergency pediatric surgery and selected clinical problems, including basic pathophysiology as well the role of the anesthesiologist in the emergency room and intensive care unit (ICU).

Anesthesia for Emergency Pediatric Surgery

Emergency anesthetic care begins with assessment of the urgency of a child's problems and an *ordering of priorities.* For example, in a child with an epidural hematoma and a closed femoral fracture, treatment of the former condition by emergency craniotomy takes precedence over setting the fracture.

History and Physical Examination

Unless the condition is so urgent that immediate resuscitation and intervention are needed, one should begin with a preop-

erative history and physical examination to assess needs, paying special attention to current medications, allergies, and any pre-existing medical or surgical conditions.

Resuscitation

For critically ill and profoundly hypotensive patients who need an immediate operation, resuscitation and the administration of anesthesia are provided simultaneously. Basic principles are applied: establish a clear airway, provide ventilation, and support hemodynamics with fluids, blood, and vasopressors as indicated. Hypnosis and analgesia should be provided as soon as the patient's condition will allow. Titrated doses of hypnotics, such as benzodiazepines or ketamine for amnesia, opioids for pain, and neuromuscular blocking agents for immobility should be used. As the patient stabilizes, inhalation anesthetics are added as tolerated. Guidelines for appropriate estimation of resuscitation drug doses for children are presented in Table 15–1 (see also Chapter 13).

Airway Control

Some urgent situations are characterized by a compromised airway, such as foreign body aspiration, epiglottitis, croup, bleeding tonsil, and facial or laryngeal trauma. In these situations, the urgency of securing the airway takes priority despite the risks associated with a "full stomach." In adults, such cases are often managed by "awake intubation," using topical anesthesia and sedation either under direct laryngoscopy or "blind" nasal intubation, or by using a flexible fiberoptic laryngoscope. Such an approach is favored in many situations because it leaves options open—that is, the patient continues breathing. Although such an approach is useful in many types of respiratory failure, it may seriously impair an already compromised airway in children who struggle during intubation attempts. An alternative approach is to anesthetize the child with a volatile agent (sevoflurane or halothane) in oxygen and with gentle cricoid pressure, maintain and assist breathing, and perform laryngoscopy with the patient under deep inhalation anesthesia. Some pediatric anesthesiologists would perform the inhalational induction of anesthesia with the patient in a left lateral decubitus position with slight Trendelenburg. This allows the tongue to fall to the left, aiding laryngoscopy; furthermore, should the patient regurgitate, pulmonary aspiration is less likely than with the patient supine. We would recom-

We acknowledge the prior contribution to this chapter by Charles B. Berde and thank Kenan Hauer for his assistance with the section on asthma.

mend this approach only if one has practiced managing the airway in this position in children without a full stomach.

Full Stomach

Children undergoing emergency surgery are considered to have a full stomach. Even those who have not eaten recently often have considerable gastric contents because of the increased acid secretion and delayed gastric emptying caused by pain, trauma, and fear. When a child's problem is not urgent, it may be appropriate to delay surgery for a period of 6 to 8 hours (using intravenous fluids to prevent deficits) to give the stomach time to empty. Provided that a patient's safety is not compromised, postponing surgery for 4 hours or longer can reduce the mean gastric residual volume by approximately 50% (see Figs. 4–1 to 4–3). This delay does not guarantee an empty stomach but may at least reduce the number of patients at risk for pulmonary aspiration of gastric contents.[1–3] Whenever it is likely that the patient has a full stomach and careful physical examination of the airway reveals no specific likelihood of a difficult intubation, it is generally best to proceed with a rapid-sequence induction. The rapid-sequence induction consists of preoxygenation, cricoid pressure, rapid administration of an induction agent such as thiopental, ketamine, or propofol, and a muscle relaxant such as succinylcholine or high-dose rocuronium, followed by laryngoscopy and tracheal intubation (see Chapter 4).[4–6] The use of succinylcholine has been questioned secondary to rare cases of dysrhythmias, including cardiac arrest. Atropine is frequently given with succinylcholine to prevent bradycardia, although the true incidence of clinically important bradycardias is unclear.[7, 8] The current adage regarding succinylcholine is "Always have it, never use it." Although this sequence is ideal for protecting against aspiration pneumonitis, it carries a number of associated risks, such as an inability to intubate the trachea, that must be weighed against the benefit of diminished risk of aspiration. As noted earlier, such an approach presumes that intubation will be straightforward or at least that ventilation with a bag and mask while maintaining cricoid pressure will be possible. It should be noted that in such a sequence, the ability to intubate is presumed, not tested. The smaller the child, the more rapidly he or she will desaturate during apnea because of the smaller ratio of functional residual capacity to oxygen consumption.[9–11] Although most adults can maintain adequate arterial oxygen saturation for up to 8 minutes of apnea following denitrogenation, newborns can become hypoxemic in less than 1 minute.[12] It is also more difficult to adequately preoxygenate and denitrogenate a frightened, struggling toddler. Additionally, rapid-sequence induction can be a considerable risk for patients with cardiovascular

Table 15–1. Guideline for Approximate Estimation of Drug Dosages in Children

Age	Fraction of Adult Dose
7 years	1/2 (0.5)
1 year	1/4 (0.25)
1 month	1/8 (0.125)
Newborn	1/10 (0.10)

issues such as hypovolemia or congenital heart disease. It is difficult to titrate the anesthetic dose to a patient's needs in a controlled fashion, and a given dose of thiopental may lead to profound hypotension due to myocardial depression and vasodilation (especially in patients who are hypovolemic or who have high levels of sympathetic tone). Conversely, severe hypertension is possible due to inadequate anesthesia during laryngoscopy. If succinylcholine is contraindicated, as in a crush injury, acute burns, myopathy, or malignant hyperthermia, a rapid induction may be accomplished by use of a nondepolarizing relaxant, usually rocuronium in a dose of 1.2 mg/kg (see Chapter 10).[6]

Some children will require endotracheal intubation but do not have an intravenous line in place. In rare circumstances, such as in children with multiple medical or surgical problems, it is nearly impossible to establish intravenous access prior to induction of anesthesia. In this circumstance, a cautious inhalation induction with sevoflurane in oxygen and cricoid pressure is a reasonable alternative. It has been shown that up to 40 cm H_2O peak inflation pressure does not cause gastric insufflation if the cricoid pressure has been properly applied.[13]

Hypovolemia and Intravascular Volume Expansion

When immediate operation is not necessary, it is advisable to replace fluid and electrolyte deficits and severe blood loss before induction of anesthesia. Mild to moderate deficits can be replaced with crystalloid solutions. In severe hypovolemia with ongoing blood loss, 5% albumin is often used as an intravascular volume expander pending blood availability. When time permits, transfusion should use fully crossmatched blood. Type-specific un-crossmatched blood has a very low incidence of transfusion reactions and in urgent situations can often be made available before crossmatched blood (see Chapters 11 and 12).[14–20]

Ketamine is often favored as an induction agent in hypovolemic patients. Ketamine is a very effective analgesic and supports blood pressure by causing the release of endogenous catecholamines.[21] In large doses, however, it may be a direct myocardial depressant.[22] Small induction doses (1–2 mg/kg IV) in moderately hypovolemic patients carry less risk. The concomitant use of benzodiazepines has been reported to diminish the incidence of bad dreams and other unpleasant emergence phenomena, but diazepam has also been reported to attenuate the catecholamine release by ketamine, and this may diminish its margin of safety in the setting of uncorrected hypovolemia.[23] Atropine (0.02 mg/kg) or scopolamine (0.01 mg/kg) is generally administered before ketamine to diminish the copious secretions stimulated by ketamine.[21]

Premedication

Premedication for emergency procedures is generally administered by the intravenous route. Opioids, when pain is present, are beneficial for children who are hemodynamically stable and have no airway compromise. Anesthetics currently in use, apart from ketamine, rarely cause profuse secretions; therefore, the use of antisialagogues before induction should be reserved for specific indications. In infants and small children, the intravenous administration of anticholinergics immediately before induction has three potential benefits: (1) maintenance of cardiac output by increasing heart rate; (2) prevention of reflex bradycardia secondary to airway manipulations; and (3) prevention of bradycardia secondary to either succinylcholine or halothane. Bradycardia is not as prevalent with the use of sevoflurane for induction compared with halothane, but this may not be true in neonates and infants.[24, 25]

Pain Management in Emergency Pediatric Surgery

Injured children are in pain at the time of arrival in the emergency department. For unstable patients and patients with evolving neurologic dysfunction, opioids must be used with caution. In many circumstances, however, injured pediatric patients are sufficiently stable to allow judicious administration of opioids. Generally, opioids free of histamine release (fentanyl) are preferable to those that release histamine (morphine) for patients who are potentially hypovolemic. Fentanyl must be titrated in small increments (0.5–1.0 μg/kg) to avoid chest wall or glottic rigidity.

In certain cases, regional nerve blocks can be used (1) to provide analgesia in the emergency department, (2) as a primary anesthetic to avoid some of the risks associated with general anesthesia, including aspiration, and (3) as a supplement to general anesthesia for postoperative analgesia.[26] For example, analgesia for patients with midshaft fractures of the femur can be provided by either a traditional femoral nerve block or the more recently described fascia iliaca compartment block,[27] diminishing pain from the femur and quadriceps muscle spasm. Similarly, an axillary block may be used for forearm fractures. Several cautions apply:

1. If sedation is used, it is essential that sedative drugs be titrated in small increments to avoid loss of airway reflexes.
2. Close communication with orthopedic and general surgical colleagues is advised so that there are no misunderstandings about the ability to perform sensory and motor examinations.
3. Occasionally, patients who appear alert with a given degree of sedation before a nerve block may become sleepier after the block, as the painful stimuli are removed. It is essential to calculate the appropriate dose in milligrams per kilogram for local anesthetics before administration (see Table 28–2).

Regional postoperative analgesia is often useful for patients with major thoracoabdominal trauma, including rib fractures. In experienced hands, thoracic epidural analgesia is an outstanding technique in this setting. Regional anesthesia and pain management are discussed in greater detail in Chapters 28 and 29.

Anxiety and Fear in Patients and Parents

Emergency surgery is a great source of fear and anxiety for children and their parents. The suddenness of the event provides little time for the patient and family to adjust to the crisis and limits the time the anesthesiologist has to develop rapport with the patient and parents. The anesthesiologist who appears calm and reassuring is of great benefit to both parties, making induction of anesthesia smoother. The importance of offering children and their parents a clear and straightforward explanation of all procedures cannot be overemphasized.

Special Problems

Airway

General Principles of Airway Management

The general principles of managing acute upper airway obstruction must be appreciated. Once the basic principles of airway management have been followed, then the specific therapy for the underlying cause may be undertaken.

Children arriving at the emergency room with acute upper airway obstruction may exhibit inspiratory stridor, tachypnea, sternal and intercostal retractions, agitation (which may be due to hypoxemia), cyanosis, and tachycardia. It is important to appreciate that they may also manifest few of these symptoms and signs yet their condition may rapidly become life threatening.

The initial response to these critically ill children should be to administer oxygen, correcting the hypoxemia, and keeping them calm to prevent dynamic collapse of the airway associated with agitation (see Fig. 7–10).[28] If a child is not cyanotic (not significantly desaturated on pulse oximetry) and has stable vital signs, then radiographic evaluation of the airway may help in clarifying the cause of the obstruction.[29] It cannot be overemphasized that it is essential that the child be stable and accompanied by a person able to manage the child's airway should problems arise. In addition, radiographs should be obtained with the child in the upright position to avoid further airway obstruction associated with the supine position.

Blood gas analysis is generally not vital; whether the arterial oxygen tension (Pa_{O_2}) is 80 mm Hg or 60 mm Hg does not alter clinical events or the response of the anesthesiologist. It is also difficult to interpret the Pa_{O_2} when the precise amount of inspired oxygen is unknown. Although the arterial carbon dioxide tension (Pa_{CO_2}) may provide a useful index of ventilatory efforts, obtaining an arterial sample may be attended by severe distress and often compromises oxygenation. The procedure to obtain the blood sample may be so disturbing to a child that severe dynamic airway collapse may precipitate worsening of the respiratory failure (see Fig. 7–10). It is thus a risk-versus-benefit issue, and the balance appears, in most situations, to swing toward the risks outweighing the benefits. In contrast, pulse oximetry provides a noninvasive, immediate, and continuous means for assessing oxygenation and is recommended as a continuous monitoring modality in all airway emergencies.

The need for inserting an intravenous line is usually not immediate. Placing an intravenous line may upset the child and may produce severe dynamic collapse of the airway. The primary focus of attention should be on the major problem, the airway. Placement of the intravenous line is therefore postponed until after induction of inhalation anesthesia in the operating room.

If there is any doubt as to whether the airway obstruction is imminently life threatening, the child is transported directly to the operating room, where a clear airway is established under controlled anesthesia and monitoring. The parents' presence in the operating room is extremely helpful for a child with severe airway compromise. The parents may be valuable in pacifying the child during the anesthetic induction phase, preventing further hypoxemia due to dynamic airway collapse that may occur with crying and agitation. Parents should be present only for the induction phase. In the operating room, our practice is to induce anesthesia with the patient in the sitting position. Halothane is an acceptable agent, but sevoflurane may be less likely to induce laryngospasm and is associated with less cardiovascular depression.[30, 31] Anesthesia is induced with a face mask technique or using one's hand to form a face mask. Once anesthesia is induced, cricoid pressure is applied to decrease the risk of aspiration.[13] If the anesthesiologist lays his or her fingers gently over the neck and gradually increases the pressure, then effective cricoid pressure can be obtained without distress to the child. It should be noted that cricoid pressure may not be necessary in patients with epiglottitis because they are usually unable to swallow (less likely to have a full stomach). Cricoid pressure may be contraindicated in patients with certain types of laryngeal foreign bodies.

With the child anesthetized and having adequate air exchange, an intravenous line is inserted and appropriate fluids and drugs administered. These children may be significantly dehydrated, especially if febrile with a prolonged period of inadequate oral intake. We therefore recommend rapid rehydration with 10 to 30 mL/kg of lactated Ringer solution or more if indicated. In addition, early administration of atropine is helpful in (1) diminishing secretions, (2) increasing heart rate and thus maintaining cardiac output in the presence of the myocardial depressant effects of the potent inhalation agents, and (3) blocking vagal reflexes associated with laryngoscopy or bronchoscopy.

The use of muscle relaxants to aid tracheal intubation is fraught with potential dangers. Once a child is paralyzed, efforts at ventilation may be ineffective. Therefore, it is vital that the anesthetic induction proceed with spontaneous respiratory efforts; this principle applies to all children with compromised or potentially compromised airways. As induction proceeds, the effectiveness of a child's respirations who demonstrates chest wall retractions may be improved by introducing continuous positive airway pressure (5 to 15 cm H_2O); this is effected by adjusting the "pop-off" valve while allowing the child to breathe spontaneously. This technique stabilizes the airway by opposing the forces of dynamic airway collapse (Fig. 15–1). As anesthesia is deepened, hypoventilation may occur, in which case the child's respirations must be assisted to prevent hypoxemia and hypercarbia. An unintubated child anesthetized with halothane is prone to cardiac dysrhythmias should hypercarbia develop.[32] This risk is less with the use of sevoflurane.[24] However, the need to administer high concentrations of inspired agent may still make halothane the agent of choice, since more MAC (minimum alveolar concentration) multiples can be delivered with a halothane vaporizer than with a sevoflurane vaporizer (see Table 8–3). The use of an end-tidal carbon dioxide monitor (shape of the expired carbon dioxide wave form) may be helpful in guiding the necessary degree of assisted ventilation, the continuous positive airway pressure, or both.

With airway obstruction and potential hypoventilation, the induction process is slow. The anesthesiologist must be aware of this, because laryngoscopy performed at a light plane may induce laryngospasm. We therefore wait until the child's eyes are centered and the rectus abdominis muscles are flaccid. Laryngoscopy is then performed, and the larynx examined; the cause of the obstruction may then be evident: the swollen red epiglottis and aryepiglottic folds. If the supraglottic structures are normal and the cause of obstruc-

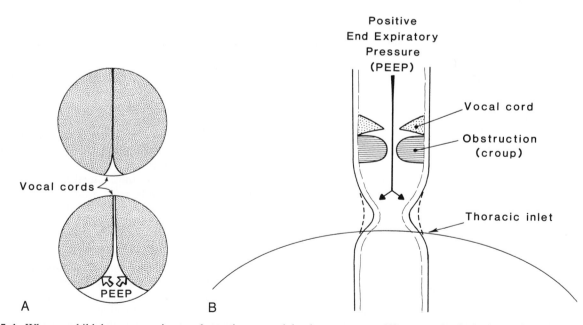

Figure 15–1. When a child has upper airway obstruction caused by laryngospasm (A) or mechanical obstruction (B), application of approximately 10 cm H_2O of positive end-expiratory pressure (PEEP; arrows) during spontaneous breathing often relieves obstruction. PEEP helps to hold the vocal cords apart (A) and the airway open (broken lines in B). (From Coté CJ: Pediatric anesthesia. In: Miller RD, ed: Anesthesia, 3rd ed. New York: Churchill Livingstone, 1990:1897–1926.)

tion remains unclear, then bronchoscopy may be indicated to establish the cause of airway obstruction beyond the glottis, such as a foreign body in the trachea or bronchus. Throughout the procedure, close attention to oxygen saturation (pulse oximetry) and the heart rate by means of a precordial stethoscope and electrocardiogram is important. Evidence of compromised oxygenation, desaturation, will become apparent before onset of bradycardia.[33] Slowing of the heart rate signals severe hypoxemia, vagal reflexes, or excessive potent anesthetic agent and requires urgent attention. Softening or loss of the heart tones as noted through a precordial stethoscope indicates severe myocardial depression.

As laryngoscopy is proceeding, a breathing patient will awaken because of redistribution and elimination of the volatile anesthetic. If the patient is allowed to "lighten" excessively, laryngospasm and other airway events are likely. It is for this reason that we change from sevoflurane to halothane once intravenous access is obtained. Pulmonary edema may complicate the sudden relief of airway obstruction and aggravate existing hypoxemia.[34–41] The primary pathogenesis of this noncardiogenic pulmonary edema is related to the marked increases in negative intrapleural pressures associated with upper airway obstruction.[35] This pulmonary edema is generally of brief duration.

When bronchoscopy is required, initial orotracheal intubation is helpful in providing a clear airway and a route for aspiration of secretions. Once a patient is stabilized, the surgeon can then perform the bronchoscopy unhurriedly and in a well-controlled situation. The procedure continues with the ventilating bronchoscope. It is important for the surgeon and anesthesiologist to have good rapport, because they are "sharing" the airway. Oxygenation, ventilation, and visualization must be adequate at all times. If a child begins to desaturate, the bronchoscope should be withdrawn into the trachea and the child oxygenated and ventilated effectively. To prevent hypoxemia, the anesthetic gas is carried in oxygen only. With the diagnostic evaluation completed, an endotracheal tube may need to be placed for therapeutic reasons or to protect the airway during awakening.

Upper Airway Obstruction

EPIGLOTTITIS. This is a life-threatening infection. In the past, epiglottitis usually affected children between the ages of 1 and 7 years and the most common pathogen was *Haemophilus influenzae*.[35, 42–44] With the advent of *H. influenzae* vaccination, the incidence of epiglottitis has diminished dramatically.[45, 46] Nevertheless, the airway skills used to manage epiglottitis are vital to the anesthesiologist and the knowledge needed to treat this entity is essential. The rapid onset and progression of this disease mandate urgent diagnosis and treatment. In addition to the symptoms of upper airway obstruction (inspiratory stridor, retractions, tachypnea), children with epiglottitis classically demonstrate drooling and difficulty with swallowing.

In all cases, our approach to epiglottitis is to establish a secure airway by means of endotracheal intubation. Tracheostomy is an alternative procedure preferred by some centers where there is less experience with stabilizing an endotracheal tube, although endotracheal intubation has become the favored approach worldwide.[47, 48]

Inspection of the epiglottis in the emergency room may increase airway obstruction by mechanisms previously discussed (dynamic airway collapse) and therefore should be avoided. Radiographic examination should be undertaken only in stable patients by skilled personnel and with adequate equipment accompanying the child to the radiographic facility. It cannot be overemphasized that radiographic examination is neither necessary nor appropriate if there is any doubt about the stability of the child's airway.

A child in severe distress is immediately moved from the emergency room to the operating room in a well-coordinated manner, under the supervision of the anesthesiologist, surgeon, and pediatrician. As described in the section on principles of management, the parents' presence during transport and induction of anesthesia is particularly valuable in this situation.

In the operating room, the child is kept calm, sitting on a parent's lap. A pulse oximeter probe and precordial stethoscope (held by an adhesive disk) are applied, and anesthesia is induced with slowly increasing concentrations of halothane or sevoflurane in oxygen with the parent assisting the anesthesiologist in gently bringing the mask to the child's face. Once the child loses consciousness, he or she is placed supine but with the head slightly up on the operating room table; the parent is ushered out of the operating room by an attendant while the anesthesia team continues the anesthetic induction.

After the child is lightly anesthetized with the volatile agent, an intravenous line is secured, rapid rehydration is begun, atropine is administered, and anesthesia is deepened. An endotracheal tube (with a stylet) is passed orally once an adequate depth of anesthesia is achieved. Spontaneous ventilation is usually maintained, as muscle relaxants may cause complete loss of the airway. Achieving a depth of anesthesia sufficient for performing laryngostomy may take longer than expected owing to shallow breathing and ventilation/perfusion ($\dot{V}/\dot{Q}$) mismatch from associated pneumonitis, atelectasis, or mucous plugs. Epiglottitis is marked by progressive swelling of the lingual surface of the epiglottis with resultant obliteration of the vallecula (Fig. 15–2A–C). Viewing the glottic opening without traumatizing the epiglottis may usually be accomplished by forcing the tip of the laryngoscope blade along the center of the base of the tongue into the vallecula, where the vallecula has been obliterated by the swollen lingual surface of the epiglottis. Lifting the base of the tongue, without directly touching the epiglottis, can then expose the glottis. A stylet within the endotracheal tube is helpful because it gives rigidity to the endotracheal tube and allows its introduction through a partially obstructed orifice. The endotracheal tube chosen should be one-half size smaller (0.5 mm internal diameter [ID]) than ordinarily selected to allow passage through the obstructed glottic opening. By choosing an endotracheal tube smaller than normal, one also lessens the risks of pressure necrosis on the mucosa.

If the anesthesiologist is unable to intubate the trachea, the trachea may be intubated with a rigid bronchoscope or, failing this, a tracheostomy or cricothyrotomy is performed (see Fig. 7–23).[49] The child is treated with appropriate antibiotics and transported to the ICU intubated, after it is made certain that accidental extubation is not possible. This will require adequate sedation and physical restraints. A blood

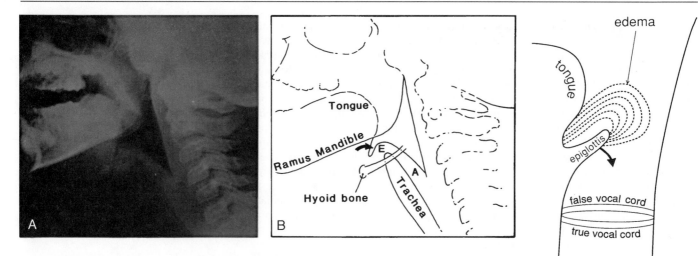

Figure 15–2. (A) Lateral neck radiograph of child with epiglottitis. Note the marked thickening of the aryepiglottic folds. (B) Schematic representation of A. Note the marked thickening of the aryepiglottic folds (A), loss ("amputation") of the vallecula (arrow), and swelling of the epiglottis (E). (C) Schematic representation of epiglottitis demonstrating progressive swelling of the lingual surface of the epiglottis, resulting in amputation of the vallecula. Progressive swelling leads to trap-door-like occlusion of the glottic opening.

culture is obtained and appropriate antibiotic therapy initiated.

Sedatives and opioids are administered, and the doses are titrated to permit the child to tolerate the endotracheal tube. Ideally, the patient should be allowed to breathe spontaneously. This increases the margin of safety if the child self-extubates. The endotracheal tube is left in place for 24 to 48 hours[50] until the airway swelling has decreased sufficiently to extubate the child.

LARYNGOTRACHEOBRONCHITIS. This is a common condition in children from 6 months to 6 years of age. It occasionally presents with life-threatening airway obstruction.[51–53] The cause is usually viral; bacterial tracheitis due to staphylococci and other organisms may present as a severe croup-like syndrome.[52, 54] The differential diagnosis includes epiglottitis or foreign body (tracheal or esophageal) aspiration.[52] The history and presentation usually are straightforward; however, radiographic evaluation may be helpful. It should be performed only when a child is stable (Fig. 15–3). In contrast to epiglottitis, the onset of laryngotracheobronchitis is insidious. An affected child demonstrates a low-grade fever and a "croupy" cough with inspiratory stridor and chest retractions. Treatment of the mild to moderate forms of croup includes cool mist and oxygen therapy; however, despite the popularity of cool mist therapy, there is no scientific evidence to support this practice.[55] When the condition is severe, the respiratory distress manifests as cyanosis in room air, severe sternal and costal retractions, and marked tachypnea and tachycardia. In this situation, in addition to administration of oxygen for the associated hypoxemia, more aggressive therapy is indicated to relieve the obstruction. At this stage, inhalation of nebulized racemic epinephrine (0.25 to 0.5 mL in 2 mL saline) with oxygen through a face mask may dramatically relieve the obstruction.[56–58] In a child who responds to racemic epinephrine inhalation, repeated treatments 1 to 4 hours apart are often necessary. The child

may experience a rebound effect, with increasing obstruction following an initial clearing of the airway. For this reason, children receiving racemic epinephrine therapy should be admitted for observation. If treatment with racemic epinephrine inhalation is unsuccessful, the underlying problem, in addition to edema, may be obstruction due to thick, inspissated secretions possibly related to bacterial superinfection, such as bacterial tracheitis.[53, 54, 59, 60] In this situation, relief of the obstruction must be obtained through endotracheal intubation, followed by pulmonary suctioning. This procedure should be performed in the operating room under controlled anesthetic conditions as for a child with epiglottitis. One large series (512 consecutive admissions in a single year) reported that approximately 6% of patients who had sternal and chest retractions on admission and failed to respond to conventional medical therapy required endotracheal intubation.[53]

In the operating room, the endotracheal tube selected should be at least one-half size smaller (0.5 mm ID) than would normally be chosen to avoid aggravating the subglottic edema and possibly causing subglottic stenosis.[61–63]

Intubated children are admitted to the ICU, and special care is given to endotracheal suctioning of inspissated secretions. The endotracheal tube is usually left in place for 3 to 5 days.

In the past, the benefits of steroid therapy had not been supported by scientific data, but newer studies and meta-analysis of numerous previous studies now suggest a potential benefit of steroid administration as part of the treatment of laryngotracheobronchitis.[64–69]

The time for extubation depends on when an air leak, indicating resolution of the subglottic pathology, develops around the endotracheal tube. With an adequate air leak (appearing at 10 to 20 cm H_2O peak inflation pressure), awake extubation may be undertaken in the pediatric ICU. Morphine given intravenously may be helpful if a child is especially anxious. In cases in which air leak is minimal (at

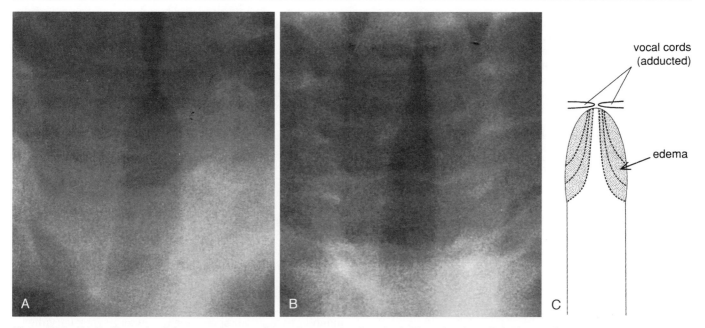

Figure 15–3. (A) Radiograph of the normal upper airway (anteroposterior view). Note that the subglottic area is rounded. (B) Laryngotracheobronchitis (croup) produces swelling (edema and inflammation), which obliterates the normal rounded subglottic area, producing the so-called sharpened pencil or steeple sign. (C) Schematic representation showing progressive swelling of the subglottic area.

pressures above 30 cm H_2O), we believe that extubation is more safely carried out in the operating room with the child under general anesthesia. When stabilized, the child is returned to the pediatric ICU. In the pediatric ICU, stridor due to glottic edema after extubation may necessitate treatment with racemic epinephrine inhalation. A single dose of steroids before extubation is thought by some investigators to protect against postextubation edema.[68]

FOREIGN BODY ASPIRATION. Any child who arrives at the emergency room with a presumptive diagnosis of foreign body aspiration requires emergency therapy. A child who is cyanotic, agitated, tachypneic, and tachycardiac requires urgent care. A history of choking and cyanosis while eating (particularly peanuts and popcorn) must arouse the strongest suspicion of foreign body aspiration. *A wheezing child may not necessarily be "asthmatic" but may have aspirated a foreign body.*[70, 71] Agitation may be misinterpreted as a state of emotional upset when it is due to serious underlying hypoxemia.

If a child is severely distressed because of partial occlusion of the airway, immediate plans should be made to remove the foreign body in the operating room. If the child is stable, then radiographic examination of the airway may be helpful in identifying and localizing the foreign body.[29] It should be appreciated, however, that most foreign bodies are not radiopaque. Hyperinflation and atelectasis are often clues to the presence of a foreign body (Fig. 15–4).

Removing the foreign body requires skilled anesthetic and surgical management (see Chapter 20). Anesthetic problems include the potential for aspiration and loss of the airway due to the presence of a full stomach. In addition, prolonged anesthetic induction must be anticipated because of the V̇/Q̇ abnormality associated with airway obstruction. The principles of anesthetic management are similar to those for epiglottitis.

The possibility of forcing the foreign body distally in the airway with assisted ventilation during anesthetic induction has caused much concern. For this reason, spontaneous ventilation is often advocated. Although spontaneous ventilation may be preferable, gentle assisted ventilation may become necessary if oxygenation and ventilation are inadequate. Topical spray of the larynx and vocal cords with 2% to 4% lidocaine may reduce the incidence of laryngospasm and coughing.

If a peanut has been aspirated, bronchoscopy should be undertaken without delay; an intense reaction to the peanut oil in the bronchus may lead to complete obstruction and

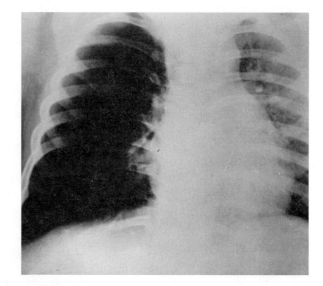

Figure 15–4. Radiograph of the chest demonstrating marked right-sided hyperinflation due to air trapping by the ball-valve effect of the foreign body.

atelectasis. Swelling of the bronchial wall makes later removal much more difficult. In a child suspected of having foreign body aspiration causing airway obstruction, one must consider the possibility that the foreign body has impacted in the esophagus and has produced airway compromise by posterior compression of the trachea (Fig. 15–5)

Lower Airway Obstruction

Anesthesiologists should be familiar with the conditions of bronchiolitis and status asthmaticus. In terms of pathology, lower airways (terminal bronchioles) are obstructed by edema, bronchiolar cellular infiltrate, mucous plugs, and various degrees of bronchospasm. In young infants with bronchiolitis, bronchospasm is thought to be less significant because of the relative lack of smooth muscle in the terminal bronchioles.[72] Bronchospasm becomes a critical factor in children with asthma.

Obstruction of the terminal airways leads to trapping of air, with hyperinflation of the chest and an increase in the physiologic dead space (Fig. 15–6A–B). The work of breathing is increased to maintain a satisfactory $PaCO_2$ with $\dot{V}/\dot{Q}$ inequality developing, leading to hypoxemia. With increased distress, respiratory failure supervenes.

Early in the course of the illness, compensation may lead to a lower than normal $PaCO_2$. Increasing severity of the disease is reflected in increasing hypoxemia, hypercarbia, and acidosis. If this trend is not checked, progression to respiratory failure will follow.

BRONCHIOLITIS. Viruses, especially respiratory syncytial virus, are the major etiologic agents of bronchiolitis. The disease usually affects infants 1 to 6 months of age. However, it may occur in children up to 12 months of age.[73–75] Former preterm infants with bronchopulmonary dysplasia are at particular risk for bronchiolitis.[76] Overall airway resistance in infants is primarily related to resistance in the peripheral airways, whereas in older children and adults, predominant resistance is in the nasopharynx.[77] In addition, an equivalent amount of inflammatory exudate within the airways more markedly affects younger infants, with their relatively smaller-diameter peripheral airways (see Fig. 7–9). The primary pathophysiologic effect of inflammation of the peripheral airways is maldistribution of ventilation and perfusion ($\dot{V}/\dot{Q}$ mismatch), leading to hypoxemia. Bronchiolitis occurs especially in epidemic form during the winter months.[73–75]

Bronchiolitis begins with an upper respiratory tract infection and fever. Tachypnea and retractions occur and are usually associated with wheezing. The chest is hyperinflated, and diffuse crepitations are heard over both lung fields. The liver is displaced downward as a result of the lung hyperinflation. Cardiac failure may occur if an infant has underlying congenital heart disease. Progressive exhaustion results in hypercarbia and respiratory failure, partly because reduced amounts of type I muscle fiber make infants prone to ventilatory fatigue (see Fig. 7–11). The diagnosis is usually established by the typical clinical picture. Detection of immunofluorescent antibodies for respiratory syncytial virus is obtained from nasopharyngeal washings.[76] The disease should not be confused with bronchopneumonia, cardiac failure, or foreign body aspiration.

The primary focus of treatment is administration of oxygen to correct hypoxemia. Pulse oximetry is a valuable indicator of the degree of hypoxemia and response to therapy. Nebulized mist is traditionally used but has not been shown to have any specific benefit.[78] Bronchodilators have not been proved to be of consistent benefit in patients with bronchiolitis. However, their use is worthy of a trial because some patients may benefit from them.[79, 80] Intravenous fluids are required for severely affected children who are unable to drink. Fluids should be carefully titrated to avoid volume overload, particularly in infants with bronchopulmonary dysplasia and cardiac failure.

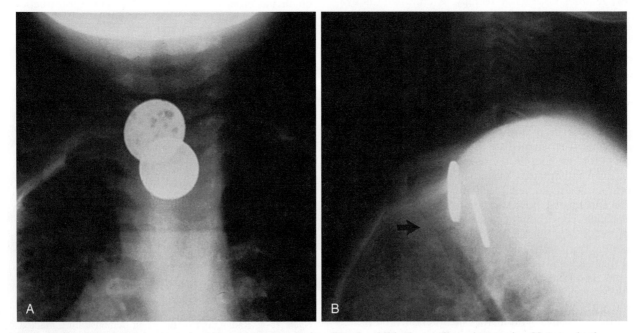

Figure 15–5. Radiograph of anterior-posterior (A) and lateral neck view (B) of a child who swallowed two coins. Note tracheal compression (arrow) due to a foreign body (coins) in the esophagus.

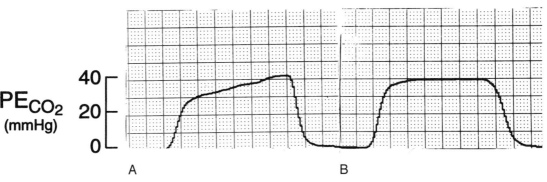

PE_{CO_2} (mmHg)

40
20
0

A   B

Figure 15–6. (A) Expired carbon dioxide tracing in the child with acute bronchospasm. Note the slowly rising expired carbon dioxide value. (B) Tracing of the same patient after administration of inhaled albuterol. Note that the expired carbon dioxide wave form now has a flat plateau indicating relief of the bronchospasm and efficient elimination of carbon dioxide from all areas of the lungs.

Ribavirin, an antiviral agent, has been used in treating infants with bronchiolitis due to respiratory syncytial virus infection, although its effectiveness has been called into question.[81, 82] In patients receiving ribavirin, special care is required in the use of mechanical ventilation because the particles tend to cause the valves of the respirator to stick, thus obstructing the ventilator. Modifications of the ventilator system and careful attention to humidity reduce this risk.[83, 84]

Assisted ventilation is required for the small number of children who develop respiratory failure. Indications for ventilation depend on the clinical picture and blood gas values. There is no absolute Pa_{CO_2} value that dictates this course of action. The outcome is usually favorable. A significant number of children will have episodes of asthma later in their lives.[85, 86]

ASTHMA AND STATUS ASTHMATICUS. Asthma is characterized by recurrent episodes of wheezing or dyspnea associated with widespread narrowing of the intrapulmonary airways. Inflammation appears to have an important role in the airway obstruction and hyper-responsiveness of asthma.[87] A cardinal feature of the disease is its reversibility, either spontaneously or with therapy.[88–93] The wheezing in asthma is predominantly expiratory. Anesthesiologists must appreciate that wheezing is not synonymous with bronchospasm. Although asthma is the most common cause of wheezing in childhood, other causes must be considered (Table 15–2).

Table 15–2. Causes of Wheezing in Children

> **Acute**
> Foreign body
> Bronchiolitis
> Inhalation injury
> **Recurrent or persistent**
> Asthma
> Foreign body
> Bronchiolitis
> Cystic fibrosis
> Recurrent pulmonary aspiration
> Mediastinal masses
> Tracheomalacia/Bronchomalacia
> Vascular ring
> Tracheal web or stenosis
> Bronchial stenosis

An asthma attack presents with increasing severity of airway obstruction. Wheezing with increasing cough and sputum production is noted. It is important to appreciate that with increasing fatigue, air movement may be so slight that wheezing is no longer audible.

PATHOPHYSIOLOGY. Airway obstruction results from the following:

1. Smooth-muscle hypertrophy and spasm of the airways
2. Inflammation and edema of the bronchial mucosa
3. Inspissated secretions.

Obstruction of the airways leads to air trapping and hyperinflation of the lungs. Lung compliance is decreased, leading to increased work of breathing. In addition, airway obstruction adversely affects $\dot{V}/\dot{Q}$ matching, leading to hypoxemia. Intrapulmonary shunting due to atelectasis contributes to hypoxemia. Dead-space ventilation is also increased, necessitating increased work of breathing to compensate. Initially, this compensation leads to hypocarbia; with increasing obstruction and muscle fatigue, the Pa_{CO_2} becomes elevated. A rising Pa_{CO_2} is a dangerous signal that heralds life-threatening ventilatory failure.[92] Increasing hypoxemia leads to metabolic acidosis, which contributes to myocardial depression, pulmonary hypertension, and right ventricular systolic overload.

MANAGEMENT. The goals of therapy are as follows:

1. Support oxygenation
2. Reduce airway obstruction
3. Support ventilation
4. Prevent complications (e.g., pneumothorax).

Medical therapy in the treatment of asthma includes inhaled and intravenous drugs (Tables 15–3 and 15–4). The

Table 15–3. Nebulized Agents for Status Asthmaticus

Drug	Onset of Action	Peak Effect	Duration of Action
Albuterol (salbutamol)	Within 5 min	1–2 hr	3–4 hr
Ipratropium bromide	10 min	1–2 hr	3–4 hr

Table 15–4. Parenteral Drug Therapy for Status Asthmaticus

Drug	Route	Dose	Adverse Effects
Beta-Adrenergic Agents			
Epinephrine aqueous 1:1000	Subcutaneous	0.01 mL/kg (=0.01 mg/kg) (maximum 0.3 mL) every 15 min × 3	Anxiety, restlessness, tremor, tachycardia
Terbutaline	Subcutaneous	0.01 mL/kg (maximum 0.25 mL) every 30 min × 2	
Terbutaline	Intravenous	Start at 0.1 μg/kg/min, titrate to effect as tolerated	
Xanthines			
Aminophylline	Intravenous	5 mg/kg loading dose over 15 min; then 0.9–1.1 mg/kg/hr; measure serum theophylline concentrations	Central nervous system stimulation: anxiety, restlessness, seizures. Cardiac: tachycardia, arrhythmias. Renal: diuresis. Gastrointestinal: nausea, vomiting
Corticosteroids			
Hydrocortisone	Intravenous	7 mg/kg immediately and 7 mg/kg/ 24 hr by continuous infusion or divided every 6 hours	Hypokalemia, hyperglycemia, fluid retention
Methylprednisolone	Intravenous	2 mg/kg immediately and 2 mg/kg/ 24 hr by continuous infusion or divided every 6 hours	
Dexamethasone	Intravenous	0.3 mg/kg immediately and 0.3 mg/ kg/24 hr	

most common drugs are the beta agonists, steroids, methylxanthines, and anticholinergics.[94-99] The role of leukotriene receptor antagonists is currently being evaluated.[100]

ANESTHESIA IN ASTHMATIC PATIENTS. In a child who is having an acute asthma attack and who requires emergency surgery, one should first attempt to control bronchospasm and optimize oxygenation. However, the urgency of the surgical problem must be taken into account. Induction of anesthesia may be carried out with standard agents. Although ketamine has bronchodilating properties,[101, 102] the secretions often associated with ketamine administration must be recognized. Avoidance of histamine-releasing agents such as morphine, curare, and thiopental may seem reasonable, although there are no scientific data to support this practice. Because rapid-sequence inductions are the rule for emergency surgery, there is a high likelihood of exacerbating bronchospasm by airway stimulation in a light plane of anesthesia.[103] Judicious premedication immediately before intubation with agents that blunt airway reflex responses, such as opioids or intravenous lidocaine, may attenuate these bronchospastic reactions. Anesthetic maintenance is aided by potent inhalation agents that dilate bronchioles and may help interrupt the efferent limb of vagus-mediated bronchospastic reflexes.[104, 105] Drying of secretions with atropine or glycopyrrolate may be useful intraoperatively, though it may exacerbate mucous plugging postoperatively.

In the operating room, wheezing during anesthesia necessitates an investigation of the underlying cause. It should be appreciated that wheezing under these circumstances may be due to mechanical problems related to the endotracheal tube, such as endobronchial intubation, plugging or kinking of the endotracheal tube, or herniation of the cuff. The markedly increased airway resistance associated with very severe status asthmaticus makes mechanical ventilation difficult. High airway pressures are required for effective ventilation, and an appropriate increase in expiratory time is necessary to prevent air trapping and the potential for pneumomediastinum and tension pneumothorax. To avoid these serious complications, mechanical ventilation is controlled so that a degree of hypercarbia is permitted, provided oxygenation is adequate and cardiac output with adequate oxygen delivery is sustained.[106, 107] This usually means limiting the peak inspiratory pressures at 40 to 45 cm H_2O and accepting a raised $Paco_2$. Note that wheezing during mechanical ventilation may have its origin in obstruction of the endotracheal tube with inspissated mucus. Once mechanical causes of wheezing have been ruled out, bronchodilator therapy may then be introduced into the anesthesia circuit. Methods of delivering the bronchodilator include nebulization and metered-dose inhalation.[108] In performing the latter procedure, it should be noted that the delivery efficiency is markedly dependent on the diameter of the endotracheal tube; smaller endotracheal tubes (<6 mm ID) lead to less efficient delivery. To overcome this problem, the bronchodilator should be introduced via a long catheter that extends to the tip of the endotracheal tube. When this is done, care should be taken in regulating the total dose of delivered drug because of the increased efficiency of drug delivery.[109] Alternatively, special adapters that allow the timing of administration of albuterol during inspiration may also allow for efficient delivery of medication. The shape of the end-tidal CO_2 wave form is often an early indicator of bronchospasm and the effectiveness of treatment (see Fig. 15–6).

For elective surgery, extubation is preferably carried out at a deeper level of anesthesia to prevent endotracheal tube–induced bronchospasm.[110] For emergency surgery in a patient with a full stomach, however, extubation should be carried out with the patient awake with intact upper airway reflexes.

Circulation

A child presenting with a surgical emergency may be in a state of shock. Shock is defined as a condition in which perfusion of blood to vital organs, with oxygen and substrates, is inadequate to meet the body's metabolic demands.[111] This inadequacy of blood flow may be due to

1. Hypovolemia (hypovolemic shock): loss of blood, plasma, electrolytes
2. Cardiac pump failure (cardiogenic shock): sepsis, hypoxemia, tamponade
3. Loss of peripheral vascular resistance (toxic shock): sepsis, drug overdose, anaphylaxis (anaphylactic shock).

In children, hypovolemia is by far the most common cause of shock. Metabolic effects of hypovolemic and cardiogenic shock include lactic acidosis produced by anaerobic metabolism due to diminished oxygen transport to the tissues. Generally, in septic shock (high-output shock), oxygen transport is not initially compromised; other factors that are not well understood account for the significant morbidity and mortality in this form of shock. The effects of inadequate perfusion on organ systems of the body are presented in Table 15–5.

Hypovolemic Shock

Blood loss due to trauma is the most common cause of shock in children. The bleeding may be "hidden," as in an intra-abdominal rupture of the liver or spleen, or retroperitoneal, as with evulsion of a kidney. It should be appreciated that in a child, compensatory mechanisms such as vasoconstriction and tachycardia to maintain perfusion are very efficient. Children may lose as much as one fourth of their blood volume without significant changes in the heart rate or blood pressure when in the supine position. In addition, an injured child may direct attention to a minor injury, overlooking a more serious one. It is therefore easy for the anesthesiologist or surgeon to underestimate the extent and gravity of the situation. Plasma loss is especially associated with burns and peritonitis; electrolyte deficiency is commonly encountered with diarrhea, vomiting, ileus, and intestinal obstruction. In sepsis, plasma proteins and electrolytes are lost via leaking capillaries (third-space loss), and hypovolemia may be a significant component of septic shock.

Management of shock requires an evaluation of the degree of hemodynamic compromise, a search for its underlying cause, and an insertion of a secure intravenous line for giving fluids rapidly.[112, 113] Intraosseous infusion of fluids is valuable in the initial management of hypovolemic shock when vascular access is difficult (see Fig. 32–4). During fluid resuscitation, attention must be paid to the adequacy of oxygenation and ventilation. Adequacy of perfusion and treatment response includes monitoring the parameters outlined in Table 15–6. The type of fluid infused remains a matter of debate, with some practitioners proponents of crystalloid resuscitation and others of colloid infusions.[114–121] Crystalloid solutions are effective in the initial management of hypovolemic shock in children. No controlled scientific studies of children have found colloid resuscitation to be superior to crystalloid. It is our practice to administer crystalloid solutions (lactated Ringer solution) as the initial resuscitation fluid. Blood should be transfused if indicated as soon as appropriate crossmatching has been carried out. However, the urgency of the situation at times demands the use of either O-negative blood or type-specific uncrossmatched blood (see Chapter 12).

Cardiogenic Shock

Cardiogenic shock is much less common in children than adults; causes include myocarditis, myocardial fibroelastosis, cardiomyopathy, sepsis, hypoxemia, pericardial tamponade (blood or air), primary heart disease, dysrhythmias, or pneumothorax with mediastinal shift and decreased venous return. Cardiac output is the product of stroke volume and heart rate; stroke volume is a function of preload, afterload, and myocardial contractility. Treatment of cardiogenic shock depends on identifying and treating the underlying cause. In addition, monitoring of preload, afterload, and contractility facilitates the choice of appropriate therapy (vasodilator, vasoconstrictor, or inotrope). The use of a flow-directed pulmonary artery (Swan-Ganz) catheter provides measurement of left-sided filling pressure, helping to guide fluid management. Thermodilution measurement of cardiac output and peripheral vascular resistance helps in assessing the effectiveness of vasoactive agents and fluid management.[122, 123]

Table 15–5. Effects of Inadequate Perfusion on Organ Systems of the Body

Respiratory failure—adult respiratory distress syndrome
Renal failure—increases morbidity and mortality
Cerebral edema—confusion and coma
Decreased liver function—depressed drug metabolism, diminished clotting factors
Gastrointestinal tract—necrosis, bleeding
Adrenal failure (uncommon)—more likely in septic shock

Table 15–6. Parameters Indicating Adequacy of Perfusion

Level of consciousness—head injury may confuse this evaluation
Perfusion of extremities—capillary refill and skin temperature
Heart rate
Blood pressure
Urine output—greater than 1 mL/kg/hr
pH—metabolic acidosis may indicate inadequate perfusion

Septic Shock

The pathophysiology of septic shock may involve several mechanisms. Sepsis causes profound vasodilation and loss of peripheral vascular resistance, leading to relative hypovolemia and, in severe cases, hypotension. Circulation is shunted away from capillary beds; therefore, despite a high cardiac output, oxygen and substrate delivery to tissue is compromised. In addition, sepsis may depress myocardial contractility. Sepsis may also lead to severe pulmonary artery hypertension and $\dot{V}/\dot{Q}$ abnormalities. Many children initially demonstrate a hyperdynamic circulation; that is, cardiac output is greater than normal. This contrasts with hypovolemic shock and cardiogenic shock, in which cardiac output is reduced. As septic shock progresses, however, the condition changes to a low-output state with a very significant increase in morbidity and mortality. Management includes identifying and eliminating the underlying cause, as in appropriate antibiotics for meningococcemia, the use of volume expanders, and administration of cardiac and vasoactive drugs (see Chapter 17).[124-126] Corticosteroids have traditionally been recommended for overwhelming shock but appear to have no beneficial effect on survival.[127]

Anaphylactic Shock

Anaphylaxis is the result of a hypersensitivity reaction to foreign substances, such as latex, insect bites, drugs (intravenous, intramuscular, oral), radiographic contrast media, and food.[128] This response is mediated through immunoglobulin E, leukotrienes, and other compounds.[129-136] Anaphylactoid reactions have a similar clinical manifestation but are not immunologically mediated. In either situation, patients may present with stridor, wheezing, urticaria, generalized swelling, profound vasodilation, and hypotension. Treatment consists of ensuring adequate ventilation and oxygenation, as well as administration of alpha-adrenergic agents (epinephrine, phenylephrine) to re-establish peripheral vascular resistance, beta agonists to relieve bronchoconstriction, corticosteroids to diminish mediator formation and release, antihistamines (H_1 and H_2 blockers) to block the effect of histamine, and fluids to support intravascular volume. Occasionally pure alpha agonists may be required to correct the peripheral vasodilation.

In patients with a history of anaphylaxis or anaphylactoid reactions, the anesthesiologist should attempt to identify the offending agent and avoid its use if possible. In addition, these patients should be treated with H_1 and H_2 blockers before anesthetic induction. Patients with severe allergic manifestations may also benefit from pretreatment with corticosteroids.[130, 134-138]

A major concern for anesthesiologists has been the marked increase in patients with latex allergy.[137-142] This is usually manifest as the sudden onset of rash, bronchospasm, and circulatory collapse. It appears to be a hypersensitivity reaction to latex or rubber products, and it is particularly common in patients with the spina bifida malformation. A reaction is most likely when there is direct contact between the latex material and mucous membranes. A history of hypersensitivity to rubber or latex materials should be sought, particularly in patients with chronic exposure to latex products, such as those who have spina bifida and perform urinary self-catheterization. Patients with a history suggesting hypersensitivity to latex or rubber products should receive pretreatment with H_1 and H_2 blockers, for example, diphenhydramine and cimetidine, and the use of latex or rubber products in these patients should be avoided. Latex-free materials should routinely be used on all meningomyelocele patients; such practice has markedly reduced the incidence of severe reactions.[143-148] Despite these precautions, severe reactions may still occur when other providers violate the latex-free procedures. Some children's hospitals now purchase only latex-free materials.

Status Epilepticus

A child is considered to be in status epilepticus when tonic-clonic movements persist for more than 20 minutes or recurrent convulsions occur without recovery of consciousness between seizures. Anesthesiologists may be called to assist in airway management. Prevention of morbidity and mortality is related to termination of increased metabolic demands (stopping the seizures) and maintenance of substrate supply by ensuring adequate oxygenation, ventilation, systemic and cerebral perfusion, and glucose stores. Status epilepticus is common in children with pre-existing seizure disorders and intercurrent infections, hypoxemic-ischemic encephalopathy (cardiac arrest), head trauma, metabolic derangements (hyponatremia and hypernatremia), viral encephalitis, intoxications, inadequate anticonvulsant drug levels, or noncompliance with anti-seizure medications. Deaths due to status epilepticus may result from compromise of ventilation and circulation by overzealous administration of anticonvulsants without adequate attention to respiratory and circulatory support.[149]

Airway and Ventilation

The initial approach to a child with prolonged seizures is to establish a patent airway, administer supplemental oxygen, and assess ventilation. For some patients, an oral or nasal airway is very helpful for establishing and maintaining airway patency. Oral airways may also serve as a bite block to help prevent injuries to the tongue and teeth. If a patient has an adequate natural airway, the oral airway is used as a bite block only, because advancement of the airway posteriorly may provoke gagging and vomiting. For many patients, oral secretions and vomitus may occlude the airway. Increased muscle tone may make it difficult to ventilate these patients adequately with a bag and mask. In this situation, tracheal intubation serves to establish a patent airway and helps protect against aspiration. The adequacy of ventilatory efforts can be difficult to assess. Tonic-clonic movements can confuse the observer's interpretations of chest wall and diaphragmatic movements and make auscultation of the chest difficult. Furthermore, these patients have a waxing and waning of their respiratory efforts. Oxygen demand and carbon dioxide production are also increased during seizures. When there is uncertainty about the patient's respiratory efforts, we recommend early intubation and assisted or controlled ventilation. The stomach should be emptied with a large-bore nasogastric tube after endotracheal intubation.

Circulation

The adequacy of blood pressure and systemic perfusion should be ensured. Patients are commonly hypertensive during seizures; hypotension should suggest causes such as drug effects (e.g., rapid administration of phenytoin), septicemia, hypovolemia, or cerebral edema and herniation.

Intravenous Access and Laboratory Studies

Intravenous access must be secured, and a blood sample taken for determination of blood glucose (dipstick), electrolytes, and ionized calcium. Depending on the circumstances, it may be appropriate to include a toxic screen, determination of the adequacy of anticonvulsant blood concentrations, and a blood culture. A bolus of glucose (0.5 g/kg) or 2 mL/kg of 25% dextrose in water should be administered when hypoglycemia is suspected.

Anticonvulsants

Intravenous administration of anticonvulsants in status epilepticus ensures the most rapid control of the seizures. One should be guided by the principle of using one drug to its maximum effect, to be followed by additional drugs if necessary. This is particularly the case for long-acting drugs such as phenobarbital and phenytoin. Drug levels are monitored to ensure therapeutic effects and avoid toxic levels in adjusting maintenance drug dosage. The main drugs used to control status epilepticus are benzodiazepines, phenytoin, and phenobarbital. In some patients, rectal administration of benzodiazepines may be initiated if intravenous access is difficult and would delay initiation of treatment.[150–152]

Anesthetic Agents and Muscle Relaxants

General anesthesia may be used in the rare case in which standard drug therapy pushed to the maximum fails to control seizures. It should be noted that muscle relaxants block the clinical manifestation of the seizure but do not affect cortical electrical discharge activity. Anesthetic agents decrease seizure discharges from the brain and reduce the brain's metabolic requirements. Agents used include pentobarbital, thiopental, and inhalation anesthetics such as isoflurane. The electroencephalogram should be monitored continuously when this form of therapy is applied. Pentobarbital coma has been successfully used in treating refractory status epilepticus. A loading dose of 4 to 8 mg/kg is followed by a maintenance dose of 1 to 3 mg/kg/hr. Blood levels of pentobarbital should be in the range of 3 to 5 mg/mL to produce burst suppression on the electroencephalogram. *CHECK DOSES.* At these high levels, respiratory and cardiovascular depression may occur, and these organ systems must be carefully monitored and supported with mechanical ventilation and vasopressor agents.[153–156]

Thiopental has also been recommended to treat refractory status epilepticus. After a loading dose of as much as 30 mg/kg, a continuous infusion is titrated to produce burst suppression on the electroencephalogram. Close monitoring of respirations and hemodynamic stability is necessary.

Isoflurane inhalation has been effective in the treatment of status epilepticus.[157] An advantage of isoflurane is its capability to suppress clinical and electroencephalographic seizure activity without significantly affecting a patient's hemodynamic status. A potential danger in this technique is that prolonged use (many hours to days) has been associated with the possible toxic levels of inorganic fluoride in the blood.[158–160]

Prevention of Injuries

Attention must be directed toward preventing injuries to the tongue, teeth, head, neck, back, and extremities that may result from tonic-clonic movements.

Poisoning

Ingestion of toxic material in childhood is a phenomenon of two age groups: children under the age of 5 years and adolescents. Children frequently ingest medications and toxic substances found around the house.[161, 162] Adolescents ingest alcohol and abuse drugs for recreation, in response to peer pressure, and as a suicide attempt or gesture.[163, 164]

In many situations, when the ingestion is recent and if the ingested substance is not caustic to the esophagus or the airway, it is possible to prevent absorption of considerable amounts of the ingested material by early use of emetics (ipecac), adsorbents (activated charcoal), and gastric lavage.[165–168] Specific antidotes (e.g., acetylcysteine for acetaminophen) are considered.

An anesthesiologist is consulted when a patient has apnea or hypoventilation and needs assisted ventilation and protection of the airway (tracheal intubation) from pulmonary aspiration of gastric contents. Depressed airway reflexes contraindicate the use of emetics; in this situation, passage of a nasogastric tube with an unprotected airway can also lead to vomiting and pulmonary aspiration. In securing the airway, the anesthesiologist should be aware that assessment of the depth of a patient's sensorial depression may be subtle. Vomiting and aspiration may be triggered by laryngoscopy and intubation attempts, even in patients who appear deeply comatose.

Before laryngoscopy, the means should be at hand for delivering positive-pressure ventilation with oxygen, as well as suction, atropine, succinylcholine, laryngoscopes, and endotracheal tubes. These patients should be preoxygenated, and cricoid pressure should be applied before intubation. Rapid changes in level of central nervous system depression may occur. Thus, if an oral endotracheal tube is inserted, it is essential that a bite block or an oral airway be placed. Our general dictum is that whenever a patient's ability to ventilate and protect his or her airway is questionable, the trachea should be intubated and ventilation assisted.

In addition to offering airway protection, an anesthesiologist may be of help in assessing and managing the hemodynamic effect of ingested medications (e.g., dysrhythmias secondary to tricyclics, myocardial depression secondary to barbiturates). Familiarity with the pharmacology of many of the agents ingested (barbiturates, opioids, anticholinergics) and facility with the clinical assessment of drug-induced depression of consciousness and cardiorespiratory reflexes make anesthesiologists particularly helpful in managing these problems.

Trauma

Trauma is a major cause of morbidity and mortality in infants and children.[169–174] It has been reported that half of all deaths in children are due to accidents, with automobile accidents accounting for 50% of traumatic deaths.[175, 176] Other causes include homicide, suicide, drowning, burns, and home accidents (falls, electrical injuries).[173, 174] The most common injury resulting in death among pediatric patients is head trauma. Effective management of major trauma requires a systematic approach to identify all injuries. Many patients have multiple injuries, some of which may not be immediately appreciated in the initial evaluation.

Emergency Room Management

Anesthesiologists should familiarize themselves with the equipment and protocols of the emergency room in their hospital, as frequently they will be asked to attend a pediatric trauma case. The rapid establishment of provisional diagnoses and ordering of priorities are essential in the emergency room management of trauma victims. Most centers use a system of a primary survey, resuscitation, a secondary survey, and definitive management.[175]

The primary survey and initial resuscitation occur at the same time and are intended to identify and stabilize those functions that are crucial to survival. This includes ensuring ventilation and stabilization of the cervical spine, supporting circulation, and controlling external hemorrhage. A rapid neurologic survey is also carried out. The Glasgow Coma Scale, modified for pediatric patients, is frequently used to follow the level of consciousness (see Tables 16–3 and 16–4).[175] Concurrently, vascular access is obtained, preferably two large-bore intravenous lines in the upper extremities. If this cannot be done quickly, a femoral line or an intraosseous line should be established.

In establishing an airway, the possibility of laryngeal, tracheal, or bronchial injury must be considered. Tracheal intubation of most patients with major trauma proceeds either with the patient awake or as a rapid sequence with appropriate sedation and muscle relaxation. When increased intracranial pressure is probable, measures to prevent further rise in intracranial pressure during intubation should be considered (see Chapter 22).

Most shock in children is due to hypovolemia, whereas cardiogenic shock, although rare, can be seen with chest trauma (Fig. 15–7). A dose of 20 mL/kg of crystalloid is the usual starting fluid bolus. Blood products should be considered when volume infusion has surpassed 80 to 100 mL/kg. During the initial resuscitation, a team member should attempt to get a history if possible. This should include the usual inquiries about allergies, medications, and past illnesses as well as the nature of the injury.[177]

Following the primary survey and resuscitation, a secondary survey is carried out. The exception is in the case of a patient who remains unstable despite ongoing resuscitation. These patients should proceed directly to the operating room

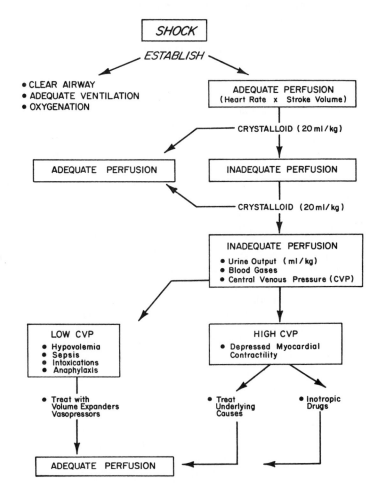

Figure 15–7. Algorithm for the management of a child in shock.

for surgical exploration. The secondary survey is a head-to-toe examination to identify additional injuries. Head examination should include visual inspection, palpation, assessment of pupillary size, reactivity, and a funduscopic examination. The cervical spine should be stabilized and assessed. Chest examination should involve inspection for wounds, palpation for tenderness and crepitance, and auscultation. Pneumothorax and hemothorax should be considered. Cardiogenic shock is unusual in children, but myocardial contusion and tamponade are possible. The abdomen should be examined, although findings can be subtle, especially in sedated or depressed patients. Direct peritoneal lavage is less frequently used to evaluate internal bleeding. Abdominal contrast-enhanced computed tomographic scanning or ultrasonography is helpful for detecting occult bleeding.[178] The extremities should be inspected for any tenderness, bruising, deformities, and vascular insufficiency.

Anesthesiologists commonly attend to respiratory and circulatory function of pediatric patients with major trauma, whereas surgical colleagues attend to diagnostic measures. Still, anesthesiologists must assess, with surgeons, the probable nature of the injuries so that they can anticipate the magnitude of bleeding, the physiologic effects of the injury, and the nature of the surgical procedures indicated. By understanding the appropriate work-up, an anesthesiologist should be able to recognize injuries that may have been overlooked and anticipate problems associated with them. The order of priorities is presented in Table 15–7.[179–181] The approach to diagnosis and treatment is dictated by the degree of urgency.

The basic principles in the management of trauma proceed along similar lines in children and adults, with some minor differences. In young children, the clinical signs of major injury may be less apparent than in older patients. Because children cannot always verbalize their complaints, clinicians must look beyond the sites of visible injury or the sites of chief complaint. For example, a child with hip pathology may complain that his or her knee hurts, and a child with major abdominal injury and a femoral fracture may complain only about the fracture. Moreover, children can often sustain major blood loss (up to 25% of their circulating blood volume) with a minimal change in vital signs; increasing pallor and sweating may be the only signs noted. A clinician may therefore have little warning before severe hypovolemic shock ensues.

The spectrum of thoracoabdominal trauma is also somewhat different for children. Abdominal trauma is much more common than thoracic trauma, and blunt trauma is much more common than penetrating trauma. Automobile accidents are the single most common cause of abdominal trauma in children.[173, 174] In thoracic trauma, hemothorax and

Table 15–7. Priorities in Emergency Trauma Management

Cardiorespiratory function
External hemorrhage
Injuries to great vessels
Retroperitoneal injury
Intraperitoneal injury
Intracranial injury
Burns and extensive soft-tissue injuries

pneumothorax are common, and chest tube placement may be life saving. The greater mobility of the mediastinum in children makes it more likely for tension pneumothorax to lead to hemodynamic compromise. Pneumothorax in children is frequently not heralded by rib fractures because of a child's compliant chest wall.

Head injury is common in childhood and is the most common cause of traumatic death.[172] Considerations related to airway and ventilatory management and intracranial pressure control are discussed in Chapter 22. The principles are similar to those in adults, with some differences. In newborns, traumatic delivery can lead to skull fractures and intracranial hematomas. In newborns and infants, unlike adults, intracranial bleeding can lead to hypovolemic shock because the head is a larger fraction of the newborn's body and the open fontanelle provides greater compliance and space for proportionately more blood loss.

Spinal cord injuries in children are relatively uncommon; they are most frequently encountered in newborns after vaginal breech deliveries and in adolescents after falls, diving, or automobile injuries. As with adults, children with potential cervical spine injuries require airway management that avoids neck flexion or extension.

Child abuse should be considered when the history of the trauma appears improbable. Funduscopic examination may disclose retinal hemorrhages, which suggest occult head injury including subdural hematomas. Examination of the skin may show bruises of various ages (see Fig. 16–5), and a skeletal survey may reveal multiple fractures of various ages, occurring most typically at the metaphyses of long bones. It is the responsibility of every physician involved, including the anesthesiologist, to be aware of the possibility of child abuse and to report all observations accurately to the appropriate authorities in the hospital. On occasion, a child who has previously been silent in the company of the parents will tell operating room or recovery room personnel about the events surrounding his or her injuries; such reports should be recorded, and appropriate referrals should be made. Abused children, particularly sexually abused children, are often terrified of painful procedures and anesthesia; the need for sensitivity and reassurance in these settings cannot be overemphasized.

Operating Room Management

Anesthetic management of pediatric trauma emergencies follows the principles outlined previously (see also Chapter 16). Establishment of the type of monitoring depends on the particular circumstance. For a child who is critically ill, surgery should proceed without delay, and the monitoring may initially include only a stethoscope, blood pressure cuff, pulse oximeter, electrocardiogram, and urinary catheter. As conditions permit, hemodynamic monitoring with arterial and central venous catheters may be established.[182, 183] Arterial catheters are helpful in situations in which there is (1) a concern about the adequacy of ventilation and a need to sample arterial blood gases; (2) a need for frequent and repeated blood sampling (severe hemorrhage or metabolic derangement); (3) hemodynamic instability; and (4) a need to alter the blood pressure rapidly. In a setting with acute blood loss, establishment of secure large-bore venous access is of higher priority than arterial access. Establishment of central venous access is often delayed until hemodynamic stability returns; rotating the neck of patients with possible cervical spine injuries must be avoided.[181]

Following initial attention to ventilation and restoration of perfusion with infused fluids, blood, and vasopressors as needed, the anesthesiologist then begins to address the less acute but important concerns. If it has not been possible to administer anesthetics or amnestics initially, they are administered in graded doses as soon as some stability is achieved. There is evidence in adult victims of major trauma that recall is very common; it is likely that this is at least as common in children.[184] Another important principle relates to maintaining body temperature. Hypothermia potentiates neuromuscular blockade and exacerbates coagulopathy. It occurs very commonly in victims of major trauma. Measures to warm the patient should be instituted as early as possible; these include warming the inspired gases, warming the blood and intravenous fluids, using warming blankets, wrapping the head and extremities (cellophane, towels, plastic bags), and increasing the room temperature (see Chapter 27).

After the surgical procedure is completed, the anesthesiologist's vigilance must continue until the patient is safely transported to the postanesthesia care unit or the ICU, where care is transferred to the appropriate physicians and nurses.

REFERENCES

1. Schurizek BA, Rybro L, Boggild-Madsen NB, et al: Gastric volume and pH in children for emergency surgery. Acta Anaesthesiol Scand 1986;30:404–408.
2. Bricker SR, McLuckie A, Nightingale DA: Gastric aspirates after trauma in children. Anaesthesia 1989;44:721–724.
3. Coté CJ: Aspiration: An overrated risk in elective patients. Adv Anesth 1992;9:1–26.
4. Sellick BA: Cricoid pressure to control regurgitation of stomach contents during induction of anaesthesia. Lancet 1961;2:404–406.
5. Salem MR, Wong AY, Fizzotti GF: Efficacy of cricoid pressure in preventing aspiration of gastric contents in paediatric patients. Br J Anaesth 1972;44:401–404.
6. Mazurek AJ, Rae B, Hann S, et al: Rocuronium versus succinylcholine: Are they equally effective during rapid-sequence induction of anesthesia? Anesth Analg 1998;87:1259–1262.
7. McAuliffe G, Bissonnette B, Boutin C: Should the routine use of atropine before succinylcholine in children be reconsidered? Can J Anaesth 1995;42:724–729.
8. Guyton DC, Scharf SM: Should atropine be routine in children? Can J Anaesth 1996;43:754–755.
9. Cross KW, Tizard JPM, Trythall DAH: The gaseous metabolism of the newborn infant. Acta Paediatr Scand 1957;46:265–285.
10. Kinouchi K, Tanigami H, Tashiro C, et al: Duration of apnea in anesthetized infants and children required for desaturation of hemoglobin to 95%. The influence of upper respiratory infection. Anesthesiology 1992;77:1105–1107.
11. Xue FS, Luo LK, Tong SY, et al: Study of the safe threshold of apneic period in children during anesthesia induction. J Clin Anesth 1996;8:568–574.
12. Gambee AM, Hertzka RE, Fisher DM: Preoxygenation techniques: Comparison of three minutes and four breaths. Anesth Analg 1987;66:468–470.
13. Moynihan RJ, Brock-Utne JG, Archer JH, et al: The effect of cricoid pressure on preventing gastric insufflation in infants and children. Anesthesiology 1993;78:652–656.
14. Hardaway RM, Adams WH: Blood clotting problems in acute care. Acute Care 1988;14–15:138–207.
15. Iserson KV, Huestis DW: Blood warming: Current applications and techniques. Transfusion 1991;31:558–571.
16. Nolan TE, Gallup DG: Massive transfusion: A current review. Obstet Gynecol Surv 1991;46:289–295.
17. Napier JA: The crossmatch. Br J Haematol 1991;78:1–4.
18. Dyke C, Sobel M: The management of coagulation problems in the surgical patient. Adv Surg 1991;24:229–257.
19. Gravlee GP: Optimal use of blood components. Int Anesthesiol Clin 1990;28:216–222.
20. Hewitt PE, Machin SJ: ABC of transfusion: Massive blood transfusion. Br Med J 1990;300:107–109.
21. White PF, Way WL, Trevor AJ: Ketamine: Its pharmacology and therapeutic uses. Anesthesiology 1982;56:119–136.
22. Schwartz DA, Horwitz LD: Effects of ketamine on left ventricular performance. J Pharmacol Exp Ther 1975;194:410–414.
23. Jackson AP, Dhadphale PR, Callaghan ML, et al: Haemodynamic studies during induction of anaesthesia for open-heart surgery using diazepam and ketamine. Br J Anaesth 1978;50:375–378.
24. Wodey E, Pladys P, Copin C, et al: Comparative hemodynamic depression of sevoflurane versus halothane in infants: An echocardiographic study. Anesthesiology 1997;87:795–800.
25. Lerman J, Sikich N, Kleinman S, et al: The pharmacology of sevoflurane in infants and children. Anesthesiology 1994;80:814–824.
26. Berde CB: Pediatric postoperative pain management. Pediatr Clin North Am 1989;36:921–940.
27. Dalens B, Vanneuville G, Tanguy A: Comparison of the fascia iliaca compartment block with the 3–in-1 block in children. Anesth Analg 1989;69:705–713.
28. Wittenborg MH, Gyepes MT, Crocker D: Tracheal dynamics in infants with respiratory distress, stridor, and collapsing trachea. Radiology 1967;88:653–662.
29. Kushner DC, Harris GB: Obstructing lesions of the larynx and trachea in infants and children. Radiol Clin North Am 1978;16:181–194.
30. Kataria B, Epstein R, Bailey A, et al: A comparison of sevoflurane to halothane in paediatric surgical patients: Results of a multicentre international study. Pediatr Anaesth 1996;6:283–292.
31. Walker SM, Haugen RD, Richards A: A comparison of sevoflurane with halothane for paediatric day case surgery. Anaesth Intensive Care 1997;25:643–649.
32. Rolf N, Coté CJ: Persistent cardiac arrhythmias in pediatric patients: Effects of age, expired carbon dioxide values, depth of anesthesia, and airway management. Anesth Analg 1991;73:720–724.
33. Coté CJ, Goldstein EA, Coté MA, et al: A single-blind study of pulse oximetry in children. Anesthesiology 1988;68:184–188.
34. Travis KW, Todres ID, Shannon DC: Pulmonary edema associated with croup and epiglottitis. Pediatrics 1977;59:695–698.
35. Lang SA, Duncan PG, Shephard DAE, et al: Pulmonary oedema associated with airway obstruction. Can J Anaesth 1990;37:210–218.
36. Kanter RK, Watchko JF: Pulmonary edema associated with upper airway obstruction. Am J Dis Child 1984;138:356–358.
37. Lee KW, Downes JJ: Pulmonary edema secondary to laryngospasm in children. Anesthesiology 1983;59:347–349.
38. Warner LO, Beach TP, Martino JD: Negative pressure pulmonary oedema secondary to airway obstruction in an intubated infant. Can J Anaesth 1988;35:507–510.
39. Hurley RM, Kearns JR: Pulmonary edema and croup. Pediatrics 1980;65:860.
40. Cozanitis DA, Leijala M, Pesonen E, et al: Acute pulmonary oedema due to laryngeal spasm. Anaesthesia 1982;37:1198–1199.
41. Frank LP, Schreiber GC: Pulmonary edema following acute upper airway obstruction. Anesthesiology 1986;65:106.
42. Emmerson SG, Richman B, Spahn T: Changing patterns of epiglottitis in children. Otolaryngol Head Neck Surg 1991;104:287–292.
43. Wurtele P: Acute epiglottitis in children and adults: A large-scale incidence study. Otolaryngol Head Neck Surg 1990;103:902–908.
44. Crysdale WS, Sendi K: Evolution in the management of acute epiglottitis: A 10–year experience with 242 children. Int Anesthesiol Clin 1988;26:32–38.
45. Adams WG, Deaver KA, Cochi SL, et al: Decline of childhood Haemophilus influenzae type b (Hib) disease in the Hib vaccine era. JAMA 1993;269:221–226.
46. Hickerson SL, Kirby RS, Wheeler JG, et al: Epiglottitis: A 9–year case review. South Med J 1996;89:487–490.
47. Oh TH, Motoyama EK: Comparison of nasotracheal intubation and tracheostomy in management of acute epiglottitis. Anesthesiology 1977;46:214–216.
48. Crockett DM, Healy GB, McGill TJ, et al: Airway management of acute supraglottitis at the Children's Hospital, Boston: 1980–1985. Ann Otol Rhinol Laryngol 1988;97:114–119.
49. Coté CJ, Eavey RD, Todres ID, et al: Cricothyroid membrane punc-

ture: Oxygenation and ventilation in a dog model using an intravenous catheter. Crit Care Med 1988;16:615–619.

50. Gonzalez C, Reilly JS, Kenna MA, et al: Duration of intubation in children with acute epiglottitis. Otolaryngol Head Neck Surg 1986; 95:477–481.

51. Davis HW, Gartner JC, Galvis AG, et al: Acute upper airway obstruction: Croup and epiglottitis. Pediatr Clin North Am 1981;28:859–880.

52. Baugh R, Gilmore BBJ: Infectious croup: A critical review. Otolaryngol Head Neck Surg 1986;95:40–46.

53. Wagener JS, Landau LI, Olinsky A, et al: Management of children hospitalized for laryngotracheobronchitis. Pediatr Pulmonol 1986; 2:159–162.

54. Jones R, Santos JI, Overall JC: Bacterial tracheitis. JAMA 1979; 242:721–726.

55. Bourchier D, Dawson KP, Fergusson DM: Humidification in viral croup: A controlled trial. Aust Paediatr J 1984;20:289–291.

56. Taussig LM, Castro O, Beaudry PH, et al: Treatment of laryngotracheobronchitis (croup). Use of intermittent positive-pressure breathing and racemic epinephrine. Am J Dis Child 1975;129:790–793.

57. Adair JC, Ring WH, Jordan WS, et al: Ten-year experience with IPPB in the treatment of acute laryngotracheobronchitis. Anesth Analg 1971;50:649–655.

58. Kilham H, Gillis J, Benjamin B: Severe upper airway obstruction. Pediatr Clin North Am 1987;34:1–14.

59. Henry RL, Mellis CM, Benjamin B: Pseudomembranous croup. Arch Dis Child 1983;58:180–183.

60. Friedman EM, Jorgensen K, Healy GB, et al: Bacterial tracheitis: Two-year experience. Laryngoscope 1985;95:9–11.

61. Downes JJ, Striker TW, Stool S: Complications of nasotracheal intubation in children with croup. N Engl J Med 1966;274:226–227.

62. McEniery J, Gillis J, Kilham H, et al: Review of intubation in severe laryngotracheobronchitis. Pediatrics 1991;87:847–853.

63. Allen TH, Steven IM: Prolonged nasotracheal intubation in infants and children. Br J Anaesth 1972;44:835–840.

64. Leipzig B, Oski FA, Cummings CW, et al: A prospective randomized study to determine the efficacy of steroids in treatment of croup. J Pediatr 1979;94:194–196.

65. Tunnessen WWJ, Feinstein AR: The steroid-croup controversy: An analytic review of methodologic problems. J Pediatr 1980;96:751–756.

66. Kairys SW, Olmstead EM, O'Connor GT: Steroid treatment of laryngotracheitis: A meta-analysis of the evidence from randomized trials. Pediatrics 1989;83:683–693.

67. Super DM, Cartelli NA, Brooks LJ, et al: A prospective randomized double-blind study to evaluate the effect of dexamethasone in acute laryngotracheitis. J Pediatr 1989;115:323–329.

68. Freezer N, Butt W, Phelan P: Steroids in croup: Do they increase the incidence of successful extubation? Anaesth Intensive Care 1990;18:224–228.

69. Anonymous: Steroids and croup. Lancet 1989;2:1134–1136.

70. Blazer S, Naveh Y, Friedman A: Foreign body in the airway: A review of 200 cases. Am J Dis Child 1980;134:68–71.

71. Cohen SR, Herbert WI, Lewis GBJ, et al: Foreign bodies in the airway: Five-year retrospective study with special reference to management. Ann Otol Rhinol Laryngol 1980;89:437–442.

72. Milner AD, Henry RL: Acute airways obstruction in children under 5. Thorax 1982;37:641–645.

73. Wohl ME, Chernick V: State of the art: Bronchiolitis. Am Rev Respir Dis 1978;118:759–781.

74. McConnochie KM, Roghmann KJ: Bronchiolitis as a possible cause of wheezing in childhood: New evidence. Pediatrics 1984;74:1–10.

75. Milner AD, Murray M: Acute bronchiolitis in infancy: Treatment and prognosis. Thorax 1989;44:1–5.

76. Groothuis JR, Gutierrez KM, Lauer BA: Respiratory syncytial virus infection in children with bronchopulmonary dysplasia. Pediatrics 1988;82:199–203.

77. Hogg JC, Williams B, Richardson JB, et al: Age as a factor in the distribution of lower-airway conductance and in the pathologic anatomy of obstructive lung disease. N Engl J Med 1970;282:1283–1287.

78. Bau SK, Aspin N, Wood DE, et al: The measurement of fluid deposition in humans following mist tent therapy. Pediatrics 1971;48:605–612.

79. Hughes DM, Lesouef PN, Landau LI: Effect of salbutamol on respiratory mechanics in bronchiolitis. Pediatr Res 1987;22:83–86.

80. O'Callaghan C, Milner AD, Swarbrick A: Nebulised salbutamol does have a protective effect on airways in children under 1 year old. Arch Dis Child 1988;63:479–483.

81. Long CE, Voter KZ, Barker WH, et al: Long-term follow-up of children hospitalized with respiratory syncytial virus lower respiratory tract infection and randomly treated with ribavirin or placebo. Pediatr Infect Dis J 1997;16:1023–1028.

82. Law BJ, Wang EE, MacDonald N, et al: Does ribavirin impact on the hospital course of children with respiratory syncytial virus (RSV) infection? An analysis using the pediatric investigators collaborative network on infections in Canada (PICNIC) RSV database. Pediatrics 1997;99:E7.

83. Outwater KM, Meissner HC, Peterson MB: Ribavirin administration to infants receiving mechanical ventilation. Am J Dis Child 1988; 142:512–515.

84. Adderley RJ: Safety of ribavirin with mechanical ventilation. Pediatr Infect Dis J 1990;9:S112–S114.

85. Rooney JC, Williams HE: The relationship between proved viral bronchiolitis and subsequent wheezing. J Pediatr 1971;79:744–747.

86. Pullan CR, Hey EN: Wheezing, asthma, and pulmonary dysfunction 10 years after infection with respiratory syncytial virus in infancy. Br Med J (Clin Res Ed) 1982;284:1665–1669.

87. Hargreave FE: Late-phase asthmatic responses and airway inflammation. J Allergy Clin Immunol 1989;83:525–527.

88. Commey JO, Levison H: Physical signs in childhood asthma. Pediatrics 1976;58:537–541.

89. Blair H: Natural history of childhood asthma: 20-year follow-up. Arch Dis Child 1977;52:613–619.

90. Williams AJ, Santiago S, Weiss EB, et al: Status asthmaticus. Acute Care 1988;14–15:208–228.

91. Soler M, Imhof E, Perruchoud AP: Severe acute asthma: Pathophysiology, clinical assessment, and treatment. Respiration 1990;57:114–121.

92. Nelson DR, Sachs MI, O'Connell EJ: Approaches to acute asthma and status asthmaticus in children. Mayo Clin Proc 1989;64:1392–1402.

93. Richards W: Hospitalization of children with status asthmaticus: A review. Pediatrics 1989;84:111–118.

94. Galant SP: Current status of beta-adrenergic agonists in bronchial asthma. Pediatr Clin North Am 1983;30:931–942.

95. Robertson CF, Smith F, Beck R, et al: Response to frequent low doses of nebulized salbutamol in acute asthma. J Pediatr 1985;106:672–674.

96. Bolte RG: Nebulized beta-adrenergic agents in the treatment of acute pediatric asthma. Pediatr Emerg Care 1986;2:250–253.

97. Jacobs M: Maintenance therapy for obstructive lung disease: How to achieve the best response with the fewest agents. Postgrad Med 1994;95:87–90.

98. Reiser J, Yeang Y, Warner JO: The effect of zaprinast (M&B 22,948, an orally absorbed mast cell stabilizer) on exercise-induced asthma in children. Br J Dis Chest 1986;80:157–163.

99. Shaw RJ, Kay AB: Nedocromil, a mucosal and connective tissue mast cell stabilizer, inhibits exercise-induced asthma. Br J Dis Chest 1985;79:385–389.

100. Drazen JM, Israel E, O'Byrne PM: Treatment of asthma with drugs modifying the leukotriene pathway. N Engl J Med 1999;340:197–206.

101. Corssen G, Gutierrez J, Reves JG, et al: Ketamine in the anesthetic management of asthmatic patients. Anesth Analg 1972;51:588–596.

102. Huber FCJ, Gutierrez J, Corssen G: Ketamine: Its effect on airway resistance in man. South Med J 1972;65:1176–1180.

103. Shnider SM, Papper EM: Anesthesia for the asthmatic patient. Anesthesiology 1961;22:886–892.

104. Hirshman CA, Bergman NA: Halothane and enflurane protect against bronchospasm in an asthma dog model. Anesth Analg 1978;57:629–633.

105. Hirshman CA, Edelstein G, Peetz S, et al: Mechanism of action of inhalational anesthesia on airways. Anesthesiology 1982;56:107–111.

106. Darioli R, Perret C: Mechanical controlled hypoventilation in status asthmaticus. Am Rev Respir Dis 1984;129:385–387.

107. Dworkin G, Kattan M: Mechanical ventilation for status asthmaticus in children. J Pediatr 1989;114:545–549.

108. Gay PC, Patel HG, Nelson SB, et al: Metered dose inhalers for bronchodilator delivery in intubated, mechanically ventilated patients. Chest 1991;99:66–71.

109. Taylor RH, Lerman J: High-efficiency delivery of salbutamol with a metered-dose inhaler in narrow tracheal tubes and catheters. Anesthesiology 1991;74:360–363.

110. Todres ID: Asthma and status asthmaticus. Semin Anesth 1984;3:98–105.

111. Witte MK, Hill JH, Blumer JL: Shock in the pediatric patient. Adv Pediatr 1987;34:139–173.

112. Presson RGJ, Haselby KA, Bezruczko AP, et al: Evaluation of a new high-efficiency blood warmer for children. Anesthesiology 1990;73:173–176.

113. Dutky PA, Stevens SL, Maull KI: Factors affecting rapid fluid resuscitation with large-bore introducer catheters. J Trauma 1989;29:856–860.

114. Virgilio RW, Rice CL, Smith DE, et al: Crystalloid vs. colloid resuscitation: Is one better? A randomized clinical study. Surgery 1979;85:129–139.

115. Kallen RJ, Lonergan JM: Fluid resuscitation of acute hypovolemic hypoperfusion states in pediatrics. Pediatr Clin North Am 1990;37:287–294.

116. Davies MJ: Crystalloid or colloid: Does it matter? J Clin Anesth 1989;1:464–471.

117. Puri VK: Colloid versus crystalloid war: A time for truce. Crit Care Med 1990;18:457–458.

118. Redl H, Krosl P, Schlag G, et al: Permeability studies in a hypovolemic traumatic shock model: Comparison of Ringer's lactate and albumin as volume replacement fluids. Resuscitation 1989;17:77–90.

119. Moss GS, Gould SA: Plasma expanders: An update. Am J Surg 1988;155:425–434.

120. Gammage G: Crystalloid versus colloid: Is colloid worth the cost? Int Anesthesiol Clin 1987;25:37–60.

121. Tranbaugh RF, Lewis FR: Crystalloid versus colloid for fluid resuscitation of hypovolemic patients. Adv Shock Res 1983;9:203–216.

122. Todres ID, Crone RK, Rogers MC, et al: Swan-Ganz catheterization in the critically ill newborn. Crit Care Med 1979;7:330–334.

123. Crone RK: Acute circulatory failure in children. Pediatr Clin North Am 1980;27:525–538.

124. Wong VK, Hitchcock W, Mason WH: Meningococcal infections in children: A review of 100 cases. Pediatr Infect Dis J 1989;8:224–227.

125. Lees MH, King DH: Cardiogenic shock in the neonate. Pediatr Rev 1988;9:258–266.

126. Perkin RM, Levin DL: Shock in the pediatric patient. Part II. Therapy. J Pediatr 1982;101:319–332.

127. Bone RC, Fisher CJJ, Clemmer TP, et al: A controlled clinical trial of high-dose methylprednisolone in the treatment of severe sepsis and septic shock. N Engl J Med 1987;317:653–658.

128. Novembre E, Cianferoni A, Bernardini R, et al: Anaphylaxis in children: Clinical and allergologic features. Pediatrics 1998;101:E8.

129. Fisher MM, Baldo BA: Acute anaphylactic reactions. Med J Aust 1988;149:34–38.

130. Fisher M: Anaphylaxis. Dis Mon 1987;33:433–479.

131. Netzel MC: Anaphylaxis: clinical presentation, immunologic mechanisms, and treatment. J Emerg Med 1986;4:227–236.

132. Goldberg M: Systemic reactions to intravascular contrast media: A guide for the anesthesiologist. Anesthesiology 1984;60:46–56.

133. Cohan RH, Dunnick NR, Bashore TM: Treatment of reactions to radiographic contrast material. AJR Am J Roentgenol 1988;151:263–270.

134. Bush WH: Treatment of systemic reactions to contrast media. Urology 1990;35:145–150.

135. Lieberman P: The use of antihistamines in the prevention and treatment of anaphylaxis and anaphylactoid reactions. J Allergy Clin Immunol 1990;86:684–686.

136. Levy JH: Allergic reactions during anesthesia. J Clin Anesth 1988;1:39–46.

137. Cremer R, Kleine-Diepenbruck U, Hoppe A, et al: Latex allergy in spina bifida patients: Prevention by primary prophylaxis. Allergy 1998;53:709–711.

138. Kwittken PL, Sweinberg SK, Campbell DE, et al: Latex hypersensitivity in children: Clinical presentation and detection of latex-specific immunoglobulin E. Pediatrics 1995;95:693–699.

139. Anonymous: Anaphylactic reactions during general anesthesia among pediatric patients: United States, January 1990–January 1991. MMWR Morb Mortal Wkly Rep 1991;40:437.

140. Swartz JS, Gold M, Braude BM, et al: Intraoperative anaphylaxis to latex: An identifiable population at risk. Can J Anaesth 1990;37:589–592.

141. Gerber AC, Jorg W, Zbinden S, et al: Severe intraoperative anaphylaxis to surgical gloves: Latex allergy, an unfamiliar condition. Anesthesiology 1989;71:800–802.

142. Axelsson IG, Eriksson M, Wrangsjo K: Anaphylaxis and angioedema due to rubber allergy in children. Acta Paediatr Scand 1988;77:314–316.

143. Birmingham PK, Dsida RM, Grayhack JJ, et al: Do latex precautions in children with myelodysplasia reduce intraoperative allergic reactions? J Pediatr Orthop 1996;16:799–802.

144. Cantani A: Latex allergy in children. J Investig Allergol Clin Immunol 1999;9:14–20.

145. Dibs SD, Baker MD: Anaphylaxis in children: A 5–year experience. Pediatrics 1997;99:E7.

146. Means LJ, Rescorla FJ: Latex anaphylaxis: Report of occurrence in two pediatric surgical patients and review of the literature. J Pediatr Surg 1995;30:748–751.

147. Pittman T, Kiburz J, Gabriel K, et al: Latex allergy in children with spina bifida. Pediatr Neurosurg 1995;22:96–100.

148. Kelly KJ, Pearson ML, Kurup VP, et al: A cluster of anaphylactic reactions in children with spina bifida during general anesthesia: Epidemiologic features, risk factors, and latex hypersensitivity. J Allergy Clin Immunol 1994;94:53–61.

149. D'Agostino J, Terndrup TE: Comparative review of the adverse effects of sedatives used in children undergoing outpatient procedures. Drug Safety 1996;14:146–157.

150. Graves NM, Kreil RL: Rectal administration of antiepileptic drugs in children. Pediatr Neurol 1987;3:321–326.

151. Uthman BM, Wilder BJ: Emergency management of seizures: An overview. Epilepsia 1989;30:S33–S37.

152. Agurell S, Berlin A, Ferngren H, et al: Plasma levels of diazepam after parenteral and rectal administration in children. Epilepsia 1975;16:277–283.

153. Young RS, Ropper AH, Hawkes D, et al: Pentobarbital in refractory status epilepticus. Pediatr Pharmacol (New York) 1983;3:63–67.

154. Rashkin MC, Youngs C, Penovich P: Pentobarbital treatment of refractory status epilepticus. Neurology 1987;37:500–503.

155. Tasker RC, Boyd SG, Harden A, et al: EEG monitoring of prolonged thiopentone administration for intractable seizures and status epilepticus in infants and young children. Neuropediatrics 1989;20:147–153.

156. Mitchell WG: Status epilepticus and acute repetitive seizures in children, adolescents, and young adults: Etiology, outcome, and treatment. Epilepsia 1996;37:S74–S80.

157. Kofke WA, Young RS, Davis P, et al: Isoflurane for refractory status epilepticus: A clinical series. Anesthesiology 1989;71:653–659.

158. Truog RD, Rice SA: Inorganic fluoride and prolonged isoflurane anesthesia in the intensive care unit. Anesth Analg 1989;69:843–845.

159. Kong KL, Tyler JE, Willatts SM, et al: Isoflurane sedation for patients undergoing mechanical ventilation: Metabolism to inorganic fluoride and renal effects. Br J Anaesth 1990;64:159–162.

160. Breheny FX: Inorganic fluoride in prolonged isoflurane sedation. Anaesthesia 1992;47:32–33.

161. Fazen LE, Lovejoy FHJ, Crone RK: Acute poisoning in a children's hospital: A 2–year experience. Pediatrics 1986;77:144–151.

162. Jaraczewska W, Kotwica M: Acute poisonings with drugs: A review of the data collected at the National Poison Information Centre during the period 1991–1995. Przegl Lek 1997;54:737–740.

163. Gawin FH, Ellinwood EHJ: Cocaine and other stimulants: Actions, abuse, and treatment. N Engl J Med 1988;318:1173–1182.

164. Cregler LL, Mark H: Medical complications of cocaine abuse. N Engl J Med 1986;315:1495–1500.

165. Berlin CMJ: Advances in pediatric pharmacology and toxicology. Adv Pediatr 1989;36:431–459.

166. Holazo AA, Colburn WA: Pharmacokinetics of drugs during various detoxification procedures for overdose and environmental exposure. Drug Metab Rev 1982;13:715–743.

167. Vertrees JE, McWilliams BC, Kelly HW: Repeated oral administration of activated charcoal for treating aspirin overdose in young children. Pediatrics 1990;85:594–598.

168. Farley TA: Severe hypernatremic dehydration after use of an activated charcoal-sorbitol suspension. J Pediatr 1986;109:719–722.

169. Newberger EH: Child abuse. In: Rosenberg ML, Fenley MA, eds: Violence in America. New York: Oxford University Press; 1991:51–78.

170. Hall JR, Reyes HM, Horvat M, et al: The mortality of childhood falls. J Trauma 1989;29:1273–1275.

171. Velcek FT, Weiss A, DiMaio D, et al: Traumatic death in urban children. J Pediatr Surg 1977;12:375–384.

172. Tepas JJ, DiScala C, Ramenofsky ML, et al: Mortality and head injury: The pediatric perspective. J Pediatr Surg 1990;25:92–95.

173. Tepas JJ, Ramenofsky ML, Barlow B, et al: National Pediatric Trauma Registry. J Pediatr Surg 1989;24:156–158.
174. Rivara FP: Traumatic deaths of children in the United States: Currently available prevention strategies. Pediatrics 1985;75:456–462.
175. Cantor RM, Leaming JM: Evaluation and management of pediatric major trauma. Emerg Med Clin North Am 1998;16:229–256.
176. Knapp JF: Practical issues in the care of pediatric trauma patients. Curr Prob Pediatr 1998;28:309–320.
177. Steichen FM: Emergency management of the severely injured child. In: Ravitch MM, Welch KJ, Benson CD, et al., eds: Pediatric Surgery. 3rd ed. Chicago: Year Book Medical Publishers; 1979:101–109.
178. Amoroso TA: Evaluation of the patient with blunt abdominal trauma: An evidence-based approach. Emerg Med Clin North Am 1999;17:63–75.
179. Fallis JC: Multiple injuries. In: Black JA, ed: Paediatric Emergencies, 2nd ed. Kent: Butterworth & Co; 1987:15–31.
180. Welsh KJ: Abdominal injuries. In: Ravitch MM, Welch KJ, Benson CD, et al., eds: Pediatric Surgery, 3rd ed. Chicago: Year Book Medical Publishers; 1979:125–148.
181. Swain A, Dove J, Baker H: ABC of major trauma: Trauma of the spine and spinal cord—I. Br Med J 1990;301:34–38.
182. Coté CJ, Jobes DR, Schwartz AJ, et al: Two approaches to cannulation of a child's internal jugular vein. Anesthesiology 1979;50:371–373.
183. Todres ID, Rogers MC, Shannon DC, et al: Percutaneous catheterization of the radial artery in the critically ill neonate. J Pediatr 1975;87:273–275.
184. Bogetz MS, Katz JA: Recall of surgery for major trauma. Anesthesiology 1984;61:6–9.

16 Pediatric Trauma

Aleksandra J. Mazurek *and* Steven C. Hall

Prehospital Care

Emergency Room Care

Initial Assessment (Primary Survey)

    A—Airway

    B—Breathing

    C—Circulation

    D—Disability

    E—Exposure

Vascular Access

    Fluid Resuscitation

Temperature Maintenance

Secondary Survey

    Organ Injury

Diagnostic Procedures and In-Hospital Transport

Interhospital Transfer

Preparation for Operative Procedure

Child Abuse

Summary

The leading cause of death in children over 1 year of age is accidents.[1] Behind this well-known fact are complex societal, governmental, and medical issues that contribute to pediatric morbidity and mortality.[2, 3] Despite the known dangers from falls, burns, violence related to drug abuse or addiction,[4–11] motor vehicle accidents, and firearms,[12–18] little effective investment has been made in the improvement of the environment that our children inhabit.[19–24] Although there are major issues in the United States, these same issues as they relate to children arise worldwide. The available tools of legislation, public education, social service agencies, medical triage systems, and research have been only sparingly used to attack these issues, with little effect on outcomes.[25]

There is a relative paucity of research in pediatric trauma.[26] Instead, the principles of adult trauma care are generally applied to the pediatric population.[27] There is also very little information on the long-term effects of trauma on physical and psychological growth and development.[28, 29]

The majority of pediatric trauma care occurs in the setting of general-purpose hospitals; regionalization of pediatric trauma care to designated pediatric centers has occurred in some major urban centers, but this is the exception rather than the rule.[30–34] Consequently, it is important for all anesthesiologists to be aware of the specific differences and needs of pediatric trauma patients compared with adult trauma patients. The epidemiology of pediatric trauma is different than that of adult trauma; this chapter describes the major differences between adult and pediatric trauma care. The management of children with burn injuries is described in Chapter 23.

The first difference between adult and pediatric trauma is that blunt trauma is much more common in children.[35–37] This demands that imaging facilities and resuscitative protocols be attuned to the nature of blunt injury evaluation in children. Second, closed head injury is more common in pediatric trauma. Mortality and morbidity increase dramatically in the presence of central nervous system (CNS) trauma, which is the predominant cause of death.[13, 38–40] Third, child abuse (sexual and physical assault) is a significant cause of pediatric trauma.[41–55] Because these children are often recognized by the medical system only after significant, sometimes repeated, injury, the mortality and morbidity of this form of trauma is high.[51–55] It is vital that all anesthesiologists be vigilant in terms of recognizing patterns of injury associated with child abuse such as extensive or unexpected bruises or burns, bite marks, welts, old rib or long bone fractures, and signs of sexual molestation.[42–49, 56–60] Lastly, the time pattern of mortality and morbidity in children is similar to that in adults.[61]

Initial mortality, comprising up to 50% of all trauma deaths, occurs at the scene of trauma from massive organ disruption or bleeding.[62] The second peak in mortality occurs 1 to 4 hours after injury, usually from progressive intracranial edema or hemorrhage, intra-abdominal and intrathoracic hemorrhage, or progressive hypoxemia from lung or airway trauma. The third peak in mortality occurs several days to weeks later, usually from sepsis and multiorgan failure. This trimodal distribution of mortality observed in adults is similar in children and is subject to the same issues for improvement of care. Rapid and efficient stabilization and transport in the field are crucial, followed by thorough in-hospital evaluation and definitive therapy, as well as meticulous periodic reexamination.

Prehospital Care

Effective care of the injured child begins at the site of injury. First aid may be administered by a witness to the accident, but initial care is often delayed until the local Emergency Medical Services (EMS) is contacted and emergency medical technicians (EMTs) arrive. The EMS response usually consists of an ambulance staffed by EMTs trained in Advanced Life Support techniques. The response time, transport time, and the level of expertise of paramedical personnel vary dramatically between locales.[63] In general, within the United States, physicians do not participate in prehospital care of the injured, but follow the military-developed principle of "scoop and run," delivering the patient to a health care facility as quickly as possible.[64] European and Canadian EMS employ physicians in the field, allowing them to provide a higher level of evaluation and treatment at the scene.[65] The two different approaches each have advantages. More extensive treatment at the scene may reverse life-threatening conditions, such as hemorrhage, in an expeditious fashion.[66, 67] However, there is a tendency to prolong the time elapsed between the accident and definitive care with this approach; this delay has been shown to be a strong factor in survival prediction of an accident victim.[68, 69] In addition, the lesser frequency of pediatric trauma (1:10) versus adult trauma provides fewer opportunities for EMTs to develop and maintain their skills in caring for the injured child.[30, 31, 70] Age- and size-appropriate equipment may not always be available.

Initial evaluation and resuscitation is often limited to the ABCs of basic life support.[71] The goal of basic life support is to ensure the adequacy of **A**-airway, **B**-breathing, and **C**-circulation. It is important to remember that the majority of out-of-hospital pediatric cardiac arrests are not primary presenting events, but the result of hemorrhage, hypoxemia, sepsis, or metabolic disorders.[72] The presence of cardiac arrest before transport to the hospital is an ominous sign. A child who is apneic and pulseless on arrival at an Emergency Department has a very high likelihood of neurologic morbidity or mortality.[73] One study has shown that an apneic and pulseless pediatric trauma victim has virtually no chance of survival if the duration of cardiac arrest exceeds 20 minutes or if more than two doses of epinephrine are required for resuscitation,[74] even if open-chest cardiopulmonary resuscitation is employed. Open-chest massage may be best reserved for penetrating chest trauma or blunt injury with vital signs present, but deteriorating in the course of resuscitation.[75, 76]

Endotracheal intubation performed on the scene, or in any emergency circumstance by non-anesthesiologists, is accompanied by a high rate of complications such as failure to intubate (2–20%), endobronchial intubation, or severe desaturation.[63, 77, 78] The success rate for endotracheal intubation at the site of the event is very dependent on the medical training and direction of the EMTs.[63] It is difficult to determine whether airway management at the site of injury is associated with more complications in pediatric patients because of the diversity of studies in the literature. EMTs also have difficulty when attempting to insert an intravenous line[67]; one paper reported a very high failure rate among EMTs when dealing with patients 1 to 18 months of age; the success rate improved after further training.[79] These studies reinforce the need for periodic retraining of EMS personnel in pediatric techniques.[80, 81] Anesthesiologists can play a key role in the education and training of EMTs in the controlled environment of the operating room.

Emergency Room Care

Pediatric trauma systems were established throughout the United States in the 1980s because evidence suggested that children did not fare well in the adult trauma systems.[82–86] Although it is preferred to transport children to a Level 1 Pediatric Trauma Center,[30] data indicate that children can do well in adult trauma centers, provided they are given competent care.[34, 87–89] This suggests that there has been improved training in the care of children in adult trauma centers. There is also indication that combined teams of adult and pediatric trauma experts can accomplish results comparable to fully staffed pediatric trauma centers.[33, 90, 91] Consequently, an emphasis should be placed on ensuring that all trauma centers are well prepared for the pediatric patient instead of necessarily establishing separate pediatric systems in each community.

The Emergency Department that accepts pediatric trauma patients should have a minimum configuration to promote effective and efficient care.[92] Dedicated trauma rooms should be set up with equipment that provides the capacity to serve as an ad hoc operating room, should the situation call for it, or to become an additional operating room in case of a disaster (Table 16–1). Suction, lighting, electrical outlets, scrub sinks, and adequate space are all important components of this facility. A rapid method for estimating drug doses and airway management devices for children of all

Table 16–1. Recommended Equipment for a Trauma Room

Airway equipment
    Appropriate sizes (newborn to adult) of endotracheal tubes, oral airways, and nasal airways
    Self-inflating ventilating device capable of administering at least 90% oxygen
    Anesthesia type bag and mask
    Difficult airway kit (see Table 7–7)
    Jet ventilator
Equipment to monitor
    Noninvasive blood pressure, with appropriately sized cuffs
    Pulse oximetry
    Capnograph or similar device to detect exhaled carbon dioxide (see Fig. 16–3)
    Temperature
    Direct arterial and central venous pressures
Surgical instruments
    Tracheostomy tray
    Thoracostomy tray
    Thoracotomy tray
    Vascular tray
Resuscitation ("crash") cart with all medications for prolonged resuscitation
Vascular access equipment, including intraosseous needles (see Fig. 16–4)
Visibly displayed charts allowing easy dosage of resuscitation medications (Broselow tape)
Pediatric Trauma Score (see Table 16–2)
Glasgow Coma Scale (see Table 16–3)
Pediatric Modified Glasgow Trauma Scale
Universal precaution equipment
Infusion pumps capable of delivering the small volumes
External warming devices
Blood warming devices

sizes is the Broselow tape; preliminary investigations suggest a possible role for this easy to use system.[93–95] These types of adjuncts for emergency care may prove to be particularly useful for emergency departments that only occasionally receive pediatric trauma patients.

The Emergency Department is the scene of highly stressful and definitive activities, the success of which depends largely on *how well the team is trained* because trauma care is a team task.[30] The roles of all participants have to be known, assigned, and rehearsed.[96] In the United States, the role of Team Leader is usually assumed by a trauma surgeon or emergency medicine physician, whereas in Europe, an anesthesiologist is often in charge. However, it is important that all involved physicians, nurses, and other personnel be incorporated in the planning, training, and re-evaluation of each member's role in the specific care of pediatric trauma patients. Such skills are, in part, gained by specially designed curricula, such as Advanced Trauma Life Support (ATLS), Pediatric Advanced Life Support (PALS), and Advanced Pediatric Life Support (APLS).[97–99] There is evidence that introducing ATLS to medical practice is making an impact on the survival of trauma victims.[100–104]

Besides readily available courses, there are sophisticated computer and video programs that offer training and preparation in decision-making paths and role rehearsal, such as the Level One Trauma Simulator being developed at the Maryland Institute for Emergency Medical Services in Baltimore.[105–107] Simulators may be able to provide an opportunity to practice the likely sequence of critical events (much like airplane pilot training) in a learning environment. Because of the erratic and seasonal nature of trauma, not everyone has the same opportunity to practice "live," making the use of a simulator a potentially important advance in training.[96, 108]

Initial Assessment (Primary Survey)

The assessment aspects of ATLS and PALS start with an initial assessment of basic life functions (the "A, B, C, D, E guide"). Only after basic life functions are satisfactorily assessed and treated (the primary survey) does further workup proceed (the secondary survey) with a head-to-toe examination of all organs. Certain procedures often occur simultaneously, such as starting an intravenous line and evaluating the airway while at the same time applying pressure on a bleeding scalp wound. This systematic approach to evaluation and reevaluation promotes observation of the most important functions that are at risk in the trauma patient. A variety of scoring systems have been developed to help predict the need for surgical interventions, intensive care, and long-term outcomes (Tables 16–2, 16–3, 16–4). Although these scoring systems have some use, *the most important principle is to continuously reevaluate patients rather than simply score the severity of their illness.*[109-117]

A—Airway

As a member of the Trauma Team, the anesthesiologist is generally responsible for airway management. Chin lift, jaw thrust, insertion of nasal or oral airways, bag and mask ventilation, and positive end expiratory pressure are the simplest recommended maneuvers to relieve airway obstruction and assure adequate oxygenation and ventilation. These should be performed without neck manipulation. Since the majority of pediatric multiple trauma victims suffer head injury (up to 95%), injury of the cervical spine must be considered present until ruled out.[111, 118, 119] Ideally, the patient's entire body should be immobilized on a spine board, a rigid cervical collar applied, and the head and neck strapped to the board between sandbags. This reduces the body mobility to 5% of normal.[120] Unfortunately, this immobilization may make bag and mask ventilation and intubation more difficult.[121] The front of the collar and strapping should be removed prior to attempted intubation and replaced with manual *in-line immobilization* (Fig. 16–1). *In-line traction is potentially harmful and should be avoided.* Direct laryngoscopy can disturb the integrity of the cervical spine. Axial traction stretches the spinal cord and has been reported to cause sudden worsening of neurologic signs.[122] Consequently, it is appropriate that trained personnel have independent responsibility to provide in-line stabilization during laryngoscopy and intubation (Fig. 16–2).

Trauma victims are assumed to have a full stomach and should be treated as such. In adults, awake intubation is a

Table 16–2. Pediatric Trauma Score

	+2	+1	−1	Score
Size	>20 kg	10–20 kg	<10 kg	
Airway	Normal	Maintainable	Unmaintainable	
Systolic Blood Pressure	>90 mm Hg	90–50 mm Hg	<50 mm Hg	
Central Nervous System	Awake	Obtunded/loss of consciousness	Comatose	
Open Wound	None	Minor	Major/penetrating	
Skeletal	None	Closed fracture	Open/multiple fracture	
			Total	

Maximum score + 12 = minor injury; minimum score − 6 = lethal injury.

Table 16–3. Glasgow Coma Scale

		Time	Field	ADM			DCHG
EYE OPENING	SPONTANEOUS	4					
	VERBAL COMMAND (to speech)	3					
	PAINFUL STIMULI (to pain only)	2					
	NO RESPONSE	1					
BEST VERBAL RESPONSE	ORIENTED (coos, babbles)	5					
	CONFUSED CONVERSATION (irritable)	4					
	INAPPROPRIATE WORDS (cries to pain)	3					
	INCOMPREHENSIBLE SOUNDS (moans to pain)	2					
	NO RESPONSE	1					
BEST MOTOR RESPONSE	OBEYS SIMPLE COMMANDS (normal movement)	6					
	LOCALIZED TO PAINFUL STIMULI	5					
	WITHDRAWS FROM PAINFUL STIMULI	4					
	ABNORMAL FLEXION RESPONSE	3					
	ABNORMAL EXTENSION RESPONSE	2					
	NO RESPONSE	1					
	TOTAL						

Total score = sum of eye opening + best motor response + best verbal response (minimum score = 3).
From Bryan J, Teasdale G: Aspects of coma after severe head injury. Lancet 1977;1:878–881.

viable option to secure the airway. Pediatric patients, especially those with head injury, changing level of consciousness, and presumed increased intracranial pressure, are *rarely* candidates for awake intubation because of the potential for raising the intracranial pressure further. Medications to reduce anxiety and pain are important adjuncts during securing of the airway. The use of drugs in emergency airway management in children by non-anesthesiologists was found to be appropriate in only 15% of cases, with sedatives and muscle relaxants often being omitted when indicated.[123, 124] Anesthesiologists should help educate EMTs and emergency medicine physicians in the use and selection of medications to facilitate endotracheal intubation (Table 16–5).[125] Only flaccid patients without vital signs can be intubated without pharmacologic aid; other children will benefit from a rapid-sequence induction. To perform rapid-sequence induction most efficiently, there may be a need for up to four people; one to intubate, one to apply cricoid pressure, one to assist with the endotracheal and suction tubes, and one to inject the drugs and watch monitors (see Fig. 16–2). Emergency endotracheal intubation performed by non-anesthesiologists carries complication rates as high as 44% in the pediatric trauma population; improvement occurs with better medical

training.[67, 77, 79, 124, 126, 127] It should be noted that although succinylcholine is the muscle relaxant with the desired combination of rapid onset and short duration, high-dose rocuronium (1.2 mg/kg) offers a reasonable alternative when succinylcholine is potentially contraindicated.[127] It should be further noted that succinylcholine and all drugs for resuscitation can be administered through an intraosseous needle when intravenous access is not available (Fig. 16–3). The onset of succinylcholine by this route is only slightly longer than following standard intravenous administration, but is much sooner than after intramuscular administration.[128]

The Emergency Department, Intensive Care Units, and Operating Room should have equipment present to deal with the potential failed intubation.[73] A "difficult airway box" containing special airway equipment, such as laryngeal mask airways, special laryngoscope blades, retrograde intubation set, and cricothyrotomy equipment for pediatric patients of all sizes and ages, should be present (see Table 7–7).

Surgical cricothyrotomy performed by non-surgeons, considered an emergency step in adults[129] in the difficult airway algorithm, is not recommended in children owing to the high incidence of laryngeal morbidity and poor success with later laryngeal reconstruction.[98] In infants, the cricothyroid mem-

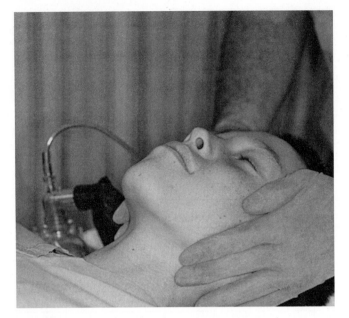

Figure 16–1. In-line stabilization prior to attempts at laryngoscopy should be made so that the head is stabilized and prevented from rotating from side to side as well as from flexing and extending. Note: no traction should be placed on the cervical spine, as this is associated with an increase in neurologic deficits in patients with proven cervical fracture.

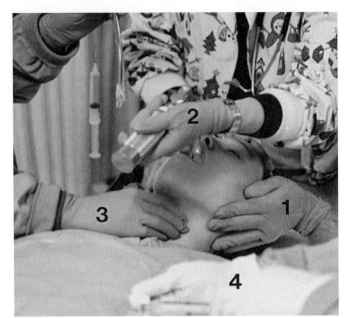

Figure 16–2. Intubation of a patient with a cervical fracture may require up to four individuals: one to provide in-line stabilization (1); a second to perform the intubation (2); a third to perform cricoid pressure and either hold the endotracheal tube or retract the cheek for the individual performing the intubation (3); and a fourth to administer the drugs (4).

brane may be very close to the sternal notch, making access difficult. Needle (intravenous catheter) cricothyrotomy is considered the procedure of choice when all other methods for providing oxygenation have failed (see Figs. 7–23 to 7–25). Cricothyroidotomy equipment, including a jet ventilator, must be readily available to be useful in the life-threatening situation of total airway obstruction.[130] Anyone who undertakes the use of such equipment must understand how it functions to avoid making a bad situation worse by causing massive subcutaneous emphysema.[131–133]

B—Breathing

Correct placement of the endotracheal tube following intubation must be ensured. The presence of bilateral, equal breath sounds and chest expansion, exhaled moisture within the endotracheal tube, the presence of exhaled CO_2 (Fig. 16–4), adequate oxygenation, and the absence of air passage sounds over the stomach confirm correct placement.[134] Unilateral absence of breath sounds demands rapid diagnosis and prompt intervention to rule out an endobronchial intubation, pneumothorax, or hemothorax.

Repeat direct laryngoscopy and adjustment of endotracheal tube position is a relatively easy task and should be carried out if there is any question about the correct placement of the endotracheal tube. A chest radiograph is ordered upon patient arrival to the Emergency Department, and al-

Figure 16–3. Examples of equipment used for intraosseous access. Note that any spinal type needle could be used for this procedure if specialized equipment is not available.

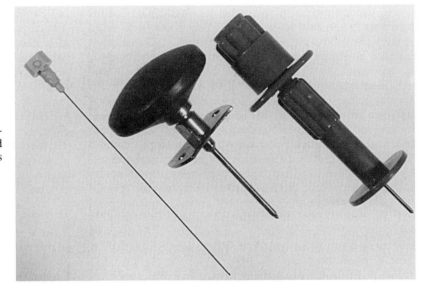

Table 16–4. Modification of Glasgow Coma Scale for Pediatric Patients

Eye Opening Response

Score	>1 Year	<1 Year
4	Spontaneous	Spontaneous
3	To verbal command	To shout
2	To pain	To pain
1	None	None

Motor Response

Score	>1 Year	<1 Year
6	Obeys commands	Spontaneous
5	Localizes pain	Localizes pain
4	Withdraws to pain	Withdraws to pain
3	Abnormal flexion to pain (decorticate)	Abnormal flexion to pain (decorticate)
2	Abnormal extension to pain (decorticate)	Abnormal extension to pain (decorticate)
1	None	None

Verbal Response

Score	>5 Years	2–5 Years	0–2 Years
5	Oriented and converses	Appropriate words, phrases	Babbles, coos appropriately
4	Confused conversation	Inappropriate words	Cries but is consolable
3	Inappropriate words	Persistent crying or screaming to pain	Persistent crying or screaming to pain
2	Incomprehensive sounds	Grunts or moans to pain	Grunts or moans to pain
1	None	None	None

Severe, <9; moderate, 9–12; mild, 13–15.

Table 16–5. Rapid Sequence Intubation Medications

Medication	Dose/Route	Use/Precautions
Atropine	0.01–0.02 mg/kg IV (0.15 mg minimum dose)	Reduces vagal response; flushed/dry skin, palpitations, mild hyperpyrexia
Lidocaine	1 mg/kg IV	Intracranial pressure control, reduces hemodynamic response to intubation
Fentanyl	1–3 μg/kg, IV	Use in combination with midazolam for analgesia during intubation and/or to help provide analgesia for surgical problems
Midazolam	0.1–0.2 mg/kg IV	Sedation, amnesia, anxiolysis; may cause hypotension when combined with opioid in hypovolemic patients
Thiopental	3–5 mg/kg IV	Sedative/hypnotic may decrease blood pressure, increase heart rate, decrease cardiac output; generally avoided in hypovolemic patients
Ketamine (in lieu of thiopental if blood pressure is unstable)	1–2 mg/kg IV	Used when central venous stability is in question; may increase intracranial pressure (not for use with head trauma); administer atropine or glycopyrrolate to avoid secretions
Succinylcholine	<4 years: 2 mg/kg IV >4 years: 1 mg/kg IV	Depolarizing, short-acting muscle relaxant; CAUTION: DO NOT USE if previous history suggests complications after its use, if potassium over 5.5, or if patient has medical problem associated with hyperkalemia, e.g. muscular dystrophy, crush or burn injury >48 hours earlier
Rocuronium	1.2 mg/kg	May be substituted for succinylcholine

Maintaining Cervical Spine Control During Intubation

The patient with a cervical spine injury requiring an artificial airway should be intubated under controlled circumstances prior to transport. A neurosurgeon or the primary trauma service physician should stabilize the head and neck during intubation. Oral intubation is the preferred route unless basilar skull fractures and facial injuries have been ruled out.

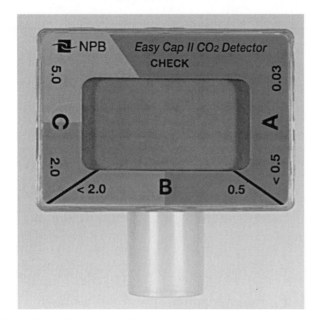

Figure 16–4. The confirmation of appropriate endotracheal intubation is best accomplished by a measurement of exhaled CO_2. When a capnograph is unavailable, portable products can be used, such as the Easy Cap II (Mallinckrodt, Inc., Pleasanton, CA), which has a dead space of 25 mL and is generally indicated for patients weighing more than 15 kg, or the PediCap (Mallinckrodt Inc., Pleasanton, CA), which has a dead space of 3 mL and is used for patients who weigh 1 to 15 kg.

ways obtained after endotracheal intubation. Pneumothorax and hemothorax are diagnosed by physical examination or chest radiograph, or both, and treated by thoracostomy.

C—Circulation

Evaluation and stabilization of the circulation implies:

1. Control of obvious hemorrhage
2. Initial evaluation of heart rate, rhythm, blood pressure, peripheral pulses, and perfusion
3. Establishment of intravenous access, in general, using at least two large-bore cannulas, with at least one in the upper extremity (should there be a laceration of the inferior vena cava).
4. Intravenous fluid administration, as needed, to restore blood pressure and heart rate to a normal range. A bolus of 10 mL/kg of balanced salt solution (without glucose) is given initially, then repeated once or twice, as needed. If there is a poor response, colloids, blood, and blood components are employed. If there is no response or an inadequate response to volume loading, vasopressors may be indicated, with epinephrine usually the first choice. A bolus of 5 to 10 µg/kg is indicated and repeated depending on the severity of hemodynamic compromise. Later, other inotropics (dopamine, dobutamine) are substituted as appropriate for the clinical situation. The patient should be repeatedly evaluated, especially if inotropics or vasopressors are needed. It should be determined why volume replacement is not, in itself, adequate to maintain adequate circulation. Factors such as undetected hemorrhages, myocardial contusion, pericardial tamponade, or pneumothorax should be considered in the child who continues to need vasopressors or inotropic support to maintain adequate blood pressure and cardiac output. A nasogastric tube should be inserted after the airway is stable and vascular access is secured to evacuate gastric contents. A urinary catheter should be inserted early in the process of resuscitation to aid in assessment of volume replacement and renal perfusion.

D—Disability

Disability refers to the abbreviated neurologic evaluation that can serve as a baseline for later assessments. ATLS recommends evaluation, as demonstrated by the acronym AVPU.

A—Awareness
V—response to Verbal stimuli
P—response to Pain
U—Unresponsive

The initial evaluation should be clearly recorded so that subsequent evaluations can use this as a baseline for comparison.

E—Exposure

Exposure refers to the necessity of removing all the garments to allow the entire body to be examined, including the posterior aspect. Great care must be exercised to turn the patient as a single unit ("log-rolling") to avoid potential spine injury.

Vascular Access

Vascular access in children, especially a child with poor perfusion, is challenging; the most difficult age group is from 0 to 18 months.[67, 79] Many techniques of obtaining central and peripheral vascular access in children have been described, but all require practice to achieve success (see Chapter 32). The intraosseous infusion technique, first used in the 1950s and later forgotten, has made a remarkable comeback in pediatric practice.[135, 136] The PALS curriculum first included it in its course in 1988, with advanced cardiac life support (ACLS) and ATLS following.[137] The 1994 revision of PALS contains the recommendation that *"intraosseous access should be established if reliable venous access cannot be achieved within three attempts or 90 seconds, whichever comes first."* The technique is simple, is easy to learn, and has a high rate of success even in the hands of nonphysicians (see Fig. 32–4).[138] It is most suitable for patients younger than the age of 6 years and is easiest to place in the anterior tibia. Intraosseous access can be used for administration of any drug or fluid needed for initial resuscitation, but should be replaced by a peripheral or central intravenous line as soon as possible.[81, 139–147] Access can be gained using specifically designed intraosseous needles, a bone marrow biopsy needle, or *any* styletted needle.

Blood should be drawn for type and crossmatch and laboratory data (complete blood count, amylase, coagulation profile, ionized calcium, glucose, electrolytes, and others, as appropriate) at the same time that venous cannulation takes place. Obtaining central venous access is not generally recommended in the *initial assessment* phase of pediatric resuscitation. Attempts at central venous cannulation bear a significant complication rate in children and should be attempted only by individuals trained in this technique (see Chapter 32).[148, 149] Consideration may be given to performing a femoral vein cutdown at the bedside if rapid access to a large vessel is needed or if, at further stages of care, central venous pressure monitoring is considered necessary. The object is to achieve effective vascular access in the most expeditious and conservative way. Peripheral venous cannulation usually best fulfills this condition.[150] Arterial blood gases are obtained as soon as an artery is cannulated and are important for ongoing evaluation of oxygenation, ventilation, and metabolic status. Portable equipment is available that can measure arterial blood gases, electrolytes, ionized calcium, hemoglobin, and glucose in less than 3 minutes with only 0.5 mL of blood.

Fluid Resuscitation

Crystalloid Solutions

Crystalloid solutions are the first intravenous fluids administered to the injured patient. However, owing to the high incidence of head injury among pediatric trauma victims, special consideration should be given to the character of administered crystalloids:

1. *Glucose content.* Experimental evidence, extrapolated to human subjects, suggests that hyperglycemia contributes to the global CNS injury.[151–153] There are limited clinical data describing poor outcome following severe brain injury or hypoxemia when the initial blood glucose levels are in excess of 200 mg/dL.[154–157] Glucose-containing solutions should not be used in the initial resuscitation phase until the presence of head injury is ruled out and hypoxemia is corrected, unless there is a need to treat hypoglycemia. Glucose-containing solutions should not be used for volume replacement but may be administered at maintenance rates to selected patients (see Chapter 11).
2. *Isotonic solutions.* Plasma hypo-osmolality increases brain water content and may cause harm.[158] Therefore, normal saline (0.9% NaCl) or other balanced salt solutions are the most appropriate fluids to administer for initial volume replacement. Administration of isotonic salt solutions, such as 0.9% NaCl, does not increase cerebral edema.[159]
3. *Hypertonic solution (HTS).* Small volumes (3–6 mL/kg) of intravenous hypertonic saline (7.5% NaCl) can be administered as a substitute for the usual 10 to 20 mL/kg lactated Ringer solution in the initial post-CNS trauma period to attract fluids from hyperemic, injured brain regions.[160–168] Fluid redistributes from the intracellular to the intravascular space, providing transient, but significant, blood pressure stabilization and improvement of cardiac performance. This modality of head trauma management (3–6 mL HTS/kg) is undergoing evaluation in the United States but has already become the standard of care for head injury patients in some countries.[160, 169] At least one study in children has demonstrated fewer inten-

sive care unit interventions in children treated with HTS.[160] Until further studies of HTS are completed, the most appropriate crystalloid to be administered to a child with head injury is normal saline, usually administered as a 10 mL/kg bolus and repeated, depending on clinical response.

Blood Products and Blood Substitutes

If the hemodynamic response to crystalloid is not satisfactory, colloids can be employed (5% albumin, Plasma-Lyte or Dextran) until type-specific compatible red blood cells are available. Type O Rh-negative packed red blood cells can be used until type-specific blood is available. Type-specific, crossmatched blood is the ideal choice for red blood cell replacement. It can be substituted by type-specific, partially crossmatched packed red blood cells, or type-specific uncrossmatched blood. However, group O Rh-negative *whole blood* should be avoided if possible. The plasma may contain high anti-A and anti-B titers that may cause hemolysis of the recipient's blood. If a significant volume of type O Rh-negative whole blood or packed red blood cells has been given and it is desired to change to the patient's blood group, anti-A and anti-B titers should be determined before administration (see Table 12–3). Patient identification, specimen labeling, and checking the blood before transfusion are essential, as is constant patient re-evaluation to detect changes secondary to mismatched transfusion at an early stage. It should be stressed that the majority (86%) of fatal hemolytic transfusion reactions are due to clerical error.[170, 171] Fresh frozen plasma, platelets, and other blood products are given only for specific indications, usually after massive transfusion and repeated coagulation profile testing. Blood substitutes (stroma-free hemoglobin and perfluorocarbons) are still undergoing experimental investigation.[172–177] Rapid transfusion requires attention as to the site of infusion, temperature of the fluids, and all the potential complications related to massive transfusion, especially ionized hypocalcemia, hyperkalemia, and hypothermia (see Chapter 12).

Temperature Maintenance

Because of their relatively large surface area, infants and children lose body heat very rapidly. Great effort must be directed at active body warming and fluid heating to prevent heat loss (see Chapter 27). Heating mattresses, heating lights, body wraps, and fluid warmers have been used[178–183]; heating respiratory gases is usually practical only in the operating room or intensive care setting. A heat-moisture exchanger ("artificial nose") between the breathing circuit and endotracheal tube can also reduce heat loss.[184] Forced-air heating devices provide the most effective means for warming patients. Similarly, high-volume intravenous fluid heating devices deliver fluids warmed close to the intravenous port. Some of these fluid-warming devices may present the potential for forming small gas bubbles in the process of fluid warming.[185] A greater likelihood of air embolism is present while using rapid infusion devices, such as Level One (SIMS Level One Technology, Inc., Rockland, MA 02370),[186–190] that must be continually monitored when in use. *Care must be taken to evacuate all air from intravenous fluid bags being administered under pressure.*

Secondary Survey

After initial resuscitation and evaluation of basic life functions, attention is rapidly directed to other potential injuries.[191, 192]

Organ Injury

In the secondary survey, an injured child undergoes a thorough, systematic physical examination from head to toe. Initially, the patient is supine for the inspection, and then "log-rolled" so that the posterior aspect of the body can be examined. Decisions regarding therapy of non-life-threatening wounds and bone fractures are made and immediate care is provided, as needed.

Head and Neck

One of the most important differences between pediatric and adult trauma is that head injury occurs in 75 to 95% of pediatric victims who suffer multiple organ trauma.[193] The cervical spine, although involved only about 10% of the time,[118, 194] is considered injured until proven otherwise. The following protocol has been useful in our institution for initial evaluation of potential cervical spine injury:

1. Cervical spine injury is viewed as "ruled out" in a responsive, 12-year-old or older patient who denies neck pain or tenderness, whose lateral cervical spine radiograph is negative, and who has no peripheral neurologic signs.
2. Patients complaining of neck pain, those who are comatose, or those who are too young to verbalize require:
   a. flexion-extension cervical radiographic series under the supervision of a neurosurgeon to identify instability that otherwise might be missed.[194]
   b. lateral radiograph that exposes the spine from C1 to C7.

The cervical spine is considered unstable until the above criteria are met, and the rigid cervical collar should remain in place.[195] Children younger than 2 years and children with Down syndrome are identified as particularly vulnerable to high C1-C2 injury due to odontoid epiphysiolysis and laxity of the ligaments.[194, 196–198]

A child's brain is poorly protected by the thin cranial bones and, therefore, is very susceptible to closed head injury. The relatively large head fixed on a relatively weak neck structure is subject to huge forces during an acceleration-deceleration event, such as a motor vehicle collision. Children can exhibit malignant brain edema, the result of post-traumatic hyperemia, which manifests within hours of injury and may cause a responsive patient to go into a deep coma within a short period of time. This means that although a child may initially appear awake and alert, there can be dramatic changes in mental status within a short time frame.[40, 199–202]

Initial treatment of the CNS-injured patient is directed at avoiding secondary injury from intracranial hypertension due to hypoxia, hypercarbia, acidosis, and hypoperfusion. Intubation and ventilation are used, as necessary. Cerebral perfusion pressure (CPP), defined as mean arterial pressure (MAP) minus central venous pressure (CVP) (CPP = MAP − CVP), is largely dependent on mean arterial pressure. Therefore, the initial goal of resuscitation is to maintain intravascular volume and central perfusion pressure, since systemic hypotension has been shown to be an important cause of morbidity and mortality in head-injured children (see Chapter 22).[203] Systemic hypotension secondary to isolated head injury is very rare, except for infants younger than 6 months of age. Blood loss from a cerebral injury either from a scalp wound or intracranial bleeding can represent a significant portion of the circulating blood volume of an infant and can cause systemic hypotension in this age group. If hypotension occurs in older children, however, a source of blood loss or cause for hypotension other than the head injury should be sought. When replacing intravascular volume, judicious attention is directed to *ensuring that one does not overhydrate the patient*, which would potentially increase cerebral edema. Previously recommended head-up tilt is now thought to be harmful because of a decrease in cerebral perfusion pressure.[204, 205]

Thorax and Abdomen

BLUNT TRAUMA VS. PENETRATING TRAUMA

Most pediatric trauma is blunt rather than penetrating in origin; it is for this reason that most pediatric patients are observed and stabilized before surgical exploration.[37] If a child has penetrating trauma (particularly of the chest), the indications for surgical intervention and exploration are similar to those in adults; a higher proportion (50% of children vs 15% of adults) will require surgical intervention.[206] Trauma centers that care for children should be equipped for the possible need for emergent chest or abdominal exploration. In urban areas, the incidence of pediatric gunshot wounds to the chest and abdomen is increasing, with half of these patients requiring surgical intervention.[207, 208] The most likely lesion that will require emergent surgery is penetrating chest trauma. Contrary to blunt injury, penetrating injury to the area below the nipple line (gunshot wound, stabbing) requires surgery in the majority of cases.[206] Although it is preferable to perform these surgical procedures in a standard operating room, it may be necessary to perform an emergency thoracotomy on admission to the Emergency Department. The Emergency Department should be equipped for this eventuality.

A review of the National Pediatric Trauma database demonstrates that the injury pattern for penetrating wounds of the liver in children differs from the pattern in adults. Of 132 pediatric patients with penetrating liver injuries, 100 injuries were the result of gunshots (76%) and 32 stabbings (24%); a high percentage of children have associated organ injury requiring surgical intervention (spleen, kidney, bowel, pancreas) compared with adults.[209] It appears that the liver provides little protection from injury to other organs compared with the same situation in adults, in whom the hepatic mass does seem to provide protection.[209]

Children with blunt trauma are generally managed conservatively. However, despite the blunt nature of the trauma, there can be clinically important hemorrhage or other damage. Hypotension can be a presenting sign of significant blood loss, myocardial contusion, pneumothorax or hemothorax, pericardial tamponade, or visceral rupture. Hypoxemia can be a presenting sign of lung contusion, airway disruption, aspiration, pneumothorax, hemothorax, or poor cardiac output.[210] The secondary survey of thorax and abdomen is used to quickly establish the likely injuries by physical examination. However, diagnostic imaging is often needed to effectively define the extent of these injuries.[211–215] Computed tomography scans are generally more sensitive than peritoneal lavage in establishing intra-abdominal injury.[216] Ultrasonography of the abdomen or echocardiography of the chest and heart is also useful for expeditious diagnosis.

Both penetrating and blunt injuries provide special problems in the pediatric patient. First, young children often are not able to articulate their complaints very well. Second, the thin and flexible chest and abdominal walls offer scant protection for the internal organs, providing little barrier to the transmission of significant force throughout these cavities. Lastly, the compliant and usually healthy heart and vascular system of the child often compensate for bleeding until there has been extraordinary blood loss, making early detection and intervention crucial. Successful diagnosis of organ injury is accomplished by frequent physical reevaluation, supported by appropriate diagnostic tests. The importance of serial examinations by the same practitioner cannot be overemphasized.

Blunt thoracic trauma can result in cardiac or lung contusion. The origin of blunt thoracic trauma in pediatric patients differs from that in adults. In children, approximately 60% are from motor vehicle accidents and 40% from automobile-pedestrian collisions, compared with 80% of cases in adults being from motor vehicle accidents.[210] The incidence of pulmonary contusion and the outcomes of pulmonary contusion are similar in pediatric and adult patients.[210, 217, 218] The lung is the most commonly injured internal chest organ in pediatric patients (50%).[219] In contrast to adult cases, most pediatric lung contusions are not accompanied by a rib fracture.[220] Of note, fracture of the first rib in children often is accompanied by major injury of large blood vessels, which requires surgical intervention.[217] Lung contusion can present as progressive hypoxemia and ventilatory failure in the hours after initial injury. This secondary injury can cause deterioration of the overall status of the child and must be detected early to institute appropriate therapy. The majority of pediatric patients with blunt cardiac injury also suffer from multiple organ injury; cardiac contusion is associated with pulmonary contusion 50% of the time and with rib fractures 23% of the time.[221] About 5% of survivors will have residual cardiac injury such as valvular (mitral or tricuspid) insufficiency.[221] This latter observation suggests the need for careful follow-up evaluation. Aortic and other vascular disruption, as well as airway disruption, are potential issues with a high mortality rate.

The majority of pediatric blunt abdominal injuries do not undergo operative therapy because the emphasis is on preservation of organ function.[222–224] Only patients with a visibly distended abdomen (secondary to continued massive bleeding or ruptured viscus) on arrival to the Emergency Department undergo immediate surgical intervention. The remainder of patients undergo observation and frequent reevaluation to preserve lacerated liver, kidney, or spleen, if possible.[225–228] A far greater percentage of adults require surgical exploration from splenic injury compared with children (59 vs. 7% in one series).[37] In addition, it appears that adult trauma surgeons treat pediatric patients similar to adult patients, with over a twofold incidence of operative intervention (52% vs. 21%) for splenic injury.[229] Aggressive fluid and blood component therapy has been used to nonoperatively treat splenic injury, with only a small minority requiring surgery.[37, 229–231]

Blunt abdominal trauma may also result in hepatic injury. Children restrained by seat belts can have significant visceral injures despite not having any external bruising or erythema over the area covered by the seat belt.[232] Children have a lower mortality rate than adults with similar hepatic injuries.[233] As with splenic injury, the majority of pediatric patients do not require surgical intervention and generally a conservative approach is taken.[226, 228, 234–237] However, as with any major injury, careful observation is critical because of the possibility of delayed hemorrhage.[238, 239] Wound packing and delayed removal with later re-exploration has been lifesaving in patients who have massive injury with the development of coagulopathy.[235, 240] Teenagers appear to have a similar injury pattern to adults in terms of organ disruption.[233]

Blunt renal trauma is another possibility that must be evaluated. Renal injuries occur more frequently in children than in adults with blunt abdominal trauma.[241, 242] Hematuria or extensive pelvic trauma is an indication for radiologic evaluation. The likelihood of injury increases in the presence of hemodynamic instability, which is also associated with multiple organ injury.[243] Extravasation of urine does not generally necessitate urgent surgical intervention unless there is ongoing blood loss.[243] Evidence suggests that percutaneous drainage of fractured kidneys increases the likelihood of organ preservation.[244] Therefore, conservative nonsurgical management is indicated for blunt renal trauma in most cases.[245, 246]

Pancreatic injury is also associated with both blunt and penetrating injuries in children and generally is managed with conservative nonsurgical interventions.[247, 248] Bicycle handle bar and seat belt injuries with or without bruising are sources of blunt trauma that can result in pancreatic injury.[232, 249] The major indications for surgical intervention are transection of the pancreatic duct and the need to preserve the spleen (distal pancreatectomy).[247, 248] In some cases, endoscopic studies can be used to determine the extent of injuries to the pancreatic duct[250]; others will be diagnosed radiologically.[215, 251]

Bowel injuries, including contusions, rupture, and transection, are associated with blunt and penetrating abdominal trauma.[249, 252, 253] As with pancreatic injury, seat belts and handle bar injuries are common even without external bruising.[232, 249] Laparoscopy may be helpful in establishing the diagnosis with a minimally invasive surgical procedure.[254] Since delayed recognition of a perforated viscus carries significant morbidity and mortality, both radiologic evaluation and frequent physical examinations are indicated.[255–257]

Diagnostic Procedures and In-Hospital Transport

The ideal hospital plan would have all diagnostic facilities close to the Emergency Department. Whenever possible, portable equipment should be brought to the bedside (radiography, echocardiography, and ultrasonography). However, it is often necessary to move the child to a computed tomography scanner, angiography suite, cardiac catheterization laboratory, or operating room. The transfer has to be performed in an expeditious manner, with monitoring and resuscitation continued throughout the transfer and the duration of the examination. Several studies have documented the frequent occurrence of mishaps during intrahospital transport (30%) that relate to the patient's condition, adequacy of monitoring, or mode of ventilation.[258–260] A review of our hospital experience found a high rate of adverse events during the transport of critically ill children to and from the operating room. These events were related to the transport equipment (including cribs), as well as the environmental obstacles such as crowded hallways. Even though patients did not suffer major complications, the events often caused a high degree of anxiety among the transporting personnel. Each institution should establish specific, written policies defining the details of internal transport, including issues such as which patients can be transported, who should be carrying out the transport (e.g., nurse, physicians), number of escorts, minimum monitoring and equipment, elevator use, and so on.[259] There should be a portable source of oxygen, self-inflating resuscitation bag, portable battery-powered multichannel monitor (the lighter the better), appropriate medications, and the necessary equipment for emergent airway management including intubation (endotracheal tube, stylet, laryngoscope, nasal and oral airways). The potential for power failure, elevator malfunction, and sudden deterioration of the patient should be addressed in the policies. Procedures for maintaining the battery power of monitors and infusion pumps (daily recharging) are vital. The ability to communicate and summon help throughout the process is an important part of an institution-wide policy.

Since trauma patients are likely to require radiologic services on a recurring basis, the capabilities for caring for these patients should be the responsibility of those working in the radiologic suites in addition to the trauma team. Areas such as the computed tomography suites that are frequently used for trauma patients should have equipment and supplies that can be used to continue the resuscitation of a trauma patient. This includes monitors, piped oxygen and suction, intravenous equipment and fluids, a resuscitation cart with medications, adequate lighting and electrical outlets, and a method of communication. The American Society of Anesthesiologists Guidelines for Nonoperating Room Anesthetizing Locations are useful in ensuring that there is proper preparation of areas that are temporarily used to care for trauma patients.[261]

Interhospital Transport

Development of current transport policies and procedures of the critically ill between institutions is the result of decades of experience. Interhospital transport of critically ill patients is associated with morbidity due to adverse events occurring in transport, such as problems with the endotracheal tube, intravenous access loss, poor neck stabilization, and so on.[262–264] One study has demonstrated better patient outcome when an injured child is accompanied by a tertiary care physician,[265] but other centers have published successful results without physicians' participation.[266, 267] End-tidal CO_2 values tend to be low during manual ventilation,[116] and there is greater variation in end-tidal CO_2 with manual than with controlled ventilation.[268]

A 1991 survey among pediatricians indicated that, even though 90% of the time they have professional services available to them, parents used the family car as the means to transfer the child to the hospital. Reasons cited were efficiency of family transport vehicle, prohibitive cost of professional services, and failure to consider it.[269] Triage personnel should be specific in their directions to families about proper transport modalities.

A National Pediatric Transport Leadership Conference formulated guidelines for pediatric interhospital critical care transport in 1990.[270] They emphasized the need for adequate team composition, direction, and continuous education. Above all, the responsibilities of both receiving and referring institutions toward the patient are stressed so there is no period of patient abandonment. The transport team is obliged to provide a level of care equal or superior to that given by the referring institution.

Preparation for Operative Procedure

Operating Room Set-Up

In busy adult trauma centers, it is a common practice to have a designated operating room for emergency trauma cases. Because pediatric trauma is almost 10 times less frequent than adult trauma and does not usually result in emergent or urgent surgery, it is uncommon to find an institution that keeps an operating room open at all times for pediatric trauma cases. Institutions that care for pediatric patients generally have a rapid case turnover so that there is usually an operating room vacant within a short time that can quickly be prepared for an emergency trauma case. After peak hours, most institutions that accept trauma patients will maintain a fully set up operating room that can be used on short notice. A standardized set-up, complete with a checklist of surgical and anesthesia equipment, which is maintained such that the equipment is organized and set up for use, serves as a guide for the personnel responsible for preparation.

In addition to standard airway and fluid administration equipment, the designated trauma room should have fluid and body warming equipment, infusion pumps, resuscitation equipment, and equipment for management of the difficult airway. A useful adjunct is portable laboratory analysis equipment that can provide laboratory data such as hemoglobin, arterial blood gas analysis, calcium, glucose, coagulation profiles, and electrolytes within minutes, using less than 0.5 mL of blood.[271, 272] In our institution, we maintain the full range of airway equipment in a single, easily viewed, and easily opened container, which allows rapid access to all sizes of endotracheal tubes, laryngoscope blades, stylets, and other airway management equipment.

Induction of Anesthesia

An injured child brought to the operating room in unstable condition arising from blunt or penetrating injury presents a challenge to the entire trauma team. The two most common clinical situations that bring a child emergently to the operating room are penetrating chest trauma and acute intracranial bleeding. In both cases, the patient may be extraordinarily unstable and require ongoing resuscitation. The anesthetic approach to such a patient depends on multiple factors.

The initial priorities in the operating room are to continue resuscitation (if needed), establish monitoring, and then proceed with induction. In most cases, the emergent nature of the procedure requires general anesthesia with a rapid-sequence induction. If the child is hemodynamically unstable, induction of anesthesia can cause vasodilation and diminished sympathetic activity, with accompanying decreased cardiac output and hypotension. Instituting positive pressure ventilation reduces venous return and further contributes to a decrease in cardiac output. The anesthesiologist needs to make the critical judgment as to whether or not the patient requires further volume administration or other measures to continue resuscitation, additional peripheral venous access, central venous access, arterial line monitoring, or to proceed with induction. It must be remembered that central venous catheters, especially multilumen catheters, are inadequate for rapid volume administration due to the marked resistance to flow through the long narrow lumen; large-bore short catheters allow much more rapid volume administration.[150, 273, 274] In some situations, the urgency of obtaining control of bleeding supersedes all other concerns. Ketamine (1–2 mg/kg) and etomidate (0.1 mg/kg) have been extensively used as induction agents because of their propensity to minimize hemodynamic changes. Ketamine, however, should be used with caution if the primary problem is increased intracranial pressure, since there is some concern that ketamine can further increase the intracranial pressure as well as increase cerebral metabolic rate for oxygen.[275–278] Both succinylcholine and rocuronium provide conditions for rapid onset of muscle relaxation that are useful during a rapid-sequence induction; high-dose rocuronium should be substituted in any patient at risk for rhabdomyolysis.[127] The maintenance anesthetic agents selected will depend on the status of the patient and associated injuries. Generally, an opioid-based anesthetic is a reasonable first choice, with inhalation agent added as tolerated. Titratable opioids with little cardiovascular effect (e.g., fentanyl), supplemented by benzodiazepines to cause amnesia (e.g., midazolam), can be given according to the patient's clinical condition. Nitrous oxide is avoided if there is potential for lung injury or pneumothorax.

During the surgical procedure, there can be significant changes in hemodynamic and ventilatory status secondary to the surgery. Usually as soon as the bleeding is surgically controlled, vital signs stabilize. Obviously all the problems associated with rapid and massive blood transfusion must be considered (see Chapter 12). However, it is crucial that the anesthesiologist remember that there may be other lesions or changes that can become manifest during the procedure.

For example, a previously undetected pneumothorax, missed during initial assessment, can rapidly expand after institution of positive pressure ventilation and may cause cardiovascular collapse. Lung contusion or aspiration pneumonitis may cause hypoxemia and hypoventilation, whereas myocardial contusion can cause unexplained decreases in cardiac contractility and hypotension. Lastly, previously undetected hemorrhage may be a cause of unexplained hypotension that will be successfully diagnosed and treated only if the anesthesiologist is vigilant in continually reexamining the patient throughout the procedure. The decision to extubate the patient at the end of the procedure is dependent on the course of the surgical procedure, anticipated complications, the nature of the injuries, the need for continued ventilatory support, and the plan for postoperative pain management (see Chapters 28 and 29).

Child Abuse

Among children younger than 5 years of age, child abuse is the second leading cause of death after unintentional injuries.[55, 59, 60, 200, 279–283] It is estimated that there are 1.5 million children abused annually in the United States, with approximately 10% of all injuries seen in the Emergency Department being abuse-related. Child abuse is not limited to the United States but is a problem that is a concern for all anesthesiologists worldwide.[284–292] The most commonly affected systems are skin and skeleton.[279, 293, 294] CNS injuries, particularly "shaken baby syndrome," carry a 15% mortality rate and a 50% morbidity rate. Head injury in a battered child is probably a late sign of child abuse, with signs of skeletal or skin injuries from previous injury often present.[13, 14, 50–54, 295, 296] Besides physical trauma, abused children demonstrate signs of hygienic, nutritional, and psychological neglect, which often leads to life-long psychological effects.[297–300] Hallmarks of diagnosis include a history inconsistent with the character and extent of injury and delay in seeking medical help. It is the responsibility of all medical professionals to understand the nature of child abuse and be especially watchful of it in the pediatric trauma patient (as well as in elective surgical patients). Several illustrative pictures of cutaneous manifestations of child abuse are presented in Figure 16–5.

SUMMARY

Although accidents remain the number one cause of pediatric mortality and morbidity, effective strategies of injury control are limited. Legislation has been directed at some of the causes of injury, specifically from motor vehicle accidents, by way of speed limits, seat belt laws, and air bag installation.[301–304] Some states have identified their own needs and designed programs addressing them, such as New Mexico's Gunshot Injury Prevention Program and Baltimore's Smoke Detector Giveaway Program.[305, 306] The changes in the child's environment, coupled with a more effective approach to pediatric trauma by the medical system, have succeeded in reducing the accident-related death rate in the United States by 30%. Injury control presents an opportunity in treatment, education, identification of hazard, screening, advocacy, and policy making.[307, 308]

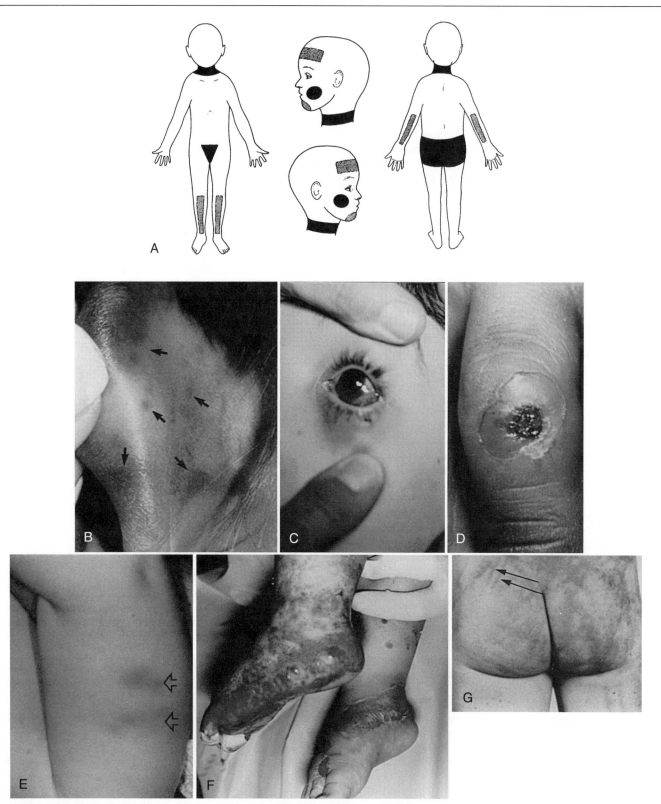

Figure 16–5. (A) Typical areas where children might present with bruises due to daily living activities. The gray areas indicate normal areas where one would expect to see bruising. The black areas are unusual areas of bruises. Any bruise in the black areas must be suspect for possible child abuse. Cutaneous manifestations of child abuse are varied. (B) Multiple bruises behind a patient's ear, indicative of a slapping of the patient (small arrows indicate multiple areas of contusion). (C) Hemorrhage of the eye, again indicating blunt trauma to the eye. (D) Classic example of a cigarette burn on the finger; these may appear anywhere on the patient's body. (E) Example of several bruises of the upper arm (open arrows) from a forceful grabbing kind of action. (F) Classic glove-like scald burn, typical of a child who was held in hot water. (G) Multiple longitudinal bruises consistent with a beating with a long narrow object such as a stick or belt. (Part A is a modification of Slide 46, Child Abuse Part 1, #7290, 1987. Medcom Inc., Garden Grove, CA 92642. Parts B, D, E, F, and G from AAP Classic Visual Diagnosis of Child Abuse. Used with permission from the American Academy of Pediatrics, Elk Grove Village, IL.)

REFERENCES

1. Peclet MH, Newman KD, Eichelberger MR, et al: Patterns of injury in children. J Pediatr Surg 1990;25:85–90.
2. Teret SP, Webster DW: Reducing gun deaths in the United States. Br Med J 1999;318:1160–1161.
3. Teret SP, Webster DW, Vernick JS, et al: Support for new policies to regulate firearms: Results of two national surveys. N Engl J Med 1998;339:813–818.
4. McGinnis JM, Foege WH: Mortality and morbidity attributable to use of addictive substances in the United States. Proc Assoc Am Phys 1999;111:109–118.
5. Bhatt RV: Domestic violence and substance abuse. Int J Gynaecol Obstet 1998;63:S25–S31.
6. Li X, Stanton B, Feigelman S: Exposure to drug trafficking among urban, low-income African American children and adolescents. Arch Pediatr Adolesc Med 1999;153:161–168.
7. Schuster MA, Halfon N, Wood DL: African American mothers in south central Los Angeles. Their fears for their newborn's future. Arch Pediatr Adolesc Med 1998;152:264–268.
8. Young NK: Effects of alcohol and other drugs on children. J Psychoactive Drugs 1997;29:23–42.
9. Brookoff D, O'Brien KK, Cook CS, et al: Characteristics of participants in domestic violence. Assessment at the scene of domestic assault. JAMA 1997;277:1369–1373.
10. Miller BA, Maguin E, Downs WR: Alcohol, drugs, and violence in children's lives. Recent Dev Alcohol 1997;13:357–385.
11. Matlock T, Slate JR, Saarnio DA: Familial variables and domestic violence. J Ark Med Soc 1995;92:222–224.
12. Wintemute GJ, Teret SP, Kraus JF, et al: When children shoot children: 88 unintended deaths in California. JAMA 1987;257:3107–3109.
13. Helfaer MA, Wilson MD: Head injury in children. Curr Opin Pediatr 1993;5:303–309.
14. Martin WS, Gussack GS: Pediatric penetrating head and neck trauma. Laryngoscope 1990;100:1288–1291.
15. Ponzer S, Bergman B, Brismar B, et al: Accidental firearm injury in childhood: A predictor of social and medical outcome? Eur J Emerg Med 1997;4:125–129.
16. Nance ML, Stafford PW, Schwab CW: Firearm injury among urban youth during the last decade: An escalation in violence. J Pediatr Surg 1997;32:949–952.
17. Nance ML, Sing RF, Branas CC, et al: Shotgun wounds in children: Not just accidents. Arch Surg 1997;132:58–61.
18. Webster DW, Gainer PS, Champion HR: Weapon carrying among inner-city junior high school students: Defensive behavior vs aggressive delinquency. Am J Public Health 1993;83:1604–1608.
19. Webster DW, Wilson ME, Duggan AK, et al: Firearm injury prevention counseling: A study of pediatricians' beliefs and practices. Pediatrics 1992;89:902–907.
20. Campbell C, Schwarz DF: Prevalence and impact of exposure to interpersonal violence among suburban and urban middle school students. Pediatrics 1996;98:396–402.
21. Dukarm CP, Holl JL, McAnarney ER: Violence among children and adolescents and the role of the pediatrician. Bull N Y Acad Med 1995;72:5–15.
22. Piessens PW, King MC, Ryan J, et al: A statewide institute to deliver professional development programs to school health personnel in Massachusetts. J Sch Health 1995;65:176–180.
23. Garcia F: The National Drug Control Strategy: The first-line approach to decreasing violence in our communities. J Health Care Poor Underserved 1995;6:177–185.
24. Wolfner GD, Gelles RJ: A profile of violence toward children: A national study. Child Abuse Negl 1993;17:197–212.
25. Vernick JS, Teret SP, Webster DW: Regulating firearm advertisements that promise home protection: A public health intervention. JAMA 1997;277:1391–1397.
26. Webster DW, Vernick JS, Ludwig J, et al: Flawed gun policy research could endanger public safety. Am J Public Health 1997;87:918–921.
27. Ramenofsky ML, Morse TS: Standards of care for the critically injured pediatric patient. J Trauma 1982;22:921–933.
28. Ewing-Cobbs L, Fletcher JM, Levin HS, et al: Academic achievement and academic placement following traumatic brain injury in children and adolescents: A two-year longitudinal study. J Clin Exp Neuropsychol 1998;20:769–781.
29. Levi RB, Drotar D, Yeates KO, et al: Posttraumatic stress symptoms in children following orthopedic or traumatic brain injury. J Clin Child Psychol 1999;28:232–243.
30. Vernon DD, Furnival RA, Hansen KW, et al: Effect of a pediatric trauma response team on emergency department treatment time and mortality of pediatric trauma victims. Pediatrics 1999;103:20–24.
31. Hulka F, Mullins RJ, Mann NC, et al: Influence of a statewide trauma system on pediatric hospitalization and outcome. J Trauma 1997;42:514–519.
32. Johnson DL, Krishnamurthy S: Send severely head-injured children to a pediatric trauma center. Pediatr Neurosurg 1996;25:309–314.
33. Schwab W, Frankel HL, Rotondo MF, et al: The impact of true partnership between a university Level I trauma center and a community Level II trauma center on patient transfer practices. J Trauma 1998;44:815–819.
34. Hall JR, Reyes HM, Meller JL, et al: The outcome for children with blunt trauma is best at a pediatric trauma center. J Pediatr Surg 1996;31:72–76.
35. Snyder CL, Jain VN, Saltzman DA, et al: Blunt trauma in adults and children: A comparative analysis. J Trauma 1990;30:1239–1245.
36. Vane D, Shedd FG, Grosfeld JL, et al: An analysis of pediatric trauma deaths in Indiana. J Pediatr Surg 1990;25:955–959.
37. Powell M, Courcoulas A, Gardner M, et al: Management of blunt splenic trauma: Significant differences between adults and children. Surgery 1997;122:654–660.
38. Colombani PM, Buck JR, Dudgeon DL, et al: One-year experience in a regional pediatric trauma center. J Pediatr Surg 1985;20:8–13.
39. Paar O, Kasperk R: The significance of multiple trauma in children. Eur J Pediatr Surg 1992;2:345–347.
40. Feickert HJ, Drommer S, Heyer R: Severe head injury in children: Impact of risk factors on outcome. J Trauma 1999;47:33–38.
41. Kini N, Lazoritz S: Evaluation for possible physical or sexual abuse. Pediatr Clin North Am 1998;45:205–219.
42. Jenny C, Hymel KP, Ritzen A, et al: Analysis of missed cases of abusive head trauma. JAMA 1999;281:621–626.
43. American Academy of Pediatrics Committee on Child Abuse and Neglect: Guidelines for the evaluation of sexual abuse of children: Subject review. Pediatrics 1999;103:186–191.
44. Hinds A, Baskin LS: Child sexual abuse: What the urologist needs to know. J Urol 1999;162:516–523.
45. Kadish HA, Schunk JE, Britton H: Pediatric male rectal and genital trauma: Accidental and nonaccidental injuries. Pediatr Emerg Care 1998;14:95–98.
46. Sinal SH, Stewart CD: Physical abuse of children: A review for orthopedic surgeons. J South Orthop Assoc 1998;7:264–276.
47. Limbos MAP, Berkowitz CD: Documentation of child physical abuse: How far have we come? Pediatrics 1998;102:53–58.
48. Paradise JE, Bass J, Forman SD, et al: Minimum criteria for reporting child abuse from health care settings. Del Med J 1997;69:357–363.
49. Ellis PS: The pathology of fatal child abuse. Pathology 1997;29:113–121.
50. Collins KA, Nichols CA: A decade of pediatric homicide: A retrospective study at the Medical University of South Carolina. Am J Forensic Med Pathol 1999;20:169–172.
51. Plunkett J: Shaken baby syndrome and the death of Matthew Eappen: A forensic pathologist's response. Am J Forensic Med Pathol 1999;20:17–21.
52. Conway EE Jr: Nonaccidental head injury in infants: "The shaken baby syndrome revisited." Pediatr Ann 1998;27:677–690.
53. Duhaime AC, Christian CW, Rorke LB, et al: Nonaccidental head injury in infants: The "shaken-baby syndrome." N Engl J Med 1998;338:1822–1829.
54. Lancon JA, Haines DE, Parent AD: Anatomy of the shaken baby syndrome. Anat Rec 1998;253:13–18.
55. Committee on Child Abuse and Neglect, 1993–1994: Shaken baby syndrome: Inflicted cerebral trauma. Del Med J 1997;69:365–370.
56. Shaw BA, Murphy KM, Shaw A, et al: Humerus shaft fractures in young children: Accident or abuse? J Pediatr Orthop 1997;17:293–297.
57. Blakemore LC, Loder RT, Hensinger RN: Role of intentional abuse in children 1 to 5 years old with isolated femoral shaft fractures. J Pediatr Orthop 1996;16:585–588.
58. Rushton FE: The role of health care in child abuse and neglect prevention. J S C Med Assoc 1996;92:133–136.
59. American Academy of Pediatrics Task Force on Adolescent Assault Victim Needs: Adolescent assault victim needs: A review of issues and a model protocol. Pediatrics 1996;98:991–1001.

60. Boyce MC, Melhorn KJ, Vargo G: Pediatric trauma documentation: Adequacy for assessment of child abuse. Arch Pediatr Adolesc Med 1996;150:730–732.
61. Furnival RA, Schunk JE: ABCs of scoring systems for pediatric trauma. Pediatr Emerg Care 1999;15:215–223.
62. Trunkey DD: Trauma: Accidental and intentional injuries account for more years of life lost in the U.S. than cancer and heart disease. Among the prescribed remedies are improved preventive efforts, speedier surgery and further research. Sci Am 1983;249:28–35.
63. Brownstein D, Shugerman R, Cummings P, et al: Prehospital endotracheal intubation of children by paramedics. Ann Emerg Med 1996;28:34–39.
64. Knight S, Vernon DD, Fines RJ, et al: Prehospital emergency care for children at school and nonschool locations. Pediatrics 1999;103:e81.
65. Suominen P, Silfvast T, Korpela R, et al: Pediatric prehospital care provided by a physician-staffed emergency medical helicopter unit in Finland. Pediatr Emerg Care 1996;12:169–172.
66. Suominen P, Baillie C, Kivioja A, et al: Prehospital care and survival of pediatric patients with blunt trauma. J Pediatr Surg 1998;33:1388–1392.
67. Su E, Mann NC, McCall M, et al: Use of resuscitation skills by paramedics caring for critically injured children in Oregon. Prehosp Emerg Care 1997;1:123–127.
68. McSwain NE Jr: Usefulness of physicians functioning as emergency medical technicians. J Trauma 1995;39:1027–1028.
69. Moront ML, Gotschall CS, Eichelberger MR: Helicopter transport of injured children: System effectiveness and triage criteria. J Pediatr Surg 1996;31:1183–1186.
70. Teanby DN, Lloyd DA, Gorman DF, et al: Regional review of blunt trauma in children. Br J Surg 1994;81:53–55.
71. Li G, Tang N, DiScala C, et al: Cardiopulmonary resuscitation in pediatric trauma patients: Survival and functional outcome. J Trauma 1999;47:1–7.
72. O'Rourke PP: Outcome of children who are apneic and pulseless in the emergency room. Crit Care Clin 1986;14:466–468.
73. Losek JD, Hennes H, Glaeser P, et al: Prehospital care of the pulseless, nonbreathing pediatric patient. Am J Emerg Med 1987;5:370–374.
74. Schindler MB, Bohn D, Cox PN, et al: Outcome of out-of-hospital cardiac or respiratory arrest in children. N Engl J Med 1996;335:1473–1479.
75. Beaver BL, Colombani PM, Buck JR, et al: Efficacy of emergency room thoracotomy in pediatric trauma. J Pediatr Surg 1987;22:19–23.
76. Sheikh A, Brogan T: Outcome and cost of open- and closed-chest cardiopulmonary resuscitation in pediatric cardiac arrests. Pediatrics 1994;93:392–398.
77. Nakayama DK, Gardner MJ, Rowe MI: Emergency endotracheal intubation in pediatric trauma. Ann Surg 1990;211:218–223.
78. Mazurek A, Noah Z, Barthel M, Reynolds M: Early management in pediatric multiple trauma victims. 6th World Congress of Emergency and Disaster Medicine, Hong Kong, 1989.
79. Losek JD, Szewczuga D, Glaeser PW: Improved prehospital pediatric ALS care after an EMT-paramedic clinical training course. Am J Emerg Med 1994;12:429–432.
80. Evans RJ, McCabe M, Thomas R: Intraosseous infusion. Br J Hosp Med 1994;51:161–164.
81. Medina FA: Rapid sequence induction/intubation using intraosseous infusion of vecuronium bromide in children. Am J Emerg Med 1992;10:359–360.
82. Haller JA Jr: Toward a comprehensive emergency medical system for children. Pediatrics 1990;86:120–122.
83. Haller JA Jr: Problems in children's trauma. J Trauma 1970;10:269–271.
84. Haller JA Jr: Pediatric trauma: The No. 1 killer of children. JAMA 1983;249:47.
85. Holmes MJ, Reyes HM: A critical review of urban pediatric trauma. J Trauma 1984;24:253–255.
86. Smith RF, Frateschi L, Sloan EP, et al: The impact of volume on outcome in seriously injured trauma patients: Two years' experience of the Chicago Trauma System. J Trauma 1990;30:1066–1075.
87. Knudson MM, Shagoury C, Lewis FR: Can adult trauma surgeons care for injured children? J Trauma 1992;32:729–737.
88. Jubelirer RA, Agarwal NN, Beyer FC III, et al: Pediatric trauma triage: Review of 1,307 cases. J Trauma 1990;30:1544–1547.
89. Bonadio WA, Wagner V: Half-strength TAC topical anesthetic for selected dermal lacerations. Clin Pediatr (Phila) 1988;27:495–498.
90. Seidel JS, Henderson DP, Ward P, et al: Pediatric prehospital care in urban and rural areas. Pediatrics 1991;88:681–690.
91. Singh R, Kissoon N, Singh N, et al: Is a full team required for emergency management of pediatric trauma? J Trauma 1992;33:213–218.
92. Doolin EJ, Browne AM, DiScala C: Pediatric trauma center criteria: An outcomes analysis. J Pediatr Surg 1999;34:885–889.
93. Lanoix R, Golden J: The facilitated pediatric resuscitation room. J Emerg Med 1999;17:363–366.
94. Davis D, Barbee L, Ririe D: Pediatric endotracheal tube selection: A comparison of age-based and height-based criteria. AANA J 1998;66:299–303.
95. Lubitz DS, Seidel JS, Chameides L, et al: A rapid method for estimating weight and resuscitation drug dosages from length in the pediatric age group. Ann Emerg Med 1988;17:576–581.
96. Mackenzie CF, Craig GR, Parr MJ, et al: Video analysis of two emergency tracheal intubations identifies flawed decision-making. The Level One Trauma Anesthesia Simulation Group. Anesthesiology 1994;81:763–771.
97. American College of Surgeons: Advance Trauma Life Support. Instructor's Manual, 5th ed. Chicago, IL: American College of Surgeons; 1993.
98. American Heart Association: Pediatric Advanced Life Support. Elk Grove Village, IL: American Academy of Pediatrics; 1994.
99. Haller A, Johnston C, Luten R, et al: Advanced Pediatric Life Support: The Pediatric Emergency Medicine Course, 2nd ed. Elk Grove Village, IL: American Academy of Pediatrics, American College of Emergency Physicians; 1993.
100. Adam R, Stedman M, Winn J, et al: Improving trauma care in Trinidad and Tobago. West Indian Med J 1994;43:36–38.
101. Ali J, Howard M: The Advanced Trauma Life Support Program in Manitoba: A 5-year review. Can J Surg 1993;36:181–183.
102. Collicott PE: Advanced Trauma Life Support (ATLS): Past, present, future. 16th Stone Lecture, American Trauma Society. J Trauma 1992;33:749–753.
103. Jacobs LM, Sinclair A, Beiser A, et al: Prehospital advanced life support: benefits in trauma. J Trauma 1984;24:8–13.
104. Schoenfeld PS, Baker MD: Management of cardiopulmonary and trauma resuscitation in the pediatric emergency department. Pediatrics 1993;91:726–729.
105. Mackenzie CF, Jefferies NJ, Hunter WA, et al: Comparison of self-reporting of deficiencies in airway management with video analyses of actual performance. LOTAS Group. Level One Trauma Anesthesia Simulation. Hum Factors 1996;38:623–635.
106. Xiao Y, Hunter WA, Mackenzie CF, et al: Task complexity in emergency medical care and its implications for team coordination. LOTAS Group. Level One Trauma Anesthesia Simulation. Hum Factors 1996;38:636–645.
107. Mackenzie CF, Hu PF, Horst RL: An audio-video system for automated data acquisition in the clinical environment. LOTAS Group. J Clin Monit 1995;11:335–341.
108. Townsend RN, Clark R, Ramenofsky ML, et al: ATLS-based videotape trauma resuscitation review: Education and outcome. J Trauma 1993;34:133–138.
109. Kaufmann CR, Maier RV, Rivara FP, et al: Evaluation of the Pediatric Trauma Score. JAMA 1990;263:69–72.
110. Lieh-Lai MW, Theodorou AA, Sarnaik AP, et al: Limitations of the Glasgow Coma Scale in predicting outcome in children with traumatic brain injury. J Pediatr 1992;120:195–199.
111. Orliaguet GA, Meyer PG, Blanot S, et al: Predictive factors of outcome in severely traumatized children. Anesth Analg 1998;87:537–542.
112. Reynolds EA: Trauma scoring and pediatric patients: Issues and controversies. J Emerg Nurs 1992;18:205–210.
113. Taylor GA, O'Donnell R, Sivit CJ, et al: Abdominal injury score: A clinical score for the assignment of risk in children after blunt trauma. Radiology 1994;190:689–694.
114. Tepas JJ III, Veldenz HC, DiScala C, et al: Pediatric risk indicator: An objective measurement of childhood injury severity. J Trauma 1997;43:258–261.
115. Yager JY, Johnston B, Seshia SS: Coma scales in pediatric practice. Am J Dis Child 1990;144:1088–1091.
116. Eichelberger MR, Gotschall CS, Sacco WJ, et al: A comparison of the trauma score, the revised trauma score, and the pediatric trauma score. Ann Emerg Med 1989;18:1053–1058.

117. Kaufmann CR, Maier RV, Kaufmann EJ, et al: Validity of applying adult TRISS analysis to injured children. J Trauma 1991;31:691–697.
118. Mazurek A: Pediatric injury patterns. Int Anesthesiol Clin 1994;32:11–25.
119. Curran C, Dietrich AM, Bowman MJ, et al: Pediatric cervical-spine immobilization: Achieving neutral position? J Trauma 1995;39:729–732.
120. Podolsky S, Baraff LJ, Simon RR, et al: Efficacy of cervical spine immobilization methods. J Trauma 1983;23:461–465.
121. Westhorpe RN: The position of the larynx in children and its relationship to the ease of intubation. Anaesth Intens Care 1987;15:384–388.
122. Hastings RH, Wood PR: Head extension and laryngeal view during laryngoscopy with cervical spine stabilization maneuvers. Anesthesiology 1994;80:825–831.
123. Nakayama DK, Waggoner T, Venkataraman ST, et al: The use of drugs in emergency airway management in pediatric trauma. Ann Surg 1992;216:205–211.
124. Redan JA, Livingston DH, Tortella BJ, et al: The value of intubating and paralyzing patients with suspected head injury in the emergency department. J Trauma 1991;31:371–375.
125. Committee on Drugs, American Academy of Pediatrics: Drugs for pediatric emergencies. Pediatrics 1998;101:E13.
126. Schwartz DE, Matthay MA, Cohen NH: Death and other complications of emergency airway management in critically ill adults: A prospective investigation of 297 tracheal intubations. Anesthesiology 1995;82:367–376.
127. Mazurek AJ, Rae B, Hann S, et al: Rocuronium versus succinylcholine: Are they equally effective during rapid-sequence induction of anesthesia? Anesth Analg 1998;87:1259–1262.
128. Moore GP, Pace SA, Busby W: Comparison of intraosseous, intramuscular, and intravenous administration of succinylcholine. Pediatr Emerg Care 1989;5:209–210.
129. Miklus RM, Elliott C, Snow N: Surgical cricothyrotomy in the field: Experience of a helicopter transport team. J Trauma 1989;29:506–508.
130. Benumof JL, Scheller MS: The importance of transtracheal jet ventilation in the management of the difficult airway. Anesthesiology 1989;71:769–778.
131. Carden E, Calcaterra TC, Lechtman A: Pneumatocele of the larynx: A complication of percutaneous transtracheal ventilation. Anesth Analg 1976;55:600–601.
132. Jorden R, Moore EE: The safety of percutaneous transtracheal ventilation (P.T.V.) in the patient with an obstructed airway remains controversial. J Trauma 1984;24:917.
133. Smith RB, Schaer WB, Pfaeffle H: Percutaneous transtracheal ventilation for anaesthesia and resuscitation: A review and report of complications. Can Anaesth Soc J 1975;22:607–612.
134. Birmingham PK, Cheney FW, Ward RJ: Esophageal intubation: A review of detection techniques. Anesth Analg 1986;65:886–891.
135. Hodge D 3d: Intraosseous infusions: a review. Pediatr Emerg Care 1985;1:215–218.
136. Spivey WH: Intraosseous infusions. J Pediatr 1987;111:639–643.
137. Zaritsky A: Pediatric resuscitation pharmacology. Members of the Medications in Pediatric Resuscitation Panel. Ann Emerg Med 1993;22:445–455.
138. Glaeser PW, Losek JD, Nelson DB, et al: Pediatric intraosseous infusions: Impact on vascular access time. Am J Emerg Med 1988;6:330–332.
139. Tighe SQ, Rudland SV, Kemp PM, et al: Paediatric resuscitation in adverse circumstances: A comparison of three routes of systemic access. J R Nav Med Serv 1993;79:75–79.
140. Ryder IG, Munro HM, Doull IJ: Intraosseous infusion for resuscitation. Arch Dis Child 1991;66:1442–1443.
141. Berg RA: Emergency infusion of catecholamines into bone marrow. Am J Dis Child 1984;138:810–811.
142. Bilello JF, O'Hair KC, Kirby WC, et al: Intraosseous infusion of dobutamine and isoproterenol. Am J Dis Child 1991;145:165–167.
143. Cilley RE: Intraosseous infusion in infants and children. Semin Pediatr Surg 1992;1:202–207.
144. Dieckmann RA, Vardis R: High-dose epinephrine in pediatric out-of-hospital cardiopulmonary arrest. Pediatrics 1995;95:901–913.
145. Driggers DA, Johnson R, Steiner JF, et al: Emergency resuscitation in children: The role of intraosseous infusion. Postgrad Med 1991;89:129–132.
146. Dubick MA, Kramer GC: Hypertonic saline dextran (HSD) and intraosseous vascular access for the treatment of haemorrhagic hypoten-

147. Hurren JS, Dunn KW: Intraosseous infusion for burns resuscitation. Burns 1995;21:285–287.
148. Helm M, Breschinski W, Lampl L, et al: Intraosseous puncture in preclinical emergency medicine. Experiences of an air rescue service. [German]. Anaesthesist 1996;45:1196–1202.
149. Brunette DD, Fischer R: Intravascular access in pediatric cardiac arrest. Am J Emerg Med 1988;6:577–579.
150. Idris AH, Melker RJ: High-flow sheaths for pediatric fluid resuscitation: A comparison of flow rates with standard pediatric catheters. Pediatr Emerg Care 1992;8:119–122.
151. Nakakimura K, Fleischer JE, Drummond JC, et al: Glucose administration before cardiac arrest worsens neurologic outcome in cats. Anesthesiology 1990;72:1005–1011.
152. D'Alecy LG, Lundy EF, Barton KJ, et al: Dextrose containing intravenous fluid impairs outcome and increases death after eight minutes of cardiac arrest and resuscitation in dogs. Surgery 1986;100:505–511.
153. Lanier WL, Stangland KJ, Scheithauer BW, et al: The effects of dextrose infusion and head position on neurologic outcome after complete cerebral ischemia in primates: Examination of a model. Anesthesiology 1987;66:39–48.
154. Metz S: Use of glucose-containing solutions during surgery. Anesthesiology 1988;68:651–652.
155. Michaud LJ, Rivara FP, Grady MS, et al: Predictors of survival and severity of disability after severe brain injury in children. Neurosurgery 1992;31:254–264.
156. Steward DJ, DaSilva CA, Flegel T: Elevated blood glucose levels may increase the danger of neurological deficit following profoundly hypothermic cardiac arrest. Anesthesiology 1988;68:653.
157. Longstreth WTJ, Diehr P, Cobb LA, et al: Neurologic outcome and blood glucose levels during out-of-hospital cardiopulmonary resuscitation. Neurology 1986;36:1186–1191.
158. Zornow MH, Scheller MS, Todd MM, et al: Acute cerebral effects of isotonic crystalloid and colloid solutions following cryogenic brain injury in the rabbit. Anesthesiology 1988;69:180–184.
159. Zornow MH, Todd MM, Moore SS: The acute cerebral effects of changes in plasma osmolality and oncotic pressure. Anesthesiology 1987;67:936–941.
160. Simma B, Burger R, Falk M, et al: A prospective, randomized, and controlled study of fluid management in children with severe head injury: Lactated Ringer's solution versus hypertonic saline. Crit Care Med 1998;26:1265–1270.
161. Shackford SR, Bourguignon PR, Wald SL, et al: Hypertonic saline resuscitation of patients with head injury: A prospective, randomized clinical trial. J Trauma 1998;44:50–58.
162. Shackford SR: Effect of small-volume resuscitation on intracranial pressure and related cerebral variables. J Trauma 1997;42:S48–S53.
163. Anderson JT, Wisner DH, Sullivan PE, et al: Initial small-volume hypertonic resuscitation of shock and brain injury: Short- and long-term effects. J Trauma 1997;42:592–600.
164. Sheikh AA, Matsuoka T, Wisner DH: Cerebral effects of resuscitation with hypertonic saline and a new low-sodium hypertonic fluid in hemorrhagic shock and head injury. Crit Care Med 1996;24:1226–1232.
165. Taylor G, Myers S, Kurth CD, et al: Hypertonic saline improves brain resuscitation in a pediatric model of head injury and hemorrhagic shock. J Pediatr Surg 1996;31:65–70.
166. Fallon WF: Trauma systems, shock, and resuscitation. Curr Opin Gen Surg 1993;2:40–45.
167. Freshman SP, Battistella FD, Matteucci M, et al: Hypertonic saline (7.5%) versus mannitol: A comparison for treatment of acute head injuries. J Trauma 1993;35:344–348.
168. Battistella FD, Wisner DH: Combined hemorrhagic shock and head injury: Effects of hypertonic saline (7.5%) resuscitation. J Trauma 1991;31:182–188.
169. Berger S, Schurer L, Hartl R, et al: Reduction of post-traumatic intracranial hypertension by hypertonic/hyperoncotic saline/dextran and hypertonic mannitol. Neurosurgery 1995;37:98–107.
170. Mercuriali F, Inghilleri G, Colotti MT, et al: Bedside transfusion errors: Analysis of 2 years' use of a system to monitor and prevent transfusion errors. Vox Sang 1996;70:16–20.
171. Linden JV, Paul B, Dressler KP: A report of 104 transfusion errors in New York State. Transfusion 1992;32:601–606.
172. Dietz NM, Joyner MJ, Warner MA: Blood substitutes: Fluids, drugs, or miracle solutions? Anesth Analg 1996;82:390–405.

146. (continued) sion in the far-forward combat arena. Ann Acad Med Singapore 1997;26:64–69.

173. Alayash AI: Hemoglobin-based blood substitutes: Oxygen carriers, pressor agents, or oxidants? Nat Biotechnol 1999;17:545–549.

174. Chang TM: Future prospects for artificial blood. Trends Biotechnol 1999;17:61–67.

175. Goodrich RP, Sowemino-Coker SO, Weinstein R: Advances in erythrocyte preservation and hemoglobin substitutes. Curr Opin Hematol 1994;1:162–169.

176. Chang TM: Modified hemoglobin blood substitutes: Present status and future perspectives. Biotechnol Annu Rev 1998;4:75–112.

177. Riess JG, Krafft MP: Fluorinated materials for in vivo oxygen transport (blood substitutes), diagnosis and drug delivery. Biomaterials 1998;19:1529–1539.

178. Borms SF, Engelen SL, Himpe DG, et al: Bair hugger forced-air warming maintains normothermia more effectively than thermo-lite insulation. J Clin Anesth 1994;6:303–307.

179. Giesbrecht GG, Ducharme MB, McGuire JP: Comparison of forced-air patient warming systems for perioperative use. Anesthesiology 1994;80:671–679.

180. Giuffre M, Finnie J, Lynam DA, et al: Rewarming postoperative patients: Lights, blankets, or forced warm air. J Post Anesth Nurs 1991;6:387–393.

181. Levison H, Linsao L, Swyer PR: A comparison of infra-red and convective heating for newborn infants. Lancet 1966;2:1346–1348.

182. Murat I, Berniere J, Constant I: Evaluation of the efficacy of a forced-air warmer (Bair Hugger) during spinal surgery in children. J Clin Anesth 1994;6:425–429.

183. Deacock S, Holdcroft A: Heat retention using passive systems during anaesthesia: Comparison of two plastic wraps, one with reflective properties. Br J Anaesth 1997;79:766–769.

184. Bissonnette B, Sessler DI: Passive or active inspired gas humidification increases thermal steady-state temperatures in anesthetized infants. Anesth Analg 1989;69:783–787.

185. Stevenson GW, Tobin M, Hall SC: Fluid warmer as a potential source of air bubble emboli. Anesth Analg 1995;80:1061.

186. Arndt M, Hofmockel R, Benad G: LEVEL 1—a new blood warming device [in German]. Anaesthesiol Reanim 1994;19:78–79.

187. Browne DA, de Boeck R, Morgan M: An evaluation of the Level 1 blood warmer series. Anaesthesia 1990;45:960–963.

188. Dunham CM, Belzberg H, Lyles R, et al: The rapid infusion system: A superior method for the resuscitation of hypovolemic trauma patients. Resuscitation 1991;21:207–227.

189. Smallman JM, Morgan M: Evaluation of the Level 1 Hotline blood warmer. Anaesthesia 1992;47:869–871.

190. Presson RGJ, Haselby KA, Bezruczko AP, et al: Evaluation of a new high-efficiency blood warmer for children. Anesthesiology 1990;73:173–176.

191. Stylianos S: Late sequelae of major trauma in children. Pediatr Clin North Am 1998;45:853–859.

192. Sobus KM, Alexander MA, Harcke HT: Undetected musculoskeletal trauma in children with traumatic brain injury or spinal cord injury. Arch Phys Med Rehabil 1993;74:902–904.

193. Tepas JJ III, DiScala C, Ramenofsky ML, et al: Mortality and head injury: The pediatric perspective. J Pediatr Surg 1990;25:92–95.

194. Pang D, Wilberger JE Jr: Spinal cord injury without radiographic abnormalities in children. J Neurosurg 1982;57:114–129.

195. Baker C, Kadish H, Schunk JE: Evaluation of pediatric cervical spine injuries. Am J Emerg Med 1999;17:230–234.

196. Davidson RG: Atlantoaxial instability in individuals with Down syndrome: A fresh look at the evidence. Pediatrics 1988;81:857–865.

197. Fuchs S, Barthel MJ, Flannery AM, et al: Cervical spine fractures sustained by young children in forward-facing car seats. Pediatrics 1989;84:348–354.

198. Keller J, Mosdal C: Traumatic odontoid epiphysiolysis in an infant fixed in a child's car seat. Injury 1990;21:191–192.

199. Stein SC, Spettell CM: Delayed and progressive brain injury in children and adolescents with head trauma. Pediatr Neurosurg 1995;23:299–304.

200. Ward JD: Pediatric issues in head trauma. New Horiz 1995;3:539–545.

201. Levin HS: Head trauma. Curr Opin Neurol 1993;6:841–846.

202. Michaud LJ, Duhaime AC, Batshaw ML: Traumatic brain injury in children. Pediatr Clin North Am 1993;40:553–565.

203. Pigula FA, Wald SL, Shackford SR, et al: The effect of hypotension and hypoxia on children with severe head injuries. J Pediatr Surg 1993;28:310–314.

204. Rosner MJ, Coley IB: Cerebral perfusion pressure, intracranial pressure, and head elevation. J Neurosurg 1986;65:636–641.

205. Patel JC, Tepas JJ III: The efficacy of focused abdominal sonography for trauma (FAST) as a screening tool in the assessment of injured children. J Pediatr Surg 1999;34:44–47.

206. Peterson RJ, Tiwary AD, Kissoon N, et al: Pediatric penetrating thoracic trauma: A five-year experience. Pediatr Emerg Care 1994;10:129–131.

207. Nance ML, Sing RF, Reilly PM, et al: Thoracic gunshot wounds in children under 17 years of age. J Pediatr Surg 1996;31:931–935.

208. Hartzog TH, Timerding BL, Alson RL: Pediatric trauma: Enabling factors, social situations, and outcome. Acad Emerg Med 1996;3:213–220.

209. Dicker RA, Sartorelli KH, McBrids WJ, et al: Penetrating hepatic trauma in children: Operating room or not? J Pediatr Surg 1996;31:1189–1191.

210. Allen GS, Cox CS Jr, Moore FA, et al: Pulmonary contusion: Are children different? J Am Coll Surg 1997;185:229–233.

211. Lowe LH, Bulas DI, Eichelberger MD, et al: Traumatic aortic injuries in children: Radiologic evaluation. AJR 1998;170:39–42.

212. Morey AF, Bruce JE, McAninch JW: Efficacy of radiographic imaging in pediatric blunt renal trauma. J Urol 1996;156:2014–2018.

213. Sivit CJ, Cutting JP, Eichelberger MR: CT diagnosis and localization of rupture of the bladder in children with blunt abdominal trauma: Significance of contrast material extravasation in the pelvis. AJR Am J Roentgenol 1995;164:1243–1246.

214. McAleer IM, Kaplan GW: Pediatric genitourinary trauma. Urol Clin North Am 1995;22:177–188.

215. Sivit CJ, Eichelberger MR, Taylor GA, et al: Blunt pancreatic trauma in children: CT diagnosis. AJR Am J Roentgenol 1992;158:1097–1100.

216. Sivit CJ, Taylor GA, Bulas DI, et al: Blunt trauma in children: Significance of peritoneal fluid. Radiology 1991;178:185–188.

217. Nakayama DK, Ramenofsky ML, Rowe MI: Chest injuries in childhood. Ann Surg 1989;210:770–775.

218. Roux P, Fisher RM: Chest injuries in children: an analysis of 100 cases of blunt chest trauma from motor vehicle accidents. J Pediatr Surg 1992;27:551–555.

219. Peterson RJ, Tepas JJ III, Edwards FH, et al: Pediatric and adult thoracic trauma: Age-related impact on presentation and outcome. Ann Thorac Surg 1994;58:14–18.

220. Nakayama DK, Copes WS, Sacco WJ: The effect of patient age upon survival in pediatric trauma. J Trauma 1991;31:1521–1526.

221. Dowd MD, Krug S: Pediatric blunt cardiac injury: Epidemiology, clinical features, and diagnosis. Pediatric Emergency Medicine Collaborative Research Committee: Working Group on Blunt Cardiac Injury. J Trauma 1996;40:61–67.

222. Cosentino CM, Luck SR, Barthel MJ, et al: Transfusion requirements in conservative nonoperative management of blunt splenic and hepatic injuries during childhood. J Pediatr Surg 1990;25:950–953.

223. Avanoglu A, Ulman I, Ergun O, et al: Blood transfusion requirements in children with blunt spleen and liver injuries. Eur J Pediatr Surg 1998;8:322–325.

224. Tepas JJ, Pickard LR, Shermeta DW, et al: Non-operative management of splenic injury. Md State Med J 1980;29:92–94.

225. Lannergren K, Tordai P, Linne T, et al: Avoiding splenectomy in the treatment of children with splenic injury. Acta Chir Scand 1990;156:359–365.

226. Gross M, Lynch F, Canty T Sr, et al: Management of pediatric liver injuries: A 13-year experience at a pediatric trauma center. J Pediatr Surg 1999;34:811–816.

227. Shafi S, Gilbert JC, Irish MS, et al: Follow-up imaging studies in children with splenic injuries. Clin Pediatr (Phila) 1999;38:273–277.

228. Bond SJ, Eichelberger MR, Gotschall CS, et al: Nonoperative management of blunt hepatic and splenic injury in children. Ann Surg 1996;223:286–289.

229. Keller MS, Vane DW: Management of pediatric blunt splenic injury: Comparison of pediatric and adult trauma surgeons. J Pediatr Surg 1995;30:221–224.

230. Emery KH, Babcock DS, Borgman AS, et al: Splenic injury diagnosed with CT: US follow-up and healing rate in children and adolescents. Radiology 1999;212:515–518.

231. Choong RK, Grattan-Smith TM, Cohen RC, et al: Splenic injury in children: A 10 year experience. J Paediatr Child Health 1993;29:192–195.

232. Tso EL, Beaver BL, Haller JA Jr: Abdominal injuries in restrained pediatric passengers. J Pediatr Surg 1993;28:915–919.

233. Shin H, Tepas JJ III, Ismail N, et al: Blunt hepatic injury in adolescents: Age makes a difference. Am Surg 1997;63:29–36.
234. Miller K, Kou D, Sivit C, et al: Pediatric hepatic trauma: Does clinical course support intensive care unit stay? J Pediatr Surg 1998;33:1459–1462.
235. Losty PD, Okoye BO, Walter DP, et al: Management of blunt liver trauma in children. Br J Surg 1997;84:1006–1008.
236. Amroch D, Schiavon G, Carmignola G, et al: Isolated blunt liver trauma: Is nonoperative treatment justified? J Pediatr Surg 1992;27:466–468.
237. Galat JA, Grisoni ER, Gauderer MW: Pediatric blunt liver injury: Establishment of criteria for appropriate management. J Pediatr Surg 1990;25:1162–1165.
238. Sjovall A, Hirsch K: Blunt abdominal trauma in children: risks of nonoperative treatment. J Pediatr Surg 1997;32:1169–1174.
239. Shilyansky J, Navarro O, Superina RA, et al: Delayed hemorrhage after nonoperative management of blunt hepatic rupture in children: A rare but significant event. J Pediatr Surg 1999;34:60–64.
240. Stylianos S: Abdominal packing for severe hemorrhage. J Pediatr Surg 1998;33:339–342.
241. Brown SL, Elder JS, Spirnak JP: Are pediatric patients more susceptible to major renal injury from blunt trauma? A comparative study. J Urol 1998;160:138–140.
242. Monstrey SJ, vander Staak FH, vanderWerken C, et al. Urinary tract injuries in children: Are they different from adults? Z Kinderchir 1988;43:31–34.
243. Thompson-Fawcett M, Kolbe A: Paediatric renal trauma: Caution with conservative management of major injuries. Aust N Z J Surg 1996;66:435–440.
244. Gill B, Palmer LS, Reda E, et al: Optimal renal preservation with timely percutaneous intervention: A changing concept in the management of blunt renal trauma in children in the 1990s. Br J Urol 1994;74:370–374.
245. Roche BG, Bugmann P, Le Coultre C: Blunt injuries to liver, spleen, kidney and pancreas in pediatric patients. Eur J Pediatr Surg 1992;2:154–156.
246. Bass DH, Semple PL, Cywes S: Investigation and management of blunt renal injuries in children: A review of 11 years' experience. J Pediatr Surg 1991;26:196–200.
247. Jobst MA, Canty TG Sr, Lynch FP: Management of pancreatic injury in pediatric blunt abdominal trauma. J Pediatr Surg 1999;34:818–823.
248. Keller MS, Stafford PW, Vane DW: Conservative management of pancreatic trauma in children. J Trauma 1997;42:1097–1100.
249. Clarnette TD, Beasley SW: Handlebar injuries in children: patterns and prevention. Aust N Z J Surg 1997;67:338–339.
250. McGahren ED, Magnuson D, Schaller RT, et al: Management of transected pancreas in children. Aust N Z J Surg 1995;65:242–246.
251. Gorenstein A, O'Halpin D, Wesson DE, et al: Blunt injury to the pancreas in children: Selective management based on ultrasound. J Pediatr Surg 1987;22:1110–1116.
252. Canty TG Sr, Canty TG Jr, Brown C: Injuries of the gastrointestinal tract from blunt trauma in children: A 12-year experience at a designated pediatric trauma center. J Trauma 1999;46:234–240.
253. Jerby BL, Attorri RJ, Morton D Jr: Blunt intestinal injury in children: The role of the physical examination. J Pediatr Surg 1997;32:580–584.
254. VanderKolk WE, Garcia VF: The use of laparoscopy in the management of seat belt trauma in children. J Laparoendosc Surg 1996;6:545–549.
255. Brown RA, Bass DH, Rode H, et al: Gastrointestinal tract perforation in children due to blunt abdominal trauma. Br J Surg 1992;79:522–524.
256. Taylor GA, Sivit CJ: Computed tomography imaging of abdominal trauma in children. Semin Pediatr Surg 1992;1:253–259.
257. Ford EG, Senac MO Jr: Clinical presentation and radiographic identification of small bowel rupture following blunt trauma in children. Pediatr Emerg Care 1993;9:139–142.
258. Braman SS, Dunn SM, Amico CA, et al: Complications of intrahospital transport in critically ill patients. Ann Intern Med 1987;107:469–473.
259. Smith I, Fleming S, Cernaianu A: Mishaps during transport from the intensive care unit. Crit Care Med 1990;18:278–281.
260. Wallen E, Venkataraman ST, Grosso MJ, et al: Intrahospital transport of critically ill pediatric patients. Crit Care Med 1995;23:1588–1595.
261. American Society of Anesthesiologists: Guidelines for nonoperating room anesthetizing locations. Park Ridge, IL: American Society of Anesthesiologists; 1994.
262. Kanter RK, Boeing NM, Hannan WP, et al: Excess morbidity associated with interhospital transport. Pediatrics 1992;90:893–898.
263. Kanter RK, Tompkins JM: Adverse events during interhospital transport: Physiologic deterioration associated with pretransport severity of illness. Pediatrics 1989;84:43–48.
264. Ridley S, Carter R: The effects of secondary transport on critically ill patients. Anaesthesia 1989;44:822–827.
265. Macnab AJ: Optimal escort for interhospital transport of pediatric emergencies. J Trauma 1991;31:205–209.
266. McCloskey KA, Johnston C: Critical care interhospital transports: Predictability of the need for a pediatrician. Pediatr Emerg Care 1990;6:89–92.
267. McCloskey KA, King WD, Byron L: Pediatric critical care transport: Is a physician always needed on the team? Ann Emerg Med 1989;18:247–249.
268. Dockery WK, Futterman C, Keller SR, et al: A comparison of manual and mechanical ventilation during pediatric transport. Crit Care Med 1999;27:802–806.
269. Baker MD, Ludwig S: Pediatric emergency transport and the private practitioner. Pediatrics 1991;88:691–695.
270. Day S, McCloskey K, Orr R, et al: Pediatric interhospital critical care transport: Consensus of a national leadership conference. Pediatrics 1991;88:696–704.
271. Connelly NR, Magee M, Kiessling B: The use of the iSTAT portable analyzer in patients undergoing cardiopulmonary bypass. J Clin Monit 1996;12:311–315.
272. Bhatia N, Silver P, Quinn C, et al: Evaluation of a portable blood gas analyzer for pediatric interhospital transport. J Emerg Med 1998;16:871–874.
273. Dutky PA, Stevens SL, Maull KI: Factors affecting rapid fluid resuscitation with large-bore introducer catheters. J Trauma 1989;29:856–860.
274. Ikeda S, Schweiss JF: Maximum infusion rates and CVP accuracy during high-flow delivery through multilumen catheters. Crit Care Med 1985;13:586–588.
275. Crumrine RS, Nulsen FE, Weiss MH: Alterations in ventricular fluid pressure during ketamine anesthesia in hydrocephalic children. Anesthesiology 1975;42:758–761.
276. List WF, Crumrine RS, Cascorbi HF, et al: Increased cerebrospinal fluid pressure after ketamine. Anesthesiology 1972;36:98–99.
277. Sari A, Okuda Y, Takeshita H: The effect of ketamine on cerebrospinal fluid pressure. Anesth Analg 1972;51:560–565.
278. Takeshita H, Okuda Y, Sari A: The effects of ketamine on cerebral circulation and metabolism in man. Anesthesiology 1972;36:69–75.
279. Dorfman DH, Paradise JE: Emergency diagnosis and management of physical abuse and neglect of children. Curr Opin Pediatr 1995;7:297–301.
280. Miller TW, Veltkamp LJ: Assessment of sexual abuse and trauma: Clinical measures. Child Psychiatry Hum Dev 1995;26:3–10.
281. Kasim MS, Cheah I, Shafie HM: Childhood deaths from physical abuse. Child Abuse Negl 1995;19:847–854.
282. Wright MS, Litaker D: Childhood victims of violence: Hospital utilization by children with intentional injuries. Arch Pediatr Adolesc Med 1996;150:415–420.
283. Kapklein MJ, Mahadeo R: Pediatric trauma. Mt Sinai J Med 1997;64:302–310.
284. Ikeda Y: Child abuse and child abuse studies in Japan. Acta Paediatr Jpn 1995;37:240–247.
285. Trocme N, McPhee D, Tam KK: Child abuse and neglect in Ontario: Incidence and characteristics. Child Welfare 1995;74:563–586.
286. Tourigny M, Bouchard C: Incidence and characteristics in identification of abused children: Cross-cultural comparison [in French]. Child Abuse Negl 1994;18:797–808.
287. Peisino MG, Vietti RM, Di Pietro P, et al: Child abuse by intoxication [in Italian]. Minerva Pediatr 1993;45:401–405.
288. Cappelleri JC, Eckenrode J, Powers JL: The epidemiology of child abuse: Findings from the Second National Incidence and Prevalence Study of Child Abuse and Neglect. Am J Public Health 1993;83:1622–1624.
289. MacKenzie G, Blaney R, Chivers A, et al: The incidence of child sexual abuse in Northern Ireland. Int J Epidemiol 1993;22:299–305.
290. Sariola H, Uutela A: The prevalence and context of family violence against children in Finland. Child Abuse Negl 1992;16:823–832.
291. Wilske J, Eisenmenger W: Unnatural causes of death in children [in German]. Offentl Gesundheitswes 1991;53:490–497.

292. Oyemade A: Child abuse and neglect: a global phenomenon. Afr J Med Sci 1991;20:5–9.

293. Jessee SA: Physical manifestations of child abuse to the head, face and mouth: A hospital survey. ASDC J Dent Child 1995;62:245–249.

294. Strouse PJ, Owings CL: Fractures of the first rib in child abuse. Radiology 1995;197:763–765.

295. O'Neill JA Jr, Meacham WF, Griffin JP, et al: Patterns of injury in the battered child syndrome. J Trauma 1973;13:332–339.

296. Chabrol B, Decarie JC, Fortin G: The role of cranial MRI in identifying patients suffering from child abuse and presenting with unexplained neurological findings. Child Abuse Negl 1999;23:217–228.

297. Schaaf KK, McCanne TR: Relationship of childhood sexual, physical, and combined sexual and physical abuse to adult victimization and posttraumatic stress disorder. Child Abuse Negl 1998;22:1119–1133.

298. Kent A, Waller G: The impact of childhood emotional abuse: An extension of the Child Abuse and Trauma Scale. Child Abuse Negl 1998;22:393–399.

299. Adams DM, Lehnert KL: Prolonged trauma and subsequent suicidal behavior: Child abuse and combat trauma reviewed. J Trauma Stress 1997;10:619–634.

300. Klein I, Janoff-Bulman R: Trauma history and personal narratives: some clues to coping among survivors of child abuse. Child Abuse Negl 1996;20:45–54.

301. Baum HM, Lund AK, Wells JK: The mortality consequences of raising the speed limit to 65 mph on rural interstates. Am J Public Health 1989;79:1392–1395.

302. Wagenaar AC, Webster DW: Preventing injuries to children through compulsory automobile safety seat use. Pediatrics 1986;78:662–672.

303. Wagenaar AC, Webster DW, Maybee RG: Effects of child restraint laws on traffic fatalities in eleven states. J Trauma 1987;27:726–732.

304. Rausch TK, Sanddal ND, Sanddal TL, et al: Changing epidemiology of injury-related pediatric mortality in a rural state: Implications for injury control. Pediatr Emerg Care 1998;14:388–392.

305. Becker TM, Olson L, Vick J: Children and firearms: A gunshot injury prevention program in New Mexico. Am J Public Health 1993;83:282–283.

306. Gorman RL, Charney E, Holtzman NA, et al: A successful city-wide smoke detector giveaway program. Pediatrics 1985;75:14–18.

307. Agran PF, Winn DG, Anderson CL, et al: The role of the physical and traffic environment in child pedestrian injuries. Pediatrics 1996;98:1096–1103.

308. Rivara FP: Traumatic deaths of children in the United States: Currently available prevention strategies. Pediatrics 1985;75:456–462.

Cardiac Physiology and Pharmacology

Francis X. McGowan, Jr, MD, *and* James M. Steven, MD

Cardiovascular Physiology
   Fetal Circulation
   Transitional Circulation
Neonatal Cardiovascular System
   Prevalence of Congenital Heart Disease
   Physiologic Categories of Congenital Heart Disease
   Postoperative Considerations
   Acquired Heart Disease
Cardiovascular Pharmacology
   Rational Use of Vasoactive Drugs
   Practical Considerations for the Use of Vasoactive Agents
   Balancing Parallel Circulations
   Vasoactive Drugs
   Antiarrhythmic Agents
Radiofrequency Catheter Ablation
Mechanical Circulatory Support
   Ventricular Assist Devices
   Extracorporeal Membrane Oxygenation
Cardiomyopathies
   Dilated Cardiomyopathy
   Hypertrophic Cardiomyopathy
   Mitochondrial Myopathies

Cardiovascular Physiology

At birth, the normal neonatal cardiovascular system rapidly undergoes major alterations in the pattern of circulation. Although these changes are most dramatic in the first hours of life, the maturation process of the heart and circulation continues over the ensuing few years. In addition to the differences in pharmacokinetics discussed elsewhere in this

We acknowledge the previous contributions of Susan L. Streltz and Paul R. Hickey.

text, neonates and infants manifest different cardiovascular pharmacodynamic responses to anesthetic drugs. An understanding of neonatal cardiovascular maturation will enable anesthesiologists caring for neonates and infants to anticipate their responses to perioperative management strategies.

Structural malformations of the cardiovascular system remain among the most common birth defects. In addition to the profound changes occurring during transitional circulation at birth, these infants are subjected to a variety of additional abnormal cardiovascular loading conditions imposed by the structural abnormality. Since congenital heart disease (CHD) often accompanies other organ system malformations, these patients may present for a variety of noncardiac procedures. In addition, early cardiac interventions have created a new population of infants and young children who have undergone major reconstructive cardiac surgery. Despite interventions designed to minimize the physiologic burdens imposed by CHD, many of these "repairs" leave significant hemodynamic residua and sequelae (see Chapter 19). Anticipating these results and their functional consequences should constitute a substantial component of anesthetic planning and management.

Acquired cardiovascular disease is significantly less common in pediatric patients than in adults. Generally these cases represent manifestations of systemic diseases that attack the integrity of cardiac structures, conduction system, or myocardium. Many cases represent progressive ailments that are significantly less amenable to surgical intervention than CHD. Nevertheless, such patients also present for a variety of cardiac and noncardiac procedures.

This chapter provides a foundation for the physiologic and pharmacologic implications germane to the anesthesiologist caring for children. The added consequences of CHD and acquired heart disease are included.

Fetal Circulation

Unlike the normal postnatal circulatory pattern, which functions as a "series" circuit of pumps (i.e., the ventricles) and resistance beds (i.e., the pulmonary and systemic circulations), the fetal circulation behaves more like a "parallel" circuit. Both the right and left ventricles provide systemic blood flow. An anatomic illustration reveals that admixture of blood occurs at a variety of fetal connections (Fig. 17–1).[1, 2] Relatively oxygenated blood returns from the placenta via the umbilical vein and crosses the ductus venosus to enter the inferior vena cava. A differential streaming effect causes much of this more saturated blood to cross the foramen ovale into the left atrium, thereby providing the most oxygenated blood for the cerebral circulation (Fig. 17–2A). Only 10% of the right ventricular output courses through the pulmonary circulation in utero (Fig. 17–2B). The remaining right ventricular output crosses the ductus arteriosus to provide the preponderance of systemic flow beyond the aortic arch.

A parallel circulatory pattern enables disparities in volume output between right and left ventricles while admixture of relatively oxygenated and deoxygenated blood occurs.

Right ventricular volume output is nearly twice the left ventricular volume output, as the left ventricle receives only the diminutive pulmonary venous return in addition to that which traverses the foramen ovale from the right atrium.[1, 3] Conversely, the right atrium receives all the systemic venous return in addition to the placental return via the umbilical vein. As a lacunar organ, the placenta does not fully oxygenate the blood passing through. Thus the highest oxygen saturation observed in the fetal circulation reaches 70 to 80%. The adaptive alterations in hemoglobin binding and other factors, such as increased 2, 3 DPG, promote adequate tissue oxygen delivery.[4]

Transitional Circulation

At birth, a variety of humoral, biochemical, and physiologic changes occur abruptly. First, the placental circulation is elim-

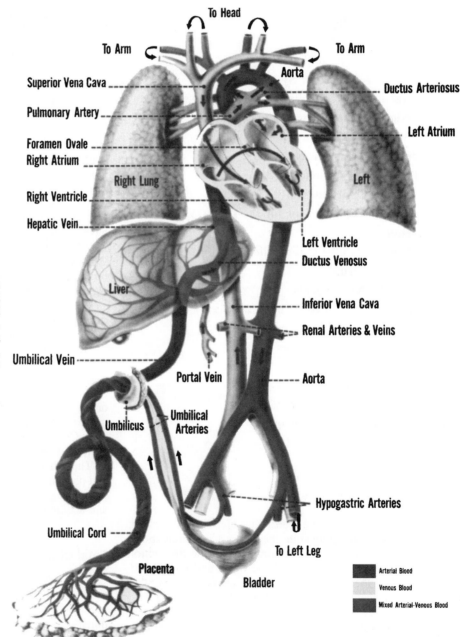

Figure 17–1. Course of the fetal circulation in late gestation. Note the selective blood flow patterns across the foramen ovale and the ductus arteriosus. (From Greeley WJ, Steven JM, Nicolson SC, et al: Anesthesia for pediatric cardiac surgery. In: Miller RD, ed: Anesthesia, Vol. 2, 5th ed. Philadelphia: Churchill Livingstone; 2000;1805–1847.)

To Head

To Arm   To Arm

Superior Vena Cava

Aorta

Ductus Arteriosus

Pulmonary Artery

Left Atrium

Foramen Ovale
Right Atrium

Right Lung   Left

Right Ventricle

Hepatic Vein

Left Ventricle

Ductus Venosus

Liver

Inferior Vena Cava

Renal Arteries & Veins

Umbilical Vein

Portal Vein   Aorta

Umbilical Arteries

Umbilicus

Hypogastric Arteries

Umbilical Cord

To Left Leg

Placenta

Bladder

Arterial Blood

Venous Blood

Mixed Arterial-Venous Blood

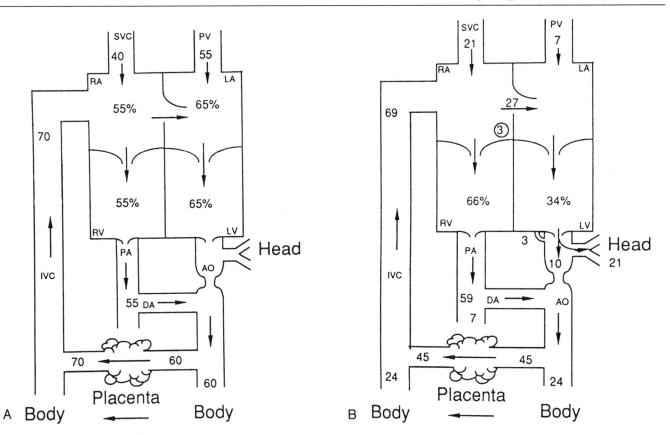

Figure 17-2. Fetal circulation in the late gestation lamb. (A) The numbers indicate the percent of oxygen saturation. The oxygen saturation is the highest in the inferior vena cava, representing flow that is primarily from the placenta. The saturation of the blood in the heart is slightly higher on the left side than on the right side. (B) The course of the circulation. The numbers represent the percentage of combined ventricular output. Some of the return from the inferior vena cava (IVC) is diverted by the crista dividens in the right atrium (RA) through the foramen ovale into the left atrium (LA), where it meets the pulmonary venous return (PV) and passes into the left ventricle (LV) and is pumped into the ascending aorta. Most of the ascending aortic flow goes to the coronary, subclavian, and carotid arteries, with only 10% of combined ventricular output passing through the aortic arch (indicated by the narrowed point in the aorta) into the descending aorta (AO). The remainder of the inferior vena cava flow mixes with return from the superior vena cava (SVC) and coronary veins (3%) and passes into the right atrium and right ventricle (RV) and is pumped into the pulmonary artery (PA). Because of the high pulmonary resistance, only 7% passes through the lungs (PV), with the rest going into the ductus arteriosus (DA) and then to the descending aorta to the placenta and lower half of the body. (Modified from Rudolph AM: Congenital Diseases of the Heart. Chicago: Year Book Publishers; 1974:1–48; from Freed MD: Fetal and transitional circulation. In: Fyler DC, ed: Nadas' Pediatric Cardiology. Philadelphia: Mosby-Year Book; 1992: 57–61.)

inated shortly after the lungs expand. Second, expansion of the lungs to a normal functional residual capacity results in optimal geometric relationship of the pulmonary microvasculature. Third, filling of the lungs with ambient atmosphere results in marked reduction in alveolar P_{CO_2} and increase in alveolar P_{O_2}. Each of these three factors acts in concert to markedly reduce pulmonary vascular resistance.[2, 5, 6] The net effect results in a substantial increase in pulmonary blood flow, thereby augmenting pulmonary venous return to the left heart. In conjunction with the elimination of the low-resistance umbilical circulation, the left ventricle is suddenly subjected to increased volume load and afterload (Table 17–1). Typically, left ventricular end-diastolic pressure and thus left atrial pressure, rises enough to exert hydrostatic pressure on the septum primum, thus closing the foramen ovale functionally. Transitional circulation is a much less stressful process for the right ventricle, since there are reductions in both pressure and volume loads.

The three fetal channels (ductus arteriosus, ductus venosus, and foramen ovale) close over a variable period. The ductus arteriosus has functionally (but not anatomically) closed in 58% of normal term infants by 2 days of life and in 98% by day 4.[7] Although many substances such as eicosanoids have been implicated, initial constriction proba-

Table 17-1. Hemodynamic Changes at Birth

Right Ventricle	Left Ventricle
Decreased afterload:	Increased afterload:
Decreased pulmonary vascular resistance	Placenta eliminated
Ductal closure	Ductal closure
Decreased volume load:	Increased volume load:
Eliminated umbilical vein return	Increased pulmonary venous return
Output diminished 25%	Output increased nearly 50%
	Transient left-to-right shunt at ductus

bly occurs primarily in response to increased arterial oxygen tension[8, 9] as well as the reduction in circulating prostaglandins that follows separation of the placenta.[3] Over the ensuing weeks, functional constriction is followed by a process of fibrosis.[10, 11] With ligation of the umbilical vein, portal pressure falls, triggering closure of the ductus venosus. This process rarely requires more than 1 to 2 weeks. The foramen ovale remains patent in the majority of infants and indeed persists when probed in 25 to 30% of adults.[12] Echocardiographic studies have confirmed right-to-left shunt via the foramen ovale in healthy infants emerging from general anesthesia, which can be a significant cause of persistent arterial desaturation at this time despite ventilation with 100% oxygen.[13]

Neonatal Cardiovascular System

The neonatal heart remains incompletely developed at birth on a variety of levels. The immature myocardium is populated by fewer, less organized myocytes. Contractile elements constitute only 30% of the fetal heart, in contrast to 60% in the adult.[14] Since the immature myocyte lacks sufficient sarcoplasmic reticulum, a vital component for rapid calcium regulation, it relies substantially more than the adult myocyte on calcium flux at the sarcolemma to initiate and terminate contraction.[15–17] These differences in myocardial cell composition and calcium transport contribute to diminished systolic and diastolic function, as compared with adults. With development to maturity, the compliance of both ventricles increases significantly (Fig. 17–3).[18] Frank-Starling curves indicate that maximal stroke volume occurs at a significantly lower atrial pressure in neonates (Fig. 17–4A and B).[19, 20] A variety of developmental changes in contractile proteins occur from fetal through early postnatal life; these include changes in pH and calcium sensitivity, as well as adenosine triphosphate (ATP) hydrolyzing activity.

The extraordinarily high metabolic rate of the neonate necessitates a proportional increase in cardiac output. Although generalizations that the neonate depends exclusively on heart rate to alter cardiac output are only partially valid, the neonatal heart functions close to maximal rate and stroke volume just to meet basic bodily demands for oxygen delivery.[21, 22] Despite structural immaturity in contractile proteins and myocardial stroma that leave the neonatal ventricle less compliant, echocardiographic studies in both the human fetus and the neonate unequivocally demonstrate the capacity to increase stroke volume (Fig. 17–5).[23] In fact, the neonate employs both tachycardia and stroke volume adjustments simply to meet metabolic demand. Thus, neonates exhibit exquisite sensitivity to pharmacologic agents that produce negative inotropic or chronotropic effects.

Immature autonomic regulation of cardiac function persists through the newborn period. Both sympathetic and parasympathetic innervation of the heart can be demonstrated at birth. However, evidence suggests that development of the sympathetic nervous system is incomplete at both the postganglionic nerve-receptor and the receptor-effector levels.[24] Sympathetic development reaches maturity by early infancy. The parasympathetic system achieves maturity within a few days of birth.[25] The relative imbalance of these two components of the autonomic nervous system at birth

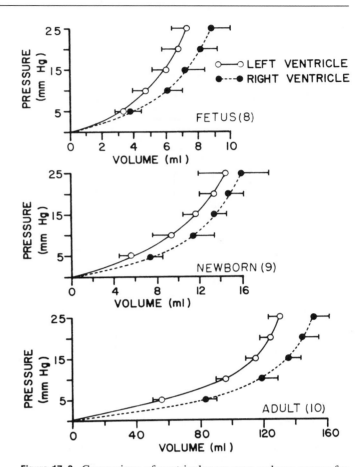

Figure 17–3. Comparison of ventricular pressure-volume curves for fetal, newborn, and adult sheep. Differences between ventricles are significant only in adult sheep. Note that the right and left ventricles have similar compliance curves in the neonates, making the physiologic relationship between ventricles more intimate (i.e., infants tend to develop biventricular failure). (From Romero T, Covell J, Friedman WF: A comparison of pressure-volume relations of the fetal, newborn and adult heart. Am J Physiol 1972;222:1285–1290.)

may account for the clinical observation that neonates are predisposed to exhibit marked vagal responses to a variety of stimuli.

At birth, pulmonary vascular development is incomplete. Lung sections demonstrate diminished numbers of arterioles, whereas the arterioles present thick medial muscularization (Fig. 17–6).[26, 27] The process of pulmonary vascular maturation occurs over the first few years of life. During that interval, arterioles proliferate faster than alveoli and the medial smooth muscle thins and extends more distally in the vascular tree. Pulmonary vascular resistance continues to fall as long as pulmonary mechanics and alveolar milieux remain favorable. However, fetal pulmonary vascular characteristics enable more profound and prolonged responses to provoking stimuli (e.g., reactive pulmonary hypertension) than might occur in the mature pulmonary vascular system.[28]

In the first days of life, neonates subjected to certain pathophysiologic conditions manifest severe, sustained increases in pulmonary vascular resistance (Table 17–2).[29, 30] The acute load imposed on the right ventricle may induce diastolic dysfunction and promote right-to-left shunt via the foramen ovale. Should pulmonary vascular resistance exceed

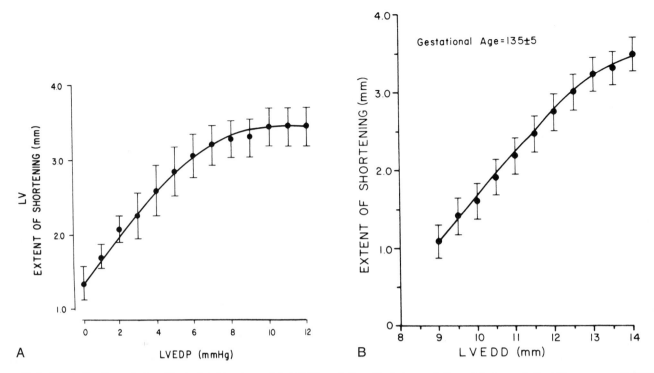

Figure 17–4. Frank-Starling relationship in fetal lamb model. (A) The relationship between left ventricular end-diastolic pressure (LVEDP) and shortening in a chronically instrumented fetal lamb model. Although myocardial performance improves with increasing LVEDP, the effect achieves a plateau at 10 mm Hg. (B) In the same model, the relationship of left ventricular end-diastolic diameter (LVEDD) to left ventricular shortening. Taken together, these experiments support the capacity, although blunted, of the fetal heart to change stroke volume on the basis of volume loading conditions. Each point and vertical bars represent mean ± SE. (From Kirkpatrick SE, Pitlick PT, Naliboff J, et al: Frank-Starling relationship as an important determinant of fetal cardiac output. Am J Physiol 1976;231:495–500.)

systemic vascular resistance, a right-to-left shunt may develop via the ductus arteriosus as well. Termed "persistent fetal circulation," this phenomenon may produce life-threatening hypoxemia that may require inhaled nitric oxide[31–34] or extracorporeal support (i.e., extracorporeal membrane oxygenation) to fulfill the placental role and sustain life.[35]

Prevalence of Congenital Heart Disease

Congenital heart disease (CHD) encompasses a wide array of structural development abnormalities of the heart and great vessels. As a group, they are among the most common congenital malformations. However, the precise incidence of CHD, both collectively and by individual anatomic subset, varies depending on definition, method of case identification, and epoch (Table 17–3). Large epidemiologic surveys place the incidence of hemodynamically significant CHD between 4 and 12 cases per 1000 live births.[36–39] Omitted from these figures are common lesions without immediate hemodynamic significance, such as mitral valve prolapse (estimated 4 to 5% prevalence in the general population), bicuspid nonstenotic aortic valve (estimated 2 to 3% prevalence), and patent ductus arteriosus in preterm neonates.

Anatomic diagnoses within the population of infants with CHD vary according to the method employed to identify cases. The Brompton data reflect the distribution of diagnoses for infants requiring hospitalization in the first year of life, collected over a decade.[39] Similarly, the New England Regional Infant Cardiac Program is a registry of patients

with CHD who died or required catheterization or surgery in the first year of life.[40] Both of these methods would introduce bias favoring more severe forms of CHD. Hoffman compiled epidemiologic reports from Western nations between 1941 and 1990.[38] Despite significant advances in diagnostic techniques during that period, the distribution of diagnoses remained relatively constant.

The increasing availability of prenatal diagnostic methods in the past decade may exert an impact on the relative prevalence of reported lesions as well as their outcome. When employing fetal echocardiography, the apparent shift toward more complex lesions may reflect technical limitations in identifying simple defects in this sample of 10,000 pregnancies at high risk for CHD.[41] In addition, evaluation in utero skews the results because it includes fatally malformed fetal subjects who will not survive to term. The prevalence of CHD among spontaneous abortions reaches 20% and remains as high as 10% in stillborn infants.[42] In this series, 50% of women whose children were given a prenatal diagnosis of CHD elected to terminate the pregnancy, particularly when presented with complex heart lesions. Thus this diagnostic capability will influence the demographic profile of CHD for future generations.

Structural cardiovascular abnormalities substantially alter the processes of fetal and neonatal maturation. Although CHD represents a nearly endless array of anatomic variants, the impact they exert on the developing cardiovascular system can be confined to a few abnormal loading conditions from a physiologic and pharmacologic perspective. Physiologic classification of CHD enables the clinician to anticipate

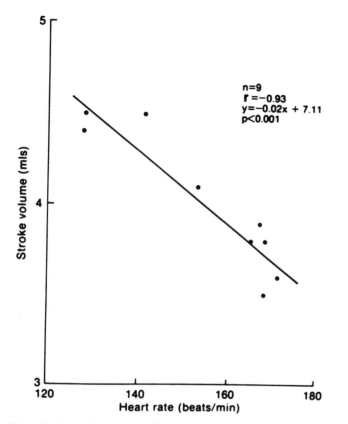

Figure 17–5. Doppler echocardiographic comparison of the effect of spontaneous changes in heart rate on stroke volume in a normal human fetus in utero, illustrating decrease in stroke volume with increases in heart rate. These observations confirm the ability of the fetal heart to change stroke volume under normal physiologic conditions. (From Kenny J, Plappert T, Doubilet P, et al: Effects of heart rate on ventricular size, stroke volume, and output in the normal human fetus: A prospective Doppler echocardiographic study. Circulation 1987;76:52–58.)

more precisely the cardiovascular response to anesthetic and surgical interventions.

Physiologic Categories of Congenital Heart Disease

Congenital heart malformations incur pathophysiologic cost by three means either alone or in combination. They inflict excess pressure loading or volume loading conditions on the myocardium, or they cause systemic hypoxemia. Conceptualizing the myriad defects in terms of these few pathophysiologic states enables the clinician to make some generalized predictions as to the response of a given patient to the perioperative manipulations and therapeutic agents to which they will be exposed.

Volume Loads

The volume substrate delivery and perfusion pressure under which blood flows to the systemic circulation are tightly regulated by an array of neurohumoral feedback mechanisms linked to metabolic demands. Structural cardiovascular defects that divert left ventricular output to the pulmonary

circulation trigger feedback mechanisms such as increased adrenal catecholamine output, increased renin and angiotensin production, expanded intravascular volume, and constriction of noncritical vascular beds to compensate for the lost systemic flow by increasing total left ventricular output.

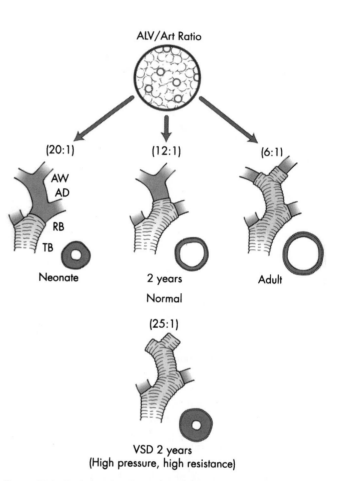

Figure 17–6. Peripheral pulmonary artery development. The normal pattern of pulmonary vascular development and that of a 2-year-old child with pulmonary vascular changes accompanying a large ventricular septal defect (VSD). Rabinovitch characterizes the pulmonary vasculature morphometrically in three respects: vessel thickness, muscular extension, and the radio of alveoli to artery seen on lung biopsy specimens. The normal neonate exhibits thick vascular smooth muscle, but this only extends as far as the arterioles accompanying the respiratory bronchiole. Neonates have an alveoli to artery ratio of 20:1. In the first few months of life, the vessels thin substantially and proliferate relative to the alveoli so that by the age of 2 years the normal child has an alveoli to artery ratio of 12:1 and thin muscles extending to the arteries associated with alveolar ducts. The normal adult has an alveoli to artery ratio of 6:1 and muscle extending all the way to the arteries in the alveolar wall. In contrast, the 2-year-old child with a large VSD has markedly diminished vessel numbers (alveoli to artery ratio 25:1) and persistent neonatal muscle thickness extending out all the way to the alveolar wall. AD, artery at alveolar duct; ALV, alveoli; AW, artery at alveolar wall; TB, artery at terminal bronchiole. (From Steven JM, Nicolson SC: Congenital heart disease. In: Atlas of Anesthesia (Miller RD, series ed), Vol VII: Pediatric Anesthesia (Greeley WJ, volume ed. p 6.6; modified from Rabinovitch M, Haworth SG, Castaneda AR, et al: Lung biopsy in congenital heart disease: A morphometric approach to pulmonary vascular disease. Circulation 1978:58:1107–1122.)

Table 17-2. Conditions Prolonging Transitional Circulation

Prematurity
Pulmonary disease
   Hypoxemia
   Hypercarbia
Congenital heart disease
Sepsis
Acidosis
Hypothermia
High altitude
Prolonged stress

Although tachycardia may represent the initial mechanism by which left ventricular output increases, ultimately stroke volume increases by dilating the left ventricle. Thus left-to-right shunts impose an added volume load on the heart.

Within the boundaries of a given heart to increase its output, the magnitude of the shunt determines the additional volume burden. Hemodynamic principles dictate the direction and magnitude of shunt. Defects at the atrial level permit shunts in proportion to the relative compliance of the ventricles and thus impose proportionally smaller volume loads than ventricular defects. The latter enable shunts in relation to differences in systolic pressure or vascular resistance in the respective pulmonary and systemic circulations. Given defects of comparable diameter, the largest volume shunts occur at the great arterial level, where left-to-right flow persists during systole and diastole.

Patients who confront excess volume loads as a result of CHD tend to exhibit clinical congestive heart failure earlier in the natural history of the disease than those subjected to additional pressure work. Differences in compensatory mechanisms may account for this distinction. Increased volume output occurs by dilation of the respective ventricle. Myocardial hypertrophy results to maintain a constant ratio of wall thickness to radius, thereby preserving systolic wall stress (Fig. 17-7).[43] This pattern of dilation and hypertrophy increases diastolic wall stress, diminishing ventricular compliance and increasing venous pressures, thus fostering the signs of congestive heart failure. In infants these include tachypnea as well as grunting respirations, nasal flaring, and/or chest retractions, poor feeding, poor growth, hepatomegaly, and diaphoresis. Clinical observations suggest that the hearts of these infants demonstrate greater vulnerability to the myocardial depressant effects of anesthetic agents than other pathophysiologic loading conditions. Another prime management goal in patients with the capacity for large left-to-right shunts is to not further compromise systemic perfusion by increasing the magnitude of the shunt (e.g., by lowering pulmonary vascular resistance).

Pressure Loads

Excess pressure loads occur when intracavitary ventricular pressure must increase to maintain sufficient flow or systemic perfusion pressure across an obstruction. Obstruction can occur in the outflow tract, semilunar valve, or great artery. Despite markedly increased intraventricular pressure, the compensatory mechanisms for pressure loads appear more effective than those for volume loads. Substantial myocardial hypertrophy develops, as does the ratio of wall thickness to radius (see Fig. 17-7).[43] This effect enables the heart to maintain normal systolic and diastolic wall stress. These children appear far less prone to the manifestations of congestive heart failure and, similarly, demonstrate more typical sensitivity to the myocardial depressant effects of anesthetic drugs. An exception to this general principle arises when an obstruction to flow develops in the dilated, volume-overloaded heart. Taken together, the combined effects of volume and pressure loading produce a fragile hemodynamic situation that is far more vulnerable than the sum of its parts.

Hypoxemia

Two distinct pathophysiologic mechanisms cause systemic hypoxemia: right-to-left shunt and admixture of systemic

Table 17-3. Incidence of Congenital Heart Disease

	Relative Incidence (percent within each study)			
	Scott et al[39]	Fyler[40]	Hoffman[38]	Allan et al[41]
Ventricular septal defect	15.4	15.7	31	5
Atrial septal defect	0.5	2.9	7.5	0
Patent ductus arteriosus	6.7	6.1	7.1	—
Pulmonary stenosis	3.0	3.3	7.0	5
Pulmonary atresia	1.9	3.1	<1	—
Coarctation of the aorta	10.5	7.5	5.6	11
Tetralogy of Fallot	9.9	8.9	5.5	3
Aortic stenosis	1.1	1.9	4.9	4
Transposition of the great arteries	10.4	9.9	4.5	2
Atrioventricular canal defect	3.9	5.0	4.4	17.5
Hypoplastic left heart syndrome	3.7	7.4	3.1	16
Tricuspid atresia	4.7	2.6	2.4	4
Single ventricle	4.3	2.4	1.5	2
Truncus arteriosus	2.1	1.4	1.4	1.5
Total anomalous pulmonary venous connection	3.6	2.6	1.4	<1
Double-outlet right ventricle	3.0	1.5	1.2	3
Ebstein's malformation	0	0	<1	7

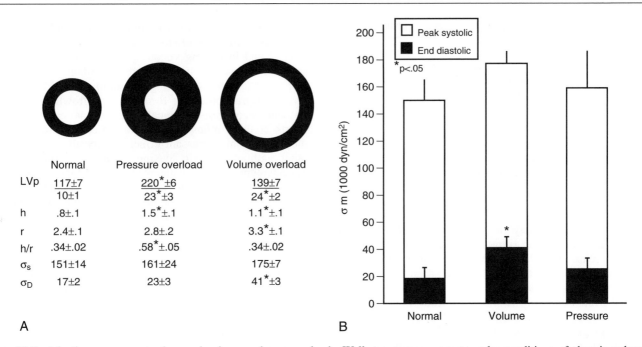

Figure 17–7. Adaptive responses to abnormal volume and pressure loads. Wall stress measurements under conditions of chronic volume or pressure overload are compared to normal. Volume overload induces dilation to facilitate larger stroke volume. The compensatory influence on the myocardial wall results in enough hypertrophy (increased thickness) to maintain a normal wall thickness to radius ratio (h/r). In contrast, chronic pressure overload induces hypertrophy significantly increasing the h/r ratio (A). Both methods of compensation act to preserve normal systolic wall stress (σ); however, chronic volume overload induces diastolic dysfunction (B). h, LV posterior myocardial wall thickness; LVp, left ventricular pressure; r, radius of the LV chamber; σ_S = peak systolic wall stress; σ_D = end-diastolic wall stress. (From Greeley WJ, Steven JM, Nicolson SC, et al: Anesthesia for pediatric cardiac surgery. In: Miller RD, ed: Anesthesia, Vol. 2, 5th ed. Philadelphia: Churchill Livingstone; 2000:1805–1847; modified from Grossman W, Jones D, McLaurin LP: Wall stress and patterns of hypertrophy in the human left ventricle. J Clin Invest 1975;56:56–64.)

and pulmonary venous return. In the former, obstruction to pulmonary arterial flow precipitates a right-to-left shunt when intracardiac or great vessel communications exist. As such, pulmonary blood flow is diminished proportional to the magnitude of the shunt. Tetralogy of Fallot represents a classic example of a right-to-left shunt lesion. However, most congenital cardiac defects that produce hypoxemia do so as a result of admixture of systemic and pulmonary venous returns. With these anomalies, pulmonary artery blood flow may be normal or even increased, yet hypoxemia ensues. The proportion of oxygenated to deoxygenated blood (i.e., pulmonary flow:systemic flow [Qp:Qs]) in the mixture determines the magnitude of systemic hypoxemia. *d*-Transposition of the great arteries (*d*-TGA) serves as an illustrative example of hypoxemia resulting from venous admixture.

Typically, lesions producing systemic hypoxemia have concomitant excess pressure or volume loads as well. Strategic anesthetic planning should seek to minimize the burden of these pathologic loading conditions while promoting optimal tissue oxygen delivery. For example, in the neonate with single-ventricle physiology, and thus complete mixing of venous returns, measures directed at lowering pulmonary vascular resistance will dramatically increase pulmonary blood flow and the proportion of oxygenated blood entering the mixture. Although systemic oxygen saturation may approach normal, the cost imposed is a dramatic increase in volume load as the heart desperately tries to sustain sufficient systemic flow despite progressive diversion of blood to the pulmonary circulation. Ultimately, the neonate with single-

ventricle physiology cannot maintain the demand for increased total cardiac output (Qp plus Qs) and systemic blood flow deteriorates, thereby compromising tissue oxygen delivery. *Clinical experience suggests that the neonate exhibits signs of better vital organ perfusion with normal systemic output at reduced saturation than diminished systemic flow of normally oxygenated blood.* From a practical standpoint (as well as through theoretical modeling) this equates to a $Q_p:Q_s$ of approximately 1.0 with oxygen saturations of approximately 75 to 85% (see further).

Postoperative Considerations

In the contemporary era of infant heart surgery, the majority of children presenting for noncardiac surgery will have already survived a cardiac intervention. The majority exhibit good functional recovery and normal "series" circulatory pattern, although some are palliated owing to anatomic or hemodynamic constraints that either preclude or defer physiologic repair. A thorough understanding of the anatomic and functional consequences of these cardiac interventions constitutes the cornerstone in planning perioperative care. Despite optimal functional recovery and normal circulatory pattern, intensive testing often reveals varying degrees of residual hemodynamic abnormalities in all but the simplest malformations (e.g., secundum atrial septal defect). Although repaired, these children's hearts may not be "normal," resulting in unanticipated responses under the perioperative stresses imposed by surgical and anesthetic interventions.[44]

The sequelae tend to occur in four broad categories: residual pathophysiologic pressure or volume loads, ventricular dysfunction, rhythm disturbances, and elevated pulmonary vascular resistance.

By definition, palliative cardiac interventions leave residual pathophysiologic conditions in the form of one or more abnormal loading conditions. Even reparative cardiac surgery may incompletely relieve obstructions, leave residual shunts, or damage valve function, resulting in residual hemodynamic pathophysiology. Impaired ventricular function may occur as a result of intraoperative myocardial injury or the long-standing effects of abnormal loading conditions.[45, 46] Although rhythm disturbances rarely accompany structural CHD in the absence of surgery, they frequently arise as a complication or sequela of specific cardiac operations. Irreversible pulmonary vascular disease develops as a consequence of protracted exposure to high pulmonary artery pressure or flow (e.g., large left-to-right shunts).[27, 47, 48] Within these broad categories, certain cardiac anomalies and specific repairs tend to predispose patients to particular sequelae. Preoperative assessment of children who have undergone these repairs should specifically evaluate each of the anticipated cardiovascular manifestations (see Chapter 19). Four common surgical interventions serve to illustrate.

Ventricular Septal Defect

Despite the simple concept that would suggest cure by closure of the communication between the ventricles, a variety of sequelae occur in patients with ventricular septal defect (VSD) even after a "perfect" operation. Echocardiographic evaluation of ventricular chamber dimension, myocardial wall thickness, and shortening fraction may all remain abnormal, particularly when the hemodynamic derangement has existed for several years (Fig. 17–8).[45, 46, 49] Whether these hearts will respond normally to the myocardial depressant effects of some anesthetic agents or the stress imposed by major surgical interventions remains speculative. Experience suggests nearly normal response to all but the most extreme conditions. As noted earlier, the patients regularly develop pulmonary vascular disease when pulmonary artery pressure and flow remain substantially elevated for years. On occasion, this process progresses, i.e., to irreversible pulmonary hypertension, despite closure of the VSD. Abnormalities in cardiac conduction also occur as a consequence of VSD closure, generally manifested immediately following the repair.

Tetralogy of Fallot

Even perfect physiologic repair of tetralogy of Fallot leaves the substrate for significant sequelae. All techniques require a right ventricular myotomy or ventriculotomy predisposing the patient to right ventricular dysfunction. This propensity is exaggerated with methods that render the pulmonary valve incompetent (e.g., transannular patch).[50] These residua rarely manifest clinically significant symptoms early unless significant pulmonary vascular obstruction persists.[51] In addi-

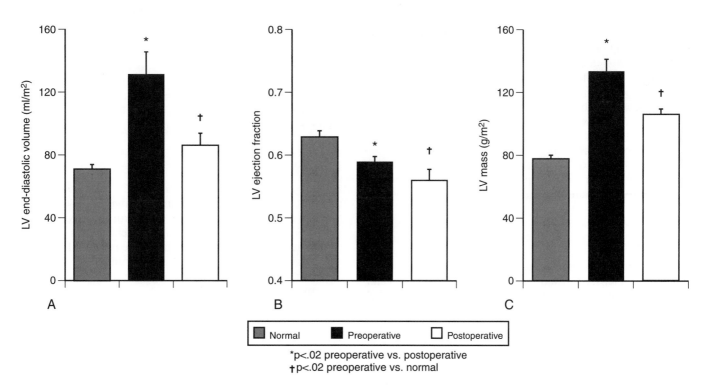

*p<.02 preoperative vs. postoperative
†p<.02 preoperative vs. normal

Figure 17–8. Postoperative changes following closure of ventricular septal defect (VSD). Echocardiographic evaluation of 23 children an average of 2 years following closure of a simple VSD. (A) Left ventricular end-diastolic volume (LVEDV). (B) Left ventricular ejection fraction (LVEF). (C) Left ventricular mass. Each graph depicts baseline values and postoperative values in the subjects as compared with normal control subjects. Although these results demonstrate a return toward normal, they remain significantly abnormal even 2 years postoperatively. (Data from Jarmakani JM, Graham TPJ, Canent RVJ: Left ventricular contractile state in children with successfully corrected ventricular septal defect. Circulation 1972;45:I102–I110; and Jarmakani JM, Graham TP Jr, Canent RV Jr, et al: The effect of corrective surgery on left heart volume and mass in children with ventricular septal defect. Am J Cardiol 1971;27:254–258.)

tion to the conduction disturbances that can accompany any VSD closure, these children may exhibit ventricular ectopy and sudden death.[52] Risk factors that predispose them to ventricular arrhythmias include residual pathophysiologic pressure or volume loading conditions that result in elevated right ventricular systolic or diastolic pressure.[53] Other risk factors for late ventricular dysfunction and sudden death may include late age at repair, residual or long-standing pressure or volume load on the right ventricle, and prior systemic-to-pulmonary palliative shunt.

Transposition of the Great Arteries

Repair of *d*-TGA has evolved substantially over the past 40 years. Early successful physiologic repair was accomplished by intra-atrial baffling procedures that redirected oxygenated blood to the right ventricle and deoxygenated blood to the left ventricle for circulation to the appropriate vascular bed (e.g., Mustard and Senning operations). The late sequelae of these procedures include arrhythmia, baffle obstruction, and right (systemic) ventricular dysfunction.[54] Followed for 15 years, virtually none of these patients remain consistently in sinus rhythm (Fig. 17–9A).[55] Sick sinus syndrome, atrial tachyarrhythmias, and sudden death constitute the most common arrhythmias in these patients.[56] Long-term outcome studies have also identified right ventricular failure in 10 to 15% of patients following intra-atrial repair of *d*-TGA (Fig. 17–9B).[57–59]

In the past 15 years, the arterial switch operation has supplanted intra-atrial repairs for *d*-TGA. Although the frequency of serious sequelae appears significantly lower, the follow-up period has not been comparable to that for Mustard or Senning operations.[60, 61] Early experience with arterial switch operation demonstrated postoperative supravalvar obstruction of the aorta or, more commonly, the pulmonary artery.[62] Reports of abnormal coronary flow patterns or coronary flow response to vasodilators have begun to emerge.[63–65] Questions have arisen regarding the long-term function of the neo-aortic valve, which was a pulmonary valve during embryologic development.[61, 65] For reasons that remain incompletely understood, patients with *d*-TGA demonstrate significantly higher risk of pulmonary vascular disease.[66] Occasionally, this serious sequela occurs despite early corrective repair.[67]

Fontan Operation

As the only physiologic repair option for children with single ventricle, the Fontan operation accomplishes several desirable objectives.[68] Systemic venous return is diverted directly into the pulmonary arteries and oxygenated blood returns to the heart for circulation to the body. As such, the Fontan operation establishes a series circulatory pattern and nearly normal systemic oxygen saturation and limits the pressure and volume load imposed on the single ventricle to that which would be expected of a normal systemic ventricle. As one might imagine, such patients exhibit marked sensitivity to any condition that might impede pulmonary blood flow. Their ability to increase cardiac output is limited to their capacity to augment pulmonary blood flow passively, requiring moderately elevated systemic venous pressure. Exercise testing confirms significant reduction in maximal ca-

pacity (Fig. 17–10B).[69, 70] Outcome studies conducted on patients who underwent the Fontan operation in the 1970s and 1980s revealed progressive deterioration in functional status (Fig. 17–10A) and ongoing mortality rates, suggesting that this procedure must be considered palliative.[71] Many modifications to the procedure have evolved during the past 20 years to improve outcome.[72–74]

Apart from their progressive deterioration in cardiac function, limited reserve, and exquisite sensitivity to factors that might impede pulmonary blood flow, patients who have survived a Fontan operation may demonstrate a variety of sequelae in the context of anesthesia and noncardiac surgery. Preservation of preload represents a central objective in preserving pulmonary blood flow and hence cardiac output. Similarly, ventilatory strategies that minimize pulmonary vascular resistance and management that preserves ventricular function act together to promote pulmonary flow. Atrial arrhythmias and sick sinus syndrome commonly complicate the outcome of patients following the Fontan operation.[56, 75] Serosal effusions of the pericardial, pleural, and peritoneal spaces may detract from optimal early and intermediate-term outcome. Taken together, these late manifestations of Fontan physiology contribute to make these patients among the most fragile candidates for subsequent noncardiac surgery.

Acquired Heart Disease

In children, acquired heart disease occurs significantly less commonly than CHD. These findings tend to represent manifestations of systemic disorders. They may accompany inherited diseases (e.g., Down syndrome and Marfan syndrome), inflammatory processes (e.g., Kawasaki disease), or infection (e.g., endocarditis). The disease process may afflict the myocardium, valves, or vasculature. As such, the anesthetic management centers on minimizing pathophysiologic hemodynamic loading conditions and preserving myocardial function and vital organ perfusion. A partial list of the more common systemic diseases follows.

Down Syndrome

At least 40% of newborns with trisomy 21 (Down syndrome) manifest CHD. The characteristic distribution of malformations reveals that nearly half are endocardial cushion defects, with VSD, tetralogy of Fallot, and patent ductus arteriosus (PDA) accounting for the majority of the rest.[76, 77] Pulmonary vascular disease may develop more rapidly in infants with Down syndrome and CHD, although the mechanism remains controversial.[78–80]

Marfan Disease

Marfan disease is an autosomal dominant connective tissue disorder that produces progressive dilation of the cardiac valve annulus structure, ultimately resulting in regurgitation.[81] Mitral valve dysfunction occurs early, ultimately affecting as many as 68% of patients with Marfan's disease.[82, 83] Functional aortic valve involvement rarely occurs prior to the second decade of life.[84] In addition, medial disruption in the aorta predisposes these children to aneurysm formation. Aortic disease can also include the coronary arteries.

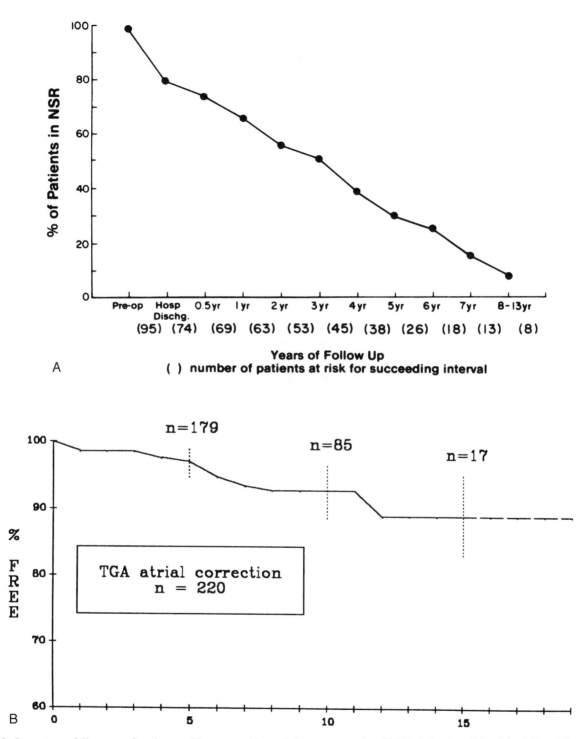

Figure 17–9. Long-term follow-up of patients with transposition of the great arteries (TGA) following "physiologic" atrial repairs. (A) Graph depicts Holter monitoring of 95 patients 3 months to 13 years following Mustard operation. The prevalence of subjects who consistently remain in sinus rhythm is less than 10% when followed more than 8 years. (From Hayes CJ, Gersony WM: Arrhythmias after the Mustard operation for transposition of the great arteries: A long term study. J Am Coll Cardiol 1986;7:133–137. (B) Kaplan-Meier graph depicting the percentage of patients from systemic (right) ventricular failure between 1 month and 20 years following a Senning operation. (From Turina MI, Siebenmann R, von Segesser L, et al: Late functional deterioration after atrial correction for transposition of the great arteries. Circulation 1989;80(suppl I):I162–I167. Reprinted with permission from the American College of Cardiology.)

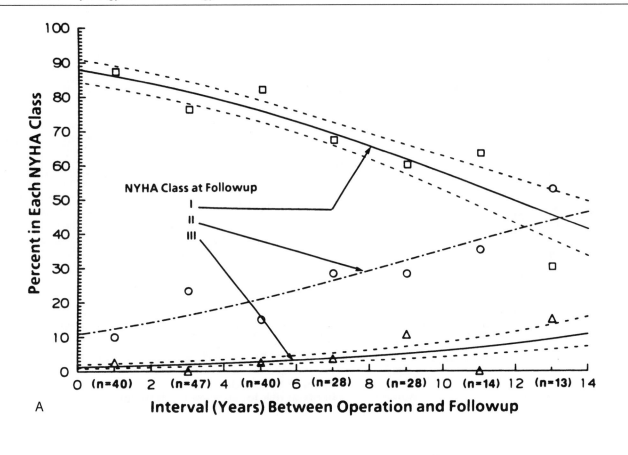

A   **Interval (Years) Between Operation and Followup**

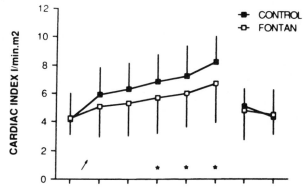

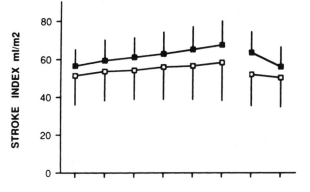

B

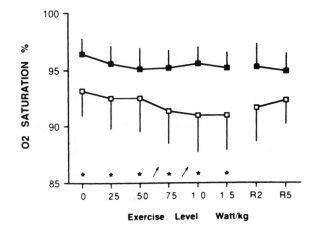

Figure 17–10. *See legend on opposite page*

Kawasaki Disease

Kawasaki disease is an acute febrile inflammatory disease that leaves residual aneurysms in a variety of vessels, including coronary arteries. Kawasaki disease has become the leading cause of acquired heart disease in children in the United States.[85] As many as 40% of children demonstrate cardiac involvement in the acute febrile stage of the illness, including myocarditis, pericardial effusion, or arrhythmia.[85–87] *Coronary aneurysms develop in 20%, causing myocardial infarction and death in as many as 3 to 4%.*[85] Although many coronary aneurysms regress over time, some produce ischemia, infarction, and occasionally rupture.[87–89]

Endocarditis

Although rheumatic heart disease is rare in the United States, it represents a predominant cause of acquired valve disease worldwide, with 85% of cases affecting the mitral valve.[90, 91] Bacterial endocarditis still occurs in association with bacteremia from a variety of sources.[92] Complex cardiac surgical procedures in young infants have dramatically changed the incidence and spectrum of patients afflicted with bacterial endocarditis.[93] Approximately 40% of endocarditis episodes develop in postoperative cardiac surgery patients, with over 80% having some pre-existing CHD or acquired cardiac disease.[94] Residual valvar dysfunction requires individual assessment.

Inflammatory Collagen-Vascular Diseases

A variety of systemic inflammatory diseases have an impact on the pericardium, myocardium, or conduction system. As many as 50% of children with systemic lupus erythematosus exhibit cardiac manifestations.[95] These include pericardial inflammation or effusion, myocarditis, valve dysfunction, and conduction system abnormalities. An inflammatory myocarditis and cardiomyopathy can also be a prominent feature of human immunodeficiency virus infection and its treatment in children.

Primary Pulmonary Hypertension

Pulmonary vascular disease that develops independent of CHD represents a particularly virulent process that progresses rapidly to death. In young children, no strong gender association emerges, although it is predominantly a disease of females from adolescence onward (4:1 ratio). Vasodilator therapy rarely provides more than brief palliation. Although lung transplantation offers some benefit, the 2-year survival rate is only 60%.[96–99]

Cardiovascular Pharmacology

Rational Use of Vasoactive Drugs

Selection of appropriate inotropic and vasopressor therapies depends on several factors, including the clinical situation, underlying cardiac abnormalities, and perfusion requirements of other organs. *The major goal is to improve oxygen delivery to the tissues.* As such, the primary focus is on improving myocardial pump function, systemic blood flow, and tissue oxygenation. Oxygen-carrying capacity (i.e., hemoglobin) should also be considered carefully in this regard. When deciding on specific agents or regimens, other factors include optimizing heart rate, contractility, and afterload. In certain congenital heart lesions, appropriate balance of systemic and pulmonary blood flow is also important (see further discussions).

Drugs that are catecholamines or have catecholamine-like effects remain the most commonly used inotropic and vasoconstrictor drugs. It is likely that improvements in cardiac output in neonates in response to drugs such as dopamine or dobutamine are due to increases in both heart rate and contractility. Some evidence exists in infants and in young children after cardiac surgery that the increases in cardiac output produced by dopamine and dobutamine may be more related to a positive chronotropic effect than to an increase in the intrinsic contractile state.[100–102] With few exceptions, drugs that primarily increase afterload, such as that provided by alpha-adrenergic agonists, have limited use in pediatric patients. This effect is mainly because large increases in afterload, without corresponding improvements in contractile state, are poorly tolerated by infants and children, particularly in the face of significant underlying contractile dysfunction.

Practical Considerations for the Use of Vasoactive Agents

Commonly used drugs, their doses, and the summary of their effects on selected cardiac functions are given in Table 17–4. Much of this information has been empirically derived from studies in adults. There is limited information about the effects of commonly used vasoactive drugs in pediatric patients at different ages and limited information about the effects of these drugs in various pathophysiologic states. Factors that are likely to provide unique responses to inotropic and vasoconstrictor drugs in neonates and infants include altered pharmacokinetics; differences in receptor types, number, and function; and variability in drug delivery. Substantial variations in measured plasma concentrations, as well as the volume of distribution, have been noted in

Figure 17–10. (A) Symptomatic outcome of 334 survivors of Fontan operation followed 1 month to 20 years. Graph illustrates the change in New York Heart Association (NYHA) classification over time. Although most patients exhibit good functional status (NYHA class I) immediately following surgery, mild functional limitations evolve over time. (Triangles indicate actual percent of patients; broken lines indicate 70% confidence intervals. (From Fontan F, Kirklin JW, Fernandez G, et al: Outcome after a "perfect" Fontan operation. Circulation 1990;81:1520–1536.) (B) Exercise studies of 42 children (2 months to 14 years) before (black columns) and following (open columns) Fontan operation compared with normal control subjects (hatched columns). Although the protocol was designed to achieve modest targets, significant differences emerged in the capacity of Fontan patients to increase cardiac output. Systemic arterial oxygen saturation remained below normal throughout. (From Gewillig MH, Lundstrom UR, Bull C, et al: Exercise responses in patients with congenital heart disease after Fontan repair: Patterns and determinants of performance. J Am Coll Cardiol 1990;15:1424–1432. Reprinted with permission from the American College of Cardiology.)

Table 17–4. Inotropics and Vasopressors

Agent	Dose (IV)	Comments
Dopamine	2–20 µg/kg min infusion	Primary effects at $beta_1$, $beta_2$, and dopamine receptors, somewhat related to dose; lower doses (2–5 µg/kg/min) can increase contractility and also have direct dopaminergic receptor effect to increase splanchnic and renal perfusion; increasing doses increase contractility via beta effects and also increase likelihood of alpha-mediated vasoconstriction; effects depend upon endogenous catecholamine stores.
Dobutamine	2–20 µg/kg/min infusion	Relatively selective $beta_1$ stimulation; also potential $beta_2$ stimulation, tachycardia, and vasodilation, especially at higher doses (>10 µg/kg/min); may be less potent than dopamine, especially in immature myocardium; no significant alpha-adrenergic effects; tachydysrhythmias perhaps more likely than with dopamine; effects independent of endogenous catecholamine stores.
Epinephrine	0.02–2.0 µg/kg/min infusion	Primary beta effects to increase contractility and vasodilation at lower (0.02–0.10 µg/kg/min) doses; increasing doses (>0.1 µg/kg/min) accompanied by increased contractility and also increased alpha-mediated vasoconstriction; may be best choice to augment contractility and perfusion, especially in situations of severely compromised ventricular function, shock, or anaphylaxis.
Isoproterenol	0.05–2.0 µg/kg/min infusion	Pure, nonselective beta-agonist; significant inotropic, chronotropic ($beta_1$ and $beta_2$) and vasodilatory ($beta_2$) effects; may be an effective pulmonary vasodilator in some patients; tachycardia and increased myocardial oxygen consumption may be dose-limiting; tachydysrhythmias may also occur; bronchodilator.
Phenylephrine	1–10 µg/kg bolus, 0.1–0.5 µg/kg/min infusion	Pure alpha-mediated vasoconstriction; no increase in contractility.
Amrinone	0.3–3 mg/kg loading dose (slowly), 5–10 µg/kg/min infusion	Increases cAMP by phosphodiesterase inhibition; positive inotropy, positive lusitropy, and smooth muscle vasorelaxation; hypotension; reversible thrombocytopenia.
Milrinone	50–100 µg/kg loading dose, 0.5–1.0 µg/kg/min infusion	Similar to amrinone (anti-platelet effects may be less).

Calcium
  Chloride
  Gluconate
	
	10–20 mg/kg/dose (slowly)
	30–100 mg/kg/dose (slowly)
		Positive inotropic and direct vasoconstricting effects; inotropy significant only if ionized calcium is low and/or ventricular function is depressed by other agents; can slow sinus node; increases electrophysiologic abnormalities from hypokalemia and digoxin.

Digoxin	Total digitalizing dose (TDD):
	  Premature: 20 µg/kg
	  Neonate: 30 µg/kg (1 month)
	  Infant: 40 µg/kg (<2 years)
	  Child: 30 µg/kg (2–5 years)
	  Over 5 years: 20 µg/kg
	  Maintenance: 5–10 µg/kg/day
	    divided q 12 hours
		TDD given in divided doses—½ TDD followed by ¼ TDD every 8–12 hr × 2 increases cardiac contractility; slows sinus node and decreases AV node conduction; long half-life (24–48 hours) that is prolonged by renal dysfunction; numerous drug interactions; toxicity includes supraventricular tachycardia, AV block, ventricular dysrhythmias; symptoms include drowsiness, nausea, vomiting; toxicity exacerbated by hypokalemia

AV, atrioventricular; cAMP, cyclic adenosine monophosphate.

pediatric patients receiving inotropics, such that as much as a 10-fold range in plasma concentrations has been noted for a given infusion rate.[103, 104]

Substantial variability can be observed in the serum concentration of a particular inotrope that is required to produce a given effect. Some of these pharmacodynamic differences are related to receptor maturation and function. It appears that, for example, beta-adrenergic receptors are at high density in the term and young infant, but their coupling to adenyl cyclase may be incomplete.[24, 105] In addition to developmental changes, controlled in part by thyroid hormone, beta-receptor and adenyl cyclase activity is diminished in response to sustained administration of exogenous beta-agonists as well as increased endogenous catecholamines. The latter is a complication of moderate to severe heart failure and other forms of severe stress such as sepsis.[106–108]

The effects of prolonged beta-adrenergic stimulation in newborn myocardium are not quite as clear. Catecholamines may up-regulate adrenergic receptor number or function, or both, in infants, perhaps in part owing to mimicking of the normal developmental program of increasing sympathetic nervous system activity as term approaches.[109] With further maturation in early postnatal life, beta-adrenergic receptor density declines. The impact of different pathophysiologic states on these processes is unclear overall. For example, congestive heart failure, cardiopulmonary bypass, and ischemic reperfusion all lead to decreased beta-receptor and adenyl cyclase expression and activity.[110–113] Higher beta-receptor density and greater receptor-stimulated adenyl cyclase activity have been shown in the myocardium of infants with tetralogy of Fallot.[114]

One must pay particular attention to technical issues when

administering vasoactive infusions to infants. Infusion preparations for infants are usually rendered in a highly concentrated form to limit the amount of volume infused and use nonstandard dilutions. Hence, the potential for dose or concentration error is substantial. One study at a tertiary care pediatric hospital demonstrated that the actual concentration of prepared solutions varied significantly.[115] The high concentration relative to patient size means that small errors (either in calculation or infusion pump flow rate) can significantly affect the actual amount of drug delivered. The corresponding slow infusion rate can also lead to a delay in drug delivery. Ensuring that the pump drive mechanism is actually delivering drug at the distal end of the infusion tubing, connecting the infusion tubing as close to the patient as possible, and using a carrier infusion delivered at constant rate are among ways to decrease variability and increase efficacy of drug infusions.

Balancing Parallel Circulations

Several groups of patients require careful attention to the balance between systemic and pulmonary blood flow (Q_p:Q_s). Examples include patients with hypoplastic left heart syndrome (who have ductal-dependent systemic blood flow), those with critical aortic coarctation (who have ductal-dependent systemic blood flow), those with large ventricular septal or atrioventricular channel defects (who have potential for left-to-right shunting and systemic hypoperfusion), and patients with palliative and surgical systemic-to-pulmonary artery shunts (e.g., Blalock-Taussig shunt).

Maintaining ductal patency with prostaglandin E_1 (see later discussion) is necessary in treatment of many of the lesions with obstruction to pulmonary or aortic blood flow. At times, atrial septostomy is also required to ensure adequate intracardiac mixing in patients with a single-ventricle physiology. *Patients with ductal-dependent systemic blood flow require careful balancing of systemic vascular resistance and pulmonary vascular resistance to maintain adequate systemic perfusion and appropriate but not excessive oxygenation.* In these patients, hyperventilation, alkalosis, and hyperoxia can decrease pulmonary vascular resistance, increase pulmonary blood flow, and lead to systemic hypoperfusion, oliguria, and metabolic acidosis. From a practical standpoint, systemic oxygen saturations of 75 to 80% and normal to mildly elevated arterial carbon dioxide tension are reasonable goals. Occasionally, reducing the inspiring oxygen concentration below 0.21 by adding nitrogen to inspired air or adding inspired carbon dioxide, requiring mechanical ventilation and heavy sedation or muscle relaxation to avoid compensatory hyperventilation, are necessary to control pulmonary blood flow in these patients. Usually, however, appropriate ventilation at low F_{IO_2} and normal to mild hypercarbia is sufficient to maintain an appropriate balance of systemic and pulmonary blood flow. Occasionally, low-dose inotropic support is also required to optimize systemic perfusion.

Similar considerations apply in patients with the potential for large left-to-right cardiac shunting. Here again, one wants to control those factors that decrease pulmonary vascular resistance to also control the magnitude of the left-to-right shunt and avoid excessive pulmonary blood flow, decreased systemic perfusion, and potential worsening of pulmonary vascular congestion.

Patients with *decreased pulmonary blood flow* resulting in cyanosis depend on the balance of pulmonary vascular resistance to systemic vascular resistance, as well as overall cardiac output, to achieve adequate oxygenation. Pulmonary blood flow will typically be through either natural (e.g., patent ductus arteriosis) or surgically created systemic-to-pulmonary arterial communications. Increased pulmonary vascular resistance or decreased systemic vascular resistance compromises pulmonary blood flow in patients with shunt-dependent pulmonary flow. In patients dependent on surgical systemic-to-pulmonary artery shunts for pulmonary blood flow, pulmonary blood flow is positively affected by increasing cardiac output and systemic vascular resistance and by decreasing pulmonary vascular resistance. Shunt size and patency are, of course, important factors as well.

Cardiac output has a direct influence on systemic arterial oxygen saturation in single-ventricle and other types of mixing lesions because of its effect on venous oxygen saturation. For example, reduced cardiac output leading to reduced venous oxygen saturation results in lower systemic arterial oxygen saturation owing to the mixing of less saturated venous blood in patients with right-to-left shunts or complete mixing lesions. Conversely, improvements in arterial oxygen saturation can be achieved in these patients by optimizing cardiac output as well as oxygen content (e.g., increasing hemoglobin in patients who are relatively anemic).

Other forms of congenital cardiac lesions can be approached with a similar level of understanding of their underlying pathophysiology. Outflow obstruction (e.g., aortic stenosis) is characterized by increased pressure work, development of chamber hypertrophy, and reduced ability to increase cardiac output in response to increased demand. Therapeutic goals for these patients include ensuring adequate preload and maintaining heart rate at a sufficiently slow rate so as to allow adequate time for chamber filling and ejection. Right ventricular outflow obstruction may benefit from reducing afterload on the right ventricle (i.e., reducing pulmonary vascular resistance). In general, systemic vascular resistance should be maintained in a setting of either right or left ventricular outflow obstruction. In the case of fixed aortic outflow, this approach is necessary to ensure adequate coronary perfusion. Right ventricular outflow obstruction leads to right ventricular hypertrophy. Adequate systemic blood pressure is necessary to ensure coronary perfusion to the hypertrophic right ventricle. It is noteworthy that a substantial percentage of total coronary flow to the right ventricle occurs during systole.

Patients with significant ventricular dysfunction, for example due to dilated cardiomyopathy (see later), are functioning at the extremes of the Laplace and Frank-Starling relationships. The practical implications are that myocardial wall tension is maximal; subendocardial perfusion is easily compromised; and even relatively minor alterations in heart rate, contractility, preload, and afterload can lead to rapid and at times irreversible myocardial decompensation. Disturbances of cardiac rhythm and conduction are also poorly tolerated in such patients. Preload augmentation may not reliably increase cardiac output and may in fact lead to further ventricular dilation and atrioventricular valve regurgitation. Either bradycardia or significant tachycardia may also be poorly tolerated. Inotropic support, along with careful afterload reduction, may improve cardiac performance in such patients with severely compromised pump function.

The effects of mechanical ventilation should also be considered.[116, 117] Pulmonary vascular resistance is increased at either very high or very low lung volumes. In the former situation, high lung volumes are associated with increased intrathoracic pressures that are transmitted to the pulmonary vasculature. Alveolar overdistention, high intrathoracic pressures, and large lung volumes compress alveolar capillaries, increasing pulmonary vascular resistance and right ventricular afterload.[118] At the other extreme, hypoventilation and significantly reduced lung volume can increase pulmonary vascular resistance by leading to hypoxia, hypercarbia, and atelectasis. Significantly impaired right ventricular function can compromise left ventricular function by the mechanism of ventricular interdependence. *Appropriate positive pressure ventilation* may improve the performance of the systemic ventricle by mechanisms that include decreased afterload, decreased work of breathing, and improvements due to better oxygenation or ventilation. These benefits may more than offset any reduction in performance due to the effects of positive pressure on venous return or other parameters.

Vasoactive Drugs

Dopamine

Dopamine continues to be the most frequently used inotropic agent in neonates, infants, and children. It has activity at alpha, beta, and dopaminergic receptors. Dopamine augments cardiac contractility through two mechanisms. First, it directly stimulates cardiac beta$_1$-receptors and provokes norepinephrine release from cardiac sympathetic nerve terminals. Second, circulating concentrations of endogenous epinephrine and norepinephrine increase significantly during dopamine infusion, leading to the suggestion that at least some of the effects of a dopamine infusion are indirectly mediated via induced release of endogenous catecholamines.[119] Because of its indirect effects, particularly to release myocardial norepinephrine stores, the response to dopamine is thought to be diminished in patients with congestive heart failure or other relatively long-standing forms of hemodynamic stress.

Activity at dopaminergic receptors in the kidney and gastrointestinal tract can lead to improved perfusion of these organ systems. The evidence that dopamine specifically and selectively leads to improved renal perfusion via stimulation of renal dopaminergic receptors (i.e., as opposed to a nonspecific and generalized improvement in cardiac output that might be seen with any positive inotrope) is conflicting.[120, 121] Regardless of mechanism, most evidence indicates that renal blood flow and perfusion are increased by dopamine therapy, even at very high concentrations.

Similar to the situation with other inotropics, pharmacokinetic studies of dopamine have shown wide variability in serum concentrations in neonates and children.[122, 123] Because of this variability in plasma concentration for a given infusion rate, as well as the wide range of serum concentrations necessary to produce a given effect, doubling (to increase) or halving (to decrease) a given dopamine infusion rate may be a logical way to approach alterations in therapy. The

frequent practice of increasing or decreasing by significantly smaller proportions, typically 5 to 10%, may not be consistent with what is currently known about the pharmacokinetics and pharmacodynamics of most inotropics.

Neonates have classically been considered to have a greater dependence on heart rate, a lower myocardial compliance, and a relative resistance to inotropic effects of exogenous catecholamines. Nonetheless, there is substantial echocardiographic evidence of increased myocardial contractility occurring at low dopamine infusion rates ($\leq 5\mu g/mg/minute$) and prior to significant increases in heart rate.[124, 125] Evidence about the effects of dopamine in sick preterm infants is also somewhat controversial. There may be a relative dissociation between its effects on the renal and mesenteric beds in these infants, such that a portion of the increase in arterial blood pressure seen with a dopamine infusion is due to mesenteric vasoconstriction and an actual decrease in mesenteric blood flow.

Although it is generally believed that vasoconstriction is significant when high infusion rates ($>10–15 \mu g/kg/minute$) of dopamine are employed, studies have shown evidence of improved cardiac output and renal blood flow even at very high doses ($\geq 20 \mu g/kg/minute$) in neonates and infants. The effects of dopamine on pulmonary vascular resistance are variable. Both minimal effect and increased pulmonary vascular resistance have been found.[100, 126–130] The effects of dopamine on pulmonary vascular resistance most likely depend on the dose as well as the underlying state of the vascular endothelium and smooth muscle. Vasoconstriction may be more likely following ischemia-reperfusion and in the presence of hypoxia. Conversely, the presence of vasodilators, such as nitroprusside, or alpha-adrenergic blockers, such as phenoxybenzamine, can prevent increased pulmonary vascular resistance in response to dopamine. Overall, dopamine remains the drug of choice in the majority of infants and children owing to its beneficial effects on mesenteric and renal blood flow, lesser chronotropic effects than some other agents, and a somewhat lower arrhythmogenic potential.[131, 132]

Dobutamine

Dobutamine is a structural analogue of isoproterenol. It was developed to provide relatively selective beta-adrenergic receptor stimulation. The inotropic effects are somewhat less potent than those of dopamine, and it has significantly less overall alpha-adrenergic potential compared with dopamine. Dobutamine does possess significant beta$_2$-adrenergic receptor agonist properties, and as such peripheral vasodilation can occur. Substantial vasodilation and tachycardia occur at higher infusion rates ($\geq 10 \mu g/kg/minute$).[133–135] The tendency toward significant tachycardia and tachyarrhythmias may be greater in neonates than in older children or adults. There is some evidence that the efficacy of dobutamine is reduced in immature animals, perhaps due to higher circulating catecholamine concentrations and alterations in beta-receptor expression and function in these immature animal models.[101, 102]

The actions of dobutamine do not depend on endogenous catecholamine stores and hence the drug may be more effective in increasing cardiac output in severe congestive heart failure and cardiogenic shock.[136, 137] In children with normal left ventricular function, dobutamine has been shown to significantly increase left ventricular relaxation. A decrease in end-systolic wall stress likely contributes to the improved diastolic relaxation caused by dobutamine.[138] As with dopamine, questions of a relative resistance in neonates have arisen, although evidence indicates that dobutamine improves left ventricular contractility in newborns with left ventricular dysfunction.[136, 139] Dobutamine does not selectively improve renal or mesenteric blood flow independently of its effects to increase cardiac output. The improvement in cardiac output seen with dobutamine is related to its effects both to increase contractility and to decrease systemic vascular resistance via vasodilation. Pulmonary vasodilation in the presence of increased pulmonary vascular resistance may also occur. As was discussed with dopamine, exponential increases in serum concentration are required to produce linear improvements in cardiac index. There is also substantial pharmacokinetic variability in dobutamine plasma concentrations.[103, 140, 141] Tolerance may occasionally develop.[142]

Isoproterenol

Isoproterenol is a pure, nonselective beta-adrenergic agonist.[143] It increases heart rate and contractility and causes vasodilation in mesenteric, renal, and skeletal muscle tissue beds. Isoproterenol is a fairly effective vasodilator of the pulmonary circulation as well.[144] Significant tachycardia almost always accompanies its use. The tachycardia and greater contractility cause significant increases in myocardial oxygen consumption that are usually well tolerated. However, these changes may be limiting in compromised hearts. The pulmonary vasodilation produced by isoproterenol may be useful in settings where tachycardia is either unimportant or in fact somewhat beneficial, such as in the newly transplanted heart.[145] Systemic vasodilation induced by isoproterenol can be sufficiently profound as to cause systemic hypotension.[129, 146] The positive chronotropic effects of isoproterenol may be useful in patients with bradycardia. Isoproterenol is also a potent bronchodilator. Prolonged use or high doses of isoproterenol and other catecholamines may be associated with the development of myocardial fibrosis.[147]

Epinephrine

Epinephrine has alpha-, beta$_1$-, and beta$_2$-adrenergic agonist effects. Based on data mainly from adult studies, lower doses of 0.02 to 0.1 µg/kg/minute are associated with predominantly beta-adrenergic effects. In this range, increases in heart rate, systolic blood pressure, and reduced diastolic blood pressure due to skeletal muscle vasodilation predominate. Doses between 0.1 and 0.2 µg/kg/minute have mixed alpha and beta effects. At higher doses, alpha-adrenergic-induced vasoconstriction is significant, and hence there is reduced skin, muscle, renal, and mesenteric blood flow. Compared with pure alpha-agonists, epinephrine provides significant inotropic effect. The effects of epinephrine do not depend on endogenous tissue catecholamine stores. Based on experience, epinephrine may be effective in patients who do not respond to dopamine or dobutamine, particularly those with significant dysfunction of the systemic ventricle in the immediate postoperative period. The addition of moderate vasoconstriction to increased contractility may be advantageous to maintain myocardial perfusion and may also increase both systemic and pulmonary blood flow in patients with shunt-dependent circulations. Important side effects include dysrhythmias (usually ventricular), and at higher doses, regional ischemia and hypoperfusion due to vasoconstriction.[101] Serum concentrations are again linearly related to infusion rate, but patient responses also display significant variability.[148]

Phenylephrine

Phenylephrine is a pure alpha-adrenergic agonist. As such, its major function is to cause peripheral vasoconstriction. It is therefore of little use in terms of supporting cardiac function, although it may be of use as a temporizing measure to acutely improve afterload, systemic blood pressure, and hence critical organ blood flow. Conversely, the acute increase in afterload produced by phenylephrine is poorly tolerated, particularly by the compromised ventricle, in the absence of inotropic support. Phenylephrine can be given to increase systemic afterload and thereby decrease right-to-left shunting in patients who have tetralogy of Fallot and experience acute right ventricular outflow tract obstruction ("Tet spell"). In cyanotic patients who depend on a systemic-to-pulmonary artery shunt for pulmonary blood flow and hence oxygenation, phenylephrine may increase the magnitude of flow through the shunt via increasing afterload and hence improve arterial oxygenation and myocardial function, despite the increase in afterload.

Phosphodiesterase Inhibitors

Phosphodiesterase inhibitors, which includes amrinone, milrinone, vesnarinone, and enoximone, are noncatecholamine, nonglycoside inhibitors of phosphodiesterase isoforms. Their primary mechanism of action is thus to increase cyclic nucleotides, primarily cyclic adenosine monophosphate (cAMP). The absence of adrenergic stimulation minimizes effects on heart rate, rhythm, and dependency on endogenous tissue catecholamine stores. In addition to positive inotropic effects, they also have significant lusitropic properties (i.e., diastolic relaxation) and promote peripheral vasodilation.[149–151] Because their mechanism of action depends on increasing cAMP by preventing its breakdown by phosphodiesterases, they may be more efficacious when administered in conjunction with agents that stimulate adenyl cyclase (e.g., beta-agonists).[152] Phosphodiesterase drugs may also have substantial anti-inflammatory properties that are not well understood at present.[153–155]

Amrinone

As with all drugs in the amrinone class, there has been debate about the relative contribution of systemic vasodilation and afterload reduction versus increased cardiac contractility as the mechanism of increased cardiac output produced by amrinone. The bulk of evidence at the present time indicates that amrinone produces significant increases in myocardial contractility and reduces ventricular afterload.[150, 156, 157] Evidence of amrinone-induced improvements in cardiac performance in neonates and infants following cardiac surgery have been demonstrated in a number of situations, including postoperative patients who have undergone the arterial switch procedure, as well as older pediatric patients undergoing the Fontan operation.[151, 156, 158] Pharmacokinetic data in children suggest that the loading and infusion doses for amrinone need to be approximately twice those reported for adults.[159] In addition to differences in volume of distribution and clearance (both higher in infants), binding of amrinone to the oxygenator membrane may be another factor that needs to be considered if the loading dose is administered during cardiopulmonary bypass.[160] Overall, these data suggest that loading doses of 2 to 4 mg/kg and infusion rates starting in the range of 10 μg/kg/minute are indicated in the neonate and infant.[160] Large bolus doses of amrinone can cause significant systemic hypotension, particularly in the period immediately following cardiac surgery. From a practical standpoint, it may be best to administer the loading dose of amrinone slowly over the period of an hour. Caution is also indicated because the elimination half-life of amrinone is quite long (3 to 15 hours). Other side effects include thrombocytopenia that is reversible, occasional drug-related fever, and increased hepatic enzymes.

Milrinone

Several studies have demonstrated improved cardiac output and overall efficacy of milrinone after cardiac surgery in neonates and infants and with other states associated with ventricular dysfunction.[161–164] Milrinone has a larger volume of distribution and higher rate of clearance in infants and children compared with adults. Adjustments to bolus dosing and infusion rates have therefore been recommended.[161, 163] Unlike amrinone, milrinone does not appear to bind to the cardiopulmonary bypass circuit. The deleterious effects on platelets have been alleged to be less with milrinone than with amrinone. Loading doses of milrinone of 50 to 100 μg/kg (typically 75 μg/mg) and starting infusion rates of 0.50 to 1.0 μg/kg/minute have been recommended.[161, 165]

Enoximone

Enoximone is a phosphodiesterase inhibitor that has been used extensively in Europe but is not currently available in the United States. Its properties are generally similar to those of the other members of its class already discussed.[149, 166] Improvements in indirect indices of cardiac function such as mixed venous oxygen saturation, ventricular filling pressures, and systemic arterial blood pressure were afforded by enoximone in infants following cardiac surgery. A shorter length of hospital stay was also observed in these infants.[167] Enoximone was also useful to support cardiac function and potentially reduce pulmonary vascular resistance in children following cardiac transplantation.[168]

Digoxin

Digoxin remains the most frequently administered oral inotropic agent. Its use in patients with congestive heart failure due to large left-to-right shunts has been questioned on the basis that it preserves apparent myocardial contractility in the presence of progressive ventricular dilatation.[169, 170] Its efficacy in improving right ventricular dysfunction due to pulmonary hypertension has also been debated.

Digoxin has both direct and indirect effects. Its direct effects are mediated via inhibition of the membrane sodium-potassium ATPase. This mechanism leads to inhibition of outward sodium ion flux. The resulting increased intracellular sodium concentration stimulates the membrane sodium-calcium exchanger, producing increased intracellular calcium and positive inotropic effect. The indirect effects of digoxin are mediated by stimulation of the parasympathetic nervous system. The parasympathetic effects of digoxin result in slowing of atrial and atrioventricular node conduction. This drug can also be given to slow the ventricular response in atrial flutter and atrial fibrillation and to treat supraventricular tachycardia (see later).

Because digoxin has a slow distribution phase following oral administration and a long elimination half-life (up to 1 to 2 days in neonates and young infants), a loading dose is usually administered (Table 17–5). Renal dysfunction can significantly prolong the elimination half-life. Therapeutic digoxin levels are between 0.5 and 2.0 ng/mL. Intravenous and oral dosing regimens are the same, although the onset of electrophysiologic effects from intravenous dosing may be much more rapid (5 to 20 minutes).

Drug interactions with digoxin are extremely numerous. It should be assumed that just about any drug administered along with digoxin would affect the absorption and clearance of digoxin, usually necessitating a *reduction in digoxin dose*. The likelihood of digoxin toxicity increases with serum levels above 3 ng/mL.[171] Symptoms of toxicity include drowsiness, nausea, and vomiting. Various conduction abnormalities and supraventricular tachycardia are the most frequent cardiac rhythm manifestations of digoxin toxicity in infants and young children. Older children and adults are more likely to experience atrioventricular block, ventricular dysrhythmias, junctional tachycardia, and premature ventricular contractions. Hypokalemia, specifically intracellular potasium depletion as would occur for example with long-standing diuretic use, exacerbates the proarrhythmic effects of digoxin.

Calcium

The role, mechanisms of action, and potential for deleterious consequences of intravenous calcium administration continue to be controversial.[172] *It is the ionized calcium concentration that is important for myocardial function.* Calcium is a positive inotrope, particularly when administered in the presence of ionized hypocalcemia. It may also improve ventricular contractility when left ventricular function is depressed by halothane, beta-adrenergic blockade, or disease (e.g., sepsis).[173, 174] In the presence of a normal myocardium and normal ionized calcium concentrations, the effects of intravenous calcium administration on contractility are much more modest.[175] Another area of controversy has to do with the effects of intravenous calcium administration on peripheral vascular resistance, with both increases and decreases in systemic vascular resistance having been found in response to intravenous calcium.[176] Calcium most likely increases *pulmonary vascular resistance.*

There is evidence in adults that the primary effect of calcium administered after cardiac surgery is to increase systemic vascular resistance and mean arterial pressure with

Table 17–5. Antihypertensives and Vasodilators*

Drug	Dose (IV)	Comments
Propranolol	0.05–0.2 mg/kg slowly	Non-selective beta-blockade; bradycardia, hypotension, worsening of myocardial pump function; AV block; hypoglycemia; bronchospasm; depression; fatigue.
Labetalol	0.1–0.4 mg/kg/dose; 0.25–1.0 mg/kg/hour infusion	Non-selective beta-blockade; selective alpha-blockade; ratio of alpha to beta blockade is 1:7 for intravenous form; doses (0.1 mg/kg) can be repeated every 5–10 minutes until desired effect achieved; side effects similar to propranolol.
Esmolol	100–500 μg/kg loading dose (over 5 minutes); 50–300 μg/kg/min infusion	Relatively selective beta blockade; short elimination half-life (7–10 minutes); hypotension, especially during bolus administration; if less than desired response after 5 minutes, can repeat or double bolus dose, followed by doubling infusion rate; non–organ-based metabolism by plasma and red blood cell esterases; infusion concentrations >10 mg/mL may predispose to venous sclerosis; dilute infusion at high rates increases risk of volume overload.
Sodium nitroprusside	Start at 0.5–1.0 μg/kg/min infusion	Maximum 6–10 μg/kg/minute; potent direct smooth muscle relaxation; dilates both arteriolar resistance and venous capacitance vessels; hypotension potentiated by hypovolemia, inhalation anesthetics, other antihypertensives; variable pulmonary vasodilation; potential cyanide toxicity; reflex tachycardia; check cyanide and thiocyanate levels if >4 μg/kg/minute infused and/or used >2–3 days.
Nitroglycerin	0.5–10 μg/kg/min infusion	Direct smooth muscle relaxation; predominantly dilates venous capacitance vessels, modest effects on arterial resistance at higher doses; weak antihypertensive effects; variable pulmonary vasodilation; used to facilitate cooling and rewarming during cardiopulmonary bypass.
Phentolamine	0.5–5 μg/kg/min infusion	Selective alpha-blocker, produces mainly arteriolar vasodilation; some direct vasodilation with mild venodilation.
Enalaprilat	5–10 μg/kg/dose q 8–24 hours	Long duration of effect; angioedema, renal failure, hyperkalemia; potential problematic hypotension with anesthetic agents (see text).
Hydralazine	0.1–0.5 mg/kg bolus 96 hours	Maximum 20 mg/dose; direct-acting smooth muscle (predominantly arteriolar) vasodilation; long effective half-life; tachyphylaxis; reflex tachycardia; lupus-like syndrome; drug fever; thrombocytopenia.
Prostaglandin E_1	0.05–0.1 μg/kg/min infusion	Direct smooth muscle relaxation, relatively specific for ductus arteriosus; variable pulmonary and systemic vasodilation; apnea in neonates

*All drugs should be started in the lower dose range and titrated to effect.

little to no effect on intrinsic myocardial contractility.[172, 177] In fact, the increase in afterload, if not accompanied by a corresponding increase in contractility, may only serve to decrease stroke volume and cardiac output. Calcium may cause or exacerbate reperfusion injury and cellular damage by mechanisms that include activation of calcium-dependent proteases and phospholipases and organellar damage due to cellular calcium overload.[178, 179] These concerns are particularly relevant in patients immediately following cardiac surgery. Intravenous calcium may also attenuate the beta-adrenergic effects of concurrently administered epinephrine.[172]

The role of intravenous calcium administration in neonates and young infants, both alone and following cardiac surgery, is more complicated. Preterm and term newborn infants have erratic calcium handling and are prone to ionized hypocalcemia.[180, 181] The neonatal myocardium is more sensitive to ionized hypocalcemia than is the adult myocardium, due to reduced intracellular calcium stores, immaturity of sarcoplasmic reticulum calcium handling mechanisms, and greater dependency on transmembrane calcium flux for excitation-contraction coupling.[182] Furthermore, the need to administer substantial volumes of citrated and albumin-containing (both of which bind calcium) blood products and other fluids in the post-cardiopulmonary bypass setting increases the likelihood of ionized hypocalcemia.[183] The most prudent approach includes awareness of the greater dependency of immature myocardium on extracellular calcium, monitoring ionized calcium concentrations, and careful administration to maintain normal or at most mildly elevated ionized calcium concentrations. This approach is particularly needed in neonates and those with diminished left ventricular function. Administration of large bolus doses of calcium immediately on reperfusion of the heart after a period of ischemia is probably ill advised because of the potential to exacerbate reperfusion injury and even cause myocardial contracture.

Extravasation of calcium can cause local venous irritation and significant tissue necrosis. It has been suggested that calcium gluconate has the potential to cause less harm in this regard than does calcium chloride. Either the gluconate or chloride form should be administered via a centrally positioned catheter whenever possible. Both calcium chloride and calcium gluconate raise ionized calcium concentrations to an equal extent when administered on the basis of equal amounts of elemental calcium.[184] Calcium may cause significant slowing of atrioventricular conduction and should be administered cautiously in patients with sinus bradycardia or junctional rhythm. Care must also be exercised when administering calcium to patients receiving digoxin, particularly in the presence of concurrent hypokalemia, as intravenous calcium will exacerbate the potential for digoxin-induced dysrhythmias in this setting.

Calcium-Sensitizing Agents

Calcium-sensitizing agents represent a relatively new class of drugs with inotropic properties that are currently under basic and applied investigation. Although their mechanism of action is not entirely clear, they appear to act by increasing the affinity of the contractile proteins for calcium or stabilizing the bond between calcium and troponin C or both. A potential advantage, therefore, over other types of inotropics is that greater myocardial contractility can be produced with minimal increase in oxygen consumption. The concept of increasing sensitivity to calcium rather than increasing cellular calcium concentrations is also attractive because of the deleterious effects of higher cytosolic calcium levels on oxygen consumption, mitochondrial function, and activation of various calcium-dependent proteases and phospholipases. There are no data available regarding their use in children or from immature animal preparations. A study in adults did demonstrate increased contractile performance and decreased systemic vascular resistance following cardiopulmonary bypass.[185] One feature confounding interpretation of their effects is that the majority of drugs with calcium sensitizing properties described thus far also have phosphodiesterase inhibiting capabilities, as well as other effects. A potential limitation to their use is that sensitizing the contractile apparatus to the effects of activator calcium is likely to be accompanied by reduced diastolic compliance (i.e., reduced relaxation). This finding is more likely to be true during ischemia and reperfusion, when myocyte calcium levels are already significantly above normal.

Beta-Blocking Agents

There are several indications for the use of beta-blockers in pediatric patients, including control of hypertension (both acutely in a perioperative period and chronically), treatment of cyanotic spells and right ventricular outflow obstruction in tetralogy of Fallot, reduction of left ventricular outflow obstruction in hypertrophic cardiomyopathy, control of heart rate in thyrotoxicosis and pheochromocytoma, and control of supraventricular tachycardia (see later).[186] Important distinctions include beta-receptor subtype selectivity, variability in half-life and metabolism, and intrinsic sympathomimetic activity. "Selective" beta-blockers lose their selectivity at higher plasma concentrations.

PROPRANOLOL. Propranolol is one of the most frequently used beta-blockers in children. Typical oral doses start at 1 to 2 mg/kg/day divided every 6 hours. A sustained release form is available for older children who are able to swallow pills. Intravenous propranolol is administered at doses of 0.05 to 0.2 mg/kg over several minutes; this may be increased if necessary. Bradycardia and hypotension can be serious problems, particularly in infants or when following intravenous administration. In addition to bradycardia, propranolol may cause conduction block at the atrioventricular node and worsen pump function in congestive heart failure. Other important side effects include fatigue, depression, and lethargy. Interactions with the beta2-receptor may exacerbate bronchospasm and predispose patients to hypoglycemia. Propranolol is primarily metabolized in the liver. Significant population variability in its kinetics has been noted. Metabolism is also affected by factors that alter the hepatic blood flow and the hepatic metabolic enzyme activity. Its major metabolite, 4-hydroxypropranolol, is also bioactive.

ATENOLOL. The use of atenolol has been increasing in pediatric patients. It is more selective for the beta1-adrenergic receptor subtype. The elimination half-life is 8 to 12 hours. There is little hepatic biotransformation, and there are no active metabolites. The typical starting dose is 1 to 2 mg/kg/day, with an upper limit in the range of 3 mg/kg/day. The drug is given once or twice daily. No intravenous form is available. Atenolol does not cross the blood-brain barrier, and thus some of the limiting side effects common to propranolol are absent. At high doses, beta1 selectivity is probably lost, leading to the potential to exacerbate bronchospasm and hypoglycemia.

ESMOLOL. Esmolol is a relatively selective beta1-adrenergic blocker. Several of its features are unique. Its onset is rapid, it can easily be titrated to a desired end point, and its effects are rapidly terminated by metabolism by red cell and plasma esterases.[187, 188] The drug has been particularly useful for the acute control of perioperative hypertension, as well as for treatment of supraventricular tachyarrhythmias (see later). Loading doses between 100 to 500 µg/kg given over 1 to 5 minutes are followed by maintenance infusions of 50 to 100 µg/kg/minute. If the desired response is not achieved, the infusion rate is then typically doubled every 5 minutes until a desired response is achieved.

Specifics on pediatric dosing are limited at present. A maximum loading dose of 500 µg/kg and infusion rates of 250 to 300 µg/kg/minute are currently suggested. A major potential side effect of esmolol administration is hypotension, particularly during bolus therapy. As noted earlier, the drug rapidly distributes and has a very short elimination half-life of 7 to 10 minutes that is unaffected by organ blood flow or disease. Thus hypotension is usually short-lived, but therapy with vasopressors may occasionally be required until it resolves.[189]

LABETALOL. Labetalol has nonselective beta-adrenergic blocking properties and is also a selective alpha-adrenergic receptor blocker. The ratio of alpha-to-beta blockade efficiency is 1:3 and 1:7 following oral and intravenous administration, respectively. The primary use of labetalol in children is to control hypertension. The drug has been given intravenously to treat hypertensive crisis, to control hypertension after aortic coarctation repair, and as an adjunct to induce controlled hypotension during surgery.[190, 191] Typical doses are 0.1 to 0.4 mg/kg given every 5 to 10 minutes until the desired effect is achieved. The elimination half-life of labetalol is 3 to 5 hours.

Vasodilators

Vasodilators are used in pediatric patients to control blood pressure during and after surgery, to treat systemic and pulmonary hypertension, and to decrease afterload on either the systemic or pulmonary ventricle, thereby improving pump function. Vasodilators are also given during cardiopulmonary bypass to reduce systemic vascular resistance to improve regional perfusion and facilitate rapid and even core cooling and rewarming.

Several different types of vasodilators are currently employed in children for these purposes. The most common are direct-acting nitrosovasodilators such as sodium nitroprusside and nitroglycerin. These drugs directly relax vascular smooth muscle to cause vasodilation. Hydralazine is another direct-acting smooth muscle vasodilator that is occasionally given to children to reduce blood pressure. Alpha-adrenergic blockers, such as phentolamine and phenoxybenzamine, are also used occasionally to acutely reduce blood pressure and systemic vascular resistance in the perioperative period. They are more frequently employed during cardiopulmonary bypass. Angiotensin-converting enzyme (ACE) inhibitors may also be useful to help control blood pressure. Prostaglandin E_1 (PGE$_1$) is a direct-acting vasodilator with the unique property of being able to dilate the ductus arteriosus and maintain its patency. Prostacyclin and inhaled nitric oxide are further additions that possess relatively selective pulmonary vasodilating capabilities.

SODIUM NITROPRUSSIDE. Sodium nitroprusside is used to reduce afterload and blood pressure before, during, and after a wide variety of procedures.[192] For example, it is provided intraoperatively and postoperatively to control systemic hypertension during and after repair of aortic coarctation and following relief of other forms of left ventricular outflow obstruction. The reduction in afterload may improve performance of a dysfunctional ventricle, particularly in combination with a positive inotropic agent.[193, 194] The ability of nitroprusside to successfully treat pulmonary hypertension is variable.[195–197]

Sodium nitroprusside is an extremely potent vasodilator that acts directly on smooth muscle to cause dilation. Its effects reduce cardiac preload as well as afterload. Onset of effect is rapid (within minutes), and offset is similarly rapid. The effect ends within 1 to 2 minutes of terminating infusion. Because of its potency, it should always be administered with an infusion pump in conjunction with direct continuous arterial pressure monitoring. The starting dosage is in the range of 0.5 to 1 µg/kg/minute. This can be increased to achieve the desired effect. The hypotensive effects of nitroprusside are potentiated by hypovolemia, inhalation anesthetics, and drugs that inhibit increases in sympathetic tone and renin release, for example, propranolol and ACE inhibitors, respectively. These effects are due to the fact that the vasodilation produced by sodium nitroprusside causes reflex increases in sympathetic tone and plasma renin activity.

Adverse effects of sodium nitroprusside include cyanide and thiocyanate toxicity, rebound hypertension, inhibition of platelet function, and increased intrapulmonary shunting. Rebound hypertension is most likely due to activation of the aforementioned reflex mechanisms. It can usually be avoided by slowly tapering the infusion rather than abruptly discontinuing it. Toxicity may occur when more than 1 mg/kg of sodium nitroprusside is administered in less than 3 hours or when more than 0.5 mg/kg/hour is administered over 24 hours. A blood cyanide level of approximately 400 µg/dL has been associated with death in a pediatric patient. Cyanide and thiocyanate toxicity are rare but may be more likely in neonates and young infants, as well as in those with impaired hepatic or renal function.[198, 199]

Cyanide production results from sodium nitroprusside metabolism. Free cyanide is then conjugated with thiosulfate by rhodanase in the liver to produce thiocyanate. A major mechanism of cyanide toxicity is via binding to cytochrome oxidase in the mitochondrial electron transport chain, thereby preventing mitochondrial respiration and adenosine triphosphate production. Signs of toxicity include tachyphylaxis to the drug, as well as elevated mixed venous oxygen saturation and metabolic acidosis. In patients who have received prolonged (greater than 24 hours) or high-dose infusions, as well as those with organ dysfunction, it may be advisable to measure serum cyanide levels. Serum thiocyanate concentrations may also be measured. Thiocyanate concentrations may increase when renal function is abnormal. Central nervous system dysfunction may occur when thiocyanate levels reach 5 to 10 mg/dL. Treatment of cyanide toxicity consists of intravenous infusion of sodium nitrite, 5 to 10 mg/kg over 5 minutes, and sodium thiosulfate, 150 to 450 mg/kg over 15 minutes. In patients with abnormal renal function in whom stimulating the production of thiocyanate from thiosulfate may be contraindicated, administration of hydroxocobalamin has been recommended.

NITROGLYCERIN. Nitroglycerin is primarily a venodilator that acts on venous capacitance vessels. It has a substantially smaller effect on arteriolar smooth muscle, and its ability to decrease elevated pulmonary vascular resistance is variable. Compared with nitroprusside, it is relatively ineffective as an antihypertensive agent. It has a short half-life and no significant toxic metabolites. Similar to nitroprusside, it may increase intrapulmonary shunting and cause platelet dysfunction. Nitroglycerin is typically administered at dosages ranging from 0.5 to 3.0 µg/kg/minute. Effects are usually seen within 2 minutes of starting the drug and resolve within 5 minutes of discontinuing it. Mild decreases in blood pressure may be observed at doses exceeding 2 to 3 µg/kg/minute.

Nitroglycerin has found some favor during cardiopulmonary bypass to facilitate rapid and effective cooling and rewarming, as well as to improve tissue blood flow. Nitroprusside and nitroglycerin may differ substantially with regard to their effects on the microcirculation. Because it primarily reduces arteriolar tone and primarily dilates precapillaries, microvascular blood flow and tissue perfusion may be more diminished by nitroprusside, particularly in the presence of reduced arterial blood pressure as seen during many phases of cardiopulmonary bypass.[200] In contrast, because nitroglycerin dilates both pre- and post-capillaries with equal efficacy, capillary perfusion is more likely to remain stable in the presence of nitroglycerin than nitroprusside.[201, 202]

PHENTOLAMINE AND PHENOXYBENZAMINE. Both of these drugs are alpha-adrenergic blocking agents with little selectively for alpha-receptor subtype. Their primary effect is to decrease resistance on the arterial side of the circulation, although both do possess weak venodilating capabilities. Phentolamine is usually administered by infusion at 0.5 to 5 µg/kg/minute. Phenoxybenzamine has a much longer half-life than phentolamine and is administered at a dose of 0.25 to 0.5 mg/kg every 6 hours. The potent arteriolar dilating effects of phenoxybenzamine and its long half-life have been found advantageous by some for use as vasodilators during cardiopulmonary bypass.

ANGIOTENSIN CONVERTING ENZYME INHIBITORS. Angiotensin converting enzyme (ACE) inhibitors are being administered with increasing frequency in pediatric patients. They may be used in the perioperative setting to help control arterial blood pressure in the context of aortic coarctation repair or relief of left ventricular outflow obstruction. They are also given on a more long-term basis to reduce afterload on the systemic ventricle and improve left ventricular performance in patients with congestive heart failure and single-ventricle physiology. Captopril, enalapril, and lisinopril are the ACE inhibitors most often used in pediatric patients at this time, but there is little information specific to pediatric patients. Side effects common to all ACE inhibitors include angioedema, acute renal failure, and hyperkalemia. A severe angioedema reaction has occasionally been fatal. Monitoring of renal function and serum potassium concentrations are indicated.

The contribution of ACE inhibitors to anesthetic-induced hypotension remains controversial. Reports on both sides of this argument can be found. It is clear that angiotensin *receptor blocking agents* such as losartan can produce significant and refractory hypotension with standard anesthetic induction techniques.[203, 204] Because of the potential risk of significant and refractory hypotension, which is usually unresponsive to volume expansion and requires substantial pressor treatment, when ACE inhibitors are present in conjunction with general anesthesia, it has been our practice to discontinue the long-acting ACE inhibitors 1 day prior to surgery.

Captopril. Captopril has a relatively short half-life (less than 2 hours), is metabolized in the liver, and is then excreted by the kidney.[205] Oral dosing in neonates is 0.1 to 0.4 mg/kg per 24 hours divided every 6 to 8 hours. Infants initially receive 0.2 to 0.3 mg/kg every 6 to 8 hours. This can be titrated toward a maximum dose of 6 mg/kg per 24 hours divided every 6 hours. Older children may receive 0.1 to 1 mg/kg per 24 hours divided every 6 to 8 hours. The short duration of effect, necessitating more frequent dosing, has led to increased use of the longer-acting ACE inhibitors (enalapril and lisinopril) in pediatric patients.

Enalapril. Enalapril is metabolized in the liver to its active form, enalaprilat. Enalapril is the only ACE inhibitor currently available in the United States that has an intravenous dosing formulation. Its safety and efficacy in infants and young children have not been established. Intravenous dosing in adults has been described at 0.6 to 1.5 mg/dose every 6 hours. Both enalapril and lisinopril are eliminated by the kidney. The duration of their hypotensive actions averages 24 hours but can last up to 30 hours.

HYDRALAZINE. Hydralazine was quite frequently used in the past to control blood pressure in children. In contrast to adults, the ability to control pulmonary hypertension in children with hydralazine was disappointing.[206] Hydralazine directly relaxes smooth muscle without known effects on receptors. It reduces cardiac afterload, but may result in significant reflex tachycardia. With long-term use, it may also cause fluid retention, requiring concurrent administration of a diuretic. Long-term oral hydralazine is given occasionally to treat systemic hypertension in children. Oral dosing is in the range of 0.75 to 3 mg/kg per 24 hours divided every 6 hours. The maximum dosage is 7.5 mg/kg per 24 hours. Its use to control systemic blood pressure and afterload in children for the long-term has largely been replaced by ACE inhibitors. It may also be administered intravenously to control blood pressure and reduce afterload. Intravenous doses are administered as a bolus of 0.1 to 0.5 mg/kg. The effects of intravenous hydralazine on pulmonary vascular resistance are also variable.[206, 207] Tachyphylaxis to the antihypertensive effects of intravenous hydralazine may occur. Important side effects include a drug-related fever, rash, pancytopenia, and lupus-like syndrome. The elimination half-life of the drug is approximately 4 hours, but the effective biologic half-life may be substantially longer owing to significant binding of the drug to vascular smooth muscle.

PROSTAGLANDIN E₁. The major use of PGE_1 is to establish or maintain patency of the ductus arteriosus. It is best able to reopen a closing ductus in neonates up to 1 to 2 weeks of age but may occasionally be effective even in older infants.[10, 208] The use of PGE_1 to establish or maintain ductal patency is beneficial when the lower body is supplied by right-to-left ductal flow, as in cases of interrupted aortic arch, critical aortic stenosis, and hypoplastic left heart syndrome. Conversely, a patent ductus arteriosus can supply pulmonary blood flow from the aorta in lesions such as pulmonary atresia, tricuspid atresia, and severe tetralogy of Fallot. Side effects of PGE_1 include systemic hypotension, apnea, increased risk of infection, and central nervous system irritability.[209] PGE_1 infusions are usually begun at 0.05 μg/kg/minute and may be increased to 0.1 μg/kg/minute or more. The risk of apnea is related to some extent to infusion rate. Intubation and ventilation are often required with infusion rates greater than 0.05 μg/kg/minute. PGE_1 has been utilized to treat primary or acquired pulmonary hypertension with varying degrees of success.[210–212]

INHALED NITRIC OXIDE. An important development in the treatment of pulmonary hypertension is inhaled nitric oxide gas, which can be delivered directly to the pulmonary circulation. Nitric oxide is made endogenously and is an endothelium-derived relaxing factor that acts on guanylate cyclase in vascular smooth muscle to produce smooth muscle relaxation.[213] Endogenous nitric oxide in the vascular system is produced by endothelial cell nitric oxide synthase. Nitric oxide synthases convert the amino acid L-arginine into nitric oxide and the byproduct L-citrulline. Nitric oxide then diffuses into the subjacent vascular smooth muscle. It produces relaxation by acting on smooth muscle guanylate cyclase to produce cyclic guanosine monophosphate, which acts on a series of protein kinases and reduces intracellular calcium levels to inhibit muscle contraction (see Fig. 14–1). Nitric oxide diffusing in the other direction from the endothelial cell into the blood vessel lumen can decrease the adhesiveness of white blood cells and platelets. Nitric oxide in the blood is rapidly bound by oxyhemoglobin, which is then oxidized to methemoglobin. From this reaction, nitric oxide is inactivated and nitrite and nitrate are released in the blood. Red blood cell methemoglobin is subsequently reduced back to hemoglobin. The rapid binding and inactivation of nitric oxide in the blood means that inhaled nitric oxide has a minimal effect on the systemic circulation and functions as a very specific pulmonary vasodilator.

Significant reductions in pulmonary vascular resistance from inhaled nitric oxide have been shown in adults with mitral stenosis, in neonates with persistent pulmonary hypertension of the neonate, in lung transplant recipients, and in patients after surgical repair of a variety of congenital heart diseases.[214–218] The efficacy of inhaled nitric oxide is in large part related to the ability to deliver it into the alveolus, which is of course in close proximity to pulmonary vascular smooth muscle. Effects on the systemic circulation are minimal because of rapid inactivation by reaction with oxyhemoglobin in the blood.

Inhaled nitric oxide has found several uses in patients with congenital heart disease. In the cardiac catheterization laboratory, it is used to assess reactivity of the pulmonary vasculature to vasodilation in patients with pulmonary hypertension. It can, therefore, help distinguish between patients with fixed pulmonary vascular obstructive disease and patients with a reversible component to pulmonary hypertension, thereby facilitating operative planning and management.

In the postoperative period following the repair of congenital heart disease, nitric oxide can be used to reduce pulmonary vascular resistance and thereby improve cardiopulmonary performance. Experience thus far suggests that patients with two ventricles who have elevated left atrial pressure or its pathophysiologic equivalents (e.g., mitral stenosis, severe congestive heart failure, cardiomyopathy, large left-to-right shunts, total anomalous pulmonary venous drainage) are the patients who will most likely respond to nitric oxide in the postoperative period with a significant decrease in pulmonary vascular resistance. Patients with single ventricle physiology may be somewhat less likely to demonstrate improvements in pulmonary blood flow and oxygenation. Interestingly, a number of patients with no response in the operating room immediately after cardiopulmonary bypass can manifest significant reductions in pulmonary vascular resistance in response to nitric oxide several hours later. The drug is administered at concentrations of 1 to 80 parts per million in oxygen with a specially adapted ventilator. Inspired gas is monitored for higher oxides of nitrogen, which are toxic. Blood methemoglobin concentrations should also be assessed while the patient is on long-term inhaled nitric oxide therapy.

Prostacyclin. Prostacyclin has shown significant promise as a pulmonary vasodilator. Compared with the other intravenous vasodilators, it is more selective in terms of its action on the pulmonary vascular bed than on the systemic circulation. It has been used in the treatment of primary pulmonary hypertension; irreversible acquired pulmonary hypertension in congenital heart disease; in patients awaiting heart, lung, or heart-lung transplantation; and in children with primary pulmonary hypertension, in neonates with persistent pulmonary hypertension, and in pulmonary hypertensive crises.[96, 97, 219–223] Inhaled prostacyclin is under experimental development.[224, 225]

Antiarrhythmic Agents

Antiarrhythmic agents have been traditionally classified in the Vaughan Williams Classification System based on presumed mechanism of action of the antiarrhythmic agent. For example, class I agents are the local anesthetics, which share an ability to block sodium channels. They are subdivided into class IA or class IB based on other effects, such as antivagal mechanisms or repolarization. Intravenous agents for pediatric patients in the United States are given in Table 17–6.

Procainamide

Procainamide is one of the most commonly used class IA agents in pediatric patients. It has sodium channel and moderate potassium channel blocking activities. Its major effect is to delay repolarization. This effect is more pronounced at faster heart rates. Intravenous procainamide can be used to treat supraventricular tachycardia associated with the Wolff-Parkinson-White syndrome, atrial flutter, and lidocaine unresponsive ventricular dysrhythmias. It may also be effective against postoperative junctional ectopic tachycardia when employed in conjunction with mild patient hypothermia.

Long-term oral therapy typically employs dosages in the range of 50 to 100 mg/kg/day, given every 4 to 6 hours. A sustained release form (administered every 8 to 12 hours) is available for older patients. For intravenous administration, a loading dose of 3 to 10 mg/kg is given over 30 to 60 minutes (for patients under 1 year of age). Substantial negative inotropic effects can occur during intravenous administration of procainamide. This effect may be more likely in the ischemic/reperfused or otherwise damaged myocardium. Older patients receive intravenous bolus doses of 5 to 15 mg/kg given over 30 to 60 minutes. Following the bolus dose, an infusion is typically started at 40 to 50 µg/kg/minute. Higher infusion rates ($\geq$ 100 µg/kg/minute) are occasionally necessary, particularly in infants. Procainamide is metabolized in the liver to N-acetyl procainamide (NAPA), which has substantial class III antiarrhythmic effects. Biotransformation of procainamide and NAPA is based on genetic acetylator status. With regard to therapeutic drug monitoring, serum procainamide levels of 4 to 8 µg/mL are required. Plasma levels of NAPA can be in a similar range. The older practice of summing procainamide and NAPA levels, however, has fallen out of favor.

The majority of procainamide-related side effects are dependent on plasma concentration and duration of therapy. The most frequent one is a systemic lupus erythematosus–like syndrome. Manifestations can include fevers, arthralgias, and rashes, and occasionally liver and kidney toxicity. A substantial number of patients demonstrate positive antinuclear antibodies with chronic therapy. This development is not necessarily an indication to discontinue therapy.

Lidocaine

Lidocaine is a member of the class IB antiarrhythmic agents. Others include mexiletine and phenytoin. One mechanism of action of these drugs is to block fast sodium channels. They also shorten action potential duration and repolarization. Like the class IA agents, their effects may be greater at faster heart rates. Lidocaine primarily affects cells below the atrioventricular node. It appears to induce an overall balancing of repolarization, as it has the greatest effects on cells with the longest action potential duration.

Lidocaine is only available in an intravenous formulation.

Table 17–6. Intravenous Antidysrhythmic Agents

Agent (Vaughan Williams Class)	Dose	Comments
Procainamide (IA; sodium, ± potassium channel blockade; antivagal effects)	3–10 mg/kg loading dose over 30 min (<1 year) 5–15 mg/kg loading dose over 30 min (>1 year) infusion 20–60 μg/kg/min (all ages)	Used to treat SVT due to WPW, atrial flutter, junctional ectopic tachycardia (with patient hypothermia), lidocaine-resistant ventricular dysrhythmias; hypotension and negative inotropy; lupus-like syndrome.
Lidocaine (IB; sodium channel blockade; speeds repolarization)	1 mg/kg bolus; then 20–50 μg/kg/min	Used for ventricular dysrhythmias; CNS toxicity (apnea, seizures, abnormal sensations).
Phenytoin (IB)	1–3 mg/kg q 5 minutes up to 15 mg/kg loading dose then 10–15 mg/kg divided q 6 hours	Drug must be infused slowly (>30 min) due to potential hypotension; similar antidysrhythmic profile to lidocaine; may be useful to treat digoxin-induced dysrhythmias.
Propranolol (II; beta-adrenergic blockade; sodium channel blockade also)	0.05–2.0 mg/kg slowly	Non-selective beta-blockade; used mainly to treat SVT; bradycardia, hypotension, worsening of myocardial pump function; AV block; hypoglycemia; bronchospasm; depression; fatigue.
Esmolol (II)	100–500 μg/kg loading dose (over 5 min); 50–250 μg/kg/min infusion	Used to treat SVT; relatively selective beta$_1$ blockade; short elimination half-life (7–10 minutes); hypotension, especially during bolus; if less than desired response after 5 minutes, can repeat or double bolus dose, followed by doubling infusion rate; non–organ based metabolism by plasma and red blood cell esterases; infusion concentrations >10 mg/mL may predispose to venous sclerosis; dilute infusion at high rates increases risk of volume overload.
Amiodarone (III; prolongs repolarization; adrenergic and calcium blockade)	1–2.5 mg/kg bolus over 5–10 min (total loading dose may be up to 5–6 mg/kg); 5–15 mg/kg/24 hour infusion	Used for resistant re-entrant atrial and ventricular dysrhythmias; may be useful for postoperative junctional ectopic tachycardia; hypotension with bolus intravenous administration; bradycardia; AV block; rare proarrhythmia and torsades de pointes; pulmonary fibrosis; hypothyroidism; controversial association with acute perioperative lung injury.
Bretylium (III)	5 mg/kg; then 10 mg/kg q 15 min (max 30 mg/kg total)	Use limited to ventricular tachycardia resistant to other therapies during cardiopulmonary resuscitation; hypotension.
Verapamil (IV; calcium channel blockade)	0.1–0.3 mg/kg bolus (maximum 5 mg)	Used for supraventricular tachycardia in older children and adults; potential for hypotension and asystole contraindicates use in patients <1 year of age; bradycardia; AV block; may increase ventricular response rate in some patients with WPW.
Adenosine	0.05–0.1 mg/kg rapid bolus followed by flush; may repeat at increasing doses of 0.05 (e.g., 0.15, 0.2, 0.25 mg/kg) q 2 minutes (maximal dose = 0.25 mg/kg or 12 mg whichever comes first)	Increases potassium channel flux and inhibits slow inward calcium current; causes transient sinus bradycardia and AV block; transient hypotension; rarely causes ventricular ectopy or atrial fibrillation; bronchospasm; used to terminate supraventricular tachycardia; used diagnostically to transiently produce AV block.
Digoxin	Total digitalizing dose (TDD): Premature: 20 μg/kg Neonate: 30 μg/kg (up to 1 month) Infant: 40 μg/kg (<2 years) Child: 30 μg/kg (2–5 years) Over 5 years: 20 μg/kg Maintenance: 5–10 μg/kg/day, divided q 12 hours	TDD given in divided doses—½ TDD followed by ¼ TDD every 8–12 hours × 2; slows sinus node and decreases AV node conduction; used to slow ventricular response in atrial flutter and fibrillation and may also treat junctional tachycardia or supraventricular tachycardia; variable effect on accessory pathways; long half-life (24–48 hours) that is prolonged by renal dysfunction; numerous drug interactions; toxicity includes supraventricular tachycardia, AV block, ventricular dysrhythmias; toxicity symptoms include drowsiness, nausea, vomiting; toxicity exacerbated by hypokalemia.
Magnesium sulfate	25–50 mg/kg bolus; 30–60 mg/kg/24 hour infusion	May be first-line therapy for torsades de pointes; also used for refractory ventricular tachycardia and ventricular fibrillation; hypotension and respiratory depression may accompany intravenous bolus dosing—intravenous calcium is an antidote.

AV, atrioventricular; CNS, central nervous system; SVT, supraventricular tachycardia; WPW, Wolff-Parkinson-White syndrome.

It is indicated for the rapid treatment of ventricular dysrhythmias. Lidocaine is initially administered as an intravenous bolus of 1 mg/kg that can be repeated once within 5 to 10 minutes. Standard lidocaine infusion rates range from 20 to 50 μg/kg/minute.

The major side effects of lidocaine administration are well known to anesthesiologists. They primarily reflect central nervous system toxicity, typically occurring at plasma levels greater than 6 to 8 μg/mL. Mental status changes, abnormal taste or other sensations, apnea, and seizures may occur. Lidocaine dosing should be reduced in patients with low cardiac output because of impairment of hepatic clearance. The administration of lidocaine to patients with atrial tachydysrhythmias or with prolongation of the QT interval can result in an increase in the ventricular response rate.

Phenytoin

Phenytoin shares many similarities to lidocaine in terms of its antiarrhythmic effects, which are also confined primarily to tissues below the atrioventricular node and His bundle. Phenytoin primarily binds to sodium channels, maintaining them in the inactivated state. Very high concentrations may also have some effect on calcium channels and automaticity. The drug is useful in treating digoxin-induced dysrhythmias, including digoxin-induced ventricular dysrhythmias.[226]

Oral dosing in infants and older children is typically 5 mg/kg per day given every 12 hours, following a total loading dose of 15 mg/kg that has been divided over 6 hours. Intravenous loading with phenytoin is accomplished by a bolus dose of 1 to 3 mg/kg. Intravenous maintenance is 10 to 15 mg/kg divided every 6 hours. Intravenous phenytoin must be administered *extremely slowly* (>30 minutes) owing to the potential for hypotension. Other side effects are similar to those seen when the drug is used for seizures and include gingival hyperplasia, aplastic anemia, ataxia, and nystagmus. The drug should be avoided in patients who are pregnant or may become pregnant because of its significant teratogenic profile (fetal hydantoin syndrome).

Flecainide and Propafenone

Flecainide and propafenone are class IC agents. As such, they have potent sodium channel blocking activity. Flecainide has been extensively evaluated in pediatric patients.[227-230] Flecainide blocks activated slow sodium channels and has less potent inhibitory effects on potassium channels. It appears to shorten the refractory time and decrease the automaticity in His-Purkinje cells. In contrast, action potential duration and refractory period are prolonged in ventricular muscle, resulting in a longer QRS duration.

Oral dosing of flecainide may be more reliable when calculated on the basis of a body surface area. Typical dosages in infants are in the range of 80 to 90 mg/m²/day, given in two doses (40–45 mg/m² q 12 hours). Older patients receive 100 to 110 mg/kg/m²/day (50–55 mg/m² q 12 hours). Loading doses are not used. Serum elimination half-life is age-dependent and is approximately 1 day in newborns, 12 hours in infants under 6 months of age, and 8 to 12 hours in older children and adults. Therapeutic trough concentrations are believed to be in the range of 200 to 1000 ng/mL. Alterations in diet can markedly affect drug absorption with

oral dosing. Intravenous flecainide is available outside of the United States. A dose of 1 to 2 mg/kg given over 5 to 10 minutes has been used. Continuous infusions are not given because of the long half-life.

Flecainide has mild to moderate negative inotropic effects. Substantial proarrhythmic effects have been observed in patients with atrial tachydysrhythmias or significant abnormalities of myocardial anatomy and function. For example, proarrhythmia was significantly increased in adult patients who received flecainide following myocardial infarction. In children and adults with paroxysmal supraventricular tachycardia, a slow but incessant SVT may result when initiating therapy. These events have led to recommendations that significant care and observation are necessary when initiating therapy with flecainide. The use of the drug is also uncertain in pediatric patients with severe myocardial dysfunction, those with myocardial injury (e.g., immediately postoperatively), and those with right-or-left-sided hypertrophy such as tetralogy of Fallot or aortic stenosis. Many electrophysiologists would avoid the use of class IC agents in patients with an abnormal or damaged myocardium.

Propafenone

The effects and risks of propafenone are quite similar to those discussed for flecainide. Propafenone administered orally is given at 150 to 200 mg/m²/day divided into three doses (50–67 mg/m² q 8 hours). Maximum dosages are 500 to 600 mg/m²/day. Propafenone has also demonstrated the ability to control dysrhythmias arising from automatic mechanisms. It may have some utility in treating postoperative junctional ectopic tachycardia. Intravenous propafenone is not available in the United States. When used, it is given as a loading dose of 0.2 to 1.0 mg/kg slowly over 10 minutes. The initial dose may be doubled to achieve a maximum 2 mg/kg total loading dose. Infusion rates of 4 to 10 μg/kg/minute have been reported.[231, 232]

Significant hypotension can occur with bolus propafenone. Hypotension is believed to be due primarily to negative inotropic effects. As discussed with flecainide, propafenone is probably contraindicated in patients with significant structural or metabolic myocardial abnormalities, such as those related to severe pressure or volume overload, ischemia-reperfusion, and myocardial infarction. Propafenone also has the potential for proarrhythmic effects as does flecainide. Propafenone is extensively metabolized in the liver, with significant intersubject variability. Its half-life has ranged from 4 hours to as long as 18 hours. Efficacy has been reported with plasma concentrations over an extremely wide range (100–2500 ng/mL).

Beta Blockers

Beta-blockers are class II antiarrhythmic agents. Their dosing and other relevant features are discussed in the section on vasoactive drugs. Their use as antiarrhythmics is briefly summarized here. The predominant beta-blockers for rhythm control in pediatric patients are propranolol, atenolol, and esmolol.

PROPRANOLOL. Propranolol is probably the most widely studied beta-blocking agent in children. It is used in this setting primarily for the acute control of supraventricular tachycardia. In addition to nonselective beta-blockade, propranolol has effects on the sodium channels and at high concentrations on calcium channels as well. It is likely that conduction tissues of neonates are more sensitive to the drug than those of older children and adults.[226, 233]

ATENOLOL. Atenolol is a commonly used longer-acting beta-blocker.[234, 235] It has more selective effects on beta-adrenergic receptors, although the risk of bronchospasm may not be completely eliminated with this drug. This beta-blocker does not cross the blood-brain barrier, which may be a reason for its lower incidence of depression, fatigue, and malaise compared with propranolol.

ESMOLOL. Esmolol is gaining in popularity for the control of perioperative tachydysrhythmias. Esmolol appears to act predominantly in the sinus node and atrioventricular node. It does not appear to have significant antiarrhythmic effects in the His-Purkinje or ventricular conducting tissues.

Class III Agents

The primary class III agents are amiodarone, sotalol, bretylium, and ibutilide. All prolong depolarization and therefore increase refractoriness. All of these drugs have numerous other properties, including membrane effect, calcium blockade, and adrenergic blockade.

AMIODARONE. In addition to prolonging refractoriness, amiodarone has sodium channel blocking and noncompetitive alpha- and beta-adrenergic receptor blocking properties. It may also interfere with potassium channels and inhibit the release of myocardial norepinephrine. Oral amiodarone is absorbed quite slowly from the gastrointestinal tract and is metabolized in the liver to an active metabolite, desethylamiodarone. Because of its high lipid solubility and large volume of distribution, tissue levels are maintained for 2 to 3 months after discontinuation of therapy. There are increasing data demonstrating the efficacy and safety of oral and intravenous amiodarone for the treatment of dysrhythmias in infants and children.[236–239] In addition to resistant re-entrant atrial and ventricular dysrhythmias, amiodarone may be effective in treating postoperative junctional ectopic tachycardia.

For oral loading, 10 to 15 mg/kg per day for 5 to 10 days is given. Following oral loading, long-term therapy is instituted with 2 to 5 mg/kg once a day. Intravenous amiodarone is usually given in 1 to 2.5 mg/kg boluses, reaching a total of 5 to 6 mg/kg, with each bolus administered over 5 to 10 minutes. In patients with resistant dysrhythmias, the average loading dose was 6.3 mg/kg, with 50% of patients requiring a continuous amiodarone infusion 10 to 15 mg/kg per 24 hours.[239]

Hypotension is the most significant acute side effect with intravenous amiodarone therapy. The effects of amiodarone may be synergistic with those of other agents that depress sinus node and atrioventricular node function. Important cardiac effects include bradycardia and atrioventricular block. Proarrhythmic effects and torsades de pointes occur rarely. Long-term oral amiodarone therapy can lead to progressive and irreversible pulmonary fibrosis. For this reason, pulmonary function tests are usually performed at regular intervals. The high iodine content of amiodarone can affect thyroid function and result in either hyperthyroidism or hypothyroidism. Other effects include drug deposits in the cornea, skin photosensitivity, and chemical hepatitis with elevated liver transaminases. Administration of amiodarone with other antiarrhythmics may lead to significant increases in the plasma concentrations of the other agents.[236, 239]

The incidence of perioperative organ dysfunction in patients who receive either acute or long-term amiodarone therapy is controversial. A syndrome with similarities to the adult respiratory distress syndrome has been described, particularly in patients exposed to high inspired oxygen concentrations undergoing thoracic surgery or cardiopulmonary bypass.[240] This finding led to the recommendation that amiodarone be discontinued for several weeks prior to elective surgery. Later studies have not shown a significantly increased incidence of lung or other organ injury in patients undergoing surgery while receiving amiodarone. Because it is most frequently given to patients with severe and life-threatening cardiac rhythm disturbances, the current recommendation is not to discontinue amiodarone before surgery. However, it may be wise to attempt to limit inspired oxygen concentration and other factors predisposing the patients receiving amiodarone to free radical and inflammatory injury.

SOTALOL. Sotalol is a newer agent available in the United States and is a class III antiarrhythmic that also has nonselective beta-adrenergic blocking effects. The beta-blocker effects predominate at lower doses, with the class III effects realized at higher concentrations. Sotalol is indicated for a number of difficult-to-control tachydysrhythmias. Oral therapy is given two or three times a day and begun at 100 mg/m^2/day. Maximum dosages are in the range of 200 mg/m^2/day. An intravenous preparation is available outside the United States, where doses between 0.2 and 1.5 mg/kg are employed. The major side effects of sotalol include mild negative inotropic responses due to its beta-blocking ability and prolongation of the QT interval and torsades de pointes due to its class III effects. Sotalol may be indicated in some patients who would otherwise receive amiodarone but whose side effects are intolerable.

BRETYLIUM. Bretylium has limited usage in pediatric patients, being primarily indicated in cardiopulmonary resuscitation for ventricular tachycardia resistant to other therapies.[241] The intravenous dose of bretylium is 5 mg/kg given as a bolus. Bretylium does have significant hypotensive properties and thus should be given slowly in patients with hemodynamically stable ventricular tachycardia. The total dose should not exceed 30 mg/kg.

IBUTILIDE. Ibutilide is one of the more recently released intravenous class III antiarrhythmic drugs. Preliminary studies are underway in patients with congenital heart disease. Ibutilide is currently indicated for the rapid pharmacologic conversion of atrial fibrillation and atrial flutter. It may be more efficacious for the latter. As with other drugs that prolong ventricular repolarization, ibutilide can prolong the QT interval and cause associated polymorphic ventricular tachycardia (torsades de pointes),[242, 243] which may occur in approximately 5 to 8% of adult patients treated with ibutilide. Because the elimination half-life of ibutilide is approximately 6 hours, the current recommendation is to observe patients for several hours after an intravenous dose. Studies thus far have used a bolus dose of 10 to 25 μg/kg administered over 10 minutes, which may be repeated once.

Verapamil

Verapamil is representative of class IV type antiarrhythmics, which are calcium channel blockers. Its greatest effect is to depress sinus node and atrioventricular node function.[244] Oral doses range from 20 to 40 mg/kg/day divided into three or four doses (5–10 mg/kg q 6 hours or 7–9 mg/kg q 8 hours). A sustained release preparation is available for older patients. Intravenous doses range from 0.1 to 0.3 mg/kg with a maximum dose of 5 mg. The most important side effect of verapamil occurs in infants and patients under 1 year of age, in whom intravenous administration can cause severe hypotension and asystole.[245] In fact, the drug is now contraindicated in patients under 1 year of age because of this complication. Other side effects include bradycardia, atrioventricular block, and increasing the ventricular response in some patients with Wolff-Parkinson-White syndrome.

Verapamil has been shown to be quite effective in terminating the majority of supraventricular tachycardias in older children and adults.[246, 247] Verapamil is also used to relieve outflow obstruction in hypertrophic cardiomyopathy[248] and as an antihypertensive in some patients. The negative inotropic and atrioventricular conduction effects of verapamil are potentiated by beta-blockers and anesthetic agents.[249, 250] Intravenous calcium and beta-adrenergic drugs such as isoproterenol have been given to reverse the depressive effects of verapamil and other calcium channel antagonists.[251, 252]

Adenosine

Intravenous adenosine is another relatively new drug that has markedly changed the therapy of supraventricular tachycardias. Its electrophysiologic effects are multiple and include increased potassium channel flux and decreased slow inward calcium current. These effects result in sinus bradycardia and transient atrioventricular block and are mediated primarily by stimulation of the A_1-purinergic receptor subtype. The onset of effects is seen within 10 to 20 seconds. Bradycardia, atrioventricular block, and hypotension last an additional 10 to 30 seconds.

The best results are achieved when the drug is administered as a bolus into the central circulation followed by a bolus of flush solution. The initial dose is 100 to 150 μg/kg given as a rapid bolus, followed by the bolus of flush solution. The dose may then be doubled up to a maximum of 300 μg/kg. The adult dose is 6 to 12 mg.[253, 254] In addition to its ability to rapidly and effectively terminate supraventricular tachycardia, the drug is useful diagnostically, because of its atrioventricular node blocking properties, to distinguish supraventricular from other dysrhythmias.

Other than the noted electrophysiologic changes, the major side effect is transient hypotension. Ventricular ectopy and atrial fibrillation may also occur. Dipyridamole and diazepam may inhibit the metabolism or cellular redistribution of adenosine. Either drug can significantly potentiate the effects of adenosine, resulting in more prolonged hypo-

tension and atrioventricular node blockade. Adenosine has been reported to cause bronchospasm, usually mild, in patients both with and without known reactive airway disease. *Intravenous aminophylline may be indicated in these patients if bronchospasm is severe, as it directly counteracts the receptor-mediated effects of adenosine.*

Digoxin

Digoxin is used for both its antiarrhythmic and its positive inotropic effects. The latter effect, along with the drug's dosing and pharmacology, was discussed previously in the section on vasoactive drugs. As an antiarrhythmic, digoxin slows both atrial and atrioventricular node conduction. It can be utilized to slow the ventricular response in atrial flutter and fibrillation and, at times, to treat patients with junctional tachycardia and supraventricular tachycardia. Digoxin may shorten or lengthen or not alter the refractory period of accessory pathways.[255, 256] As such and because sudden death does occur occasionally in patients with Wolff-Parkinson-White syndrome and other accessory pathway syndromes, digoxin may be contraindicated in these conditions. Digoxin does easily cross the placenta, and it remains the primary treatment for termination of fetal supraventricular tachycardia.[257]

Digoxin dosing in infants and children must be done carefully. Infants have higher myocellular levels of digoxin than adults.[169, 258–260] The dosing schedule of digoxin, based on age, is shown in Table 17–6. Intravenous and oral dosing are essentially the same. The onset of effect is more rapid with intravenous (5 to 10 minutes) then it is with oral dosing (1 to 2 hours). The half-life of digoxin is quite long, approaching 1 to 2 days in young infants. Significant renal dysfunction prolongs the half-life, as does significant congestive heart failure. There are no active metabolites of digoxin. Therapeutic digoxin levels are 0.7 to 2.0 ng/mL. Samples to measure digoxin concentration should be obtained either just prior to a dose or at least 6 hours after the preceding dose.

Cardiac injury, such as ischemia-reperfusion and myocarditis, may increase sensitivity to digoxin. Toxicity is more likely in patients whose plasma levels exceed 3 ng/mL.[171] Signs of toxicity include proarrhythmia, nausea, vomiting, and drowsiness. Infants and young children frequently manifest digoxin toxicity as supraventricular tachycardia and atrioventricular node conduction disturbances, whereas adult patients seem to be more prone to ventricular arrhythmias, premature ventricular contractions, atrioventricular blocks, and junctional tachycardias. Hypokalemia exacerbates the risk of digoxin toxicity. The interactions of other drugs with digoxin are extremely numerous. In general, administration of other drugs is likely to require a reduction in digoxin dosing.

Radiofrequency Catheter Ablation

Over the last 10 years, radiofrequency energy delivered via catheter to ablate abnormal conduction pathways and automatic foci has largely replaced other forms of catheter and surgical dysrhythmia treatments. Improvements in catheter design, computer-aided electrophysiologic mapping techniques, and underlying electrophysiologic knowledge have led to substantial increases in the safety and efficacy of these procedures. As a result, complex antiarrhythmic regimens, or even single drugs with significant side effects, continue to decrease. Radiofrequency catheter ablation (RFCA) is becoming the first line treatment for symptomatic tachydysrhythmias arising from accessory pathways such as Wolff-Parkinson-White syndrome and atrioventricular node re-entry tachycardias. With added experience and ability, improved results are also being achieved for more complicated ventricular dysrhythmias, as well as the ablation of atrial flutter and fibrillation. Knowledge and success are also increasing when dysrhythmias occur in the setting of complicated underlying anatomy, such as Fontan, Mustard, or Senning types of surgical repairs of congenital heart disease.

Indications for RFCA include patient preference, life-threatening symptoms, adverse drug effects, patient noncompliance with drug regimens, and tachycardia-induced ventricular dysfunction. The overall success rate for accessory pathway ablation overall in a multicenter study was 83%, with a complication rate of under 5%.[261] In our institutions, the success rate for accessory pathway ablations is well over 90%, with a complication rate of 2% or less. The high success rate and low complication rate for accessory pathways in particular may make RFCA the preferred mode of therapy compared with pharmacologic therapy for these lesions. Providing RFCA prior to complicated elective surgery is another indication that we have used to perform RFCA in patients with significant tachydysrhythmias.

Numerous reports have described the effects of anesthetic agents on both normal and accessory pathway conduction.[262–265] In these studies, propofol and sevoflurane have been shown to have minimal or no effect on normal sinoatrial or atrioventricular node function and no significant effect on conduction via the accessory pathway in Wolff-Parkinson-White syndrome. Other inhaled anesthetics such as isoflurane and halothane have varying effects on measured electrophysiologic conduction that, although statistically significant, do not appear to be clinically relevant in terms of electrophysiologic mapping. No inhalation or intravenous agent used in any of these studies prevented induction of the underlying dysrhythmia. There is, however, widespread belief that anesthetic agents may hinder attempts to induce and map some automatic (as opposed to re-entrant) tachycardias.

Mechanical Circulatory Support

Mechanical methods of providing circulatory support during reversible myocardial failure, as a means of cardiopulmonary support before and after cardiac surgery and as a bridge to cardiac transplantation, have become increasingly important over the past 5 to 10 years.[266, 267] Contrary to the situation in adults, in which a variety of short-term and long-term assist devices and implantable heart-type devices are available, the need for miniaturization and a range of sizes has limited the development of such devices for children. At the present time, essentially three modalities are available for neonates, infants, and small children: extracorporeal membrane oxygenation (ECMO), ventricular assist devices (VADs), and intra-aortic balloon counterpulsation.

Ventricular Assist Devices

A VAD may be the preferred choice in infants with primary single (either right or left) ventricular dysfunction because VADs are relatively simple in design, require less time and volume to prime than ECMO circuits, and usually require less technical assistance once employed. The most common VAD-type device is a centrifugal pump, although roller pumps and newer impeller-type pumps are also used. Bleeding complications and the requirements for blood products and platelet transfusions are generally lower in patients on a VAD compared with those on an ECMO. The requirement for systemic heparinization is also proportionately less. Because of the lower technical difficulty and complication rate, a VAD may be more suitable for long-term support as a bridge to cardiac transplantation in the patient with failure confined to one ventricle. VADs also improve left ventricular drainage and unloading, and hence improve potential for myocardial recovery. Available experience indicates that a left VAD, right VAD, or double VAD can successfully support the circulation that has been compromised by cardiomyopathy or postcardiotomy ventricular failure. The majority of experience in VAD in the setting of congenital heart disease has occurred (1) in patients with recovering postischemic myocardium following repair of an anomalous origin of the left coronary artery from the pulmonary artery, and (2) in patients with transposition of the great vessels following the arterial switch procedure in whom the VAD was useful to "adapt" the poorly prepared left ventricle to pumping against systemic afterload.[268–272] When a VAD is used, the function of the nonsupported ventricle and decompression of the supported ventricle must be closely monitored. In addition to continuous arterial pressure monitoring, both left atrial and right atrial pressure monitoring is also recommended.

Extracorporeal Membrane Oxygenation

More than 200 pediatric patients per year were reported in 2000 to the Extracorporeal Life Support Organization registry (ELSO, 2000) in whom ECMO was used for cardiac indications. Common indications for ECMO in cardiac patients include preoperative resuscitation, inability to wean from cardiopulmonary bypass following cardiac surgery, postoperative cardiopulmonary failure, myocarditis, and acute fulminant cardiomyopathy. ECMO is also utilized as a bridge to cardiac transplantation and for treatment of irreversible cardiac failure in any of the aforementioned situations.[266, 267, 273–278]

In the preoperative period, ECMO or occasionally VAD may be beneficial for critically ill patients prior to cardiac surgery. This situation can be viewed as a means to facilitate preoperative stabilization and recovery of end organ dysfunction. The success of ECMO to wean patients (i.e., patients without any period of hemodynamic stability or the ability to separate from cardiopulmonary bypass) directly from cardiopulmonary bypass continues to be poor. Reported survival rates in this specific situation range between 10 and 30%, with irreversible cardiac disease and bleeding among the major issues.

In contrast, ECMO is a more effective option for infants and children who have had a period of relative stability after termination of cardiopulmonary bypass and who have had residual cardiac defects excluded. Myocardial or respiratory failure and postsurgical cardiac arrest are the most frequent indications for ECMO in this group. Survival rates are quite good (60–70%) provided ECMO is instituted rapidly and effectively. Witnessed arrest followed by cardiopulmonary resuscitation times of as long as 1 hour prior to instituting ECMO have been associated with good outcome in the postcardiotomy situation.[279]

Although it is impossible to make definitive recommendations, in general, inability to regain substantial myocardial function after 48 to 72 hours of ECMO for postcardiotomy failure usually indicates that there is little likelihood of recovering substantial myocardial function subsequently. This finding also appears to be true for patients in whom ECMO was instituted for acute fulminant myocarditis and severe dilated cardiomyopathy. In this latter group, the proper institution of ECMO may allow sufficient resuscitation and stabilization to limit end-organ dysfunction while awaiting potential myocardial recovery or serving as a bridge to transplantation.

Complications of ECMO in the cardiac patient population include hemorrhage, renal insufficiency, neurologic injury, infection, and technical problems with the ECMO circuit. Overall, the survival rate to hospital discharge across institutions and indications is approximately 40% when ECMO is utilized in pediatric cardiac patients. Failure to survive is most often due to residual and often unrecognized or irreparable cardiac defects, irreversible severe myocardial dysfunction, or significant noncardiac end-organ injury sustained prior to the institution of ECMO. Other issues include pulmonary hypertension, severe hypoxemia, and refractory dysrhythmias. Hemorrhagic complications are particularly problematic in the group in whom ECMO is instituted as a means to terminate cardiopulmonary bypass.

The presence of a systemic-to-pulmonary artery shunt is another factor that limits appropriate physiologic resuscitation by ECMO. The shunt can contribute to excessive pulmonary blood flow and hence low systemic blood flow. Completely occluding the shunt may lead to ischemic lung injury and reperfusion injury of the lung when blood flow is reestablished during ECMO weaning. Judicious narrowing of the shunt to allow a small, controlled amount of pulmonary blood flow has occasionally been successful in this situation.

In summary, mechanical assist devices are an important addition to pharmacologic means to support the failing circulation in patients with severe cardiomyopathy (i.e., acute, fulminant, or chronic) and severe myocardial dysfunction following cardiac surgery and as a bridge to cardiac transplantation. Because of improved techniques and reported good outcomes, ECMO has probably "moved up the list" of therapies to be employed in witnessed pediatric in-hospital cardiac arrest from any cause. The approach at our institution is that if circulation cannot be effectively restored within 15 minutes following witnessed cardiac arrest, preparations to begin ECMO are made. The success in patients with reversible myocardial dysfunction (e.g., approximately one third of patients with acute fulminant myocarditis, and 40 to 70% of patients following cardiac surgery or heart transplantation) suggests that the ability to perform extracorporeal circulatory support quickly and effectively is now a requirement of programs engaged in pediatric cardiac surgery and transplantation.

Cardiomyopathies

Cardiomyopathies in children are divided into two broad categories, primary/idiopathic, when no known underlying disease is responsible, and secondary, when they occur in association with an underlying disorder. Depending on their functional and morphologic characteristics, cardiomyopathies of either the primary or secondary sort are usually classified as dilated, hypertropic, or restrictive (Table 17–7).

Dilated Cardiomyopathy

Dilated cardiomyopathy is the most frequent type of cardiomyopathy found in children. Most cases of primary dilated cardiomyopathy are believed to result from an underlying viral or inflammatory process, although definitive proof is often lacking. Familial dilated cardiomyopathy is another important cause.[280] Factors associated with poor prognosis include severe cardiomegaly, low cardiac output, severely depressed ejection fraction (<0.3), and dysrhythmias.[281] Ventricular dilation may be severe enough to cause functional mitral or tricuspid regurgitation. Children with the diagnosis of dilated cardiomyopathy under 2 years of age have the worst prognosis. Overall, mortality rates in children may be greater than 50% within 1 year of diagnosis.[282, 283] The functional profile of dilated cardiomyopathy includes decreased ejection fraction and stroke volume, increased ven-

Table 17–7. Pediatric Cardiomyopathies

Anatomic types:	dilated, hypertrophic, restrictive (rare)
Infectious:	viral, bacterial, fungal, protozoal, rickettsial
Endocrine:	diabetes, hypo- or hyperthyroidism, catecholamine-induced
Storage diseases:	mucopolysaccharidoses, glycogen storage diseases, sphingolipidoses
Hereditary:	muscular dystrophies, mitochondrial myopathies, Friedreich's ataxia
Collagen-vascular:	Kawasaki disease, systemic lupus erythematosus, juvenile rheumatoid arthritis
Toxic:	anthracyclines; irradiation, human immunodeficiency viral protease inhibitors; hemachromatosis
Infiltrative:	leukemia
Nutritional:	carnitine deficiency, thiamine deficiency, phosphate deficiency, protein-calorie malnutrition; beta-ketothiolase deficiency
Miscellaneous:	hemolytic-uremic syndrome, Reye's syndrome, tachydysrhythmias, congenital heart disease with chronic volume and/or pressure overload

tricular volume and filling pressure, and normal or decreased ventricular compliance. Death typically results from progressive heart failure and related organ dysfunction, or sudden death due to cardiac dysrhythmias.

Combinations of diuretics, inotropics, and vasodilators may improve symptoms and clinical status. In patients who present with acute fulminant myocarditis, a subgroup may experience complete or significant resolution of myocardial dysfunction and its associated symptoms if they survive. Intensive therapy, which may include mechanical cardiac support (see earlier discussion), is often necessary for these patients.

Another important cause of dilated cardiomyopathy in children is the anthracycline anticancer agents, such as doxorubicin, which are cardiotoxic. Acute toxicity occurring during or shortly after anthracycline administration typically manifests as electrocardiographic and cardiac conduction disturbances. A subacute reaction consisting of myocarditis and pericarditis may develop within 2 to 4 weeks after administration. Long-term toxicity manifests primarily as left ventricular dysfunction. The major risk factor for the development of this complication, which is irreversible, is total administered dose. The likelihood increases at doses over 250 mg/m². Ventricular dysfunction may occur in as many as 25 to 30% of patients who receive greater than 500 mg/m².[284, 285]

In addition to dose, other risk factors for the development of ventricular dysfunction following Adriamycin administration include young age at the time of administration and perhaps female gender.[286] Available data suggest that in patients who received anthracyclines when they were very young, the risk of cardiomyopathy is progressive with age and body growth. The echocardiographic finding of increased afterload and decreased left ventricular wall thickness may precede reduction in systolic function as measured by shortening fraction or ejection fraction.[286, 287] The significance of these earlier changes when not accompanied by reductions in systolic function on anesthetic risk or anesthetic-induced myocardial depression are not certain. Intraoperative and postoperative complications have been reported in children who have received Adriamycin.[288–290] It appears that a reduction in shortening fraction or ejection fraction, or a history of congestive heart failure, or any combination of these, can be predictive of anesthetic-related cardiovascular complications. A recent chest radiograph, electrocardiogram, and echocardiogram are indicated. As in other patients with myocardial dysfunction, the history that is obtained regarding functional status may not be completely reliable due to patient self-limitation. Formal exercise testing, when possible, can be useful to gauge functional reserve.

The principles of anesthetic management in patients with dilated cardiomyopathy are focused on their reduced systolic function.[291] General recommendations include preserving ventricular filling and intravascular volume status, minimizing drug-induced myocardial depression, and avoiding significant increases in afterload. Circulation times may be prolonged, and hence the onset of intravenous agents may be delayed. Although opioids and benzodiazepines given individually are well tolerated, the combination of the two can result in significant myocardial depression.[292, 293] In the poorly compensated or uncompensated patient with symptoms of congestive heart failure, drugs such as ketamine

may serve primarily to increase afterload and thereby reduce stroke volume and cardiac output.[294, 295] Once adequate filling volumes are ensured, intraoperative hypotension may best be treated with agents that have beneficial effects on contractility (ephedrine or dobutamine) without significantly increasing afterload. For this reason, agents with pure alpha-adrenergic effects are probably best avoided. Continuous monitoring of arterial and ventricular filling pressures may be helpful to guide therapy in patients with severe ventricular dysfunction. These patients may also benefit from the institution of measures to optimize ventricular performance and systemic perfusion, such as inotropic and "inodilator" (e.g., amrinone and milrinone) therapy, in a "prophylactic" fashion, prior to inducing anesthesia. "Tune-ups" prior to major surgery of several days of low-dose inotropic or inotropic plus "inodilator" regimens, gentle diuresis, and optimized nutritional status may be beneficial, although formal proof of this is lacking.

Hypertrophic Cardiomyopathy

Hypertropic cardiomyopathy is the other anatomic type of cardiomyopathy that is frequently seen in pediatric patients.[296] It is often hereditary, transmitted as an autosomal dominant trait. It usually occurs as asymmetric hypertrophy of the interventricular septum, leading to the newer terminology of asymmetric septal hypertrophy. However, it may occasionally be concentric. Left ventricular outflow tract obstruction and diastolic dysfunction are common. In its most severe form, the ventricle becomes massively thickened and elongated and the outflow tract dramatically narrowed. In spite of these features, the ejection fraction is usually normal or even high (≥ 0.7), reflecting underlying systolic hypercontractility. This number may be misleading, however, as the predominant pathophysiologic issues are basal or dynamic left ventricular outflow tract obstruction and the potential for severe diastolic dysfunction. Ventricular tachycardia or fibrillation is the most frequent cause of sudden death in these patients. Risk factors for sudden death include young age at presentation, family history of hypertrophic cardiomyopathy, and syncopal or pre-syncopal symptoms.[297–299] Neither symptom severity nor the severity of left ventricular outflow obstruction appears to be a factor that helps to predict the risk of sudden death.

Surgical procedures to resect obstructing left ventricular tissue relieve the outflow obstruction and improve the symptoms but do not appear to influence the risk of sudden death due to ventricular dysrhythmias.[300] This finding may in part be due to an underlying abnormality of myocyte ion channels that likely are part of the pathophysiologic basis of the disorder. Both calcium channel antagonists and beta-adrenergic blockers have been successful in reducing shortness of breath and improving exercise tolerance.[301] However, as is the case with surgical relief of outflow obstruction, neither these therapies nor antiarrhythmic agents have been shown to reduce mortality. In contrast, there may be some survival benefit from implantable cardiac defibrillators in these patients.

The most frequent symptoms in patients with hypertropic cardiomyopathy include angina, syncope or presyncope, tachydysrhythmias, and pulmonary edema. Tachydysrhythmias are poorly tolerated due to the decrease in diastolic filling time, which increases the degree of left ventricular outflow tract obstruction. The presence of a new systolic murmur in a child or young adult who has had previous good medical care should raise the suspicion of the development of asymmetric septal hypertrophy or hypertrophic cardiomyopathy.

The electrocardiogram may show evidence of left ventricular hypertrophy, or Q waves indicative of septal hypertrophy. Echocardiography usually defines the small, hyperdynamic left ventricular chamber and asymmetric hypertrophy of the interventricular septum and provides Doppler measurement of the magnitude of the gradient across the left ventricular outflow tract. Mitral regurgitation may also be present. Echocardiography is relatively insensitive for the detection of diastolic dysfunction, the presence of which should be assumed in this disorder. The presence of markedly elevated left ventricular end-diastolic pressure at cardiac catheterization is far more useful in this regard. Because of the potential dynamic aspect of the obstruction, provocative maneuvers such as exercise testing may help quantify the severity of the obstruction and may also provide useful information regarding the influence of factors such as tachycardia and blood pressure on the degree of obstruction.

As was the case with dilated cardiomyopathy, anesthetic management is directed at factors that influence myocardial contractility, preload, and afterload. Patients with severe hypertrophy may develop myocardial ischemia or critically increased outflow obstruction, or both, from even modest degrees of systemic hypotension or tachycardia. In general, events or agents that increase outflow obstruction (and thus should be avoided) include (1) those that increase myocardial contractility (e.g., catecholamines, tachycardia), (2) those that decrease preload (hypovolemia, hemorrhage, vasodilators, tachycardia, excessive positive pressure ventilation), and (3) those that decrease afterload. Conversely, factors that may improve outflow obstruction include (1) agents that decrease myocardial contractility (e.g., halothane, beta-blockers, or calcium channel blockers), (2) those that increase effective preload (decreased heart rate, volume expansion), and (3) those that moderately increase afterload.

Maintenance of normal sinus rhythm is important to preserve ventricular filling and limit outflow obstruction. Tachycardia may be carefully treated with beta-blockers, such as esmolol and propranolol, with care taken to avoid systemic hypotension. The patients are often sensitive to reduced afterload because of its effects in decreasing perfusion of the hypertrophied myocardium and because of the increase in outflow tract obstruction that accompanies the decrease in afterload. Maintaining both high filling pressures with volume administration and afterload with agents such as phenylephrine have been helpful. Volume administration must be carefully titrated owing to the propensity to pulmonary edema as a result of markedly reduced ventricular compliance.

Mitochondrial Myopathies

Disorders of mitochondrial function, formerly thought to be uncommon, are now considered to be one of the most frequent types of metabolic disease. Overall, mitochondrial disorders are believed to result from faulty oxidative phosphorylation and result in deficiencies in energy production. These diseases are frequently due to specific defects in the mitochondrial electron transport chain that carries out oxidative phosphorylation to produce mitochondrial ATP. They may also be caused by defects in substrate transport or usage, such as abnormalities in the pyruvate dehydrogenase complex or Krebs cycle.

The majority of these abnormalities are believed to be genetic in origin. Most mitochondrial proteins are encoded by the nuclear genes. These nuclear genes encode for the majority of the protein subunits that are part of the respiratory chain. However, a distinct mitochondrial genome encodes a smaller number of essential subunits of the respiratory chain, as well as the ribonucleic acids and enzymes necessary for intramitochondrial translation of mitochondrial DNA. Because inheritance can thus be mendelian or maternal (e.g., in mitochondrial genes), or a combination of the two, the inheritance pattern and modes of phenotypic expression of the mitochondrial diseases can be extremely variable. Point mutations have currently been described in the MELAS (mitochondrial encephalopathy, lactic acidosis, and stroke-like episodes), LHON (Leber's hereditary optic neuropathy, cardiomyopathy, and deafness), and NARP (neuropathy, ataxia, retinitis pigmentosa) syndromes.[302, 303]

The central nervous system is typically involved in all children with mitochondrial disorders. Nervous system manifestations include encephalopathy, mental retardation, acute intermittent metabolic decompensation with encephalopathy, spastic paraplegias, skeletal muscle myopathy, central apnea, and autonomic dysfunction. Anemia, recurrent infection, and hypoglycemia are also found.

Cardiac manifestations include either dilated or hypertrophic cardiomyopathy, intracardiac conduction effects or dysrhythmias, and autonomic dysfunction resulting in abnormal regulation of blood pressure.[302] One or more of these cardiac abnormalities may be present in a third or more of patients with a mitochondrial defect.

Although formal studies are not available, and would be difficult given the diverse molecular pathogenesis of these disorders, the general impression is that patients with mitochondrial disorders are extremely susceptible to decompensation at times of stress, infection, surgery, and anesthesia.[304] The mechanisms underlying this response are not at all clear but likely are related to the limited and defective nature of mitochondrial energy production. Products of the systemic response to stress, ischemia-reperfusion, and infection include substances such as tumor necrosis factor-alpha and oxyradicals, which can reduce mitochondrial function, mitochondrial electron transport, and substrate utilization. Thus, one can speculate that minimizing the stress and inflammatory responses to surgery might be beneficial in these patients.

Evidence in the *Caenorhabditis elegans* nematode suggests that a potential site of inhaled anesthetic action is a subunit of complex I in the mitochondrial electron transport chain.[305] Whether the mechanism of inhaled anesthetic action depends directly on this complex I subunit or instead is related to secondary effects at other sites is not clear. Nonetheless, this information is intriguing with regard to the potential deleterious effect of inhaled anesthetic agents on patients with underlying mitochondrial disorders who have pre-existing defects in oxidative phosphorylation. Anesthetics may exacerbate the underlying mitochondrial defect. In practice, anesthetic experience with these disorders is limited. Recommendations are further limited by the diversity of the underlying molecular defect and phenotypic expression patterns. Patients with known or presumed myopathy should be suspected of and evaluated for an underlying mitochondrial disorder. Abnormalities, including cardiomyopathy and severe neurologic and metabolic decompensation at times of stress, infection, and surgery, should be anticipated.

REFERENCES

1. Rudolph AM: In: Rudolph AM, ed: Congenital Diseases of the Heart. Chicago: Year Book Publishers; 1974.
2. Teitel DF, Iwamoto HS, Rudolph AM: Effects of birth-related events on central blood flow patterns. Pediatr Res 1987;22:557–566.
3. Heymann MA: Fetal and postnatal circulations: Pulmonary circulation. In: Emmanouilides GC, Riemenschneider TA, Allen HD, et al., eds: Moss and Adams Heart Disease in Infants, Children, and Adolescents Including the Fetus and Young Adult, 5th ed. Baltimore: Williams & Wilkins; 1995:41–59.
4. Sacks LM, Delivoria-Papadopoulos M: Hemoglobin-oxygen interactions. Semin Perinatol 1984;8:168–183.
5. Cassin S, Dawes GS, Mott JC, et al: The vascular resistance of the foetal and newly ventilated lung of the lamb. J Physiol 1964;171:61–79.
6. Rudolph AM, Yuan S: Response of the pulmonary vasculature to hypoxia and H$^+$ ion concentration changes. J Clin Invest 1966;45:399–411.
7. Reller MD, Ziegler ML, Rice MJ, et al: Duration of ductal shunting in healthy preterm infants: An echocardiographic color flow Doppler study. J Pediatr 1988;112:441–446.
8. Kovalik V: The response of the isolated ductus arteriosus to oxygen and anoxia. J Physiol 1963;169:185–197.
9. McMurphy DM, Heymann MA, Rudolph AM, et al: Developmental changes in constriction of the ductus arteriosus: Responses to oxygen and vasoactive agents in the isolated ductus arteriosus of the fetal lamb. Pediatr Res 1972;6:231–238.
10. Clyman RI, Mauray F, Roman C, et al: Factors determining the loss of ductus arteriosus responsiveness to prostaglandin E. Circulation 1983;68:433–436.
11. Fay FS, Cooke PH: Guinea pig ductus arteriosus. II. Irreversible closure after birth. Am J Physiol 1972;222:841–849.
12. Hagen PT, Scholz DG, Edwards WD: Incidence and size of patent foramen ovale during the first 10 decades of life: An autopsy study of 965 normal hearts. Mayo Clin Proc 1984;59:17–20.
13. Moorthy SS, Haselby KA, Caldwell RL, et al: Transient right-left interatrial shunt during emergence from anesthesia: Demonstration by color flow Doppler mapping. Anesth Analg 1989;68:820–822.
14. Baum VC, Palmisano BW: The immature heart and anesthesia. Anesthesiology 1997;87:1529–1548.
15. Hoerter J, Mazet F, Vassort G: Perinatal growth of the rabbit cardiac cell: Possible implications for the mechanism of relaxation. J Mol Cell Cardiol 1981;13:725–740.
16. Jarmakani JM, Nakanishi T, George BL, et al: Effect of extracellular calcium on myocardial mechanical function in the neonatal rabbit. Dev Pharmacol Ther 1982;5:1–13.
17. Nayler WG, Fassold E: Calcium accumulating and ATPase activity of cardiac sarcoplasmic reticulum before and after birth. Cardiovasc Res 1977;11:231–237.
18. Romero T, Covell J, Friedman WF: A comparison of pressure-volume relations of the fetal, newborn, and adult heart. Am J Physiol 1972;222:1285–1290.
19. Kirkpatrick SE, Pitlick PT, Naliboff J, et al: Frank-Starling relationship as an important determinant of fetal cardiac output. Am J Physiol 1976;231:495–500.
20. Thornburg KL, Morton MJ: Filling and arterial pressures as determinants of RV stroke volume in the sheep fetus. Am J Physiol 1983;244:H656–H663.
21. Teitel DF, Sidi D, Chin T, et al: Developmental changes in myocardial contractile reserve in the lamb. Pediatr Res 1985;19:948–955.
22. Winberg P, Jansson M, Marions L, et al: Left ventricular output during postnatal circulatory adaptation in healthy infants born at full term. Arch Dis Child 1989;64:1374–1378.
23. Kenny J, Plappert T, Doubilet P, et al: Effects of heart rate on ventricular size, stroke volume, and output in the normal human fetus: A prospective Doppler echocardiographic study. Circulation 1987;76:52–58.
24. Papp JG: Autonomic responses and neurohumoral control in the human early antenatal heart. Basic Res Cardiol 1988;83:2–9.
25. Sachis PN, Armstrong DL, Becker LE, et al: Myelination of the human vagus nerve from 24 weeks postconceptional age to adolescence. J Neuropathol Exp Neurol 1982;41:466–472.
26. Hislop A, Reid L: Pulmonary arterial development during childhood: Branching pattern and structure. Thorax 1973;28:129–135.
27. Rabinovitch M, Haworth SG, Castaneda AR, et al: Lung biopsy in congenital heart disease: A morphometric approach to pulmonary vascular disease. Circulation 1978;58:1107–1122.
28. James LS, Rowe RD: The pattern of response of pulmonary and systemic arterial pressures in newborn and older infants to short periods of hypoxia. J Pediatr 1957;51:5–11.
29. Abman SH: Abnormal vasoreactivity in the pathophysiology of persistent pulmonary hypertension of the newborn [electronic citation]. Pediatr Rev 1999;20:e103–e109.
30. Levin DL, Heymann MA, Kitterman JA, et al: Persistent pulmonary hypertension of the newborn infant. J Pediatr 1976;89:626–630.
31. Davidson D, Barefield ES, Kattwinkel J, et al: Inhaled nitric oxide for the early treatment of persistent pulmonary hypertension of the term newborn: A randomized, double-masked, placebo-controlled, dose-response, multicenter study. The I-NO/PPHN Study Group. Pediatrics 1998;101:325–334.
32. Wessel DL, Adatia I: Clinical applications of inhaled nitric oxide in children with pulmonary hypertension. Adv Pharmacol 1995;34:475–504.
33. Wessel DL, Adatia I, Van Marter LJ, et al: Improved oxygenation in a randomized trial of inhaled nitric oxide for persistent pulmonary hypertension of the newborn [electronic citation]. Pediatrics 1997;100:e7.
34. Wessel DL, Adatia I, Giglia TM, et al: Use of inhaled nitric oxide and acetylcholine in the evaluation of pulmonary hypertension and endothelial function after cardiopulmonary bypass. Circulation 1993;88:2128–2138.
35. Bartlett RH, Gazzaniga AB, Toomasian J, et al: Extracorporeal membrane oxygenation (ECMO) in neonatal respiratory failure: 100 cases. Ann Surg 1986;204:236–245.
36. Gillum RF: Epidemiology of congenital heart disease in the United States. Am Heart J 1994;127:919–927.
37. Hoffman JI: Congenital heart disease: Incidence and inheritance. Pediatr Clin North Am 1990;37:25–43.
38. Hoffman JI: Incidence of congenital heart disease: I. Postnatal incidence. Pediatr Cardiol 1995;16:103–113.
39. Scott DJ, Rigby ML, Miller GA, et al: The presentation of symptomatic heart disease in infancy based on 10 years' experience (1973–82): Implications for the provision of services. Br Heart J 1984;52:248–257.
40. Fyler DC: Report of the New England Regional Infant Cardiac Program. Pediatrics 1980;65:375–461.
41. Allan LD, Sharland GK, Milburn A, et al: Prospective diagnosis of 1,006 consecutive cases of congenital heart disease in the fetus. J Am Coll Cardiol 1994;23:1452–1458.
42. Hoffman JI: Incidence of congenital heart disease: II. Prenatal incidence. Pediatr Cardiol 1995;16:155–165.
43. Grossman W, Jones D, McLaurin LP: Wall stress and patterns of hypertrophy in the human left ventricle. J Clin Invest 1975;56:56–64.
44. Stark J: Do we really correct congenital heart defects? J Thorac Cardiovasc Surg 1989;97:1–9.
45. Jarmakani JM, Graham TPJ, Canent RVJ: Left ventricular contractile state in children with successfully corrected ventricular septal defect. Circulation 1972;45:I102–I110.
46. Jarmakani JM, Graham TP Jr, Canent RV Jr, et al: The effect of corrective surgery on left heart volume and mass in children with ventricular septal defect. Am J Cardiol 1971;27:254–258.
47. Heath D, Edwards JE: The pathology of hypertensive pulmonary vascular disease: Descriptions of six grades of structural changes in the pulmonary arteries with special reference to congenital cardiac septal defects. Circulation 1958;18:533–547.
48. Hoffman JI, Rudolph AM, Heymann MA: Pulmonary vascular disease with congenital heart lesions: Pathologic features and causes. Circulation 1981;64:873–877.

49. Cordell D, Graham TPJ, Atwood GF, et al: Left heart volume characteristics following ventricular septal defect closure in infancy. Circulation 1976;54:294–298.

50. Nollert G, Fischlein T, Bouterwek S, et al: Long-term survival in patients with repair of tetralogy of Fallot: 36-year follow-up of 490 survivors of the first year after surgical repair. J Am Coll Cardiol 1997;30:1374–1383.

51. Kirklin JK, Kirklin JW, Blackstone EH, et al: Effect of transannular patching on outcome after repair of tetralogy of Fallot. Ann Thorac Surg 1989;48:783–791.

52. Cullen S, Celermajer DS, Franklin RC, et al: Prognostic significance of ventricular arrhythmia after repair of tetralogy of Fallot: A 12-year prospective study. J Am Coll Cardiol 1994;23:1151–1155.

53. Murphy JG, Gersh BJ, Mair DD, et al: Long-term outcome in patients undergoing surgical repair of tetralogy of Fallot. N Engl J Med 1993;329:593–599.

54. Kirjavainen M, Happonen JM, Louhimo I: Late results of Senning operation. J Thorac Cardiovasc Surg 1999;117:488–495.

55. Hayes CJ, Gersony WM: Arrhythmias after the Mustard operation for transposition of the great arteries: A long-term study. J Am Coll Cardiol 1986;7:133–137.

56. Gelatt M, Hamilton RM, McCrindle BW, et al: Risk factors for atrial tachyarrhythmias after the Fontan operation. J Am Coll Cardiol 1994;24:1735–1741.

57. Hurwitz RA, Caldwell RL, Girod DA, et al: Right ventricular systolic function in adolescents and young adults after Mustard operation for transposition of the great arteries. Am J Cardiol 1996;77:294–297.

58. Turina MI, Siebenmann R, von Segesser L, et al: Late functional deterioration after atrial correction for transposition of the great arteries. Circulation 1989;80:I162–I167.

59. Wilson NJ, Clarkson PM, Barratt-Boyes BG, et al: Long-term outcome after the mustard repair for simple transposition of the great arteries: 28-year follow-up. J Am Coll Cardiol 1998;32:758–765.

60. Haas F, Wottke M, Poppert H, et al: Long-term survival and functional follow-up in patients after the arterial switch operation. Ann Thorac Surg 1999;68:1692–1697.

61. Massin MM: Midterm results of the neonatal arterial switch operation: A review. J Cardiovasc Surg (Torino) 1999;40:517–522.

62. Williams WG, Quaegebeur JM, Kirklin JW, et al: Outflow obstruction after the arterial switch operation: A multi-institutional study. Congenital Heart Surgeons Society. J Thorac Cardiovasc Surg 1997;114:975–987.

63. Bengel FM, Hauser M, Duvernoy CS, et al: Myocardial blood flow and coronary flow reserve late after anatomical correction of transposition of the great arteries. J Am Coll Cardiol 1998;32:1955–1961.

64. Bonnet D, Bonhoeffer P, Piechaud JF, et al: Long-term fate of the coronary arteries after the arterial switch operation in newborns with transposition of the great arteries. Heart 1996;76:274–279.

65. Massin MM, Nitsch GB, Dabritz S, et al: Angiographic study of aorta, coronary arteries, and left ventricular performance after neonatal arterial switch operation for simple transposition of the great arteries. Am Heart J 1997;134:298–305.

66. Newfeld EA, Paul MM, Muster AJ, et al: Pulmonary vascular disease in complete transposition of the great arteries: A study of 200 patients. Am J Cardiol 1974;34:75–82.

67. Rivenes SM, Grifka RG, Feltes TF: Development of advanced pulmonary vascular disease in D-transposition of the great arteries after the neonatal arterial switch operation. Tex Heart Inst J 1998;25:201–205.

68. Fontan F, Baudet E: Surgical repair of tricuspid atresia. Thorax 1971;26:240–248.

69. Durongpisitkul K, Driscoll DJ, Mahoney DW, et al: Cardiorespiratory response to exercise after modified Fontan operation: determinants of performance. J Am Coll Cardiol 1997;29:785–790.

70. Gewillig MH, Lundstrom UR, Bull C, et al: Exercise responses in patients with congenital heart disease after Fontan repair: Patterns and determinants of performance. J Am Coll Cardiol 1990;15:1424–1432.

71. Fontan F, Kirklin JW, Fernandez G, et al: Outcome after a "perfect" Fontan operation. Circulation 1990;81:1520–1536.

72. Gentles TL, Mayer JE Jr, Gauvreau K, et al: Fontan operation in five hundred consecutive patients: Factors influencing early and late outcome. J Thorac Cardiovasc Surg 1997;114:376–391.

73. Mahle WT, Wernovsky G, Bridges ND, et al: Impact of early ventricular unloading on exercise performance in preadolescents with single ventricle Fontan physiology. J Am Coll Cardiol 1999;34:1637–1643.

74. Rosenthal M, Bush A, Deanfield J, et al: Comparison of cardiopulmonary adaptation during exercise in children after the atriopulmonary and total cavopulmonary connection Fontan procedures. Circulation 1995;91:372–378.

75. Gardiner HM, Dhillon R, Bull C, et al: Prospective study of the incidence and determinants of arrhythmia after total cavopulmonary connection. Circulation 1996;94:II17–II21.

76. Spicer RL: Cardiovascular disease in Down syndrome. Pediatr Clin North Am 1984;31:1331–1343.

77. Tandon R, Edwards JE: Cardiac malformations associated with Down's syndrome. Circulation 1973;47:1349–1355.

78. Clapp S, Perry BL, Farooki ZQ, et al: Down's syndrome, complete atrioventricular canal, and pulmonary vascular obstructive disease. J Thorac Cardiovasc Surg 1990;100:115–121.

79. Levine OR, Simpser M: Alveolar hypoventilation and cor pulmonale associated with chronic airway obstruction in infants with Down syndrome. Clin Pediatr (Phila) 1982;21:25–29.

80. Yamaki S, Yasui H, Kado H, et al: Pulmonary vascular disease and operative indications in complete atrioventricular canal defect in early infancy. J Thorac Cardiovasc Surg 1993;106:398–406.

81. Pyeritz RE, McKusick VA: The Marfan syndrome: Diagnosis and management. N Engl J Med 1979;300:772–777.

82. Pyeritz RE, Wappel MA: Mitral valve dysfunction in the Marfan syndrome: Clinical and echocardiographic study of prevalence and natural history. Am J Med 1983;74:797–807.

83. Sisk HE, Zahka KG, Pyeritz RE: The Marfan syndrome in early childhood: Analysis of 15 patients diagnosed at less than 4 years of age. Am J Cardiol 1983;52:353–358.

84. Phornphutkul C, Rosenthal A, Nadas AS: Cardiac manifestations of Marfan syndrome in infancy and childhood. Circulation 1973;47:587–596.

85. Rowley AH, Shulman ST: Kawasaki syndrome. Pediatr Clin North Am 1999;46:313–329.

86. Fujiwara H, Hamashima Y: Pathology of the heart in Kawasaki disease. Pediatrics 1978;61:100–107.

87. Newburger JW, Burns JC: Kawasaki disease. Vasc Med 1999;4:187–202.

88. Burns JC, Shike H, Gordon JB, et al: Sequelae of Kawasaki disease in adolescents and young adults. J Am Coll Cardiol 1996;28:253–257.

89. Koutlas TC, Wernovsky G, Bridges ND, et al: Orthotopic heart transplantation for Kawasaki disease after rupture of a giant coronary artery aneurysm. J Thorac Cardiovasc Surg 1997;113:217–218.

90. Kaplan S: Chronic rheumatic heart disease. In: Adams FH, Emmanouilides GC, eds: Heart Disease in Infants, Children and Adolescents, 3rd ed. Baltimore: Williams & Wilkins; 1983:522–564.

91. Stollerman GH: Rheumatic fever. Lancet 1997;349:935–942.

92. Brook MM: Pediatric bacterial endocarditis: Treatment and prophylaxis. Pediatr Clin North Am 1999;46:275–287.

93. Ashkenazi S, Levy O, Blieden L: Trends of childhood infective endocarditis in Israel with emphasis on children under 2 years of age. Pediatr Cardiol 1997;18:419–424.

94. Van Hare GF, Ben Shachar G, Liebman J, et al: Infective endocarditis in infants and children during the past 10 years: A decade of change. Am Heart J 1984;107:1235–1240.

95. Moder KG, Miller TD, Tazelaar HD: Cardiac involvement in systemic lupus erythematosus. Mayo Clin Proc 1999;74:275–284.

96. Barst RJ: Pharmacologically induced pulmonary vasodilatation in children and young adults with primary pulmonary hypertension. Chest 1986;89:497–503.

97. Barst RJ: Recent advances in the treatment of pediatric pulmonary artery hypertension. Pediatr Clin North Am 1999;46:331–345.

98. Boucek MM, Novick RJ, Bennett LE, et al: The Registry of the International Society of Heart and Lung Transplantation: Second Official Pediatric Report—1998. J Heart Lung Transplant 1998;17:1141–1160.

99. Bridges ND: Lung transplantation in children. Curr Opin Cardiol 1998;13:73–77.

100. Lang P, Williams RG, Norwood WI, et al: The hemodynamic effects of dopamine in infants after corrective cardiac surgery. J Pediatr 1980;96:630–634.

101. Bohn DJ, Poirier CS, Edmonds JF, et al: Hemodynamic effects of dobutamine after cardiopulmonary bypass in children. Crit Care Med 1980;8:367–371.

102. Berner M, Rouge JC, Friedli B: The hemodynamic effect of phentolamine and dobutamine after open-heart operations in children: Influence of the underlying heart defect. Ann Thorac Surg 1983;35:643–650.

103. Banner W Jr, Vernon DD, Minton SD, et al: Nonlinear dobutamine pharmacokinetics in a pediatric population. Crit Care Med 1991;19:871–873.

104. Eldadah MK, Schwartz PH, Harrison R, et al: Pharmacokinetics of dopamine in infants and children. Crit Care Med 1991;19:1008–1011.

105. Artman M, Kithas PA, Wike JS, et al: Inotropic responses change during postnatal maturation in rabbit. Am J Physiol 1988;255:H335–H342.

106. Bristow MR, Ginsburg R, Minobe W, et al: Decreased catecholamine sensitivity and beta-adrenergic-receptor density in failing human hearts. N Engl J Med 1982;307:205–211.

107. Pracyk JB, Slotkin TA: Thyroid hormone differentially regulates development of beta-adrenergic receptors, adenylate cyclase and ornithine decarboxylase in rat heart and kidney. J Dev Physiol 1991;16:251–261.

108. Zeiders JL, Seidler FJ, Iaccarino G, et al: Ontogeny of cardiac beta-adrenoceptor desensitization mechanisms: Agonist treatment enhances receptor/G-protein transduction rather than eliciting uncoupling. J Mol Cell Cardiol 1999;31:413–423.

109. Giannuzzi CE, Seidler FJ, Slotkin TA: Beta-adrenoceptor control of cardiac adenylyl cyclase during development: Agonist pretreatment in the neonate uniquely causes heterologous sensitization, not desensitization. Brain Res 1995;694:271–278.

110. Reithmann C, Reber D, Kozlik-Feldmann R, et al: A post-receptor defect of adenylyl cyclase in severely failing myocardium from children with congenital heart disease. Eur J Pharmacol 1997;330:79–86.

111. Owen VJ, Burton PB, Michel MC, et al: Myocardial dysfunction in donor hearts: A possible etiology. Circulation 1999;99:2565–2570.

112. Feldman MD, Copelas L, Gwathmey JK, et al: Deficient production of cyclic AMP: Pharmacologic evidence of an important cause of contractile dysfunction in patients with end-stage heart failure. Circulation 1987;75:331–339.

113. Schwinn DA, Leone BJ, Spahn DR, et al: Desensitization of myocardial beta-adrenergic receptors during cardiopulmonary bypass: Evidence for early uncoupling and late downregulation. Circulation 1991;84:2559–2567.

114. Sun LS, Du F, Quaegebeur JM: Right ventricular infundibular beta-adrenoceptor complex in tetralogy of Fallot patients. Pediatr Res 1997;42:12–16.

115. Allen EM, Van Boerum DH, Olsen AF, et al: Difference between the measured and ordered dose of catecholamine infusions. Ann Pharmacother 1995;29:1095–1100.

116. Badke FR: Left ventricular dimensions and function during right ventricular pressure overload. Am J Physiol 1982;242:H611–H618.

117. Kaul S: The interventricular septum in health and disease. Am Heart J 1986;112:568–581.

118. Calvin JE Jr: Acute right heart failure: pathophysiology, recognition, and pharmacological management. J Cardiothorac Vasc Anesth 1991;5:507–513.

119. Stopfkuchen H, Racke K, Schworer H, et al: Effects of dopamine infusion on plasma catecholamines in preterm and term newborn infants. Eur J Pediatr 1991;150:503–506.

120. Seri I, Tulassay T, Kiszel J, et al: Cardiovascular response to dopamine in hypotensive preterm neonates with severe hyaline membrane disease. Eur J Pediatr 1984;142:3–9.

121. Wenstone R, Campbell JM, Booker PD, et al: Renal function after cardiopulmonary bypass in children: Comparison of dopamine with dobutamine. Br J Anaesth 1991;67:591–594.

122. Bhatt-Mehta V, Nahata MC, McClead RE, et al: Dopamine pharmacokinetics in critically ill newborn infants. Eur J Clin Pharmacol 1991;40:593–597.

123. Padbury JF, Agata Y, Baylen BG, et al: Pharmacokinetics of dopamine in critically ill newborn infants. J Pediatr 1990;117:472–476.

124. DiSessa TG, Leitner M, Ti CC, et al: The cardiovascular effects of dopamine in the severely asphyxiated neonate. J Pediatr 1981;99:772–776.

125. Padbury JF, Agata Y, Baylen BG, et al: Dopamine pharmacokinetics in critically ill newborn infants. J Pediatr 1987;110:293–298.

126. Driscoll DJ, Gillette PC, Ezrailson EG, et al: Inotropic response of the neonatal canine myocardium to dopamine. Pediatr Res 1978;12:42–45.

127. Furman WR, Summer WR, Kennedy TP, et al: Comparison of the effects of dobutamine, dopamine, and isoproterenol on hypoxic pulmonary vasoconstriction in the pig. Crit Care Med 1982;10:371–374.

128. Harris WH, Van Petten GR: The effects of dopamine of blood pressure and heart rate of the unanesthetized fetal lamb. Am J Obstet Gynecol 1978;130:211–215.

129. Mentzer RM, Alegre CA, Nolan SP: The effects of dopamine and isoproterenol on the pulmonary circulation. J Thorac Cardiovasc Surg 1976;71:807–814.

130. Privitera PJ, Loggie JM, Gaffney TE: A comparison of the cardiovascular effects of biogenic amines and their precursors in newborn and adult dogs. J Pharmacol Exp Ther 1969;166:293–298.

131. Stephenson LW, Edmunds LHJ, Raphaely R, et al: Effects of nitroprusside and dopamine on pulmonary arterial vasculature in children after cardiac surgery. Circulation 1979;60:104–110.

132. Williams DB, Kiernan PD, Schaff HV, et al: The hemodynamic response to dopamine and nitroprusside following right atrium-pulmonary artery bypass (Fontan procedure). Ann Thorac Surg 1982;34:51–57.

133. Bhatt-Mehta V, Nahata MC: Dopamine and dobutamine in pediatric therapy. Pharmacotherapy 1989;9:303–314.

134. Lopez SL, Leighton JO, Walther FJ: Supranormal cardiac output in the dopamine- and dobutamine-dependent preterm infant. Pediatr Cardiol 1997;18:292–296.

135. Martinez AM, Padbury JF, Thio S: Dobutamine pharmacokinetics and cardiovascular responses in critically ill neonates. Pediatrics 1992;89:47–51.

136. Perkin RM, Levin DL, Webb R, et al: Dobutamine: A hemodynamic evaluation in children with shock. J Pediatr 1982;100:977–983.

137. Schranz D, Stopfkuchen H, Jungst BK, et al: Hemodynamic effects of dobutamine in children with cardiovascular failure. Eur J Pediatr 1982;139:4–7.

138. Harada K, Tamura M, Ito T, et al: Effects of low-dose dobutamine on left ventricular diastolic filling in children. Pediatr Cardiol 1996;17:220–225.

139. Stopfkuchen H, Schranz D, Huth R, et al: Effects of dobutamine on left ventricular performance in newborns as determined by systolic time intervals. Eur J Pediatr 1987;146:135–139.

140. Berg RA, Donnerstein RL, Padbury JF: Dobutamine infusions in stable, critically ill children: Pharmacokinetics and hemodynamic actions. Crit Care Med 1993;21:678–686.

141. Schwartz PH, Eldadah MK, Newth CJ: The pharmacokinetics of dobutamine in pediatric intensive care unit patients. Drug Metab Dispos 1991;19:614–619.

142. Unverferth DA, Blanford M, Kates RE, et al: Tolerance to dobutamine after a 72 hour continuous infusion. Am J Med 1980;69:262–266.

143. Reyes G, Schwartz PH, Newth CJ, et al: The pharmacokinetics of isoproterenol in critically ill pediatric patients. J Clin Pharmacol 1993;33:29–34.

144. Daoud FS, Reeves JT, Kelly DB: Isoproterenol as a potential pulmonary vasodilator in primary pulmonary hypertension. Am J Cardiol 1978;42:817–822.

145. Jaccard C, Berner M, Rouge JC, et al: Hemodynamic effect of isoprenaline and dobutamine immediately after correction of tetralogy of Fallot: Relative importance of inotropic and chronotropic action in supporting cardiac output. J Thorac Cardiovasc Surg 1984;87:862–869.

146. Driscoll DJ, Gillette PC, Lewis RM, et al: Comparative hemodynamic effects of isoproterenol, dopamine, and dobutamine in the newborn dog. Pediatr Res 1979;13:1006–1009.

147. Maguire JF, O'Rourke PP, Colan SD, et al: Cardiotoxicity during treatment of severe childhood asthma. Pediatrics 1991;88:1180–1186.

148. Fisher DG, Schwartz PH, Davis AL: Pharmacokinetics of exogenous epinephrine in critically ill children. Crit Care Med 1993;21:111–117.

149. Hausdorf G, Friedel N, Berdjis F, et al: Enoximone in newborns with refractory postoperative low-output states (LOS). Eur J Cardiothorac Surg 1992;6:311–317.

150. Ovadia M, Thoele D, Gersony WM: Amrinone: Efficacy and safety in infants and children. Circulation 1988;78(suppl II):II293.

151. Wessel DL, Triedman JK, Wernovsky G, et al: Pulmonary and systemic hemodynamic effects of amrinone in neonates following cardiopulmonary bypass. Circulation 1989;80(suppl II):II488.

152. Gage J, Rutman H, Lucido D, et al: Additive effects of dobutamine and amrinone on myocardial contractility and ventricular performance in patients with severe heart failure. Circulation 1986;74:367–373.

153. Matsumori A, Ono K, Sato Y, et al: Differential modulation of cytokine production by drugs: Implications for therapy in heart failure. J Mol Cell Cardiol 1996;28:2491–2499.

154. Takeuchi K, del Nido PJ, Ibrahim AE, et al: Vesnarinone and amrinone reduce the systemic inflammatory response syndrome. J Thorac Cardiovasc Surg 1999;117:375–382.

155. Takeuchi K, del Nido PJ, Ibrahim AE, et al: Increased myocardial calcium cycling and reduced myofilament calcium sensitivity in early endotoxemia. Surgery 1999;126:231–238.

156. Bailey JM, Miller BE, Kanter KR, et al: A comparison of the hemodynamic effects of amrinone and sodium nitroprusside in infants after cardiac surgery. Anesth Analg 1997;84:294–298.

157. Konstam MA, Cohen SR, Salem DN, et al: Effect of amrinone on right ventricular function: predominance of afterload reduction. Circulation 1986;74:359–366.

158. Sorensen GK, Ramamoorthy C, Lynn AM, et al: Hemodynamic effects of amrinone in children after Fontan surgery. Anesth Analg 1996;82:241–246.

159. Lawless S, Burckart G, Diven W, et al: Amrinone pharmacokinetics in neonates and infants. J Clin Pharmacol 1988;28:283–284.

160. Williams GD, Sorensen GK, Oakes R, et al: Amrinone loading during cardiopulmonary bypass in neonates, infants, and children. J Cardiothorac Vasc Anesth 1995;9:278–282.

161. Bailey JM, Miller BE, Lu W, et al: The pharmacokinetics of milrinone in pediatric patients after cardiac surgery. Anesthesiology 1999;90:1012–1018.

162. Chang AC, Atz AM, Wernovsky G, et al: Milrinone: Systemic and pulmonary hemodynamic effects in neonates after cardiac surgery. Crit Care Med 1995;23:1907–1914.

163. Ramamoorthy C, Anderson GD, Williams GD, et al: Pharmacokinetics and side effects of milrinone in infants and children after open heart surgery. Anesth Analg 1998;86:283–289.

164. Skoyles JR, Sherry KM, Price C: Intravenous milrinone in patients with severe congestive cardiac failure awaiting heart transplantation. J Cardiothorac Vasc Anesth 1992;6:222–225.

165. Lindsay CA, Barton P, Lawless S, et al: Pharmacokinetics and pharmacodynamics of milrinone lactate in pediatric patients with septic shock. J Pediatr 1998;132:329–334.

166. Boldt J, Kling D, Moosdorf R, et al: Enoximone treatment of impaired myocardial function during cardiac surgery: Combined effects with epinephrine. J Cardiothorac Anesth 1990;4:462–468.

167. Cossolini M, Ferri F, Giupponi A, et al: Enoximone in the treatment of postoperative low cardiac output syndrome in pediatric heart surgery: Open study in tetralogy of Fallot. [in Italian]. Minerva Anestesiol 1997;63:213–219.

168. Bauer J, Dapper F, Demirakca S, et al: Perioperative management of pulmonary hypertension after heart transplantation in childhood. J Heart Lung Transplant 1997;16:1238–1247.

169. Berman WJ, Yabek SM, Dillon T, et al: Effects of digoxin in infants with congested circulatory state due to a ventricular septal defect. N Engl J Med 1983;308:363–366.

170. White RD, Lietman PS: Commentary: A reappraisal of digitalis for infants with left-to-right shunts and "heart failure". J Pediatr 1978;92:867–870.

171. Smith TW: Digitalis toxicity: Epidemiology and clinical use of serum concentration measurements. Am J Med 1975;58:470–476.

172. Butterworth JF, Strickland RA, Mark LJ, et al: Calcium does not augment phenylephrine's hypertensive effects. Crit Care Med 1990;18:603–606.

173. Denlinger JK, Kaplan JA, Lecky JH, et al: Cardiovascular responses to calcium administered intravenously to man during halothane anesthesia. Anesthesiology 1975;42:390–397.

174. Drop LJ, Laver MB: Low plasma ionized calcium and response to calcium therapy in critically ill man. Anesthesiology 1975;43:300–306.

175. Drop LJ, Geffin GA, O'Keefe DD, et al: Relation between ionized calcium concentration and ventricular pump performance in the dog under hemodynamically controlled conditions. Am J Cardiol 1981;47:1041–1051.

176. Scheidegger D, Drop LJ, Schellenberg JC: Role of the systemic vasculature in the hemodynamic response to changes in plasma ionized calcium. Arch Surg 1980;115:206–211.

177. Royster RL, Butterworth JF, Prielipp RC, et al: A randomized, blinded, placebo-controlled evaluation of calcium chloride and epinephrine for inotropic support after emergence from cardiopulmonary bypass. Anesth Analg 1992;74:3–13.

178. Zaloga GP, Chernow B: The multifactorial basis for hypocalcemia during sepsis: Studies of the parathyroid hormone–vitamin D axis. Ann Intern Med 1987;107:36–41.

179. Malcolm DS, Holaday JW, Chernow B, et al: Calcium and calcium antagonists in shock and ischemia. In: Chernow B, ed: The Pharmacologic Approach to the Critically Ill Patient, 2nd ed. Baltimore: Williams & Wilkins; 1988:889–895.

180. Mizrahi A, London RD, Gribetz D: Neonatal hypocalcemia: Its causes and treatment. N Engl J Med 1968;278:1163–1165.

181. Tsang RC, Donovan EF, Steichen JJ: Calcium physiology and pathology in the neonate. Pediatr Clin North Am 1976;23:611–626.

182. Chin TK, Friedman WF, Klitzner TS: Developmental changes in cardiac myocyte calcium regulation. Circ Res 1990;67:574–579.

183. Coté CJ, Drop LJ, Hoaglin DC, et al: Ionized hypocalcemia after fresh frozen plasma administration to thermally injured children: Effects of infusion rate, duration, and treatment with calcium chloride. Anesth Analg 1988;67:152–160.

184. Coté CJ, Drop LJ, Daniels AL, et al: Calcium chloride versus calcium gluconate: Comparison of ionization and cardiovascular effects in children and dogs. Anesthesiology 1987;66:465–470.

185. Nijhawan N, Nicolosi AC, Montgomery MW, et al: Levosimendam enhances cardiac performance after cardiopulmonary bypass: A prospective, randomized placebo-controlled trial. J Cardiovasc Pharmacol 1999;34:219–228.

186. Ponce FE, Williams LC, Webb HM, et al: Propranolol palliation of tetralogy of Fallot: experience with long-term drug treatment in pediatric patients. Pediatrics 1973;52:100–108.

187. Kaplan JA: Dupont critical care lecture: Role of ultrashort-acting β-blockers in the perioperative period. J Cardiothor Anaesth 1988;2:683–691.

188. Nussbaum J, Zane EA, Thys DM: Esmolol for the treatment of hypercyanotic spells in infants with tetralogy of Fallot. J Cardiothorac Anesth 1989;3:200–202.

189. Trippel DL, Wiest DB, Gillette PC: Cardiovascular and antiarrhythmic effects of esmolol in children. J Pediatr 1991;119:142–147.

190. Bojar RM, Weiner B, Cleveland RJ: Intravenous labetalol for the control of hypertension following repair of coarctation of the aorta. Clin Cardiol 1988;11:639–641.

191. Jones SE: Coarctation in children: Controlled hypotension using labetalol and halothane. Anaesthesia 1979;34:1052–1055.

192. Przybylo HJ, Stevenson GW, Schanbacher P, et al: Sodium nitroprusside metabolism in children during hypothermic cardiopulmonary bypass. Anesth Analg 1995;81:952–956.

193. Beekman RH, Rocchini AP, Dick M, et al: Vasodilator therapy in children: Acute and chronic effects in children with left ventricular dysfunction or mitral regurgitation. Pediatrics 1984;73:43–51.

194. Miller DC, Stinson EB, Oyer PE, et al: Postoperative enhancement of left ventricular performance by combined inotropic-vasodilator therapy with preload control. Surgery 1980;88:108–117.

195. Brent BN, Berger HJ, Matthay RA, et al: Contrasting acute effects of vasodilators (nitroglycerin, nitroprusside, and hydralazine) on right ventricular performance in patients with chronic obstructive pulmonary disease and pulmonary hypertension: A combined radionuclide-hemodynamic study. Am J Cardiol 1983;51:1682–1689.

196. Knapp E, Gmeiner R: Reduction of pulmonary hypertension by nitroprusside. Int J Clin Pharmacol Biopharm 1977;15:75–80.

197. Rich S, Brundage BH, Levy PS: The effect of vasodilator therapy on the clinical outcome of patients with primary pulmonary hypertension. Circulation 1985;71:1191–1196.

198. Davies DW, Kadar D, Steward DJ, et al: A sudden death associated with the use of sodium nitroprusside for induction of hypotension during anaesthesia. Can Anaesth Soc J 1975;22:547–552.

199. Davies DW, Greiss L, Kadar D, et al: Sodium nitroprusside in children: Observations on metabolism during normal and abnormal responses. Can Anaesth Soc J 1975;22:553–560.

200. Kuipers JR, Sidi D, Heymann MA, et al: Effects of nitroprusside on cardiac function, blood flow distribution, and oxygen consumption in the conscious young lamb. Pediatr Res 1984;18:618–626.

201. Franke N, Endrich B, Messmer K: Changes in microcirculation by the administration of sodium nitroprusside and nitroglycerin. [in German]. Schweiz Med Wochenschr 1981;111:1017–1020.

202. Hauss J, Schonleben K, Spiegel HU, et al: Nitroprusside- and nitroglycerin-induced hypotension: Effects on hemodynamics and on the microcirculation. World J Surg 1982;6:241–250.

203. Coriat P, Richer C, Douraki T, et al: Influence of chronic angiotensin-converting enzyme inhibition on anesthetic induction. Anesthesiology 1994;81:299–307.

204. Woodside J Jr, Garner L, Bedford RF, et al: Captopril reduces the dose requirement for sodium nitroprusside induced hypotension. Anesthesiology 1984;60:413–417.

205. Chatterjee K, Parmley WW, Cohn JN, et al: A cooperative multicenter study of captopril in congestive heart failure: Hemodynamic effects and long-term response. Am Heart J 1985;110:439–447.

206. Beekman RH, Rocchini AP, Rosenthal A: Hemodynamic effects of hydralazine in infants with a large ventricular septal defect. Circulation 1982;65:523–528.

207. Artman M, Parrish MD, Boerth RC, et al: Hemodynamic effects of acute hydralazine in infants with atrioventricular canal defects. Circulation 1982;66(suppl II):II112.

208. Freed MD, Heymann MA, Lewis AB, et al: Prostaglandin E₁ in infants with ductus arteriosus–dependent congenital heart disease. Circulation 1981;64:899–905.

209. Lewis AB, Freed MD, Heymann MA, et al: Side effects of therapy with prostaglandin E₁ in infants with critical congenital heart disease. Circulation 1981;64:893–898.

210. Fonger JD, Borkon AM, Baumgartner WA, et al: Acute right ventricular failure following heart transplantation: Improvement with prostaglandin E₁ and right ventricular assist. J Heart Transplant 1986;5:317–321.

211. Szczeklik J, Dubiel JS, Mysik M, et al: Effects of prostaglandin E₁ on pulmonary circulation in patients with pulmonary hypertension. Br Heart J 1978;40:1397–1401.

212. Watkins WD, Peterson MB, Crone RK, et al: Prostacyclin and prostaglandin E₁ for severe idiopathic pulmonary artery hypertension. Lancet 1980;1:1083.

213. Roberts JD Jr, Chen TY, Kawai N, et al: Inhaled nitric oxide reverses pulmonary vasoconstriction in the hypoxic and acidotic newborn lamb. Circ Res 1993;72:246–254.

214. Frostell C, Fratacci MD, Wain JC, et al: Inhaled nitric oxide: A selective pulmonary vasodilator reversing hypoxic pulmonary vasoconstriction. Circulation 1991;83:2038–2047.

215. Miller OI, Celermajer DS, Deanfield JE, et al: Very-low-dose inhaled nitric oxide: A selective pulmonary vasodilator after operations for congenital heart disease. J Thorac Cardiovasc Surg 1994;108:487–494.

216. Roberts JD Jr, Lang P, Bigatello LM, et al: Inhaled nitric oxide in congenital heart disease. Circulation 1993;87:447–453.

217. Adatia I, Perry S, Landzberg M, et al: Inhaled nitric oxide and hemodynamic evaluation of patients with pulmonary hypertension before transplantation. J Am Coll Cardiol 1995;25:1656–1664.

218. Journois D, Pouard P, Mauriat P, et al: Inhaled nitric oxide as a therapy for pulmonary hypertension after operations for congenital heart defects. J Thorac Cardiovasc Surg 1994;107:1129–1135.

219. Bush A, Busst C, Knight WB, et al: Modification of pulmonary hypertension secondary to congenital heart disease by prostacyclin therapy. Am Rev Respir Dis 1987;136:767–769.

220. Bush A, Busst CM, Knight WB, et al: Comparison of the haemodynamic effects of epoprostenol (prostacyclin) and tolazoline. Br Heart J 1988;60:141–148.

221. Wax D, Garofano R, Barst RJ: Effects of long-term infusion of prostacyclin on exercise performance in patients with primary pulmonary hypertension. Chest 1999;116:914–920.

222. Curling PE, Zaidan JR, Murphy DA, et al: Treatment of pulmonary hypertension after human orthotopic heart transplantation. Anesth Analg 2000;66:S37.

223. Bush A, Busst C, Booth K, et al: Does prostacyclin enhance the selective pulmonary vasodilator effect of oxygen in children with congenital heart disease? Circulation 1986;74:135–144.

224. Pappert D, Busch T, Gerlach H, et al: Aerosolized prostacyclin versus inhaled nitric oxide in children with severe acute respiratory distress syndrome. Anesthesiology 1995;82:1507–1511.

225. Zwissler B, Rank N, Jaenicke U, et al: Selective pulmonary vasodilation by inhaled prostacyclin in a newborn with congenital heart disease and cardiopulmonary bypass. Anesthesiology 1995;82:1512–1516.

226. Klitzner TS, Friedman WF: Cardiac arrhythmias: The role of pharmacologic intervention. Cardiol Clin 1989;7:299–318.

227. Fish FA, Gillette PC, Benson DW Jr: Proarrhythmia, cardiac arrest and death in young patients receiving encainide and flecainide. The Pediatric Electrophysiology Group. J Am Coll Cardiol 1991;18:356–365.

228. Perry JC, McQuinn RL, Smith RT Jr, et al: Flecainide acetate for resistant arrhythmias in the young: Efficacy and pharmacokinetics. J Am Coll Cardiol 1989;14:185–191.

229. Perry JC, Garson A Jr: Encainide and flecainide in children: Separating the wheat from the chaff. J Am Coll Cardiol 1991;18:366–367.

230. Wren C, Campbell RW: The response of paediatric arrhythmias to intravenous and oral flecainide. Br Heart J 1987;57:171–175.

231. Garson A Jr, Moak JP, Smith RT Jr, et al: Usefulness of intravenous propafenone for control of postoperative junctional ectopic tachycardia. Am J Cardiol 1987;59:1422–1424.

232. Janousek J, Paul T, Reimer A, et al: Usefulness of propafenone for supraventricular arrhythmias in infants and children. Am J Cardiol 1993;72:294–300.

233. Shand DG, Sell CG, Oates JA: Hypertrophic obstructive cardiomyopathy in an infant-propranolol therapy for three years. N Engl J Med 1971;285:843–844.

234. Trippel DL, Gillette PC: Atenolol in children with ventricular arrhythmias. Am Heart J 1990;119:1312–1316.

235. Trippel DL, Gillette PC: Atenolol in children with supraventricular tachycardia. Am J Cardiol 1989;64:233–236.

236. Figa FH, Gow RM, Hamilton RM, et al: Clinical efficacy and safety of intravenous amiodarone in infants and children. Am J Cardiol 1994;74:573–577.

237. Garson A Jr, Gillette PC, McVey P, et al: Amiodarone treatment of critical arrhythmias in children and young adults. J Am Coll Cardiol 1984;4:749–755.

238. Perry JC, Knilans TK, Marlow D, et al: Intravenous amiodarone for life-threatening tachyarrhythmias in children and young adults. J Am Coll Cardiol 1993;22:95–98.

239. Perry JC, Fenrich AL, Hulse JE, et al: Pediatric use of intravenous amiodarone: Efficacy and safety in critically ill patients from a multicenter protocol. J Am Coll Cardiol 1999;27:1246–1250.

240. Rady MY, Ryan T, Starr NJ: Preoperative therapy with amiodarone and the incidence of acute organ dysfunction after cardiac surgery. Anesth Analg 1997;85:489–497.

241. Koch-Weser J: Drug therapy: Bretylium. N Engl J Med 1979;300:473–477.

242. Ellenbogen KA, Stambler BS, Wood MA, et al: Efficacy of intravenous ibutilide for rapid termination of atrial fibrillation and atrial flutter: A dose-response study. J Am Coll Cardiol 1996;28:130–136.

243. Murray KT: Ibutilide. Circulation 1998;97:493–497.

244. Singh BN, Ellrodt G, Peter CT: Verapamil: A review of its pharmacological properties and therapeutic use. Drugs 1978;15:169–197.

245. Epstein ML, Kiel EA, Victoria BE: Cardiac decompensation following verapamil therapy in infants with supraventricular tachycardia. Pediatrics 1985;75:737–740.

246. Greco R, Musto B, Arienzo V, et al: Treatment of paroxysmal supraventricular tachycardia in infancy with digitalis, adenosine-5′-triphosphate, and verapamil: A comparative study. Circulation 1982;66:504–508.

247. Soler-Soler J, Sagrista-Sauleda J, Cabrera A, et al: Effect of verapamil in infants with paroxysmal supraventricular tachycardia. Circulation 1979;59:876–879.

248. Spicer RL, Rocchini AP, Crowley DC, et al: Hemodynamic effects of verapamil in children and adolescents with hypertrophic cardiomyopathy. Circulation 1983;67:413–420.

249. Reves JG, Kissin I, Lell WA, et al: Calcium entry blockers: Uses and implications for anesthesiologists. Anesthesiology 1982;57:504–518.

250. Schulte-Sasse U, Hess W, Markschies-Hornung A, et al: Combined effects of halothane anesthesia and verapamil on systemic hemodynamics and left ventricular myocardial contractility in patients with ischemic heart disease. Anesth Analg 1984;63:791–798.

251. Hariman RJ, Mangiardi LM, McAllister RGJ, et al: Reversal of the cardiovascular effects of verapamil by calcium and sodium: Differences between electrophysiologic and hemodynamic responses. Circulation 1979;59:797–804.

252. Hattori VT, Mandel WJ, Peter D: Calcium for myocardial depression from verapamil. N Engl J Med 1982;306:238.

253. Overholt ED, Rheuban KS, Gutgesell HP, et al: Usefulness of adenosine for arrhythmias in infants and children. Am J Cardiol 1988;61:336–340.

254. Till J, Shinebourne EA, Rigby ML, et al: Efficacy and safety of adenosine in the treatment of supraventricular tachycardia in infants and children. Br Heart J 1989;62:204–211.

255. Byrum CJ, Wahl RA, Behrendt DM, et al: Ventricular fibrillation associated with use of digitalis in a newborn infant with Wolff-Parkinson-White syndrome. J Pediatr 1982;101:400–403.

256. Wellens HJ, Durrer D: Effect of digitalis on atrioventricular conduction and circus-movement tachycardias in patients with Wolff-Parkinson-White syndrome. Circulation 1973;47:1229–1233.

257. Kleinman CS, Copel JA, Weinstein EM, et al: In utero diagnosis and treatment of fetal supraventricular tachycardia. Semin Perinatol 1985;9:113–129.

258. Johnson GL, Desai NS, Pauly TH, et al: Complications associated with digoxin therapy in low-birth-weight infants. Pediatrics 1982;69:463–465.

259. Pinsky WW, Jacobsen JR, Gillette PC, et al: Dosage of digoxin in premature infants. J Pediatr 1979;94:639–642.

260. Wettrell G, Andersson KE: Clinical pharmacokinetics of digoxin in infants. Clin Pharmacokinet 1977;2:17–31.

261. Kugler JD, Danford DA, Deal BJ, et al: Radiofrequency catheter ablation for tachyarrhythmias in children and adolescents. The Pediatric Electrophysiology Society. N Engl J Med 1994;330:1481–1487.

262. Lavoie J, Walsh EP, Burrows FA, et al: Effects of propofol or isoflurane anesthesia on cardiac conduction in children undergoing radiofrequency catheter ablation for tachydysrhythmias. Anesthesiology 1995; 82:884–887.

263. Sharpe MD, Cuillerier DJ, Lee JK, et al: Sevoflurane has no effect on sinoatrial node function or on normal atrioventricular and accessory pathway conduction in Wolff-Parkinson-White syndrome during alfentanil/midazolam anesthesia. Anesthesiology 1999;90:60–65.

264. Sharpe MD, Dobkowski WB, Murkin JM, et al: The electrophysiologic effects of volatile anesthetics and sufentanil on the normal atrioventricular conduction system and accessory pathways in Wolff-Parkinson-White syndrome. Anesthesiology 1994;80:63–70.

265. Sharpe MD, Dobkowski WB, Murkin JM, et al: Propofol has no direct effect on sinoatrial node function or on normal atrioventricular and accessory pathway conduction in Wolff-Parkinson-White syndrome during alfentanil/midazolam anesthesia. Anesthesiology 1995;82:888–895.

266. Karl TR: Extracorporeal circulatory support in infants and children. Semin Thorac Cardiovasc Surg 1994;6:154–160.

267. Pennington DG, Swartz MT: Circulatory support in infants and children. Ann Thorac Surg 1993;55:233–237.

268. del Nido PJ, Duncan BW, Mayer JE Jr, et al: Left ventricular assist device improves survival in children with left ventricular dysfunction after repair of anomalous origin of the left coronary artery from the pulmonary artery. Ann Thorac Surg 1999;67:169–172.

269. Karl TR, Sano S, Horton S, et al: Centrifugal pump left heart assist in pediatric cardiac operations: Indication, technique, and results. J Thorac Cardiovasc Surg 1991;102:624–630.

270. Konertz W: Mechanical circulatory assist in pediatric patients. Int J Artif Organs 1997;20:681–683.

271. Loebe M, Muller J, Hetzer R: Ventricular assistance for recovery of cardiac failure. Curr Opin Cardiol 1999;14:234–248.

272. Sidiropoulos A, Hotz H, Konertz W: Pediatric circulatory support. J Heart Lung Transplant 1998;17:1172–1176.

273. Delius RE, Zwischenberger JB, Cilley R, et al: Prolonged extracorporeal life support of pediatric and adolescent cardiac transplant patients. Ann Thorac Surg 1990;50:791–795.

274. Duncan BW, Hraska V, Jonas RA, et al: Mechanical circulatory support in children with cardiac disease. J Thorac Cardiovasc Surg 1999;117:529–542.

275. Duncan BW, Ibrahim AE, Hraska V, et al: Use of rapid-deployment extracorporeal membrane oxygenation for the resuscitation of pediatric patients with heart disease after cardiac arrest. J Thorac Cardiovasc Surg 1998;116:305–311.

276. Kanter KR, Pennington G, Weber TR, et al: Extracorporeal membrane oxygenation for postoperative cardiac support in children. J Thorac Cardiovasc Surg 1987;93:27–35.

277. Pennington DG, McBride LR, Kanter KR, et al: Bridging to heart transplantation with circulatory support devices. J Heart Transplant 1989;8:116–123.

278. Pennington DG, Swartz MT: Mechanical circulatory support prior to cardiac transplantation. Semin Thorac Cardiovasc Surg 1990;2:125–134.

279. del Nido PJ, Dalton HJ, Thompson AE, et al: Extracorporeal membrane oxygenator rescue in children during cardiac arrest after cardiac surgery. Circulation 1992;86:II300–II304.

280. Michels VV, Moll PP, Miller FA, et al: The frequency of familial dilated cardiomyopathy in a series of patients with idiopathic dilated cardiomyopathy. N Engl J Med 1992;326:77–82.

281. Matitiau A, Perez-Atayde A, Sanders SP, et al: Infantile dilated cardiomyopathy: Relation of outcome to left ventricular mechanics, hemodynamics, and histology at the time of presentation. Circulation 1994;90:1310–1318.

282. Chen SC, Nouri S, Balfour I, et al: Clinical profile of congestive cardiomyopathy in children. J Am Coll Cardiol 1990;15:189–193.

283. Griffin ML, Hernandez A, Martin TC, et al: Dilated cardiomyopathy in infants and children. J Am Coll Cardiol 1988;11:139–144.

284. McQuillan PJ, Morgan BA, Ramwell J: Adriamycin cardiomyopathy: Fatal outcome of general anaesthesia in a child with adriamycin cardiomyopathy. Anaesthesia 1988;43:301–304.

285. Unverferth DV, Magorien RD, Leier CV, et al: Doxorubicin toxicity. Cancer Treat Rev 1982;9:149–164.

286. Lipshultz SE, Lipsitz SR, Mone SM, et al: Female sex and drug dose as risk factors for late cardiotoxic effects of doxorubicin therapy for childhood cancer. N Engl J Med 1995;332:1738–1743.

287. Lipshultz SE, Colan SD, Gelber RD, et al: Late cardiac effects of doxorubicin therapy for acute lymphoblastic leukemia in childhood. N Engl J Med 1991;324:808–815.

288. Borgeat A, Chiolero R, Baylon P, et al: Perioperative cardiovascular collapse in a patient previously treated with doxorubicin. Anesth Analg 1988;67:1189–1191.

289. Burrows FA, Hickey PR, Colan S: Perioperative complications in patients with anthracycline chemotherapeutic agents. Can Anaesth Soc J 1985;32:149–157.

290. Caviale P, McClellan EL: Adriamycin toxicity: Effects in subsequent anesthesia and surgery. J Kansas Med Soc 1981;82:553–554.

291. Waterman PM, Bjerke R: Rapid-sequence induction technique in patients with severe ventricular dysfunction. J Cardiothor Anaesth 1988;2:602–606.

292. Reves JG, Kissin I, Fournier SE, et al: Additive negative inotropic effect of a combination of diazepam and fentanyl. Anesth Analg 1984;63:97–100.

293. Burtin P, Daoud P, Jacqz-Aigrain E, et al: Hypotension with midazolam and fentanyl in the newborn. Lancet 1991;337:1545–1546.

294. Gutzke GE, Shah KB, Glisson SN, et al: Cardiac transplantation: A prospective comparison of ketamine and sufentanil for anesthetic induction. J Cardiothorac Anesth 1989;3:389–395.

295. Berman W Jr, Fripp RR, Rubler M, et al: Hemodynamic effects of ketamine in children undergoing cardiac catheterization. Pediatr Cardiol 1990;11:72–76.

296. Maron BJ, Roberts WC, Epstein SE: Sudden death in hypertrophic cardiomyopathy: A profile of 78 patients. Circulation 1982;65:1388–1394.

297. Maron BJ, Tajik AJ, Ruttenberg HD, et al: Hypertrophic cardiomyopathy in infants: Clinical features and natural history. Circulation 1982;65:7–17.

298. Maron BJ, Bonow RO, Cannon RO III, et al: Hypertrophic cardiomyopathy: Interrelations of clinical manifestations, pathophysiology, and therapy (1). N Engl J Med 1987;316:780–789.

299. McKenna W, Deanfield J, Faruqui A, et al: Prognosis in hypertrophic cardiomyopathy: Role of age and clinical, electrocardiographic and hemodynamic features. Am J Cardiol 1981;47:532–538.

300. Fighali S, Krajcer Z, Leachman RD: Septal myomectomy and mitral valve replacement for idiopathic hypertrophic subaortic stenosis: Short- and long-term follow-up. J Am Coll Cardiol 1984;3:1127–1134.

301. Wigle ED, Sasson Z, Henderson MA, et al: Hypertrophic cardiomyopathy. The importance of the site and the extent of hypertrophy. A review. Prog Cardiovasc Dis 1985;28:1–83.

302. Nissenkorn A, Zeharia A, Lev D, et al: Multiple presentation of mitochondrial disorders. Arch Dis Child 1999;81:209–214.

303. Zeviani M, Tiranti V, Piantadosi C: Mitochondrial disorders. Medicine (Baltimore) 1998;77:59–72.

304. Casta A, Quackenbush EJ, Houck CS, et al: Perioperative white matter degeneration and death in a patient with a defect in mitochondrial oxidative phosphorylation. Anesthesiology 1997;87:420–425.

305. Kayser EB, Morgan PG, Sedensky MM: GAS-1: A mitochondrial protein controls sensitivity to volatile anesthetics in the nematode Caenorhabditis ellegans. Anesthesiology 1999;90:545–554.

18 Anesthesia for Children Undergoing Heart Surgery

Robert W. Reid, Frederick A. Burrows, *and* Paul R. Hickey

Preanesthetic Evaluation
  History
  Physical Examination
  Laboratory Evaluation
Specific Perioperative Challenges in Pediatric Cardiac Anesthesia
  Cyanosis
  Intracardiac Shunting
  Impaired Hemostasis
Anesthetic Management
  Planning
  Premedication
  Monitoring
  Induction of Anesthesia
  Maintenance of Anesthesia
  Control of Systemic and Pulmonary Vascular Resistance During Anesthesia
Choice of Anesthetic Agents
  Inhalation Agents
  Intramuscular and Intravenous Anesthetics
  Muscle Relaxants
Management of Cardiopulmonary Bypass
  Separation from Cardiopulmonary Bypass
Managing Impaired Hemostasis Following Separation from Bypass
  Conventional Replacement Strategies
  Effect of Hemofiltration and Modified Ultrafiltration upon Hemostasis
  Antifibrinolytic Therapy
Stress Response to Cardiac Surgery
Anesthetic Considerations in Specific Cardiac Defects
  Atrial Septal Defect
  Ventricular Septal Defect
  Tetralogy of Fallot
  Coarctation of the Aorta
  Patent Ductus Arteriosus
Principles of Postoperative Cardiac Care
Anesthesia for Cardiac Catheterization
  General Considerations
  Patient Management
  Postcatheterization Management
Outcome of Anesthesia in Children with Heart Disease

Each year, 30,000 infants are born with congenital heart disease in the United States. Advances in surgical technique and perioperative management have allowed earlier definitive repair to be performed. One half of these infants will undergo surgery during their first year of life.[1] The perioperative management of children with complex cardiac defects requires a dedicated team of anesthesiologists, cardiologists, intensivists, surgeons, perfusionists, and nurses. Anesthesiologists caring for these patients are challenged by some of the greatest physiologic aberrations encountered in clinical medicine. The most important consideration when anesthetizing children with heart disease is the necessity for individualized care. Every congenital heart defect is polymorphic and may be clinically manifest across a broad clinical spectrum. For example, a child with tetralogy of Fallot may present with severe cyanosis and congestive failure in the first months of life or may exhibit virtually normal growth and few symptoms during childhood. "Cookbook" approaches to the care of children with heart disease are fraught with inaccuracy. The anesthetic management of these infants and children is based on the principles of pediatric anesthetic care outlined in previous chapters of this text, as well as on the physiologic and pharmacologic considerations of the pediatric cardiovascular system as described in Chapter 17.

Preanesthetic Evaluation

History

Evaluation before surgery is based on the classic triad of history, physical examination, and laboratory investigation. Specific areas in the history must be explored in detail. Cyanosis, whether intermittent or continuous, as well as squatting, sweating, and syncope all are important cardiac symptoms and signs useful in evaluating clinical status. Exercise and feeding intolerance, tachypnea, and failure to thrive early in life are major manifestations of congestive heart failure in young children.

Because children are medically treated with beta-blockers, calcium channel blockers, digoxin, and diuretics, past and current cardiac medications are important aspects of the history. Past episodes of congestive heart failure requiring hospitalization must be carefully reviewed, as must any major systemic disease. Previous surgical procedures and the anesthesia records should be reviewed in detail. If cardiac surgical procedures have been previously performed, evidence for residual cardiac dysfunction and rhythm disturbance must be carefully sought out. Associated cardiac and non-cardiac anomalies and their status must be precisely defined.

Physical Examination

Much useful information is gained by physical examination, although specific anatomic diagnoses of congenital heart disease may be difficult to make by physical examination alone. Evaluation of respiratory rate and pattern, including associated signs of respiratory distress such as nasal flaring, retractions, and grunting, is helpful in assessing cardiac function and providing a baseline for the judgment of adequacy of ventilation before postoperative extubation.

Pulses and their quality in all extremities provide clinical evidence of coarctation or previous sacrifice of a subclavian artery (e.g., Blalock-Taussig shunt or coarctation repair). When coupled with pulse pressure, palpation of the pulses may reveal aortic incompetence or patent ductus arteriosus (PDA). Respiratory variations in pulse pressure may indicate hypovolemia or cardiac tamponade.

The general activity level, oxygen saturation, presence of cyanosis at rest or during crying, nutritional status, height and weight percentile, pedal temperature, presence of hepatomegaly or splenomegaly, and fullness of the anterior fontanelle all give the clinician useful information about a child's circulatory status and cardiovascular reserve. The presence of scars on the chest from previous procedures should be noted. In addition to these observations, the preanesthetic examination includes examination of the airway and venous access, as well as assessment of the patients' behavior and their relationship with their parents.

Laboratory Evaluation

Laboratory data, including echocardiography and cardiac catheterization, are important for understanding the cardiac pathophysiology. Electrolyte disturbances secondary to chronic diuretic therapy or renal dysfunction should be sought. Hematologic evaluation should include hemoglobin determination and screening coagulation tests. The hemoglobin level is often the best indicator of right-to-left shunting magnitude and chronicity. Children with cyanotic heart defects should have an arterial blood gas measurement and pulse oximetry measurement to determine the baseline oxygenation and ventilation status. The electrocardiogram should be reviewed for the presence of underlying conduction disturbances, ventricular hypertrophy or strain pattern, and myocardial ischemia. The chest radiograph will provide useful information regarding the cardiac size, pulmonary vascular congestion, airway distortion, atelectasis, and possible pulmonary infection. Absence of a thymic shadow may suggest the presence of DiGeorge syndrome and the need for special blood product preparation. The lateral film should be carefully examined in children who have undergone prior cardiac surgery, and the position of major vessels in relationship to the sternum should be noted. A pulmonary homograft or aorta that is immediately adherent to the sternum will alert the surgeon and anesthesiologist to the potential for disaster during sternotomy and may suggest the need for presternotomy cannulation of femoral vessels.

Cardiac catheterization data must be carefully evaluated for right- and left-sided pressures, the site and magnitude of shunting, pressure gradients indicating obstructive lesions, evidence of regurgitant lesions, systemic oxyhemoglobin saturation, and myocardial function. The response of the pulmonary vasculature to 100% inspired oxygen during catheterization is important, especially in patients with pulmonary hypertension. Decreases in pulmonary artery pressure with 100% oxygen indicate that the pulmonary vasculature is reactive and that pulmonary vascular obstructive disease, if present, is potentially reversible. Pressure measurements must be evaluated in the context of flow. In cases in which pulmonary flow is several times the systemic flow despite pulmonary hypertension of more than half the systemic pressure level, pulmonary hypertension is unlikely to persist after repair of a defect through which significant left-to-right shunt is occurring. When normal levels of pulmonary flow are restored, pulmonary pressures generally return to normal. Pressure gradients are dependent on cardiac output. For instance, in coarctation of the aorta, a small pressure gradient is misleading if cardiac output is low at the time of measurement, and the apparent degree of coarctation and obstruction will be underestimated.

Although catheterization data are important, they may be misleading in a patient who is heavily sedated, anesthetized, or receiving supplemental oxygen during the catheterization study. Furthermore, these data may be months old, thus bearing little relation to the current clinical status in the rapidly changing cardiovascular system of a child. Raw data obtained during a catheterization are subject to different interpretations. Wide variations in calculated shunts, pulmonary-to-systemic flow ratios, and vascular resistance are possible, depending on how the raw data are manipulated. For these reasons, catheterization data require careful interpretation and integration with the clinical picture. Catheterization data that do not fit the current clinical status of a child should be critically viewed.

Developments in two-dimensional echocardiography and Doppler flow mapping have proven valuable in the evaluation of congenital cardiac lesions. In many defects, effective echocardiography supplants the need for cardiac catheterization. Echocardiography may provide critical information regarding the configuration and size of cardiac chambers, presence of septal defects and shunts, patency of the ductus arteriosus, orientation and function of cardiac valves, and assessment of ventricular function. Although transthoracic imaging is generally acceptable, certain defects, including valve abnormalities, are more readily imaged via transesophageal approach. The cardiac anesthesiologist may be consulted to provide sedation or anesthesia during transesophageal echocardiography or cardiac catheterization.

Specific Perioperative Challenges in Pediatric Cardiac Anesthesia

Cyanosis

Children with cyanotic cardiac defects compensate for chronic hypoxia with increased erythropoiesis, increased circulating blood volume, vasodilation, and metabolic adjustments of factors such as circulating 2,3-diphosphoglycerate. These physiologic adjustments allow greater tissue delivery of oxygen. The increase in blood viscosity with polycythemia leads to increased vascular resistance and sludging, which have resulted in renal, pulmonary, and cerebral thromboses, especially in dehydrated children.[2] Long periods without oral intake both preoperatively and postoperatively should therefore be avoided in children with hematocrits greater than 50%, unless adequate intravenous hydration is provided.

Pulmonary vascular resistance (PVR) increases more than systemic vascular resistance (SVR) as the hematocrit rises, further decreasing pulmonary blood flow in patients who already have compromised pulmonary circulation.[3, 4] Coagulopathies are common in children with cyanotic congenital heart disease and may influence surgical hemostasis.[5-7] When the hematocrit is greater than 65%, excessive viscosity impairs microvascular perfusion and outweighs the advantages of increased oxygen-carrying capacity. Reduction of red blood cell volume has been shown to correct the coagulopa-

thy and also to improve hemodynamics when hematocrit elevations are extreme.[8]

Intracardiac Shunting

In congenital heart disease, much of the pathophysiology involves communications between chambers or vessels that are normally separate, resulting in shunting of blood between ventricles, atria, the great arteries, or a combination of these, depending on the nature of the lesion. Management of shunting is a major consideration during anesthesia and requires an understanding of the factors that control shunting.

Dependent and Obligatory Shunts

Rudolph's distinction between dependent and obligatory shunting is very useful for understanding control of intracardiac shunting (Table 18–1).[9] Dependent shunts are those in which size and direction of shunting through abnormal cardiac communications depend on the relationship between PVR and SVR and are thus variable. Dependent shunting occurs between two structures having pressures that are nearly equal or at least having the same order of magnitude. Dependent shunts include PDA, simple atrial or ventricular septal defects (ASD or VSD), aortopulmonary windows, and other systemic-to-pulmonary shunts, such as a Blalock-Taussig shunt.

In contrast, obligatory shunts are those in which shunting is relatively independent of the relationship between PVR and SVR. Resistances tend to be fixed, and blood flow occurs between structures having pressures differing by an order of magnitude. Obligatory shunting occurs between the left ventricle and the right atrium in common atrioventricular canal defects and between systemic arteries and veins in peripheral arteriovenous fistulas.

Special forms of obligatory shunts occur in complex heart disease when partial or complete obstruction to blood flow occurs along with communications between chambers. In

Table 18–1. Types of Intracardiac Shunts

Type	Hemodynamic Characteristics	Magnitude and Control	Clinical Examples
Dependent shunt	Large, unrestricted shunt between two structures having pressures that are nearly equal	Variable shunting that is dependent on the balance between PVR and SVR (more subject to control)	Large ASD, VSD, or PDA; aortopulmonary windows; systemic-to-pulmonary arterial shunt (e.g., Blalock-Taussig shunt)
Obligatory shunt	Large, unrestricted shunt between two structures having pressures that differ by an order of magnitude	Relatively fixed, high-volume shunting that is independent of PVR and SVR (less subject to control)	Left ventricle to right atrium in complete atrioventricular canal; peripheral arteriovenous fistula
Restrictive shunt	Small, restrictive shunt between two structures without regard to pressure difference	Relatively fixed, low to moderate volume shunting that is independent of PVR and SVR (less subject to control)	Small, minimally significant ASD, VSD, or PDA; VSD with pulmonic stenosis or coarctation; tetralogy of Fallot with pulmonary atresia

ASD, atrial septal defect; PDA, patent ductus arteriosus; PVR, pulmonary vascular resistance; SVR, systemic vascular resistance; VSD, ventricular septal defect.

tricuspid or mitral atresia, obligatory shunting occurs between the atria because there is no atrial outlet on the side of the atresia. In aortic or pulmonary atresia, likewise, obligatory shunting occurs between either the atria or the ventricles because there is no ventricular outlet. Although these special types of obligatory shunts are independent of vascular resistances, they can only occur simultaneously with a dependent type of shunt at another level; such an example is a PDA, which provides either pulmonary blood flow in pulmonary atresia or systemic flow in aortic atresia.

When partially obstructive lesions occur simultaneously with communications between chambers, as in pulmonary stenosis with PDA or tetralogy of Fallot, the distinctions between the two types of shunts blur. Similarly, when the pressure differential on two sides of a dependent shunt becomes very great, it takes on the characteristics of an obligatory shunt. However, except in the most complex forms of congenital heart disease, knowledge of the distinctions between various types of shunting described earlier is sufficient when anesthetizing most children with congenital heart disease. These distinctions predict how any particular stress or anesthetic manipulations will alter shunts.

Restrictive Shunts

The foregoing discussion assumes that the intracardiac and great vessel communications are relatively large and nonrestrictive. When communications are small, the size of the defect itself limits shunting, and considerations of relative PVR and SVR become correspondingly smaller in determining the amount of shunting. Whenever there is a large pressure differential at the same level of the circulation on either side of a communication, the communication is restrictive; flow is limited across the defect, and other factors determining shunt flow become less important. This is usually the situation in children with mild heart disease that is asymptomatic or minimally symptomatic, such as small ASDs and VSDs or a small PDA.

Dependent Shunting During Anesthesia

In children with dependent shunts, the direction and amount of intracardiac shunting are determined by the circulatory dynamics. Control of circulatory dynamics to minimize the shunt is one major goal of anesthetic management. Because shunting in these children is dependent on the relationship between SVR and PVR, anesthetic management often revolves around control of relative vascular resistances.

In children with dependent right-to-left shunts, decreases in SVR or increases in PVR increase the shunt. In children with dependent left-to-right shunts, increases in SVR and decreases in PVR increase the shunt. In children with bidirectional or balanced shunting, any change in either vascular resistance increases the net shunt away from the side with elevated vascular resistance.

For practical purposes, acute increases in left-to-right shunts during anesthesia are of clinical importance in a number of situations. A substantial "steal" of systemic blood flow by the pulmonary circulation can occur whenever there is parallel circulation, for example, in atrioventricular

canal, truncus arteriosus, and hypoplastic left heart syndrome.[10]

Left-to-right shunting is generally well tolerated, except when pulmonary steal leads to systemic hypotension and resultant insufficient coronary perfusion. Shunting from right to left, because it is accompanied by at least some degree of arterial oxygen desaturation, is relatively poorly tolerated and is much more frequently a problem during anesthesia.

Impaired Hemostasis

The combination of immature coagulation factor synthesis and dramatic hemodilution during bypass leads to impaired hemostasis following bypass in infants and children. At birth, the levels of vitamin K–dependent coagulation factors in healthy term-infants are only 40 to 66% of adult values. During the first month of life, these levels increase to 53 to 90% of adult values.[11] However, children with congenital heart defects, especially those with cyanosis or systemic hypoperfusion, often continue to have depressed factor levels secondary to impaired hepatic protein synthesis. Although antithrombin III levels are also low, true heparin resistance is rare in infants because of the equal decrease in coagulation factors. At the onset of cardiopulmonary bypass, the introduction of the prime volume, which is two to three times greater than the child's blood volume, dilutes the factor levels to 50% and platelet count to 30% of pre-bypass levels. This degree of dilution occurs even when the pump circuit is primed with whole blood. Greater dilution is seen at centers, which use packed erythrocytes in the priming volume. Thus, at the conclusion of neonatal bypass, the activity of factors is often as low as one third of adult values, fibrinogen is frequently below 100 mg/dL, and the platelet count is 50 to 80 $\times$ 10^9 per liter.[12] In addition to these quantitative changes, platelets undergo functional changes during bypass. Extracorporeal circulation causes a loss of platelet adhesion receptors, activation of platelets, and formation of leukocyte-platelet conjugates. Platelet adhesion receptors are more depressed in children with cyanotic versus acyanotic cardiac defects.[7] Heparin also impairs platelet function independent of cardiopulmonary bypass.[13] Lastly, cardiac surgery is associated with significant activation of the fibrinolytic system.[14] Because of this multifactorial coagulopathy, blood losses greater than one blood volume are not uncommon in neonatal patients following separation from bypass.

Anesthetic Management

Planning

After a thorough preanesthetic evaluation, the anesthesiologist should identify the most critical areas of the child's pathophysiology and determine the physiologic goals of the perioperative and postoperative periods. A cooperative team approach and open communication facilitates management of children with complex cardiac defects. The anesthesiologist should meet with the cardiologists, surgeons, and intensivists prior to surgery to discuss the management goals and potential complications, which are anticipated. Special concerns regarding the need for blood components may be discussed with the transfusion pathologist. It is important also to be mindful of questions and concerns that parents have during this preoperative period.

Children with shunting as their primary problem are categorized as those with right-to-left and those with left-to-right shunts. The concern in management of these children is to maintain adequate perfusion of both the pulmonary and systemic circulations. Defects with either large dependent shunts or complete mixing must be delicately and deliberately managed so as to maintain an appropriate balance between PVR and SVR. In these cases, one should initially try to maintain the same ventilation and oxygenation status as that present prior to induction of anesthesia. Unintended hyperventilation or excessive oxygenation may result in systemic hypoperfusion and acidosis secondary to excessive pulmonary blood flow at the expense of the systemic circulation. On the other hand, hypoventilation or hypovolemia may lead to hypoxia secondary to inadequate pulmonary blood flow. Children with restrictive shunts and inadequate pulmonary blood flow may require aggressive hyperventilation with 100% oxygen to minimize PVR and maintain adequate pulmonary blood flow. If pulmonary hypertension is present, then anesthetic management is directed at minimizing fluctuations in pulmonary artery pressure. In defects that are primarily obstructive (e.g., congenital valvular obstruction, obstruction in the great vessels, or acquired valvular obstruction) or in regurgitant lesions, the concerns of filling pressure, perfusion pressure, and heart rate become paramount. When primary myocardial dysfunction is a critical problem, avoiding myocardial depression, implementing inotropic support, and maintaining appropriate filling pressure are essential.

Premedication

Recommendations for specific premedications in pediatric patients with heart disease are legion. We generally omit premedications for infants less than 6 months of age and often prescribe little or no premedication for older, healthier children who show little anxiety and with whom good preoperative rapport can be established. In children with severe congestive heart failure or with cyanosis, heavy premedication is generally avoided. Supplemental premedication, administered under the direct supervision of the anesthesiologist in the preoperative facility, provides for a calm child and gentle separation from the parents. Oxygen, ventilation bag and mask, and pulse oximetry should be immediately available. If an intravenous line is in place, intravenous midazolam may be titrated in small increments. If intravenous access is not yet available, the oral midazolam formulation (0.75 to 1.0 mg/kg) may be administered with a small cup or with a syringe.[15] If the child is anticipated to be particularly uncooperative, ketamine 2 to 4 mg/kg in combination with oral atropine 0.02 mg/kg (to decrease the risk of secretions and laryngospasm due to the ketamine) may be mixed with the oral midazolam.[16, 17] A child who will not accept oral premedication may be premedicated with a single intramuscular injection of ketamine 1 to 2 mg/kg, midazolam 0.2 mg/kg, and glycopyrrolate 0.02 mg/kg. Unsupervised premedication of the infant or young child on the ward is avoided, as it may exacerbate the blunted ventilatory response to hypoxia that is often encountered in congenital heart disease.[18]

Monitoring

Noninvasive monitoring during pediatric cardiac surgery includes pulse oximetry, five-lead electrocardiography, an automated blood pressure cuff, a precordial or esophageal stethoscope, continuous airway manometry, real-time inspired and expired capnography, anesthetic gas and oxygen analysis, multiple-site temperature measurement, and volumetric urine collection. Because the pulse oximeter is especially vital when managing children with congenital cardiac disease, at least two probes should be placed on different limbs in the event that one should fail during the procedure. In children with cyanotic congenital heart disease, conventional pulse oximetry overestimates arterial oxygen saturation as saturation decreases.[19] This error tends to be worse with severe hypoxemia.[20] When monitoring children with shunting across the ductus arteriosus, a probe should be placed on a right hand digit to measure pre-ductal oxygenation and a second probe should be placed on a toe or foot to measure post-ductal oxygenation. Children undergoing repair of coarctation of the aorta should be monitored with a pulse oximeter on the right upper limb, as it may be the only reliable monitor during the repair; and both pre- and post-coarctation blood pressure cuffs should be placed. These two cuffs may be cycled, and the differential noted, before and after surgical correction.

Monitoring end-tidal carbon dioxide tension ($PETCO_2$) is of value in most patients. However, in children with cyanotic-shunting cardiac lesions, $PETCO_2$ measurement may be unreliable because of significant ventilation-perfusion mismatching.[21] Arterial blood gases are the most accurate measure of the adequacy of ventilation and oxygenation. To provide for rapid decision-making, it is very helpful to have the blood gas analysis machine located in or immediately near the cardiac operating room.[22]

Monitoring of ionized calcium levels in arterial blood is essential during cardiac surgery or other surgical procedures in which significant quantities of citrated blood are infused rapidly or when entire blood volumes are replaced. Neonatal patients are especially prone to disturbance of their ionized calcium level when citrated blood is infused, and those with limited cardiac reserve tolerate ionized hypocalcemia poorly because of greater sensitivity to the myocardial effects of citrate infusion.[23] The total serum calcium value by itself is misleading in this regard.

Temperature monitoring during cardiopulmonary bypass is a critical guide to adequate brain cooling and to appropriate rewarming prior to separation from bypass. Because it is not practical to measure brain temperature directly, surrogate measuring sites are utilized. The tympanic membrane, esophagus, and rectum should all be monitored. Of these sites, the esophagus most closely matches (whereas the tympanum and rectum overestimate) the true brain temperature.[24] The rectal temperature is a useful guide during the rewarming phase.

After induction of anesthesia, an arterial catheter should be placed in those patients who will undergo cardiopulmonary bypass. The radial artery may generally be percutaneously cannulated with relative ease even in infants. Prior arterial cannulation, prior placement of a Blalock-Taussig shunt, or coarctation of the aorta may interfere with accurate radial artery pressure measurements. Children with trisomy 21 may have radial anomalies that make cannulation of the radial artery challenging. The femoral artery may be easily and safely cannulated in children older than 1 month. However, in neonatal patients, femoral artery cannulation is associated with a significant rate of perfusion-related complications.[25, 26] Catheters placed in the dorsalis pedis or posterior tibial artery often provide inaccurate hemodynamic data, especially after separation from bypass, and it may even become difficult to sample blood from for laboratory testing. In the rare circumstance that peripheral arterial cannulation cannot be accomplished, the surgeon may place a catheter in the internal mammary artery after sternotomy and a sterile monitoring line may be passed over the drapes.

Central venous lines can be very useful in children with cardiac disease. For cardiac surgical procedures, there are two commonly used methods of obtaining central access; the decision of which to use may be determined in part by institutional bias. In the first method, the cardiac surgeons usually expose the heart quickly and have it available for inspection and estimation of filling pressures. Central lines can be readily established from the field and handed off to the anesthesia team. These transthoracic central lines are useful but still carry a small amount of risk.[27] The use of the second method, percutaneous insertion of central venous lines, may again reflect institutional bias, but the method is particularly indicated for long, complex procedures, especially when access to the infant is limited or the heart is not exposed. Percutaneous cannulation of the central circulation through either the internal jugular approach or the subclavian approach has been demonstrated to be safe.[28] However, it is important to appreciate that insertion of central venous lines through the internal jugular or subclavian route may fail or may be associated with pneumothorax, hemorrhage, and hematoma formation after puncture of major arteries.[28–30] Cannulation of the external jugular vein may avoid some of these serious complications when the catheter can be successfully threaded into the central circulation (59% in one study of children).[31] In children with unrestrictive ventricular or atrial septal defects, including hearts with a single ventricle or single atrium, the central venous pressure is equivalent to left ventricular filling pressure. Cannulation of vessels draining into the superior vena cava should be approached with caution in children with univentricular anatomy who may undergo the Fontan procedure, since thrombosis of the superior vena cava can be a devastating complication in these children.

In neonates and infants with persistent fetal circulation or respiratory failure and in children who have primary myocardial disease or valvular disease and otherwise normal hearts, thermodilution pulmonary arterial lines can be of great value. However, pulmonary arterial lines in children with intracardiac defects usually provide little more information than a simple central line, are difficult to insert without fluoroscopy, and may not provide meaningful measurements of cardiac output.

Contractility and cardiac output can be assessed in a number of ways without having a thermodilution catheter. If the chest is open, one may look directly at the heart to see how well it is contracting. Two-dimensional echocardiography provides more direct quantitative and qualitative information regarding ventricular filling and contractility. Arterial blood pressure is also a reliable indicator of cardiac output, as is urine output. However, there is a group of cardiac patients who have significantly elevated SVR, usually due to the use of moderate to high doses of vasopressors. These patients may have adequate arterial oxygenation and adequate arterial pressure because of the vasopressors; however, cardiac output may be low, as indicated by metabolic acidosis and low mixed venous oxygen pressure. A normal venous oxygen tension value is 40 mm Hg. Some children with congenital cardiac lesions have an arterial oxygen tension (Pao_2) only slightly higher than 40 mm Hg. However, they chronically compensate with polycythemia. A mixed venous oxygen tension of significantly less than 40 mm Hg and a progressive metabolic acidosis, despite moderate to high inotropic support, may well herald a poor outcome.

Transesophageal echocardiography (TEE) has proved very helpful during the intraoperative management of specific children undergoing cardiac surgery. Those children undergoing closure of a ventricular septal defect or repair of a cardiac valve benefit most from intraoperative TEE monitoring because adequacy of the repair may be confirmed immediately upon separating from bypass. If a significant residual defect is detected, cardiopulmonary bypass may be reinstituted and additional repair undertaken. It is generally best to insert the TEE probe shortly after endotracheal intubation and before the surgical drapes are placed. Endotracheal tube placement via the nares provides for greater stability during TEE probe manipulation. The endotracheal tube should be carefully secured and held to prevent tracheal extubation. The cardiologist may choose to perform a brief echocardiographic examination prior to onset of bypass, to confirm the preoperative evaluation and to more easily evaluate the post-repair results. Anteflexion of the probe may compress the left atrium and cause hemodynamic instability, especially in the neonatal patient. If unexplained hemodynamic deterioration occurs during TEE manipulation, the probe should be advanced into the stomach or removed from the patient. During cardiopulmonary bypass, the anesthesiologist should confirm that the echocardiographic machine has been turned off or the probe has been disconnected, because an electrically active probe may cause heating of the esophagus and surrounding tissues.

Induction of Anesthesia

An intravenous induction is preferable for children with severe cardiac defects. If a patent intravenous line is not in place on arrival at the operating room, the majority of children with *less severe* cardiac defects tolerate an inhalation induction. The most common inhalation agents used are halothane or sevoflurane in oxygen, with or without nitrous oxide. The odor of isoflurane is too pungent for a smooth inhalation induction in children. Concentrations of no greater than 50% nitrous oxide are used if a child has a cyanotic lesion. Under these circumstances, the child requires extremely close observation to ensure that cyanosis does not worsen. Pulse oximetry is particularly valuable during induction and should be the first monitor placed.

An inhalation induction should never be forced on any

patient. A child usually responds to being held in one's arms, with the mask close to his or her face (or initially using a cupped hand to channel the gases from the circuit if the mask is poorly tolerated). If a frightened child does not tolerate an inhalation induction, it is best to stop and comfort the child. After an expeditious intramuscular injection of ketamine 3 to 5 mg/kg, midazolam 0.2 to 0.3 mg/kg, and atropine 0.02 mg/kg, the child will gradually calm down and accept the mask for an inhalation induction.

It is important to allow a minute or two of inhalation of nitrous oxide and oxygen before slowly advancing the inspired concentration up to no greater than 2% for halothane or 5% for sevoflurane. The electrocardiogram should be observed closely for changes in the P wave, such as conversion to a retrograde P wave or transformation to a junctional rhythm. Such a change may indicate that the child is becoming too deeply anesthetized.

Many pediatric cardiac lesions require adequate mixing for maintenance of satisfactory oxygen saturation. Transposition of the great vessels with intact ventricular septum is a good example. If systemic pressure declines, hypoxemia will quickly follow. If hypoxemia, airway compromise, or hypotension develop, one should have a low threshold for administration of 100% oxygen and an intramuscular injection of ketamine 3 to 5 mg/kg, succinylcholine 5 mg/kg or rocuronium 1.5 to 2.0 mg/kg, and atropine 0.02 mg/kg. Maintenance of the airway is critical. Once the child is adequately anesthetized, an intravenous line and additional invasive monitoring catheters may be inserted.

Maintenance of Anesthesia

Maintenance of anesthesia in pediatric heart patients depends on the preoperative status and the response to induction. Whether inhalation agents, additional opioids, or other intravenous agents are used for maintenance depends on the tolerance of the individual patient and postoperative plans for ventilatory management. If a primary opioid-based anesthetic is chosen, additional opioid should be administered upon initiation of cardiopulmonary bypass to offset dilution from the pump prime and maintain adequate opioid plasma levels. Awareness during adult cardiac surgery has been reported when amnestic agents are not utilized. Although children may be unable to describe such events, the potential for awareness during pediatric cardiac surgery should not be underestimated. To prevent awareness, isoflurane may be administered via the membrane oxygenator with an anesthetic vaporizer, or intravenous midazolam 0.15 to 0.2 mg/kg may be administered.

Control of Systemic and Pulmonary Vascular Resistance During Anesthesia

In a child with a congenital heart defect, intraoperative changes in cardiac shunting represent a unique problem during maintenance of anesthesia. Although it is not always clear whether deterioration in clinical condition in these patients is due to changes in shunting or to primary myocardial dysfunction, the intraoperative events and progress of the anesthetic usually suggest a cause. Decreases in arterial oxygenation or in systemic blood flow may be due to alterations in intracardiac shunting. When circulating blood volume is adequate, either pharmacologic support or techniques of managing intracardiac shunting by modifying the balance between PVR and SVR can be used.

Manipulation of SVR during anesthesia is useful for adult cardiac patients. However, during anesthesia for congenital heart disease, there is the additional need to manipulate PVR, which may prove very difficult. The reasons for this are that (1) control of PVR is poorly understood, (2) vasoactive drugs usually are distributed on both sides of the circulation, and (3) pharmacologic attempts to modify shunting have produced unpredictable results.[32–34]

Despite these problems, a number of techniques have proved useful in manipulating relative PVR and SVR (Table 18–2). Potent inhalation anesthetics appear to reduce SVR more than PVR. PVR is decreased in children by increasing inspired oxygen to 100% and by hyperventilation to a pH of 7.6 or greater.[35, 36] Positive end-expiratory pressure, acidosis, hypothermia, and the use of 30% or less inspired oxygen can increase PVR. Vasoconstrictors such as phenylephrine increase SVR more than PVR and therefore are acutely effective in reducing right-to-left shunting and increasing left-to-right shunting in the operating room.

During cardiac surgical procedures, a direct method of selectively increasing PVR or SVR is to have the surgeon place partially obstructing tourniquets around pulmonary arteries or the aorta to increase resistance so that flow to the opposite side of the circulation increases. SVR can be increased similarly during abdominal surgery with aortic clamps if higher systemic pressures are needed to perfuse the lungs through a systemic-to-pulmonary-artery shunt. Although these are only temporary measures, they may be useful to re-establish a better relative balance of resistances and a more normal physiology in a deteriorating clinical situation.

Choice of Anesthetic Agents

Inhalation Agents

Conventional inhalation induction, when administered cautiously, can be used safely in children with minor cardiac

Table 18–2. Techniques to Manipulate Relative Vascular Resistances

Vascular Resistance	Increases	Decreases
Pulmonary	PEEP	Avoid PEEP
	High airway pressure	Low airway pressure
	Atelectasis	Normal FRC
	Low FIO_2	High FIO_2
	Acidosis and hypercapnia	Alkalosis and hypocapnia
	Increased hematocrit	Low hematocrit
	Sympathetic stimulation	Blunted stress response
	Direct surgical manipulation	Nitric oxide
		? Other vasodilators
Systemic	Vasoconstrictors	Potent inhalation agents
	Direct manipulation	Vasodilators

FIO_2, fraction concentration of inspired oxygen; FRC, functional residual capacity; PEEP, positive end-expiratory pressure.

defects. However, in children with moderate or severe heart disease, use of the potent inhalation agents considerably narrows the margin of safety and probably should be avoided. Although theoretical differences exist in uptake and distribution of inhalation anesthetics in children with intracardiac shunting, these considerations are of little practical importance in clinical anesthesia, as has been shown in children with left-to-right shunts.[37]

Halothane

Studies have shown a significant incidence of hypotension with bradycardia in infants with normal cardiovascular systems during induction with halothane.[38] During halothane induction in normal infants, halothane decreases the cardiac index to 73% of awake values at 1.0 minimum alveolar concentration (MAC) and 59% at 1.5 MAC.[39] Uptake of halothane in infants less than 3 months of age has been demonstrated to be considerably more rapid than in adults. Thus, anesthetic concentration probably increases more rapidly in the myocardium of an infant as well.[40] Although the effects of halothane on the human neonatal myocardium are unknown, it has been shown that young rats have a reduced cardiovascular tolerance for halothane but require greater amounts for anesthesia.[41] The MAC for halothane in infants 1 to 6 months of age also has been shown to be the highest of any age group.[42] This increased anesthetic requirement in infants, combined with the immaturity of their cardiovascular system, partly explains the relative cardiovascular intolerance for halothane in infants. Atropine has been used intramuscularly before induction to partially compensate for the myocardial depression of halothane by reducing bradycardia and hypotension.[38] Intravenous atropine 0.02 mg/kg increases cardiac index by 21% at 1.5 MAC.[39] Although halothane may produce some degree of hypotension, an increase in arterial saturation in children with cyanotic congenital heart disease may occur.[43]

Sevoflurane

In healthy infants and children, sevoflurane provides a smooth induction of anesthesia because it has a pleasant odor and is not irritating to the airway. In contrast to halothane, sevoflurane causes no reduction in heart rate at 1.0 and 1.5 MAC in healthy children compared with awake values.[44, 45] In the absence of nitrous oxide, sevoflurane also causes less depression of myocardial contractility than halothane during induction of anesthesia in children.[45] Sevoflurane does cause a mild decrease in systemic vascular resistance. This anesthetic has not been evaluated in children with cardiac disease; however, unless there is a concern for balancing SVR and PVR, it would seem to offer a reasonable alternative to halothane.

Isoflurane

At equipotent levels, isoflurane causes similar hemodynamic depression in neonates and infants when compared with halothane.[39] Isoflurane is generally not used for induction of anesthesia because of a high incidence of laryngospasm (greater than 20%).[46] Inadequate ventilation because of laryngospasm or other causes quickly leads to large increases

in PVR secondary to hypoxemia and hypercarbia. This increase in PVR and the resulting pulmonary hypertension is poorly tolerated in small children with heart disease, especially in the presence of right-to-left shunting.

A slow induction with halothane or sevoflurane may be well tolerated in children with mild to moderate heart disease. However, the cited studies along with our clinical experience suggest that potent inhalation agents may be an unwise choice for induction in young infants with severe cardiac disease. In children of any age with marginal cardiovascular reserve and in those with severe desaturation of systemic arterial blood due to right-to-left shunting, the myocardial depression and systemic hypotension due to potent inhalation agents are poorly tolerated. A more appropriate use of these anesthetic agents in children with severe heart disease is the addition of low concentrations of the inhalation agent to control hypertensive responses after induction.

Nitrous Oxide

The use of nitrous oxide for anesthetic maintenance in congenital heart disease is controversial because of the risk of enlarging intravascular air emboli and the potential to increase PVR. Nitrous oxide may cause microbubbles and macrobubbles to expand, thus increasing obstruction to blood flow in arteries and capillaries. In all children with shunts, the potential exists for these bubbles to be shunted directly into the systemic circulation. Thus, routine use of air traps in intravenous lines in patients with known intracardiac defects should be combined with careful purging of air bubbles from all intravenous lines. The outcome following coronary air embolism is made worse by nitrous oxide.[47] Additionally, the hemodynamic effects of venous air embolism are increased by nitrous oxide, even without paradoxical embolization.[48] In patients with pre-existing right-to-left shunts, paradoxical air embolism is clearly a potential problem; but even patients with large left-to-right shunts can transiently reverse their shunts. This is especially true during coughing or a Valsalva maneuver, when the normal transatrial pressure gradient is reversed. Several studies have demonstrated right-to-left shunting of microbubbles of air after injection of saline into the right atrium during these maneuvers.[49–51] Because coughing and Valsalva maneuvers may occur during anesthetic induction, even the most rigorous attention to air bubbles in intravenous lines may not prevent some small amounts of air from reaching the systemic circulation. Microbubbles have also been observed following cardiopulmonary bypass.[52]

Nitrous oxide is reported to increase PVR in adults.[53, 54] However, it does not seem to affect PVR or pulmonary artery pressure in infants at 50% concentration.[55] Nitrous oxide does mildly decrease cardiac output at this concentration.[55, 56] It has been suggested that the use of nitrous oxide should be avoided in children with limited pulmonary blood flow, pulmonary hypertension, or depressed myocardial function. In the well-compensated patient who does not require 100% inspired oxygen, nitrous oxide (generally at concentrations of 50%) may be used during induction but then discontinued prior to tracheal intubation. If reduced inspired oxygen is indicated to maintain an appropriate balance between

PVR and SVR following intubation, air may be added to the inspired gas mixture.

Intramuscular and Intravenous Anesthetics

Intravenous and intramuscular induction techniques are safe and effective in neonates and infants with severe cardiac disease. They are also useful in older children with severely diminished functional cardiac reserve.

Ketamine

When intravenous access is a problem, intramuscular ketamine 5 mg/kg is well tolerated even by sick children with cyanosis or congestive heart failure.[57, 58] Concomitant intramuscular succinylcholine 5 mg/kg or rocuronium 1.5 to 2.0 mg/kg is used to facilitate control of the airway. Atropine or glycopyrrolate is administered to offset the secretions often produced by ketamine. Although increases in PVR have been reported in adults following ketamine, in well-premedicated children, ketamine causes no change in PVR when the airway is maintained and ventilation is supported.[59, 60] In children with congenital heart disease, the ejection fraction is well preserved during ketamine anesthesia.[60, 61] Our clinical experience with intramuscular ketamine has been excellent in most forms of heart disease, including those with limited pulmonary blood flow and cyanosis, when arterial oxygen saturation usually improves with ketamine.[43]

When intravenous access is available in patients with marginal cardiac reserve, several techniques may be used for induction. Intravenous ketamine 1 to 2 mg/kg is an excellent induction agent in most forms of congenital heart disease. Relative contraindications to the use of ketamine may be coronary insufficiency caused by anomalous coronary artery, severe critical aortic stenosis, or hypoplastic left-heart syndrome with aortic atresia and hypoplasia of the ascending aorta. These patients are prone to ventricular fibrillation because of relative coronary insufficiency. Tachycardia and catecholamine release following ketamine administration may predispose the patients in this group to ventricular fibrillation. In these particular patients, the use of a high-dose fentanyl technique in doses of up to 75 μg/kg, given with pancuronium, may provide greater stability.

Opioids

As in adults with severe cardiac disease, high-dose intravenous fentanyl administered with pancuronium and with 100% oxygen, or air and oxygen, is an excellent induction technique in very sick children with all forms of congenital heart disease. In neonates and infants, the use of high-dose opioid anesthesia provides excellent hemodynamic stability, with suppression of the hormonal and metabolic stress response.[62] When fentanyl or other opioids are used with nitrous oxide, the negative inotropic effects of nitrous oxide may appear, especially in sicker patients.[53, 63] The high-dose fentanyl technique is effective in premature neonates undergoing ligation of a PDA.[64] In high-risk full-term neonates and in older infants with severe congenital heart disease, use of the high-dose fentanyl technique in doses of up to 75 μg/kg, given with pancuronium, results in minimal hemodynamic response to induction, intubation, and surgical incision.[65] Oxygen saturation levels are well maintained and often improve during induction, even in cyanotic children.[66] Changes in cardiac index, SVR, and PVR in infants given 25 μg/kg of fentanyl have been shown to be insignificant.[67] The use of pancuronium with the high-dose fentanyl technique is recommended, because the vagolytic effects of pancuronium offset the vagotonic effects of fentanyl. The hemodynamic stability reported in infants with high-dose fentanyl and pancuronium may not be found when other muscle relaxants are used.[68]

Sufentanil (5–20 μg/kg) is an alternative to fentanyl. The use of high-dose opioid technique (fentanyl or sufentanil) necessitates continuous postoperative ventilatory support. Alfentanil has limited use in cardiac surgical procedures requiring significant postoperative analgesia because of its short duration of action. However, alfentanil is a useful anesthetic adjunct in the cardiac catheterization laboratory.

Thiopental and Propofol

Intravenous induction with thiopental and propofol generally is not used in patients with severe cardiac defects. A reduced dose of thiopental 1 to 2 mg/kg or propofol 1 to 1.5 mg/kg may be safe for induction in patients with moderate defects and may result in improved arterial oxygen saturation in cyanotic patients.[66] In pediatric patients with minimal cardiac defects, intravenous induction with larger doses (thiopental 3 to 5 mg/kg or propofol 2 to 3 mg/kg) is usually well tolerated, provided the patient is euvolemic.

Muscle Relaxants

Pancuronium has been well studied in children with congenital heart disease and causes no change in heart rate or blood pressure when administered over 60 to 90 seconds.[69] An intubating bolus dose of pancuronium may produce tachycardia and an increase in cardiac output. This bolus dose effect is sometimes desirable to support cardiac output in infants in congestive heart failure, because their stroke volume is fixed. Pancuronium may be the muscle relaxant of choice when high-dose opioid techniques are used to oppose the vagotonic effects of opioids such as fentanyl.

Management of Cardiopulmonary Bypass

The management of any patient during cardiopulmonary bypass (CPB) involves the external control of three factors: pump flow rate, temperature, and hemodilution. Most physiologic mechanisms in the pediatric patient are different from the adult and CPB management must accommodate these differences. In the management of pediatric patients it may be necessary to alter each of these three factors to a greater extent than in the management of adults.

Perfusion flow rate requirements are relatively greater when compared with adults. This is due to the higher metabolic rate and increased demand for oxygen in pediatric patients. Recommended flow rates at normothermia are 2.4 to 3.2 L/min/m² or 130 to 150 mL/kg with perfusion pressures of 30 to 50 mm Hg. The higher flow rate requirements can make surgery difficult. Moderate to profound hypothermia reduces the cerebral metabolic rate for oxygen (CMR_{O_2})

and allows for low-flow cardiopulmonary bypass or profound hypothermic circulatory arrest techniques to be utilized.[70] As children become older, lower flows are used. The standard adult flows of 50 to 70 mL/kg/min are used in children weighing more than 50 kg. As a child ages, perfusion pressures generally increase.

A good indication of perfusion during bypass in children is the rate of cooling or warming in various parts of the body. Core temperature, as measured by distal esophageal temperature, generally changes most quickly, followed by a lag of several degrees of the nasopharyngeal and tympanic temperatures. A somewhat longer lag is noted in the rectal and skin temperatures, because these measurements reflect more peripheral perfusion. Temperature gradients between these areas decrease as a steady state is achieved. The same gradients generally are observed in reverse order during rewarming.

Profound hypothermic circulatory arrest or low-flow cardiopulmonary bypass are frequently employed for the surgical repair of complex neonatal cardiac defects.[71] Animal experiments and clinical experience have shown apparent safety of hypothermia to 15° to 20°C.[72] Cerebral hypothermia markedly reduces the CMRo$_2$ by nonspecifically slowing biochemical reactions. During ischemia, hypothermia prolongs the time to terminal depolarization, delays the depletion of high-energy phosphates,[73, 74] and reduces the rate of excitatory amino acid release.[75, 76] Additional mechanisms of cerebral protection during hypothermic ischemia includes an alkaline shift in intracellular pH[77] and protection against reperfusion injury including the no-reflow phenomenon (when the vascular supply to an area of brain becomes irreversibly occluded during the circulatory arrest period and perfusion to that area does not recover), calcium influx, and free radical damage.[71] The primary determinants of complete and uniform brain cooling are the uniformity of blood flow to the brain, the temperature of this blood, and the duration of cooling.[78] If short cooling times are utilized (i.e., less than 20 min), the brain is less likely to be adequately cooled. It is desirable to wait until the target surrogate temperature has been reached and then to wait an additional 5 to 10 minutes before low-flow bypass or circulatory arrest is begun.[79] Ice packs may be placed around the head prior to arrest. Surface cooling does not speed brain cooling[78]; however, ice packs may prevent slight brain warming during circulatory arrest.

Barbiturates also reduce CMRo$_2$ by specifically stabilizing active synaptic membranes when activity of these membranes has not already been suppressed by hypothermia alone.[80] Even at temperatures below 18°C, over 50% of infants still have cerebral electrical activity at the onset of circulatory arrest when barbiturates are not administered.[81, 82] Thus barbiturate administration can be expected to provide additional CMRo$_2$ suppression beyond that provided by hypothermia alone.[80] There are reasons why barbiturate administration *early* in the cooling phase might be disadvantageous. First, barbiturates increase cerebral vascular resistance[83] and may interfere with effective brain cooling if administered early. Second, early barbiturate administration hinders the increase in cerebral energy state normally observed during cooling and results in decreased brain energy state during circulatory arrest in an animal model.[84] However, once hypothermic levels have been reached, thiopental 10 mg/kg may be administered to ablate any residual cerebral activity, particularly if a prolonged period of low-flow bypass or circulatory arrest is anticipated.[85]

The hemodilution effects of CPB, apparent in adult patients as a consequence of the pump prime, are magnified in the pediatric patient. For example, a neonate weighing 2500 g has a blood volume of about 200 mL and the smallest CPB circuit has a priming volume of 450 to 600 mL. Therefore, the ratio of prime-to-patient volume is about 2:1 to 3:1.[70] During CPB it has been suggested that hematocrits of 18 to 22% be maintained during profound hypothermia.[70] The diminished oxygen-carrying capacity of the depleted red blood cell concentration is offset by the increased capillary flow rates achieved as a result of lower viscosity. The lower viscosity from hemodilution will also offset the increase in viscosity that results from low perfusion temperatures.[70] Furthermore, hypothermia increases the hemoglobin oxygen affinity and markedly impairs oxygen transfer to the plasma. Thus, during profound hypothermia, dissolved oxygen in the plasma provides nearly all of the brain's oxygen requirements.[86] With hemodilution, the blood concentration of plasma proteins, formed blood elements, and drugs is diluted and significantly lowered.[12, 87] These changes reduce osmotic and oncotic pressure, which may cause a progressive increase in extracellular water, which in turn can compromise ventricular and respiratory function, intestinal motility, and wound healing.[88, 89] Physiologic processes such as coagulation can be impaired, and replacement of platelets and coagulation factors is often necessary following separation from bypass.[12] The reduction in drug levels with the establishment of CPB has been noted previously and supplementation of anesthetic agents is required to attenuate the stress response, to prevent movement, and to maintain amnesia.[62, 87, 90]

Separation from Cardiopulmonary Bypass

Weaning from CPB involves decreasing the venous return by clamping of the venous cannulae and gradual filling of the heart through the arterial cannula. Adequacy of blood volume is assessed by direct visualization and by measuring right or left atrial filling pressures. The arterial cannula is left in place so that a slow infusion of residual pump blood can be used to optimize filling pressures. Myocardial function is assessed by direct visualization, and also by measurement of right or left atrial pressure, or by the use of intraoperative epicardial or transesophageal echocardiography. In corrected physiology, the pulse oximeter can be used to assess the adequacy of cardiac output.[91] Low saturations or the inability of the oximeter probe to register a pulse may be a sign of very low output and high systemic resistance or vasoconstriction due to inhomogeneous rewarming.[92]

Difficulty in weaning from CPB can usually be attributed to one or more of the following factors: (1) a poor surgical result, (2) right or left ventricular dysfunction, or (3) pulmonary artery hypertension. To determine the cause of difficulty in weaning a patient from CPB, an intraoperative cardiac catheterization can be performed to assess isolated chamber hemodynamics. Pull-back pressures may be measured to assess for residual pressure gradients between chambers, across valves or outflow tracts, and through repaired sites of stenosis or conduits. Intracardiac oxygen saturation measurements may be determined to look for residual shunts.[27] The use of epicardial or transesophageal echocardiography has also proved useful in providing an intraoperative assessment of the structure of the repaired heart and in identifying abnormalities that may require further repair prior to leaving the operating room.[93–95]

Left and right ventricular dysfunction can be treated by optimizing preload and heart rate, by increasing coronary perfusion pressure, by correcting ionized calcium levels, by adding inotropic support, and by decreasing afterload. In neonates with shunt physiology, the use of primary alpha agonists or inotropics whose alpha effects predominate in higher doses (e.g., dopamine and epinephrine) should be minimized. These agents may substantially increase pulmonary blood flow, thereby increasing, rather than reducing, cardiac work.

It is often impossible to separate neonates and infants with pulmonary hypertension or pulmonary hypertensive crisis from CPB because of right ventricular failure due to the elevated PVR. Pharmacologic management of pulmonary hypertension has proved difficult. Administration of traditional vasodilators such as nitroglycerin, sodium nitroprusside, hydralazine, and nifedipine has been used with variable success.[55, 96–99] Prostaglandin E₁ has been used to treat pulmonary hypertensive crisis with varying degrees of success.[100] Drugs such as isoproterenol, amrinone, nitroglycerin, tolazoline, and adenosine have been used for their effects on the pulmonary vasculature.[98, 101, 102] These agents decrease SVR as well as the PVR and may result in a systemic hypotension that can limit their clinical use. Ventilatory manipulations have proved to be only variably effective.[98] Inhaled nitric oxide (NO), a selective pulmonary vasodilator, has proved to be of clinical benefit in the management of acute pulmonary hypertension in some children with congenital heart disease and undergoing surgical repair.[103, 104] Synthesized from the amino acid L-arginine by NO synthetase, NO is rapidly inactivated by oxidation to inorganic nitrite and nitrate in the presence of oxyhemoglobin or oxymyoglobin.[105] Thus, NO-dependent vasodilator tone is likely entirely locally regulated.[106] The concentrations of NO required for selective pulmonary vasodilation (less than 80 parts per million) appear to be without direct toxic effects when administered for short periods of time. The short half-life of exogenously administered NO in combination with its rapid inactivation by hemoglobin is likely to account for the pulmonary vascular selectivity.[107]

Once adequate hemodynamics are achieved, protamine is administered and coagulation abnormalities are addressed. Doses of protamine vary between institutions, but a dose of 1 mg of protamine per 100 units of heparin administered initially should bring the activated clotting time close to the baseline measurement. The chest is closed when hemostasis is satisfactory and the patient is returned to the intensive care unit. Although the primary influence on outcome is the execution of the operation and intraoperative events, postoperative intensive care is clearly an important factor.

Managing Impaired Hemostasis Following Separation from Bypass

Conventional Replacement Strategies

In an effort to normalize factors and platelets to effective levels, many centers utilize fresh whole blood. In adult patients[108] and an in vitro aggregation study,[109] transfusion of fresh whole blood provided equal or greater hemostatic and functional benefit versus transfusion of platelet concentrates. In children, transfusion of fresh whole blood less than 48 hours from harvest is associated with less blood loss compared with transfusion of reconstituted whole blood (packed erythrocytes, fresh frozen plasma, and platelets).[110] However, fresh whole blood is often difficult to obtain. Furthermore, the units must be refrigerated for 24 to 48 hours while donor screening is performed and this storage causes significant platelet injury. Platelets that are stored at 4°C for even 30 minutes undergo irreversible shape and functional changes,[111] referred to as the "cold storage lesion." This injury involves rapid polymerization of actin monomers in the platelet cytoskeleton.[112] Insistence on fresh whole blood places tremendous pressures on the transfusion service and donor center to coordinate the matching of donor types with often unanticipated recipient needs. Alternatively, reconstituted whole blood, "modified whole blood," or individual component therapy may be utilized. In "modified whole blood," the plasma and erythrocytes from the same donor are retained together, but the platelets are separated and stored at room temperature for optimal survival. If individual component therapy is utilized and rapid-response coagulation testing is unavailable, a rational approach is to transfuse platelets *first* when abnormal hemostasis is noted and then follow with cryoprecipitate if continued microvascular bleeding is observed. In the majority of cases, platelets alone will normalize whole blood coagulation and viscoelastic parameters.[113] Cryoprecipitate is preferable to fresh frozen plasma, especially in the infant, because fibrinogen levels are more readily restored with less volume. Use of fresh frozen plasma in the infant may result in excessive dilution of red cell mass and platelets.

Effect of Hemofiltration and Modified Ultrafiltration upon Hemostasis

Cytokines and complement are released during rewarming. Cytokines are subsequently known to activate coagulation and fibrinolysis.[114] By removing these inflammatory mediators during rewarming, high-volume, zero-balance hemofiltration has been shown to improve hemostasis, hemodynamics, oxygenation, and pulmonary function following bypass.[115–117] The molecular cut-off weight of hemoconcentration units is 65,000 Daltons. No major changes in coagulation factor levels have been observed following hemofiltration.

Antifibrinolytic Therapy

The fibrinolytic system is activated during cardiac surgery and is probably a significant cause of post-bypass bleeding.[14, 118, 119] Children undergoing *repeat* cardiac surgery are potentially at most risk for fibrinolytic bleeding. Plasminogen is activated by tissue plasminogen activator and converted to plasmin. Plasmin binds to fibrin at lysine-binding sites and cleaves the polymer. Plasminogen also exerts an adverse effect on platelet function.[120] Three antifibrinolytic agents are clinically available: ε-aminocaproic acid, tranexamic acid, and aprotinin. ε-Aminocaproic acid and tranexamic acid are synthetic lysine analogues, which inhibit plasminogen conversion and plasmin activity. Tranexamic acid is 7 to 10 times more potent than ε-aminocaproic acid. Both synthetic agents are renally eliminated, largely unchanged, through glomerular filtration. Aprotinin is a naturally occurring nonspecific serine protease inhibitor. It has a basic polypeptide structure including 58 amino acids. Aprotinin is a potent inhibitor of plasmin and kallikrein. It also affects the contact phase of coagulation, modulates complement activation, and preserves platelet adhesion receptors.[121] Aprotinin is taken up with high affinity by the renal proximal tubular epithelial cells and excreted mostly unchanged.

Tranexamic Acid and Aminocaproic Acid

Pharmacokinetic data are limited and pharmacodynamic data are unstudied for the antifibrinolytic agents in the pediatric population. The recommended initial bolus for tranexamic acid ranges from 10 mg/kg[122] to 100 mg/kg.[123, 124] We commonly administer tranexamic acid as 100 mg/kg for the initial bolus before skin incision, followed by 10 mg/kg/hr by continuous infusion, and an additional 100 mg/kg in the pump prime to offset the dilutional effect. It may be particularly important to administer the second bolus following onset of bypass in children because of the large alteration in circulating blood volume when the bypass circuit is introduced. Since tranexamic acid is more potent than ε-aminocaproic acid, some prefer to use tranexamic acid in children because it is easier to provide the high-dose regimen without excessive volume. When ε-aminocaproic acid is used, the initial bolus and prime addition are typically 100 to 150 mg/kg followed by an infusion of 25 to 50 mg/kg/hr.

Aprotinin

The recommended aprotinin regimen, in children with a body surface area less than 1.16 m², includes an initial load and prime addition of 240 mg/m² and an infusion of 56 mg/m²/hr.[125, 126] *Because of the risk for anaphylaxis, a 1 mL test dose must be administered prior to the initial loading dose.* There is no evidence that aprotinin is more efficacious in reducing blood loss than tranexamic acid.[127–129] However, aprotinin may offer some advantage over synthetic antifibrinolytics because it is a potent kallikrein inhibitor and may modulate the post-bypass inflammatory response.[130, 131] Whether these anti-inflammatory effects translate to improved patient outcome in children has yet to be proven. Aprotinin may cause anaphylactoid and anaphylactic reactions because of its polypeptide structure and bovine extraction. The risk of anaphylactoid reaction in adults receiving aprotinin is estimated to be 1 in 200 on first exposure and up to 1 in 11 on second exposure.[132, 133] Fortunately, the incidence of hypersensitivity reactions to aprotinin in children may be much less than that in adults. Nevertheless, children with complex cardiac defects often require multiple staged procedures, and caution should be exercised when re-exposing these children to aprotinin. However, because of its effectiveness in decreasing bleeding following cardiopulmonary bypass and its additional actions of modulating the post-bypass inflammatory response, the agent remains a valuable drug in our armamentarium. Anaphylactic reactions to ε-aminocaproic acid or tranexamic acid have not been reported.

Thrombosis

An increased incidence of perioperative myocardial infarction and postoperative renal dysfunction has been reported in adults receiving aprotinin.[134] Since this report, there has been a continued concern that antifibrinolytic agents might promote a hypercoagulable state. In adults, cases of cerebral,[135–137] pulmonary,[138] aortic,[139] mesenteric,[140] and retinal[141] thrombosis have been reported in association with antifibrinolytic therapy. Although the pediatric efficacy studies to date have not shown an increased incidence of thrombotic complications, these studies have not had the statistical power necessary to detect subtle or devastating complications of these agents. Children undergoing the fenestrated Fontan procedure, bidirectional Glenn shunt, pulmonary unifocalization, or other procedures involving low-velocity pathways may be at most risk for potential thrombotic complications. The use of antifibrinolytic therapy in children undergoing profound hypothermic circulatory arrest is a special area of concern.[142–146]

Stress Response to Cardiac Surgery

Cardiac surgery and cardiopulmonary bypass are altered physiologic conditions associated with exaggerated stress responses characterized by the release of a large number of metabolic and hormonal substances, which include catecholamines, cortisol, growth hormone, prostaglandins, complement, glucose, insulin, and beta-endorphins.[62, 147, 148] The cause of the elaboration of these compounds is multifactorial and includes contact of blood with foreign surfaces, low perfusion pressure, anemia, hypothermia, myocardial ischemia, low levels of anesthesia, and nonpulsatile flow. Other factors contributing to the elevation of stress hormones include delayed renal and hepatic clearance and exclusion of the pulmonary circulation during extracorporeal circulation.[149]

Neonatal infants of all viable gestational ages, as well as older infants and children, have nociceptive systems that are sufficiently developed and integrated with brain stem cardiovascular control centers to produce both humoral and circulatory responses to pain and stress.[150] Substantial humoral, metabolic, and cardiovascular responses to painful and stressful stimulation during surgery have been documented in newborns of various gestational ages and older infants.[62, 90, 149, 151] Hormonal stress responses in neonates subjected to cardiac[62] and noncardiac[151] operations have been found to be three to five times greater than adult responses to similar operations.[62] Circulatory responses to stressful stimuli in children include systemic and pulmonary hypertension.

Humoral stress responses are particularly extreme during and after cardiac surgery and are characterized by increases in circulating catecholamines, glucagon, cortisol, beta-endorphins, growth hormone, and insulin.[62, 90, 149, 151] In these studies, circulating levels of catecholamines increased by as much as 400% over baseline preoperative levels. This is evidence of massive activation of sympathetic outflow in response to surgical stimulation. Some of these responses may continue for several days postoperatively.

It has been suggested that such extreme stress responses and neuroendocrine activation may be associated with greater mortality and morbidity during the postoperative period.[90] In adult studies, intraoperative adrenergic activation of 50% above baseline is associated with significant postoperative alterations in beta-adrenergic receptor function, including increased beta-receptor density and decreased receptor affinity. Mortality among adults with severe congestive failure is associated with increased levels of hormones regulating cardiovascular function including aldosterone, epinephrine, and norepinephrine.[152] In neonatal patients undergoing cardiac surgery, elevated stress hormones have been associated with increased hospital mortality.[90]

The metabolic response to stress in children includes increased oxygen consumption, glycogenolysis, gluconeogenesis, and lipolysis. These metabolic responses cause substantial intraoperative and postoperative catabolism. The metabolic stress responses following comparable operative stresses are greater in magnitude in newborns than in adult patients and result in substantial alterations in metabolic balance and levels of various metabolic substrates.[62, 90, 149–151] These metabolic alterations are usually related to changes in plasma cortisol, catecholamines, and other counter-regulatory hormones such as glucagon and growth hormone.[62, 90, 149] The most prominent effects seen clinically as a result of stimulation of these processes are perioperative hypoglycemia and hyperglycemia, lactic acidemia, and negative nitrogen balance extending well into the postoperative period.[90] Neonates and infants tolerate such metabolic derangements poorly. This impaired tolerance is due to a relative lack of endogenous reserves of carbohydrates, proteins, and fats, the high metabolic cost of rapid growth, a high obligate requirement for glucose by the relatively large brain, the immature hormonal control of intermediary metabolism, and the limited functional capabilities of immature enzyme systems in the metabolic organs. Thus severe stress responses superimposed on the "normal" neonatal and infant physiology may be poorly tolerated. However, it is still unclear whether or not these metabolic alterations might provide some beneficial effects toward mobilizing the bodily resources to provide a metabolic milieu for healing tissues or whether they are purely maladaptive, resulting in detrimental effects on postoperative outcome.

Another factor to consider is the potential effect of stress-induced hyperglycemia on neurologic outcome. Neonates and young infants are capable of substantial rates of glucose production, mainly from glycogenolysis and gluconeogenesis, during stress. This can result in substantial hyperglycemia during major surgery in neonates. Such hyperglycemic response may be associated with poorer neurologic outcome, particularly after a period of cerebral ischemia.[153] The use of high doses of fentanyl (greater than 50 μg/kg) has been shown to reduce the hormonal stress response and resultant hyperglycemia and may lessen the risk of neurologic injury.[154]

In sufficient doses, opioids can blunt the stress responses in neonates, infants, and adults.[155–158] This blunting results in a more normal, homeostatic humoral and metabolic milieu in the circulation by reducing neuroendocrine activation and levels of regulating hormones.[156–158] In infants, the use of high-dose opioids for major surgical procedures and postoperative sedation substantially attenuates the neuroendocrine response to surgically induced pain and stress.[62, 90, 149, 151] Catecholamine release resulting from intraoperative stress

responses may predispose the vulnerable myocardium to dysrhythmias. In neonates with hypoplastic left heart syndrome, sudden ventricular fibrillation occurred in a large proportion (50%) of neonates during surgical manipulation until high doses of fentanyl were used as the primary anesthetic agent.[159] With the use of high-dose opioids, intraoperative ventricular fibrillation has virtually disappeared as a problem in this group of neonates.[10] In several studies, opioids have been shown to increase the ventricular fibrillation threshold in isolated cardiac Purkinje fibers and to alter action potential duration similar to that with class III antiarrhythmic agents.[160, 161] Thus even electrophysiologic events in the neonatal heart, in addition to humoral and hemodynamic responses, may be altered by using high-dose fentanyl anesthesia to attenuate the effect of pain and stress in neonates.

Anesthetic Considerations in Specific Cardiac Defects

Specific discussion of anesthetic considerations for various repairs (Table 18–3) of each form of congenital heart disease is beyond the scope of this chapter.[162] However, a brief discussion of the problems that may be encountered during repair of the more common congenital heart lesions is presented. These include atrial septal defect (ASD), ventricular septal defect (VSD), tetralogy of Fallot, coarctation of the aorta, and patent ductus arteriosus (PDA).

Atrial Septal Defect

Atrial septal defects are relatively benign in childhood, and except for rare large defects, affected children are usually asymptomatic or mildly symptomatic. Even with the larger ostium primum defects, symptoms tend to be mild unless

Table 18–3. Distribution of Surgical Procedures at a Major Pediatric Cardiac Surgical Center

Procedure	Percent of Total
Repair of septal defects	22
atrial septal defect, ventricular septal defect, atrioventricular canal	
Systemic outflow reconstruction	21
transposition of the great arteries, interrupted aortic arch, coarctation of the aorta, hypoplastic left-heart syndrome, subaortic stenosis, etc.	
Pulmonary outflow reconstruction	18
tetralogy of Fallot repair, right ventricular conduit placement or revision, etc.	
Cavopulmonary anastomosis	13
bidirectional Glenn shunt, fenestrated Fontan procedure	
Patent ductus arteriosus ligation	6
Pacemaker placement or replacement	6
Other	14
Total	100

Cardiac surgical procedures and their frequency at Children's Hospital, Boston. Cumulative data from 1992 to 1995, inclusive (Peter C. Laussen; personal communication).

associated with moderate to severe mitral regurgitation; in that case, the lesion is properly termed an *incomplete atrioventricular canal.*

When an isolated ASD is repaired during childhood, most anesthetic agents are well tolerated. PVR usually remains normal during childhood, and pulmonary artery pressures are only mildly elevated as a result of moderate left-to-right shunting. The shunt is not large because the gradient across the atrial septum is small. Transient reversal of this gradient, and thus shunting, is possible with coughing and Valsalva maneuver or with events such as loss of the airway and severe hypoventilation (hypoxemia causing pulmonary hypertension). Systemic air embolization or arterial desaturation can result. Eisenmenger physiology, in which high pulmonary blood flow results in markedly elevated PVR and permanent reversal of atrial shunting, is rarely observed, because surgical repair is now being performed at a younger age.

Surgical repair is straightforward, except when a sinus venosus type of septal defect is encountered and the septal patch must be placed to baffle pulmonary venous return from the right lung into the left atrium. If not appreciated and corrected, this defect results in a continued left-to-right shunt and volume overload on the right side of the heart as pulmonary venous blood from the right lung returns to the right atrium.

Cardiopulmonary bypass time is short and separation from bypass is usually uncomplicated. If the anesthetic is managed carefully by limiting the amount of narcotic administered, for example, fentanyl 10 µg/kg, and using primarily inhalational agents, patients can often be extubated in the operating room or in the intensive care unit shortly after arrival.[163, 164] Transfusion of nonautologous blood can frequently be avoided.

Ventricular Septal Defect

In early childhood, a VSD may be a serious problem, primarily because the pressure gradient between the two communicating chambers tends to be high. As PVR decreases during early infancy, right ventricular pressure declines, and thus the amount of dependent shunting across the ventricular septum becomes large, with resulting volume overload of the left ventricle. This situation can lead to congestive failure, which if severe enough results in failure to thrive. Severe pulmonary hypertension in childhood is a possibility if large lesions are uncorrected.

When the VSD is small, the lesion behaves more like an ASD. After the initial physiologic reduction in PVR during infancy, PVR often remains low early in childhood, although pulmonary artery pressures are somewhat elevated because of the large left-to-right shunt and correspondingly high pulmonary blood flows. If repair is delayed until late in childhood, pulmonary vascular disease may develop from the high flow and pressure. In that event, PVR may remain elevated even after flow has decreased to normal following repair.

When defects are large with elevated right-sided pressures, pulmonary to systemic flow ratios greater than 2:1, and presence of congestive failure, problems may be encountered on induction of anesthesia. Only low concentrations of potent inhalation agents can be tolerated without significant systemic hypotension. Intravenous induction techniques, such as ketamine or fentanyl, maintain systemic arterial pressure and are generally safer. In patients with a large VSD, it is important to limit the inspired oxygen concentration administered during induction and maintenance of anesthesia to just that necessary to maintain a normal room air oxygen saturation. The use of a high inspired oxygen concentration can result in a rapid decrease in PVR and increased left-to-right shunting. If right ventricular pressures are close to systemic pressures, relatively mild systemic hypotension can cause the dependent shunt to reverse; the left-to-right shunt then becomes right-to-left, with systemic desaturation and further myocardial dysfunction, leading to progressive hypotension.

If the defect is small, such that the heart is able to support the shunting without congestive failure, and right-sided pressures are only mildly elevated, a cautious inhalation induction, bearing in mind the limited cardiac reserve, may be well tolerated. Regardless of induction technique and size of VSD, if the airway becomes obstructed or if alveolar hypoventilation occurs, PVR will increase markedly, increasing right ventricular pressure and possibly reversing the dependent shunt, even when systemic pressures are maintained. The degree of airway obstruction or hypoventilation tolerated depends on resting levels of right ventricular pressure.

If shunt reversal should occur and the child becomes cyanotic, establishment of the airway, hyperventilation with 100% oxygen, and use of an alpha-adrenergic agent (such as phenylephrine) to support systemic pressure usually results in return to baseline pulmonary arterial and right ventricular systolic pressure, with resumption of left-to-right shunting. In clinical practice, the tendency should be to err on the side of using techniques that lower PVR and maintain SVR, tending to increase slightly the left-to-right shunt. The higher the probability of right-to-left shunting, the more important this approach becomes.

Once induction is accomplished, maintenance of anesthesia is generally smooth until cardiopulmonary bypass. Although VSD repair is often straightforward, a number of problems can occur. Outflow tract obstruction in either the left or right ventricle can sometimes result when the VSD is subvalvular or malaligned so that closure of the defect crowds either the pulmonary or the aortic valve orifice. A redundant outflow patch can cause the same problem.

Injury to the bundle of His, with complete heart block, may require pacemaker support to allow weaning from bypass. A more common problem is residual muscular VSDs that are undiagnosed preoperatively. These may be difficult to find among the trabeculated interior of the right ventricle, even when specifically sought. The resulting residual left-to-right shunting may make weaning from bypass difficult and may complicate the anesthetic course after bypass and the postoperative course in the intensive care unit because of low cardiac output. If problems are encountered after the repair, drawing a pulmonary artery blood sample and comparing its saturation with a simultaneous mixed venous sample from the right atrium will reveal any significant increase in oxygen saturation in the right ventricle, indicating a residual shunt. The presence of a residual VSD is best evaluated with intraoperative two-dimensional epicardial or transesophageal echocardiography, thus allowing correction before leaving the operating room.[165]

Children having small defects, with short bypass times and benign intraoperative courses, can be extubated in the operating room. If defects are larger and bypass times lengthen, extubation may be safer if delayed by several hours. In the more severe forms of VSD, with marked congestive failure, prolonged bypass times, profound hypothermic circulatory arrest, and possible intraoperative ventriculotomy, extubation must be guided by the postoperative clinical course and is often delayed until the next day.

Tetralogy of Fallot

Tetralogy of Fallot varies widely in its severity. Infants may become cyanotic and have frequent hypercyanotic episodes ("Tet spells") in the first 6 months of life, requiring palliation with a systemic-to-pulmonary arterial shunt or repair during infancy. In its milder forms, no palliation is needed, and children may remain largely asymptomatic and acyanotic through early childhood. In the more severe forms, significant outflow obstruction of the right ventricle rapidly leads to systemic pressures in that chamber, with right-to-left shunting intermittently or continuously through the VSD. Stress may lead to increases in both right ventricular outflow obstruction and PVR, increasing right-to-left shunting and resulting in severe cyanosis. PVR is usually normal because the pulmonic stenosis and right-to-left shunting protect the vascular bed of the lungs from both the high pressure in the right ventricle and high flow present in VSDs with left-to-right shunts.

Maintenance of systemic pressures and a patent airway are critical during induction of anesthesia. If patients are extremely cyanotic and polycythemic, adequate preoperative hydration is necessary. In severe cases, techniques using 100% oxygen, with fentanyl and pancuronium as the baseline anesthetic agents, are satisfactory. Ketamine also is an excellent induction agent if the airway is maintained and ventilation is controlled. Increases in PVR associated with ketamine in children probably are secondary effects of the respiratory depression with hypoventilation and loss of airway patency.[60]

If a cyanotic spell develops during induction or before initiation of cardiopulmonary bypass, especially during manipulation and cannulation of the great vessels of the heart, initial treatment should be as outlined for reversal of shunt in VSDs. This includes hyperventilation with 100% oxygen, a bolus of phenylephrine 1 µg/kg followed by an infusion of 0.1 µg/kg/min, increasing as necessary to maintain a clinically satisfactory oxygen saturation, and initial volume infusion of at least 10 to 20 mL/kg. As an alternative or an addition to the steps mentioned, treatment with intravenous beta-blockers such as propranolol (5 µg/kg initially, then increasing as required) or esmolol (100 to 200 µg/kg/min as a constant infusion without a loading dose) has been advocated.[166, 167] Morphine 0.1 to 0.2 mg/kg has also been used to abort Tet spells, although it may not be as useful in a well-anesthetized patient.

Most patients with tetralogy of Fallot have residual ventricular dysfunction after repair. Pulmonary insufficiency of some degree and right ventricular dysfunction resulting from right ventriculotomy and cardiopulmonary bypass are always present. Some patients may also have a right bundle branch block. If residual pulmonic obstruction, shunting, or peripheral pulmonic stenosis is added, right ventricular function can be severely compromised, requiring significant inotropic support. Pulmonary artery hemoglobin oxygen saturations of greater than 80% during ventilation with 50% inspired oxygen generally indicate a significant residual left-to-right shunt.[168] Residual shunts of this magnitude may complicate the post-bypass intraoperative course and the postoperative course in the intensive care unit.

Because of these problems, children undergoing surgery for tetralogy of Fallot are generally not extubated until the day after the operation, unless the defects are mild and the intraoperative course has been totally benign.

Coarctation of the Aorta

Coarctation of the aorta has a wide range of presentations, from the sick, acidotic newborn with critical coarctation in which the ductus arteriosus supplies the great majority of the systemic perfusion to the lower half of the body, to the asymptomatic older child whose coarctation is discovered incidentally and who has only minimal upper extremity hypertension.

Neonates with critical coarctation require prostaglandin E$_1$ infusion to maintain ductal patency, improve systemic perfusion, and correct acidosis. Induction must be carefully carried out to maintain cardiovascular stability in the presence of a large right-to-left shunt to the lower half of the body. Some stability is provided by the more normal arterial saturations in the upper half of the body perfused by the left ventricle, but myocardial depressant anesthetics are still poorly tolerated. Asymptomatic older children tolerate a smooth induction by any of a number of techniques. The potential for shunting is virtually nil, and cardiac reserve is usually good.

It is preferable to place an arterial line in the right radial artery. The blood pressure cuff is usually placed on one of the legs for comparison of the gradient. Pulse oximeters are usually placed on both the right hand and a lower extremity.

Intraoperative problems related to the procedure are different when comparing neonatal with older patients. Retraction of the lung in the lateral decubitus position may have profound consequences on arterial oxygenation, especially in a neonate whose transitional circulation is still unstable. Use of the subclavian flap angioplasty technique for repair renders the left arm useless for intraoperative blood pressure measurements.

Cross-clamping of the aorta is generally well tolerated by neonates, because the isthmus of the aorta has little flow through it. In older children, especially those with pre-existing hypertension of the upper extremity, cross-clamping of the aorta may result in systolic pressures in the upper half of the body approaching 200 mm Hg. Although aggressive treatment of this may appear indicated, the anesthesiologist should be aware that when the thoracic aorta is cross-clamped, perfusion of renal, hepatic, and especially spinal cord vascular beds is dependent on high arterial pressures in the upper half of the body and collateral flow. Lowering arterial pressures in the upper half of the body to less than preanesthetic values may predispose the kidneys and the spinal cord to ischemic damage. Studies of animals confirm that although use of vasodilators such as nitroprusside may improve the circulation above the occlusion, the mean arterial pressure and organ perfusion below the occlusion decrease. This effect has been associated with paraplegia in dogs.[169, 170] Mild hypothermia to 34°C may prove helpful in preventing ischemic injury by reducing metabolic demand.

In children with coarctation, especially after a short cross-clamp time, the decline in arterial pressure with removal of the cross-clamp is usually mild to moderate, and the pressure quickly rises again if central blood volume is adequate. More severe decrements in pressure may be treated with partial reapplication of the clamp and gradual removal. Reactive hypertension in the intraoperative and postoperative period frequently responds to judicious use of labetalol and hydralazine. Extubation in the operating room for older patients with coarctation is routine, whereas sick neonates and infants are usually ventilated at least overnight.

Patent Ductus Arteriosus

A PDA may vary greatly in its hemodynamic consequences. A large PDA in a newborn may cause congestive failure and ventilator dependence, particularly in a premature infant. A small PDA may remain undetected during early childhood in asymptomatic children.

Considerations on induction are similar to those in coarctation of the aorta in patients of similar age and preoperative condition, except that left-to-right shunting with pulmonary overperfusion and systemic underperfusion must be considered. Low diastolic pressure and pulmonary steal from the systemic circulation can result in decreased organ perfusion. In neonatal lambs with left-to-right ductal shunting, perfusion of the myocardium, gastrointestinal tract, and even the brain increases significantly when the ductus is obliterated.[171] Elevated pulmonary artery pressures with the potential for reversal of shunting are rarely encountered in patients with this lesion, except in older patients with end-stage pulmonary vascular obstructive disease and a large PDA. Transient reversal of shunting across the ductus with desaturation of blood flowing to the lower half of the body can occur, as it does in neonates with transitional fetal circulation.

Although surgical repair has traditionally been performed via left thoracotomy, PDA ligation may also be performed via video-assisted thoracoscopy technique.[172, 173] Transesophageal echocardiography is helpful to confirm interruption of the flow after clip placement when the video-assisted thoracoscopy technique is utilized.[174] If the child is too small for a TEE probe to be safely placed, an esophageal stethoscope may be positioned at the point of maximal murmur amplitude, and complete cessation of this murmur should be noted after clipping.

Principles of Postoperative Cardiac Care

Children who undergo cardiopulmonary bypass or who required inotropic support during non-bypass procedures require intensive care postoperatively. Transport of these patients to the intensive care unit should be accomplished expeditiously, with monitoring appropriate to the length of the transport and the patient's condition before transport. Continuation of inotropic support is essential during trans-

port, especially because children who require this support are prone to become unstable. The stresses involved in transport and the often unavoidable changes in the rate of administration of drugs and intravenous fluids during transport make this a particularly vulnerable period. Portable battery-operated infusion pumps must be used for long transports, especially when inotropic agents are required. The utmost vigilance must be maintained during preparations for transfer, as well as during and after transfer into the intensive care unit. Frequent interruptions in monitoring and an urgent need for therapeutic interventions during transport have been reported in children following cardiothoracic surgery.[175] In our experience, hypovolemia is the most frequent problem during and immediately after transport, and immediate availability of blood and blood products is imperative during this period.

After cardiac surgical procedures, the rapidity with which cardiac tamponade may cause cardiovascular collapse must be appreciated. Tamponade may occur even with apparently adequate drainage from chest and mediastinal tubes. In young children, the small volume of the pericardial space leads to rapid onset of tamponade with few preliminary warning signs. The small-caliber drainage tubes used in infants are easily clotted or sequestered from the area of tamponade so that they become ineffective.

Reasonable attempts must be made to limit the number of exposures to blood products. Infusion of platelets, cryoprecipitate, and other blood components should follow documented need based on coagulation study parameters such as the prothrombin time and partial thromboplastin time. The minimum acceptable hematocrit for corrected cardiac lesions such as an uncomplicated ASD or VSD is approximately 20% in the postoperative period. More complex lesions with some degree of continuing cyanosis require a higher hematocrit.

The use of adequate sedation to prevent movement has been shown to decrease oxygen consumption in the postoperative period.[176] The use of muscle relaxants may not further reduce oxygen consumption significantly in patients who are not actively moving, but these agents often facilitate control of ventilation to optimize oxygenation and shunting. The use of fentanyl with muscle paralysis and use of pancuronium as a continuation of anesthesia postoperatively for hours or days have been reported to help control pulmonary hypertension and shunting after repair of congenital diaphragmatic hernia.[177] Other forms of sedation are also reported to control pulmonary hypertension postoperatively. The use of high-dose fentanyl with muscle relaxant technique has also been applied to the postoperative care of neonates and infants with highly reactive pulmonary circulations after repair of congenital heart disease. Inhaled nitric oxide may be delivered postoperatively to assist with the treatment of severe pulmonary hypertension.[178] The use of moderately high doses of fentanyl to blunt the stress responses of the pulmonary circulation to noxious stimuli such as endotracheal suctioning has been demonstrated to be effective in infants.[155]

The timing of extubation is based on the preoperative assessment of a child's cardiopulmonary status, the surgical procedure performed, and the hemodynamic status following repair. Following an uncomplicated secundum ASD repair, the trachea may often be extubated in the operating room or immediately upon arrival to the intensive care unit.[163, 164] Children who have undergone the Fontan procedure benefit from early resumption of spontaneous ventilation, as long as normocarbia is maintained, because positive pressure ventilation impairs pulmonary blood flow in the post-Fontan physiology. When a ventriculotomy has been performed, when continued inotropic support is required, or when postoperative pulmonary hypertension is anticipated, extubation should be delayed. Children with significant potential for right-to-left shunting, limited pulmonary blood flow, or pulmonary hypertension have little tolerance for hypoventilation and should be wide awake with an unobstructed airway before extubation. Even mild hypoventilation secondary to residual anesthetic in the postoperative period may result in hypoxic vasoconstriction and increases in PVR.

Anesthesia for Cardiac Catheterization

Cardiac catheterization procedures are indicated for both diagnostic and therapeutic purposes. Angiographic imaging remains an essential component in defining the anatomy of structures that are beyond the hilum of the lung and in patients in whom echocardiographic imaging is suboptimal due to poor acoustic windows. However, advances in noninvasive cardiac imaging that have occurred over the last 10 years have produced a shift in emphasis in the cardiac catheterization laboratory such that invasive studies are now performed primarily to obtain hemodynamic information and/or for the purpose of therapeutic transcatheter intervention.

Therapeutic cardiac catheterization can be divided into four major categories (Table 18–4), which carry certain predictable risks. Understanding of the interventionist's equipment and of the basic approach to interventions allows the anesthesiologist to anticipate those portions of the procedures that carry the greatest risk to the patient.[179] Such understanding also enables the recognition of when an untoward event is the result of the interventionist's actions. Close cooperation and communication between the cardiologist and the anesthesiologist facilitate such recognition.

General Considerations

For many procedures, such as dilations and device placement, success of the procedure depends on achieving a stable position of a stiff wire that ends in or passes through the heart. Stretching of the right heart produced by a stiff wire or sheath passing through to the pulmonary artery can result in bradycardia, tricuspid insufficiency, and pulmonic insufficiency. Passage of a retrograde wire into the left ventricle often results in ventricular ectopy, consisting of a few premature ventricular contractions or a short run of ventricular ectopy and occasionally ventricular fibrillation. Passage of a wire, sheath, or catheter through the right heart or retrograde into the left heart will, on occasion, result in complete heart block.

The use of large, long sheaths that extend from the neck or groin into the thorax is associated with the risk of embolism of air or thrombus.[180] These events are prevented only by meticulous attention to technique on the part of the interventionist. The risk of air embolism is significantly reduced by the use of positive pressure ventilation, and that of thromboembolism is reduced by adequate anticoagulation.[181]

Angioplasty balloons, which are rigid and straight when inflated, are often positioned in curved structures, such as the right ventricular outflow tract or a pulmonary artery. Inflation of the balloon can result in distortion of the heart or in rupture of the heart or vessel. In addition, a balloon may traverse several structures, in which case inflation of the balloon may result in unintended dilation of a valve, vessel, or septum. Balloon inflation may also result in a transient elimination of or severe diminution of cardiac output.

Any implantable device is a potentially embolic device. Keeping the patient immobile facilitates prevention of device embolization. Stimuli such as oral or endotracheal suctioning, blood pressure cuff inflation, or loud conversation should be avoided in the presence of a sedated patient at the time that an implantable device is being positioned in the heart or vasculature.

Patient Management

Cardiac catheterization procedures require routine patient monitoring, including electrocardiogram, blood pressure, arterial oxygen saturation, and temperature. End-tidal carbon dioxide pressure is monitored continuously, either with nasal prongs in the spontaneously breathing patient or via a side port in the breathing circuit in anesthetized patients. Secure intravenous access is established to provide additional sedation or a means for resuscitation. Once the cardiologist has arterial and venous catheters in place, beat-to-beat monitoring of the arterial pressure, measurements of filling pressure, and arterial blood-gas analysis are readily available.

Table 18–4. Common Procedures Performed in the Cardiac Catheterization Laboratory

Category	Example
Diagnostic	Hemodynamic catheterization
	Angiographic catheterization
Therapeutic	
Dilations	Atrial septectomy (Rashkind procedure)
	Valvular dilation (pulmonary artery stenosis)
	Vessel dilation (coarctation of the aorta)
Occlusions	
Device occlusion	Patent ductus arteriosus
	Atrial septal defects
	Ventricular septal defects
Coil occlusion	Patent ductus arteriosus
	Aortopulmonary collaterals
Foreign body retrieval	Embolized devices
	Retained intracardiac lines
Radiofrequency ablation	Accessory pathways (Wolff-Parkinson-White syndrome)
	Ectopic atrial foci (ectopic atrial tachycardia)
	Ectopic ventricular foci (ectopic ventricular tachycardia)

Patient positioning is important. Many of these procedures are of prolonged duration and particular attention must be paid to padding pressure points to minimize the risk of pressure injury. Similarly, brachial plexus injury is a risk, as the arms are positioned above the head to facilitate imaging. Once the patient is anesthetized, the risk of such nerve injury can be minimized by frequent passive movement of the arms.[182–184]

Antibiotic coverage (cefazolin 30 mg/kg, administered in the catheterization laboratory and repeated every 6 hours for two additional doses) is provided for interventional procedures involving device or coil placement.[185]

The management of patients undergoing diagnostic or therapeutic cardiac catheterizations may require no anesthesia or sedation, monitored anesthetic care, or general anesthesia. Certain procedures may require combinations of the above techniques. For routine diagnostic catheterizations, the cardiologist will generally prefer that the patient breathe spontaneously without supplemental oxygen so as to obtain the most realistic assessment of the patient's usual hemodynamic state. However, if a normal pH and partial pressure of carbon dioxide are not maintained, the hemodynamic findings may be meaningless. Normal ventilation achieved with mechanical assistance is preferable to respiratory acidosis with a natural airway. For some catheterizations, hemodynamic measurements may be limited to answer a few pertinent questions, after which a therapeutic procedure may be performed. The cardiologist may request a spontaneously breathing, minimally sedated patient while the hemodynamic assessment is being performed and then a fully anesthetized patient for the therapeutic portion of the catheterization. Thus, the decision to intubate or refrain from intubating the trachea must be individualized, and the decision must be arrived at mutually between the anesthesiologist and the cardiologist.

Sedation schedules vary among institutions and the agents used range from chloral hydrate, pentobarbital, meperidine, midazolam, morphine, and "lytic cocktail." This last compound is composed of meperidine 25 mg, promethazine 6.25 mg, and chlorpromazine 6.25 mg per milliliter and is administered via intramuscular injection, to a maximum dose of 0.11 mL/kg or 2.0 mL. In all sedation cases, local anesthesia is administered at the site of the catheter insertion.

When monitored anesthetic care is provided, most anesthesiologists utilize a combination of opioids and benzodiazepines in titrated doses. Both ketamine and propofol by intermittent bolus and by continuous infusion have been successfully used. Propofol has some myocardial depressant action and should be reserved for patients with good myocardial function, whereas ketamine has been demonstrated to have minimal effect on the hemodynamics and respiratory function of patients undergoing catheterization.[61, 186] Sedation and monitored anesthetic care techniques carry a small but definite risk of respiratory compromise.[184, 187]

In considering those patients selected to receive general anesthesia, the anesthetic technique is determined primarily by the myocardial function of the patient. Most children will tolerate induction of anesthesia with sodium thiopental followed by maintenance with inhalational anesthetics (isoflurane) and opioids (fentanyl 3–10 μg/kg). Children with depressed myocardial function can be induced with ketamine 1 to 2 mg/kg. If combined with fentanyl, pancuro-

nium has a minimal effect on heart rate, and, in many young children, the relative tachycardia may be an advantage because the cardiac output is rate dependent. In older children in whom an increase in heart rate may be detrimental, vecuronium can be used, because it lacks a vagolytic effect. In children with near terminally depressed myocardial function and depleted catecholamine stores, ketamine may be contraindicated, acting as a direct myocardial depressant. In these patients, careful titration with fentanyl and midazolam for induction or, alternatively, etomidate may be used. The use of caudal blockade has been proposed as an adjunct for cardiac catheterization. However, this technique does not sedate the child who may have to lie still for several hours, and it may alter hemodynamics. Additionally, it does not facilitate insertion of a subclavian or internal jugular vein catheter. However, such techniques may prove useful for postprocedural analgesia.

Transcatheter ablation of accessory pathways or automatic foci, using radiofrequency energy, has become an effective method for treating many re-entrant and automatic dysrhythmias. The anesthetic management of patients undergoing radiofrequency ablation differs in some respects from the previously described procedures. Radiofrequency energy is a low-power, high-frequency current that enables controlled injury by creating heat at the tip of the catheter. In contrast to direct current, which can cause intense retrosternal pain, radiofrequency ablation is virtually painless. Although most often used in structurally normal hearts as an alternate to surgery, radiofrequency ablation is also used preoperatively and postoperatively to abolish dysrhythmias that occur in children with structural congenital heart disease.[188, 189]

Although there is an extensive body of literature addressing anesthetic agents and their cardiovascular effects, there is little information concerning the effects of these agents on the normal conduction system. Most studies have been performed in adults, using surface electrocardiograph, and have been limited to the proarrhythmic properties of anesthetic agents in combination with endogenous and exogenous catecholamines. Studies of intravenous agents demonstrate that fentanyl, alfentanil, and midazolam had no effect on the accessory pathway refractory period in patients with Wolff-Parkinson-White syndrome, whereas droperidol increases the refractory period.[190] A similar study performed during surgical ablation of accessory pathways in patients with Wolff-Parkinson-White syndrome examined the effects of volatile anesthetic agents and alfentanil.[191] Sufentanil 20 μg/kg, combined with lorazepam 0.06 mg/kg, also had no clinically significant effect on the accessory pathway. A study of volatile agents demonstrated that enflurane (strongest effect), then isoflurane, and halothane (least effect) increased the refractory period within the accessory and normal pathways.[192] A recent study comparing the effects of isoflurane and propofol with those of baseline anesthesia (alfentanil–nitrous oxide–pancuronium) in 20 children with supraventricular tachycardia demonstrated no effect on electrophysiologic measurements.[193]

Postcatheterization Management

Postprocedural management of patients who have undergone interventional procedures is dependent on the hemodynamic status of the patient. A small number of patients will require postprocedural admission to an intensive care facility.[194] Most patients, however, may be recovered in a post-anesthetic care unit for 30 to 60 minutes, where they can be monitored during emergence from anesthesia as well as for possible adverse events related to the procedure. Discomfort, particularly that resulting from the femoral cannulation site and the need for pressure dressing, can be considerable and can be treated with opioids. Nausea and vomiting can be a problem that requires rapid treatment, as the straining may disrupt the femoral cannulation sites.

Outcome of Anesthesia in Children with Heart Disease

Children with heart disease have an increased incidence of cardiovascular complications during anesthesia and surgery, but the magnitude of this risk has not been well documented. In 1966, a 3% anesthetic mortality rate was reported in infants less than 1 year of age undergoing cardiac surgery.[195] Few data are available to document modern mortality from anesthesia in children with heart disease, but a well-managed anesthetic should rarely contribute to mortality and little to morbidity even in the sickest children with cardiac disease.[196]

REFERENCES

1. Benson DWJ: Changing profile of congenital heart disease. Pediatrics 1989;83:790–791.
2. Phornphutkul C, Rosenthal A, Nadas AS, et al: Cerebrovascular accidents in infants and children with cyanotic congenital heart disease. Am J Cardiol 1973;32:329–334.
3. Lister G, Hellenbrand WE, Kleinman CS, et al: Physiologic effects of increasing hemoglobin concentration in left-to-right shunting in infants with ventricular septal defects. N Engl J Med 1982;306:502–506.
4. Fouron JC, Hebert F: The circulatory effects of hematocrit variations in normovolemic newborn lambs. J Pediatr 1973;82:995–1003.
5. Ekert H, Sheers M: Preoperative and postoperative platelet function in cyanotic congenital heart disease. J Thorac Cardiovasc Surg 1974;67:184–190.
6. Kontras SB, Sirak HD, Newton WAJ: Hematologic abnormalities in children with congenital heart disease. JAMA 1966;195:611–615.
7. Rinder CS, Gaal D, Student LA, et al: Platelet-leukocyte activation and modulation of adhesion receptors in pediatric patients with congenital heart disease undergoing cardiopulmonary bypass. J Thorac Cardiovasc Surg 1994;107:280–288.
8. Maurer HM, McCue CM, Robertson LW, et al: Correction of platelet dysfunction and bleeding in cyanotic congenital heart disease by simple red cell volume reduction. Am J Cardiol 1975;35:831–835.
9. Rudolph AM: Congenital Diseases of the Heart. Chicago: Year Book Medical Publishers; 1974.
10. Hansen DD, Hickey PR: Anesthesia for hypoplastic left heart syndrome: Use of high-dose fentanyl in 30 neonates. Anesth Analg 1986;65:127–132.
11. Andrew M, Paes B, Milner R, et al: Development of the human coagulation system in the full-term infant. Blood 1987;70:165–172.
12. Kern FH, Morana NJ, Sears JJ, et al: Coagulation defects in neonates during cardiopulmonary bypass. Ann Thorac Surg 1992;54:541–546.
13. Khuri SF, Valeri CR, Loscalzo J, et al: Heparin causes platelet dysfunction and induces fibrinolysis before cardiopulmonary bypass. Ann Thorac Surg 1995;60:1008–1014.
14. Tabuchi N, de Haan J, Boonstra PW, et al: Activation of fibrinolysis in the pericardial cavity during cardiopulmonary bypass. J Thorac Cardiovasc Surg 1993;106:828–833.
15. Levine MF, Hartley EJ, Macpherson BA, et al: Oral midazolam premedication for children with congenital cyanotic heart disease undergoing cardiac surgery: A comparative study. Can J Anaesth 1993;40:934–938.
16. Stewart KG, Rowbottom SJ, Aitken AW, et al: Oral ketamine premedication for paediatric cardiac surgery: A comparison with intramuscular morphine (both after oral trimeprazine). Anaesth Intensive Care 1990;18:11–14.
17. Warner DL, Cabaret J, Velling D: Ketamine plus midazolam, a most effective paediatric oral premedicant. Pediatr Anaesth 1995;5:293–295.
18. Edelman NH, Lahiri S, Braudo L, et al: The blunted ventilatory response to hypoxia in cyanotic congenital heart disease. N Engl J Med 1970;282:405–411.
19. Praud JP, Carofilis A, Bridey F, et al: Accuracy of two wavelength pulse oximetry in neonates and infants. Pediatr Pulmonol 1989;6:180–182.
20. Fanconi S: Pulse oximetry for hypoxemia: A warning to users and manufacturers. Intensive Care Med 1989;15:540–542.
21. Lazzell VA, Burrows FA: Stability of the intraoperative arterial to end-tidal carbon dioxide partial pressure difference in children with congenital heart disease. Can J Anaesth 1991;38:859–865.
22. Stewart FC, Morana NJ, Sears JJ, et al: Anesthesia laboratory for the pediatric operating room. Int Anesthesiol Clin 1992;30:177–188.
23. Rebeyka IM, Yeh TJ, Hanan SA, et al: Altered contractile response in neonatal myocardium to citrate-phosphate-dextrose infusion. Circulation 1990;82:IV367–IV370.
24. Stone JG, Young WL, Smith CR, et al: Do standard monitoring sites reflect true brain temperature when profound hypothermia is rapidly induced and reversed? Anesthesiology 1995;82:344–351.
25. Adar R, Rubinstein N, Blieden L: Immediate complications and late sequelae of arterial catheterization in children with congenital heart disease. Pediatr Cardiol 1983;4:25–28.
26. Glenski JA, Beynen FM, Brady J: A prospective evaluation of femoral artery monitoring in pediatric patients. Anesthesiology 1987;66:227–229.
27. Gold JP, Jonas RA, Lang P, et al: Transthoracic intracardiac monitoring lines in pediatric surgical patients: A ten-year experience. Ann Thorac Surg 1986;42:185–191.
28. Prince SR, Sullivan RL, Hackel A: Percutaneous catheterization of the internal jugular vein in infants and children. Anesthesiology 1976;44:170–174.
29. Groff DB, Ahmed N: Subclavian vein catheterization in the infant. J Pediatr Surg 1974;9:171–174.
30. Groff DB: Complications of intravenous hyperalimentation in newborns and infants. J Pediatr Surg 1969;4:460–464.
31. Humphrey MJ, Blitt CD: Central venous access in children via the external jugular vein. Anesthesiology 1982;57:50–51.
32. Beekman RH, Rocchini AP, Rosenthal A: Hemodynamic effects of nitroprusside in infants with a large ventricular septal defect. Circulation 1981;64:553–558.
33. Beekman RH, Rocchini AP, Rosenthal A: Hemodynamic effects of hydralazine in infants with a large ventricular septal defect. Circulation 1982;65:523–528.
34. Linday LA, Levin AR, Klein AA, et al: Acute effects of vasodilators on left-to-right shunts in infants and children. Pediatr Pharmacol (New York) 1981;1:267–278.
35. Morray JP, Lynn AM, Mansfield PB: Effect of pH and Pco_2 on pulmonary and systemic hemodynamics after surgery in children with congenital heart disease and pulmonary hypertension. J Pediatr 1988;113:474–479.
36. Morgan P, Lynn AM, Parrot C, et al: Hemodynamic and metabolic effects of two anesthetic techniques in children undergoing surgical repair of acyanotic congenital heart disease. Anesth Analg 1987;66:1028–1030.
37. Tanner GE, Angers DG, Barash PG, et al: Effect of left-to-right, mixed left-to-right, and right-to-left shunts on inhalational anesthetic induction in children: A computer model. Anesth Analg 1985;64:101–107.
38. Friesen RH, Lichtor JL: Cardiovascular depression during halothane anesthesia in infants: Study of three induction techniques. Anesth Analg 1982;61:42–45.
39. Murray DJ, Forbes RB, Mahoney LT: Comparative hemodynamic depression of halothane versus isoflurane in neonates and infants: An echocardiographic study. Anesth Analg 1992;74:329–337.
40. Brandom BW, Brandom RB, Cook DR: Uptake and distribution of halothane in infants: In vivo measurements and computer simulations. Anesth Analg 1983;62:404–410.
41. Cook DR, Brandom BW, Shiu G, et al: The inspired median effective

dose, brain concentration at anesthesia, and cardiovascular index for halothane in young rats. Anesth Analg 1981;60:182–185.

42. Lerman J, Robinson S, Willis MM, et al: Anesthetic requirements for halothane in young children 0–1 month and 1–6 months of age. Anesthesiology 1983;59:421–424.

43. Greeley WJ, Bushman GA, Davis DP, et al: Comparative effects of halothane and ketamine on systemic arterial oxygen saturation in children with cyanotic heart disease. Anesthesiology 1986;65:666–668.

44. Lerman J, Sikich N, Kleinman S, et al: The pharmacology of sevoflurane in infants and children. Anesthesiology 1994;80:814–824.

45. Holzman RS, van der Velde ME, Kaus SJ, et al: Sevoflurane depresses myocardial contractility less than halothane during induction of anesthesia in children. Anesthesiology 1996;85:1260–1267.

46. Friesen RH, Lichtor JL: Cardiovascular effects of inhalation induction with isoflurane in infants. Anesth Analg 1983;62:411–414.

47. Tuman KJ, McCarthy RJ, Spiess BD, et al: Effects of nitrous oxide on coronary perfusion after coronary air embolism. Anesthesiology 1987;67:952–959.

48. Mehta M, Sokoll MD, Gergis SD: Effects of venous air embolism on the cardiovascular system and acid base balance in the presence and absence of nitrous oxide. Acta Anaesthesiol Scand 1984;28:226–231.

49. Banas JSJ, Meister SG, Gazzaniga AB, et al: A simple technique for detecting small defects of the atrial septum. Am J Cardiol 1971;28:467–471.

50. Kronik G, Mosslacher H: Positive contrast echocardiography in patients with patent foramen ovale and normal right heart hemodynamics. Am J Cardiol 1982;49:1806–1809.

51. Lynch JJ, Schuchard GH, Gross CM, et al: Prevalence of right-to-left atrial shunting in a healthy population: Detection by Valsalva maneuver contrast echocardiography. Am J Cardiol 1984;53:1478–1480.

52. Topol EJ, Humphrey LS, Borkon AM, et al: Value of intraoperative left ventricular microbubbles detected by transesophageal two-dimensional echocardiography in predicting neurologic outcome after cardiac operations. Am J Cardiol 1985;56:773–775.

53. Schulte-Sasse U, Hess W, Tarnow J: Pulmonary vascular responses to nitrous oxide in patients with normal and high pulmonary vascular resistance. Anesthesiology 1982;57:9–13.

54. Lappas DG, Buckley MJ, Laver MB, et al: Left ventricular performance and pulmonary circulation following addition of nitrous oxide to morphine during coronary-artery surgery. Anesthesiology 1975;43:61–69.

55. Hickey PR, Hansen DD, Strafford M, et al: Pulmonary and systemic hemodynamic effects of nitrous oxide in infants with normal and elevated pulmonary vascular resistance. Anesthesiology 1986;65:374–378.

56. Murray DJ, Forbes RB, Dull DL, et al: Hemodynamic responses to nitrous oxide during inhalation anesthesia in pediatric patients. J Clin Anesth 1991;3:14–19.

57. Levin RM, Seleny FL, Streczyn MV: Ketamine-pancuronium-narcotic technic for cardiovascular surgery in infants: A comparative study. Anesth Analg 1975;54:800–805.

58. Vaughan RW, Stephen CR: Ketamine for corrective cardiac surgery in children. South Med J 1973;66:1226–1230.

59. Gassner S, Cohen M, Aygen M, et al: The effect of ketamine on pulmonary artery pressure: An experimental and clinical study. Anaesthesia 1974;29:141–146.

60. Hickey PR, Hansen DD, Cramolini GM, et al: Pulmonary and systemic hemodynamic responses to ketamine in infants with normal and elevated pulmonary vascular resistance. Anesthesiology 1985;62:287–293.

61. Morray JP, Lynn AM, Stamm SJ, et al: Hemodynamic effects of ketamine in children with congenital heart disease. Anesth Analg 1984;63:895–899.

62. Anand KJ, Hansen DD, Hickey PR: Hormonal-metabolic stress responses in neonates undergoing cardiac surgery. Anesthesiology 1990;73:661–670.

63. Motomura S, Kissin I, Aultman DF, et al: Effects of fentanyl and nitrous oxide on contractility of blood-perfused papillary muscle of the dog. Anesth Analg 1984;63:47–50.

64. Robinson S, Gregory GA: Fentanyl-air-oxygen anesthesia for ligation of patent ductus arteriosus in preterm infants. Anesth Analg 1981;60:331–334.

65. Hickey PR, Hansen DD: Fentanyl- and sufentanil-oxygen-pancuronium anesthesia for cardiac surgery in infants. Anesth Analg 1984;63:117–124.

66. Laishley RS, Burrows FA, Lerman J, et al: Effect of anesthetic induction regimens on oxygen saturation in cyanotic congenital heart disease. Anesthesiology 1986;65:673–677.

67. Hickey PR, Hansen DD, Wessel DL, et al: Pulmonary and systemic hemodynamic responses to fentanyl in infants. Anesth Analg 1985;64:483–486.

68. Salmenpera M, Peltola K, Takkunen O, et al: Cardiovascular effects of pancuronium and vecuronium during high-dose fentanyl anesthesia. Anesth Analg 1983;62:1059–1064.

69. Maunuksela EL, Gattiker RI: Use of pancuronium in children with congenital heart disease. Anesth Analg 1981;60:798–801.

70. Gruenwald CE, Andrew M, Burrows FA, et al: Cardiopulmonary bypass in the neonate. In: Karp RB, Laks H, Wechsler AS, eds: Advances in Cardiac Surgery. Chicago: Mosby Year Book; 1993:137–156.

71. Hickey PR, Andersen NP: Deep hypothermic circulatory arrest: A review of pathophysiology and clinical experience as a basis for anesthetic management. J Cardiothorac Anesth 1987;1:137–155.

72. Coselli JS, Crawford ES, Beall ACJ, et al: Determination of brain temperatures for safe circulatory arrest during cardiovascular operation. Ann Thorac Surg 1988;45:638–642.

73. Norwood WI, Norwood CR, Ingwall JS, et al: Hypothermic circulatory arrest: 31–phosphorus nuclear magnetic resonance of isolated perfused neonatal rat brain. J Thorac Cardiovasc Surg 1979;78:823–830.

74. Swain JA, McDonald TJJ, Griffith PK, et al: Low-flow hypothermic cardiopulmonary bypass protects the brain. J Thorac Cardiovasc Surg 1991;102:76–83.

75. Nakashima K, Todd MM, Warner DS: The relation between cerebral metabolic rate and ischemic depolarization: A comparison of the effects of hypothermia, pentobarbital, and isoflurane. Anesthesiology 1995;82:1199–1208.

76. Nakashima K, Todd MM: Effects of hypothermia on the rate of excitatory amino acid release after ischemic depolarization. Stroke 1996;27:913–918.

77. Norwood WI, Norwood CR, Castaneda AR: Cerebral anoxia: Effect of deep hypothermia and pH. Surgery 1979;86:203–209.

78. Dexter F, Hindman BJ: Computer simulation of brain cooling during cardiopulmonary bypass. Ann Thorac Surg 1994;57:1171–1178.

79. Hindman BJ, Dexter F: Estimating brain temperature during hypothermia. Anesthesiology 1995;82:329–330.

80. Steen PA, Newberg L, Milde JH, et al: Hypothermia and barbiturates: Individual and combined effects on canine cerebral oxygen consumption. Anesthesiology 1983;58:527–532.

81. Reilly EL, Brunberg JA, Doty DB: The effect of deep hypothermia and total circulatory arrest on the electroencephalogram in children. Electroencephalogr Clin Neurophysiol 1974;36:661–667.

82. Weiss M, Weiss J, Cotton J, et al: A study of the electroencephalogram during surgery with deep hypothermia and circulatory arrest in infants. J Thorac Cardiovasc Surg 1975;70:316–329.

83. Woodcock TE, Murkin JM, Farrar JK, et al: Pharmacologic EEG suppression during cardiopulmonary bypass: Cerebral hemodynamic and metabolic effects of thiopental or isoflurane during hypothermia and normothermia. Anesthesiology 1987;67:218–224.

84. Siegman MG, Anderson RV, Balaban RS, et al: Barbiturates impair cerebral metabolism during hypothermic circulatory arrest. Ann Thorac Surg 1992;54:1131–1136.

85. Reid RW, Warner DS: Pro: arguments for use of barbiturates in infants and children undergoing deep hypothermic circulatory arrest. J Cardiothorac Vasc Anesth 1998;12:591–594.

86. Dexter F, Kern FH, Hindman BJ, et al: The brain uses mostly dissolved oxygen during profoundly hypothermic cardiopulmonary bypass. Ann Thorac Surg 1997;63:1725–1729.

87. Greeley WJ, de Bruijn NP, Davis DP: Sufentanil pharmacokinetics in pediatric cardiovascular patients. Anesth Analg 1987;66:1067–1072.

88. Das JB, Eraklis AJ, Jones JE: Water and solute excretion following cardiopulmonary bypass with hemodilution: The effects of the osmolarity of the perfusion prime. J Thorac Cardiovasc Surg 1969;58:789–794.

89. Bevan DR: Colloid osmotic pressure. Anaesthesia 1980;35:263–270.

90. Anand KJ, Hickey PR: Halothane-morphine compared with high-dose sufentanil for anesthesia and postoperative analgesia in neonatal cardiac surgery. N Engl J Med 1992;326:1–9.

91. Oshita S, Uchimoto R, Oka H, et al: Correlation between arterial blood pressure and oxygenation in tetralogy of Fallot. J Cardiothorac Anesth 1989;3:597–600.

92. Severinghaus JW, Spellman MJJ: Pulse oximeter failure thresholds in hypotension and vasoconstriction. Anesthesiology 1990;73:532–537.

93. Ungerleider RM, Greeley WJ, Sheikh KH, et al: The use of intraoperative echo with Doppler color flow imaging to predict outcome after repair of congenital cardiac defects. Ann Surg 1989;210:526–533.

94. Ungerleider RM, Greeley WJ, Sheikh KH, et al: Routine use of intraoperative epicardial echocardiography and Doppler color flow imaging to guide and evaluate repair of congenital heart lesions: A prospective study. J Thorac Cardiovasc Surg 1990;100:297–309.

95. Greeley WJ, Ungerleider RM: Echocardiography during surgery for congenital heart disease. In: deBruijn NP, Clements FM, eds: Intraoperative Use of Echocardiography. Philadelphia: J B Lippincott Company; 1991:29–156.

96. Lee KY, Molloy DW, Slykerman L, et al: Effects of hydralazine and nitroprusside on cardiopulmonary function when a decrease in cardiac output complicates a short-term increase in pulmonary vascular resistance. Circulation 1983;68:1299–1303.

97. Ziskind Z, Pohoryles L, Mohr R, et al: The effect of low-dose intravenous nitroglycerin on pulmonary hypertension immediately after replacement of a stenotic mitral valve. Circulation 1985;72:64–69.

98. Burrows FA, Klinck JR, Rabinovitch M, et al: Pulmonary hypertension in children: Perioperative management. Can Anaesth Soc J 1986;33:606–628.

99. Prielipp RC, Rosenthal MH, Pearl RG: Hemodynamic profiles of prostaglandin E_1, isoproterenol, prostacyclin, and nifedipine in vasoconstrictor pulmonary hypertension in sheep. Anesth Analg 1988;67:722–729.

100. Heymann MA, Hoffman JIE: Persistent pulmonary hypertension in the newborn. In: Weir EK, Reeves JT, eds: Pulmonary Hypertension. Mount Kisco, New York: Futura Publishing Company; 1984:45–72.

101. Hines R: Post-cardiac surgery pulmonary hypertension. J Cardiothorac Vasc Anesth 1993;7(Suppl):8–11.

102. Morgan JM, McCormack DG, Griffiths MJ, et al: Adenosine as a vasodilator in primary pulmonary hypertension. Circulation 1991;84:1145–1149.

103. Frostell C, Fratacci MD, Wain JC, et al: Inhaled nitric oxide: A selective pulmonary vasodilator reversing hypoxic pulmonary vasoconstriction. Circulation 1991;83:2038–2047.

104. Fratacci MD, Frostell CG, Chen TY, et al: Inhaled nitric oxide: A selective pulmonary vasodilator of heparin-protamine vasoconstriction in sheep. Anesthesiology 1991;75:990–999.

105. Ignarro LJ: Endothelium-derived nitric oxide: actions and properties. FASEB J 1989;3:31–36.

106. Moncada S, Palmer RM, Higgs EA: Nitric oxide: physiology, pathophysiology, and pharmacology. Pharmacol Rev 1991;43:109–142.

107. Yoshimura T: Spectral properties of nitric oxide complexes of cytochrome C' from Alcaligenes sp. NCIB 11015. Biochemistry 1986;25:2436–2442.

108. Mohr R, Martinowitz U, Lavee J, et al: The hemostatic effect of transfusing fresh whole blood versus platelet concentrates after cardiac operations. J Thorac Cardiovasc Surg 1988;96:530–534.

109. Lavee J, Martinowitz U, Mohr R, et al: The effect of transfusion of fresh whole blood versus platelet concentrates after cardiac operations: A scanning electron microscope study of platelet aggregation on extracellular matrix. J Thorac Cardiovasc Surg 1989;97:204–212.

110. Manno CS, Hedberg KW, Kim HC, et al: Comparison of the hemostatic effects of fresh whole blood, stored whole blood, and components after open heart surgery in children. Blood 1991;77:930–936.

111. Golan M, Modan M, Lavee J, et al: Transfusion of fresh whole blood stored (4 degrees C) for short period fails to improve platelet aggregation on extracellular matrix and clinical hemostasis after cardiopulmonary bypass. J Thorac Cardiovasc Surg 1990;99:354–360.

112. Winokur R, Hartwig JH: Mechanism of shape change in chilled human platelets. Blood 1995;85:1796–1804.

113. Miller BE, Mochizuki T, Levy JH, et al: Predicting and treating coagulopathies after cardiopulmonary bypass in children. Anesth Analg 1997;85:1196–1202.

114. van der Poll T, Levi M, Hack CE, et al: Elimination of interleukin 6 attenuates coagulation activation in experimental endotoxemia in chimpanzees. J Exp Med 1994;179:1253–1259.

115. Journois D, Pouard P, Greeley WJ, et al: Hemofiltration during cardiopulmonary bypass in pediatric cardiac surgery: Effects on hemostasis, cytokines, and complement components. Anesthesiology 1994;81:1181–1189.

116. Naik SK, Knight A, Elliott M: A prospective randomized study of a modified technique of ultrafiltration during pediatric open-heart surgery. Circulation 1991;84:422–431.

117. Journois D, Israel-Biet D, Pouard P, et al: High-volume, zero-balanced hemofiltration to reduce delayed inflammatory response to cardiopulmonary bypass in children. Anesthesiology 1996;85:965–976.

118. Kucuk O, Kwaan HC, Frederickson J, et al: Increased fibrinolytic activity in patients undergoing cardiopulmonary bypass operation. Am J Hematol 1986;23:223–229.

119. Petaja J, Peltola K, Sairanen H, et al: Fibrinolysis, antithrombin III, and protein C in neonates during cardiac operations. J Thorac Cardiovasc Surg 1996;112:665–671.

120. Adelman B, Rizk A, Hanners E: Plasminogen interactions with platelets in plasma. Blood 1988;72:1530–1535.

121. Tabuchi N, de Haan J, Boonstra PW, et al: Aprotinin effect on platelet function and clotting during cardiopulmonary bypass. Eur J Cardiothorac Surg 1994;8:87–90.

122. Horrow JC, Van Riper DF, Strong MD, et al: The dose-response relationship of tranexamic acid. Anesthesiology 1995;82:383–392.

123. Karski JM, Dowd NP, Joiner R, et al: The effect of three different doses of tranexamic acid on blood loss after cardiac surgery with mild systemic hypothermia (32 degrees C). J Cardiothorac Vasc Anesth 1998;12:642–646.

124. Reid RW, Zimmerman AA, Laussen PC, et al: The efficacy of tranexamic acid versus placebo in decreasing blood loss in pediatric patients undergoing repeat cardiac surgery. Anesth Analg 1997;84:990–996.

125. Royston D: High-dose aprotinin therapy: a review of the first five years' experience. J Cardiothorac Vasc Anesth 1992;6:76–100.

126. D'Errico CC, Shayevitz JR, Martindale SJ, et al: The efficacy and cost of aprotinin in children undergoing reoperative open heart surgery. Anesth Analg 1996;83:1193–1199.

127. Brown RS, Thwaites BK, Mongan PD, Bouska GW: Aprotonin (AP) offers no advantage over tranexamic acid (TA) in high risk cardiac surgery. Anesthesiology 1995;83:A97.

128. Wong BI, McLean RF, Fremes SE, Harrington EM, Lee E: Aprotinin & tranexamic acid for complex open-heart surgery. Anesth Analg 1995;80:SCA13.

129. Murkin JM, McKenzie FN, White S, Shannon NA, Adams SJ: A comparison of complications of different antifibrinolytics in cardiac surgical patients undergoing repeat median sternotomy. Anesth Analg 1995;80:SCA132.

130. Aoki M, Jonas RA, Nomura F, et al: Effects of aprotinin on acute recovery of cerebral metabolism in piglets after hypothermic circulatory arrest. Ann Thorac Surg 1994;58:146–153.

131. Royston D: Serine protease inhibition prevents both cellular and humoral responses to cardiopulmonary bypass. J Cardiovasc Pharmacol 1996;27(Suppl):1–9.

132. Freeman JG, Turner GA, Venables CW, et al: Serial use of aprotinin and incidence of allergic reactions. Curr Med Res Opin 1983;8:559–561.

133. Diefenbach C, Abel M, Limpers B, et al: Fatal anaphylactic shock after aprotinin reexposure in cardiac surgery. Anesth Analg 1995;80:830–831.

134. Cosgrove DM, Heric B, Lytle BW, et al: Aprotinin therapy for reoperative myocardial revascularization: A placebo-controlled study. Ann Thorac Surg 1992;54:1031–1036.

135. Agnelli G, Gresele P, De Cunto M, et al: Tranexamic acid, intrauterine contraceptive devices and fatal cerebral arterial thrombosis: Case report. Br J Obstet Gynaecol 1982;89:681–682.

136. Davies D, Howell DA: Tranexamic acid and arterial thrombosis. Lancet 1977;1:49.

137. Rydin E, Lundberg PO: Tranexamic acid and intracranial thrombosis. Lancet 1976;2:49.

138. Woo KS, Tse LK, Woo JL, et al: Massive pulmonary thromboembolism after tranexamic acid antifibrinolytic therapy. Br J Clin Pract 1989;43:465–466.

139. Hocker JR, Saving KL: Fatal aortic thrombosis in a neonate during infusion of epsilon-aminocaproic acid. J Pediatr Surg 1995;30:1490–1492.

140. Razis PA, Coulson IH, Gould TR, et al: Acquired C_1 esterase inhibitor deficiency. Anaesthesia 1986;41:838–840.

141. Parsons MR, Merritt DR, Ramsay RC: Retinal artery occlusion associated with tranexamic acid therapy. Am J Ophthalmol 1988;105:688–689.

142. Goldstein DJ, DeRosa CM, Mongero LB, et al: Safety and efficacy

of aprotinin under conditions of deep hypothermia and circulatory arrest. J Thorac Cardiovasc Surg 1995;110:1615–1621.

143. Regragui IA, Bryan AJ, Izzat MB, et al: Aprotinin use with hypothermic circulatory arrest for aortic valve and thoracic aortic surgery: Renal function and early survival. J Heart Valve Dis 1995;4:674–677.

144. Hornick P, Taylor KM: Is aprotinin safe when used in the context of profound hypothermia and circulatory arrest? A literary review. J Heart Valve Dis 1995;4:669–673.

145. Smith CR, Mongero LB, DeRosa CM, et al: Safety of aprotinin in profound hypothermia and circulatory arrest. Ann Thorac Surg 1994;58:606–608.

146. Sundt TM, Kouchoukos NT, Saffitz JE, et al: Renal dysfunction and intravascular coagulation with aprotinin and hypothermic circulatory arrest. Ann Thorac Surg 1993;55:1418–1424.

147. Hindmarsh KW, Sankaran K, Watson VG: Plasma beta-endorphin concentrations in neonates associated with acute stress. Dev Pharmacol Ther 1984;7:198–204.

148. Greeley WJ, Leslie JB, Su M, Davis DP, Xuan T, Watkins WD: Plasma atrial natriuretic peptide release during pediatric cardiovascular anesthesia and surgery. Anesthesiology 1986;65:A414.

149. Anand KJS, Sippell WG, Aynsley-Green A: Randomized trial of fentanyl anaesthesia in preterm babies undergoing surgery: Effects on the stress response. Lancet 1987;1:62–66.

150. Anand KJ, Hickey PR: Pain and its effects in the human neonate and fetus. N Engl J Med 1987;317:1321–1329.

151. Anand KJ, Sippell WG, Schofield NM, et al: Does halothane anaesthesia decrease the metabolic and endocrine stress responses of newborn infants undergoing operation? Br Med J (Clin Res Ed) 1988; 296:668–672.

152. Swedberg K, Eneroth P, Kjekshus J, et al: Hormones regulating cardiovascular function in patients with severe congestive heart failure and their relation to mortality. CONSENSUS Trial Study Group. Circulation 1990;82:1730–1736.

153. Steward DJ, DaSilva CA, Flegel T: Elevated blood glucose levels may increase the danger of neurological deficit following profoundly hypothermic cardiac arrest. Anesthesiology 1988;68:653.

154. Ellis DJ, Steward DJ: Fentanyl dosage is associated with reduced blood glucose in pediatric patients after hypothermic cardiopulmonary bypass. Anesthesiology 1990;72:812–815.

155. Hickey PR, Hansen DD, Wessel DL, et al: Blunting of stress responses in the pulmonary circulation of infants by fentanyl. Anesth Analg 1985;64:1137–1142.

156. Haxholdt OS, Kehlet H, Dyrberg V: Effect of fentanyl on the cortisol and hyperglycemic response to abdominal surgery. Acta Anaesthesiol Scand 1981;25:434–436.

157. Giesecke K, Hamberger B, Jarnberg PO, et al: High- and low-dose fentanyl anaesthesia: Hormonal and metabolic responses during cholecystectomy. Br J Anaesth 1988;61:575–582.

158. Walsh ES, Paterson JL, O'Riordan JB, et al: Effect of high-dose fentanyl anaesthesia on the metabolic and endocrine response to cardiac surgery. Br J Anaesth 1981;53:1155–1165.

159. Hickey PR, Hansen DD: High-dose fentanyl reduces intraoperative ventricular fibrillation in neonates with hypoplastic left heart syndrome. J Clin Anesth 1991;3:295–300.

160. Blair JR, Pruett JK, Introna RP, et al: Cardiac electrophysiologic effects of fentanyl and sufentanil in canine cardiac Purkinje fibers. Anesthesiology 1989;71:565–570.

161. Saini V, Carr DB, Hagestad EL, et al: Antifibrillatory action of the narcotic agonist fentanyl. Am Heart J 1988;115:598–605.

162. Hickey PR, Wessel DL: Anesthesia for treatment of congenital heart disease. In: Kaplan JA, ed. Cardiac Anesthesia, vol. 2, 2nd ed. New York: Grune & Stratton; 1987:635–724.

163. Burrows FA, Taylor RH, Hillier SC: Early extubation of the trachea after repair of secundum-type atrial septal defects in children. Can J Anaesth 1992;39:1041–1044.

164. Laussen PC, Reid RW, Stene RA, et al: Tracheal extubation of children in the operating room after atrial septal defect repair as part of a clinical practice guideline. Anesth Analg 1996;82:988–993.

165. de Bruijn NP, Clements FM, Kisslo JA: Intraoperative transesophageal color flow mapping: Initial experience. Anesth Analg 1987;66:386–390.

166. Nussbaum J, Zane EA, Thys DM: Esmolol for the treatment of hypercyanotic spells in infants with tetralogy of Fallot. J Cardiothorac Anesth 1989;3:200–202.

167. Geary V, Thaker U, Chalmers P, et al: Esmolol in tetralogy of Fallot. J Cardiothorac Anesth 1989;3:524–526.

168. Lang P, Chipman CW, Siden H, et al: Early assessment of hemodynamic status after repair of tetralogy of Fallot: A comparison of 24 hour (intensive care unit) and 1 year postoperative data in 98 patients. Am J Cardiol 1982;50:795–799.

169. Gelman S, Reves JG, Fowler K, et al: Regional blood flow during cross-clamping of the thoracic aorta and infusion of sodium nitroprusside. J Thorac Cardiovasc Surg 1983;85:287–291.

170. Symbas PN, Pfaender LM, Drucker MH, et al: Cross-clamping of the descending aorta: Hemodynamic and neurohumoral effects. J Thorac Cardiovasc Surg 1983;85:300–305.

171. Baylen BG, Ogata H, Ikegami M, et al: Left ventricular performance and regional blood flows before and after ductus arteriosus occlusion in premature lambs treated with surfactant. Circulation 1983;67:837–843.

172. Burke RP: Video-assisted thoracoscopic surgery for patent ductus arteriosus. Pediatrics 1994;93:823–825.

173. Lavoie J, Burrows FA, Hansen DD: Video-assisted thoracoscopic surgery for the treatment of congenital cardiac defects in the pediatric population. Anesth Analg 1996;82:563–567.

174. Lavoie J, Javorski JJ, Donahue K, et al: Detection of residual flow by transesophageal echocardiography during video-assisted thoracoscopic patent ductus arteriosus interruption. Anesth Analg 1995;80:1071–1075.

175. Sudan N, Kosarussavadi B, Rothstein P, et al: Transport of children following cardiothoracic surgery. Anesthesiology 1985;55:A337.

176. Palmisano BW, Fisher DM, Willis M, et al: The effect of paralysis on oxygen consumption in normoxic children after cardiac surgery. Anesthesiology 1984;61:518–522.

177. Vacanti JP, Crone RK, Murphy JD, et al: The pulmonary hemodynamic response to perioperative anesthesia in the treatment of high-risk infants with congenital diaphragmatic hernia. J Pediatr Surg 1984;19:672–679.

178. Wessel DL, Adatia I, Thompson JE, et al: Delivery and monitoring of inhaled nitric oxide in patients with pulmonary hypertension. Crit Care Med 1994;22:930–938.

179. Javorski JJ, Hansen DD, Laussen PC, et al: Paediatric cardiac catheterization: Innovations. Can J Anaesth 1995;42:310–329.

180. Wessel DL, Keane JF, Parness I, et al: Outpatient closure of the patent ductus arteriosus. Circulation 1988;77:1068–1071.

181. Grady RM, Eisenberg PR, Bridges ND: Rational approach to use of heparin during cardiac catheterization in children. J Am Coll Cardiol 1995;25:725–729.

182. Bridges ND, Lock JE, Castaneda AR: Baffle fenestration with subsequent transcatheter closure: Modification of the Fontan operation for patients at increased risk. Circulation 1990;82:1681–1689.

183. Bridges ND, Perry SB, Keane JF, et al: Preoperative transcatheter closure of congenital muscular ventricular septal defects. N Engl J Med 1991;324:1312–1317.

184. Hickey PR, Wessel DL, Streitz SL, et al: Transcatheter closure of atrial septal defects: Hemodynamic complications and anesthetic management. Anesth Analg 1992;74:44–50.

185. Dajani AS, Taubert KA, Wilson W, et al: Prevention of bacterial endocarditis. Recommendations by the American Heart Association. JAMA 1997;277:1794–1801.

186. Smith I, White PF, Nathanson M, et al: Propofol: An update on its clinical use. Anesthesiology 1994;81:1005–1043.

187. Malviya S, Burrows FA, Johnston AE, et al: Anaesthetic experience with paediatric interventional cardiology. Can J Anaesth 1989; 36:320–324.

188. Van Hare GF, Lesh MD, Stanger P: Radiofrequency catheter ablation of supraventricular arrhythmias in patients with congenital heart disease: Results and technical considerations. J Am Coll Cardiol 1993;22:883–890.

189. Levine JC, Walsh EP, Saul JP: Radiofrequency ablation of accessory pathways associated with congenital heart disease including heterotaxy syndrome. Am J Cardiol 1993;72:689–693.

190. Gomez-Arnau J, Marquez-Montes J, Avello F: Fentanyl and droperidol effects on the refractoriness of the accessory pathway in the Wolff-Parkinson-White syndrome. Anesthesiology 1983;58:307–313.

191. Sharpe MD, Dobkowski WB, Murkin JM, et al: Alfentanil-midazolam anaesthesia has no electrophysiological effects upon the normal conduction system or accessory pathways in patients with Wolff-Parkinson-White syndrome. Can J Anaesth 1992;39:816–821.

192. Sharpe MD, Dobkowski WB, Murkin JM, et al: The electrophysiologic effects of volatile anesthetics and sufentanil on the normal atrioventricular conduction system and accessory pathways in Wolff-Parkinson-White syndrome. Anesthesiology 1994;80:63–70.

193. Lavoie J, Walsh EP, Burrows FA, et al: Effects of propofol or isoflurane anesthesia on cardiac conduction in children undergoing radiofrequency catheter ablation for tachydysrhythmias. Anesthesiology 1995;82:884–887.

194. Laussen PC, Hansen DD, Perry SB, et al: Transcatheter closure of ventricular septal defects: Hemodynamic instability and anesthetic management. Anesth Analg 1995;80:1076–1082.

195. Strong MJ, Keats AS, Cooley DA: Anesthesia for cardiovascular surgery in infancy. Anesthesiology 1966;27:257–265.

196. Hickey PR, Hansen DD, Norwood WI, et al: Anesthetic complications in surgery for congenital heart disease. Anesth Analg 1984;63:657–664.

19

Management of the Patient with Repaired or Palliated Congenital Heart Disease

Maureen A. Strafford

Repaired Congenital Heart Disease

   Definitive Repair

   Palliative Repair

   Interventional Cardiac Catheterization Repair

Outcome After Repair

Preoperative Factors Influencing Outcome After Cardiac Repair

   Age at Time of Repair

   Preoperative Cyanosis and Polycythemia

   Preoperative Congestive Heart Failure

   Preoperative Dysrhythmias

   Preoperative Pulmonary Hypertension

Potential Issues of Concern in the Repaired Congenital Heart Disease Patient

   Associated Noncardiac Defects

   Monitoring Concerns

   Psychosocial Concerns

   Endocarditis Risk

Surgical Repairs and Natural History Studies Defining Long-Term Outcome

   Patent Ductus Arteriosus

   Coarctation of the Aorta

   Atrial Septal Defect

   Ventricular Septal Defect

   Atrioventricular Septal Defect

   Tetralogy of Fallot

   Transposition of the Great Arteries

Nonsurgical Repairs (Interventional Cardiac Catheterization) and Natural History Studies Defining Long-Term Outcome

   Valvular Lesions: Dilatation

   Vascular Angioplasties

   Coarctation of the Aorta

   Pulmonary Artery Stenosis

   Systemic Venous Obstructions

   Cardiovascular Stents

   Opening of Atrial Communications

   Closure of Communications: Intracardiac and Extracardiac

   Risk Assessment

Perioperative Evaluation of Repaired Congenital Heart Disease

The child with congenital heart disease (CHD) is no longer a rare clinical challenge for the pediatric anesthesiologist. Patients with CHD have benefited from advances in pediatric medicine and surgery; survival for patients with even the most complex lesions is now a real possibility. The American Heart Association in 1996 estimated that 300,000 children under the age of 21 had CHD and approximately 1,000,000 children and adults are alive with CHD. At least 35 different congenital cardiac defects are recognized. Thirty-eight percent of patients under 21 years of age with CHD have undergone one or more cardiac surgical procedures. From 1986 to 1996, death rates for congenital cardiovascular defects declined 25%. Every year, approximately 32,000 infants are born with CHD, many requiring immediate neonatal intervention.[1-3] Table 19–1 presents common abbreviations to describe the spectrum of congenital heart lesions.

Table 19–1. Common Abbreviations for Anatomic Terms

Abbreviation	Term
AoDT	Descending truck of the aorta
AsAo	Ascending aorta
ASD	Atrial septal defect (1° = primum, 2° = secundum)
AVVR	Atrioventricular valvular regurgitation
CAVC	Complete atrioventricular canal (an endocardial cushion defect)
CoA	Coarctation of the aorta
CS	Coronary sinus
DILV	Double inlet left ventricle
DORV	Double outlet right ventricle
HLHS	Hypoplastic left heart syndrome
IVC	Inferior vena cava
IVS	Intact ventricular septum
MCA	Multiple congenital anomalies
LVOTO	Left ventricular outflow tract obstruction
PA	Pulmonary artery *or* pulmonic atresia
PDA	Patent ductus arteriosus
PFC	Persistent fetal circulation
PFO	Patent foramen ovale
PS	Pulmonic stenosis
SCA	Subclavian artery
SI	Situs inversus
SV	Single ventricle
SVC	Superior vena cava
TA	Tricuspid atresia
TAPVR	Total anomalous pulmonary venous return; same as TAPVC (C = connection). Also PAPVR/PAPVC (P = partial)
TGA	Transposition of the great arteries; sometimes TGV (V = vessels)
TOF	Tetralogy of Fallot
VSD	Ventricular septal defect

A better understanding of the dynamic nature of neonatal cardiac physiology, advances in cardiac surgery, better perfusion techniques, improved perioperative and anesthetic care (e.g., advanced ventilatory strategies and improved pharmacologic agents), and major advances in the techniques of interventional cardiac catheterization are just a few of the factors that have resulted in a large, and an increasing, cohort of CHD patients who survive the critical neonatal and infant period, often after complex cardiac surgical procedures. Every year, an increasing number of patients with complex congenital heart lesions reach adulthood in good health. As we follow this group of patients over time, we have gained additional perspective from numerous natural history studies in the fields of pediatric cardiology and cardiac surgery. For several congenital heart defects, these studies and the insights gained from them have directly led to new surgical and medical approaches that result in improved survival as well as improved long-term lifespan, quality of life, and cardiac function.

In light of this optimistic situation, does the *repaired* CHD patient present any concerns for the pediatric anesthesiologist? Unlike the child with *unrepaired* CHD, in whom symptoms of cyanosis, dysrhythmias, or congestive heart failure alert the anesthesiologist to an altered and potentially unstable hemodynamic situation, the repaired CHD patient is often asymptomatic and appears well. Nevertheless, subtle but important abnormalities in cardiac physiology may be unmasked by the stress of surgery and anesthesia. This chapter addresses important issues associated with the anesthetic evaluation and management of children with repaired CHD. In many ways, this chapter serves to introduce the pediatric anesthesiologist to an overview of the ever-increasing long-term natural history literature that spans several decades. In addition, the information outlined in this chapter provides important background so that effective consultation with pediatric cardiologists and pediatric cardiac surgeons can be made. Although it is impossible to review all the lesions that can occur in CHD patients, it is the aim of this chapter to review the more common lesions. In addition, the long-term outcome in patients who are repaired nonsurgically, that is, an increasing number of patients who have undergone repair in the interventional cardiac catheterization laboratory, are reviewed. The wealth of natural history data for specific lesions is informative, but over several decades we also have learned that there are some general conclusions about long-term outcome that can be applied to all lesions. Factors that influence long-term outcome are reviewed and may serve as a helpful algorithm in preanesthetic evaluation and perioperative management.

Repaired Congenital Heart Disease

Definitive Repair

When we discuss the CHD patient who has undergone *definitive repair*, we assume that the patient has undergone cardiac surgical repair that results in normal physiology (although not necessarily normal anatomy) and that the patient will experience an improved quality of life and lifespan. In addition, further cardiac surgical intervention is not anticipated. The improvement in quality of life in the definitively repaired patient is often dramatic and immediate. Cardiac symptoms resolve. Exercise tolerance improves. Children undergo growth spurts and function as healthy children. However, the improvement in lifespan, especially for more complicated defects, may be less well defined. Aggressive neonatal cardiac surgical repair for many lesions has only been performed for two to three decades, and long-term comprehensive follow-up data are studied closely. Natural history studies therefore are an extremely valuable source of information for pediatric cardiologists and cardiac surgeons. Analysis of these data has led to dramatic changes in the initial surgical and medical approaches when problems are identified over long-term follow-up. The best example of this is the current management of transposition of the great arteries. Transposition of the great arteries was considered an unrepairable defect for many infants even 40 years ago. Intra-atrial repair, such as the Mustard and Senning operations, transformed the dismal prognosis into dramatic survival rates. However, follow-up studies (which are further detailed in another part of this chapter) revealed a disturbing pattern of dysrhythmias, ventricular failure, and other abnormalities as patients survived decades after repair. As a result of these natural history studies, an entirely different approach to repair, the arterial switch operation, became the standard for neonatal repair of transposition of the great arteries. Even early and mid-term follow-up studies of the arterial switch operation are confirming that this shift in surgical technique has been a wise choice for patients with transposition of the great arteries.

Palliative Repair

In contrast to definitive repair, *palliative repair* implies that future procedures are anticipated and necessary to restore the patient to a state of normal physiology and to improve lifespan. Certain lesions do not lend themselves to final definitive repair. The group of patients with single ventricle physiology is an example of this type of patient. Patients with single ventricle physiology have complete admixture of systemic venous and pulmonary venous blood. The Fontan procedure was originally used for patients with tricuspid atresia but has now been applied to a variety of other lesions, including hypoplastic left heart syndrome. The goal of the Fontan procedure is to separate the mixing of the pulmonary venous and systemic venous circulations. As a result, the right atrium becomes the "pumping chamber" for systemic venous blood and the remaining ventricle (it may be a left or right ventricle depending on the defect) becomes the systemic ventricle. After the Fontan procedure, future definitive procedures are not anticipated, but the defect in these patients is best considered palliated rather than definitively repaired. This group of patients represents an ever-increasing group of patients who present for management of noncardiac surgery (see later discussion). Many of these patients appear well and are asymptomatic. However, their underlying physiology presents important challenges under the stress of anesthesia and surgery.

Interventional Cardiac Catheterization Repair

In view of the dramatic advances in the interventional cardiac catheterization laboratory, many patients with CHD are now amenable to definitive repair in the cardiac catheterization laboratory and survive without the mark of a sternal or thoracotomy scar. Natural history follow-up data for this group of patients are also being collected and carefully reviewed.

Outcome After Repair

Every cardiac procedure carries inherent risk. Even after the immediate risk of surgery has passed, the patient may still have cardiac residua, sequelae, or complications as a result of the procedure. Knowledge of the surgical procedure and the potential residua, sequelae, and complications may not be readily known to the anesthesiologist who is evaluating a patient with repaired CHD. This chapter reviews some of the more common cardiac surgical procedures and the potential residua, sequelae, and complications of those procedures. As a result, the pediatric anesthesiologist will have a more informed perspective from which to create a safe and effective anesthetic plan.

Residua are defined as abnormalities that were part of the original defect that are still present after surgical repair. For example, it is often surgically difficult to close multiple small muscular ventricular septal defects; therefore, the patient may be left with a small residual ventricular septal defect. The residual ventricular septal defect is considered a residuum of the procedure. If it is hemodynamically significant, it may require further intervention. In general, residua should be surgically avoidable.

In contrast, the *sequelae* of an operation may not be avoidable. The sequelae of an operation may be of minimal concern or ultimately a major concern. For example, a patient with transposition of the great arteries who undergoes a Mustard or Senning procedure has a rerouting of blood at the atrial level. This is an unavoidable sequela of choosing an atrial procedure for transposition of the great arteries repair. As a result, the right ventricle after a Mustard or Senning procedure becomes the systemic ventricle. Long-term studies after Mustard or Senning repair revealed a disturbing increase in right ventricular (i.e., systemic ventricular) failure over time.

A *complication* of a procedure is considered an avoidable problem. For example, the left anterior descending coronary artery may cross the right ventricular outflow tract in a patient with tetralogy of Fallot. Since patients undergoing tetralogy of Fallot repair most often require a right ventriculotomy across the right ventricular outflow tract, failure to recognize the left anterior descending coronary vessel in the right ventricular outflow tract may result in the serious complication of left anterior descending coronary vessel compromise, which could cause myocardial infarction.

Preoperative Factors Influencing Outcome After Cardiac Repair

Natural history studies have provided information about specific cardiac lesions after repair as well as some general conclusions regarding outcome for all CHD patients. For example, certain preoperative factors appear to influence both short-term and long-term outcome after definitive repair. These historical facts are important to elicit from the patient, parents, and pediatric cardiologist or cardiac surgeon and by a thorough review of the medical record.

Age at Time of Repair

Prior to the availability of bypass and the possibility of the repair of intracardiac defects, closed heart procedures for repair of patent ductus arteriosus (PDA) and coarctation of the aorta and the Blalock-Taussig shunt for cyanotic heart disease had been pioneering surgical events. The era of modern open-heart cardiac surgery was ushered in with the advent of cardiopulmonary bypass techniques. Despite these major advances, neonatal and infant repair did not seem plausible for many years. The introduction of deep hypothermic circulatory arrest, better perfusion equipment and techniques, improved surgical and anesthetic techniques, advances in neonatal and pediatric intensive care medicine, including ventilatory and monitoring equipment, and safer pharmacologic agents all contributed to advances in earlier repair (i.e., in a neonate or infant). Nevertheless, definitive surgical repair during the neonatal and infant periods remained controversial. For example, many centers advocated a multistaged approach to surgical repair of certain lesions (e.g., the cyanotic neonate/infant with tetralogy of Fallot would undergo a palliative procedure such as a Blalock-Taussig [systemic artery to pulmonary artery] shunt as a first-stage repair). Cyanosis would be improved although not eliminated, and the child would undergo a definitive repair at a later date. Other more aggressive pediatric cardiac surgical centers advocated a one-stage neonatal or infant repair rather then a multistaged palliative repair. Over the last decade, natural history studies have confirmed the advantages of early, definitive infant repair for many lesions. Cardiac abnormalities such as cyanosis, polycythemia, pulmonary hypertension, and dysrhythmias may clinically improve or resolve after repair, but the long-term effects on the cardiovascular system may, in fact, be more significant and become more clinically overt as time passes after repair. For example, a one-stage repair of tetralogy of Fallot in a patient younger than 1 year of age has been shown to improve the incidence of long-term dysrhythmia risk when compared with children who underwent repair after 1 year of age.

Preoperative Cyanosis and Polycythemia

The goal of any definitive cardiac repair is to eliminate cyanosis and the body's compensatory response of polycythemia. Both cyanosis and polycythemia have subtle, important, but still not completely well understood effects on cardiac function and pulmonary vascular hemodynamics that cause long-term effects. It is well known that cyanosis leads to polycythemia as the body's response to an increased need for tissue oxygen delivery. However, there is a price to pay with the increasing hematocrit. Hyperviscosity of blood as a result of high hematocrits (in the 60–75 % range) has deleterious secondary effects acutely, chronically, and even after repair and resumption of normal hematocrits. Both systemic and pulmonary vascular resistances increase exponentially as blood viscosity increases and coronary arterial blood flow decreases. The presence of polycythemia, coupled with the increased risk of thrombus formation at high hematocrits, may increase the risk of coronary artery insufficiency even with normal coronary artery anatomy. This relative coronary artery insufficiency may be asymptomatic, although angina and myocardial infarction have been described in polycythemic patients. It may be that chronic polycythemia results in asymptomatic subendocardial ischemia and eventually subendocardial fibrosis over time. The duration and degree of hypoxemia and polycythemia that the patient experienced are important historical factors for the evaluation of possible long-term residual cardiac muscle blood flow abnormalities.

Preoperative Congestive Heart Failure

The heart's response to increased volume or pressure work is well understood (see also Chapter 17). The neonatal heart is in many ways a more dynamic organ than the fully mature heart. Research in the area of neonatal cardiac response to pressure or volume overload has resulted in a better understanding of the age-dependent mechanisms in normal cardiac growth and pressure-induced left ventricular hypertrophy. Unlike in the adult or older child, normal postnatal myocardial growth is dramatically affected by hemodynamic factors. There is an initial early hyperplastic phase that includes myocytes and capillaries and then a myocyte hypertrophic phase. Of interest, the neonate who has a pressure overload imposed will have the induction of both myocyte hyperplasia and hypertrophy. In contrast, only myocyte hy-

pertrophy is observed at a later age. Multiple factors influence these observed changes. Importantly, the capacity to develop hyperplasia is age-related, being greater in the neonate and young infant. As the child ages, a more adult model of hypertrophy is observed. Clinically, this has been well demonstrated in the neonate and young infant in the arterial switch operation, in which the left ventricle can be prepared for systemic work before the switch by having a pulmonary artery band placed. The left ventricle hypertrophies and can accept systemic work within a matter of days, usually less than a week.[4, 5]

Preoperative Dysrhythmias

Dysrhythmias may be present in many CHD patients before definitive repair and may reflect the effects of chronic chamber enlargement or an intrinsic risk of rhythm disturbances associated with specific lesions. While dysrhythmias often improve or resolve after definitive repair, follow-up studies indicate that over time the patient with preoperative dysrhythmias is at higher risk for the long-term reappearance of a rhythm disturbance. Some patients may be at risk for a dysrhythmia even with minimal hemodynamic compromise. For example, the patient with an atrial septal defect usually has minimal cardiovascular dysfunction both preoperatively and postoperatively. Nevertheless, over time, despite an excellent surgical result and normal cardiac function, these patients appear to be at greater risk of atrial dysrhythmias over their lifespan. In addition, surgical repair, especially with prosthetic materials such as intracardiac patches, presents a possible focus for dysrhythmias as fibrosis occurs along suture lines. It is important to note that the diagnosis of a dysrhythmia may not be obvious on surface electrocardiograph (ECG) alone and that more comprehensive diagnostic testing, such as Holter monitoring, event monitoring, exercise testing, and invasive electrophysiologic studies, may be more revealing. In certain groups at higher risk for dysrhythmias, such as patients with postoperative tetralogy of Fallot and transposition of the great arteries (following Mustard or Senning procedures), these tests may be routinely ordered. Any patient who is at risk for a postoperative dysrhythmia may first manifest this abnormality under the stress of surgery. Infants and young children are not able to provide a history of palpitations or chest discomfort at the time of a dysrhythmia. Usually, a dysrhythmia must be sustained or significantly impair cardiac function to be detected in this age group. If a patient who is at risk for a dysrhythmia after cardiac surgery reports a symptom, such as dizziness or near syncope, that may be due to an undiagnosed dysrhythmia, this information is worthy of thorough preoperative evaluation. *Even a brief dysrhythmia without cardiovascular compromise in certain patients during anesthesia may be indicative of an underlying problem worthy of further investigation postoperatively.* It is therefore important to convey such information to the cardiology team caring for the patient in follow-up. Tables 19–2 and 19–3[6] summarize the incidence of arrhythmias in patients with preoperative congenital heart defects as well as the incidence in patients following surgical repair. Table 19–4 presents a commonly used grading system for severity of dysrhythmias.[7]

Table 19–2. Incidence of Arrhythmias in Patients with Unrepaired Congenital Heart Defects

Cardiac Defect	Atrial Flutter Fibrillation	PSVBs	Sinus Bradycardia, Junctional Rhythm	Wolff Parkinson White Syndrome	Supraventricular Tachycardia	AV Block	PVBs	Ventricular Tachycardia, Sudden Death
Sinus venosus and secundum ASD	+ to +++,*		+ to ++	**	**	0 to +,*		
Ebstein's anomaly	+ to ++,*			++	++			**,†
Pulmonary valve stenosis		++						
VSD		++		**	**		++	+
AVSD				**	**			
PDA	0 to +++,*			**	+	**	+	
Tetralogy of Fallot				**	+		0 to +++,*	
Aortic valve stenosis	0 to +++,*	+		**	+ to ++		+ +,†	**,†
Coarctation of the aorta				**	**/**,†			**,†
d-TGA	0 to +	0 to +	+ to +++ (intermittent)		**	+ to ++		0 to +
l-TGA	‡			**	++	+ to ++		++ to +++
Polysplenia	‡		+ to +++,*	**	**	++		
Asplenia	‡		+	**	**	**		
Tricuspid atresia	‡			+	+			
Eisenmenger physiology			**,† (paroxysxmal)				+++	++

PSVBs, premature supraventricular beats exceeding normal for age; PVBs, premature ventricular beats exceeding normal for age; +, up to 10% incidence; ++, 10–40% incidence; +++, 40–60% incidence; ++++, 60–90% incidence; *, progressive incidence with age; **, reported but incidence not established; †, progressive incidence with advancement of hemodynamic abnormality; ‡, related to highly prevalent associated abnormalities; ASD, atrial septal defect; VSD, ventricular septal defect; AVSD, atrioventricular septal defect; PDA, patent ductus arteriosus; TGA, transposition of the great arteries.
From Kanter RJ: Syncope and sudden death. In: Garson A Jr, Bricker JT, Fisher DJ, Neish SR, eds: The Science and Practice of Pediatric Cardiology, 2nd ed, Vol. II. Baltimore: Williams & Wilkins; 1998:2172.

Preoperative Pulmonary Hypertension

The presence of pulmonary hypertension preoperatively can influence the morbidity and mortality in the immediate postoperative period. In fact, improved neonatal surgical outcome is in many ways a direct result of improved management of this clinical challenge both intraoperatively and postoperatively. Prolonged pulmonary hypertension preoperatively, even if only for the first few months or years of life, may result in permanent structural changes in the pulmonary arterial bed that may have long-lasting effects, even in the face of improved clinical status after repair. The level of severity of pulmonary hypertension and the length of time that pulmonary hypertension existed before definitive repair are both factors that may influence residual problems after repair.

Potential Issues of Concern in the Repaired Congenital Heart Disease Patient

Associated Noncardiac Defects

Up to 25% of children with CHD have an associated extracardiac malformation, often as part of a multiple malformation syndrome.[8] These noncardiac defects may require surgical repair either before or after definitive surgical repair of the cardiac lesion. Airway abnormalities that may stress the potent and important interaction of the cardiopulmonary systems deserve special attention. Certain surgical procedures (e.g., compared to noncongenital heart disease patients, CHD patients have a higher incidence of scoliosis that requires surgical repair) with the stress of large blood loss, positional changes, and long operative time may create problems even for the asymptomatic post-repair CHD patient.

Monitoring Concerns

The repaired CHD patient may have undergone one or more predefinitive repair procedures. Obtaining venous and arterial access may be difficult in the patient who has had multiple surgical procedures, vascular cutdowns, and catheterization procedures. The patient who has had a Blalock-Taussig shunt (subclavian artery to pulmonary artery shunt), commonly utilized for palliative treatment of many cyanotic lesions, may have an inaccurate blood pressure reading on the side of the upper extremity where the shunt was placed. The patient who has had a right Blalock-Taussig shunt may have an inaccurate blood pressure reading on the right arm, even after takedown of the shunt at the time of definitive repair. In coarctation of the aorta, the left subclavian artery may arise at or beyond the narrowed coarctation area. As a result, these patients may have a lower blood pressure on the left upper extremity, since the left subclavian may arise beyond the narrowed coarctation area. A difference between right and left arm blood pressure readings in patients who have had coarctation of the aorta repair may reflect the presence of a residual coarctation or re-coarctation. Patients who have undergone Fontan repair may be at increased risk for superior vena cava thrombus. For this reason, central venous pressure monitoring via the right internal jugular vein may be contraindicated or, if needed, used for the shortest possible time perioperatively.

Psychosocial Concerns

Most children who have undergone multiple hospitalizations and procedures will present unique psychosocial issues at

Table 19–3. Incidence of Chronic Arrhythmias in Postoperative Repaired Congenital Heart Defect Patients

Procedure	Atrial Flutter Fibrillation	Sinus, Junctional Bradycardia	SVPBs	Complete AV Block	Pacemaker Requirement	VPBs	Ventricular Tachycardia	Sudden Death
Mustard, Senning operation	++ to +++	+++ to ++++++,*		+ to ++	+++		+++,†	++ to ++++++,†
Fontan operation	++++	**		**	+++ to +++++		+++,†	++
Tetralogy of Fallot	+++,##			++	**	Up to +++++*/†‡	Up to ++++,†/##	++
Ebstein's anomaly		++	Up to ++++					++ to +++,##
Pulmonic stenosis						Up to +++ to ++++	Up to +++,*	+
Atrial septal defect	+ to ++++++,‡			**	Up to ++			
Ventricular septal defect							Up to ++++++,†	++
Aortic stenosis						Up to +++++,†	+++ to +++++,†	++ to +++

SVPBs, supraventricular premature beats; VPBs, ventricular premature beats; *, related to time since surgery; **, reported, but incidence not established; †, highest with longer time since surgery; #, includes ventricular tachycardia inducibility during electrophysiology study; ##, highest with hemodynamic compromise; ‡, related to presence of preoperative arrhythmia; +, 0–1% incidence; ++, 1–5% incidence; +++, 5–10% incidence; ++++, 10–20% incidence; +++++, 20–60% incidence.

From Kanter RJ: Syncope and sudden death. In: Garson A Jr, Bricker JT, Fisher DJ, Neish SR, eds: The Science and Practice of Pediatric Cardiology, 2nd ed, Vol. II. Baltimore: Williams & Wilkins; 1998:2172.

Table 19–4. Arrhythmia Severity Scoring System

Lown Arrhythmia Score	Arrhythmia
0	No ventricular ectopic beats
1	Occasional isolated ventricular premature beats
2	Frequent ventricular premature beats (> 1/min or 30/hour)
3	Multiform ventricular premature beats
4	Repetitive ventricular premature beats
a	Couplets
b	Salvos
5	Early ventricular premature beats

From Lown V, Calvert AF, Armington R, Ryan M: Monitoring for serious arrhythmias and high risk of sudden death. Circulation 1975;51–52:III189–III198.

the time of a repeat surgical procedure, even if it is a minor procedure in a healthy child with minimal anticipated risk. Despite good health, parents may still experience increased anxiety and separation issues at the time of surgery. In addition, parents may be concerned when the healthy child who has undergone definitive CHD repair is still considered at increased risk; thus the discussion of anesthetic risk must be sensitively addressed. Although many parents are quite knowledgeable about the status of their child's cardiac function and follow-up, it is nevertheless essential to consult with the cardiology team regarding details of the child's history.

Endocarditis Risk

Children with CHD, even after definitive repair, are still at risk for bacterial endocarditis; however, the exact risk and incidence are not well defined. One study reviewed the 30-year incidence of infective endocarditis after surgery for CHD of all Oregon residents who had surgical repair for 1 of 12 major CHD lesions at the age of 18 years or younger from 1958 to 1998.[9] At 25 years after surgery, the cumulative

incidence of endocarditis was 1.3% for tetralogy of Fallot, 2.7% for isolated ventricular septal defects, 3.5% for coarctation of the aorta, 13.3% for valvular aortic stenosis, and 2.8% for primum atrial septal defects. At 20-year follow-up, transposition of the great arteries had a 4.0% incidence. At 10 years, complete atrioventricular canal defects had a 1.1% incidence, whereas the rate was 5.3% for pulmonary atresia with intact ventricular septum and 6.4% for pulmonary atresia with ventricular septal defect. In this cohort, no children with secundum atrial septal defects, PDA, or pulmonic stenosis had infective endocarditis after surgery. The American Heart Association guidelines for subacute bacterial endocarditis (infective endocarditis) prophylaxis are outlined in Tables 19–5 to 19–8.[10]

Surgical Repairs and Natural History Studies Defining Long-Term Outcome

Congenital heart disease is often complex, with multiple lesions present in combination; the surgical approach may be modified depending on the unique combination of lesions. It is impossible to review all anatomic defects and medical and surgical approaches since these are so numerous and treatment continues to evolve. However, an overview of the most common lesions, especially those for which natural history data are most extensively available, will enable the anesthesiologist to have a more informed perspective from which to implement a safe and effective anesthetic plan.

Patent Ductus Arteriosus

Patent ductus arteriosus can be present in isolation or in association with virtually all other congenital heart defects. In the neonate with a critical cardiac malformation, pulmonary or systemic blood flow may be dependent on the continued patency of the ductus arteriosus. The premature neonate with lung disease may also maintain patency of the ductus. These "ducts" are in many cases "physiologic" ducts, and the patency responds to different levels of oxygen tension

Table 19–5. Cardiac Conditions Associated with Endocarditis

Endocarditis Prophylaxis Recommended	Endocarditis Prophylaxis Not Recommended

High-risk category
  Prosthetic cardiac valves, including bioprosthetic and homograft valves
  Previous bacterial endocarditis
  Complex cyanotic congenital heart disease (e.g., single ventricle states, transposition of the great arteries, tetralogy of Fallot)
  Surgically constructed systemic pulmonary shunts or conduits
Moderate-risk category
  Most other congenital cardiac malformations (other than above and below)
  Acquired valvular dysfunction (e.g., rheumatic heart disease)
  Hypertrophic cardiomyopathy
  Mitral valve prolapse with valvar regurgitationa and/or thickened leaflets*
	Negligible-risk category (no greater risk than the general population)
	  Isolated secundum atrial septal defect
	  Surgical repair of atrial septal defect, ventricular septal defect, or patent ductus arteriosus (without residua beyond 6 months)
	  Previous coronary artery bypass graft surgery
	  Mitral valve prolapse without valvular regurgitation*
	  Physiologic, functional, or innoent heart murmurs*
	  Previous Kawasaki disease without valvular dysfunction
	  Previous rheumatic fever without valvular dysfunction
	  Cardiac pacemakers (intravascular and epicardial) and implanted defibrillators

*See references for further details.
From Dajani AS, Taubert KA, Wilson W, et al: Prevention of bacterial endocarditis. Recommendations by the American Heart Association. JAMA 1997;227:1794–1801. Copyright 1997, American Medical Association.

Table 19–6. Nondental Procedures and Endocarditis Prophylaxis

Endocarditis Prophylaxis Recommended	Endocarditis Prophylaxis Not Recommended

Respiratory tract
  Tonsillectomy and/or adenoidectomy
  Surgical operations that involve respiratory mucosa
  Bronchoscopy with a rigid bronchoscope
Gastrointestinal tract*
  Sclerotherapy for esophageal varices
  Esophageal stricture dilation
  Endoscopic retrograde cholangiography with biliary obstruction
  Biliary tract surgery
  Surgical operations that involve intestinal mucosa
Genitourinary tract
  Prostatic surgery
  Cystoscopy
  Urethral dilation
	Respiratory tract
	  Endotracheal intubation
	  Bronchoscopy with a flexible bronchoscope, with or without biopsy†
	  Tympanostomy tube insertion
	Gastrointestinal tract
	  Transesophageal echocardiography†
	  Endoscopy with or without gastrointestinal biopsy†
	Genitourinary tract
	  Vaginal hysterectomy†
	  Vaginal delivery†
	  Cesarean section
	  In uninfected tissue
	    Urethral catheterization
	    Uterine dilatation and curettage
	    Therapeutic abortion
	    Sterilization procedures
	    Insertion or removal of intrauterine devices
	Other
	  Cardiac catheterization, including balloon angioplasty
	  Implanted cardiac pacemakers, implanted defibrillators, and coronary stents
	  Incision or biopsy of surgically scrubbed skin
	  Circumcision

*Prophylaxis is recommended for high-risk patients; optional for medium-risk patients.
†Prophylaxis is optional for high-risk patients.
From Dajani AS, Taubert KA, Wilson W, et al: Prevention of bacterial endocarditis: Recommendations by the American Heart Association. JAMA 1997;277:1794–1801. Copyright 1997, American Medical Association.

as well as prostaglandins and other humoral influences. However, the true anatomic PDA does not close normally during the first days of life, and, when isolated as a lesion, it may remain asymptomatic in the infant and child until a continuous murmur is detected.

Surgical Repair

The modern era of cardiac surgery was heralded when Gross reported the first successful surgical procedure for a congeni-

tal heart defect with the ligation of a PDA in a child in 1938.[11] This was considered an innovative, heroic, and pioneering surgical procedure (Fig. 19–1). Today, because of major advances in interventional catheterization procedures, patients with an isolated PDA now routinely undergo transcatheter closure in the catheterization laboratory rather than surgical closure via a thoracotomy (see later discussion). Nevertheless, in many ways, patients who have undergone definitive surgical repair of a PDA remain among the group of patients with the least risk of residua, sequelae, and

Table 19–7. Prophylactic Regimens for Dental, Oral, Respiratory Tract, or Esophageal Procedures

Situation	Agent	Regimen*
Standard general prophylaxis	Amoxicillin	Adults: 2.0 g; children: 50 mg/kg orally 1 h before procedure
Unable to take oral medications	Ampicillin	Adults: 2.0 g IM or IV; children: 50 mg/kg IM or IV within 30 min before procedure
Allergic to penicillin	Clindamycin *or*	Adults: 600 mg; children: 20 mg/kg orally 1 h before procedure
	Cephalexin† or Cefadroxil† *or*	Adults: 2.0 g; children: 50 mg/kg orally 1 h before procedure
	Azithromycin or Clarithromycin	Adults: 500 mg; children: 15 mg/kg orally 1 h before procedure
Allergic to penicillin and unable to take oral medications	Clindamycin *or*	Adults: 600 mg; children: 20 mg/kg IV within 30 min before procedure
	Cefazolin†	Adults: 1.0 g; children: 25 mg/kg IM or IV within 30 min before procedure

IM = intramuscular; IV = intravenous.
*Total children's dose should not exceed adult dose.
†Cephalosporins should not be used in individuals with immediate-type hypersensitivity reaction (urticaria, angioedema, or anaphylaxis) to penicillins.
From Dajani AS, Taubert KA, Wilson W, et al: Prevention of bacterial endocarditis: Recommendations by the American Heart Association. JAMA 1997;277:1794–1801. Copyright 1997, American Medical Association.

Table 19–8. Prophylactic Regimens for Genitourinary and Gastrointestinal (Excluding Esophageal) Procedures

Situation	Agents*	Regiment†*
High-risk patients	Ampicillin plus gentamicin	Adults: ampicillin 2.0 g IM or IV plus gentamicin 1.5 mg/kg (not to exceed 120 mg) within 30 min of starting the procedure; 6 h later, ampicillin 1 g IM/IV or amoxicillin 1 g orally Children: ampicillin 50 mg/kg IM or IV (not to exceed 2.0 g) plus gentamicin 1.5 mg/kg within 30 min of starting the procedure; 6 h later, ampicillin 25 mg/kg IM/IV or amoxicillin 25 mg/kg orally
High-risk patients allergic to ampicillin/amoxicillin	Vancomycin plus gentamicin	Adults: vancomycin 1.0 g IV over 1–2 h plus gentamicin 1.5 mg/kg IV/IM (not to exceed 120 mg); complete injection/infusion within 30 min of starting the procedure Children: vancomycin 20 mg/kg IV over 1–2 h plus gentamicin 1.5 mg/kg IV/IM; complete injection/infusion within 30 min of starting the procedure
Moderate-risk patients	Amoxicillin or ampicillin	Adults: amoxicillin 2.0 g orally 1 h before procedure, or ampicillin 2.0 g IM/IV within 30 min of starting the procedure Children: amoxicillin 50 mg/kg orally 1 h before procedure, or ampicillin 50 mg/kg IM/IV within 30 min of starting the procedure
Moderate-risk patients allergic to ampicillin/amoxicillin	Vancomycin	Adults: vancomycin 1.0 g IV over 1–2 h; complete infusion within 30 min of starting the procedure Children: vancomycin 20 mg/kg IV over 1–2 h; complete infusion within 30 min of starting the procedure

IM = intramuscular; IV = intravenous.
*Total children's dose should not exceed adult dose.
†No second dose of vancomycin or gentamicin is recommended.
From Dajani AS, Taubert A, Wilson W, et al: Prevention of bacterial endocarditis: Recommendations by the American Heart Association. JAMA 1997;277:1794–1801. Copyright 1997, American Medical Association.

complications after cardiac surgery.[12–15] Except for the premature infant who has ligation (without routine division) of a duct, the standard surgical procedure is ligation and division of the ductus.

Residua

Residua include the rare possibility of recanalization or incomplete initial ligation; these problems, though rare, are seen after ligation procedures only.

Sequelae

After successful surgical repair, the sequelae of PDA closure are rare. If a PDA is undiagnosed and goes untreated into adulthood, pulmonary hypertension, congestive heart failure, infective endocarditis, and even pulmonary vascular disease may be seen in later life. The sequela of this prolonged abnormal physiology is the possibility of pulmonary hypertension persisting after ligation (in adulthood). Today, however, it is an extremely rare occurrence for a PDA to remain

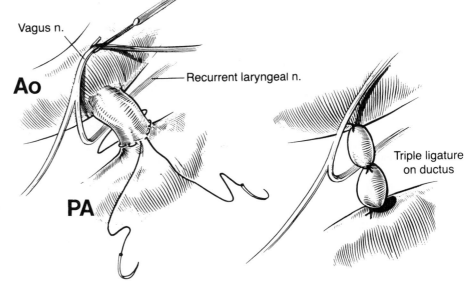

Figure 19–1. Ligation of patent ductus arterious (PDA). This schematic representation of ligation of PDA illustrates the close proximity of the recurrent laryngeal nerve and the vagus nerve. Division of the PDA is also performed, except in the premature infant. Ao, aorta; PA, pulmonary artery. (Modified from Castaneda AR, Jonas RA, Mayer JE Jr, Hanley FL: Patent ductus arteriosus. In: Castaneda AR, Jonas RA, Mayer JE Jr, Hanley FL, eds: Cardiac Surgery of the Neonate and Infant. Philadelphia: W.B. Saunders; 1994: 209.)

undiagnosed. Almost uniformly, the isolated PDA is diagnosed and the patient undergoes successful treatment within the first few years of life and can be expected to live a normal, healthy life without cardiovascular compromise. With respect to anesthetic risk, these children post-repair should be treated as healthy children and do not even require endocarditis prophylaxis (the exception being those patients who undergo device closure in the catheterization laboratory, see later).

Complications

Complications of the procedure include injury to the recurrent laryngeal nerve or disruption of the thoracic duct with resultant chylothorax. More serious complications include incorrect ligation of nearby structures such as the left pulmonary artery, the descending aorta, or even the carotid artery. These are usually immediately evident and catastrophic complications.[9-12]

Coarctation of the Aorta

Coarctation of the aorta accounts for 7.5% of critically ill infants with heart disease and 5 to 10% of congenital cardiac lesions. Coarctation of the aorta is often associated with other cardiac and noncardiac lesions and in congenital syndromes such as Turner syndrome.[16-19] Approximately 50% of patients with coarctation of the aorta have associated cardiac lesions, most commonly left-sided obstructive or hypoplastic defects and ventricular septal defects.[20] A bicommissural aortic valve is found in 85% of these patients.[21] In addition to Turner syndrome, noncardiac abnormalities in the musculoskeletal, respiratory, genitourinary, and gastrointestinal systems are described in about 25% of patients.[22] Berry aneurysms of the circle of Willis occur in 3 to 10% of patients.[23] *Patients with coarctation of the aorta should be suspected to have multisystem abnormalities even after repair.*

Coarctation of the aorta is a narrowing of the lumen of the aorta and has been classically divided into *infantile* and *adult* forms. This pathologic description may be somewhat artificial. A long-segment diffuse narrowing, including hypoplasia and underdevelopment of the aortic arch and isthmus of the aorta, is seen in the infantile form. The adult form is described as a discrete narrowing in the region of the insertion of the ductus arteriosus into the aorta (Fig. 19–2). Eighty-five percent of neonates with coarctation of the aorta will have a major associated cardiac lesion that often causes significant hemodynamic compromise. On the other hand, the discrete narrowing of the adult form may be an isolated lesion and may escape detection in the neonatal and infancy periods, since upper extremity hypertension may be the only symptom of the isolated coarctation of the aorta. With routine blood pressure screening in early childhood, coarctation of the aorta should usually be detected on routine physical examination in infancy and no later than early childhood.

Surgical Repair

In 1945, Crafoord and Nylin[24] and Gross and Hufnagel[25] reported successful repair of coarctation of the aorta via resection of the narrowed site and end-to-end anastomosis of the aorta. More than 50 years later and even though modifications have been performed, this surgical approach remains the preferred method for treating the adult or discrete form of coarctation of the aorta and is advocated in the infant form as well in certain situations. Figure 19–3 illustrates alternative surgical approaches for coarctation of the aorta repair, which include patch aortoplasty, left subclavian flap angioplasty, extended resection and anastomosis, and reverse subclavian flap aortoplasty. Many of the modifications that have developed over the past 50 years have been developed to address the difficult management of the infantile coarctation anatomy and the risk of re-coarctation. The diffuse, narrowed isthmus and hypoplasia of the aortic arch make a resection and end-to-end anastomosis more technically difficult for the infantile form of coarctation. Some centers have advocated a modification of this surgical approach called an extended resection and anastomosis. In addition, one of the important goals of neonatal/infant coarctation repair is to enhance normal growth of the aorta so that the risk for re-coarctation is minimized.

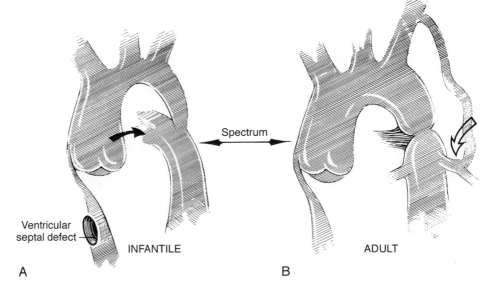

Figure 19–2. Infantile and adult forms of coarctation of the aorta. The infantile form of coarctation of the aorta (A) shows a more diffuse hypoplasia of the aortic arch. In fact, the ductus arteriosus can be larger than the aortic arch at the area of the coarctation (solid curved arrow). In contrast, the adult form of coarctation (B) is more discrete. Collaterals (open curved arrow) can form as illustrated in the adult form diagram (B) and will be seen as rib-notching on routine chest radiograph. (From Castaneda AR, Jonas RA, Mayer JE Jr, Hanley FL: Aortic coarctation. In: Castaneda AR, Jonas RA, Mayer JE Jr, Hanley FL, eds: Cardiac Surgery of the Neonate and Infant. Philadelphia: W.B. Saunders; 1994: 334.)

Ventricular septal defect

INFANTILE

A

Spectrum

ADULT

B

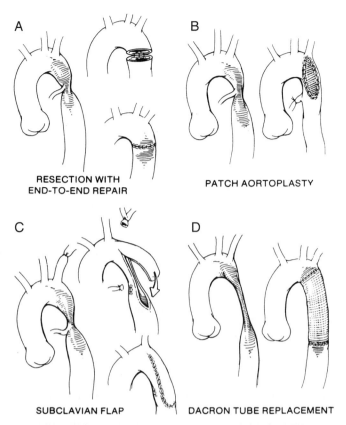

Figure 19-3. Surgical repair of coarctation of the aorta. There are a variety of technical approaches to coarctation repair, depending on the age of the child as well as the underlying anatomy: (A) Resection with end-to-end repair, (B) patch aortoplasty, (C) subclavian flap. In addition, repair of re-coarctation may be approached differently with a Dacron tube placement (D). (From Morriss MJH, McNamara DG: Coarctation of the aorta and interrupted aortic arch. In: Garson A Jr, Bricker JT, McNamara DG, eds: The Science and Practice of Pediatric Cardiology. Philadelphia: Lea & Febiger; 1990: 1334.)

Left subclavian patch aortoplasty was reported by Waldhausen and Nahrwold in 1966 (see Fig. 19–3).[26] This approach uses the left subclavian artery as a native patch. The subclavian artery is ligated and divided distally and then turned down. As a result, the narrowed area of the aorta is enlarged, native vascular tissue is used, and a circumferential suture line is avoided. The vertebral artery is ligated to avoid subclavian steal and the left subclavian is also sacrificed.

Interposition grafts bridging the ascending and descending aorta can bypass the coarctation. Obviously, this prosthetic material does not grow and presents the additional risk of calcification and narrowing. These bridging grafts have been used in patients who have had serious multiple episodes of re-coarctation.

Since coarctation of the aorta has been amenable to surgical repair for more than 50 years, there is a significant body of literature on the natural history of this defect after surgical repair. We now know that even after successful coarctation repair, patients still carry an increased risk of long-term residua, sequelae, and complications. For example, the long-term clinical course of 646 patients repaired at the Mayo Clinic between 1946 and 1981 was reviewed. Of these

patients, 571 were available for long-term follow-up. The survival rate was 91% at 10, 84% at 20, and 72% at 30 years after surgery. The most common cause of death was premature coronary artery disease, followed by sudden death, heart failure, cerebrovascular accidents, and ruptured aortic aneurysm. In this group of patients, age at repair was an important predictor of survival. The 20-year survival rate was 91% for those operated on before 14 years of age but only 79% for patients operated on after 14 years.[27–30] Additional studies have reinforced the important role of early repair in decreasing long-term cardiovascular morbidity and mortality. Clearly, patients with unrepaired coarctation with sustained upper extremity hypertension experience negative cardiovascular function when followed long-term. Age at time of repair also influences long-term outcome (see later discussion).

Residua

The obvious residua associated with this repair are the risk of residual or recurrent coarctation. *Age at the time of repair* and *type of surgical procedure* affect the risk of re-coarctation. A review of several surgical series reveals a wide range of overall risk of re-coarctation (3% to 41%).[27, 31–33] In one series, infants had a 26% risk of re-coarctation compared with 3% for all patients.[27] Another paper reported a 19% restenosis rate for neonates and 5% for infants.[32] Backer's series revealed a 50% rate in infants younger than 1 month and 4% for patients older than 1 month,[31] whereas another study revealed that patients operated on before 2 years of age had a 13% restenosis risk, compared with a 0.7% risk after 2 years of age.[33]

The *type of surgical repair* is also a predictor for re-coarctation risk. Some centers reported a lower rate of re-coarctation after subclavian flap aortoplasty (11%) compared with end-to-end anastomosis (23%) and patch aortoplasty (27%).[34] On the other hand, results vary from center to center and may reflect surgical preference and experience as well as patient selection.[28, 35, 36] It is clear that no single technique can be declared superior to the others in minimizing re-coarctation risk. An alternative to surgical repair, namely interventional cardiac catheterization angioplasty, has added a further area of discussion to this risk assessment, since many centers advocate interventional angioplasty for initial and re-coarctation repair (see later discussion).

Sequelae

The patient who has undergone coarctation repair still has an abnormal aorta and may have significant abnormalities in cardiac function and vascular reactivity even if successful relief of stenosis has been achieved. Although 97 to 98% of long-term survivors of coarctation repair have New York Heart Association (NYHA) class I disease and report no cardiovascular symptoms, abnormalities are sometimes present.[29, 37] Even in the face of a successful hemodynamic result, echocardiographic studies have shown persistence of myocardial hypertrophy with impaired diastolic left ventricular function. Left ventricular systolic function is often normal or hyperdynamic. Premature coronary artery disease, myocardial infarction, and congestive heart failure are seen in 12% of patients 11 to 15 years after surgery; most notably these are patients who underwent repair in late childhood or early adulthood.[38]

Hypertension can be seen in patients following coarctation repair even with an apparent excellent surgical repair. An upper extremity blood pressure reading in the post-repair patient cannot be interpreted without a corresponding lower extremity measurement to assess the possibility of a gradient across the coarctation site. In addition, the absence of a gradient measured at rest does not rule out the possibility of a residual gradient during exercise or with stress. This exercise-induced gradient may over time contribute to the observed abnormalities in left ventricular function and left ventricular hypertrophy.[39–43] Finally, the post-repair patient might only demonstrate such a gradient during the stress of surgery, with perioperative pain or anxiety. *Hypertension in such a patient might be the first opportunity to recognize a gradient and should not be ignored.*

One of the major risk factors for persistent hypertension over a long-term period is the duration of preoperative hypertension. Several studies have suggested an increased incidence of systemic hypertension with increasing length of follow-up: 13% at 8 years, 49% at 17 years, and 68% at 30 years.[28, 44] As a result, most pediatric cardiologists recommend early elective repair; some advocating repair in the first year of life rather than in the school-aged child as was the recommendation a decade ago.

Complications

The immediate complications of coarctation of the aorta repair include damage to the recurrent laryngeal nerve, the phrenic nerve, or the thoracic duct. Rebound or paradoxical hypertension can be seen in the immediate postoperative period, probably due to a baroreceptor-mediated increase in sympathetic activity and a reflex vasospasm in the vascular beds distal to the coarctation. Vasopressin increases and atrial natruretic factor decreases immediately after coarctation repair.[45–47] Post-coarctectomy syndrome (abdominal pain and bowel dysfunction) is also seen acutely and may represent mesenteric arteritis. Finally, the most serious complication of coarctation repair is spinal cord injury due to compromised or interrupted spinal cord arterial blood flow, seen in 0.5% of patients.[48]

Atrial Septal Defect

Historically, atrial septal defect, like PDA and coarctation of the aorta, is also one of the earliest surgically repaired lesions. Therefore, it is a congenital lesion for which many long-term natural history studies exist. In the early 1940s and 1950s, surgeons attempted various closed (non-bypass) methods for closure, followed by open heart repairs and eventually repair using cardiopulmonary bypass.[49–53] There are several different anatomic forms of ASD (Fig. 19–4).[54] Risk factors for postoperative residua, sequelae, and complications vary depending on the anatomic defect. Most patients with an ASD are relatively asymptomatic from the cardiovascular standpoint both preoperatively and postoperatively. Nevertheless, the nature of the surgical repair and the intrinsic defect can predispose these patients to certain long-term problems, even in the presence of an asymptomatic cardiovascular status. In addition, many types of ASDs are amenable to device closure in the cardiac catheterization laboratory (see later discussion).[55]

The four types of ASDs are ostium secundum, sinus venosus, coronary sinus, and ostium primum. These are different anatomic defects but present with similar pathophysiology; namely, a communication between the right and left atrium that results in a left-to-right shunt and increased pulmonary blood flow. Left unrepaired, excessive pulmonary blood flow over decades may lead to pulmonary vascular obstructive disease. Atrioventricular canal defects, or ostium primum ASD, are discussed in a separate section because atrioventricular canal defects often have major abnormalities of the atrioventricular valves and the ventricular septum. ASDs are also commonly seen in association with other cardiac defects; this discussion focuses on those patients who have an ASD as the major defect and the consequences

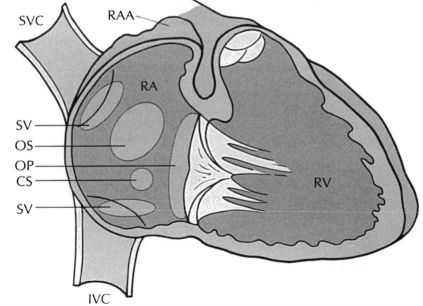

Figure 19–4. Diagrammatic representation of the sites of communication between the atria, shown from the perspective of the right atrium. The ostium secundum (OS) defect is typically located in the area of the fossa ovalis, the most common site for an atrial communication, and results from a deficiency in the septum primum. The ostium primum (OP) defect is adjacent to the atrioventricular valve. The sinus venosus (SV) defect is adjacent to the superior vena cava (SVC) or the inferior vena cava (IVC). The coronary sinus septum can be deficient and result in a coronary sinus (CS) defect. RA, right atrium; RV, right ventricle. (From Silverman N: The secundum atrial septal defect and atrioventricular septal defects. In: Freedom RM, Braunwald E, eds: Atlas of Heart Diseases, Congenital Heart Disease, Vol. XII, St. Louis: Mosby; 1997: 12.2.)

of that lesion on follow-up. Patients with an isolated ASD have a high incidence of associated cardiac defects. For example, right ventricular enlargement may cause a leftward shift of the ventricular septum; this geometric change causes mitral valve prolapse.

OSTIUM SECUNDUM ATRIAL SEPTAL DEFECT. The most common of ASDs, the ostium secundum defect, is located in the area of the fossa ovalis. Depending on the size and whether multiple defects, or fenestrations, are present, this type of ASD has also been treated with interventional device closure in the catheterization laboratory.

SINUS VENOSUS ATRIAL SEPTAL DEFECT. Sinus venosus defects are located in the atrial septum near the superior vena cava orifice. Because the right upper and middle lobe pulmonary veins usually attach to the low superior vena cava or superior vena cava–right atrium junction, partial anomalous pulmonary venous return may be seen with a sinus venosus defect.

CORONARY SINUS ATRIAL SEPTAL DEFECT. The common wall between the coronary sinus and the left atrium is either partially or completely absent in coronary sinus defects; a persistent superior vena cava is also frequently present.

OSTIUM PRIMUM ATRIAL SEPTAL DEFECT. The atrioventricular septum is absent in ostium primum ASD. In this condition, the ASD occurs anterior to the fossa ovalis (and the anterior limbus). This type of defect often is associated with abnormalities of the mitral valve and may include a ventricular component as well. This abnormality is discussed in detail under the section on atrioventricular septal defects.

Preoperative Factors Influencing Outcome After Repair

A patient with an ASD has increased pulmonary blood flow as a result of left-to-right shunting. Congestive heart failure and pulmonary artery hypertension are rare before repair, but if they are left uncorrected, as time passes, the incidence of these abnormalities increases. The rate at which elevated pulmonary vascular resistance occurs is variable. Some patients with large shunts may survive into the sixth or seventh decade of life without pulmonary vascular obstructive disease, but pulmonary vascular obstructive disease has been described in children as young as 2 years of age.[56] Other factors may contribute to the variability of progression to pulmonary vascular obstructive disease in patients with ASD. For example, a biologically deficient form of von Willebrand factor may contribute to an accelerated form of pulmonary vascular obstructive disease in patients with CHD, including ASD.[57] Patients who live at high altitudes or in certain areas of the world (Vellore, India) may be at greater risk of developing pulmonary hypertension early in life.[58, 59]

Although congestive heart failure, pulmonary artery hypertension, and pulmonary vascular obstructive disease are rare in the preoperative ASD patient, the incidence of dysrhythmias is not. *The presence of preoperative dysrhythmias may indicate an increased risk of postoperative dysrhythmias,* even with excellent repair and normal cardiovascular status. In a study of 108 preoperative ASD patients (age

range, 3 to 63 years), patients with large left-to-right shunts had an increased incidence of atrial dysrhythmias.[60] Large shunt and advanced age were predictive of risk for atrial dysrhythmias. Patients with pulmonary to systemic blood flow ratios (Qp/Qs) of 2:1 or less had an 11% incidence of preoperative atrial dysrhythmias, but patients with a Qp/Qs of 3:1 or greater had a 38% incidence of preoperative atrial dysrhythmias.

Age at time of repair is clearly a risk factor for preoperative atrial dysrhythmias. Fifty percent of patients over the age of 30 years at the time of repair had atrial dysrhythmias, whereas only 25% of patients under 30 years of age exhibited atrial dysrhythmias preoperatively. The presence or absence of pulmonary hypertension was not predictive of the risk of atrial dysrhythmias. Serious atrial dysrhythmias may be symptomatic (e.g., atrial fibrillation, atrial flutter, and supraventricular tachycardia) and clearly predominate in the unrepaired older patient.[61] Patients younger than 18 years at the time of repair have a much lower risk for preoperative atrial dysrhythmias; in one study, only 2% of 204 younger patients exhibited preoperative atrial dysrhythmias.[62] In a study of 123 patients who had undergone secundum or sinus venosus atrial septal defect repair, 4% required pacemakers and two developed complete atrioventricular block. On late follow-up (27 to 32 years), atrial flutter or fibrillation increased with an increase in age at repair from 4% if repair occurred before the age of 11 years up to 59% if surgery occurred after the age of 41 years.[63] Symptomatic sinus node dysfunction was described in 7.5% of 269 patients after ASD repair.[64]

Surgical Repair

Surgical repair is indicated in patients with large secundum ASDs, although noninvasive repair with a closure device is increasingly an option. Closure of the defect may be suture closure alone if the anatomy lends itself to such closure or with a patch closure of most defects. The closure of small defects or of a patent foramen ovale is more controversial. Since any potential communication between the right and left side of the heart carries the risk of paradoxical right-to-left shunting and stroke, closure of small defects or patent foramen ovale is advocated by some. For example, an association has been described between patent foramen ovale and cryptogenic stroke. In addition, patients with a patent foramen ovale have undergone catheter closure because of a history of paradoxical embolic phenomena.[65–67]

Residua and Sequelae

The most obvious residuum after ASD repair is a residual atrial shunt. In addition, cardiac enlargement and ECG evidence of right ventricular hypertrophy may also be considered a residuum after surgery. Despite asymptomatic cardiac status, most children with ASD have cardiac enlargement on chest radiograph and right ventricular hypertrophy on ECG preoperatively. Although most children have resolution of these abnormalities in follow-up, complete resolution is not the rule. A follow-up study of 71 children operated on for ASD secundum repair demonstrated that only 65% had a normal chest radiograph 2 years after repair. Twenty-seven percent showed persistence of cardiac enlargement on chest radiograph after many years. Eighty-six percent of children had a normalization of the ECG, showing fewer right ventricular forces and less rightward axis deviation within a short period after surgery. However, 4% of children did show persistence of right ventricular hypertrophy on ECG over the long term.[68] When right ventricular size is examined by echocardiogram in ASD secundum patients, both preoperatively and postoperatively, 80% of children had evidence of right ventricular dilatation for a period of up to 5 years.[63] The finding of persistent right ventricular dilatation has also been confirmed at cardiac catheterization when preoperative and 1-year postoperative right ventricular volumes were examined.[56, 69]

Ventricular Septal Defect

Ventricular septal defect (VSD) is the most common cardiac defect found in children and is often found in combination with other lesions or in more complex cardiac malformations. This section focuses on patients with isolated VSD who require surgical repair. In surveys of large pediatric cardiac clinics, 20 to 29% of patients have VSD.[70–72] Not all patients with VSD require surgical repair, since approximately 35 to 40% of small defects spontaneously close and do not require surgical intervention. Closure usually occurs before 2 years of age, and 80% of isolated muscular defects in the trabecular septum close spontaneously.[72–80]

The nomenclature describing the anatomy of VSD has changed over recent decades, mainly because of an improved ability to visualize and define the anatomy more precisely with angiographic and echocardiographic studies. The precise definition of VSD location and size is essential for accurate and complete surgical repair. In addition, the surgeon must be aware of the location of the VSD in relation to the conduction system and the best possible surgical approach to close the VSD completely without injury to the conduction system. If at all possible, a transatrial approach through the right atrium is preferred, primarily because a ventriculotomy is avoided. Other approaches include through the great vessels. Because of the trabeculated anatomy of the right ventricular septum, muscular VSDs are often surgically difficult to approach via a transatrial or right ventriculotomy. Obviously the least desirable approach is through a left ventriculotomy, especially in the small neonatal or infant heart. A patient who undergoes a ventriculotomy has an area of ventricular scarring and fibrosis that over time may contribute to decreased ventricular performance or act as an area for the genesis of a dysrhythmia. The closure of any VSD carries the risk of conduction system injury or damage. Figure 19–5[81] schematically demonstrates the anatomic location of the conduction system and its close proximity to important conduction system landmarks. Figure 19–6[82] describes the regions of the ventricular septum and the location of various types of VSDs as seen from both the right ventricular and the left ventricular aspect.

The patient with a large VSD has increased pulmonary blood flow as a result of a large left-to-right shunt, and the resultant pulmonary hypertension causes congestive heart failure. Medical management of congestive heart failure is often only a short-term intervention in the neonate or young infant with severe congestive heart failure. The risk of permanent pulmonary arterial bed remodeling and the development of irreversible pulmonary vascular obstructive disease are life-threatening possibilities. Pulmonary vascular obstructive disease has been observed in patients with a large left-to-right shunt and pulmonary hypertension within the first 2 years of life.[71, 75, 77, 83–85] Once pulmonary vascular obstructive disease has developed, the patient is inoperable. For this reason, repair of a large VSD is strongly advocated within the first 2 years of life. Current management of the patient with a large VSD and pulmonary hypertension is aggressive surgical management during infancy if medical management of congestive heart failure is ineffective.

Preoperative Factors Influencing Outcome After Repair

Patients with VSDs that require surgical repair clinically demonstrate the symptoms of a well-understood pathophysiology: a large left-to-right shunt that results in elevated pulmonary blood flow, pulmonary hypertension, and, if left unrepaired, the potential for developing irreversible pulmo-

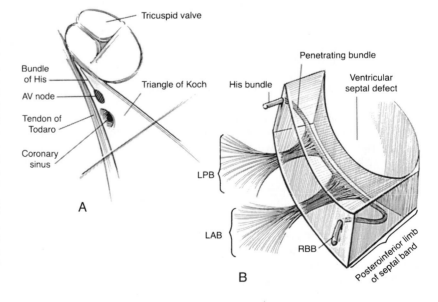

Figure 19–5. Schematic representation of the conduction system in ventricular septal defect. The atrioventricular (AV) node is within the triangle of Koch, which is close to orifice of the coronary sinus and between the annulus of the tricuspid valve and the tendon of Todaro (A). The bundle of His, originating from the AV node, extends toward the tricuspid valve and penetrates along the margin of the membranous septum across the muscular ventricular septum, giving rise to the left posterior branch (LPB) and left anterior branch (LAB) (B). The right bundle branch (RBB) then travels back along the ventricular septum toward the right ventricular septal surface. (From Castaneda AR, Jonas RA, Mayer JE Jr, Hanley FL: Ventricular septal defect. In: Castaneda AR, Jonas RA, Mayer JE Jr, Hanley FL, eds: Cardiac Surgery of the Neonate and Infant. Philadelphia: W.B. Saunders; 1994: 189.)

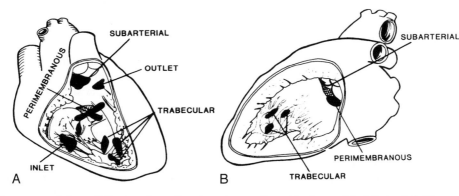

Figure 19–6. Schematic representation of the location of various types of ventricular septal defects. (A) View of VSDs from the right ventricular outflow tract. (B) View from the left ventricle. (From Gumbiner CH, Takao A: Ventricular septal defect. In: Garson A Jr, Bricker JT, Fisher DJ, Neish SR, eds: The Science and Practice of Pediatric Cardiology. Baltimore: Williams & Wilkins; 1998: 1121.)

nary vascular obstructive disease, even within the first 2 years of life. Perhaps the greatest factor that influences outcome after repair over the long term is the *age at repair*, the age at which the abnormal physiology is corrected and ventricular function and pulmonary artery pressure are returned to normal levels.

Therefore, the anesthetic evaluation and assessment of any patient who has undergone VSD repair must include how old the patient was at the time of repair. As with other lesions, it appears that successful repair within the first year of life results in an improved long-term outcome. For example, although most long-term survivors are asymptomatic and well,[77, 86–93] exercise performance may nevertheless be mildly diminished, although less in the group undergoing repair in the first year of life.[88, 94–97] In addition, the degree as well as the duration of preoperative pulmonary hypertension is important. Most patients who are repaired before 2 years of age have a return to normal pulmonary vascular resistance.[77, 84, 98, 99] However, patients with moderately elevated pulmonary vascular resistance who are repaired after 2 years of age may have a subsequent rise in pulmonary vascular resistance.[77, 84, 87, 90, 91, 100, 101] These patients rarely progress to irreversible pulmonary vascular obstructive disease.[87]

Surgical Repair

Historically, closure of VSDs ranks among one of the earliest successful surgical repairs. In 1955, Lillehei reported the first successful closure using cross-circulation with direct visualization of the defect.[102] In the early years of surgical repair, the risks of primary definitive repair were high enough to warrant a two-stage palliative approach to management. Infants with a large VSD, pulmonary hypertension, and congestive heart failure often underwent pulmonary artery banding to control the amount of left-to-right shunting and avoid the progression of pulmonary vascular obstructive disease. Despite the successful management of congestive heart failure with this palliative approach, especially in small infants with large VSDs, multiple problems have been described with the two-stage palliative approach to VSD repair. Since as many as 8% of large defects close spontaneously by the age of 2 years,[77] some patients whose VSD had closed spontaneously after pulmonary artery banding were

nevertheless required to undergo open heart surgical removal of the pulmonary artery band and repair of the stenotic area at the pulmonary artery band site. Other disadvantages of the two-stage approach included increased combined operative mortality, technical problems of debanding, and risk for the development of subaortic stenosis (possibly due to changes in intracardiac turbulent flow dynamics and subsequent distortion of the septal wall).[103, 104] Advances in all areas of diagnostic and therapeutic perioperative management have led to decreased risk with a one-stage primary repair, even in neonates and small infants. As a result, the majority of pediatric cardiac surgical centers now advocate a one-stage repair[104–108] except for certain high-risk patients, such as patients with multiple VSDs, VSDs requiring a left ventriculotomy, and premature neonates or infants with concomitant pulmonary disease.[105, 109, 110]

Indications for surgical repair are now fairly standard (Table 19–9),[82] except that the age at which primary repair is performed is younger than it was 15 to 20 years ago. In addition to these well-accepted indications, patients with subaortic VSD who are at risk for aortic cusp prolapse or those patients with a perimembranous VSD with aortic regurgitation are referred for surgical repair even in the face of a smaller shunt because of the well-described risk of progression to aortic valve regurgitation.[111–118]

As outlined earlier, the surgical approach to VSD repair has implications for long-term postoperative outcome. The

Table 19–9. Indications and Contraindications for Surgical Repair of Ventricular Septal Defect

Indications	Contraindications
Age	
Under 6 months: uncontrolled congestive heart failure	Absolute: Rp/Rs>1:1
6 to 24 months: pulmonary hypertension or symptoms	Relative: Rp/Rs>0.75
Over 24 months: Qp/Qs>2:1	

Qs, systemic blood flow; Qp, pulmonary blood flow; Rp, pulmonary vascular resistance; Rs, systemic vascular resistance.
From Gumbiner CH, Takao A: Ventricular septal defects. In Garson A Jr, Bricker JT, Fisher DJ, Neish SR, eds: The Science and Practice of Pediatric Cardiology, 2nd ed, Vol 1. Baltimore: Williams & Wilkins; 1998:1133.

majority of perimembranous defects can be repaired via a transatrial approach, avoiding the problems associated with a ventriculotomy.[119–122] Defects located in the inlet septum may require detachment of the septal leaflet of the tricuspid valve for optimal surgical exposure. Muscular defects are best approached via a left ventriculotomy, and the risks of left ventriculotomy must be weighed against the risks of leaving behind residual defects when exposure is suboptimal via an alternative approach.[123–125] Defects in the outlet septum may be approached via the pulmonary artery.

In a study of 50 patients who underwent VSD repair, 29 patients had repair via a right ventriculotomy at an average age of 4.4 years with an average of 15.1 years of follow-up post-repair. Twenty-one patients had repair via an atriotomy route at an older age, 6.6 years, with 12.1 years of follow-up. Right bundle branch block was more frequent (62%) in the group whose VSD closure was approached through a ventriculotomy versus those whose repair was approached through an atriotomy (33%). Late complete atrioventricular block was observed in two patients who underwent repair through an atriotomy. Disorders of supraventricular excitability were seen in one patient repaired via ventriculotomy and two patients repaired via an atriotomy. On Holter monitoring, 34% of the ventriculotomy group had serious ventricular dysrhythmias (≥ Lown grade 2; see Table 19–4) compared with 26.5% of the atriotomy group. The occurrence of ventricular arrhythmias in the patient population as a whole increased significantly with age at surgery and age at follow-up evaluation.[126]

It is clear that the need for ventriculotomy increases the risk for serious dysrhythmias. For example, sudden death occurs in 1 to 2% of postoperative VSD patients who required a right ventriculotomy.[127] As previously outlined in Tables 19–2 and 19–3,[128] all patients with VSD are at risk of pre-repair and post-repair dysrhythmias. In addition to serious ventricular dysrhythmias, which are more common in the ventriculotomy group, atrioventricular block and conduction abnormalities may be seen because of the close proximity of the conduction system during patch closure of the defect and subsequent scarring and fibrosis in the area of the patch that occur over time.

Residua and Sequelae

The most obvious residuum of a VSD closure is a residual septal defect. The improvements in preoperative diagnosis and the use of intraoperative pulmonary artery monitoring and transesophageal echocardiography have reduced the incidence of residual defects. Patients operated on within the last decade can be expected to have a lower incidence of residual defects when compared with patients operated on decades ago in the early years of surgical therapy. In one study, 148 infants whose defects were repaired in the first year of life underwent follow-up cardiac catheterization 1 year postoperatively; 98% of these infants had complete or virtual closure of the defect. Two infants had residual shunts that were large enough to warrant reoperation (Qp/Qs > 2:1).[129]

Two natural history studies of CHD patients have been conducted at the national level.[87] Review of patients with VSDs included patients managed both medically and surgically. In the First Natural History Study of Congenital Heart Defects (NHS-1), the original cohort consisted of 1280 patients, with 1099 alive at completion of NHS-1.[130] New data were obtained on 976 (76.3%) of the original cohort. The probability of 25-year survival was 87%. Of the 860 patients managed medically during NHS-1, 245 subsequently required surgical closure of the VSD. Only 5.5% of patients who had surgical closure required a second operation. On follow-up, there was a higher-than-normal prevalence of serious arrhythmias, even with small defects.[131]

As part of the Second Natural History Study of Congenital Heart Defects (NHS-2), 24-hour ambulatory ECG monitoring was performed for full participants in the study. At least 15.5 hours of monitoring was required for inclusion in the analysis. This was achieved for 755 (90.6%) of the patients. Multiform premature ventricular contractions, ventricular couplets, and ventricular tachycardia were considered "serious arrhythmias." For patients with VSDs, the variables associated with "serious arrhythmias" were different for medically and surgically managed patients. For medically managed patients, higher mean pulmonary artery pressure on admission to NHS-1 and older age on admission to NHS-2 were associated with the presence of serious arrhythmias. For surgically managed patients, higher NYHA functional class and cardiomegaly were associated with serious arrhythmias. The prevalence of "serious arrhythmias" was second highest for patients with VSD, who had the second highest incidence of sudden death. Furthermore, isolated dysrhythmias, especially ventricular dysrhythmias, have very serious implications in patients who also have coexistent abnormalities in ventricular performance. Bacterial endocarditis occurred rarely. Nevertheless, patients after repair of VSD are still at risk of endocarditis, especially those with small residual defects, and should receive proper treatment when indicated (see Tables 19–5 to 19–8). Of patients with small VSDs, 94.1% were in NYHA functional class I. With the exception of those who were unoperated and who went on to develop pulmonary vascular obstructive disease or Eisenmenger's syndrome, most patients had a final clinical status that was excellent or good.[87] As discussed previously, if successful closure of the defect occurs, then the risk of residual pulmonary hypertension on long-term follow-up is very low. Those patients with residual defects or repair after the age of 2 years are at greater risk for having residual pulmonary hypertension.

When a ventriculotomy is performed, the surface ECG commonly shows a right bundle branch block (RBBB) pattern. However, the surface ECG cannot define the location of the RBBB. Distal RBBB that occurs because the ventriculotomy affects distal Purkinje fibers has less serious implications and represents the majority of RBBB seen in patients after a ventriculotomy. Proximal RBBB is less common and is more ominous because of the risk for the development of more advanced block, especially in the setting of left axis deviation. Any patient with a RBBB on surface ECG may further present difficulties in diagnosis if a supraventricular tachycardia occurs, since supraventricular tachycardia with RBBB may resemble ventricular tachycardia on ECG and make it difficult to differentiate between supraventricular tachycardia and ventricular tachycardia. The presence of postoperative RBBB is common (62%) but does not appear to be associated with adverse effects.[129, 131–133] In one study, 9% of postoperative patients had bifascicular block (RBBB and left axis deviation), which has been suggested as a risk factor for sudden death in patients following tetralogy of Fallot repair. Sudden death or syncopal or near syncopal symptoms were not seen in this group of patients with bifascicular block after VSD repair. However, the long-term implications of this ECG pattern need to be followed.

Ventricular performance after VSD repair has been studied; patients with large VSDs have increased left ventricular preload and increased stroke volume with normal contractility.[134] Left ventricular dilatation and hypertrophy is also usually present. The right ventricle may be mildly dilated but returns to normal size after repair. If repair is undertaken in the first 2 years of life, the left ventricle also returns to normal size and there is normal left ventricular wall mass and contractility. If repair is delayed or performed in later childhood, left ventricular dilatation, hypertrophy, and contractility may remain abnormal. When these abnormalities persist, symptoms may be present only during exercise. Therefore, the stress of surgery and anesthesia may potentially unmask these abnormalities.

Complications

Closure of a VSD carries with it the risk of complete heart block. Since the 1960s,[98, 104, 135] however, a better understanding of the location and course of the conduction system has decreased the incidence of surgically induced atrioventricular block, and in most centers the incidence is now less than 2% in patients with simple VSD.[136, 137]

Atrioventricular Septal Defect

Atrioventricular septal defects describe a group of malformations with a range of pathologic features.[138] A central feature of these defects is the presence of an atrial septal defect in addition to a defect in the ventricular septum and one or both atrioventricular valves. Because of the range and variety of defects, this group of patients should be evaluated more extensively for risks after surgical repair. In general, several terms have been used to describe this group of congenital heart lesions, including endocardial cushion defect, atrioven-

tricular canal defect, atrioventricular septal defect, canalis atrioventricularis communis, and persistent atrioventricular ostium. Since atrioventricular septal defects consist of a spectrum of abnormalities, they are often described as complete or incomplete atrioventricular septal defects (Fig. 19–7). Figure 19–8 schematically represents the different levels of communication that are possible in atrioventricular septal defects.[54] Finally, atrioventricular septal defects have been classified on the basis of the location and attachments of the anterosuperior bridging leaflet of the atrioventricular valve.[138] It is clear that the anterior or aortic leaflet of the mitral valve is abnormal in most hearts with atrioventricular septal defects. Both anterior and posterior components of the leaflet are present but separated by a cleft or gap. It is in fact *a hallmark of atrioventricular septal defects that the atrioventricular valves are abnormal; this finding distinguishes this group of lesions from other VSDs and other ASDs.* "Balanced" defects are those in which the atrioventricular valves overlie both ventricles equally (Fig. 19–9). In more complex atrioventricular septal defects, there may be associated hypoplasia of one of the ventricles as a result of relationship of the atrioventricular orifice to the underlying ventricular mass. The "unbalanced" atrioventricular septal defects (in which the atrioventricular valves do not lie equally over both ventricles and one predominates, i.e., right or left dominant) present additional challenges to surgical repair and long-term outcome. Finally, the defective atrioventricular septum in atrioventricular septal defects is associated with abnormalities in the placement of the atrioventricular conduction system that are not normally found in other VSDs and ASDs. This abnormal placement has important surgical implications, making injury during repair more likely. The finding of a superior leftward axis on ECG is a reflection of the abnormal location of the conduction system in this group of defects.

Preoperative Factors Influencing Outcome After Repair

The physiology of atrioventricular septal defects is similar to the physiology seen in large ASDs and VSDs. When the

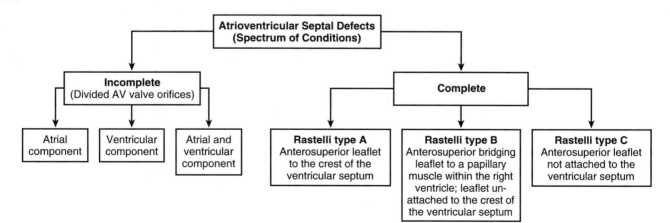

Figure 19–7. Atrioventricular septal defects: levels of communication. The spectrum of conditions seen in patients with atrioventricular septal defects (AVSDs). In the complete form of the defect, the atrioventricular (AV) valve resembles an embryonic "AV valve" and has five leaflets with anterosuperior and posteroinferior bridging leaflets straddling the septa, a mural leaflet at the left margin, and a posterior and anterior leaflet making up the rest of the right margin of the common orifice. (Modified from Silverman N: The secundum atrial septal defect and atrioventricular septal defects. In: Freedom RM, Braunwald E, eds: Atlas of Heart Diseases, Congenital Heart Disease, Vol. XII. St. Louis: Mosby; 1997: 12.4.)

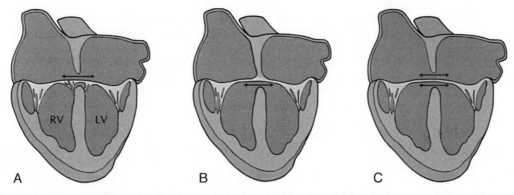

Figure 19–8. Atrioventricular septal defects: levels of communication. (A) Purely atrial level of communication. The atrioventricular (AV) valves are adherent to the ventricular septum, and there is no communication at the ventricular level. (B) Only ventricular communication. The AV valves have fused with the lower edge of the atrial septum, obliterating the ostium primum defect, and only the interventricular level shunt is present here. This defect is often called a ventricular septal defect of the AV canal type. (C) Combined levels of communication above and below the AV valves. Arrows indicate the levels of communication. (From Silverman N: The secundum atrial septal defect and atrioventricular septal defects. In: Freedom RM, Braunwald E, eds: Atlas of Heart Diseases, Congenital Heart Disease, Vol. XII. St. Louis: Mosby, 1997: 12.5.)

atrial defect is the only defect, the physiology will be similar to a large secundum defect, except that the presence of mitral regurgitation may worsen symptoms. Similarly, an atrioventricular septal defect with only a ventricular component will present with symptoms of congestive heart failure and pulmonary hypertension and be further complicated if significant atrioventricular valve regurgitation is present. When both a significant atrial and ventricular defect are present, in association with atrioventricular valve regurgitation, the patient will have significant symptoms of congestive heart failure and pulmonary hypertension that is often refractory to medical management in the young infant. In addition, this group of patients with complete atrioventricular septal defect may have a more accelerated course to pulmonary vascular obstructive disease. For example, lung biopsies obtained in patients with complete atrioventricular septal defect between 6 months and 1 year of age (either open biopsy or at autopsy) revealed pulmonary vascular changes, including medial hypertrophy in infants younger than 6 months of age. After 1 year of age, most of these unrepaired patients with complete atrioventricular septal defects had evidence of severe pulmonary vascular changes, including evidence of pulmonary vascular obstructive disease.[139] Patients with Down syndrome have a high incidence of atrioventricular septal defects, which is complicated by a tendency for Down syndrome patients to develop early and severe pulmonary vascular obstructive disease.[140, 141] Obviously, concern about early pulmonary vascular obstructive disease creates urgency for repair for many patients with atrioventricular septal defects; however, surgical repair of this group of patients is often complicated by the abnormal atrioventricular valve. Valvuloplasty may not result in a perfectly functioning valve, but it is clearly preferable to valve replacement in the young infant or child. In fact, artificial valve replacement in the young infant may be technically difficult. In small infants, the placement of an artificial mitral valve may contribute to left ventricular outflow tract obstruction. Therefore, the choice of valvuloplasty rather than valve replacement may result in residual mitral valve regurgitation that may eventually lead to reoperation or valve replacement. Control of congestive heart failure and pulmonary hypertension may

be attempted with a two-stage palliative approach, using pulmonary artery banding as the first-stage palliation. However, primary repair in mid-infancy is still advocated in most centers today.[142] Early primary repair eliminates the volume and pressure overload on the ventricles and, over the long term, may result in improved ventricular function.

Preoperative factors such as congestive heart failure, degree and duration of pulmonary hypertension, and dysrhythmias influence outcome, as in patients with large VSDs. In addition, abnormalities in the atrioventricular valves and the possibility of residual valvar regurgitation add an important factor to long-term follow-up and outcome.

Surgical Repair

The approach to surgical repair varies, and, in many ways, each patient must have an individualized approach. In addition, different centers advocate different approaches. A single Dacron patch can be used to close the atrial and ventricular defects. This approach requires a resuspension of the right and left portions of the common atrioventricular valve. Other centers use a two-patch technique and sandwich the leaflet tissue between the two patches.[143–146] There is also surgical controversy over the approach to repairing the left atrioventricular valve.[147, 148] The timing of surgery clearly takes into account the degree, duration, and effects of congestive heart failure and pulmonary hypertension weighed against the risks and outcome associated with mitral valvuloplasty and mitral valve replacement in the young infant.

Residua and Sequelae

In addition to the obvious residua of residual atrial or ventricular septal defects, residual mitral valve regurgitation remains a serious problem that may necessitate reoperation or mitral valve replacement in the long term. A 20-year review of repair of atrioventricular septal defects showed that reoperation for mitral regurgitation has decreased significantly over time but in recent years has stabilized at about 7%.[142]

When analyzing long-term outcome in patients with atrio-

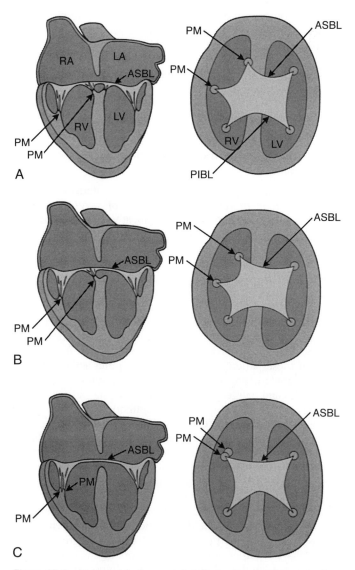

Figure 19–9. Atrioventricular septal defects: levels of communication. The Rastelli classification of the different types of complete atrioventricular (AV) canal defects is based on the morphology of the anterosuperior bridging leaflet (ASBL). Two-dimensional echocardiography confirms Rastelli's surgically based classification. This diagram illustrates the types of AV valve attachments of the ASBL as seen by echocardiography. The left column is a series of four-chamber views and the right column is a series of subcostal short axis or parasternal short axis views. (A) Rastelli type A defect. Here the ASBL is attached to the papillary muscle lying on the crest of the septum between the left ventricle (LV) and right ventricle (RV). In the subcostal view, the posteroinferior bridging leaflet (PIBL) is attached to the crest of the septum. (B) Rastelli type B defect. The ASBL is not attached to the septum but to the papillary muscle (PM) arising from the right ventricle. (C) Rastelli type C defect. The ASBL is attached to the papillary muscle, which also supports the other leaflet of the tricuspid valve yielding a free-floating non-attached leaflet. The arrows in the right-sided figures indicate how the papillary muscle attachment is from a septally attached (type A) to right ventricle–originating papillary muscle (type B) and a papillary muscle fused with the anterior papillary muscle within the right ventricle (type C). LA, left atrium; RA, right atrium. (From Silverman N: The secundum atrial septal defect and atrioventricular septal defects. In: Freedom RM, Braunwald E, eds: Atlas of Heart Diseases, Vol. XII. St. Louis: Mosby; 1997: 12.6.)

ventricular septal defects, it is best to remember that there is a continuum of problems within the diagnosis of atrioventricular septal defects. The presence or absence of a ventricular defect is probably a reasonable way to approach categorizing the different pathologic findings and hemodynamic results. In a large study examining the outcome of 719 patients over 20 years who underwent repair of atrioventricular septal defects at Children's Hospital in Boston, the long-term results were analyzed according to the presence or absence of a ventricular communication that required surgical intervention. In this study, 258 patients did not require repair of a ventricular defect. They presented for surgery at an older age, with 197 patients being repaired after age 2 years. Two of these patients died secondary to severe hypoplasia of the left ventricle and both patients had significant mitral regurgitation. Eight of the 61 patients whose defects were repaired at an age younger than 2 years died and were noted to have severe mitral regurgitation and other anomalies. Long-term follow-up of the entire 258 patients without a ventricular defect describes three additional late deaths.[149] In the group with a ventricular communication, 461 patients underwent repair and there were 62 (13.4%) early deaths in this group. Nevertheless, there has been a significant decrease in mortality over time, from 25% to 2.9%, even at a time when more complex lesions were repaired. Reoperation occurred for residual defects, residual hemodynamically significant mitral regurgitation, and pacemaker implantation for complete atrioventricular block. Of the 394 survivors, follow-up data were available for 217 and there were 7 late deaths in this group.[149]

Complications

The pathology of atrioventricular septal defects also includes an abnormal and vulnerable position of the conduction system that demands close surgical attention during repair. There has been a decline over the last decade in the incidence of postoperative atrioventricular block in all surgeries because surgeons have become aware of the location of the atrioventricular node and the His bundle and how to avoid it at the time of repair. Nevertheless, this complication can still occur. When atrioventricular block is observed in the operating room in the immediate post-bypass period, both atrial and ventricular wires are placed and used. Contusion and edema of the area near the atrioventricular node may contribute to this early postoperative block, which may resolve within the first few postoperative days. Nevertheless, many electrophysiologists in major cardiac centers advocate the placement of a permanent pacemaker in any post-surgical patient who has complete atrioventricular block that lasts beyond 10 to 14 postoperative days.[150]

Tetralogy of Fallot

Tetralogy of Fallot was first described in 1672, and the "tetrad" consists of four pathologic characteristics: a ventricular septal defect, infundibular pulmonic stenosis, right ventricle hypertrophy, and dextroposition of the aorta. Other associated anomalies include multiple VSDs in about 3% of patients and various coronary artery anomalies, most notably an anterior descending coronary artery that crosses the right ventricular outflow tract at the usual place for an outflow tract patch.

It is important to realize that there is a well-described spectrum of obstruction to right ventricular outflow in tetralogy of Fallot patients, which includes infundibular obstruction, pulmonary valve stenosis, and hypoplasia of both the pulmonary annulus and the pulmonary trunk. The degree of right ventricular outflow tract obstruction varies however; therefore, the clinical symptoms of cyanosis and the potential for hypercyanotic spells ("Tet spells") may also vary. The obstruction to pulmonary blood flow consists of a "fixed" component (the narrowed infundibulum, the stenotic pulmonary valve, and the stenotic or hypoplastic pulmonary arteries) as well as a "dynamic" component of infundibular muscular narrowing. It is the dynamic infundibular spasm that many believe contributes to a marked decrease in pulmonary blood flow that occurs during a hypercyanotic spell. Patients with tetralogy of Fallot and pulmonary atresia represent a very different pathologic subset. There is a wide range of origin, size, and distribution of the pulmonary blood supply in patients with tetralogy of Fallot with pulmonary atresia. In addition, there has been a significant change in surgical and therapeutic approach to this complex group of patients over the last decade.

Another variant of tetralogy of Fallot is tetralogy of Fallot with absent pulmonary valve that is pathologically and physiologically quite different from tetralogy of Fallot and tetralogy of Fallot with pulmonary atresia. Neither tetralogy of Fallot with pulmonary atresia nor tetralogy of Fallot with absent pulmonary valve are discussed in this chapter. Although some extrapolation of long-term data from the classic tetralogy of Fallot group of patients can be made to these other groups, tetralogy of Fallot with pulmonary atresia and tetralogy of Fallot with absent pulmonary valve are sufficiently more complex and varied with respect to anatomy, surgical management, and long-term follow-up to warrant a separate, more complex discussion. In addition, surgical management, especially of the patients with tetralogy of Fallot with pulmonary atresia, is an evolving area of study and research.

Historically, classic tetralogy of Fallot patients represent a group of patients with much long-term outcome data. The first surgical intervention for patients with tetralogy of Fallot was the Blalock-Taussig shunt (subclavian artery to pulmonary artery anastomosis) in 1945. Other palliative procedures followed in the years and decades to follow, including the Waterston shunt (ascending aorta to right pulmonary artery), the Potts shunt (descending aorta to left pulmonary artery), and the Brock pulmonary valvotomy and infundibulotomy as a closed heart procedure.[151–154] The first open-heart procedure took place in 1954 when Lillehei and collaborators used controlled cross-circulation in a 10-month-old child to do the first intracardiac repair of tetralogy of Fallot with VSD closure and relief of right ventricular outflow tract obstruction.[155] This landmark report was also notable for the fact that half of these patients were under 2 years of age.

Despite initial reports of successful infant repairs, subsequent papers reported high mortality, and many centers abandoned this approach in favor of a two-stage palliation with shunt followed by definitive repair and shunt takedown later in childhood. This question of definitive versus palliative repair remained a controversial area. Eventually selected centers adopted an aggressive one-stage repair approach, including infants less than 3 months old. Children's Hospital in Boston began such an approach in 1972 while this one-stage plan was still controversial among cardiac centers.[156] Over the last almost three decades, however, the long-term follow-up data on these early definitively repaired infants have resulted in an impressive body of data to support this one-stage repair approach.

Preoperative Factors Influencing Outcome After Repair

Two factors stand out as indicators of long-term outcome: the *age at time of repair* and the *type of surgical repair*, including specifically the need for a right ventricular outflow tract patch across the pulmonary annulus. Additionally, although preoperative dysrhythmias are not common, conduction abnormalities and dysrhythmias in the postoperative period have implications on long-term follow-up of these patients. Tetralogy of Fallot patients may also be at risk for sudden death if they possess a certain constellation of electrophysiologic and conduction abnormalities.[157–159] Long-term follow-up of patients with more complex congenital heart lesions, such as tetralogy of Fallot, have found that many of these patients are clinically well and asymptomatic but nevertheless are at risk for cardiac compromise under anesthesia and surgery. More than 90% of patients with tetralogy of Fallot will survive to adulthood with good functional long-term results. Other residua, sequelae, or complications of the procedure may be well tolerated or may have some deleterious effect on long-term outcome.[160] Late results of children who underwent repair during infancy reveal a decreased incidence of dysrhythmias in the younger age group when followed long term. Only 2 of 184 patients had ventricular ectopy on ECG, and Holter data from 41 patients revealed 1 with sinus node dysfunction, 12 with Lown grade 1 ectopy, and 1 with Lown grade 2 ectopy or greater (see Table 19–4).[161] Other preoperative factors that may influence outcome include the presence of a small hypoplastic pulmonary annulus that may require a transannular patch and carry with it important long-term implications, that is, pulmonary valve regurgitation. Obviously, chronic preoperative cyanosis and hypoxemia present problems with any patient, as discussed earlier.

Surgical Repair

Improved surgical morbidity and mortality for tetralogy of Fallot patients is a direct result of close collaboration among surgeons, cardiologists, and pathologists over several decades. Congenital heart disease pathologists have added tremendously to the surgeon's understanding of critical issues in the repair of tetralogy of Fallot. Even during the 1950s, Lillehei recognized the essential need for adequate enlargement of the right ventricular infundibulum with a patch, as well as the need for the patch to extend beyond the pulmonary valve annulus in certain cases.[162] A transannular patch usually results in a regurgitant pulmonary valve after repair. The implications of these sequelae of transannular patch are discussed later. In addition to adequate relief of right ventricular outflow tract obstruction, delineation of the VSD anatomy and its relationship to the conduction system was an important milestone in collaboration between surgeons and pathologists. Insights gained over several decades have therefore decreased the incidence of residual VSD and conduction abnormalities and have resulted in an overall improved surgical repair.[163] Figure 19–10 illustrates the anatomic malformation and Figure 19–11 illustrates the surgical approach to closure of the VSD and right ventricular outflow tract obstruction repair (either with a right ventricular outflow tract patch or transannular patch), with special emphasis on the location of the conduction system and how the surgeon can avoid damage during VSD patch placement.[164]

Residua and Sequelae

The most obvious residuum of tetralogy of Fallot repair is a *residual VSD*, either because of incomplete closure of a VSD or because an additional VSD is undiagnosed and therefore left unrepaired. The frequency of residual VSDs (of any size) has been described to be as high as 20%.[160, 165] Precise localization of a VSD with echocardiography both preoperatively and intraoperatively and post-bypass in the operating room have resulted in a decrease in the incidence of residual VSDs.[166] Nevertheless, some VSDs, such as those in the trabecular muscular septum, are technically very challenging, even when identified preoperatively. Small residual VSDs with small shunts ($Q_P/Q_S < 1.5:1$) may be well tolerated. In

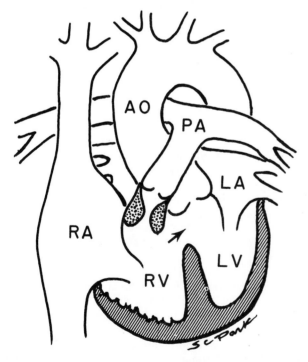

Figure 19–10. Schematic representation of the anatomic abnormalities of tetralogy of Fallot. The arrow indicates the location of the ventricular septal defect (VSD) and the over-riding of the aorta. The stippled area illustrates the infundibular pulmonary stenosis. Ao, aorta; LA, left atrium; LV, left ventricle; PA, pulmonary artery; RA, right atrium; RV, Right ventricle. (From Neches WH, Park SC, Ettedgui JA: Tetralogy of Fallot and tetralogy of Fallot with pulmonary atresia. In: Garson A Jr, Bricker JT, Fisher DJ, Neish SR, eds: The Science and Practice of Pediatric Cardiology, 2nd ed, Vol. 1. Baltimore: Williams & Wilkins; 1998: 1384.)

general, patients with larger shunts with a Q_P/Q_S ratio greater than 1.5:1 will require reoperation.[160, 167]

Residual and right ventricular outflow tract obstruction is another residuum that may be caused by residual pulmonic stenosis at the level of the pulmonary valve or annulus. In addition, pulmonary artery stenosis, either at the pulmonary artery bifurcation or more distally, is another site of residual obstruction, especially in those patients who had a two-stage repair with placement of a subclavian to pulmonary artery anastomosis and subsequent takedown at the time of definitive repair. It has been estimated that most patients after repair of tetralogy of Fallot have some degree of residual pulmonary stenosis, which is nevertheless trivial or mild (right ventricular pressure is less than 50% of systemic) so that further intervention is not expected. About 10% of patients will have excessive right ventricular hypertension; that is, right ventricular pressure greater than 75% of systemic pressure that requires surgical repair.[160, 165, 167, 168]

Two well-recognized sequelae of tetralogy of Fallot repair have long-term implications: *pulmonary valve regurgitation* and *right ventriculotomy*. *Pulmonary regurgitation* can occur after pulmonary valvectomy or, more commonly, after placement of a transannular outflow patch. Even severe "wide-open" pulmonary regurgitation can be hemodynamically well tolerated if no other abnormalities are present.[160, 165, 168] Nevertheless, the apparent "benign" nature of pulmonary regurgitation in surgically repaired tetralogy of Fallot patients is being re-examined. Chronic volume load on the right ventricle as a result of chronic pulmonary regurgitation may negatively affect ventricular function over the long term, and early valved right ventricle to pulmonary artery conduit repair is being advocated by some centers.[169] Patients with chronic pulmonary regurgitation have cardiomegaly on chest radiograph and larger right ventricular volumes[170]; other studies have demonstrated reduced exercise capacity and an increased incidence of ventricular arrhythmias.[168] These patients are typically clinically asymptomatic from the cardiovascular standpoint but are nevertheless emblematic of the type of well-appearing postoperative cardiac patient who may exhibit "unexpected" problems during anesthesia, especially for surgery that involves major blood loss, volume shifts, alterations in airway mechanics, or other hemodynamic stressors.

Right ventriculotomy may result in sequelae in most tetralogy of Fallot repairs, since closure of the VSD and relief of right ventricular outflow tract obstruction is optimally approached through the right ventricle. As discussed previously, a ventriculotomy scar carries with it the risk of long-term dysrhythmias as fibrosis and scarring occur at the site of the ventriculotomy. In addition, closure of the VSD through the right ventricle also necessitates suturing in close proximity to the conduction system (see Fig. 19–11), which may also lead to dysrhythmias.[164]

There is a large body of literature characterizing the postoperative dysrhythmias following tetralogy of Fallot repair. Ventricular arrhythmias, conduction abnormalities, and the risk of sudden death are the major concerns for patients after tetralogy of Fallot repair. An important conclusion to be drawn from these data, collected from many centers over several decades, is that residual hemodynamic abnormalities worsen the *risk* for dysrhythmias as well as the *type* of dysrhythmia. In fact, clinical and experimental studies have

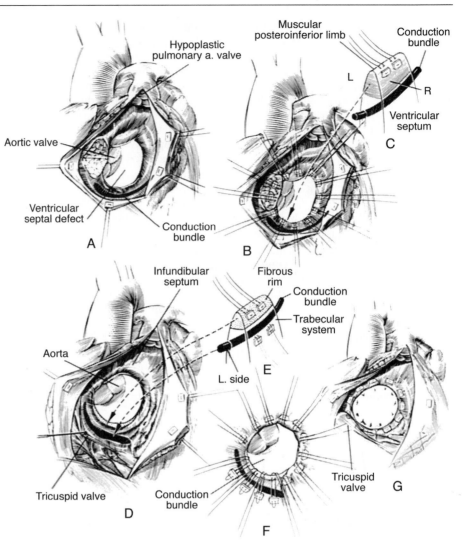

Figure 19–11. Tetralogy of Fallot: Ventricular septal defect (VSD) closure and conduction system. A review of the diagram makes it clear why the surgeon must be knowledgeable about the placement of sutures in patch closure of the malalignment VSD in tetralogy of Fallot, since the conduction bundle may be at risk for damage with the placement of sutures in the area (C & E). (From Castaneda AR, Jonas RA, Mayer JE Jr, Hanley FL: Tetralogy of Fallot. In: Cardiac Surgery of the Neonate and Infant. Philadelphia: W.B. Saunders; 1994: 224.)

suggested that residual abnormalities, especially those that result in increased right ventricular wall stress, increase the risk of ventricular arrhythmia and even sudden death.[171, 172] On routine electrocardiograms, 10% of patients have premature ventricular arrhythmias (PVCs) and 30% have PVCs when exercised. Children with normal hearts usually suppress PVCs with exercise. However, exercise-suppression of benign PVCs is not a reliable finding in tetralogy patients.[173, 174] Isolated PVCs may be benign, but more serious ventricular dysrhythmias such as frequent or multiform PVCs, ventricular tachycardia, or ventricular fibrillation may occur. As more invasive studies are done, the ability to diagnose serious dysrhythmias increases. For example, on Holter monitoring, 50% of postoperative tetralogy of Fallot patients exhibit ventricular arrhythmias and 9% have nonsustained or sustained ventricular tachycardia.[173, 175–187] Finally, in a more complex electrophysiologic protocol, 17% of patients had nonsustained and 9% had sustained ventricular tachycardia. Electrophysiologic mapping of these foci has found multiple sites of origin; these include the area of the ventriculotomy, the area of the infundibular resection, and areas near the VSD patch. The presence of premature ventricular beats on resting or exercise electrocardiogram may be a harbinger of more serious ventricular arrhythmias and

sudden death.[157–159] Certainly *their appearance during anesthesia should not be ignored or attributed primarily to benign causes.*

The overall incidence of sudden death in tetralogy of Fallot patients after repair is about 0.3% per patient year after surgical repair.[186] Postoperative tetralogy of Fallot is the most common diagnosis in all children with sudden death between the ages of 1 and 16 years.[187, 188] Early repair in infancy may reduce this incidence.[161, 189] Many patients with repaired tetralogy of Fallot who are at risk for sudden death do not usually exhibit warning symptoms; in one study only 18% of patients with sudden death had prior symptoms.[185] Some studies have shown that 25% of postoperative patients have abnormalities of atrioventricular conduction.[190, 191] RBBB commonly appears on surface ECG and is considered benign. However, it is impossible to define the level of the RBBB. The patient with transient atrioventricular block in the postoperative period who later demonstrates bifascicular block (left axis deviation with RBBB) may be manifesting a warning sign of later complete heart block.

Although earlier follow-up studies implicated bifascicular block with progression to complete heart block as the cause of sudden death in postoperative tetralogy patients, it is now widely accepted that sudden death is more commonly caused by serious ventricular dysrhythmias.[157–159] Furthermore, the combination of ventricular dysrhythmias with residual right ventricular hypertension is ominous and should be aggressively evaluated and treated. In an animal model, it has been shown that as heart rate increases in a hypertensive right ventricle, the resultant decrease in cardiac output, myocardial oxygen delivery, and increase in catecholamine levels decrease the threshold for ventricular fibrillation.[172, 192]

In general, a good correlation has been found between abnormal hemodynamics and the presence of inducible non-sustained or sustained ventricular tachycardia at electrophysiologic study.[179, 185, 187] Age at operation and increased time since surgery are important factors that may help predict risk for serious dysrhythmias, but many pediatric cardiologists nevertheless raise serious concerns, based on multiple studies, that there may be an increased risk of developing ventricular dysrhythmias in *all* postoperative tetralogy of Fallot patients. Therefore there is a need for continued attention to this problem in long-term follow-up.[184–186, 193] Radiofrequency ablation and implantable antitachycardia devices, as well as medical anti-arrhythmia therapy have been used successfully in patients at risk. Natural history studies will continue to define appropriate diagnostic and therapeutic strategies for this group of tetralogy of Fallot patients. *The informed anesthesiologist who is aware of the dysrhythmia risk in asymptomatic tetralogy of Fallot patients may play a role in diagnosing latent rhythm abnormalities that first manifest during the stress of anesthesia and surgery.*

Abnormalities in ventricular function may be considered a sequela of the effects of preoperative chronic cyanosis and hypoxemia on ventricular function, as well as a sequela of the surgical repair; that is, right ventriculotomy, residual and right ventricular outflow tract obstruction, residual VSD, and pulmonary valvular regurgitation. Even if a VSD is completely closed, patients with tetralogy of Fallot are known to have significant systemic-to-pulmonary artery collaterals[194] that may also cause a left-to-right shunt. These collaterals may be dealt with intraoperatively with ligation, or, if they are unreachable surgically, occlusion in the catheterization laboratory can be carried out preoperatively or postoperatively.[195–197] Right ventricular dysfunction may be secondary to a volume load from a residual VSD or pulmonary regurgitation or secondary to a pressure load from residual right ventricular outflow tract obstruction. Follow-up cardiac catheterization 1 to 2 years postoperatively demonstrates normal right ventricular end-diastolic and right atrial pressures when these abnormalities are not present.[134, 165, 198]

Complications

Patients with tetralogy of Fallot may have an anomalous or accessory anterior descending coronary artery that arises from the right coronary artery and crosses the right ventricular outflow tract at exactly the site where the surgeon may place a vertical ventriculotomy for repair of tetralogy of Fallot. If this anomalous coronary artery is not diagnosed preoperatively or recognized at the time of surgery and is injured or transected, serious left ventricular dysfunction may compromise immediate postoperative survival as well as long-term ventricular function. Fortunately, this serious problem can be anticipated and diagnosed preoperatively.

Either a horizontal ventriculotomy or a right ventricular-to-pulmonary artery conduit may be used to bypass the area and relieve right ventricular outflow tract obstruction.

Transposition of the Great Arteries

The medical and surgical management of patients with transposition of the great arteries over the last 50 years serves as an example of how advances in all areas of pediatric cardiac medicine and surgery have changed the outcome and lives of thousands of patients with CHD. Patients with transposition of the great arteries were once considered inoperable, and 90% died during infancy.[199–202] Since the diagnosis of transposition of the great arteries represents 5 to 7% of all CHD patients, this was a devastating diagnosis for a large group of patients.[17, 74, 199]

Historically, the changing surgical management also parallels the better understanding of the pathology, the physiology, and the long-term problems after repair. The current management of neonates with transposition of the great arteries represents the culmination of progress in all areas of pediatric cardiac medicine and surgery, including surgical techniques, pharmacologic innovation, angiography, and interventional catheterization procedures, advances in bypass and intensive care unit management of critically ill neonates, and finally the ongoing natural history data that compelled re-examination and eventually implementation of new surgical approaches. As a result, patients with transposition of the great arteries are now expected to have markedly improved lifespans, perhaps even normal in length, with a marked decrease in the residua and sequelae that impaired cardiac function and ultimately quality of life and lifespan in previous decades. Table 19–10 gives a brief historical overview of advances in diagnosis and management and how today's modern treatment plan has evolved.[203, 204]

In patients with transposition of the great arteries, the aorta and pulmonary artery connect to inappropriate ventricles (right ventricle to aorta and left ventricle to pulmonary artery). The atrioventricular valves are connected to the usual ventricle (mitral valve to left ventricle and tricuspid valve to right ventricle) and the aorta and aortic valve (with coronary ostia) arises as usual from the left ventricle and the pulmonary valve and pulmonary artery from the right ventricle (Fig. 19–12). The result of this rearrangement is that the circulatory system is set as a parallel circuit rather than a series circuit (Fig. 19–13). Clearly such a circulatory pattern is incompatible with life without some communication between the pulmonary and systemic circulations.[204] Typically, at birth this communication is the PDA, which must remain patent rather than closed, as normally happens within the first few days of life. In about 40 to 45% of patients with transposition of the great arteries, a coexisting VSD is present (although one third of these VSDs are small and have little hemodynamic importance). The presence of a VSD therefore provides a channel for mixing and communication of the two circuits.[205, 206]

Historically, surgical approaches to management initially dealt with palliation, especially the critical need for a more reliable mixing communication between the right and left side of the neonate's cardiac circulation. The atrial septectomy operation (Blalock-Hanlon procedure) described in 1950[207] gave critically ill infants a chance at surviving the

Table 19–10. Major Milestones in the History of Diagnosis and Treatment of Transposition of the Great Arteries

Presurgical: Before 1950

1945:	Blalock-Taussig and Potts anastomoses

Palliative surgical: 1950–1963

1950:	Blalock-Hanlon atrial septectomy
1952:	Pulmonary artery banding
1956:	Baffes procedure
1959:	Senning operation
1962:	Waterston-Cooley anastomosis

Surgical repair: 1964–1973

1964:	Mustard operation
1966:	Rashkind balloon septostomy
1969:	Rastelli operation
1970–1973:	Profound hypothermia

Repair during infancy: 1974–1983

1975:	Park blade septostomy
1976:	Jatene arterial switch operation
1977:	Prostaglandin E_1
1977:	Senning operation (revival)

Current era of management: 1984–present

Arterial switch operation

From Neches WH, Park SC, Ettedgui JA: Transposition of the great arteries. In: Garson A Jr, Bricker JT, Fisher DJ, Neish SR, eds: The Science and Practice of Pediatric Cardiology. Baltimore: Williams & Wilkins; 1998:1490.

neonatal period by surgically creating an atrial septal defect, as a site for communication, albeit with significant perioperative morbidity and mortality. The Rashkind procedure, or the creation of an atrial septal defect using a balloon atrial septostomy in the catheterization laboratory, described in 1966, heralded the advent of interventional catheterization as a key component to management.[208] The introduction of prostaglandin in the late 1970s offered a pharmacologic alternative to maintaining ductal patency while stabilizing the sick neonate prior to a more definitive procedure, such as the Rashkind procedure.

In the 1950s and 1960s, attempts at more definitive repair were made. Of interest, Mustard first approached repair of transposition of the great arteries via an arterial switch procedure in which the left coronary artery was the only transferred artery. This procedure used monkey lungs as oxygenators and all seven patients died. Other attempts at anatomic repair were also unsuccessful.[209–212] Abandoning this more anatomically correct switch procedure, Senning and Mustard implemented surgical *atrial switch* procedures that created a series circulation by "switching" or redirecting blood at the atrial level via an intra-atrial baffle, thus resulting in a "physiologic" repair. Anatomically, the right ventricle became the systemic ventricle after these procedures.[213, 214]

The long-term sequelae of atrial switch repair were dismaying, especially as natural history follow-up data accumulated. It was clear that the development of dysrhythmias (felt secondary to significant suturing and eventual fibrosis at the site of the atrial baffle) and right ventricular failure (i.e., systemic ventricular failure) were serious concerns. The new

era of surgical treatment for transposition of the great arteries began in the late 1970s and early 1980s with a new surgical approach to a more anatomically and physiologically correct repair, namely the *arterial switch operation*.[215] This procedure was eventually applied successfully to neonates with transposition of the great arteries.[216] The ongoing collection of natural history data on patients who have undergone the arterial switch procedure is now moving into two decades of follow-up from some centers, and the data are encouraging for an optimistic long-term outcome.

Since there are such different issues and outcomes in patients who have undergone an atrial switch procedure (Mustard or Senning) compared with an arterial switch procedure, it is really more reasonable and practical to discuss postoperative issues in patients with transposition of the great arteries from these two different perspectives.

Preoperative Factors Influencing Outcome After Mustard or Senning (Atrial Switch) Repair

The typical clinical scenario for a patient with transposition of the great arteries who was born in the decades preceding adoption of the arterial switch procedure was fairly predictable. The neonate with transposition of the great arteries was typically undiagnosed before birth (prenatal echocardiography was unavailable or not used routinely). At birth, when ductal patency began to be compromised, cyanosis, metabolic acidosis, and eventual cardiac collapse would ensue.

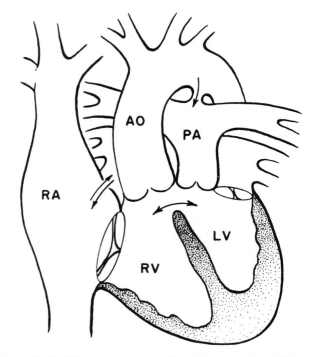

Figure 19–12. Schematic representation of transposition of the great arteries. Arrows indicate possible areas for mixing of systemic and pulmonary venous blood (atrial level, ventricular level, and/or level of ductus arteriosus). Ao, aorta; LV, left ventricle; PA, pulmonary artery; RA, right atrium; RV, right ventricle. (From Neches WH, Park SC, Ettedgui JA: Transposition of the great arteries. In: Garson A Jr, Bricker JT, Fisher DJ, Neish SR, eds: The Science and Practice of Pediatric Cardiology, 2nd ed, Vol. 1. Baltimore: Williams & Wilkins; 1998: 1470.)

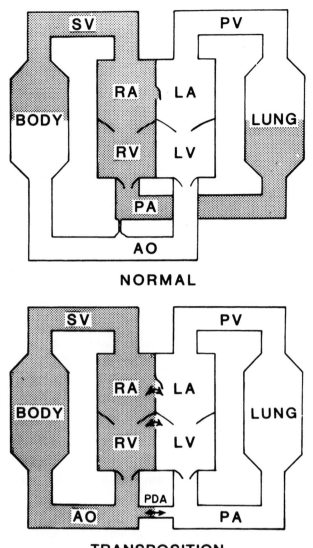

Figure 19–13. Transposition of the great arteries. A schematic representation of blood flow in transposition of the great arteries compared with normal anatomy. Ao, aorta; LA, left atrium; LV, left ventricle; PA, pulmonary artery; PDA, patent ductus arteriosus; PV, pulmonary vein; RA, right atrium; RV, right ventricle; SV, systemic vein. (From Neches WH, Park SC, Ettedgui JA: Transposition of the great arteries. In: Garson A Jr, Bricker JT, Fisher DJ, Neish SR, eds: The Science and Practice of Pediatric Cardiology, 2nd ed, Vol. 1. Baltimore: Williams & Wilkins; 1998: 1470.)

In the early surgical era, a Blalock-Hanlon atrioseptectomy was the only surgical option to create a communication for mixing. This procedure carried significant risks, especially since it was performed in a critically ill infant with a closing PDA. With the introduction of the Rashkind procedure (balloon atrial septostomy), a nonsurgical alternative to ASD creation, the outcome for these sick, cyanotic neonates improved considerably. Finally, the introduction in the late 1970s of prostaglandin to maintain ductal patency permitted clinical stabilization of the cyanotic neonate before proceeding to the Rashkind procedure in the cardiac catheterization laboratory, thus further improving outcome during the critical neonatal period.[217] Infants with a significant VSD escaped

deterioration in the first few days of life because of a site (VSD) for mixing. However, mild cyanosis would be present in these patients, and within a few weeks as pulmonary vascular resistance fell, symptoms of congestive heart failure would begin to cause clinical deterioration.

Both groups of neonates (those without a VSD who require an urgent neonatal Rashkind procedure and those with a VSD who may not) would be cyanotic but would have survived the critical neonatal period and were then candidates for atrial diversion (a Mustard or Senning procedure) at some later date in infancy. The timing of this definitive surgery became important because of several factors. It was recognized that patients with transposition of the great arteries were at risk for developing early (often as young as 3 months of age) and rapidly progressive pulmonary vascular obstructive disease. Multiple causes have been proposed for this serious risk and include increased pulmonary blood flow, elevated pulmonary artery pressure, systemic hypoxemia, polycythemia, microthrombi, and enlarged aortopulmonary collateral arteries. Therefore, early definitive Senning repair was advocated by some centers to avoid this ominous complication of pulmonary vascular obstructive disease.[218] As more patients with transposition of the great arteries underwent atrial switch operations, the natural history data made it clear within several years that several potential long-term problems existed with the Mustard and Senning atrial switch procedures (see later discussion). Some centers felt that the Senning operation had advantages over the Mustard operation. Since the Senning operation used little or no prosthetic material, concerns about the role of prosthetic material in late venous obstruction seemed to theoretically present less of a risk. It was also hoped that long-term problems with dysrhythmias would be ameliorated. Furthermore, the group of patients with transposition of the great arteries and VSD were at particular risk for higher perioperative mortality and morbidity with a Mustard or Senning procedure plus VSD closure.

Any patient who has undergone a Mustard or Senning procedure must be evaluated for a host of long-term residua or sequelae. Of most concern in terms of influencing outcome is the presence of pulmonary vascular disease preoperatively. Since calculation of pulmonary vascular resistance is difficult preoperatively in the patient with transposition of the great arteries, prolonged time before reversal of cyanosis, polycythemia, and increased pulmonary blood flow may have a negative effect on long-term outcome and the potential for residual pulmonary hypertension and vascular changes. Therefore, there are two preoperative factors that influence long-term outcome in the Mustard/Senning group: the degree and duration of cyanosis and polycythemia preoperatively and the patient's age at which definitive repair was performed, with earlier repair aimed at alleviating the risk for pulmonary vascular changes and pulmonary vascular obstructive disease.

Surgical Repair: Mustard or Senning (Atrial Switch)

Senning first described an atrial diversion via placement of an intra-atrial baffle in 1959 (Fig. 19–14).[204, 213] Poor surgical results did not make it a popular surgical approach. In 1964, Mustard's atrial operation was described and became the most popular procedure for patients with transposition of the

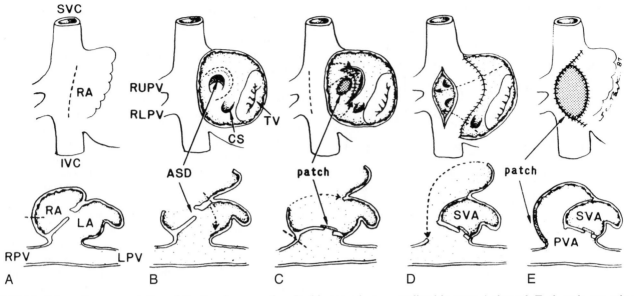

Figure 19–14. Schematic representation of the Senning operation. In this procedure, as outlined in steps A through E, there is extensive use of right atrial tissue to create the pulmonary venous atrium. Some patch material is used, often pericardial tissue, to complete the procedure. At completion, the pulmonary veins enter the newly created pulmonary venous atrium. The use of patch material is less when compared with the Mustard procedure (see Fig. 19–15). However, use of less patch material did not significantly affect the long-term problems with dysrhythmias, as was initially hoped. The top row is surgical views through the right atrium and the bottom row is cross-sectional views of each sequence of the repair. ASD, atrial septal defect; CS, coronary sinus; IVC, inferior vena cava; LA, left atrium; LPV, left pulmonary vein; PVA, pulmonary venous atrium; RA, right atrium; RLPV, right lower pulmonary vein; RPV, right pulmonary vein; RUPV, right upper pulmonary vein; SVA, systemic venous atrium; SVC, superior vena cava; TV, tricuspid valve. (From Neches WH, Park SC, Ettedgui JA; Transposition of the great arteries. In: Garson A Jr, Bricker JT, Fisher DJ, Neish SR, eds: The Science and Practice of Pediatric Cardiology, 2nd ed, Vol. 1. Baltimore: Williams & Wilkins; 1998: 1495.)

great arteries (Fig. 19–15).[204, 214] Both the Mustard and the Senning procedures use an intra-atrial baffle to redirect the systemic venous inflow across the mitral valve and left ventricle to the pulmonary circulation and the pulmonary venous blood across the tricuspid valve and right ventricle to the aorta and systemic circulation.

The main difference between the Mustard and Senning procedures is that the atrial septum is completely excised in the Mustard procedure and prosthetic material is used to create the baffle. The Senning procedure uses a flap of atrial septum to form part of the baffle. The Senning procedure was initially felt to be more technically challenging, and for most of the 1960s and 1970s, the Mustard procedure was the primary choice of surgery. However, as advances in infant surgery progressed, the Senning procedure replaced the Mustard procedure as the surgery of choice, and by the mid-1980s a survival rate of over 95% was expected for infants with transposition of the great arteries in most centers.[219–224] Many centers believed that using atrial tissue in the Senning procedure would help decrease problems with atrial dysrhythmias and sinus node problems that were becoming increasingly evident in postoperative Mustard patients.[225–227]

Natural history studies therefore played an extremely crucial role in the reassessment of the atrial diversion operations. In addition to serious and progressive problems with dysrhythmias and baffle obstruction problems, the Mustard and Senning procedures, as physiologic repair, also resulted in the right ventricle becoming the systemic ventricle. The long-term prospect of right ventricular (systemic ventricle)

failure was an ominous problem that became increasingly evident as time from surgery elapsed.

Residua, Sequelae, and Complications of Mustard or Senning Operations (Atrial Switch)

Both Mustard and Senning *atrial baffle procedures* result in a physiologic repair that nevertheless is anatomically quite different from the result after the *arterial switch procedure*. After the Mustard or Senning procedure, the placement of the atrial baffle results in systemic venous blood flow across the mitral valve into the left ventricle, across the pulmonary valve, and finally into the pulmonary circulation. At the same time, pulmonary venous blood is directed across the tricuspid valve and into the right ventricle and ultimately across the aortic valve, into the aorta and the systemic circulation. The creation of the intra-atrial baffle results in the potential for several problems: (1) pulmonary venous obstruction, (2) systemic venous obstruction, and (3) sinus node dysfunction from baffle suturing near the high right atrial border or secondary to cannulation of the superior vena cava near the sinus node.

After the Mustard operation, 10 to 20% of patients had significant systemic venous obstruction. Many of these patients are clinically asymptomatic or have subtle symptoms (e.g., early morning facial edema),[228–231] but some required reoperation. On the other hand, pulmonary venous obstruction, though less common, can be seen as a late complication and may impose more of a cardiovascular burden. Mustard patients show this more serious complication about 5 to 10%

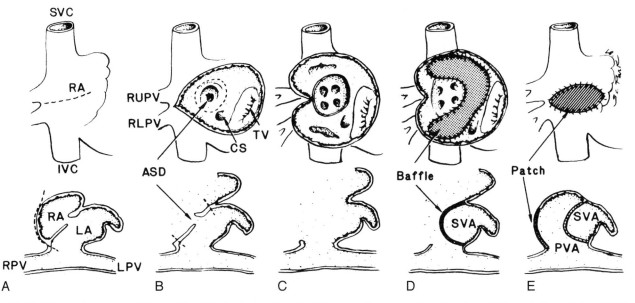

Figure 19–15. Schematic representation of the Mustard operation. In this procedure, as outlined in steps A through E, an intra-atrial baffle is created using prosthetic material or pericardial tissue. This intra-atrial baffle is placed so that pulmonary and venous blood is directed into the appropriate circulation. However, the placement of the intra-atrial baffle resulted in extensive suture lines, which later became a source of fibrosis, obstruction, and/or foci for dysrhythmias. The top row is surgical views through the right atrium and the bottom row is a cross-sectional view of each sequence of the repair. ASD, atrial septal defect; CS, coronary sinus; IVC, inferior vena cava; LA, left atrium; LPV, left pulmonary vein; PRV, right pulmonary vein; PVA, pulmonary venous atrium; RA, right atrium; RLPV, right lower pulmonary vein; RUPV, right upper pulmonary vein; SVA, systemic venous atrium; SVC, superior vena cava; TV, tricuspid valve. (From Neches WH, Park SC, Ettedgui JA: Transposition of the great arteries. In: Garson A Jr, Bricker JT, Fisher DJ, Neish SR, eds: The Science and Practice of Pediatric Cardiology, 2nd ed, Vol. 1. Baltimore: Williams & Wilkins; 1998: 1494.)

of the time and reoperation is more often required than with the Senning procedure.[230–233] Technical changes in baffle placement, baffle size, and baffle material seemed to offer an improved long-term outcome. The adoption of the Senning procedure with the use of native atrial tissue was seen as a solution to many long-term Mustard procedure–related problems. In addition, the Senning procedure was technically easier to perform in the neonate and young infant than the Mustard procedure. Many centers advocated the Senning procedure and good results were reported.[218, 223, 224, 234–237] Nevertheless, problems with baffle obstruction, while fewer, did not disappear. Furthermore, the long-term outcome with respect to dysrhythmias and the Senning procedure was less than optimal (see Table 19–3).[238, 239]

Dysrhythmias were also an extremely important long-term problem for Mustard patients. In the immediate postoperative period, sinus rhythm problems were commonly seen and were believed to be secondary to bypass cannulation and surgical problems such as damage to the sinus node artery or the sinus node itself at the time of surgery. The region between the coronary sinus and the tricuspid valve was also an area at risk for atrioventricular node damage.[226, 240–246] Atrial arrhythmias and sick sinus syndrome were seen and continued to increase in frequency as follow-up time postoperatively increased. Surgical manipulations and technical changes seemed to improve the immediate problem, and the incidence of acute postoperative dysrhythmias decreased. Nevertheless, as natural history data accumulated, it became clear that patients undergoing the Senning procedure also did not escape long-term problems with dysrhythmias.[6, 247] At postoperative cardiac catheterization, sinus node recovery abnormalities (30% incidence), and junctional

rhythm were present.[238, 239] Table 19–3[248] summarizes the dysrhythmias in multiple studies on Mustard and Senning procedures. Ten-year follow-up studies predict a 50% incidence of atrial dysrhythmias for all patients after Mustard and Senning procedures. The loss of sinus rhythm as time elapsed (40% in sinus rhythm 20 years postoperatively) and an increasing incidence of atrial flutter and sudden death in one 30-year follow-up study of Mustard patients raised ongoing concerns.[249] The significant risk for dysrhythmias created a need for surgical reassessment, despite the low rate of acute operative morbidity and mortality that had been achieved with the Mustard and Senning procedures.

Since the tricuspid valve becomes the "systemic atrioventricular valve" after a Mustard or Senning procedure, any problems with tricuspid valve insufficiency might raise long-term concerns. In many studies, tricuspid valve insufficiency was rarely seen (<5%)[250] but did seem to be related to VSD closure through the tricuspid valve.[228, 230, 231, 251] Some investigators felt that tricuspid valve insufficiency was associated with postoperative dysrhythmias.[252]

The most obvious sequela of atrial switch procedures is that the right ventricle becomes the systemic ventricle. Whether the right ventricle can do systemic work for a normal lifespan is a question that cannot be definitively answered, since the first patients to survive an atrial baffle procedure are entering their third and fourth decade of follow-up. However, studies suggest that about 10% of Mustard or Senning patients will suffer from systemic ventricular failure in long-term follow-up.[253] The conclusion from many studies over decades is that systemic right ventricular function in Mustard patients is below normal, even though these patients are asymptomatic and doing well.[254–257] There are many factors that may influence the incidence of ventricular dysfunction, however, and these include the type of atrial switch (Senning patients had better function than Mustard patients),[258] age at operation (younger age showing better long-term function), better preoperative ventricular function, and better myocardial protection.[206, 259, 260]

Those patients who suffer from severe right ventricular failure may be considered candidates for a two-staged arterial switch procedure in which pulmonary artery banding and systemic-to-pulmonary artery shunt are placed to prepare the left ventricle to become the systemic ventricle and perform systemic work. This is not a low-risk alternative for patients with systemic ventricular failure after Mustard or Senning procedures, but it may offer an alternative surgical option to cardiac transplantation.[261]

Preoperative Factors Influencing Outcome After Arterial Switch Operation

Because definitive repair is performed soon after birth with the one-stage arterial switch procedure, many of the long-term problems associated with chronic hypoxemia, cyanosis, polycythemia, and congestive heart failure are avoided. The presence of a VSD or especially multiple VSDs, other congenital heart anomalies such as coarctation, or atrioventricular valve abnormalities may influence immediate outcome in the neonatal postoperative period. Probably the most important preoperative factor that influences outcome in patients undergoing an arterial switch is the pattern of coronary artery distribution. The origin, proximal course, and branching of the coronary arteries is very variable in transposition of the great arteries. Since the coronary arteries are transplanted during an arterial switch procedure, the location of the coronary arteries determines the surgical difficulty with such a switch. Even with a large variety of coronary artery anatomy, (all of which may be "switchable"), certain coronary patterns have been shown to significantly increase the risk of arterial switch operations.[262-272] These risk patterns include a left coronary artery that has a retropulmonary course and intramural course of the left coronary artery. Table 19–11[273] summarizes the risk factors for death after the arterial switch operation, which is an overview of a multi-institutional study from the Congenital Heart Surgeons Society. An interesting risk factor is an earlier calendar date of surgery. It was clear in the late 1980s that surgeons experienced a learning curve for this operation.[204, 215, 274]

Surgical Repair: Arterial Switch Repair

The arterial switch operation consists of transection of both great arteries, removal of the coronary arteries with a "button" of tissue around the coronary ostium, and transplantation of the coronary arteries above the "neo-aortic" valve (the pulmonary valve before the switch) (Fig. 19–16).[216] The initial approach to the arterial switch procedure was a two-stage repair: an initial "banding" of the pulmonary artery so that the low-pressure left ventricle would become "prepared" to do systemic work, and placement of a Blalock-Taussig shunt to counteract the limitation of pulmonary blood flow that the band would impose. The band and the shunt therefore put a volume and pressure load on the left

Table 19–11. Risk Factors for Death After the Arterial Switch Operation*

Anatomic

Coronary artery abnormalities
  Retropulmonary course of the LCA
  Intramural course of the LCA
Multiple ventricular septal defects
Dextrocardia

Procedural/Support-Related

Surgical augmentation of the aortic arch
Longer global myocardial ischemic time
Longer total circulatory arrest time

Other

(Earlier) calendar date of surgery
(Older) age at surgery (for TGA/IVS)

*As assessed by data from Boston Children's Hospital from 1983 to 1993 (n = 580). LCA, left coronary artery; IVS, intact ventricular septum; TGA, transposition of the great vessels.
From Wernovsky G, Freed MD: Transposition of the great arteries: Results and outcome of the arterial switch operation. In: Freedom RM, Braunwald E, eds: Atlas of Heart Diseases, Vol. XII. St. Louis: Mosby; 1997.

ventricle. Several months after stage 1, debanding, takedown of the shunt, and the arterial switch would be performed.[271]

In 1984, Castaneda reported a one-stage arterial switch approach in neonates; this approach has been adopted over the last 16 years for a majority of neonates with transposition of the great arteries. Because it is a one-stage neonatal repair, the residua, sequelae, and complications of banding, shunt placement, and takedown are avoided.[275]

Residua and Sequelae and Complications of the Arterial Switch Procedure

Long-term sequelae of the arterial switch operation are summarized in Table 19–12.[276] It is well recognized that supravalvar pulmonary stenosis is a widely recognized sequela of the arterial switch operation. Re-intervention has been needed in 5 to 30% of patients, with a peak need for re-intervention at about 6 months post procedure. Many of these patients can be treated in the interventional cardiac catheterization laboratory with dilatation of the pulmonic stenosis. Risk factors for supravalvular pulmonic stenosis are listed in Table 19–13.[261, 275, 277-281] The risk of dysrhythmias after Mustard and Senning procedures was a major determinant in changing the surgical approach to transposition of the great arteries. Mid-term data support this change, since the incidence of dysrhythmias appears to be significantly less after arterial switch operations; sinus rhythm is uniformly present, with rare exceptions.[244, 271, 275, 282-285] Figure 19–17 illustrates the results of the Boston Children's Hospital experience comparing the arterial switch operation with Mustard procedure for correction of transposition of the great arteries.[284] Electrophysiologic studies have confirmed these good conduction system results with normal sinus node and normal atrioventricular conduction in patients after the arterial switch operation. Ischemia or exercise-induced ventricular ectopy is also rare.[275, 286] Table 19–3 summarizes the immediate postoperative data and follow-up data using Holter monitoring in a large group of patients who under-

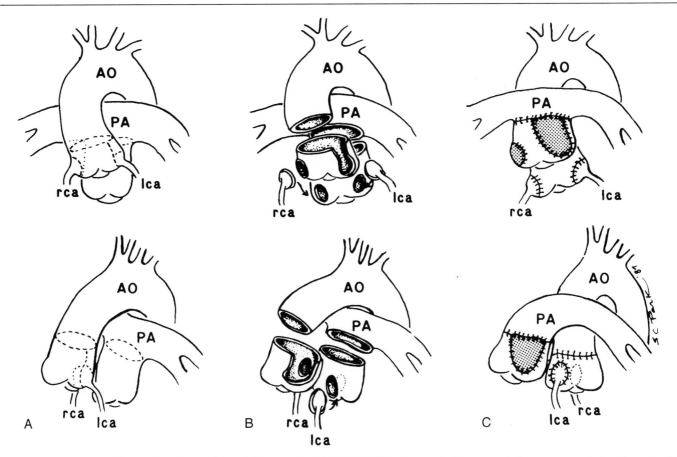

Figure 19–16. Diagram illustrating the arterial switch operation (ASO). (A) The abnormal placement of the great vessels is schematically demonstrated. (B) The transection of the great vessels and reimplantation of the coronary arteries. (C) The completed arterial switch procedure. As a result of the arterial switch, the original pulmonary valve is now a neo-aortic valve and the aortic valve is the neo-pulmonary valve. The extensive supravalvular suture lines raise the possibility of long-term concerns about fibrosis and supravalvular stenosis. Top, Frontal view. Bottom, Sagittal view. Ao, aorta; LCA, left coronary artery; PA, pulmonary artery; RCA, right coronary artery. (From Neches WH, Park SC, Ettedgui JA: Transposition of the great arteries. In: Garson A Jr, Bricker JT, Fisher DJ, Neish SR, eds: The Science and Practice of Pediatric Cardiology, 2nd ed, Vol 1. Baltimore: Williams & Wilkins; 1998: 1498.)

went the arterial switch operation.[287] Neo-aortic regurgitation with a range of severity has been described following arterial switch operations.[265, 288–290] A much higher incidence has been described after the two-stage repair.[291–293]

Cardiac function shows excellent preservation in midterm results after arterial switch operations.[282] In a study examining myocardial perfusion, function, and exercise tolerance, the patients were physically well and asymptomatic, and they had normal exercise tolerance. However, resting radionuclide myocardial perfusion was abnormal in almost all patients, although there was improvement with exercise.[294]

The most important, and as yet unanswered, question is the fate of coronary artery growth and the potential for coronary artery ostial stenosis or kinking as fibrosis and scarring occur over the years following surgery. A small subgroup of patients (1–3%) have asymptomatic occlusion

Table 19–12. Long-Term Sequelae of the Arterial Switch Operation

Supravalvular pulmonary stenosis
  Anastomosis, branch pulmonary arteries
  Neo-aortic regurgitation
  Neo-aortic root dilatation
Coronary abnormalities
Arrhythmia
  Ectopy, sinus node dysfunction, atrioventricular block
Enlarged bronchial collateral arteries
Supravalvular aortic stenosis
Left ventricular dysfunction

From Wernovsky G, Freed MD: Transposition of the great arteries: Results and outcome on the arterial switch operation. In: Freedom RM, Braunwald E, eds: Atlas of Heart Diseases, Vol. XII. St Louis: Mosby; 1997.

Table 19–13. Risk Factors for Supravalvular Pulmonary Stenosis After the Arterial Switch Operation

Lower weight at operation
"Rapid" two-stage arterial switch operation
Preoperative right ventricular outflow tract obstruction
  (subaortic [neopulmonic] stenosis)
"Inverted" right and circumflex coronary arteries
Earlier calendar year of surgery

From Wernovsky G, Freed MD: Transposition of the great arteries: Results and outcome of the arterial switch operation. In: Freedom RM, Braunwald E, eds: Atlas of Heart Diseases, Vol. XII. St Louis: Mosby; 1997.

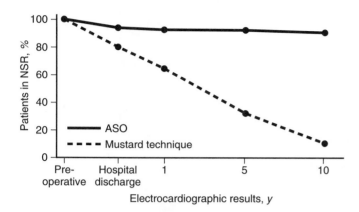

Figure 19–17. Postoperative arrhythmias: arterial switch operation (ASO) versus Mustard operation. This chart illustrates the dramatic difference in patients with normal sinus rhythm between patients after the arterial switch operation or after the Mustard operation (Boston Children's Hospital experience). It is clear that the mid-term results illustrated here are encouraging for patients with ASO: normal sinus rhythm persists over time. NSR, normal sinus rhythm; Y, years after repair. (From Wernovsky G, Freed MD: Transposition of the great arteries: Results and outcome of the arterial switch operation. In: Freedom RM, Braunwald E, eds: Atlas of Heart Diseases, Congenital Heart Diseases, Vol. XII. St. Louis: Mosby; 1997: 16.7.)

of the coronary arteries.[268, 282, 283] Many of these patients develop collateral arteries, implying that the occlusion occurs gradually. Late death secondary to myocardial infarction has been reported in 1% to 2% of hospital survivors.[282, 283, 295] Clearly, long-term issues with coronary artery stenosis will be defined over the next several decades. In general, ongoing data support the excellent short-term and long-term outcomes for arterial switch operation patients, the promise of excellent cardiac function, and freedom from serious dysrhythmias.

Fontan Procedure

The Fontan procedure was originally described by Fontan and Baudet in 1971 as a surgical treatment for patients with tricuspid atresia.[296] The absence of a tricuspid valve and the inability of systemic venous blood to reach the pulmonary circulation mandates that systemic venous and pulmonary venous blood mix completely at the atrial level. As a result of this mandatory mixing, the left ventricle receives an excessive volume load of desaturated blood that circulates to the systemic circulation as well as the pulmonary circulation via a mandatory downstream shunt such as a VSD, PDA, or surgically created systemic-to-pulmonary artery shunt. The Fontan procedure results in a separation of the mixed systemic and pulmonary venous blood, relieving cyanosis and decreasing the volume loading of the left ventricle.

The initial Fontan procedure included a direct right atrial to pulmonary artery anastomosis so that the right atrium became the "pumping chamber" for systemic venous return to reach the pulmonary artery (Fig. 19–18). A classic Glenn shunt in which the superior vena cava is anastomosed end-to-end to the right pulmonary artery was part of the original procedure.[296] Central venous pressure is the driving force for pulmonary blood flow. For hemodynamic stability to be

maintained, the right atrium cannot face any anatomic obstruction or increase in pulmonary resistance without dire cardiovascular consequences. For this reason, the Fontan procedure cannot be a realistic option in the neonate because the pulmonary vascular resistance is high in neonates.

Other "right-heart" bypass procedures such as the Glenn shunt and multiple modifications of the original Fontan procedure have resulted in the application of the Fontan procedure to a wider array of complex congenital heart lesions than the initial experience with tricuspid atresia patients. In recent decades, a diverse group of patients with single-ventricle physiology have benefited from the Fontan procedure, most notably patients with hypoplastic left heart syndrome who were offered no therapeutic alternative until the mid 1980s.

Why should patients who have undergone the Fontan procedure be included in a discussion of management of the definitively repaired CHD patient? In many ways, the Fontan patient is a "definitively" palliated patient in whom no further procedures are anticipated. Many of these patients appear quite well and are often asymptomatic.[297–299] They are, however, emblematic of how asymptomatic status should not give the pediatric anesthesiologist a false sense of security about cardiovascular stability. Every Fontan patient is at risk for cardiovascular compromise if the underlying physiology is not well understood when the stress of surgery and anesthesia intervenes.

Finally, the term *Fontan procedure* now encompasses multiple surgical modifications of the original procedure, and it is worth reviewing some of these different modifications. Nevertheless, management of the single ventricle patient has been a dramatic and evolving clinical challenge. Fontan procedures now carry less risk and better outcomes, despite being offered to more high-risk patients with complicated conditions. This improved outcome is a direct result of minimizing the risk factors found historically to be associated with poor outcome.

Preoperative Factors Influencing Outcome After Repair

A clear understanding of the physiology of the Fontan circulation elucidates why certain risk factors must be eliminated or minimized to improve immediate and long-term outcome. As noted, after the Fontan procedure, central venous pressure drives pulmonary blood flow. Systemic output comes from pulmonary venous return. Individual pressure gradients combine to elevate the central venous pressure. For example, if there is an elevation of the gradient between systemic vein and pulmonary atrium, the central venous pressure and restrictive ventricular preload will be elevated beyond clinically tolerated levels. Cardiac output will be severely reduced and cardiovascular collapse may ensue. It is obvious then why *ventilatory strategies must address minimizing the development of gradients such as acute rises in pulmonary vascular resistance*. Other significant risk factors for problems after Fontan repair include poor ventricular function with elevated end-diastolic pressure, atrioventricular valve insufficiency, elevated pulmonary vascular resistance, pulmonary artery obstruction, and stenosis of the systemic venous to pulmonary artery connection.[300–302] Many of the important advances in surgical modifications and the timing

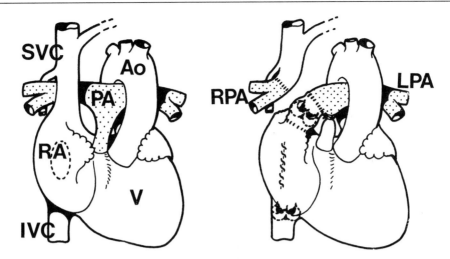

Figure 19–18. Schematic representation of original description of the Fontan repair. The superior vena cava (SVC) is anastomosed end-to-end to the right pulmonary artery (RPA) (classic Glenn shunt) and the right atrium is anastomosed to the left pulmonary artery (right figure). The Fontan and related procedures were initially described as right heart bypass procedures and were applied to patients with right heart obstruction, such as the tricuspid atresia pictured here (left figure). The goal was to achieve as closely as possible a normal circulatory pattern. Desaturated systemic venous blood is routed to pulmonary arteries, where central venous pressure drives the blood through the lungs. The fully saturated pulmonary venous blood returns to the single ventricle, where it is pumped to the body. Fontan anatomy separates the systemic and pulmonary venous return, relieving cyanosis. Pulmonary blood flow is provided by central venous pressure rather than through a banded pulmonary artery or a systemic to pulmonary artery shunt. The single ventricle is thus relieved of the volume load of pulmonary blood flow. This procedure with its modifications was later applied to any congenital heart disease with single ventricle physiology. Ao, aorta; IVC, inferior vena cava; LPA, left pulmonary artery; PA, pulmonary artery; RA, right atrium, RPA, right pulmonary artery; V, ventricle (either right or left). (Modified from Fontan F, Baudet E: Surgical repair of tricuspid atresia. Thorax 1971; 26:240–248. With permission of the BMJ Publishing Group.)

of different surgical procedures have been directed at minimizing these preoperative risk factors.

Surgical Repair

Surgical intervention varies according to the specific anatomy and physiology of the single ventricle. Patients with single-ventricle physiology include a wide array of lesions, including some of the more complicated constellations of anatomic abnormalities. However, as an overview, it is more useful to approach these patients with the underlying physiology in mind.

Most patients with single-ventricle physiology fall into one of three categories:

1. *Unobstructed systemic outflow with obstruction to pulmonary blood flow.* These neonates are cyanotic and require a systemic-to-pulmonary artery shunt to urgently deal with severe cyanosis in the neonatal period. The placement of the shunt is crucial, so that distortion and possible stenosis at the site of shunt placement are minimized. Pulmonary artery stenosis at the time of the Fontan procedure is a major contributor to early failure.
2. *No obstructions to either systemic or pulmonary blood flow.* This group of neonates may be mildly cyanotic but clinically compensated until pulmonary vascular resistance begins to fall and excessive pulmonary blood flow ensues. As a result, congestive heart failure symptoms will predominate and pulmonary artery banding may be indicated to control these symptoms.
3. *Obstructed systemic blood flow with unobstructed pulmonary blood flow.* This group of patients typically exhibits a spectrum of systemic obstruction. On one extreme is the hypoplastic left heart syndrome that must be managed

by the Norwood procedure as stage I (creation of a neo-aorta, a right-sided modified Blalock-Taussig shunt, and an atrial septectomy; Fig. 19–19),[303] followed later by modifications of the Fontan operation. Less extreme obstruction to pulmonary blood flow may be handled with the Damus-Stansel-Kaye operation, in which the unobstructed pulmonary outflow is used to give relief of systemic outflow tract obstruction. Pulmonary blood flow comes from a systemic-to-pulmonary artery shunt or a bidirectional cavopulmonary anastomosis (Fig. 19–20).[304] The key to management of the neonate with one of these clinical scenarios is to achieve the goal of a balanced circulation without excessive pulmonary blood flow but enough flow to avoid severe cyanosis. Most neonates need some surgical intervention, as described earlier.

Several modifications of the surgical approach were aimed at (1) minimizing pulmonary artery distortion long term (which would create serious problems at the time of final Fontan procedure) and (2) enhancing normal growth and development of the pulmonary arteries from the neonatal period until the time of the Fontan operation. A significant advance in this area was the application of the bidirectional cavopulmonary anastomosis or bidirectional Glenn shunt (superior vena cava anastomosis end-to-end to the right pulmonary artery) to patients as a staged approach to the final Fontan repair. Figure 19–21[305] illustrates the bidirectional Glenn shunt as a staging procedure in the management of tricuspid atresia. The bidirectional Glenn shunt and the classic Glenn shunt (superior vena cava to right pulmonary artery anastomosis) have beneficial results. The bidirectional Glenn shunt allows for optimal pulmonary artery growth without significant risk of pulmonary artery distortion. Physiologically, the single ventricle is relieved of the volume and

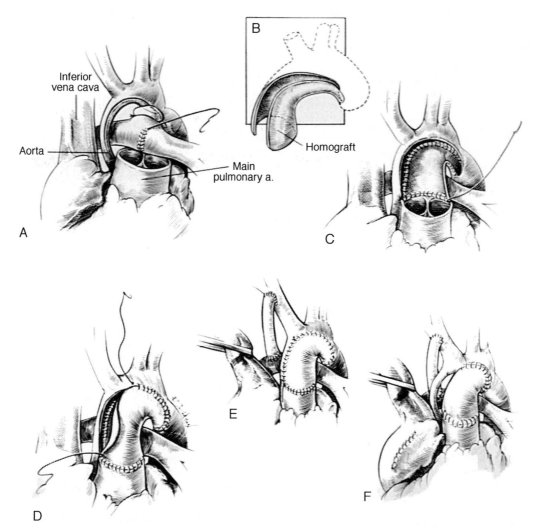

Figure 19–19. Stage I Norwood procedure for hypoplastic left heart syndrome. First stage palliation for hypoplastic left heart syndrome. (A) Incisions used for the procedure, incorporating a cuff of arterial wall allograft. The distal divided main pulmonary artery may be closed by direct suture or with a patch. (B) Dimensions of the cuff of the arterial wall allograft. (C) The arterial wall allograft is used to supplement the anastomosis between the proximal divided main pulmonary artery and the ascending aorta, aortic arch, and proximal descending aorta. (D & E) The procedure is completed by an atrial septectomy and a 3.5 mm modified right Blalock shunt. (F) When the ascending aorta is particularly small, an alternative procedure involves placement of a complete tube of arterial allograft. The tiny ascending aorta may be left in situ, as indicated, or implanted into the side of the neoaorta. (From Castaneda AR, Jonas RA, Mayer JE Jr, Hanley FL: Hypoplastic left heart syndrome. In: Cardiac Surgery of the Neonate and Infant. Philadelphia: W.B. Saunders; 1994: 371.)

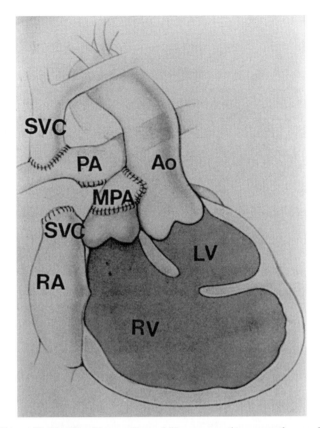

Figure 19–20. The Damus-Stansel-Kaye operation uses the unobstructed pulmonary outflow tract to provide relief of systemic outflow obstruction. The main pulmonary artery (MPA) is anastomosed to the aorta (Ao). Pulmonary blood flow is provided with a systemic to pulmonary artery shunt or bidirectional cavopulmonary anastomoses. LV, left ventricle; PA, pulmonary artery; RA, right atrium; RV, right ventricle; SVC, superior vena cava. (Modified from Laks H, Gates RN, Elami A, et al: Damus-Stansel-Kaye procedure: Technical modifications. Ann Thorac Surg 1992; 54:169–172, with permission from the Society of Thoracic Surgeons.)

pressure load of the pulmonary circulation and as a result, cyanosis dramatically improves.[306–308] Reducing ventricular volume load is an important preventive step toward preserving ventricular function long term as well as lowering the risk of atrioventricular valve insufficiency. The bidirectional Glenn shunt can be carried out in infants as young as 1 month,[309] although it is typically performed in the infant 6 months of age or older. Inferior vena cava blood returns directly to the heart so that sudden changes in pulmonary vascular resistance are less likely to lead to cardiovascular compromise, although cyanosis may increase.

Alternatively, the bidirectional superior vena cava to pulmonary artery anastomosis can be performed as a hemi-Fontan procedure (Fig. 19–22).[310] Patients can then move to the final palliation, which is now called the "completion Fontan." Originally, the Fontan procedure consisted of a direct right atrium to pulmonary artery anastomosis. Studies over the last decade have demonstrated that avoiding turbulence in the Fontan connection is essential so that maximal flow is reached with a minimal pressure drop.[311] As a result of this understanding, a new modification, the lateral tunnel Fontan procedure, was developed (Fig. 19–23).[312] The lateral

tunnel channels inferior vena caval blood flow through the atrium in a lateral, cylindrical, linear pathway. Improved outcomes have been observed secondary to the superior flow dynamics through the lateral tunnel. Another important modification was fenestration of the intra-atrial baffle, which significantly improved the rates of morbidity and mortality in the immediate postoperative period, when elevations of pulmonary vascular resistance can result in a life-threatening decrease in cardiac output (Fig. 19–24).[313, 314] The fenestration permits right-to-left shunting and results in a lower central venous pressure, increased left ventricular preload, and improved cardiac output even in the presence of a mild degree of systemic desaturation. At a later date, the fenestration can be closed using a device in the catheterization laboratory.[313]

Residua, Sequelae, and Complications

The evolving surgical management of the patient with single-ventricle physiology makes it difficult to compare early cohorts of patients who have undergone surgery with those who have benefited from many of the modifications described. Large series of patients operated on in the early era showed a 5-year survival rate between 63% and 79%.[297, 299] However, a recent study reported an 80% survival rate for

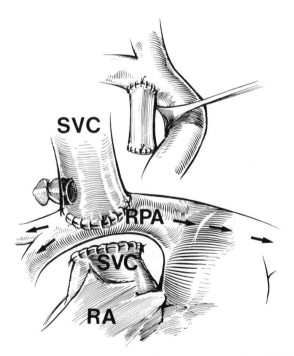

Figure 19–21. Bidirectional cavopulmonary anastomosis. A bidirectional cavopulmonary anastomosis can be constructed as a bidirectional Glenn shunt in which the superior vena cava (SVC) is anastomosed to the confluent pulmonary arteries (RPA), allowing blood flow to both right and left pulmonary arteries (arrows). In contrast, the classic Glenn shunt results in superior vena cava blood going into the right pulmonary artery, which has been transected and removed from the main pulmonary artery and left pulmonary artery (see Fig. 19–18). (Modified from Castaneda AR, Jonas RA, Mayer JE, Hanley FL: Single ventricle tricuspid atresia. In: Cardiac Surgery of the Neonate and Infant. Philadelphia: W.B. Saunders; 1994:262.)

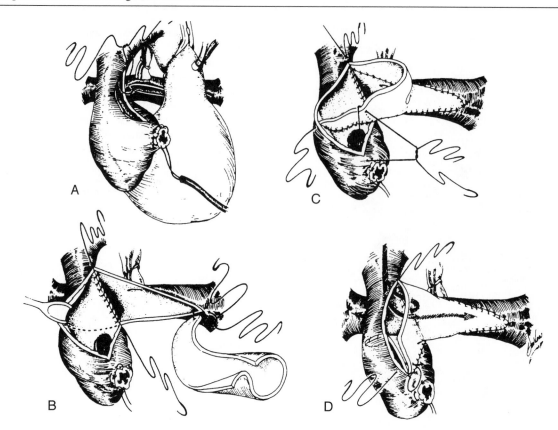

Figure 19–22. The Hemi-Fontan operation. The bidirectional cavopulmonary anastomosis (BDCPA) can also be constructed as a Hemi-Fontan. A large anastomosis is constructed between the superior vena cava and the confluent pulmonary arteries (A). Cavoatrial continuity is maintained and the pulmonary arteries are augmented (B & C). A dam, constructed of homograft and continuous with the pulmonary artery augmentation, completely diverts the superior vena cava flow into the pulmonary arteries (D). Subsequent completion Fontan is simplified because a large connection between the pulmonary arteries and atrium is already present. The dam is excised and the lateral tunnel is constructed (see Fig. 19–23). (From Jacobs ML: Hypoplastic left heart syndrome. In: Kaiser LR, Kron IL, Spray TL, eds: Mastery of Cardiothoracic Surgery. Philadelphia: Lippincott-Raven; 1998: 863.)

Figure 19–23. Lateral tunnel Fontan operation. After creation of a bidirectional cavopulmonary anastomosis (BDCPA), a follow-up surgical procedure is the construction of a lateral tunnel Fontan. A tube graft of polytetrafluoroethylene (PTFE) is incised longitudinally and used to route the inferior vena cava (IVC) blood to the confluent pulmonary arteries. Only a strip of atrial muscle, necessary for growth, is exposed to the increased venous pressure. The lateral tunnel Fontan minimizes turbulence, thus decreasing loss of energy in the Fontan connection. The result is more pulmonary blood flow and therefore systemic cardiac output at lower central venous pressure. In addition, atrial dilatation and hypertension, a risk factor for development of atrial arrhythmias, is avoided. (From Kirklin JW, Barrett-Boyes BG: Tricuspid atresia and the Fontan procedures. In: Cardiac Surgery, 2nd ed. New York: Churchill Livingstone; 1993: 1070.)

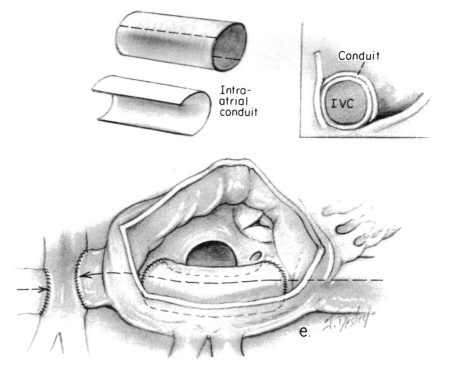

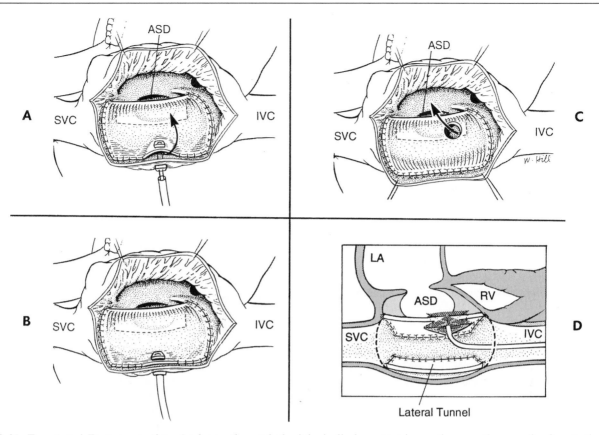

Figure 19–24. Fenestrated Fontan operation. An innovative and physiologically important innovation was the use of a fenestration at the time of Fontan repair. The risk of early ventricular failure has been shown to be decreased by the use of a fenestrated Fontan procedure. The defect in the lateral tunnel connection allows for right-to-left shunting. The fenestration ameliorates the impact of elevation of pulmonary vascular resistance and myocardial dysfunction; cardiac output is maintained and central venous pressure is lowered by the right-to-left shunt, although the patient has mild arterial desaturation. The fenestrated Fontan repair can be constructed with a snare (A). The end of the snare is commonly placed in a subcutaneous space in the upper abdomen at the end of the sternotomy incision. The fenestration can be closed by accessing the snare in the subcutaneous tissue rather than an open procedure (B). The fenestration can be constructed without a snare (C) and a catheter-delivered closure device can be used for occlusion (D). ASD, atrial septal defect; IVC, inferior vena cava; LA, left atrium; RV, right ventricle; SVC, superior vena cava. (From Kopf GS: Tricuspid atresia. In: Mavroudis C, Backer CL, eds: Pediatric Cardiac Surgery. St. Louis: Mosby; 1994: 394.)

patients operated on after 1988 and 90% for those operated on after 1990.[315]

Patients who have had these procedures are at risk for several serious long-term problems. These include a decline in functional status, deteriorating ventricular function, dysrhythmias, protein-losing enteropathy, and death.[297–299, 315] The need for a persistently elevated central venous pressure as part of Fontan physiology is responsible for many of these long-term problems. Protein-losing enteropathy is the loss of gastrointestinal tract protein. This complication may develop in previously well Fontan patients. The elevated central venous pressure leads to bowel edema, malabsorption, and malnutrition. Length of survival may be a risk factor. In one study, 2.5% of 363 patients followed for 5.4 years had protein-losing enteropathy.[298] When follow-up was extended to 10 years in another group of patients, 13.4% of patients were noted to develop protein-losing enteropathy.[316]

Dysrhythmias are common. Sinus node dysfunction was seen in 13% of patients, and 16% had atrial flutter in one study. Importantly, the risk for atrial flutter increased as the postoperative period increased, with 40% of patients having atrial flutter at 10 years.[317] Some of these long-term problems

may decrease as natural history data are collected on the Fontan population that has benefited from modifications since Fontan's original description in 1971. The data are not yet clear and continue to be reviewed. At the same time, it must also be kept in mind that these successful modifications also led to the application of the Fontan procedure to groups of patients with single ventricle physiology with increasingly more complex conditions.[297, 315]

Nonsurgical Repairs (Interventional Cardiac Catheterization) and Natural History Studies Defining Long-Term Outcome

The cardiac catheterization laboratory has played a pivotal role in the half century of advances in the management of CHD. An accurate anatomic diagnosis, coupled with precise hemodynamic measurements, was best obtained in the cardiac catheterization laboratory. These measurements were considered the "gold standard" for diagnosis. Surgeons and cardiologists could then make a more informed and appropriate plan. In addition, routine postoperative cardiac catheterizations followed by complex electrophysiologic studies in CHD patients contributed valuable information to the natural history databank. As has been described previously, Rashkind and Miller revolutionized the management of transposition of the great arteries with the first and most successful interventional procedure, the Rashkind balloon septostomy.

In the late 1970s, two-dimensional echocardiography was added to the diagnostic armamentarium of the pediatric cardiologist and in some ways threatened the supremacy of the cardiac catheterization laboratory. More patients, including neonates, could be diagnosed with great accuracy, so that a preoperative cardiac catheterization was deemed not necessary. Postoperative cardiac catheterizations were replaced with routine echocardiographic follow-up.

Nevertheless, over the last decade, the focus of the cardiac catheterization laboratory has changed dramatically and remains in the forefront of management of CHD. Today, the catheterization laboratory plays a major therapeutic role in the management of CHD, such that certain patients routinely undergo interventional procedures for the repair of their defect rather than surgery. In addition, interventional techniques may be part of a staged approach to repair or may be crucial in the repair of postoperative residua, sequelae, or complications of surgery. In the same way that surgery may be definitive or palliative, interventional techniques may also be definitive or palliative. This section briefly reviews the indications for interventional therapy, especially with those lesions that are no longer routinely treated with surgery. Table 19–14 summarizes the different lesions that may be amenable to interventional procedures in the catheterization laboratory.

Table 19–14. Congenital Heart Defects Amenable to Interventional Cardiac Catheterization Repair

Dilation of Valvular Lesions
- Dilation of the pulmonary valve
- Dilation of the aortic valve
- Dilation of the mitral valve
- Dilation of bioprosthetic valves

Vascular Angioplasties
- Dilation of coarctation of the aorta
- Dilation of pulmonary artery stenosis
- Dilation of systemic venous obstructions

Endovascular Stents

Opening of Atrial Communications
- Balloon atrial septostomy
- Blade septostomy

Closure of Extracardiac and Intracardiac Communications
- Closure of aortopulmonary collaterals
- Closure of surgical systemic to pulmonary shunts
- Closure of arteriovenous malformations
- Closure of venovenous connections
- Closure of patent ductus arteriosus
- Closure of atrial septal defect
- Closure of ventricular septal defect

Valvular Lesions: Dilatation

Pulmonary Valve

Since the first report of successful pulmonary valvuloplasty, catheterization laboratory dilatation is now considered the treatment of choice for moderate to severe pulmonary valve stenosis and for critical pulmonary valve stenosis in neonates.[318–320] A gradient of 50 mm Hg or more with normal cardiac output is an indication for relief of obstruction. Long-term outcomes include residual stenosis or pulmonary regurgitation and the consequent pressure or volume work that these derangements cause on the right ventricle. In a multi-institution study (22 institutions) from the Valvuloplasty and Angioplasty of Congenital Anomalies group, 74% of the total of 533 patients were deemed successfully treated (i.e., gradients < 36 mm Hg). At the 3-year follow-up, 23% had a suboptimal gradient.[321]

Aortic Valve

Aortic stenosis, treated with valvuloplasty, has shown good results in children with this lesion. The indications for valvuloplasty are the same as for surgical intervention: (1) peak-to-peak gradients of 70 mm Hg, (2) 50 mm Hg gradient with associated symptoms, and (3) ST-T wave changes on the ECG indicative of myocardial ischemia at rest or with exercise. The success rate for balloon valvuloplasty has been 87% to 97%,[322–325] with average gradient relief of 55% to 70%.[323, 326] Aortic regurgitation and coronary arterial occlusion are recognized complications but are rare.[327, 328] Studies have demonstrated no significant differences in mortality, morbidity, or need for reintervention within 1 year when surgery is compared to interventional valvuloplasty.[322, 328] Follow-up studies show that at 4 years' follow-up, 75% do not need re-intervention and 50% are also free of need for re-intervention at 8 years.[323, 327]

Neonatal aortic stenosis has a different outcome profile. Neonates suffer more morbidity, but studies now demonstrate that interventional dilatation is as safe as surgery in neonates, with an early mortality of 11%.[329] The rate of both morbidity and mortality in neonates has decreased considerably.[330] Neonates are more likely to require re-intervention within 10 years when compared with older infants and children.[331]

Mitral Valve

Congenital mitral stenosis is rare and is often associated with other left-sided heart defects such as coarctation of the aorta and hypoplasia of the left ventricle. These symptomatic infants have high rates of morbidity and mortality. Obviously, avoiding valve replacement in a small neonate is beneficial and dilatation can postpone this surgical event.[332–334] Complications can be serious and include left ventricular perforation, complete atrioventricular block, mitral valve leaflet injury, and severe mitral regurgitation.[333]

Bioprosthetic Valve

Bioprosthetic valves, most commonly those placed in a conduit, can become calcified and have a high failure rate in children (>40% at 3 to 5 years).[335-337] Balloon dilatation has demonstrated an average 40% gradient reduction in most patients, although increased valve incompetence can result.[338] The pulmonary valve in a conduit is the most commonly dilated valve, although all other valves have been treated.

Vascular Angioplasties

The American Heart Association has made a statement that balloon angioplasty is indicated in patients with recoarctation of the aorta, systemic vein stenosis, or pulmonary artery stenosis. Other patients may also be treated with angioplasty, including children older than 6 months with native coarctation and systemic-to-pulmonary-artery shunts; pulmonary vein stenosis is not as well treated with this technique.[339]

Coarctation of the Aorta

Because surgery for recurrent coarctation of the aorta is technically challenging and therefore carries an increased risk for morbidity and mortality,[340] angioplasty has become the treatment of choice. The data on follow-up in several large studies shows an immediate success rate of 65 to 100% with a low procedure mortality rate from 0% to 2.5%. The rate of recurrent stenosis is about 30% in patients with a re-coarctation.[341-348]

Balloon angioplasty for the neonate with coarctation is more controversial. Neonates have a much higher rate of restenosis compared to children who undergo the procedure after 1 year.[349] In a multi-institutional review of 25 centers from the Valvuloplasty and Angioplasty of Congenital Anomalies Registry, 907 procedures (422 coarctation of the aorta and 548 recoarctation of the aorta) had an acute success rate of 81% for native coarctation of the aorta and 75% for recoarctation, with a low procedure-related mortality rate of 0.7%.

The most noteworthy sequela of balloon angioplasty is the possibility of aneurysm formation as a result of intimal tears and aortic wall weakening. The rate of developing aneurysms varies from 0 to 14% in patients with recoarctation and 2 to 6% for native coarctation.[341-343, 347-350] Aneurysms, however, can also be seen after surgical repair (5–21% after 10 years).[351, 352]

Pulmonary Artery Stenosis

Pulmonary artery stenosis can be present from a variety of causes and, depending on the location, can be surgically difficult or impossible to repair. At the same time, even mild degrees of pulmonary stenosis can be poorly tolerated in certain patients (e.g., Fontan patients, tetralogy of Fallot patients). Balloon dilatation carries a low morbidity and mortality rate (1–2%).[353] However, long-term clinical benefit is seen in less than 35% of patients, with 15 to 20% having significant restenosis.[354, 355]

Systemic Venous Obstructions

Systemic venous obstruction can be seen in patients who have undergone baffle intra-atrial repairs for transposition of the great arteries. These lesions are highly amenable to dilatation with little risk.[356, 357]

Cardiovascular Stents

Because of the concern that vascular dilatation carries with it a risk of restenosis, various intravascular stent devices have been used to prevent this sequela. Congenital or postoperative branch pulmonary stenosis represents the largest group of patients treated with cardiovascular stents. Surgery is technically challenging and the incidence of restenosis after surgery is high. In a multi-institutional study of 121 stents in 85 patients, all patients were shown to be hemodynamically improved, especially with an increase in blood flow to the affected lung.[358] Since balloon angioplasty alone is less than ideal (50% initial success rate and 17% restenosis), stent placement results are encouraging, with 100% vessel enlargement and a low medium-term restenosis rate.[354, 359]

Opening of Atrial Communications

The Rashkind procedure in 1966 heralded the era of interventional catheterization laboratory procedures. Blade septostomy is needed when an atrial communication is desired in older infants beyond 1 month of age when the septum is too thick to use a balloon.

Closure of Communications: Intracardiac and Extracardiac

Closure of congenital or acquired anomalous vascular connections is an area of active investigation and treatment. Gianturco et al.[196] described transcatheter occlusion more than 20 years ago, and Gianturco coils remain the most commonly used occlusion devices for CHD. Aortopulmonary collaterals, surgical systemic-to-pulmonary shunts, arteriovenous malformations, coronary artery fistulas, venovenous connections, and PDA have all been successfully closed with a variety of occlusion devices.[360-365]

Finally, intracardiac defect closure dates back to the 1970s with the use of a double-umbrella device for closure of an atrial septal defect.[366] At present a number of different devices are available for ASD closure. The resolution of shunting is immediate, and after 1 year, hemodynamically significant leaks are seen in only 5 to 10% of patients.[367-369] Complications are rare but include damage to other intracardiac structures, such as atrioventricular valves, systemic or pulmonary veins, or perforation. The closure of ventricular septal defects has also been attempted. Several devices have been used to close defects, especially complicated ones such as muscular defects in small infants.[370-374]

Risk Assessment

Every patient and parent deserves a fair assessment of the risks associated with the anesthetic procedure. In addition, historical information on risk can inform the anesthesiologist and the surgeon about potential problems. Dramatic improvements in anesthetic risk for CHD patients undergoing cardiac surgery were well described over the last decade.[375]

On the other hand, risk assessment for the CHD patient

Table 19–15. Evaluation of the Repaired Congenital Heart Disease Patient

- Review underlying CHD anatomy and physiology.
- Review the surgical procedure(s) and understand the anatomy and physiology that results.
- Identify potential residua, sequelae, and complications of the procedure(s).
- Identify the presence of prerepair factors influencing long-term outcome.
  - Age at time of repair
  - Preoperative cyanosis and polycythemia
  - Preoperative CHF
  - Preoperative dysrhythmias
  - Preoperative pulmonary hypertension
- Identify potential cardiac alterations that may manifest with surgery/anesthesia.
- Identify risk of dysrhythmia and plan possible diagnostic and therapeutic regimens. This includes a thorough review of treatment options with the pediatric cardiology team, including aids to diagnosis of unusual dysrhythmias, and guidelines for cardioversion if possibly anticipated. Finally, develop an understanding and plan for intraoperative use of pacemaker and reprogramming, if necessary.
- Identify risk of ventricular dysfunction becoming symptomatic and plan for appropriate inotropic support if indicated.
- Identify risk of pulmonary hypertension becoming symptomatic. Plan for effective ventilatory strategies to minimize a rise in pulmonary artery pressure.
- Identify need for endocarditis and plan appropriately.
- Consult with pediatric cardiologists and cardiac surgeons and discuss need for possible preoperative testing by cardiology team, as indicated. Plan for postoperative monitoring.
- Assess anesthetic risk.

who undergoes noncardiac surgery has only recently been examined by some centers. The data on this group of patients typically examine risk for all CHD patients, repaired and unrepaired. Not surprisingly, the unrepaired or palliated patient presents a greater risk. In addition, the more complex and stressful the surgical procedure, the greater the risk of anesthetic problems as well. No study examines the risk of anesthesia for just the definitively repaired patient, although examination of outcome from studies examining postoperative outcome after general surgical procedures do include them. In such a study, 27 deaths were observed among 226 procedures, with minor procedures having a 3% mortality rate (2 of 70 procedures) compared with 16% for major procedures (25 of 156 procedures). When a logistic analysis was performed, previous corrective surgery (definitive or palliative) did not alter postoperative outcome. Risk factors such as high American Society of Anesthesiologists (ASA) status, age less than 6 months, low weight, and emergency surgery were associated with increased risk.[376] Another study from the Mayo Perioperative Outcome Group reviewed 276 patient outcomes (patients less than 50 years of age with CHD) who underwent 480 procedures. The overall frequency of anesthetic complications was 5.8%, with only one intraoperative death. Surgery on the respiratory or nervous system had a high frequency of complications. Ambulatory surgical procedures had a low risk of 1.7%. Patients with unrepaired defects and the presence of cyanosis, congestive heart failure, high ASA status, and young age at surgery were at greatest risk.[377]

Perioperative Evaluation of Repaired Congenital Heart Disease

This chapter has introduced the pediatric anesthesiologist to a body of information that is essential when an anesthetic plan must be formulated in the surgically repaired CHD patient (Table 19–15). This chapter has also introduced the emerging literature on interventional cardiac catheterization repair as a path to definitive repair.

We fully expect that the anesthesiologist caring for the adult with acquired heart disease who has undergone surgical repair such as coronary artery bypass or valve replacement will be quite knowledgeable and fluent in the cardiac residua, sequelae, and complications of those disease states, even if the adult patient is asymptomatic and appears well. Despite the complexity of CHD and the large array of lesions, these children deserve the same knowledgeable approach to anesthetic planning as the adult after cardiac surgery. The definitively repaired patient who appears well and has no complaints referable to the cardiovascular system nevertheless may be at risk for manifesting an array of potential abnormalities that may be clinically asymptomatic at the time of preoperative evaluation. From this overview, general principles emerge to guide the pediatric anesthesiologist in the formulation of a safe and effective anesthetic perioperative plan.

References

1. Perloff JK: Medical center experiences. J Am Coll Cardiol 1991;18:315–318.
2. Wilson NJ, Neutze JM: Adult congenital heart disease: principles and management guidelines—Part I. Aust N Z J Med 1993;23:498–503.
3. Congenital heart disease after childhood: an expanding patient population. 22nd Bethesda Conference, Maryland, October 18–19, 1990. J Am Coll Cardiol 1991;18:311–342.
4. Izumo S, Nadal-Ginard B, Mahdavi V: Protooncogene induction and reprogramming of cardiac gene expression produced by pressure overload. Proc Natl Acad Sci U S A 1988;85:339–343.
5. Di Donato RM, Fujii AM, Jonas RA, et al: Age-dependent ventricular response to pressure overload. Considerations for the arterial switch operation. J Thorac Cardiovasc Surg 1992;104:713–722.
6. Kanter RJ, Garson A: Arrhythmia in congenital heart disease. In: Podrid PJ, Kowey PR, eds: Cardiac Arrhythmias: Mechanisms, Diagnoses, and Management. Baltimore: Williams & Wilkins; 1995.
7. Lown B, Calvert AF, Armington R, et al: Monitoring for serious arrhythmias and high risk of sudden death. Circulation 1975;52:III189–III198.
8. Greenwood RD, Rosenthal A, Parisi L, et al: Extracardiac abnormalities in infants with congenital heart disease. Pediatrics 1975;55:485–492.
9. Morris CD, Reller MD, Menashe VD: Thirty-year incidence of infective endocarditis after surgery for congenital heart defect. JAMA 1998;279:599–603.
10. Dajani AS, Taubert KA, Wilson W, et al: Prevention of bacterial endocarditis. Recommendations by the American Heart Association. JAMA 1997;277:1794–1801.
11. Gross RE, Hubbard JP: Landmark article Feb 25, 1939: Surgical ligation of a patent ductus arteriosus. Report of first successful case. JAMA 1984;251:1201–1202.
12. Panagopoulos PG, Tatooles CJ, Aberdeen E, et al: Patent ductus arteriosus in infants and children. A review of 936 operations (1946–69). Thorax 1971;26:137–144.
13. Bickford BJ: Surgical aspects of patent ductus arteriosis: a review of 228 cases. Arch Dis Child 1960;35:92–96.
14. Trusler GA: Surgery for patent ductus arteriosus—1979. In: Jones JC, Tucker BL, Lindesmith GG, eds: First Clinical Conference on Congenital Heart Disease. New York: Grune & Stratton; 1979:39–45.

15. Jones JC: Twenty-five years' experience with surgery of the patent ductus arteriosus. J Cardiovasc Surg 1965;50:149–165.
16. Samanek M, Slavik Z, Zborilova B, et al: Prevalence, treatment, and outcome of heart disease in live-born children: a prospective analysis of 91,823 live-born children. Pediatr Cardiol 1989;10:205–211.
17. Fyler DC: Report of the New England Regional Infant Cardiac Program. Pediatrics 1980;65:375–461.
18. Tikkanen J, Heinonen OP: Risk factors for coarctation of the aorta. Teratology 1993;47:565–572.
19. Fyler DC: Coarctation of the Aorta. In: Fyler DC, ed: Nadas' Pediatric Cardiology. Philadelphia: Hanley & Belfus; 1992:535–556.
20. Beekman RH: Coarctation of the aorta. In: Emmanouilides GC, Riemenschneider TA, Allen HD, et al., eds: Moss and Adams Heart Disease in Infants, Children, and Adolescents Including the Fetus and Young Adult, 5th ed. Baltimore: Williams & Wilkins; 1995:1111–1133.
21. Morriss MJH, McNamara DG: Coarctation of the aorta and interrupted aortic arch. In: Garson A Jr, Brinker JT, McNamara DG, eds: The Science and Practice of Pediatric Cardiology. Philadelphia: Lea & Febiger; 1990:1317–1346.
22. Becker AE, Becker MJ, Edwards JE: Anomalies associated with coarctation of aorta: Particular reference to infancy. Circulation 1970;41:1067–1075.
23. Hodes HL, Steinfeld L, Blumenthal S: Congenital cerebral aneurysms and coarctation of the aorta. Arch Pediatr 1959;76:28–43.
24. Crafoord C, Nylin G: Congenital coarctation of the aorta and its surgical treatment. J Thoracic Surg 1945;14:347–361.
25. Gross RE, Hufnagel CA: Coarctation of the aorta: Experimental studies regarding its surgical correction. N Engl J Med 1945;233:287–293.
26. Waldhausen JA, Nahrwold DL: Repair of coarctation of the aorta with a subclavian flap. J Thorac Cardiovasc Surg 1966;51:532–533.
27. Cohen M, Fuster V, Steele PM, et al: Coarctation of the aorta: Long-term follow-up and prediction of outcome after surgical correction. Circulation 1989;80:840–845.
28. Presbitero P, Demarie D, Villani M, et al: Long term results (15–30 years) of surgical repair of aortic coarctation. Br Heart J 1987;57:462–467.
29. Brouwer RM, Erasmus ME, Ebels T, et al: Influence of age on survival, late hypertension, and recoarctation in elective aortic coarctation repair: Including long-term results after elective aortic coarctation repair with a follow-up from 25 to 44 years. J Thorac Cardiovasc Surg 1994;108:525–531.
30. Venturini A, Papalia U, Chiarotti F, et al: Primary repair of coarctation of the thoracic aorta by patch graft aortoplasty: A three-decade experience and follow-up in 60 patients. Eur J Cardiothorac Surg 1996;10:890–896.
31. Backer CL, Paape K, Zales VR, et al: Coarctation of the aorta: Repair with polytetrafluoroethylene patch aortoplasty. Circulation 1995;92:132–136.
32. Pfammatter JP, Ziemer G, Kaulitz R, et al: Isolated aortic coarctation in neonates and infants: Results of resection and end-to-end anastomosis. Ann Thorac Surg 1996;62:778–782.
33. Koller M, Rothlin M, Senning A: Coarctation of the aorta: Review of 362 operated patients. Long-term follow-up and assessment of prognostic variables. Eur Heart J 1987;8:670–679.
34. Zehr KJ, Gillinov AM, Redmond JM, et al: Repair of coarctation of the aorta in neonates and infants: A thirty-year experience. Ann Thorac Surg 1995;59:33–41.
35. Rostad H, Abdelnoor M, Sorland S, et al: Coarctation of the aorta, early and late results of various surgical techniques. J Cardiovasc Surg (Torino) 1989;30:885–890.
36. Fenchel G, Steil E, Seybold-Epting W, et al: Repair of symptomatic aortic coarctation in the first three months of life: Early and late results after resection and end-to-end anastomosis and subclavian flap angioplasty. J Cardiovasc Surg (Torino) 1988;29:257–263.
37. Sarioglu T, Kinoglu B, Sarioglu A, et al: Early and moderate long-term results of a new surgical technique for repair of aortic coarctation. Eur J Cardiothorac Surg 1996;10:884–888.
38. Maron BJ, Humphries JO, Rowe RD, et al: Prognosis of surgically corrected coarctation of the aorta: A 20-year postoperative appraisal. Circulation 1973;47:119–126.
39. Kimball TR, Reynolds JM, Mays WA, et al: Persistent hyperdynamic cardiovascular state at rest and during exercise in children after successful repair of coarctation of the aorta. J Am Coll Cardiol 1994;24:194–200.
40. Krogmann ON, Rammos S, Jakob M, et al: Left ventricular diastolic dysfunction late after coarctation repair in childhood: Influence of left ventricular hypertrophy. J Am Coll Cardiol 1993;21:1454–1460.
41. Moskowitz WB, Schieken RM, Mosteller M, et al: Altered systolic and diastolic function in children after "successful" repair of coarctation of the aorta. Am Heart J 1990;120:103–109.
42. Johnson MC, Gutierrez FR, Sekarski DR, et al: Comparison of ventricular mass and function in early versus late repair of coarctation of the aorta. Am J Cardiol 1994;73:698–701.
43. Sigurdardottir LY, Helgason H: Echocardiographic evaluation of systolic and diastolic function in postoperative coarctation patients. Pediatr Cardiol 1997;18:96–100.
44. Katz G, Uretzky G, Beer G, et al: Long-term results of surgical repair of coarctation of the aorta: Evaluation by exercise test. Cardiology 1987;74:465–473.
45. Rathi L, Keith JD: Postoperative blood pressures in coarctation of the aorta. Br Heart J 1964;26:671–678.
46. Benedict CR, Grahame-Smith DG, Fisher A: Changes in plasma catecholamines and dopamine beta-hydroxylase after corrective surgery for coarctation of the aorta. Circulation 1978;57:598–602.
47. Stewart JM, Gewitz MH, Woolf PK, et al: Elevated arginine vasopressin and lowered atrial natriuretic factor associated with hypertension in coarctation of the aorta. J Thorac Cardiovasc Surg 1995;110:900–908.
48. Brewer LA III, Fosburg RG, Mulder GA, et al: Spinal cord complications following surgery for coarctation of the aorta: A study of 66 cases. J Thorac Cardiovasc Surg 1972;64:368–381.
49. Lewis FJ, Taufic M: Closure of atrial septal defects with the aid of hypothermia: Experimental accomplishments and the report of one successful case. Surgery 1953;33:52–59.
50. Bailey CP, Nichols HT, Bolton HE, et al: Surgical treatment of forty-six interatrial septal defects by atrio-septo-pexy. Ann Surg 1954;140:805–820.
51. Søndergaard T: Closure of atrial septal defects: Report of three cases. Acta Chir Scand 1954;107:492–498.
52. Gross RE, Pomeranz AA, Watkins E Jr, et al: Surgical closure of defects of the interauricular septum by use of an atrial well. N Engl J Med 1952;247:455–460.
53. Gibbon JH Jr: Application of a mechanical heart and lung apparatus to cardiac surgery. Minn Med 1954;171:171–185.
54. Silverman NH: The secundum atrial septal defect and atrioventricular septal defects. In: Freedom RM, Braunwald E, eds: Atlas of Heart Diseases Congenital Heart Disease, Vol XXII. St. Louis: Mosby; 1997:12.1–12.10.
55. Bridges ND, Hellenbrand W, Latson L, et al: Transcatheter closure of patent foramen ovale after presumed paradoxical embolism. Circulation 1992;86:1902–1908.
56. Graham TP Jr, Jarmakani JM, Atwood GF, et al: Right ventricular volume determinations in children: Normal values and observations with volume or pressure overload. Circulation 1973;47:144–153.
57. Rabinovitch M, Andrew M, Thom H, et al: Abnormal endothelial factor VIII associated with pulmonary hypertension and congenital heart defects. Circulation 1987;76:1043–1052.
58. Cherian G, Uthaman CB, Durairaj M, et al: Pulmonary hypertension in isolated secundum atrial septal defect: High frequency in young patients. Am Heart J 1983;105:952–957.
59. Dalen JE, Haynes FW, Dexter L: Life expectancy with atrial septal defect: Influence of complicating pulmonary vascular disease. JAMA 1967;200:442–446.
60. Sealy WC, Farmer JC, Young WG Jr, et al: Atrial dysrhythmia and atrial secundum defects. J Thorac Cardiovasc Surg 1969;57:245–250.
61. Brandenburg RO Jr, Holmes DR Jr, Brandenburg RO, et al: Clinical follow-up study of paroxysmal supraventricular tachyarrhythmias after operative repair of a secundum type atrial septal defect in adults. Am J Cardiol 1983;51:273–276.
62. Bink-Boelkens MT, Velvis H, van der Heide JJ, et al: Dysrhythmias after atrial surgery in children. Am Heart J 1983;106:125–130.
63. Murphy JG, Gersh BJ, McGoon MD, et al: Long-term outcome after surgical repair of isolated atrial septal defect: Follow-up at 27 to 32 years. N Engl J Med 1990;323:1645–1650.
64. Bricker TJ, Gillette PC, Cooley DA, et al: Dysrhythmias after repair of atrial septal defect. Tex Heart Inst J 1986;13:203–208.
65. Lewis FJ: High defects of the atrial septum. J Thorac Cardiovasc Surg 1958;36:1–11.
66. Lechat P, Mas JL, Lascault G, et al: Prevalence of patent foramen ovale in patients with stroke. N Engl J Med 1988;318:1148–1152.

67. Webster MW, Chancellor AM, Smith HJ, et al: Patent foramen ovale in young stroke patients. Lancet 1988;2:11–12.
68. Young D: Later results of closure of secundum atrial septal defect in children. Am J Cardiol 1973;31:14–22.
69. Meyer RA, Korfhagen JC, Covitz W, et al: Long-term follow-up study after closure of secundum atrial septal defect in children: an echocardiographic study. Am J Cardiol 1982;50:143–148.
70. Fyler DC: Ventricular septal defect. In: Fyler DC, ed: Nadas' Pediatric Cardiology. Philadelphia: Hanley & Belfus; 1992:435–457.
71. Graham TP Jr, Gutgesell HP: Ventricular septal defects. In: Emmanouilides GC, Reimenschneider TA, Allan HD, et al., eds: Moss and Adams Heart Disease in Infants, Children, and Adolescents Including the Fetus and Young Adult, 5th ed. Baltimore: Williams & Wilkins; 1995:724–746.
72. Mitchell SC, Korones SB, Berendes HW: Congenital heart disease in 56,109 births: Incidence and natural history. Circulation 1971;43:323–332.
73. Sutherland GR, Godman MJ, Smallhorn JF, et al: Ventricular septal defects. Two dimensional echocardiographic and morphological correlations. Br Heart J 1982;47:316–328.
74. Hoffman JI, Christianson R: Congenital heart disease in a cohort of 19,502 births with long-term follow-up. Am J Cardiol 1978;42:641–647.
75. Hoffman JI, Rudolph AM: The natural history of ventricular septal defects in infancy. Am J Cardiol 1965;16:634–653.
76. Meberg A, Otterstad JE, Froland G, et al: Increasing incidence of ventricular septal defects caused by improved detection rate. Acta Paediatr 1994;83:653–657.
77. Weidman WH, Blount SG Jr, DuShane JW, et al: Clinical course in ventricular septal defect. Circulation 1977;56:I156–I169.
78. Trowitzsch E, Braun W, Stute M, et al: Diagnosis, therapy, and outcome of ventricular septal defects in the 1st year of life: a two-dimensional colour-Doppler echocardiography study. Eur J Pediatr 1990;149:758–761.
79. Alpert BS, Cook DH, Varghese PJ, et al: Spontaneous closure of small ventricular septal defects: Ten-year follow-up. Pediatrics 1979;63:204–206.
80. Hiraishi S, Agata Y, Nowatari M, et al: Incidence and natural course of trabecular ventricular septal defect: Two-dimensional echocardiography and color Doppler flow imaging study. J Pediatr 1992;120:409–415.
81. Castaneda AR, Jonas RA, Mayer JE Jr, et al: Ventricular septal defect. In: Castaneda AR, Jonas RA, Mayer JE Jr, et al., eds: Cardiac Surgery of the Neonate and Infant. Philadelphia: WB Saunders Co; 1994:187–199.
82. Gumbiner CH, Takao A: Ventricular septal defect. In: Garson A Jr, Bricker JT, Fisher DJ, et al., eds: The Science and Practice of Pediatric Cardiology, 2nd ed. Baltimore: Williams & Wilkins; 1998:1119–1140.
83. DuShane JW, Weidman WH, Ritter DG: Influence of the natural history of large ventricular septal defects on management of patients. Birth Defects 1972;8:63–68.
84. DuShane JW, Krongrad E, Ritter DG, et al: The fate of raised pulmonary vascular resistance after surgery in ventricular septal defect. In: Kidd BSL, Rowe RD, eds: The Child With Congenital Heart Disease After Surgery. Mount Kisco: Futura Publishing Co; 1976:299–312.
85. DuShane JW, Kirklin JW: Selection for surgery of patients with ventricular septal defect and pulmonary hypertension. Circulation 1960;21:13–20.
86. Van Hare GF, Soffer LJ, Sivakoff MC, et al: Twenty-five-year experience with ventricular septal defect in infants and children. Am Heart J 1987;114:606–614.
87. Kidd L, Driscoll DJ, Gersony WM, et al: Second natural history study of congenital heart defects: Results of treatment of patients with ventricular septal defects. Circulation 1993;87:I38–I51.
88. Maron BJ, Redwood DR, Hirshfeld JW Jr, et al: Postoperative assessment of patients with ventricular septal defect and pulmonary hypertension: Response to intense upright exercise. Circulation 1973;48:864–874.
89. Gersony WM, Hayes CJ, Driscoll DJ, et al: Second natural history study of congenital heart defects: Quality of life of patients with aortic stenosis, pulmonary stenosis, or ventricular septal defect. Circulation 1993;87:I52–I65.
90. Moller JH, Patton C, Varco RL, et al: Late results (30 to 35 years) after operative closure of isolated ventricular septal defect from 1954 to 1960. Am J Cardiol 1991;68:1491–1497.
91. Meijboom F, Szatmari A, Utens E, et al: Long-term follow-up after surgical closure of ventricular septal defect in infancy and childhood. J Am Coll Cardiol 1994;24:1358–1364.
92. Otterstad JE, Erikssen J, Froysaker T, et al: Long term results after operative treatment of isolated ventricular septal defect in adolescents and adults. Acta Med Scand Suppl 1986;708:1–39.
93. McNamara DG, Latson LA: Long-term follow-up of patients with malformations for which definitive surgical repair has been available for 25 years or more. Am J Cardiol 1982;50:560–568.
94. Driscoll DJ, Wolfe RR, Gersony WM, et al: Cardiorespiratory responses to exercise of patients with aortic stenosis, pulmonary stenosis, and ventricular septal defect. Circulation 1993;87:I102–I113.
95. Graham TP Jr, Cordell GD, Bender HW Jr: Ventricular function following surgery. In: Kidd BSL, Rowe RD, eds: The Child With Congenital Heart Disease After Surgery. Mount Kisco: Futura Publishing Co; 1976:277–293.
96. Otterstad JE, Froysaker T, Eriksson J, et al: Long-term results in isolated ventricular septal defect surgically repaired after age 10. Comparison with the natural course in similarly-aged patients. Scand J Thorac Cardiovasc Surg 1985;19:221–229.
97. Jarmakani JM, Graham TP Jr, Canent RV Jr, et al: The effect of corrective surgery on left heart volume and mass in children with ventricular septal defect. Am J Cardiol 1971;27:254–258.
98. Kirklin JW, DuShane JW: Indications for repair of ventricular septal defects. Am J Cardiol 1963;12:75–79.
99. Hallidie-Smith KA, Hollman A, Cleland WP, et al: Effects of surgical closure of ventricular septal defects upon pulmonary vascular disease. Br Heart J 1969;31:246–260.
100. Wallgren CG, Boccanelli A, Zetterqvist P, et al: Late results after surgical closure of ventricular septal defect in children. Scand J Thorac Cardiovasc Surg 1980;14:145–151.
101. Fuster V, Ritter DG, McGoon DC: Medical and surgical long-term followup of ventricular septal defect with pulmonary vascular obstructive disease. Am J Cardiol 1979;43:346.
102. Lillehei CW, Cohen M, Warden HE, et al: The results of direct vision closure of ventricular septal defects in eight patients by means of controlled cross circulation. Surg Gynecol Obstet 1955;101:447–466.
103. Arciniegas E, Farooki ZQ, Hakimi M, et al: Surgical closure of ventricular septal defect during the first twelve months of life. J Thorac Cardiovasc Surg 1980;80:921–928.
104. Kirklin JW, Appelbaum A, Bargeron LM Jr: Primary repair versus banding for ventricular septal defects in infants. In: Kidd BSL, Rowe RD, eds: The Child with Congenital Heart Disease After Surgery. Mount Kisco: Futura Publishing; 1976:3–9.
105. Richardson JV, Schieken RM, Lauer RM, et al: Repair of large ventricular septal defects in infants and small children. Ann Surg 1982;195:318–322.
106. McGrath LB: Methods for repair of simple isolated ventricular septal defect. J Card Surg 1991;6:13–23.
107. Chang AC, Hanley FL, Lock JE, et al: Management and outcome of low birth weight neonates with congenital heart disease. J Pediatr 1994;124:461–466.
108. Hardin JT, Muskett AD, Canter CE, et al: Primary surgical closure of large ventricular septal defects in small infants. Ann Thorac Surg 1992;53:397–401.
109. Gomez R, Sanchez PA, Martinez R, et al: Ventricular septal defect in infancy: Surgical criteria and experience. Jpn Heart J 1983;24:699–710.
110. Parenzan L, Bianchi T, Crupi G, et al: Ventricular septal defect: Indications for corrective surgery and results. In: Doyle EF, Engle MA, Gersony WM, et al., eds: Proceedings of the Second World Congress of Pediatric Cardiology. New York: Springer-Verlag; 1986:531–535.
111. Keane JF, Plauth WH Jr, Nadas AS: Ventricular septal defect with aortic regurgitation. Circulation 1977;56:I172–I177.
112. Otterstad JE, Ihlen H, Vatne K: Aortic regurgitation associated with ventricular septal defects in adults: Clinical course, haemodynamic, angiographic and echocardiographic findings. Acta Med Scand 1985;218:85–96.
113. Lue H-C, Wang T-K, Hou S-H, et al: Natural history of aortic valve prolapse in subpulmonic ventricular septal defect in Chinese people. In: Doyle EF, Engle MA, Gersony WM, et al., eds: Proceedings of the Second World Congress in Pediatric Cardiology. New York: Springer-Verlag; 1986:1277.
114. Hitchcock JF, Suijker WJ, Ksiezycka E, et al: Management of ventric-

ular septal defect with associated aortic incompetence. Ann Thorac Surg 1991;52:70–73.

115. Umebayashi Y, Yuda T, Fukuda S, et al: Surgery for ventricular septal defect with aortic regurgitation. [in Japanese]. Kyobu Geka 1993;46:1013–1016.

116. Ishikawa S, Morishita Y, Sato Y, et al: Frequency and operative correction of aortic insufficiency associated with ventricular septal defect. Ann Thorac Surg 1994;57:996–998.

117. Rhodes LA, Keane JF, Keane JP, et al: Long follow-up (to 43 years) of ventricular septal defect with audible aortic regurgitation. Am J Cardiol 1990;66:340–345.

118. Backer CL, Idriss FS, Zales VR, et al: Surgical management of the conal (supracristal) ventricular septal defect. J Thorac Cardiovasc Surg 1991;102:288–295.

119. Backer CL, Winters RC, Zales VR, et al: Restrictive ventricular septal defect: How small is too small to close? Ann Thorac Surg 1993;56:1014–1018.

120. Subramanian S: Ventricular septal defect: Problems of repair in infancy. In: Kidd BSL, Rowe RD, eds: The Child with Congenital Heart Disease After Surgery. Mount Kisco: Futura Publishing; 1976:11–26.

121. Guo JQ, Xue GX, Zhu XD, et al: Surgical treatment of congenital ventricular septal defect: A 21 year experience in 1,187 patients. Chin Med J (Engl) 1983;96:323–329.

122. Henze A, Koul BL, Wallgren G, et al: Repair of ventricular septal defect in the first year of life. Scand J Thorac Cardiovasc Surg 1984;18:151–154.

123. Kirklin JK, Castaneda AR, Keane JF, et al: Surgical management of multiple ventricular septal defects. J Thorac Cardiovasc Surg 1980;80:485–493.

124. Serraf A, Lacour-Gayet F, Bruniaux J, et al: Surgical management of isolated multiple ventricular septal defects: Logical approach in 130 cases. J Thorac Cardiovasc Surg 1992;103:437–442.

125. Griffiths SP, Turi GK, Ellis K, et al: Muscular ventricular septal defects repaired with left ventriculotomy. Am J Cardiol 1981;48:877–886.

126. Vaksmann G, Fournier A, Chartrand C, et al: Arrhythmia disorders after repair of ventricular septal defects. Comparison of atrial and ventricular approaches. [in French]. Arch Mal Coeur Vaiss 1989;82:731–735.

127. Moller JH, Patton C, Varco RL, et al: Post-operative ventricular septal defect: Twenty-four-to-thirty year follow-up of 245 patients. Proceedings of the Second World Congress of Pediatric Cardiology. New York: Springer-Verlag; 1986:1278–1279.

128. Kanter RJ: Syncope and sudden death. In: Garson A Jr, Bricker JT, Fisher DJ, et al., eds: The Science and Practice of Pediatric Cardiology, 2nd ed. Baltimore: Williams & Wilkins; 1998:2169–2199.

129. Yeager SB, Freed MD, Keane JF, et al: Primary surgical closure of ventricular septal defect in the first year of life: Results in 128 infants. J Am Coll Cardiol 1984;3:1269–1276.

130. Mitchell SC, Korones SB, Berendes HW: Congenital heart disease in 56,109 births. Incidence and natural history. Circulation 1971;43:323–332.

131. Wolfe RR, Driscoll DJ, Gersony WM, et al: Arrhythmias in patients with valvar aortic stenosis, valvar pulmonary stenosis, and ventricular septal defect: Results of 24-hour ECG monitoring. Circulation 1993;87:I89–I101.

132. Gumbiner CH: Bundle branch and fascicular block. In: Gillette PC, Gartner JC Jr, eds: Pediatric Cardiac Dysrhythmias. New York: Grune & Stratton; 1981:405–420.

133. van Lier TA, Harinck E, Hitchcock JF, et al: Complete right bundle branch block after surgical closure of perimembranous ventricular septal defect: Relation to type of ventriculotomy. Eur Heart J 1985;6:959–962.

134. Graham TP Jr: Ventricular performance in congenital heart disease. Circulation 1991;84:2259–2274.

135. Lev M, Fell EH, Arcilla R, et al: Surgical injury to the conduction system in ventricular septal defect. Am J Cardiol 1964;14:464–476.

136. Yeager SB, Freed MD, Keane JF, et al: Primary surgical closure of ventricular septal defect in the first year of life: Results in 128 infants. J Am Coll Cardiol 1984;3:1269–1276.

137. Doty DB, McGoon DC: Closure of perimembranous ventricular septal defect. J Thorac Cardiovasc Surg 1983;85:781–790.

138. Rastelli G, Kirklin JW, Titus JL: Anatomic observations on complete form of persistent common atrioventricular canal with special reference to atrioventricular valves. Mayo Clin Proc 1966;41:296–308.

139. Newfeld EA, Sher M, Paul MH, et al: Pulmonary vascular disease in complete atrioventricular canal defect. Am J Cardiol 1977;39:721–726.

140. Cooney TP, Thurlbeck WM: Pulmonary hypoplasia in Down's syndrome. N Engl J Med 1982;307:1170–1173.

141. Chi TPL: The pulmonary vascular bed in children with Down syndrome. J Pediatr 1975;86:533–538.

142. Hanley FL, Fenton KN, Jonas RA, et al: Surgical repair of complete atrioventricular canal defects in infancy: Twenty-year trends. J Thorac Cardiovasc Surg 1993;106:387–394.

143. Chin AJ, Keane JF, Norwood WI, et al: Repair of complete common atrioventricular canal in infancy. J Thorac Cardiovasc Surg 1982;84:437–445.

144. McGoon DC, Puga FJ, Danielson GK: Atrioventricular canal. In: Sabiston DC Jr, Spencer DC, eds: Gibbon's Surgery of the Heart. Philadelphia: WB Saunders; 1983:1051–1066.

145. Pacifico AD: Atrioventricular septal defects. In: Stark J, de Leval M, eds: Surgery for Congenital Heart Defects. London: Grune & Stratton; 1983:285–300.

146. Kirklin JW, Pacifico AD, Kirklin JK: The surgical treatment of atrioventricular canal defects. In: Arciniegas E, ed: Pediatric Cardiac Surgery. Chicago: Year Book Medical Publishers; 1985:155–170.

147. Carpentier A: Surgical anatomy and management of the mitral component of atrioventricular canal defects. In: Anderson RH, Shinebourne EA, eds: Paediatric Cardiology 1977. Edinburgh: Churchill Livingstone; 1978:477–490.

148. Rastelli GC, Ongley PA, Kirklin JW, et al: Surgical repair of the complete form of persistent common atrioventricular canal. J Thorac Cardiovasc Surg 1968;55:299–308.

149. Castaneda A, Jonas RA, Mayer JE Jr, et al: Atrioventricular canal defect. In: Castaneda A, Jonas RA, Mayer JE Jr, et al, eds: Cardiac Surgery of the Neonate and Infant. Philadelphia: WB Saunders; 1994:167–186.

150. Gillette PC, Shannon C, Blair H, et al: Transvenous pacing in pediatric patients. Am Heart J 1983;105:843–847.

151. Blalock A, Taussig HB: The surgical treatment of malformations of the heart in which there is pulmonary stenosis or pulmonary atresia. JAMA 1945;128:189–202.

152. Brock RC: Pulmonary valvulotomy for the relief of congenital pulmonary stenosis. Report of 3 cases. Br Med J 1948;I:1121–1126.

153. Potts WJ, Smith S, Gibson S: Anastomosis of the aorta to a pulmonary artery: Certain types in congenital heart disease. JAMA 1946;132:627–631.

154. Waterston D: Leceni Fallotovy tetralogie u deti do jednoho roku veku. Rozhl Chir 1962;XLI:3–6.

155. Lillehei CW, Cohen M, Warden HE, et al: Direct vision intracardiac surgical correction of the tetralogy of Fallot, pentalogy of Fallot and pulmonary atresia defects. Ann Surg 1955;142:418–444.

156. Murphy JD, Freed MD, Keane JF, et al: Hemodynamic results after intracardiac repair of tetralogy of Fallot by deep hypothermia and cardiopulmonary bypass. Circulation 1980;62:I168.

157. Quattlebaum TG, Varghese J, Neill CA, et al: Sudden death among postoperative patients with tetralogy of Fallot: A follow-up study of 243 patients for an average of twelve years. Circulation 1976;54:289–293.

158. James FW, Kaplan S, Chou TC: Unexpected cardiac arrest in patients after surgical correction of tetralogy of Fallot. Circulation 1975;52:691–695.

159. Gillette PC, Yeoman MA, Mullins CE, et al: Sudden death after repair of tetralogy of Fallot: Electrocardiographic and electrophysiologic abnormalities. Circulation 1977;56:566–571.

160. Poirier RA, McGoon DC, Danielson GK, et al: Late results after repair of tetralogy of Fallot. J Thorac Cardiovasc Surg 1977;73:900–908.

161. Walsh EP, Rockenmacher S, Keane JF, et al: Late results in patients with tetralogy of Fallot repaired during infancy. Circulation 1988;77:1062–1067.

162. Gott VL: C. Walton Lillehei and total correction of tetralogy of Fallot. Ann Thorac Surg 1990;49:328–332.

163. Di Donato RM, Jonas RA, Lang P, et al: Neonatal repair of tetralogy of Fallot with and without pulmonary atresia. J Thorac Cardiovasc Surg 1991;101:126–137.

164. Casteneda AR, Jonas RA, Mayer JE Jr, et al: Tetralogy of Fallot. In: Casteneda AR, Jonas RA, Mayer JE Jr, et al, eds: Cardiac Surgery of the Neonate and Infant. Philadelphia: WB Saunders; 1994:215–234.

165. Ruzyllo W, Nihill MR, Mullins CE, et al: Hemodynamic evaluation

of 221 patients after intracardiac repair of tetralogy of Fallot. Am J Cardiol 1974;34:565–576.

166. Ungerleider RM, Greeley WJ, Sheikh KH, et al: Routine use of intraoperative epicardial echocardiography and Doppler color flow imaging to guide and evaluate repair of congenital heart lesions: A prospective study. J Thorac Cardiovasc Surg 1990;100:297–309.

167. Uretzky G, Puga FJ, Danielson GK, et al: Reoperation after correction of tetralogy of Fallot. Circulation 1982;66:I202–I208.

168. Joransen JA, Lucas RV Jr, Moller JH: Postoperative haemodynamics in tetralogy of Fallot: A study of 132 children. Br Heart J 1979;41:33–39.

169. Warner KG, Anderson JE, Fulton DR, et al: Restoration of the pulmonary valve reduces right ventricular volume overload after previous repair of tetralogy of Fallot. Circulation 1993;88:II189–II197.

170. Fuster V, McGoon DC, Kennedy MA, et al: Long-term evaluation (12 to 22 years) of open heart surgery for tetralogy of Fallot. Am J Cardiol 1980;46:635–642.

171. Marie PY, Marcon F, Brunotte F, et al: Right ventricular overload and induced sustained ventricular tachycardia in operatively "repaired" tetralogy of Fallot. Am J Cardiol 1992;69:785–789.

172. Dreyer WJ, Paridon SM, Fisher DJ, et al: Rapid ventricular pacing in dogs with right ventricular outflow tract obstruction: insights into a mechanism of sudden death in postoperative tetralogy of Fallot. J Am Coll Cardiol 1993;21:1731–1737.

173. Garson A Jr, Gillette PC, Gutgesell HP, et al: Stress-induced ventricular arrhythmia after repair of tetralogy of Fallot. Am J Cardiol 1980;46:1006–1012.

174. Garson A Jr, Gillette PC, Porter CJ: Electrophysiologic induction of ventricular dysrhythmias in 152 children with normal or abnormal hearts. J Am Coll Cardiol 1983;1:614–616.

175. Deanfield JE, McKenna WJ, Presbitero P, et al: Ventricular arrhythmia in unrepaired and repaired tetralogy of Fallot: Relation to age, timing of repair, and haemodynamic status. Br Heart J 1984;52:77–81.

176. Deanfield JE, Franklin R, McKenna WJ, et al: Prognostic significance of ventricular arrhythmias after repair of tetralogy of Fallot: A prospective study. Proceedings of the Second World Congress of Pediatric Cardiology. New York: Springer-Verlag; 1986:467–468.

177. Matina D, Mouly A, Massol J, et al: Ventricular arrhythmia following repair of Fallot's tetralogy. Apropos of 59 cases. [in French]. Arch Mal Coeur Vaiss 1985;78:103–110.

178. Sullivan ID, Presbitero P, Gooch VM, et al: Is ventricular arrhythmia in repaired tetralogy of Fallot an effect of operation or a consequence of the course of the disease? A prospective study. Br Heart J 1987;58:40–44.

179. Deal BJ, Scagliotti D, Miller SM, et al: Electrophysiologic drug testing in symptomatic ventricular arrhythmias after repair of tetralogy of Fallot. Am J Cardiol 1987;59:1380–1385.

180. Kugler JD, Pinsky WW, Cheatham JP, et al: Sustained ventricular tachycardia after repair of tetralogy of Fallot: New electrophysiologic findings. Am J Cardiol 1983;51:1137–1143.

181. Fukushige J, Shimomura K, Harada T, et al: Incidence and severity of ventricular arrhythmia in patients after repair of tetralogy of Fallot. Jpn Heart J 1988;29:795–800.

182. Kori Y, Suwa K, Shiroma K: Ventricular premature contraction after repair of tetralogy of Fallot: The influence of postoperative factors, particularly the right ventricular regional wall motion. Jpn Circ J 1989;53:213–218.

183. Chandar JS, Wolff GS, Garson A Jr, et al: Ventricular arrhythmias in postoperative tetralogy of Fallot. Am J Cardiol 1990;65:655–661.

184. Vaksmann G, Fournier A, Davignon A, et al: Frequency and prognosis of arrhythmias after operative "correction" of tetralogy of Fallot. Am J Cardiol 1990;66:346–349.

185. Garson A Jr: Ventricular arrhythmias after repair of congenital heart disease: Who needs treatment? Cardiol Young 1991;1:177–181.

186. Cullen S, Celermajer DS, Franklin RC, et al: Prognostic significance of ventricular arrhythmia after repair of tetralogy of Fallot: A 12-year prospective study. J Am Coll Cardiol 1994;23:1151–1155.

187. Garson A Jr, McNamara DG: Sudden death in a pediatric cardiology population, 1958 to 1983: Relation to prior arrhythmias. J Am Coll Cardiol 1985;5:134B–137B.

188. Harris P, Alexson C, Lewis E, et al: Sudden unexpected death in adolescence. In: Doyle EF, Engle MA, Gersony WM, et al., eds: Proceedings of the Second World Congress of Pediatric Cardiology. New York: Springer-Verlag; 1986:1183–1185.

189. Joffe H, Georgakopoulos D, Celermajer DS, et al: Late ventricular arrhythmia is rare after early repair of tetralogy of Fallot. J Am Coll Cardiol 1994;23:1146–1150.

190. Neches WH, Park SC, Mathews RA, et al: Tetralogy of Fallot: postoperative electrophysiologic studies. Circulation 1977;56:713–719.

191. Friedli B, Bolens M, Taktak M: Conduction disturbances after correction of tetralogy of Fallot: Are electrophysiologic studies of prognostic value? J Am Coll Cardiol 1988;11:162–165.

192. Dreyer WJ, Paridon SM, Varughes A, Fisher DJ, Garson A: Serum norepinephrine elevation in dogs with high right ventricular pressure during simulated ventricular tachycardia. Am J Cardiol. 2000;60:639.

193. Garson A Jr, Randall DC, Gillette PC, et al: Prevention of sudden death after repair of tetralogy of Fallot: Treatment of ventricular arrhythmias. J Am Coll Cardiol 1985;6:221–227.

194. Rocchini AP, Rosenthal A, Freed M, et al: Chronic congestive heart failure after repair of tetralogy of Fallot. Circulation 1977;56:305–310.

195. Zuberbuhler JR, Dankner E, Zoltun R, et al: Tissue adhesive closure of aortic-pulmonary communications. Am Heart J 1974;88:41–46.

196. Gianturco C, Anderson JH, Wallace S: Mechanical devices for arterial occlusion. Am J Roentgenol Radium Ther Nucl Med 1975;124:428–435.

197. Grinnell VS, Mehringer CM, Hieshima GB, et al: Transaortic occlusion of collateral arteries to the lung by detachable valved balloons in a patient with tetralogy of Fallot. Circulation 1982;65:1276–1278.

198. Rosing DR, Borer JS, Kent KM, et al: Long-term hemodynamic and electrocardiographic assessment following operative repair of tetralogy of Fallot. Circulation 1977;58:I209–I216.

199. Liebman J, Cullum L, Belloc NB: Natural history of transposition of the great arteries: Anatomy and birth and death characteristics. Circulation 1969;40:237–262.

200. Campbell M: Incidence of cardiac malformations at birth and later, and neonatal mortality. Br Heart J 1973;35:189–200.

201. Shahar RM: Complete Transposition of the Great Arteries. New York: Academic Press; 1973.

202. Esscher E, Michaelsson M, Smedby B: Cardiovascular malformation in infant deaths. 10-year clinical and epidemiological study. Br Heart J 1975;37:824–829.

203. Sauer U, Gittenberger-de Groot AC: Transposition of the great arteries: anatomic types and coronary artery patterns. In: Freedom RM, Braunwald E, eds: Atlas of Heart Diseases. Congenital Heart Disease, Vol XII. St. Louis: Mosby; 1997:15.1–15.12.

204. Neches WH, Park SC, Ettedgui JA: Transposition of the great arteries. In: Gartner JC Jr, Brinker JT, Fisher DJ, et al, eds: The Science and Practice of Pediatric Cardiology, 2nd ed. Baltimore: Williams & Wilkins; 1998:1463–1503.

205. Kirklin JW, Barratt-Boyes BG: Complete transposition of the great arteries. In: Kirklin JW, Barratt-Boyes BG, eds: Cardiac Surgery, 2nd ed. New York: Churchill Livingstone; 1993:1383–1468.

206. Fyler DC: D-Transposition of the great arteries. In: Fyler DC, ed: Nadas' Pediatric Cardiology. Philadelphia: Hanley & Belfus; 1992:557–575.

207. Blalock A, Hanlon CR: The surgical treatment of complete transposition of the aorta and the pulmonary artery. Surg Gynecol Obstet 1950;90:1–15.

208. Rashkind WJ, Miller WW: Creation of an atrial septal defect without thoracotomy: A palliative approach to complete transposition of the great arteries. JAMA 1966;196:991–992.

209. Idriss FS, Goldstein IR, Grana L, et al: A new technique for complete correction of transposition of the great vessels: An experimental study with a preliminary clinical report. Circulation 1961;24:5–11.

210. Albert HM: Surgical correction of transposition of the great vessels. Surg Forum 1954;5:74–77.

211. Baffes TG: A new method for surgical correction of transposition of the aorta and pulmonary artery. Surg Gynecol Obstet 1956;102:227–233.

212. Mustard WT, Chute AL, Keith JD, et al: A surgical approach to transposition of the great vessels with extracorporeal circuit. Surgery 1954;36:39–51.

213. Senning A: Surgical correction of transposition of the great vessels. Surgery 1959;45:966–980.

214. Mustard WT: Successful two-stage correction of transposition of the great vessels. Surgery 1964;55:469–472.

215. Jatene AD, Fontes VF, Paulista PP, et al: Successful anatomic correction of transposition of the great vessels: A preliminary report. Arq Bras Cardiol 1975;28:461–464.

216. Castaneda AR, Norwood WI, Jonas RA, et al: Transposition of the

great arteries and intact ventricular septum: Anatomical repair in the neonate. Ann Thorac Surg 1984;38:438–443.

217. Lang P, Freed MD, Bierman FZ, et al: Use of prostaglandin E₁ in infants with d-transposition of the great arteries and intact ventricular septum. Am J Cardiol 1979;44:76–81.

218. deLeon VH, Hougen TJ, Norwood WI, et al: Results of the Senning operation for transposition of the great arteries with intact ventricular septum in neonates. Circulation 1984;70:t-5.

219. Stark J, Leval MD, Waterston DJ, et al: Corrective surgery of transposition of the great arteries in the first year of life: Results in 63 infants. J Thorac Cardiovasc Surg 1974;67:673–681.

220. Kawabori I, Guntheroth WG, Morgan BC, et al: Surgical correction in infancy to reduce mortality in transposition of the great arteries. Pediatrics 1977;60:83–85.

221. Bailey LL, Jacobson JG, Merritt WH, et al: Mustard operation in the 1st month of life. Am J Cardiol 1982;49:766–770.

222. Piccoli GP, Wilkinson JL, Arnold R, et al: Appraisal of the Mustard procedure for the physiological correction of "simple" transposition of the great arteries: Eighty consecutive cases, 1970–1980. J Thorac Cardiovasc Surg 1981;82:436–446.

223. Mahony L, Turley K, Ebert P, et al: Long-term results after atrial repair of transposition of the great arteries in early infancy. Circulation 1982;66:253–258.

224. Marx GR, Hougen TJ, Norwood WI, et al: Transposition of the great arteries with intact ventricular septum: Results of Mustard and Senning operations in 123 consecutive patients. J Am Coll Cardiol 1983;1:476–483.

225. Edwards WD, Edwards JE: Pathology of the sinus node in d-transposition following the Mustard operation. J Thorac Cardiovasc Surg 1978;75:213–218.

226. Beerman LB, Neches WH, Fricker FJ, et al: Arrhythmias in transposition of the great arteries after the Mustard operation. Am J Cardiol 1983;51:1530–1534.

227. El-Said G, Rosenberg HS, Mullins CE, et al: Dysrhythmias after Mustard's operation for transposition of the great arteries. Am J Cardiol 1972;30:526–532.

228. Park SC, Neches WH, Mathews RA, et al: Hemodynamic function after the Mustard operation for transposition of the great arteries. Am J Cardiol 1983;51:1514–1519.

229. Stark J, Silove ED, Taylor JF, et al: Obstruction to systemic venous return following the Mustard operation for transposition of the great arteries. J Thorac Cardiovasc Surg 1974;68:742–749.

230. Hagler DJ, Ritter DG, Mair DD, et al: Clinical, angiographic, and hemodynamic assessment of late results after Mustard operation. Circulation 1978;57:1214–1220.

231. Arciniegas E, Farooki ZQ, Hakimi M, et al: Results of the Mustard operation for dextro-transposition of the great arteries. J Thorac Cardiovasc Surg 1981;81:580–587.

232. Berman MA, Barash PS, Hellenbrand WE, et al: Late development of severe pulmonary venous obstruction following the Mustard operation. Circulation 1977;56:II91–II94.

233. Driscoll DJ, Nihill MR, Vargo TA, et al: Late development of pulmonary venous obstruction following Mustard's operation using a Dacron baffle. Circulation 1977;55:484–488.

234. Quaegebeur JM, Rohmer J, Brom AG: Revival of the Senning operation in the treatment of transposition of the great arteries. Preliminary report on recent experience. Thorax 1977;32:517–524.

235. Parenzan L, Locatelli G, Alfieri O, et al: The Senning operation for transposition of the great arteries. J Thorac Cardiovasc Surg 1978;76:305–311.

236. Bender HW Jr, Graham TP Jr, Boucek RJ Jr, et al: Comparative operative results of the Senning and Mustard procedures for transposition of the great arteries. Circulation 1980;62:I197–I203.

237. Matherne GP, Razook JD, Thompson WM Jr, et al: Senning repair for transposition of the great arteries in the first week of life. Circulation 1985;72:840–845.

238. Byrum CJ, Bove EL, Sondheimer HM, et al: Hemodynamic and electrophysiologic results of the Senning procedure for transposition of the great arteries. Am J Cardiol 1986;58:138–142.

239. George BL, Laks H, Klitzner TS, et al: Results of the Senning procedure in infants with simple and complex transposition of the great arteries. Am J Cardiol 1987;59:426–430.

240. Rodriguez-Fernandez HL, Kelly DT, Collado A, et al: Hemodynamic data and angiographic findings after Mustard repair for complete transposition of the great arteries. Circulation 1972;46:799–808.

241. Gillette PC, el Said GM, Sivarajan N, et al: Electrophysiological abnormalities after Mustard's operation for transposition of the great arteries. Br Heart J 1974;36:186–191.

242. Gillette PC, Kugler JD, Garson A Jr, et al: Mechanisms of cardiac arrhythmias after the Mustard operation for transposition of the great arteries. Am J Cardiol 1980;45:1225–1230.

243. Sunderland CO, Henken DP, Nichols GM, et al: Postoperative hemodynamic and electrophysiologic evaluation of the interatrial baffle procedure. Am J Cardiol 1975;35:660–666.

244. Hayes CJ, Gersony WM: Arrhythmias after the Mustard operation for transposition of the great arteries: A long-term study. J Am Coll Cardiol 1986;7:133–137.

245. Vetter VL, Tanner CS, Horowitz LN: Electrophysiologic consequences of the Mustard repair of d-transposition of the great arteries. J Am Coll Cardiol 1987;10:1265–1273.

246. Kirjavainen M, Happonen JM, Louhimo I: Late results of Senning operation. J Thorac Cardiovasc Surg 1999;117:488–495.

247. Gelatt M, Hamilton RM, McCrindle BW, et al: Arrhythmia and mortality after the Mustard procedure: A 30-year single-center experience. J Am Coll Cardiol 1997;29:194–201.

248. Yacoub MH, Radley-Smith R, Maclaurin R: Two-stage operation for anatomical correction of transposition of the great arteries with intact interventricular septum. Lancet 1977;1:1275–1278.

249. Clarkson PM, Neutze JM, Barratt-Boyles BG, et al: Late postoperative hemodynamic results and cineangiocardiographic findings after Mustard atrial baffle repair for transposition of the great arteries. Circulation 1976;53:525–532.

250. Tynan M, Aberdeen E, Stark J: Tricuspid incompetence after the Mustard operation for transposition of the great arteries. Circulation 1972;45:I111–I115.

251. Chang AC, Wernovsky G, Wessel DL, et al: Surgical management of late right ventricular failure after Mustard or Senning repair. Circulation 1992;86:II140–II149.

252. Murphy JH, Barlai-Kovach MM, Mathews RA, et al: Rest and exercise right and left ventricular function late after the Mustard operation: Assessment by radionuclide ventriculography. Am J Cardiol 1983;51:1520–1526.

253. Jarmakani JM, Canent RV Jr: Preoperative and postoperative right ventricular function in children with transposition of the great vessels. Circulation 1974;50:II39–II45.

254. Graham TP Jr, Atwood GF, Boucek RJ Jr, et al: Abnormalities of right ventricular function following Mustard's operation for transposition of the great arteries. Circulation 1975;52:678–684.

255. Hagler DJ, Ritter DG, Mair DD, et al: Right and left ventricular function after the Mustard procedure in transposition of the great arteries. Am J Cardiol 1979;44:276–283.

256. Graham TP Jr, Burger J, Bender HW, et al: Improved right ventricular function after intra-atrial repair of transposition of the great arteries. Circulation 1985;72:II45–II51.

257. Warnes CA, Somerville J: Transposition of the great arteries: Late results in adolescents and adults after the Mustard procedure. Br Heart J 1987;58:148–155.

258. Neukermans K, Sullivan TJ, Pitlick PT: Successful pregnancy after the Mustard operation for transposition of the great arteries. Am J Cardiol 1988;62:838–839.

259. Clarkson PM, Wilson NJ, Neutze JM, et al: Outcome of pregnancy after the Mustard operation for transposition of the great arteries with intact ventricular septum. J Am Coll Cardiol 1994;24:190–193.

260. Wernovsky G, Giglia TM, Jonas RA, et al: Course in the intensive care unit after 'preparatory' pulmonary artery banding and aortopulmonary shunt placement for transposition of the great arteries with low left ventricular pressure. Circulation 1992;86:II133–II139.

261. Wernovsky G, Hougen TJ, Walsh EP, et al: Midterm results after the arterial switch operation for transposition of the great arteries with intact ventricular septum: Clinical, hemodynamic, echocardiographic, and electrophysiologic data. Circulation 1988;77:1333–1344.

262. Hourihan M, Colan SD, Wernovsky G, et al: Growth of the aortic anastomosis, annulus, and root after the arterial switch procedure performed in infancy. Circulation 1993;88:615–620.

263. Yamaguchi M, Hosokawa Y, Imai Y, et al: Early and midterm results of the arterial switch operation for transposition of the great arteries in Japan. J Thorac Cardiovasc Surg 1990;100:261–269.

264. Tsuda E, Imakita M, Yagihara T, et al: Late death after arterial switch operation for transposition of the great arteries. Am Heart J 1992;124:1551–1557.

265. Sidi D, Planche C, Kachaner J, et al: Anatomic correction of simple transposition of the great arteries in 50 neonates. Circulation 1987;75:429–435.

266. Serraf A, Lacour-Gayet F, Bruniaux J, et al: Anatomic repair of Taussig-Bing hearts. Circulation 1991;84:III200–III205.

267. Norwood WI, Dobell AR, Freed MD, et al: Intermediate results of the arterial switch repair: A 20-institution study. J Thorac Cardiovasc Surg 1988;96:854–863.

268. Day RW, Laks H, Drinkwater DC: The influence of coronary anatomy on the arterial switch operation in neonates. J Thorac Cardiovasc Surg 1992;104:706–712.

269. Vogel M, Smallhorn JF, Gilday D, et al: Assessment of myocardial perfusion in patients after the arterial switch operation. J Nucl Med 1991;32:237–241.

270. Vetter VL, Tanner CS: Electrophysiologic consequences of the arterial switch repair of d-transposition of the great arteries. J Am Coll Cardiol 1988;12:229–237.

271. Wernovsky G, Freed MD: Transposition of the great arteries: results and outcome of the arterial switch operation. In: Freedom RM, Braunwald E, eds: Atlas of Heart Diseases, Vol XII. St. Louis: Mosby; 1997:16.1–16.10.

272. Jatene AD, Fontes VF, Souza LC, et al: Anatomic correction of transposition of the great arteries. J Thorac Cardiovasc Surg 1982;83:20–26.

273. Bical O, Hazan E, Lecompte Y, et al: Anatomic correction of transposition of the great arteries associated with ventricular septal defect: midterm results in 50 patients. Circulation 1984;70:891–897.

274. Trusler GA, Castaneda AR, Rosenthal A, et al: Current results of management in transposition of the great arteries, with special emphasis on patients with associated ventricular septal defect. J Am Coll Cardiol 1987;10:1061–1071.

275. Wernovsky G, Mayer JE Jr, Jonas RA, et al: Factors influencing early and late outcome of the arterial switch operation for transposition of the great arteries. J Thorac Cardiovasc Surg 1995;109:289–301.

276. Wernovsky G, Sanders SP: Coronary artery anatomy and transposition of the great arteries. Coron Artery Dis 1993;4:148–157.

277. Nakanishi T, Matsumoto Y, Seguchi M, et al: Balloon angioplasty for postoperative pulmonary artery stenosis in transposition of the great arteries. J Am Coll Cardiol 1993;22:859–866.

278. Nogi S, McCrindle BW, Boutin C, et al: Fate of the neopulmonary valve after the arterial switch operation in neonates. J Thorac Cardiovasc Surg 1998;115:557–562.

279. Santoro G, Di Carlo D, Formigari R, et al: Late onset pulmonary valvar stenosis after arterial switch operation for transposition of the great arteries. Heart 1998;79:311–312.

280. Castaneda A: Arterial switch operation for simple and complex TGA: Indication criteria and limitations relevant to surgery. Thorac Cardiovasc Surg 1991;39:151–154.

281. Castaneda AR, Trusler GA, Paul MH, et al: The early results of treatment of simple transposition in the current era. J Thorac Cardiovasc Surg 1988;95:14–28.

282. Gittenberger-de Groot AC, Sauer U, Quaegebeur J: Aortic intramural coronary artery in three hearts with transposition of the great arteries. J Thorac Cardiovasc Surg 1986;91:566–571.

283. Lange PE, Pulss W, Sievers HH, et al: Cardiac rhythm and conduction after two-stage anatomic correction of simple transposition of the great arteries. Thorac Cardiovasc Surg 1986;34:22–24.

284. Rhodes LA, Wernovsky G, Keane JF, et al: Arrhythmias and intracardiac conduction after the arterial switch operation. J Thorac Cardiovasc Surg 1995;109:303–310.

285. Martin RP, Radley-Smith R, Yacoub MH: Arrhythmias before and after anatomic correction of transposition of the great arteries. J Am Coll Cardiol 1987;10:200–204.

286. Jenkins KJ, Hanley FL, Colan SD, et al: Function of the anatomic pulmonary valve in the systemic circulation. Circulation 1991; 84:III173–III179.

287. Gibbs JL, Qureshi SA, Grieve L, et al: Doppler echocardiography after anatomical correction of transposition of the great arteries. Br Heart J 1986;56:67–72.

288. Martin RP, Ladusans EJ, Parsons JM, et al: Incidence, importance and determinants of aortic regurgitation after anatomical correction of transposition of the great arteries. Br Heart J 1988;59:120–121.

289. Gibbs JL, Qureshi SA, Wilson N, et al: Doppler echocardiographic comparison of haemodynamic results of one- and two-stage anatomic correction of complete transposition. Int J Cardiol 1988;18:85–92.

290. Sievers HH, Lange PE, Arensman FW, et al: Influence of two-stage anatomic correction on size and distensibility of the anatomic pulmonary/functional aortic root in patients with simple transposition of the great arteries. Circulation 1984;70:202–208.

291. Yacoub M, Bernhard A, Lange P, et al: Clinical and hemodynamic results of the two-stage anatomic correction of simple transposition of the great arteries. Circulation 1980;62:I190–I196.

292. Weindling SN, Wernovsky G, Colan SD, et al: Myocardial perfusion, function and exercise tolerance after the arterial switch operation. J Am Coll Cardiol 1994;23:424–433.

293. Tanel RE, Wernovsky G, Landzberg MJ, et al: Coronary artery abnormalities detected at cardiac catheterization following the arterial switch operation for transposition of the great arteries. Am J Cardiol 1995;76:153–157.

294. Allada V, Jarmakani JM, Yeatman L: Percutaneous transluminal coronary angioplasty in an infant with coronary artery stenosis after arterial switch operation. Am Heart J 1991;122:1464–1465.

295. Haas F, Wottke M, Poppert H, et al: Long-term survival and functional follow-up in patients after the arterial switch operation. Ann Thorac Surg 1999;68:1692–1697.

296. Fontan F, Baudet E: Surgical repair of tricuspid atresia. Thorax 1971;26:240–248.

297. Cetta F, Feldt RH, O'Leary PW, et al: Improved early morbidity and mortality after Fontan operation: The Mayo Clinic experience, 1987 to 1992. J Am Coll Cardiol 1996;28:480–486.

298. Gentles TL, Gauvreau K, Mayer JE Jr, et al: Functional outcome after the Fontan operation: Factors influencing late morbidity. J Thorac Cardiovasc Surg 1997;114:392–403.

299. Gentles TL, Mayer JE Jr, Gauvreau K, et al: Fontan operation in five hundred consecutive patients: Factors influencing early and late outcome. J Thorac Cardiovasc Surg 1997;114:376–391.

300. Choussat A, Fontan F, Besse P, et al: Selection criteria for Fontan's procedure. In: Anderson RH, Shinebourne EA, eds: Paediatric Cardiology 1977. New York: Churchill Livingstone; 1978:559–566.

301. Kirklin JK, Blackstone EH, Kirklin JW, et al: The Fontan operation. Ventricular hypertrophy, age, and date of operation as risk factors. J Thorac Cardiovasc Surg 1986;92:1049–1064.

302. Knott-Craig CJ, Danielson GK, Schaff HV, et al: The modified Fontan operation: An analysis of risk factors for early postoperative death or takedown in 702 consecutive patients from one institution. J Thorac Cardiovasc Surg 1995;109:1237–1243.

303. Castaneda AR, Jonas AJ, Mayer JE Jr, et al: Hypoplastic left heart syndrome. In: Castaneda AR, Jonas AJ, Mayer JE Jr, et al., eds: Cardiac Surgery of the Neonate and Infant. Philadelphia: WB Saunders; 1994:363–385.

304. Laks H, Gates RN, Elami A, et al: Damus-Stansel-Kaye procedure: Technical modifications. Ann Thorac Surg 1992;54:169–172.

305. Castaneda AR, Jonas RA, Mayer JE Jr, et al: Single-ventricle tricuspid atresia. In: Castaneda AR, Jonas RA, Mayer JE Jr, et al., eds: Cardiac Surgery of the Neonate and Infant. Philadelphia: WB Saunders; 1994:249–272.

306. Bridges ND, Jonas RA, Mayer JE, et al: Bidirectional cavopulmonary anastomosis as interim palliation for high-risk Fontan candidates: Early results. Circulation 1990;82:IV170–IV176.

307. Hopkins RA, Armstrong BE, Serwer GA, et al: Physiological rationale for a bidirectional cavopulmonary shunt. A versatile complement to the Fontan principle. J Thorac Cardiovasc Surg 1985;90:391–398.

308. Lamberti JJ, Spicer RL, Waldman JD, et al: The bidirectional cavopulmonary shunt. J Thorac Cardiovasc Surg 1990;100:22–29.

309. Reddy VM, Liddicoat JR, Hanley FL: Primary bidirectional superior cavopulmonary shunt in infants between 1 and 4 months of age. Ann Thorac Surg 1995;59:1120–1125.

310. Jacobs ML: Hypoplastic left heart syndrome. In: Kaiser LR, Kron IL, Spray TL, eds: Mastery of Cardiothoracic Surgery. Philadelphia: Lippincott-Raven; 1998:858–866.

311. de Leval MR, Kilner P, Gewillig M, et al: Total cavopulmonary connection: A logical alternative to atriopulmonary connection for complex Fontan operations. Experimental studies and early clinical experience. J Thorac Cardiovasc Surg 1988;96:682–695.

312. Kirklin JW, Barratt-Boyes BG: Tricuspid atresia and the Fontan procedure. In: Kirklin JW, Barratt-Boyes BG, eds: Cardiac Surgery, 2nd ed. New York: Churchill Livingstone; 1993:1055–1104.

313. Bridges ND, Lock JE, Castaneda AR: Baffle fenestration with subsequent transcatheter closure: Modification of the Fontan operation for patients at increased risk. Circulation 1990;82:1681–1689.

314. Kopf GS: Tricuspid atresia. In: Mavroudis C, Backer CL, eds: Pediatric Cardiac Surgery, 2nd ed. St. Louis: Mosby; 1994:379–400.

315. Driscoll DJ, Offord KP, Feldt RH, et al: Five- to fifteen-year follow-up after Fontan operation. Circulation 1992;85:469–496.

316. Feldt RH, Driscoll DJ, Offord KP, et al: Protein-losing enteropathy after the Fontan operation. J Thorac Cardiovasc Surg 1996;112:672–680.

317. Fishberger SB, Wernovsky G, Gentles TL, et al: Factors that influence the development of atrial flutter after the Fontan operation. J Thorac Cardiovasc Surg 1997;113:80–86.

318. Kan JS, White RI Jr, Mitchell SE, et al: Percutaneous balloon valvuloplasty: A new method for treating congenital pulmonary-valve stenosis. N Engl J Med 1982;307:540–542.

319. Caspi J, Coles JG, Benson LN, et al: Management of neonatal critical pulmonic stenosis in the balloon valvotomy era. Ann Thorac Surg 1990;49:273–278.

320. Gildein HP, Kleinert S, Goh TH, et al: Treatment of critical pulmonary valve stenosis by balloon dilatation in the neonate. Am Heart J 1996;131:1007–1011.

321. McCrindle BW: Independent predictors of long-term results after balloon pulmonary valvuloplasty: Valvuloplasty and Angioplasty of Congenital Anomalies (VACA) Registry Investigators. Circulation 1994;89:1751–1759.

322. Gatzoulis MA, Rigby ML, Shinebourne EA, et al: Contemporary results of balloon valvuloplasty and surgical valvotomy for congenital aortic stenosis. Arch Dis Child 1995;73:66–69.

323. Moore P, Egito E, Mowrey H, et al: Midterm results of balloon dilation of congenital aortic stenosis: Predictors of success. J Am Coll Cardiol 1996;27:1257–1263.

324. Rocchini AP, Beekman RH, Ben Shachar G, et al: Balloon aortic valvuloplasty: Results of the Valvuloplasty and Angioplasty of Congenital Anomalies Registry. Am J Cardiol 1990;65:784–789.

325. Saiki K, Kato H, Suzuki K, et al: Balloon valvuloplasty for congenital aortic valve stenosis in an infant and children. Acta Paediatr Jpn 1992;34:433–440.

326. Kuhn MA, Latson LA, Cheatham JP, et al: Management of pediatric patients with isolated valvar aortic stenosis by balloon aortic valvuloplasty. Cathet Cardiovasc Diagn 1996;39:55–61.

327. Hawkins JA, Minich LL, Shaddy RE, et al: Aortic valve repair and replacement after balloon aortic valvuloplasty in children. Ann Thorac Surg 1996;61:1355–1358.

328. Justo RN, McCrindle BW, Benson LN, et al: Aortic valve regurgitation after surgical versus percutaneous balloon valvotomy for congenital aortic valve stenosis. Am J Cardiol 1996;77:1332–1338.

329. Mosca RS, Iannettoni MD, Schwartz SM, et al: Critical aortic stenosis in the neonate: A comparison of balloon valvuloplasty and transventricular dilation. J Thorac Cardiovasc Surg 1995;109:147–154.

330. Magee AG, Nykanen D, McCrindle BW, et al: Balloon dilation of severe aortic stenosis in the neonate: comparison of anterograde and retrograde catheter approaches. J Am Coll Cardiol 1997;30:1061–1066.

331. Gaynor JW, Bull C, Sullivan ID, et al: Late outcome of survivors of intervention for neonatal aortic valve stenosis. Ann Thorac Surg 1995;60:122–125.

332. Grifka RG, O'Laughlin MP, Nihill MR, et al: Double-transseptal, double-balloon valvuloplasty for congenital mitral stenosis. Circulation 1992;85:123–129.

333. Moore P, Adatia I, Spevak PJ, et al: Severe congenital mitral stenosis in infants. Circulation 1994;89:2099–2106.

334. Spevak PJ, Bass JL, Ben Shachar G, et al: Balloon angioplasty for congenital mitral stenosis. Am J Cardiol 1990;66:472–476.

335. Gundry SR, Razzouk AJ, Boskind JF, et al: Fate of the pericardial monocusp pulmonary valve for right ventricular outflow tract reconstruction: Early function, late failure without obstruction. J Thorac Cardiovasc Surg 1994;107:908–912.

336. Kopf GS, Geha AS, Hellenbrand WE, et al: Fate of left-sided cardiac bioprosthesis valves in children. Arch Surg 1986;121:488–490.

337. Miller DC, Stinson EB, Oyer PE, et al: The durability of porcine xenograft valves and conduits in children. Circulation 1982;66:I172–I185.

338. Waldman JD, Schoen FJ, Kirkpatrick SE, et al: Balloon dilatation of porcine bioprosthetic valves in the pulmonary position. Circulation 1987;76:109–114.

339. Allen HD, Beekman RH, III, Garson A Jr, et al: Pediatric therapeutic cardiac catheterization: A statement for healthcare professionals from the Council on Cardiovascular Disease in the Young, American Heart Association. Circulation 1998;97:609–625.

340. Beekman RH, Rocchini AP, Behrendt DM, et al: Reoperation for coarctation of the aorta. Am J Cardiol 1981;48:1108–1114.

341. Anjos R, Qureshi SA, Rosenthal E, et al: Determinants of hemodynamic results of balloon dilation of aortic recoarctation. Am J Cardiol 1992;69:665–671.

342. Cooper SG, Sullivan ID, Wren C: Treatment of recoarctation: Balloon dilation angioplasty. J Am Coll Cardiol 1989;14:413–419.

343. Hellenbrand WE, Allen HD, Golinko RJ, et al: Balloon angioplasty for aortic recoarctation: Results of Valvuloplasty and Angioplasty of Congenital Anomalies Registry. Am J Cardiol 1990;65:793–797.

344. Hijazi ZM, Fahey JT, Kleinman CS, et al: Balloon angioplasty for recurrent coarctation of aorta. Immediate and long-term results. Circulation 1991;84:1150–1156.

345. McCrindle BW, Jones TK, Morrow WR, et al: Acute results of balloon angioplasty of native coarctation versus recurrent aortic obstruction are equivalent. Valvuloplasty and Angioplasty of Congenital Anomalies (VACA) Registry Investigators. J Am Coll Cardiol 1996;28:1810–1817.

346. Rao PS, Wilson AD, Chopra PS: Immediate and follow-up results of balloon angioplasty of postoperative recoarctation in infants and children. Am Heart J 1990;120:1315–1320.

347. Witsenburg M, The SH, Bogers AJ, et al: Balloon angioplasty for aortic recoarctation in children: Initial and follow up results and midterm effect on blood pressure. Br Heart J 1993;70:170–174.

348. Yetman AT, Nykanen D, McCrindle BW, et al: Balloon angioplasty of recurrent coarctation: A 12-year review. J Am Coll Cardiol 1997;30:811–816.

349. Fletcher SE, Nihill MR, Grifka RG, et al: Balloon angioplasty of native coarctation of the aorta: Midterm follow-up and prognostic factors. J Am Coll Cardiol 1995;25:730–734.

350. Mendelsohn AM, Lloyd TR, Crowley DC, et al: Late follow-up of balloon angioplasty in children with a native coarctation of the aorta. Am J Cardiol 1994;74:696–700.

351. Ho SY, Somerville J, Yip WC, et al: Transluminal balloon dilation of resected coarcted segments of thoracic aorta: Histological study and clinical implications. Int J Cardiol 1988;19:99–105.

352. Isner JM, Donaldson RF, Fulton D, et al: Cystic medial necrosis in coarctation of the aorta: A potential factor contributing to adverse consequences observed after percutaneous balloon angioplasty of coarctation sites. Circulation 1987;75:689–695.

353. Ovaert C, Benson LN, Nykanen D, et al: Transcatheter treatment of coarctation of the aorta: A review. Pediatr Cardiol 1998;19:27–44.

354. Hosking MC, Thomaidis C, Hamilton R, et al: Clinical impact of balloon angioplasty for branch pulmonary arterial stenosis. Am J Cardiol 1992;69:1467–1470.

355. O'Laughlin MP: Catheterization treatment of stenosis and hypoplasia of pulmonary arteries. Pediatr Cardiol 1998;19:48–56.

356. Mullins CE, Latson LA, Neches WH, et al: Balloon dilation of miscellaneous lesions: Results of Valvuloplasty and Angioplasty of Congenital Anomalies Registry. Am J Cardiol 1990;65:802–803.

357. Musewe NN, Robertson MA, Benson LN, et al: The dysplastic pulmonary valve: Echocardiographic features and results of balloon dilatation. Br Heart J 1987;57:364–370.

358. O'Laughlin MP, Slack MC, Grifka RG, et al: Implantation and intermediate-term follow-up of stents in congenital heart disease. Circulation 1993;88:605–614.

359. Trant CA Jr, O'Laughlin MP, Ungerleider RM, et al: Cost-effectiveness analysis of stents, balloon angioplasty, and surgery for the treatment of branch pulmonary artery stenosis. Pediatr Cardiol 1997;18:339–344.

360. Perry SB, Radtke W, Fellows KE, et al: Coil embolization to occlude aortopulmonary collateral vessels and shunts in patients with congenital heart disease. J Am Coll Cardiol 1989;13:100–108.

361. Perry SB, Rome J, Keane JF, et al: Transcatheter closure of coronary artery fistulas. J Am Coll Cardiol 1992;20:205–209.

362. Siblini G, Rao PS: Coil embolization in the management of cardiac problems in children. J Invasive Cardiol 1996;8:332–340.

363. Rothman A: Pediatric cardiovascular embolization therapy. Pediatr Cardiol 1998;19:74–84.

364. Terry PB, White RI Jr, Barth KH, et al: Pulmonary arteriovenous malformations: Physiologic observations and results of therapeutic balloon embolization. N Engl J Med 1983;308:1197–1200.

365. Vance MS: Use of platinum microcoils to embolize vascular abnormal-

ities in children with congenital heart disease. Pediatr Cardiol 1998;19:145–149.

366. King TD, Thompson SL, Steiner C, et al: Secundum atrial septal defect: Nonoperative closure during cardiac catheterization. JAMA 1976;235:2506–2509.

367. Boutin C, Musewe NN, Smallhorn JF, et al: Echocardiographic follow-up of atrial septal defect after catheter closure by double-umbrella device. Circulation 1993;88:621–627.

368. Justo RN, Nykanen DG, Boutin C, et al: Clinical impact of transcatheter closure of secundum atrial septal defects with the double umbrella device. Am J Cardiol 1996;77:889–892.

369. Latson LA: Per-catheter ASD closure. Pediatr Cardiol 1998;19:86–93.

370. Bridges ND, Perry SB, Keane JF, et al: Preoperative transcatheter closure of congenital muscular ventricular septal defects. N Engl J Med 1991;324:1312–1317.

371. Fishberger SB, Bridges ND, Keane JF, et al: Intraoperative device closure of ventricular septal defects. Circulation 1993;88:II205–II209.

372. Lock JE, Block PC, McKay RG, et al: Transcatheter closure of ventricular septal defects. Circulation 1988;78:361–368.

373. Rigby ML, Redington AN: Primary transcatheter umbrella closure of perimembranous ventricular septal defect. Br Heart J 1994;72:368–371.

374. Sideris EB, Walsh KP, Haddad JL, et al: Occlusion of congenital ventricular septal defects by the buttoned device: "Buttoned device" Clinical Trials International Register. Heart 1997;77:276–279.

375. Hickey PR, Hansen DD, Norwood WI, et al: Anesthetic complications in surgery for congenital heart disease. Anesth Analg 1984;63:657–664.

376. Hennein HA, Mendeloff EN, Cilley RE, et al: Predictors of postoperative outcome after general surgical procedures in patients with congenital heart disease. J Pediatr Surg 1994;29:866–870.

377. Warner MA, Lunn RJ, O'Leary PW, et al: Outcomes of noncardiac surgical procedures in children and adults with congenital heart disease. Mayo Perioperative Outcomes Group. Mayo Clin Proc 1998;73:728–734.

20

Anesthesia for Otorhinolaryngology Procedures

Lynne R. Ferrari *and* Susan A. Vassallo

Adenoidectomy and Tonsillectomy
  Obstructive Sleep Apnea
  Preoperative Evaluation
  Anesthetic Management
  Peritonsillar Abscess
  Complications and Postoperative Considerations
Stridor
  Bronchoscopy
Endoscopic Laser Surgery
  Tracheostomy
Ear Surgery
  Myringotomy and Tube Insertion
  Middle Ear and Mastoid Surgery

Anesthesiologists care for children undergoing a wide variety of otolaryngology procedures. It is imperative that the physiologic and anatomic considerations be fully understood to provide safe anesthetic management and ideal conditions for both patients and surgeons.

Adenoidectomy and Tonsillectomy

Adenoidectomy is usually performed in conjunction with tonsillectomy; however, in some situations only adenoidectomy is performed. Indications for adenoidectomy alone include chronic or recurrent purulent adenoiditis (despite adequate medical therapy) and recurrent otitis media with effusion secondary to adenoidal hyperplasia. Advanced degrees of adenoidal hyperplasia may lead to nasopharyngeal obstruction, obligate mouth breathing, poor feeding resulting in failure to thrive, speech disorders, and sleep disturbances. Long-standing nasal obstruction can result in orofacial abnormalities with a narrowing of the upper airway and dental abnormalities, which may be avoided by removal of hypertrophied adenoid tissue.

Tonsillectomy with or without adenoidectomy is still one of the most commonly performed pediatric surgical procedures.[1] Chronic or recurrent tonsillitis and obstructive tonsillar hyperplasia are the major indications for surgical removal, although other indications do exist (Table 20–1).[2, 3] Surgical treatment is required when tonsillitis recurs despite adequate medical therapy or when it is associated with peritonsillar abscess or acute airway obstruction. Halitosis, persistent pharyngitis, and cervical adenitis may accompany chronic tonsillitis. Tonsillar hyperplasia may lead to chronic airway obstruction resulting in sleep apnea, carbon dioxide (CO_2) retention, cor pulmonale, failure to thrive, swallowing disorders, and speech abnormalities. Many of these adverse effects are reversible with surgical excision of the tonsils. Children with cardiac valvular disease are at risk for endocarditis due to recurrent streptococcal bacteremia secondary to infected tonsils.

Obstructive Sleep Apnea

Obstruction of the oropharyngeal airway by hypertrophied tonsils leading to apnea during sleep is an important clinical

Table 20–1. Indications for Tonsillectomy and/or Adenoidectomy

Infection

    Acute tonsillitis or adenoiditis
    Recurrent tonsillitis or adenoiditis
    Chronic tonsillitis or adenoiditis
    Peritonsillar abscess

Obstruction

    Nasal airway (adenoids)
    Pharyngeal airway (tonsils)
    Sleep apnea
    Cyanosis
    Failure to thrive
    Cor pulmonale due to airway obstruction

Mass Lesion

    Tonsillar/adenoidal
    Benign
    Malignant

syndrome requiring surgical treatment (Table 20–2). These patients have difficulty breathing while awake despite only mild to moderate tonsillar enlargement on visual inspection. Airway obstruction and apnea, however, do occur during sleep. Apnea is defined as cessation of respiratory flow for at least 10 seconds for older infants and children and 15 seconds for infants less than 52 weeks post-conceptual age.[4]

The diagnosis of sleep apnea syndrome is made with the use of polysomnography (a graphic recording of respiratory activity during natural sleep). To confirm the diagnosis of obstructive sleep apnea syndrome, one of the following findings is required: (1) apnea confirmed by airflow cessation diagnosed on auscultation and oxygen desaturation to less than 90%, as measured by pulse oximetry; (2) obstructive apnea identified by the absence of ventilatory gas exchange for at least 10 seconds accompanied by paradoxic movement of the rib cage and abdomen; (3) upper airway obstruction documented by nasopharyngoscopy or cinefluoroscopy or both. The two most frequent levels of obstruction during sleep are at the soft palate and base of the tongue.[5]

Both anatomic and physiologic factors are responsible for the pathogenesis of obstructive sleep apnea. Hypertrophied tonsils obstruct the upper airway during inspiration and lead to labored respiration, which worsens with the administration of sedatives as well as during natural sleep. Anatomic abnormalities that narrow the aperture of the nasopharyngeal airway allow the tongue to be displaced posteriorly and predispose susceptible individuals to airway obstruction (Table 20–3). Obesity is present in 66% of patients.[6] Fatty infiltration of the abdomen and neck limit the normal excursion of the lower jaw, leading to protrusion of the tongue during sleep. The oropharyngeal space becomes restricted, and the possibility of obstruction is increased. Nearly half of patients with obstructive sleep apnea syndrome are found to have neurologic dysfunction, including behavioral disturbances and primary central nervous system disorders. Central nervous system disease affecting brainstem regions that control upper airway musculature results in occlusion of the oropharynx when the collapsing force of negative inspiratory pressure exceeds the dilating force of pharyngeal muscular contraction, resulting in obstructive apnea. Asphyxial brain damage secondary to obstructive sleep apnea can lead to seizure disorders.

Common associated findings in children with obstructive sleep apnea syndrome include hypoxemia, hypercarbia, and partial airway obstruction while awake. The goals of treatment are to relieve airway obstruction and increase the cross-sectional area of the pharynx.[7] Because hypertrophied tonsils

Table 20–2. Clinical Presentation of Obstructive Sleep Apnea Syndrome in Children Aged 2 to 6 Years

Snoring
Somnolence
Apnea
Failure to thrive
Developmental delay
Recurrent respiratory tract infections
Craniofacial dysmorphism
Cor pulmonale
Cardiac dysrhythmias

Table 20–3. Anatomic Abnormalities Associated with Obstructive Sleep Apnea

Enlarged tonsils and/or adenoids
Cleft palate repair
Micrognathia
Pierre Robin syndrome
Treacher Collins syndrome
Temporomandibular joint ankylosis
Arthrogryposis multiplex congenita
Goldenhar syndrome
Generalized facial abnormalities
Crouzon syndrome
Larsen syndrome
Trisomy 21
Acromegaly
Prader-Willi syndrome
Neuromuscular malformations
Chiari malformation
Syringobulbia
Cerebral palsy

are the most frequent cause of upper airway obstruction, tonsillectomy is effective in relieving obstructive sleep apnea in 66% of cases.[4]

Increased airway resistance secondary to hypertrophied tonsils and adenoids can cause alveolar hypoventilation; cor pulmonale can be found in children with long-standing hypoxemia and hypercarbia (Fig. 20–1).[8, 9] These patients have electrocardiographic (ECG) and echocardiographic evidence of right ventricular hypertrophy, and one third have chest radiographs consistent with cardiomegaly.[4, 10] Patients with cor pulmonale can develop ventricular dysfunction and cardiac dysrhythmias from repeated apneic episodes that occur during sleep; pulmonary artery pressure progressively increases with each apneic episode, resulting in clinically important systemic and pulmonary artery hypertension. Digitalization is required in some patients and surgical removal of the tonsils and adenoids can reverse these progressive cardiovascular changes in most cases.[9]

In some patients with obstructive sleep apnea syndrome, other factors predispose them to the development of cor pulmonale. These patients often are mentally handicapped and have some degree of central nervous system dysfunction within the medulla or hypothalamus. They have a persistently elevated arterial CO_2 tension even after relief of airway obstruction and are insensitive to hypercapnia despite hypoxemia. This situation may eventually progress to respiratory failure. It is thought that a hyperreactive pulmonary vascular bed exists in this subgroup of patients. The increased pulmonary vascular resistance and myocardial depression in response to hypoxia, hypercarbia, and acidosis is far greater than what is expected for a similar degree of physiologic alteration in the normal population.[10] Some of these patients may require nasal constant positive airway pressure during sleep; rarely, others will require a tracheostomy to relieve the chronic upper airway obstruction.

Preoperative Evaluation

Because children requiring tonsillectomy and adenoidectomy have frequent infections, the presence of recent upper respi-

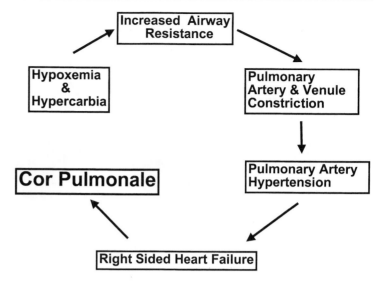

Figure 20–1. Patients with chronic tonsillar hypertrophy may have long-standing hypoxemia and hypercarbia, which can lead to cor pulmonale.

ratory infection (URI) or tonsillitis may alter the anesthetic management. Parents should be questioned about a child's current use of antibiotics, antihistamines, or other medicines. A history of sleep apnea should be specifically sought.

The physical examination should begin with observation of the patient. The presence of audible respiration, mouth breathing, nasal quality of the speech, and chest retractions are consistent with clinically important upper airway obstruction. Mouth breathing may be the result of nasopharyngeal obstruction due to chronic adenoidal hypertrophy. The facies should be noted because children with chronic oropharyngeal obstruction often have a longer face, a retrognathic mandible, and a high arched palate resulting from long-standing mouth breathing.[11] Finally, the oropharynx should be inspected for evaluation of tonsillar size to determine the degree of airway obstruction and to identify patients with the potential for difficulty with mask ventilation and intubation (Fig. 20–2).

A thorough examination of the chest by auscultation should be performed. Wheezing or rales may be present as a result of lower respiratory extension of pharyngitis or tonsillitis. Inspiratory stridor or prolongation of the expiratory phase of respiration may indicate partial airway obstruction due to hypertrophied tonsils or adenoids.

A complete blood count should be obtained for assessment of hemoglobin and for white blood cell count elevation, indicating recent or current infection. Because tonsillectomy and adenoidectomy are accompanied by blood loss, determination of platelet count, prothrombin time, partial thromboplastin time, or other appropriate measure of coagulation may also be indicated, although not all pediatric otolaryngologists obtain these screening studies. Many over-the-counter "cold" medications and antihistamines contain aspirin, which may affect platelet function; therefore, assessment of bleeding time may also be part of the preoperative laboratory evaluation. A chest radiograph and an ECG are not routinely ordered and are necessary only if a specific history of abnormalities in these organ systems is elicited, such as recent pneumonia, bronchitis, URI, or history consistent with cor pulmonale. If cor pulmonale is suspected, an echocardiogram may also be indicated to confirm the diagnosis.

Anesthetic Management

The anesthetic goals for tonsillectomy and adenoidectomy are: (1) to provide a smooth atraumatic induction; (2) to provide the surgeon with optimal operating conditions; (3) the establishment of intravenous access to provide a route for volume expansion and medications should they be necessary; and (4) to provide rapid emergence so that the patient is awake and able to protect the recently instrumented airway. The need for a premedication is determined during the preanesthetic evaluation. *Children who have a history of sleep apnea or intermittent airway obstruction or who have very large tonsils should not receive sedative premedications unless they are directly under supervision by the anesthesia care team.*

Anesthesia is usually induced with halothane or sevoflurane, oxygen, and nitrous oxide by mask. A parent's presence in the operating room during inhalation induction is often helpful in an anxious, unpremedicated child. Endotracheal intubation is accomplished under deep inhalation anesthesia or aided by a short-acting nondepolarizing muscle relaxant. Preformed endotracheal tubes such as the RAE tube (Mallinckrodt Medical, Inc., St. Louis, MO 63134) are particularly useful. An antisialagogue is usually administered to minimize secretions in the operative field. Blood in the pharynx can enter the trachea during the surgical procedure; for this reason, the supraglottic region immediately above the vocal cords and around the endotracheal tube should be packed with surgical gauze. Alternatively, a cuffed endotracheal tube may be used, provided there is a leak around the cuff between 20 and 40 cm H_2O peak inflation pressure. Monitoring consists of a precordial stethoscope, ECG, temperature probe, automated blood pressure cuff, pulse oximeter, and inspired oxygen and end-tidal CO_2 measurement.

The use of the laryngeal mask airway (LMA) for adenotonsillectomy was described in 1990, however it was not until the widespread availability of a model with a flexible spiral-metallic reinforced shaft that it was widely utilized.[12, 13] The wide, rigid tube of the original model did not fit under the mouth gag and was easily compressed or dislodged during full mouth opening. The newer, flexible model has a soft, reinforced shaft, which easily fits under

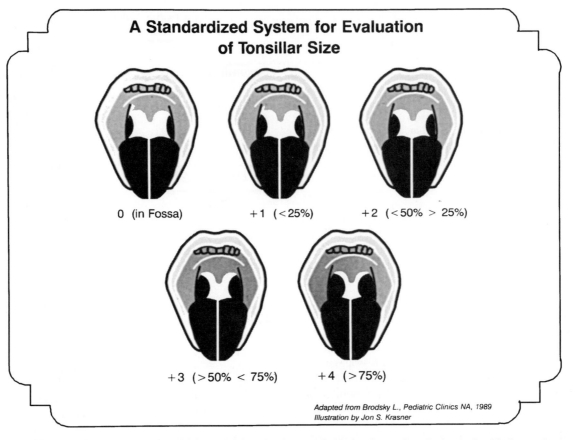

Figure 20–2. Classifying tonsil size may be helpful in evaluating the degree of airway obstruction. Patients classified as +3 or greater (i.e., having more than 50% of the pharyngeal area occupied by hypertrophied tonsils) are at an increased risk of developing airway obstruction during anesthetic induction. (Modified from Brodsky L: Modern assessment of tonsils and adenoids. Pediatr Clin North Am 1989;36:1551–1569; illustration by Jon S. Krasner.)

the mouth gag without becoming dislodged or compressed. Adequate surgical access can be achieved and the lower airway is reasonably well protected from exposure to blood during the procedure.[14, 15]

The same depth of anesthesia should be obtained during insertion of the LMA as would be required for performing laryngoscopy and endotracheal intubation. Greater anesthetic depth is certainly required when placing the LMA than when inserting an oral airway. Insertion is possible after either the intravenous administration of 3.5 mg/kg propofol or when sufficient depth of anesthesia is achieved using a volatile agent administered by mask.[16] It has been recommended that the LMA only be inserted into the spontaneously breathing child and positive pressure ventilation be avoided, although gentle assisted ventilation is both safe and effective if peak inspiratory pressure is kept below 20 cm H_2O.[17] The leak fraction produced during ventilation with the LMA increases with increasing airway pressure. The frequency of gastric insufflation ranges from 2% at a peak inspiratory pressure of 15 cm H_2O to 35% at 30 cm H_2O.[18] Ventilation using the LMA is adequate if airway resistance and pulmonary compliance are normal, but insufflation of air into the stomach will occur in the presence of increased ventilatory pressure, thus increasing the risk of regurgitation of gastric contents. Tonsillar enlargement can make LMA insertion difficult, so care in placement is essential.[19] Maneuvers to overcome this difficulty include increased head extension,

lateral insertion of the mask, anterior displacement of the tongue, pressure on the tip of the LMA using the index finger as it negotiates the pharyngeal curve, or use of the laryngoscope if all else fails.[20] Dislodgment of the device does not occur during extreme head extension, assuming that good position and ventilation were obtained prior to changes in head position.[21] Advantages of the LMA over traditional endotracheal intubation may be a decrease in the incidence of postoperative stridor and laryngospasm and an increase in immediate postoperative oxygen saturation.[22] Recovery may be improved overall and fewer episodes of airway obstruction have been noted.[15] The LMA is useful only in patients who can tolerate spontaneous respirations; it is our practice not to use controlled ventilation with the LMA. *The LMA should be viewed as a useful adjunct to airway management, never a substitute for endotracheal intubation.* If the child is breathing spontaneously at a regular rate and depth, the LMA may be removed prior to the patient's emergence from anesthesia. The oropharynx should be gently suctioned with a soft flexible catheter, the LMA deflated and removed, an oral airway inserted, and the respirations assisted with 100% oxygen delivered by mask. It is often distressing for young children to awaken with the LMA still in place and although the device is an appropriate substitute for oral airway in the adult population, the same is not so in children. If the practitioner wishes to remove the LMA when the child has emerged from anesthesia, it should be deflated and removed as soon as possible after the return to consciousness. The use of the LMA for tonsillectomy must balance possible benefits with possible risks; the decision to use the LMA for this procedure is an individual decision.

Blood and secretions may be present in the oropharynx at the conclusion of surgery and should be carefully suctioned prior to emergence from anesthesia. Emptying the stomach with an orogastric tube may be helpful in preventing emesis. If adenoidectomy has been performed, the nasal route for nasogastric tube insertion should not be used because unremoved adenoids may be dislodged, or bleeding at the surgical site may be induced. It is preferable to wait for the child to be "awake" and able to clear blood and secretions as efficiently as possible before removing the endotracheal tube. Extubation in the lateral position with the head slightly down may allow blood and secretions to pool in the dependent cheek rather than around the laryngeal inlet. Intact airway and pharyngeal reflexes are of utmost importance in preventing aspiration, laryngospasm, and airway obstruction. Following surgery, patients are placed in the lateral position and transported to the recovery room for careful observation

and monitoring. Opioids are generally required to provide adequate analgesia. The presence of blood in the stomach and the need for opioids are a potent stimulus to vomiting, as are swelling and inflammation of the posterior pharynx and uvula. The incidence of emesis after tonsillectomy can be as great as 60%.[23] Some practitioners may consider this operation an indication for the prophylactic use of an antiemetic because of this high incidence of emesis.

Peritonsillar Abscess

Peritonsillar abscess (quinsy tonsil) is a condition that may require immediate surgical intervention to relieve potential or existing airway obstruction. An acutely infected tonsil may undergo abscess formation, producing a large mass in the lateral pharynx that may interfere with swallowing and breathing (Fig. 20–3A–C). Fever and pain are present. Trismus is often an accompanying finding and is caused by compression of nerves by the tense peritonsillar mass and inflammation of the muscles of the face and neck. Treatment consists of surgical drainage of the abscess with or without tonsillectomy, plus intravenous antibiotic therapy.

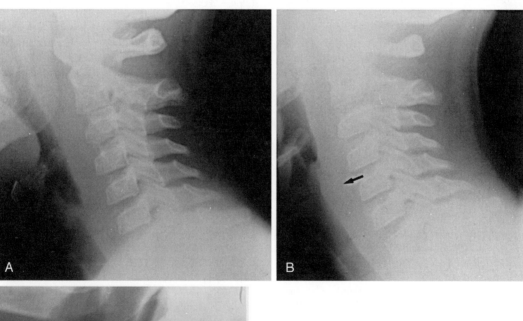

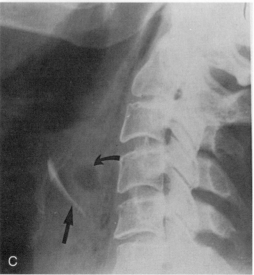

Figure 20–3. Retropharyngeal abscess in a young pediatric patient. (A) Initial presentation. (B) Thirty-six hours after onset of symptoms. Note widening of the prevertebral space (arrow). (C) Retropharyngeal abscess surrounding a foreign body (straight arrow). Note the presence of gas pockets within the abscess (curved arrow).

Although the airway may seem compromised, the peritonsillar abscess is most often in a fixed location in the lateral pharynx and does not usually interfere with ventilation of the patient by mask after induction of general anesthesia. Visualization of the vocal cords is usually not impaired because the pathology is supraglottic and well above the laryngeal inlet. Laryngoscopy must be carefully approached to avoid excessive manipulation of the larynx and surrounding structures. Intubation should be gentle, however, because the tonsillar area is tense and friable and unintended rupture of the abscess can occur, leading to spillage of purulent material into the trachea.

Complications and Postoperative Considerations

The most serious complication of tonsillectomy is postoperative hemorrhage, which occurs at a frequency of 0.1 to 8.1%.[24–26] Approximately 75% of postoperative tonsillar hemorrhages occur within 6 hours of surgery. The majority of the remaining 25% occurs within the first 24 hours after surgery, although bleeding may be noted until the sixth postoperative day. Sixty-seven percent of cases of postoperative bleeding originate in the tonsillar fossa, 27% in the nasopharynx, and 7% in both.[27] Initial attempts to control bleeding may be made using pharyngeal packs and cautery. If this fails, patients must return to the operating room for exploration and surgical hemostasis. With the advent of new, more potent antiemetics, the vomiting that occurs when blood enters the stomach may be suppressed or masked. It is therefore prudent to note if an antiemetic was given during the initial anesthetic since there may have been more bleeding than noted by observation of hematemesis alone.[28]

Large volumes of blood that are not appreciated by the patient, parent, or surgeon may originate from the tonsillar bed and be swallowed. Patients thus affected must be considered to have a full stomach, and anesthetic precautions addressing this problem must be taken. Before induction, it is important that the blood pressure be checked in both the erect and supine positions ("tilt test"), looking for orthostatic changes resulting from decreases in intravascular volume because the amount of blood swallowed is often unknown and can be considerable. Intravenous access must be established and volume replacement initiated. The hematocrit must be determined, and a blood sample for type and cross-match sent to the blood bank before induction. A rapid-sequence induction accompanied by cricoid pressure and intubation with a styletted endotracheal tube are essential. Various laryngoscope blades, handles, and endotracheal tubes should be available. Suction apparatus should be prepared in duplicate because blood in the airway may impair visualization of the vocal cords and cause plugging of the endotracheal tube or suction apparatus; if one suction becomes blocked with a blood clot, another is readily available.

Acute postoperative pulmonary edema is an infrequent but potentially life-threatening complication seen when chronic airway obstruction is suddenly relieved. One proposed mechanism is that during inspiration in the chronically obstructed child prior to adenotonsillectomy, the negative intrapleural pressure that is generated causes an increase in venous return, enhancing pulmonary blood volume. During exhalation, a positive intrapleural and alveolar pressure is generated, which decreases pulmonary blood volume. The rapid relief of obstruction during the postoperative period results in a decreased airway pressure, an increase in venous return, an increase in pulmonary hydrostatic pressure, hyperemia, and finally edema.[29] The prevention of this situation may be attempted during induction of anesthesia by applying moderate amounts of continuous positive pressure to the airway, thus allowing time for circulatory adaptation to take place.[30] This physiologic sequence is similar to that seen in patients with severe acute airway obstruction during epiglottitis or laryngospasm.[31]

Nausea and vomiting may occur in up to 60% of tonsillectomy patients. It is unclear whether the cause is irritation due to blood in the stomach, interference with the gag reflex by inflammation and edema at the surgical site, or administration of opioids. There is some evidence to suggest that certain analgesic agents, especially meperidine, might increase the probability of post-tonsillectomy emesis and other analgesic agents should be substituted.[24] Antiemetic agents such as droperidol (50–75 µg/kg) and metoclopramide (0.15 mg/kg) have been effective in controlling postoperative emesis.[32, 33] There have been many reports of the successful use of ondansetron in controlling postoperative nausea and vomiting by antagonism of serotonin receptors. The incidence is reduced from 40% to 10% when 0.1 mg/kg is administered intravenously prior to incision or orally during the immediate preoperative period.[34, 35] Other data suggest that an intravenous dose of 0.15 mg/kg lowered the incidence from 62% to 27%; however, droperidol combined with metoclopramide was just as effective.[36, 37] Even intravenous administration of as little as 0.05 mg/kg of ondansetron has been shown to provide highly effective prophylaxis.[38] An intravenous dose of 0.1 mg/kg has been shown to be a superior rescue medication administered once vomiting has begun.[39] The cost of ondansetron precludes universal administration and perhaps it should be administered prophylactically to those patients who have an increased risk of postoperative nausea and vomiting and for use as a rescue medication in the postoperative period in other patients. The optimal antiemetic may prove to be a combination of several medications, each having a unique pharmacologic effect. Several papers have reported a clinically important reduction in the incidence of nausea and vomiting following the administration of dexamethasone (0.5 mg/kg); at least one paper found more prolonged benefit when compared with ondansetron.[40]

Post-tonsillectomy dehydration secondary to poor oral intake as a result of nausea, vomiting, or pain occurs in 1.1% of cases.[25] Vigorous intravenous hydration during surgery can offset the physiologic effects of postoperative decreases in fluid intake.

Pain after adenoidectomy is usually minimal, but pain after tonsillectomy is severe and contributes to poor fluid intake. An increased requirement for postoperative pain medications has been noted in patients who have had laser or electrocautery used as part of the operative tonsillectomy compared with those who had sharp surgical dissection and ligation of blood vessels to achieve hemostasis.[41] Administration of intraoperative corticosteroids may decrease edema formation and subsequent discomfort.[42] Infiltration of the peritonsillar space with local anesthetic and epinephrine has been shown to be effective in reducing intraoperative blood loss and decreasing postoperative pain.[43] The pre-incision infiltration of each tonsillar pillar with 3 to 5 mL of 0.25% bupivacaine with epinephrine 1:200,000 substantially diminished immediate as well as long-term post-tonsillectomy pain. An explanation for the long-term pain relief may be that neural blockade prevents nociceptive stimulus impulses from entering the central nervous system during and immediately following surgery, thus suppressing the formation of a sustained hyperexcitable state, which is responsible for the maintenance of postoperative pain.[44–46]

The administration of high-dose acetaminophen administered rectally may be an effective analgesic in some patients. Doses of up to 40 mg/kg have been advocated to achieve serum levels that will provide adequate analgesia after tonsillectomy.[47] There has been a great deal of discussion surrounding the use of ketorolac as an analgesic after tonsillectomy. It has been proven to be an effective treatment for post-tonsillectomy pain with the potential of minimizing associated respiratory depression, nausea, and vomiting following opioid administration. The effect of the nonsteroidal anti-inflammatory agents on coagulation has led to controversy regarding the advisability of their use with a surgical procedure that is associated with bleeding complications. Although there is some evidence to suggest that the intravenous administration of 1 mg/kg of ketorolac prior to achieving surgical hemostasis increases the incidence of post-surgical bleeding, there are others who have demonstrated no increase in bleeding when a single dose of the drug is administered at the conclusion of the surgery after hemostasis has been obtained.[48–52] The use of ketorolac for prevention and treatment of post-tonsillectomy pain should be discussed with the surgeon and a joint decision should be made.

Patients undergoing adenoidectomy may be safely discharged on the same day, after recovering from surgery and anesthesia. Tonsillectomy has traditionally been a procedure that warranted postoperative admission for observation, administration of analgesics, and hydration. Many centers are discharging tonsillectomy patients on the day of surgery without an apparent increase in adverse outcomes.[25, 27, 41, 53] It is recommended that patients be observed for early hemorrhage for a minimum of 6 hours, have adequate oral fluid intake, and be free from severe nausea, vomiting, and pain prior to discharge. If children cannot take oral fluids because of pain or vomiting, or if vomiting is so severe that it requires frequent administration of antiemetics, admission to the hospital is necessary. Patients with sleep apnea, either with or without cor pulmonale, should be admitted to the hospital after tonsillectomy for monitoring of cardiorespiratory function. As a result of changes in third-party reimbursement, many patients who require hospital admission after tonsillectomy are not covered by their insurance carriers. To circumvent this problem, some centers have established 23-hour observation units.

There are situations in which overnight admission to the hospital is essential. The American Academy of Otolaryngology has identified the following patients as being high risk and requiring postoperative admission to the hospital[54]:

- Age under 3 years
- Abnormal measurement of coagulation, with or without an identifiable bleeding disorder
- Obstructive sleep apnea

- Systemic medical disorders that render the patient an increased anesthetic and surgical risk
- Craniofacial abnormality
- Acute peritonsillar abscess
- Geographic or social conditions that prevent easy and rapid return to the medical facility in the event of a complication

Stridor

Noisy breathing due to obstructed airflow is known as stridor. Inspiratory stridor results from upper airway obstruction, expiratory stridor results from lower airway obstruction, and biphasic stridor is present with midtracheal lesions (see Chapter 7). The evaluation of a child with stridor begins with taking a thorough history. The age of symptom onset helps suggest a cause; for instance, laryngotracheomalacia and vocal cord paralysis are usually present at or shortly after birth, whereas cysts or mass lesions develop later in life (Table 20–4). Information indicating positions that make the stridor better or worse should be obtained, since placing a child in a position that allows gravity to aid in reducing obstruction can be of benefit during anesthetic induction.

Physical examination reveals the general condition of a child or infant as well as the degree of the airway compromise. Laboratory examination may include assessment of hemoglobin, a chest radiograph, and barium swallow, which can aid in identifying lesions that may be compressing the trachea. Computed tomography, magnetic resonance imaging scan and tomograms may be indicated in isolated instances but are not routinely ordered. Specific note of the signs and symptoms listed in Table 20–5 should be made.

Laryngomalacia is the most common cause of stridor in infants and is most often due to a long epiglottis that pro-

Table 20–4. Causes of Stridor

Supraglottic Airway

Choanal atresia
Cyst
Mass
Large tonsils
Large adenoids
Craniofacial abnormalities
Foreign body

Larynx

Laryngomalacia
Vocal cord paralysis
Subglottic stenosis
Hemangiomas
Cysts
Laryngocele
Infection (tonsillitis, peritonsillar abscess)
Foreign body

Subglottic Airway

Tracheomalacia
Vascular ring
Foreign body
Infection (croup, epiglottitis)
Hemangiomas

Table 20–5. Signs and Symptoms Specifically Examined in Patients with Stridor

Respiratory rate	Chest retractions
Heart rate	Nasal flaring
Wheezing	Level of consciousness
Cyanosis	

lapses posteriorly and prominent arytenoid cartilages with redundant aryepiglottic folds that prolapse into the glottic opening during inspiration.[55] The definitive diagnosis is obtained by direct laryngoscopy and by rigid or flexible bronchoscopy.

Preliminary examination is usually carried out in the surgeon's office. A small flexible fiberoptic bronchoscope is inserted through the nares into the oropharynx, and the movement of the vocal cords is observed. Alternatively, it may be accomplished in the operating room before anesthetic induction in an awake patient or in a lightly anesthetized patient during spontaneous respiration. Patients must be spontaneously breathing so that the vocal cords move freely. After deepening anesthesia and topicalization of the laryngeal structures, a rigid bronchoscope is inserted through the vocal cords and the subglottic area is inspected; the lower trachea and bronchi are evaluated with a rigid or flexible fiberoptic bronchoscope.

Bronchoscopy

Small infants may be brought into the operating room unpremedicated; older children may experience respiratory depression and worsening of airway obstruction if heavy premedication is administered. The airway must be protected from aspiration of gastric contents during prolonged airway manipulation; therefore, premedication with the full regimen of acid aspiration prophylaxis may be indicated in some patients.

The goals of anesthesia are analgesia, an unconscious patient, and a "quiet" surgical field.[56] Coughing, bucking, or straining during instrumentation with the rigid bronchoscope may cause difficulty for the surgeon and result in damage to the patient's airway. At the conclusion of the procedure, patients should be returned to consciousness quickly with airway reflexes intact to protect the recently instrumented airway.

For most patients, a pulse oximeter, blood pressure cuff, ECG, and precordial stethoscope are applied before induction. Inhalation induction by mask is accomplished with 100% oxygen and a volatile agent (usually halothane or sevoflurane) administered in increasing concentrations. Patients should be placed in the position that produces the least adverse effect on airway symptoms (often the sitting position). Alternatively, in those patients who have intravenous access established prior to anesthesia, intravenous induction may be accomplished with propofol, followed by mask ventilation with a volatile agent.

After sufficient depth of anesthesia has been obtained, an intravenous line is inserted, the patient vigorously hydrated to make up for intravascular volume deficits, and the depth of anesthesia increased. An antisialagogue (atropine or glycopyrrolate) should be administered intravenously to decrease secretions that may impair the view through the bronchoscope. At this time, topicalization of the vocal cords should occur to decrease the incidence of coughing or bucking during instrumentation, which might result in damage to the vocal cords and accessory structures. Lidocaine, either 2 or 4%, is the most frequently utilized local anesthetic on the vocal cords. It may be applied to the vocal cords either by atomizer or sprayed with a 3 mL syringe fitted with a 22-gauge IV catheter (without the needle). The volume of local anesthetic should be limited by the toxic dose, since complete absorption via mucosal surfaces occurs. Local anesthetic should *never* be applied through a non-Luer-lock syringe fitted with a needle at the end, since the needle may become loose and be catapulted under the pressure of injection through the vocal cords down into the lower airway.

It is wise to ask the surgeon if movement of the vocal cords will be observed at the conclusion of the procedure or if tracheal or bronchial dynamics will be evaluated during the procedure so that the anesthetic may be planned accordingly (i.e., spontaneous respirations preserved during light levels of anesthesia versus no respiratory efforts and the use of short-acting muscle relaxants). If evaluation of vocal cord movement is required, the surgeon may choose to begin the procedure with a flexible bronchoscope. In the neonate or young infant, this is best accomplished by nasal insertion of the bronchoscope with the patient in the sitting position while awake. Nasal insertion provides an excellent view of the moving vocal cords. In some patients, topicalization of the nasopharynx with lidocaine facilitates passage of the nasal pharyngoscope or bronchoscope. Administration of 50% nitrous oxide also provides additional analgesia. In the child who vigorously objects to awake nasal instrumentation, anesthesia may be induced by mask with a volatile agent (halothane is still the best agent for this) in 100% oxygen. In both situations, the patient must maintain spontaneous respiration. The non-paralyzed child may go into laryngospasm, so it is prudent to administer 100% oxygen at all times until the airway has been secured.

After completion of flexible pharyngoscopy/bronchoscopy, the surgeon will generally proceed to rigid bronchoscopy. The size of a rigid bronchoscope refers to the internal diameter. Because the external diameter may be significantly greater than that of an endotracheal tube of similar size (Table 20–6), care must be taken to select a bronchoscope of proper external diameter to avoid damage to the laryngeal structures. A rigid bronchoscope can be used for ventilation during examination of the airway. It is often most useful to paralyze the patient with a fixed lesion, which diminishes the risk of vocal cord injury secondary to movement. For non-fixed lesions, such as aspirated foreign body, and for assessment for bronchomalacia or tracheomalacia, it is safest to proceed with spontaneous ventilation, deep level of anesthesia, and good topical anesthesia of the vocal cords. It should be noted that airway instrumentation in the non-paralyzed patient is most effective with halothane as the primary volatile agent. The newer volatile agents, desflurane and sevoflurane, although tempting because of their decreased solubility, have not yet been shown to be effective as the sole anesthetic agent in this situation. Desflurane causes too much respiratory irritation and is not recommended for use in unintubated pediatric patients, and sevoflurane even at maximal concentrations does not always

Table 20–6. External Diameter of Standard Endotracheal Tube Versus Rigid Bronchoscope

Internal Diameter (mm)	Endotracheal Tube* External Diameter (mm)	Rigid Bronchoscope† External Diameter (mm)
2.0	2.9	
2.5	3.6	4.2
3.0	4.3	5.0
3.5	4.9	5.7
3.7 (bronchoscope)		6.3
4.0	5.6	6.7
5.0	6.9	7.8
6.0	8.2	8.2

*Mallinckrodt Medical, Inc., Saint Louis, MO.
†Karl Storz Endoscopy-America, Inc., Culver City, CA.

produce a motionless patient.[57] The rigid bronchoscope is inserted through the vocal cords, and ventilation is accomplished through a side port attached to the anesthetic circuit with a flexible extension. During ventilation of the patient with the telescope in place, high resistance may be encountered as a result of partial occlusion of the lumen. High fresh gas flow rates, large tidal volumes with high inflation pressures, and high inspired volatile anesthetic concentrations are often necessary to compensate for leaks around the ventilating bronchoscope and the high resistance encountered when the viewing telescope is in place. Hand ventilation at higher than normal rates is most effective in achieving adequate ventilation. Adequate time for exhalation must be provided for passive recoil of the chest.

An alternative method of ventilation utilizes the Sanders jet ventilation technique. The principle of jet ventilation involves intermittent bursts of oxygen delivered under a pressure of 50 psi through a 16-gauge catheter attached to a rigid bronchoscope.[58] Intermittent flow is accomplished by depressing the lever of an on-off valve. A jet of oxygen is released at the tip of the 16-gauge catheter, creating a Venturi effect that entrains room air into the bronchoscope. This jet of oxygen and room air allows inflation of the lungs to occur; however, there is the possibility of hypoxemia in some patients, because oxygen delivered to the trachea is diluted by entrained room air. The use of jet ventilation techniques is associated with the additional risks of pneumothorax or pneumomediastinum due to rupture of alveolar blebs or a bronchus.[59]

Because ventilation may be intermittent and at times is suboptimal, it is recommended that 100% oxygen be used as the carrier gas during bronchoscopic examination. For the same reason, an inhalation-based anesthetic should be supplemented with intravenous adjunct to maintain an adequate depth of anesthesia. A background infusion of propofol (75–150 μg/kg/min) is ideal, since intravenous agents that cause excessive respiratory depression should be avoided.

At the conclusion of rigid bronchoscopy, an endotracheal tube is usually placed in the trachea to control the airway during recovery from anesthesia. Insertion of an endotracheal tube is particularly important if muscle relaxants have been used, because passive regurgitation of gastric contents is more likely to occur in paralyzed patients. One additional advantage of placing an endotracheal tube at the conclusion of rigid bronchoscopy is that should the surgeon wish to examine the distal airways, a small flexible fiberoptic bronchoscope can be passed through the endotracheal tube. Another reason to intubate the trachea at the conclusion of bronchoscopy is to size the larynx and determine the degree of airway obstruction. A standard endotracheal tube is inserted beyond the narrowest portion of the obstructed airway while maintaining a leak between 10 and 25 cm H_2O. The leak is measured by applying positive pressure to the airway via the endotracheal tube and listening with a stethoscope for an air leak around the endotracheal tube at the level of the suprasternal notch. The outer diameter of the appropriate endotracheal tube is compared to the diameter of the child's trachea and the percentage of obstruction is calculated. Grade I obstruction involves up to 50% of the airway, grade II from 51% to 70%, and grade III is greater than 70% (Fig. 20–4A & B).[60]

Endoscopic Laser Surgery

A laser (an acronym for *Light Amplified by Stimulated Emission of Radiation*) is sometimes used for surgical procedures on the airway. The laser consists of a tube with reflective mirrors at either end and an amplifying medium between them to generate electron activity, resulting in the production of light.[61]

The CO_2 laser is the most widely used in medical practice, having particular application in the treatment of laryngeal or vocal cord papillomas, laryngeal webs, and resection of subglottic tissue and hemangiomas. A laser is useful for endoscopic procedures because the beam may be directed down open-tube endoscopes and is invisible, thereby affording the surgeon an unobstructed view of the lesion during resection. The energy emitted by a CO_2 laser is absorbed by water or the water contained in blood and tissues. Human tissue is 80% water, and laser energy is absorbed by this tissue water, rapidly raising its temperature, denaturing protein, and causing vaporization of the target tissue. The thermal energy of the laser beam cauterizes capillaries as it vaporizes tissues; therefore, bleeding is minimal and very little postoperative edema occurs.

These properties give the laser a high degree of specificity; however, they also supply the route by which a misdirected laser beam may cause injury to a patient or to unprotected operating room personnel.[62] Laser radiation increases the temperature of absorbent material; therefore, flammable objects, such as surgical drapes, must be kept away from the path of the laser beam. Unprotected surfaces, such as skin, can be burned by the laser beam and thus must be shielded. Wet towels should be applied to cover the skin of the face and neck of the patient when the laser is being used to avoid burns from deflected beams.

The eyes are especially vulnerable to laser damage. The CO_2 laser can burn the cornea; the neodymium:yttrium aluminum garnet laser can damage both the anterior and posterior chambers of the eye as well as the cornea and retina; and the argon, ruby, and helium-neon lasers can cause retinal damage. To avoid eye damage, wet gauze pads are applied

Percent Subglottic Stenosis by Endotracheal Tube Size (mm ID)

Age ↓	ETT →	2	2.5	3	3.5	4	4.5	5	5.5	6
Preterm		40								
Preterm		58	30							
0-3 mon		68	48	26		No obstruction				
3-9 mon	No Detectable Lumen	75	59	41	22					
9 mon-2 yr		80	67	53	38	20				
2 yr		84	74	62	50	35	19			
4 yr		86	78	68	57	45	32	17		
6 yr		89	81	73	64	54	43	30	16	
	Grade IV	Grade III			Grade II		Grade I			

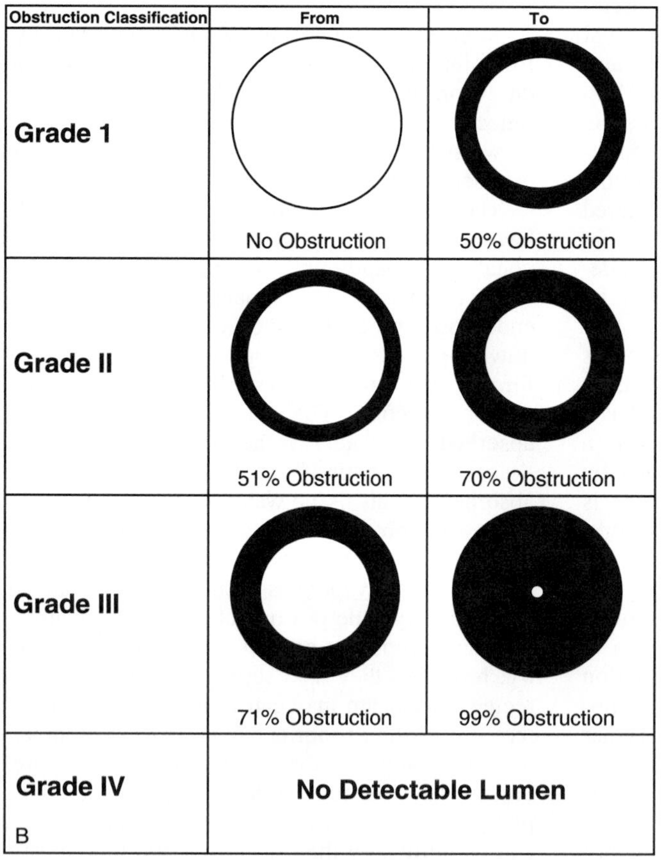

A

Obstruction Classification	From	To
Grade 1	No Obstruction	50% Obstruction
Grade II	51% Obstruction	70% Obstruction
Grade III	71% Obstruction	99% Obstruction
Grade IV	No Detectable Lumen	

B

Figure 20–4. (A) Method of determining percentage of airway obstruction. After easy passage of an endotracheal tube, a manometer is placed at the connection of the elbow of the anesthesia circuit and the endotracheal tube. A stethoscope is placed over the larynx and the circuit is slowly pressurized. The size endotracheal tube with which a leak occurs at 20 cm H_2O peak inflation pressure is matched with the age of the patient to assess the degree of airway narrowing (e.g., a 3.0 mm IO tube that leaks at 20 cm H_2O peak inflation pressure in a 2-year-old indicates approximately 62% narrowing). It should be noted that this chart is based on one institution's experience and that the manufacturer of the endotracheal tubes was not described, thus the actual external diameter of the endotracheal tubes used is unknown. (B) Schematic representation of subglottic stenosis classification system. (Modified from Myer CM III, O'Connor DM, Cotton RT: Proposed grading system for subglottic stenosis based on endotracheal tube sizes. Ann Otol Laryngol 1994;103:319–323.)

over the closed eyes of the anesthetized patient and a towel is wrapped around the head, covering the eyes and keeping the gauze pads in place. Any stray beam is absorbed by the wet gauze, preventing penetration into the eyes. All operating room personnel should wear special protective goggles with side shields to protect their eyes from the laser beam.

Most anesthetic techniques are suitable for laser surgery provided that patients are totally immobile and the laser beam can be directed at a target that is entirely still. A muscle relaxant and controlled ventilation with small tidal volumes are usually required. Both oxygen and nitrous oxide support combustion, so the primary gas for anesthetic maintenance should consist of blended oxygen and air. The in-

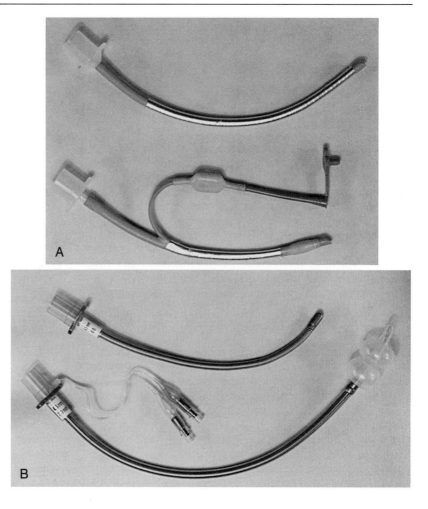

Figure 20–5. (A) Cuffed and uncuffed red rubber endotracheal tubes wrapped with reflective metallic tape for use during laser airway surgery. Note that this metallic tape is not approved by the Food and Drug Administration for this application. (B) Cuffed and uncuffed flexible metal endotracheal tubes for use during laser airway surgery.

spired oxygen content should be reduced to 30% or as close to this level as possible. A pulse oximeter is particularly helpful in this situation. Cuffed endotracheal tubes should have the cuff filled with sterile saline or water rather than air, so that a spark striking the cuff and burning a hole in it will be immediately extinguished.[63] If ignition of an endotracheal tube does occur, saline should be flushed down the tube, which should be immediately removed, and the patient ventilated with 100% oxygen.

The choice of endotracheal tube used during laser surgery can affect the safety of the technique. All standard polyvinyl-chloride endotracheal tubes are flammable and can ignite and vaporize when in contact with a laser beam. Red rubber endotracheal tubes do not vaporize but instead deflect the laser beam when wrapped with metallic tape; however, the metallic tape can only be applied up to the cuff and not around it, so the area below the vocal cords may still be vulnerable (Fig. 20–5A). Endotracheal tubes have been manufactured specifically for use during laser surgery. Some have a double cuff to ensure protection of the airway in the event that one cuff is pierced by the laser beam. Others have a special matte finish that is effective in deflecting the laser beam throughout its entire length. Nonreflective flexible metal endotracheal tubes are also specifically manufactured for use during laser surgery (Fig. 20–5B). The outer diameter of the metal laser tube is considerably greater than the polyvinyl-chloride counterpart, especially in the small sizes. Thus they may not be appropriate for very small infants or

for children with a severely narrowed airway (Table 20–7). Although these endotracheal tubes offer some advantage, they are considerably more expensive than metallic tape–wrapped red rubber endotracheal tubes.

Some surgeons prefer an apneic technique when working on the airway of small infants and children. The advantage of this technique is the absence of an endotracheal tube that may interfere with the small surgical field. In this circumstance, a child is anesthetized and rendered immobile either by administration of a muscle relaxant or by deep inhalation of a volatile agent. The trachea is not intubated,

Table 20–7. External Diameter of Standard Plastic Versus Metal Endotracheal Tube*

Internal Diameter (mm)	External Diameter (mm)	
	Plastic	**Metal**
3.0	4.3	5.2
3.5	4.9	5.7
4.0	5.5	6.1
4.5	6.2	7.0 (Cuffed)
5.0	6.8	7.5
5.5	7.5	7.9
6.0	8.2	8.5

*Mallinckrodt Medical, Inc., St. Louis, MO.

and the airway is given over to the surgeon, who uses the laser for very brief periods. In between laser applications, the patient may be ventilated by mask or intermittent insertion of a small endotracheal tube. Because apnea is a component of this technique, it is prudent for the patient to be ventilated with 100% oxygen. Although this technique has been widely used with safety, there is a greater potential for debris and resected material to enter the trachea.

A modification of the apneic technique that does not require endotracheal intubation but does provide for oxygenation during laser surgery utilizes a jet ventilator. The operating laryngoscope may be fitted with a catheter through which air is entrained and the patient intermittently ventilated by the jet. The advantage of this technique is twofold. The surgical field is extremely quiet because large excursions of the diaphragm are eliminated and ventilation of the patient is uninterrupted. In morbidly obese patients and those with severe small-airway disease, effective ventilation is not accomplished with this technique and an alternate technique should be used.[64]

A technique of spontaneous ventilation without an endotracheal tube may also be employed. To utilize this method, a suspension laryngoscope (usually a Benjamin or Lindholm) that has an oxygen insufflation side port is fitted with an endotracheal tube adapter and inserted into the larynx (Fig. 20–6). The volatile anesthetic gas is mixed with oxygen and administered via the side port lumen, which has its distal opening at the end of the blade. Anesthesia is maintained without muscle relaxant in the spontaneously breathing patient. A propofol infusion may be added in a dose of 75 to 150 μg/kg/min and the concentration of volatile anesthetic may be decreased. The vocal cords are sprayed with 4% lidocaine to decrease their reactivity, paying close attention to the toxic dose of local anesthetic agent.[65] The advantage to this technique is that long periods of uninterrupted laser application may be provided. Unlike techniques that require paralysis, the spontaneously breathing patient will effectively

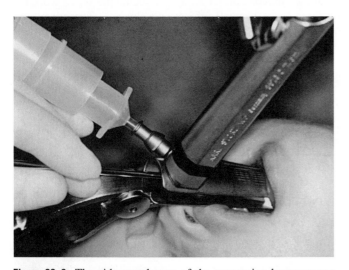

Figure 20–6. The side port lumen of the suspension laryngoscope, which opens at the distal end of the blade, is fitted with an endotracheal tube adapter. The anesthesia circuit is attached to the endotracheal tube adapter, thereby providing oxygen and volatile anesthetic gas immediately proximal to the trachea, which will be inhaled by the spontaneously breathing patient.

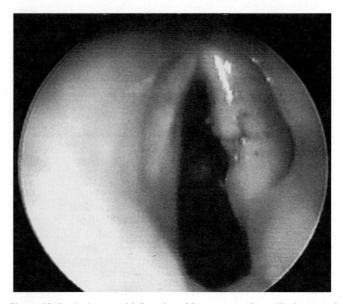

Figure 20–7. A 4-year-old female with recurrent juvenile laryngeal papillomatosis. Note the papilloma originating from the right true vocal cord.

eliminate CO_2, thereby avoiding the hypercarbia associated with other techniques. When this technique is used during laser treatment of laryngeal papilloma, viral particles are not propelled into the lower airway. Disadvantages include the absence of complete control of the airway, the possibility of laryngospasm, the presence of some vocal cord movement, and inadequate scavenging of anesthetic gases. It is important that both the surgeon and anesthesiologist agree that in the event of an airway complication during the use of this or other techniques without an endotracheal tube, that the patient may require paralysis, intubation, and controlled ventilation.

The most common indications for laser surgery in infants and children are for correction of congenital or acquired glottic web or for treatment of laryngeal papillomatosis. Juvenile laryngeal papillomatosis is the most common laryngeal tumor occurring in the pediatric population and the only effective treatment is surgical excision of the papilloma lesions (Fig. 20–7). The human papilloma virus is the etiology of the tumors, and although they are rarely malignant or invasive, significant morbidity is encountered due to airway obstruction secondary to tumor growth. If left untreated, symptoms of aphonia, respiratory distress, hoarseness, stridor, right ventricular hypertrophy, and cor pulmonale may occur.[66] Large lesions may be surgically excised, but the mainstay of surgical treatment is by either carbon dioxide (CO_2) or titanyl phosphate (KTP) laser vaporization.[67] The condition is characterized by numerous relapses and recurrences despite adequate resection. Patients may return to the operating room as frequently as every 4 to 6 weeks. Laryngeal scarring, edema, fibrosis, and glottic web formation have been reported in patients who have had laser treatment of laryngeal papillomatosis.[68] A complete evaluation of airway dynamics and function is essential in each patient each time he or she presents for general anesthesia, since review of prior anesthetic records may not accurately predict the respiratory status or the anatomy since the last procedure.

Tracheostomy

Tracheostomy in infants and children is usually performed electively in a controlled manner, although the occasional emergency situation is encountered. Lesions such as congenital or acquired vocal paralysis, central hypoventilation syndrome (Ondine's Curse), craniofacial abnormalities (such as Pierre Robin malformation), persistent laryngotracheomalacia, and congenital or acquired subglottic stenosis are some of the conditions requiring elective tracheostomy. These children have usually had a period of watchful waiting, which later results in the need for tracheostomy due to persistent hypoxemia, hypercarbia, or intermittent obstruction that cannot be eliminated with the natural airway. Other children have acute deterioration of the airway and require tracheostomy on an emergent basis. Children with severe epiglottitis or children with partially obstructed airways in whom adequate ventilation and oxygenation become impossible on induction of anesthesia may require emergency tracheostomy.

Children requiring elective tracheostomy more often than not can be intubated. Ideally the child should come to the operating room unpremedicated to avoid pharmacologically induced respiratory depression, but this is not always feasible. In selected cases, parental presence may be beneficial during induction, and in others judicial use of a benzodiazepine such as oral midazolam is acceptable. In either case, the child is brought to the operating room, monitors are applied, and anesthesia is induced by mask with increasing concentrations of a volatile agent such as halothane or sevoflurane in oxygen. Early use of assisted manual ventilation delivering 3 to 5 cm H_2O and occasionally even higher levels of positive end-expiratory pressure is helpful in "stenting" open the airway. As the depth of anesthesia is increased, controlled manual ventilation is introduced. After securing intravenous access, an antisialagogue is administered and the child may be paralyzed with a short-acting nondepolarizing agent if controlled ventilation is easily accomplished and if the larynx may be visualized by direct laryngoscopy. Topical local anesthesia (lidocaine) is applied by atomizer or syringe. The patient is then intubated. Children with subglottic stenosis may require intubation with an endotracheal tube much smaller than calculated for age; therefore a wide variety of sizes as well as stylets should be available.

Anesthesia is maintained with volatile agents so that early spontaneous ventilation and recovery of airway reflexes are present at the conclusion of surgery. One hundred percent oxygen should be administered throughout the procedure since the airway may be lost at any time. Intravenous narcotic agents or local anesthetics, or both, to the incision should be utilized to manage postoperative pain. A thrashing, crying child who is in pain will compromise the integrity of newly established surgical airway.

Children who cannot be intubated may undergo an "awake" tracheostomy with sedation and local anesthesia. Ketamine, although an attractive alternative, does produce secretions that may further compromise an already marginal airway. Children who can be anesthetized with a volatile agent administered by mask but who cannot be intubated due to severe subglottic stenosis or inability to visualize the vocal cords by direct laryngoscopy may have the airway maintained with spontaneous ventilation and a face mask or an LMA until a surgical airway is obtained.

Once the trachea has been entered, a portion of the delivered tidal volume is lost through the incision, and adequate ventilation may be difficult to provide. There are two philosophies regarding paralysis at this juncture: If the surgeon (such as an otolaryngologist who is very familiar with the airway) is certain that a tracheostomy tube can be placed, then paralysis is appropriate to provide adequate muscle relaxation and prevention of coughing during tracheostomy tube insertion. If the surgeon is less experienced with the airway (such as some general and plastic surgeons perform tracheostomies as part of a larger surgical procedure), it is prudent to not administer any muscle relaxation and allow spontaneous respiration. Therefore, if the airway is not immediately cannulated, the patient can maintain spontaneous respirations. The insertion of the tracheostomy inner cannula into a false tracheal passage may occur, in which case effective ventilation becomes impossible. If the patient had been intubated, it is prudent to leave the endotracheal tube within the lumen of the trachea but pulled back to just proximal to the tracheal incision so that it can be readily advanced should difficulty be encountered with passage of the tracheotomy tube. Once the tracheotomy tube is safely inserted, the endotracheal tube is removed, the anesthesia circuit is attached to the tracheotomy tube, and the wound is closed. In the event of the tracheostomy tube becoming dislodged or removed, the tracheal incision will close and attempts at reinsertion may result in bleeding, the creation of a false passage, or trauma to the tracheal wall. The tracheal lumen is identified by internal traction sutures, which are placed by the surgeon at the end of the surgical procedure (Fig. 20–8A). By the surgeon's pulling up on the external ends of these sutures, the tracheal incision is identified and tracheotomy opened so that safe reinsertion of an artificial airway is accomplished (Fig. 20–8B). The patient should not leave the operating room without the potentially life-saving sutures in place and properly identified. Flexible fiberoptic bronchoscopy through the new tracheostomy tube is usually performed to confirm appropriate location of the tip of the tracheostomy tube above the carina.

Ear Surgery

The ear and its associated structures are target organs for many pathologic conditions frequently found in children. Recurrent otitis media resulting in impairment of hearing and cholesteatoma formation are common conditions requiring surgical intervention.

Myringotomy and Tube Insertion

Chronic serous otitis media in children can lead to hearing loss. Drainage of accumulated fluid in the middle ear is effective treatment for this condition. Myringotomy creates an opening in the tympanic membrane through which fluid can drain. It may be performed alone; however, when the incision heals, the drainage path is occluded. Therefore, it is frequently accompanied by tube placement. A small plastic tube inserted in the tympanic membrane serves as a stent for the ostium and allows for continued drainage of the mid-

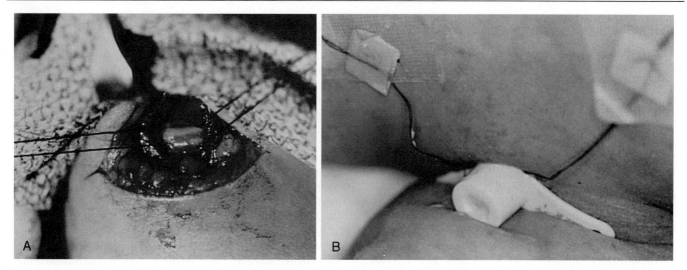

Figure 20–8. (A) Intraoperative placement of sutures will identify and expose the tracheal lumen. The head is located at the bottom of the picture and the feet toward the top. Note that stay sutures are placed through the lateral walls of the trachea prior to incision of the tracheal rings. After surgical incision of the tracheal rings, lateral traction will pull the strap muscles laterally, open the tracheal incision and expose the site for tracheostomy tube insertion. (B) Postoperative view of the stay sutures, which are identified and stabilized by tape as they emerge from the wound at the conclusion of surgery.

dle ear until the tubes are naturally extruded in 6 months to a year or surgically removed at an appropriate time (Fig. 20–9).

Myringotomy with tube insertion is a very short procedure, and anesthesia may be effectively accomplished with a potent inhalation agent, oxygen, and nitrous oxide administered by mask. Most patients can be managed safely without intravenous access. If unanticipated difficulty arises, intravenous access is usually quickly established and medications or fluids administered. Premedication is not generally recommended because most sedative drugs used for premedication outlast the duration of the surgical procedure. Discomfort after myringotomy and tube insertion is minimal and acetaminophen is usually sufficient. Since the procedure is so brief and intravenous access usually has not been obtained, administration of acetaminophen, either via the oral preoperatively or the rectal route immediately after induction, provides good postoperative analgesia. The recommended dose of oral acetaminophen is 10 to 20 mg/kg but the initial rectal dose is generally higher (40 mg/kg).[47] Patients with chronic otitis frequently have an accompanying recurrent URI. Eradication of middle ear fluid often resolves the concomitant URI. Because the anesthetic is administered by mask and endotracheal intubation is not required, the criteria for cancellation of surgery and anesthesia may be altered. No significant differences in perioperative complications between asymptomatic children and children fulfilling criteria for a mild URI have been found. Morbidity is not increased in children presenting for minor surgery with acute uncomplicated URI (Table 20–8) if they did not require endotracheal intubation.[69, 70] It is recommended that children with URI symptoms have oxygen saturation measured before induction

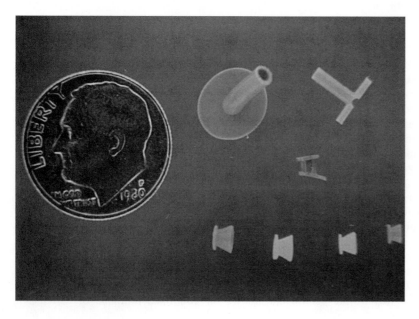

Figure 20–9. Lateral and cross-sectional views of beveled and T myringotomy tubes compared with a dime; the conduit at the center of the myringotomy tube allows drainage of middle ear fluid. (Courtesy of Dr. Michael Cunningham, Boston, MA.)

Table 20–8. Criteria for Mild Upper Respiratory Tract Infection*

Sore throat	Nonproductive cough
Sneezing	Temperature < 38.3°C (101°F)
Rhinorrhea	Laryngitis
Congestion	Malaise

*At least two symptoms must be present.
Abstracted from Tait AR, Knight PR: The effects of general anesthesia on upper respiratory tract infections in children. Anesthesiology 1987;67:930–935.

of general anesthesia, and supplemental oxygen should be administered postoperatively to those patients who have oxygen saturation less than 93%.[71]

Middle Ear and Mastoid Surgery

Tympanoplasty and mastoidectomy are two of the most common major ear operations performed on children. Surgical identification and preservation of the facial nerve are necessary because of its proximity to the surgical field. The nerve must be isolated and its function verified by means of electrical stimulation. Therefore, paralysis with muscle relaxants is usually avoided and a volatile agent is used as the primary anesthetic. If a narcotic-relaxant technique is chosen, at least 30% of muscle response, as determined by a twitch monitor, should be preserved.

To gain access to the surgical site, the head is positioned on a headrest, which may be lower than the operating table. In addition, extreme degrees of lateral rotation may be required. The anesthesiologist and surgeon must be extremely vigilant in ensuring that nerves, muscles, and bony structures are not injured. Extreme tension should not be placed on the heads of the sternocleidomastoid muscle, and this limiting factor determines a safe degree of lateral head rotation. The laxity of the ligaments of the cervical spine as well as immaturity of the odontoid process in children makes them especially prone to C1-C2 subluxation. *Fifteen to 31% of patients with Down syndrome or achondroplasia may have atlantoaxial instability.*[72–75] Care in anterior-posterior positioning can avoid injury in this area.

Bleeding must be kept to a minimum during surgery of the small structures of the middle ear. Relative hypotension, keeping the mean arterial pressure 25% below baseline, is effective (see Chapter 12). Injection of concentrated epinephrine solution, often 1:8000, is performed in the area of the tympanic vessels to produce vasoconstriction. Close attention should be paid to the dose of injected epinephrine to avoid arrhythmias and wide variations in blood pressure. The maximum dosage is 10 μg/kg per 30 min.

The middle ear and sinuses are air-filled, nondistensible cavities. An increase in the volume of gas contained within these structures results in an increase in pressure. When inhaled nitrous oxide is used, inspired, alveolar, and blood concentrations equilibrate. Nitrous oxide diffuses along a concentration gradient into air-filled middle ear spaces more rapidly than nitrogen moves out, because nitrous oxide is 30 times more soluble than nitrogen in the blood. The middle ear is vented through the opening of the eustachian tube. Normal passive venting of the eustachian tube occurs at 20 to 30 cm H_2O pressure. It has been shown that use of nitrous oxide results in pressures that exceed the ability of the

eustachian tube to vent the middle ear within 5 minutes, leading to pressure buildup.[76] If eustachian tube function is interfered with during the surgical procedure, then pressure in the middle ear can increase further. Venting of the middle ear occurs intermittently, leading to constant changes in middle ear pressure, which in turn cause movement of the tympanic membrane.[77] During procedures in which the tympanic membrane is replaced or a perforation is patched, nitrous oxide should be discontinued or, if this is not possible, limited to a maximum of 50% before the application of the tympanic membrane graft to reduce the potential for pressure-related displacement.[78]

After nitrous oxide is discontinued, it is quickly reabsorbed, creating a void in the middle ear, with resulting negative pressure. This negative pressure may result in serous otitis, disarticulation of the ossicles in the middle ear (especially the stapes), and hearing impairment, which may last up to 6 weeks postoperatively. The use of nitrous oxide may cause a high incidence of postoperative nausea and vomiting, which are a direct result of negative middle ear pressure during recovery. The negative pressure created by the reabsorption of nitrous oxide stimulates the vestibular system by producing traction on the round window. Although all patients have the potential for nausea and vomiting postoperatively, children less than 8 years of age seem to be most affected.[79] If the use of nitrous oxide cannot be avoided, administration of antiemetics is warranted. Local infiltration of the great auricular nerve can provide pain relief equivalent to that of opioids and reduce the incidence of vomiting.[80]

REFERENCES

1. Brodsky L: Modern assessment of tonsils and adenoids. Pediatr Clin North Am 1989;36:1551–1569.
2. Berkowitz RG: Tonsillectomy in children under 3 years of age. Arch Otolaryngol Head Neck Surg 1990;116:685–686.
3. Potsic WP: Tonsillectomy and adenoidectomy. Int Anesthesiol Clin 1988;26:58–60.
4. Brouillette RT, Fernbach SK, Hunt CE: Obstructive sleep apnea in infants and children. J Pediatr 1982;100:31–40.
5. Chaban R, Cole P, Hoffstein V: Site of upper airway obstruction in patients with idiopathic obstructive sleep apnea. Laryngoscope 1988;98:641–647.
6. Guilleminault C: Obstructive sleep apnea: The clinical syndrome and historical perspective. Med Clin North Am 1985;69:1187–1203.
7. Leiberman A, Tal A, Brama I, et al: Obstructive sleep apnea in young infants. Int J Pediatr Otorhinolaryngol 1988;16:39–44.
8. Noonan JA: Reversible cor pulmonale due to hypertrophied tonsils and adenoids: Studies in two cases (P). Circulation 1965;31[Supplement II]:164.
9. Cayler GG, Johnson EE, Lewis BE, et al: Heart failure due to enlarged tonsils and adenoids: The cardiorespiratory syndrome of increased airway resistance. Am J Dis Child 1969;118:708–717.
10. Bland JWJ, Edwards FK: Pulmonary hypertension and congestive heart failure in children with chronic upper airway obstruction: New concepts of etiologic factors. Am J Cardiol 1969;23:830–837.
11. Smith RM, Gonzalez C: The relationship between nasal obstruction and craniofacial growth. Pediatr Clin North Am 1989;36:1423–1434.
12. Alexander CA: A modified Intavent laryngeal mask for ENT and dental anaesthesia. Anaesthesia 1990;45:892–893.
13. Haynes SR, Morton NS: The laryngeal mask airway: A review of its use in paediatric anaesthesia. Paediatr Anaesth 1993;3:65–73.
14. Nair I, Bailey PM: Review of uses of the laryngeal mask in ENT anaesthesia. Anaesthesia 1995;50:898–900.
15. Williams PJ, Bailey PM: Comparison of the reinforced laryngeal mask airway and tracheal intubation for adenotonsillectomy. Br J Anaesth 1993;70:30–33.

16. Allsop E, Innes P, Jackson M, et al: Dose of propofol required to insert the laryngeal mask airway in children. Paediatr Anaesth 1995;5:47–51.

17. Pennant JH, White PF: The laryngeal mask airway: Its uses in anesthesiology. Anesthesiology 1993;79:144–163.

18. Devitt JH, Wenstone R, Noel AG, et al: The laryngeal mask airway and positive-pressure ventilation. Anesthesiology 1994;80:550–555.

19. Mason DG, Bingham RM: The laryngeal mask airway in children. Anaesthesia 1990;45:760–763.

20. O'Neill B, Templeton JJ, Caramico L, et al: The laryngeal mask airway in pediatric patients: Factors affecting ease of use during insertion and emergence. Anesth Analg 1994;78:659–662.

21. Goudsouzian NG, Cleveland R: Stability of the laryngeal mask airway during marked extension of the head. Paediatr Anaesth 1993;3:117–119.

22. Webster AC, Morley-Forster PK, Dain S, et al: Anaesthesia for adenotonsillectomy: A comparison between tracheal intubation and the armoured laryngeal mask airway. Can J Anaesth 1993;40:1171–1177.

23. Ferrari LR, Donlon JV: Metoclopramide reduces the incidence of vomiting after tonsillectomy in children. Anesth Analg 1992;75:351–354.

24. Carithers JS, Gebhart DE, Williams JA: Postoperative risks of pediatric tonsilloadenoidectomy. Laryngoscope 1987;97:422–429.

25. Colclasure JB, Graham SS: Complications of outpatient tonsillectomy and adenoidectomy: A review of 3,340 cases. Ear Nose Throat J 1990;69:155–160.

26. Chiang TM, Sukis AE, Ross DE: Tonsillectomy performed on an outpatient basis: Report of a series of 40,000 cases performed without a death. Arch Otolaryngol 1968;88:307–310.

27. Crysdale WS, Russel D: Complications of tonsillectomy and adenoidectomy in 9409 children observed overnight. CMAJ 1986;135:1139–1142.

28. Hamid SK, Selby IR, Sikich N, et al: Vomiting after adenotonsillectomy in children: A comparison of ondansetron, dimenhydrinate, and placebo. Anesth Analg 1998;86:496–500.

29. Feinberg AN, Shabino CL: Acute pulmonary edema complicating tonsillectomy and adenoidectomy. Pediatrics 1985;75:112–114.

30. Galvis AG, Stool SE, Bluestone CD: Pulmonary edema following relief of acute upper airway obstruction. Ann Otol Rhinol Laryngol 1980;89:124–128.

31. McColley SA, April MM, Carroll JL, et al: Respiratory compromise after adenotonsillectomy in children with obstructive sleep apnea. Arch Otolaryngol Head Neck Surg 1992;118:940–943.

32. Broadman LM, Ceruzzi W, Patane PS, et al: Metoclopramide reduces the incidence of vomiting following strabismus surgery in children. Anesthesiology 1990;72:245–248.

33. Lin DM, Furst SR, Rodarte A: A double-blinded comparison of metoclopramide and droperidol for prevention of emesis following strabismus surgery. Anesthesiology 1992;76:357–361.

34. Ummenhofer W, Frei FJ, Urwyler A, et al: Effects of ondansetron in the prevention of postoperative nausea and vomiting in children. Anesthesiology 1994;81:804–810.

35. Splinter WM, Baxter MR, Gould HM, et al: Oral ondansetron decreases vomiting after tonsillectomy in children. Can J Anaesth 1995;42:277–280.

36. Furst SR, Rodarte A: Prophylactic antiemetic treatment with ondansetron in children undergoing tonsillectomy. Anesthesiology 1994;81:799–803.

37. Lawhorn CD, Bower C, Brown RE Jr, et al: Ondansetron decreases postoperative vomiting in pediatric patients undergoing tonsillectomy and adenoidectomy. Int J Pediatr Otorhinolaryngol 1996;36:99–108.

38. Watcha MF, Bras PJ, Cieslak GD, et al: The dose-response relationship of ondansetron in preventing postoperative emesis in pediatric patients undergoing ambulatory surgery. Anesthesiology 1995;82:47–52.

39. Khalil S, Rodarte A, Weldon BC, et al: Intravenous ondansetron in established postoperative emesis in children. S3A–381 Study Group. Anesthesiology 1996;85:270–276.

40. Splinter W, Roberts DJ: Prophylaxis for vomiting by children after tonsillectomy: Dexamethasone versus perphenazine. Anesth Analg 1997;85:534–537.

41. Linden BE, Gross CW, Long TE, et al: Morbidity in pediatric tonsillectomy. Laryngoscope 1990;100:120–124.

42. Fairbanks DN: Uvulopalatopharyngoplasty complications and avoidance strategies. Otolaryngol Head Neck Surg 1990;102:239–245.

43. Broadman LM, Patel RI, Feldman BA, et al: The effects of peritonsillar infiltration on the reduction of intraoperative blood loss and post-tonsillectomy pain in children. Laryngoscope 1989;99:t-81.

44. Goldsher M, Podoshin L, Fradis M, et al: Effects of peritonsillar infiltration on post-tonsillectomy pain: A double-blind study. Ann Otol Rhinol Laryngol 1996;105:868–870.

45. Jebeles JA, Reilly JS, Gutierrez JF, et al: Tonsillectomy and adenoidectomy pain reduction by local bupivacaine infiltration in children. Int J Pediatr Otorhinolaryngol 1993;25:149–154.

46. Johansen M, Harbo G, Illum P: Preincisional infiltration with bupivacaine in tonsillectomy. Arch Otolaryngol Head Neck Surg 1996;122:261–263.

47. Birmingham PK, Tobin MJ, Henthorn TK, et al: Twenty-four-hour pharmacokinetics of rectal acetaminophen in children: An old drug with new recommendations. Anesthesiology 1997;87:244–252.

48. Judkins JH, Dray TG, Hubbell RN: Intraoperative ketorolac and post-tonsillectomy bleeding. Arch Otolaryngol Head Neck Surg 1996;122:937–940.

49. Gallagher JE, Blauth J, Fornadley JA: Perioperative ketorolac tromethamine and postoperative hemorrhage in cases of tonsillectomy and adenoidectomy. Laryngoscope 1995;105:606–609.

50. Sutters KA, Levine JD, Dibble S, et al: Analgesic efficacy and safety of single-dose intramuscular ketorolac for postoperative pain management in children following tonsillectomy. Pain 1995;61:145–153.

51. Splinter WM, Rhine EJ, Roberts DW, et al: Preoperative ketorolac increases bleeding after tonsillectomy in children. Can J Anaesth 1996;43:560–563.

52. Hall SC: Tonsillectomies, ketorolac, and the march of progress. Can J Anaesth 1996;43:544–548.

53. Guida RA, Mattucci KF: Tonsillectomy and adenoidectomy: An inpatient or outpatient procedure? Laryngoscope 1990;100:491–493.

54. Brown OE, Cunningham MJ: Am Acad Otolaryngol-Head Neck Surg Bulletin 1996;15:13–15.

55. Zalzal GH: Stridor and airway compromise. Pediatr Clin North Am 1989;36:1389–1402.

56. Woods AML: Pediatric bronchoscopy, bronchography, and laryngoscopy. In: Berry FA Jr, ed: Anesthetic Management of Difficult and Routine Pediatric Patients. New York: Churchill Livingstone; 1986:189–250.

57. Zwass MS, Fisher DM, Welborn LG, et al: Induction and maintenance characteristics of anesthesia with desflurane and nitrous oxide in infants and children. Anesthesiology 1992;76:373–378.

58. Sanders RB: Two ventilating attachments for bronchoscopes. Del Med 1967;July:170–192.

59. Steward DJ: Percutaneous transtracheal ventilation for laser endoscopic procedures in infants and small children. Can J Anaesth 1987;34:429–430.

60. Myer CM 3rd, O'Connor DM, Cotton RT: Proposed grading system for subglottic stenosis based on endotracheal tube sizes. Ann Otol Rhinol Laryngol 1994;103:319–323.

61. Hermens JM, Bennett MJ, Hirshman CA: Anesthesia for laser surgery. Anesth Analg 1983;62:218–229.

62. Sosis MB: Anesthesia for laser surgery. Anesth Clin N Am 1993;11:537–552.

63. Sosis MB, Dillon FX: Saline-filled cuffs help prevent laser-induced polyvinylchloride endotracheal tube fires. Anesth Analg 1991;72:187–189.

64. Weeks DB: Laboratory and clinical description of the use of jet-venturi ventilator during laser microsurgery of the glottis and subglottis. Anesth Rev 1985;12:32–36.

65. Quintal MC, Cunningham MJ, Ferrari LR: Tubeless spontaneous respiration technique for pediatric microlaryngeal surgery. Arch Otolaryngol Head Neck Surg 1997;123:209–214.

66. Hawkins DB, Udall JN: Juvenile laryngeal papillomas with cardiomegaly and polycythemia. Pediatrics 1979;63:156–157.

67. Rimell FL, Shapiro AM, Mitskavich MT, et al: Pediatric fiberoptic laser rigid bronchoscopy. Otolaryngol Head Neck Surg 1996;114:413–417.

68. Wetmore SJ, Key JM, Suen JY: Complications of laser surgery for laryngeal papillomatosis. Laryngoscope 1985;95:798–801.

69. Tait AR, Knight PR: The effects of general anesthesia on upper respiratory tract infections in children. Anesthesiology 1987;67:930–935.

70. Tait AR, Pandit UA, Voepel-Lewis T, et al: Use of the laryngeal mask airway in children with upper respiratory tract infections: A comparison with endotracheal intubation. Anesth Analg 1998;86:706–711.

71. DeSoto H, Patel RI, Soliman IE, et al: Changes in oxygen saturation following general anesthesia in children with upper respiratory infection signs and symptoms undergoing otolaryngological procedures. Anesthesiology 1988;68:276–279.

72. Williams JP, Somerville GM, Miner ME, et al: Atlanto-axial subluxation and trisomy-21: Another perioperative complication. Anesthesiology 1987;67:253–254.

73. Pueschel SM, Scola FH, Perry CD, et al: Atlanto-axial instability in children with Down syndrome. Pediatr Radiol 1981;10:129–132.

74. Moore RA, McNicholas KW, Warran SP: Atlantoaxial subluxation with symptomatic spinal cord compression in a child with Down's syndrome. Anesth Analg 1987;66:89–90.

75. Kalla GN, Fening E, Obiaya MO: Anaesthetic management of achondroplasia. Br J Anaesth 1986;58:117–119.

76. Casey WF, Drake-Lee AB: Nitrous oxide and middle ear pressure: A study of induction methods in children. Anaesthesia 1982;37:896–900.

77. Patterson ME, Bartlett PC: Hearing impairment caused by intratympanic pressure changes during general anesthesia. Laryngoscope 1976;86:399–404.

78. Munson ES: Transfer of nitrous oxide into body air cavities. Br J Anaesth 1974;46:202–209.

79. Montgomery CJ, Vaghadia H, Blackstock D: Negative middle ear pressure and postoperative vomiting in pediatric outpatients. Anesthesiology 1988;68:288–291.

80. Suresh S, Barcelona SL, Young N, et al: Postoperative pain management in children undergoing tympanomastoid surgery: Is a local block better than intravenous opioid? Anesthesiology 1999;91:A1281.

21

Anesthesia for Ophthalmology

Susan A. Vassallo *and* Lynne R. Ferrari

Pathophysiology
  Intraocular Pressure
  Oculocardiac Reflex
  Effects of Anesthesia on Intraocular Pressure
Anesthetic Management
  Preoperative Evaluation
  Premedication
  Monitors
  Induction and Intubation
  Anesthetic Maintenance
Systemic Effects of Ophthalmologic Drugs
  Topical Anesthetics
  Mydriatics
  Cycloplegics
Drugs Used in Glaucoma Therapy
  Direct-Acting Cholinergic (Parasympathomimetic) Drugs
  Indirect-Acting Irreversible Anticholinergic Drugs
  Adrenergic (Sympathomimetic) Drugs
  Beta-Adrenergic-Blocking Drugs
  Carbonic Anhydrase Inhibitors
  Hypertonic Solutions
  Corticosteroids
  Intraocular Gases (Air, Sulfur Hexafluoride, Carbon Octofluorine)
Specific Pediatric Ophthalmologic Problems and Operations
  Congenital Cataracts
  Glaucoma
  Strabismus
  Retinopathy of Prematurity
"Open Eye Injury and Full Stomach" Controversy

Ophthalmic surgery encompasses a broad spectrum of procedures ranging from a simple lacrimal duct exploration to the more complicated vitreoretinal repair. This chapter reviews the essential points of ocular anatomy and physiology and outlines the effects of anesthetic drugs and manipulations on intraocular dynamics.

Pathophysiology

Intraocular Pressure

Intraocular pressure (IOP) is measured by either applanation or Schiotz tonometry, techniques that calculate the amount of force needed to indent or flatten the cornea. The normal range for IOP is 10 to 24 mm Hg; three factors are responsible for this value:

1. Internal pressure generated by the fluid and semisolid contents of the eye (aqueous humor, blood, lens)
2. External pressure on the eye generated by surrounding ocular muscles and orbital venous pressure
3. The pressure generated by the sclera itself

The volume of aqueous humor is the most important determinant of IOP (Fig. 21–1). The aqueous humor is synthesized by the ciliary body in the posterior chamber of the eye. After flowing through the pupil into the anterior chamber, where it first enters the spaces of Fontana and then the canal of Schlemm, it eventually drains into the venous outflow of the head. Thus, an equilibrium exists between aqueous humor production and absorption.

Aqueous humor formation is described in terms of fluid mechanics by the following equation:

$$IOP = K \left[(OP_{aq} - OP_{pl}) + P_c \right]$$

where K = coefficient of outflow, OP_{aq} = osmotic pressure of aqueous humor, OP_{pl} = osmotic pressure of plasma, and P_c = capillary pressure.

A clinical application of this formula is the administration of mannitol to lower IOP; this hypertonic solution acutely increases the OP_{pl} and increases the gradient between OP_{aq} and OP_{pl}, thereby causing water to exit the aqueous humor and thus lowering the IOP.

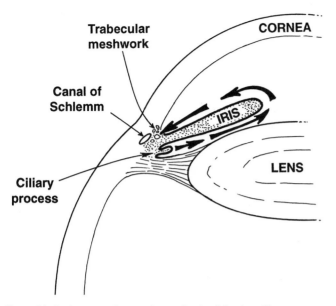

Figure 21–1. Aqueous humor is synthesized in the ciliary process; it then circulates around the iris, past the lens, and into the anterior chamber (arrows). After flowing through the trabecular meshwork, aqueous humor enters the canal of Schlemm, which drains into the episcleral venous system. Pathologic conditions that increase venous pressure, obstruct the canal of Schlemm, or increase aqueous humor production may cause an increase in intraocular pressure.

The absorption of aqueous humor is mathematically described by a modification of the Poiseuille law:

$$A = [(P_{iop} - P_v) \times r^4]/(8n \times l)$$

where A = volume of aqueous outflow per time units (microliters per minute), P_{iop} = IOP, P_v = venous pressure, r = radius of the Fontana spaces, n = viscosity of the aqueous humor, and l = length of the Fontana spaces. Systemic venous pressure increases with coughing, vomiting, a Valsalva maneuver, or straining and therefore decreases aqueous humor absorption. A second implication of the previous equation is the effect of miotics, which enlarge the spaces of Fontana (r) and hence are often prescribed to increase aqueous humor outflow (A) and reduce IOP.

The relationship between arterial pressure and IOP is less well defined. In studies of animals, a primitive type of autoregulation has been found to maintain a stable IOP throughout a wide range of systemic pressures.[1] A study conducted in humans in the setting of induced hypotension demonstrated that IOP increased as the arterial pressure increased only if the initial measurement was low (i.e., IOP less than 11 mm Hg).[2] It appears that arterial pressure is a less significant determinant of IOP than central venous pressure.

Oculocardiac Reflex

The oculocardiac reflex is a trigeminovagal reflex and most commonly presents as sinus bradycardia (Fig. 21–2). However, other dysrhythmias, including junctional bradycardia, ventricular bigeminy, and sinus arrest, may occur. The reflex is initiated by mechanical stimulation, such as traction on the extraocular muscles, direct pressure on the globe, or ocular trauma. Retrobulbar injection of local anesthetic can occasionally trigger this reflex. Both the long and short ciliary nerves carry afferent impulses to the ciliary ganglion; these fibers then join the ophthalmic division of the trigeminal nerve (cranial nerve V), pass through the gasserian ganglion, and synapse in the main sensory nucleus of cranial nerve V, which is located in the floor of the fourth ventricle. The efferent limb of this pathway begins in the dorsal nucleus of the vagus nerve (cranial nerve X), just below the fourth ventricle. Activation of this nucleus causes increased vagal output to the sinoatrial node, resulting in bradycardia or other dysrhythmias. The diving reflex seen in mammals is a similar trigeminovagal reflex, only it is elicited by facial immersion in cold water. Here, bradycardia is an adaptive technique that minimizes oxygen demand during diving.[3]

The incidence of the oculocardiac reflex depends on specific characteristics of the study population, such as age or type of operation.[4, 5] The reflex occurs more frequently in younger patients, usually during strabismus or orbital surgery. Early clinical observations reported that traction on the medial rectus muscle was the most potent stimulus for this reflex. Later studies did not confirm this finding; tugging on any of the extraocular muscles can evoke the oculocardiac reflex. Although various techniques to prevent or blunt this reflex have been proposed, their efficacy is controversial. In general, though, it is agreed that preoperative intramuscular administration of an anticholinergic drug does not reliably abolish this reflex.[6]

There are many approaches to management of the oculocardiac reflex. If a dysrhythmia occurs, one can ask the surgeon to release traction on the muscle and wait for restoration to a normal sinus rhythm. An anticholinergic drug (atropine, 0.01–0.02 mg/kg or glycopyrrolate, 0.01 mg/kg) can be given if the bradycardia is persistent or worrisome. Some practitioners prefer to give atropine or glycopyrrolate intravenously before any manipulation of the eye. Finally, retrobulbar anesthesia may ablate the oculocardiac reflex, but this intervention also may elicit a dysrhythmia.

In our practice, we routinely administer atropine to children undergoing strabismus surgery. The drug is administered intravenously in an initial dose of 0.01 to 0.02 mg/kg before manipulation of the eye. In a limited study, glycopyrrolate (0.01 mg/kg) administered intravenously before surgery proved as effective as atropine in preventing the bradycardia associated with strabismus correction.[7] If an anticholinergic is not administered, the choice of muscle relaxant may also be important; pancuronium has been shown to reduce the incidence and severity of bradycardia.[8] If the oculocardiac reflex occurs during other types of eye procedures, the first response is to ask the surgeon to remove the stimulus; the reflex fatigues quickly, and the pulse usually increases within seconds. If it does not, then intravenous atropine is immediately administered.

Effects of Anesthesia on Intraocular Pressure

Almost every drug in an anesthesiologist's pharmacopeia affects IOP. The mechanism of action varies, but the outcome can usually be predicted by applying the formulas discussed in the previous section.

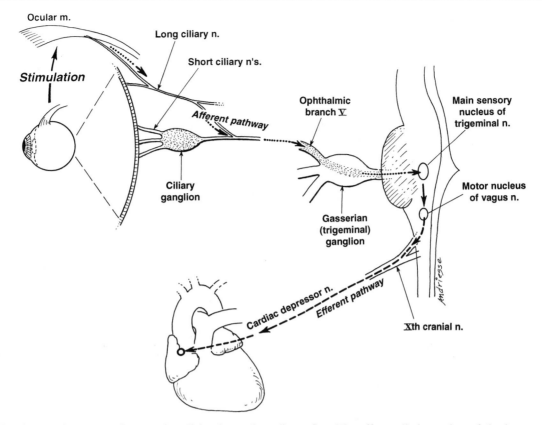

Figure 21–2. Traction on the extraocular muscles elicits the oculocardiac reflex. The afferent limb consists of the long and short ciliary nerves, which synapse in the ciliary ganglion (dotted lines with arrows). The ophthalmic division of the trigeminal nerve (cranial nerve V) carries the impulse to the gasserian ganglion; the arc continues to the sensory nucleus of cranial nerve V in the brainstem. Fibers in the reticular formation synapse with the nucleus of the vagus nerve (cranial nerve X) (dashed lines with arrows). Efferent fibers from the vagus nerve terminate in the heart (dashed lines with arrows).

Volatile Anesthetics

In spontaneously breathing patients, halothane, enflurane, and isoflurane all decrease IOP by 20 to 30% from awake baseline values.[9] This phenomenon is dose related and occurs throughout a concentration range of 1 to 5%. The decrease in IOP results from a combination of an increase in aqueous humor outflow and a decrease in extraocular muscle tone. Studies of animals have proposed a central IOP control center located in the diencephalon[10]; this region may determine resting IOP. The generalized inhibition of synaptic activity caused by inhalation anesthetics may depress this center's output, resulting in decreased IOP. It appears that desflurane and sevoflurane have similar effects on IOP as the other potent inhalation agents.[11–14]

Measurement of IOP in awake infants and children is difficult; hence, the next logical concern is the optimal time during anesthesia to record IOP. In a study evaluating the effects of an oxygen-nitrous oxide-halothane (O_2:N_2O:halothane) mask anesthetic on IOP in patients between the ages of 6 months and 12 years, IOP remained constant for 10 minutes after the eyes returned to a neutral midline position.[15] IOP did not decrease in a dose-related manner when the end-tidal halothane concentration was increased from 0.5 to 1.0%. However, tracheal intubation after atracurium administration (0.5 mg/kg) was associated with a 5 to 6 mm Hg rise in IOP. This investigation supports the premise that IOP measurements can be reliably compared during a stan-

dard O_2:N_2O:halothane anesthetic before intubation. This is likely true for sevoflurane as well.[13]

Benzodiazepines, Barbiturates, Etomidate, Propofol, Opioids

When administered intravenously as premedicants, both diazepam and midazolam decrease IOP[16, 17]; this effect is not observed with oral diazepam (0.2 mg/kg).[18] The barbiturates sodium thiopental and methohexital are thought to reduce IOP by their effects on a control center in the hypothalamus. Specific evaluation of sodium thiopental (3 mg/kg) confirmed this observation in adult men scheduled for elective nonophthalmic surgery.[19] Despite pronounced myoclonus, etomidate lowers IOP when used as an induction agent and during continuous infusion.[20] Propofol in an induction dose of 2.1 mg/kg lowers IOP by approximately 40% (12 to 7 mm Hg), which is similar to the decrease produced by an equivalent dose of sodium thiopental (4.9 mg/kg).[21] Intramuscular and intravenous morphine lower IOP, as does intravenous fentanyl and its analogues, alfentanil and sufentanil.[22, 23] In adults, clonidine (5 μg/kg), a central alpha-adrenergic antagonist, lowers IOP by as much as 35% and systemic blood pressure by 10%.[24]

Ketamine

Ketamine maintains a unique position in the class of general anesthetics with respect to IOP. An early study using Schiotz indentation tonometry concluded that intramuscular ketamine (5 mg/kg) increased IOP by a maximum of 37% compared with preinjection values.[25] This protocol studied children between the ages of 4 and 7 years and thus required a preoperative training session to prepare them for awake examination. Within 30 minutes of injection, IOP returned to baseline values. However, this investigation did not have a control group (e.g., using saline) to assess the changes in IOP that might accompany the "stress" associated with an intramuscular injection. Another study demonstrated that intramuscular ketamine reduces IOP in children.[26] Blepharospasm and nystagmus secondary to the tonic contraction of extraocular muscles are distracting to many ophthalmologists. Nevertheless, some pediatric ophthalmologists conduct eye examinations using ketamine sedation/anesthesia.

Neuromuscular Relaxants

Of the nondepolarizing drugs, *d*-tubocurarine has been studied most extensively with respect to IOP. A decrease in IOP has been found when *d*-tubocurarine is administered in a dose adequate for intubation.[27] This effect on IOP may relate to autonomic ganglionic blockade and systemic hypotension associated with *d*-tubocurarine administration. Despite its vagolytic properties, pancuronium also lowers IOP.[28] The intermediate-acting neuromuscular relaxants atracurium and vecuronium are associated with no change or a decrease in IOP.[29–32] Rocuronium is similar to atracurium or vecuronium.

Succinylcholine increases IOP when administered in the dose range of 1 to 2 mg/kg.[33, 34] In anesthetized humans, the average rise in IOP is 8 to 10 mm Hg and occurs within 4 minutes of an intravenous bolus. IOP then returns to a control or baseline value 6 minutes after administration. This observation was initially attributed to the fast tonic contractions of the twitch-type fibers found in extraocular muscles.[35] However, an increase in IOP following succinylcholine has been demonstrated in a completely isolated animal's eye.[36, 37] It was postulated that orbital smooth-muscle contraction is responsible for the elevation in IOP. The effect of intramuscular succinylcholine on IOP has not been examined; IOP presumably is increased in a similar fashion. The intensity of muscle fasciculation does not predict the degree to which IOP increases.

Various induction techniques have been proposed in an attempt to avoid the rise in IOP associated with succinylcholine. Early strategies in adults advocated the administration of a small dose of a nondepolarizing relaxant (either 3 mg of curare or 20 mg of gallamine) at least several minutes before succinylcholine administration.[38] Decades later, however, other investigators negated this claim in both children and adults; IOP increased an average of 12 mm Hg after succinylcholine administration despite pretreatment with curare (0.09 mg/kg) or gallamine (0.3 mg/kg).[39] When comparing these results, it is important to note that indentation tonometry was the standard method of IOP measurement until the mid-1970s. Thereafter, applanation tonometry assumed such a role; the latter technique is a more sensitive indicator of IOP.

The effects of lidocaine, succinylcholine, and tracheal intubation on IOP have been examined in a select pediatric population.[40] Children who were between the ages of 18 months and 7 years and were scheduled for strabismus surgery received an oral premedication mix of atropine (0.02 mg/kg), promethazine (0.8 mg/kg), and chloral hydrate (25 mg/kg) 1 hour before the procedure. Baseline IOP was measured 7 minutes after an $O_2:N_2O$:halothane mask induction. Patients were randomly assigned to one of three study protocols: group 1 received lidocaine (2 mg/kg IV) followed by placebo and tracheal intubation; group 2, placebo followed by succinylcholine (1 mg/kg IV) and tracheal intubation; group 3, lidocaine (2 mg/kg IV) and succinylcholine (1 mg/kg IV) followed by tracheal intubation. The authors concluded that lidocaine (2 mg/kg IV) causes an insignificant increase in IOP, after which tracheal intubation also increases IOP slightly. Together, lidocaine, laryngoscopy, and tracheal intubation are associated with a small but significant increase in IOP from baseline (mean increase of 2 mm Hg). Succinylcholine alone (1 mg/kg) results in a statistically significant rise in IOP; the actual value remains elevated at least 30 minutes after succinylcholine administration. Tracheal intubation 75 seconds after the bolus dose does not exacerbate the increase in IOP. Most importantly, the combination of lidocaine (2 mg/kg IV) and succinylcholine (1 mg/kg IV) is not associated with a lower IOP. That is, the increase in IOP that follows both succinylcholine administration and tracheal intubation cannot be abolished by prior lidocaine use. However, at 30 minutes after injection, the mean IOP in the lidocaine-succinylcholine group was closer to baseline values.

Since endotracheal intubation is the major source of a rise in IOP, anesthetic techniques that minimize cardiovascular responses to laryngoscopy and intubation will help reduce the potential for increases in IOP.[23, 41] Use of a laryngeal mask airway (LMA) has been shown to have less of an effect on IOP than insertion of an endotracheal tube,[42] but the patient population at risk, that is, patients with open globe injury, would still require an endotracheal tube, since most of these patients will have a full stomach (see later).

Metabolic and Physiologic Effects on Intraocular Pressure

Hypoxia and hypercapnia are associated with an increase in IOP; these changes are presumably caused by retinal vasodilation, which occurs in conjunction with cerebral vasodilation.[43] Hypothermia decreases aqueous humor production and thus ultimately lowers IOP. Increases in central venous pressure due to coughing, a head-down position, or venous congestion will increase IOP. Laryngoscopy and endotracheal intubation can also increase IOP if they cause a significant increase in systemic arterial pressure or are associated with coughing.

Anesthetic Management

Preoperative Evaluation

An ocular defect can occur as an isolated problem in an otherwise healthy child, or it may be one manifestation of a multisystemic disease process. The preoperative evaluation should include a thorough assessment of a patient's functional status. Infants with retinopathy of prematurity often have other conditions associated with prematurity, such as immature or abnormal lungs (respiratory dysfunction, bronchopulmonary dysplasia), apnea and bradycardia, patent ductus arteriosus, intraventricular hemorrhage, hydrocephalus, subglottic stenosis, very low birth weight, and failure to thrive (see Chapters 2, 4, and 14). Congenital cataracts frequently occur in infants with inborn errors of metabolism or intrauterine infection. For these reasons, taking a prenatal history is essential; the mother should be questioned specifically with respect to preterm labor, illnesses during pregnancy, medications, and the use of cigarettes, alcohol, and recreational drugs. An account of the delivery is also crucial; was fetal distress or maternal hemorrhage present? Parents can often recite their infant's birth weight, post-conceptual age, and Apgar scores. A premature infant may remain hospitalized for a serious problem such as respiratory distress syndrome or may simply require additional time for feeding and growing.

Was the infant discharged to the care of his or her parents with special equipment such as an apnea monitor or supplemental oxygen? Does the infant take medications other than vitamins? Has the infant steadily gained weight? Has the infant recently had an infection of the upper respiratory tract or ears? The functional status of an older child can often be readily assessed by asking the parents about hospitalizations since birth. A family history pertinent to general health and possible anesthetic complications is helpful.

Premedication

The goals of premedication are to

1. Decrease the child's anxiety while awaiting surgery
2. Facilitate the separation between child and parents
3. Decrease anesthetic requirements during induction
4. Decrease salivary secretions when indicated
5. Decrease gastric volume and increase gastric pH when indicated
6. Decrease postoperative nausea and vomiting

The concept of premedication has a special connotation for each person participating in the care of a child. Although the patient should remain the center of attention, the parents, anesthesiologist, surgeon, and operating room nurses are also affected by the method of premedication. For example, most ophthalmologists instill a mydriatic before the eye examination. Although these eye drops are not painful, their administration can be frightening and difficult for a squirming toddler. Many parents frequently ask, "Why don't you give the drops once my child is asleep?" In this situation, the parents' goal is to minimize stressful activities and the surgeon's goal is to optimize examination conditions. Our usual response to such a question is to explain briefly to the parents the operative protocol. Because adequate pupillary dilation occurs 15 to 20 minutes after application, a delay in eye drop placement prolongs the entire anesthetic time. With few exceptions, parents accept this approach as rational and in the child's best interest.

Infants less than 9 months of age rarely require a sedative before surgery. After this age, children may experience anxiety and distress when separated from their parents. For a brief procedure, such as lacrimal duct probing, the best "premedication" often is to allow parents to be present for the induction of anesthesia. A familiar face and voice are often successful in allaying fears. Similarly, once emergence

is complete, parents are encouraged to sit by the child during the recovery room stay. The key to this approach is a calm and reassuring nursing staff. Parents need to be carefully instructed as to what they might observe during their child's anesthetic induction and forewarned of their child's postanesthesia drowsiness and possible nausea (see Chapter 4). Equally important, older children should be told they will wake up with a patch over one eye. This point requires frequent reiteration during the recovery period.

If preoperative sedation is indicated, the most common premedication choice is oral midazolam.[44] Oral administration of midazolam (0.25–0.50 mg/kg) results in sedation within 10 to 15 minutes and usually lasts 30 to 45 minutes; higher doses (up to 1.0 mg/kg) are associated with more rapid onset but may prolong recovery.[45] Nasal administration of midazolam (0.2–0.3 mg/kg) is an alternative but it has a bitter taste and is not generally recommended.[46–48]

Rectal methohexital (25 mg/kg) induces sleep within 7 to 10 minutes; this method results in a peaceful separation from the parents.[49, 50] A mask induction (e.g., O_2:N_2O:sevoflurane or halothane) is then performed. We do not advocate rectal methohexital for procedures scheduled for less than 30 minutes (i.e., simple eye examination, suture removal), because its duration of action may surpass the surgical time. Methohexital may be administered intramuscularly (10 mg/kg) if a child is extremely uncooperative. Ketamine is not recommended because of its propensity to cause nystagmus and blepharospasm.[51]

After the age of 6 or 7 years, many children can participate in a mask induction without prior sedation. At the conclusion of the preoperative assessment, it is customary to give an anesthesia mask to children so that they can become familiar with it. A brief description of the equipment (e.g., hoses, breathing bag, pulse oximeter) also facilitates the induction. Thereafter, children can practice holding the mask in the waiting area in the presence of their parents.

By the age of 9 years, children can often be offered a choice between a mask or intravenous induction (see Chapters 3 and 9). Many older children prefer the simplicity and speed of an intravenous approach. The use of 50% nitrous oxide combined with subcutaneous lidocaine is another alternative for older children. Topical local anesthesia with lidocaine prilocaine cream (EMLA or eutectic mixture of local anesthesia) has facilitated intravenous placement in children and adolescents.[52, 53] For maximal efficacy, it must be applied 45 to 60 minutes prior to intravenous placement; two sites are chosen in case the first attempt is unsuccessful. If there is a delay between the preoperative evaluation and the induction of anesthesia, we place a heparin lock in the presence of the parents and then let the child return to the playroom-waiting area. However, if a child becomes more anxious while awaiting surgery, then intravenous sedation such as midazolam is administered. Children must be carefully observed by skilled nursing staff following intravenous sedation. The parents are allowed to remain at the stretcher side or securely holding their child once medication has been administered.

Monitors

The essential monitoring devices used during pediatric ophthalmic surgery include a precordial or esophageal stethoscope, pulse oximeter, electrocardiogram, blood pressure device, capnograph (end-tidal carbon dioxide), oxygen analyzer, and thermometer. If neuromuscular relaxation is used, then a blockade monitor with a train-of-four stimulus is applied. For infants, a heated or passive humidifier, warming blanket, hot air warming blanket, or radiant heater are also used. During eye surgery, most of the head and torso is covered with both plastic and cloth drapes. Once surgery has begun, we reset the warming blanket to a lower temperature. Because it is rare to infuse large quantities of intravenous solutions, a fluid warmer is not necessary.

Induction and Intubation

Placement of an intravenous line and either an LMA or endotracheal intubation accompanies almost all but the simplest pediatric eye procedures. In an infant or small child, even an examination under anesthesia can last 45 minutes because of the time a surgeon spends drawing and photographing retinal fields. It is awkward and sometimes nearly impossible to share an infant's limited head area with another pair of hands and an operating microscope. Once the intravenous catheter is placed, glycopyrrolate or atropine may be administered if indicated and anesthesia deepened. In the past, endotracheal intubation was seen as the safest method to secure the airway. However, as anesthesiologists gain familiarity with the LMA, this method of airway management will have an increased role in pediatric eye surgery. The LMA is suitable for examinations under anesthesia, as well as suture removal. Its placement is not associated with a significant increase in IOP.[42] The LMA has been used in infants and children with bronchopulmonary dysplasia undergoing follow-up examination for retinopathy of prematurity as a means for avoiding bronchospasm, which may follow endotracheal intubation.[54]

The decision to administer an anticholinergic drug depends on several factors. If the heart rate is slow after an O_2:N_2O:inhalation induction in a young infant scheduled for strabismus correction, it is reasonable to administer an anticholinergic drug before intubation or manipulation of the eye. Intubation can be accomplished under inhalation anesthesia alone or after neuromuscular relaxation. Atracurium (0.5 mg/kg), cisatracurium (0.1–0.2 mg/kg), rocuronium (0.5–0.6 mg/kg), or vecuronium (0.1 mg/kg) may be administered if the latter method is chosen. If an uncuffed endotracheal tube is used, a leak at 20 to 30 cm H_2O during positive-pressure ventilation confirms correct endotracheal tube size. Because excess gases from this leak exit close to the operative field, we usually place a moistened oral pack around the endotracheal tube to minimize the amount of anesthetic drug that reaches the surgeon. A cuffed endotracheal tube offers an advantage in that gas leaks are avoided. One can adjust the cuff volume if a child's tracheal diameter falls between endotracheal tube sizes. In our practice, we use uncuffed tubes for infants and young children and cuffed tubes for older children unless there is a history of post-intubation edema. The stomach is emptied with a suction catheter. Small gauze strips are placed in each nostril to prevent secretions from seeping under the drapes into an opened eye. Finally, the entire oronasal area is covered with a plastic drape directed away from the surgical site.

Anesthetic Maintenance

For brief procedures such as cataract extraction or strabismus repair, anesthesia can be maintained with O_2:N_2O:inhalation agent. These procedures cause some postoperative pain, similar to the uncomfortable sensation of a grain of sand in the eye. It is advisable to mention this point to older children before surgery. For longer procedures such as correction of a retinal detachment, neuromuscular relaxation supplemented by narcotic or inhalation anesthesia guarantees an immobile eye. This technique is especially appropriate in small infants with retinopathy of prematurity. These babies frequently are in the lowest percentile for weight ($<$ 5% of expected weight); the concentration of inhalation anesthetic necessary to prevent reflex eye movement may produce hypotension or bradycardia. Even after replacement of fluid deficits, some infants may still not tolerate even low concentrations of halothane. Because sevoflurane and desflurane cause less myocardial depression, these drugs may be especially useful if the child has cardiovascular disease or is frail. It should be noted that desflurane is only used for maintenance of anesthesia and not for induction because of the propensity toward laryngospasm.[55]

A smooth emergence is a goal common to all types of surgery, although pediatric ophthalmologists understandably feel quite protective of a delicate retinal repair. The stomach is again emptied with a suction catheter before return of pharyngeal reflexes. The bandage and eye shield are properly secured. If neuromuscular blockade still exists, as determined by both clinical assessment and the twitch monitor, then neostigmine (0.06 mg/kg) and either glycopyrrolate (0.01 mg/kg) or atropine (0.02 mg/kg) are administered through the intravenous port closest to the patient. Once spontaneous ventilation has returned, the trachea may be extubated in a lateral position before full awakening. This method minimizes coughing and straining on the endotracheal tube; it is not appropriate in children whose airway was difficult to maintain before intubation, nor is it appropriate in patients with gastroesophageal reflux or a patient with a full stomach. In contrast, extubation of premature or developmentally delayed infants does not occur until emergence is complete. Purposeful movements, grimacing, and spontaneous eye opening are signs that correlate well with full return of airway reflexes.

If an infant, either premature or full term, has a history of apnea or bradycardia, he or she is cared for in the recovery area and in the unit with both an oxygen saturation monitor and apnea monitor. Former premature infants who are less than 55 weeks of post-conceptual age are monitored postoperatively for a minimum of 24 hours, even if apnea or bradycardia was not present before the procedure. Former preterm infants who are anemic (hematocrit $<$ 30%), those with ongoing apnea at home, and those with an apnea spell in recovery are also admitted and monitored even if older than 55 weeks of post-conceptual age.[56]

Systemic Effects of Ophthalmologic Drugs

The pharmacopeia of ophthalmologists contains medications both familiar and foreign to anesthesiologists. It is imperative that the ocular and systemic effects of these medications be appreciated. Topically applied drugs reach the systemic vasculature slowly by absorption through the ocular conjunctiva. Drugs that reach the nasal mucosa via the nasolacrimal duct are rapidly absorbed systemically. Holding pressure on the inner canthi of the eyes may impede a solution's flow into the nasolacrimal duct and thus localize it to the conjunctival tissue. A note of caution is appropriate here: many of these drugs are prescribed intentionally to alter pupillary size. Therefore, clinicians should not rely on this physical sign as an indicator of depth of anesthesia.

Topical Anesthetics

Proparacaine Hydrochloride

Preparation: 0.5% solution
Dose: 1 to 2 drops before examination
Onset: 30 seconds
Duration: 15 to 20 minutes

Proparacaine hydrochloride is used in older children who present for suture removal or for follow-up eye examination after recent surgery. It provides anesthesia quickly and has a brief duration.

Cocaine Hydrochloride

Preparation: 4% solution
Dose: 1 to 2 sprays
Onset: 30 seconds
Duration: 30 minutes

Cocaine is no longer applied directly to the eye because it can injure the cornea. However, its vasoconstrictive property is useful during nasolacrimal duct procedures if the drug is used properly.[57] A gauze pack moistened with cocaine and placed in the nasal passages before instrumentation reduces capillary oozing.

Mydriatics

A mydriatic dilates the pupil and thus facilitates ophthalmoscopy.

Phenylephrine Hydrochloride

Preparation: 2.5% solution
Dosage: 1 to 2 drops in each eye before examination
Onset: 30 minutes
Duration: 2 to 3 hours

Phenylephrine hydrochloride dilates the pupil and vasoconstricts capillaries. Absorption is believed to occur via conjunctival tissues, and effects are usually limited to the eyes. However, if a large dose is administered or if the drug is applied directly to open blood vessels, systemic effects such as hypertension can occur.[58–61] Because a relative overdose is possible in a small infant, only the 2.5% concentration is used in pediatric patients.

Cycloplegics

A cycloplegic dilates the pupil and prevents the lens from accommodating by paralyzing the ciliary muscle. Lens accommodation is vigorous in the child and young adult and it weakens with age. "Cycloplegic refraction" is an important component of the pediatric eye examination since it can uncover refractive errors compensated by accommodation. Retinal disease can cause visual loss and strabismus; cycloplegia optimizes funduscopy because the pupil is dilated maximally.

Cyclopentolate Hydrochloride

Preparation: 0.5% and 1% solutions
Dose: 1 drop in each eye every 5 minutes × 2 doses before examination
Onset: 30 to 45 minutes
Duration: 8 to 24 hours

Cyclopentolate hydrochloride is one of the most common medications administered before eye examination. It has minimal systemic effects when used in the recommended dose range. The 0.5% solution is used for young infants and the 1% solution is used thereafter. Proparacaine drops are instilled prior to cyclopentolate because proparacaine minimizes reflex tearing. Cyclopentolate is often administered in combination with phenylephrine (2.5%), which does not have a cycloplegic effect. However, two case reports describe seizure activity in children who received 2% cyclopentolate (one drop in each eye), although one of these patients had a prior history of epilepsy.[62]

Tropicamide

Preparation: 0.5% to 1% solution
Dose: 1 drop every 5 minutes × 2 doses before examination
Onset: 30 to 45 minutes
Duration: 4 to 8 hours

Tropicamide (1%) is also used in combination with phenylephrine (2.5%) but it is a less effective cycloplegic in children than cyclopentolate.

Atropine

Preparation: 0.5% to 1% solution or ointment
Dose: 1 drop tid × 3 days before examination
Onset: maximum dilation occurs in 1 to 2 days
Duration: 1 to 2 weeks

Atropine is a potent cycloplegic that may cause prolonged blurring. Systemic toxicity can occur and may present as fever, dry mouth, flushing of the face, tachycardia, nausea, and delirium ("central cholinergic syndrome"). Physostigmine antagonizes both the central and the peripheral systemic effects of atropine. In the past, atropine was the preferred cycloplegic for children, especially for those with strabismus. Now, atropine is reserved for children who have an inadequate cycloplegic effect from repeated doses of cyclopentolate.

Drugs Used in Glaucoma Therapy

Several classes of drugs are used in the treatment of glaucoma. Each type lowers IOP, although the mechanism of action may be different. In essence, though, there are two approaches to this problem: either decrease the formation of aqueous humor or increase the drainage of aqueous humor.

Direct-Acting Cholinergic (Parasympathomimetic) Drugs

Pilocarpine Hydrochloride

Preparation: 0.25% and 0.5% to 2% solutions
Dosage: 1 to 2 drops in each eye several times a day
Onset: 20 minutes
Duration: 4 to 6 hours

Pilocarpine hydrochloride is a first-line drug in the treatment of glaucoma. It acts to constrict the pupils and thus increases the size of the canals of Schlemm, facilitating aqueous humor outflow.

Indirect-Acting Irreversible Cholinergic Drugs

Echothiophate Iodide

Preparation: 0.125% solution
Dosage: 1 to 2 drops in each eye twice a day
Onset: 4 to 8 hours
Duration: days to weeks

Echothiophate iodide (and anti-cholinesterase) is the longest-acting miotic, and it causes extreme pupillary constriction. Its prescription is limited to those patients with glaucoma that is refractory to pilocarpine or epinephrine therapy. Significant systemic absorption occurs and results in low levels of plasma cholinesterase. The clinical implication of this event is of paramount importance to pediatric anesthesiologists. The metabolism of succinylcholine and mivacurium is greatly reduced, and prolonged paralysis may occur in patients receiving echothiophate iodine. Early pharmacologic studies measured plasma cholinesterase activity at 5% of normal range.[63] Full enzyme function does not recover until 4 to 6 weeks after the drug is discontinued. Thus succinylcholine or mivacurium should either be avoided or used with caution, as in much lower doses than normal, in patients taking echothiophate.[64, 65]

Adrenergic (Sympathomimetic) Drugs

Epinephrine Hydrochloride

Preparation: 0.25%, 0.5%, 1.0%, and 2.0% solutions
Dosage: 1 to 2 drops in each eye twice a day
Onset: 30 minutes
Duration: 12 to 72 hours

Epinephrine hydrochloride has a long duration of action and does not produce miosis. It acts to decrease aqueous humor formation and increase its drainage. Systemic effects such as tachycardia and hypertension can occur. Epinephrine is rarely used in the therapy of pediatric glaucoma.[66, 67]

Beta-Adrenergic-Blocking Drugs

Timolol Maleate

Preparation: 0.25% and 0.5% solutions
Dosage: 1 drop in each eye one to two times a day
Onset: 30 minutes
Duration: 12 to 24 hours

Timolol maleate blocks both beta$_1$- and beta$_2$-adrenergic receptors and it lowers IOP by decreasing the production of aqueous humor. It does not affect pupil size or visual acuity. Signs of systemic beta-blocking activity have been reported in adults and include exacerbation of asthma and symptomatic sinus bradycardia.[68, 69] In the pediatric population, timolol has rarely been associated with apnea.[70, 71] For this reason, its use in neonates is limited.

Betaxolol Hydrochloride

Preparation: 0.25% and 0.5% solutions
Dose: 1 drop one to two times a day
Onset: 30 minutes
Duration: 12 to 72 hours

Betaxolol is equally effective as timolol in the therapy of glaucoma. It is more selective for beta$_1$ receptors and therefore is less likely to cause bronchoconstriction in children with asthma. Other nonselective beta receptor antagonists include levobunolol hydrochloride, metipranolol hydrochloride, and carteolol hydrochloride.

Carbonic Anhydrase Inhibitors

The secretion of aqueous humor is an energy-dependent process that uses the sodium pump mechanism. Aqueous humor formation is greatly reduced by inhibiting the carbonic anhydrase enzyme in the ciliary body.

$$H_2O + CO_2 = H_2CO_3 = H^+ + HCO_3^-$$

Carbonic anhydrase inhibitors are sulfonamide derivatives and are used commonly in the medical management of childhood glaucoma.

Acetazolamide (Diamox)

Preparation: oral suspension, 15 mg/mL; intravenous, 100 mg/mL
Dosage: oral, 10 to 15 mg/kg PO qid; intravenous, 5 to 10 mg/kg IV every 4 to 6 hours
Onset: oral, 30 to 40 minutes; intravenous, 2 to 10 minutes
Duration: 4 to 6 hours

The intravenous preparation of acetazolamide is especially useful in the treatment of acute open-angle glaucoma. Infants may develop a metabolic acidosis that is treated by adding sodium bicarbonate (1 mEq/kg/day) to the regimen. Prolonged administration is associated with other systemic effects such as hypokalemia and renal stone formation.[72–75]

Dorzolamide Hydrochloride

Preparation: 2% solution
Dose: 1 drop bid to qid
Onset: 60 minutes
Duration: 6 to 8 hours

This drug is used in combination with other glaucoma medications and is not associated with the systemic effects of acetazolamide (e.g., metabolic acidosis).

Hypertonic Solutions

By increasing plasma osmotic pressure, hypertonic solutions (urea, mannitol, and glycerin) reduce IOP by decreasing the volume of aqueous humor; water leaves the anterior chamber and enters the plasma. These drugs are used in the management of acute (angle-closure) glaucoma and in the perioperative period when it may be necessary to rapidly lower IOP.

Mannitol

Preparation: 25% solution in water
Dosage: 0.25 to 1.0 g/kg
Onset: 30 minute
Duration: 5 to 6 hours

Mannitol is an inert sugar with an osmolality of 1.4 mOsm/mL. Its hemodynamic effects occur in two phases. Immediately, a relative hypervolemia exists; within 30 to 60 minutes, renal loss of water with subsequent sodium and potassium excretion occurs. At this stage, hypotension due to hypovolemia may result. Mannitol is most often administered preoperatively to lower IOP acutely. Administration should occur over several minutes rather than as an intravenous bolus because rapid administration causes acute vasodilation and may result in transient hypotension.[76]

Corticosteroids

Topical corticosteroids are provided in eye drop form and ointment for treatment of inflammatory conditions such as conjunctivitis, scleritis, or uveitis. Topical steroids can increase the activity of the herpes simplex virus and may cause fungal infections or open-angle glaucoma. Intravenous steroids are also administered intraoperatively during procedures such as "open-sky" vitrectomy. The usual choice is hydrocortisone, 1 to 5 mg/kg as a single dose. In this setting, steroid therapy is believed to reduce postoperative scarring of retinal tissue.

Intraocular Gases (Air, Sulfur Hexafluoride, Carbon Octofluorine)

Occasionally a small gas bubble is injected intraocularly during retinal detachment surgery. Nitrous oxide will diffuse into this volume-limited space; IOP will increase and may impair retinal perfusion. If N_2O is used during retinal surgery, it should be discontinued 15 minutes before intraocular gas injection. N_2O must not be used in the postoperative period for the same reason. The time period for avoidance depends on the solubility of the specific gas in blood. N_2O should not be used for 5 days after air injection, for 10 days after sulfur hexafluoride injection, and for at least 30 days after octofluorine injection.

Specific Pediatric Ophthalmologic Problems and Operations

Congenital Cataracts

A congenital cataract is defined as any lens opacity that is present at birth. A cataract distorts image formation by hindering the passage of light to the retina. Because cataracts do not regress with age, surgical removal is necessary. It is crucial to perform this procedure in early infancy to provide for optimal stimulation of the retina during the critical period of visual development.[77-79] Maternal rubella during the first trimester of gestation is a well-known cause of congenital cataracts. Other associated conditions include chromosomal disorders (e.g., trisomies 13, 18, and 21) and metabolic disorders such as galactosemia and Wilson disease. At least half of all congenital cataracts occur spontaneously. In certain conditions (e.g., Marfan syndrome or homocystinuria), the lens is subluxed at birth (ectopia lentis). The dislocated lens eventually becomes cloudy and must be removed.

After instillation of a cycloplegic, an incision is made near the limbus (junction of sclera and cornea). The lens is aspirated after emulsification. Complications of this procedure include retinal detachment, both early and late in the healing phase.

Glaucoma

Glaucoma can occur primarily as a developmental problem or it can appear as a secondary lesion after eye injury or cataract surgery.[80-85] Infantile glaucoma is present at birth or during the first 3 years of life and is probably transmitted as an autosomal recessive trait.[81] Juvenile glaucoma has an onset between the ages of 4 and 30 years. Several anomalies are associated with glaucoma; the most notable are Sturge-Weber syndrome, von Recklinghausen syndrome, and craniofacial malformations. Anesthetic considerations therefore must also involve an understanding of the child's other medical conditions or congenital malformations.

Congenital glaucoma is due to inadequate outflow of aqueous humor. An infant's eye is more compliant than an adult's. Therefore, as IOP increases, the eye enlarges, a condition termed *buphthalmos*. The edematous cornea is hazy; afflicted infants have tearing, photophobia, and blepharospasm. Measurement of IOP, gonioscopy (examination of the anterior chamber angle), and funduscopic evaluation of the optic disk confirm the diagnosis. For this procedure, mask induction of general anesthesia is appropriate. IOP measurements should be obtained before laryngoscopy and tracheal intubation because these events raise IOP. In small infants, this requires coordination between the anesthesiologist and surgeon. Once the IOP is determined, intubation is performed because this maneuver does not interfere with gonioscopy or funduscopy. A laryngeal mask airway is an alternative to endotracheal intubation for periodic glaucoma examinations.[42] These procedures can be lengthy if photography is used to document the pathology.

Although open-angle glaucoma of the adult type is initially managed medically with miotics, infantile glaucoma must be treated surgically. Miotic eye drops are prescribed preoperatively until the definitive operation is performed. Goniotomy facilitates drainage of aqueous humor through normal channels and has a 70 to 80% cure rate. A filtering procedure directs aqueous humor from the anterior chamber into the canals of Schlemm. These two operations are less effective in the treatment of secondary glaucoma. In this case, cyclocryotherapy is used: A cryoprobe is applied to the conjunctiva and cooled to $-70°C$. A vascular reaction and subsequent fibrosis in the nearby ciliary body hinder aqueous humor formation and ultimately decrease IOP. A fourth procedure, known as *trabeculotomy*, is performed in cases of unsuccessful medical treatment, goniotomy, or filtering. This operation obliterates a portion of the trabeculum between the anterior chamber and the canal of Schlemm. A more direct route for aqueous humor drainage is established.

Strabismus

Strabismus is a deviation of one eye relative to the visual axis of the other eye. The deviation can occur in one eye and results in either esophoria, the tendency of one eye to turn inward, or exophoria, the tendency of one eye to turn outward. Esotropia, or convergent strabismus, is the inward deviation of both eyes; "crossed eyes" is the colloquial term given to this condition. Strabismus occurs in 2 to 3% of children. If left uncorrected, unilateral strabismus leads to amblyopia exanopsia; to prevent diplopia, the image from the deviated eye is suppressed, and retinal development is hindered. Because visual maturation occurs by age 5, it is imperative to realign the deviated eye early in childhood. Therefore, the goals of strabismus therapy are threefold:

1. To maintain visual acuity in the deviated eye
2. To provide binocular vision
3. To improve the child's appearance

The last goal is extremely important in the development of a child's self-esteem.

The surgical correction of strabismus is essentially a repositioning of the extraocular muscles. To strengthen a muscle a resection is performed, and to weaken a muscle a recession is performed. For example, a mild esotropia or inward deviation is corrected by weakening the medial rectus muscle. This allows the eye to return to a midline position. A more severe deviation may require both a recession of the medial rectus muscle and a resection or strengthening of the lateral rectus muscle. Strabismus surgery is generally performed in an ambulatory setting. On awakening, the child may complain of a gritty sensation in the eye, which is usually relieved with rectal acetaminophen (30 to 40 mg/kg) administered at the beginning of surgery so as to have an adequate blood level at the time of awakening.[86, 87]

The incidence of postoperative nausea and vomiting after strabismus correction is high (40–85%) when compared with other ambulatory procedures. This complication occasionally delays discharge and overshadows an essentially minor procedure. Although the explanation for excessive nausea and vomiting is still unknown, many prophylactic measures have been proposed. These include: droperidol (20–75 μg/kg)[88–90]; lidocaine (1.5 mg/kg)[91]; metoclopramide (0.15 mg/kg)[92]; propofol (0.15–0.30/mg/kg/min)[93–95]; propofol-fentanyl[96]; ondansetron (0.075–0.15 mg/kg)[97]; granisetron (40 μg/kg)[98]; clonidine (0.004 mg/kg)[99]; and acupressure at the P6 site.[100]

It is difficult to assess the efficacy of each measure, since the anesthetic techniques across studies vary greatly. For example, both inhalation and intravenous drugs are used for induction and maintenance of anesthesia. Gastric suctioning may or may not have been performed. Medications such as atropine, benzodiazepines, or narcotics may or may not have been given. Furthermore, the study end points differ: Did vomiting occur in the first 8 hours or first 24 hours? Did retching without vomiting occur? Did vomiting or excessive sedation delay hospital discharge?

In our institution, we have found that replacement of the entire fluid deficit during the intraoperative and early recovery period decreases postoperative nausea and vomiting. Anesthesia is maintained with O_2:N_2O:halothane, sevoflurane or isoflurane, and all patients undergo gastric emptying before extubation. We administer ondansetron (0.15 mg/kg) before manipulation of the eyes. Fluids are not forced, but apple juice is offered once a child complains of thirst.[101] Children are not aroused forcefully in the post-anesthesia care unit but are allowed to sleep quietly. We inform parents of the high chance of nausea and vomiting associated with strabismus surgery. We also give parents an emesis basin and towel at discharge and caution them that the car ride may incite vomiting. We also tell parents that children undergoing this procedure seem to sleep a great deal for the first 24 to 48 hours postoperatively.

Retinopathy of Prematurity

Retinopathy of prematurity (ROP) is an abnormal proliferation of vascular tissue; it occurs principally in low birth weight infants. The condition was observed initially in 1942 and later given the name *retrolental fibroplasia*.[102] In 1951, oxygen (O_2) therapy was implicated in the pathogenesis of acute neonatal retinopathy.[103] In 1987, the Committee on the Classification of Retinopathy of Prematurity agreed to rename and redefine the disease according to the stage of retinal disruption.[104]

Normal retinal development begins with the outward migration of mesenchyme from the optic disk. The nasal edge is closer and matures earlier during gestation. The temporal retina does not reach full maturation until 44 weeks after conception, and it is in this region that ROP most frequently occurs. As the mesenchyme advances, it differentiates into a fine capillary network. Current models of ROP propose a mechanism of injury in which the capillary bed is obliterated and supplanted by a mesenchymal arteriovenous shunt[105]; this structure is the hallmark of ROP. Spontaneous regression of the disease occurs in 85% of cases and results from eventual differentiation of shunt cells into capillaries. Persistent ROP is due to the proliferation of undifferentiated primitive mesenchymal cells. Growth of these cells past the internal limiting membrane of the retina and into the vitreous body can ultimately cause a traction retinal detachment. At this stage of the disease, visual function is significantly compromised.

Studies have now identified a population at risk for ROP. The most important variable is birth weight; infants weighing less than 1000 g have a 45% chance of developing ROP.[106] Gestational age is a correlate because it determines the degree of retinal development. The role of oxygen is controversial. In 1951, an Australian pediatrician first described oxygen therapy as a factor in the pathogenesis of ROP.[103] She noted a higher incidence of retinal problems in the private nursery where oxygen was readily available. The premature babies of poorer families, cared for in the ward nursery where oxygen was less readily available, had a lower incidence of ROP. Later studies suggested that the risk for ROP was thought to be associated with an arterial oxygen tension greater than 100 mm Hg.[107] More recent studies have implicated the free radicals O_2^- and OH^-, as well as hydrogen peroxide in the genesis of ROP.[108–111] Normally, enzymes such as superoxide dismutase and cytochrome oxidase protect susceptible cell membranes against these injurious products of oxygen-mediated reactions. The immature retina may be deficient in these enzyme systems and thus more vulnerable to the effects of hyperoxia.[112] Studies now suggest a changing oxygen environment as a contributing factor in ROP. Some reports describe premature infants who did not receive supplemental oxygen but who nonetheless developed ROP.[113] Finally, the disease has occurred in full-term infants of normal birth weight, in infants with cyanotic heart disease,[114, 115] and in infants who suffered severe intrauterine bleeding due to placental abruption.[116]

The treatment of ROP is directed at preventing its progression and repair of existing retinal defects.[117, 118] The immature avascular retina probably secretes an angiogenic factor in response to its hypoxic environment. This factor then stimulates a vasoproliferative reaction in the leading edge of the vascular retina. Ablation of the avascular retina should inhibit the release of angiogenic factor and thus minimize the neovascularization. Cryotherapy or application of a cooled probe destroys the avascular retina. This procedure is moderately successful in limiting the extent of retinal disease. It is not uniformly effective in preventing eventual retinal detachment.

A scleral buckling procedure is indicated for a posterior retinal detachment. A silicone prosthesis is implanted in the sclera to secure the retina against the globe. If neovascularization has progressed into the vitreous, a scleral buckle alone is insufficient. Vitrectomy is performed through either a "closed" approach or an "open-sky" approach. The latter procedure has gained popularity in the treatment of ROP. Surgical exposure is improved by the surgeon's removing the cornea and preserving it in tissue solution during the operation. The lens is removed, revealing the abnormal retrolental membranes, vascular vitreous, and detached retina. The membranes and vitreous are finely cut and aspirated, thus allowing the retina to be repositioned against the choroid. The cornea is then reattached; saline injection serves to re-establish the fluid nature of the anterior chamber. Bedside cryotherapy under general anesthesia for very low birth weight infants is an option in some neonatal intensive care units.[119]

The American Academies of Pediatrics and Ophthalmology have recommended a screening examination of premature infants for retinopathy of prematurity.[120, 121] In summary, these guidelines call for a dilated indirect ophthalmoscopic examination of infants with a birth weight less than 1500 g or gestational age less than 28 weeks. Infants who are over 1500 g or 28 weeks should also be examined if clinical suspicion is present. This examination should occur between 31 and 33 weeks of post-conceptual age. Follow-up examinations at 1- to 2-week intervals are indicated for infants with mild retinal disease. Ablative surgery for infants with moderate-to-severe retinal disease should occur within 72 hours of diagnosis if the baby will tolerate surgery.

"Open Eye Injury and Full Stomach" Controversy

In the scenario of a patient with an open eye injury and a full stomach, a clinician has two goals during the induction of general anesthesia: (1) protection of the airway and avoidance of pulmonary aspiration of gastric contents and (2) maintenance of nearly normal IOP. The concern for avoiding increases in IOP stems from a case report describing the loss of vitreous humor after the use of succinylcholine.[122] The mechanism of action presumed a sudden rise in IOP from baseline value, which then accentuated the pressure gradient between intraocular contents and the environment. Since this account, the essential question remains whether there is a preferred anesthetic plan.

A child who presents with an eye injury requires a prompt evaluation that includes a complete physical examination. This approach ensures that other injuries, especially neurologic, are not overlooked. If a child has suffered a scleral laceration from a foreign body, early placement of an intravenous catheter is not an absolute requirement. However, if a child has both ocular and orthopedic injuries (e.g., due to a car accident), fluid replacement in the emergency room is essential. In either instance, the child may benefit from a histamine (H_2) receptor antagonist (e.g., cimetidine, 7.5 mg/kg PO or IV, ranitidine, 15 mg/kg) at least 45 minutes before surgery.[123] Ideally, once the child has arrived in the operating room, intravenous catheter placement should be attempted. The most adept person should make the first attempt at intravenous catheter placement. If placement fails (several unsuccessful attempts on an agitated patient), then an alternative plan must be devised. Two possibilities include sedation with rectal methohexital (25 mg/kg) or an O_2:N_2O:halothane or sevoflurane induction accompanied by cricoid pressure applied by a skilled assistant. As soon as the intravenous catheter is inserted, the anesthesiologist must decide whether intubation should proceed with or without the aid of a neuromuscular relaxant.

In our opinion, use of a relaxant provides optimal conditions for intubation. If the depth of anesthesia is misjudged and laryngoscopy precipitates coughing, IOP is elevated even during a halothane or sevoflurane induction. The use of succinylcholine as opposed to a nondepolarizing relaxant may still be a controversial issue. Succinylcholine has the most rapid onset and is usually the drug of choice in patients with a full stomach. A strategy to blunt the elevation in IOP caused by succinylcholine includes the intravenous use of atropine (0.02 mg/kg) and curare (0.1 mg/kg), followed by sodium thiopental (5–6 mg/kg) or propofol (2–3 mg/kg), combined with lidocaine (1.5 mg/kg), and succinylcholine (1.5–2.0 mg/kg). This induction sequence has been followed at our institution for several years and has not been associated with expulsion of intraocular tissue.

Early reports on the use of the intermediate-acting relaxants atracurium and vecuronium contained suggestions designed to shorten the onset time. The "priming technique" was applied to both drugs and consisted of administering a small dose (atracurium, 0.05 mg/kg, or vecuronium, 0.01 mg/kg), waiting 4 minutes, and then administering an induction dose of sodium thiopental and an intubating dose of atracurium (0.5 mg/kg) or vecuronium (0.1 mg/kg).[124, 125] This plan shortened the onset time to 90 seconds for both drugs. Another option is to administer a very large dose of vecuronium (0.2 mg/kg) as a single bolus during induction.[126] This approach shortens the time to onset but considerably lengthens the duration of action (from 45 minutes to 2 hours). High-dose rocuronium (1.2 mg/kg or 2 × ED$_{95}$) has been demonstrated to be an alternative to succinylcholine and will provide about 60 minutes or more of neuromuscular blockade.[127] Some patients, however, may cough if laryngoscopy is attempted at 30 seconds following administration. If a contraindication to succinylcholine use exists (e.g., family history of malignant hyperthermia, burn injury), these induction methods are certainly appropriate. Once intubation is accomplished, the stomach should be emptied with suction while the patient is still paralyzed. A gag reflex elicited by a gastric tube also increases IOP and should be avoided until the eye is closed. The usual precautions regarding extubation still apply: the child should be awake and have intact airway reflexes.

REFERENCES

1. Macri FJ: Vascular pressure relationships and the intraocular pressure. Arch Ophthalmol 1961;65:571–574.
2. Tsamparlakis J, Casey TA, Howell W, et al: Dependence of intraocular pressure on induced hypotension and posture during surgical anaesthesia. Trans Ophthalmol Soc U K 1980;100:521–526.
3. Reis DJ, Golanov EV, Galea E, et al: Central neurogenic neuroprotection: Central neural systems that protect the brain from hypoxia and ischemia. Ann N Y Acad Sci 1997;835:168–186.
4. Berler DK: The oculocardiac reflex. Am J Ophthalmol 1963;56:954–959.
5. Taylor C, Wilson FM, Roesch R, et al: Prevention of the oculo-cardiac reflex in children. Anesthesiology 1963;24:646–649.
6. Mirakhur RK, Clarke RS, Dundee JW, et al: Anticholinergic drugs in anaesthesia: A survey of their present position. Anaesthesia 1978;33:133–138.
7. Meyers EF, Tomeldan SA: Glycopyrrolate compared with atropine in prevention of the oculocardiac reflex during eye-muscle surgery. Anesthesiology 1979;51:350–352.
8. Loewinger J, Friedmann-Neiger I, Cohen M, et al: Effects of atracurium and pancuronium on the oculocardiac reflex in children. Anesth Analg 1991;73:25–28.
9. Ausinsch B, Graves SA, Munson ES, et al: Intraocular pressures in children during isoflurane and halothane anesthesia. Anesthesiology 1975;42:167–172.
10. Moses RA, Hart WM Jr: Adler's Physiology of the Eye: Clinical Application. St. Louis: C.V. Mosby; 1987.
11. Sator S, Wildling E, Schabernig C, et al: Desflurane maintains intraocular pressure at an equivalent level to isoflurane and propofol during unstressed non-ophthalmic surgery. Br J Anaesth 1998;80:243–244.
12. Artru AA, Momota Y: Trabecular outflow facility and formation rate of aqueous humor during anesthesia with sevoflurane-nitrous oxide or sevoflurane-remifentanil in rabbits. Anesth Analg 1999;88:781–786.
13. Yoshitake S, Sendaya K, Mizutani A, et al: The changes of intraocular pressure during sevoflurane anesthesia in children [in Japanese]. Masui 1993;42:52–55.
14. Artru AA: Rate of anterior chamber aqueous formation, trabecular outflow facility, and intraocular compliance during desflurane or halothane anesthesia in dogs. Anesth Analg 1995;81:585–590.
15. Watcha MF, Chu FC, Stevens JL, et al: Effects of halothane on intraocular pressure in anesthetized children. Anesth Analg 1990;71:181–184.
16. Ferrari LR, Donlon JV: A comparison of propofol, midazolam, and methohexital for sedation during retrobulbar and peribulbar block. J Clin Anesth 1992;4:93–96.
17. Fragen RJ, Hauch T: The effect of midazolam maleate and diazepam on intraocular pressure in adults. Arzneimittelforschung 1981;31:2273–2275.
18. Al-Abrak MH: Diazepam and intraocular pressure. Br J Anaesth 1978;50:866.
19. Joshi C, Bruce DL: Thiopental and succinylcholine: Action on intraocular pressure. Anesth Analg 1975;54:471–475.
20. Thomson MF, Brock-Utne JG, Bean P, et al: Anaesthesia and intraocular pressure: A comparative of total intravenous anaesthesia using etomidate with conventional inhalation anaesthesia. Anaesthesia 1982;37:758–761.
21. Mirakhur RK, Shepherd WF, Darrah WC: Propofol or thiopentone: Effects on intraocular pressure associated with induction of anaesthe-

sia and tracheal intubation (facilitated with suxamethonium). Br J Anaesth 1987;59:431–436.
22. Leopold IH, Comroe JH Jr: Effect of intramuscular administration of morphine, atropine, scopolamine, and neostigmine on the human eye. Arch Ophthalmol 1948;40:285–290.
23. Mostafa SM, Lockhart A, Kumar D, et al: Comparison of effects of fentanyl and alfentanil on intra-ocular pressure: A double-blind controlled trial. Anaesthesia 1986;41:493–498.
24. Ghignone M, Noe C, Calvillo O, et al: Anesthesia for ophthalmic surgery in the elderly: The effects of clonidine on intraocular pressure, perioperative hemodynamics, and anesthetic requirement. Anesthesiology 1988;68:707–716.
25. Yoshikawa K, Murai Y: The effect of ketamine on intraocular pressure in children. Anesth Analg 1971;50:199–202.
26. Ausinsch B, Rayburn RL, Munson ES, et al: Ketamine and intraocular pressure in children. Anesth Analg 1976;55:773–775.
27. Al-Abrak MH, Samuel JR: Effects of general anaesthesia on the intraocular pressure in man: Comparison of tubocurarine and pancuronium in nitrous oxide and oxygen. Br J Ophthalmol 1974;58:806–810.
28. Litwiller RW, DiFazio CA, Rushia EL: Pancuronium and intraocular pressure. Anesthesiology 1975;42:750–752.
29. Schneider MJ, Stirt JA, Finholt DA: Atracurium, vecuronium, and intraocular pressure in humans. Anesth Analg 1986;65:877–882.
30. Murphy DF, Eustace P, Unwin A, et al: Atracurium and intraocular pressure. Br J Ophthalmol 1985;69:673–675.
31. Maharaj RJ, Humphrey D, Kaplan N, et al: Effects of atracurium on intraocular pressure. Br J Anaesth 1984;56:459–463.
32. Polarz H, Bohrer H, von Tabouillot W, et al: Comparative effects of atracurium and vecuronium on intraocular pressure. Ger J Ophthalmol 1995;4:91–93.
33. Pandey K, Badola RP, Kumar S: Time course of intraocular hypertension produced by suxamethonium. Br J Anaesth 1972;44:191–196.
34. Metz HS, Venkatesh B: Succinylcholine and intraocular pressure. J Pediatr Ophthalmol Strabismus 1981;18:12–14.
35. Peachey L, Huxley AF: Structural identification of twitch and slow striated muscle fibers of the frog. J Cell Biol 1962;13:177–180.
36. Katz RL, Eakins KE: Mode of action of succinylcholine on intraocular pressure. J Pharmacol Exp Ther 1968;162:1–9.
37. Kelly RE, Dinner M, Turner LS, et al: Succinylcholine increases intraocular pressure in the human eye with the extraocular muscles detached. Anesthesiology 1993;79:948–952.
38. Miller RD, Way WL, Hickey RF: Inhibition of succinylcholine-induced increased intraocular pressure by non-depolarizing muscle relaxants. Anesthesiology 1968;29:123–126.
39. Meyers EF, Krupin T, Johnson M, et al: Failure of nondepolarizing neuromuscular blockers to inhibit succinylcholine-induced increased intraocular pressure, a controlled study. Anesthesiology 1978;48:149–151.
40. Warner LO, Bremer DL, Davidson PJ, et al: Effects of lidocaine, succinylcholine, and tracheal intubation on intraocular pressure in children anesthetized with halothane-nitrous oxide. Anesth Analg 1989;69:687–690.
41. Zimmerman AA, Funk KJ, Tidwell JL: Propofol and alfentanil prevent the increase in intraocular pressure caused by succinylcholine and endotracheal intubation during a rapid sequence induction of anesthesia. Anesth Analg 1996;83:814–817.
42. Watcha MF, White PF, Tychsen L, et al: Comparative effects of laryngeal mask airway and endotracheal tube insertion on intraocular pressure in children. Anesth Analg 1992;75:355–360.
43. Aboul-Eish E: Physiology of the eye pertinent to anesthesia. In Smith RB (ed): Anesthesia in Ophthalmology, pp 1–31. Boston, Little, Brown & Co, 1973.
44. Kain ZN, Mayes LC, Bell C, et al: Premedication in the United States: A status report. Anesth Analg 1997;84:427–432.
45. Suresh S, Cohen IJ, Matuszczak M, et al: Dose ranging, safety, and efficacy of a new oral midazolam syrup in children. Anesthesiology 1998;89:A1313.
46. Karl HW, Rosenberger JL, Larach MG, et al: Transmucosal administration of midazolam for premedication of pediatric patients: Comparison of the nasal and sublingual routes. Anesthesiology 1993;78:885–891.
47. Davis PJ, Tome JA, McGowan FX Jr, et al: Preanesthetic medication with intranasal midazolam for brief pediatric surgical procedures: Effect on recovery and hospital discharge times. Anesthesiology 1995;82:2–5.

48. Committee on Drugs, American Academy of Pediatrics: Alternate routes of drug administration: Advantages and disadvantages. Pediatrics 1997;100:143–152.

49. Liu LM, Gaudreault P, Friedman PA, et al: Methohexital plasma concentrations in children following rectal administration. Anesthesiology 1985;62:567–570.

50. Liu LM, Goudsouzian NG, Liu PL: Rectal methohexital premedication in children, a dose-comparison study. Anesthesiology 1980;53:343–345.

51. White PF: Clinical uses of intravenous anesthetic and analgesic infusions. Anesth Analg 1989;68:161–171.

52. Bjerring P, Arendt-Nielsen L: Depth and duration of skin analgesia to needle insertion after topical application of EMLA cream. Br J Anaesth 1990;64:173–177.

53. Gajraj NM, Pennant JH, Watcha MF: Eutectic mixture of local anesthetics (EMLA) cream. Anesth Analg 1994;78:574–583.

54. Ferrari LR, Goudsouzian NG: The use of the laryngeal mask airway in children with bronchopulmonary dysplasia. Anesth Analg 1995;81:310–313.

55. Zwass MS, Fisher DM, Welborn LG, et al: Induction and maintenance characteristics of anesthesia with desflurane and nitrous oxide in infants and children. Anesthesiology 1992;76:373–378.

56. Coté CJ, Zaslavsky A, Downes JJ, et al: Postoperative apnea in former preterm infants after inguinal herniorrhaphy: A combined analysis. Anesthesiology 1995;82:809–822.

57. Altman AJ, Albert DM, Fournier GA: Cocaine's use in ophthalmology: Our 100-year heritage. Surv Ophthalmol 1985;29:300–306.

58. Samantary S, Thomas A: Systemic effects of topical phenylephrine. Indian J Ophthalmol 1975;23:16–17.

59. Wilensky JT, Woodward HJ: Acute systemic hypertension after conjunctival instillation of phenylephrine hydrochloride. Am J Ophthalmol 1973;76:156–157.

60. Merritt JC, Kraybill EN: Effect of mydriatics on blood pressure in premature infants. J Pediatr Ophthalmol Strabismus 1981;18:42–46.

61. Wellwood M, Goresky GV: Systemic hypertension associated with topical administration of 2.5% phenylephrine HCl. Am J Ophthalmol 1982;93:369–370.

62. Kennerdell JS, Wucher FP: Cyclopentolate associated with two cases of grand mal seizure. Arch Ophthalmol 1972;87:634–635.

63. De Roeth A Jr, Dettbarn W-D, Rosenberg P, et al: Effect of phospholine iodine on blood cholinesterase levels of normal and glaucoma subjects. Am J Ophthalmol 1965;59:586–592.

64. Donati F, Bevan DR: Controlled succinylcholine infusion in a patient receiving echothiophate eye drops. Can Anaesth Soc J 1981;28:488–490.

65. Cavallaro RJ, Krumperman LW, Kugler F: Effect of echothiophate therapy on the metabolism of succinylcholine in man. Anesth Analg 1968;47:570–574.

66. Everitt DE, Avorn J: Systemic effects of medications used to treat glaucoma. Ann Intern Med 1990;112:120–125.

67. Nelson ME, Andrzejowski AZ: Systemic hypertension in patients receiving dipivalyl adrenaline for glaucoma. Br Med J 1988;297:741–742.

68. Nelson WP: Adverse respiratory and cardiovascular events attributed to timolol ophthalmic solution, 1978–1985. Am J Ophthalmol 1987;104:97–98.

69. Fraunfelder FT, Meyer SM: Systemic side effects from ophthalmic timolol and their prevention. J Ocul Pharmacol 1987;3:177–184.

70. Bailey PL: Timolol and postoperative apnea in neonates and young infants. Anesthesiology 1984;61:622.

71. Olson RJ, Bromberg BB, Zimmerman TJ: Apneic spells associated with timolol therapy in a neonate. Am J Ophthalmol 1979;88:120–122.

72. Wistrand PJ: The use of carbonic anhydrase inhibitors in ophthalmology and clinical medicine. Ann N Y Acad Sci 1984;429:609–619.

73. Gabay EL: Metabolic acidosis from acetazolamide therapy. Arch Ophthalmol 1983;101:303–304.

74. Kass MA, Kolker AE, Gordon M, et al: Acetazolamide and urolithiasis. Ophthalmology 1981;88:261–265.

75. Epstein DL, Grant WM: Carbonic anhydrase inhibitor side effects: Serum chemical analysis. Arch Ophthalmol 1977;95:1378–1382.

76. Coté CJ, Greenhow DE, Marshall BE: The hypotensive response to rapid intravenous administration of hypertonic solutions in man and in the rabbit. Anesthesiology 1979;50:30–35.

77. Calhoun JH: Cataracts in children. Pediatr Clin North Am 1983;30:1061–1069.

78. Enoch JM, Campos EC: Helping the aphakic neonate to see. Int Ophthalmol 1985;8:237–248.

79. Lambert SR, Drack AV: Infantile cataracts. Surv Ophthalmol 1996;40:427–458.

80. Franks W, Taylor D: Congenital glaucoma: A preventable cause of blindness. Arch Dis Child 1989;64:649–650.

81. Mandal AK: Current concepts in the diagnosis and management of developmental glaucomas. Indian J Ophthalmol 1993;41:51–70.

82. Russell-Eggitt I, Zamiri P: Review of aphakic glaucoma after surgery for congenital cataract. J Cataract Refract Surg 1997;23(Suppl):664–668.

83. Chew E, Morin JD: Glaucoma in children. Pediatr Clin North Am 1983;30:1043–1060.

84. Kwitko ML: Secondary glaucoma in infants and children. Trans Ophthalmol Soc U K 1978;98:105–110.

85. Richardson KT: Glaucoma in children. Int Ophthalmol Clin 1977;17:183–186.

86. Birmingham PK, Tobin MJ, Henthorn TK, et al: Twenty-four-hour pharmacokinetics of rectal acetaminophen in children: An old drug with new recommendations. Anesthesiology 1997;87:244–252.

87. Birmingham PK, Tobin MJ, Henthorn TK, et al: "Loading" and subsequent dosing of rectal acetaminophen in children: A 24 hour pharmacokinetic study of new dosing recommendations. Anesthesiology 1996;85:A1105.

88. Abramowitz MD, Oh TH, Epstein BS, et al: The antiemetic effect of droperidol following outpatient strabismus surgery in children. Anesthesiology 1983;59:579–583.

89. Lerman J, Eustis S, Smith DR: Effect of droperidol pretreatment on postanesthetic vomiting in children undergoing strabismus surgery. Anesthesiology 1986;65:322–325.

90. Brown RE Jr, James DJ, Weaver RG, et al: Low-dose droperidol versus standard-dose droperidol for prevention of postoperative vomiting after pediatric strabismus surgery. J Clin Anesth 1991;3:306–309.

91. Christensen S, Farrow-Gillespie A, Lerman J: Incidence of emesis and postanesthetic recovery after strabismus surgery in children: A comparison of droperidol and lidocaine. Anesthesiology 1989;70:251–254.

92. Broadman LM, Ceruzzi W, Patane PS, et al: Metoclopramide reduces the incidence of vomiting following strabismus surgery in children. Anesthesiology 1990;72:245–248.

93. Weir PM, Munro HM, Reynolds PI, et al: Propofol infusion and the incidence of emesis in pediatric outpatient strabismus surgery. Anesth Analg 1993;76:760–764.

94. Watcha MF, Simeon RM, White PF, et al: Effect of propofol on the incidence of postoperative vomiting after strabismus surgery in pediatric outpatients. Anesthesiology 1991;75:204–209.

95. Reimer EJ, Montgomery CJ, Bevan JC, et al: Propofol anaesthesia reduces early postoperative emesis after paediatric strabismus surgery. Can J Anaesth 1993;40:927–933.

96. Larsson S, Asgeirsson B, Magnusson J: Propofol-fentanyl anesthesia compared with thiopental-halothane with special reference to recovery and vomiting after pediatric strabismus surgery. Acta Anaesthesiol Scand 1992;36:182–186.

97. Davis A, Krige S, Moyes D: A double-blind randomized prospective study comparing ondansetron with droperidol in the prevention of emesis following strabismus surgery. Anaesth Intensive Care 1995;23:438–443.

98. Fujii Y, Saitoh Y, Tanaka H, et al: Comparison of granisetron and droperidol in the prevention of vomiting after strabismus surgery or tonsillectomy in children. Paediatr Anaesth 1998;8:241–244.

99. Mikawa K, Nishina K, Maekawa N, et al: Oral clonidine premedication reduces vomiting in children after strabismus surgery. Can J Anaesth 1995;42:977–981.

100. Yentis SM, Bissonnette B: Ineffectiveness of acupuncture and droperidol in preventing vomiting following strabismus repair in children. Can J Anaesth 1992;39:151–154.

101. Schreiner MS, Nicolson SC, Martin T, et al: Should children drink before discharge from day surgery? Anesthesiology 1992;76:528–533.

102. Terry TL: Extreme prematurity and fibroblastic overgrowth of persistent vascular sheath behind each crystalline lens: I. preliminary report. Am J Ophthalmol 1942;25:203–204.

103. Campbell K: Intensive oxygen therapy as a possible cause of retrolental fibroplasia: A clinical approach. Med J Aust 1951;2:48–50.

104. The International Committee for the Classification of the Late Stages of Retinopathy of Prematurity: An international classification of reti-

nopathy of prematurity. II. The classification of retinal detachment. Arch Ophthalmol 1987;105:906–912.

105. Flynn JT, Bancalari E, Bachynski BN, et al: Retinopathy of prematurity. Diagnosis, severity, and natural history. Ophthalmology 1987;94:620–629.

106. Flynn JT: Acute proliferative retrolental fibroplasia: Multivariate risk analysis. Trans Am Ophthalmol Soc 1983;81:549–591.

107. Kinsey VE, Hemphill FM: Etiology of retrolental fibroplasia: Preliminary report of a co-operative study of retrolental fibroplasia. Am J Ophthalmol 1955;40:116–174.

108. Inder TE, Clemett RS, Austin NC, et al: High iron status in very low birth weight infants is associated with an increased risk of retinopathy of prematurity. J Pediatr 1997;131:541–544.

109. Rao NA, Wu GS: Oxygen free radicals and retinopathy of prematurity. Br J Ophthalmol 1996;80:387.

110. Kelly FJ: Free radical disorders of preterm infants. Br Med Bull 1993;49:668–678.

111. Saugstad OD: Oxygen toxicity in the neonatal period. Acta Paediatr Scand 1990;79:881–892.

112. Patz A: The role of oxygen in retrolental fibroplasia. Trans Am Ophthalmol Soc 1968;66:940–985.

113. Adamkin DH, Shott RJ, Cook LN, et al: Nonhyperoxic retrolental fibroplasia. Pediatrics 1977;60:828–830.

114. Brockhurst RJ, Chishti MI: Cicatricial retrolental fibroplasia: Its occurrence without oxygen administration and in full term infants. Albrecht Von Graefes Arch Klin Exp Ophthalmol 1975;195:113–128.

115. Kalina RE, Hodson WA, Morgan BC: Retrolental fibroplasia in a cyanotic infant. Pediatrics 1972;50:765–768.

116. Jandeck C, Kellner U, Kossel H, et al: Retinopathy of prematurity in infants of birth weight > 2000 g after haemorrhagic shock at birth. Br J Ophthalmol 1996;80:728–731.

117. Hirose T, Lou PL: Retinopathy of prematurity. Int Ophthalmol Clin 1986;26:1–23.

118. Flynn JT: Oxygen and retrolental fibroplasia: update and challenge. Anesthesiology 1984;60:397–399.

119. Sullivan TJ, Clarke MP, Tuli R, et al: General anesthesia with endotracheal intubation for cryotherapy for retinopathy of prematurity. Eur J Ophthalmol 1995;5:187–191.

120. American Academy of Pediatrics Committee on Practice and Ambulatory Medicine, Section on Ophthalmology: Eye examination and vision screening in infants, children, and young adults. Pediatrics 1996;98:153–157.

121. American Academy of Pediatrics, the American Association for Pediatric Ophthalmology and Strabismus, and the American Academy of Ophthalmology: Screening examination of premature infants for retinopathy of prematurity: A joint statement. Pediatrics 1997;100:273.

122. Lewallen WM Jr: The use of succinylcholine in ocular surgery. Am J Ophthalmol 1960;49:773–780.

123. Goudsouzian NG, Coté CJ, Liu LM, et al: The dose-response effects of oral cimetidine on gastric pH and volume in children. Anesthesiology 1981;55:53–56.

124. Naguib M, Abdulatif M, Gyasi HK, et al: Priming with atracurium: Improving intubating conditions with additional doses of thiopental. Anesth Analg 1986;65:1295–1299.

125. Taboada JA, Rupp SM, Miller RD: Refining the priming principle for vecuronium during rapid-sequence induction of anesthesia. Anesthesiology 1986;64:243–247.

126. Abbott MA, Samuel JR: The control of intra-ocular pressure during the induction of anaesthesia for emergency eye surgery: A high-dose vecuronium technique. Anaesthesia 1987;42:1008–1012.

127. Mazurek AJ, Rae B, Hann S, et al: Rocuronium versus succinylcholine: Are they equally effective during rapid-sequence induction of anesthesia? Anesth Analg 1998;87:1259–1262.

22 Pediatric Neurosurgical Anesthesia

Elizabeth A. Eldredge, Sulpicio G. Soriano, *and* Mark A. Rockoff

Pathophysiology
    Intracranial Compartments
    Intracranial Pressure
    Cerebral Blood Volume and Cerebral Blood Flow
    Cerebrovascular Autoregulation
Anesthetic Management
    Preoperative Evaluation
    Premedication
    Monitoring
    Induction
    Airway Management and Intubation
    Muscle Relaxants
    Positioning
    Local Anesthesia
    Maintenance
    Blood and Fluid Management
    Temperature Control
    Venous Air Emboli
    Emergence
Special Procedures
    Trauma
    Craniotomy
    Hydrocephalus
    Craniosynostosis
    Craniofacial Reconstruction
    Congenital Anomalies
    Neuroradiologic Procedures

Children requiring neurosurgical procedures present special challenges to anesthesiologists. In addition to addressing problems common to general pediatric anesthesia practice, special considerations must be given to the effects of anesthesia on the central nervous system of children with neurologic disease. This chapter emphasizes a clinical approach to the evaluation and management of these patients.

Pathophysiology

Intracranial Compartments

The skull can be compared to a rigid container with nearly incompressible contents. Under normal conditions, the intracranial space is occupied by the brain and its interstitial fluid (80%), cerebrospinal fluid (CSF) (10%), and blood (10%). In pathologic states, space-occupying lesions such as edema, tumor, hematoma, or abscess may be present. The Monro-Kellie hypothesis, elaborated in the 19th century, states that the sum of all intracranial volumes is constant. Thus, an increase in volume of one compartment must be accompanied by an approximately equal decrease in volume of the other compartments, except when the cranium can expand to accommodate a larger volume, such as in infants with open sutures, or intracranial pressure (ICP) will become elevated.[1] To a limited extent, in the nonacute situation, the brain can compensate for pathologic increases in intracranial volume by intracellular dehydration and reduction of interstitial fluid.[2–4] However, the compensatory mechanisms provided by the other compartments (CSF and blood) can be more readily altered in acute situations and are better understood.

Under normal conditions, CSF exists in dynamic equilibrium, with absorption balancing production. The rate of CSF production in adults is approximately 0.35 mL/min or 500 mL/day.[5] The average adult has approximately 100 to 150 mL of CSF distributed throughout the brain and subarachnoid space. Thus, CSF is replaced several times each day. Children have correspondingly smaller volumes of CSF, but the rate of CSF production is similar to that of adults.[5, 6] In infants with obstruction of CSF pathways, more than 100 mL/day of CSF is frequently obtained with extraventricular drainage.[7]

Production occurs primarily in the choroid plexus of the lateral, third, and fourth ventricles. Active transport of ions (sodium) occurs across the epithelial membrane of the choroid plexus into the ventricular cavities. The passive transport of water re-establishes osmotic equilibrium and results in accumulation of intraventricular CSF. Normally, CSF circulates through the aqueducts of Sylvius, the fourth ventricle, and the foramina of Luschka and Magendie, and into the subarachnoid space. Production of CSF is only slightly affected by the alterations of ICP and is usually unchanged in children with hydrocephalus.[6] Some drugs, including acetazolamide, furosemide, and steroids, are mildly effective in temporarily decreasing CSF production.[1,8, 9] There is an inverse relationship between the rate of CSF production and serum osmolality; an increase in serum osmolality causes a decrease in CSF production. Choroid plexus papillomas causing overproduction of CSF are rare, but are more likely to occur during childhood.

Absorption of CSF is not well understood, but arachnoid villi appear to be important sites for reabsorption of CSF into the venous system. One-way valves that appear to be open at about 5 mm Hg exist between the subarachnoid space and the sagittal sinus. Some reabsorption may also occur from the spinal subarachnoid space and the ependymal lining of the ventricles. Reabsorption increases with elevation of ICP. However, pathologic processes that obstruct arachnoid villi or interfere with CSF flow result in decreased CSF absorption. Such conditions include intracranial hemorrhage, infection, tumor, and congenital malformations.[10]

Translocation of CSF initially compensates for increases in intracranial volume and minimizes elevation of ICP. This translocation occurs through the foramen magnum to the distensible spinal subarachnoid space. A new equilibrium is then temporarily achieved by a decrease in the production of CSF or an increase in the rate of absorption. However, when intracranial volume surpasses these compensatory mechanisms, ICP rises precipitously, resulting in rapid clinical deterioration. Distortion of normal anatomy may obstruct CSF pathways and venous drainage, and herniation of brain tissue eventually occurs. In the presence of open fontanelles or open cranial sutures, this pathologic process may be partially attenuated by increasing head circumference. It is important to note, however, that herniation can still occur in patients with open fontanelles when severe increases in ICP develop acutely.

Intracranial Pressure

Increased ICP causes secondary brain injury by producing cerebral ischemia and ultimately herniation. Ischemia occurs when ICP increases and cerebral perfusion pressure (CPP) decreases. As cerebral blood flow (CBF) and the supply of nutrients are curtailed, cell damage and death occur, leading to increased intracellular and extracellular water and further increases in ICP. When ICP exceeds blood pressure (BP), CPP decreases, the brain becomes ischemic, and cell death occurs (Fig. 22–1).[11]

Herniation Syndromes

Several herniation syndromes exist. The most common is *transtentorial* herniation in which the uncus of the temporal lobe is displaced from the supratentorial to the infratentorial space. Compression of the third cranial nerve and brainstem results in pathognomonic signs of pupillary dilatation, hemiparesis, and loss of consciousness. If this compression is not promptly relieved, apnea, bradycardia, and death occur.

In *cerebellar* herniation, the cerebellar tonsils herniate through the foramen magnum from the posterior fossa to the cervical spinal space. Compression of the brainstem results in cardiorespiratory failure and death.

Cingulate subfalcial herniation is the most subtle herniation syndrome. An expanding hemispheric lesion creates a pressure gradient and eventually pushes brain tissue underneath the falx cerebri into the opposite hemispheric space. The displaced brain tissue compresses one or both anterior cerebral arteries, causing ischemia. These patients frequently present with loss of bladder control and contralateral lower extremity weakness, both of which are not discernible in anesthetized or comatose patients.

Herniation may also occur through an open *skull defect*, such as occurs after surgery or trauma. Bulging open fontanelles may be a manifestation of herniation in young infants.

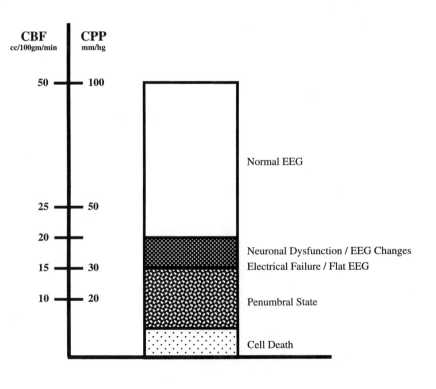

Figure 22–1. Cerebral blood flow (CBF), cerebral perfusion pressure (CPP), and brain ischemia. Changes in CBF and CPP affecting neuronal synaptic function and cellular integrity. When CBF decreases to approximately 15 to 20 mL/100 g/min, there is distinct neuronal dysfunction on the electroencephalogram (EEG). At 15 mL/100 g/min, the EEG is essentially flat, and electrical activity ceases to function. At 6 to 15 mL/100 g/min, a penumbral state occurs in which there is energy for cellular integrity but insufficient energy for synaptic function. Neuronal survival is unlikely if this low CBF is allowed to occur for more than an ill-defined but critical period of time. At less than 6 mL/100 g/min, there is no energy for cellular membrane integrity. Infarction occurs at this stage unless reperfusion is accomplished immediately.

Signs of Increased Intracranial Pressure

In children, the clinical signs of increased ICP are highly variable. Papilledema, pupillary dilatation, hypertension, and bradycardia may be absent despite intracranial hypertension, or they may occur with normal ICP.[10, 12] When associated with elevated ICP, they are usually late and dangerous signs.[13] Chronic increases in ICP are often manifested by complaints of headache, irritability, and vomiting, particularly in the morning. Papilledema may not be present even in children dying as a result of intracranial hypertension.[14] A diminished level of consciousness and abnormal motor responses to painful stimuli are frequently associated with an elevated ICP.[10] Computed tomography (CT) or magnetic resonance imaging (MRI) can reveal small or obliterated ventricles or basilar cisterns, hydrocephalus, intracranial masses, or midline shifts. Diffuse cerebral edema is a common finding when increased ICP is associated with closed head injury, encephalopathy, or encephalitis.

Monitoring Intracranial Pressure

Techniques to monitor ICP in adults have been successfully used in children.[15–17] Ventricular catheters are generally accepted as the most accurate and reliable means of measurement. They also permit removal of CSF for diagnostic or therapeutic indications. The major risks of intraventricular catheters are infection and hemorrhage, which, though rare, may cause devastating complications. In addition, these catheters may be difficult to insert precisely in the conditions in which they are needed most, as in severe cerebral edema with small ventricles. In comparison with intraventricular catheters, subarachnoid bolts can be placed when the ventricles are obliterated. This procedure minimizes trauma to brain tissue and poses less risk of serious infection and hemorrhage. The major disadvantages are that subarachnoid bolts may underestimate ICP, particularly in areas distant from their insertion site, and they are difficult to stabilize in infants with a thin calvarium. Epidural monitors that do not require a fluid interface can be implanted outside of the dura, thus avoiding the risks of CSF contamination and the limitations of fluid-dependent systems.[18, 19] Most epidural systems correlate well with intraventricular measurements, but they cannot be recalibrated once inserted. Epidural monitors have also been secured noninvasively to the open anterior fontanelle of infants and appear to reflect changes in ICP. Fiberoptic catheters with self-contained transducers can also be used to measure ICP from intraventricular, subarachnoid, or intraparenchymal sites. These monitors avoid some of the problems of external fluid-filled transducers but, like epidural transducers, cannot be recalibrated once inserted.

Normal values for ICP are generally accepted as less than 15 mm Hg. In full-term neonates, normal ICP is 2 to 6 mm Hg and is probably lower in premature infants. Children with intracranial pathology but normal ICP occasionally exhibit pressure waves, which are considered abnormal.[10] In the presence of open fontanelles, ICP may remain normal despite significant intracranial pathology; increasing head circumference may be the first clinical sign. Furthermore, bulging fontanelles may not develop, especially when the process evolves slowly.

Intracranial Compliance

The absolute value of ICP does not indicate how much compensation is possible. Clearly, if ICP is significantly elevated, compensatory mechanisms have failed. However, pathologic states may be present despite an ICP within normal range. Intracranial compliance (the change in pressure relative to the change in volume) is a valuable concept when applied to intracranial dynamics. Figure 22–2 presents a schematic relationship between the addition of volume to intracranial compartments and ICP. The actual shape of the curve depends on the time over which the volume increases and the relative size of the compartments. At normal intracranial volumes (point 1), ICP is low but compliance is high and remains so despite small increases in volume. When volume increases rapidly, compensatory abilities are surpassed; further increases in volume are reflected as increases in pressure. This can occur when the actual ICP is still within normal limits but the compliance is low (point 2). When ICP is already high, further volume expansion results in rapid ICP elevation (point 3). In clinical practice, compliance can be evaluated with a ventriculostomy catheter or by observing the response of ICP to external stimulation, for instance tracheal suction, coughing, and agitation.

Intracranial compliance is notably lower in children when compared with adults. Several physiologic and mechanical factors such as a higher ratio of brain water content, less CSF volume, and higher ratio of brain content to intracranial capacity, all contribute to a relatively decreased intracranial compliance in children.[2] Thus, pediatric patients may be at increased risk of herniation compared with adults when similar relative increases in ICP have occurred. Infants, on the other hand, if faced with a slowly increasing ICP, may have a higher compliance due to their open fontanelles and sutures.

Cerebral Blood Volume and Cerebral Blood Flow

In addition to CSF, cerebral blood volume (CBV) represents another compartment in which compensatory mechanisms influence ICP. Although the CBV occupies only a small proportion (10%) of the intracranial space, changes related to dynamic blood volume occur, often initiated by anesthesia

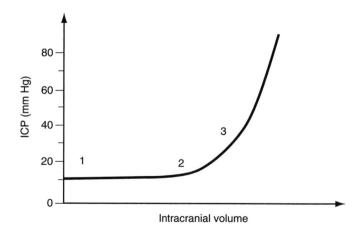

Figure 22–2. Idealized intracranial compliance curve (see text for details).

or intensive care procedures. As with other vascular beds, most intracranial blood is contained in the low-pressure, high-capacitance venous system. Increases in intracranial volume are initially met by decreases in CBV. This response is apparent in hydrocephalic infants in whom venous blood shifts from intracranial to extracranial vessels produce distended scalp veins.[20] Ultimately, increased CBV results in elevated ICP.

In a normal adult, CBF is approximately 55 mL/100 g of brain tissue per minute.[21-23] This represents almost 15% of the cardiac output for an organ that accounts for only 2% of body weight. Estimates of CBF are less uniform in the pediatric population. Normal CBF in healthy awake children is approximately 100 mL per 100 g of brain tissue per minute and can represent up to 25% of cardiac output.[24, 25] Neonates and premature infants appear to have a lower CBF (approximately 40 mL/100 g per minute) than children and adults.[26, 27] In infants, CBF is subject to modification by sleep states and feeding.[28]

Cerebral blood flow is regulated to meet the metabolic demands of the brain. In adults, the cerebral metabolic rate for oxygen ($CMRO_2$) is approximately 3.5 to 4.5 mL O_2 per 100 g per minute; in children, it is higher.[24] General anesthesia can depress $CMRO_2$ as much as 50%.[29] The coupling of CBF and $CMRO_2$ is probably mediated by the effect of local hydrogen ion concentration on cerebral vessels. Conditions that result in acidosis (hypoxemia, hypercarbia, ischemia) cause cerebrovascular dilation, which augments both CBF and CBV. Similarly, a reduction in brain metabolism ($CMRO_2$) normally reduces CBF and CBV. When autoregulation is impaired, CBF is determined by factors other than metabolic demand. When CBF exceeds metabolic requirements, luxury perfusion or hyperemia is said to exist. Many pharmacologic agents act directly on the cerebral vasculature to alter CBF and CBV.

Cerebral Perfusion Pressure

At present, CBF determinations are difficult to perform, require expensive equipment, and are limited to investigational centers. Transcranial Doppler ultrasonography appears promising but is not widely available. However, CPP is a helpful guide to the adequacy of the cerebral circulation. CPP is defined as the pressure gradient across the brain and is the difference between mean systemic arterial pressure ($\overline{BP}$) at the entrance to the brain minus mean exit pressure (mean central venous pressure). When ICP is elevated, it replaces venous pressure in the calculation of CPP. In supine patients, mean CPP can, for practical purposes, be considered to equal $\overline{BP}$ minus the mean ICP ($CPP = \overline{BP} - \overline{ICP}$). If the brain and heart are positioned at different levels, all pressures should be referenced at the level of the head (external auditory meatus).

Cerebrovascular Autoregulation

Effects of Blood Pressure

In adults, CBF remains relatively constant within a $\overline{\overline{BP}}$ range of 50 to 150 mm Hg (Fig. 22–3). Autoregulation enables brain perfusion to remain stable despite moderate changes in $\overline{BP}$ or ICP. Normally, with low ICP and low venous

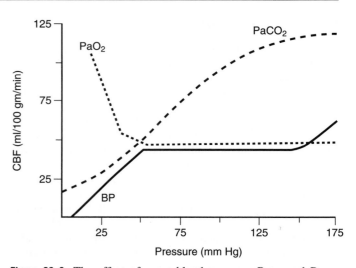

Figure 22–3. The effect of mean blood pressure, PaO_2, and $PaCO_2$ on cerebral blood flow (CBF) in the normal brain. (From Shapiro HM: Intracranial hypertension: Therapeutic and anesthetic considerations. Anesthesiology 1975;43:447.)

pressure, $\overline{BP}$ approximates CPP. Beyond the range of autoregulation, CBF becomes pressure dependent. In chronic hypertensive cases, both the upper and lower limits of autoregulation are elevated. Cerebral autoregulation is abolished by acidosis, tumor, cerebral edema, vascular malformations, and various drugs, even at sites far removed from a discrete lesion.[21]

Autoregulation is partially mediated by myogenic control of arteriolar resistance. When CPP decreases, cerebral vessels dilate to maintain CBF, thereby increasing CBV. When CPP increases, cerebral vasoconstriction occurs and CBF is maintained with a lower CBV. Outside the limits of autoregulation, CBF becomes passively dependent on changes in CPP. Even small BP decreases may then result in ischemia, whereas BP elevations increase CBF and, therefore, ICP. Abrupt elevations in BP disrupt autoregulatory mechanisms and result in vasodilation, increased CBF, and cerebral edema. The duration of this breakthrough and the rate at which normal autoregulation is re-established vary greatly.

The limits of autoregulation are not known for normal infants and children; autoregulation probably occurs at lower absolute values than in adults.[30] Although the lower limit of autoregulation in adults is approximately 50 mm Hg, this BP is not usually reached until the first weeks of life. Intact autoregulatory mechanisms have been demonstrated within lower BP ranges in newborn animals when compared with those in mature animals.[31] Cerebral autoregulation may be abolished in critically ill humans.[32]

Effects of Oxygen

Cerebral blood flow remains constant within a wide range of oxygenation. When the partial pressure of arterial O_2 (PaO_2) falls below 50 mm Hg, CBF increases exponentially in adults such that at a PaO_2 of 15 mm Hg, CBF is approximately four times normal (see Fig. 22–3).[33] The resultant increase in CBV causes a marked elevation in ICP when intracranial compliance is low; the lower limit for PaO_2 is probably less in neonates. It is important to remember that O_2 delivery is more important than actual PaO_2 level. Evidence suggests that hyperoxia decreases CBF. Early studies by Kety and Schmidt demonstrated only a 10% decrease in CBF in adults breathing 100% O_2; however, decreases of 33% have been reported in neonates.[34, 35]

Effects of Carbon Dioxide

There is a linear relationship between the arterial partial pressure of carbon dioxide ($PaCO_2$) and CBF (see Fig. 22–3). In adults, a 1 mm Hg increase in $PaCO_2$ increases CBF approximately 2 mL/100 g/min.[34] More importantly, these changes in the magnitude and direction of CBF have been demonstrated to parallel those of CBV. The ability of CBF and therefore of CBV to change with $PaCO_2$ is the basis for hyperventilation to reduce ICP. Likewise, increases in $PaCO_2$ result in elevated CBF, although it appears that the limits at which this occurs in neonates differ from the limits in adults.[36] Similarly, there is little information about the extent and duration of cerebrovascular responsiveness to hyperventilation in brain-injured and critically ill patients, particularly in the pediatric population. Moderate hyperventilation is, however, frequently utilized to lower ICP acutely, although prolonged hyperventilation may be detrimental, at least in head-injured patients.[37, 38]

It has been suggested that extreme hyperventilation to $PaCO_2$ less than 20 mm Hg may be associated with regional or global ischemia by reducing CBF to levels below that required for adequate cerebral perfusion.[39] Others maintain that there is no recognized lower limit for $PaCO_2$. There are certainly anecdotal reports of children in the intensive care setting who appear to benefit acutely by hyperventilation to a $PaCO_2$ in the range of 15 to 20 mm Hg to control ICP. Whatever the extent of hyperventilation and hypercarbia, it is important to maintain hemodynamic stability and adequate perfusion pressure, because systemic hypotension, often associated with extreme hyperventilation, can compromise CBF.

Autoregulation of CBF is impaired in areas of damaged brain.[40] Blood vessels in an ischemic zone are subject to hypoxemia, hypercarbia, and acidosis, which are potent stimuli for vasodilation. These vessels develop maximally reduced cerebrovascular tone or vasomotor paralysis. Furthermore, small localized lesions may result in impaired autoregulation in areas far removed from the site of injury.[21] The extent of autoregulatory impairment is variable in brain-damaged patients. Techniques that measure global CBF may not detect localized changes. CBF determinations have shown that a common response to head injury in pediatric patients is early hyperemia and increased CBF. Although ICP may be initially normal, intracranial compliance is significantly reduced.

To summarize, a normal brain has several regulatory mechanisms that match cerebral blood supply to metabolic demand. Loss of regional or global autoregulation is common in a wide variety of pathologic processes. An injured brain is less able to compensate for increases in intracranial volume. Knowledge of normal brain physiology and the changes that occur during pathologic states forms the basis for the safe anesthetic management of pediatric neurosurgical patients.

Anesthetic Management

Preoperative Evaluation

History

Preoperative evaluation of pediatric patients is discussed in Chapter 4. However, certain aspects of this evaluation are of special relevance to neurosurgical patients. The duration and severity of illness often vary greatly. Some patients have a history of multiple surgical procedures and complex medical problems. Significant developmental delays or neuromuscular impairments are also common in this patient population. Others have been completely healthy until the onset of their symptoms. The anesthetic plan, including postoperative care, needs to consider the particulars of each patient and disease state.

A history of food or drug allergies, eczema, or asthma may provide a warning of an adverse reaction to contrast agents frequently used in neuroradiologic procedures. Special attention should be given to symptoms of allergy to latex products, such as lip swelling after blowing up a balloon, because anaphylaxis has been reported in a number of children who have undergone multiple previous operations, especially patients with meningomyeloceles.[41]

Pediatric diseases that may influence anesthetic decisions should be sought. For example, the choice of induction method may be modified by a history of severe asthma or symptomatic esophageal reflux. Recurrent croup may influence the choice of endotracheal tube size. Enlarged adenoids make nasotracheal intubation more difficult, and a history of obstructive sleep apnea has important implications for postoperative monitoring. Protracted vomiting, anorexia, enuresis, or excessive urination should prompt careful evaluation of hydration and electrolytes. Diabetes insipidus and inappropriate secretion of antidiuretic hormone are common in this population. A history of the use of aspirin or aspirin-containing remedies for headaches or respiratory tract infections is information that is not usually spontaneously offered by parents yet has important implications for operative and postoperative bleeding. Steroids are often initiated at the time of diagnosis of intracranial tumors; they need to be continued and often augmented in the perioperative period. Therapeutic levels of anticonvulsants should be verified preoperatively and maintained perioperatively. Patients on long-term anticonvulsants may develop toxicity, especially if seizures are difficult to control; this is frequently manifest with abnormalities in hematologic or hepatic function, or both. Patients on chronic anticonvulsant therapy may also require increased amounts of sedatives, nondepolarizing muscle relaxants, and narcotics because of enhanced metabolism of these drugs.[42–44]

Physical Examination

The physical examination should include a brief neurologic evaluation, including level of consciousness, motor and sensory function, normal and pathologic reflexes, integrity of the cranial nerves, and signs and symptoms of intracranial hypertension. Examination of pupillary size and responsiveness can detect benign anisocoria. Preoperative respiratory assessment should specifically include the effects of motor weakness, impaired gag and swallowing mechanisms, and evidence of active pulmonary disease such as aspiration pneumonia. Evidence of muscle atrophy and weakness should be noted, since up-regulation of acetylcholine receptors may precipitate sudden hyperkalemia following succinylcholine administration and induce resistance to nondepolarizing muscle relaxants in the affected limbs.[45] Body weight should be accurately measured to guide the administration of drugs, fluids, and blood products. Physical signs of dehydration (see Table 11–9) should be noted, especially in patients who have been chronically ill or receiving osmotic or diuretic agents.

Laboratory and Radiologic Evaluation

In all but the most minor procedures, laboratory data should include a hematocrit determination. Blood typing and cross-matching should be performed for any major procedure. The need for additional studies, such as evaluation of coagulation parameters, serum electrolyte levels and osmolality, and blood urea nitrogen and creatinine values, as well as arterial blood gas analysis, chest radiograph, or electrocardiogram are made on an individual basis. Liver function tests and a hematologic profile should be obtained if not recently reviewed in children taking long-term anticonvulsants. Specific neuroradiologic studies are usually obtained by the neurosurgeon and should also be reviewed by the anesthesiologist. For example, the anesthesiologist should know which children with a ventriculoperitoneal shunt have "slit ventricles," since these patients have special risks in the perioperative period[46] (see section on hydrocephalus). In addition, the amount of sedation necessary to perform radiologic studies may also be helpful in planning the induction of anesthesia. Preoperative neurophysiologic studies, including electroencephalography and evoked potentials, may provide a baseline for comparison for intraoperative and postoperative evaluations.

Preoperative Discussions

Once a patient has been fully assessed, it is important to discuss the case with the entire surgical team involved—the neurosurgeons, nurses, and, when appropriate, neurophysiologists. Each part of the team has their own concerns such as position of the patient during surgery, equipment needed, type of anesthetic technique to be used, and so on. Communication is important so that everyone understands what is planned.

It is also vital to have a thorough and candid discussion with the patient's parents (and with the patient, when age-appropriate). They should be able to confirm their understanding of the planned procedure, including the site of operation, and be aware, when applicable, of the specific needs for invasive monitoring, blood products, and postoperative intensive care. They should have an opportunity to have all their questions answered and understand the consent form they are asked to sign.

Premedication

Children are usually frightened by their illness, the hospital environment, and disruption of their routines; they are most readily consoled by their parents. Preschoolers may have only a superficial cognitive understanding of their condition and may respond to the anxiety of their parents. Older children and adolescents are likely to be appropriately nervous about the surgical procedure and its long-term implications. Sedation is usually withheld from pediatric neurosurgical patients until they arrive in the preoperative area to avoid the problem of an oversedated, neurologically impaired patient with inadequate supervision. An exception is the rare child with an intracranial aneurysm or arteriovenous malformation that has recently bled in whom premedication may be warranted to avoid agitation. Narcotics are best withheld preoperatively, since they may cause nausea or respiratory depression, especially in patients with increased ICP; sedatives alone are generally adequate to relieve anxiety. Atropine is not usually administered because its vagolytic effect often dissipates by the time of induction and its drying effect is disturbing to patients.

Sedatives are administered in the parents' presence to facilitate a smooth separation and induction. Midazolam (0.5–1.0 mg/kg) may be given orally; it usually requires 5 to 20 minutes to take effect. Alternatively, an intravenous catheter can be inserted following application of EMLA cream. Incremental doses of intravenous midazolam may then be carefully titrated. Another method is to administer barbiturates rectally (methohexital, 20–30 mg/kg, given as a 10% solution in sterile water or saline). Rectal barbiturates probably lower ICP in a manner similar to intravenous barbiturates, provided that airway obstruction is avoided. Methohexital lowers the seizure threshold in patients with psychomotor and temporal lobe epilepsy and is best avoided in these situations.[47] Rectal thiopental in the same dose is a reasonable alternative in these circumstances. The risk of severe respiratory depression may be increased in patients who have myelodysplasia and are given rectal methohexital; special caution should be exercised in these patients.[48]

Monitoring

Minimal monitoring for pediatric neuroanesthesia includes a stethoscope (precordial or esophageal), electrocardiogram, pulse oximeter, blood pressure (by auscultation, palpation, oscillometry, Doppler, automated electronic method, invasive arterial catheter), capnogram, and temperature. Neuromuscular blockade monitoring is also important, but nerve stimulators may give misleading information about the extent of relaxation if applied to a denervated extremity. When paresis is present, nerve stimulation should be at a site of normal neurologic function. A precordial Doppler monitor should be used in patients undergoing craniotomy, because the relatively large head size of children places them at particular risk for air emboli. Monitoring devices for ICP are used for the same indications as in adults. Intraoperative electroencephalogram and electrophysiologic (EP) monitoring require advanced coordination among the neurosurgeon, anesthesiologist, and neurophysiologist. Urinary output should be quantitated during prolonged procedures, in cases with anticipated large blood loss, and when diuretics or osmotic agents are administered. An infant feeding tube may be substituted for a urinary catheter in small infants; collection into a syringe may facilitate assessment of hourly output.

In general, an arterial catheter is placed for all craniotomies because of the potential for sudden and severe hemodynamic changes. *Small patient size should not preclude the use of invasive monitoring and may actually be an indication for a more aggressive approach.* An increase in the paradox in the arterial pressure waveform with positive pressure ventilation is often the best indication of intravascular volume deficiency and the need for fluid replacement (see Fig. 12–7). Intra-arterial catheters (22- to 24-gauge) can be placed percutaneously in the radial, dorsalis pedis or posterior tibial arteries even in small infants; it is rarely necessary to resort to surgical cutdown. The arterial transducer should be zeroed at the level of the head if the head and heart positions differ so that CPP can accurately be assessed. The lateral corner of the eye or the external auditory meatus approximate the level of the foramen of Monro and are convenient landmarks. In the first days of life, both the umbilical artery and the umbilical vein can be cannulated. These catheters should be discontinued as soon as alternative access is established because of the potential for serious complications.

Central venous cannulation may be indicated for procedures involving major blood loss or possible air emboli. Percutaneous central venous cannulation (external or internal jugular, femoral, or subclavian veins) using the Seldinger technique is possible even in the smallest infants. However, in children undergoing neurosurgical resections, it is often best to access the femoral vein, thereby avoiding the Trendelenburg position and the risk of accidental carotid artery puncture and hematoma formation, which could compromise both cerebral blood flow and venous drainage. Cannulation of antecubital veins may also provide central venous access but is technically difficult in small patients. When rapid blood loss is a consideration in a small child in whom adequate peripheral venous access is difficult to obtain, a single-lumen, large-bore catheter is most commonly inserted in a femoral vein. Multilumen central venous catheters are inadequate for rapid blood transfusion. All central catheters should be removed as soon as possible after the procedure to minimize the risk of central venous thrombosis developing.

Induction

Pediatric neurosurgical patients present various clinical problems that may appear to have contradictory solutions. These include decreased intracranial compliance, increased risk of regurgitation and aspiration, a potentially difficult airway and intravenous access, and poor cooperation. Careful evaluation of the severity of each problem helps the anesthesiologist prioritize concerns and decide on the safest method of induction. In the presence of decreased intracranial compliance, the primary goal during induction is to minimize severe increases in ICP. In general, most intravenous drugs decrease CBF and metabolism and, therefore, ICP.[49] Barbiturates are usually the induction agents of choice because they do not cause pain with injection in small intravenous catheters. Thiopental (4–8 mg/kg) is most frequently used. Propofol (2–5 mg/kg) appears to have similar cerebral properties, plus an antiemetic effect; however, its antiemetic effect is usually not relevant for lengthy procedures. Etomidate, a possible neuroprotective agent, can also be used if hemodynamic stability is a concern.[50–52] Ketamine should be avoided because of its known ability to increase cerebral metabolism,

CBF, and ICP. Sudden increases in ICP have been reported following ketamine administration, especially in infants and children with hydrocephalus.[53, 54]

Other measures to lower ICP during induction include controlled hyperventilation and administration of fentanyl and supplemental barbiturates before laryngoscopy and intubation. Lidocaine (1.0–1.5 mg/kg) has also been shown to limit elevation of ICP when administered several minutes before laryngoscopy.[55] However, it is probably no more effective than additional barbiturate or narcotic and may lower the seizure threshold.

Rectal barbiturates are particularly useful in children younger than 5 years who resist separation from their parents. Alternatively, oral midazolam is an effective anxiolytic without causing the same degree of sedation as methohexital. Once consciousness is blunted, an intravenous catheter is placed or an inhalation induction is performed.

Sevoflurane has replaced halothane for inhaled inductions because of its more rapid onset and high patient acceptability. It rarely may be associated with bradycardia or cardiovascular depression when administered to small infants. In cases in which the ICP is elevated but the patient is not considered to have a "true" full stomach, that is, they have been without oral intake for many hours, and yet intravenous access is very difficult, inhalation of sevoflurane to light levels of anesthesia may be used to facilitate insertion of an intravenous catheter. Similar to isoflurane in its cerebral physiologic effects, sevoflurane with hyperventilation appears to blunt the increase in ICP secondary to cerebral vasodilatation from volatile anesthetic agents alone.[56–58] Sevoflurane may offer an additional advantage because it causes less myocardial depression compared with halothane.[59] Finally, any patient in whom succinylcholine is contraindicated should not undergo an inhalational induction, since laryngospasm is always a possibility. Inhalational inductions should be avoided in these patients until a nondepolarizing agent with a very rapid onset that can be administered intramuscularly is developed.

A common problem is an uncooperative toddler who has an intracranial tumor and moderately decreased intracranial compliance, yet is agitated and resistant to separation from parents. Some clinicians advocate the use of rectal barbiturates with meticulous attention to airway maintenance to avoid obstruction and resultant hypercarbia and hypoxemia. Others would argue that a crying, agitated child has demonstrated a tolerance to increased ICP and that intravenous induction is safer. Fortunately (for the anesthesiologist, though not for the patient), patients who have severe intracranial hypertension generally have a decreased level of consciousness and it becomes easier to insert an intravenous catheter in those situations when it is most necessary.

Airway Management and Intubation

It is crucial that airway management be effective and smooth to avoid the ICP-increasing effects of hypoxemia, hypercarbia, and coughing. Controlled hyperventilation, narcotic administration, and supplemental barbiturates before intubation improve cerebral compliance and minimize increases in ICP caused by laryngoscopy and intubation.

Oral intubation is often preferred because it is expeditious and minimizes airway stimulation and duration of apnea; it certainly is the technique of choice when a rapid-sequence induction is indicated. Once the airway is secured and an adequate depth of anesthesia ensured, an oral endotracheal tube can be readily exchanged for a nasotracheal tube. Nasotracheal intubation offers the advantage of increased stability and increased comfort for patients when postoperative intubation is necessary. Nasotracheal tubes are usually used for pediatric patients who will be in the prone position and whose airway will be inaccessible during the surgical procedure (such as a posterior fossa craniotomy).

Contraindications to nasal intubation include choanal stenosis, potential basilar skull fracture, transphenoidal procedures, and risk for sinusitis. If nasotracheal intubation is planned, it is advantageous to prepare the nares with topical vasoconstrictors to minimize the risk of bleeding. Vasoconstrictors should not be sprayed into the nose, since they are rapidly and effectively absorbed and can produce hypertension. Placing a few drops of 0.25% phenylephrine (Neo-Synephrine) on cotton-tipped applicators and positioning them in the nares, against the nasal mucosa, will prevent overdosages and has the added benefit of helping gauge the patency of the nasal passage once sleep has been induced. Whichever route is chosen for intubation, it is important to secure the endotracheal tube with liberal amounts of tincture of benzoin and waterproof tape; waterproof adhesive dressings can also protect the tape from surgical preparation solutions. If an oral endotracheal tube is used, it should be placed on the side of the mouth that will be upward so that draining oral secretions will not loosen the tape.

In prolonged combined neurosurgical and craniofacial reconstructions, the endotracheal tube may be sutured to the nasal septum or wired to the teeth. A nasogastric or orogastric tube is inserted after intubation to decompress the stomach and evacuate gastric contents; leaving it open to gravity drainage during the case will prevent positive pressure from building up in the stomach should air leak around an uncuffed endotracheal tube. Finally, the patient's eyes should be closed and covered with a large, clear, waterproof dressing. Placing lubricant in the eyes prior to this has not been shown to reduce the risk of corneal abrasions.[60] In children, application of lubricant to the eyes may actually increase the risk of corneal abrasions, since pediatric patients will often scratch their eyes in the postoperative period if their vision has been blurred by lubricating ointments.

Muscle Relaxants

Because of its rapid onset and brief duration of action, succinylcholine is frequently used to facilitate intubation in patients with a full stomach. The intubating dose is 1 to 2 mg/kg IV or 3 to 5 mg/kg IM.[61] In children it is safest to precede this with atropine (0.01–0.02 mg/kg, minimum dose 0.1 mg) to prevent bradycardia. Increases in ICP due to succinylcholine usually are not clinically significant[62]; they may be minimized by pretreatment with a nondepolarizing muscle relaxant.[63] However, this may make succinylcholine less effective, even when the dose of succinylcholine is increased. Succinylcholine is contraindicated in those situations when it may induce life-threatening hyperkalemia in the presence of denervation injuries due to various causes, including severe head trauma, crush injury, burns, spinal

cord dysfunction, encephalitis, multiple sclerosis, stroke, and tetanus.[64]

Alternatively, nondepolarizing muscle relaxants such as rocuronium, pancuronium, cisatracurium, or vecuronium may be used but most have a slower onset than succinylcholine. However, when rocuronium is administered in sufficiently large doses (1.2 mg/kg), the onset of action is hastened and approaches that of succinylcholine.[65] Careful application of cricoid pressure to occlude the esophagus during manual hyperventilation may be used when succinylcholine is contraindicated. Pancuronium is particularly useful in infants, because its vagolytic properties increase heart rate and maintain cardiac output, especially when fentanyl is also administered. Other nondepolarizing muscle relaxants can also be used when combined with fentanyl but may be associated with bradycardia unless atropine is administered. If the neurosurgeon plans direct nerve stimulation, muscle relaxants should be allowed to dissipate after induction. As noted earlier, the amount of most nondepolarizing muscle relaxants necessary to maintain paralysis is increased in patients receiving chronic anticonvulsant medications, although cisatracurium, like atracurium, has not shown this tendency, probably because of its unique metabolism with Hoffman elimination.[66]

Positioning

Positioning is an especially important consideration in pediatric neuroanesthesia. Children with increased ICP should be transported to the preoperative holding area and operating room with the head elevated in the midline position to maximize cerebral venous drainage.

Once a patient is in the operating room, the neurosurgeons and anesthesiologists all must have adequate access to the patient. In infants and small children, slight displacement of the endotracheal tube can result in extubation or endobronchial intubation. During prolonged procedures, it is important for the anesthesiologist to be able to visually inspect the endotracheal tube and circuit connections, and to suction the endotracheal tube when necessary. Using proper draping and a flashlight, one can create a "tunnel" to ensure access to the airway. It is also important to position the head to avoid soft tissue and ischemic nerve damage. Generally this is not a problem since patients are often placed in pins in a Mayfield head holder. It can be a concern, however, when patients are positioned on a cerebellar headrest. Adequate padding should be used in such situations (Figs. 22–4 and 22–5). Extreme head flexion can cause brainstem compression in patients with posterior fossa pathology, such as mass lesions or an Arnold-Chiari malformation. Extreme flexion can also cause high cervical spinal cord ischemia, endotracheal tube obstruction by kinking, displacement of the endotracheal tube to the carina, or its movement into the right mainstem bronchus.[67]

Intravascular catheters should also be accessible for visual inspection. Luer-lock connections are recommended because unobserved disconnection may result in exsanguination. Intravascular catheters may infiltrate, causing local soft tissue damage and extravascular administration of fluids, blood products, and medications. The patient's eyes should be closed and covered with a waterproof dressing. Additional protective padding such as gauze pads or foam can be

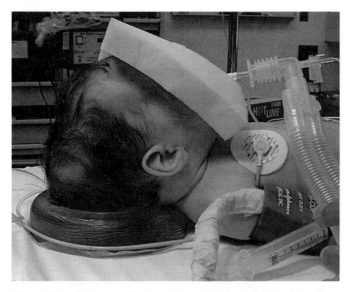

Figure 22–4. Protective foam padding placed on the face after intubation but prior to prone positioning.

placed over the face and eyes if necessary. In combined craniofacial-neurosurgical reconstructions, the eyelids may be sutured closed. Extremities should be secured in a neutral position and well padded. It is important to avoid stretching peripheral nerves and to prevent skin and soft tissue pressure injury due to direct contact with surgical accessories such as instrument stands and grounding wires (see Fig. 22–5). It is also important to ensure that any extremities that are not directly visible to the anesthesiologist (such as those on the opposite side of the operating room table) cannot fall off the table during the procedure, even if the position of the table is changed during surgery. In older children and adolescents undergoing prolonged procedures, the legs may be wrapped to prevent venous pooling or pneumatic stockings may be utilized.

Prone Position

The prone position is commonly used for posterior fossa and spinal cord surgery. Extensive padding is necessary to prevent a wide spectrum of compression and stretch injuries. The torso is usually supported by padding under the chest

and pelvis. It is important to ensure free abdominal wall motion because increased intra-abdominal pressure may impair ventilation, cause vena cava compression, and increase epidural venous pressure and bleeding. The easiest way to do this is to place "jelly" rolls or rolled blankets laterally on each side of the patient's chest running from the shoulders toward the pelvis. A separate jelly roll or rolled blanket under the pelvis may occasionally be necessary in larger children. It is important to be sure that these rolls do not press into the flexed hips or compress the femoral nerve or the genitalia. Placing the rolls in this position should also allow a transthoracic Doppler monitor to be easily placed on the anterior chest without undue pressure.

There are several different ways to position the head. It may simply be rotated and supported by padding, with care taken to avoid direct pressure on the eyes and nose and to keep the pinna of the ears flat. For infants and toddlers, a cerebellar head frame is another alternative when the cranium is too thin for pins. In this situation, the child's forehead and cheeks rest on a well-padded head frame and the eyes are free in the center of the horseshoe-shaped support. Most surgeons prefer head pins and a head frame for older patients. A nasotracheal tube can enhance stability, especially in the prone position. One should ensure that the nasotracheal tube is properly positioned (after taping) and does not cause a mainstem intubation during positioning for surgery. This can be ensured by flexing the patient's head onto the chest while the patient is still in the supine position. Care should be taken that the upper nares are free from pressure caused by an upturned endotracheal or nasogastric tube, and the tape used to hold other tubes (gastric, esophageal) should not adhere to the endotracheal tube tape so that accidental dislodgment of these other devices does not result in extubation. The breathing circuit should be suspended from the operating table and all connections reinforced. One should always have an emergency plan to turn the patient to the supine position should this suddenly become necessary; therefore, the patient's bed should always be readily available.[68]

Significant airway edema may develop in a patient who is in the prone position for a lengthy period of time. Oral airways are best avoided for this reason since they can also result in significant edema of the tongue. Rarely, prophylactic postoperative intubation may be necessary if a great deal of facial swelling has developed during a lengthy operation

Figure 22–5. Patient positioned prone prior to surgery.

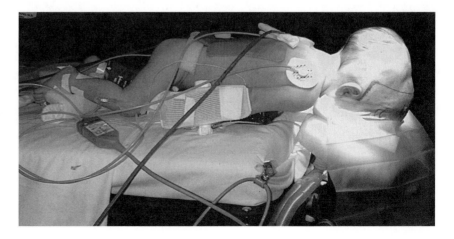

and no air leak can be heard around an endotracheal tube when the cuff is deflated.

Modified Lateral Position

Insertion or revision of ventriculoperitoneal shunts may require that the supine patient be rotated to a semilateral position. This is accomplished by placing rolls under the patient's shoulder and side. The dependent shoulder and arm should be placed in a neutral position to avoid injury to the brachial plexus and peripheral nerves. The knees are supported in a slightly flexed position and the heels padded. This position is also used for some temporal and parietal craniotomies.

Sitting Position

Fortunately, the sitting position is used less commonly in pediatric neurosurgical procedures and is rarely used in children younger than 3 years of age. When it is used, however, all precautions to prevent hypotension and air embolism must be meticulously followed. The lower extremities are wrapped in elastic bandages, and positioning is undertaken gradually with continuous monitoring. The head must be carefully flexed to avoid kinking the endotracheal tube, advancing it into a bronchial position, or compressing the chin on the chest (which can block venous and lymphatic drainage of the tongue). Extreme flexion can also result in brainstem or cervical spinal cord ischemia, or both. As in the prone position, nasotracheal tubes are often inserted because they are more secure. The patient's upper extremities are supported and padded in the patient's lap. All pressure points and extremities must be well-padded to prevent peripheral nerve (especially sciatic, brachial plexus, and peroneal) damage and to avoid pressure sores. Control levers to lower the head position should be easily accessible to the anesthesiologist and unencumbered by wires and drapes (Fig. 22–6).

Local Anesthesia

It is helpful for the neurosurgeon to infiltrate local anesthesia into the scalp prior to incision. This not only aids the anesthesiologist by providing some degree of analgesia, but the epinephrine contained within the solution will reduce scalp blood loss. If 0.25% bupivacaine with 1:200,000 epinephrine is utilized, a dose of 0.5 mL/kg is safe to administer. This will deliver 1.25 mg/kg of bupivacaine and 2.5 μg/kg of epinephrine, both well within the safe range, even if some of the drug is accidentally administered intravenously. When greater volumes are required, the solution can be diluted with an equal volume of normal saline. This still is effective for both vasoconstriction and a prolonged sensory block in the postoperative period. Specific nerve blocks of the supraorbital and supratrochlear nerves may provide analgesia to the frontal area to the mid-coronal portion of the occiput.[69] Blockade of the greater occipital nerve will provide analgesia to the posterior of the occiput to the mid-coronal area of the occiput (see Figs. 28–12 to 28–14).[70, 71]

Maintenance

General anesthesia is required for most therapeutic as well as many diagnostic procedures. Ventilation is controlled whenever intracranial hypertension is a concern, and in all infants. Although spontaneous ventilation provides another indication of brainstem function, its disadvantages (hypoventilation, increased potential for air embolism) are outweighed by the safety of controlled hyperventilation.

Maintenance of general anesthesia can be accomplished using inhalation anesthetics, intravenous infusions, or a combination of these. Agents that decrease ICP and $CMRO_2$ and maintain CPP are most desirable (Table 22–1). The commonly used volatile agents generally uncouple CBF and $CMRO_2$ such that CBF increases while $CMRO_2$ decreases. All potent inhalation agents are cerebral vasodilators (thus causing increases in both CBF and ICP). Low doses of

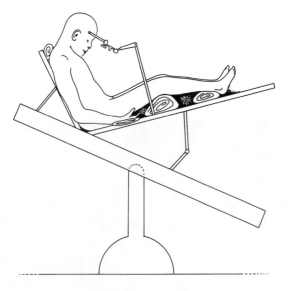

OPERATIVE POSITION

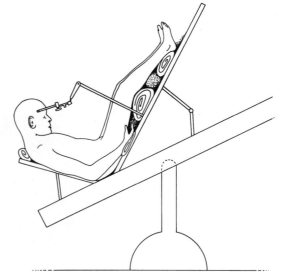

RESUSCITATION POSITION

Figure 22–6. Resuscitation from the modified standard sitting position. Normal operative position (A), and resuscitation position (B). Note that the position can be expeditiously changed by one control of the operating table.

Table 22–1. Neurophysiologic Effects of Common Anesthetic Agents

	MAP	CBF	CPP	ICP	CMRO$_2$	CSF Production	CSF Absorption	SSEP Amplitude	SSEP Latency
Nitrous Oxide	Ø/↓	↑-↑↑	↓	↑-↑↑	↓↑	↑↓	↑↓	↓	↑-Ø
Volatile Agents									
Halothane	↓↓	↑↑↑	↑↑	↑↑	↓↓	↑↓	Ø/↓	↓	↑
Enflurane	↓↓	↑↑	↑↑	↑↑	↓↓	↑	↓	↓	↑
Isoflurane	↓↓	↑	↑↑	↑	↓↓↓	↓↑	↑	↓	↑
Sevoflurane	↓↓	↑	↑	↑	↓↓↓		↑	↓	↑
Desflurane	↓↓	↑	↑	↑	↓	↑	↓	↓	↑
Hypnotics									
Thiopental	↓↓	↓↓↓	↑↑↑	↓↓↓	↓↓↓	↑↓	↑	↓	↑
Propofol	↓↓↓	↓↓↓	↑↑	↓↓	↓↓↓			↑	↑
Etomidate	Ø/↓	↓↓↓	↑↑	↓↓↓	↓↓↓	↑↓	↑	↑	Ø
Ketamine	↑↑	↑↑↑	↑↑↑	↑↑↑	↑	↑↓	↓	↑	Ø
Benzodiazepine	Ø/↓	↓↓	↑	Ø/↓	↓↓	↑↓	↑	↓	Ø-↑
Narcotics	Ø/↓	↓	↑↓	Ø/↓	↓	↑↓	↑	↓	↑
Droperidol	↓↓	↓	↑	↓	Ø/↓				

CBF, cerebral blood flow; CMRO$_2$, cerebral metabolic rate for oxygen; CPP, cerebral perfusion pressure; CSF, cerebrospinal fluid; ICP, intracranial pressure; MAP, mean arterial pressure; Ø, no change; SSEP, somatosensory evoked potential.

isoflurane, sevoflurane, or desflurane, combined with hyperventilation, cause minimal changes in CBF and ICP.[56, 57, 72] Isoflurane is usually the volatile agent of choice in maintenance of neuroanesthesia. At two times the minimum alveolar concentration (MAC), it can induce a level of anesthesia associated with an isoelectric EEG while, unlike several other volatile agents, still maintaining hemodynamic stability. Enflurane is rarely used because it may be epileptogenic, especially when combined with hyperventilation.[73] One controlled study has demonstrated a similar effect with sevoflurane and hyperventilation, but the clinical implications of this are yet to be defined.[74] When induction is completed and the airway controlled, isoflurane is most commonly used for maintenance because it is relatively inexpensive, especially when used with low-flow anesthesia. It can be discontinued during surgical closure, permitting early awakening and neurologic examination.

All halogenated agents cause dose-dependent myocardial depression, some degree of peripheral vasodilatation, and systemic hypotension. These effects make their use in the sitting position more hazardous. Nitrous oxide is usually used in combination with a low-dose volatile agent and opioids. Nitrous oxide is contraindicated, however, if the patient has undergone a recent craniotomy (within the past few weeks) since air can remain in the head for prolonged periods following previous surgery.[75] In this situation, high-dose opioid combined with an anxiolytic (benzodiazepine) or a higher dose volatile agent in oxygen may be used initially and nitrous oxide added once the dura is opened to avoid the risk of a tension pneumocephalus.

Fentanyl is generally administered when a narcotic technique is chosen because it is easily titratable with minimal side effects. A common loading dose is 10 μg/kg, although it is best to give this amount in divided doses (part at induction and part before incision) because of the delay generally associated with neurosurgical preparation. A dose of 2 μg/kg/hour is then usually adequate for maintenance, although some children, particularly those receiving chronic anticonvulsants, may require more (>3 μg/kg/hr). An ultra-short-acting narcotic such as remifentanil may also be used, but must be administered by continuous infusion (see Chapter 8). Short-acting narcotics have minimal postoperative effects, and thus hypertension due to the onset of pain can rapidly develop when these infusions are discontinued unless other longer-acting narcotics have been administered in advance.[76]

Blood and Fluid Management

Blood loss is difficult to estimate accurately in neurosurgical procedures, because much of the loss is absorbed by the operative drapes and the surgical field is difficult for the anesthesiologist to visualize. Irrigation solutions also confuse sponge weights and suction measurements. Accuracy can be improved if all suctioned blood is collected in calibrated containers visible to the anesthesiologist. Much blood loss occurs during the initial surgical exposure because of the scalp's marked vascularity. Although bleeding from bone is difficult to control, blood loss from the scalp can be decreased by the subcutaneous infiltration of dilute local anesthetic and epinephrine solutions prior to surgical incision.

Blood and fluid management is discussed in Chapters 11 and 12. However, disruption of the blood-brain barrier by underlying pathologic processes, trauma, or surgery predisposes neurosurgical patients to cerebral edema, which may be exacerbated by excessive administration of intravenous fluids. Intravenous fluid administration concerns in neurosurgical anesthesia involve (1) cerebral perfusion, (2) cerebral edema, (3) water and sodium homeostasis, and (4) serum glucose concentration.

When large blood loss is expected and blood transfusion is highly likely, it is best to begin blood transfusions at the beginning of surgery rather than to wait until the patient becomes severely anemic. In such situations, blood replacement on a milliliter for milliliter basis is appropriate. In most cases, however, blood transfusions are not anticipated and attempts should be made to avoid administration of blood products with their associated risks. In such situations, crystalloid solutions are administered. Although there remains controversy based on conflicting studies regarding the use of crystalloid versus colloid solutions in neurosurgical patients, most investigators believe that osmotic pressure gradients are more important than oncotic pressure gradients when trying to avoid cerebral edema. Thus, unless indicated by a specific situation, crystalloid solutions are the main intravenous solutions administered during most neurosurgical procedures. Lactated Ringer solution is not considered a truly isotonic solution, since its osmolality is 273 mOsm/L (normal being 285 to 290 mOsm/L). Normal saline is slightly hypertonic (308 mOsm/L) and is generally the fluid of choice since reduction of serum osmolality is not desirable. However, rapid infusion of normal saline in large amounts has been associated with hyperchloremic metabolic acidosis.[77] Should there be large fluid requirements for a case, alternating bags of lactated Ringer solution with normal saline will minimize the risk of hypernatremia and acidosis and still avoid hypoosmolality.

Inducing dehydration with osmotic and loop diuretics is a useful strategy to minimize cerebral edema and provide an optimal surgical field. However, one must be aware of the potential for hypotension and rebound effects associated with their use. Rapid administration of hypertonic solutions can cause profound but transient hypotension due to peripheral vasodilation.[78] Glucose-containing solutions are generally unnecessary during neurosurgical procedures and are probably best avoided except in situations in which hypoglycemia is a concern, such as in diabetic patients, patients receiving hyperalimentation, premature and newborn infants, and malnourished or debilitated children. In such situations, it is important to administer the glucose solutions at or slightly below maintenance (by constant infusion pump) and to monitor serum glucose periodically throughout surgery to avoid extreme glucose fluctuations. Blood glucose levels are usually well-maintained even in small children in the absence of intravenous glucose administration during typical (balanced) neurosurgical anesthetics. The potential association of cerebral infarct size with hyperglycemia (blood glucose values in excess of 250 mg/dL) during ischemia is of significant concern.[79]

Meticulous management of fluids and blood products to minimize cerebral edema is a cornerstone of pediatric neuroanesthesia. It is important to keep in mind the potential for unexpected hemorrhage. Although cerebral hemorrhage is fortunately a rare event, when it does occur it can be sudden and catastrophic. Therefore, all patients should have secure, large-bore intravenous access and blood products and the means for warming this blood should be immediately available during most craniotomies.

Temperature Control

The importance of thermal homeostasis and the particular vulnerability of infants are discussed in Chapter 27. Because the head accounts for a large proportion of an infant's body surface area, infants are particularly susceptible to heat loss during neurosurgical procedures. Special attention should be focused on maintaining normal temperature from the time the patient is brought into the operating room. Ambient room temperature should be high during positioning, preparation, and draping. Infrared warming lights may be helpful for infants, but they should be used at the distance recommended by the manufacturer because they can cause cutaneous burns. Warming blankets are also helpful, particularly in patients weighing less than 10 kg; they may also be useful in a larger patient whose body is completely covered with surgical drapes. Heated or passive humidifiers can be included in the airway circuit and will assist in maintenance of body temperature as well. Forced hot air warming mattresses are the most effective means of maintaining body temperature.[80]

Occasionally hypothermia can be utilized as a method of neural protection. For every degree Celsius decrease in body temperature, there is approximately a 7% decrease in $CMRO_2$.[81] Therefore, induced hypothermia may be advantageous in special situations, such as intracranial neurovascular surgery, when there is a strong likelihood of a period of temporary cerebral ischemia occurring. In such situations, the temperature should not be allowed to drop below 30°C due to the potential for cardiac arrhythmias at temperatures below 30°C. Rewarming should occur before the patient is awakened to avoid shivering, unless the patient is going to be kept sedated and paralyzed in the intensive care unit postoperatively.

Venous Air Emboli

Venous air emboli (VAE) are a potential danger whenever the operative site is elevated above the heart, and the risk increases as the height difference increases.[82] Intracranial venous sinuses have dural attachments that impede their ability to collapse. Other potential air entry sites include bone, bridging veins, and spinal epidural veins. When air enters the central circulation, right ventricular output may be reduced. As air moves peripherally into the pulmonary circulation, pulmonary edema and bronchoconstriction occur and may progress to acute cor pulmonale, cardiovascular collapse, and death. Air may gain access to the systemic circulation through right-to-left intracardiac shunts, as in patent foramen ovale, atrial or ventricular septal defects, and others. Potential cardiac shunts exist in many otherwise healthy infants and children and may become clinically significant if pulmonary hypertension develops acutely after a large air embolism. Paradoxical air emboli may cause cerebral or coronary artery obstruction with subsequent cerebral infarction or ventricular fibrillation.

Although the incidence of VAE is greatest in the sitting position, the lateral, supine, and prone positions also pose significant risks. VAE have also been observed during craniotomy for craniosynostosis even when the operating room table is flat. The incidence of VAE in children undergoing suboccipital craniotomy in the sitting position is not significantly different from that in adults, but children appear to have a higher incidence of hypotension and a lower likelihood of successful aspiration of central (intravascular) air.[83]

Prompt recognition of VAE is crucial to successful management. Precordial Doppler ultrasonography has been demonstrated to be the earliest and most sensitive indicator of intracranial air (Fig. 22–7).[84] It enables diagnosis before the pathologic consequences occur. The precordial Doppler device is usually placed over the fourth or fifth intercostal

AIR EMBOLISM

Relative Sensitivity

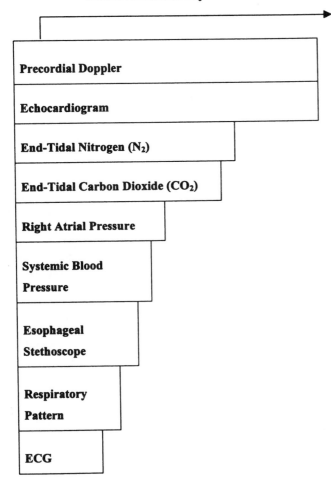

Figure 22–7. Relative sensitivity of air embolism–monitoring modalities.

space at the right sternal border where it best detects right heart tones. Appropriate Doppler positioning can be confirmed by listening for the characteristic change in sounds after rapid administration of a few milliliters of saline into a central or peripheral venous catheter. When VAE occurs, there is reflex pulmonary vasoconstriction and ventilation/perfusion mismatch caused by the air blocking passage of blood; this results in increased dead space ventilation and causes a sudden decrease in end-tidal CO_2 concentration. Monitoring the end-tidal CO_2 concentration is very useful in making the diagnosis and can be used to monitor the severity and duration of air emboli (Fig. 22–8). An increase in end-tidal nitrogen concentration during continuous monitoring is a specific sign of air emboli, but is usually of such small magnitude that it is frequently difficult to detect with devices currently available in clinical practice. Increases in right atrial and pulmonary artery pressures correlate with the size of emboli, but these delayed findings should not be relied upon alone for monitoring and diagnosis. Echocardiography (transthoracic or transesophageal) may be the most specific method for detecting small air emboli but is not easily used intraoperatively especially in small infants and children.[85–87]

Several authors have recommended a preoperative echocardiographic screening for patent foramen ovale in any patient being considered for a sitting craniotomy; some feel that a patent foramen ovale is an absolute contraindication to a sitting position.[86, 88]

Aspiration of air from a central venous catheter is rarely successful unless massive amounts have been entrained. If small VAE are detected by other devices (e.g., Doppler, end-tidal CO_2), the value of central venous catheter aspiration for air is quite limited. When central venous pressure catheters are necessary, such as when the patient is going to be in the seated position or when massive blood loss is anticipated, an attempt should be made to place the tip at the junction of the superior vena cava and right atrium just above the right atrium. This location provides the optimal location for aspiration of entrained air. More importantly, a central venous catheter is useful to estimate maintenance of circulating blood volume and to rapidly administer fluids and resuscitative medications when necessary. The position of a central venous catheter near the heart should be confirmed by radiograph, by transducing CVPs, or with the aid of electrocardiographic monitoring. Central venous catheters that will remain in the postoperative period should have definitive radiographic confirmation to ensure that they do not migrate into the heart. Erosion of the catheter tip through the heart causing fatal pericardial tamponade has occurred up to days following surgery in small children.[89, 90]

As soon as a change in Doppler sounds is noted during surgery (and not felt to be due to administration of intravenous medications), the surgeon should be informed and nitrous oxide and inhalation agents discontinued. Attempts should immediately be made to identify and occlude the site of air entry either by flooding the operative field with saline when appropriate (such as during a posterior fossa craniotomy) or by applying bone wax to bone edges. The head of the table can be lowered if necessary and this will have the effect of increasing cerebral venous pressure and stopping entrainment of air, as well as augmenting the patient's peripheral venous return and increasing systemic blood pressure. Jugular veins can be compressed manually, although great care must be taken to avoid simultaneous compression of the carotid arteries. Attempts can be made to aspirate air through a central venous catheter if one is in place. The application of positive end-expiratory pressure increases cen-

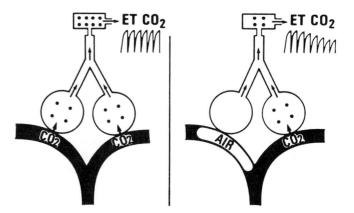

Figure 22–8. Mechanism of decreased end-tidal CO_2 following an air embolus. (Courtesy of Dr. J. Drummond.)

tral venous pressure but also decreases cardiac filling pressure, cardiac output, and blood pressure; extreme increases in positive end-expiratory pressure are usually unwarranted. One must be prepared to provide vasopressor support and fluid resuscitation.

Once the patient has been stabilized, the procedure is resumed and a revised anesthetic plan is instituted. The decision to administer nitrous oxide after successful treatment of VAE is controversial. If reinstitution of nitrous oxide is associated with another decrease in end-tidal CO_2 concentration or clinical deterioration, then residual air bubbles are likely present and nitrous oxide should be discontinued. If no changes occur, many clinicians reinstitute nitrous oxide unless repeated episodes of VAE occur.

Emergence

Protecting the brain is always a major goal of anesthetic management during neurosurgical procedures (Table 22–2). However, emergence and extubation should be smooth and controlled to prevent fluctuations in ICP and venous and arterial pressures.[91] Because vomiting may be a problem in this regard, as well as an uncomfortable and distressing experience for the patient, a variety of antiemetics are often used. Unfortunately, despite this, the incidence of nausea and vomiting is very high in postoperative neurosurgical patients. This is likely because blood in the CSF is a potent emetic and because narcotics are often used to treat postoperative headache. Although ondansetron has not been shown to be effective for prophylaxis in children undergoing a craniotomy,[92] it is often given as a rescue agent after other antiemetics such as Decadron (dexamethasone) and metoclopramide have failed. Droperidol is very effective, but is best administered after the patient awakens from anesthesia and

neurologic function can be assessed. Large (70 μg/kg) doses are sedating, while small doses (10–15 μg/kg) generally are not. Combinations of antiemetics may be more effective than any single agent alone.

Intravenous lidocaine (1.0–1.5 mg/kg) before extubation can help suppress coughing and straining on the endotracheal tube, but a supplemental dose of fentanyl appears equally effective and may even be less sedating. Labetalol, an alpha- and beta-adrenergic blocking agent, can be incrementally administered for the control of blood pressure during the acute period of emergence, but this is rarely necessary in children who have received adequate amounts of narcotics prior to the end of the surgery. When needed (generally for adolescents), labetalol (up to 3 mg/kg total dose) may be necessary, but this usually does not have to be repeated in the postoperative period.

Neuromuscular blockade should be pharmacologically reversed because even the slightest residual weakness is poorly tolerated and may confuse the neurologic examination. Adequate spontaneous ventilation and oxygenation and an awake mental status should be demonstrated before extubation. The exception to this may be after neurovascular surgery, when it is frequently possible to avoid even brief periods of hypertension by extubating the patient "deep." If there is danger of postoperative intracranial hypertension or if the patient does not meet respiratory or neurologic criteria for extubation, the endotracheal tube should remain in place and additional sedation should be administered before transport to the intensive care unit.

Repeated neurologic examinations are important in assessing postoperative progress. Deteriorating status is often one of the earliest signs of intracranial hemorrhage. For this reason, it is desirable to have a child as fully alert as possible immediately after the operation. In unconscious patients, ICP

Table 22–2. Maneuvers of Neuroprotection

Goals	Avoid cerebral edema
	Avoid cerebral hypoxia
	Avoid cerebral hypoperfusion
	Avoid cerebral hypermetabolism
	Avoid neuronal membrane damage
Maneuver	**Function**
Head of bed at 30 degrees in midline	Increases cerebral venous drainage while maintaining CPP
Steroids	Improve outcome in spinal cord injury
	Decrease vasogenic cerebral edema in patients with tumors
	Stabilize neuronal membranes
	Free-radical scavengers
Controlled ventilation	Maintains Pa_{CO_2} at normal to slightly low levels → prevents cerebral vasodilation, prevents increased ICP
Muscle paralysis	Avoids coughing, straining, patient movement, and other causes of increased ICP
Ventricular drainage	Decreases ICP
Antihypertensives	Prevent further cerebral edema, ischemia and/or cerebral hemorrhage
	Severe hypotension can significantly decrease CPP
Anticonvulsants	Prevent seizure activity and increased ICP
Hypothermia	Decreases $CMRO_2$ and CMRglu consumption
Barbiturate coma	Membrane-stabilizing effect
	Decreases CBF and $CMRO_2$

CBF, cerebral blood flow; CMRglu, cerebral metabolic rate for glucose; $CMRO_2$, cerebral metabolic rate for oxygen; CPP, cerebral perfusion pressure; ICP, intracranial pressure; Pa_{CO_2}, partial pressure of arterial carbon dioxide.

can be monitored invasively. CT scans are extremely helpful in evaluating the cause of a rising ICP or deteriorating mental status.

Pain is generally not severe following a craniotomy, although morphine is often necessary the first postoperative night. Ketorolac may best be avoided in the initial postoperative period because of its propensity to alter platelet function. Oral acetaminophen can be begun as soon as the patient is able to take medicine by mouth, or it may be given rectally.[93]

Diabetes insipidus or inappropriate secretion of antidiuretic hormone may complicate postoperative fluid and electrolyte management, particularly when surgery is in the region of the hypothalamus and pituitary gland. Careful observation of fluid status and repeated laboratory evaluation of blood and urine for osmolality and sodium values are important in these situations. When diabetes insipidus does develop, it can be managed with a continuous infusion of dilute aqueous vasopressin (1–10 mU/kg/hr; 0.001–0.01 U/kg/hr). In such circumstances, it is especially important to avoid administering large amounts of hypotonic intravenous solutions that may result in a rapid and dangerous fall in serum sodium and osmolality. In general, if postoperative fluids are administered as normal saline in strictly limited amounts, aqueous vasopressin can be effective in treating patients with diabetes insipidus until they are able to take oral fluids, at which time intranasal desmopressin (synthetic vasopressin) can be administered instead. Diabetes insipidus, when it does develop following surgery in the pituitary region (such as for a craniopharyngioma), may only be transient and it is important to continuously assess the ongoing need for vasopressin.

Portable EEGs and evoked auditory, somatosensory, and, less commonly, visual potentials may be helpful in assessing patients who are deeply sedated or paralyzed. Observation in an intensive care unit capable of managing children is vital for the prevention or early detection and treatment of postoperative complications. CT scans and MRI scans are often obtained in the day or two following a craniotomy; maintaining patency of the intravenous catheters throughout this time will provide a route for sedation for these procedures when necessary.

Special Procedures

Trauma

Head Injury

Trauma is the primary cause of death in children, and head injuries produce the majority of the mortality and much of the morbidity in survivors.[94–96] Motor vehicle accidents continue to be the most frequent preventable cause of head injury, although domestic violence and sports are also common causes of trauma in children. Assaults and suicide attempts have become increasingly common in adolescents. Anesthesiologists may be involved in caring for injured children during the earliest stages of stabilization, resuscitation, and evaluation and throughout the surgical and postoperative period.

Children with head trauma may have minimal neurologic abnormalities at the time of initial evaluation. However,

increased ICP and neurologic deficits may progressively develop. This is because brain injuries are thought to occur in two stages. The primary insult is due to biomechanical forces that disrupt the cranium, neural tissue, and vasculature at the time of impact. Secondary injury is a result of parenchymal damage caused by pathologic sequelae subsequent to the primary insult. This can be a result of hypotension, hypoxia, cerebral edema, or intracranial hypertension. Whereas prevention of primary injuries must be addressed in a sociopolitical forum, such as by seatbelt laws, sports injury prevention, and domestic violence legislation, anesthesiologists are instrumental in preventing or minimizing secondary injury (see also Chapter 16).

There are significant differences between children and adults in the pattern of injuries sustained. While intracranial hematomas (epidural, subdural, or intraparenchymal) are common in adults, they are less frequent in children. In contrast, diffuse cerebral edema occurs more often in pediatric patients than in adults following blunt head trauma.[97]

Scalp Injuries

One of the most commonly encountered operative head injuries in the pediatric patient is a scalp laceration. Most of these can be managed in the emergency room setting, but more serious injuries may need to be repaired in the operating room to provide patient immobility and comfort. Children can lose a significant amount of their blood volume from a scalp injury, since a larger portion of the cardiac output goes to the head compared with adults. Infants less than 1 year of age can even become hemodynamically unstable due to blood loss from a subgaleal hematoma alone, as in a closed scalp injury, so hypovolemia should always be considered and treated prior to induction of anesthesia. Good intravascular access and blood products should always be available. In addition, co-existing intracranial or other injuries need to be considered and preoperative CT scanning may be warranted.

Skull Fractures

Skull fractures are a common manifestation of pediatric head trauma. The vast majority are linear and do not require surgical treatment. They are of concern primarily because the force required to produce them may damage the underlying brain and vasculature. A linear fracture over a major blood vessel (such as the middle meningeal artery) or a large dural sinus may result in intracranial hemorrhage. Fortunately, most children have an uneventful course after sustaining a simple skull fracture. A small minority develop a leptomeningeal cyst or growing fracture that eventually requires surgical treatment. Multiple skull fractures in the absence of documented major trauma should always raise the suspicion of child abuse.

Depressed skull fractures often require surgical repair. These may occur even in the absence of a scalp laceration. However, displacement of the inner table of the skull requires greater force than that needed to produce a simple linear fracture and has greater potential to damage underlying tissues. Approximately one third of all depressed fractures are uncomplicated, another third are associated with dural lacerations, and the remaining third are associated with cortical lacerations. The extent of cortical injury is the primary determinant of morbidity and mortality. Surgical débridement and elevation are usually performed as soon as possible after the injury.

Basilar skull fractures are less common in children. Despite the force needed to produce these fractures, they have an excellent prognosis and rarely require surgical intervention. However, the possibility of a basilar skull fracture should be considered when caring for children with altered mental status, seizures, or associated trauma requiring surgery. Findings include periorbital ecchymoses ("raccoon eyes"), retroauricular ecchymosis (Battle sign), hemotympanum, clear rhinorrhea, or otorrhea. Unless absolutely necessary (e.g., in mandibular wiring), nasotracheal intubation or passage of a nasogastric tube is best avoided because the cribriform plate is very thin and easily disrupted. Complications of basilar skull fracture include meningitis from a CSF leak, cranial nerve damage, and anosmia.

Epidural Hematoma

Epidural hematomas most commonly develop in the temporoparietal region due to arterial bleeding from an injured middle meningeal artery. They can also develop in the posterior fossa as a result of bleeding from a venous sinus. Epidural hematomas are not necessarily associated with an overlying skull fracture. The classic natural history in adults is a "lucid interval" between the initial loss of consciousness and later neurologic deterioration. Infants and children may not have any altered mental status in the early stages following the injury. However, as the hematoma expands, it can result in the development of unconsciousness, hemiparesis, and pupillary dilatation. This deterioration can be quite rapid once a mass effect occurs. Treatment is prompt surgical evacuation, because delays are associated with increased morbidity. Medical therapy directed at decreasing ICP should be instituted as soon as a diagnosis is suspected. Children generally recover well, although morbidity is usually a reflection of underlying brain injury.

Subdural Hematoma

Subdural hematomas are usually associated with cortical damage resulting from either direct parenchymal contusion or laceration of blood vessels. Acute subdural hematomas are almost always traumatic and frequently a result of abuse (shaking of small children, particularly those less than 1 year of age). The shaken baby syndrome, a well-known entity, occurs when an infant is shaken so vigorously that significant neuronal disruption occurs, as well as tears in the cortical bridging veins, which cause subdural hematomas.[98-100] These infants suffer significant brain damage, complicated by episodes of apnea and further hypoxic insult.

Subdural hematomas also occasionally occur secondary to birth trauma within the first hours of life. Vitamin K deficiency, congenital coagulopathies, and disseminated intravascular coagulopathy are all considerations in this group of patients. Great force is necessary to produce a subdural hematoma, whether by direct impact, laceration of blood vessels, or traumatic separation of the brain and overlying dura. Aggressive resuscitation and medical management are instituted simultaneously with preparation for surgical evacuation. Cerebral edema, uncontrolled intracranial hypertension, and persistent neurologic deficits often characterize the postoperative course. Chronic subdural hematomas or effusions may also develop in infancy, although these children do not usually present with acute symptoms. They are often diagnosed when the child is noted to be irritable and vomiting or develops an increase in head circumference. Chronic subdural hematomas can increase in size, causing slow but significant increases in ICP. Although a craniotomy is sometimes performed, most patients undergo some kind of drainage or shunting procedure as definitive treatment.

Intracerebral Hematoma

Intracerebral hematomas are fortunately rare but have a poor prognosis. Deep parenchymal hematomas are most often extensions of cortical contusions in a patient with severe neurologic injury. Rarely a localized hematoma may be appropriate for surgical evacuation to decompress the brain. In general, however, intraparenchymal hematomas are not evacuated for fear of damaging viable brain tissue. Anticonvulsants are usually administered prophylactically and it is safest in the initial period after injury to avoid any medications that interfere with coagulation (such as ketorolac or heparin).

Spinal Injury

Although isolated cervical spine injuries are uncommon in the pediatric population, all children with severe head trauma should initially be assumed to have a cervical spine injury.[101, 102] Different causes of spinal injuries seem to be associated with specific age groups. Motor vehicle accidents produce the largest number of injuries in older children and adolescents, while birth injuries and falls are the most common cause of problems in infants and young children.[103] Spinal cord injury itself may be caused by a variety of forces including hyperflexion, hyperextension, rotation, vertical compression, flexion rotation, and shearing. The injury may involve bony, ligamentous, cartilaginous, vascular, or neural components of the spine or adjacent structures. The biomechanics and functional anatomy of the pediatric spine also vary depending on the age of the child. Older children and teenagers are more likely to sustain injuries in the thoracolumbar region of the spine, while infants and younger children are more likely to suffer injuries in the high cervical region, particularly in the atlantoaxial region. The cervical spine is at higher risk in the infant and younger child because of the relatively weak and flexible neck that supports a proportionally large and heavy head, with the atlanto-occipital area acting as a pivot point. Atlanto-occipital dislocations are generally the most devastating neurologic injuries, leaving children neurologically destroyed but not necessarily dead.

As with brain injury, spinal cord injury occurs in two phases. The primary insult results from biomechanical forces and bony fragments directly impacting the spinal cord. Secondary injury results from the pathologic sequelae of the primary injury: edema and ischemia due to cortical compression, hypotension, hypoxia, and so on. Inappropriate manipulation of a patient with an unstable fracture can exacerbate both primary and secondary injuries. Anesthesiologists caring for a child with a potential cervical spine injury should know that spinal cord injuries in children commonly occur without actual evidence of spinal bone fractures on plain cervical radiographs. These injuries are known as SCIWORA (spinal cord injuries without radiologic abnormality).[104] Injuries to the cervical spine in particular are often difficult to recognize but may sometimes be identified by odontoid displacement or prevertebral swelling on radiograph. As a result, CT is frequently indicated when a spinal injury is initially suspected in a child with trauma. Once a child with a potential spine injury is determined to be medically stable, these studies should be obtained as soon as possible. However, the patient's airway and cardiorespiratory function must be continuously and closely monitored until a spinal cord injury can be ruled out. Sometimes, as with brain injury, there can be a delay in the onset of neurologic deficits with SCIWORA injuries.[105]

Respiratory failure is the most common cause of death after isolated cervical spine injury; impaired respiratory function is a major cause of morbidity. The level of injury determines the degree of impairment. The phrenic nerve originates primarily from C4 but receives contributions of fibers from C3 and C5. Lesions at C5 leave partial diaphragmatic innervation but impair abdominal and intercostal accessory muscles. Lesions between C6 and T7 preserve diaphragmatic innervation but diminish accessory muscle function.

Children with a cervical spine injury may rapidly develop respiratory failure due to decreased vital capacity, increased dead space, retention of secretions, and respiratory muscle fatigue. Resultant hypercarbia and hypoxia aggravate the secondary injury to both brain and spinal cord. Respiratory status may be further impaired by associated trauma to the chest, causing pulmonary contusion or pneumothorax, or by aspiration of gastric contents.

Prompt airway management is critical to avoid hypoxia, ensure adequate respiratory mechanics, preserve neural function, and prevent extension of spinal injury. The head and neck must be immediately immobilized; restraint of the extremities may also be required. During airway manipulation, an assistant should maintain the head and neck in a neutral position (see Figs. 16–1 and 16–2). Various endotracheal tubes and laryngoscope blades should be available, as well as equipment and personnel for an emergency tracheostomy. Small fiberoptic bronchoscopes are available that can fit through infant-sized endotracheal tubes. Retrograde intubation using a guide wire introduced through the cricothyroid membrane may be useful in larger children or adolescents (see Chapter 7). Insertion of a laryngeal mask airway may be lifesaving until a more secure airway can be achieved with fiberoptic or other means.[106–111] However, an unstable infant or child whose airway cannot be secured by conventional means is probably best managed by an emergency tracheostomy. As a temporizing measure, a cricothyroidotomy can be performed using a large (14-gauge) catheter to which an adaptor from a 3 mm internal diameter endotracheal tube is attached (see Fig. 7–23).[112] This permits oxygenation (though inadequate ventilation) until personnel and equipment for tracheostomy are assembled.

Hemodynamic instability may also be a problem due to hypovolemia from concurrently bleeding injuries or severe head trauma. Patients with spinal shock exhibit loss of vasomotor tone or loss of normal neurocardiac function with associated bradycardia and decreased myocardial contractility. Intravenous fluid and vasopressors may be necessary for management.

Although there are currently few data regarding children, steroids are usually administered to patients with spinal injuries as soon as possible after the initial trauma in the hopes of reducing neurologic injury. The most commonly used drug is methylprednisolone, 30 mg/kg, administered over the first 15 minutes, followed by an infusion of 5.4 mg/kg/hr for the following 23 hours.[113, 114] Methylprednisolone is felt to be effective via multiple mechanisms including improved spinal blood flow, inhibition of the arachidonic acid cascade, and modulation of the local immune response.[115] In addition, some evidence suggests that GM1-ganglioside, with or without methylprednisolone, may be advantageous in decreasing demyelination and promoting neurologic recovery if administered soon after a spinal injury.[116–122]

If the spinal cord injury is greater than 24 hours old, succinylcholine should not be administered, since it can result in massive hyperkalemia.[123] In addition, physiologic changes may occur due to autonomic hyperreflexia, which frequently develops following cervical or high thoracic spinal lesions. This autonomic hyperreflexia is capable of producing severe, even life-threatening, vasomotor instability with hypertension and arrhythmias.[124, 125]

Craniotomy

Tumors

Brain tumors are the most common solid tumors in children, exceeded only by the leukemias as the most common pediatric malignancy.[126] Approximately 1500 to 2000 new brain tumors are diagnosed in children each year in the United States. Unlike the situation in adults, the majority of brain tumors in children are infratentorial, in the posterior fossa. These include medulloblastomas, cerebellar astrocytomas, brainstem gliomas, and ependymomas of the fourth ventricle. Because posterior fossa tumors usually obstruct CSF flow, increased ICP occurs early. Presenting signs and symptoms include early morning vomiting and irritability or lethargy. Cranial nerve palsies and ataxia are also common findings with respiratory and cardiac irregularities usually occurring late. Sedation or general anesthesia may be required for radiologic evaluation or radiation therapy.

Surgical resection of a posterior fossa tumor presents a number of anesthetic challenges. Children are usually positioned prone, although the lateral or sitting positions are utilized by some neurosurgeons. In any case, the head will be flexed, and the position and patency of the endotracheal tube must be meticulously ensured. A nasotracheal tube is preferred when the patient is prone, since it is easier to secure and less likely to be dislodged. Proper positioning of the endotracheal tube is initially done by confirmation of clear bilateral breath sounds with the head flexed as much as possible while the patient is still supine after intubation is performed. Care should be taken to ensure that all other nasal and oral tubes (e.g., gastric, esophageal) do not cause pressure on the nares or lips, which, after lengthy procedures, can lead to edema or erosion.

Arrhythmias and acute blood pressure changes may occur during surgical exploration, especially when the brainstem is manipulated, so careful observation of the electrocardiogram and arterial waveform tracing is important. Altered respiratory control is generally masked by muscle relaxants and mechanical ventilation. Intracranial compliance is presumed to be decreased even when ICP is only marginally elevated and precautions to minimize increases in ICP should be taken. If ICP is markedly elevated or acutely worsens, a ventricular catheter may be inserted by the neurosurgeon prior to tumor resection to permit emergent drainage of CSF. VAE is a potentially serious complication that is not eliminated by the use of the prone or lateral position because head-up gradients of 10 to 20 degrees are frequently used to improve cerebral venous drainage. In infants and toddlers, large head size relative to body size accentuates this problem.

Tumors in the midbrain include craniopharyngiomas, optic gliomas, pituitary adenomas, and hypothalamic tumors and account for approximately 15% of intracranial tumors. Hypothalamic tumors (hamartomas, gliomas, and teratomas) frequently present with precocious puberty in children who are large for their chronological age. Craniopharyngiomas are the most common perisellar tumors in children and adolescents and may be associated with hypothalamic and pituitary dysfunction. Symptoms often include growth failure, visual impairment, and endocrine abnormalities.

Signs and symptoms of hypothyroidism should be sought and thyroid function tests measured. Steroid replacement (dexamethasone or hydrocortisone) is generally administered since the integrity of the hypothalamic-pituitary-adrenal axis may be uncertain. In addition, diabetes insipidus occurs preoperatively in some patients and is a common postoperative problem. A careful history usually reveals this condition preoperatively, especially if attention is focused on nocturnal drinking and enuresis. Evaluation of serum electrolytes and osmolality, urine-specific gravity, and urine output is helpful since hypernatremia and hyperosmolality, along with dilute urine, are typical findings. If diabetes insipidus does not exist preoperatively, it usually does not develop until the postoperative period. This is because there appears to be an adequate reserve of antidiuretic hormone in the posterior pituitary gland capable of functioning for many hours even when the hypothalamic-pituitary stalk is damaged intraoperatively.

Postoperative diabetes insipidus is marked by a sudden large increase in dilute urine output associated with a rising serum sodium concentration and osmolality. Treatment can initially be with dilute crystalloid solutions to replace the urine output with careful attention to electrolyte measurements. However, urine output is usually so prodigious (up to 1 L/hr in an adult) that an infusion of aqueous vasopressin (1–10 mU/kg/hr) is best utilized with fluid input then carefully restricted to match urine replacement and estimates of insensible losses. If diabetes insipidus persists, intranasal desmopressin can be used to replace intravenous pitressin, since desmopressin generally needs to be administered only twice daily. Return of antidiuretic hormone activity a few days postoperatively may cause a marked decrease in urinary output, water intoxication, seizures, and cerebral edema if desmopressin is not discontinued and fluid administration not adjusted appropriately.

Transsphenoidal surgery is generally only performed in adolescents and older children with pituitary adenomas; however, it should be treated like other midbrain tumors in terms of monitoring and vascular access. Patients are usually intubated orally to give the surgeon optimal access to the nasopharynx, and preparations for an emergent craniotomy should be anticipated in case unexpected massive bleeding develops. Since nasal packs are inserted at the end of surgery, patients should be fully awake prior to tracheal extubation.

Gliomas of the optic pathways occur with increased frequency in patients with neurofibromatosis. Presenting symptoms include visual changes and proptosis; increased ICP and hypothalamic dysfunction are usually late findings. There are two main forms of neurofibromatosis: type 1, also known as peripheral or von Recklinghausen neurofibromatosis, and type 2, also known as central or bilateral acoustic neurofibromatosis. Type 1 neurofibromatosis is associated with other tumors, including pheochromocytomas, neuroblastomas, leukemia, sarcomas, and Wilms tumors. Neurofibromas tend to be highly vascular and thus the anesthesiologist should be prepared for significant blood loss.

Approximately 25% of intracranial tumors in children involve the cerebral hemispheres. These are primarily astrocytomas, oligodendrogliomas, ependymomas, and glioblastomas. Neurologic symptoms are more likely to include a seizure disorder or focal deficits. Succinylcholine should be avoided if motor weakness is present since it can cause sudden massive hyperkalemia. Nondepolarizing muscle relaxants and narcotics may be metabolized more rapidly than usual in patients receiving chronic anticonvulsants. Choroid plexus papillomas are rare but occur most often in children younger than 3 years of age. They usually arise from the choroid plexus of the lateral ventricle and produce early hydrocephalus as a result of increased production of CSF and obstruction of CSF flow. Hydrocephalus usually resolves with surgical resection. When lesions lie near the motor or sensory strip, a special type of somatosensory evoked potential monitoring called "phase reversal" may also be used to delineate these locations.[127] If cortical stimulation is planned to help identify motor areas, muscle relaxants must be permitted to wear off. Nitrous oxide and narcotics are usually sufficient to prevent patient movement during these periods.

Stereotactic biopsies or craniotomies present special concerns regarding airway accessibility. Newer head frames are available that have adjustable anterior positions so that the airway is readily accessible (Fig. 22–9). It is more comfortable and less distressing for the patient to have anesthesia induced before the head frame is applied, even though this means the anesthesiologist must induce anesthesia in the radiology suite and then transport the patient from the CT scanner to the operating room. The wrench that is used to apply (and remove) the head frame should be taped to the frame itself, so that it is always readily available should emergent removal of the head frame become necessary.

Vascular Anomalies

Arteriovenous Malformations

Arteriovenous malformations consist of large arterial feeding vessels, dilated communicating vessels, and large draining veins carrying arterialized blood. Large malformations, especially those involving the posterior cerebral artery and vein

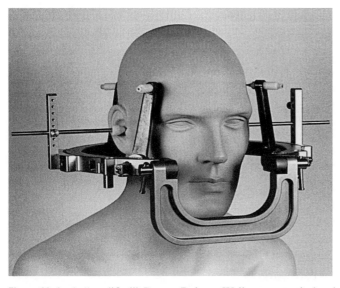

Figure 22-9. A "modified" Brown-Roberts-Wells stereotactic head frame with an adjustable face piece that provides enhanced access to the airway. (From Stokes MA, Soriano SG, Tarbell NJ, et al: Anesthesia for stereotactic radiosurgery in children. J Neurosurg Anesthesiol 1995;7:100–108.)

of Galen, may present as congestive heart failure (high output heart failure, often with pulmonary hypertension) in the newborn period. The prognosis for these types of arteriovenous malformations is generally quite poor. Saccular dilation of the vein of Galen may present itself later in infancy or childhood as hydrocephalus secondary to obstruction of the aqueduct of Sylvius. Malformations not large enough to produce congestive heart failure usually remain clinically silent unless they cause seizures or a stroke or until the acute rupture of a communicating vessel results in subarachnoid or intracerebral hemorrhage.[128] Intracranial bleeds are the most common presentation in this population, and mortality when this occurs is estimated at 25%.

Treatment usually consists of embolization or radiation of deep malformations, surgical excision (usually of the more superficial ones), or a combination of these modalities. Anesthetic management for elective embolic procedures usually involves a standard general anesthetic with muscle relaxants and secure intravenous access; moderate hyperventilation may actually enhance visualization of abnormal blood vessels that do not respond with vasoconstriction. The anesthesiologist should be knowledgeable about the types of embolic agents that will be used and their potential complications. Anticonvulsant therapy is routine. Newborns in cardiac failure may be receiving several inotropic agents. Bleeding, especially from the femoral arterial puncture site (which cannot always be visualized), should always be a consideration. Fluid overload can occur due to the large amounts of contrast agents administered, especially in a young infant who may already be in high output cardiac failure. One should always be prepared for the possibility of an emergency craniotomy should a vessel rupture occur.

Aneurysms

Intracranial aneurysms are most often due to a congenital malformation in an arterial wall. Patients with coarctation of the aorta or polycystic kidney disease have an increased incidence of these aneurysms. They usually remain asymptomatic during childhood; most ruptures that occur in childhood are fatal. Symptoms of subarachnoid or intracerebral hemorrhage frequently appear suddenly in a previously healthy young adult. When technically feasible, surgical ligation or clipping constitute the treatment of choice.[129]

Anesthesia for surgical resection of vascular malformations and aneurysms in children presents unique challenges, especially if the diagnosis has been preceded by an intracranial hemorrhage. These are some of the few situations in pediatric neuroanesthesia in which deep preoperative sedation may be beneficial to avoid sudden hypertensive episodes. Blood products should be in the operating room and verified before the start of the procedure. Ensuring adequate depth of anesthesia before any invasive maneuver prevents precipitous hypertension. Adequate venous access to deal with sudden and massive blood loss is crucial but can generally be established after induction. A means of warming blood, such as a rapid transfusion device, should be immediately available. The use of hypothermia may be of benefit in certain situations.

Controlled hypotension may also be valuable in some situations for brief periods of time to reduce tension in the abnormal blood vessels and improve the safety of surgical manipulation.[130] It is not clear, however, whether the benefits of controlled hypotension are worth the risks, especially in small children (see Chapter 12). Controlled hypotension should not be used in the presence of increased ICP, however, because of the risk of causing decreased cerebral perfusion pressure with resulting ischemia and further increased ICP. Controlled hypotension may be induced with potent inhalation agents combined with vasodilators (nitroprusside or nitroglycerin) when necessary. Intermediate-acting adrenergic antagonists (labetalol, esmolol) are also effective. Ganglionic blockers are generally avoided because their propensity to dilate pupils can confuse postoperative evaluation. Although the absolute limits of acceptable hypotension are unknown, a mean blood pressure greater than 40 mm Hg (for infants) and 50 mm Hg (for older children) generally appear safe. At the conclusion of the procedure and before closing the dura, the operative site should be inspected after the blood pressure has been permitted to return to normal to assure adequate hemostasis.

Hemodynamic stability is also important during emergence to avoid bucking, coughing, straining, and hypertension during extubation. Excessive hypertension should be avoided to prevent postoperative bleeding, although in most cases of aneurysm clipping, a slightly elevated BP may be desirable postoperatively to minimize the risk of vasospasm. Postoperatively, following resection of an arteriovenous malformation, there can be serious complications due to cerebral edema with increased ICP or hemorrhage. This is generally called normal perfusion pressure breakthrough and is believed to be caused by hyperemia of the areas surrounding the previous arteriovenous malformation site where vessels suffer from continued vasomotor paralysis and cannot vasoconstrict. Treatment is controversial but generally involves therapy for increased ICP (diuretics, moderate hyperventilation, head elevation) in addition to judicious use of moderate hypotension (while maintaining CPP) and moderate hypothermia. Once surgery is completed, it is particularly important that patients be able to cooperate with a neurologic examination and that careful control of BP and postoperative intensive care be available.

Moyamoya Disease

Moyamoya disease is an anomaly that results in progressive and life-threatening occlusion of intracranial vessels, primarily the internal carotid arteries near the circle of Willis.[131] An abnormal vascular network of collaterals develops at the base of the brain, giving rise to the Japanese name (translated roughly as "puff of smoke") associated with the angiographic appearance of this condition (Fig. 22–10). In the congenital form, the dysplastic process may involve systemic (especially renal) arteries as well. The acquired variety may be associated with meningitis, neurofibromatosis, chronic inflammation, connective tissue diseases, certain hematologic disorders, or prior intracranial radiation. For reasons that are unknown, this disease appears to be more common in children of Japanese ancestry. Associated intracranial aneurysms are rare in children but may occur in more than 10% of adult patients. Abnormal electrocardiographic findings have also been described with this syndrome in adults. Moyamoya disease usually presents as transient ischemic attacks progressing to strokes and fixed neurologic deficits in children. The attacks may be precipitated by hyperventilation.[132] There is a high morbidity and mortality rate if left untreated. Medical management consists of antiplatelet therapy, such as aspirin or calcium channel blockers. The most common surgical operation for correction in the pediatric population is pial synangiosis, which involves suturing a scalp artery (usually the superficial temporal artery) onto the pial surface of the brain to enhance revascularization.[133]

Careful and continuous monitoring of end-tidal CO_2 concentration is essential to anesthetic management.[134] Patients with moyamoya disease have reduced hemispheric blood flow in both hemispheres, and hyperventilation may also further reduce regional blood flow and cause significant EEG and neurologic changes.[135] Thus, it is crucial that normocapnia be maintained throughout the procedure. In effect, this may be one of the only conditions in pediatric neuroanesthesia in which mild hyperventilation is inappropriate.[136] Adequate hydration and maintenance of baseline BP are also

therefore extremely important. The majority of these patients has intravenous catheters inserted the night before surgery and are given one and a half times maintenance fluids to avoid dehydration during the perioperative period. There may be benefit in EEG monitoring during these procedures to detect and potentially treat ischemia that appears to be a result of cerebral vasoconstriction in response to direct surgical manipulation of the brain itself. Normothermia is maintained, particularly at the end of the procedure, to avoid postoperative shivering and stress response. As in most neurosurgical procedures, a smooth extubation without hypertension or crying is desirable. Although very little literature exists regarding intraoperative and postoperative complications during moyamoya surgery, it appears that most complications (strokes) occur postoperatively and are associated with dehydration and crying (hyperventilation) episodes.[137]

Seizure Surgery

Epilepsy is one of the most common neurologic disorders of childhood. Although most patients are successfully treated with anticonvulsant medications, some are resistant to such therapy or develop unacceptable side effects. In recent years, surgery has become a feasible option in select patients to control intractable seizures.[138]

The preoperative evaluation should seek potential side effects from anticonvulsant medications. These generally manifest as abnormalities of hematologic function (abnormal coagulation, depression of red or white blood cell or platelet counts) or hepatic function. Specific anticonvulsant levels should be determined to detect over- or under-medication. It is also worth noting that many anticonvulsants enhance metabolism of nondepolarizing muscle relaxants and narcotics, thereby leading to an increase (up to 50%) in the amount of these drugs needed during a surgical procedure. The preoperative evaluation should also detect underlying conditions that are causing the seizures, as well as disabilities that can result from progressive neurologic dysfunction.

One of the major concerns of the neurosurgeon is to avoid resection of brain tissue that controls vital functions, such as motion, sensation, speech, and memory, especially if a seizure focus lies near cortical areas controlling these

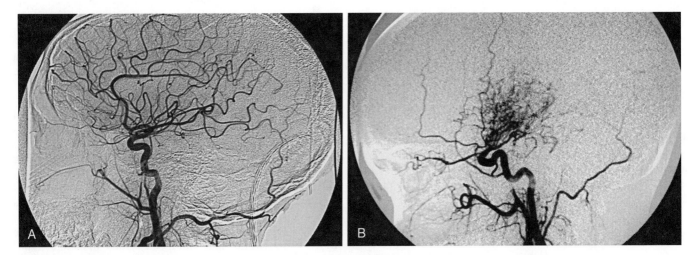

Figure 22–10. Moyamoya disease. Lateral angiogram of the common carotid vasculature in (A) a normal patient, and (B) a patient with Moyamoya disease. Note lack of cortical vessels and "hazy" collateral flow in the disease state.

functions. Cooperative adolescents and adults can assist in determination of the limits of safe cortical resection if they can be assessed during the surgical procedure. These "awake" craniotomies are usually carried out using short-acting sedatives and analgesics, such as propofol and fentanyl, to induce unconsciousness for instillation of local anesthetics, insertion of monitoring catheters, and skull opening.[139] Subsequently, patients can be allowed to awaken for determining whether the seizure focus is near the "eloquent" cortex (the cortex that controls vital functions) during surgical resection. They can then have sedative and narcotic agents reinstituted for the craniotomy closure.

Younger children (generally less than 10 years of age) or uncooperative patients of any age generally will not tolerate this approach and will require general anesthesia throughout. In such circumstances, intraoperative electrophysiologic studies, such as somatosensory evoked potentials, EEG, and motor stimulation, may be used to help localize and determine the function of the site of planned resection. If EEG studies are to be performed, a nitrous oxide/narcotic technique enables all potent volatile agents that depress cerebral electrical activity to be eliminated by the time of study. If direct cortical motor stimulation is planned, muscle relaxants must be permitted to wear off as well. Occasionally, a seizure focus is difficult to identify intraoperatively. In these situations, hyperventilation or methohexital (in small doses, 0.25–0.5 mg/kg) may be helpful in producing EEG seizure activities.[140, 141]

In some patients, seizures are so generalized that detecting the site of origin is difficult. When this occurs, evaluation with intracranial EEG monitoring ("grids and strips") may be accomplished by direct electrocorticography (Fig. 22–11). These leads are placed on the surface of the cortex following a craniotomy under general anesthesia. Intraoperative EEG monitoring is limited during these procedures merely to ensure that all leads are functional; the actual monitoring for seizures takes place over the next several days to see if a "focus" can be identified that is amenable to resection. These patients need to be observed carefully in the postoperative period, since complications can develop from having intracranial electrodes in place. Since air frequently persists in the skull for up to 3 weeks following a craniotomy,[75] these patients should not have nitrous oxide administered for their subsequent procedures (to resect a seizure focus and/or remove the electrocorticography leads) until their dura has been opened to prevent the development of tension pneumocephalus. We have found it is helpful to insert a peripheral intravenous central catheter in children undergoing these procedures, since antibiotic therapy is administered while the electrodes are in place (approximately 1 week), and this avoids the need for multiple peripheral intravenous catheter insertions.

When a focal resection is not possible, a lobectomy or corpus callosotomy may be attempted. It should be noted, however, that children undergoing this latter procedure are often somnolent for the first few postoperative days, especially if a "complete" callosotomy is performed. Occasionally, small children will undergo a hemispherectomy because their seizures are attributed to an abnormal hemisphere that is usually already severely dysfunctional, as when a hemiparesis is already present. These can be very challenging cases for the anesthesiologist, since much blood can be lost (from one half to multiples of the estimated blood volume).[142]

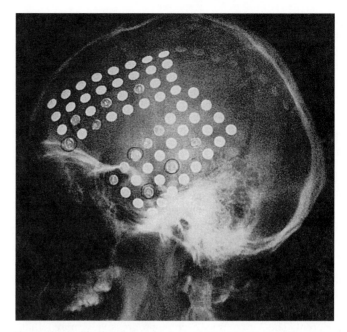

Figure 22–11. Skull radiograph of a patient with intracranial electrocorticography grids in place.

Since this procedure is usually performed when patients are very young (to permit the other hemisphere to "take over" function of both sides), ensuring adequate intravenous access can be challenging. Frequently, a large-bore catheter inserted into a femoral vein is helpful in these cases to facilitate rapid replacement of blood, crystalloid solutions, and medications.

One advancement in epilepsy treatment has been the development of the vagal nerve stimulator. Although the exact mechanism of how it functions is not understood at this time, it appears to inhibit seizure activity at the brainstem or cortical levels.[143, 144] It is becoming a popular form of treatment since it has shown benefit with minimal side effects in many patients who are disabled by intractable seizures. Large, randomized patient trials are currently underway to determine the overall efficacy of this new treatment. At this time, there are few published series of vagal nerve stimulation studies in children, but it is estimated that there is a 60 to 70% improvement in seizure control in children receiving vagal nerve stimulation, with the best results in those with drop attacks.[145, 146]

The vagal nerve stimulator device is a programmable stimulator similar to a cardiac pacemaker placed subcutaneously under the left anterior chest wall. Bipolar platinum stimulating electrodes, which are implanted around the left vagus nerve, are connected to the generator via subcutaneously tunneled wires. The procedure usually takes about 2 hours. The device automatically activates for up to 30 seconds every 5 minutes. Although stimulation of the vagal nerve in this manner may affect vocal cord function, sudden bradycardia or other side effects are uncommon.

Hydrocephalus

Hydrocephalus is a condition involving a mismatch of CSF production and absorption resulting in an increased intracranial CSF volume. It can be caused by a variety of pathologic processes. Except for rare instances of excess CSF production, such as in choroid plexus papillomas, the majority of cases of hydrocephalus are secondary to some type of obstruction or inability to absorb CSF appropriately. Commonly, this is a result of hemorrhage (neonatal intraventricular or subarachnoid), congenital problems (aqueductal stenosis) trauma, infection, or tumors (especially in the posterior fossa). Hydrocephalus can be classified as nonobstructive/communicating or obstructive/noncommunicating based on the ability of CSF to flow around the spinal cord in its usual manner.

Intracranial hypertension or a decrease in intracranial compliance almost always accompanies untreated hydrocephalus in children. How much intracranial compliance exists and how acutely hydrocephalus develops are both instrumental in how severe the signs and symptoms of hydrocephalus will be. In the young infant, if hydrocephalus develops slowly, the skull will expand and the cerebral cortical mantle will stretch until massive craniomegaly (often with irreversible neurologic damage) occurs. However, if the cranial bones are fused or the cranium cannot expand fast enough, neurologic signs and symptoms rapidly become apparent. The patient may become progressively more lethargic and develop vomiting, cranial nerve dysfunction ("setting sun" sign), bradycardia, and ultimately brain herniation and death.

Unless the etiology of the hydrocephalus can be definitively treated, treatment entails surgical placement of an extracranial shunt. Most shunts transport CSF from the lateral ventricles to the peritoneal cavity (ventriculoperitoneal shunts). Occasionally the distal end of the shunt must be placed in the right atrium or pleural cavity, usually due to problems with the ability of the peritoneal cavity to absorb CSF. Newer shunt systems with "programmable" valves are being tried to reduce the need for shunt revisions.[147]

The use of a percutaneous flexible neuroendoscope through a burr hole in the skull has provided an alternative to extracranial shunt placement.[148] During these procedures, a ventriculostomy may be made to bypass an obstruction (such as aqueductal stenosis) by forming a communicating hole from one area of CSF flow to another using a blunt probe inserted through the neuroendoscope. Common locations for a ventriculostomy are through the septum pellucidum (so the lateral ventricles can communicate) or through the floor of the third ventricle into the adjacent CSF cisterns. Complications such as damage to the basilar artery or its branches or neural injuries can be life threatening when they occur, and the anesthesiologist should be prepared for an emergency craniotomy during these procedures.

The anesthetic plan in a patient with hydrocephalus should be directed at controlling ICP and relieving the obstruction as soon as possible. Often, in the presence of increased ICP, these patients have been vomiting and at risk for pulmonary aspiration, in which case a rapid-sequence induction and tracheal intubation with cricoid pressure should be performed. Ketamine is a particularly dangerous agent to use in these situations because it can lead to sudden massive intracranial hypertension. Therefore, barbiturates are generally used for induction. Hydrocephalus often produces large dilated scalp veins in infants, and these can be used for induction of anesthesia if necessary. If intravenous access cannot be established, then an inhalation induction with sevoflurane and gentle cricoid pressure may be an alterna-

tive, though less desirable, method of induction.[149] This method results in venodilation and generally facilitates establishment of intravenous access. Once an intravenous catheter is inserted, hyperventilation should be instituted, the patient may be paralyzed, the trachea intubated, the inhalation agent decreased or discontinued, and the remainder of the anesthetic maintained with a balanced nitrous oxide/narcotic technique or low concentrations of isoflurane. The possibility of VAE during placement of the distal end of a ventriculoatrial shunt should always be kept in mind. Postoperatively, patients should be observed carefully because an altered mental status and recent peritoneal incision place them at high risk for pulmonary aspiration once feedings are begun.

There are a few special situations involving shunts that anesthesiologists should be familiar with. Children who develop a shunt infection usually have their entire shunt system removed and external ventricular drainage established. They return to the operating room for placement of a new system several days later after their infection has been treated with antibiotics. While an external drain is in place, one must be careful not to dislodge the ventricular tubing. In addition, the height of the drainage bag should not be changed in relationship to the patient's head to avoid sudden changes in ICP. For example, suddenly lowering an open drainage bag can siphon CSF rapidly from the patient, resulting in collapse of the ventricles and rupture of cortical veins. When transporting patients with CSF drainage, or when moving them from a stretcher to an operating room table, it is best to close off the ventriculostomy tubing during these brief periods.

Anesthesiologists should also be aware of a special condition known as slit ventricle syndrome (Fig. 22–12). This situation develops in approximately 5 to 10% of patients with CSF shunts and is associated with overdrainage of CSF and small, "slit-like" lateral ventricular spaces. Patients with this condition do not have the usual amount of intracranial CSF to compensate for alterations in brain or intracranial blood volume. Thus, special attention should be paid to patients in whom CT scans indicate the presence of this condition. In particular, it is probably safest to avoid the administration of excess or hypotonic intravenous solutions in these situations in the intraoperative and postoperative periods to minimize the chances of brain swelling developing. These patients cannot seem to accommodate to situations that otherwise healthy children would easily tolerate. Episodes of postoperative cerebral herniation have been reported after uneventful surgical procedures.[46]

Craniosynostosis

Craniosynostosis is a congenital anomaly in which one or more cranial sutures close prematurely. It occurs in approximately one of every 2000 births, with males affected more frequently than females. The craniosynostosis may be simple, involving one suture, or it may be very complex and be associated with a variety of syndromes. The head may assume various shapes depending on which sutures are involved. If uncorrected, the deformed cranium can result in increased ICP and compression of brain, with potential neurologic sequelae including blindness.[150] However, repair is frequently undertaken to improve a child's appearance. Surgical correction is usually performed within the first

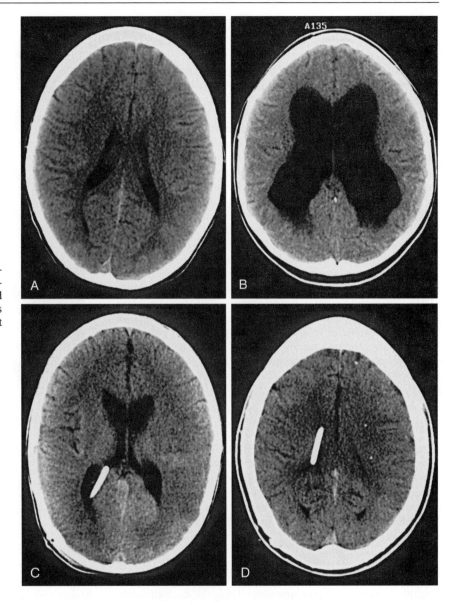

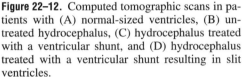

Figure 22–12. Computed tomographic scans in patients with (A) normal-sized ventricles, (B) untreated hydrocephalus, (C) hydrocephalus treated with a ventricular shunt, and (D) hydrocephalus treated with a ventricular shunt resulting in slit ventricles.

months of life to achieve the best cosmetic results. This is because brain growth is very rapid during infancy, "pushing" the skull into a normal shape. Repair of craniosynostosis may involve removal of one small strip of bone from the skull, or it may entail multiple craniectomies or even complete reconstruction of the calvarium.

Although these operations are extradural procedures, they nonetheless can entail significant blood loss from the scalp and cranium. It is therefore important to establish adequate venous access for rapid blood administration, especially if multiple sutures are involved. Central venous access to follow cardiac filling pressures and an arterial line for continuous blood pressure monitoring are often indicated depending on the severity of the deformity. It is prudent to have blood products readily available in the operating room, since they are often required. Generally, knowing the sutures to be repaired and the neurosurgeon involved, the anesthesiologist can anticipate which infants will usually require a blood transfusion before they become profoundly anemic. In such situations, it is often safest to begin transfusion of blood right from the beginning of surgery (to replace blood lost on

a milliliter for milliliter basis); this is especially true for patients presenting with physiologic anemia of infancy.

The incidence of VAE is also significant during these procedures.[82, 151] Precordial Doppler ultrasonography and end-tidal CO_2 monitoring are useful for early detection of VAE. Placing bone "wax" on the open edges of cut bone, treatment with additional fluids, and if necessary lowering the head of the table may prevent small episodes of VAE from progressing to major air entrainment and cardiovascular collapse. Blood loss may continue into the postoperative period, usually in the subgaleal space; careful observation and repeat hematocrit determinations are warranted.[152]

Craniofacial Reconstruction

Craniofacial deformities pose many challenges to pediatric anesthesiologists. The number of syndromes is vast and includes maxillofacial deformities, mandibular abnormalities, and malformations of the extremities. Often hydrocephalus and spinal anomalies (including Chiari malformations) and other major systemic anomalies co-exist. Detailed descriptions are beyond the scope of this chapter, and readers are referred to various compendia of birth defects. These patients frequently require multiple surgical procedures throughout childhood, often combining neurosurgical, plastic, otorhinolaryngologic, dental, and maxillofacial teams. They may be difficult to fit with a mask, frequently have obstructed nasal passages, and may be difficult to intubate. Various pediatric masks, airways (including laryngeal mask airways), and laryngoscope blades should be available (see Chapter 7). An anterior commissure laryngoscope or fiberoptic bronchoscope may be helpful as well. Tracheostomy may sometimes be a necessary component of the procedure.

As with any prolonged complex surgical procedure, massive blood loss, intravascular fluid shifts, and heat conservation assume paramount importance. Blood loss can occur acutely or slowly during the procedure in the form of ongoing oozing. With extensive bony repairs, VAE may occur with catastrophic results. Manipulation of intracranial volume can improve access to orbital and maxillary structures, especially if intracranial hypertension is of concern. This may be accomplished by hyperventilation, CSF drainage, or the use of osmotic or loop diuretics. Postoperative intubation is often appropriate, because deaths in the postoperative period associated with these procedures have often been the result of compromise of the airway resulting in impairment of oxygenation and ventilation.

Congenital Anomalies

Congenital anomalies of the central nervous system generally occur as midline defects. This dysraphism may occur anywhere along the neural axis, involving the head (encephalocele) or spine (meningomyelocele) (Fig. 22–13). The defect may be relatively minor and affect only superficial bony and membranous structures or may include a large segment of malformed neural tissue.

Encephalocele

Encephaloceles can occur anywhere from the occiput to the frontal area. They can even appear as nasal "polyps" if they protrude through the cribriform plate. Rarely they are filled with so much CSF that the defect can be nearly as large as the head itself. Large defects may present challenges to endotracheal intubation. Much blood loss can develop, especially if venous sinuses are entered. Adequate intravenous access should be ensured and blood products be available.

Myelodysplasia

Defects in the spine are known as spina bifida. If a bulge containing CSF without spinal tissue exists, it is called a meningocele. When neural tissue is also present within the lesion, the defect is called a meningomyelocele. Open neural tissue is known as rachischisis. Hydrocephalus is usually present when paralysis occurs below the lesion and is usually associated with an Arnold-Chiari malformation (see later).

Most patients with a meningomyelocele present for primary closure within the first day or two of life to minimize the risk of infection. Many are now scheduled electively before birth for repair, because the defect is usually apparent on prenatal ultrasonography. Many neurosurgeons prefer to

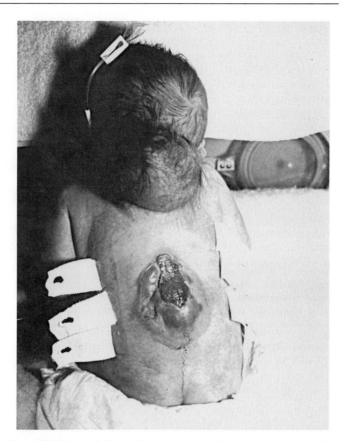

Figure 22–13. An infant with both encephalocele and myelomeningocele defects. Note the large exposed surface areas that make this patient prone to dehydration. Difficulty may be encountered in positioning for induction of anesthesia, and significant loss of blood and cerebrospinal fluid during surgical correction should be anticipated.

insert a ventriculoperitoneal shunt at the time of initial surgery. Alternatively, a shunt may be inserted a few days later or even occasionally deferred if there is no evidence of hydrocephalus at birth. A major anesthetic consideration is positioning the neonate for induction at surgery. In most cases, tracheal intubation can be performed with the infant in the supine position and the uninvolved portion of the patient's back supported with towels (or a "donut" ring) so there is no direct pressure on the meningomyelocele. For very large defects, it is occasionally necessary to place the infant in the lateral position for induction and intubation. Succinylcholine is rarely necessary in these situations, but does not appear to cause problems with hyperkalemia, probably because the defect develops early in gestation.[153] Airway management, mask fit, and intubation may be difficult in infants with massive hydrocephalus or very large defects. In such cases, awake intubation after administration of atropine may occasionally be the safest alternative. Blood loss may be considerable during repair of a meningomyelocele when large amounts of skin are to be undermined to cover the defect. Repair of a meningomyelocele can be done with spinal anesthesia, but general anesthesia is often preferred, especially if a ventriculoperitoneal shunt is also indicated.[154]

Patients with myelodysplasia are at high risk of developing allergic reactions to latex.[41] This is likely a result of repeated exposures to latex products encountered during surgery, including non-neurosurgical procedures required to correct co-existing orthopedic and urologic problems, or repeated bladder catheterizations. Therefore, from birth these patients are best managed in as latex-free an environment as possible to minimize the chances of sensitization.[155] Interestingly, patients who develop latex allergy appear to have an increased incidence of allergic reactions to other substances, including some antibiotics and foods, so anaphylaxis should always be anticipated in these situations.

Postoperatively, respiratory status should be carefully assessed. Pulse oximetry is valuable during recovery from anesthesia because of difficulty with breathing after a tight closure, and because ventilatory responses to hypoxia are often diminished or absent in these patients when a Chiari malformation co-exists.[156] Intrauterine surgery is currently being investigated as a way of diminishing the degree of damage caused by myelodysplasia.[157, 158]

Chiari Malformations

There are four types of Chiari malformations (Table 22–3). The Arnold-Chiari malformation (type II) almost always co-exists in children with myelodysplasia. This defect consists of a bony abnormality in the posterior fossa and upper cervical spine with caudal displacement of the cerebellar vermis, fourth ventricle, and lower brainstem below the plane of the foramen magnum. Medullary cervical cord compression can occur (Fig. 22–14). Vocal cord paralysis with stridor and respiratory distress, apnea, abnormal swallowing and pulmonary aspiration, opisthotonos, and cranial nerve deficits may be associated with the Arnold-Chiari malformation and usually present during infancy. Patients with vocal cord paralysis or a diminished gag reflex may require tracheostomy and gastrostomy to secure the airway and minimize chronic aspiration. Patients of any age may have abnormal responses to hypoxia and hypercarbia because of cranial nerve and brainstem dysfunction.[156, 159] Extreme head flexion may cause brainstem compression in otherwise asymptomatic patients.

Chiari malformations (type I) can occur in healthy children without myelodysplasia. These defects involve caudal displacement of the cerebellar tonsils below the foramen magnum but patients generally have much milder symptoms, sometimes presenting only with headache or neck pain.[160] Surgical treatment usually involves a decompressive suboccipital craniectomy with cervical laminectomies.

Table 22–3. Types of Chiari Malformations

Type I: Caudal displacement of cerebellar tonsils below the plane of the foramen magnum
Type II: (Arnold-Chiari; associated with myelomeningocele): Caudal displacement of the cerebellar vermis, fourth ventricle, and the lower brainstem below the plane of the foramen magnum. Dysplastic brainstem with characteristic "kink," elongation of the fourth ventricle, "beaking" of the quadrigeminal plate, hypoplastic tentorium with small posterior fossa, polymicrogyria, enlargement of the massa intermedia
Type III: Caudal displacement of the cerebellum and brainstem into a high cervical meningocele
Type IV: Cerebellar hypoplasia

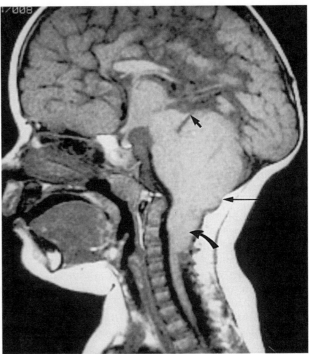

Figure 22–14. Magnetic resonance image of a patient with a Chiari II malformation. The small posterior fossa results in both upward and downward herniation of brain tissue. The short arrow indicates a "beaked" tectum showing upward herniation while the curved arrow indicates downward herniation of the cerebellar tonsils through the foramen magnum (thin arrow).

Other Spinal Defects

Other spinal anomalies (lipomeningoceles, lipomyelomeningoceles, diastematomyelias, and dermoid tracts) may manifest themselves as tethered cords. Skin defects, generally over the lower lumbar region, may present as dural sinus tracks or lipomeningoceles. Hair tufts, skin dimples, or fatty pads may all be associated with spinal defects. Sometimes these anomalies present when toilet training or ambulation is noted to be abnormal or later in childhood when patients complain of back pain. Children who have had a meningomyelocele repaired after birth may also develop an ascending neurologic deficit from a tethered spinal cord as growth occurs. Early detection of a tethered cord is now more common with magnetic resonance imaging. Prophylactic surgical untethering is common. Anesthetic management for surgical release of a tethered cord usually entails monitoring the innervation of the lower extremities and bowel and bladder with nerve stimulators and rectal electromyelograms or manometry. Thus, muscle relaxants must be avoided or permitted to wear off prior to intraoperative assessment.

Neuroradiologic Procedures

A wide variety of neuroradiologic procedures are performed in children. Anesthesiologists are often needed to provide immobilization and relief of the patient's anxiety. Anesthetic considerations for neurodiagnostic procedures (e.g., CT, MRI) are discussed elsewhere in this book (see Chapter 25), but certain therapeutic neuroradiologic procedures are worth noting here.

Embolization of arterial malformations or aneurysms can be performed during angiography, and the anesthesiologist needs to be aware of the embolic material being injected (e.g., coils, glue, alcohol), since complications can develop. Stereotactic head frames may also be placed prior to neurologic procedures, since this may be helpful in localizing surgery or radiation therapy. Anesthesia should be induced before the head frame is applied, not only for patient comfort, but also so that the airway may be easily secured with an endotracheal tube before the head frame limits airway access. A modified head frame has been developed (see Fig. 22–9) that has a moveable piece over the face and is safer to use than the conventional "rigid" stereotactic head frame, which often protrudes over the patient's nose or mouth.[161] Anesthesia is maintained after the initial radiologic procedures are performed, keeping the child asleep in the recovery room if necessary, until surgery or radiosurgery is completed and the head frame is removed.

An operating room has been built within an MRI machine, enabling surgery to be performed with unlimited and instantaneous access to MRI scans (Fig. 22–15). These procedures present special challenges to both neurosurgeons and anesthesiologists, since all equipment must be non-ferromagnetic in this environment. As with anesthesia for diagnostic MRI scans, special monitors and an MRI-compatible anesthesia machine must be utilized. However, it is much more challenging to do an entire craniotomy within this environment, especially since these procedures take many hours and are associated with blood loss, and access to the patient is severely limited. Some monitoring equipment generally utilized in conventional operating rooms during these procedures (such as precordial Doppler ultrasonogram, temperature probe, fluid warmers) are not yet compatible with this environment. Nevertheless, we have safely performed many craniotomies in children in this MRI operating room, and the equipment for these procedures is rapidly evolving.

REFERENCES

1. Shapiro HM: Intracranial hypertension: Therapeutic and anesthetic considerations. Anesthesiology 1975;43:445–471.
2. Arieff AI, Ayus JC, Fraser CL: Hyponatraemia and death or permanent brain damage in healthy children. Br Med J 1992;304:1218–1222.
3. Ayus JC, Arieff AI: Pathogenesis and prevention of hyponatremic encephalopathy. Endocrinol Metab Clin North Am 1993;22:425–446.
4. Trachtman H: Cell volume regulation: a review of cerebral adaptive mechanisms and implications for clinical treatment of osmolal disturbances. I. Pediatr Nephrol 1991;5:743–750.
5. Minns RA, Brown JK, Engleman HM: CSF production rate: "Real time" estimation. Z Kinderchir 1987;42:36–40.
6. Blomquist HK, Sundin S, Ekstedt J: Cerebrospinal fluid hydrodynamic studies in children. J Neurol Neurosurg Psychiatry 1986;49:536–548.
7. Rosman NP: Increased intracranial pressure in childhood. Pediatr Clin North Am 1974;21:483–499.
8. Rubin RC, Henderson ES, Ommaya AK, et al: The production of cerebrospinal fluid in man and its modification by acetazolamide. J Neurosurg 1966;25:430–436.
9. Clasen RA, Pandolfi S, Casey DJ: Furosemide and pentobarbital in cryogenic cerebral injury and edema. Neurology 1974;24:642–648.
10. Bruce DA, Berman WA, Schut L: Cerebrospinal fluid pressure monitoring in children: Physiology, pathology and clinical usefulness. Adv Pediatr 1977;24:233–290.
11. Jones TH, Morawetz RB, Crowell RM, et al: Thresholds of focal cerebral ischemia in awake monkeys. J Neurosurg 1981;54:773–782.
12. Marshall LF, Smith RW, Shapiro HM: The influence of diurnal rhythms in patients with intracranial hypertension: Implications for management. Neurosurgery 1978;2:100–102.
13. McDowall DG: Monitoring the brain. Anesthesiology 1976;45:117–134.
14. Chaves-Carballo E, Gomez MR, Sharbrough FW: Encephalopathy and fatty infiltration of the viscera (Reye-Johnson syndrome): A 17-year experience. Mayo Clin Proc 1975;50:209–215.
15. Hanlon K: Description and uses of intracranial pressure monitoring. Heart Lung 1976;5:277–282.
16. Lundberg N, Troupp H, Lorin H: Continuous recording of the ventricular-fluid pressure in patients with severe acute traumatic brain injury: A preliminary report. J Neurosurg 1965;22:581–590.
17. Coroneos NJ, McDowall DG, Pickerodt VW, et al: A comparison of intracranial extradural pressure with subarachnoid pressure. Br J Anaesth 1971;43:1198.
18. Ream AK, Silverberg GD, Corbin SD, et al: Epidural measurement of intracranial pressure. Neurosurgery 1979;5:36–43.
19. Levin AB, Kahn AR, Bahr DE: Epidural intracranial pressure monitoring: A new system. Med Instrum 1983;17:293–296.
20. Di Rocco C, McLone DG, Shimoji T, et al: Continuous intraventricular cerebrospinal fluid pressure recording in hydrocephalic children during wakefulness and sleep. J Neurosurg 1975;42:683–689.
21. Lassen NA, Christensen MS: Physiology of cerebral blood flow. Br J Anaesth 1976;48:719–734.
22. Lassen NA, Hoedt-Rasmussen K: Human cerebral blood flow measured by two inert gas techniques: Comparison of the Kety-Schmidt method and the intra-arterial injection method. Circ Res 1966;19:681–694.

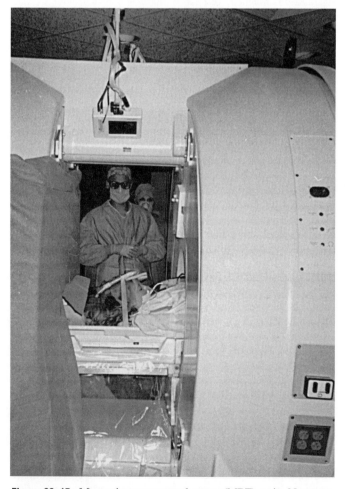

Figure 22–15. Magnetic resonance therapy (MRT) unit. Neurosurgeons are preparing a pediatric patient for a craniotomy. The technical difficulties both from a neurosurgical as well as an anesthesiology perspective are self-explanatory.

23. Kety SS, Schmidt CF: The nitrous oxide method for the quantitative determination of cerebral blood flow in man: Theory, procedure, and normal values. J Clin Invest 1948;27:476–483.

24. Kennedy C, Sokoloff L: An adaptation of the nitrous oxide method to the study of cerebral circulation in children: Normal values for cerebral blood flow and cerebral metabolic rate in childhood. J Clin Invest 1957;36:1130–1137.

25. Mehta S, Kalsi HK, Nain CK, et al: Energy metabolism of brain in human protein-calorie malnutrition. Pediatr Res 1977;11:290–293.

26. Cross KW, Dear PR, Hathorn MK, et al: An estimation of intracranial blood flow in the new-born infant. J Physiol (Lond) 1979;289:329–345.

27. Younkin DP, Reivich M, Jaggi J, et al: Noninvasive method of estimating human newborn regional cerebral blood flow. J Cereb Blood Flow Metab 1982;2:415–420.

28. Milligan DW: Cerebral blood flow and sleep state in the normal newborn infant. Early Hum Dev 1979;3:321–328.

29. Settergren G, Lindblad BS, Persson B: Cerebral blood flow and exchange of oxygen, glucose, ketone bodies, lactate, pyruvate and amino acids in infants. Acta Paediatr Scand 1976;65:343–353.

30. Luerssen TG: Intracranial pressure: Current status in monitoring and management. Semin Pediatr Neurol 1997;4:146–155.

31. Hernandez MJ, Brennan RW, Bowman GS: Autoregulation of cerebral blood flow in the newborn dog. Brain Res 1980;184:199–202.

32. Lou HC, Lassen NA, Friis-Hansen B: Impaired autoregulation of cerebral blood flow in the distressed newborn infant. J Pediatr 1979;94:118–121.

33. Cohen PJ, Alexander SC, Smith TC, et al: Effects of hypoxia and normocarbia on cerebral blood flow and metabolism in conscious man. J Appl Physiol 1967;23:183–189.

34. Kety SS, Schmidt CF: The effects of altered arterial tensions of carbon dioxide and oxygen on cerebral blood flow and cerebral oxygen consumption in normal young men. J Clin Invest 1948;27:484–492.

35. Rahilly PM: Effects of 2% carbon dioxide, 0.5% carbon dioxide, and 100% oxygen on cranial blood flow of the human neonate. Pediatrics 1980;66:685–689.

36. Rogers MC, Nugent SK, Traystman RJ: Control of cerebral circulation in the neonate and infant. Crit Care Med 1980;8:570–574.

37. Marion DW, Firlik A, McLaughlin MR: Hyperventilation therapy for severe traumatic brain injury. New Horiz 1995;3:439–447.

38. Skippen P, Seear M, Poskitt K, et al: Effect of hyperventilation on regional cerebral blood flow in head-injured children. Crit Care Med 1997;25:1402–1409.

39. Kennealy JA, McLennan JE, Loudon RG, et al: Hyperventilation-induced cerebral hypoxia. Am Rev Respir Dis 1980;122:407–412.

40. Lassen NA: Control of cerebral circulation in health and disease. Circ Res 1974;34:749–760.

41. Holzman RS: Clinical management of latex-allergic children. Anesth Analg 1997;85:529–533.

42. Tempelhoff R, Modica PA, Spitznagel ELJ: Anticonvulsant therapy increases fentanyl requirements during anaesthesia for craniotomy. Can J Anaesth 1990;37:327–332.

43. Alloul K, Whalley DG, Shutway F, et al: Pharmacokinetic origin of carbamazepine-induced resistance to vecuronium neuromuscular blockade in anesthetized patients. Anesthesiology 1996;84:330–339.

44. Soriano SG, Kaus SJ, Sullivan LJ, et al: Onset and duration of action of rocuronium in children receiving chronic anticonvulsant therapy. Paediatr Anaesth 2000;10:133–136.

45. Melton AT, Antognini JF, Gronert GA: Prolonged duration of succinylcholine in patients receiving anticonvulsants: Evidence for mild up-regulation of acetylcholine receptors? Can J Anaesth 1993;40:939–942.

46. Eldredge EA, Rockoff MA, Medlock MD, et al: Postoperative cerebral edema occurring in children with slit ventricles. Pediatrics 1997;99:625–630.

47. Rockoff MA, Goudsouzian NG: Seizures induced by methohexital. Anesthesiology 1981;54:333–335.

48. Yemen TA, Pullerits J, Stillman R, et al: Rectal methohexital causing apnea in two patients with meningomyeloceles. Anesthesiology 1991;74:1139–1141.

49. Shapiro HM, Galindo A, Wyte SR, et al: Rapid intraoperative reduction of intracranial pressure with thiopentone. Br J Anaesth 1973;45:1057–1062.

50. Modica PA, Tempelhoff R: Intracranial pressure during induction of anaesthesia and tracheal intubation with etomidate-induced EEG burst suppression. Can J Anaesth 1992;39:236–241.

51. Tulleken CA, van Dieren A, Jonkman J, et al: Clinical and experimental experience with etomidate as a brain protective agent. J Cereb Blood Flow Metab 1982;2:S92–S97.

52. Milde LN, Milde JH: Preservation of cerebral metabolites by etomidate during incomplete cerebral ischemia in dogs. Anesthesiology 1986;65:272–277.

53. Lockhart CH, Jenkins JJ: Ketamine-induced apnea in patients with increased intracranial pressure. Anesthesiology 1972;37:92–93.

54. Crumrine RS, Nulsen FE, Weiss MH: Alterations in ventricular fluid pressure during ketamine anesthesia in hydrocephalic children. Anesthesiology 1975;42:758–761.

55. Abou-Madi MN, Keszler H, Yacoub JM: Cardiovascular reactions to laryngoscopy and tracheal intubation following small and large intravenous doses of lidocaine. Can Anaesth Soc J 1977;24:12–19.

56. Baker KZ: Desflurane and sevoflurane are valuable additions to the practice of neuroanesthesiology: pro. J Neurosurg Anesthesiol 1997;9:66–68.

57. Tempelhoff R: The new inhalational anesthetics desflurane and sevoflurane are valuable additions to the practice of neuroanesthesia: con. J Neurosurg Anesthesiol 1997;9:69–71.

58. Scheller MS, Tateishi A, Drummond JC, et al: The effects of sevoflurane on cerebral blood flow, cerebral metabolic rate for oxygen, intracranial pressure, and the electroencephalogram are similar to those of isoflurane in the rabbit. Anesthesiology 1988;68:548–551.

59. Holzman RS, van der Velde ME, Kaus SJ, et al: Sevoflurane depresses myocardial contractility less than halothane during induction of anesthesia in children. Anesthesiology 1996;85:1260–1267.

60. Roth S, Thisted RA, Erickson JP, et al: Eye injuries after nonocular surgery. A study of 60,965 anesthetics from 1988 to 1992. Anesthesiology 1996;85:1020–1027.

61. Liu LM, DeCook TH, Goudsouzian NG, et al: Dose response to intramuscular succinylcholine in children. Anesthesiology 1981;55:599–602.

62. Kovarik WD, Mayberg TS, Lam AM, et al: Succinylcholine does not change intracranial pressure, cerebral blood flow velocity, or the electroencephalogram in patients with neurologic injury. Anesth Analg 1994;78:469–473.

63. Minton MD, Grosslight K, Stirt JA, et al: Increases in intracranial pressure from succinylcholine: prevention by prior nondepolarizing blockade. Anesthesiology 1986;65:165–169.

64. Cooperman LH: Succinylcholine-induced hyperkalemia in neuromuscular disease. JAMA 1970;213:1867–1871.

65. Mazurek AJ, Rae B, Hann S, et al: Rocuronium versus succinylcholine: Are they equally effective during rapid-sequence induction of anesthesia? Anesth Analg 1998;87:1259–1262.

66. Spacek A, Neiger FX, Spiss CK, et al: Atracurium-induced neuromuscular block is not affected by chronic anticonvulsant therapy with carbamazepine. Acta Anaesthesiol Scand 1997;41:1308–1311.

67. Todres ID, deBros F, Kramer SS, et al: Endotracheal tube displacement in the newborn infant. J Pediatr 1976;89:126–127.

68. Meridy HW, Creighton RE, Humphreys RP: Complications during neurosurgery in the prone position in children. Can Anaesth Soc J 1974;21:445–453.

69. Lorenc ZP, Ivy E, Aston SJ: Neurosensory preservation in endoscopic forehead plasty. Aesthetic Plast Surg 1995;19:411–413.

70. Pinosky ML, Fishman RL, Reeves ST, et al: The effect of bupivacaine skull block on the hemodynamic response to craniotomy. Anesth Analg 1996;83:1256–1261.

71. Becser N, Bovim G, Sjaastad O: Extracranial nerves in the posterior part of the head: Anatomic variations and their possible clinical significance. Spine 1998;23:1435–1441.

72. Scheller MS, Nakakimura K, Fleischer JE, et al: Cerebral effects of sevoflurane in the dog: Comparison with isoflurane and enflurane. Br J Anaesth 1990;65:388–392.

73. Neigh JL, Garman JK, Harp JR: The electroencephalographic pattern during anesthesia with Ethrane: Effects of depth of anesthesia, PaCO2, and nitrous oxide. Anesthesiology 1971;35:482–487.

74. Yli-Hankala A, Vakkuri A, Sarkela M, et al: Epileptiform electroencephalogram during mask induction of anesthesia with sevoflurane. Anesthesiology 1999;91:1596–1603.

75. Reasoner DK, Todd MM, Scamman FL, et al: The incidence of pneumocephalus after supratentorial craniotomy: Observations on the disappearance of intracranial air. Anesthesiology 1994;80:1008–1012.

76. Baker KZ, Ostapkovich N, Sisti MB, et al: Intact cerebral blood flow reactivity during remifentanil/nitrous oxide anesthesia. J Neurosurg Anesthesiol 1997;9:134–140.

77. Scheingraber S, Rehm M, Sehmisch C, et al: Rapid saline infusion produces hyperchloremic acidosis in patients undergoing gynecologic surgery. Anesthesiology 1999;90:1265–1270.

78. Coté CJ, Greenhow DE, Marshall BE: The hypotensive response to rapid intravenous administration of hypertonic solutions in man and in the rabbit. Anesthesiology 1979;50:30–35.

79. Wass CT, Lanier WL: Glucose modulation of ischemic brain injury: Review and clinical recommendations. Mayo Clin Proc 1996;71:801–812.

80. Murat I, Berniere J, Constant I: Evaluation of the efficacy of a forced-air warmer (Bair Hugger) during spinal surgery in children. J Clin Anesth 1994;6:425–429.

81. Rosomoff H, Holaday D: Cerebral blood flow and cerebral oxygen consumption during hypothermia. Am J Physiol 1954;179:85–88.

82. Harris MM, Yemen TA, Davidson A, et al: Venous embolism during craniectomy in supine infants. Anesthesiology 1987;67:816–819.

83. Cucchiara RF, Bowers B: Air embolism in children undergoing suboccipital craniotomy. Anesthesiology 1982;57:338–339.

84. Albin MS, Carroll RG, Maroon JC: Clinical considerations concerning detection of venous air embolism. Neurosurgery 1978;3:380–384.

85. Furuya H, Suzuki T, Okumura F, et al: Detection of air embolism by transesophageal echocardiography. Anesthesiology 1983;58:124–129.

86. Schwarz G, Fuchs G, Weihs W, et al: Sitting position for neurosurgery: Experience with preoperative contrast echocardiography in 301 patients. J Neurosurg Anesthesiol 1994;6:83–88.

87. Mammoto T, Hayashi Y, Ohnishi Y, et al: Incidence of venous and paradoxical air embolism in neurosurgical patients in the sitting position: Detection by transesophageal echocardiography. Acta Anaesthesiol Scand 1998;42:643–647.

88. Porter JM, Pidgeon C, Cunningham AJ: The sitting position in neurosurgery: A critical appraisal. Br J Anaesth 1999;82:117–128.

89. Pesce C, Mercurella A, Musi L, et al: Fatal cardiac tamponade as a late complication of central venous catheterization: a case report. Eur J Pediatr Surg 1999;9:113–115.

90. van Engelenburg KC, Festen C: Cardiac tamponade: A rare but life-threatening complication of central venous catheters in children. J Pediatr Surg 1998;33:1822–1824.

91. Bruder N, Ravussin P: Recovery from anesthesia and postoperative extubation of neurosurgical patients: A review. J Neurosurg Anesthesiol 1999;11:282–293.

92. Furst SR, Sullivan LJ, Soriano SG, et al: Effects of ondansetron on emesis in the first 24 hours after craniotomy in children. Anesth Analg 1996;83:325–328.

93. Birmingham PK, Tobin MJ, Henthorn TK, et al: Twenty-four-hour pharmacokinetics of rectal acetaminophen in children: An old drug with new recommendations. Anesthesiology 1997;87:244–252.

94. Kissoon N, Dreyer J, Walia M: Pediatric trauma: Differences in pathophysiology, injury patterns and treatment compared with adult trauma. Can Med Assoc J 1990;142:27–34.

95. Pascucci RC: Head trauma in the child. Intensive Care Med 1988;14:185–195.

96. Bruce DA, Raphaely RC, Goldberg AI, et al: Pathophysiology, treatment and outcome following severe head injury in children. Childs Brain 1979;5:174–191.

97. Bruce DA, Alavi A, Bilaniuk L, et al: Diffuse cerebral swelling following head injuries in children: The syndrome of "malignant brain edema." J Neurosurg 1981;54:170–178.

98. American Academy of Pediatrics Committee on Child Abuse and Neglect: Shaken baby syndrome: Inflicted cerebral trauma. Pediatrics 1993;92:872–875.

99. Duhaime AC, Christian CW, Rorke LB, et al: Nonaccidental head injury in infants: The "shaken-baby syndrome." N Engl J Med 1998;338:1822–1829.

100. Conway EE Jr: Nonaccidental head injury in infants: "The shaken baby syndrome revisited." Pediatr Ann 1998;27:677–690.

101. Hamilton MG, Myles ST: Pediatric spinal injury: Review of 174 hospital admissions. J Neurosurg 1992;77:700–704.

102. Hamilton MG, Myles ST: Pediatric spinal injury: Review of 61 deaths. J Neurosurg 1992;77:705–708.

103. Osenbach RK, Menezes AH: Pediatric spinal cord and vertebral column injury. Neurosurgery 1992;30:385–390.

104. Osenbach RK, Menezes AH: Spinal cord injury without radiographic abnormality in children. Pediatr Neurosci 1989;15:168–174.

105. Pang D, Wilberger JE Jr: Spinal cord injury without radiographic abnormalities in children. J Neurosurg 1982;57:114–129.

106. Tunkel DE, Fisher QA: Pediatric flexible fiberoptic bronchoscopy through the laryngeal mask airway. Arch Otolaryngol Head Neck Surg 1996;122:1364–1367.

107. Badr A, Tobias JD, Rasmussen GE, et al: Bronchoscopic airway evaluation facilitated by the laryngeal mask airway in pediatric patients. Pediatr Pulmonol 1996;21:57–61.

108. Bahk JH, Han SM, Kim SD: Management of difficult airways with a laryngeal mask airway under propofol anaesthesia. Paediatr Anaesth 1999;9:163–166.

109. Haynes SR, Morton NS: The laryngeal mask airway: A review of its use in paediatric anaesthesia. Paediatr Anaesth 1993;3:65–73.

110. Martens P: The use of the laryngeal mask airway by nurses during cardiopulmonary resuscitation: Results of a multicentre trial. Anaesthesia 1994;49:3–7.

111. Reinhart DJ, Simmons G: Comparison of placement of the laryngeal mask airway with endotracheal tube by paramedics and respiratory therapists. Ann Emerg Med 1994;24:260–263.

112. Coté CJ, Eavey RD, Todres ID, et al: Cricothyroid membrane puncture: Oxygenation and ventilation in a dog model using an intravenous catheter. Crit Care Med 1988;16:615–619.

113. Bracken MB, Collins WF, Freeman DF, et al: Efficacy of methylprednisolone in acute spinal cord injury. JAMA 1984;251:45–52.

114. Bracken MB, Shepard MJ, Collins WF, et al: A randomized, controlled trial of methylprednisolone or naloxone in the treatment of acute spinal-cord injury. Results of the Second National Acute Spinal Cord Injury Study. N Engl J Med 1990;322:1405–1411.

115. Hall ED: The neuroprotective pharmacology of methylprednisolone. J Neurosurg 1992;76:13–22.

116. Geisler FH: Clinical trials of pharmacotherapy for spinal cord injury. Ann N Y Acad Sci 1998;845:374–381.

117. Zeidman SM, Ling GS, Ducker TB, et al: Clinical applications of pharmacologic therapies for spinal cord injury. J Spinal Disord 1996;9:367–380.

118. Constantini S, Young W: The effects of methylprednisolone and the ganglioside GM1 on acute spinal cord injury in rats. J Neurosurg 1994;80:97–111.

119. Nobile-Orazio E, Carpo M, Scarlato G: Gangliosides: Their role in clinical neurology. Drugs 1994;47:576–585.

120. Geisler FH, Dorsey FC, Coleman WP: Past and current clinical studies with GM-1 ganglioside in acute spinal cord injury. Ann Emerg Med 1993;22:1041–1047.

121. Geisler FH: GM-1 ganglioside and motor recovery following human spinal cord injury. J Emerg Med 1993;11:49–55.

122. Skaper SD, Leon A: Monosialogangliosides, neuroprotection, and neuronal repair processes. J Neurotrauma 1992;9:S507–S516.

123. Gronert GA, Theye RA: Pathophysiology of hyperkalemia induced by succinylcholine. Anesthesiology 1975;43:89–99.

124. Amzallag M: Autonomic hyperreflexia. Int Anesthesiol Clin 1993;31:87–102.

125. Colachis SC III: Autonomic hyperreflexia with spinal cord injury. J Am Paraplegia Soc 1992;15:171–186.

126. Pollack IF: Brain tumors in children. N Engl J Med 1994;331:1500–1507.

127. Young WL, Solomon RA, Pedley TA, et al: Direct cortical EEG monitoring during temporary vascular occlusion for cerebral aneurysm surgery. Anesthesiology 1989;71:794–799.

128. Millar C, Bissonnette B, Humphreys RP: Cerebral arteriovenous malformations in children. Can J Anaesth 1994;41:321–331.

129. Ostergaard JR, Voldby B: Intracranial arterial aneurysms in children and adolescents. J Neurosurg 1983;58:832–837.

130. Salem MR, Wong AY, Bennett EJ, et al: Deliberate hypotension in infants and children. Anesth Analg 1974;53:975–981.

131. Suzuki J, Takaku A: Cerebrovascular "moyamoya" disease: Disease showing abnormal net-like vessels in base of brain. Arch Neurol 1969;20:288–299.

132. Sunder TR, Erwin CW, Dubois PJ: Hyperventilation induced abnormalities in the electroencephalogram of children with Moyamoya disease. Electroencephalogr Clin Neurophysiol 1980;49:414–420.

133. Adelson PD, Scott RM: Pial synangiosis for moyamoya syndrome in children. Pediatr Neurosurg 1995;23:26–33.

134. Soriano SG, Sethna NF, Scott RM: Anesthetic management of children with moyamoya syndrome. Anesth Analg 1993;77:1066–1070.

135. Takeuchi S, Tanaka R, Ishii R, et al: Cerebral hemodynamics in patients with moyamoya disease: A study of regional cerebral blood flow by the 133Xe inhalation method. Surg Neurol 1985;23:468–474.

136. Iwama T, Hashimoto N, Yonekawa Y: The relevance of hemodynamic factors to perioperative ischemic complications in childhood moyamoya disease. Neurosurgery 1996;38:1120–1125.

137. Sakamoto T, Kawaguchi M, Kurehara K, et al: Postoperative neurological deterioration following the revascularization surgery in children with moyamoya disease. J Neurosurg Anesthesiol 1998;10:37–41.

138. Vickrey BG, Hays RD, Rausch R, et al: Outcomes in 248 patients who had diagnostic evaluations for epilepsy surgery. Lancet 1995;346:1445–1449.

139. Soriano SG, Eldredge EA, Wang FK, et al: The effect of propofol on intraoperative electrocorticography and cortical stimulation during awake craniotomies in children. Paediatr Anaesth 2000;10:29–34.

140. Modica PA, Tempelhoff R, White PF: Pro- and anticonvulsant effects of anesthetics (Part II). Anesth Analg 1990;70:433–444.

141. Ford EW, Morrell F, Whisler WW: Methohexital anesthesia in the surgical treatment of uncontrollable epilepsy. Anesth Analg 1982;61:997–1001.

142. Carson BS, Javedan SP, Freeman JM, et al: Hemispherectomy: A hemidecortication approach and review of 52 cases. J Neurosurg 1996;84:903–911.

143. McLachlan RS: Vagus nerve stimulation for intractable epilepsy: A review. J Clin Neurophysiol 1997;14:358–368.

144. Schachter SC, Saper CB: Vagus nerve stimulation. Epilepsia 1998;39:677–686.

145. FineSmith RB, Zampella E, Devinsky O: Vagal nerve stimulator: A new approach to medically refractory epilepsy. N J Med 1999;96:37–40.

146. Hornig GW, Murphy JV, Schallert G, et al: Left vagus nerve stimulation in children with refractory epilepsy: An update. South Med J 1997;90:484–488.

147. Black PM, Hakim R, Bailey NO: The use of the Codman-Medos Programmable Hakim valve in the management of patients with hydrocephalus: Illustrative cases. Neurosurgery 1994;34:1110–1113.

148. Goumnerova LC, Frim DM: Treatment of hydrocephalus with third ventriculocisternostomy: Outcome and CSF flow patterns. Pediatr Neurosurg 1997;27:149–152.

149. Moynihan RJ, Brock-Utne JG, Archer JH, et al: The effect of cricoid pressure on preventing gastric insufflation in infants and children. Anesthesiology 1993;78:652–656.

150. Virtanen R, Korhonen T, Fagerholm J, et al: Neurocognitive sequelae of scaphocephaly. Pediatrics 1999;103:791–795.

151. Faberowski LW, Black S, Mickle JP: Incidence of venous air embolism during craniectomy for craniosynostosis repair. Anesthesiology 2000;92:20–23.

152. Faberowski LW, Black S, Mickle JP: Blood loss and transfusion practice in the perioperative management of craniosynostosis repair. J Neurosurg Anesthesiol 1999;11:167–172.

153. Dierdorf SF, McNiece WL, Rao CC, et al: Failure of succinylcholine to alter plasma potassium in children with myelomeningocoele. Anesthesiology 1986;64:272–273.

154. Viscomi CM, Abajian JC, Wald SL, et al: Spinal anesthesia for repair of meningomyelocele in neonates. Anesth Analg 1995;81:492–495.

155. Birmingham PK, Dsida RM, Grayhack JJ, et al: Do latex precautions in children with myelodysplasia reduce intraoperative allergic reactions? J Pediatr Orthop 1996;16:799–802.

156. Oren J, Kelly DH, Todres ID, et al: Respiratory complications in patients with myelodysplasia and Arnold-Chiari malformation. Am J Dis Child 1986;140:221–224.

157. Sutton LN, Adzick NS, Bilaniuk LT, et al: Improvement in hindbrain herniation demonstrated by serial fetal magnetic resonance imaging following fetal surgery for myelomeningocele. JAMA 1999;282:1826–1831.

158. Bruner JP, Tulipan N, Paschall RL, et al: Fetal surgery for myelomeningocele and the incidence of shunt-dependent hydrocephalus. JAMA 1999;282:1819–1825.

159. Ward SL, Nickerson BG, van der Hal A, et al: Absent hypoxic and hypercapneic arousal responses in children with myelomeningocele and apnea. Pediatrics 1986;78:44–50.

160. Putnam PE, Orenstein SR, Pang D, et al: Cricopharyngeal dysfunction associated with Chiari malformations. Pediatrics 1992;89:871–876.

161. Stokes MA, Soriano SG, Tarbell NJ, et al: Anesthesia for stereotactic radiosurgery in children. J Neurosurg Anesthesiol 1995;7:100–108.

23 Anesthesia for Children with Burn Injuries

S. K. Szyfelbein, J. A. Jeevendra Martyn, Robert L. Sheridan, *and* Charles J. Coté

Pathophysiology
  Cardiac
  Pulmonary
  Renal
  Hepatic
  Central Nervous System
  Hematologic
  Gastrointestinal
  Skin
  Metabolic
  Calcium Homeostasis
Pharmacology
Resuscitation and Initial Evaluation
  Airway and Oxygenation
  Carbon Monoxide Poisoning
  Adequacy of Circulation
  Associated Injury
  Circumferential Burns
  Electrical Burns
Guidelines to Anesthetic Management
  General Principles
  Special Considerations
  Awakening
Pain Management
Hyperbaric Oxygenation
Summary

Every year in the United States, about 1.25 million people are treated for burns. Of these burned patients, 500,000 are hospitalized, with an 11% mortality rate.[1, 2] Children account for at least 25% of these patients. These patients are well managed only when their care providers thoroughly understand the physiologic and pharmacologic abnormalities associated with burn injury.[3] These abnormalities include metabolic derangements, neurohumoral responses, massive fluid shifts, sepsis, and the systemic effects of massive tissue destruction. This chapter discusses the pathophysiology, the initial evaluation and resuscitation, the anesthetic management, and the pain management of pediatric patients with burn injury. Some of the principles presented are derived from experiences with adult patients and applied to children, whereas others are the result of more than 25 years of experience in caring for children with burn injuries.

Pathophysiology

A burn is unique among traumatic injuries. It destroys skin, the largest organ of the body, upon which we depend for thermal regulation, fluid and electrolyte homeostasis, and protection against bacterial infection. It is important to appreciate that even minor, localized burn injuries are associated with systemic responses.[4–11] Several mediators released from the burned areas activate the inflammatory response and cause the edema. Complements, arachidonic acid metabolites, and oxygen radicals are involved in this response.[12] Cytokines seem to be the main mediators of the systemic effects.[13] Endotoxins are frequently detected in the immediate post-burn period and usually correlated to burn size and are predictive of the development of multiple organ failure and the subsequent demise of the patient.[12] Nitric oxide levels are also increased in these patients.[14] The clinical symptoms and pathologic changes are relatively more severe in children, and, unfortunately, the gravity of the injury is often underestimated because of their greater ratio of body surface area to weight (Fig. 23–1).

Soon after injury, massive fluid shifts occur from the vascular compartment into the burned tissue, resulting in sequestration of fluid, even in nonburned areas, causing significant hemoconcentration.[4, 9, 15–17] Despite the massive fluid loss, systemic blood pressure may be maintained as a result of the outpouring of catecholamines and antidiuretic hormone.[18, 19] In the first 4 days after a burn of moderate size or larger, an amount of albumin equal to approximately twice the total body plasma content is lost through the

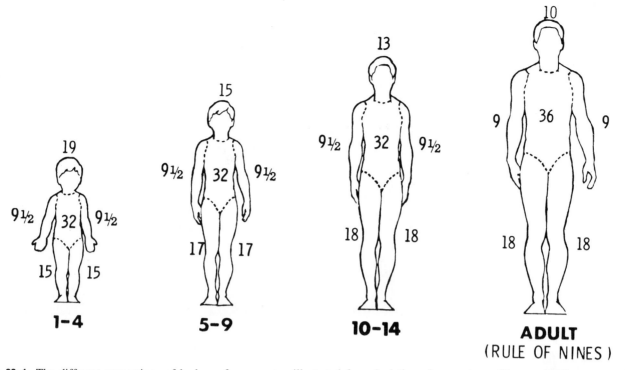

Figure 23–1. The different proportions of body surface area are illustrated for calculation of percentage of burn according to a patient's age. Note the large proportion of body surface area that the head and face account for in an infant. (From Carvajal HF, Goldman AS: Burns. *In* Vaughan VC III, McKay RJ, Nelson WE, eds.: Nelson's Textbook of Pediatrics. Philadelphia: WB Saunders, 1975:281.)

wound. Half of this albumin remains sequestered in the extravascular space for 3 weeks or more.[4] In addition to the direct effects of the burn (thrombosis, increased capillary permeability), changes in vascular integrity occur in areas remote from the injury resulting in tissue edema.[17, 20–23] In the pulmonary capillary network, these changes may be life threatening; severe pulmonary edema and vascular congestion may result.

Cardiac

Immediately after injury, cardiac output is strikingly reduced.[24–27] This decrease is often related to the rapid reduction in circulating blood volume or to the severe compressive effects of circumferential burns on the abdomen and chest, impairing venous return.[26] Despite adequate cardiac filling pressures, however, some patients continue to have a reduced cardiac output. This finding suggests other contributing factors, such as a direct myocardial depression from the burn injury. Some investigators have described circulating myocardial depressant factors such as interleukins, tumor necrosis factors, or oxygen free radicals existing in subjects with extensive third-degree burns.[28–33]

Three to 5 days after a burn injury, patients develop a hypermetabolic state. This may result in a two- to threefold increase in cardiac output, which persists for weeks to months, depending on the extent of the injury and the length of time needed for wound closure. Gram-negative sepsis, however, may cause a depressed cardiac output. Closure of the burn wound usually decreases metabolic demand, resulting in a concomitant reduction in cardiac output.[34]

Pulmonary

Pulmonary function may be adversely affected from the upper airway to terminal alveoli. The upper airway is an excellent heat exchanger; just as it warms cold air, it cools hot air. The cooling of hot inspired air may result in heat destruction of laryngeal tissues; the air in a closed space (e.g., house or automobile fire) may reach 538°C (1000°F) 2 feet above floor level. Inspiration of superheated air damages the upper airway; airway obstruction occurs as a result of massive edema formation involving all airway structures above the carina.[35, 36] The proximal bronchi may suffer heat destruction of the ciliated epithelium and mucosa. The distal bronchi and alveoli may be damaged by inhalation of toxic fumes, such as nitrogen dioxide and sulfur dioxide, which combine with water in the tracheobronchial tree to form nitric and sulfuric acids. Upper airway damage is therefore usually related to a heat injury, whereas lower airway injury is usually related to chemical or toxic effects. Acid gases such as hydrochloric, sulfuric, and phosgene penetrate deeply, thereby damaging the alveolar membranes and surfactants.[37] Wool and cotton combustion result in aldehyde formation; aldehyde inhalation may cause pulmonary edema in concentrations as low as 10 parts per million.[35, 36] Combustion of synthetic materials (insulation, wall paneling) releases hydrogen cyanide. Although it is apparently rare,[38] cyanide poisoning can lead to histotoxic hypoxia and death.[39–53] Inhalation of hydrogen cyanide is an often unrecognized cause of immediate death.

The overall effect of a pulmonary inhalation injury is necrotizing bronchitis, bronchial swelling, alveolar destruction, exudation of protein, loss of surfactant, loss of the

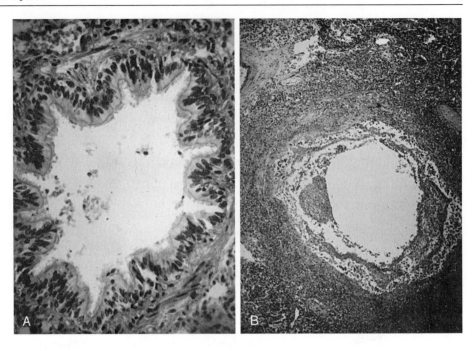

Figure 23–2. Cross section of a normal bronchiole (A). Note the ciliated epithelial layer. Compare with a cross section of a distal bronchiole from a patient who died from an inhalation injury (B). Note the marked thickening of the bronchial wall, the massive inflammatory cell infiltrate, the sloughing of the mucosa, and the total destruction of the ciliated columnar epithelium.

protective bronchial lining, and bronchospasm, all of which contribute to the development of bronchopneumonia (Fig. 23–2A&B). Inhalation of particulate matter (smoke, soot) and lower airway edema also result in mechanical airway obstruction. Edema of the bronchi, combined with loss of integrity of the pulmonary capillary endothelium, results in decreased pulmonary compliance. Chest wall compliance may also be diminished by circumferential chest burns, which have a tourniquet-like effect.[26, 53, 54] All of these injuries lead to clinically important ventilation/perfusion abnormalities, with resultant hypoxemia and hypercarbia. Victims of severe smoke inhalation may not often have any direct burn injury to tissue.[55]

Extrapulmonary factors such as changes in cardiac output can also contribute to hypoxemia. Measurement of blood gases alone may not indicate these factors. Rational therapy of reduced arterial oxygen saturation requires evaluation of both extrapulmonary and intrapulmonary factors contributing to arterial desaturation.[56, 57] Measurements that discriminate extrapulmonary and intrapulmonary factors include cardiac output, mixed venous oxygen content or saturation, and shunt fraction.[56] In general, the prognosis of cutaneous burn is compounded by the simultaneous occurrence of a pulmonary burn. It is estimated that the presence of an inhalational injury doubles the mortality rate from cutaneous burns.[37]

Renal

Renal function may be adversely affected soon after injury as a result of myoglobinuria and hemoglobinuria.[58] The former is most common after electrical injury, whereas the latter is encountered after severe cutaneous burns. Hypovolemia, hypotension, and hypoxemia may further aggravate renal dysfunction, resulting in acute tubular necrosis. Increased production of catecholamines, angiotensin, vasopressin, and aldosterone lead to systemic vasoconstriction compounding the renal insufficiency.[59] Release of vasoactive peptides such as endothelin-1 may cause acute vasoconstric-

tion that may also have adverse effects on renal function.[31] Fluid retention generally occurs during the first 5 days after injury, and diuresis begins after this. Thus there may be impairment of renal function soon after injury, which may also delay drug excretion. Three to 7 days after the burn injury, glomerular filtration rate increases pari passu with cardiac output and increased metabolic rate.[60–62] The serum half-life of many antibiotics as well as other medications excreted through glomerular filtration may be altered as a result of changes (increased or decreased) in glomerular filtration rate.[62–66] Patients suffering a burn that covers more than 40% of their body surface area demonstrate renal tubular dysfunction, mainly an inability to concentrate the urine.[18, 59, 60] Even during hyperosmolar states, antidiuresis is not observed, suggesting an inadequate renal response to antidiuretic hormone and aldosterone. Thus it is possible to observe adequate urine output even in the presence of hypovolemia.[67] Episodic or persistent hypertension is frequent in children; it may in part be mediated by increased renin and catecholamine production.[19, 68] If hypertension is persistent, then treatment should be instituted to avoid excessive stress on the cardiovascular system.

Hepatic

The liver may be damaged by hypoxemia, by hypoperfusion during the early post-burn phase as a result of hypovolemia or hypotension, and by inhaled or absorbed chemical toxins.[69, 70] Hepatic dysfunction may later result from drug toxicity, sepsis, or blood transfusions. Studies in adults have found increased hepatic blood flow, increased protein synthesis and breakdown, and increased hepatic gluconeogenesis during the hypermetabolic phase of burn injury. With the onset of sepsis, hepatic glucose output and alanine uptake may decrease sharply, but hepatic blood flow and oxygen utilization can remain elevated.[69] Fatty infiltration of the liver has also been reported.[70, 71] Sustained increases in hepatic blood flow deliver more drug to the liver; this effect, combined with drug-induced enzyme induction, may result in a reduced drug half-life.[72] Although all studies of animals suggest a depressed clearance of drugs after burn injury, clinical studies of the capacity of the liver to metabolize drugs are conflicting, even for the same class of drugs.[73–78] The magnitude of the burn, the time after injury, and the effects of co-administered drugs each may have a role in these conflicting reports.

Central Nervous System

The central nervous system may be adversely affected by inhalation of neurotoxic chemicals or by hypoxic encephalopathy; other contributing factors include sepsis, hyponatremia, and hypovolemia.[79] The central nervous system dysfunction includes hallucinations, personality changes, delirium, seizures, abnormal neurologic symptoms, and coma.[80] These effects may be due to the burn injury itself or to the administration of drugs necessary for sedation/anxiolysis/analgesia.[81] Such effects usually clear after several weeks. Abnormalities of central nervous system neurotransmitters have been postulated to mediate the anorexia associated with extensive burn injury.[82] The possibility of cerebral edema and increased intracranial pressure must also be considered during the initial phases of burn injury. Under such circumstances, the usual measures for treating increased intracranial pressure would be instituted (see Chapter 22). Data suggest that rapid overcorrection of hyponatremia may be associated with cerebral injury.[83]

Hematologic

Blood viscosity may increase as a result of hemoconcentration secondary to fluid shifts and because of alterations in plasma protein content.[4, 15] The hematopoietic system is also adversely affected; an ongoing hemolytic anemia secondary to the burn injury is common.[84, 85] An inhibitor of erythroid stem cells has also been found in the sera of burn patients; it may in part contribute to the anemia of burn injury.[86] Another study has demonstrated a normal erythropoietin response to anemia in patients with burn injury.[87] The half-life of red blood cells is diminished in burn patients and many laboratory tests are necessary; these factors also contribute to the development of anemia.[88, 89] The possible role of artificial erythropoietin for the care of burned patients has yet to be defined.[90, 91]

In the early stage, thrombocytopenia, secondary to increased platelet aggregation and trapping of platelets in the lungs, is followed by an increase in platelet count 10 to 14 days after burn injury. This elevation persists for several months.[85, 88, 92] An increase in fibrin split products (disseminated intravascular coagulopathy), which lasts for 3 to 5 days, may occur.[92] Factors V, VII, and VIII and fibrinogen are also increased several-fold over baseline for the first 3 months after severe injury uncomplicated by sepsis.[92, 93] We have observed a number of patients who had elevated platelet counts and who experienced a marked reduction in platelet count with the onset of sepsis. The sudden onset of thrombocytopenia calls for an evaluation for sepsis.

Gastrointestinal

Gastrointestinal function is diminished immediately after thermal injury secondary to the development of gastric and intestinal ileus.[94] Because of the danger of pulmonary aspiration of gastric contents during this time, the stomach should be adequately vented and appropriate gastric acid prophylaxis instituted. Approximately 48 to 72 hours after a burn, with diminishing of the generalized edema, gastrointestinal function is usually restored. Enteral feeding should be established at this time to provide calories, to attenuate the hypermetabolic response, and to prevent gluconeogenesis and stress ulceration.[15, 16, 95, 96] Early enteral feeding has the added advantage that it can diminish muscle catabolism and even reduce bacterial translocation through the intestinal mucosa.[97]

In patients unable to tolerate enteral feeding, parenteral nutrition must be initiated.[95, 96, 98] Stress ulcers (Curling ulcers) are associated with any burn injury and may be life threatening; however, the incidence has decreased in critically ill patients, perhaps in part as a result of better pharmacologic control of gastric acidity.[99, 100] Prospective studies of pediatric and adult burn victims and patients in intensive care indicate that cimetidine in the usual doses may not adequately protect seriously ill patients from increases in gastric acidity.[66, 101, 102] This increased requirement is related to pharmacokinetic or pharmacodynamic alterations.[66, 103] Therefore, frequent feedings when tolerated, the liberal use of antacids, combined with larger or more frequent doses of H2-receptor antagonists, may be required to help prevent the development of stress ulceration.[15, 94, 103]

Skin

Extensive skin destruction results in the inability to regulate body heat, to conserve fluids and electrolytes, and to protect against bacterial invasion. Permeability of burned tissues is markedly increased and proportional to the number of layers of tissue damaged.[104] Since children have a much greater ratio of body surface area to weight compared with adults, they are even more prone to dangerous hypothermia and fluid and electrolyte imbalances (see Fig. 23–1). It is important to keep these patients covered as much as possible; to elevate the environmental temperature; and to use radiant warmers, plastic wrap around extremities, reflective insulated blankets, warm inspired respiratory gases, and hot air heating blankets. Late complications affecting the skin include progressive scar formation, which results in movement-restricting contractures.[26, 54] Topical antibiotic and antibacterial therapy is necessary to prevent burn wound sepsis.[105, 106]

Metabolic

Many metabolic alterations follow extensive burn injury. Increased utilization of glucose, fat, and protein result in greater oxygen demand and increased carbon dioxide production.[2, 5, 7, 8, 10, 11, 15, 69, 95, 107–109] Mediators that have been implicated in these metabolic changes include interleukin-1, tumor necrosis factor, catecholamines, prostanoids, and other stress hormones.[2, 16] Centrally mediated or sepsis-induced hyperthermia also increases oxygen consumption and carbon dioxide production. Some of these abnormalities may persist even after complete closure of the burn wounds, when metabolic demand is already reduced.[34] Intravenous alimentation, particularly with high glucose concentrations, may increase carbon dioxide production and therefore increase ventilatory requirements.[95, 110] Increase in oxygen demand and carbon dioxide production must be compensated for during controlled mechanical ventilation.

Calcium Homeostasis

Many acutely burned patients demonstrate an abnormally low ionized calcium Ca^{++} level. Marked abnormalities in the indices of calcium metabolism in both acute and recovery phases may persist for as long as 7 weeks after injury (Fig. 23–3).[111] Hypophosphatemia and hypermagnesemia revert toward normal during the latter phase of recovery from the acute injury. The usual reciprocal relationship between calcium and inorganic phosphate is not evident in patients with major burn injury. Therefore, supplemental calcium therapy is extremely important in the management of severely burned patients, particularly during extensive surgical procedures, in which ionized hypocalcemia may have adverse cardiovascular effects. In general, frequent small boluses would be safer and more effective than intermittent large boluses (see Figs. 12–4 and 12–5).[112] A dose of 2.5 mg/kg calcium chloride or 7.5 mg/kg calcium gluconate ionize at equivalent rates and produce equivalent increases in Ca^{++}.

Pharmacology

Subsequent to any major thermal injury, many changes in hepatic, renal, and pulmonary function take place. Uptake and clearance of drugs may be decreased because of impaired organ perfusion during the hypovolemic period.[2, 72, 74, 75, 113, 114] After the immediate post-burn period, the patient becomes hypermetabolic.[2] During the hypermetabolic phase, because of increased blood flow and enzyme induction, the activity of the clearing organs may be enhanced.[60–63, 66, 69, 72, 77, 103, 113–116] The massive edema present in the burned and nonburned areas and the loss of drug through burn wound can result in an apparent increase in the central or total volume of distribution.

Many drugs are highly bound by plasma proteins. The activity of such drugs is likely to depend more on the unbound than total drug concentrations. The two major binding proteins, alpha$_1$-acid glycoprotein and albumin, increase and decrease, respectively, after burn injury, resulting in either decreased or increased free fractions of those drugs with which they bind.[72, 114, 116] For example, the clearance of morphine and meperidine seems to be enhanced or impaired, depending on the size of the burn, with a tendency for a bigger burn to have reduced morphine or meperidine clearance compared with moderate burns. Burned patients, however, tend to have higher clearances than do patients without burn injury.[74–76, 117, 118] Similarly, pharmacokinetic studies of lorazepam and diazepam indicate depressed clearance of the former and enhanced clearance of the latter.[77, 78]

There is evidence that burn injury, with its complications and hormonal responses, may cause changes in receptor numbers in tissues.[78, 82, 113, 116, 119–125] It is therefore not surprising to hear reports of aberrant responses to drugs acting on adrenergic and cholinergic receptors. These include altered sensitivity to succinylcholine at the neuromuscular junction, increased sensitivity to dopamine in the pulmonary circulation, and decreased sensitivity to nondepolarizing relaxants.[72, 114, 119–123, 126, 127] Other examples of drugs affected by burn-induced kinetic and dynamic changes include aminoglycoside antibiotics, diazepam, and cimetidine. Burn-induced alterations in kinetics and dynamics make the clinical response to any medication unpredictable. Therefore, clinical effects should always be closely monitored and plasma concentrations, protein binding, and clearance evaluated whenever possible.[63, 65, 72, 103, 114, 128–130]

Resuscitation and Initial Evaluation

Resuscitation of patients with a burn injury must give priority to the establishment of a clear airway, as well as maintenance of adequate oxygenation and circulating blood volume. The diagnosis and evaluation of associated injuries must also be considered.

Airway and Oxygenation

All patients with burn injuries, especially those with inhalation injuries, must be considered hypoxemic; many suffer from carbon monoxide (CO) poisoning. Therefore, during transport to the hospital and on admission, administration of a high inspired oxygen concentration is mandatory pending evaluation for the severity of CO poisoning or pulmonary injury.[131] Direct injury to the airway and alveoli occurs in patients who have sustained pulmonary injury due to the inhalation of smoke, flames, noxious gases, heated air, or

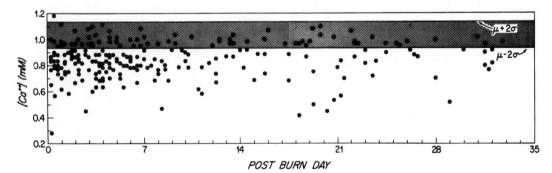

Figure 23–3. Ionized calcium values from burned children and adults are plotted for the first 35 days after burn injury. Note that the majority of values are abnormally low. (From Szyfelbein SK, Drop LJ, Martyn JA: Persistent ionized hypocalcemia during resuscitation and recovery phases of body burns. Crit Care Med 1981;9:454–458.)

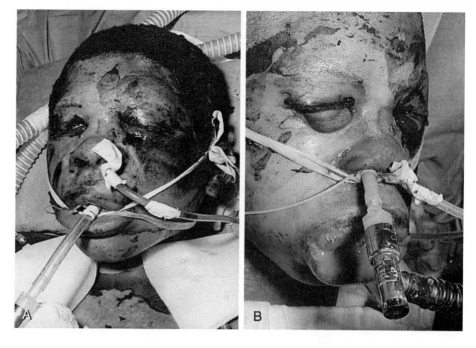

Figure 23–4. A young child who had just sustained a facial burn in a closed space (A). Note the early onset of facial edema. The same patient several hours later (B) shows massive edema formation that extends into the oropharynx, larynx, and trachea (similar to the combined effects of macroglossia, epiglottitis, and laryngotracheobronchitis). Early prophylactic intubation is mandatory in any facial burn or in any patient when there is potential for inhalation injury. Note that the endotracheal tube was changed from an oral to a nasal position and that it is secured with cloth tape rather than adhesive tape.

steam.[16, 17, 35, 36, 39–54, 132, 133] When a patient is burned in an enclosed space (house, automobile) or if thermal burns or carbonaceous materials are evident about the mouth and nose, respiratory involvement is probable.[49, 134] Upper airway obstruction caused by edema of the lips, nose, tongue, pharynx, or glottis is very common. The resultant airway obstruction can be compared with the combined effects of acute macroglossia, epiglottitis, and laryngotracheobronchitis. The decreasing patency of the airway by rapidly increasing edema, beginning in the first hours after the injury and lasting several days, makes delayed intubation hazardous if not impossible (Fig. 23–4A&B). Prophylactic intubation should be performed in any case of severe facial burns or when pulmonary burn and upper airway inhalation injury are suspected. Severity of adverse outcome is related to the presence or absence of inhalation injury.[135]

Control of the airway in pediatric patients is usually accomplished under general anesthesia. In the case of pure inhalational injury without facial or upper airway burns, the need for intubation should be considered on a case-by-case basis. Clinical experience shows that endotracheal tubes can be left in place in these patients for weeks with fewer risks than the alternative, tracheostomy.[136, 137] Tracheostomy in thermally injured patients is associated with high mortality rates; in one pediatric series, the death rate approached 100%.[138] In general, it is taught that uncuffed endotracheal tubes are preferred in infants and children. In some of these patients, however, high inspiratory pressures are necessary, which may require the use of cuffed endotracheal tubes. Low-pressure cuffed endotracheal tubes have been successfully used in the intensive care and operating room setting.[139, 140] Tracheostomy should be considered only in extreme situations in which intubation is technically impossible. Another means of reducing barotrauma in these patients is permissive hypercarbia.[141]

Carbon Monoxide Poisoning

Carboxyhemoglobin is produced by the combination of CO with the iron of the heme radical, the oxygen-binding site. CO combines more slowly with hemoglobin than oxygen but is bound more than 200 times more firmly.[142, 143] Inhalation of 1% CO for 2 minutes can result in carboxyhemoglobin values of 30%.[144] The toxic effects of CO poisoning are due to tissue hypoxia from decreased oxygen delivery. Decreased delivery occurs because CO reduces oxygen binding capacity, and, even in small amounts, carboxyhemoglobin shifts the oxygen-dissociation curve to the left (Fig. 23–5).[36, 131, 143, 145–148]

The majority of smoke inhalation victims have CO poisoning. Direct measurement of carboxyhemoglobin is an important guide to the adequacy of treatment. Estimates of the carboxyhemoglobin concentration may be derived by measuring (not calculating) oxygen saturation or arterial oxygen content. The half-life of carboxyhemoglobin is approximately 4 hours when the patient is breathing room air but decreases to 30 minutes when 100% oxygen is administered with mechanical ventilation.[36] Immediate administration of oxygen is therefore essential to achieve the highest possible level of oxygen in the blood; positive-pressure ventilation may be indicated in severe cases.[147, 149, 150] Pulse oximeters do not differentiate between oxyhemoglobin and carboxyhemoglobin; in contrast, transcutaneous oxygen analyzers are useful.[151] Pulse oximetry cannot be used to monitor the oxygenation of patients with CO poisoning because carboxyhemoglobin produces an overestimation of oxygen saturation. The photo detector is "fooled" into interpreting carboxyhemoglobin as oxyhemoglobin.[151–153] The usefulness of hyperbaric oxygen for the treatment of CO poisoning has not been clearly established in humans.[131, 154–156] However, it is reasonable to conclude that burned patients with mild exposure, as evidence by carboxyhemoglobin levels less than 30% without neurologic symptoms, can be treated with high oxygen concentrations. Comatose patients with carboxyhemoglobin levels of greater than 30% at the time of hospital admission can benefit from hyperbaric oxygenation (see later discussion).[148] If cyanide poisoning is confirmed by measurement of its level in blood, the administration of hydroxoco-

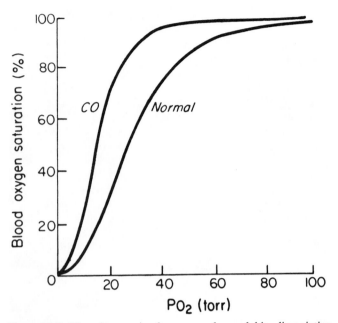

Figure 23–5. The changes in the oxygen-hemoglobin dissociation curve that occur with carbon monoxide poisoning. The oxygen-hemoglobin dissociation curve is altered in shape and is shifted to the left. Therefore, less oxygen is available for delivery to tissues, and the oxygen carried by hemoglobin is more tightly bound. (From Fein A, Leff A, Hopewell PC: Pathophysiology and management of the complications resulting from fire and the inhaled products of combustion: review of the literature. Crit Care Med 1980;8:94–98.)

balamin, sodium thiosulfate, nitrates, or a combination of these is warranted (see Chapter 12).[157]

Adequacy of Circulation

The various formulas for determining fluid replacement are estimates and often need modification, depending on clinical and laboratory findings.[2–4, 15, 16, 19, 20, 158–169] The most widely accepted fluid protocols in current use are the Parkland (Baxter) and Brooke formulas. It is important to remember that all formulas are only guides to fluid therapy; they should be modified for individual patients, depending on the response (Table 23–1). The most important response is maintenance of good urine output (0.5–1 ml/kg/h).

Either formula gives the estimated resuscitation volume, in addition to the calculated normal maintenance fluid requirement for each day. *These formulas are of great value*

Table 23–1. Parkland and Brooke Formulas

	Fluid Therapy		
	Crystalloid (mL/kg)	Colloid (mL/kg)	
Parkland	4.0	+ 0	× percent burn × wt (kg)
Brooke	0.5	+ 1.5	× percent burn × wt (kg)

Note: Half this volume is administered during the first 8 hours and the remainder during the next 16 hours. Infants who weigh ≤10 kg may have even greater fluid requirements (see text).

in guiding the fluid resuscitation of older patients; however, serious underestimation may occur if applied to infants weighing less than 10 kg. In such patients, it is reasonable to estimate the normal hourly maintenance fluid requirements and then add to this the fluid volume of the Parkland or Brooke formula.[2] Alternatively, the crystalloid fluid regimen for resuscitation can be increased to 6 mL/kg times the percent surface area burn per 24 hours.[170, 171]

The degree of edema formation is dependent on the volume and composition of the resuscitation fluid administered. Therefore, some burn centers use colloids or hypertonic saline (with or without albumin) during early burn wound resuscitation. These modified regimens are reported to be particularly useful in the very young and the elderly.[2, 15, 16, 167–169, 172] The purported advantage is less tissue edema. It is of interest that the overall morbidity, mortality, and incidence of renal failure are the same as with standard burn resuscitation fluid protocols. Consequently, only crystalloids are used for all burn patients in our institution because of their simplicity, reduced cost, and similar outcomes. Further work is required before routinely advocating hypertonic fluid regimens in children.[173]

The syndrome of hyperosmolar hyperglycemic nonketotic coma (severe dehydration, marked hyperglycemia, serum hyperosmolality, and coma in the absence of ketoacidosis) may be associated with burns and has a high mortality.[4] The need to control the use of glucose-containing solutions at all times, particularly during the initial volume resuscitation, and the need for frequent serum glucose measurement is thus emphasized.

The general appearance of the patient and his or her sensorium provide important guides to the effectiveness of the resuscitative therapy. In addition, urine output is usually a helpful indicator of the need for fluid replacement, bearing in mind the possible increase in antidiuretic hormone secretion and occasional tubular dysfunction.[18, 60] Every effort must be made to protect the kidneys by providing adequate fluid replacement.[2, 174] Renal failure in the presence of major burns is virtually tantamount to death. However, overly vigorous fluid therapy may result in pulmonary edema and excessive tissue edema. Therefore, the volume resuscitation of a burned child necessitates careful titration of all fluids to replace the circulating blood volume. Commonly used end points of satisfactory fluid resuscitation include heart rate, systemic arterial blood pressure, urinary output, central venous pressure, arterial oxygenation, and pH. In more severely ill patients, cardiac performance is appraised by pulmonary artery flow-directed catheters and measurement of cardiac output.[24, 25, 27] Multiple factors, including ventricular compliance, pulmonary artery hypertension, and positive end-expiratory airway pressure, distort measured atrial filling pressures. Using the thermodilution principle, mean pulmonary artery pressure, pulmonary capillary wedge pressure, central venous pressure, ventricular volume, and ejection fraction have been measured in burned young adults and adolescents as a guide to the adequacy of fluid therapy.[25, 27, 57] End-diastolic ventricular volume may be superior to the conventional measures in predicting the adequacy of circulating blood volume. Cardiovascular function estimated by echocardiography and ^{99}Tc ventriculography may be of value in critically ill patients.[57, 175] These advanced cardiac evalua-

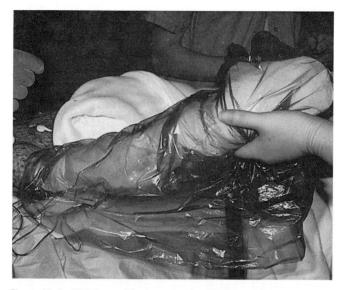

Figure 23–6. Children with extensive burn injury can be kept warm by having the extremities wrapped with sterile plastic bags. Covering the head is also an important method of heat preservation.

tions are not required in most children; they are mostly useful when there is pre-trauma cardiovascular compromise.

In a child, the evaporative fluid losses exceed 4000 mL/m^2 of burn surface each day, compared with only 2500 mL/m^2 in an adult.[169, 176] Concomitantly, for each square meter of burn surface, 2500 to 4000 kcal of heat is lost each day. Minimizing caloric expenditure and providing caloric supplementation simultaneously are the only ways to prevent catabolism of body tissues. The tendency for children to be poikilothermic, particularly in the absence of protective skin as a result of the burn injury, causes profound temperature derangements. Efforts to maintain a normal body temperature involve active warming by a warming blanket, elevated ambient room temperatures, laminar flow room, and warmed intravenous fluids, as well as prevention of heat loss by keeping patients covered with forced air warming devices even in the intensive care unit. These measures are especially important during the initial volume resuscitation and in the operating room when dressings are taken down for examination and excision (Fig. 23–6).

Associated Injury

Associated injuries such as a tension pneumothorax, a ruptured spleen or liver, long bone fractures, or head injury are easy to overlook, especially during the early phase of burn wound fluid resuscitation. Taking a detailed history, especially from the emergency medical personnel and family, combined with a careful physical examination, is mandatory during the initial resuscitation because such injuries may compound or be hidden by the need for an increased volume of resuscitation fluids.

Circumferential Burns

There are immediate adverse cardiovascular and respiratory responses to circumferential burns of the chest, abdomen, and extremities.[2, 26, 53, 54] Circumferential burns of the thorax can contribute to respiratory failure due to decreased chest wall compliance. Functional residual capacity is reduced with airway closure and atelectasis, resulting in profound hypoxemia.[35, 36, 39–54] Deep circumferential burns of the chest and abdomen may generate excessive intrathoracic and intra-abdominal pressure, which, in addition to restricting diaphragmatic movement, may reduce the already low cardiac output by impairing venous return (Fig. 23–7A&B).[26, 53, 54] When this occurs, both extrapulmonary and intrapulmonary factors can contribute to arterial desaturation.[56]

The edema of damaged tissues can also generate severe compressive forces, restricting or occluding the blood flow to burned extremities; the result may be ischemia, which, if left untreated, may necessitate partial or total amputation. Escharotomies of circumferential burns of the chest, abdomen, and extremities must be performed urgently, because impaired hemodynamics and respiratory mechanics can cause irreversible damage within hours after the burn injury.

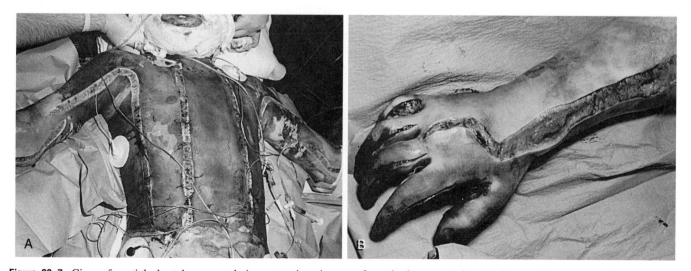

Figure 23–7. Circumferential chest burns result in severe impairment of respirations secondary to the tourniquet effect of the shrinking eschar and subcutaneous edema (A). The widely separated escharotomy lines indicate the severity of the constriction. Similar effects occur in circumferentially burned extremities (B). Early escharotomy may help to preserve blood flow and obviate amputation.

Escharotomy often may be accomplished without the need for general anesthesia, because a full-thickness burn destroys all skin innervation.

Electrical Burns

Electrical burns occur with household voltage (electric cords/sockets) and non-household high-voltage current (power line/lightening). High-voltage injuries are often associated with loss of limbs and other injuries that are not immediately obvious.[177-180] The extent of the injury is unpredictable. The surface injury is often small, but the extent of underlying tissue damage and necrosis is massive. Such an injury is a combination of electrical and thermal damage.[180, 181] Victims often have concurrent injuries such as fractures of vertebrae or long bones, ruptured organs, myocardial injury, or numerous contusions. Even patients with low-voltage injuries may have abnormalities of cardiac conduction.[179] Patients with electrical burns may be admitted in a coma with seizures. Muscle tissue surrounding bone is usually more affected than superficial muscles because electrical current tends to travel along neurovascular bundles. Early fasciotomy is needed to preserve the blood flow to extremities. It necessitates general anesthesia during the first day of injury at the time when fluid shifts, hyperkalemia, and myoglobinuria are maximal. Massive myonecrosis and hemolysis may result in hyperkalemia, as well as myoglobinuria and hemoglobinuria. In the presence of hemoglobinuria or myoglobinuria, an increased urine flow (>1 mL/kg/hr) should be ensured by the administration of increased fluids and mannitol.[182] Alkalization of urine may prevent the precipitation of these proteins in the renal tubules. Follow-up of patients with electrical injuries often reveals unpredictable sequelae, which may manifest months to years later; these injuries may occur in organs or areas that do not appear abnormal during the acute course of illness. These late complications most frequently include neurologic dysfunction, ocular damage, damage to the gastrointestinal tract, changes in the electrocardiogram, and delayed hemorrhage from large vessels.[181, 182]

Guidelines to Anesthetic Management

Anesthetic management of pediatric patients with severe thermal injury begins with the initial resuscitation and continues for many years through reconstructive surgery. Knowledge and understanding of the pathophysiology of burn injury enable anesthesiologists to plan appropriate anesthetic management and to recognize and treat complications arising as a result of burn injury or its therapy (Table 23-2).[2, 183]

Table 23-2. Systemic Effects of Burn Injury

System	Early	Late
Cardiovascular	↓ CO due to decreased circulating blood volume, myocardial depressant factor	↑ CO due to sepsis ↑ CO 2-3 times > baseline for months (hypermetabolism) Hypertension
Pulmonary	Upper airway obstruction due to edema Lower airway obstruction due to edema, bronchospasm, particulate matter ↓ FRC ↓ Pulmonary compliance ↓ Chest wall compliance	Bronchopneumonia Tracheal stenosis ↓ Chest wall compliance
Renal	↓ GFR a) Secondary to ↓ circulating blood volume b) Myoglobinuria c) Hemoglobinuria Tubular dysfunction	↑ GFR 2° to ↑ CO Tubular dysfunction
Hepatic	↓ Function due to ↓ circulating blood volume, hypoxia, hepatotoxins	Hepatitis ↑ Function due to hypermetabolism, enzyme induction, ↑ CO ↓ Function due to sepsis, drug interactions
Hematopoietic	↓ Platelets ↑ Fibrin split products, consumptive coagulopathy, anemia	↑ Platelets ↑ Clotting factors Possible AIDS, hepatitis
Neurologic	Encephalopathy Seizures ↑ ICP	Encephalopathy Seizures ICU psychosis
Skin	↑ Heat, fluid, electrolyte loss	Contractures, scar formation
Metabolic	↓ Ionized calcium	↑ Oxygen consumption ↑ Carbon dioxide production ↓ Ionized calcium ↑ Tolerance to narcotics, sedatives
Pharmacokinetics	Altered volume of distribution Altered protein binding Altered pharmacokinetics Altered pharmacodynamics	Enzyme induction, altered receptors Drug interaction

↓, Decrease in; ↑, increase in; AIDS, acquired immunodeficiency syndrome; CO, cardiac output; FRC, functional residual capacity; GFR, glomerular filtration rate; ICP, intracranial pressure; ICU, intensive care unit.

General Principles

Patients coming to the operating room for burn wound excision and grafting must be properly prepared physiologically and psychologically, and specific equipment must be available in the operating room. This preparation is discussed in the paragraphs that follow.

- *Psychological support* must be provided by parents, nurses, physicians, and trained psychologists. It is important for anesthesiologists to understand that a great deal of psychological stress and guilt are felt by the families of children who have sustained a severe burn injury. This stress may be transferred to anger at the physicians, nurses, and other members of the burn care team. The parents are angry that their child has sustained a devastating injury and occasionally vent this anger and frustration. It is therefore vital that the entire burn care team understand this familial response, spend as much time as possible listening to parents' concerns, and emphasize all that is being done to ensure the very best for their child. Specific nurses and physicians should be designated to communicate with the family to avoid misunderstandings and confusion about issues of patient care. The anesthesia care team, while explaining the risks of anesthesia, must emphasize the extensive monitoring and the central role that anesthesiologists have in assuring the well-being of their child. Special emphasis must be placed on methods for minimizing physical and psychological pain during transport, in the operating room, and postoperatively.

- *Adequate sedation and pain control* are necessary before moving patients to the operating room; this move is painful, both physically and emotionally. Intravenous narcotics, such as fentanyl, which has minimal histamine release, are particularly helpful; intravenous midazolam is also helpful for its sedative and amnestic properties. Drug doses should not be based on standard doses used in patients without thermal injury. Burned patients develop tolerance to most narcotics and sedatives, thus requiring higher doses over time to achieve a satisfactory clinical response.[184, 185] The dose of sedative or narcotic should be titrated to effect while the patient is carefully observed and monitored.

- *Correction of intravascular volume* before induction of anesthesia may require fluid boluses during and after sedation and before transport.

- It is critically important to *minimize heat loss* and maintain patient euthermia. This is difficult because of the massive evaporative heat loss that occurs through open wounds. Operating room temperatures during extensive excisions are commonly maintained near 37°C.[16] Attention must be paid to minimize heat loss both during transport and in the operating room. Multiple blankets or thermal reflective covers are helpful. Special equipment is used to maintain body temperature, including a warming blanket, radiant warmer, blood warmer, heated humidifier, and forced hot air warmers. Simply wrapping the extremities in sterile plastic bags and covering the head with plastic or thermal insulation material markedly reduces heat and fluid losses (see Fig. 23–6). Although a hot operating room is uncomfortable for staff, maintaining the patient's temperature may be helpful in maintaining

normal blood clotting. Each calorie that does not have to be spent to maintain body temperature is one more that can be used in the healing process.

- *Adequate monitoring* for major blood loss and fluid shifts includes arterial and central venous cannulas, a urinary catheter, an electrocardiogram, a pulse oximeter, a capnograph, and an esophageal stethoscope. In more critically ill patients, catheters to measure left heart filling pressures are useful. A secure intravenous route for volume infusion is essential. If the potential for rapid blood loss exists, multilumen catheters may not be adequate because of their high-flow resistance. Rapid infusion devices may be particularly helpful.[186-188] The femoral veins may be useful for large volume lines, which are removed at the completion of surgery.

- *Specific anesthetic equipment* is used, including various sterilized laryngoscope blades, endotracheal tubes, airways, and blood pressure cuffs. A ventilator is essential to free the anesthesiologist's hands.

Invasive arterial and central venous pressure monitoring may be established after induction of anesthesia in most pediatric patients. Thiopental or propofol in incremental doses is usually well tolerated, provided there is adequate intravascular volume. Studies in children long recovered from acute burn injury found a 40% increase in the thiopental dose needed to ablate the lid reflex, compared with children without burn injury (Fig. 23–8).[189] Ketamine may on occasion be preferred if the adequacy of intravascular volume is in question or if invasive monitoring lines must be inserted before anesthetic induction; tolerance to ketamine

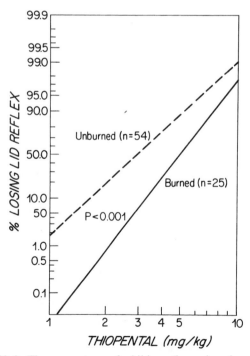

Figure 23–8. The percentage of children (burned and unburned) who lost the lid reflex is compared with the intravenous bolus dose of thiopental. Note the marked shift in the dose-response curve. (From Coté CJ, Petkau AJ: Thiopental requirements may be increased in children reanesthetized at least one year after recovery from extensive thermal injury. Anesthesiology 1981;55:S338.)

with repeated administration has been reported.[176, 190] High-dose fentanyl or morphine combined with nitrous oxide for those patients who will be ventilated postoperatively is also an acceptable anesthetic technique. Generally an inhalation agent is titrated to clinical effect to supplement the narcotic-based anesthetic. One must be observant for chest wall rigidity if a large bolus of fentanyl is administered. Other methods of induction include rectal methohexital or thiopental for infants and small children. A slow inhalation induction is preferable for patients with a compromised airway, bearing in mind the potential for cardiovascular depression.

Succinylcholine is contraindicated in burned patients because of potentially lethal efflux of potassium ions from muscle.[119, 122] This abnormal response probably occurs because the entire muscle membrane, rather than just the myoneural junction, is occupied by acetylcholine receptors. *The muscle tissue of burn victims can thus be resistant to nondepolarizing muscle relaxants and can have an abnormal response to depolarizing muscle relaxants.*[122] The duration of this dangerous response to succinylcholine is unknown. However, we have observed a child who demonstrated marked resistance to nondepolarizing relaxants 463 days after burn injury; this response indirectly suggests that sensitivity to succinylcholine may persist long after the acute injury phase.[191] The nondepolarizing muscle relaxants are therefore the relaxants of choice in patients with a burn injury. It has been found that after burns over more than 25% of body surface area, both the total dose of *d*-tubocurarine administered and the serum concentration necessary to attain

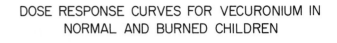
DOSE RESPONSE CURVES FOR VECURONIUM IN NORMAL AND BURNED CHILDREN

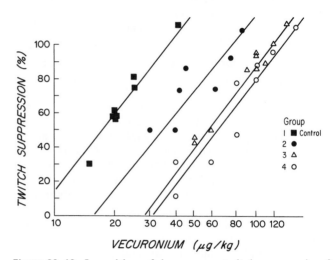

Figure 23–10. Logarithm of dose versus twitch suppression for vecuronium in control subjects and burned children. In the presence of acute injury, the vecuronium effective dose values increased with increasing burn size. The slopes of the curves were not different, but the intercepts were significantly different ($P<0.01$). Solid squares, children without burn injury; solid circles, children with <40% burn injury; open triangle, children with 40–60% burn injury; open circles, children with >60% burn injury. (From Mills AK, Martyn JAJ: Neuromuscular blockade with vecuronium in paediatric patients with burn injury. Br J Clin Pharm 1989;28:155–159.)

a given degree of muscle twitch depression are three to five times greater than in subjects without burn injury (Figs. 23–9 and 23–10).[72, 113–115, 122, 129, 130] If rapid intubation is needed and one is confident that the patient can be ventilated, high doses of rocuronium can be used.[192] Recovery from neuromuscular blockade has been observed at serum concentrations that would cause 100% twitch depression in patients without burn injury. Studies with nondepolarizing muscle relaxants indicate that the hyposensitivity is highly correlated to the magnitude of burn (r = 0.88).[130, 193–195] Protein binding and pharmacokinetic studies with *d*-tubocurarine indicate that these two factors contribute little to the enhanced muscle relaxant requirements.[72, 113–115, 122] An increase in the number of acetylcholine receptors at the neuromuscular junction and an altered affinity for the relaxant by those receptors have a major role in the elevated demand for nondepolarizing muscle relaxants.[120, 121] Pharmacologic reversal of neuromuscular blockade, however, poses no special problem in burned patients. Studies with intermediate and short-acting nondepolarizing relaxants have shown resistance but not as pronounced as has been observed with the long-acting relaxants. With mivacurium, the effects are rather similar to those in normal children; the resistance is partially compensated by decreased hydrolysis because of the lower plasma cholinesterase levels.

Maintenance of anesthesia is usually accomplished with nitrous oxide, oxygen, a muscle relaxant, and a narcotic or inhalation agent. All the commonly used anesthetic agents can be administered to burned patients. Sevoflurane offers

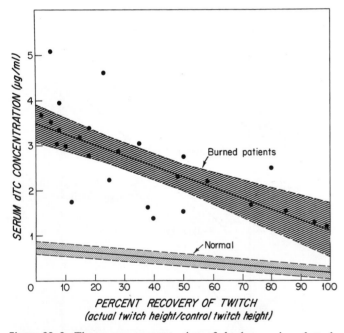

Figure 23–9. The serum concentration of *d*-tubocurarine plotted against the percentage of recovery of the response to electrical twitch stimulation. Shaded areas represent 95% confidence limits. Note the marked increase in requirements for burned patients; they may completely recover from neuromuscular blockade despite serum concentrations that would result in complete paralysis in unburned patients. (From Martyn JAJ, Szyfelbein SK, Ali HH, et al: Increased *d*-tubocurarine requirement following major thermal injury. Anesthesiology 1980;52:353–355.)

an advantage of smooth inhalation induction; isoflurane or halothane can be used for maintenance. There are no data that repeated halothane anesthetics in burned children cause hepatotoxicity. All anesthetics cause concentration-dependent depression of cardiac output. In very ill patients, anesthetic doses—but not muscle relaxant requirements—are drastically reduced; in this situation, high-dose fentanyl-oxygen anesthesia or neuroleptanesthesia appear to be well tolerated. Ketamine may be the anesthetic agent of choice in specific circumstances, such as to avoid airway manipulation after application of fresh facial grafts or for very brief procedures. A number of burn centers use ketamine as the sole anesthetic and find it to be quite satisfactory; we rarely use ketamine as the sole anesthetic agent. The postoperative analgesia and somnolence for prolonged periods produced by ketamine may be considered an advantage in some instances in which postoperative agitation might dislodge fresh skin grafts. Conversely, prolonged somnolence will delay reinstitution of critical enteral nutrition.

The inspired oxygen concentration is regulated according to the arterial blood gases and oxygen saturation. A pulse oximeter may not function properly on tissue discolored with silver nitrate; scraping the fingernail and cleaning the skin allow proper transmission and reception of the pulse oximeter light.[196] Pulse oximetry has a vital role in identifying developing hypoxemia before the desaturation becomes life threatening.[197] A pulse oximeter probe generally can function even on burned digits. If a patient's digits are swollen or vasoconstriction prevents normal pulse oximeter function, then alternative sites must be sought. Alternative sites include the earlobe, nasal septum, and tongue. We have found the tongue to be particularly valuable; an additional benefit is that the tissues of the mouth apparently direct the interfering electrons of the electrocautery unit away from the pulse oximeter probe placed on the tongue (i.e., minimal electrocautery artifact). We have been able to use as many as three simultaneous electrocautery units without disrupting pulse oximetry monitoring.[198] A sealed oximeter probe that prevents electrical current leakage and leaching of adhesive can be easily modified (Fig. 23–11A–D).[198, 199] Newer reflectance oximeters may also have a role in the care of burned patients.[200]

Because of increased metabolic rate, increased carbon dioxide production, and inhalation injury, an increase in alveolar ventilation compared with healthy patients is often required. Blood gas analysis must therefore be assessed early and frequently throughout the anesthetic procedure. Constant monitoring of expired carbon dioxide is very helpful during intraoperative management; however, one must be cognizant of the possibility of significant differences between arterial and expired carbon dioxide values as a result of shunting and dead-space ventilation in patients with severe pulmonary injury. *In this circumstance, an expired carbon dioxide monitor may be used for trending and as a disconnect alarm but*

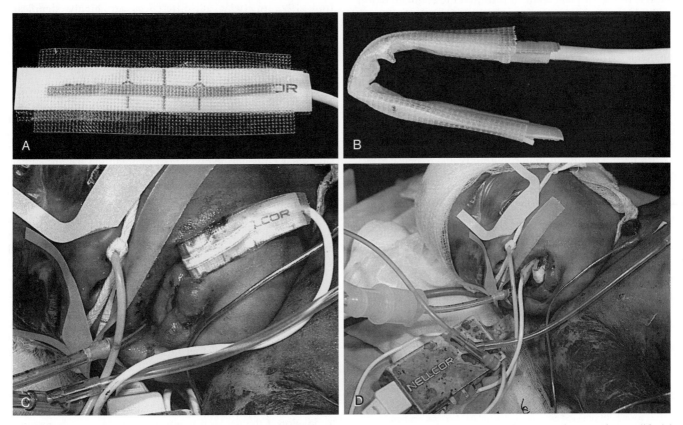

Figure 23–11. In patients with severe vasoconstriction or inadequate peripheral blood flow, a pulse oximeter probe may be modified by taping the malleable metal nosepiece from a paper operating room mask on the back side (A), shaping it into a horseshoe (B). Care must be taken not to occlude either the transmitting or receiving light module with the tape. The oximeter is then placed around the edge of the cheek (C) or the tongue (D). (Note: The manufacturer may not approve of these modifications; a sealed probe may be preferable to a standard oximeter probe since this would diminish the possibility of electrical current leakage and leaching of adhesive.)

should not be relied on to adjust and assess the adequacy of ventilation. The endotracheal tube must be secured with tracheostomy tape because standard adhesive tape does not stick to burned tissue and wet dressings. Electrocardiographic leads also do not adhere and for this reason are placed under dependent portions of the body or sutured onto the skin after the patient is anesthetized. The standard measures for protecting the cornea from drying and for positioning the limbs to prevent nerve compression must be observed.

The most important feature of the intraoperative course is monitoring and replacing a patient's blood loss. For this reason, invasive intravascular monitoring is essential. The Seldinger approach has proved particularly valuable for central venous cannulation and may also be of value should there be a need to use the femoral artery for monitoring.[201, 202] Patients may lose one to three blood volumes during each burn excision. One must therefore be familiar with the surgical approach to burn excision. During a tangential excision, a patient might lose three to five times more blood than during excisions down to fascia (Table 23–3). The liberal use of very dilute concentrations of epinephrine (500 µg/L in normal saline) injected subcutaneously in both donor and excision sites markedly reduces surgical blood loss.[203] As much as 10 µg/kg epinephrine per 20 minutes may be injected even during halothane anesthesia.[204] In practice, we often begin transfusion even before harvesting a skin graft or burn excision. Blood loss is also quite dependent on the expertise of the surgical team. It is difficult to estimate blood and fluid loss despite accurate weighing of surgical sponges because of significant losses hidden by the surgical drapes and evaporation. Other indicators of circulating blood volume, such as urine output, central venous pressure, arterial pressure, and shape of the arterial waveform, must be closely monitored.

Early excision of full-thickness burns has improved survival and shortened hospital stays.[205–207] It has been observed that 5% of the blood volume was lost for every 1% of the body surface excised and grafted.[208, 209] This extensive blood loss has been a source of major morbidity and expense.[210, 211] During the last several years, effective blood conserving techniques for excision have been developed that can drastically reduce intraoperative blood loss. These techniques include (1) clearly planning the excision to be performed prior to its initiation; (2) performing all extremity excisions under pneumatic tourniquet, exsanguinating the extremity prior to

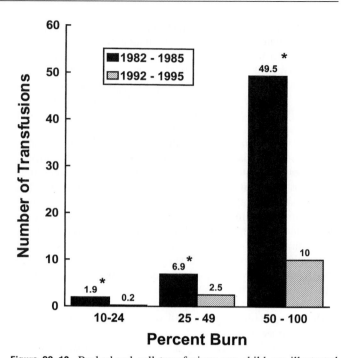

Figure 23–12. Packed red cell transfusions per child are illustrated for well matched groups of children managed during two intervals: 1982–1985 and 1992–1995. During the second interval, blood conservation techniques during excision were routinely employed. Patients are stratified by burn size: 10–24%, 25–50%, and 50–100%. Note the nearly fivefold reduction in red blood cell transfusions from 1992 to 1995; all differences are highly significant (*$P < 0.001$).

tourniquet inflation, and wrapping the extremity in a hemostatic dressing prior to tourniquet deflation; (3) conducting all fascial excisions with coagulating electrocautery; (4) performing major layered excisions as early as possible after injury, prior to the development of significant wound hyperemia; (5) executing all layered torso excisions after subeschar epinephrine clysis; (6) maintaining patient euthermia, primarily through maintaining a hot operating room (near 37°C); and (7) subcutaneous injection of diluted epinephrine in donor areas.

Large doses of epinephrine are well tolerated and markedly diminish bleeding. In a series of 25 consecutive children undergoing extensive layered excision, we utilized a total dose of epinephrine averaging 25 ± 3 µg/kg without complication.[203] Based on preoperative and postoperative hematocrit and known volume of transfusion, the percent of the total blood volume lost per percent of total wound excised, generated an average 0.98 ± 0.19% of the blood volume per percent of the body surface excised (Fig. 23–12). This was about one fifth of that typically seen with this type of excision.[212, 213] Operating with epinephrine clysis or tourniquets requires the surgeon to have the ability to accurately determine wound bed viability in the absence of free bleeding. This is an important acquired skill that may be difficult to develop if the surgeon is not performing these procedures frequently.

Chronic ionized hypocalcemia is commonly observed with major thermal injury. Prophylactic intermittent administration of calcium chloride or calcium gluconate is strongly

Table 23–3. Approximate Expected Blood Loss for Burn Excision as a Percentage of Body Surface Area*

Procedure	Estimated Blood Loss (mL/cm²)
Fascial excision	1.5†
Tangential excision	4†

*These calculations are based on the measurement of blood loss during surgical procedures at the Shriner's Burn Institute (unpublished data). These guidelines have been used for over 10 years and have proved to be useful in clinical practice.
†This includes percentage of body surface area (BSA) of burn excised and area of skin harvested. For example, if a 10 kg child with BSA of 0.45 m² (4500 cm²) has a 10% harvest and a 10% excision, for a total of 20%, we get 0.2 × 4500 = 900 cm². Therefore, tangential procedures would result in 900 × 4 = 3600 mL estimated blood loss, and fascial procedures would result in 900 × 1.5 = 1350 mL estimated blood loss.

recommended during the rapid infusion of citrated blood products (see Fig. 12–5).[214–217] We have observed that a number of children suffer electromechanical dissociation or even cardiac arrest during the rapid administration of fresh frozen plasma (FFP). This observation prompted a controlled prospective study in which highly significant reductions in Ca^{++} were found whenever FFP was administered at a rate of 1 mL/kg/min or greater (see Fig. 12–5).[217] Interestingly, there was no relation between adverse cardiovascular responses, rate of FFP infusion, or Ca^{++}. A careful review of the previous cases of cardiac arrest revealed that all children were anesthetized with halothane, whereas in our prospective study, most were anesthetized with "balanced" techniques. We then studied dogs using two concentrations of halothane anesthesia and administered intravenous sodium citrate in a concentration equivalent to 1 mL/kg/min FFP. Significant reductions in Ca^{++} were found during both levels of halothane anesthesia; however, greater adverse cardiovascular responses were observed during deep (1.5 × the minimum alveolar concentration [MAC] of halothane) anesthesia. In fact, several dogs suffered cardiac arrest when ionized hypocalcemia was combined with halothane anesthesia (1.5 MAC).[218] These studies suggest that the myocardial depression induced by ionized hypocalcemia is potentiated by the halothane-induced myocardial depression. Hypocalcemia or halothane anesthesia by themselves do not appear to produce cardiovascular instability as significant as the combination. It is therefore vital to maintain normal Ca^{++} values when citrated blood products are rapidly administered, particularly during halothane anesthesia. For patients weighing less than 10 kg, 10 mg of calcium chloride is administered every 15 to 30 minutes. Additional exogenous calcium is administered during rapid infusion of FFP or citrated whole blood (see Chapter 12).[217]

It is our clinical impression that the rapid administration of FFP or citrated whole blood through a central line, without additional exogenous calcium, may be more likely to induce severe hypotension, bradycardia, and electrical mechanical dissociation. Our experience has been that rapid administration of citrated blood products is safer through peripheral lines. Rapid administration of washed packed or citrated packed red blood cells does not cause ionized hypocalcemia. It would also seem advantageous to administer exogenous calcium through a peripheral line to avoid high concentrations in coronary vessels. However, one must also bear in mind that calcium administered simultaneously in the same intravenous line with FFP or citrated blood products may result in clot formation unless the calcium is rapidly flushed through the intravenous system.

Special Considerations

Pharmacologic Responses

As a general rule, patients with burn injuries require larger than normal doses of all medications, including antibiotics, cimetidine, muscle relaxants, opioids, benzodiazepines, and anesthetic drugs.[2, 62, 65, 66, 72, 76–78, 103, 114–118, 122, 128–130, 189, 193–195] In general, the cardiovascular response to catecholamines is attenuated because of a reduced affinity of beta-adrenergic receptors for ligands and diminished second messenger production.[219] Pharmacokinetic studies in acutely burned pa-

tients indicate that the increased requirement for antibiotics and cimetidine is due in part to leakage through the burn wound, rapid urinary excretion, and altered volume of distribution.[72, 114] Pharmacokinetic studies of d-tubocurarine demonstrate an increased central volume of distribution, normal total volume of distribution, and increased urinary excretion, as well as increased plasma binding. These studies did not find losses of d-tubocurarine through the burn wound. Thermal injuries of more than 30% of body surface area cause an up-regulation of acetylcholine receptors and consequent resistance to nondepolarizing relaxants.[120–122, 124, 125, 220] In addition, there appears to be increased tolerance to sedatives and narcotics. A pharmacokinetic study of diazepam in adult burn victims demonstrated a significantly higher free fraction (pharmacologically active component), whereas the clearance of free diazepam was reduced. An increased tolerance to diazepam despite a higher fraction of pharmacologically active drug and decreased clearance suggests resistance at tissue receptors similar to that observed for muscle relaxants at the neuromuscular junction.[78] A similar tolerance has been observed with narcotics despite decreased metabolic clearance.[78, 184] The persistence of such changes in requirements for both muscle relaxants and anesthetic drugs long after recovery from burn injury must be kept in mind and doses titrated according to needs.[65, 72, 114, 189, 191]

The pharmacology of many medications commonly used in burned patients remains to be investigated.[65] In general, one must be aware of the alterations in distribution volume, protein binding, excretion, and increased or decreased metabolism. Furthermore, these patients are frequently taking multiple medications, and therefore drug interactions, potentiations, and incompatibilities must be considered. Of particular importance in this context are the H_2-receptor antagonists, which are commonly used in burned patients and are known to inhibit the clearance of many other medications (see Chapter 8).

Methemoglobinemia

A less common but important source of intraoperative cyanosis and hypoxemia is the development of methemoglobinemia. In burns treated with silver nitrate dressings, the presence of some strains of gram-negative bacteria, which are capable of reducing nitrates to nitrites, creates a situation in which the nitrites diffuse into the bloodstream, converting hemoglobin into methemoglobin.[4, 105, 106] The methemoglobin decreases the available oxygen-carrying capacity and increases the affinity of the unaltered hemoglobin for oxygen, thereby further impairing the delivery of oxygen; as a result, the oxygen/hemoglobin P50 curve is shifted to the left. Methemoglobinemia should therefore be considered in the differential diagnosis of cyanosis. Approximately 5 g of deoxyhemoglobin for each deciliter of blood are necessary to produce visible cyanosis, but a comparable skin color is produced by 1.5 to 2.0 g of methemoglobin for each deciliter of blood. Blood that contains more than approximately 10% methemoglobin usually appears dark red or even brown, despite a high oxygen tension, and does not change color even with vigorous agitation in room air. Measured oxygen saturation or content is low. However, pulse oximetry, although demonstrating a decrease in saturation, provides a falsely elevated value.[152, 153] Treatment consists of removing the toxic agent, administration of methylene blue (2 mg/kg), oxygen inhalation, and possibly hemodialysis.

Endotracheal Tube Size

Because burned patients frequently undergo multiple anesthetic procedures, special considerations must be given to endotracheal tube type and size. When appropriate, uncuffed endotracheal tubes should be used and a record maintained of the size of endotracheal tube and peak inflation pressure at which leakage occurs around the endotracheal tube for each anesthetic procedure. It is common to note the use of smaller endotracheal tubes as weeks go by, heralding the development of a subglottic lesion (stenosis, granuloma, polyps), which should be investigated with bronchoscopy. If cuffed endotracheal tubes must be used, then a high-volume, low-pressure variety is recommended. The low-pressure cuffed endotracheal tube seems to be as safe as uncuffed tubes in children. When nitrous oxide is used, the intraoperative cuff pressure should be checked to avoid excessive pressure on the tracheal mucosa. We generally inflate the cuff to the minimum pressure that allows controlled ventilation.

Hyperalimentation

Hyperalimentation fluids are frequently administered to burned patients.[96, 98] These fluids should be continued intraoperatively; however, we generally reduce the rate of infusion to one half to two thirds of the initial infusion rate, because metabolic rate is usually decreased as a result of anesthetic drugs as well as reduced body temperature. These fluids should be administered with a constant-infusion pump to avoid accidental over- or underinfusion. If the hyperalimentation fluids must be terminated (e.g., to permit blood transfusion), then monitoring of blood glucose levels is recommended. Dangerous rebound hypoglycemia may occur if infusion of these solutions is abruptly interrupted and no compensation is made with other glucose-containing solutions. It should be noted that most blood products, particularly whole blood and FFP, provide a significant glucose load.

Awakening

In the immediate postoperative period, oxygen consumption increases even in the absence of shivering.[221] If oxygen debt develops (metabolic acidosis), appropriate measures must be taken to correct it. Special consideration must also be given to the likelihood of severe pain. Analgesic drugs should be administered in increasingly liberal doses because of increased drug tolerance. Adequacy of air exchange and patency of the airway, however, must be given first priority. In patients with lower extremity donor sites or even upper abdominal donor sites, we have used "single-shot" caudal blockade (see Chapter 28). This block must only be used when the caudal area is free of burn injury and the patient is not septic.

Pain Management

The treatment of pain in the intensive care unit and operating room before and after surgery is a major concern for anesthe-siologists.[184] Nearly every modality used to help patients recover from the injury (burn dressing changes, physical therapy, weighing the patient, skin grafting, skin donation) is associated with pain. The difficulty in treating this pain results in part from the variability of the stimulus (baseline constant discomfort to very painful burn dressing changes) and the great psychological overlay because the patient anticipates the pain. Our experience has been that the amount of pain is directly proportional to the size of the thermal injury.

Evidence suggests that communication with a patient, carefully explaining why certain treatments are necessary despite the pain caused, decreases the analgesic requirements.[184, 222–224] In the past, the treatment of pain with narcotics was limited for fear of creating "addiction"; however, no studies of pediatric patients have documented addiction, and studies of adults reveal a very low addiction rate.[225–229] There are some data to suggest that in the early stages of burn injury there may be an increased potency of analgesic medications[230] but that later in the burn injury there is a marked increase in analgesic requirements. Our experience has been that the "background" pain is well treated with either a very long-acting narcotic (e.g., methadone) or with constant intravenous infusions of narcotics (e.g., morphine).[73, 75, 184] These infusions can also be supplemented with oral acetaminophen.[231] Another method that we have found particularly useful for providing background analgesia is the administration of MS Contin (slow-release morphine tablets) orally, twice daily.[74] Intramuscular injections are avoided. Short-acting narcotics can then be titrated intravenously as indicated for the painful procedures.

When poorly controlled, pain and anxiety have adverse psychologic[232–234] and physiologic[12] effects. Post-traumatic stress disorder has been reported to occur in up to 30% of those with serious burns,[235] and may be related to both the accident and the treatment, particularly in the setting of inadequate control of pain and anxiety. An inconsistent approach to pain and anxiety will be associated with inappropriate degrees of patient discomfort, nonuniform drug selection with inconsistent dosing of unfamiliar drugs, varying tolerance of patient discomfort by different staff members, and bedside disagreements over management of patient distress.

To address this issue, a pain and anxiety guideline should be developed by all facilities treating burned patients routinely.[236–239] We developed one such guideline that we have followed for several years, which is briefly described in Table 23–4.[185] The ideal characteristics of such a guideline include (1) safety and efficacy over the broad range of ages and injury acuities seen in the particular unit; (2) explicit recommendations for drug selection, dosing, and escalation of dosing; (3) a limited formulary that generates staff familiarity with agents used; and (4) regular assessment of pain and anxiety levels and guidance for intervention as needed through dose ranging. We have found this structured approach to management of this predictable problem to be very effective over the broad range of injury severity and patient ages seen in our unit. Substantial escalation of drug doses, particularly in patients with large injuries, is commonly required; doses should be titrated to patient needs. When the patient is being weaned toward extubation, background medications should be tapered toward a sensorium consistent with airway protection; many patients are safely

Table 23–4. Pain Treatment Plan

Clinical State	Background Anxiety	Background Pain	Procedural Anxiety	Procedural Pain	Transition to Next Clinical State
Mechanically ventilated acute burn	Midazolam infusion	Morphine sulfate infusion	Midazolam intravenous titration	Morphine sulfate intravenous titration	Wean infusions 10–20% per day and substitute nonmechanically ventilated acute guideline
Nonmechanically ventilated acute burn	Scheduled enteral lorazepam	Scheduled enteral morphine sulfate	Lorazepam intravenous titration or enteral dose	Morphine sulfate enteral or intravenous titration	Wean scheduled drugs 10–20% per day and substitute chronic acute guideline
Chronic acute burn	Scheduled enteral lorazepam	Scheduled enteral morphine sulfate	Lorazepam enteral dose	Morphine sulfate enteral dose	Wean scheduled and bolus drugs 10–20% per day to outpatient requirements and pruritus medications
Reconstructive surgical patient	Scheduled enteral lorazepam	Scheduled enteral morphine sulfate	Lorazepam enteral dose	Morphine sulfate enteral dose	Wean scheduled drugs and bolus drugs to outpatient requirement

extubated while still receiving opiate and benzodiazepine infusions. Finally, it is essential to emphasize that the most effective of all analgesics and anxiolytics is prompt, definitive wound closure.

Tolerance to narcotics occurs over time and must be considered so that adequate analgesia is provided throughout the recovery period. It is common to observe patients who receive 1 mg/kg of morphine at the beginning of a 2-hour operative procedure to be ready for extubation but to require additional narcotic for continued pain relief postoperatively. In burned victims, we have found a significant reduction in the distribution and excretion phases of most narcotics, with the half-life reduced to 37 minutes for morphine, compared with the half-life of 126 minutes in children without thermal injury (Fig. 23–13). Thus, an increased rate of excretion and degradation may influence the effect of some narcotics. We have observed some adolescents to require as much as 8000 μg of fentanyl per burn dressing change. As a child recovers, the painful stimuli diminish and the narcotic requirements are gradually reduced. This is generally such a prolonged process that withdrawal is not an issue. Anesthesiologists can have a central role in the treatment of the pain of thermal injuries and, with an understanding of pharmacology, pharmacokinetics, and pharmacodynamics, are a vital resource for the care of these patients (see Chapter 29).

Hyperbaric Oxygenation

There is no compelling evidence that the hyperbaric oxygen treatment modality has a role in the management of burn wounds.[15, 240] The most common indication for hyperbaric therapy in burned patients is concomitant carbon monoxide (CO) poisoning.[36, 154] CO binds avidly to hemoglobin[241] and other iron-containing enzymes, such as intramitochondrial cytochromes, interfering with the delivery and utilization of oxygen respectively.[147, 242] Patients suffering significant CO exposure are at risk of developing both acute and delayed neurologic sequelae. The pathophysiology of neurologic sequelae is not known, although imaging studies suggest a potentially reversible demyelinating process.[243] Data support-

ing the use of hyperbaric oxygen to prevent and treat these complications may be weak,[244] but cannot be discounted given the seriousness of these sequelae.

The important practical question is whether hyperbaric treatment will decrease the frequency and severity of delayed neurologic sequelae in burn patients with concomitant CO poisoning. This is a difficult question because the incidence of delayed sequelae is not known, and determining the severity of an individual exposure is often not possible. Delayed sequelae include headaches, irritability, personality changes, confusion, loss of memory, and gross motor deficits. The frequency with which those exposed develop these symptoms is not known with certainty, but they are reported to occur in approximately 10% of patients with serious exposures.[145, 245] A symptom-free interval of several days is commonly reported. Delayed hyperbaric treatment may relieve symptoms, and spontaneous resolution of delayed sequelae may be expected in up to 75% of patients within 1 year.[246–253] The severity of CO poisoning is often difficult to know, as there is a poor correlation between serum carboxyhemoglobin and degree of CO exposure.[254, 255] Neuropsychiatric testing has been proposed as a more accurate way to determine this,[256] but such detailed examinations are difficult in burned patients secondary to pain medications and hemodynamic instability. Some clinicians feel that a history of unconsciousness indicates that an exposure has been severe enough to warrant treatment.[245, 246, 255, 256] One randomized prospective study of 60 patients with relatively mild CO poisoning noted an incidence of delayed neuropsychiatric symptoms discernible by special testing in patients treated with 100% oxygen compared with none in those treated with hyperbaric oxygen.[145, 247] Using overt neurologic symptoms as an end point, the value of hyperbaric oxygen was examined in a group of 629 patients with CO poisoning.[257] In patients without initial impairment of consciousness, there was no difference between outcome with 6 hours of normobaric 100% oxygen and 2 hours of hyperbaric oxygen at 2 atmospheres. In patients with impairment of consciousness (and presumably more serious exposures), there was no difference in outcome between those treated with one session and those treated with two sessions of hyperbaric oxygen

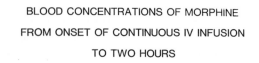

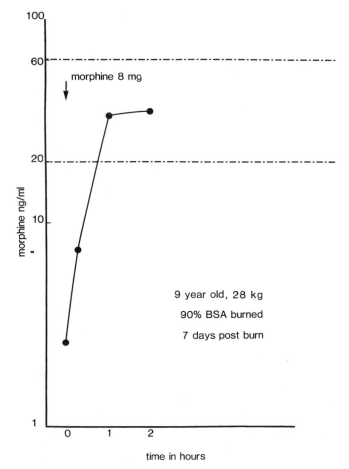

Figure 23–13. Changes in serum morphine values in a 9-year-old child who suffered 90% burn injury and received 0.3 mg/kg IV. Note the shortened half-life and rapid decline in effective blood values (i.e., <20 ng/mL). Altered pharmacokinetics may contribute in part to the increased narcotic requirements observed in some patients with extensive burn injury. (From Osgood PF, Szyfelbein SK: Management of pain. In Martyn JAJ, ed: Acute Management of the Burned Patient. Philadelphia: WB Saunders, 1990.)

at 2 atmospheres. Recovery from serious CO poisoning is possible, as demonstrated by limited uncontrolled case series.[149, 258] Hyperbaric oxygen treatment is not without expense, inconvenience, and risk,[148, 254] and the indications for treatment of burned patients with concomitant CO poisoning is debated.[156, 259] One study described complications seen during treatment of a heterogeneous groups of patients: emesis (6%), seizures (5%), agitation requiring restraints or sedation (2%), cardiac dysrhythmias or arrests (2%), arterial hypotension (2%), and tension pneumothorax (1%).[156] Complications may be expected more frequently in the critically ill.[260] Hyperbaric oxygen treatment is probably appropriate in burned patients with documented or strongly suspected serious carbon monoxide poisoning who are hemodynamically stable, not requiring an ongoing burn resuscitation, not wheezing or air trapping, and in whom such treatment does not require interfacility transport inconsistent with good general burn treatment.

Summary

The care of burned patients involves detailed knowledge of the early and late effects of burn injury on the respiratory, cardiac, renal, central nervous system, hepatic, gastrointestinal, hematopoietic, and metabolic systems. An awareness of altered pharmacokinetics and pharmacodynamics in relation to anesthetic agents, combined with an understanding of the problems of massive blood transfusion, also contributes to safe anesthetic care. Finally, the importance of adequate analgesia, sedation, and concern for the psychological well-being of these devastatingly injured children cannot be overemphasized. Knowledge of all of these factors combines to produce a successful outcome.

REFERENCES

1. Brigham PA, McLoughlin E: Burn incidence and medical care use in the United States: Estimates, trends, and data sources. J Burn Care Rehabil 1996;17:95–107.
2. MacLennan N, Heimbach DM, Cullen BF: Anesthesia for major thermal injury. Anesthesiology 1998;89:749–770.
3. Monafo WW: Initial management of burns. N Engl J Med 1996;335:1581–1586.
4. Moncrief JA: Burns. N Engl J Med 1973;288:444–454.
5. Cone JB, Wallace BH, Caldwell FT Jr: The effect of staged burn wound closure on the rates of heat production and heat loss of burned children and young adults. J Trauma 1988;28:968–972.
6. Braquet M, Lavaud P, Dormont D, et al: Leukocytic functions in burn-injured patients. Prostaglandins 1985;29:747–765.
7. Jahoor F, Desai M, Herndon DN, et al: Dynamics of the protein metabolic response to burn injury. Metabolism 1988;37:330–337.
8. Vaughan GM, Becker RA, Unger RH, et al: Nonthyroidal control of metabolism after burn injury: Possible role of glucagon. Metabolism 1985;37:637–641.
9. Bergstrom JP, Larsson J, Nordstrom H, et al: Influence of injury and nutrition on muscle water and electrolytes: Effect of severe injury, burns and sepsis. Acta Chir Scand 1987;153:261–266.
10. Aulick LH, McManus AT, Mason ADJ, et al: Effects of infection on oxygen consumption and core temperature in experimental thermal injury. Ann Surg 1986;204:48–52.
11. Wolfe RR, Herndon DN, Jahoor F, et al: Effect of severe burn injury on substrate cycling by glucose and fatty acids. N Engl J Med 1987;317:403–408.
12. Youn YK, Lalonde C, Demling R: The role of mediators in the response to thermal injury. World J Surg 1992;16:30–36.
13. Arturson G: Pathophysiology of the burn wound and pharmacological treatment. The Rudi Hermans Lecture, 1995. Burns 1996;22:255–274.
14. Preiser JC, Reper P, Vlasselaer D, et al: Nitric oxide production is increased in patients after burn injury. J Trauma 1996;40:368–371.
15. Demling RH: Burns. N Engl J Med 1985;313:1389–1398.
16. Deitch EA: The management of burns. N Engl J Med 1990;323:1249–1253.
17. Pitt RM, Parker JC, Jurkovich GJ, et al: Analysis of altered capillary pressure and permeability after thermal injury. J Surg Res 1987;42:693–702.
18. Morgan RJ, Martyn JA, Philbin DM, et al: Water metabolism and antidiuretic hormone (ADH) response following thermal injury. J Trauma 1980;20:468–472.
19. Wilmore DW, Long JM, Mason AD Jr, et al: Catecholamines: Mediator of the hypermetabolic response to thermal injury. Ann Surg 1974;180:653–669.
20. Martyn JA, Burke JF: Is there a selective increase in pulmonary capillary permeability following cutaneous burns? Chest 1979;76:374–375.
21. Harms BA, Bodai BI, Kramer GC, et al: Microvascular fluid and

protein flux in pulmonary and systemic circulations after thermal injury. Microvasc Res 1982;23:77–86.

22. Harms BA, Kramer GC, Bodai BI, et al: Effect of hypoproteinemia on pulmonary and soft tissue edema formation. Crit Care Med 1981;9:503–508.

23. Demling RH, Smith M, Bodai B, et al: Comparison of postburn capillary permeability in soft tissue and lung. J Burn Care Rehabil 1981;1:86–92.

24. Aikawa N, Martyn JA, Burke JF: Pulmonary artery catheterization and thermodilution cardiac output determination in the management of critically burned patients. Am J Surg 1978;135:811–817.

25. Martyn JA, Snider MT, Farago LF, et al: Thermodilution right ventricular volume: A novel and better predictor of volume replacement in acute thermal injury. J Trauma 1981;21:619–626.

26. Turbow ME: Abdominal compression following circumferential burn: Cardiovascular responses. J Trauma 1973;13:535–541.

27. Martyn JA, Snider MT, Szyfelbein SK, et al: Right ventricular dysfunction in acute thermal injury. Ann Surg 1980;191:330–335.

28. Moati F, Sepulchre C, Miskulin M, et al: Biochemical and pharmacological properties of a cardiotoxic factor isolated from the blood serum of burned patients. J Pathol 1979;127:147–156.

29. Kremer B, Allgower M, Graf M, et al: The present status of research in burn toxins. Intensive Care Med 1981;7:77–87.

30. Mueller M, Sartorelli K, DeMeules JE, et al: Effects of fluid resuscitation on cardiac dysfunction following thermal injury. J Surg Res 1988;44:745–753.

31. Huribal M, Cunningham ME, D'Aiuto ML, et al: Endothelin-1 and prostaglandin E2 levels increase in patients with burns. J Am Coll Surg 1995;180:318–322.

32. Weiss SM, Lakshminarayan S: Acute inhalation injury. Clin Chest Med 1994;15:103–116.

33. Kaufman TM, Horton JW: Burn-induced alterations in cardiac beta-adrenergic receptors. Am J Physiol 1992;262:H1585–H1591.

34. Lalonde C, Demling RH: The effect of complete burn wound excision and closure on postburn oxygen consumption. Surgery 1987;102:862–868.

35. Trunkey DD: Inhalation injury. Surg Clin North Am 1978;58:1133–1140.

36. Fein A, Leff A, Hopewell PC: Pathophysiology and management of the complications resulting from fire and the inhaled products of combustion: Review of the literature. Crit Care Med 1980;8:94–98.

37. Tredget EE, Shankowsky HA, Taerum TV, et al: The role of inhalation injury in burn trauma. A Canadian experience. Ann Surg 1990;212:720–727.

38. Barillo DJ, Goode R, Esch V: Cyanide poisoning in victims of fire: Analysis of 364 cases and review of the literature. J Burn Care Rehabil 1994;15:46–57.

39. Davies JW: Toxic chemicals versus lung tissue: An aspect of inhalation injury revisited. The Everett Idris Evans Memorial Lecture—1986. J Burn Care Rehabil 1986;7:213–222.

40. Green GM, Jakab GJ, Low RB, et al: Defense mechanisms of the respiratory membrane. Am Rev Respir Dis 1977;115:479–514.

41. Nieman GF, Clark WR, Wax SD, et al: The effect of smoke inhalation on pulmonary surfactant. Ann Surg 1980;191:171–181.

42. Shimazu T, Yukioka T, Hubbard GB, et al: A dose-responsive model of smoke inhalation injury: Severity-related alteration in cardiopulmonary function. Ann Surg 1987;206:89–98.

43. Herndon DN, Barrow RE, Traber DL, et al: Extravascular lung water changes following smoke inhalation and massive burn injury. Surgery 1987;102:341–349.

44. Nieman GF, Clark WRJ, Goyette D, et al: Wood smoke inhalation increases pulmonary microvascular permeability. Surgery 1989;105:481–487.

45. Narita H, Kikuchi I, Ogata K, et al: Smoke inhalation injury from newer synthetic building materials: A patient who survived 205 days. Burns 1987;13:147–152.

46. Desai MH, Rutan RL, Herndon DN: Managing smoke inhalation injuries. Postgrad Med 1989;86:69–76.

47. Stothert JC Jr, Herndon DN, Lubbesmeyer HJ, et al: Airway acid injury following smoke inhalation. Prog Clin Biol Res 1988;264:409–413.

48. Pruitt BA Jr, Erickson DR, Morris A: Progressive pulmonary insufficiency and other pulmonary complications of thermal injury. J Trauma 1975;15:369–379.

49. Wroblewski DA, Bower GC: The significance of facial burns in acute smoke inhalation. Crit Care Med 1979;7:335–338.

50. Stone HH: Pulmonary burns in children. J Pediatr Surg 1979;14:48–52.

51. Zawacki BE, Jung RC, Joyce J, et al: Smoke, burns, and the natural history of inhalation injury in fire victims: A correlation of experimental and clinical data. Ann Surg 1977;185:100–110.

52. Stephenson SF, Esrig BC, Polk HCJ, et al: The pathophysiology of smoke inhalation injury. Ann Surg 1975;182:652–660.

53. Demling RH: Postgraduate course: respiratory injury. Part III: Pulmonary dysfunction in the burn patient. J Burn Care Rehabil 1986;7:277–284.

54. Quinby WC Jr: Restrictive effects of thoracic burns in children. J Trauma 1972;12:646–655.

55. Hantson P, Butera R, Clemessy JL, et al: Early complications and value of initial clinical and paraclinical observations in victims of smoke inhalation without burns. Chest 1997;111:671–675.

56. Martyn JA, Aikawa N, Wilson RS, et al: Extrapulmonary factors influencing the ratio of arterial oxygen tension to inspired oxygen concentration in burn patients. Crit Care Med 1979;7:492–496.

57. Martyn JA, McKusick K, Strauss HW, et al: Ventricular volume and ejection fraction in the diagnosis of the aetiology of low cardiac output in burned patients. Anaesthesia 1986;41:511–515.

58. Gupta KL, Kumar R, Sekhar MS, et al: Myoglobinuric acute renal failure following electrical injury. Ren Fail 1991;13:23–25.

59. Aikawa N, Wakabayashi G, Ueda M, et al: Regulation of renal function in thermal injury. J Trauma 1990;30:S174–S178.

60. Eklund J, Granberg PO, Liljedahl SO: Studies on renal function in burns. I. Renal osmolal regulation, glomerular filtration rate and plasma solute composition related to age, burned surface area and mortality probability. Acta Chir Scand 1970;136:627–640.

61. Ciaccio EI, Fruncillo RJ: Urinary excretion of D-glucaric acid by severely burned patients. Clin Pharmacol Ther 1979;25:340–344.

62. Loirat P, Rohan J, Baillet A, et al: Increased glomerular filtration rate in patients with major burns and its effect on the pharmacokinetics of tobramycin. N Engl J Med 1978;299:915–919.

63. Garrelts JC, Peterie JD: Altered vancomycin dose vs. serum concentration relationship in burn patients. Clin Pharmacol Ther 1988;44:9–13.

64. Luterman A, Dacso CC, Curreri PW: Infections in burn patients. Am J Med 1986;81:45–52.

65. Bonate PL: Pathophysiology and pharmacokinetics following burn injury. Clin Pharmacokinet 1990;18:118–130.

66. Martyn JA, Greenblatt DJ, Abernethy DR: Increased cimetidine clearance in burn patients. JAMA 1985;253:1288–1291.

67. Schiavon M, Di Landro D, Baldo M, et al: A study of renal damage in seriously burned patients. Burns Incl Therm Inj 1988;14:107–112.

68. Falkner B, Roven S, DeClement FA, et al: Hypertension in children with burns. J Trauma 1978;18:213–217.

69. Wilmore DW, Goodwin CW, Aulick LH, et al: Effect of injury and infection on visceral metabolism and circulation. Ann Surg 1980;192:491–504.

70. Czaja AJ, Rizzo TA, Smith WR Jr, et al: Acute liver disease after cutaneous thermal injury. J Trauma 1975;15:887–894.

71. Herndon DN, Stein MD, Rutan TC, et al: Failure of TPN supplementation to improve liver function, immunity, and mortality in thermally injured patients. J Trauma 1987;27:195–204.

72. Martyn J: Clinical pharmacology and drug therapy in the burned patient. Anesthesiology 1986;65:67–75.

73. Kart T, Christrup LL, Rasmussen M: Recommended use of morphine in neonates, infants and children based on a literature review: Part 2—Clinical use. Pediatr Anaesth 1997;7:93–101.

74. Herman RA, Veng-Pedersen P, Miotto J, et al: Pharmacokinetics of morphine sulfate in patients with burns. J Burn Care Rehabil 1994;15:95–103.

75. Furman WR, Munster AM, Cone EJ: Morphine pharmacokinetics during anesthesia and surgery in patients with burns. J Burn Care Rehabil 1990;11:391–394.

76. Cederholm I, Bengtsson M, Bjorkman S, et al: Long term high dose morphine, ketamine and midazolam infusion in a child with burns. Br J Clin Pharm 1990;30:901–905.

77. Martyn J, Greenblatt DJ: Lorazepam conjugation is unimpaired in burn trauma. Clin Pharmacol Ther 1988;43:250–255.

78. Martyn JA, Greenblatt DJ, Quinby WC: Diazepam kinetics in patients with severe burns. Anesth Analg 1983;62:293–297.

79. Sepulchre C, Moati F, Miskulin M, et al: Biochemical and pharmacological properties of a neurotoxic protein isolated from the blood serum of heavily burned patients. J Pathol 1979;127:137–145.

80. Antoon AY, Volpe JJ, Crawford JD: Burn encephalopathy in children. Pediatrics 1972;50:609–616.

81. Sheridan RL, McEttrick M, Bacha G, et al: Midazolam infusion in pediatric patients with burns who are undergoing mechanical ventilation. J Burn Care Rehabil 1994;15:515–518.

82. Chance WT, Berlatzky Y, Minnema K, et al: Burn trauma induces anorexia and aberrations in CNS amine neurotransmitters. J Trauma 1985;25:501–507.

83. McKee AC, Winkelman MD, Banker BQ: Central pontine myelinolysis in severely burned patients: Relationship to serum hyperosmolality. Neurology 1988;38:1211–1217.

84. Curreri PW, Hicks JE, Aronoff RJ, et al: Inhibition of active sodium transport in erythrocytes from burned patients. Surg Gynecol Obstet 1974;139:538–540.

85. Heideman M: The effect of thermal injury on hemodynamic, respiratory, and hematologic variables in relation to complement activation. J Trauma 1979;19:239–247.

86. Wallner SF, Vautrin R: The anemia of thermal injury: Mechanism of inhibition of erythropoiesis. Proc Soc Exp Biol Med 1986;181:144–150.

87. Vasko SD, Burdge JJ, Ruberg RL, et al: Evaluation of erythropoietin levels in the anemia of thermal injury. J Burn Care Rehabil 1991;12:437–441.

88. Lawrence C, Atac B: Hematologic changes in massive burn injury. Crit Care Med 1992;20:1284–1288.

89. Housinger TA, Warden GD, Shouse J: Ordering of laboratory work in the management of pediatric burn patients: Technical note. J Trauma 1993;34:139–141.

90. Still JMJ, Belcher K, Law EJ, et al: A double-blinded prospective evaluation of recombinant human erythropoietin in acutely burned patients. J Trauma 1995;38:233–236.

91. Poletes GP, Miller SF, Finley RK, et al: Blood use in the burn unit: A possible role for erythropoietin. J Burn Care Rehabil 1994;15:37–41.

92. Simon TL, Curreri PW, Harker LA: Kinetic characterization of hemostasis in thermal injury. J Lab Clin Med 1977;89:702–711.

93. Cullen JJ, Murray DJ, Kealey GP: Changes in coagulation factors in patients with burns during acute blood loss. J Burn Care Rehabil 1989;10:517–522.

94. Munster AM: The early management of thermal burns. Surgery 1980;87:29–40.

95. Burke JF, Wolfe RR, Mullany CJ, et al: Glucose requirements following burn injury. Parameters of optimal glucose infusion and possible hepatic and respiratory abnormalities following excessive glucose intake. Ann Surg 1979;190:274–285.

96. Sheridan RL, Yu YM, Prelack K, et al: Maximal parenteral glucose oxidation in hypermetabolic young children: A stable isotope study. JPEN J Parenter Enteral Nutr 1998;22:212–216.

97. Deitch EA, Rutan R, Waymack JP: Trauma, shock, and gut translocation. New Horiz 1996;4:289–299.

98. Phillips GD: Total parenteral nutrition in acute illness. Anaesth Intensive Care 1985;13:288–299.

99. Czaja AJ, McAlhany JC, Andes WA, et al: Acute gastric disease after cutaneous thermal injury. Arch Surg 1975;110:600–605.

100. Pingleton SK: Complications of acute respiratory failure. Am Rev Respir Dis 1988;137:1463–1493.

101. Martyn JA: Cimetidine and/or antacid for the control of gastric acidity in pediatric burn patients. Crit Care Med 1985;13:1–3.

102. Priebe HJ, Skillman JJ, Bushnell LS, et al: Antacid versus cimetidine in preventing acute gastrointestinal bleeding: A randomized trial in 75 critically ill patients. N Engl J Med 1980;302:426–430.

103. Martyn JA, Greenblatt DJ, Hagen J, et al: Alteration by burn injury of the pharmacokinetics and pharmacodynamics of cimetidine in children. Eur J Clin Pharmacol 1989;36:361–367.

104. Gardner GG, Martin CJ: The mathematical modelling of thermal responses of normal subjects and burned patients. Physiol Meas 1994;15:381–400.

105. Monafo WW, Freedman B: Topical therapy for burns. Surg Clin North Am 1987;67:133–145.

106. Monafo WW, West MA: Current treatment recommendations for topical burn therapy. Drugs 1990;40:364–373.

107. Baxter CR: Problems and complications of burn shock resuscitation. Surg Clin North Am 1978;58:1313–1322.

108. Kien CL, Rohrbaugh DK, Burke JF, et al: Whole body protein synthesis in relation to basal energy expenditure in healthy children and in children recovering from burn injury. Pediatr Res 1978;12:211–216.

109. Aulick LH, Wilmore DW: Increased peripheral amino acid release following burn injury. Surgery 1979;85:560–565.

110. Mushambi MC, Bailey SM, Trotter TN, et al: Effect of alcohol on gastric emptying in volunteers. Br J Anaesth 1993;71:674–676.

111. Szyfelbein SK, Drop LJ, Martyn JAJ, et al: Persistent ionized hypocalcemia in patients during resuscitation and recovery phases of body burns. Crit Care Med 1981;9:454–458.

112. Coté CJ, Drop LJ, Daniels AL, et al: Calcium chloride versus calcium gluconate: Comparison of ionization and cardiovascular effects in children and dogs. Anesthesiology 1987;66:465–470.

113. Martyn JA, Matteo RS, Greenblatt DJ, et al: Pharmacokinetics of d-tubocurarine in patients with thermal injury. Anesth Analg 1982;61:241–246.

114. Martyn JAJ: Clinical pharmacology and therapeutics in burns. In: Martyn JAJ, ed: Acute Management of Burn Trauma. Philadelphia: WB Saunders; 1990:180–200.

115. Leibel WS, Martyn JA, Szyfelbein SK, et al: Elevated plasma binding cannot account for the burn-related d-tubocurarine hyposensitivity. Anesthesiology 1981;54:378–382.

116. Martyn JA, Abernethy DR, Greenblatt DJ: Plasma protein binding of drugs after severe burn injury. Clin Pharmacol Ther 1984;35:535–539.

117. Bloedow DC, Goodfellow LA, Marvin J, et al: Meperidine disposition in burn patients. Res Commun Chem Pathol Pharmacol 1986;54:87–99.

118. Denson DD, Concilius RR, Warden G, et al: Pharmacokinetics of continuous intravenous infusion of methadone in the early post-burn period. J Clin Pharmacol 1990;30:70–75.

119. Gronert GA, Theye RA: Pathophysiology of hyperkalemia induced by succinylcholine. Anesthesiology 1975;43:89–99.

120. Kim C, Fuke N, Martyn JA: Burn injury to rat increases nicotinic acetylcholine receptors in the diaphragm. Anesthesiology 1988;68:401–406.

121. Kim C, Martyn J, Fuke N: Burn injury to trunk of rat causes denervation-like responses in the gastrocnemius muscle. J Appl Physiol 1988;65:1745–1751.

122. Martyn J, Goldhill DR, Goudsouzian NG: Clinical pharmacology of muscle relaxants in patients with burns. J Clin Pharmacol 1986;26:680–685.

123. Aprille JR, Aikawa N, Bell TC, et al: Adenylate cyclase after burn injury: Resistance to desensitization by catecholamines. J Trauma 1979;19:812–818.

124. Ward JM, Martyn JA: Burn injury–induced nicotinic acetylcholine receptor changes on muscle membrane. Muscle Nerve 1993;16:348–354.

125. Kim C, Hirose M, Martyn JA: d-Tubocurarine accentuates the burn-induced upregulation of nicotinic acetylcholine receptors at the muscle membrane. Anesthesiology 1995;83:309–315.

126. Cone JB, Ransom JM, Tucker WE, et al: The effect of dopamine on postburn myocardial depression. J Trauma 1982;22:1019–1020.

127. Martyn J, Wilson RS, Burke JF: Right ventricular function and pulmonary hemodynamics during dopamine infusion in burned patients. Chest 1986;89:357–360.

128. Glew RH, Moellering RC Jr, Burke JF: Gentamicin dosage in children with extensive burns. J Trauma 1976;16:819–823.

129. Martyn JA, Goudsouzian NG, Matteo RS, et al: Metocurine requirements and plasma concentrations in burned paediatric patients. Br J Anaesth 1983;55:263–268.

130. Martyn JA, Liu LM, Szyfelbein SK, et al: The neuromuscular effects of pancuronium in burned children. Anesthesiology 1983;59:561–564.

131. Ernst A, Zibrak JD: Carbon monoxide poisoning. N Engl J Med 1998;339:1603–1608.

132. Hollingsed TC, Saffle JR, Barton RG, et al: Etiology and consequences of respiratory failure in thermally injured patients. Am J Surg 1993;166:592–596.

133. Rue LW, Cioffi WG, Mason AD, et al: Improved survival of burned patients with inhalation injury. Arch Surg 1993;128:772–778.

134. Brown DL, Archer SB, Greenhalgh DG, et al: Inhalation injury severity scoring system: A quantitative method. J Burn Care Rehabil 1996;17:552–557.

135. Ryan CM, Schoenfeld DA, Thorpe WP, et al: Objective estimates of the probability of death from burn injuries. N Engl J Med 1998;338:362–366.

136. Sheridan R, Remensnyder J, Prelack K, et al: Treatment of the seriously burned infant. J Burn Care Rehabil 1998;19:115–118.

137. Morrow SE, Smith DL, Cairns BA, et al: Etiology and outcome of pediatric burns. J Pediatr Surg 1996;31:329–333.

138. Eckhauser FE, Billote J, Burke JF, et al: Tracheostomy complicating massive burn injury: A plea for conservatism. Am J Surg 1974;127:418–423.

139. Khine HH, Corddry DH, Kettrick RG, et al: Comparison of cuffed and uncuffed endotracheal tubes in young children during general anesthesia. Anesthesiology 1997;86:627–631.

140. Deakers TW, Reynolds G, Stretton M, et al: Cuffed endotracheal tubes in pediatric intensive care. J Pediatr 1994;125:57–62.

141. Sheridan RL, Kacmarek RM, McEttrick MM, et al: Permissive hypercapnia as a ventilatory strategy in burned children: Effect on barotrauma, pneumonia, and mortality. J Trauma 1995;39:854–859.

142. Haldane J, Loraine-Smith J: The absorption of oxygen by the lungs. J Physiol 1897;22:231–258.

143. Douglas CG, Haldane JS, Haldane JBS: The laws of combination of hemoglobin with carbon monoxide and oxygen. J Physiol 1912;44:275–304.

144. Stewart RD, Stewart RS, Stamm W, et al: Rapid estimation of carboxyhemoglobin level in fire fighters. JAMA 1976;235:390–392.

145. Ginsberg MD: Carbon monoxide intoxication: clinical features, neuropathology and mechanisms of injury. J Toxicol Clin Toxicol 1985;23:281–288.

146. Gorman DF, Runciman WB: Carbon monoxide poisoning. Anaesth Intensive Care 1991;19:506–511.

147. Hardy KR, Thom SR: Pathophysiology and treatment of carbon monoxide poisoning. J Toxicol Clin Toxicol 1994;32:613–629.

148. Keenan HT, Bratton SL, Norkool DM, et al: Delivery of hyperbaric oxygen therapy to critically ill, mechanically ventilated children. J Crit Care 1998;13:7–12.

149. Meert KL, Heidemann SM, Sarnaik AP: Outcome of children with carbon monoxide poisoning treated with normobaric oxygen. J Trauma 1998;44:149–154.

150. Walker AR: Emergency department management of house fire burns and carbon monoxide poisoning in children. Curr Opin Pediatr 1996;8:239–242.

151. Barker SJ, Tremper KK: The effect of carbon monoxide inhalation on pulse oximetry and transcutaneous PO$_2$. Anesthesiology 1987;66:677–679.

152. Barker SJ, Tremper KK, Hyatt J: Effects of methemoglobinemia on pulse oximetry and mixed venous oximetry. Anesthesiology 1989;70:112–117.

153. Tremper KK, Barker SJ: Pulse oximetry. Anesthesiology 1989;70:98–108.

154. Grim PS, Gottlieb LJ, Boddie A, et al: Hyperbaric oxygen therapy. JAMA 1990;263:2216–2220.

155. Olson KR, Seger D: Hyperbaric oxygen for carbon monoxide poisoning: Does it really work? Ann Emerg Med 1995;25:535–537.

156. Tibbles PM, Perrotta PL: Treatment of carbon monoxide poisoning: A critical review of human outcome studies comparing normobaric oxygen with hyperbaric oxygen. Ann Emerg Med 1994;24:269–276.

157. Silverman SH, Purdue GF, Hunt JL, et al: Cyanide toxicity in burned patients. J Trauma 1988;28:171–176.

158. Pruitt BA Jr: Fluid and electrolyte replacement in the burned patient. Surg Clin North Am 1978;58:1291–1312.

159. Wisnicki JL, Sato RM, Baxter CR: Current concepts in burn care. Ann Plast Surg 1986;16:242–249.

160. Baxter C: Fluid resuscitation, burn percentage, and physiologic age. J Trauma 1979;19(Suppl):864–865.

161. Baxter CR: Fluid volume and electrolyte changes of the early postburn period. Clin Plast Surg 1974;1:693–703.

162. Caldwell FT, Bowser BH: Critical evaluation of hypertonic and hypotonic solutions to resuscitate severely burned children: a prospective study. Ann Surg 1979;189:546–552.

163. Moylan JA Jr, Reckler JM, Mason AD Jr: Resuscitation with hypertonic lactate saline in thermal injury. Am J Surg 1973;125:580–584.

164. Jelenko C 3d, Williams JB, Wheeler ML, et al: Studies in shock and resuscitation, I: use of a hypertonic, albumin-containing, fluid demand regimen (HALFD) in resuscitation. Crit Care Med 1979;7:157–167.

165. Monafo WW, Chuntrasakul C, Ayvazian VH: Hypertonic sodium solutions in the treatment of burn shock. Am J Surg 1973;126:778–783.

166. Boswick JA Jr, Thompson JD, Kershner CJ: Critical care of the burned patient. Anesthesiology 1977;47:164–170.

167. Carvajal HF, Parks DH: Optimal composition of burn resuscitation fluids. Crit Care Med 1988;16:695–700.

168. Bowser-Wallace BH, Caldwell FT Jr: A prospective analysis of hypertonic lactated saline v. Ringer's lactate-colloid for the resuscitation of severely burned children. Burns Incl Therm Inj 1986;12:402–409.

169. Bowser-Wallace BH, Caldwell FT Jr: Fluid requirements of severely burned children up to 3 years old: Hypertonic lactated saline vs. Ringer's lactate-colloid. Burns Incl Therm Inj 1986;12:549–555.

170. Graves TA, Cioffi WG, McManus WF, et al: Fluid resuscitation of infants and children with massive thermal injury. J Trauma 1988;28:1656–1659.

171. Merrell SW, Saffle JR, Sullivan JJ, et al: Fluid resuscitation in thermally injured children. Am J Surg 1986;152:664–669.

172. Horton JW, White J, Baxter CR, et al: Hypertonic saline dextran resuscitation of thermal injury. Ann Surg 1990;211:301–311.

173. Yim JM, Vermeulen LC, Erstad BL, et al: Albumin and nonprotein colloid solution use in US academic health centers. Arch Intern Med 1995;155:2450–2455.

174. Shirani KZ, Vaughan GM, Mason AD Jr, et al: Update on current therapeutic approaches in burns. Shock 1996;5:4–16.

175. Hoffman MJ, Greenfield LJ, Sugerman HJ, et al: Unsuspected right ventricular dysfunction in shock and sepsis. Ann Surg 1983;198:307–319.

176. Wilson RD: Anesthesia and the burned child. Int Anesthesiol Clin 1975;13:203–217.

177. Zubair M, Besner GE: Pediatric electrical burns: management strategies. Burns 1997;23:413–420.

178. Wallace BH, Cone JB, Vanderpool RD, et al: Retrospective evaluation of admission criteria for paediatric electrical injuries. Burns 1995;21:590–593.

179. Garcia CT, Smith GA, Cohen DM, et al: Electrical injuries in a pediatric emergency department. Ann Emerg Med 1995;26:604–608.

180. Hammond JS, Ward CG: High-voltage electrical injuries: Management and outcome of 60 cases. South Med J 1988;81:1351–1352.

181. Solem L, Fischer RP, Strate RG: The natural history of electrical injury. J Trauma 1977;17:487–492.

182. Dixon GF: The evaluation and management of electrical injuries. Crit Care Med 1983;11:384–387.

183. Lamb JD: Anaesthetic considerations for major thermal injury. Can Anaesth Soc J 1985;32:84–92.

184. Osgood PF, Szyfelbein SK: Management of burn pain in children. Pediatr Clin North Am 1989;36:1001–1013.

185. Sheridan RL, Hinson M, Nackel A, et al: Development of a pediatric burn pain and anxiety management program. J Burn Care Rehabil 1997;18:455–459.

186. Browne DA, de Boeck R, Morgan M: An evaluation of the Level 1 blood warmer series. Anaesthesia 1990;45:960–963.

187. Presson RGJ, Haselby KA, Bezruczko AP, et al: Evaluation of a new high-efficiency blood warmer for children. Anesthesiology 1990;73:173–176.

188. Rothen HU, Lauber R, Mosimann M: An evaluation of the Rapid Infusion System. Anaesthesia 1992;47:597–600.

189. Coté CJ, Petkau AJ: Thiopental requirements may be increased in children reanesthetized at least one year after recovery from extensive thermal injury. Anesth Analg 1985;64:1156–1160.

190. White PF, Way WL, Trevor AJ: Ketamine: Its pharmacology and therapeutic uses. Anesthesiology 1982;56:119–136.

191. Martyn JA, Matteo RS, Szyfelbein SK, et al: Unprecedented resistance to neuromuscular blocking effects of metocurine with persistence after complete recovery in a burned patient. Anesth Analg 1982;61:614–617.

192. Mazurek AJ, Rae B, Hann S, et al: Rocuronium versus succinylcholine: Are they equally effective during rapid-sequence induction of anesthesia? Anesth Analg 1998;87:1259–1262.

193. Mills AK, Martyn JA: Neuromuscular blockade with vecuronium in paediatric patients with burn injury. Br J Clin Pharmacol 1989;28:155–159.

194. Mills AK, Martyn JA: Evaluation of atracurium neuromuscular blockade in paediatric patients with burn injury. Br J Anaesth 1988;60:450–455.

195. Satwicz PR, Martyn JA, Szyfelbein SK, et al: Potentiation of neuromuscular blockade using a combination of pancuronium and dimethyltubocurarine: Studies in children following acute burn injury or during reconstructive surgery. Br J Anaesth 1984;56:479–484.

196. Coté CJ, Goldstein EA, Fuchsman WH, et al: The effect of nail polish on pulse oximetry. Anesth Analg 1988;67:683–686.

197. Coté CJ, Goldstein EA, Coté MA, et al: A single-blind study of pulse oximetry in children. Anesthesiology 1988;68:184–188.

198. Coté CJ, Daniels AL, Connolly M, et al: Tongue oximetry in children with extensive thermal injury: Comparison with peripheral oximetry. Can J Anaesth 1992;39:454–457.

199. Jobes DR, Nicolson SC: Monitoring of arterial hemoglobin oxygen saturation using a tongue sensor. Anesth Analg 1988;67:186–188.

200. Sheridan RL, Prelack KM, Petras LM, et al: Intraoperative reflectance oximetry in burn patients. J Clin Monit 1995;11:32–34.

201. Coté CJ, Jobes DR, Schwartz AJ, et al: Two approaches to cannulation of a child's internal jugular vein. Anesthesiology 1979;50:371–373.

202. Seldinger SI: Catheter replacement of the needle in percutaneous arteriography. Acta Radiol 1953;39:368–376.

203. Sheridan RL, Szyfelbein SK, Petras L, Lydon M: Staged high dose epinephrine clysis in pediatric burn excisions. J Burn Care Rehabil 1998;19:S199.

204. Karl HW, Swedlow DB, Lee KW, et al: Epinephrine-halothane interactions in children. Anesthesiology 1983;58:142–145.

205. Sheridan RL, Hurley J, Smith MA, et al: The acutely burned hand: management and outcome based on a ten-year experience with 1047 acute hand burns. J Trauma 1995;38:406–411.

206. Tompkins RG, Remensnyder JP, Burke JF, et al: Significant reductions in mortality for children with burn injuries through the use of prompt eschar excision. Ann Surg 1988;208:577–585.

207. Sheridan RL, Tompkins RG, Burke JF: Management of burn wounds with prompt excision and immediate closure. J Intensive Care Med 1994;9:6–19.

208. Moran KT, O'Reilly TJ, Furman W, et al: A new algorithm for calculation of blood loss in excisional burn surgery. Am Surg 1988;54:207–208.

209. Housinger TA, Lang D, Warden GD: A prospective study of blood loss with excisional therapy in pediatric burn patients. J Trauma 1993;34:262–263.

210. Rutan RL, Bjarnason DL, Desai MH, et al: Incidence of HIV seroconversion in paediatric burn patients. Burns 1992;18:216–219.

211. Morris JAJ, Wilcox TR, Reed GW, et al: Safety of the blood supply: Surrogate testing and transmission of hepatitis C in patients after massive transfusion. Ann Surg 1994;219:517–525.

212. Desai MH, Herndon DN, Broemeling L, et al: Early burn wound excision significantly reduces blood loss. Ann Surg 1990;211:753–759.

213. Budny PG, Regan PJ, Roberts AH: The estimation of blood loss during burns surgery. Burns 1993;19:134–137.

214. Kahn RC, Jascott D, Carlon GC, et al: Massive blood replacement: Correlation of ionized calcium, citrate, and hydrogen ion concentration. Anesth Analg 1979;58:274–278.

215. Stulz PM, Scheidegger D, Drop LJ, et al: Ventricular pump performance during hypocalcemia: Clinical and experimental studies. J Thorac Cardiovasc Surg 1979;78:185–194.

216. Denlinger JK, Nahrwold ML, Gibbs PS, et al: Hypocalcaemia during rapid blood transfusion in anaesthetized man. Br J Anaesth 1976;48:995–1000.

217. Coté CJ, Drop LJ, Hoaglin DC, et al: Ionized hypocalcemia after fresh frozen plasma administration to thermally injured children: Effects of infusion rate, duration, and treatment with calcium chloride. Anesth Analg 1988;67:152–160.

218. Coté CJ: Depth of halothane anesthesia potentiates citrate-induced ionized hypocalcemia and adverse cardiovascular events in dogs. Anesthesiology 1987;67:676–680.

219. Wang C, Martyn JA: Burn injury alters beta-adrenergic receptor and second messenger function in rat ventricular muscle. Crit Care Med 1996;24:118–124.

220. Marathe PH, Dwersteg JF, Pavlin EG, et al: Effect of thermal injury on the pharmacokinetics and pharmacodynamics of atracurium in humans. Anesthesiology 1989;70:752–755.

221. Demling RH, Lalonde C: Oxygen consumption is increased in the postanesthesia period after burn excision. J Burn Care Rehabil 1989;10:381–387.

222. Kavanagh C: A new approach to dressing change in the severely burned child and its effect on burn-related psychopathology. Heart Lung 1983;12:612–619.

223. Kavanagh C: Psychological intervention with the severely burned child: Report of an experimental comparison of two approaches and their effects on psychological sequelae. J Am Acad Child Adolesc Psychiatry 1983;22:145–156.

224. Perry S, Heidrich G: Management of pain during debridement: a survey of U.S. burn units. Pain 1982;13:267–280.

225. Porter J, Jick H: Addiction rare in patients treated with narcotics. N Engl J Med 1980;302:123.

226. Goodman JE, McGrath PJ: The epidemiology of pain in children and adolescents: A review. Pain 1991;46:247–264.

227. McGrath PJ, Finley GA: Attitudes and beliefs about medication and pain management in children. J Palliat Care 1996;12:46–50.

228. McGrath PJ, Frager G: Psychological barriers to optimal pain management in infants and children. Clin J Pain 1996;12:135–141.

229. Schechter NL, Allen D: Physicians' attitudes toward pain in children. J Dev Behav Pediatr 1986;7:350–354.

230. Silbert BS, Lipkowski AW, Cepeda MS, et al: Enhanced potency of receptor-selective opioids after acute burn injury. Anesth Analg 1991;73:427–433.

231. Meyer WJ, Nichols RJ, Cortiella J, et al: Acetaminophen in the management of background pain in children post-burn. J Pain Symptom Manage 1997;13:50–55.

232. Foertsch CE, O'Hara MW, Stoddard FJ, et al: Treatment-resistant pain and distress during pediatric burn-dressing changes. J Burn Care Rehabil 1998;19:219–224.

233. Stoddard FJ: Coping with pain: A developmental approach to treatment of burned children. Am J Psychiatry 1982;139:736–740.

234. Stoddard FJ, Martyn J, Sheridan R: Psychiatric issues in pain of burn injury. Curr Rev Pain 1997;1:130–136.

235. Roca RP, Spence RJ, Munster AM: Posttraumatic adaptation and distress among adult burn survivors. Am J Psychiatry 1992;149:1234–1238.

236. Schechter NL, Blankson V, Pachter LM, et al: The ouchless place: No pain, children's gain. Pediatrics 1997;99:890–894.

237. Weisman SJ, Schechter NL: The management of pain in children. Pediatr Rev 1991;12:237–243.

238. Walco GA, Cassidy RC, Schechter NL: Pain, hurt, and harm: The ethics of pain control in infants and children. N Engl J Med 1994;331:541–544.

239. Zeltzer LK, Anderson CT, Schechter NL: Pediatric pain: current status and new directions. Curr Probl Pediatr 1990;20:409–486.

240. Brannen AL, Still J, Haynes M, et al: A randomized prospective trial of hyperbaric oxygen in a referral burn center population. Am Surg 1997;63:205–208.

241. Buehler JH, Berns AS, Webster JR, et al: Lactic acidosis from carboxyhemoglobinemia after smoke inhalation. Ann Intern Med 1975;82:803–805.

242. Tibbles PM, Edelsberg JS: Hyperbaric-oxygen therapy. N Engl J Med 1996;334:1642–1648.

243. Chang KH, Han MH, Kim HS, et al: Delayed encephalopathy after acute carbon monoxide intoxication: MR imaging features and distribution of cerebral white matter lesions. Radiology 1992;184:117–122.

244. Seger D, Welch L: Carbon monoxide controversies: Neuropsychologic testing, mechanism of toxicity, and hyperbaric oxygen. Ann Emerg Med 1994;24:242–248.

245. Thom SR, Keim LW: Carbon monoxide poisoning: A review of epidemiology, pathophysiology, clinical findings, and treatment options including hyperbaric oxygen therapy. J Toxicol Clin Toxicol 1989;27:141–156.

246. Myers RA, Snyder SK, Emhoff TA: Subacute sequelae of carbon monoxide poisoning. Ann Emerg Med 1985;14:1163–1167.

247. Thom SR, Taber RL, Mendiguren II, et al: Delayed neuropsychologic sequelae after carbon monoxide poisoning: prevention by treatment with hyperbaric oxygen. Ann Emerg Med 1995;25:474–480.

248. Werner B, Back W, Akerblom H, et al: Two cases of acute carbon monoxide poisoning with delayed neurological sequelae after a "free" interval. J Toxicol Clin Toxicol 1985;23:249–265.

249. Schwartz A, Hennerici M, Wegener OH: Delayed choreoathetosis following acute carbon monoxide poisoning. Neurology 1985;35:98–99.

250. Myers RA, Snyder SK, Linberg S, et al: Value of hyperbaric oxygen in suspected carbon monoxide poisoning. JAMA 1981;246:2478–2480.

251. Mathieu D, Nolf M, Durocher A, et al: Acute carbon monoxide poisoning: Risk of late sequelae and treatment by hyperbaric oxygen. J Toxicol Clin Toxicol 1985;23:315–324.

252. Choi IS: Delayed neurologic sequelae in carbon monoxide intoxication. Arch Neurol 1983;40:433–435.

253. Neufeld MY, Swanson JW, Klass DW: Localized EEG abnormalities in acute carbon monoxide poisoning. Arch Neurol 1981;38:524–527.

254. Myers RA, Britten JS: Are arterial blood gases of value in treatment decisions for carbon monoxide poisoning? Crit Care Med 1989;17:139–142.

255. Norkool DM, Kirkpatrick JN: Treatment of acute carbon monoxide poisoning with hyperbaric oxygen: A review of 115 cases. Ann Emerg Med 1985;14:1168–1171.

256. Jefferson JW: Subtle neuropsychiatric sequelae of carbon monoxide intoxication: Two case reports. Am J Psychiatry 1976;133:961–964.

257. Raphael JC, Elkharrat D, Jars-Guincestre MC, et al: Trial of normobaric and hyperbaric oxygen for acute carbon monoxide intoxication. Lancet 1989;2:414–419.

258. Weaver LK, Hopkins RO, Larson-Lohr V: Neuropsychologic and functional recovery from severe carbon monoxide poisoning without hyperbaric oxygen therapy. Ann Emerg Med 1996;27:736–740.

259. Grube BJ, Marvin JA, Heimbach DM: Therapeutic hyperbaric oxygen: Help or hindrance in burn patients with carbon monoxide poisoning? J Burn Care Rehabil 1988;9:249–252.

260. Sloan EP, Murphy DG, Hart R, et al: Complications and protocol considerations in carbon monoxide–poisoned patients who require hyperbaric oxygen therapy: Report from a ten-year experience. Ann Emerg Med 1989;18:629–634.

24 Anesthesia for Organ Transplantation

Marla S. Gendelman, Mateen Raazi, Peter J. Davis, *and* Erich A. Everts, Jr.

Cardiac Transplantation
    Changing Patient Demographics and Indications
    Contraindications
    Donor Selection
    Preoperative Evaluation
    Surgical Technique
    Operative Management
    Postoperative Management
    Rejection and Its Management
    Outcomes Following Pediatric Heart Transplantation
Heart-Lung and Lung Transplantation
    Indications for Lung Transplantation
    Heart-Lung Versus Lung Transplantation
    Single Versus Double Lung Transplantation
    Lobar Transplantation and Retransplantation
    Xenotransplantation and Bridge-to-Transplantation Devices
    Recipient Evaluation
    Donor Evaluation
    Operative Technique
    Anesthetic Management
    Postoperative Management
    Complications from Pediatric Lung and Heart-Lung Transplantation
Liver Transplantation
    Cardiovascular and Respiratory Issues
    Renal and Metabolic Issues
    Hematology and Coagulation Issues
    Operative Technique
    Anesthetic Management
    Intraoperative Concerns
    Patient Outcome
Renal Transplantation
    Preoperative Considerations
    Preoperative Evaluation
    Operative Technique
    Anesthetic Management
    Postoperative Management
Bone Marrow Transplantation
    Recipient Preparation
    Transplant Procedure
    Anesthetic Management
    Post-Transplant Management

Cardiac Transplantation

The number of cardiac transplantations performed in children has steadily increased since the first procedure by Kantrowitz in 1967[1] and is now limited mainly by the availability of donor organs. The indications for pediatric cardiac transplantation have expanded resulting in the inclusion of children with a wider range of age and diagnoses. Recipients of pediatric heart transplants are living longer with a vastly improved quality of life. This is due in part to the use of better immunosuppressive regimens with significantly fewer side effects. Still, rejection of the donor heart by the recipient remains a major threat and the principal cause of post-transplant mortality.

Changing Patient Demographics and Indications

At its inception, heart transplantation in children was an extension of the adult cardiac transplantation programs. As such, most of the transplants were performed in older children and adolescents in whom the diagnostic indication was a cardiomyopathy (most commonly dilated, but also ischemic, hypertrophic, and secondary to chemotherapeutic agents). As the indications for pediatric heart transplantation have broadened, an increasing number of younger children with congenital heart disease are undergoing the procedure.

In fact, congenital heart disease, including hypoplastic left heart syndrome and other complex congenital cardiac lesions, has overtaken cardiomyopathy as the leading cause of cardiac transplantation in younger children. Other indications for transplantation include life-threatening arrhythmias not amenable to ablative techniques,[2] myocarditis, cardiac angiosarcoma, and rare disorders of endomyocardial morphogenesis.[3]

Contraindications

The contraindications to pediatric cardiac transplantation include the presence of active infection, increased pulmonary vascular resistance greater than 10 Woods units,[4] irreversible noncardiac organ damage, severe systemic disease, pulmonary emboli or infarction, and active malignancy. In addition, severe psychosocial problems that could impair postoperative care, and lack of reliable caretakers and a stable family structure are also critical issues in pediatric cardiac transplantation.

Donor Selection

Traditionally, selection criteria used for adult donors (Table 24–1) are applied to pediatric heart donors. Recently there has been some concern that these criteria do not correlate well with myocardial pathologic findings in infants and children and may falsely limit the availability of donor organs in the pediatric age group.[5] More accurate predictors of donor suitability in children are needed.

It is important for myocardial preservation to minimize the ischemia time of the donor heart to less than 6 hours and preferably less than 4 hours. However, there is some evidence to suggest that ischemia times up to nearly 8½ hours may be well tolerated by pediatric hearts without any adverse consequences.[6] Donor-recipient heart size matching is another critical issue for successful pediatric heart transplantation. It has been suggested, however, that the use of an oversized donor may be beneficial, particularly in patients with pretransplantation pulmonary hypertension. The use of an undersized donor should be strongly discouraged, as it is associated with a higher rate of donor heart failure.[7]

Preoperative Evaluation

Patients considered for cardiac transplantation demonstrate impaired cardiac performance and various degrees of dysfunction of other major organ systems secondary to their low cardiac output. A thorough history must be obtained,

Table 24–1. Donor Selection Criteria Used for Adults: Factors That Make the Donor Heart Not Suitable

---

Identified pre-existing heart disease
Strongly suspected or proved major infection
Prolonged cardiac arrest (>15 min)
Prolonged high-dose inotropic support (>10 μg/kg/min dopamine or dobutamine, for >12 hours)
Major chest trauma
History of drug abuse
Extracranial malignancy

---

with particular attention to exercise tolerance, and the need for inotropic agents. Investigations to be reviewed include an electrocardiogram (ECG), chest radiographs, and an echocardiogram. A review of the cardiac catheterization data is extremely helpful in formulating a safe anesthetic plan. Valuable data gained from such a review include assessment of left ventricular function, left ventricular end-diastolic pressure, and pulmonary artery pressures and resistance, and analysis of any dysrhythmias provoked during catheterization and the response to any medications, including oxygen, or to pacing.

Laboratory investigations should include serum electrolytes, hemoglobin and hematocrit, assessment of coagulation status (prothrombin time [PT], partial thromboplastin time [PTT], and platelet count) and an analysis of baseline respiratory status. The anesthetic plan should take into account all medications that a patient is receiving and their potential interactions with anesthetic agents. Consultation with the child's cardiologist is valuable, given the cardiologist's intimate knowledge of the patient's medical and psychological condition and his or her long-standing relationship with the patient and family.

Surgical Technique

Although the technique of pediatric heart transplantation is basically similar to that used in adults, greater technical difficulty and risk of hemorrhage is to be expected; this is true especially of patients with prior cardiac surgery and those patients with complex congenital heart disease. Hypothermic cardiopulmonary bypass is utilized. A period of deep hypothermia with circulatory arrest may be used, especially in younger infants and those requiring significant aortic or other vascular reconstruction. The period of circulatory arrest is usually less than 30 to 45 minutes. Longer circulatory arrest times may increase the risk of postoperative neurologic injury.[8]

After a median sternotomy and initiation of cardiopulmonary bypass, the ascending aorta is cross-clamped, the venae cavae are snared about the venous cannula, and the aorta and the main pulmonary artery are divided at the level of their respective semilunar valves. The ventricles of the recipient are separated from the atria along the atrioventricular groove and removed. The donor atria are then anastomosed to the recipient atria. Several measures are used to aid in myocardial preservation of the donor heart. These include the instillation of an iced solution in the chest cavity, irrigation of the left ventricular cavity with a cold saline solution, and strict avoidance of left ventricular distension. After completion of the aortic anastomosis, the aortic cross-clamp is removed and the aorta and the left-sided chambers are vented of air. The pulmonary artery anastomosis is then completed and cardiopulmonary bypass is discontinued after the return of cardiac function. Epicardial pacing wires are routinely applied to the heart, mediastinal chest tubes are positioned for drainage, and the sternum is closed.

Operative Management

Anesthetic preparation must include medications available for intraoperative manipulation of the myocardium and vascular system. Infusions of vasoactive drugs, including epinephrine, isoproterenol, dopamine, dobutamine, nitroprusside, amrinone, and nitroglycerine, must be readily available. After coordination with the donor team, the patient is transported to the operating room. If the patient was previously receiving supplemental oxygen, this is continued in the pre-induction period. Before induction, monitoring devices are applied; these include a precordial stethoscope, ECG, noninvasive blood pressure cuff, and pulse oximeter. After induction, central venous and arterial catheters are inserted in addition to temperature probes (esophageal, rectal, tympanic) and a urinary catheter. Although the use of a pulmonary artery catheter is not universal, its use with a new donor heart may be helpful in the post-bypass period as well as in the early perioperative periods. Because transthoracic intracardiac catheters are often placed at the termination of cardiopulmonary bypass, preoperative placement of a pulmonary artery catheter may not be necessary. In patients who have undergone multiple cardiac procedures, potential risks of sternotomy and reoperation should be addressed and include the need for adequate volume infusion lines, blood products in the operating room, and preparation for emergency femoral bypass.

The contractile state of the myocardium in patients with end-stage cardiac disease is already at its critical limit; therefore, any further decrease, as occurs with many potent anesthetic agents, electrolyte imbalance, or arrhythmias, will be very poorly tolerated. Stroke volume remains relatively fixed and significantly reduced; maintenance of sinus rhythm is critically important.[9] Preload must be maintained within a very narrow range; small fluctuations in circulating blood volume produce exaggerated responses. For any given increase in afterload in these patients, one may see a precipitous decrease in stroke volume compared with patients with a normal heart. In patients with increased pulmonary vascular resistance, one must avoid conditions that predispose to further increases in pulmonary resistance, such as hypoxemia, hypercarbia, acidosis, or increased adrenergic tone secondary to light anesthesia, which may precipitate terminal right- or left-sided heart failure.[10]

Because most patients have minimal cardiovascular reserve and borderline function, anxiolytic premedicant drugs are best administered in a monitored setting such as the preoperative area or in the operating room itself. To limit donor ischemic time and because donor availability is not predictable, these operations are considered emergency procedures. Various induction techniques have been used, depending on the nature of the cardiac disease and the degree of risk for pulmonary aspiration. The myocardium in end-stage disease is unusually sensitive to the depressant effects of various anesthetic drugs and to subtle changes in the hemodynamic balance that exists in the factors controlling cardiac output, such as contractility, cardiac output, preload, and afterload. If a rapid-sequence induction is required, the patient is denitrogenated with 100% oxygen, cricoid pressure is applied, and a combination of atropine (0.02 mg/kg), etomidate (0.2 mg/kg), and succinylcholine (1–2 mg/kg) is intravenously administered.[11]

Following induction, anesthesia is usually maintained with fentanyl (50–100 μg/kg or sufentanil 10–15 μg/kg administered in incremental doses), followed by pancuronium (0.1 mg/kg).[12, 13] The use of potent inhaled anesthetics is contraindicated because of their myocardial depressant effect. Although nitrous oxide has been shown to increase pulmonary vascular resistance in adults, studies in children with repaired congenital heart defects have not observed this effect.[14]

In pediatric patients, cardiac replacement takes place under cardiopulmonary bypass at temperatures of 26° to 28°C; whereas in newborn or young infants, this procedure is often performed at 18° to 20°C under total hypothermic circulatory arrest. As the anastomoses are completed, patients are slowly rewarmed. Hemodynamic conditions must be fully optimized before cardiopulmonary bypass is terminated. Of primary concern is the status of the pulmonary circulation, as one must avoid conditions that increase pulmonary vascular resistance and thereby cause undue stress on the donor right ventricle. Factors that increase pulmonary artery pressure include hypoxia, acidosis, hypothermia, increased adrenergic tone with light anesthesia, and polycythemia. Therefore, it is imperative to ensure adequate ventilation and oxygenation with the tendency toward hyperventilation and hyperoxia, normothermia, and adequate anesthesia. The narrow range of afterload with which the donor right ventricle can function cannot be overemphasized. If these efforts fail to decrease pulmonary vascular resistance to acceptable levels, further measures are undertaken with pharmacologic agents; these include prostaglandin E_1, amrinone, and nitric oxide. Because systemic hypotension may occur, it may be necessary to support the systemic circulation with the addition of a vasopressor, most often dopamine, dobutamine, or, rarely, epinephrine.

Dysrhythmias are common during the post-bypass period. The ECG is unique in demonstrating two independent P waves, one from the donor right atrium and the other from the recipient right atrial remnant. It is only the donor sino-atrial node, however, that transmits impulses to the ventricles. This chronic denervation has several implications. The lack of direct innervation eliminates the baroreceptor reflex; therefore, the donor heart is unable to respond acutely to changes in arterial pressure with circulating blood volume alterations. In this situation, cardiac output becomes primarily dependent on venous return and the effects of circulating catecholamines, which act directly on the myocardium.

Coronary arteries are no longer innervated, and with loss of resting sympathetic tone, coronary flow increases. However, evidence suggests that cardiac adrenergic signals play an important role in regulating myocardial blood flow with increases in coronary blood flow in response to sympathetic stimulation.[15] Of prime importance is the fact that when considering pharmacotherapy, one must remember that the donor heart will not respond to drugs that act through the autonomic nervous system (ephedrine, mephentermine, metaraminol) but only to those that exert direct cardiac effects (phenylephrine, epinephrine, dopamine). For drugs that exert both direct and indirect effects (ephedrine, metaraminol), only the direct effects will be observed. Dysrhythmias secondary to acute denervation and ischemia are common. Junctional and nodal rhythms are the most common abnormal rhythms, but because of the abnormal ECG associated with the presence of two sinoatrial nodes, the diagnosis of these rhythms is often only confirmed by direct observation of the donor heart. In the setting of nodal rhythm in a heart with limited stroke volume, isoproterenol is titrated to maintain heart rates in the high normal range. In some cases, temporary pacing may be required. Because of the peripheral vasodilator effects of isoproterenol, should additional inotropic support be required, the addition of dopamine or dobutamine in dosage ranges of 5 to 10 μg/kg/min may be useful. Once hemodynamic stability is confirmed, protamine sulfate is carefully administered and the heart decannulated. The chest is closed after favorable hemostatic control is obtained. Sternal closure may compromise fragile hemodynamics, especially when donor-recipient heart size is not exact. In addition, any compression of the right ventricular outflow tract during sternal closure may result in unanticipated and deleterious increases in right ventricular pressure. Therefore, in some cases, closure at sternotomy is staged.

Postoperative Management

All pharmacotherapy must be withdrawn very gradually because the donor myocardium is unusually sensitive to hemodynamic changes. Particular attention should be directed at maintaining stable pulmonary artery pressures, because acute increases in pulmonary vascular resistance could severely compromise right ventricular function. Normal acid-base status must be maintained and adequate analgesia ensured. Arrhythmias may be an early sign of rejection. These patients may generally be extubated approximately 24 to 36 hours postoperatively. Postoperative complications include cardiac failure, arrhythmias, infection, and rejection. Side effects of immunosuppressant therapy may stress already compromised organ systems.

Rejection and Its Management

Rejection is the most common cause of death after pediatric heart transplantation. Donor-recipient mismatch for gender, race, blood type, Rh factor, and HLA typing do not correlate with rejection history. Older age at transplantation and cytomegalovirus disease, however, are correlated with more frequent rejection episodes.[16] Excellent medium-term follow-up results have been obtained with a rejection management and surveillance protocol that emphasizes both the minimum use of long-term oral steroids and noninvasive techniques for diagnosing rejection.

Outcome Following Pediatric Heart Transplantation

Survival for pediatric heart transplant recipients 1 year of age or older is comparable to survival after adult heart transplantation. Risk factors for death include the need for assist devices, nonidentical ABO blood types, and younger age.[17] Infants and young children tend to have a higher early mortality rate than do older children. Survival rates at 2- and 5-year follow-up of 79% and 75%, respectively, have been reported for pediatric heart transplant recipients, making transplantation a viable option for selected pediatric patients.[18]

Heart-Lung and Lung Transplantation

Long-term survival of lung, heart, and heart-lung transplant recipients has been enhanced by improvements in donor and recipient selection, organ harvest and preservation, preoperative and postoperative care, surgical technique, and the control of rejection through the use of FK-506 and cyclosporine A. Although it has been more than 13 years since the introduction of heart-lung and lung transplantation, less than 5% of the total number of transplants have been performed in the pediatric age group.[19] The scarcity of suitable donor organs for pediatric patients is the major limiting factor in pediatric transplantation.

Indications for Lung Transplantation

Lung transplantation is indicated for progressive, irreversible end-stage pulmonary failure. The indications for lung transplantation in children are significantly different from those in adults. Most adult lung transplants are performed for emphysema, cystic fibrosis, or pulmonary hypertension. In children, however, pulmonary fibrosis and pulmonary vascular diseases are the primary reasons for lung transplantation (Table 24-2). Potential indications for lung transplantation in infancy include congenital diaphragmatic hernia, surfactant protein deficiency, pulmonary vein stenosis or atresia, or primary pulmonary hypoplasia. In contrast with lung transplantation, the indications for heart-lung transplantation are quite similar in both the pediatric and the adult population. The major causes for heart-lung transplantation include cystic fibrosis and pulmonary vascular disease of either the primary or secondary type.

Heart-Lung Versus Lung Transplantation

The actuarial survival rate for bilateral single lung transplant recipients has been reported as 75% at 1 year, 56% at 2 years, and 36% at 3 years,[20] which is comparable to that of heart and lung transplant recipients. This would imply that there would be little advantage to heart-lung transplantation over lung transplantation for most patients whose heart is otherwise normal or correctable. From the standpoint of

Table 24-2. Pediatric Indications for Lung Transplantation

Pulmonary fibrosis
    Usual interstitial fibrosis
    Desquamative interstitial fibrosis (rare)
    Pulmonary alveolar proteinosis
    Idiopathic pulmonary alveolar microlithiasis
    Cystic fibrosis
    Radiation-induced pulmonary fibrosis
    Obliterative bronchiolitis
    Bronchopulmonary dysplasia
    Congenital surfactant deficiencies
    Collagen vascular disease
Pulmonary vascular disease
    Primary pulmonary hypertension
    Pulmonary hypertension after corrected congenital heart
        disease
    Pulmonary hypertension and correctable congenital heart
        disease (Eisenmenger syndrome)
    "Inadequate" pulmonary vascular bed
    Pulmonary atresia, ventricular septal defect, no central
        pulmonary arteries
    Congenital diaphragmatic hernia

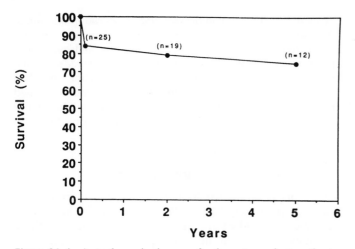

Figure 24–1. Actual survival curve for lung transplant patients. (From Slaughter MS, Braunlin E, Bowman RM 3d, et al:. Pediatric heart transplantation: Results of 2- and 5-year follow-up. J Heart Lung Transplant 1994;13:627.)

optimal use of scarce donor organs, it may be advisable to utilize lung transplantation and save the donor heart for another recipient.

Single Versus Double Lung Transplantation

The 1-year and 2-year survival rates for single and double lung transplant recipients are not significantly different (Fig. 24–1). However, there are situations in which bilateral sequential lung transplantation might be superior to single lung transplantation. This is most evident for cases in which chronic infections of the lungs are present, such as in cystic fibrosis. Although it has been suggested that long-term results might be better with bilateral lung transplantation in patients with pulmonary hypertension, the 1- and 2-year survival rates between bilateral and single transplantation for pulmonary hypertension are essentially the same: 54 versus 58% and 50 versus 56%, respectively.[19] However, because of the nature of their underlying disease, pediatric patients typically do not receive single lung transplants.

Lobar Transplantation and Retransplantation

Because of the relative donor organ shortage, pulmonary lobar transplantation from living related donors has become a feasible option to ease the pediatric organ shortage. Although there are no reported series of lobar transplantation, a small number of reduced-size lung transplants have been performed in children (V. A. Starnes, personal communication, 1993). The mortality rate for children with congenital diaphragmatic hernia remains in the 20 to 60% range despite the use of extracorporeal membrane oxygenation.[19] Children with congenital diaphragmatic hernia with pulmonary hypoplasia and pulmonary hypertension who require extracorporeal membrane oxygenation therapy potentially stand to gain significantly from lobar transplantation.

Xenotransplantation and Bridge-to-Transplantation Devices

In view of the severe shortage of donor organs, xenotransplantation (organs from animals) has become another alterna-

tive. The long-term results of such transplantation have so far been poor, however. The only currently available bridge-to-transplantation device is extracorporeal membrane oxygenation, which is associated with significant complications.

Recipient Evaluation

Evaluation of patients as potential lung transplant recipients is mainly concerned with their pulmonary and cardiovascular status. Pulmonary evaluation typically includes a chest radiograph, pulmonary function tests, ventilation-perfusion scans, and exercise testing; however, pulmonary function and exercise testing are often not possible in pediatric patients. In single lung transplants, ventilation and perfusion scans help determine the optimal side for transplantation, that is, that with more severe disease.[21] Computed tomography and magnetic resonance imaging may also provide additional information. The cardiac evaluation focuses on right ventricular performance. A two-dimensional echocardiogram and radionuclide ventriculogram are performed to evaluate the degree of pulmonary hypertension and right ventricular dysfunction. If the results of these tests are inconclusive, catheterization of the right side of the heart is performed. If evidence of significant pulmonary hypertension is noted, the response to vasodilators is assessed. In older children, oxygen saturation is recorded at rest and during exercise with administration of supplemental oxygen. With this thorough preoperative cardiopulmonary evaluation, patient reserves and the need for cardiopulmonary bypass are determined. Preoperative indicators suggesting the need for cardiopulmonary bypass include the need for oxygen at rest, oxygen desaturation with exercise despite supplemental oxygen, severe pulmonary artery hypertension (greater than one half systemic), or evidence of right heart decompensation (ejection fraction < 25%).

The goal of pretransplant evaluation is to identify those patients who may or may not be suitable candidates for the procedure (Table 24–3) and to optimize their overall condition in advance. Patients are evaluated by a social worker and a psychologist for potential psychosocial problems and by a dietitian to review their nutritional status. Because these patients are frequently undernourished, they are placed on high-calorie intake in preparation for transplantation. During this initial hospitalization, the parents and patient are informed of the details of the anesthetic and the surgical

Table 24–3. Selection Criteria for Suitable Lung Transplant Recipients

Failure of maximum medical therapy
Good right ventricular function
Absence of systemic disease, particularly renal and hepatic damage
Minimal or no chronic steroid therapy
Good nutritional status
Absence of contraindications to immunosuppression
Medically compliant
Absence of significant psychiatric illness
Good psychosocial support system
No active infection
No active malignancy
No severe chest wall deformities

plans, because the urgency of surgery precludes any in-depth discussion on the day of surgery. These patients are critically ill, making continued re-evaluation necessary while they await donor organ availability; worsening in the overall physical condition is the norm. Particular attention is given to the development of right heart failure, which would make a recipient unsuitable for isolated lung transplantation. In these patients, the possibility of combined heart-lung transplantation should be considered.

Donor Evaluation

The scarcity of donor organs continues to be the major obstacle in lung transplantation. For various reasons, only 10% of the available lung and heart-lung blocs were recovered in the pediatric age group according to the 1991 United Network for Organ Sharing Data.[19] In addition, pediatric donor lungs can be given to an adult recipient but adult lungs are unlikely to be given to a pediatric recipient because there are many more adults than children awaiting lung transplantation in the United States.

The donor criteria (Table 24–4) include ABO compatibility and size matching within 10% as measured by horizontal and vertical measurements of the donor and the recipient on chest radiographs. However, it has recently been suggested that with the elective use of cardiopulmonary bypass and aggressive postoperative support, a broad size range can be used.[22]

Operative Technique

In single lung procedures, the patient is positioned in the standard decubitus position for a right or left thoracotomy. If partial cardiopulmonary bypass is anticipated, the ipsilateral femoral vessels are also prepared. Revascularization of the donor lung to the recipient involves anastomosis of pulmonary veins to a cuff of left atrium isolated in a vascular clamp, end-to-end anastomosis of the pulmonary artery, and end-to-end bronchial anastomosis. The re-established airway is examined with the fiberoptic bronchoscope to ensure that there is no bronchial stenosis.

En bloc double lung transplantation involves anastomoses of the trachea, left atrium, and pulmonary artery, necessitating the use of cardiopulmonary bypass. The complexity of this procedure makes it less suitable for more debilitated patients. The need for heparinization with cardiopulmonary bypass predisposes to significant hemorrhage in patients with known pleural adhesions, such as cystic fibrosis. The proce-

Table 24–4. Donor Criteria for Lung Transplantation

No pre-existing lung disease
Minimal ventilatory support
Negative bacterial cultures from tracheal aspirates
No history of intravenous drug abuse or neoplastic disease
Arterial oxygen tension greater than 25 mm Hg with 100%
    inspired oxygen and positive end-expiratory pressure of 5 cm
    H_2O
ABO compatibility
Appropriate size match
Physical proximity to recipient (transport time)

dure for bilateral sequential transplant is actually two single-lung transplants, one performed immediately after the other.[23] It has become the preferred method when bilateral transplantation is indicated, because cardiopulmonary bypass may or may not be necessary, bronchial anastomoses heal better, and arrest of the heart is not required. After the lung with the poorer function is replaced, patients are maintained on their newly transplanted lung while the transplant is performed on the other side. For these procedures, either a bronchial blocker or a left-sided endobronchial tube may be used. In children, because of the technical difficulty in isolating one lung, coupled with the hemodynamic instability frequently associated with one-lung ventilation, many centers perform bilateral sequential lung transplants with the aid of cardiopulmonary bypass.

Anesthetic Management

Intraoperative management of patients undergoing lung transplantation begins with preparation of the necessary equipment. As with any high-risk cardiopulmonary procedure, extensive monitoring and resuscitative capabilities are required. In addition to the standard monitors, the use of a pulmonary artery catheter with the ability to measure right ventricular ejection fraction is helpful, because the ability of the right ventricle to tolerate increases in afterload must be continually assessed. This application is currently available only for adolescent and adult patients. In addition, equipment to isolate ventilation must be available. This includes an assortment of double-lumen tubes in addition to bronchial blockers for smaller patients for whom double-lumen tubes are not available. A fiberoptic bronchoscope of appropriate size is necessary to confirm proper endotracheal tube or bronchial blocker position and to assess the bronchial reconstruction at the end of the procedure. A ventilator and anesthesia circuit of low compression volume are used, and a continuous positive-pressure system may be necessary. Medications that may be required include vasodilators for the pulmonary circulation prostaglandin E_1, nitroglycerin, sodium nitroprusside, and nitric oxide. In addition, vasoactive medications to support the systemic circulation are necessary (dopamine, dobutamine, and epinephrine). Cardiopulmonary bypass must be readily available.

Anesthetic management of adult patients undergoing lung transplantation has been described.[11, 24–26] Because of the scarcity of donor organs and the minimal ischemic times that must be maintained, lung transplantation is an urgent procedure. Patients are quickly re-evaluated for progression of the disease before being transported to the operating room with supplemental oxygen. Sedative preanesthetic medication, if needed, should be used cautiously as these patients have virtually no pulmonary reserve. This is often a challenge in younger patients who exhibit increased anxiety. Because the urgent nature of the procedure often does not allow sufficient time for gastric emptying, prophylactic measures (including H_2 blockers, metoclopramide, and so on) should be undertaken to reduce the risk of pulmonary aspiration of gastric contents.

After the patient is positioned on the operating room table, standard monitoring is applied. Because of the nature of their disease, these patients often cannot lie flat and are maintained in the head-up position as long as possible, with supplemental oxygen continuously administered. Infection is always a major concern in transplant recipients; strict aseptic techniques should always be observed. Because time constraints limit the allowable travel time, patients are prepared in the operating room while awaiting assessment of the donor organs by the harvest team. Two large-bore venous cannulas are placed in the upper extremities. A radial or femoral arterial catheter is placed for blood sampling and direct measurement of arterial pressure. In some centers, pediatric patients undergoing bilateral sequential lung transplants are positioned supine with their arms suspended above their heads; in these patients, a femoral arterial catheter and adequate intravenous access in the lower extremities are placed. A pulmonary artery catheter is placed but is positioned in the nontransplanted lung during single lung transplants and in the main pulmonary artery during double lung transplantation. In patients with elevated pulmonary artery pressure, the risk of arterial rupture may be greater when the catheter is placed more distally.

For patients in whom a pulmonary artery catheter cannot be placed, a multiport central venous catheter is placed for direct measurement of central ventral pressure (CVP) and for infusion of vasoactive drugs. *Extreme care must be taken to prevent air entrainment when central venous catheterization is performed in nonanesthetized patients, since these patients generate extremely high negative intrathoracic pressures to maintain ventilation.*

Once it has been determined by direct inspection that the donor organs are suitable for transplantation, the recipient is anesthetized. In many younger patients, the placement of invasive monitors is not possible without general anesthesia; therefore, this process begins only after suitability of donor organs has been confirmed. After adequate denitrogenation with 100% oxygen, a rapid or modified rapid sequence intravenous induction is performed; most patients are at risk for the aspiration of gastric contents because of the unscheduled nature of the procedure. In patients with very limited cardiopulmonary reserves, it is important to avoid even mild myocardial depression. Induction is achieved with the intravenous administration of etomidate, fentanyl, and succinylcholine or rocuronium. In adults, ketamine is avoided because it potentially increases pulmonary vascular resistance. In children, however, ketamine has little effect on pulmonary vascular resistance.[27]

The method of securing the airway depends on the proposed surgical procedure. If the patient's size permits, a left-sided double-lumen tube is placed, as the margin of safety with it appears greater than with a right-sided tube, especially with changes in the patient's position.[28] In children, when appropriately sized double-lumen endotracheal tubes are not available, a bronchial blocker may be used. Whatever type of endotracheal tube is used, care must be taken to ensure proper cuff inflation; overdistention of the cuff exerts undue pressure on the tracheal or bronchial mucosa, thereby compromising blood flow. Fiberoptic bronchoscopy is used to confirm proper endotracheal tube or bronchial blocker position.

After induction and intubation, a urinary catheter and temperature probe are placed and all pressure points are padded. Anesthesia is maintained with a combination of agents, such as fentanyl, sufentanil, and a muscle relaxant, titrated to effect. Because of the nitrogen-splinting effects in maintaining alveolar patency, an air-oxygen mixture is used if 100% oxygen is not required. Although volatile anesthetic agents may result in an increased alveolar-arterial gradient (from blunting of hypoxic pulmonary vasoconstriction response) and hemodynamic compromise, nonetheless, low inspired concentrations of inhaled agents may be useful to decrease the afterload on the right ventricle when the pulmonary artery is cross-clamped.

Positioning of the patient is dictated by the proposed transplant procedure. For single-lung transplants, the lateral decubitus thoracotomy position is used and adequate padding must be applied to avoid pressure on all neurovascular structures and bony prominences. For en bloc bilateral transplants, the patient is positioned as for a median sternotomy. Patients undergoing bilateral sequential procedures are positioned supine with their arms secured over their head to expose the entire anterior and lateral chest walls. This position allows bilateral anterolateral thoracotomies. Extreme care is taken to avoid damage due to overextension of or pressure on vital axillary structures.

During the operation, predictable problems may be encountered at certain stages. The idea of performing a pneumonectomy in a patient with end-stage pulmonary failure is alarming in itself. The success of the procedure hinges on the ability of the patient to tolerate one-lung ventilation and the ability of the right ventricle to tolerate an acute increase in afterload with clamping of the pulmonary artery before pneumonectomy. The ability to tolerate one-lung ventilation is assessed early in the operative procedure. With the patient in the supine position, ventilation to the transplant side is interrupted, and pulmonary artery pressure, cardiac index, arterial blood gas tensions, and oxygen saturation are assessed. Indications for cardiopulmonary bypass include marked and persistent elevations in pulmonary artery pressure, arterial oxygen desaturation, hypercarbia, and evidence of right heart failure. Acute increases in pulmonary artery pressure are initially treated with vasodilators (prostaglandin E$_1$, nitroprusside, nitroglycerin, or nitric oxide). If a therapeutic response does not occur, preparation is made for bypass.

With the patient placed in the thoracotomy position, proper endotracheal tube placement is again confirmed with a fiberoptic bronchoscope. During the lateral thoracotomy, one-lung ventilation is instituted to facilitate surgical exposure. Hypoxemia may develop from the resultant shunt secondary to perfusion in the absence of ventilation; with limited pulmonary reserve, carbon dioxide retention may also occur. Initial therapy involves increasing the inspired oxygen concentration (if not already 100%) and increasing minute ventilation. If the initial therapy is unsuccessful, an attempt is made to recruit the nonventilated lung with the application of positive end-expiratory pressure to the dependent lung and continuous positive airway pressure to the nondependent lung. High-frequency ventilation has been advocated as a method that causes less surgical interference. If these maneuvers are unsuccessful, preparation is made for cardiopulmonary bypass.

The most critical period occurs when the ipsilateral pulmonary artery is clamped, before pneumonectomy. The outcome is determined by the ability of the recipient's right ventricle to tolerate this sudden rise in afterload. Methods used to assess the performance of the right ventricle during this critical period include measurements of pulmonary artery pressure and cardiac index, serial measurements of right ventricular ejection fraction, and direct visual inspection of the performance of the right side of the heart. If right-sided failure is observed, the combination of a vasodilator to unload the right side of the heart (nitroprusside or nitroglycerine), together with inotropic support (dopamine), may often be required. Prostaglandin E_1 has also been used for its vasodilator effect. Although this increase in pulmonary pressure is sudden, it usually is not sustained, because vascular resistance in the native lung decreases, taking some strain off the right ventricle. If right-sided heart failure results despite these measures, cardiopulmonary bypass is instituted.

Once the patient is stabilized, a vascular clamp is applied across the left atrium to provide an adequate cuff for attaching the donor pulmonary veins. This may severely impair left atrial and ventricular filling and further increase right-sided afterload. Inotropic support may be required to maintain cardiovascular stability. In the past, to reduce total ischemia time, blood flow to the donor organ was restored before bronchial anastomosis and re-establishment of ventilation to the transplanted lung; this produced profound hypoxemia secondary to the large created shunt. To avoid this problem, every attempt is made to restore ventilation to the transplanted lung with 100% oxygen before reperfusion. After confirmation of airway integrity by fiberoptic bronchoscopy, the chest is closed. The patient is placed supine, and if a double-lumen tube was used, it is changed to a standard single-lumen tube.

Fluid management of these patients entails severe restriction to keep them as "dry" as possible, although patients with cystic fibrosis frequently have large fluid requirements after unclamping. Blood loss is generally not severe unless extensive adhesions are encountered during initial dissection. It has been suggested that the use of aprotinin may reduce the amount of perioperative hemorrhage in pediatric patients at high risk for bleeding after lung transplantations; these include patients with cystic fibrosis and those with previous cardiothoracic operations.[29] Total crystalloid input is restricted and blood volume is maintained by infusing 5% albumin or blood products as needed. Because of severe fluid restriction and the use of nephrotoxic agents for immunosuppression, low-dose dopamine is used to promote an adequate urine output.

Postoperative Management

Postoperatively, these patients generally require ventilatory support for the first 8 to 72 hours. Fluid administration must be kept to a minimum because pulmonary congestion occurs easily and may be difficult to eradicate. Diuretics are used judiciously. In addition, the transplanted lung is maintained in a nondependent position. Cardiac output is maintained with the use of inotropic support, although high levels of vasopressors may decrease bronchial blood flow, contributing to the potential for airway necrosis. Analgesia is usually achieved with the use of a thoracic epidural catheter, which is usually placed in the early postoperative period.

Complications from Pediatric Lung and Heart-Lung Transplantation

As more pediatric patients undergo lung and heart-lung transplantation, specific categories of post-transplant complications are becoming evident. These complications can be categorized as (1) anatomic and surgical, (2) infectious, (3) rejection, (4) post-transplant lymphoproliferative disease, (5) drug related, and (6) chronic pain.[30] Reimplantation injury and vascular obstruction with thrombus formation occur early in the post-transplant period. In contrast, stenosis at tracheal and bronchial anastomotic sites develops more slowly. Post-transplant infections are common, contributed to in major part by the immunosuppressive therapy used. These include all varieties of bacterial, viral, fungal, and protozoal infections, with cytomegaloviral infection being particularly lethal. Rejections may be acute or chronic, with frequent episodes of acute rejection increasing the chances of chronic rejection. Chronic rejection is characterized most ominously by obliterative bronchiolitis. While there has been little improvement in the treatment of obliterative bronchiolitis, it has been suggested that treatment early in the course of the disease may improve the long-term outcome.[19] Differentiation of rejection from infection is based on tissue diagnosis, requiring either a transbronchial or an open-lung biopsy. Post-transplant lymphoproliferative disease, related to Epstein-Barr virus infection, is common in children and difficult to treat. Immunosuppressive drugs used in pediatric transplant recipients include cyclosporine or FK-506 together with azathioprine and steroids. These drugs have significant systemic toxicity that adds considerably to post-transplant morbidity.

Liver Transplantation

Liver transplantation is now a mainstay of therapy in pediatric patients with end-stage liver disease. With the advent of newer immunosuppressive agents, the 1-year survival approaches 90%. General indications for liver transplantation in pediatric patients include patients with (1) primary liver disease that is expected to worsen and result in hepatic failure, (2) nonprogressive liver disease whose risks outweigh the risks of liver transplantation, (3) metabolic disease, (4) primary hepatic malignancies, and (5) fulminant hepatic failure. For pediatric patients, the disease-specific indications differ from those of adults. Biliary atresia, biliary hypoplasia, and Alagilles syndrome are the most frequent causes (60%) for orthotopic liver transplantation (OLT) in children. Inborn errors of metabolism (tyrosinemia, glycogen storage disease, urea cycle defects) and metabolic disorders (α_1-antitrypsin, Wilson's disease, and cystic fibrosis) are the other major categories.

Many physiologic alterations are associated with end-stage liver disease (Table 24–5) and their symptomatology is consistent with acute hepatocellular failure or chronic hepatocellular dysfunction. In general, most pediatric patients present with symptoms of chronic hepatocellular dysfunction.

Cardiovascular and Respiratory Issues

Due to the effects of anemia, cirrhosis, and portal hypertension, the cardiovascular system is often in a hyperdynamic state. Cardiac output is increased as a result of both increased heart rate and stroke volume. Peripheral arteriovenous shunting, decreased systemic vascular resistance, decreased

Table 24–5. Pathophysiologic Changes Associated with End-Stage Liver Failure

System	Change
Cardiovascular	Hyperdynamic circulation
	Low peripheral vascular resistance
	Portal hypertension
	Pericardial effusion
Pulmonary	Hypoxemia
	Restrictive lung disease
	Arteriovenous shunting
Hematologic	Anemia
	Thrombocytopenia
	Coagulopathy
Metabolic	Decreased pseudocholinesterase
	Hypoglycemia
	Hyperglycemia
	Hypokalemia
	Alkalosis or acidosis
Renal	Prerenal azotemia
	Hepatorenal syndrome
Gastrointestinal	Delayed gastric emptying
	Esophageal varices
Neurologic	Cerebral edema
	Encephalopathy

arterial blood pressure, and arterial oxygen desaturation may be observed. The presence of arteriovenous shunting coupled with a hyperdynamic state also results in a high mixed venous saturation. In spite of the hyperdynamic state, the effective blood volume in patients with end-stage liver disease is decreased. In children with familial hypercholesterol syndromes, hypercholesterolemia can lead to signs and symptoms of ischemic heart disease or congestive heart failure.

Hypoxemia is a frequent occurrence in children with end-stage liver disease. Hypoxemia may be secondary to restrictive lung disease from massive ascites or hepatosplenomegaly. In addition, intrinsic pulmonary disease or intrapulmonary and extrapulmonary arteriovenous shunting can contribute to hypoxemia. In most patients with chronic end-stage liver disease, diffusion and ventilation/perfusion defects are the most common causes of hypoxemia. In these patients, supplemental oxygen corrects the hypoxemia.

Although pulmonary hypertension is associated with end-stage liver disease, its prevalence in patients with end-stage liver disease is less than 1%.[31] The etiology of pulmonary hypertension in patients with end-stage liver disease is unclear but may be related to thromboemboli, hyperkinetic systemic circulation, or humoral pulmonary vasoconstrictors. Pulmonary hypertension appears to be variable with respect to its etiology, its response to pharmacologic interventions, and its effect on survival in patients undergoing liver transplantation.[32, 33] The adult respiratory distress syndrome is observed in some patients with end-stage liver.[34–38] In patients with acute respiratory distress syndrome and impaired hepatocellular function, systemic and pulmonary defenses are compromised; mortality in these patients is very high.[36, 39]

Renal and Metabolic Issues

Abnormalities of glucose metabolism are common in hepatic failure, and patients must be assessed for their preoperative and intraoperative glucose requirements. Hypoglycemia may be observed in acute fulminant hepatic failure. Contributing factors include decreased glucose production, glucagon resistance, and decreased oral intake. Hyperglycemia due to insulin resistance may also develop in some patients. Hypoalbuminemia is often present with advanced disease. Decreased oncotic pressure manifesting as ascites or peripheral edema is common. Drug distribution and elimination are affected by the combined effects of altered protein binding, altered metabolic pathways, or hepatic blood flow.

Common fluid and electrolyte abnormalities include hyponatremia, hypokalemia, hyperphosphatemia, hypomagnesemia, and hypocalcemia. These electrolyte abnormalities are often exacerbated by chronic diuretic therapy. Renal abnormalities secondary to hepatorenal syndrome, prerenal azotemia, or acute renal failure may also be observed. Patients requiring perioperative dialysis have a poorer prognosis.[40]

Hematology and Coagulation Issues

All patients exhibit some degree of anemia. Anemia in liver failure patients usually results from underlying coagulopathies, chronic occult blood loss, and nutritional deficiencies. Of primary concern in the preoperative preparation and intraoperative management of these patients are the coagulation abnormalities. Etiologic factors include reduced synthesis of the liver-dependent factors (I, II, V, VII, IX, X), thrombocytopenia secondary to the hypersplenism of portal hypertension, and underlying nutritional deficiencies secondary to poor absorption of fat-soluble vitamins necessary for coagulation such as vitamin K. Rarely, chronic disseminated intravascular coagulopathy or fibrinolysis is observed. Preoperative evaluation includes measurements of PT, PTT, platelet count, and fibrinogen. Elevations of PT and PTT greater than 30% of normal are common. Management of this coagulopathy with transfusion of large quantities of factor-enriched blood products (fresh frozen plasma, cryoprecipitate), although tolerated well by adolescent and adult patients, may pose a clinically important problem for infants and small children, who may be subject to acute volume overload with congestive heart failure and pulmonary edema. In this situation, plasmapheresis or, in a small infant, exchange transfusion may be beneficial.[41]

Operative Technique

The operative methods for liver transplantation include auxiliary and orthotopic techniques. In the auxiliary technique, the native liver remains in place and an additional whole liver or liver segment is grafted into the recipient. In the OLT, the native liver is removed and a cadaveric whole liver, cadaveric reduced-size liver, or a living related left lateral segment graft is used. Because there exists a relative organ shortage for pediatric patients, efforts to increase the pediatric donor pool have resulted in the more frequent use of liver segments, particularly from living related donors, in lieu of whole liver grafts.

Although many surgical variations may be considered, depending on the donor's and recipient's anatomy (especially with a segmental transplant), the operative technique is generally divided into three stages. Patients are prepared from the clavicles to the groin, and a wide subcostal incision is made. It may be extended through the xiphoid process. During stage 1, the liver is isolated and dissected to its vascular pedicle. Blood loss during this stage is influenced by the patient's underlying coagulation state, the presence of adhesions resulting from previous intra-abdominal procedures, and collateral venous circulation. The second stage or anhepatic stage occurs when the diseased liver is removed from the circulation. The initial description of the operation involved clamping the suprahepatic inferior vena cava (IVC), the infrahepatic IVC, the portal vein, and the hepatic artery. The liver was then removed along with its infrahepatic and suprahepatic vena cava segments. Revascularization of the donor liver took place in the following order: the suprahepatic IVC was anastomosed; the infrahepatic IVC was partially reanastomosed; the organ was flushed via the portal vein to remove the preservative solution and air; the infrahepatic IVC and the portal vein anastomosis were then completed; and finally, the clamps on these vessels were released, thereby restoring venous circulation to the donor organ. More recently, the piggy-back technique has been used (Fig. 24–2A&B).[42] In this technique, the IVC is preserved, and the donor's suprahepatic vena cava is anastomosed to the recipient's hepatic veins. The infrahepatic segment of the donor vena cava is oversewn. Thus, venous return to the heart from the recipient's femoral area is maintained throughout the operative procedure. A temporary portacaval shunt may be used during the procedure to augment venous return from the splanchnic bed.[43] The third stage, or revascularization stage, involves re-establishment of hepatic artery inflow and subsequent biliary anastomosis. If the hepatic artery is extremely small, it may be necessary to graft the donor artery onto the infrarenal aorta. In this situation, a conduit is often necessary, requiring cross-clamping of the recipient's abdominal aorta. Biliary anastomosis is accomplished by attachment of the donor common duct to a limb of recipient jejunum with a Roux anastomosis (Fig. 24–3).

A cholecystectomy is routinely performed. After hemostasis is achieved, the abdomen is closed.

Reduced-Size Cadaveric Livers

Reduced-size liver transplants include reduced cadaveric transplants, split-liver transplants, and partial grafts from living-related donors.[44–54] With reduced-size liver transplants, the eligible donor pool for pediatric patients can be expanded to include donors 10 times the weight of the patient. In addition, Ryckman et al.[51] noted that the use of reduced-size grafts allowed for a redistribution of the donor source to smaller recipients and a reduction in the death rate of children listed for transplantation. Thus, adult-size donors can be used even for small children. The surgical technique, as described by Bismuth and Houssin,[44] involves transecting the liver parenchyma along the insertion of the falciform ligament and using the left lobe of the liver (segments II, III, or II–IV) as the donor graft. Vascular anastomoses are end-to-end and the bile duct is anastomosed end-to-end in a roux-en-Y to the recipient's jejunum (Fig. 24–4). In essence, the advantage of this technique is that it allows adult organs to be used in children.

Split-Liver Grafts

Split-liver grafts take place when a single donor liver is divided in such a way as to provide two viable grafts for transplantation into two different recipients.[47, 50] In this technique, the donor liver is split such that the right lobe contains all of the structures (i.e., portal vein, celiac trunk, common bile duct, and inferior vena cava). Thus, the placement of the right lobe graft in the recipient is similar to placement in the standard liver transplant. The left lobe graft, however, uses the left lobar branches to constitute its vascular and biliary structures. The hepatic vein anastomosis is generally made to the common trunk of the middle and

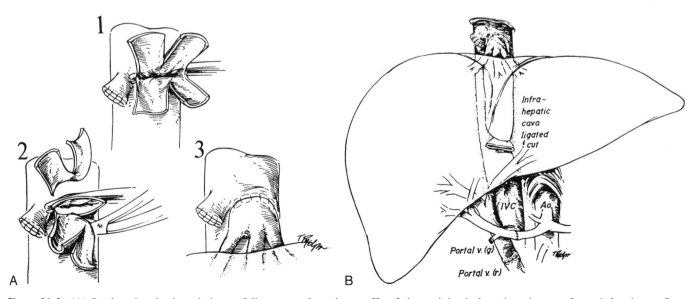

Figure 24–2. (A) In the piggyback technique of liver transplantation, cuffs of the recipient's hepatic veins are formed for the outflow anastomosis with the donor's suprahepatic vena cava. (B) The final appearance, such that the recipient's hepatic veins are anastomosed to the donor suprahepatic vena cava and the donor infrahepatic vena cava is oversewn. (From Tzakis A, Todo S, Starzl TE: Orthotopic liver transplantion with preservation of the inferior vena cava. Ann Surg 1989;210:649–652.)

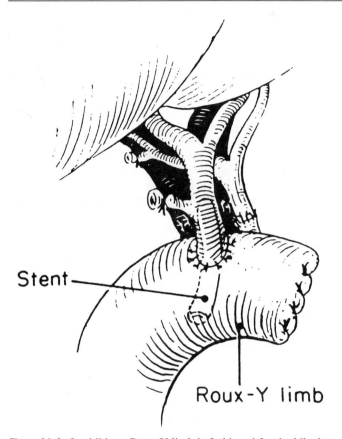

Figure 24–3. In children, Roux-Y limb is fashioned for the bile duct anastomosis. (Modified from Busuttil R, Klintman G: Transplantation of the Liver. Philadelphia: WB Saunders, 1996.)

left hepatic veins of the recipient. The portal vein is sewn end-to-end but frequently requires an interposition graft, and the arterial supply frequently requires an interposed iliac artery graft. The biliary system is completed with a roux-en-Y cholangiojejunostomy.

Living-Related Donors

The use of living-related organ donors had undergone considerable ethical and medical consideration before its introduction for children with end-stage liver disease.[54–61] The major medical and ethical concerns with this technique are the risks to the donor. The technique for this procedure involves transplantation of the left lateral segment. The results of the procedure vary from institution to institution as well as with the severity of the recipient's underlying liver disease. The incidence of complications in the donor has decreased since the surgical technique was changed from a full left hepatectomy to a left lateral segmentectomy.

Anesthetic Management

The anesthetic management of patients undergoing liver transplantation requires an understanding of the patient's hepatic dysfunction in addition to emphasis on conditions that place a particular patient at increased risk. Most patients are considered to have a full stomach and may be at risk for

pulmonary aspiration. Contributory factors include the urgent nature of the procedure, which does not allow sufficient time for gastric emptying; prolonged gastric emptying; significant abdominal distention secondary to ascites and hepatosplenomegaly, which increased intra-abdominal pressure; and recent bleeding from esophageal varices. In the majority of patients, therefore, induction of anesthesia is most often accomplished with an intravenous rapid-sequence technique. Thiopental (4–6 mg/kg), ketamine (1–2 mg/kg), and etomidate (0.2 mg/kg) are the preferred hypnotic induction agents, with etomidate reserved for patients with cardiovascular dysfunction. Succinylcholine (1–2 mg/kg), rocuronium (1–2 mg/kg), or vecuronium (0.2–0.5 mg/kg) are administered to facilitate endotracheal intubation. An oral endotracheal tube is placed to rapidly secure the patient's airway.

Maintenance of anesthesia is achieved using a potent inhalation agent, narcotics, and nondepolarizing muscle relaxants. Isoflurane is the most commonly used potent inhalation anesthetic because of its low degree of metabolism and biologic activity, its ability to maintain cardiovascular stability, and its ability to maintain the relationship of hepatic oxygen supply to oxygen demand in states of mild hypoxia. Muscle relaxation is usually achieved with a long-acting nondepolarizing agent such as pancuronium. Ventilation is maintained with an air-oxygen mixture. Nitrous oxide should be avoided because it may cause excessive bowel distention and complicate surgical closure, especially in infants.

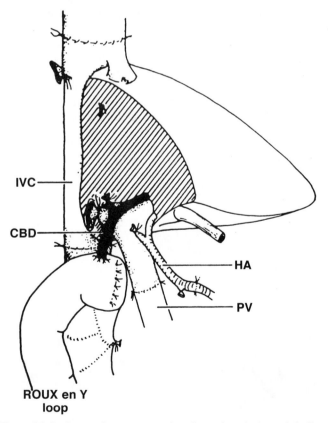

Figure 24–4. Anatomic reconstruction for reduced size adult liver graft. CBD, common bile ducts; IVC, inferior vena cava; HA, hepatic artery; PV, portal vein. (From Bismuth H, Houssin D: Reduced-sized orthotopic liver graft in hepatic transplantation in children. Surgery 1984;95:367–370.)

After induction, further intravascular access is established with large-bore catheters. Because of concerns about infection in immunosuppressed patients, strict aseptic technique is essential. Several large-bore catheters are placed in the upper extremities. Direct arterial pressure measurement is essential. Placement of the arterial catheter in the upper extremities is preferred, but in small infants femoral artery catheters may be used. Central venous access is achieved either by percutaneous placement of an internal jugular or subclavian double lumen catheter. The double lumen catheter allows for both central venous pressure monitoring and a route for fluid and drug administration but is not relied upon for volume administration. Although pulmonary artery catheterization is considered routine in adult patients, it is generally not necessary in pediatric patients. A nasogastric tube, urinary catheter, esophageal stethoscope, and esophageal and rectal temperature probes are also placed.

The patient is positioned supine on a hot air warming mattress. Both arms are abducted and flexed at the elbows to allow easy access to the arterial cannula and assessment of the upper extremity intravenous sites. Pressure points are well padded, and the head and legs are wrapped to minimize heat loss. Throughout the procedure, proper patient positioning must be continually ensured, particularly over pressure points. In some patients, a second hot air warming mattress is placed around the head.

Patient monitoring is essential for successful outcome. Cardiovascular assessment includes an ECG, direct arterial pressure measurement, CVP measurement, and, in rare situations, pulmonary artery pressure and cardiac output assessment. Laboratory analysis includes serial measurements of arterial blood gas tensions, hematocrit, blood glucose, and serum levels of sodium, potassium, and ionized calcium. Frequent evaluation of the coagulation system may be necessary. Coagulation evaluation usually requires measurement of PT, PTT, platelet count, and fibrinogen levels. Bedside assessment with the thromboelastogram is helpful.[62, 63] The thromboelastogram repeatedly measures the shear elasticity of a blood clot from the time when fibrin strands are formed to the completion of the clot formation, including fibrinolysis. An oscillating cup contains 0.36 mL of whole blood kept at 37°C (Fig. 24–5). A pin, suspended by a torsion wire, is lowered into the blood specimen in the cup. While the blood remains fluid, the container motion does not influence the pin. Once the clot begins to form, the fibrin strands gradually strengthen their hold on the cup and pin. Therefore, the cup is coupled to the pin; and the shear elasticity of the blood clot, which is transmitted to the pin, is recorded on thermal paper (see further).

Intraoperative Concerns

Maintaining nearly normal physiologic parameters is a challenge during liver transplantation. The major problems encountered during liver transplantation include cardiovascular instability, metabolic abnormalities, coagulation defects, renal insufficiency, hypothermia, and the problems associated with massive blood transfusion (see Chapter 12).[63–68]

Cardiovascular Instability

Unique cardiovascular changes occur during the various stages of the transplant operation. Significant hypotension

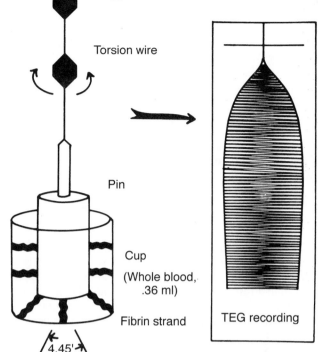

Figure 24–5. The thromboelastogram set-up with normal tracing (see text for details). (From Kang YG, Martin DJ, Marquez J, et al.: Intraoperative changes in blood coagulation and thromboelastographic monitoring in liver transplantation. Anesth Analg 1985;64: 888–896.)

may be observed during stage 1. Hypotension may be caused by various factors: drainage of ascites, surgical manipulation with compression of hilar vessels, blood loss, and electrolyte abnormalities, particularly ionized hypocalcemia, associated with rapid transfusion of reconstituted blood, whole blood, or fresh frozen plasma. Pre-existing myocardial disease rarely contributes to hypotension during transplantation in pediatric patients. With further dissection, surgical manipulation results in compression of the hilar vessels, impeding venous return and leading to hypotension. Previous operative procedures may create intra-abdominal adhesions, or extensive collateral venous blood vessels may exacerbate blood loss. Preoperative coagulation defects with elevation in PT and PTT are a further predisposing factor that can exacerbate blood loss.[69] Thrombocytopenia encountered with hypersplenism or intraoperative dilutional coagulopathy further contributes to increased blood loss.

Cardiovascular instability also occurs during stage 2. In the initial description of the operation, occlusion of the suprahepatic and infrahepatic IVC and portal vein produces a precipitous decline in venous return and hypotension. In pediatric patients with significant portal hypertension and adequate collateral blood flow, vena caval occlusion is well tolerated. For those patients with insufficient collaterals, cross-clamping the vena cava results in a low cardiac output. In these patients, the veno-veno bypass system is necessary. With veno-veno bypass, blood from the portal veins and infrahepatic IVC via the femoral vein is delivered to the superior vena cava via the axillary or internal jugular vein. This system uses a centrifugal pump system, heparin-bonded shunt tubing, and no systemic heparinization.[70] To prevent thrombus formation, flow rates greater than 1000 mL/min must be maintained; therefore, use of this system in patients less than 20 kg is not possible. With the surgical evolution of the piggy-back technique, hemodynamic instability during stage 2 has been minimized.

Reperfusion of the grafted liver marks the onset of stage 3 of the procedure. Significant hemodynamic alterations may be noted with the unclamping of the hepatic vessels (reperfusion syndrome).[71] The hemodynamic changes of the reperfusion syndrome include hypotension, bradycardia, ventricular arrhythmias, and, rarely, cardiac arrest. The etiology of these disturbances includes severe hyperkalemia, hypocalcemia, or metabolic acidosis, resulting from the release of stagnant circulation or from the direct effects of the preservative solution. To minimize the effect of the preservative solution, an effort is made to back-flush the system before completion of the caval anastomosis. Prophylactic treatment to prevent hyperkalemia, hypocalcemia, and acidosis is generally not necessary, although calcium chloride, sodium bicarbonate, glucose, and insulin should be readily available and administered promptly if indicated. Significant air embolism occurring with revascularization, although rare, may be devastating.

Metabolic Abnormalities

The occurrence of hypoglycemia has been overstated in the literature, whereas hyperglycemia is more commonly noted (Fig. 24–6). Hyperglycemia is most pronounced on reperfusion of the liver graft and is related to glucose release from damaged hepatocytes. Hyperglycemia may also be secondary to administration of glucose-containing blood products, such as citrate-phosphate-dextrose preservative, or a decrease in glucose utilization. Persistent hyperglycemia may be secondary to marked ischemic damage and denotes a poor prognosis.[72]

Derangements in both acid-base and electrolyte balance are common during liver replacement. Metabolic acidosis may be caused by rapid transfusion of acidic blood products,

decreased metabolism of citrate and lactic acids, or the release of acidic blood from stagnant tissues on reperfusion. This acidosis is treated with hyperventilation and titration with sodium bicarbonate. On reperfusion of a functioning graft, metabolic alkalosis may be encountered secondary to the conversion of citrate and lactate to bicarbonate.

Frequent measurements of ionized calcium and serum potassium levels are required because electrolyte imbalances are common.[73] Serum ionized calcium concentrations are inversely proportional to serum citrate levels. With transfusion of stored blood products and inadequate hepatic metabolism, serum citrate levels rise progressively and serum ionized calcium levels decrease proportionately and resolve only after reperfusion of the liver graft.

Coagulation Defects

The sequence of changes in coagulation during OLT is unique.[62, 63, 74] Although changes in the coagulation profile as assessed by the thromboelastogram (Fig. 24–7A&B) in adults and children undergoing OLT are similar (e.g., poor preoperative coagulation and severe coagulopathy on reperfusion), the changes in coagulation in children appear to be less severe than those in adults.[75]

With the exception of factor VIII, all other coagulation factors are synthesized in the liver. Defective synthesis of essential factors and inadequate clearance of activated factors by the recipient's diseased liver account for a significant portion of abnormal bleeding. Factor VIII and fibrinogen levels are usually normal or increased, although an abnormal fibrinogen is often synthesized.[76] Thrombocytopenia occurs in over 50% of the patients. A low-grade fibrinolysis, a consequence of low antiplasmin levels and diminished clearance of tissue plasminogen activator, often is present before OLT.

During both the preanhepatic and the anhepatic stages, a dilutional coagulopathy resulting from the massive administration of blood exacerbates the existing coagulopathy as a direct consequence of the liver's inability to metabolize

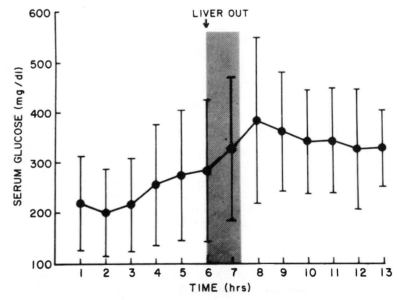

Figure 24–6. Intraoperative glucose versus time (mean and SD represented). Shaded area represents the anhepatic phase. (From Borland LM, Roule M, Cook DR: Anesthesia for pediatric orthotopic liver transplantation. Anesth Analg 1985;64:117.)

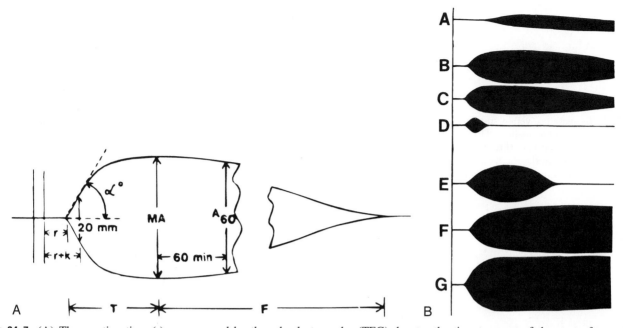

Figure 24–7. (A) The reaction time (r) as measured by thromboelastography (TEG) denotes the time to onset of the start of coagulation and should be approximately 6 to 8 minutes. It represents the rate of thromboplastin formation. Prolongation of this portion of TEG usually represents factor deficiency and is treated with the administration of fresh frozen plasma (FFP). The coagulation time (r + k) is the period between the start of the TEG recording and the time to the generation of an amplitude of 20 mm. It is a measurement of the speed of solid clot formation. The clot formation rate is measured by the alpha angle and normally is greater than 50 degrees. Abnormalities of the alpha angle represent platelet function, fibrinogen, and the intrinsic pathway. Alpha-angle abnormalities are usually corrected by cryoprecipitate administration. The maximum amplitude (MA) is most indicative of platelet function and normally measures between 50 and 70 mm. (B) Abnormalities of coagulation noted prior to surgery. A: There is prolongation of the r time and a diminution of the alpha angle as well as the MA. B: Improved coagulation during stage 1 is noted as there is administration of FFP and platelets as the surgery progresses. Note the improved MA and r time. There is also an improved alpha angle. C: TEG representative of the continued coagulopathy seen during stage 2 of the surgery. Note the progressive diminution of the MA and the progressive tapering of the MA, which suggest possible fibrinolysis. D: A classic representation of fibrinolysis seen in stages 1 and 2. E: Fibrinolysis on graft reperfusion. Note that in this case the clot formed takes somewhat longer before dissolution occurs. F: Amicar-treated TEG, demonstrating dramatic improvement of the fibrinolytic stage. Note the improved MA, r time, and alpha angle. G: The end TEG showing a normal coagulation profile, which is representative of normal liver function from the graft as well as continued administration of coagulation factors. (From Scott V, Davis PJ: Autologous transfusion in orthotopic liver transplantation. In: Salem MR, ed: Blood Conservation in the Surgical Patient. Philadelphia: Williams & Wilkins 1996:340.)

tissue plasminogen activator. The underlying coagulopathy may be exacerbated by continued blood replacement.

Changes in coagulation at the onset of stage 3 are common and multifactorial. Continued blood loss and massive transfusion requirements result in diminution in platelets and in levels of factors V and VIII. With graft reperfusion, primary fibrinolysis thought to be secondary to the release of tissue plasminogen activator from the grafted liver also occurs.

Renal Insufficiency

The maintenance of normal renal function may be challenging during liver transplantation. Oliguria is common, and many factors are contributory. Renal perfusion is reduced during the anhepatic phase. Prompt diuresis generally occurs on revascularization of the graft. Pre-existing hepatorenal syndrome and the nephrotoxic effects of cyclosporine A and FK-506 may also be contributory. It is unclear whether the use of intraoperative low-dose dopamine is effective in protecting renal function.[77, 78]

Hypothermia

Hypothermia almost invariably occurs (Fig. 24–8). The causes include prolonged exposure of intra-abdominal contents, rapid transfusion of inadequately warmed blood products, the use of cold lactated Ringer solution to flush the donor graft, and reduced heat production. All efforts should be made to minimize hypothermia. Appropriate measures include plastic draping of the head and extremities, a heated humidifier and hot air warming blankets, appropriate high-capacity blood-warming devices, warmed irrigating solutions, and a warm ambient temperature in the operating room.

Massive Blood Transfusion Side Effects

Problems associated with massive transfusion include hyperkalemia, ionized hypocalcemia secondary to citrate intoxication, dilutional coagulopathy, hypothermia, and volume overload.[79-87] Some problems associated with blood transfusion are unique to patients undergoing organ transplantation. Of primary concern in any patient who is immunosuppressed is the risk of infection. Cytomegalovirus (CMV) is prevalent

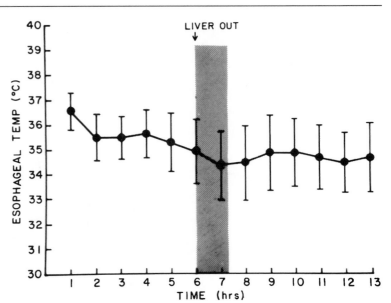

Figure 24–8. Temperature versus time in pediatric patients undergoing liver transplantation. The shaded area represents the anhepatic period. (From Borland LM, Roule M, Cook DR: Anesthesia for pediatric orthotopic liver transplantation, Anesth Analg 1985;64:117.)

in the adult population; however, many infants and children are CMV negative. CMV antibody-negative transplant recipients are at risk for seroconversion after transfusion of CMV-positive blood products; therefore, an attempt is made to provide CMV-negative blood. The blood products most likely to transmit disease include whole blood, packed red blood cells (PRBCs), and platelets. Because CMV is transmitted within white blood cells and because fresh frozen plasma is free of these cells, fresh frozen plasma remains safe regardless of the status of the donor. If CMV-negative blood is unavailable, a blood filter capable of removing white blood cells should be used.

Patient Outcome

Changes in surgical techniques and procurement procedures as well as improvements in immunosuppression and postoperative care have all had an impact on patient survival (Fig. 24–9). Patient age, size, underlying medical status, and type

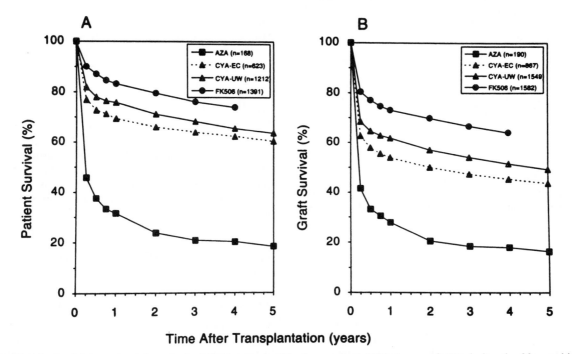

Figure 24–9. The Kaplan-Meier actuarial survival of 3394 patients (A) who received 4188 liver graft (B) during the 30-year history of the program at the Universities of Colorado (1963–1980) and Pittsburgh (1981–1993). The dates of case accrual from bottom to top curves were 1963–1979 (group I), 1980–1987 (group II), 1987–1989 (group III), and 1989–1993 (group IV). The difference in survival between group III (CyA) and group IV (FK-506) was statistically significant ($P<0.0001$). (From Todo S, Fung J, Starzyl TE, et al: Single center experience with primary orthotopic liver transplantation under FK-506 immunosuppression. Ann Surg 1994;220:297–308.)

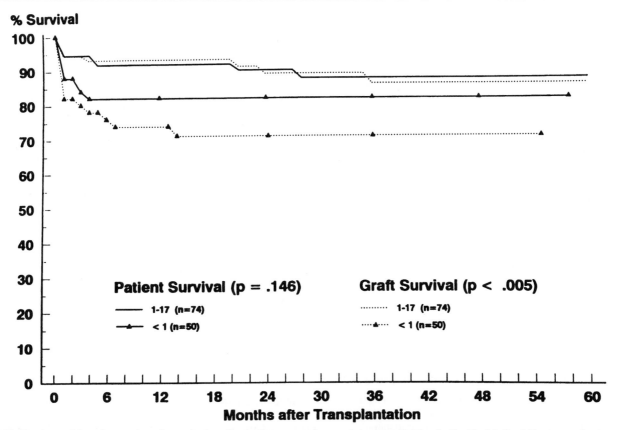

Figure 24–10. Actuarial patient and graft survival pediatric liver transplant recipients at California Pacific Medical Center: patients younger than 1 year (infants compared with those older than 1 year). Most of the grafts lost were full-size livers. (From Esquivel C: Results: Survival and quality of life after orthotopic liver transplantation in children. In: Busuttil R, Klintmalm G, eds: Transplantation of the Liver. Philadelphia: WB Saunders, 1996:238–243.)

of surgical procedure are all factors thought to influence patient and graft survival.

In the early years of liver transplantation, age was thought to be a risk factor, with children under 1 year having higher mortality rates than older children and adults.[88] More recent statistics suggest, however, that age does not affect patient survival (Fig. 24–10). The severity of a patient's illness (i.e., United Network for Organ Sharing classification) can affect survival. Although an early report by Malatack et al.[89] noted no correlation between patient survival and severity of illness, more recent data suggest that the severity of illness influences survival (Fig. 24–11). The type of surgical procedure (e.g., whole graft, slit graft) performed in the donor also affects survival in infants. In infants, reduced-size grafts have significantly improved survival statistics compared with whole-graft transplants (Fig. 24–12).

Renal Transplantation

Renal transplantation is the most well-established of all the organ transplantation procedures and has been performed in pediatric patients since 1963. Improvements in perioperative management, immunosuppression, surgical techniques, and vascular access for hemodialysis have contributed to long-term survival of pediatric renal transplant recipients. The mean incidence of end-stage renal disease in children is approximately 1 to 5 per million young children and in-

creases in the teenage years to 7 to 8 per million,[90] with more than half of these cases secondary to congenital or hereditary disorders (Table 24–6).[91, 92] An adult's kidney is often used, resulting in shorter waiting periods and better donor-recipient matching because of the scarcity of pediatric donors. The potential number of pediatric renal transplant recipients is greater than the supply and has hastened the development of living-related kidney donations. Problems associated with long-term dialysis, such as complex access problems, growth deficiencies, irreversible central nervous system injury associated with uremia, and psychosocial maladjustment, can thus be avoided.[93] Optimum medical management of renal failure in pediatric patients can still result in inadequate growth and development,[94] making early renal transplantation the treatment of choice over medical management in children with end-stage renal disease. Studies show that children successfully transplanted early in life return to normal growth and development rates and can even experience accelerated or "catch-up" growth.[94] Transplantation is more cost-effective than long-term hemodialysis in the pediatric population. The results of graft and patient survival for cadaveric renal transplantation in infants less than 1 year of age are poor and should probably not be attempted. These children can usually be managed successfully with peritoneal dialysis until transplantation at an older age.[90] Absolute and relative contraindications to transplantation include metastatic malignancy, active infection, human immunodeficiency virus infection, ABO incompatibility, thrombosis of the vena

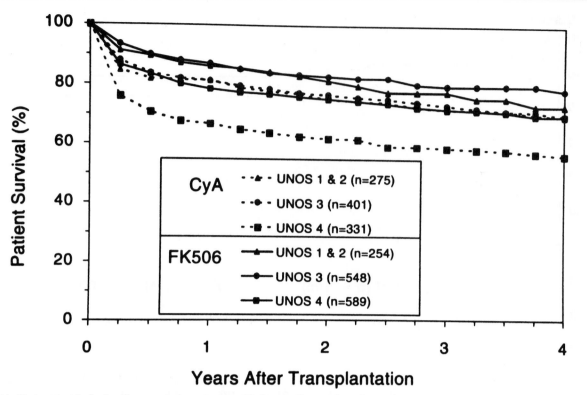

Figure 24–11. Patient survival after liver transplantation stratified according to the primary immunosuppressant and the medical urgency for surgery as defined by the standard criteria of the United Network for Organ Sharing (UNOS). (From Abu-Elmagd K, Todo S, Fung J, et al: Hepatic transplantation at the University of Pittsburgh: New horizons and paradigms after 30 years of experience. In: Terasaki PJ, Cecka JM, eds: Clinical Transplants. Los Angeles, CA: UCLA Tissue Typing Laboratory, 1994:137–156. Munksgaard International Publishers Ltd., Copenhagen, Denmark. Copyright © 1994.)

cava and iliac veins, psychiatric problems, drug abuse, brain injury, severe mental retardation, and active autoimmune process.

Preoperative Considerations

Renal failure is a multisystem disease influencing many physiologic parameters (Table 24–7). The cardiovascular system is affected as a result of volume overload and anemia, which result in increased cardiac output and hyperdynamic circulation.[95] Patients often are hypertensive because of their expanded intravascular volume and, in some instances, hyper-reninemia (10–15%). Postural hypotension is common from a variety of causes, including antihypertensive agents, autonomic neuropathy, and hypovolemia post-dialysis. Although uncommon in the pediatric population, pericarditis secondary to uremia may also be observed; this is rarely hemorrhagic pericarditis. Anemia is universal in end-stage renal disease and is usually normocytic and normochromic.

Table 24–6. Etiology of End-Stage Renal Failure in Children

Glomerulonephritis	Hereditary interstitial nephritis
Obstructive nephropathy	Cystinosis
Pyelonephritis	Oxalosis
Dysplasia-hypoplasia	Hemolytic uremic syndrome
Medullary cystic disease	Lupus nephritis
Polycystic disease	Anaphylactoid purpura nephritis
Alport syndrome	Nephrotic syndrome

The etiology includes a decrease in erythropoietin production, direct effects of uremia on bone marrow, deficiency of folic acid and vitamins B_6 and B_{12}, increases in red blood cell turnover, hemolysis from dialysis, and frequent phlebotomy. This chronic anemia is well tolerated because these

Table 24–7. Pathophysiologic Changes Associated with End-Stage Renal Failure

System	Change
Cardiovascular	Increased cardiac output
	Arrhythmias
	Hypertension
	Cardiomyopathy
	Pericarditis
Hematologic	Anemia
	Platelet dysfunction
Fluids/electrolytes	Volume overload
	Hyperkalemia
	Hyperphosphatemia
	Hypocalcemia
	Hypermagnesemia
	Hyponatremia
	Hyperglycemia
	Metabolic acidosis
Gastrointestinal	Delayed gastric emptying
Neurologic	Peripheral neuropathy
	Autonomic dysfunction
	Encephalopathy
	Disequilibrium syndrome

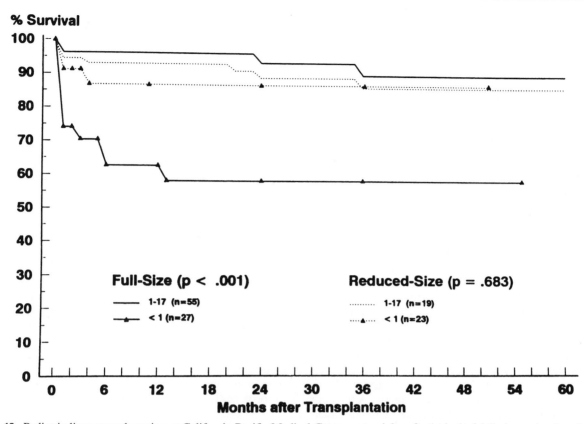

Figure 24–12. Pediatric liver transplantation at California Pacific Medical Center: actuarial graft survival of full-size and reduced-size livers in patients younger than 1 year compared with that in patients between 1 and 17 years of age. In the patients younger than 1 year, graft survival of the reduced-size livers was significantly better than that of the full-size livers ($P = 0.0268$). (From Esquivel C: Results: Survival and quality of life after orthotopic liver transplantation in children. In: Busuttil R, Klintmalm G, eds: Transplantation of the Liver. Philadelphia: WB Saunders, 1996:243.)

patients compensate with increased cardiac output and increased levels of 2,3-diphosphoglycerate, with a resultant rightward shift in the oxygen-hemoglobin dissociation curve.[96] These patients often have received recombinant erythropoietin therapy before transplantation, which may decrease their need for transfusion of PRBCs and decrease their potential for antigenic mismatches. Provided a patient is well compensated and hematocrit values are greater than 18 to 20%, preoperative PRBC transfusion is generally not indicated and may pose the risk of volume overload. However, the use of donor-specific transfusions has led to improved survival when transplanting from living-related or cadaver donors.[97, 98]

Other physiologic parameters that can be altered include coagulation, fluid and electrolyte balance, glucose tolerance, and central nervous system function. Coagulation may be impaired as a result of deficient platelet function due to the accumulation of guanidinosuccinic acid, heparin effect following hemodialysis, increased factor VIII and fibrinogen, and decreased antithrombin III levels. Fluid and electrolyte imbalances such as hypervolemia, hyperkalemia, hyponatremia, hyperphosphatemia, hypocalcemia, hypermagnesemia, and metabolic acidosis can be observed and are usually reversed with dialysis.[99, 100] Hyperparathyroidism may occur secondary to chronic hypocalcemia and may result in subsequent osteomalacia; in severe cases, pretransplant parathyroidectomy may be indicated. Glucose intolerance with insu-

lin resistance is common. Patients with end-stage renal disease often exhibit delayed gastric emptying and increased gastric residual volume with hyperacidity and should be treated as having a "full stomach." Central nervous system dysfunction may be mild to severe and includes a progressive encephalopathy secondary to uremia, peripheral neuropathy, seizures, and autonomic dysfunction. Uremic encephalopathy must be corrected in the pretransplantation period with dialysis. Pulmonary problems can include pulmonary edema secondary to volume overload or cardiomyopathy and uremic pneumonitis. Many patients are hepatitis positive; strict universal precautions should be followed in caring for these patients.

Although the native kidney is often preserved to facilitate erythropoietin and vitamin D production, pretransplant native nephrectomy may be performed for renal malignancy, severe hypertension unresponsive to antihypertensive agents, or chronic infection. This procedure is generally performed weeks or months before transplantation.

Most patients with end-stage renal failure are maintained preoperatively with peritoneal dialysis or hemodialysis. The goals of dialysis are maintenance of an euvolemic state, normal acid-base status, normal serum electrolytes, and improved growth and development. Complications of hemodialysis include hypotension secondary to blunted sympathetic responses, disequilibrium syndrome with rapid hemodialysis, and, less commonly, air embolism, nausea, aluminum intoxication, and febrile reactions caused by endotoxin-contaminated dialysate. Complications of peritoneal dialysis include peritonitis, bowel perforation, pleural effusion, atelectasis, protein loss, and hyperglycemia.

Preoperative Evaluation

Preoperative evaluation focuses on the fluid and electrolyte status of the patient and identification of coexisting disease. Patients undergoing renal transplantation can be subdivided into two categories: those receiving grafts from living-related donors and those receiving cadaver organs. Patients receiving living-related donor grafts undergo transplantation electively at a time when their hydration, electrolyte, metabolic, and nutritional status is optimized. Although patients undergoing chronic dialysis are usually stable, for patients receiving cadaver organs, optimal physiologic balance may not be achievable at the time they are notified of the availability of a suitable donor organ. With current preservation techniques, renal transplantation has become an urgent rather than an emergent procedure. Kidneys can be preserved for 48 to 72 hours in modern preservative solutions. Therefore, there is ample time for preoperative dialysis should it be indicated. A patient's dialysis history should be reviewed. The time of last dialysis should be noted, because hypovolemia immediately following dialysis and hypervolemia and hyperkalemia just before the next dialysis therapy are common. A patient's dry weight is that minimum weight achieved without vascular instability, generally achieved at the conclusion of dialysis. Comparisons of present weight with the post-dialysis dry weight help estimate a patient's current fluid volume. Serum levels of electrolytes and creatinine, blood urea nitrogen, hematocrit, platelet count, PT, PTT, and acid-base status should be obtained in the immediate preoperative period. Ideally, patients should be hemodialyzed within 24 hours before surgery to ensure normal serum electrolytes and an euvolemic state.

Patients with end-stage renal disease can be hypertensive as a direct reflection of fluid balance or secondary to hyper-reninemia. Although dialysis may ensure normotension in the majority of patients, other patients, such as those with hyper-reninemic hypertension, are controlled with antihypertensive agents. These antihypertensive agents should be continued in the preoperative period. Following bilateral nephrectomy, blood pressure is a direct reflection of plasma volume.

On physical examination, of special note is the degree of hydration. Vascular access shunts are seldom used in children, but, if they are present, these vascular access shunts need to be protected during the perioperative period, should poor graft function require postoperative hemodialysis.

Patients undergoing living-related kidney transplantation should be made NPO for 8 hours preoperatively. Patients undergoing cadaveric transplantation are made NPO as soon as they are made aware the transplant is going to occur. Premedication can be given to very anxious patients. If a patient has no vascular access, oral midazolam may be given. Although oral diazepam has been used extensively, its half-life is markedly prolonged in patients with end-stage renal disease. In many situations after vascular access has been established, small doses of midazolam, with its relatively short half-life, may be administered intravenously in the preoperative area and titrated to effect.[101] For patients who undergo surgery on a more urgent basis, such as those receiving cadaveric transplants, preoperative administration of an H_2 blocker, metoclopramide, and sodium citrate should be considered to decrease the risk of aspiration pneumonitis.

Operative Technique

The surgical procedure for kidney transplantation is performed in three stages, which include (1) exposure and preparation of the iliac vessels in larger children and adults or the aorta and inferior vena cava in small children and infants, (2) revascularization of the donor kidney, and (3) construction of the urinary drainage system. Surgical technique is governed by practical size considerations. In older children and adults, a crescent-shaped lower abdominal incision is made; with an extraperitoneal approach, a donor kidney is placed in the iliac fossa, generally on the right side. Venous anastomosis to the recipient's iliac vein is achieved in an end-to-end or end-to-side fashion. Arterial continuity is achieved by anastomosis to the iliac or hypogastric artery in the recipient. This may result in ischemia to the lower extremities for a period of time. In infants and small children (<15 kg), a midline abdominal incision is made and the kidney is placed either retroperitoneally or intra-abdominally. Venous anastomosis to the recipient's inferior vena cava is achieved in an end-to-side fashion. Arterial continuity is accomplished by anastomosis to the recipient aorta. This requires total or partial cross-clamping of the aorta and inferior vena cava for up to 60 minutes and may cause ischemia distally. Multiple or complex vascular anastomoses may be required in some instances. After completion of the vascular anastomoses, venous and arterial clamps are released, resulting in reperfusion of the grafted kidney and lower extremities. Cold hyperkalemic preservative solution and lactic acid from the lower extremities can cause hypotension and hyperkalemia with potential cardiac depression. This is more pronounced in infants and small children in whom an adult-size organ may require a large percent of the child's cardiac output for it to be adequately perfused. Urinary drainage in both infants and older children is achieved by either a direct anastomosis between the donor ureter and the recipient ureter or, more commonly, by ureteral implantation into the recipient's bladder.[102]

Anesthetic Management

As with routine anesthetics, monitors placed before induction include an ECG, precordial stethoscope, pulse oximeter, and a noninvasive blood pressure device. After induction, an esophageal temperature probe, train-of-four neuromuscular stimulator, and urinary catheter are placed. CVP may be monitored with either percutaneous insertion or, when long-term access is desirable, by surgical placement, such as with a Broviac or Hickman catheter. Invasive blood pressure monitoring is generally avoided to spare arterial vessels that may be necessary if future hemodialysis is required. Exceptions are found in infants receiving an adult kidney, as more cardiovascular instability may be anticipated because of the large volume shifts, and direct arterial measurement may be beneficial (placed in the upper extremities because the arterial anastomosis requires cross-clamping of the recipient aorta). Intraoperative laboratory parameters to be monitored include serial determinations of acid-base status (arterial or venous blood gases), serum electrolytes, and hematocrit.

The method of anesthetic induction must take into consideration the fluid balance of the patient, serum levels of electrolytes (most notably potassium), the presence of hypertension, cardiovascular status, and the risk of regurgitation and aspiration. An intravenous induction is the method of choice for the majority of patients. Thiopental is most commonly used and is tolerated well by most adults and children. Ketamine or etomidate are reasonable alternatives in the hemodynamically unstable recipient. In renal failure, the albumin concentration may be significantly reduced, thereby increasing the unbound fraction of drug that binds to albumin. This effect, however, is somewhat offset by the greater volume of distribution observed in renal failure; therefore, dosing requirements may be only modestly reduced. In patients with renal failure, alpha-1-acid glycoprotein levels increase and inhibitors may also be present, and this can also influence the protein binding characteristics of narcotics and induction agents.[103] All induction agents and narcotics should be titrated to effect, because the volume and metabolic status of this group of patients may vary markedly. The choice of muscle relaxant depends on the need to achieve rapid endotracheal intubation and the concentration of serum potassium. For patients who are believed to be at significant risk for regurgitation and whose serum potassium is in the normal range (<5 mEq/L), succinylcholine, with its rapid onset of action, remains the agent of choice. After its administration, serum potassium increases up to 0.75 to 1.0 mEq/L may be expected, although this increase may be exaggerated in patients exhibiting evidence of uremic neuropathy.[104, 105] For patients with documented or suspected hyperkalemia, a modified rapid-sequence induction with intubation doses of cis-atracurium or rocuronium avoids the potential complications associated with succinylcholine-induced hyperkalemia. Rarely, patients present for transplantation before the need for dialysis. In the pediatric patient undergoing living-related donor transplantation, assuming normal electrolyte values and adequate fasting times, inhalation induction techniques may be considered before the establishment of intravenous access. Halothane or sevoflurane may be used for mask induction of infants and small children without vascular access and is usually well-tolerated.

For maintenance of anesthesia, the use of the nondepolarizing relaxant atracurium or cis-atracurium can be used. Atracurium and cis-atracurium have the ideal pharmacokinetic properties for patients with renal failure, because elimination is through nonrenal pathways (Hoffmann degradation and ester hydrolysis). Significant hypotension may result from histamine release when using atracurium, especially when used in the higher doses (>0.5 mg/kg) necessary for endotracheal intubation.[106] Vecuronium and rocuronium also produce neuromuscular blockade of short duration without adverse cardiovascular effects, and because the primary route of excretion is in the bile, the effect of a single bolus appears unchanged in anephric patients.[107, 108] Rocuronium pharmacokinetics in patients with renal failure demonstrate decreased rates of clearance and longer mean residence times, but no significant differences in onset time or clinical

duration of action.[108] Although several studies have demonstrated a cumulative effect when repeated doses are administered, neuromuscular reversal is usually not problematic.[109] In renal failure, the action of these agents may be potentiated by acidosis, hypocalcemia, hypermagnesemia, hypothermia, and hypovolemia. The use of a neuromuscular blockade monitor is particularly helpful, because dosing requirements vary from patient to patient.

The recipient is positioned supine, often with a roll under the flank where the kidney will be placed. Caution should be taken to ensure proper positioning and padding of all extremities. Special attention should be directed to extremities where a hemodialysis access shunt may be present, and continuous monitoring of patency by palpation or Doppler is necessary throughout the procedure.

Maintenance of anesthesia generally includes a mixture of air and oxygen or nitrous oxide and oxygen, a potent inhalation agent, a nondepolarizing muscle relaxant, and an intravenous narcotic. All potent inhalation agents must be carefully titrated in this patient population; halothane has the most potent calcium channel blocking properties and may cause severe myocardial depression in hypocalcemic patients; isoflurane may be a reasonable choice for most patients but is more likely to provoke airway irritation; sevoflurane may be the most desirable agent because its hemodynamic profile is like that of isoflurane but it is not irritating to the airways. The anesthesiologist must balance the risks and benefits of each potent inhalation agent according to the needs of each individual patient.

The narcotic of choice is usually fentanyl. Fentanyl has no active metabolites that contribute significant opioid action, but is significantly protein-bound (84%). Initial doses of 5 to 10 μg/kg followed by 1 to 2 μg/kg/hr may be used. Morphine is metabolized in the liver to morphine-3-glucuronide and morphine-6-glucuronide. The morphine-6 metabolite is metabolically active and the metabolites are excreted by the kidney. Morphine metabolites accumulate in renal failure and can exert a significant respiratory depressant effect. Morphine is less protein-bound than the other opioid drugs (30%), and is bound mainly to albumin. Morphine should be used cautiously in the setting of renal failure. Meperidine has active metabolites (normeperidine, meperidinic acid, and normeperidinic acid) that can accumulate in the setting of renal failure. Normeperidine has some narcotic properties and can produce seizures. Meperidine is protein-bound mainly to alpha-1-acid glycoproteins rather than albumin. Cumulative doses of meperidine should be avoided in renal failure patients because they can produce overdosage, seizures, and toxicity. In some centers, if the patient is free of a coagulopathy, the placement of an epidural catheter allows a combined regional/general anesthesia technique, thereby reducing intraoperative anesthetic requirements and providing a means for postoperative pain management.

Ventilation is controlled and patients maintained in the normocarbic range. Although hypoventilation resulting in increasing acidosis may increase extracellular potassium, hyperventilation is also detrimental because the leftward shift in the oxygen-hemoglobin dissociation curve results in decreased oxygen availability in patients with decreased reserve secondary to anemia.

Monitoring fluid status in anephric patients is challenging because the fluid balance of individual patients varies greatly. Fluid management during renal transplantation must consider preoperative fluid status (most often a reflection of the dialysis schedule), basal fluid requirements, intraoperative losses, and fluid shifts associated with perfusion of the new graft or translocation into "third-space" compartments. Preoperative fluid status is estimated by review of current weight in relation to dry weight and blood pressure response with administration of anesthetic medications. Serial measurement of CVP, systemic blood pressure, and acid-base balance is paramount in fluid management. These patients often are hypertensive despite a low intravascular volume, that is, hyper-reninemia. Others may exhibit volume-dependent hypertension. In addition, uremic patients may demonstrate autonomic dysfunction with heart rate changes independent of changes in circulating blood volume.

In an effort to avoid unnecessary administration of potassium, the use of potassium-containing solutions such as lactated Ringer solution is avoided; 5% dextrose with 0.45% sodium chloride is commonly administered to replace hourly deficits, but normal saline should be used to replace third-space and blood loss. Patients with no urine output require approximately 400 to 500 mL/m²/day. It is generally accepted that maximal recipient hydration achieved before unclamping during the transplant procedure (CVP of 12 to 18 mm Hg) aids in decreasing the risk of acute tubular necrosis in the postoperative period.[110] This is achieved with a liberal use of warm crystalloid or colloid infusion. Intraoperative blood loss is generally not excessive and, when necessary, responds to the administration of 5% albumin or PRBCs. A progressive decrease in hematocrit secondary to both blood loss and hemodilution with volume expansion and increasing acidosis determines the need for increasing oxygen-carrying capacity with the transfusion of PRBCs. If transfusion is indicated, washed PRBCs should be used to minimize fluid volume and potassium administered. In addition, as with any immunosuppressed patient, all blood products should be irradiated to eliminate the risk of graft-versus-host disease and white blood cell filters used to remove CMV if the recipient is seronegative.[111–113]

Before revascularization of the donor kidney, consideration must be given to each institution's individual protocols for the administration of specific medications. These drugs should be readily available for administration with the dosage calculated in advance. Although protocols vary between centers, most include furosemide, mannitol, and methylprednisolone sodium succinate. Immunosuppressive therapy with azathioprine or cyclosporine or both is administered.

When the vascular clamps are released, various hemodynamic changes may be encountered. Although hypertension may occur as a result of the release of renin from the ischemic donor kidney, hypotension is much more common. This hypotension may be due to a combination of factors, including reduced circulating blood volume secondary to the volume required to perfuse the newly transplanted kidney (especially an adult's kidney transplanted into an infant), blood loss from anastomotic leaks, or a sudden decrease in peripheral vascular resistance due to stagnant blood and preservative solution entering the circulation when the inferior vena cava cross-clamp is released. Blood volume and blood pressure must be maintained during this critical period. In an infant receiving an adult's organ, 25 to 40% of the patient's blood volume may be sequestered in the new organ,

often necessitating rapid volume infusion. Additionally, the normal blood pressure in an infant may be significantly less than the pressure that the transplanted adult's organ is normally accustomed to; therefore, it may be desirable to achieve a mean arterial pressure closer to adult values in these recipients. These patients generally require red cell transfusion. Other, more remote, causes of inadequate perfusion include vascular steal phenomena secondary to vascular dialysis shunts close to the transplanted kidney, as well as anastomotic complications. With adequate perfusion, a new kidney takes on its characteristic firm, red appearance and begins to function immediately, with the formation of urine. After reperfusion, renal function follows one of several courses. With living-related transplantation, a brisk diuresis often ensues, necessitating continued generous replacement of fluids and electrolytes. Other patterns observed resemble early acute tubular necrosis, in which waste products accumulate despite what appears to be adequate urine output. After periods of prolonged preservation and ischemia, an oliguric or anuric pattern may be observed. In this last pattern, temporary hemodialysis may be required until renal function recovers.

On completion of the procedure, neuromuscular blockade is reversed. Standard doses of reversal agents are administered because their clearance is prolonged to a similar degree to that of the nondepolarizing muscle relaxants. Once adequate neuromuscular reversal and ventilation have been confirmed, the trachea may be extubated in the operating room. Exceptions are small infants with adult donor kidneys, whose ventilation may be compromised as a result of the increase in intra-abdominal pressure due to the large kidney; these patients often require assisted ventilation for 24 to 36 hours postoperatively.

Postoperative Management

All patients are observed postoperatively in an intensive care unit or a specific organ transplantation unit. Fluid balance and electrolyte levels are monitored closely. Therapy is guided by measurement of urine output, serum and urine electrolytes, and arterial and CVP measurements. Fluid replacement is most often accomplished by administration of 2.5% dextrose with 0.45% sodium chloride, and continued electrolyte replacement is dictated by serial measurement of blood and urine values. Renal perfusion and function are initially assessed with baseline radionuclide scans. Suitable analgesia is usually achieved with intravenous administration of narcotics, although epidural analgesia has been utilized. Early postoperative complications include pulmonary insufficiency, severe fluid or electrolyte imbalance, infection, and kidney rejection.

Bone Marrow Transplantation

Bone marrow transplantation is an accepted form of therapy for patients with a wide range of nonmalignant and malignant disorders (Table 24–8).[114] The application of bone marrow transplantation therapy is currently limited by the number of suitable donors. As the donor pool increases with the use of national marrow registries, so will the number of bone marrow transplants. In cases of nonmalignant disease

Table 24–8. Indications for Bone Marrow Transplantation

Nonmalignant disorders
    Aplastic anemia
    Congenital immunodeficiency syndromes
    Thalassemia
    Lysosomal storage diseases (e.g., Hurler syndrome)
    Sickle cell anemia
Malignant disorders
    Leukemias (acute lymphocytic, acute myelogenous, chronic myelogenous)
    Refractory lymphomas (Hodgkin, non-Hodgkin)
    Solid tumors (stage IV neuroblastoma)

such as Hurler syndrome, aplastic anemias, hemoglobinopathies, and severe immunodeficiencies, bone marrow transplantation is pursued in the hope that new bone marrow stem cells will replace the dysfunctional marrow cells with normal marrow stem cells. This may allow the bone marrow to produce deficient enzymes or normal cellular elements such as erythrocytes, platelets, leukocytes, lymphocytes, macrophages, and monocytes. Eventually even the hepatic Kupffer cells, pulmonary alveolar macrophages, osteoclasts, and neural glial cells can be shown to be of donor origin. The most widespread application for bone marrow transplantation in the pediatric population is for treatment of malignant disease, including the leukemias. In children with acute lymphocytic leukemia, chemotherapy alone may induce remission and prolong survival. Acute myelogenous and chronic myelogenous leukemia carry a poor prognosis with bone marrow transplantation as the only curative option. Refractory lymphomas and some solid tumors may also benefit from bone marrow transplantation. For malignant diseases, bone marrow transplantation is performed to replace deficient or defective myeloid or lymphoid stem cells and enzymes with those from normal donor marrow. High-dose chemotherapy and radiotherapy used in the treatment of malignant disease produces lethal myelosuppressive effects from which bone marrow transplantation serves as a "rescue." Documentation of the disease status is important in the treatment of malignant disease because the incidence of relapse is higher if patients are transplanted during a disease relapse. Additional benefit may be achieved by the so-called graft-versus-leukemia effect, in which the donor graft has an immunologic response against recipient leukemia cells that were not eradicated by the intense chemoradiotherapy.[115]

Bone marrow transplants may be classified into three types, which are determined by the donor-recipient relationship (Table 24–9). An *allogeneic* transplant occurs between two genetically different individuals of the same species. Donor and recipient are identified according to their major human leukocyte antigens. They may be related (parents, siblings) or unrelated. A related, perfect match is termed a *genetic match*. Mismatched transplants demonstrate an increased incidence of graft-versus-host disease. In a *syngeneic* transplant, an identical twin serves as the donor. For an *autologous* transplant, a patient donates his or her own marrow to be later reinfused for rescue.

Recipient Preparation

Recipient preparation varies depending on whether the patient is being transplanted for malignant or nonmalignant disease. Patients undergoing bone marrow transplantation are generally admitted to the hospital in advance of the actual transplantation. Central venous access lines are inserted to facilitate transfusion and blood sampling during the transplantation and engraftment period. Before the actual harvest and transplant procedure, various preparative conditioning regimens are followed. The function of these regimens is to empty out recipient marrow, thereby creating space for transplanted stem cell engraftment; to provide immunosuppression, to prevent rejection with allogeneic transplants; and to eradicate residual tumor cells in the recipient. The regimens may involve total body irradiation or administration of alkylating agents, such as cyclophosphamide (Cytoxan). Total body irradiation is a potent antitumor method utilized commonly in many bone marrow transplant protocols. Total body irradiation may be delivered as a single dose or in fractional doses given up to twice daily for 4 to 5 days. The use of fractional total body irradiation allows for a higher total amount of radiation to be used with less toxicity to the eyes (cataracts), lungs (interstitial pneumonitis), and gastrointestinal tract (mucositis). For pediatric patients who may be unable to cooperate, brief general anesthesia is often required to render them motionless while being irradiated. Radiotherapy sessions can be facilitated with the intravenous administration of methohexital, ketamine, or propofol. Because the anesthesiologist cannot be present during these sessions owing to the significant radiation exposure, patients are monitored by video camera in addition to ECG, automated blood pressure measurement, capnography, and pulse oximetry. These sessions can last from 2 to 20 minutes and may be scheduled as a twice-a-day regimen. Patients are maintained NPO for solids but are allowed to have clear liquids up until 2 hours before the scheduled radiotherapy session. Nausea and vomiting are treated with intravenous fluid hydration and ondansetron as needed.

Transplant Procedure

The actual harvest procedure takes place in the operating room with the patient under general or regional anesthesia. A healthy allogeneic donor has often predonated blood before the harvest procedure with the intent of autologous transfusion during the marrow aspiration procedure.[116] Autologous donors are not usually able to predonate blood for transfusion. The allogeneic donors are usually admitted the morning of surgery and are discharged the following day. Marrow is aspirated by multiple punctures of the posterior iliac spine and iliac crest. Because only small amounts are

Table 24–9. Classification of Bone Marrow Transplants

Category	Definition
Autologous	Patient predonates own bone marrow for reinfusion, following chemotherapy/radiotherapy for malignant disease
Syngeneic	Transplantation between identical twins
Allogeneic	Donor and recipient are of different genetic origin but are identified with histocompatibility testing

obtained with any single puncture, numerous aspirations are performed. It is occasionally necessary to use the anterior iliac crest and, rarely, the sternum. The amount of marrow required is variable and depends on the weight of the bone marrow transplant recipient. Approximately 10 mL of marrow per kilogram body weight should be obtained for the recipient. This large number of cells is necessary because no currently available method is able to select only the pluripotential stem cells necessary. The marrow is then placed into a beaker containing heparin without preservatives.

The type of post-harvest processing depends largely on the type of transplant to be performed. With syngeneic donation, the marrow is merely filtered to remove potential emboli before infusion. In allogeneic transfusions, donor marrow may undergo T-cell depletion techniques to reduce the risk of graft-versus-host disease, mediated by immunocompetent T-cell lymphocytes. With autologous transplants, depending on the nature of the disease, the marrow is treated with monoclonal antibody and complement to eradicate remaining malignant cells, then cryopreserved for later infusion. The actual marrow transplantation involves simple intravenous infusion of marrow cells into the recipient.[115]

Anesthetic Management

When considering anesthesia for marrow transplantation, patients fall into two categories: autologous donors and allogeneic donors. With the exception of an autologous transplantation, marrow donors are generally in good health. Although the risks of the procedure may be minimal, a thorough history and physical examination must be reviewed in light of the fact that the procedure is of no direct benefit to the allogeneic donor. Preoperative assessment includes determination of hematocrit and possibly obtaining a coagulation profile, should a regional anesthetic be preferred. Preoperative autologous donation eliminates the risk of homologous transfusion, should a transfusion be necessary for the donor. This technique, however, has limited application in very young donors.

The presentation of autologous donors may be varied. Previous surgical interventions must be carefully reviewed in addition to any chemotherapy or radiotherapy that was previously administered. The anesthetic implications of cancer chemotherapy have been extensively reviewed.[117, 118] Prior anthracycline therapy (Adriamycin, daunomycin, and doxorubicin) can result in cardiac toxicity and recent preoperative echocardiography and electrocardiogram will reveal decreases in ejection fraction, shortening fraction, heart block, or arrhythmias. Any history of heart failure puts the patient at risk for occurrence of sudden and unpredictable cardiac decompensation during general anesthesia. The effects of chemotherapy on the pulmonary system are potentiated by total body irradiation and can result in radiation pneumonitis. A preoperative chest radiograph should be obtained to evaluate the possibility of pulmonary metastases. Patients who have received preoperative chemotherapy known to be toxic to the pulmonary system (such as bleomycin, busulfan, carmustine, and methotrexate) should be evaluated extensively, particularly if they have underlying lung disease. Renal dysfunction secondary to chemotherapy agents is common. Drugs such as cisplatin and amphotericin

B (particularly when given together) are common offending agents. Kidney function must be evaluated prior to autologous marrow retrieval by examining serum electrolytes, blood urea nitrogen, creatinine, and creatinine clearance. Patients for autologous donation are usually severely immunocompromised secondary to cancer chemotherapy agents and radiation therapy. Extraordinary care must therefore be taken in maintaining strict aseptic technique with all invasive procedures, including vascular access and airway management. Prudence requires proper skin preparation before intravenous catheter placement, the use of sterilized airway equipment, and the use of bacterial filters on the breathing circuit.

Diagnostic bone marrow aspiration may be performed under local anesthesia with sedation, but bone marrow donation requires multiple aspirations (up to 100 punctures), may take 2 to 3 hours, and causes patients various degrees of discomfort. For these reasons, most of these procedures are performed under general anesthesia or, on occasion, with regional anesthesia.

Induction of anesthesia is determined by physical status and the patient's ability to cooperate. Various methods have been used with equal success. Noninvasive monitors include an ECG, automated blood pressure measurement, pulse oximeter, capnograph, temperature probe, and precordial or esophageal stethoscope. *Rectal temperature instrumentation and rectal induction techniques are avoided in immunocompromised patients (i.e., autologous donors) because of the risk of infection.* Adequate intravenous access is established for administering blood products. The decision about whether to place a urinary catheter is determined by the anticipated volume of marrow aspirated (related to donor blood volume), anticipated fluid shifts, and duration of the procedure. The patient's trachea is intubated, and the patient is placed in the prone position for aspiration of the posterior iliac crest. Anesthetic maintenance consists of a volatile inhalation agent or a "balanced" anesthetic technique with nitrous oxide and opioids.

For selected patients, regional anesthesia should be considered. Autologous donors by definition have undergone various regimens for eradication of disease and marrow preparation. Although it may be prudent to perform coagulation studies on all patients undergoing regional anesthetic techniques, these patients in particular often have various degrees of hepatic involvement. Therefore, a preoperative coagulation profile (PT, PTT, platelet count, and bleeding time) should be obtained. For older allogeneic donors, the use of spinal or epidural anesthesia should be considered. The use of a caudal regional technique (with or without narcotic) in combination with general anesthesia can provide postoperative pain control in the younger bone marrow donors.

Fluid management in these patients requires communication with the hematologist, accurate measurement of volumes aspirated, and ongoing physiologic assessment. Because fluid replacement may be significant, all fluids administered should be prewarmed. Many allogenic patients predonate because transfusion is often necessary. If transfusion is necessary in immunocompromised patients and autologous blood is unavailable, blood should be irradiated because of the concern for the development of graft-versus-host disease. In addition, if blood donors are CMV positive, a white blood

Table 24–10. Risk Factors for Graft Rejection

Sensitization from previous transfusion
HLA mismatch
Abnormal microenvironment, e.g., marrow fibrosis
Use of T-cell depletion techniques

cell filter should be used, because CMV is carried within leukocytes.

Post-Transplant Management

Intensive supportive care is required during the engraftment period. As mentioned, all recipients undergo measures to ensure functional marrow ablation before transplantation. As a result, these patients are severely immunocompromised. Protective isolation and aseptic technique are therefore required both before and after transplantation, and broad-spectrum antibiotics are often administered. Engraftment generally occurs 14 to 21 days after infusion, with the granulocytic response occurring predictably in 14 to 21 days and the red blood cell and platelet response occurring much later (up to 3 to 5 weeks after transplantation). During this time, frequent red blood cell and platelet transfusions are necessary. Serial measurements of peripheral blood counts and bone marrow sampling ultimately confirm engraftment.

Engraftment rates range from 90 to 98%; however, there are several risk factors for graft rejection (Table 24–10). Additional post-transplantation problems include graft-versus-host disease, delayed immune reconstitution, relapse of malignancy, and late effects such as delayed growth and development. Graft-versus-host disease, mediated by immunocompetent T lymphocytes in the donor marrow, occurs in 30 to 40% of bone marrow transplant recipients and can be fatal in one third of patients afflicted. It occurs on infusion, when an immunologic response develops, involving not only cytotoxic injury but also the release of other lymphokines, such as interleukin-2 and tumor necrosis factor. Graft-versus-host disease may occur in acute or chronic forms. Prophylaxis includes a short course of immunosuppression with methotrexate, cyclosporine A, and prednisone, often in combination. Risk factors for graft-versus-host disease include HLA disparity, increased age, and sex mismatch (female donor into male recipient). Also, sensitization from a previous pregnancy and an antibody response to the Y antigen have been theorized as possible causes. In marrow transplant recipients at greater risks, in vitro T-cell depletion has been effective in reducing the incidence and severity of graft-versus-host disease.[115]

Since the majority of these patients develop stomatitis or mucositis, post-transplantation management usually includes patient-controlled analgesia.

REFERENCES

1. Kantrowitz A: Frontiers in heart surgery. R I Med 1967;50:470–479.
2. Anderson TM: Indications and candidacy for heart transplantation in children. In: Dunn JF, Donner RM, eds: Heart Transplantation in Children. Mount Kisco, NY: Futura; 1990:7–15.
3. Carrel T, Neth J, Pasic M, et al: Should cardiac transplantation for congenital heart disease be delayed until adult age? Eur J Cardiothorac Surg 1994;8:462–468.
4. McGowan FX Jr, Bailey PL: Heart, lung, and heart-lung transplantation. In: Cook DR, Davis PJ, eds: Anesthetic Principles for Organ Transplantation. New York: Raven Press; 1994:87.
5. Doroshow RW, Ashwal S, Saukel GW: Availability and selection of donors for pediatric heart transplantation. J Heart Lung Transplant 1995;14:52–58.
6. Kawauchi M, Gundry SR, de Begona JA, et al: Prolonged preservation of human pediatric hearts for transplantation: correlation of ischemic time and subsequent function. J Heart Lung Transplant 1993;12:55–58.
7. Tamisier D, Vouhe P, Le Bidois J, et al: Donor-recipient size matching in pediatric heart transplantation: A word of caution about small grafts. J Heart Lung Transplant 1996;15:190–195.
8. Eke CC, Gundry SR, Baum MF, et al: Neurologic sequelae of deep hypothermic circulatory arrest in cardiac transplant infants. Ann Thorac Surg 1996;61:783–788.
9. Clark NJ, Martin RD: Anesthetic considerations for patients undergoing cardiac transplantation. J Cardiovasc Anesth 1988;2:519–542.
10. Lowe DA: Anesthetic considerations in pediatric cardiac transplantation. In: Dunn JF, Donner RM, eds: Heart Transplantation in Children. Mount Kisco, NY: Futura; 1990:39–69.
11. Triantafillou AN, Heerdt PM: Lung transplantation. Int Anesthesiol Clin 1991;29:87–109.
12. Hickey PR, Hansen DD: Fentanyl- and sufentanil-oxygen-pancuronium anesthesia for cardiac surgery in infants. Anesth Analg 1984;63:117–124.
13. Demas K, Wyner J, Mihm FG, et al: Anaesthesia for heart transplantation: A retrospective study and review. Br J Anaesth 1986;58:1357–1364.
14. Hickey PR, Hansen DD, Strafford M, et al: Pulmonary and systemic hemodynamic effects of nitrous oxide in infants with normal and elevated pulmonary vascular resistance. Anesthesiology 1986;65:374–378.
15. Di Carli MF, Tobes MC, Mangner T, et al: Effects of cardiac sympathetic innervation on coronary blood flow. N Engl J Med 1997;336:1208–1215.
16. Chinnock RE, Baum MF, Larsen R, et al: Rejection management and long-term surveillance of the pediatric heart transplant recipient: The Loma Linda experience. J Heart Lung Transplant 1993;12:S255–S264.
17. Shaddy RE, Naftel DC, Kirklin JK, et al: Outcome of cardiac transplantation in children: Survival in a contemporary multi-institutional experience. Pediatric Heart Transplant Study. Circulation 1996;94(Suppl):II69–II73.
18. Slaughter MS, Braunlin E, Bolman RM 3d, et al: Pediatric heart transplantation: Results of 2- and 5-year follow-up. J Heart Lung Transplant 1994;13:624–630.
19. Spray TL: Projections for pediatric heart-lung and lung transplantation. J Heart Lung Transplant 1993;12:S337–S343.
20. Metras D, Kreitmann B, Riberi A, et al: Bilateral single-lung transplantation in children. Ann Thorac Surg 1995;60(Suppl):S578–S581.
21. Hurford WE, Kolker AC, Strauss HW: The use of ventilation/perfusion lung scans to predict oxygenation during one-lung anesthesia. Anesthesiology 1987;67:841–844.
22. Lillehei CW, Shamberger RC, Mayer JE Jr, et al: Size disparity in pediatric lung transplantation. J Pediatr Surg 1994;29:1152–1155.
23. Pasque MK, Cooper JD, Kaiser LR, et al: Improved technique for bilateral lung transplantation: Rationale and initial clinical experience. Ann Thorac Surg 1990;49:785–791.
24. Conacher ID, McNally B, Choudhry AK, et al: Anaesthesia for isolated lung transplantation. Br J Anaesth 1988;60:588–591.
25. Conacher ID: Isolated lung transplantation: A review of problems and guide to anaesthesia. Br J Anaesth 1988;61:468–474.
26. Gayes JM, Giron L, Nissen MD, et al: Anesthetic considerations for patients undergoing double-lung transplantation. J Cardiothorac Anesth 1990;4:486–498.
27. Hickey PR, Hansen DD, Cramolini GM, et al: Pulmonary and systemic hemodynamic responses to ketamine in infants with normal and elevated pulmonary vascular resistance. Anesthesiology 1985;62:287–293.
28. Benumof JL, Partridge BL, Salvatierra C, et al: Margin of safety in positioning modern double-lumen endotracheal tubes. Anesthesiology 1987;67:729–738.
29. Jaquiss RD, Huddleston CB, Spray TL: Use of aprotinin in pediatric lung transplantation. J Heart Lung Transplant 1995;14:302–307.
30. Kurland G, Orenstein DM: Complications of pediatric lung and heart-lung transplantation. Curr Opin Pediatr 1994;6:262–271.

31. Lebrec D, Capron JP, Dhumeaux D, et al: Pulmonary hypertension complicating portal hypertension. Am Rev Respir Dis 1979;120:849–856.

32. Cheng EY, Woehlck HJ: Pulmonary artery hypertension complicating anesthesia for liver transplantation. Anesthesiology 1992;77:389–392.

33. Prager MC, Cauldwell CA, Ascher NL, et al: Pulmonary hypertension associated with liver disease is not reversible after liver transplantation. Anesthesiology 1992;77:375–378.

34. Matuschak GM, Rinaldo JE: Organ interactions in the adult respiratory distress syndrome during sepsis: role of the liver in host defense. Chest 1988;94:400–406.

35. Matuschak GM, Rinaldo JE, Pinsky MR, et al: Effects of end-stage liver failure on the incidence and resolution of the adult respiratory distress syndrome. J Crit Care 1987;2:162–173.

36. Matuschak GM, Shaw BW Jr: Adult respiratory distress syndrome associated with acute liver allograft rejection: Resolution following hepatic retransplantation. Crit Care Med 1987;15:878–881.

37. Pinsky MR: Multiple systems organ failure: malignant intravascular inflammation. Crit Care Clin 1989;5:195–198.

38. Montgomery AB, Stager MA, Carrico CJ, et al: Causes of mortality in patients with the adult respiratory distress syndrome. Am Rev Respir Dis 1985;132:485–489.

39. Ali M, Wall WJ: Resolution of the adult respiratory distress syndrome following colectomy and liver transplantation. Chest 1990;98:1032–1034.

40. Ellis D, Avner ED, Starzl TE: Renal failure in children with hepatic failure undergoing liver transplantation. J Pediatr 1986;108:393–398.

41. Munoz SJ, Ballas SK, Moritz MJ, et al: Perioperative management of fulminant and subfulminant hepatic failure with therapeutic plasmapheresis. Transplant Proc 1989;21:3535–3536.

42. Tzakis A, Todo S, Starzl TE: Orthotopic liver transplantation with preservation of the inferior vena cava. Ann Surg 1989;210:649–652.

43. Tzakis AG, Reyes J, Nour B, et al: Temporary end to side portacaval shunt in orthotopic hepatic transplantation in humans. Surg Gynecol Obstet 1993;176:180–182.

44. Bismuth H, Houssin D: Reduced-sized orthotopic liver graft in hepatic transplantation in children. Surgery 1984;95:367–370.

45. Broelsch CE, Emond JC, Whitington PF, et al: Application of reduced-size liver transplants as split grafts, auxiliary orthotopic grafts, and living related segmental transplants. Ann Surg 1990;212:368–375.

46. Broelsch CE, Whitington PF, Emond JC, et al: Liver transplantation in children from living related donors: Surgical techniques and results. Ann Surg 1991;214:428–437.

47. Emond JC, Whitington PF, Thistlethwaite JR, et al: Transplantation of two patients with one liver: Analysis of a preliminary experience with 'split-liver' grafting. Ann Surg 1990;212:14–22.

48. Esquivel CO, Nakazato P, Cox K, et al: The impact of liver reductions in pediatric liver transplantation. Arch Surg 1991;126:1278–1285.

49. Heffron TG, Emond JC, Whitington PF, et al: Biliary complications in pediatric liver transplantation: A comparison of reduced-size and whole grafts. Transplantation 1992;53:391–395.

50. Otte JB, de Ville de Goyet J, Alberti D, et al: The concept and technique of the split liver in clinical transplantation. Surgery 1990;107:605–612.

51. Ryckman FC, Flake AW, Fisher RA, et al: Segmental orthotopic hepatic transplantation as a means to improve patient survival and diminish waiting-list mortality. J Pediatr Surg 1991;26:422–427.

52. Stevens LH, Emond JC, Piper JB, et al: Hepatic artery thrombosis in infants. A comparison of whole livers, reduced-size grafts, and grafts from living-related donors. Transplantation 1992;53:396–399.

53. Tan KC, Yandza T, de Hemptinne B, et al: Hepatic artery thrombosis in pediatric liver transplantation. J Pediatr Surg 1988;23:927–930.

54. Thistlethwaite JR Jr, Emond JC, Heffron TG, et al: Innovative use of organs for liver transplantation. Transplant Proc 1991;23:2147–2151.

55. Otte JB, de Ville de Goyet J, Sokal E, et al: Size reduction of the donor liver is a safe way to alleviate the shortage of size-matched organs in pediatric liver transplantation. Ann Surg 1990;211:146–157.

56. Strong RW, Lynch SV: Ethical issues in living related donor liver transplantation. Transplant Proc 1996;28:2366–2369.

57. Strong RW, Lynch SV, Ong TH, et al: Successful liver transplantation from a living donor to her son. N Engl J Med 1990;322:1505–1507.

58. Emond JC, Rosenthal P, Roberts JP, et al: Living related donor liver transplantation: The UCSF experience. Transplant Proc 1996;28:2375–2377.

59. Heffron TG, Langnas AN, Fox IJ, et al: Living related donor liver transplantation at the University of Nebraska Medical Center (1996). Transplant Proc 1996;28:2382.

60. Kitai T, Higashiyama H, Takada Y, et al: Pulmonary embolism in a donor of living-related liver transplantation: estimation of donor's operative risk. Surgery 1996;120:570–573.

61. Otte JB, de Ville de Goyet J, Reding R, et al: Living related donor liver transplantation in children: The Brussels experience. Transplant Proc 1996;28:2378–2379.

62. Kang YG, Martin DJ, Marquez J, et al: Intraoperative changes in blood coagulation and thrombelastographic monitoring in liver transplantation. Anesth Analg 1985;64:888–896.

63. Kang YG, Freeman JA, Aggarwal S, et al: Hemodynamic instability during liver transplantation. Transplant Proc 1989;21:3489–3492.

64. Borland LM, Roule M, Cook DR: Anesthesia for pediatric orthotopic liver transplantation. Anesth Analg 1985;64:117–124.

65. Carmichael FJ, Lindop MJ, Farman JV: Anesthesia for hepatic transplantation: Cardiovascular and metabolic alterations and their management. Anesth Analg 1985;64:108–116.

66. Davis PJ, Cook DR: Anesthetic problems in pediatric liver transplantation. Transplant Proc 1989;21:3493–3496.

67. Estrin JA, Belani KG, Ascher NL, et al: Hemodynamic changes on clamping and unclamping of major vessels during liver transplantation. Transplant Proc 1989;21:3500–3505.

68. Kalpokas M, Bookallil M, Sheil AG, et al: Physiological changes during liver transplantation. Anaesth Intensive Care 1989;17:24–30.

69. Lichtor JL, Emond J, Chung MR, et al: Pediatric orthotopic liver transplantation: Multifactorial predictions of blood loss. Anesthesiology 1988;68:607–611.

70. Griffith BP, Shaw BW Jr, Hardesty RL, et al: Veno-venous bypass without systemic anticoagulation for transplantation of the human liver. Surg Gynecol Obstet 1985;160:270–272.

71. Aggarwal S, Kang Y, Freeman JA, et al: Postreperfusion syndrome: cardiovascular collapse following hepatic reperfusion during liver transplantation. Transplant Proc 1987;19(Suppl 3):54–55.

72. Mallett SV, Kang Y, Freeman JA, et al: Prognostic significance of reperfusion hyperglycemia during liver transplantation. Anesth Analg 1989;68:182–185.

73. Martin TJ, Kang Y, Robertson KM, et al: Ionization and hemodynamic effects of calcium chloride and calcium gluconate in the absence of hepatic function. Anesthesiology 1990;73:62–65.

74. Lewis JH, Bontempo FA, Awad SA, et al: Liver transplantation: intraoperative changes in coagulation factors in 100 first transplants. Hepatology 1989;9:710–714.

75. Kang Y, Borland LM, Picone J, et al: Intraoperative coagulation changes in children undergoing liver transplantation. Anesthesiology 1989;71:44–47.

76. Martinez J, Palascak JE, Kwasniak D: Abnormal sialic acid content of the dysfibrinogenemia associated with liver disease. J Clin Invest 1978;61:535–538.

77. Polson RJ, Park GR, Lindop MJ, et al: The prevention of renal impairment in patients undergoing orthotopic liver grafting by infusion of low dose dopamine. Anaesthesia 1987;42:15–19.

78. Swygert TH, Roberts LC, Valek TR, et al: Effect of intraoperative low-dose dopamine on renal function in liver transplant recipients. Anesthesiology 1991;75:571–576.

79. Miller RD: Complications of massive blood transfusions. Anesthesiology 1973;39:82–93.

80. Collins JA: Problems associated with the massive transfusion of stored blood. Surgery 1974;75:274–295.

81. Benson RE, Isbister JP: Massive blood transfusion. Anaesth Intensive Care 1980;8:152–157.

82. Zauder HL: Massive transfusion. Int Anesthesiol Clin 1982;20:157–170.

83. Coté CJ: Blood, colloid, and crystalloid therapy. Anesth Clin North Am 1991;9:865–884.

84. Coté CJ: Depth of halothane anesthesia potentiates citrate-induced ionized hypocalcemia and adverse cardiovascular events in dogs. Anesthesiology 1987;67:676–680.

85. Coté CJ, Drop LJ, Daniels AL, et al: Calcium chloride versus calcium gluconate: Comparison of ionization and cardiovascular effects in children and dogs. Anesthesiology 1987;66:465–470.

86. Coté CJ, Drop LJ, Hoaglin DC, et al: Ionized hypocalcemia after fresh frozen plasma administration to thermally injured children: Effects of infusion rate, duration, and treatment with calcium chloride. Anesth Analg 1988;67:152–160.

87. Coté CJ, Liu LM, Szyfelbein SK, et al: Changes in serial platelet counts following massive blood transfusion in pediatric patients. Anesthesiology 1985;62:197–201.

88. Iwatsuki S, Starzl TE, Todo S, et al: Experience in 1,000 liver transplants under cyclosporine-steroid therapy: A survival report. Transplant Proc 1988;20(Suppl 1):498–504.

89. Malatack JJ, Schaid DJ, Urbach AH, et al: Choosing a pediatric recipient for orthotopic liver transplantation. J Pediatr 1987;111:479–489.

90. Fine RN, Salusky IB, Ettenger RB: The therapeutic approach to the infant, child, and adolescent with end-stage renal disease. Pediatr Clin North Am 1987;34:789–801.

91. Lum CT, Wassner SJ, Martin DE: Current thinking in transplantation in infants and children. Pediatr Clin North Am 1985;32:1203–1232.

92. Najarian JS, So SK, Simmons RL, et al: The outcome of 304 primary renal transplants in children (1968–1985). Ann Surg 1986;204:246–258.

93. Sheldon CA, Geary DF, Shely EA, et al: Surgical considerations in childhood end-stage renal disease. Pediatr Clin North Am 1987;34:1187–1207.

94. McGraw ME, Haka-Ikse K: Neurologic-developmental sequelae of chronic renal failure in infancy. J Pediatr 1985;106:579–583.

95. Santos F, Friedman BI, Chan JC: Management of chronic renal failure in children. Curr Probl Pediatr 1986;16:237–301.

96. Dodds A, Nicholls M: Haematological aspects of renal disease. Anaesth Intensive Care 1983;11:361–368.

97. Opelz G, Terasaki PI: Dominant effect of transfusions on kidney graft survival. Transplantation 1980;29:153–158.

98. Salvatierra O Jr, Vincenti F, Amend WJ Jr, et al: The role of blood transfusions in renal transplantation. Urol Clin North Am 1983;10:243–252.

99. Di Minno G, Martinez J, McKean ML, et al: Platelet dysfunction in uremia: Multifaceted defect partially corrected by dialysis. Am J Med 1985;79:552–559.

100. Kasiske BL, Kjellstrand CM: Perioperative management of patients with chronic renal failure and postoperative acute renal failure. Urol Clin North Am 1983;10:35–50.

101. Vinik HR, Reves JG, Greenblatt DJ, et al: The pharmacokinetics of midazolam in chronic renal failure patients. Anesthesiology 1983;59:390–394.

102. Miller LC, Lum CT, Bock GH, et al: Transplantation of the adult kidney into the very small child: Technical considerations. Am J Surg 1983;145:243–247.

103. Davis PJ, Stiller RL, McGowan FX, et al: Decreased protein binding of alfentanil in plasma from children with kidney or liver failure. Paediatr Anaesth 1993;3:19–22.

104. Powell DR, Miller R: The effect of repeated doses of succinylcholine on serum potassium in patients with renal failure. Anesth Analg 1975;54:746–748.

105. Walton JD, Farman JV: Suxamethonium hyperkalaemia in uraemic neuropathy. Anaesthesia 1973;28:666–668.

106. Fahey MR, Rupp SM, Fisher DM, et al: The pharmacokinetics and pharmacodynamics of atracurium in patients with and without renal failure. Anesthesiology 1984;61:699–702.

107. Fahey MR, Morris RB, Miller RD, et al: Pharmacokinetics of Org NC45 (norcuron) in patients with and without renal failure. Br J Anaesth 1981;53:1049–1053.

108. Cooper RA, Mirakhur RK, Wierda JM, et al: Pharmacokinetics of rocuronium bromide in patients with and without renal failure. Eur J Anaesthesiol Suppl 1995;11:43–44.

109. Starsnic MA, Goldberg ME, Ritter DE, et al: Does vecuronium accumulate in the renal transplant patient? Can J Anaesth 1989;36:35–39.

110. Carlier M, Squifflet JP, Pirson Y, et al: Confirmation of the crucial role of the recipient's maximal hydration on early diuresis of the human cadaver renal allograft. Transplantation 1983;36:455–456.

111. Ferrara JL, Deeg HJ: Graft-versus-host disease. N Engl J Med 1991;324:667–674.

112. Napier JA: Blood Transfusion Therapy. New York: John Wiley & Sons; 1987.

113. Leitman SF, Holland PV: Irradiation of blood products: Indications and guidelines. Transfusion 1985;25:293–303.

114. Kadota RP, Smithson WA: Bone marrow transplantation for diseases of childhood. Mayo Clin Proc 1984;59:171–184.

115. Tabbara IA: Allogeneic bone marrow transplantation: Acute and late complications. Anticancer Res 1996;16:1019–1026.

116. Filshie J, Pollock AN, Hughes RG, et al: The anaesthetic management of bone marrow harvest for transplantation. Anaesthesia 1984;39:480–484.

117. Chung F: Cancer, chemotherapy and anaesthesia. Can Anaesth Soc J 1982;29:364–371.

118. Selvin BL: Cancer chemotherapy: Implications for the anesthesiologist. Anesth Analg 1981;60:425–434.

Anesthesia Outside the Operating Room

Charles J. Coté

Patient Evaluation

Facilities Evaluation

Equipment

Monitoring

Goals of Anesthesia

Specific Procedures

    Computed Tomography

    Myelography and Polytomography

    Invasive Radiology and Angiography

    Embolization Procedures

    Magnetic Resonance Imaging

    Cardiac Catheterization

    Radiation Therapy

Emergency Room Patients

Mentally Handicapped Children

Post-study Care

Radiation Protection

One of the most difficult tasks anesthesiologists face is to anesthetize an infant or a child in a room other than an operating room. This experience may be uncomfortable because anesthesia must be provided in an unfamiliar environment while working with individuals who may not be able to respond to the special needs of an anesthesiologist, particularly if an emergency should arise. In addition, the facility may not be designed for providing safe anesthesia.

The most common area requesting anesthesia for children outside of the operating room environment is the radiology suite; requirements range from simple sedation to general anesthesia with complete control of respiration and movement. The challenge faced by anesthesiologists is to provide the ideal conditions necessary for the proposed interventional study or radiologic procedure while not compromising a patient's safety or the quality of anesthetic care. Because it is not feasible for an anesthesiologist to be present with every sedated child, anesthesiologists will become increasingly involved in developing sedation protocols and monitoring guidelines so that other subspecialists are able to safely care for routine "healthy" pediatric patients (see Chapter 26).[1, 2]

Patient Evaluation

Patients scheduled for a radiologic, endoscopic, or other procedure requiring anesthesia or sedation *require the same careful preanesthesia evaluation as any surgical patient.* This evaluation mandates a careful medical history, necessary consultations with subspecialists if indicated, and appropriate laboratory evaluation. Children and their parents require the same careful explanation of general anesthesia, the risks, and the level of anesthetic monitoring to avoid unnecessary anxiety (see Chapters 1, 3, and 4). The reason general anesthesia is required often has not been adequately explained to the parents.

The need for premedication, the timing of premedication, the necessity of continuing current medications, the indication for acid aspiration prophylaxis, and appropriate fasting guidelines are assessed during the preoperative visit (see Chapters 4 and 11). The anesthesiologist must have a clear understanding of the proposed procedure so that a patient's safety is balanced with the needs of the individual performing the procedure. The success of a study depends on the appropriate planning, understanding, and communication between specialists. Specific details must be sought regarding issues such as the position of the patient, the geographic relationship of the patient and the anesthesiologist, the need for an intravenous line for administering contrast material, the need for a urinary catheter, or the need for special anesthesia circuits to accommodate the changes in a patient's position relative to the anesthesia machine.

Facilities Evaluation

It is extremely helpful to examine the radiologic, endoscopic, or other facility before providing anesthesia. Many facilities have unique geographic configurations that may prevent an anesthesia machine, an equipment cart, the anesthesiologist, and the patient from remaining in close proximity. Overhead radiologic monitors may prevent positioning a fully configured anesthesia machine close to the patient. Logistical problems such as the location of suction, scavenging, and oxygen hoses, the presence or absence of piped-in nitrous oxide and oxygen, electrical outlets that can be used by operating room equipment, and the appropriate number of such outlets all are important factors to be addressed before anesthetizing a patient. Is the environment air-conditioned to prevent radiologic equipment malfunction due to overheating, thus necessitating the use of methods to keep the patient normothermic? Air-conditioning can make a patient, particularly an infant, susceptible to hypothermia (see Chapter 27). The radiologic table is often limited in mobility and rarely is equipped to provide the Trendelenburg position or to allow a patient to be positioned so that the head is appropriately oriented in relation to the anesthesia machine and anesthesiologist. Will the anesthesiologist be able to observe the radiology monitors from within the location they are forced to remain? In the cardiac catheterization laboratory, will the invasive pressure tracings be available for viewing by the anesthesiologist? These factors are particularly important in older facilities, which were never designed to provide for the needs of an anesthesiologist. All of these concerns should be adequately addressed with the appropriate members of the endoscopic, cardiology, or radiologic team to solve logistical, monitoring, and environmental problems before they become a source of irritation and conflict.

In addition, it is important to work out a mechanism for scheduling such procedures at a mutually convenient time to prevent unnecessary delays. Patient safety and optimal care are the first priority. With increased awareness on the part of the individual who is performing the procedure of the potential for disaster when a child is sedated, anesthesiologists will become increasingly involved in sedating or anesthetizing infants and children for radiologic, endoscopic, and emergency room procedures.[3–5] It is vitally important that anesthesiologists aggressively intervene in the architectural design of any new facility to ensure an operating room type of environment. This is particularly true for magnetic resonance imaging (MRI), which requires specific modifications to provide safe anesthesia care.

Equipment

Anesthesiologists must assume that the equipment necessary to conduct safe anesthesia will not be provided by the individuals in the procedure suite. Therefore, a fully configured anesthesia machine or a cart with all of the necessary monitors must be available. A mobile cart with the supplies to conduct anesthesia is helpful (see Table 31–1). This cart should be stocked with intravenous, airway, and suction equipment, as well as all the drugs necessary to maintain anesthesia and sustain life should an emergency arise. The need to correct the cardiovascular effects of anaphylaxis in particular must always be anticipated, especially when contrast material or antibiotics are to be administered.[6–13] Using the same "pediatric cart" in the operating room and outside of the operating room provides all individuals anesthetizing children with a familiar setup for supplies.

Warming devices, such as a heated humidifier or warming blanket, are essential for maintaining thermal stability in the cold environment of a radiologic suite, provided that the coils of the warming blanket do not interfere with the radiologic procedure. Forced hot air blankets are particularly useful in this venue.[14, 15] Infants are likely to lose body heat during the course of a procedure because they have a very high body surface area to weight ratio. Children with neurologic dysfunction are also prone to problems with thermoregulation.[16, 17] Covering an infant's head and minimizing exposure to the cold environment help reduce convective and radiation heat losses (see Chapter 27).

Monitoring

It is mandatory that all anesthetized or heavily sedated patients be monitored to the same extent as in the operating room.[1, 2, 4, 5, 18, 19] Standard monitoring of pediatric cases includes an electrocardiogram (ECG), a blood pressure monitor, a precordial or esophageal stethoscope (if the anesthesiologist is to remain in the room with the patient or if the stethoscope will not interfere with the procedure), and monitors of continuous oxygen saturation (pulse oximetry), inspired oxygen concentrations, and expired carbon dioxide. If the anesthesiologist is not able to remain in the room with the patient, then some means of continuous observation must be established (glass window or remote camera) to allow simultaneous observation of the patient and the monitors.

Goals of Anesthesia

The primary goal for all procedures is to anesthetize or sedate the patient safely while providing optimal conditions for a successful study or treatment. The superb resolution of many radiologic procedures is dependent on complete absence of movement. Cerebral angiographic procedures in particular may be affected by the slightest movement, even motions related to respiration; alterations in cerebral blood flow secondary to the choice of anesthetic technique or the constancy and value of arterial carbon dioxide pressure ($PaCO_2$) may alter the quality of the results.[20–23] Some procedures require a subject to be motionless for a matter of seconds (radiation therapy); lack of motion is essential to prevent damage to normal tissues while destroying the target tissues. Although ketamine has been successfully used, we believe that it may not be appropriate for radiation therapy because purposeless movement may occur.[24–27] Because ketamine causes nystagmus, this agent may complicate the targeting of a radiation therapy treatment for retinoblastoma. Ketamine may also not be appropriate in patients with increased intracranial pressure because it increases both cerebral blood flow and cerebral metabolic rate for oxygen ($CMRO_2$).[23] In addition, ketamine has been demonstrated to increase cerebrospinal fluid pressure in children with hydrocephalus and has been associated with apnea in a child with increased intracranial pressure.[28–30]

Also of concern is the fact that some patients will return for a whole series of treatments or the study may be conducted in preparation for a surgical procedure. It is therefore important to develop expertise with methods of induction that are minimally traumatic to a patient's psyche and to use medications that may produce amnesia.[31, 32]

Studies that do not require contrast media usually do not cause pain; sedation may be more efficacious than general anesthesia for such studies (e.g., computed tomography [CT] scans or radiation therapy). Other procedures may be painful either because of the procedure itself (e.g., in angiography, pain due to insertion of the catheters and injection of the contrast material) or because of the position required; in these situations, general anesthesia is preferable to sedation. Endotracheal intubation is required for most procedures to have complete control of respiration, particularly when a patient is placed in an unusual position or if the anesthesiologist will not have direct access to the airway. The laryngeal mask airway is a very useful adjunct to airway management in patients who do not require endotracheal intubation.[33, 34]

Specific Procedures

Computed Tomography

General anesthesia or deep sedation is usually required for children less than 6 years of age and for children with a mental handicap to prevent movement during the CT scan; this procedure requires immobilization but is painless.[4, 35] CT scans on a child younger than 3 months (without contrast) can generally be accomplished while the infant is sucking on a bottle of formula; if the child has just been fed, he or she may sleep through the entire procedure.[26, 27] Most "healthy" children are sufficiently cooperative to have a CT scan without the need for sedation if contrast is not required. However, for children between 6 months and 6 years of age, rectal methohexital (10%) administered in a dose of 30 mg/kg is a safe and reliable method of deep sedation.[36–38] This dose is slightly higher than for the induction of anesthesia; however, it provides a reasonably deep

level of sedation within 7 to 10 minutes in the majority of patients, and the sedation generally lasts slightly longer than the CT scan procedure. Patients are usually sedated so that they fall asleep in their parent's arms, thus avoiding a traumatic separation.[31] Children taking seizure medications may require slightly higher doses, such as 40 mg/kg.[39] It should be noted that this method of deep sedation/anesthetic induction is being used with increased frequency by nonanesthesiologists.[40, 41]

A theoretic problem with methohexital is that oxybarbiturates may induce seizures in patients who have temporal lobe epilepsy; in practice, this is an extremely rare occurrence.[42] The seizures induced by methohexital are usually self-limiting. A further concern is that patients who develop a seizure after methohexital may be in a postictal state and may therefore require prolonged monitoring after the CT scan. Thiopental (10%) may be substituted for methohexital in children with known temporal lobe epilepsy, with the anticipation that they may remain sedated for a slightly longer period of time. As with any drug administered rectally, there is considerable patient-to-patient variability in drug absorption and the duration of the sedation produced.

Once a child is appropriately sedated, it is important to place him or her in the scanning device in a position that prevents airway obstruction. This is generally accomplished by placing a folded towel or padding beneath the shoulders so that the head is slightly extended at the atlanto-occipital junction (Fig. 25–1). The head is held in position with sandbags or padding and the adequacy of air exchange observed. The majority of patients who develop airway obstruction after rectal methohexital administration is due to the head flexing forward; simply extending the head generally relieves this obstruction.[43] A pulse oximeter probe is applied to a toe, a blood pressure cuff is applied, electrocardiographic (ECG)

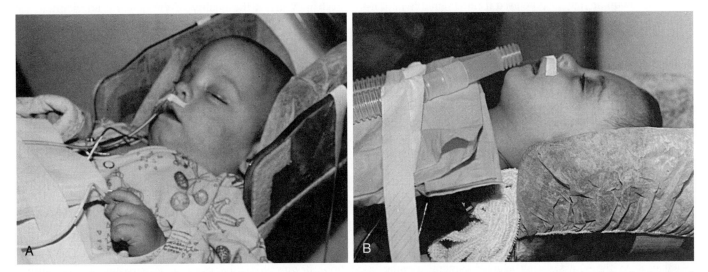

Figure 25–1. (A) Placing an infant or young child flat on the typical gantry for computed tomography causes the patient's head to be flexed forward, resulting in airway obstruction. Taping a sample line of a side-stream carbon dioxide analyzer to the nares provides evidence of each respiration. (B) Placing a folded towel or pad beneath the shoulders allows appropriate position to maintain airway patency; high-flow oxygen can be delivered by taping the Y piece of an anesthesia circuit near the mouth and nares. This method for monitoring respiration can be used for any sedated patient. After sedating the patient and applying all monitoring devices (oximetry, capnography, automated blood pressure, electrocardiography), the anesthesiologist can turn the monitors so that they face the observation window. To reduce radiation exposure, the anesthesiologist can then remain outside of the scanning room while having complete monitoring data immediately available.

leads are appropriately placed, and a catheter to sample expired carbon dioxide is taped close to the nares. Carbon dioxide monitoring does not provide an accurate end-tidal carbon dioxide value but certainly demonstrates that a patient is breathing.

Oxygen can be administered by "enriching" the environment near a patient's face or by using nasal oxygen cannulas. Care must be taken not to stimulate the patient excessively while applying nasal cannulas, especially if the patient is lightly sedated. All monitors are turned so that they face the leaded window of the CT scanner; the anesthesiologist can thus avoid radiation from the scanner while being able to diagnose airway obstruction or desaturation immediately.[44-47]

If an intravenous catheter is necessary to administer contrast material, a small skin wheal of local anesthetic with a 27-gauge needle is used. A patient who is sedated with methohexital generally cries slightly or withdraws the hand or foot in response to this painful stimulus. After a few moments, the hand or foot relaxes, and the catheter can easily be inserted through the anesthetized skin without further upsetting the patient. An alternative is to insert a 25-gauge Butterfly-type device (Abbott Hospitals, Inc., Chicago IL). This method is rapid, is relatively painless, and provides a means of supplementing the sedation should the procedure outlast the duration of the rectal methohexital. If supplementation is required, small increments of intravenous thiopental (0.5–1.0 mg/kg), methohexital (0.25–0.5 mg/kg of a 1% solution), or propofol (0.5–1.0 mg/kg) provide the necessary sedation without producing apnea.

If only sedation is required, a number of sedation methods have efficacy for this procedure.[48-50] If the sedation is prescribed by nonanesthesiologists, then it is important to have a rigorous safety program in place so as to ensure patient safety.[1, 2, 51-53] A uniform hospital-wide system for monitoring and vigilance should be in place (see Chapter 26).[1, 2] Intramuscular ketamine may also be used if intracranial hypertension is not a problem; however, any injection is painful and may be associated with sterile abscess formation.[54] Oral or rectal chloral hydrate (50–75 mg/kg) is another method of sedation primarily used in small infants.[48-50] This drug has been used with great safety for many years. However, children under chloral hydrate sedation can develop airway obstruction due to large tonsils, depression of genioglossus muscle function, or to inadequate positioning; care must always be taken to ensure a patent airway.[55-57] Theoretic concerns about potential generation of carcinogens from breakdown products may make chloral hydrate a less popular choice, but single-day administration still seems appropriate until this concern is further clarified.[58-60] Oral, intramuscular, or intravenous midazolam is another acceptable technique for sedating children but must be used with caution when combined with other medications that may depress ventilation.[61-63] Midazolam may not be a very effective choice when used as the sole sedating agent.[64] General anesthesia is rarely necessary.

Myelography and Polytomography

Myelography and polytomography procedures involve placing contrast material into the neuraxis through a spinal tap; these procedures are associated with a great deal of patient motion and are often performed with the patient prone.

The endotracheal tube position must be constantly observed because with extreme head flexion or change in head position, accidental endobronchial intubation or extubation may result. The esophageal stethoscope and all intravenous lines must be secure; pulse oximetry and capnography may provide an early warning of airway or circulatory compromise.[44-46, 65-67] The majority of these procedures are carried out in conjunction with a CT scan, usually in patients with lower spinal cord deformities such as a tethered spinal cord.

Invasive Radiology and Angiography

Any angiographic or invasive radiology procedure is painful; therefore, general anesthesia or very deep sedation is usually required in children.[68] It is particularly important to have a clear understanding of the underlying pathologic condition being studied, because anesthetic agents and the control of ventilation can have profound effects on regional blood flow.

If a patient has a cerebral aneurysm or arteriovenous malformation, specific anesthetic consideration is given to control of hemodynamic responses during airway manipulation and injection of contrast material as well as to the potential for paradoxic embolization.[69-72] Wide swings in systemic blood pressure could be dangerous, leading to rupture of the aneurysm or exacerbation of bleeding. Patients should be adequately anesthetized to avoid a rapid rise in blood pressure during and after laryngoscopy. Conversely, patients should not be allowed to become hypotensive, because this might compromise blood flow to areas supplied by the aneurysm. At the end of the procedure, an opioid helps blunt pressor responses immediately before extubation. If intracranial hypertension exists, appropriate measures for controlling intracranial hypertension should be utilized (see Chapter 22). The anesthetic technique and arterial carbon dioxide tension are important variables to control, because each may affect the quality of the cerebral arteriogram.[20-23] Communication with the angiographer often helps determine which anesthetic technique would be of greatest help in providing the clearest images. Potent anesthetic agents dilate cerebral blood vessels, thus increasing cerebral blood flow, cerebral blood volume, and intracranial pressure; this latter effect would ordinarily be of concern only if a patient had pre-existent problems with intracranial hypertension. Increased cerebral blood flow would decrease the transit time of the contrast material, however. One report suggests better definition of small vessels when halothane was avoided; this finding may be related to the fact that the halothane group was allowed to breathe spontaneously (i.e., they may have had an elevated $PaCO_2$).[20, 21] Higher-quality images have been obtained when $PaCO_2$ is kept between 25 and 35 mm Hg; this is another reason to monitor expired carbon dioxide levels and to use controlled ventilation to maintain a constant $PaCO_2$.[20-22] Anesthesia using a combination of nitrous oxide, oxygen, a narcotic, and a muscle relaxant usually provides suitable conditions for most arteriograms. This technique provides the least pharmacologic effect on cerebral blood vessels, a light plane of anesthesia from which the patient will rapidly awaken, and pain relief during the wake-up process. It also permits the administration of low concentrations of a potent inhalation agent to control hemodynamic responses without adversely affecting the quality of the angiogram.

During angiographic procedures, the angiography table is frequently moved to assess the position of catheters and guide wires. The security of the endotracheal tube must be carefully guarded, and constant communication between the angiographer and the anesthesia team is mandatory to avoid accidental extubation or dislodgment of intravenous catheters. Using extra-long anesthesia breathing hoses and securing the breathing circuit at a fixed point on the angiography table may help prevent such complications.

During highly magnified cerebral angiography, it is often necessary to stop all movement completely, even motion due to respiration. In this situation, the angiographer and anesthesiologist must coordinate the period of apnea. This is generally accomplished with the use of nondepolarizing muscle relaxants and by physically disconnecting the ventilator from the circuit during the 10 to 20 seconds required for injecting contrast material and performing the angiogram.

If a large number of injections are probable, consideration must be given to the effects of a large osmotic load on urine output. It is reasonable in very long procedures to insert a urinary catheter to avoid overdistension of the bladder. Intravenous fluid replacement therapy must take into account the forced osmotic diuresis that results, and additional fluid should be administered to compensate for urinary losses. A further concern is the possibility of arrhythmias during the injection, as well as a brief period of hypotension (vasodilation) immediately after the injection of high-osmolality contrast material.[73] Low-ionic contrast materials have fewer adverse cardiovascular side effects.[74-77]

The total dose of contrast material administered is of great importance. Infants and small children have an increased blood volume per kilogram of body weight compared with adults and may require slightly larger contrast doses on a weight basis. However, it is possible for the radiologist to administer higher than recommended doses, given the frequent increments of contrast material required to obtain satisfactory studies. In most cases, this only requires compensation with increased intravenous fluid therapy; however, some contrast materials can be nephrotoxic.[78, 79] It is therefore helpful to discuss the total "safe" dose of contrast material for each patient and to record the volume of contrast material administered so that the radiologist is aware of approaching maximum safe limits. This is particularly important when studying multiple vessels, each in two views, and when studying patients with compromised cardiac or renal function. It is advisable to calculate pediatric guidelines for both volume and total osmotic load before the procedure.

Contrast materials are generally divided into two categories: (1) high-osmolality contrast media (e.g., diatrizoate [Hypaque, Renografin], iothalamate [Conray]; osmolality 1400 to 1500 mOsm/L) and (2) low-osmolality contrast media (e.g., ioxaglate [Hexabrix], iopamidol [Isovue], iohexol [Omnipaque]; osmolality 600 to 700 mOsm/L).[74, 75, 80-84] The high-osmolality contrast media are associated with a greater incidence of adverse reactions, including life-threatening reactions.[76, 85] Low-osmolality contrast agents thus would be advantageous in patients with a prior history of contrast agent reaction, however even low-ionic agents are associated with life-threatening reactions.[86] There is conflicting evidence of the value of one agent over the other in terms of renal toxicity.[79, 87] Because the low-osmolality contrast media often cost more than the high-osmolality contrast

media, specific indications are usually listed for the use of the more expensive low-osmolality media.[77, 85, 88] One further concern is that the low-osmolality contrast media have significantly fewer anticoagulant properties than the high-osmolality agents, thus increasing their propensity for causing clot formation within the catheters and flush syringes. Frequent flushing of all catheters and syringes is required to prevent microembolization.[85, 89, 90]

Flush solutions used by the angiographer and the total dose of administered heparin should also be recorded. It is possible for the angiographer to administer an excessive dose of heparin in flush solutions. Because 100 units of heparin per kilogram increase the activated clotting time to three times normal, it would be reasonable to measure the activated clotting time whenever the total dose of heparin exceeds 20 U/kg.[91] Infants and children apparently require more heparin per kilogram and have a shorter heparin half-life than adults.[91, 92] Nevertheless, measurement of the activated clotting time can be useful in quantifying the systemic effects of heparin and the reversal of this effect with protamine should that be necessary.

The wake-up should be as smooth as possible, because coughing or straining can dislodge the clot at the angiography site and result in unobserved bleeding. After wake-up, patients should remain as quiet as possible because movement may also dislodge the clot. It is important to maintain pressure on the arterial puncture site during the move from the radiology table to the recovery room stretcher and from the recovery room stretcher to the patient's bed. Placing a pulse oximeter probe on a toe on the same side as the arterial puncture is a useful means of avoiding the potential for arterial thrombosis due to excessive compression of the puncture site; loss of the oximeter signal implies no arterial blood flow. Lifting a patient from one bed to another, rather than allowing the patient to move independently, helps prevent dislodgment of the clot. The puncture site must be inspected to ensure that bleeding is not occurring each time that a patient is moved or if a patient suddenly moves the leg with the arterial puncture.

Embolization Procedures

Embolization procedures generally require prolonged anesthesia and pose the potential for serious complications. The type and severity of complication depend on the structures being embolized and the site of the pathology.[93-95] Any type of cerebral embolization procedure presents the risk of stroke, whereas procedures in other locations run the risk of damage to surrounding normal tissues.[93, 96, 97] Most procedures in children are for ablation of arteriovenous malformations; all of these patients are at risk for paradoxic emboli.

Patients are increasingly brought to the radiology suite to embolize active arterial bleeding.[98-100] Such cases are perhaps the most difficult for an anesthesiologist because the patients are critically ill and have ongoing blood loss. If the radiologist has difficulty in passing the catheter to the appropriate vessel or if there are multiple "feeding" vessels, a prolonged volume resuscitation can result. In a non-operating room location, this event can be particularly anxiety-producing because the individuals who staff angiography facilities are not generally accustomed to managing massive blood loss. In this circumstance, one must have the capability of transducing arterial and cardiac filling pressures; it is important to have adequate skilled support personnel available (i.e., another anesthesiologist or nurse anesthetist). Additionally, constant-infusion pumps for the administration of vasopressors must be available. A "runner" to expeditiously deliver laboratory test results (e.g., blood gases, hematocrit, electrolytes, ionized calcium, coagulation profiles) and coordination with the blood bank to obtain blood products are necessary and potentially lifesaving. It is also important to have excellent communication with the angiographer so that if a patient becomes critically hypovolemic and it is difficult to maintain intravascular volume, then everyone is prepared to move rapidly to the operating room to gain surgical control of the bleeding.

Magnetic Resonance Imaging

The major advantages of the MRI to patients are that there is no exposure to radiation and the MRI scans are uniquely sensitive for imaging of the spinal cord, brain, and joints. In addition, the need for contrast material is sometimes avoided.[101-103] Unfortunately, this device has significant disadvantages (i.e., its images are easily degraded by outside radiofrequency, thus the need for placing the scanner inside a large Faraday cage). Conversely, the radiofrequencies emitted and the powerful magnetic field generated by the scanner create a technologic nightmare for anesthesiologists because they can affect nearly every monitoring device.[104-110]

The magnetic fields generated by an MRI scanner can be divided into three types: (1) the static magnetic field, (2) the rapidly varying magnetic field during scanning, and (3) the radiofrequency magnetic field generated during scanning.[111-115] Each of these creates problems with monitoring devices and raises issues regarding safety for the patient and anesthesiologist.

One must be aware of the effects the magnetic fields may have on the anesthesiologist and the patient.[111-118] Safety guidelines are available for industrial exposure to magnetic fields[119, 120] and must also be considered for the MRI.[114] Surgical clips, pins, shrapnel, ferromagnetic foreign bodies of the eye, any type of ferromagnetic implant, connections on some tissue expanders, and artificial joints may be attracted to the magnet by the static magnetic field; in addition, ferromagnetic materials may heat up as a result of the radiofrequency magnetic field generated during scanning.[104, 111-118, 121-126] Nonferromagnetic materials such as stainless steel wires, titanium, and Vitallium (cobalt-chromium alloy) plates will cause artifacts on the scans (stainless steel > Vitallium > titanium) but apparently do not move or heat up.[127] Pacemakers fail, and the implanted wires offer potential for electrical currents generated by the radiofrequency field or the rapidly varying magnetic field to be carried directly to the heart.[111, 113-116] Even newer model pacemakers are susceptible to alteration in function during scanning with low-power (0.5 tesla) magnets.[128] One paper postulates the possibility for transesophageal pacing during "low radiofrequency exposure."[129] It is therefore vitally important to obtain a complete history from patients, especially regarding prior surgical procedures (surgical vascular clips, implants, tissue expanders, prosthetic heart valves, pacemaker), foreign bodies of the eye, or pieces of shrapnel. Catastrophic damage to the eye, motion of cerebral aneurysm clips, and

heating of implanted metallic devices have been reported.[111-118, 121-124] Some centers routinely screen their patients with a metal detector, and others perform a simple radiographic evaluation before MRI scanning to diagnose the presence of metallic foreign bodies.[111, 113-115] It appears that metallic foreign bodies in vital areas (brain, cardiac valve, inner ear implant, eye) are the most likely to cause damage as a result of attraction by the magnet. Metallic devices that have been placed in less vital areas and that have been fibrosed over (surgical clips on the mesentery) are unlikely to cause damage.[111, 113-115] It is not the anesthesiologist's responsibility, however, to clear patients for MRI scanning.

There is little information about the safety of prolonged or repeated exposure to powerful magnetic fields, but short-term exposure appears to be safe.[111, 113-115, 130, 131] Data suggest a possible increased incidence of malignancies in populations living near high-tension wires or working in power-generating facilities.[130, 132] Ongoing studies are addressing the safety of working near MRI devices on a daily basis.[115] ECG changes (ST segments) have been reported in normal individuals exposed to the more powerful 1.5 T units, but these are apparently transient in nature and not associated with arrhythmias or clinically important symptoms.[115, 133] On a practical note, watches may be ruined and magnetic coding signatures stripped off credit cards.[118]

Although this technology is purported to be safe, it should be noted that it does not have a long track record. It is therefore reasonable for the anesthesiologist to approach exposure cautiously (i.e., limit the amount of time spent in close proximity to the magnet).[119, 120] It is reasonable to develop methods that provide a safely anesthetized or sedated patient while maintaining a "safe" distance from the magnet.[104-107, 111, 115, 134-139]

The Faraday cage that surrounds the magnet is there to protect the magnet from radiofrequency interference in the local environment, not to shield individuals from the magnetic field. The static magnetic field generated by the magnet usually extends beyond the boundaries set by the Faraday cage that houses the magnet. The engineers who installed the magnet can mark the strength of the magnetic field on the floor outside the MRI scanner room (Fig. 25-2). The strength of the magnetic field is proportional to the distance from the magnet to the third power.[115]

The radiofrequency emitted by the scanner prevents standard operating room pulse oximeters from functioning during scanning, and the powerful magnet may interfere with the ventilator, noninvasive automated blood pressure machine, ECG, infusion pumps, and other monitors.[104, 106, 111, 113-115] The magnetic field may exert a powerful attraction on an anesthesia machine that has a high ferromagnetic mass (e.g., standard oxygen and nitrous oxide tanks). Thus either a stripped down anesthesia machine with aluminum tanks or a special MRI compatible but more expensive anesthesia machine is advisable.

A major disadvantage for the anesthesiologist is that a patient, especially an infant or child, is positioned out of reach during the scanning procedure (Fig. 25-3).[104, 106, 111] Because any movement destroys the clarity of MRI images and the duration of such studies is unpredictable, I usually use general anesthesia. Even adults or older children may become claustrophobic and require a general anesthetic or sedation to achieve a successful scan.[104, 140-142] New open

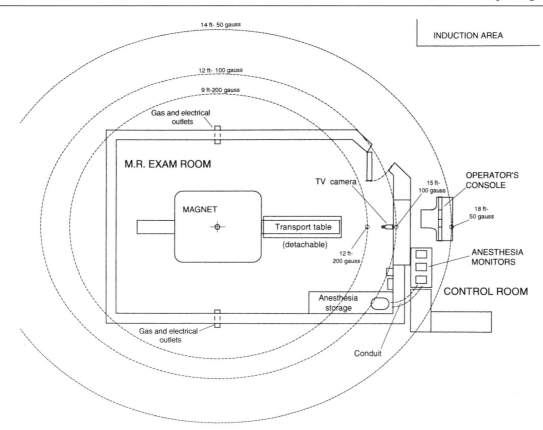

Figure 25–2. Floor plan of a magnetic resonance imaging (MRI) facility specifically designed to meet the special needs of the anesthesiologist. Note that provisions must be made to allow monitoring cables and devices to pass through the walls of the Faraday cage without compromising its integrity to be able to transmit data out of the MRI scanner room. A solid-state camera and incandescent spotlight directed down the lumen of the MRI scanner allow observation of the patient on a remote monitor. The intensity of the magnetic field is inversely proportional to the distance cubed from the magnet and the orientation of the magnet; note that the magnetic field extends beyond the walls of the Faraday cage, indicating the continued need to be concerned about the effects of magnetic fields. Separate induction areas as well as indicated areas of intense magnetic field are helpful for the safety of the patient and anesthesiologist. (Modified from drawings of a new MRI facility by Hoskins Scott & Partners, Inc., Boston, MA.)

configuration machines have a lower incidence of claustrophobia.

Of central concern for anesthesiologists is how to safely anesthetize or sedate patients in this technologically hostile environment (see Figs. 25–2 and 25–3). The strength of the magnetic field creates problems with any ferromagnetic material,[104, 111, 113–115] thus mandating the use of an MRI-compatible anesthesia machine, brass or aluminum laryngoscope blades and handles, plastic or aluminum stethoscopes, plastic connectors for the stethoscope, nonferromagnetic intravenous poles and clipboards for the anesthesia record, and intravenous catheters that do not contain a metal hub. Ferromagnetic materials cannot be carried in pockets. I have observed clipboards, pens, scissors, oxygen tanks, anesthesia machines, patients' stretchers, a patient's cane, and other materials pulled into or toward the magnet. The batteries within laryngoscope handles may be attracted to the magnet.[104] One anecdotal report describes a fatal injury resulting from an unsecured ferromagnetic oxygen tank striking a patient in the head. It is therefore mandatory that all equipment be modified or secured to avoid being attracted to the magnet. Oxygen tanks must be full before bringing the anesthesia machine into the MRI scanner and *only aluminum tanks can be used.*

Traditional circle systems are not long enough to reach from the anesthesia machine to the patient during scanning. An extra-long circle circuit made of noncompliant material can be used on a machine outside of the scanner or specially long circle circuits used on machines brought into the scanning room. An alternative is to use a nonrebreathing anesthesia circuit (Mapleson D arm with a scavenger device) attached to a nonferromagnetic intravenous pole with a long fresh gas hose (usually 15 to 20 feet). The anesthesia machine, which is stripped of most ferromagnetic materials, is located as far from the magnet as reasonably feasible.[104, 134–139] Patients are generally anesthetized or sedated at a distance from the magnet and then brought into the scanner room (see Fig. 25–2); newer units have a gantry that can be separated from the MRI scanner to facilitate this process. The intense magnetic field produced by the more powerful 1.5 T units makes a separate induction room strongly advisable because the equipment necessary to perform endotracheal intubation can be attracted to the magnet (batteries in the laryngoscope). In addition, because the greatest period of cardiovascular and airway instability is during induction, it is vital that all monitors function perfectly without interference from the magnetic field. The trade-off is that anesthetizing patients in a separate location then introduces risks in

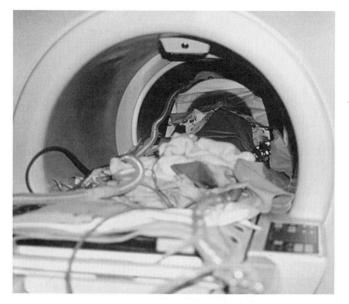

Figure 25–3. A typical pediatric patient is completely out of reach or view during magnetic resonance (MR) scanning, thus mandating the use of techniques that provide continuous monitoring of oxygen saturation, capnography, and blood pressure. A remote solid-state camera and incandescent spotlight aimed down the barrel of the MR scanner can provide the ability to observe a portion of the patient (toes, feet) on a remote monitor.

transporting them and positioning them in the MRI scanner room.

Useful techniques have been high-dose rectal thiopental, inhalation, or intravenous induction followed by a propofol infusion, or spontaneous respirations with low concentration of inhalation agent and nitrous oxide.[143, 144] Rectal methohexital and oral chloral hydrate have also been used.[41, 145] Some anesthesiologists prefer endotracheal intubation whereas others use a laryngeal mask airway.[34]

If a ventilator is to be used, then care must be taken to ensure that the magnet does not affect proper function (special ventilators are available).[110] Generally, an extra-long respiratory hose is required to connect the ventilator on the anesthesia machine to the anesthesia circuit attached to the intravenous pole; these respiratory circuits should be of low compliance to minimize compression volume losses.[109, 137, 139] When controlling ventilation, a Mapleson D circuit with fresh gas flow of one times the minute ventilation prevents clinically important rebreathing.[146] I have anesthetized 100 kg patients with only 7 L/min of fresh gas flow using a Mapleson D circuit with controlled ventilation.

The most important concern of anesthesiologists is to be able to continuously and appropriately monitor patients even *during the scanning procedure.* The phosphors of standard ECG screens are generally distorted by the magnetic field and the radiofrequency generated by the scanner. With these systems the ECG is usually of little value other than to diagnose the fact that the heart is generating electrical activity; even the rhythm may be difficult to determine.[111, 115] A number of patients have been reported to suffer a burn injury from ECG leads, possibly as a result of the ECG wires acting as antennae for the radiofrequency magnetic field generated by the magnet during scanning, therefore causing

a radiofrequency burn.[147] Alternatively, the burn injury may be due to coiling of the ECG wires, thereby generating electrical current secondary to the rapid changes in the direction of the magnetic field.[148] Whatever the mechanism, it appears that ECG monitoring during MRI poses a potential danger to patients; therefore, using standard ECG monitoring may be contraindicated during scanning. All ECG wires must be removed from the patient during scanning unless they are absolutely necessary. If there is a need to keep the ECG wires connected (cardiac scans, gated scans), then *meticulous attention to avoid coiling the wires, minimal contact with the patient's body, ECG leads with the least possible wire, using graphite ECG leads, and braiding the wires together may reduce the potential for burn injury.*[111, 114, 115, 148–153] Newer systems use a single pad placed beneath the patient, which then only has a single shielded cable connecting it to the monitor (Invivo Research, Inc., Orlando, FL).

An automated blood pressure machine is limited by the distance it can be placed from an infant because the algorithm built into the machine is dependent on the length and size of the tubing. Blood pressure thus must often be monitored manually (i.e., "bounce" pressure with a mercury manometer, Doppler, or Korotkoff sounds).[104, 106, 154] However, during scanning, it is difficult to hear Korotkoff sounds. A special extra-long blood pressure tubing that does not significantly affect the accuracy of the blood pressure determination can be used for older patients. The automated blood pressure device can then be placed outside of the scanner room, away from the effects of the magnetic field. In some infants, we have also used larger blood pressure cuffs placed on the thigh rather than the arm, allowing compatibility with the longer tubing used for older patients. It should be noted that these pressures are only useful for trending and may not correlate well with upper extremity blood pressure measurements.[155]

Because patients are so far removed from reach and because the inside of the magnet is dark and narrow, it is difficult to monitor patients visually.[111] Fluorescent lighting may affect the scan, so an incandescent light source must be provided. The use of a remote, shielded, solid-state camera may allow visualization of the patient if an incandescent light is directed down the barrel of the scanner; usually only the toes are readily seen.

The use of a side-stream carbon dioxide monitor with a very long sampling tube extending out of the MRI scanner room allows breath-to-breath monitoring of respirations (not accurate measurement) and the rhythm of ventilation. For sedated patients, a change in respiratory pattern may indicate that they require additional sedation. Interruption of carbon dioxide sensing may indicate apnea or airway obstruction and can provide an early warning before a patient develops oxygen desaturation.[46] The extra-long sample tubing may, however, result in a greater lag time between the event taking place and the time of its detection.

Pulse oximetry is perhaps the most important monitor because it provides real-time information about the status of ventilation, circulation, and oxygenation. Pulse oximetry gives early warning of developing desaturation before the point at which this desaturation becomes dangerous.[44, 45] This early warning of desaturation is particularly vital during MRI scanning because patients are completely out of view and in a dark environment. The major technologic problem is how to monitor safely so that the radiofrequency generated by the pulse oximeter does not interfere with the scan image and so that the radiofrequency generated by the MRI scanner does not interfere with the oximeter. *The majority of standard operating room pulse oximeters function between scanning modes but do not function continuously throughout the scanning procedure.* A number of pulse oximeters specifically designed to minimize the radiofrequency produced (thereby minimizing radiofrequency artifact on the MRI scan) are available. Special modifications such as reducing the number of computer chips, shortening the length of connections within the unit that can act like antennae, and using battery power have markedly reduced the radiofrequency signals generated by the oximeter unit. In addition, some models use multiple shielding layers wrapped around the sensor cable and several radiofrequency "chokes" minimize radiofrequency magnetic field signals that can travel along the length of the cable. The use of fiberoptic cables also prevents this problem. These modifications eliminate radiofrequency interference from the magnet reaching the oximeter and radiofrequency from the oximeter reaching the magnet. Severe burn injuries from pulse oximeter probes have been attributed to coiling of the oximeter cable, resulting in the formation of a conductive loop.[156, 157] Therefore, even with this specially designed pulse oximeter, *it is extremely important to place the probe as close as possible to the edge of the magnet (e.g., on a toe), to prevent any of the cable from touching the patient, and to avoid creating any loops in the cable.*[111, 113–115, 156]

The combination of a solid-state camera focused on the patient to be able to observe the patient, pulse oximetry to continuously monitor oxygen saturation, expired carbon dioxide monitoring to document respiration, and automated blood pressure measurement allows these patients to be cared for safely without the need for the anesthesiologist to remain in the room with them. Use of a camera focused on the pulse oximeter (which remains in the scanning room) provides an image on a remote monitor placed next to the capnograph and automated blood pressure device (which are outside of the scanning room); this arrangement allows the anesthesiologist to monitor patients carefully while avoiding prolonged close exposure to the powerful magnetic field. MRI scanning facilities designed to accommodate the needs of anesthesiologists have special built-in conduits that allow the appropriate cables and tubings to be extended outside the Faraday cage without compromising its integrity. To retrofit such modifications can be extremely expensive. Figure 25–2 presents a solution to this problem. It is unacceptable not to monitor oxygen saturation and expired carbon dioxide in the MRI scanner, because the proper technology to monitor despite the powerful magnetic field is available.

My practice had been to intubate nearly all patients scheduled for MRI because of the distance from the anesthesia machine and the fact that patients are essentially out of reach. However, the laryngeal mask airway provides the necessary safety net of maintaining a clear airway while circumventing the need for endotracheal intubation.[33, 158, 159] A patient with increased intracranial pressure, however, would benefit from endotracheal intubation, controlled ventilation, and avoidance of high-dose potent inhalation agents.

Obviously patients with a full stomach also require endotracheal intubation.

Cardiac Catheterization

Because the decision for surgical intervention is often based on hemodynamic data obtained at the time of cardiac catheterization, it is important to be aware of possible anesthetic-induced variables that may affect the catheterization data. Certainly, the negative inotropic effects of most potent inhalation agents, the effects of oxygenation and arterial carbon dioxide variations on pulmonary artery pressure and pulmonary artery blood flow, and the positive inotropic effects of some agents such as ketamine or pancuronium should be considered but are occasionally overlooked. It is for this reason that some pediatric cardiologists prefer to heavily sedate rather than "anesthetize" these patients. It is important to monitor these patients, just as for general anesthesia, to be able to diagnose adverse events and intervene in a timely manner. Obviously all the equipment, medications, and monitors used in the operating room should be available to safely anesthetize these patients (see also Chapters 17 to 19).

Radiation Therapy

Patients undergoing radiation therapy must remain perfectly motionless for the brief duration of the treatment. Since the anesthesiologist is not able to remain with the patient because of the radiation, monitoring with pulse oximetry, an ECG, an automated blood pressure device, and expired carbon dioxide sampling (a catheter is taped close to the nares as for CT scans; see Fig. 25–1) are used. Two cameras are required: One focuses on the patient to observe for movement, and the other focuses on the monitors that are in the room with the patient.[160, 161]

Rectal barbiturates have been useful for these treatments; however, a gaseous induction and maintenance of spontaneous respiration with gas insufflation constitute a reliable alternative technique.[36, 37, 39, 162] If a child is scheduled for a long series of treatments, inserting a Broviac or Hickman type of catheter facilitates the rapidity of induction and minimizes psychological trauma due to repeated mask or rectal inductions. In this circumstance, a continuous infusion of propofol is particularly valuable because patients remain motionless and rapidly awaken. The induction and maintenance dose must be individualized. These patients are usually cared for on an outpatient basis, and with appropriate use of available anesthetic techniques, most are ready for discharge within 1 hour of concluding the procedure. Neonates and infants continue to gain weight despite 4 to 5 weeks of almost daily radiation therapy treatments.[163]

Emergency Room Patients

Anesthesiologists will be increasingly consulted to sedate or anesthetize children in the emergency room for reduction of a fracture, suture of lacerations, or diagnostic radiologic studies. The main concern in this circumstance is the lack of appropriate fasting or the effects of the injury on gastric motility. The decision about when and how deeply to sedate such a child must be individualized; however, the risk of pulmonary gastric fluid aspiration is ever present. This risk may be reduced by delaying the procedure if it is not urgent or by taking advantage of the full retinue of acid aspiration prophylaxis.

A study of children requiring emergency surgery investigated the gastric residual volume in children who had been in the hospital for 1 to 4 hours before anesthetic induction versus those who had been in the hospital for 4 to 8 hours or longer.[164] The mean gastric residual volume was 1.1 mL/kg (range 0.35 to 2.98 mL/kg) for the group who had fasted for less than 4 hours, but this was reduced to a mean of 0.51 mL/kg (range 0.13 to 1.36 mL/kg) for children fasting for 4 to 8 hours. Children who had fasted for more than 8 hours had a mean gastric residual volume of 0.28 mL/kg (range 0.11 to 0.86 mL/kg). The mean gastric residual volume after 4 hours of fasting is similar to that of children scheduled for elective surgical procedures.[165] In addition, the appropriate use of medications that increase gastric emptying and decrease gastric acid production, as well as the administration of oral antacids (nonparticulate), would potentially further reduce this risk.[166] This does not imply that these patients are not at risk if the procedure is delayed or gastric aspiration prophylaxis measures instituted; rather, it only suggests that the danger may be diminished. Obviously, the danger of postponing treatment or radiologic evaluation must be balanced against the benefits of reduced risk for aspiration.

Once a decision has been made to sedate such a patient, the level of sedation must be carefully titrated to minimize the potential for the loss of consciousness or protective airway reflexes.[1, 4] The combination of a local anesthetic, a regional nerve block (e.g., axillary block to set a fracture), and minimal levels of sedation can be very efficacious. Ketamine in high doses has been demonstrated to result in the loss of protective airway reflexes, as has the administration of 50% nitrous oxide.[167, 168] Low-dose ketamine (0.25–0.5 mg/kg IV) combined with low dose midazolam (25–50 μg/kg IV) can be very effective The combination of nitrous oxide with any other sedative or hypnotic may produce a state of general anesthesia, necessitating appropriate measures to protect the airway (endotracheal intubation).[169]

It is essential that such patients be carefully observed after the procedure, until the full return of protective airway reflexes and the ability to maintain a patent airway are assured. It is not unusual to have patients who appear to be minimally affected by sedatives or opioids during the procedure (because of stress and pain) become much more deeply sedated when the procedure is completed.

Mentally Handicapped Children

Anesthesiologists are frequently consulted to sedate or anesthetize patients with mental or motor handicaps when they are to undergo procedures that ordinarily would not require such measures. In this circumstance, it is vital that all available medical and anesthesia records be obtained to have a complete understanding of underlying medical or surgical conditions (e.g., seizure disorders, gastroesophageal reflux, the presence of hydrocephalus). This information facilitates appropriate management of current medications, premedication, and design of the anesthetic prescription.

Even though the chronologic age of a patient may be 20 to 30 years, the mental age may be 5 years. Such a patient must be managed just as one would a 5-year-old. Fear of injections, needles, masks, and separation from parents or guardians are all of vital importance to these patients. The induction or sedation techniques must be similar to those indicated for younger children. If an intravenous line cannot be inserted without significant upset to a patient, a mask induction with the help and consolation of a parent or special guardian may be of particular value. Rectal or oral sedation is also a reasonable alternative. I have anesthetized such adult patients while they were being held and consoled by their parents. Such management is very rewarding for the patient and the anesthesiologist.

Post-study Care

As with any patient undergoing general anesthesia or being heavily sedated, one must always be vigilant for airway compromise. These patients, even those sedated but not anesthetized, must be monitored in an appropriate recovery facility. Because the recovery room is often remote from the site of study, patients should have intact airway reflexes and a stable airway before departure or should be transported with an endotracheal tube in place. Portable oxygen and a means of delivering positive-pressure ventilation are important; a battery-powered transport pulse oximeter is essential for diagnosing desaturation during the transfer to recovery.

Radiation Protection

The risk of x-ray exposure is a concern for anesthesiologists. Anesthesiologists should take appropriate precautions, always keeping a lead apron between themselves and the source of radiation.[47, 152] A thyroid protector may also be indicated. Most currently used radiographic equipment is designed to minimize the patient's, radiologist's, and anesthesiologist's exposure; however, the continued need for protection should not be underestimated, particularly if one frequently works in these locations. One should always minimize unnecessary exposure and design the anesthetic technique to allow patients to breathe spontaneously or have a ventilator present so that the anesthesiologist can step out of the immediate vicinity during periods of increased exposure (e.g., during rapidly taken radiographs with dye injection). The anesthesiologist's exposure is affected by the duration of exposure, the distance from the x-ray source, and the protective shielding being used. Increasing the distance from the source of ionizing radiation markedly reduces exposure. A lead screen suspended between the x-ray tube and the angiographer and anesthesia team also reduces exposure.

REFERENCES

1. Committee on Drugs American Academy of Pediatrics: Guidelines for monitoring and management of pediatric patients during and after sedation for diagnostic and therapeutic procedures. Pediatrics 1992;89:1110–1115.
2. Gross JB, Bailey PL, Caplan RA, et al: Practice guidelines for sedation and analgesia by non-anesthesiologists: A report by the American

Society of Anesthesiologists Task Force on Sedation and Analgesia by Non-anesthesiologists. Anesthesiology 1996;84:459–471.

3. Coté CJ: Sedation protocols: Why so many variations? Pediatrics 1994;94:281–283.

4. Coté CJ: Sedation for the pediatric patient: A review. Pediatr Clin North Am 1994;41:31–58.

5. Coté CJ: Monitoring guidelines: Do they make a difference? AJR Am J Roentgenol 1995;165:910–912.

6. Kurkchubasche AG, Fendya DG, Tracy TFJ, et al: Blunt intestinal injury in children: Diagnostic and therapeutic considerations. Arch Surg 1997;132:652–657.

7. Ridley LJ: Allergic reactions to oral iodinated contrast agents: Reactions to oral contrast. Australas Radiol 1998;42:114–117.

8. Shehadi WH: Death following intravascular administration of contrast media. Acta Radiol Diagn (Stockh) 1985;26:457–461.

9. Goldberg M: Systemic reactions to intravascular contrast media: A guide for the anesthesiologist. Anesthesiology 1984;60:46–56.

10. Shehadi WH, Toniolo G: Adverse reactions to contrast media: A report from the Committee on Safety of Contrast Media of the International Society of Radiology. Radiology 1980;137:299–302.

11. Cohan RH, Dunnick NR, Bashore TM: Treatment of reactions to radiographic contrast material. AJR Am J Roentgenol 1988;151:263–270.

12. Lasser EC, Berry CC, Mishkin MM, et al: Pretreatment with corticosteroids to prevent adverse reactions to nonionic contrast media. AJR Am J Roentgenol 1994;162:523–526.

13. Lasser EC, Berry CC, Talner LB, et al: Protective effects of corticosteroids in contrast material anaphylaxis. Invest Radiol 1988;23(Suppl 1):S193–S194.

14. Murat I, Berniere J, Constant I: Evaluation of the efficacy of a forced-air warmer (Bair Hugger) during spinal surgery in children. J Clin Anesth 1994;6:425–429.

15. Borms SF, Engelen SL, Himpe DG, et al: Bair hugger forced-air warming maintains normothermia more effectively than thermo-lite insulation. J Clin Anesth 1994;6:303–307.

16. Bissonnette B, Sessler DI, LaFlamme P: Intraoperative temperature monitoring sites in infants and children and the effect of inspired gas warming on esophageal temperature. Anesth Analg 1989;69:192–196.

17. Bissonnette B, Sessler DI, LaFlamme P: Passive and active inspired gas humidification in infants and children. Anesthesiology 1989;71:350–354.

18. Eichhorn JH: Effect of monitoring standards on anesthesia outcome. Int Anesthesiol Clin 1993;31:181–196.

19. Eichhorn JH, Cooper JB, Cullen DJ, et al: Standards for patient monitoring during anesthesia at Harvard Medical School. JAMA 1986;256:1017–1020.

20. Du Boulay G, Edmonds-Seal J, Bostick T: The effect of intermittent positive pressure ventilation upon the calibre of cerebral arteries in spasm following subarachnoid haemorrhage: A preliminary communication. Br J Radiol 1968;41:46–48.

21. Edmonds-Seal J, Du Boulay G, Bostick T: The effect of intermittent positive pressure ventilation upon cerebral angiography with special reference to the quality of the films: A preliminary communication. Br J Radiol 1967;40:957–958.

22. Dallas SH, Moxon CP: Controlled ventilation for cerebral angiography. Br J Anaesth 1969;41:597–602.

23. Smith AL, Wollman H: Cerebral blood flow and metabolism: Effects of anesthetic drugs and techniques. Anesthesiology 1972;36:378–400.

24. Lo JN, Buckley JJ, Kim TH, et al: Anesthesia for high-dose total body irradiation in children. Anesthesiology 1984;61:101–103.

25. Amberg HL, Gordon G: Low-dose intramuscular ketamine for pediatric radiotherapy: A case report. Anesth Analg 1976;55:92–94.

26. Aidinis SJ, Zimmerman RA, Shapiro HM, et al: Anesthesia for brain computer tomography. Anesthesiology 1976;44:420–425.

27. Ferrer-Brechner T, Winter J: Anesthetic considerations for cerebral computer tomography. Anesth Analg 1977;56:344–347.

28. Crumrine RS, Nulsen FE, Weiss MH: Alterations in ventricular fluid pressure during ketamine anesthesia in hydrocephalic children. Anesthesiology 1975;42:758–761.

29. List WF, Crumrine RS, Cascorbi HF, et al: Increased cerebrospinal fluid pressure after ketamine. Anesthesiology 1972;36:98–99.

30. Lockhart CH, Jenkins JJ: Ketamine-induced apnea in patients with increased intracranial pressure. Anesthesiology 1972;37:92–93.

31. Coté CJ: Induction techniques in pediatric anesthesia. ASA Refresher Courses in Anesthesiology 1989;17:43–57.

32. Twersky RS, Hartung J, Berger BJ, et al: Midazolam enhances anterograde but not retrograde amnesia in pediatric patients. Anesthesiology 1993;78:51–55.

33. Brain AI: The laryngeal mask: A new concept in airway management. Br J Anaesth 1983;55:801–805.

34. Goudsouzian NG, Denman W, Cleveland R, et al: Radiologic localization of the laryngeal mask airway in children. Anesthesiology 1992;77:1085–1089.

35. Broennle AM, Cohen DE: Pediatric anesthesia and sedation. Curr Opin Pediatr 1993;5:310–314.

36. Goresky GV, Steward DJ: Rectal methohexitone for induction of anaesthesia in children. Can Anaesth Soc J 1979;26:213–215.

37. Liu LMP, Goudsouzian NG, Liu P: Rectal methohexital premedication in children: A dose comparison study. Anesthesiology 1980;53:343–345.

38. Bjorkman S, Gabrielsson J, Quaynor H, et al: Pharmacokinetics of I.V. and rectal methohexitone in children. Br J Anaesth 1987;59:1541–1547.

39. Griswold JD, Liu LM: Rectal methohexital in children undergoing computerized cranial tomography and magnetic resonance imaging scans. Anesthesiology 1987;67:A494.

40. Manuli MA, Davies L: Rectal methohexital for sedation of children during imaging procedures. AJR Am J Roentgenol 1993;160:577–580.

41. Glasier CM, Stark JE, Brown R, et al: Rectal thiopental sodium for sedation of pediatric patients undergoing MR and other imaging studies. AJNR Am J Neuroradiol 1995;16:111–114.

42. Rockoff MA, Goudsouzian NG: Seizures induced by methohexital. Anesthesiology 1981;54:333–335.

43. Daniels AL, Coté CJ, Polaner DM: Continuous oxygen saturation monitoring following rectal methohexitone induction in paediatric patients. Can J Anaesth 1992;39:27–30.

44. Coté CJ, Goldstein EA, Coté MA, et al: A single-blind study of pulse oximetry in children. Anesthesiology 1988;68:184–188.

45. Coté CJ, Rolf N, Liu LM, et al: A single-blind study of combined pulse oximetry and capnography in children. Anesthesiology 1991;74:980–987.

46. Coté CJ, Liu LM, Szyfelbein SK, et al: Intraoperative events diagnosed by expired carbon dioxide monitoring in children. Can Anaesth Soc J 1986;33:315–320.

47. Henderson KH, Lu JK, Strauss KJ, et al: Radiation exposure of anesthesiologists. J Clin Anesth 1994;6:37–41.

48. Vade A, Sukhani R, Dolenga M, et al: Chloral hydrate sedation in children undergoing CT and MR imaging: Safety as judged by American Academy of Pediatrics (AAP) Guidelines. Am J Rad 1995;165:905–909.

49. Cook BA, Bass JW, Nomizu S, et al: Sedation of children for technical procedures: Current standard of practice. Clin Pediatr (Phila) 1992;31:137–142.

50. Greenberg SB, Faerber EN, Aspinall CL: High dose chloral hydrate sedation for children undergoing CT. J Comput Assist Tomogr 1991;15:467–469.

51. Frush DP, Bisset GS, Hall SC: Pediatric sedation in radiology: The practice of safe sleep. AJR Am J Roentgenol 1996;167:1381–1387.

52. Egelhoff JC, Ball WSJ, Koch BL, et al: Safety and efficacy of sedation in children using a structured sedation program. AJR Am J Roentgenol 1997;168:1259–1262.

53. Frush DP, Bisset GS: Sedation of children in radiology: time to wake up. AJR Am J Roentgenol 1995;165:913–914.

54. Reich DL, Silvay G: Ketamine: An update on the first twenty-five years of clinical experience. Can J Anaesth 1989;36:186–197.

55. Biban P, Baraldi E, Pettenazzo A, et al: Adverse effect of chloral hydrate in two young children with obstructive sleep apnea. Pediatrics 1993;92:461–463.

56. Fishbaugh DF, Wilson S, Preisch JW, et al: Relationship of tonsil size on an airway blockage maneuver in children during sedation. Pediatr Dent 1997;19:277–281.

57. Hershenson M, Brouillette RT, Olsen E, et al: The effect of chloral hydrate on genioglossus and diaphragmatic activity. Pediatr Res 1984;18:516–519.

58. Salmon AG, Kizer KW, Zeise L, et al: Potential carcinogenicity of chloral hydrate: A review. J Toxicol Clin Toxicol 1995;33:115–121.

59. Smith MT: Chloral hydrate warning. Science 1990;250:359.

60. American Academy of Pediatrics, Committee on Drugs, Committee on Environmental Health: Use of chloral hydrate for sedation in children. Pediatrics 1993;92:471–473.

61. Tolia V, Fleming SL, Kauffman RE: Randomized, double-blind trial of midazolam and diazepam for endoscopic sedation in children. Dev Pharmacol Ther 1990;14:141–147.

62. Alexander CM, Gross JB: Sedative doses of midazolam depress hypoxic ventilatory responses in humans. Anesth Analg 1988;67:377–382.

63. Yaster M, Nichols DG, Deshpande JK, et al: Midazolam-fentanyl intravenous sedation in children: Case report of respiratory arrest. Pediatrics 1990;86:463–467.

64. McCarver-May DG, Kang J, Aouthmany M, et al: Comparison of chloral hydrate and midazolam for sedation of neonates for neuro-imaging studies. J Pediatr 1996;128:573–576.

65. Partridge BL: Use of pulse oximetry as a noninvasive indicator of intravascular volume status. J Clin Monit 1987;3:263–268.

66. Wippermann CF, Schranz D, Huth RG: Evaluation of the pulse wave arrival time as a marker for blood pressure changes in critically ill infants and children. J Clin Monit 1995;11:324–328.

67. Wallace CT, Baker JD 3d, Alpert CC, et al: Comparison of blood pressure measurement by Doppler and by pulse oximetry techniques. Anesth Analg 1987;66:1018–1019.

68. Cotsen MR, Donaldson JS, Uejima T, et al: Efficacy of ketamine hydrochloride sedation in children for interventional radiologic procedures. AJR Am J Roentgenol 1997;169:1019–1022.

69. Lassen NA, Christensen MS: Physiology of cerebral blood flow. Br J Anaesth 1976;48:719–734.

70. Shapiro HM, Aidinis SJ: Neurosurgical anesthesia. Surg Clin North Am 1975;55:913–928.

71. Holden AM, Fyler DC, Shillito J Jr, et al: Congestive heart failure from intracranial arteriovenous fistula in infancy: Clinical and physiologic considerations in eight patients. Pediatrics 1972;49:30–39.

72. Hood JB, Wallace CT, Mahaffey JE: Anesthetic management of an intracranial arteriovenous malformation in infancy. Anesth Analg 1977;56:236–241.

73. Coté CJ, Greenhow DE, Marshall BE: The hypotensive response to rapid intravenous administration of hypertonic solutions in man and in the rabbit. Anesthesiology 1979;50:30–35.

74. Gertz EW, Wisneski JA, Chiu D, et al: Clinical superiority of a new nonionic contrast agent (iopamidol) for cardiac angiography. J Am Coll Cardiol 1985;5:250–258.

75. Wisneski JA, Gertz EW, Neese RA, et al: Absence of myocardial biochemical toxicity with a nonionic contrast agent (iopamidol). Am Heart J 1985;110:609–617.

76. Caro JJ, Trindade E, McGregor M: The risks of death and of severe nonfatal reactions with high- vs low-osmolality contrast media: a meta-analysis. AJR Am J Roentgenol 1991;156:825–832.

77. Latchaw RE: The use of nonionic contrast agents in neuroangiography: A review of the literature and recommendations for clinical use. Invest Radiol 1993;28:S55–S59.

78. Port FK, Wagoner RD, Fulton RE: Acute renal failure after angiography. Am J Roentgenol Radium Ther Nucl Med 1974;121:544–550.

79. Brezis M, Epstein FH: A closer look at radiocontrast-induced nephropathy. N Engl J Med 1989;320:179–181.

80. McClennan BL: Adverse reactions to iodinated contrast media: Recognition and response. Invest Radiol 1994;29(Suppl 1):S46–S50.

81. Stolberg HO, McClennan BL: Ionic versus nonionic contrast use. Curr Probl Diagn Radiol 1991;20:47–88.

82. McClennan BL, Stolberg HO: Intravascular contrast media. Ionic versus nonionic: Current status. Radiol Clin North Am 1991;29:437–454.

83. McClennan BL: Low-osmolality contrast media: Premises and promises. Radiology 1987;162:1–8.

84. Cohan RH, Dunnick NR: Intravascular contrast media: Adverse reactions. AJR Am J Roentgenol 1987;149:665–670.

85. King BF, Hartman GW, Williamson B Jr, et al: Low-osmolality contrast media: A current perspective. Mayo Clin Proc 1989;64:976–985.

86. Thomsen HS, Bush WHJ: Treatment of the adverse effects of contrast media. Acta Radiol 1998;39:212–218.

87. Schwab SJ, Hlatky MA, Pieper KS, et al: Contrast nephrotoxicity: A randomized controlled trial of a nonionic and an ionic radiographic contrast agent. N Engl J Med 1989;320:149–153.

88. Jacobson PD, Rosenquist CJ: The introduction of low-osmolar contrast agents in radiology: Medical, economic, legal, and public policy issues. JAMA 1988;260:1586–1592.

89. Grabowski EF, Head C, Michelson AD: Nonionic contrast media: Procoagulants or clotting innocents? Invest Radiol 1993;28(Suppl 5):S21–S24.

90. Grabowski EF: A hematologist's view of contrast media, clotting in angiography syringes and thrombosis during coronary angiography. Am J Cardiol 1990;66:23F–25F.

91. Dauchot PJ, Berzina-Moettus L, Rabinovitch A, et al: Activated coagulation and activated partial thromboplastin times in assessment and reversal of heparin-induced anticoagulation for cardiopulmonary bypass. Anesth Analg 1983;62:710–719.

92. McDonald MM, Hathaway WE: Anticoagulant therapy by continuous heparinization in newborn and older infants. J Pediatr 1982;101:451–457.

93. Low DW: Hemangiomas and vascular malformations. Semin Pediatr Surg 1994;3:40–61.

94. Hubbard AM, Fellows KE: Pediatric interventional radiology: Current practice and innovations. Cardiovasc Intervent Radiol 1993;16:267–274.

95. Kaye RD, Grifka RG, Towbin R: Intervention in the thorax in children. Radiol Clin North Am 1993;31:693–712.

96. Fox AJ, Pelz DM, Lee DH: Arteriovenous malformations of the brain: Recent results of endovascular therapy. Radiology 1990;177:51–57.

97. Brown KT, Friedman WN, Marks RA, et al: Gastric and hepatic infarction following embolization of the left gastric artery: Case report. Radiology 1989;172:731–732.

98. Allison DJ, Jordan H, Hennessy O: Therapeutic embolization of the hepatic artery: A review of 75 procedures. Lancet 1985;1:595–599.

99. Lang EV, Picus D, Marx MV, et al: Massive upper gastrointestinal hemorrhage with normal findings on arteriography: Value of prophylactic embolization of the left gastric artery. AJR Am J Roentgenol 1992;158:547–549.

100. Lang EV, Picus D, Marx MV, et al: Massive arterial hemorrhage from the stomach and lower esophagus: Impact of embolotherapy on survival. Radiology 1990;177:249–252.

101. Hanigan WC, Wright SM, Wright RM: Clinical utility of magnetic resonance imaging in pediatric neurosurgical patients. J Pediatr 1986;108:522–529.

102. Lipper EG, Ross GS, Heier L, et al: Magnetic resonance imaging in children of very low birth weight with suspected brain abnormalities. J Pediatr 1988;113:1046–1049.

103. Packer RJ, Zimmerman RA, Bilanuik LT, et al: Magnetic resonance imaging of lesions of the posterior fossa and upper cervical cord in childhood. Pediatrics 1985;76:84–90.

104. Nixon C, Hirsch NP, Ormerod IE, et al: Nuclear magnetic resonance: Its implications for the anaesthetist. Anaesthesia 1986;41:131–137.

105. Barnett GH, Ropper AH, Johnson KA: Physiological support and monitoring of critically ill patients during magnetic resonance imaging. J Neurosurg 1988;68:246–250.

106. McArdle CB, Nicholas DA, Richardson CJ, et al: Monitoring of the neonate undergoing MR imaging: Technical considerations. Work in progress. Radiology 1986;159:223–226.

107. Shellock FG: Monitoring during MRI: An evaluation of the effect of high-field MRI on various patient monitors. Med Electron 1986;17:93–97.

108. Keeler EK, Casey FX, Engels H, et al: Accessory equipment considerations with respect to MRI compatibility. J Magn Reson Imaging 1998;8:12–18.

109. Rotello LC, Radin EJ, Jastremski MS, et al: MRI protocol for critically ill patients. Am J Crit Care 1994;3:187–190.

110. Tobin JR, Spurrier EA, Wetzel RC: Anaesthesia for critically ill children during magnetic resonance imaging. Br J Anaesth 1992;69:482–486.

111. Shellock FG, Crues VJ: Safety considerations in magnetic resonance imaging. Magn Reson Imaging Decisions 1988;2:25–30.

112. Budinger TF: Nuclear magnetic resonance (NMR) in vivo studies: Known thresholds for health effects. J Comput Assist Tomogr 1981;5:800–811.

113. Shellock FG, Morisoli S, Kanal E: MR procedures and biomedical implants, materials, and devices: 1993 update. Radiology 1993;189:587–599.

114. Kanal E, Shellock FG, Talagala L: Safety considerations in MR imaging. Radiology 1990;176:593–606.

115. Shellock FG: Biological effects and safety aspects of magnetic resonance imaging. Magn Reson Q 1989;5:243–261.

116. Laptook AR: Magnetic resonance: Safety considerations and future directions. Semin Perinatol 1990;14:189–192.

117. Dujovny M, Kossovsky N, Kossowsky R, et al: Aneurysm clip motion during magnetic resonance imaging: In vivo experimental study with metallurgical factor analysis. Neurosurgery 1985;17:543–548.

118. Fowler JR, ter Penning B, Syverud SA, et al: Magnetic field hazard. N Engl J Med 1986;314:1517.

119. Bailey WH, Su SH, Bracken TD, et al: Summary and evaluation of guidelines for occupational exposure to power frequency electric and magnetic fields. Health Phys 1997;73:433–453.

120. Miller G: Exposure guidelines for magnetic fields. Am Ind Hyg Assoc J 1987;48:957–968.

121. Duffy FJJ, May JWJ. Tissue expanders and magnetic resonance imaging: the "hot" breast implant. Ann Plast Surg 1995;35:647–649.

122. Gold JP, Pulsinelli W, Winchester P, et al: Safety of metallic surgical clips in patients undergoing high-field-strength magnetic resonance imaging. Ann Thorac Surg 1989;48:643–645.

123. Barrafato D, Henkelman RM: Magnetic resonance imaging and surgical clips. Can J Surg 1984;27:509–510.

124. Kelly WM, Paglen PG, Pearson JA, et al: Ferromagnetism of intraocular foreign body causes unilateral blindness after MR study. AJNR Am J Neuroradiol 1986;7:243–245.

125. Kanal E, Shellock FG: The value of published data on MR compatibility of metallic implants and devices. AJNR Am J Neuroradiol 1994;15:1394–1396.

126. Kanal E, Shellock FG, Lewin JS: Aneurysm clip testing for ferromagnetic properties: Clip variability issues. Radiology 1996;200:576–578.

127. Sullivan PK, Smith JF, Rozzelle AA: Cranio-orbital reconstruction: Safety and image quality of metallic implants on CT and MRI scanning. Plast Reconstr Surg 1994;94:589–596.

128. Sommer T, Lauck G, Schimpf R, et al: MRI in patients with cardiac pacemakers: In vitro and in vivo evaluation at 0.5 tesla. [in German]. Rofo Fortschr Geb Rontgenstr Neuen Bildgeb Verfahr 1994;168:36–43.

129. Hofman MB, de Cock CC, van der Linden JC, et al: Transesophageal cardiac pacing during magnetic resonance imaging: Feasibility and safety considerations. Magn Reson Med 1996;35:413–422.

130. Beers GJ: Biological effects of weak electromagnetic fields from 0 Hz to 200 MHz: A survey of the literature with special emphasis on possible magnetic resonance effects. Magn Reson Imaging 1989;7:309–331.

131. Anonymous: Magnetic resonance imaging of the cardiovascular system. Present state of the art and future potential. Council on Scientific Affairs. Report of the Magnetic Resonance Imaging Panel. JAMA 1988;259:253–259.

132. Youngson JH, Clayden AD, Myers A, et al: A case/control study of adult haematological malignancies in relation to overhead power lines. Br J Cancer 1991;63:977–985.

133. Weikl A, Moshage W, Hentschel D, et al: ECG changes caused by the effect of static magnetic fields of nuclear magnetic resonance tomography using magnets with a field power of 0.5 to 4.0 Telsa. [in German]. Z Kardiol 1989;78:578–586.

134. Smith DS, Askey P, Young ML, et al: Anesthetic management of acutely ill patients during magnetic resonance imaging. Anesthesiology 1986;65:710–711.

135. Roth JL, Nugent M, Gray JE, et al: Patient monitoring during magnetic resonance imaging. Anesthesiology 1985;62:80–83.

136. Geiger RS, Cascorbi HF: Anesthesia in an NMR scanner. Anesth Analg 1984;63:622–623.

137. Boutros A, Pavlicek W: Anesthesia for magnetic resonance imaging. Anesth Analg 1987;66:367.

138. Rao CC, McNiece WL, Emhardt J, et al: Modification of an anesthesia machine for use during magnetic resonance imaging. Anesthesiology 1988;68:640–641.

139. Ramsay JG, Gale L, Sykes MK: A ventilator for use in nuclear magnetic resonance studies. Br J Anaesth 1986;58:1181–1184.

140. Flaherty JA, Hoskinson K: Emotional distress during magnetic resonance imaging. N Engl J Med 1989;320:467–468.

141. Quirk ME, Letendre AJ, Ciottone RA, et al: Anxiety in patients undergoing MR imaging. Radiology 1989;170:463–466.

142. Fishbain DA, Goldberg M, Labbe E, et al: Long-term claustrophobia following magnetic resonance imaging. Am J Psychiatry 1988;145:1038–1039.

143. Beekman RP, Hoorntje TM, Beek FJ, et al: Sedation for children undergoing magnetic resonance imaging: Efficacy and safety of rectal thiopental. Eur J Pediatr 1996;155:820–822.

144. Vangerven M, Van Hemelrijck J, Wouters P, et al: Light anaesthesia with propofol for paediatric MRI. Anaesthesia 1992;47:706–707.

145. Marti-Bonmati L, Ronchera-Oms CL, Casillas C, et al: Randomized double-blind clinical trial of intermediate- versus high-dose chloral hydrate for neuroimaging of children. Neuroradiology 1995;37:687–691.

146. Badgwell JM, Wolf AR, McEvedy BA, et al: Fresh gas formulae do not accurately predict end-tidal PCO_2 in paediatric patients. Can J Anaesth 1988;35:581–586.

147. Brown TR, Goldstein B, Little J: Severe burns resulting from magnetic resonance imaging with cardiopulmonary monitoring: Risks and relevant safety precautions. Am J Phys Med Rehabil 1993;72:166–167.

148. Kanal E, Shellock FG: Burns associated with clinical MR examinations. Radiology 1990;175:585.

149. Kanal E, Shellock FG: Patient monitoring during clinical MR imaging. Radiology 1992;185:623–629.

150. Dimick RN, Hedlund LW, Herfkens RJ, et al: Optimizing electrocardiograph electrode placement for cardiac-gated magnetic resonance imaging. Invest Radiol 1987;22:17–22.

151. Wendt RE 3d, Rokey R, Vick GW 3d, et al: Electrocardiographic gating and monitoring in NMR imaging. Magn Reson Imaging 1988;6:89–95.

152. Wong WF, Rokey R, Wendt RE 3d, et al: An electrocardiograph-respiration gating device for MR studies. J Magn Reson Imaging 1992;2:233–235.

153. Rokey R, Wendt RE, Johnston DL: Monitoring of acutely ill patients during nuclear magnetic resonance imaging: Use of a time-varying filter electrocardiographic gating device to reduce gradient artifacts. Magn Reson Med 1988;6:240–245.

154. Sellden H, de Chateau P, Ekman G, et al: Circulatory monitoring of children during anaesthesia in low-field magnetic resonance imaging. Acta Anaesthesiol Scand 1990;34:41–43.

155. Crapanzano MS, Strong WB, Newman IR, et al: Calf blood pressure: Clinical implications and correlations with arm blood pressure in infants and young children. Pediatrics 1996;97:220–224.

156. Shellock FG, Slimp GL: Severe burn of the finger caused by using a pulse oximeter during MR imaging. AJR Am J Roentgenol 1989;153:1105.

157. Bashein G, Syrory G: Burns associated with pulse oximetry during magnetic resonance imaging. Anesthesiology 1991;75:382–383.

158. Brodrick PM, Webster NR, Nunn JF: The laryngeal mask airway: A study of 100 patients during spontaneous breathing. Anaesthesia 1989;44:238–241.

159. Grebenik CR, Ferguson C, White A: The laryngeal mask airway in pediatric radiotherapy. Anesthesiology 1990;72:474–477.

160. Bashein G, Russell AH, Momii ST: Anesthesia and remote monitoring for intraoperative radiation therapy. Anesthesiology 1986;64:804–807.

161. Friesen RH, Morrison JEJ, Verbrugge JJ, et al: Anesthesia for intraoperative radiation therapy in children. J Surg Oncol 1987;35:96–98.

162. Brett CM, Wara WM, Hamilton WK: Anesthesia for infants during radiotherapy: An insufflation technique. Anesthesiology 1986;64:402–405.

163. Griswold JD, Vacanti FX, Goudsouzian NG: Twenty-three sequential out-of-hospital halothane anesthetics in an infant. Anesth Analg 1988;67:779–781.

164. Schurizek BA, Rybro L, Boggild-Madsen NB, et al: Gastric volume and pH in children for emergency surgery. Acta Anaesthesiol Scand 1986;30:404–408.

165. Coté CJ, Goudsouzian NG, Liu LM, et al: Assessment of risk factors related to the acid aspiration syndrome in pediatric patients-gastric pH and residual volume. Anesthesiology 1982;56:70–72.

166. Coté CJ: NPO after midnight for children: A reappraisal. Anesthesiology 1990;72:589–592.

167. Carson IW, Moore J, Balmer JP, et al: Laryngeal competence with ketamine and other drugs. Anesthesiology 1973;38:128–133.

168. Nishino T, Takizawa K, Yokokawa N, et al: Depression of the swallowing reflex during sedation and/or relative analgesia produced by inhalation of 50% nitrous oxide in oxygen. Anesthesiology 1987;67:995–998.

169. Litman RS, Berkowitz RJ, Ward DS: Levels of consciousness and ventilatory parameters in young children during sedation with oral midazolam and nitrous oxide. Arch Pediatr Adolesc Med 1996;150:671–675.

26 Pediatric Sedation for Diagnostic and Therapeutic Procedures Outside the Operating Room

Richard F. Kaplan, Myron Yaster, Maureen A. Strafford, *and* Charles J. Coté

Definition of Levels of Sedation

Goals of Sedation

Risks and Complications Associated with Sedation

Guidelines

    Before Sedation

    During Sedation

    Post-Sedation Care

Implementation of Successful Sedation Guidelines

    Institution-Wide

    Department-Wide

Specific Sedation Techniques

    Local Anesthetics

    Anxiolytics

    Systemic Anesthetics

Establishment of a Sedation Service

Sedation and analgesia for diagnostic and therapeutic procedures performed by anesthesiologists and nonanesthesiologists outside of the operating room has dramatically increased.[1] Great progress has been made in the understanding of sedation and analgesia within and outside of the operating room.[2] The mere restraint of a child for a frightening or painful procedure is clearly unjustified.[3–6] Opioids and nonopioids, local anesthetics, and regional techniques are commonly used for the treatment of acute intraoperative and postoperative pain.[7–9] Procedures performed outside of the operating room require the same attention to anxiolysis, analgesia, and sedation as procedures performed in the operating room. Painful procedures that frequently are performed outside of the operating room (bone marrow aspiration, lumbar puncture, repair of minor surgical wounds, insertion of arterial or venous catheters, burn dressing changes, fracture reduction, bronchoscopy, endoscopy) require analgesia and often sedation, which may reach deep sedation or general anesthesia levels.

Sedation and immobility are often required for nonpainful procedures. Patients undergoing diagnostic studies (computed tomography, magnetic resonance imaging, positron emission tomography, electroencephalography, electromyelography) or who require high doses of ionizing radiation must be absolutely motionless and immobile for 10 to 90 minutes, or longer.[10] Young children, as well as the developmentally and medically handicapped, are simply unable to remain motionless for even short periods of time. Many older children and adults are unable to enter the confined space and often frightening environment of a diagnostic imaging scanner. The fear and anxiety associated with procedures is difficult to control and may be exacerbated by parental anxiety, separation from parents, and the pain or anticipation of pain from the procedure. Although distraction, guided imagery, and the use of videos and music have clear and documented benefit, they are often not enough to efficiently and successfully complete procedures.[11–14]

Another reason for the increase in procedures outside of the operating room that require sedation and analgesia is the emphasis by managed care providers on lowering costs. It is assumed that sedation and analgesia for diagnostic and therapeutic procedures can be provided more cheaply, conveniently, and "efficiently" outside of the operating room. Thus, procedures in children such as central line placement, bone marrow aspiration, bronchoscopy, and endoscopy, which in the past may have been performed in an operating or recovery room under sedation or general anesthesia by an anesthesiologist, are now performed in offices or special procedure rooms, often without the direct supervision of an anesthesiologist.

These new environments and new expectations of sedation and analgesia for diagnostic and therapeutic procedures outside the operating room require appropriate definitions, goals, guidelines, monitoring, and adequate personnel to decrease the risk for pediatric patients. Since anesthesiologists are usually consulted to help develop within-institution guidelines for sedation as required by the Joint Commission on Accreditation of Healthcare Organizations (JCAHO), this chapter includes a number of tables and figures that can be used as templates of information for properly trained nonanesthesiologists.[15]

Definition of Levels of Sedation

Sedation and analgesia for procedures represent a continuum of consciousness to unconsciousness with three levels most commonly described: conscious sedation, deep sedation, and general anesthesia. Sedation and analgesia for procedures is a continuum (Fig. 26–1); a patient may easily pass from a light level of sedation to general anesthesia.[16, 17] A clear understanding of the definition of sedation is mandatory to recognize when the child has progressed from sedation and analgesia (conscious sedation) to deep sedation or from deep sedation to general anesthesia. Recognition of this transition allows escalation of monitoring and care to avoid complications. The American Academy of Pediatrics (AAP) formalized and defined the concepts of conscious sedation, deep sedation, and general anesthesia as follows[16, 17]:

Conscious sedation: a medically controlled state of depressed consciousness that (1) allows protective reflexes to be maintained; (2) retains the ability to

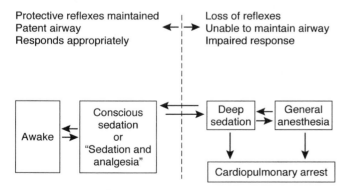

Figure 26–1. The sedation continuum: A patient may readily pass from a light level of sedation to deep sedation. Health care providers must be prepared to increase vigilance and intensity of monitoring consistent with the depth of sedation. One must consider all children under the age of 6 years as deeply sedated, since "conscious sedation" in this age group for most patients is an oxymoron.

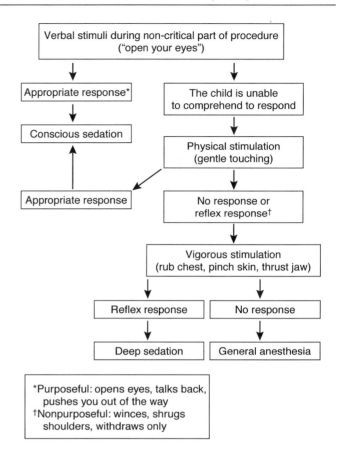

Figure 26–2. Sedated patients must be continuously evaluated for depth of sedation and appropriateness of response. As diagrammed in Figure 26–1, sedation is a continuum. A child should only be considered "consciously sedated" if he or she is able to make a purposeful response, not a reflex withdrawal from a painful stimulus.

maintain a patent airway independently and continuously; and (3) permits appropriate responses by the patient to physical stimulation or verbal commands, e.g., "Open your eyes."

Deep sedation: a medically controlled state of depressed consciousness or unconsciousness from which the patient is not easily aroused. It may be accompanied by a partial or complete loss of protective reflexes, and includes the inability to maintain a patent airway independently and respond purposefully to physical stimulation or verbal command.

General anesthesia: a medically controlled state of unconsciousness accompanied by a loss of protective reflexes, including the inability to maintain an airway independently and respond purposefully to physical stimulation or verbal command.

The assessment of the depth of sedation based on response to stimulation is illustrated in Figure 26–2. A common problem with the assessment of the sedated child is to interpret any movement in response to pain as "appropriate" and therefore a sign of "conscious sedation." A child who is consciously sedated should respond to pain by saying "ouch," pushing your hand away, and pulling the covers over himself or herself. Reflex withdrawal from pain is considered a sign of deep sedation and not conscious sedation and should lead to escalation of care of the patient, since respiratory depression may occur.[1, 18–20] To reduce confusion surrounding these definitions, the American Society of Anesthesiologists (ASA) specifically rephrased *conscious sedation* to *sedation and analgesia*.[21]

Many, if not most, procedures in children requiring sedation can be carried out only during deep sedation.[1, 20] The achievement of a state of anxiolysis and immobility during a painful or frightening procedure in small children using "conscious" sedation is extremely difficult. Furthermore, small children can quickly move from conscious to deep sedation with loss of airway reflexes. It should therefore be assumed that children less than 6 years old will require a level of vigilance consistent with that required for deep sedation.[20] We view the phrase "conscious sedation" to be an oxymoron for children younger than 6 years of age.

Goals of Sedation

The goals of pediatric sedation can be summarized as follows[20]:

- Guard the patient's safety and welfare
- Minimize physical discomfort or pain
- Minimize negative psychological responses to treatment by providing analgesia and anxiolysis and maximize the potential for amnesia
- Control behavior
- Return the patient to a state in which safe discharge is possible.

Risks and Complications Associated with Sedation

The foremost goal is to optimize patient safety by minimizing complications. There are numerous case reports describing pediatric sedation complications but few hard data on the frequency of adverse events (numerator) compared to the total number of sedations (denominator).

$$\text{Risk} = \frac{\text{Numerator}}{\text{Denominator}} = \frac{\text{Number of Adverse Events}}{\text{Number of Patients Sedated}}$$

It is likely that the cases of adverse outcome reported represent the tip of the pyramid (Fig. 26–3). Inherent problems with these calculations include age of patient, underlying disease, level of sedation, type of drug, monitors, personnel, guidelines used for sedation, severity of event, and experience and type of practitioner.

One of the most extensive surveys on risks in sedation involving pediatric dentistry was carried out in 1982.[22] Three thousand questionnaires given to pediatric dentists were reviewed for sedation complications. Seventy-four percent of adverse reactions did not require hospitalization, whereas 26% required intubation and life support. The overall incidence of adverse events was 1 in 5000 if narcotics were administered and 1 in 20,000 for patients sedated with non-narcotics. Death and morbidity was 1 in 10,000 when narcotics were administered and less when non-narcotics were administered.

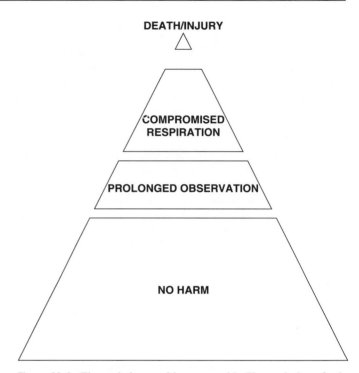

Figure 26–3. The sedation accident pyramid: The majority of adverse sedation events result in no harm. A smaller number result in no harm but require prolonged observation. An even smaller number result in the need for some intervention, usually related to respirations (repositioning the head, a jaw thrust, bag/mask respirations/intubation). A very small number result in injury or death because the sentinel event was missed or inadequately treated. The latter cases are the types that occasionally are reported in newspapers, but generally they go unreported. The reported cases likely represent just the tip of the pyramid in terms of events that could have indicated a developing problem.

Additional studies have used the guidelines of the AAP[17] and focus on the more common signs of patient compromise such as the incidence of respiratory and cardiovascular complications.

Radiologic procedures with sedation (computed tomography or magnetic resonance imaging) were studied in 400 children less than 4 years old.[23] Chloral hydrate, chloral hydrate plus hydroxyzine, and meperidine in typical doses were used and the AAP guidelines were followed. Mild hypoxia (90–95% SaO_2) occurred in 5% of children 1 to 4 years old and 9% of children less than 1 year old. Severe hypoxia ($< 90\%$ SaO_2) occurred in 0.5% of patients. There was no permanent disability. Another study showed a 50% incidence of SaO_2 less than 90% in newborns given chloral hydrate (75 mg/kg PO) or midazolam (0.2 mg/kg IV).[24]

A *pediatric emergency department* retrospectively studied 487 patients given the classic "lytic cocktail," Demerol, Phenergan, and Thorazine (DPT) (2:1:1 mg/kg, respectively).[25] A 0.6% incidence of severe respiratory depression requiring naloxone was observed.

Upper *gastrointestinal endoscopy* in 34 patients (age, 2 months to 18 years) has also been studied.[26] Children were given meperidine, diazepam, or midazolam or a combination of these. Monitoring included pulse oximetry and electrocardiography (ECG). Sixty-eight percent of normal patients had hemoglobin saturations less than 90%; 75% of normal patients had arrhythmias. No adverse outcomes were reported.

One study has reviewed contributing factors from adverse sedation events.[27] Adverse sedation event information was derived from the Food and Drug Administration's adverse drug event self-reporting system,[28] the U.S. Pharmacopoeia Reports of Adverse Events, and a survey of over 1000 pediatric specialists (pediatric anesthesiologists, intensivists, and emergency physicians). One hundred eighteen incidents from hospital and non-hospital settings were reviewed and consensus agreement as to contributory causes was found on 95 cases. Outcomes included death (51), neurologic injury (9), prolonged hospital stay (21), and no harm (14). The initial adverse events were respiratory (80%) in both hospital- and non-hospital-based settings. Other causes of adverse sedation events included drug-drug interactions, inadequate monitoring, inadequate medical evaluation, lack of an independent observer, and inadequate management of resuscitation. There were more cardiac arrests as a second event, more neurologic injury, and more deaths in the non-hospital-based settings compared with hospital settings despite the fact that non-hospital-based adverse events occurred in older and healthier patients (lower ASA status) (Table 26–1). Successful outcome was related to the use of pulse oximetry compared with patients without any monitoring. Seventy-eight percent of adverse outcomes in patients who were not monitored resulted in death or neurologic injury, whereas 24% of patients who were monitored with pulse oximetry died or had neurologic injury. All patients monitored with pulse oximetry in a hospital-based venue were rescued without injury.

Conclusions from the above studies include the following:

- ALL classes of drugs (sedatives, barbiturates, benzodiazepines, and narcotics) have been associated with problems even when administered in "recommended doses."
- ALL areas using sedation have reported adverse events.
- Children 1 to 6 years of age are at greatest risk. Most had no severe underlying disease.
- Respiratory depression, airway obstruction, desaturation, and apnea are the most frequently encountered initial adverse events.

Table 26–1. Adverse Sedation Events: Hospital-Based Versus Non-Hospital-Based Events in Children Sedated by Nonanesthesiologists

Adverse Events	Hospital-Based	Non-Hospital-Based
Age ± SD (years)	3.8 ± 3.82	6.97 ± 5.75
ASA physical status I & II (%)	56	89
Primary event—respiratory (%)	80	80
Secondary event—cardiac arrest (%)	14	54
Inadequate resuscitation (%)	2	57
Outcome—death or neurologic injury (%)	37	92

Abstracted from Coté CJ, Notterman DA, Karl HW, et al: Adverse sedation events in pediatrics: A critical incident analysis of contributory factors. Pediatrics 2000;105:805–814.

- Adverse events involved multiple drugs (especially three or more sedating medications), drug errors or overdose, inadequate medical evaluation, inadequate monitoring, inadequate practitioner skills, and premature discharge.
- Most complications from sedation were avoidable.
- Uniform guidelines for both in-hospital and out-of-hospital sedation must include appropriate personnel skilled in airway management and resuscitation.
- Health-care personnel who sedate children for procedures must have advanced airway and resuscitation skills so as to successfully manage complications and rescue the patient.

It is clear that a dramatic decrease in risk has occurred with the initiation of guidelines but that more progress in the areas listed above must continue. In particular, rigid application of the AAP guidelines combined with advanced airway and resuscitation skills would likely improve outcomes of adverse sedation-related events in all venues and in particular, non-hospital-based venues. Pediatric anesthesiologists must become more involved with training and education of our nonanesthesiology colleagues who sedate children. More importantly, we must help develop screening processes that will divert all high-risk patients (ASA physical status 3 or 4) to the care of an anesthesiologist or other health-care providers with the necessary training, skills, and experience.

Guidelines

Many professional societies have established practice guidelines for the care of children and adults who are being sedated for diagnostic or therapeutic procedures outside of the operating room. These organizations include the ASA,[21] the American Academy of Pediatric Dentistry,[29–31] the American College of Emergency Physicians,[32] the American College of Radiologists,[33] and the AAP.[16, 17]

The guidelines vary in their definitions, monitoring, and personnel requirements. In 1992, the Committee on Drugs of the AAP updated its sedation policy and placed emphasis on monitoring and a systematic approach, hence the revised title: "Guidelines for Monitoring and Management of Pediatric Patients During and After Sedation for Diagnostic and Therapeutic Procedures."[17] The guidelines are directed toward nonanesthesiologists who provide sedation outside of the operating room since operating room practice by anesthesiologists is guided by guidelines and practice parameters of the ASA. The AAP guidelines were established with the consultation of the Section on Anesthesiology of the AAP, the Committee on Standards of the ASA, the Committee on Pediatric Anesthesiology of the ASA, and the Society for Pediatric Anesthesia. The AAP definitions and guidelines were the first sedation guidelines developed, have been endorsed by all of the subspecialty committees of the AAP, and are the most widely used guidelines for sedation.[16, 17] They are the most consistent with recent JCAHO requirements for sedation.[15] They also, in the opinion of the authors, provide the largest safety margin for pediatric patients and have appropriate recommendations for escalation of care of the deeply sedated child. The guidelines also acknowledge the fine line between deep sedation and general anesthesia. The AAP guidelines present a systematic approach to sedation, which includes presedation medical evaluation with a focused airway examination, informed consent, appropriate fasting, appropriate laboratory testing, procedural monitoring, and continuation of that monitoring through recovery, age- and size-appropriate equipment, adequate personnel, and strict discharge criteria. The AAP guidelines therefore are recommended and elaborated upon in this chapter. The guidelines were meant to establish a *uniform* level of care throughout all subspecialties providing pediatric sedation. The AAP guidelines are divided into before sedation, during sedation, and post-sedation categories.[17] Anesthesiologists are encouraged to use the AAP guidelines as a template for their own institutional guidelines.

Before Sedation

Facilities, personnel, and equipment must be immediately available to treat emergency situations arising from sedation.[17] These complications include vomiting, aspiration, seizures, anaphylaxis, respiratory depression, airway obstruction, apnea, and cardiac arrest. A protocol for *back-up emergency services* shall be clearly identified. In non-hospital environments, ambulance services must be assured. *On-site* equipment of appropriate sizes must be immediately available and include the following:

- Positive-pressure O_2 delivery system (90% O_2 for $\geq$ 60 min) (checked before each sedation)
- Suction and catheters
- Noninvasive blood pressure measurement equipment
- Pulse oximetry
- Emergency cart with age- and size-appropriate drugs and equipment

Sedatives should not be administered at home or in an area unsupervised by medically trained personnel, since unrecognized complications may lead to disaster. There are anecdotal reports of children who have been injured or died when they were given appropriate doses of chloral hydrate or midazolam at home in anticipation of a procedure in an office.[27] One child, placed in a car seat during transport, apparently became deeply sedated, had airway obstruction, and died. Sedatives should be administered only by appropriately trained health-care providers and only in a facility where appropriate monitoring and personnel are available.

Documentation before sedation must include the following[17]:

1. Informed consent in accordance with local, state, and institutional guidelines.
2. Verbal and written instructions to the responsible person. These shall include the objectives of sedation, anticipated changes in behavior, discharge instructions, and a 24-hour telephone number for follow-up. Examples of presedation (phone and written) instructions used in radiology and dentistry are presented in Figures 26–4 and 26–5.
3. *Dietary precautions* must be clearly stated and documented for elective sedation (Table 26–2). Elective patients at risk for aspiration (e.g., uncontrolled gastroesophageal reflux, obesity, pregnancy) may benefit from drugs to decrease gastric volume and/or acidity. In emergency situations in which appropriate NPO status cannot

Table 26–2. Recommended Preprocedural Sedation Fasting

Age (mo)	Recommendation
0–5	No milk or solids for 4 hours*
6–36	No milk or solids for 6 hours*
>36	No milk or solids for 8 hours*

*Clear liquids (water, apple juice, Jell-O, etc.) may continue for up to 2 hours before the procedure.

Breast milk is considered "milk" and should be withheld for 4 hours before the procedure.

Data from Committee on Drugs, American Academy of Pediatrics: Guidelines for monitoring and management of pediatric patients during and after sedation for diagnostic and therapeutic procedures. Pediatrics 1992;89:1110–1115.

be established, the lightest effective level of sedation should be used. An emergency patient may require intubation to protect the airway before sedation.

4. A *health evaluation* performed by a licensed practitioner must be done. The evaluation must include the following:
   - Age and weight
   - Health history: allergies, drug usage, relevant diseases, physical abnormalities, pregnancy status, history of sedation or general anesthesia, relevant family history
   - Review of systems: especially note airway problems (loud snoring and obstructive sleep apnea, recent colds, croup), poorly controlled asthma, cyanosis, congestive heart failure, central nervous system abnormalities, and seizure history
   - Physical examination, especially a focused airway examination looking for anatomic airway abnormalities (large tonsils, hypoplastic mandible, midfacial hypoplasia, cervical spine abnormalities) is required
   - Vital signs: heart rate, blood pressure, respiratory rate, and temperature
   - ASA physical status classification.

A detailed health evaluation is critical in identifying children whose underlying medical conditions may place them at increased risk for sedation complications. These patients should be referred to an anesthesiologist or other qualified specialist for sedation. Of particular concern is upper airway obstruction that would likely become worse with the administration of sedatives.[27] Tonsil and adenoid hypertrophy are common in this age group and associated with loud snoring or obstructive sleep apnea. Parents will frequently tell the practitioner that their child snores loudly and then "stops breathing." These children are at increased risk for airway obstruction and should be referred to an airway specialist (anesthesiologist, pediatric intensivist, pediatric emergency medicine specialist) for procedures requiring any sedation.[34, 35] Problems for which consultation with an anesthesiologist is suggested are as follows:

1. Medical problems
   - ASA III or IV status
   - Pulmonary-airway obstruction (tonsils/adenoids): loud snoring, obstructive sleep apnea; poorly controlled asthma
   - Morbid obesity ($\geq$ two times ideal body weight)
   - Cardiovascular conditions: cyanosis, congestive heart failure

DEPARTMENT OF PEDIATRIC RADIOLOGY

PATIENT SEDATION PHONE CALL FORM

Exam Name _____ completed by _____

Exam Date _____ Time _____ message by _____

Patient Name _____ Age _____ Phone Number _____

Diagnosis _____

Interpreter services needed _____ yes or _____ no

Quick review of current medical history:

1)   Any current cold symptoms fever or rash? _____

2)   Any history of reflux, snoring and/or apnea? _____ Is your child on any monitor at night?

3)   Any prior sedation(s) _____ When? _____ Medication(s) used? _____

4)   Any history of developmental delay, behavior problems, and/or autism? _____

5)   Any significant medical/surgical/respiratory history? (such as asthma) or heart disease? _____

6)   Current medications? (may take medications with a sip of water) _____

Pre-exam instructions given to: _____ Date _____

1)   Since this procedure has been scheduled with sedation, you will need to sign in at the MRI/CT reception desk no later than _____ (*2 hours early for CT Abdomen) to avoid having your child's exam delayed or rescheduled.

2)   In preparation for the exam, your child may not have any milk or milk products, formula or solid foods after _____. He/she is not to have anything by mouth after _____.

3)   We require the presence and signature of a parent or legal guardian for all procedures.

4)   You will need to arrange to be here with your child for a minimum of 3-4 hours for the testing and recovery phase. Please note that other children are not permitted in the testing area for safety reasons.

5)   If your child has a stuffy nose, fever, productive cough, or any significant medical/surgical or respiratory history such as: heart disease, asthma, or any other breathing problems we may not be able to proceed with the sedation as scheduled. Please call to speak with a Radiology Nurse for further instructions. To reschedule an exam please call.

6)   Please remember to bring your Insurance Card, referral and/or authorization #, if required, to avoid having your child's exam delayed or rescheduled.

7)   Thank you for your time and we look forward to seeing you tomorrow at _____ (arrival time).

8)   Picc Lines Only: Consent signed or parent present or # where parents can be reached _____
                *(If parent is present have them come to MRI area so consent can be obtained)

9)   Inpatients Only: must have working IV _____ any precautions? _____ how do they travel? _____
                We will need parent present or phone number where parent can be reached for consent _____

	NPO TIMES vs. AGE GROUPS				NPO TIMES vs. AGE GROUPS		
	0-5M	6-36M	>36M		0-5M	6-36M	>36M
EXAM TIME				**EXAM TIME**			
0700	0300	0100	2300	1045	0645	0445	0245
0745	0345	0145	2345	1100	0700	0500	0300
0800	0400	0200	2400	1130	0730	0530	0330
0830	0430	0230	2430	1200 & 1215	0800	0600	0400
0900 & 0915	0500	0300	0100	1300	0900	0700	0500
1000	0600	0400	0200	1345	0945	0745	0545
1030	0630	0430	0230	1400	1000	0800	0600
				1500	1100	0900	0700

Figure 26–4. Sample patient sedation phone call form. (Courtesy of Children's National Medical Center, Washington, DC.)

DEPARTMENT OF PEDIATRIC DENTISTRY

PREOPERATIVE INSTRUCTIONS FOR DENTAL TREATMENT UNDER SEDATION

1.   WHAT IS SEDATION?

Your child needs to receive a mild sedative prior to receiving dental treatment. This sedative is given as a liquid by mouth or as a suppository one-half to one hour prior to the scheduled dental appointment.

2.   HISTORY AND PHYSICAL EXAM

Your child needs a complete physical examination within one month of the sedation appointment. The examination is performed by your primary care physician, who must fill out completely the Short Hospital Admission Form that we give you. You are responsible for bringing to us the completed Short Hospital Admission Form. WITHOUT THE COMPLETED FORM, THE SEDATION APPOINTMENT WILL BE CANCELED.

3.   NO SOLID FOOD BY MOUTH AFTER MIDNIGHT BEFORE THE SURGERY

Your child may drink clear liquids (apple juice, water, Kool-aid ™) until 4 hours before the procedure.

4.   IF YOUR CHILD BECOMES ILL

If your child has any signs of a cold, such as a runny nose, cough or congestion, please call the clinic at (202) 884-2160. Please also call us if your child is exposed to any communicable disease such as measles, mumps or chicken pox within 3 weeks of the sedation appointment.

5.   AFTER THE SEDATION APPOINTMENT

After the sedation appointment, please expect your child to be drowsy and require support. Someone should be available to drive the patient home. Plan on limited activity. You will need to give your child water, clear fluids and soft foods until he/she is able to tolerate a normal diet.

6.   PLEASE ARRIVE AT THE DENTAL CLINIC PROMPTLY AT _____ ON _____,
_____.

You must plan on remaining in the Dental Clinic during your child's entire dental appointment.

Figure 26–5. Sample preoperative instruction sheet for dental treatment performed on a sedated patient. (Courtesy of Children's National Medical Center, Washington, DC.)

- Prematurity, less than 60 weeks of post-conceptual age: residual pulmonary, cardiovascular, gastrointestinal, neurologic problems
- Neurologic conditions: poorly controlled seizures, central apnea
- Gastrointestinal conditions: uncontrolled gastroesophageal reflux

2. Procedures requiring deep sedation in patients with a full stomach
3. Management problems
   - Severe developmental delay
   - Patients who are difficult to control
   - History of failed sedation
   - Oversedation
   - Hyperactive (paradoxical) response to sedatives

It is important to review the child's presedation medications. Particular note must be made of the use of protease inhibitors by many patients with human immunodeficiency virus infection. These protease inhibitors (e.g., nelfinavir, ritonavir, saquinavir) are potent inhibitors of the cytochrome P450 CYP3A metabolic pathway. This pathway is responsible for the metabolism of many sedatives, including midazolam and may markedly prolong its duration of action and may lead to life-threatening respiratory depression. Erythromycin and some calcium channel blockers may also inhibit the cytochrome system and delay metabolism of midazolam.[36-38]

During Sedation

The AAP guidelines require a minimum of two persons during sedation.[17] The practitioner must be competent to use and administer sedatives, provide appropriate monitoring, and manage complications. Training in pediatric basic life support is required. Pediatric advanced life support is strongly recommended. The second person (assistant) is responsible for monitoring and assisting in supportive care and resuscitation. The assistant is encouraged to have pediatric basic life support training. *If the child becomes deeply sedated, one person must have as his or her sole responsibility the role of constantly observing the patient's vital signs, airway patency, and adequacy of ventilation.*

Documentation should occur on a time-based "sedation flow sheet" similar to an anesthesia record. An example of a sedation flow sheet is given in Figure 26–6. The sedation flow sheet should be uniform throughout the institution and designed to be easy to use, complete, and comprehensive such that filling out the form will ensure that all aspects of the AAP guidelines (presedation, sedation, post-sedation) are followed. The flow sheet should have guidelines and instructions on the back, which answer questions that are commonly asked regarding the sedation process.

Baseline vital signs shall be documented on the sedation flow sheet. The name, route, time of administration, and dosage of all drugs administered must be recorded. There must be continuous quantitative monitoring of oxygen saturation and heart rate, such as by pulse oximetry. The time-based sedation flow sheet must contain intermittent recording of respiratory rate, heart rate, oxygen saturation, and blood pressure as well as the patient's level of consciousness and responsiveness. Although not specified, the typical time interval for recording data during sedation and analgesia (conscious sedation) is every 15 minutes unless this interferes with the procedure (e.g., inappropriate time for response to stimulation). *If the child becomes deeply sedated, then vital signs must be documented at least every 5 minutes.* A summary of monitoring, documentation, personnel, and equipment during sedation is given in Table 26–3.

Post-Sedation Care

The child must recover in a facility that has a functioning suction apparatus and the capacity to deliver 90% or greater

Table 26–3. Recommended Intensity of Monitoring, Documentation, Personnel, and Equipment for Different Levels of Sedation

	Conscious Sedation	Deep Sedation
Monitoring	Pulse oximetry continuous Heart rate continuous Respiratory rate every 15 min Level of consciousness every 15 min (if possible)	Pulse oximetry continuous Heart rate continuous Respiratory rate every 5 min Blood pressure every 15 min Level of consciousness every 5 min (if possible)
Documentation	Pulse oximetry every 15 min Heart rate every 15 min Respiratory rate every 15 min Blood pressure every 15 min Level of consciousness every 15 min, if possible	Pulse oximetry every 15 min Heart rate every 5 min Respiratory rate every 5 min Blood pressure every 5 min Level of consciousness every 5 min, if possible
Personnel	Same individual may observe patient and assist with procedure.	*Dedicated independent observer—may not assist with procedure.*
Equipment	Pulse oximeter Blood pressure device Stethoscope	Pulse oximeter Blood pressure device Stethoscope Electrocardiographic monitor and defibrillator immediately available
Airway Equipment	Age- and size-appropriate	Age- and size-appropriate

Data from Committee on Drugs, American Academy of Pediatrics: Guidelines for monitoring and management of pediatric patients during and after sedation for diagnostic and therapeutic procedures. Pediatrics 1992;89:1110–1115.

SEDATION FLOWSHEET   ADDRESSOGRAPH

Pertinent Information   Guidelines: See Reverse Side

Date _____ Diagnosis _____ Procedure _____

Physician_____   Referring Physician_____

Consent Obtained   ❑Yes ❑No   Sedation/Procedure Explained ❑Yes ❑No

   Allergies_____   Patient Weight_____

   NPO Time (solids) _____ (liquids) _____ Precautions_____

Current Medications: _____ Special Considerations: _____

*Signature/Title*_____   _____

Pre-Sedation History and Physical Assessment

ASA Classification_____

❑ Fever   ❑ Nasal congestion   ❑Apnea/Snoring   ❑ Facial Anomalies / Abnormal Airway

❑Asthma/Respiratory   ❑Other_____

If Deep Sedation Anticipated (Only Cardiac Cath, Upper Endoscopy, Bronchoscopy)   ❑NA

1. Airway: Oropharynx, Jaw, Neck - Normal   ❑Yes ❑No

2. Personal or Family Hx of Anesthesia Problems   ❑Yes ❑No

                                         *Comments*_____

*Physician/LIP Signature*_____   _____

Procedure / Patient Monitoring

Sedation Medications / Dose / Time:

1. _____ 3. _____

2. _____ 4. _____

Key:	LOC:		(A) Awake,	(CR) Crying,	(L) Lethargic	(SL) Sleeping		
	Response to Stimulation:		**(V) Voice,**	**(T) Tactile**	**(P) Painful**	**(D) Inappropriate** *Deep Sedation*		
Time	**Temp**	**HR**	**RR**	**BP**	**SaO2**	**LOC**	**Response to Stimulation**	**Comments /Meds**	**Initials**
								Pre-Sedation	

Comments:

Initials	Signature/Title

Discharge Criteria: See Reverse side for documentation

Figure 26–6. *See legend on opposite page*

Post Sedation Discharge Criteria: For all patients receiving sedation

Vitals Signs WNL for age	❏Yes	❏No	❏NA	Discharge Instruction Reviewed
Absence of respiratory distress	❏Yes	❏No	❏NA	❏Yes ❏No
Supplemental O2 ≤ pre-sedation level	❏Yes	❏No	❏NA	
Absence of nausea / vomiting	❏Yes	❏No	❏NA	
Awake and responsive to command	❏Yes	❏No	❏NA	Instruction Given To:
Able to Speak	❏Yes	❏No	❏NA	
Able to sit, stand, walk with help	❏Yes	❏No	❏NA	_____
Absence of respiratory distress	❏Yes	❏No	❏NA	

Discharge Instruction Received By: _____

(Parent/Legal Guardian Signature)

Discharged By: _____**Time:**_____

(Signature/Title)

Guidelines for Completing Sedation Flowsheet:

- The department performing the procedure will initiate the Sedation Flow Sheet.
- Consent is mandatory for all sedative drugs given by any route (Oral, IV, Nasal, IM, etc.).
- For Inpatients, refer to History and Physical, Nursing Database, Pediatric Flow Sheet and Medication Administration Record (MAR) for relevant information. Record all pertinent information on the Sedation Flow Sheet.

Pertinent Information   Per Nurse

- Complete all areas as applicable with signature and title.

Pre-Sedation History and Physical Assessment   Per Physician or Licensed Independent Practitioner (LIP)

- Complete all areas as applicable with signature and title.

- ASA Classification: *Must be assigned by the physician ordering the sedation.*

Class I	A normally healthy patient
Class II	A patient with mild systemic disease
Class III	A patient with severe systemic disease
Class IV	A patient with severe systemic disease that is a constant threat to life
Class V	A moribund patient who is not expected to survive without life operation

  ≥ASA Class III patients require consultation

Deep Sedation

- *Must be anticipated during Cardiac Cath, Bronchoscopy, and Upper Endoscopy.*
- *Airway assessment and history of personal or family problems related to anesthesia must be assessed per Physician.*
- *One patient care provider must monitor and continuously assess the patient as their sole responsibility.*
- *Record VS every 5 minutes.*

Procedure / Patient Monitoring   (Use Key for patient monitoring).

- Write in name, dosage and time of medications ordered.
- Patient monitoring must include: HR, Respirations, SaO2, LOC, Response to Stimulation.
- Write any comments or medications in the appropriate column.
- Entries should be made every 15 minutes for conscious sedation. Monitoring and documentation will continue until the child responds to gentle stimulation or voice. If stimulation associated with monitoring interferes with the procedure, it should be done when appropriate.
- Provider who completes any portion of the flow sheet must sign their name and initials in designated areas.

Post Sedation Discharge Criteria

- All age appropriate discharge criteria must be met before child can be sent back to unit or discharged home.
- Discharge instructions must be reviewed and given to parent/legal guardian prior to discharge home with appropriate signature(s) and date.

Figure 26–6 *Continued.* Sample sedation flow sheet. (Courtesy of Children's National Medical Center, Washington, DC.)

oxygen via a bag and mask. Patient's vital signs should be recorded at specific intervals. Recording usually occurs every 15 minutes unless the child is still deeply sedated, in which case vital signs should be recorded every 5 minutes. In some hospitals, as part of ensuring uniformity of care throughout the institution, this may best be accomplished in the same recovery room as for the operating room.

Recommended discharge criteria include the following[17]:

1. Cardiovascular function and airway patency are stable and satisfactory.
2. Child is easily aroused and protective reflexes are intact.
3. Patient can speak (if age appropriate).
4. Patient can sit up (if age appropriate) or walk with assistance.
5. Presedation level of consciousness is achieved, or as close as possible to normal level for very young or handicapped children.
6. Adequate state of hydration exists.

Examples of post-sedation follow-up instructions and phone calls from radiology and dentistry departments of the Children's National Medical Center are given in Figures 26–7 and 26–8.

DEPARTMENT OF PEDIATRIC RADIOLOGY

POST-EXAM CALL

PATIENT NAME: _____   PHONE # _____

Post-exam call made to: _____   Date _____

Sedation Type _____   Staff Notes _____

Hello. This is _____ (full name), from the Children's Hospital Radiology Department. This is a follow-up call regarding the (MRI or CT) exam that _____ (child's name) had on _____ (date).

How is your child feeling today?

Do you feel that your child experienced any unexpected reaction following his/her exam?

Do you have any questions or concerns that we could help you with?

Thank you for your time. We would like to thank you for choosing Children's National Medical Center.

COMPLETED BY: _____

IF YOU GET AN ANSWERING MACHINE PLEASE USE FORM BELOW:

Hello. This is _____ (full name), from the Children's Hospital Radiology Department. This is a follow-up call regarding the (MRI or CT) exam that _____ (child's name) had on _____ (date).

This is follow-up phone call to that exam. We hope your child is feeling well today.

If you feel that your child experienced any unexpected reaction following his/her exam, or if you have questions or concerns that we could help you with please call us at 202-884-2526 and ask to speak with one of the Radiology Nurses.

We would like to thank you for choosing Children's National Medical Center.

MESSAGE LEFT BY: _____

Figure 26–7. Sample post-examination call form. (Courtesy of Children's National Medical Center, Washington, DC.)

DEPARTMENT OF PEDIATRIC DENTISTRY

POSTOPERATIVE INSTRUCTIONS FOLLOWING
DENTAL TREATMENT UNDER SEDATION

1.   OBSERVATION

Carefully observe your child until all sedative effects have disappeared. Watch your child closely for signs of breathing difficulty.

2.   DIET

You may give your child small amounts of water and clear fluids (broth, soda or juices), or soft foods (jello, sherbet) until he/she appears hungry and able to tolerate his/her regular diet. Remember that your child's lip and tongue will be numb – wait for the numbness to wear off before allowing your child to eat.

3.   ACTIVITY

Your child should remain fairly quiet and rest for the remainder of today. Avoid any strenuous activity. He/she may resume regular activities tomorrow.

4.   MEDICATION

Pain medication is usually not necessary but Tylenol may be given for minor discomfort.

5.   CALL THE DENTAL CLINIC IF:

    a.   temperature over 101 degrees
    b.   persistent vomiting
    c.   persistent drowsiness or dizziness
    d.   difficulty with breathing
    e.   unusual bleeding
    f.   any other concern

YOUR CHILD'S FOLLOWUP APPOINTMENT IS AT _____ ON
_____.

Figure 26–8. Sample postoperative instruction sheet for dental treatment performed on a sedated patient. (Courtesy of Children's National Medical Center, Washington, DC.)

Implementation of Successful Sedation Guidelines

Institution-Wide

The implementation of a successful institution-wide policy involves organization, education, record-keeping, enforcement, and continuing quality improvement.[39-41] A sedation committee must be carefully organized and involves many departments, practitioners, and geographic areas within the institution. The goal of the committee must be to create a sedation policy that can facilitate patient care without placing undo burden on practitioners. An overly burdensome policy may foster the avoidance of sedation and analgesia altogether or circumvention of the policy. Ideally, the committee should be composed of representatives from at least one and preferably two to three sedation practitioner services (e.g., endoscopist, intensivist, dentist, surgeon, or emergency medicine practitioner), anesthesiology, nursing, pharmacy, hospital administration, and risk management. The responsibilities of the sedation committee include the creation of hospital (institution)-wide sedation policies, determination of hospital (institution)-wide personnel and equipment needs, creation of educational programs, monitoring of sedation problems, and modification of policies as needed. Involving risk management should protect all against discovery from legal professionals.

Department-Wide

The Department of Anesthesiology Chairman (or designate) plays a pivotal if not central role. The Department of Anesthesiology must help formulate policy, educate nonanesthesiology sedation practitioners, act as consultant on difficult patients, and determine when sedation by a nonanesthesiologist is inappropriate. The Department of Anesthesiology should approve sedation flow sheets and records and be involved, along with the committee and the institution's risk management department in periodic review of the records and compliance with documentation and institutional policies and procedures. A member of the Department of Anesthesiology should also serve in the process of continuous quality improvement. Continuous quality improvement is needed to review complications, incident reports, and sedation flow sheets to ensure compliance with policy, and recommend changes to the sedation committee. Sedation and analgesia require a treatment plan. The Department of Anesthesiology must play a decisive role in determining which sedatives, hypnotics, general anesthetics, and analgesics can be safely used alone and in combination in each institution. Several drugs in particular can easily produce deep sedation or general anesthesia, airway obstruction, an unprotected airway, and cardiorespiratory collapse—namely, methohexital, thiopental, nitrous oxide (when combined with other sedating medications), ketamine, propofol, and remifentanil. Whether these drugs can or should be administered by nonanesthesiologists and, if so, under what conditions, must be determined on an institution-by-institution basis.

There are many studies purporting the safety of these drugs when administered by nonanesthesiologists.[23, 42-54] There are a number of case reports documenting catastrophes as well.[55-60] The problem with all of these studies is that a true sedation disaster is rare and the number of patients involved in these studies is relatively small. This does not allow sufficient numbers to truly interpret the safety of any of these methods of sedation. The study of rare events requires thousands of cases and it is for this reason that more common events such as desaturation, airway obstruction, apnea, or other respiratory event can be used as a surrogate marker for the more serious but rare events such as death or neurologic injury (see Fig. 26-3).[61-70]

Education is vital to maintain safety. An ongoing institution-wide educational program on sedation emphasizing physician (or dentist) responsibility, nursing responsibility, and guidelines and pharmacology of drugs should be given frequently enough to train the staff and to accommodate staff turnover (usually one to two times a year). Teaching modules, videos, and handouts should supplement this program.[20] Education must also emphasize the limits of sedation by the nonanesthesiologist and criteria for a sedation consult or sedation by an anesthesiologist.

The role of the Department of Nursing cannot be minimized.[40] The institution's sedation teaching module should be reviewed by newly employed nurses during their orientation. Registered nurses should be encouraged to attend the hospital course on sedation once every 2 years or to review a nursing module. Nurses should be encouraged to fill out a yearly education profile that includes progress on sedation education.

Physician, dentist, and nurse compliance with the sedation policy as well as a system for continuous quality improvement are the final pieces of the puzzle. Compliance can be monitored by the Medical and Dental Staff Office and the Department of Nursing, as well as by a committee charged with the responsibility of continuing quality improvement. *This committee should fall under the purview of risk management.* Staff privileges for practitioners to administer sedation should require attendance at educational programs, for example, every 2 years, and some form of life-support credentialing, such as Basic or Advanced Life Support, Pediatric Advanced Life Support, Advanced Pediatric Life Support, or Advanced Cardiac Life Support. Every 6 months, the Medical Staff Office should report to the department chairman and nursing office a list of individual staff members who need to take an educational course. It is the responsibility of the department chairman and nursing supervisors to secure individual staff compliance. Failure of the individual physician or nurse to meet educational requirements should result in review of institutional sedation privileges and possible termination of privileges for administering procedural sedation.

Variance reports should be reported and generated when sedation policy is not followed or when a critical incident occurs. The appropriate institutional review committee reviews the incident and reports to the sedation committee. Educational and corrective action should take place as quickly as possible. This committee should not be viewed as "sedation police" but rather as a resource to objectively and unemotionally review critical sedation-related events. The committee can then determine where the "system" broke down to define what went wrong and why, for example, inadequate history taking combined with sedation, inadequate monitoring combined with delay in problem recognition, or inadequate recovery procedures combined with a resedation at home. This critical incident analysis then allows recommendations to be made for future prevention.[61, 64, 69]

The development of a systematic approach to sedation creates a safety net that will protect children while providing sedation and analgesia for procedures. Although differing patient needs, practice requirements, and location limitations produce problems that are individual and specific, the "systems approach" solution to the problem of pediatric sedation and analgesia as outlined in this chapter is eminently feasible. Perhaps more importantly, it can be accomplished in a way that compromises neither patient safety nor comfort. Anesthesiologists are central to this process.

Specific Sedation Techniques

A *sedation treatment plan* analyzing the requirements for analgesics, anxiolytics, or both is necessary for each patient and will vary depending on the procedure and the anxiety of the patient and family. Psychological techniques to allay anxiety (cuddling, parental support, warm blankets, a gentle reassuring voice, and hypnosis) are extraordinarily useful adjuncts to the sedation plan.[11-14]

Many drugs used for sedation and analgesia are not approved by the Food and Drug Administration (FDA) for use in young children (e.g., fentanyl in children < 2 years; morphine < 12 years, bupivacaine < 12 years, propofol < 12 years). The lack of "approval" by the FDA does not imply that a drug should not be used, rather it only means that the manufacturer never carried out the appropriate studies to gain FDA approval.[1, 71-74] A ruling by the FDA in 1994 stated that pediatric labeling must be more complete for drugs used in pediatrics. Drug companies had two years to comply.[75] Although some sedative drugs (e.g., Fentanyl Oralet, midazolam) developed pediatric labeling guidelines, many others did not. In 1997, the FDA passed the FDA Modernization Act.[76] The act states that if a drug company studies an already adult-approved drug in children, it will receive a patent extension or exclusive rights for an additional 6 months. It has been reported (Wall Street Journal, February 23, 1999) that an average clinical trial costs $250,000 to $1 million. The average 6-month profit for a drug is $50 million. This economic incentive is expected to greatly improve studies and labeling in drugs for children. In 1998, the Final Rule was passed by Congress[77]; this law empowers the FDA to require that pediatric studies be conducted on all new drug applications if there will be a pediatric indication.[77] Previous to this new legislation, the FDA was only able to request rather than require studies.[72] It is hoped that these two new legislative efforts will improve the safety of drugs in children by encouraging pediatric drug research and the development of pediatric formulations.[72, 78-82] Unfortunately, these legislative efforts do not apply to the old drugs that are no longer patent-protected, so drug labeling will still be deficient for the use of these drugs in children.

The main classes of drugs used for sedation and analgesia for diagnostic and therapeutic procedures are as follows:

- Local anesthetics
- Anxiolytics and sedatives
- Barbiturates
- Opioid analgesics
- Systemic anesthetics

Local Anesthetics

Local anesthetics play a critical role in analgesia for painful procedures and greatly reduce requirements for systemic narcotics. Applications of local anesthetics to skin and mucous membranes as well as local and regional blocks (including Bier blocks) are easily performed. Epinephrine (1:100,000–10 µg/mL) is used as a vasoconstrictor and lengthens the duration of nerve blocks, decreases bleeding, and reduces systemic toxicity by decreasing vascular uptake. The toxicity of local anesthetics is additive when used in combination. No more than the maximum amount (mg/kg) should be drawn up in a syringe so as to avoid accidental overdose (Table 26–4). Epinephrine solutions can cause tissue ischemia and are contraindicated in end-arterial areas (digits, ear, and penis). Specific blocks used in the sedated child are subcutaneous infiltration, field blocks, and intravenous regional anesthesia. A discussion of these topics and treatment of local anesthetic toxicity is found in Chapter 28.

Topical administration of local anesthetics is useful in the sedated patient. EMLA cream is a *E*utectic *M*ixture of *L*ocal *A*nesthetics (lidocaine 2.5% and prilocaine 2.5%). When placed on the skin for 60 minutes[83, 84] it is useful for reducing the pain of skin incision, intravenous insertions, lumbar punctures, and circumcision.[85-87] Absorption of large amounts of prilocaine can cause methemoglobinuria. It should only be applied to normal intact skin in appropriate doses[20] (for patients < 10 kg, apply to a maximum of approximately 100 cm^2 surface area; 10–20 kg, apply to a maximum of approximately 600 cm^2; > 20 kg, apply to a maximum of approximately 2000 cm^2). The duration of action is 1 to 2 hours after the cream is removed. Adverse reactions include skin blanching, erythema, itching, rash, and methemoglobinemia. It is contraindicated in children younger than 1 month of age, in patients with congenital or idiopathic methemoglobinemia, and in infants receiving methemoglobinemia-inducing drugs (e.g., phenytoin, phenobarbital, acetaminophen, and sulfonamides).

TAC is a mixture of *T*etracaine (1%), *A*drenaline (1:4,000), and *C*ocaine (4%). Original mixtures that included

Table 26–4. Maximum Recommended Doses and Duration of Local Anesthetics

Local Anesthetic	Maximum Dose (mg/kg)		Approximate Duration (min)
	Without Epinephrine	*With Epinephrine*	
Procaine	7.0	10.0	60–90
2-Chloroprocaine	15.0	20.0	30–60
Tetracaine	1.0	1.5	180–600
Lidocaine	5.0	7.0	90–200
Mepivacaine	5.0	7.0	120–240
Bupivacaine	2.0	3.0	180–600
Ropivacaine	3.0	—	180–600

From Coté CJ, Strafford MA: The Principles of Pediatric Sedation. Boston: Tufts University School of Medicine, 1998.

up to 11.8% cocaine are not recommended, since 4% cocaine is equally effective and less toxic.[88] The vasoconstriction and local anesthetic properties of cocaine in combination with the other ingredients make this solution useful in repairing skin lacerations. TAC is not commercially available and is made in individual hospital pharmacies. Systemic toxic reactions and deaths have occurred in children because of excessive doses or mucosal absorption.[89, 90] Cocaine dysrhythmias are due to catecholamine reuptake blockade as well as coronary artery spasm and are difficult to treat. The recommended maximum dose is 1.5 mL/10 kg.[1, 20] Half the solution is placed on the wound while half is held on the surface with a bandage. Analgesia and vasoconstriction are maximal in 10 to 15 minutes. It should not be applied to the digits, nose, ear, penis, mucous membranes, or skin flap. Other mixtures of local anesthetics and vasoconstrictors have been created to avoid the toxicity of TAC. *Tetracaine (1%) Adrenalin (0.4%)* and *Lidocaine (4%)* (TAL), as well as *Bupivacaine (0.5%)* and *Norepinephrine (1:26,000)* (BN) topical solutions appear as effective as TAC.[91, 92] Another equally effective and potentially less toxic topical anesthetic is prilocaine (3.5%) and phenylephrine (0.1%) (Prilophen).[93]

Anxiolytics

The most commonly used anxiolytics and sedatives in pediatric sedation are chloral hydrate, diazepam, and midazolam.

Chloral hydrate is one of the most widely used sedatives in neonates and children less than 3 years of age (Table 26–5).[50, 94–96] Although it has a long safety record, it can cause respiratory depression due to airway obstruction, and deaths have been associated with its use alone and when combined with other sedating medications.[23, 27, 35, 97–99] It can be given orally or rectally. Onset of sedation is 30 to 60 minutes and the usual clinical duration is 1 hour. The active metabolite, trichloroethanol, has a half-life of 10 hours in toddlers, 18 hours in term infants, and 40 hours in preterm infants (see Fig. 9–3).[100] The unpredictable onset and active metabolites dictate that this drug (as well as all sedatives for sedation) be given only in facilities capable of resuscitation (AAP guidelines) and that discharge occur when sedation is clearly lessening and the child meets discharge criteria. Table 26–5 lists doses, routes, onset, duration, adverse reactions, drug interactions, and contraindications. Chloral hydrate should be considered a drug with a long duration of action

Table 26–5. Chloral Hydrate

Dose and Route of Administration	*Oral:* 25 to 100 mg/kg up to 1 g/dose (maximum of 2 g in two divided doses) *Rectal:* 25 to 100 mg/kg up to 1 g/dose (maximum of 2 g in two divided doses)
Onset of Action/ Time to Peak Effect	Onset: 15 to 30 minutes Peak effect: 30 to 60 minutes
Duration of Action	60 minutes **(residual sedation may persist for 10 or more hours in toddlers, but 20 hours or more in neonates)**
Adverse Reactions	Desaturation Respiratory depression and airway obstruction	Reported in patients with anatomic airway anomalies, large tonsils, and patients with significant cardiopulmonary, neurologic, or hepatorenal disorders
	Agitation Ataxia Vomiting Cardiac arrhythmias	Associated with excessive or repetitive dosing, patients with cardiac disease
	Increased risk of direct and indirect hyperbilirubinemia and kernicterus in newborns Metabolic acidosis with repeat administration, particularly in neonates	Not recommended for repeat use in neonates; single dose will produce prolonged sedation in preterm infants and full-term infants younger than 1 month of age
Drug Interactions	Concomitant administration with other sedatives or opioids increases the risk of respiratory complications May alter the rate of metabolism of warfarin or warfarin-related anticoagulants	
Special Concerns	Dose should be decreased in high-risk or debilitated patients Metabolite (trichloroethanol) is responsible for most, if not all, of the sedative effects Because of a longer half-life, prolonged sedation is possible in neonates Contraindicated in patients with hepatic failure and in neonates except for single-dose administration Most effective in children under 4 years of age	
Contraindications	Preterm and term neonates (repeat dosing) Should not be used on a chronic basis Patients with significant hepatic or renal disease Patients with cardiac dysrhythmias Patients who have previously exhibited an idiosyncrasy or hypersensitivity to chloral hydrate Oral dose contraindicated in patients with gastritis Patients with porphyria	
Antagonist	None available	

From Coté CJ, Strafford MA: Principles of Pediatric Sedation. Boston: Tufts University School of Medicine, 1998.

because of the very long half-life. Therefore, infants sedated with chloral hydrate might benefit from prolonged observation after meeting standard discharge criteria, since resedation (especially after stimulation is stopped) is possible. Airway obstruction and death have occurred after chloral hydrate sedation in a child who was in a car seat in the back of a car while going home following procedural sedation.[27]

The benzodiazepines (*diazepam* and *midazolam*) are commonly used in pediatric sedation and exert their effects by interacting with gamma-aminobutyric acid receptors in the central nervous system. The sedated child usually becomes compliant but does not lose consciousness. Children frequently move, and another agent such as a narcotic may be necessary if the patient must not move for the procedure to be successfully accomplished. Although many children initially act disinhibited and "drunk" following small doses of benzodiazepines, some patients have a true paradoxical response and become more agitated with higher doses.[101] It is wiser to switch to a different sedative drug in these patients, since increasing the dose of benzodiazepines may lead to severe agitation followed by unconsciousness and respiratory compromise. The benzodiazepines have the advantage of antegrade amnesia in a significant number of patients.[102, 103] Benzodiazepines produce mild respiratory depression and upper airway obstruction.[104–106] Respiratory depression may become severe in compromised patients or children with tonsil hypertrophy. The combination of benzo-

diazepines and narcotics can produce a "superadditive effect" on respiratory depression in which the total depressant effect from the combination of drugs is much greater than the sum of their anticipated individual effects.[107] Diazepam is more fat soluble than midazolam and has twice the duration of sedative effect, but intravenous administration can be painful. The onset of intravenous diazepam is approximately three times faster than that of intravenous midazolam (see Fig. 9–2),[108, 109] whereas the onset of oral midazolam is faster than that of oral diazepam. The markedly prolonged and variable elimination half-life and active metabolite of diazepam (desmethyl-diazepam) make midazolam a superior sedative drug in children, particularly infants.[110–115] Midazolam is the only drug in this class approved for neonates. Midazolam can be given intravenously, intranasally, sublingually, orally, or rectally. The oral route has become very popular and is well tolerated. A manufactured oral cherry-flavored form is now available. Nasal administration causes burning and should be avoided.[116, 117] Rectal administration is usually well tolerated in children who have not been toilet trained (age $\approx$ < 1 year), but absorption may be irregular owing to many factors, including superior versus inferior hemorrhoidal vein absorption within the rectum. The use of diazepam and midazolam is detailed in Tables 26–6 and 26–7.

Flumazenil is a specific benzodiazepine antagonist and will rapidly reverse the sedative and respiratory effects of benzodiazepines.[118–122] In patients who are taking benzodiaz-

Table 26–6. Diazepam (Valium)

Dose and Route of Administration	*Oral*: 0.1 to 0.3 mg/kg *Intravenous*: 0.1 to 0.3 mg/kg (maximum single dose 10 mg; titrate to effect) *Intramuscular*: **not recommended** due to low, erratic absorption (< 60% of administered dose) *Rectal*: 0.2 to 0.3 mg/kg, mg/kg, **not recommended** due to erratic absorption
Time of Peak Effect	*Intravenous*: 1 to 2 minutes *Oral*: 60 minutes
Duration of Action	*Intravenous*: 2 to 6 hours—dose related (elimination half-life 20 to 40 hours)
Adverse Reactions	Respiratory depression — Dose-related, more pronounced with IV route; may be exacerbated by rapid administration and coadministration of other CNS depressant medications Ataxia Paradoxic excitation Pain and phlebitis at injection site — Slow administration, preferable in largest possible vein Hypotension — Increased risk of hypotension with rapid IV administration
Drug Interactions	Concomitant administration with opioids, barbiturates, or other CNS depressant medications increases the risk of respiratory depression and apnea. When administered with opioids, the initial dose should be reduced by at least 25 to 33% Use with other CNS depressant medications prolongs the recovery time Clearance can be delayed when administered in association with cimetidine (Tagamet)
Special Concerns	Elimination prolonged (half-life as long as 100 hours) in premature neonates; prolonged sedation may result Because of the possibility of impaired metabolism, caution should be used in patients with severe hepatic dysfunction Pharmacologically active metabolite, desmethyl-diazepam, has a half-life of 30 to 219 hours Dose should be decreased in high-risk or debilitated patients
Contraindications	Patients with known sensitivity to benzodiazepines, patients with acute narrow-angle glaucoma, or those with open-angle glaucoma who are not receiving therapy
Antagonist	Flumazenil (10 μg/kg over 15 seconds every 1 to 2 minutes up to 1 mg); **observe at least 2 hours for resedation**

CNS, central nervous system; IV, intravenous.

Reproduced with permission from Coté CJ, Strafford MA: The Principles of Pediatric Sedation. Boston: Tufts University School of Medicine, 1998.

Table 26–7. Midazolam (Versed)

Dose and Route of Administration	*Oral*: 0.25 to 0.75 mg/kg *Sublingual*: 0.25 to 0.3 mg/kg *Nasal*: 0.2 to 0.3 mg/kg; not recommended (see text) *Intravenous*: 0.05 to 0.15 mg/kg; titrate to effect *Intramuscular*: 0.05 to 0.15 mg/kg *Rectal*: 0.5 to 0.75 mg/kg
Time of Peak Effect	*Intravenous*: 3 to 5 minutes *Intranasal*: 10 to 15 minutes *Sublingual*: 10 to 15 minutes *Oral*: 10 to 30 minutes *Rectal*: 10 to 20 minutes
Duration of Action	*Intravenous*: 20 to 60 minutes (dose-related) (elimination half-life 1.5 to 2.5 hours) *Oral and rectal*: 60 minutes (dose-related)

Adverse Reactions		
	Respiratory depression	Dose- and rate-related, more pronounced with IV route; more likely when coadministered with other CNS depressant medications. Reduce initial dose by at least 25% to 33% when coadministered with an opioid.
	Ataxia	
	Paradoxical excitation	
	Hypotension	Rapid administration in neonates, coadministration of fentanyl in neonates
	Myoclonic, seizure-like activity	Rapid administration in neonates
	Nasal burning	Following nasal administration

Drug Interactions	Concomitant administration with opioids, barbiturates, or other CNS depressant medications increases the risk of respiratory depression and apnea. When administered with opioids, the initial dose should be reduced by at least 25% to 33%. Use with other CNS depressant medications prolongs the recovery time. Erythromycin and calcium channel blockers delay metabolism through cytochrome P450 enzyme inhibition. Titrate slowly to effect in HIV patients taking protease inhibitors (due to cytochrome P450 inhibition). Neonates are particularly susceptible to hypotension with rapid IV administration or concomitant administration of fentanyl.
Special Concerns	Dose should be decreased in high-risk or debilitated patients. Nasal administration is associated with burning sensation; potential for direct neurotoxicity (theoretic concern). Elimination may be prolonged in patients with congestive heart failure, in neonates, and in patients receiving vasopressors. Midazolam is known to cause airway obstruction by reducing hypopharyngeal airway patency.
Antagonist	Flumazenil (10 µg/kg over 15 seconds every 1 to 2 minutes up to 1 mg); **observe at least 2 hours for resedation**.

CNS, central nervous system; HIV, human immunodeficiency virus; IV, intravenous.
From Coté CJ, Strafford MA: The Principles of Pediatric Sedation. Boston: Tufts University School of Medicine, 1998.

epines for seizures or drug dependency, those symptoms may recur if flumazenil is given.[123] The recommended dose of flumazenil is 10 µg/kg up to 1 mg intravenously. Antagonism begins within 1 to 2 minutes and lasts approximately 1 hour. Since resedation after 1 hour may occur, the patient must be carefully monitored for at least 2 hours. Repeat flumazenil may be necessary. It should be noted that flumazenil will not antagonize the respiratory depression secondary to opioids[124]; in that situation an opioid antagonist is also required. Flumazenil should not be administered for the routine reversal of the sedative effects of benzodiazepines but reserved for reversal of respiratory depression.

Pentobarbital is the most commonly used intermediate-acting barbiturate for sedation. It has a long history of use during radiologic procedures. Studies have shown a low incidence of respiratory obstruction and transient desaturation.[125] The barbiturates tend to make children more sensitive to pain and should be combined with analgesics when used during painful procedures. Pentobarbital's relatively long duration (1–2 hours) and slow recovery sometimes leaves

children in a prolonged disinhibited state that necessitates prolonged recovery and restraint. Newer, shorter-acting, faster recovery drugs are quickly replacing pentobarbital. Details of pentobarbital use are given in Table 26–8.

Opioid analgesics are rarely used alone for diagnostic and therapeutic procedures in children. Although the opioids provide some sedation, the sedation produced is usually inadequate, therefore requiring combination with a sedative. The "super-additive" respiratory depressant effects of the combination of narcotics and sedatives must be reemphasized[107, 126] and vigilance must be heightened. This is especially true in infants and children with upper airway obstruction (e.g., tonsil/adenoid hypertrophy, trisomy 21, mucopolysaccharidosis). Infants less than 3 months of age and former preterm infants have a very large patient-to-patient drug metabolism variability and are more susceptible to narcotic-induced respiratory depression.[127] Other serious effects of narcotics include bradycardia, hypotension, seizures, and opioid-induced glottic and chest wall rigidity.

The newest rapid-acting narcotic is *remifentanil*. This

rapid-onset, extremely potent, short-duration narcotic is associated with too high an incidence of apnea and chest wall rigidity to be used by the nonanesthesiologist for pediatric sedation.[128]

Morphine may be considered for painful procedures (over 1 hour) or in situations in which the child will also be in pain after the procedure. The duration of action is 3 to 5 hours after intravenous administration.[127] Morphine may be given orally (0.2–0.5 mg/kg), intravenously (0.05–0.1 mg/kg; maximum, 0.3 mg/kg) or intramuscularly (0.1–0.2 mg/kg). Rectal administration may cause delayed respiratory depression from erratic absorption and should be abandoned.[129] Time to peak effect for oral, intravenous, or intramuscular administration is 60 minutes, 3 to 5 minutes, and 10 to 30 minutes, respectively. Adverse reactions in addition to respiratory depression include hypotension (in part histamine related), dysphoria, delirium, nausea, vomiting, smooth muscle spasm (biliary, ureteral), urinary retention, and pruritus. Special precautions are required for its use in neonates, debilitated patients, and children with airway obstruction or asthma.

Meperidine (Demerol) is also useful in longer procedures, since its clinical duration of action is 2 to 4 hours.[20] Meperidine is not recommended in neonates because its elimination half-life is 3 to 59 hours.[130] It may be given orally (1–2 mg/kg), intravenously (0.5–1.0 mg/kg; maximum 3 mg/kg), or intramuscularly (1–2 mg/kg). The rectal route is not recommended. Time of peak effect for meperidine is 30 to 90 minutes for oral and intramuscular administration and 1 to 3 minutes for intravenous administration. In addition to respiratory depression, the active metabolite of meperidine (normeperidine) may cause seizures. Meperidine should not be used long-term or in patients with poor renal clearance.[131]

Other adverse reactions include delirium, nausea, vomiting, urinary retention, pruritus, smooth muscle spasm, and hypotension (histamine induced). Special considerations include avoidance in patients taking monaminoxidase inhibitors (serotonin-induced hyperpyrexia and cardiovascular instability). Central nervous system toxicity may occur in patients taking tricyclic antidepressants and phenothiazines. Patients taking phenytoin (Dilantin) may have a lesser analgesic effect. Naloxone or nalmefene reversal of meperidine-induced respiratory depression may precipitate seizures caused by normeperidine.

Meperidine (Demerol, 25 mg/mL) in the past was commonly mixed as a "lytic cocktail" with promethazine (Phenergan, 6.25 mg/mL) and chlorpromazine (Thorazine, 6.25 mg/mL). The mixture, called DPT, is still used despite warnings of its long sedation duration (7–19 hours), hypotension, seizures, extrapyramidal reactions, and severe, prolonged life-threatening respiratory depression.[25, 50, 132–134] *It is the opinion of the authors that DPT should be abandoned*

Table 26–8. Pentobarbital (Nembutal)

Dose and Range of Administration	*Oral*: 4 to 5 mg/kg
	Intravenous: 1 to 2 mg/kg up to 7.5 mg/kg, not to exceed 50 mg/min—titrate every 5 minutes; titrate to effect
	Intramuscular: 2 to 6 mg/kg not to exceed 100 mg
	Rectal suppository: 4 to 5 mg/kg
	    2 months to 1 year: One 30 mg suppository
	    1 to 4 years: One 30 mg or one 60 mg suppository
	    5 to 12 years: One 60 mg suppository
	    12 to 14 years: One 60 mg or one 120 mg suppository

Onset of Action	*Oral*: dose-related, 20 to 60 minutes *Intravenous*: dose-related, 2 to 5 minutes with peak at 5 to 10 minutes *Intramuscular*: dose-related, 2 to 5 minutes with peak at 15 minutes *Rectal*: dose-related, 20 to 60 minutes
Adverse Reactions	Apnea Hypoventilation Hypotension Hallucinations Anxiety Ataxia Laryngospasm
Drug Interactions	Lowers level of oral anticoagulants Enhances metabolism of steroids Impairs absorption of oral griseofulvin Shortens half-life of doxycycline Sodium valproate and valproic acid increase half-life of barbiturates Monoamine oxidase inhibitors increase barbiturate half-life
Special Concerns	Respiratory depression, apnea, and airway obstruction as well as prolonged recovery when co-administered with other CNS depressant medications
Contraindications	Patients with known sensitivity to barbiturates; patients with porphyria

CNS, central nervous system.
From Coté CJ, Strafford MA: The Principles of Pediatric Sedation. Boston: Tufts University School of Medicine, 1998.

altogether, but certainly because of its very long half-life and clinical depression, it is not recommended for outpatient procedures.[25, 133-138]

Fentanyl is rapidly replacing morphine and meperidine as the narcotic of choice for analgesia and sedation for procedures in children. Fentanyl (Sublimaze) is available in parenteral form, oral transmucosal delivery form (Oralet), and in a transdermal patch delivery form (Duragesic). *Duragesic is not to be used for sedation and analgesia during procedures and is therefore beyond the scope of this chapter.*

The Oralet is the only narcotic currently approved by the FDA for sedation and analgesia during procedures in children. It is fentanyl in a sweetened, raspberry-flavored matrix. Approximately 35% of the fentanyl dose is absorbed via the oral mucosa as the child sucks on the lozenge. The swallowed part of the lozenge is poorly absorbed in the stomach and intestine.[139] Administration usually takes 10 to 15 minutes. The Oralet has been useful in mildly painful and anxiety-producing situations such as burn dressing changes[140] and skin laceration repair.[141] The 2 to 3 hours' duration of analgesia with Oralet also helps with post-procedure pain relief (see Fig. 9–4). The incidence of nausea and vomiting is similar to that of other opioid analgesics.[139]

Intravenous fentanyl in doses of 0.25 µg/kg to 0.5 µg/kg have a near immediate onset. Doses must be given in small aliquots and carefully titrated to avoid chest wall and glottic rigidity. The duration of action is 30 to 45 minutes. Close post-procedure observation is required, since respiratory depression can outlast analgesia. Adverse effects of both oral and intravenous forms are similar and summarized in Table 26–9 along with drug interactions and special concerns.

Opioid antagonists specifically reverse the respiratory and analgesic effects of narcotics and should be readily available when narcotics are used. Naloxone (Narcan) is the most commonly used antagonist.[142] Nalmefene (Revex) has a longer half-life (approximately 10 hours) than naloxone, but pediatric experience is limited.[143] *Opioid antagonists should not be used for routine reversal of the sedative effects of narcotics but reserved for reversal of respiratory depression or respiratory arrest.* Naloxone may be given intravenously, intramuscularly, or subcutaneously. The initial dose for respiratory depression is 1 to 2 µg/kg titrated to effect every 2 to 3 minutes. A dose of 10 to 100 µg/kg up to 2 mg may be required for respiratory arrest. Adverse reactions from reversal of analgesia include nausea, vomiting, tachycardia, hypertension, delirium, and pulmonary edema.[144-146] Patients

Table 26–9. Fentanyl (Sublimaze)

Dose and Route of Administration	*Oral transmucosal (Fentanyl Oralet):* 0.005 to 0.015 mg/kg (5 to 15 µg/kg) ≥ 2 years of age and ≥ 10 kg *Intravenous:* 0.25 to 0.5 µg/kg up to 2 to 3 µg/kg (slowly titrate)	
Onset of Action/ Time to Peak Effect	*Intravenous:* 2 to 3 minutes; **onset immediate** *Intramuscular:* onset 7 to 15 minutes *Oral transmucosal (Fentanyl Oralet):* onset 15 to 30 minutes, peak 10 to 15 minutes **following completion**	
Duration of Action	*Intravenous:* 30 to 45 minutes *Oral transmucosal (Fentanyl Oralet):* 2 to 3 hours	
Adverse Reactions	Respiratory depression	More common in infants with rapid infusion of drug, and when coadministered with other CNS depressant medications.
	Bradycardia Dysphoria Delirium Nausea Vomiting Pruritus Urinary retention Smooth muscle spasm	
	Chest wall and glottic rigidity	Risk decreased with slow infusion and small doses; **chest wall and glottic rigidity may be reversed by succinylcholine or naloxone.** May occur with doses as low as 1 to 2 µg/kg.
	Hypotension	Neonates receiving midazolam; patients who are hemodynamically unstable.
Drug Interactions	Concomitant administration of other respiratory depressants, including benzodiazepines, increases the risk of respiratory depression.	
Special Concerns	Dose should be decreased in high-risk or debilitated patients. Elimination may be prolonged in neonates, especially those with impaired hepatic blood flow. The respiratory depressant effects may last considerably longer than the opioid effects. Pharmacokinetics and pharmacodynamics of oral transmucosal delivery are affected by administration time. Use with caution in patients at risk for biliary cholelithiasis. Delayed excretion in patients with impaired hepatic blood flow. **The transdermal delivery system is not recommended for routine pediatric use; should be used only in pediatric patients receiving long-term opioid therapy under the supervision of a pain specialist.**	
Antagonist	Naloxone (see text) Nalmefene (see text)	

CNS, central nervous system.
From Coté CJ, Strafford MA: The Principles of Pediatric Sedation. Boston: Tufts University School of Medicine, 1998.

on long-term narcotics should be given narcotic reversal agents in low doses and with extreme caution, since withdrawal seizures and delirium may occur. Patients given naloxone may renarcotize after 1 hour. *If naloxone is used, then the patient should be observed for a minimum of 2 hours.* Repeat naloxone may be necessary.

Systemic Anesthetics

Systemic anesthetics—ketamine, propofol, methohexital, and N_2O—traditionally have been used in the operating room by anesthesiologists to produce a state of deep sedation (i.e., monitored anesthesia care) or general anesthesia. With appropriate monitoring and personnel, these agents can be safely used outside of the operating room for diagnostic and therapeutic procedures. These drugs are extremely difficult if not impossible to titrate in children so that only a state of "conscious sedation" is produced. The child may quickly become deeply sedated and develop airway compromise. *These drugs should be used only by anesthesiologists or other practitioners who have specific training in the use of these drugs and have advanced airway management skills since airway obstruction, apnea, and cardiovascular instability may quickly and unpredictably occur.* The use of these agents in the operating room for monitored anesthesia care and general anesthesia by anesthesiologists is discussed elsewhere. The following discussion will emphasize the use of these drugs for sedation outside the operating room when an anesthesiologist may not be directly involved.

Ketamine has been available for over 20 years and in low doses can cause intense analgesia with minimal respiratory and cardiovascular depression (Table 26–10). Typical starting doses[147] are 1 to 2 mg/kg IM, 0.25 to 0.5 mg/kg IV, or 4 to 6 mg/kg PO.[148–150] The intramuscular onset is 2 to 5 minutes with a peak of 20 minutes; duration can be 30 to 120 minutes. Intravenous onset occurs in less than 1 minute, with a peak effect in several minutes and duration of action of approximately 15 minutes. Oral doses of 4 to 6 mg/kg

are usually combined with atropine and have an effect in 30 minutes and last up to 120 minutes.[20] Higher doses or supplementation with other sedatives or narcotics may produce deep sedation or general anesthesia. Ketamine should always be administered with an antisialagogue (atropine 0.02 mg/kg or glycopyrrolate 0.01 mg/kg), since copious secretions from ketamine alone may induce laryngospasm.[151] Although initially thought to maintain airway reflexes, this is not the case; ketamine will not protect against aspiration.[152] Cardiovascular stability and pulmonary vascular resistance is usually maintained if normocarbia is present.[153] Ketamine is associated with dysphoric reactions and hallucinations during emergence (up to 12%) and should generally be administered with a benzodiazepine, although this may deepen and prolong sedation. Ketamine is also associated with nonpurposeful motion, which limits its usefulness when immobility is necessary (i.e., computed tomographic scans). Ketamine can markedly increase cerebral blood flow and is contraindicated in patients with increased intracranial pressure. Other contraindications include head injury, open globe injury, hypertension, and psychosis. Ketamine can induce apnea in neonates as well as a decreased response to hypercarbia, laryngospasm, and coughing. There is no antagonist available.

Propofol is a short-acting sedative hypnotic in an intralipid formulation. It has no analgesic properties, but it does have antiemetic and antipruritic properties. Although small doses of propofol (25–50 µg/kg/min) can provide "conscious sedation" in adults, deep sedation and airway obstruction quickly occur in pediatric patients. It is generally best administered by titration with an infusion pump by individuals with advanced airway skills. As discussed previously, there has been much interest in using this agent outside of the operating room, especially in pediatric intensive care units. Cases of fatal metabolic acidosis, myocardial failure, and lipemic serum have been reported in children who received several days of propofol treatment.[154–156] Other studies[157] have not found a strong correlation. Short-term propo-

Table 26–10. Ketamine

Dose and Route of Administration	*Oral*: 4–6 mg/kg combined with atropine (0.02–0.03 mg/kg); may also be combined with low dose midazolam (0.05 mg/kg) for more profound sedation. *Intravenous*: 0.25–1.0 mg/kg (combined with atropine 0.01–0.02 mg/kg) **Start with 0.25–0.5 mg/kg titrating doses at 3- to 5-minute intervals.** *Intramuscular*: 1–2 mg/kg (combined with atropine (0.02 mg/kg) *Rectal*: 4–6 mg/kg (combined with atropine 0.02 mg/kg) *Nasal*: **not recommended** *Warning:* ketamine can produce a state of general anesthesia. **Note: concomitant administration of low dose benzodiazepine, e.g., 0.025–0.05 mg/kg midazolam, will improve the level of sedation, reduce the propensity for dreaming, and reduce the total dose of ketamine. This also allows at least one component of the sedation regimen to be reversible (flumazenil) should a problem arise.**
Onset of Action/ Time to Peak Effect	*Intravenous*: < 1 minute (maximum effect several minutes) titration of low doses (0.25–0.5 mg/kg) is highly recommended to avoid a state of general anesthesia *Intramuscular*: 2–5 minutes (peak effect 20 minutes—dose-dependent) *Oral and rectal*: > 5 minutes (peak effect 30 minutes—dose-dependent)
Duration of Action	Larger doses associated with a longer duration, general anesthesia *Intravenous*: 15 minutes *Intramuscular*: 30 to 120 minutes *Oral and rectal*: 30 to 120 minutes

Table continued on following page

Table 26–10. Ketamine *Continued*

Adverse Reactions	Rare respiratory depression	Risk increased with rapid bolus injections. Neonates are particularly at increased risk.
	Decreased response to hypercarbia	
	Laryngospasm, coughing	Especially patients with upper respiratory tract infections and infants less than 3 months of age.
	Apnea	In infants less than 3 months of age and/or with rapid injection.
	Stimulation of salivary and tracheobronchial secretions	May be minimized by coadministration of an antisialagogue.
	Mild-to-moderate increases in blood pressure, heart rate and cardiac output	May be exaggerated by rapid intravenous administration.
	Emergence phenomenon, hallucinations (up to 12% of patients)	More common in adults than children and with IV compared with intramuscular administration. May be reduced with coadministration of a benzodiazepine.
	Paradoxical hypotension in critically ill patients	
	Skeletal muscle hypotonicity	
	Rigidity	
	Mild disequilibrium	
	Ataxia	
	Random movements of head or extremities	
	Elevates intracranial pressure and cerebral metabolic rate.	Contraindicated in patients with intracranial hypertension
	Nystagmus	Usually indicates onset of drug effect
	Vomiting	
	Increases intraocular pressure	Contraindicated in patients with glaucoma or open globe injury
	Transient erythematous rash	
	May cause loss of protective reflexes; aspiration of gastric contents may occur in patients with a full stomach.	Use the lowest effective dose in patients at risk for pulmonary aspiration of gastric contents.
Drug Interactions	Half-life may be prolonged if given concomitantly with other drugs that undergo hepatic metabolism.	
	Coadministration with benzodiazepines or opioids may reduce the incidence of dreaming but also prolong recovery.	
Special Concerns	Should be used with caution in patients with a full stomach since it may impair protective laryngeal reflexes.	
	Not recommended for children with an active upper respiratory tract infection.	
	Not recommended without concomitant administration of an antisialagogue.	
Contraindications	Contraindications include head injury associated with loss of consciousness or altered mental status, increased intracranial pressure, open globe injury, hypertension, prior adverse reaction to ketamine, and psychosis.	
Antagonist	None available	

Modified with permission from Coté CJ, Strafford MA: The Principles of Pediatric Sedation. Boston: Tufts University School of Medicine, 1998.

fol sedation has not been associated with such problems. Typical doses, time to peak effect, adverse reactions, and concerns are listed in Table 26–11.

Methohexital is a short-acting oxybarbiturate that is rapidly metabolized and redistributed and has a rapid recovery.[158] Induction of anesthesia occurs with intravenous doses of 1 to 2 mg/kg. Apnea, hiccoughs, and rare cases of methohexital-induced seizures in patients with temporal lobe epilepsy have been reported.[159] Methohexital has been used intramuscularly in doses of 8 to 10 mg/kg but has a prolonged onset[160] and is not generally recommended. Rectal methohexital (20–25 mg/kg, 100 mg/mL solution) can induce deep sedation in 7 to 11 minutes[161] with a duration of sedation of about 30 minutes.[162] Absorption through the rectal route is erratic.[163] The variability of absorption, tendency to deep sedation, and airway problems have decreased the use of methohexital in favor of newer drugs. This medication should be used only by individuals with advanced airway skills, since upper airway obstruction and apnea may readily occur.[164]

Nitrous oxide (N_2O) is a potent inhalation analgesic with a peak effect in 3 to 5 minutes and very rapid return to

Table 26–11. Propofol (Diprivan)

Dose and Range of Administration	*Intravenous:* 0.05 to 0.2 mg/kg/minute (50–200 µg/kg/min) as an infusion **Warning: Propofol produces a state of general anesthesia. Bolus dose of 2 mg/kg is an induction dose. This drug should only be administered by individuals with advanced airway skills and is best administered using a constant infusion pump. Lower doses should be used initially and titrated to effect when coadministered with other CNS depressant medications.**
Time to Peak Effect	Intravenous: very rapid (< 30 seconds)
Duration of Action	~8 minutes
Adverse Reactions	Pain on injection — May be ameliorated by prior use of lidocaine, administration into large veins, or concomitant administration of an opioid Respiratory depression and apnea — Dose and rate of administration related. More likely when coadministered with other CNS depressant medications Hypotension — Associated with rapid injection Increased salivary and tracheobronchial secretions Anaphylactoid reactions and bacterial contamination — Attributed to lipid emulsion delivery form Metabolic acidosis Myoclonic movements
Drug Interactions	Concomitant administration of other respiratory depressants may increase the risk of respiratory depression.
Special Concerns	Dose should be decreased in high-risk or debilitated patients. Dose should be decreased in patients who are hemodynamically unstable. Strict aseptic technique required, since propofol supports the growth of microorganisms.
Antagonist	None available

CNS, central nervous system.

From Coté CJ, Strafford MA: The Principles of Pediatric Sedation. Boston: Tufts University School of Medicine, 1998.

baseline when discontinued. A premixed tank of no more than 50% N₂O is available (Entonox). Administration of N₂O must follow the AAP guidelines,[17, 20] which state that (1) only ASA-physical status I or II patients may receive N₂O without direct anesthesia supervision, (2) inhalation equipment must have the capacity to deliver 100% oxygen and never less than 25% oxygen, (3) a calibrated oxygen analyzer must be used.[17, 20] Although N₂O in 50% concentration with oxygen usually produces "conscious sedation," the addition of any sedatives or hypnotics may rapidly produce deep sedation or general anesthesia and require increased monitoring and vigilance.[98, 104] Adverse reactions, drug interactions, and special concerns are listed in Table 26–12.

Establishment of a Sedation Service

The safe sedation of children requires a systematic approach, as described in the preceding sections. However, even though anesthesiologists (ourselves included) feel that our specialty is best trained and equipped to perform this service, the reality at the moment is that we have insufficient resources and the monetary return is so variable that we as a profession are unable to provide this service for all children. Therefore, it is vital that anesthesiologists copartner with hospital administration, nursing administration, and colleagues in other specialties to help develop appropriate methods of sedation, training, and education, so as to create a within-institution system that is safe and efficient and provides the appropriate safety net for children. Since the major source of morbidity and mortality associated with sedation

of children is the effect of sedating medications upon respirations, practitioners who sedate children must have advanced airway skills to successfully manage airway obstruction, hypoventilation, laryngospasm, or apnea.[27] The other specialists with this type of expertise include emergency medicine specialists and intensive care specialists.

A committee made up of physicians and nursing specialists from the specialty areas that require sedation services (radiology, oncology, gastroenterology, dental, emergency medicine, cardiology, pulmonary) plus representatives from hospital administration, anesthesiology, quality care, the code committee, risk management, and others should review current within-hospital policies and procedures for all areas sedating children. Once this information is gathered (what population, special needs of that population, medications utilized, venue of recovery, monitoring during and after sedation, presedation screening, the consent process), a global picture can be made of the institution's and the specialists' needs. Generally this process rapidly reveals areas with inadequate equipment, inadequate monitoring, inadequate screening, and so on, which need to be corrected. This discovery process often reveals areas where sedation was being administered but that had been virtually unrecognized and therefore not standardized.

Once this process is completed, then the committee and the hospital administration can begin deciding how best to meet the demands of providing sedation efficiently, safely, and in a cost-effective manner. This may require the establishment of a sedation service directed by an anesthesiologist, an intensivist, or an emergency medicine physician. It may require the cooperation of the anesthesia department to allow all sedated children to recover in the centralized recov-

Table 26–12. Nitrous Oxide

Dose and Route of Administration	**A mixture of no greater than 50% nitrous oxide in oxygen administered as the sole sedating agent**	
Time of Peak Effect	3 to 5 minutes	
Duration of Action	Washout of nitrous oxide is very rapid and generally accomplished within several minutes of breathing 100% oxygen	
Adverse Reactions	Decreases in cardiac output and blood pressure	Issue in patients with myocardial dysfunction
	Depresses ventilatory response to hypoxia	Generally not a problem because it is administered with oxygen
	Alters cerebral blood flow and increases intracranial pressure	Potentially a problem in patients with head trauma; should not be administered to this population by nonanesthesiologists
	Loss of consciousness	Generally not a problem unless other sedating agents have been coadministered
	Aspiration	Generally not a problem unless other sedating medications have been coadministered
Drug Interactions	Deep sedation may occur if used in conjunction with opioids or other sedatives and may progress to a state of deep sedation/general anesthesia.	
Contraindications	Patients with respiratory failure Patients with altered mental status Patients with otitis media Patients with bowel obstruction Patients with pneumothorax	
Special Concerns	Pollution of the environment; adequate gas scavenging must be ensured	
Antagonist	None available—rapidly washed out when breathing 100% oxygen	

From Coté CJ, Strafford MA: The Principles of Pediatric Sedation. Boston: Tufts University School of Medicine, 1998.

ery room with the anesthesia department available to consult on recovery issues. It may require the hospital administration to financially support the salaries of a number of trained nursing specialists and even to subsidize the salaries of the physicians in charge of the sedation service so as to ensure the presence of highly trained quality individuals for the care of sedated children. It might involve the development of a centralized sedation area where many common procedures could be scheduled as in the operating room (e.g., bone marrow aspirations, suture removal, eye examinations, simple dental procedures, endoscopic procedures, echocardiograms). The bottom line is that there needs to be a creative and nonterritorial approach to this issue so that the right thing is done to ensure that children undergo procedures with proper anxiolysis, analgesia, and care, so that their safety is protected. No child should suffer unnecessary pain or distress. It is up to us as health-care providers to help develop the system to provide the appropriate safety net.

REFERENCES

1. Coté CJ: Sedation for the pediatric patient: A review. Pediatr Clin North Am 1994;41:31–58.
2. Schecter NL, Berde CB, Yaster M: Pain in Infants, Children and Adolescents. Baltimore. Williams & Wilkins; 1993.
3. Anand KJ, Sippell WG, Aynsley-Green A: Randomized trial of fentanyl anaesthesia in preterm babies undergoing surgery: effects on the stress response. Lancet 1987;1:62–66.
4. Anand KJ, Hickey PR:Halothane-morphine compared with high-dose sufentanil for anesthesia and postoperative analgesia in neonatal cardiac surgery. N Engl J Med 1992;326:1–9.
5. Anand KJ, Hansen DD, Hickey PR: Hormonal-metabolic stress responses in neonates undergoing cardiac surgery. Anesthesiology 1990;73:661–670.
6. Grunau RV, Whitfield MF, Petrie JH, et al: Early pain experience, child and family factors, as precursors of somatization: A prospective study of extremely premature and fullterm children. Pain 1994;56:353–359.
7. Yaster M, Tobin JR, Fisher QA, et al: Local anesthetics in the management of acute pain in children. J Pediatr 1994;124:165–176.
8. Zeltzer LK, Bush JP, Chen E, et al: A psychobiologic approach to pediatric pain: Part II. Prevention and treatment. Curr Probl Pediatr 1997;27:264–284.
9. Yaster M, Deshpande JK: Management of pediatric pain with opioid analgesics. J Pediatr 1988;113:421–429.
10. Yaster M, Krane EJ, Kaplan RF, et al: Pediatric Pain Management and Sedation Handbook, 1st ed. St. Louis: Mosby–Year Book; 1997.
11. Kazak AE, Penati B, Brophy P, et al: Pharmacologic and psychologic interventions for procedural pain. Pediatrics 1998;102:59–66.
12. Ellis JA, Spanos NP: Cognitive-behavioral interventions for children's distress during bone marrow aspirations and lumbar punctures: a critical review. J Pain Symptom Manage 1994;9:96–108.
13. Gonzalez JC, Routh DK, Armstrong FD: Effects of maternal distraction versus reassurance on children's reactions to injections. J Pediatr Psychol 1993;18:593–604.
14. Schechter NL: Pain and pain control in children. Curr Probl Pediatr 1985;15:1–67.
15. Joint Commission on Accreditation of Healthcare Organizations: Oakbrook Terrace, IL: Accreditation Manual for Hospitals, 1999.
16. Committee on Drugs, Section on Anesthesiology, American Academy of Pediatrics: Guidelines for the elective use of conscious sedation, deep sedation, and general anesthesia in pediatric patients. Pediatrics 1985;76:317–321.
17. Committee on Drugs, American Academy of Pediatrics: Guidelines for monitoring and management of pediatric patients during and after sedation for diagnostic and therapeutic procedures. Pediatrics 1992;89:1110–1115.
18. Coté CJ: Monitoring guidelines: Do they make a difference? AJR Am J Roentgenol 1995;165:910–912.

19. Coté CJ: Sedation protocols: Why so many variations? Pediatrics 1994;94:281–283.

20. Coté CJ, Strafford MA: The Principles of Pediatric Sedation. Boston: Tufts University School of Medicine; 1998.

21. Gross JB, Bailey PL, Caplan RA, et al: Practice guidelines for sedation and analgesia by non-anesthesiologists: A report by the American Society of Anesthesiologists Task Force on Sedation and Analgesia by Non-anesthesiologists. Anesthesiology 1996;84:459–471.

22. Aubuchon RW: Sedation liabilities in pedodontics. Pediatr Dent 1982;4:171–180.

23. Vade A, Sukhani R, Dolenga M, et al: Chloral hydrate sedation in children undergoing CT and MR imaging: Safety as judged by American Academy of Pediatrics (AAP) Guidelines. AJR Am J Roentgenol 1995;165:905–909.

24. McCarver-May DG, Kang J, Aouthmany M, et al: Comparison of chloral hydrate and midazolam for sedation of neonates for neuroimaging studies. J Pediatr 1996;128:573–576.

25. Terndrup TE, Cantor RM, Madden CM: Intramuscular meperidine, promethazine, and chlorpromazine: Analysis of use and complications in 487 pediatric emergency department patients. Ann Emerg Med 1989;18:528–533.

26. Gilger MA, Jeiven SD, Barrish JO, et al: Oxygen desaturation and cardiac arrhythmias in children during esophagogastroduodenoscopy using conscious sedation. Gastrointest Endosc 1993;39:392–395.

27. Coté CJ, Notterman DA, Karl HW, et al: Adverse sedation events in pediatrics: A critical incident analysis of contributory factors. Pediatrics 2000;105:805–814.

28. Food and Drug Administration, Subcommittee of the Anesthetic & Life Support Drugs Advisory Committee on Pediatric Sedation, 1994.

29. American Academy of Pediatric Dentistry: Guidelines for the elective use of conscious sedation, deep sedation, and general anesthesia in pediatric patients. ASDC J Dent Child 1986;53:21–22.

30. American Academy of Pediatric Dentistry: Guidelines for the elective use of pharmacologic conscious sedation and deep sedation in pediatric dental patients. Pediatr Dent 1993;15:297–299.

31. American Academy of Pediatric Dentistry: Guidelines for the elective use of pharmacologic conscious sedation and deep sedation in pediatric dental patients. Pediatr Dent 1997;19:48–52.

32. American College of Emergency Physicians: The use of pediatric sedation and analgesia. Ann Emerg Med 1997;29:834–835.

33. Nelson MD Jr: Guidelines for the monitoring and care of children during and after sedation for imaging studies. AJR Am J Roentgenol 1994;160:581–582.

34. Fishbaugh DF, Wilson S, Preisch JW, et al: Relationship of tonsil size on an airway blockage maneuver in children during sedation. Pediatr Dent 1997;19:277–281.

35. Biban P, Baraldi E, Pettenazzo A, et al: Adverse effect of chloral hydrate in two young children with obstructive sleep apnea. Pediatrics 1993;92:461–463.

36. Olkkola KT, Aranko K, Luurila H, et al: A potentially hazardous interaction between erythromycin and midazolam. Clin Pharmacol Ther 1993;53:298–305.

37. Hiller A, Olkkola KT, Isohanni P, et al: Unconsciousness associated with midazolam and erythromycin. Br J Anaesth 1990;65:826–828.

38. Backman JT, Olkkola KT, Aranko K, et al: Dose of midazolam should be reduced during diltiazem and verapamil treatments. Br J Clin Pharmacol 1994;37:221–225.

39. Dlugose D: Risk management considerations in conscious sedation. Crit Care Nurs Clin North Am 1997;9:429–440.

40. Ross PJ, Fochtman D: Conscious sedation: A quality management project. J Pediatr Oncol Nurs 1995;12:115–121.

41. Rayhorn N: Sedating and monitoring pediatric patients: Defining the nurse's responsibilities from preparation through recovery. MCN Am J Matern Child Nurs 1998;23:76–85.

42. Cotsen MR, Donaldson JS, Uejima T, et al: Efficacy of ketamine hydrochloride sedation in children for interventional radiologic procedures. AJR Am J Roentgenol 1997;169:1019–1022.

43. Lowrie L, Weiss AH, Lacombe C: The pediatric sedation unit: a mechanism for pediatric sedation. Pediatrics 1998;102:E30.

44. Lund N, Papadakos PJ: Barbiturates, neuroleptics, and propofol for sedation. Crit Care Clin 1995;11:875–886.

45. Parker RI, Mahan RA, Giugliano D, et al: Efficacy and safety of intravenous midazolam and ketamine as sedation for therapeutic and diagnostic procedures in children. Pediatrics 1997;99:427–431.

46. Vade A, Sukhani R: Ketamine hydrochloride for interventional radiology in children: Is it sedation or anesthesia by the radiologist? AJR Am J Roentgenol 1998;171:265–266.

47. Freyer DR, Schwanda AE, Sanfilippo DJ, et al: Intravenous methohexital for brief sedation of pediatric oncology outpatients: Physiologic and behavioral responses. Pediatrics 1997;99:E8.

48. Bloomfield EL, Masaryk TJ, Caplin A, et al: Intravenous sedation for MR imaging of the brain and spine in children: Pentobarbital versus propofol. Radiology 1993;186:93–97.

49. Swanson ER, Seaberg DC, Mathias S: The use of propofol for sedation in the emergency department. Acad Emerg Med 1996;3:234–238.

50. Cook BA, Bass JW, Nomizu S, et al: Sedation of children for technical procedures: Current standard of practice. Clin Pediatr (Phila) 1992;31:137–142.

51. Dachs RJ, Innes GM: Intravenous ketamine sedation of pediatric patients in the emergency department. Ann Emerg Med 1997;29:146–150.

52. Egelhoff JC, Ball WSJ, Koch BL, et al: Safety and efficacy of sedation in children using a structured sedation program. AJR Am J Roentgenol 1997;168:1259–1262.

53. Frush DP, Bisset GS, Hall SC: Pediatric sedation in radiology: the practice of safe sleep. AJR Am J Roentgenol 1996;167:1381–1387.

54. Green SM, Wittlake WA, Petrack EM: Meeting the guidelines and standards for pediatric sedation and analgesia. Pediatr Emerg Med Rep 1997;2:67–78.

55. Litman RS: Apnea and oxyhemoglobin desaturation after intramuscular ketamine administration in a 2-year-old child. Am J Emerg Med 1997;15:547–548.

56. Roelofse JA, Roelofse PG: Oxygen desaturation in a child receiving a combination of ketamine and midazolam for dental extractions. Anesth Prog 1997;44:68–70.

57. Mitchell RK, Koury SI, Stone CK: Respiratory arrest after intramuscular ketamine in a 2-year-old child. Am J Emerg Med 1996;14:580–581.

58. Crane M: The medication errors that get doctors sued. Med Economics, Nov 22, 1993, 36–41.

59. Kaufman E, Jastak JT: Sedation for outpatient dental procedures. Compend Contin Educ Dent 1995;16:462–480.

60. Krippaehne JA, Montgomery MT: Morbidity and mortality from pharmacosedation and general anesthesia in the dental office. J Oral Maxillofac Surg 1992;50:691–698.

61. Flanagan JF: The critical incident technique. Psychol Bull 1954;51:327–358.

62. Runciman WB, Webb RK, Lee R, et al: The Australian Incident Monitoring Study. System failure: An analysis of 2000 incident reports. Anaesth Intensive Care 1993;21:684–695.

63. Leape LL: The preventability of medical injury. In Bogner MS (ed): Human Error in Medicine. Hillsdale, NJ: Lawrence Erlbaum Associates; 1994, pp 13–25.

64. Moray N: Error reduction as a systems problem. In: Bogner MS, ed: Human Error in Medicine. Hillsdale, NJ: Lawrence Erlbaum Associates; 1994, pp 67–91.

65. Cooper JB, Newbower RS, Kitz RJ: An analysis of major errors and equipment failures in anesthesia management: considerations for prevention and detection. Anesthesiology 1984;60:34–42.

66. Leape LL, Lawthers AG, Brennan TA, et al: Preventing medical injury. QRB Qual Rev Bull 1993;19:144–149.

67. Cooper JB, Newbower RS, Long CD, et al: Preventable anesthesia mishaps: A study of human factors. Anesthesiology 1978;49:399–406.

68. Gaba DM: Human error in anesthetic mishaps. Int Anesthesiol Clin 1989;27:137–147.

69. Bogner MS: Human Error in Medicine. Hillsdale, NJ: Lawrence Erlbaum Associates; 1994.

70. Reason J: Human Error. Cambridge: Cambridge University Press; 1990.

71. Committee on Drugs, American Academy of Pediatrics: Unapproved uses of approved drugs: The physician, the package insert, and the FDA. Pediatrics 1996;98:143–145.

72. Coté CJ, Kauffman RE, Troendle GJ, et al: Is the "therapeutic orphan" about to be adopted? Pediatrics 1996;98:118–123.

73. Coté CJ: Unapproved uses of approved drugs. Paediatr Anaesth 1997;7:91–92.

74. Coté CJ: "Off-label" use of drugs in pediatric anesthesia: Legal, clinical, and policy considerations. Curr Op Anaesth 1999;12:325–327.

75. U.S. Department of Health and Human Services, Food and Drug Administration. Federal Registrar, 64240–64250 (1994). 21 CFR Part 201.

76. U.S. Food and Drug Administration Modernization Act. Pub. L. 105–115, Section 111 of (21 U.S.C. 355A) (1997).

77. U.S. Food and Drug Administration. Regulations requiring manufacturers to assess the safety and effectiveness of new drugs and biological products in pediatric patients. 21 CFR Parts 201, 312, 314, and 601 [Docket No. 97N–0165] (1998).

78. Kauffman RE: Drug trials in children: Ethical, legal, and practical issues. J Clin Pharmacol 1994;34:296–299.

79. Kauffman RE: Fentanyl, fads, and folly: Who will adopt the therapeutic orphans? J Pediatr 1991;119:588–589.

80. Kauffman RE: Status of drug approval processes and regulation of medications for children. Curr Opin Pediatr 1995;7:195–198.

81. Wilson JT, Kearns GL, Murphy D, et al: Paediatric labelling requirements: Implications for pharmacokinetic studies. Clin Pharmacokinet 1994;26:308–325.

82. Wilson JT: Pediatric pharmacology: The path clears for a noble mission. J Clin Pharm 1993;33:210–212.

83. Bjerring P, Arendt-Nielsen L: Depth and duration of skin analgesia to needle insertion after topical application of EMLA cream. Br J Anaesth 1990;64:173–177.

84. Gajraj NM, Pennant JH, Watcha MF: Eutectic mixture of local anesthetics (EMLA) cream. Anesth Analg 1994;78:574–583.

85. Taddio A, Nulman I, Goldbach M, et al: Use of lidocaine-prilocaine cream for vaccination pain in infants. J Pediatr 1994;124:643–648.

86. Wolf SI, Shier JM, Lampl KL, et al: EMLA cream for painless skin testing: A preliminary report. Ann Allerg 1994;73:40–42.

87. Benini F, Johnston CC, Faucher D, et al: Topical anesthesia during circumcision in newborn infants. JAMA 1993;270:850–853.

88. Smith SM, Barry RC: A comparison of three formulations of TAC (tetracaine, adrenalin, cocaine) for anesthesia of minor lacerations in children. Pediatr Emerg Care 1990;6:266–270.

89. Dailey RH: Fatality secondary to misuse of TAC solution. Ann Emerg Med 1988;17:159–160.

90. Daya MR, Burton BT, Schleiss MR, et al: Recurrent seizures following mucosal application of TAC. Ann Emerg Med 1988;17:646–648.

91. Ernst AA, Marvez-Valls E, Nick TG, et al: LAT (lidocaine-adrenaline-tetracaine) versus TAC (tetracaine- adrenaline-cocaine) for topical anesthesia in face and scalp lacerations. Am J Emerg Med 1995;13:151–154.

92. Smith GA, Strausbaugh SD, Harbeck-Weber C, et al: Comparison of topical anesthetics without cocaine to tetracaine-adrenaline-cocaine and lidocaine infiltration during repair of lacerations: Bupivacaine-norepinephrine is an effective new topical anesthetic agent. Pediatrics 1996;97:301–307.

93. Smith GA, Strausbaugh SD, Harbeck-Weber C, et al: Prilocaine-phenylephrine and bupivacaine-phenylephrine topical anesthetics compared with tetracaine-adrenaline-cocaine during repair of lacerations. Am J Emerg Med 1998;16:121–124.

94. Temme JB, Anderson JC, Matecko S: Sedation of children for CT and MRI scanning. Radiol Technol 1990;61:283–285.

95. Greenberg SB, Faerber EN, Aspinall CL, et al: High-dose chloral hydrate sedation for children undergoing MR imaging: Safety and efficacy in relation to age. AJR Am J Roentgenol 1993;161:639–641.

96. Greenberg SB, Faerber EN, Aspinall CL: High dose chloral hydrate sedation for children undergoing CT. J Comput Assist Tomogr 1991;15:467–469.

97. Moore PA, Mickey EA, Hargreaves JA, et al: Sedation in pediatric dentistry: A practical assessment procedure. J Am Dent Assoc 1984;109:564–569.

98. Litman RS, Kottra JA, Verga KA, et al: Chloral hydrate sedation: The additive sedative and respiratory depressant effects of nitrous oxide. Anesth Analg 1998;86:724–728.

99. Wilson S: Chloral hydrate and its effects on multiple physiological parameters in young children: A dose-response study. Pediatr Dent 1992;14:171–177.

100. Mayers DJ, Hindmarsh KW, Sankaran K, et al: Chloral hydrate disposition following single-dose administration to critically ill neonates and children. Devel Pharmacol Therapeutics 1991;16:71–77.

101. Doyle WL, Perrin L: Emergence delirium in a child given oral midazolam for conscious sedation. Ann Emerg Med 1994;24:1173–1175.

102. Payne KA, Coetzee AR, Mattheyse FJ: Midazolam and amnesia in pediatric premedication. Acta Anaesthiol Belg 1991;42:101–105.

103. Twersky RS, Hartung J, Berger BJ, et al: Midazolam enhances antgrograde but not retrograde amnesia in pediatric patients. Anesthesiology 1993;78:51–55.

104. Litman RS, Berkowitz RJ, Ward DS: Levels of consciousness and ventilatory parameters in young children during sedation with oral midazolam and nitrous oxide. Arch Pediatr Adolesc Med 1996;150:671–675.

105. Alexander CM, Gross JB: Sedative doses of midazolam depress hypoxic ventilatory responses in humans. Anesth Analg 1988;67:377–382.

106. Drummond GB: Comparison of sedation with midazolam and ketamine: Effects on airway muscle activity. Br J Anaesth 1996;76:663–667.

107. Yaster M, Nichols DG, Deshpande JK, et al: Midazolam-fentanyl intravenous sedation in children: Case report of respiratory arrest. Pediatrics 1990;86:463–467.

108. Buhrer M, Maitre PO, Hung O, et al: Electroencephalographic effects of benzodiazepines. I. Choosing an electroencephalographic parameter to measure the effect of midazolam on the central nervous system. Clin Pharmacol Ther 1990;48:544–554.

109. Buhrer M, Maitre PO, Crevoisier C, et al: Electroencephalographic effects of benzodiazepines. II. Pharmacodynamic modeling of the electroencephalographic effects of midazolam and diazepam. Clin Pharmacol Ther 1990;48:555–567.

110. Klotz U, Avant GR, Hoyumpa A, et al: The effects of age and liver disease on the disposition and elimination of diazepam in adult man. J Clin Invest 1975;55:347–359.

111. Mandelli M, Tognoni G, Garattini S: Clinical pharmacokinetics of diazepam. Clin Pharmacokinet 1978;3:72–91.

112. Greenblatt DJ, Allen MD, Harmatz JS, et al: Diazepam disposition determinants. Clin Pharmacol Ther 1980;27:301–312.

113. Burtin P, Jacqz-Aigrain E, Girard P, et al: Population pharmacokinetics of midazolam in neonates. Clin Pharmacol Ther 1994;56:615–625.

114. Jacqz-Aigrain E, Burtin P: Clinical pharmacokinetics of sedatives in neonates. Clin Pharmacokinet 1996;31:423–443.

115. Jacqz-Aigrain E, Daoud P, Burtin P, et al: Pharmacokinetics of midazolam during continuous infusion in critically ill neonates. Eur J Clin Pharmacol 1992;42:329–332.

116. Karl HW, Keifer AT, Rosenberger JL, et al: Comparison of the safety and efficacy of intranasal midazolam or sufentanil for preinduction of anesthesia in pediatric patients. Anesthesiology 1992;76:209–215.

117. Connors K, Terndrup TE: Nasal versus oral midazolam for sedation of anxious children undergoing laceration repair. Ann Emerg Med 1994;24:1074–1079.

118. Blouin RT, Conard PF, Perreault S, et al: The effect of flumazenil on midazolam-induced depression of the ventilatory response to hypoxia during isohypercarbia. Anesthesiology 1993;78:635–641.

119. Flogel CM, Ward DS, Wada DR, et al: The effects of large-dose flumazenil on midazolam-induced ventilatory depression. Anesth Analg 1993;77:1207–1214.

120. Flumazenil Study Group: Reversal of central nervous system effects by flumazenil after intravenous conscious sedation with midazolam: Report of a multicenter study. Clin Ther 1992;14:861–877.

121. Jones RDM, Lawson AD, Andrew LJ, et al: Antagonism of the hypnotic effect of midazolam in children: A randomized, double-blind study of placebo and flumazenil administered after midazolam-induced anaesthesia. Br J Anaesth 1991;66:660–666.

122. Sugarman JM, Paul RI: Flumazenil: A review. Pediatr Emerg Care 1994;10:37–43.

123. McDuffee AT, Tobias JD: Seizure after flumazenil administration in a pediatric patient. Pediatr Emerg Care 1995;11:186–187.

124. Weinbrum A, Geller E: The respiratory effects of reversing midazolam sedation with flumazenil in the presence or absence of narcotics. Acta Anaesthesiol Scand 1990;34(Suppl 92):65–69.

125. Strain JD, Harvey LA, Foley LC, et al: Intravenously administered pentobarbatal sodium for sedation on pediatric CT. Radiology 1986;161:105–108.

126. Neidhart P, Burgener MC, Schwieger I, et al: Chest wall rigidity during fentanyl- and midazolam-fentanyl induction: Ventilatory and haemodynamic effects. Acta Anaesthesiol Scand 1989;33:1–5.

127. Olkkola KT, Hamunen K, Maunuksela EL: Clinical pharmacokinetics and pharmacodynamics of opioid analgesics in infants and children. Clin Pharmacokinet 1995;28:385–404.

128. Rosow C: Remifentanil: A unique opioid analgesic. Anesthesiology 1993;79:875–876.

129. Gourlay GK, Boas RA: Fatal outcome with use of rectal morphine for postoperative pain control in an infant. Br Med J 1992;304:766–767.

130. Pokela ML, Olkkola KT, Koivisto M, et al: Pharmacokinetics and

pharmacodynamics of intravenous meperidine in neonates and infants. Clin Pharmacol Ther 1992;52:342–349.

131. Hagmeyer KO, Mauro LS, Mauro VF: Meperidine-related seizures associated with patient-controlled analgesia pumps. Ann Pharmacother 1993;27:29–32.

132. Agency for Health Care Policy and Research, U.S. Public Health Service: Acute pain management guideline panel, acute pain management: Operative or medical procedures and trauma. Clinical practice guideline, 1992. Rockville MD: U.S. Department of Health and Human Services.

133. Terndrup TE, Dire DJ, Madden CM, et al: A prospective analysis of intramuscular meperidine, promethazine, and chlorpromazine in pediatric emergency department patients. Ann Emerg Med 1991;20:31–35.

134. Snodgrass WR, Dodge WF: Lytic/"DPT" cocktail: Time for rational and safe alternatives. Pediatr Clin North Am 1989;36:1285–1291.

135. Yeung PK, Hubbard JW, Korchinski ED, et al: Pharmacokinetics of chlorpromazine and key metabolites. Eur J Clin Pharmacol 1993;45:563–569.

136. Loo JC, Midha KK, McGilveray IJ: Pharmacokinetics of chlorpromazine in normal volunteers. Commun Psychopharmacol 1980;4:121–129.

137. Terndrup TE, Dire DJ, Madden CM, et al: Comparison of intramuscular meperidine and promethazine with and without chlorpromazine: A randomized, prospective, double-blind trial. Ann Emerg Med 1993;22:206–211.

138. American Academy of Pediatrics, Committee on Drugs: Reappraisal of lytic cocktail/demerol, phenergan, and thorazine (DPT) for the sedation of children. Pediatrics 1995;95:598–602.

139. Dsida RM, Wheeler M, Birmingham PK, et al: Premedication of pediatric tonsillectomy patients with oral transmucosal fentanyl citrate. Anesth Analg 1998;86:66–70.

140. Sharar SR, Bratton SL, Carrougher GJ, et al: A comparison of oral transmucosal fentanyl citrate and oral hydromorphone for inpatient pediatric burn wound care analgesia. J Burn Care Rehabil 1998;19:516–521.

141. Schutzman SA, Burg J, Liebelt E, et al: Oral transmucosal fentanyl citrate for premedication of children undergoing laceration repair. Ann Emerg Med 1994;24:1059–1064.

142. Perry HE, Shannon MW: Diagnosis and management of opioid- and benzodiazepine-induced comatose overdose in children. Curr Opin Pediatr 1996;8:243–247.

143. Glass PS, Jhaveri RM, Smith LR: Comparison of potency and duration of action of nalmefene and naloxone. Anesth Analg 1994;78:536–541.

144. Prough DS, Roy R, Bumgarner J, et al: Acute pulmonary edema in healthy teenagers following conservative doses of intravenous naloxone. Anesthesiology 1984;60:485–486.

145. Chamberlain JM, Klein BL: A comprehensive review of naloxone for the emergency physician. Am J Emerg Med 1994;12:650–660.

146. Bowdle TA: Clinical pharmacology of antagonists of narcotic-induced respiratory depression: A brief review. Acute Care 1988;12(Suppl 1):70–76.

147. Hannallah RS, Patel RI: Low-dose intramuscular ketamine for anesthesia pre-induction in young children undergoing brief outpatient procedures. Anesthesiology 1989;70:598–600.

148. Gutstein HB, Johnson KL, Heard MB, et al: Oral ketamine preanesthetic medication in children. Anesthesiology 1992;76:28–33.

149. Tobias JD, Phipps S, Smith B, et al: Oral ketamine premedication to alleviate the distress of invasive procedures in pediatric oncology patients. Pediatrics 1992;90:537–541.

150. Reinemer HC, Wilson CF, Webb MD: A comparison of two oral ketamine-diazepam regimens for sedating anxious pediatric dental patients. Pediatr Dent 1996;18:294–300.

151. Gingrich B: Difficulties encountered in a comparative study of orally administered midazolam and ketamine. Anesthesiology 1994;80:1414–1415.

152. Carson IW, Moore J, Balmer JP, et al: Laryngeal competence with ketamine and other drugs. Anesthesiology 1973;38:128–133.

153. Hickey PR, Hansen DD, Cramolini GM, et al: Pulmonary and systemic hemodynamic responses to ketamine in infants with normal and elevated pulmonary vascular resistance. Anesthesiology 1985;62:287–293.

154. Parke TJ, Stevens JE, Rice AS, et al: Metabolic acidosis and fatal myocardial failure after propofol infusion in children: five case reports. Br Med J 1992;305:613–616.

155. Hanna JP, Ramundo ML: Rhabdomyolysis and hypoxia associated with prolonged propofol infusion in children. Neurology 1998;50:301–303.

156. Strickland RA, Murray MJ: Fatal metabolic acidosis in a pediatric patient receiving an infusion of propofol in the intensive care unit: Is there a relationship? Crit Care Med 1995;23:405–409.

157. Pepperman ML, Macrae D: A comparison of propofol and other sedative use in paediatric intensive care in the United Kingdom. Paediatr Anaesth 1997;7:143–153.

158. Bjorkman S, Gabrielsson J, Quaynor H, et al: Pharmacokinetics of I.V. and rectal methohexitone in children. Br J Anaesth 1987;59:1541–1547.

159. Rockoff MA, Goudsouzian NG: Seizures induced by methohexital. Anesthesiology 1981;54:333–335.

160. Jeffries G: Radiotherapy and children's anaesthesia. Anaesthesia 1988;43:416–417.

161. Manuli MA, Davies L: Rectal methohexital for sedation of children during imaging procedures. AJR Am J Roentgenol 1993;160:577–580.

162. Liu LM, Goudsouzian NG, Liu PL: Rectal methohexital premedication in children, a dose-comparison study. Anesthesiology 1980;53:343–345.

163. Liu LM, Gaudreault P, Friedman PA, et al: Methohexital plasma concentrations in children following rectal administration. Anesthesiology 1985;62:567–570.

164. Daniels AL, Coté CJ, Polaner DM: Continuous oxygen saturation monitoring following rectal methohexitone induction in paediatric patients. Can J Anaesth 1992;39:27–30.

27

Temperature Regulation: Normal and Abnormal (Malignant Hyperthermia)

Bruno Bissonnette *and* John F. Ryan

Normal Thermoregulation in Infants and Children: Physiologic Mechanisms

    Afferent Thermal Sensing

    Central Regulation

    Efferent Responses

Thermoregulation in the Newborn

Perioperative Hypothermia: Physiologic Modifications

    Internal Redistribution of Heat

    Thermal Imbalance

    Thermal Steady-State (Plateau or Rewarming)

Effects of Anesthetic Medications on Thermoregulation

Perioperative Hyperthermia

    Physiologic Considerations

    Clinical Implications

Malignant Hyperthermia

    Incidence

    Genetics

    Pathophysiology

    Diagnosis

    Differential Diagnosis

    Masseter Spasm, Masseter Muscle Rigidity, Masseter Tetany

    Muscle Biopsy Testing

    Patients with Malignant Hyperthermia Susceptibility

    Management of a Malignant Hyperthermia Crisis

    Actions of Dantrolene

    Subsequent Anesthetic Procedures

    The Family

Temperature Monitoring

    Indications for Temperature Monitoring

    Thermometers

    Temperature Monitoring Sites

Prevention of Hypothermia

    Preventing Redistribution Hypothermia

    Operating Room Temperature

    Warming Devices

    Airway Humidification

    Intravenous Fluid Warming

Conclusions

Under normal circumstances, central body temperature is maintained within 0.4°C of its set point of 37°C. Drugs and illness affect the efficiency of the thermoregulatory system. Hypothermia is common during anesthesia and surgery because of anesthetic-induced inhibition of thermoregulatory mechanisms and patient exposure to a cold operating room environment. This chapter describes the normal and abnormal physiologic mechanisms of thermoregulation, including malignant hyperthermia and the effects of anesthetic agents on this system.

Normal Thermoregulation in Infants and Children: Physiologic Mechanisms

The thermoregulatory system is similar to other physiologic control systems in that the brain uses negative feedback to

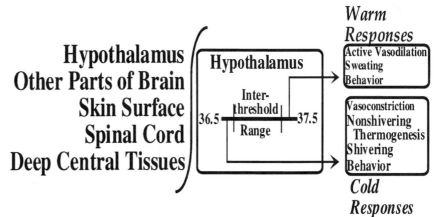

Figure 27–1. The thermoregulatory model. Thermal inputs received from a variety of tissues including the brain, skin surface, spinal cord, and deep core structures are integrated by the hypothalamus, which determines the mean body temperature. The "inter-threshold range" is the mean body temperature during which no effector responses are triggered. On either side of this inter-threshold range are triggered thermoregulatory responses (warm responses or cold responses). (Adapted from Sessler DI: Temperature monitoring. In: Miller RD, ed.: Anesthesia, 4th ed. New York: Churchill Livingstone, 1994:1363–1382.)

keep variations from normal values to a minimum.[1] Intraoperative hypothermia provokes peripheral vasoconstriction.[2–4] The principal site of temperature regulation is the hypothalamus, which interprets signals derived from other parts of the brain, the spinal cord, the central core tissues, and the skin surface. The processing of thermoregulatory information occurs in three stages: (1) afferent thermal sensing, (2) central regulation, and (3) efferent response.

Afferent Thermal Sensing

The hypothalamus receives information from thermally sensitive cells throughout the body. In the periphery, anatomically distinct warm and cold receptors detect the ambient temperature; each receptor type transmits the information through afferent nerve conduction pathways. The intensity of the stimulus rather than the type of nerve fiber influences the speed of transmission. The thermal information obtained by the cold-sensitive cells is transmitted to the hypothalamus by A-delta fibers. The thermal information obtained from the warm receptors is carried by unmyelinated C fibers. The C fibers also detect and convey pain, which is why intense heat cannot be distinguished from sharp pain.[5, 6] Most ascending thermal information travels along the spinothalamic tracts in the anterior spinal cord, but no single spinal tract is solely responsible for conveying thermal information.[7]

Central Regulation

Central regulation by the hypothalamus occurs by comparing integrated thermal inputs from the skin surface, neuraxis, and deep tissues with threshold temperatures for heat and cold. Other structures in the brain and spinal cord also possess some thermoregulatory capacity; however, the extent to which these "lower" structures contribute to overall regulation is not known. When the integrated input from all sources exceeds the upper threshold or falls below the lower threshold, efferent responses are initiated from the hypothalamus to maintain body temperature (higher or lower) (Fig. 27–1). The inter-threshold range, that is, the temperature range over which no regulatory responses occur, is quite narrow in the awake state (approximately 0.2°C) but much broader during anesthesia (approximately 3.5°C) (Fig. 27–2). The inter-threshold range is also wider in the hypothermic state than in the hyperthermic state. Although the brain presumably detects temperature changes within the inter-

threshold range, these changes do not trigger regulatory responses until one of the threshold temperatures is reached. This physiologic system behaves as an "all or none" phenomenon. The mechanism by which the body determines absolute threshold temperatures is not known, but it appears that the thresholds are influenced by many factors such as circadian rhythm, exercise, food intake, thyroid function, anesthetics, and other drugs, as well as cold and warm adaptation. Central regulation is intact from infancy but may be impaired in elderly or extremely ill patients. Thermoregulatory responses are triggered by integrated sampling of thermal signals from nearly every tissue in the body (the mean body temperature) and not simply central core temperature.

Mean body temperature, that is, the temperature of all body tissues, is a physiologically weighted average reflecting the thermoregulatory importance of various tissues. The different efferent responses in humans, such as behavioral responses, are the result of integrated thermal inputs, which are determined almost exclusively by skin-surface tempera-

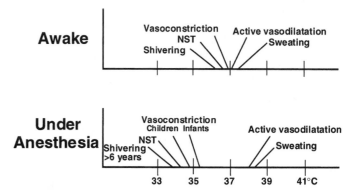

Figure 27–2. Schematic diagram illustrating thermoregulatory thresholds and gains in awake and anesthetized infants and children. Vertical lines represent the maximal intensity of the effector responses. The horizontal lines represent the mean body temperature. The mean body temperature that triggers the response is the threshold and the slope indicates the gain of that response. The sensitivity of the thermoregulatory system is the distance between the first cold response (vasoconstriction) and the first warm response (active vasodilatation). (From Bissonnette B: Thermoregulation and paediatric anaesthesia. Curr Opin Anesthesiol 1993;6:537–542.)

ture, not by tissue heat content, cutaneous heat flux, or central temperature.[8, 9]

Efferent Responses

A thermal steady state is actively maintained when the hypothalamus responds to thermal changes—temperatures exceeding the appropriate high or low threshold. Thus, thermal deviations from the threshold temperature initiate efferent responses that increase metabolic heat production (non-shivering and shivering thermogenesis), decrease environmental heat loss (active vasoconstriction and behavioral maneuvers, e.g., covering up with a blanket), or increase heat loss (active vasodilation, sweating and behavioral maneuvers, e.g., removing clothing). Behavioral responses to environmental temperatures outside the thermoneutral range (approximately 28°C for unclothed adult humans) are quantitatively the most important thermoregulatory effectors in humans (e.g., heating a home, putting on a sweater).

Cutaneous vasoconstriction is the first and most consistent thermoregulatory response to hypothermia. Digital skin blood flow has two components, nutritional (capillary) and thermoregulatory (arteriovenous shunts). Thermoregulatory-induced decreases in cutaneous blood flow are greatest (up to 100-fold) in arteriovenous shunts of the hands, feet, ears, lips, and nose.[10] Shunts are typically 100 μm in diameter, which means that one can divert as much as 10,000 times more blood than a comparable length of 10 μm diameter capillary.[11] Shunt blood flow is primarily mediated by norepinephrine released by presynaptic adrenergic terminals that are sensitized by local cooling and inhibited by temperatures equal to or exceeding 35°C[12]; flow also decreases in the more numerous capillaries.[13] Despite impressive decreases in cutaneous perfusion resulting from thermoregulatory vasoconstriction, heat loss from the whole body is reduced only 25%.[14]

The ability to produce heat by increasing metabolic rate and oxygen consumption is the other component of thermal regulation.[15] Heat production is achieved by three mechanisms: voluntary muscle activity, involuntary muscle activity (shivering), and non-shivering thermogenesis. Voluntary muscle activity for heat production is obliterated during the operative period. Of the two remaining mechanisms for heat production, non-shivering thermogenesis is the major component in the newborn versus shivering thermogenesis for heat production in the older child and adult. The contribution of non-shivering thermogenesis in adults is debatable.[16] The time course and relation of non-shivering thermogenesis to shivering thermogenesis (see Fig. 27–2) and factors involved in the developmental aspects of switching on and switching off of the non-shivering thermogenesis mechanism remain to be elucidated.[15] Non-shivering thermogenesis is the infant's primary response to hypothermia, but it compensates poorly for ineffective shivering and limited vasoconstriction compared with adults. Premature or small for gestational age infants have an exceptionally large skin-surface area compared with body mass and therefore lose proportionately more heat through skin than adults.[17, 18] The combination of proportionally increased heat loss, diminished ability to produce endogenous heat, and a diminished thermoregulatory response efficacy makes infants particularly vulnerable to developing hypothermia.

Non-shivering thermogenesis is an increase in metabolic heat production without increases in mechanical muscular work. Non-shivering thermogenesis occurs principally through metabolism of brown fat but can also occur at a lesser degree in skeletal muscle, liver, brain, and white fat.[19] Brown fat differentiates in the human fetus at 26 to 30 weeks of gestational age. Brown fat constitutes 2 to 6% of the infant's total body weight and is located mainly in six areas: between the scapulae, in small masses around blood vessels in the neck, in large deposits in the axillae, in medium-sized masses in the mediastinum, around the internal mammary vessels in the mediastinum, and around the adrenal glands or kidneys. Morphologically, brown fat contains multinucleated cells with numerous mitochondria. The mitochondria appear densely packed with cristae and have increased respiratory chain components.[20] Brown fat is a highly specialized tissue with both an abundant vascular supply and rich innervation of the sympathetic nervous system. It is activated primarily by beta-sympathetic stimulation, which uncouples oxidative phosphorylation.[16, 21, 22] With cold stress, there are increases in norepinephrine production leading to brown fat metabolism.[23] In addition to norepinephrine, glucocorticoids and thyroxine also have been implicated as factors in non-shivering thermogenesis.[16, 24, 25] The heat produced by non-shivering thermogenesis is primarily a by-product of fatty acid metabolism, but it also can result from glucose metabolism and gluconeogenesis. Non-shivering thermogenesis can be inhibited surgically by sympathectomy and pharmacologically by ganglionic and beta blockade, and by inhalation agents.[26–29]

Shivering is characterized by high-frequency, irregular muscular activity that begins in upper body muscles. Typically, tremor spasms wrack the body, producing a "waxing and waning" electromyographic pattern.[30] It is believed that shivering only occurs after maximal vasoconstriction, when non-shivering thermogenesis and behavioral maneuvers have proven to be insufficient to maintain an adequate mean body temperature and/or perhaps spinal cord temperature.[31–34] With increasing age, shivering thermogenesis assumes a more prominent role in thermoregulation. Vigorous shivering can briefly increase metabolic heat production fourfold but will sustain only twofold increases. Oxygen consumption ($\dot{V}O_2$) will be proportionally increased.[16, 35–37] In healthy patients, this increase in $\dot{V}O_2$ is met by an increase in cardiac output without any hemodynamic compromise. In patients with limited myocardial reserve, however, this increase in $\dot{V}O_2$ can result in a decreased mixed venous oxygen content that, under a less than perfect ventilation-perfusion ($\dot{V}/\dot{Q}$) ratio, can decrease arterial oxygen content and, consequently, decrease tissue oxygen delivery.

The efficacy of the thermoregulatory mechanisms determines the range of tolerable thermal environments. Extremes of age, illness, or drug effect can provoke thermal disturbances despite normal ambient temperatures and can produce aberrant or inadequate response to environmental temperature deviations.

Thermoregulation in the Newborn

The neonate's thermoregulatory range is limited and easily overwhelmed by environmental influences. The lower temperature limit of thermal regulation in adults is 0°C, whereas in newborns it is 22°C. Newborns, infants, and small children are more sensitive to hypothermia because their efferent mechanisms are less effective, they have an increased surface-area-to-volume ratio, they have increased thermal conductance, and they lose proportionately more metabolic heat through their skin.

The neutral thermal environment is defined as the range of ambient temperatures at which metabolic rate is minimal and temperature regulation is achieved by nonevaporative physical processes alone. The range of the neutral thermal environment is limited in infants. In general, the maintenance of a core temperature in cool environments results in an increase in oxygen consumption and the development of metabolic acidosis. In full-term infants, oxygen consumption does not correlate with rectal temperature but rather increases directly with the skin-surface-to-environmental temperature gradient.[38] Increases in oxygen consumption are minimal at skin-surface-to-environmental temperature gradients of 2°C to 4°C. Thus, at environmental temperatures of 32 to 34°C and abdominal skin temperatures of 36°C, the resting newborn infant is usually in a state of minimal increased oxygen consumption, that is, the neutral thermal state. Thus, normal rectal temperatures do not imply a state of minimal increased oxygen consumption. However, during anesthesia, infants do respond actively to a decrease in mean body temperature by showing a strong cutaneous vasoconstrictive response and intraoperative warming. Studies have not yet determined the thermoregulatory response of premature newborn or small for gestational age infants.

Perioperative Hypothermia: Physiologic Modifications

General anesthesia decreases the temperature threshold at which the body initiates thermoregulation in response to cold stress (see Fig. 27–2). Mild intraoperative hypothermia 1 to 3°C below normal is common and results from a combination of events: (1) an approximately 20% reduction in metabolic heat production during halothane anesthesia[28]; (2) increased environmental exposure; (3) anesthetic-induced central thermoregulatory inhibition[31, 39, 40]; and (4) redistribution of heat within the body.[8] Hypothermia has a typical profile during general anesthesia and usually develops in three phases (Fig. 27–3): (1) internal redistribution of heat; (2) thermal imbalance (heat loss to the environment); and (3) thermal steady-state (plateau or rewarming).

Internal Redistribution of Heat

The first phase of general anesthesia–induced hypothermia is a rapid cooling of the central core (vessel-rich organs) temperature during the first 30 to 45 minutes (Fig. 27–4). The peripheral compartment (the other tissues but not skin) acts as a dynamic buffer that functions to accommodate any changes in core temperature by vasodilation or vasoconstriction. The skin compartment (or "shell") is the barrier between the environment and the core and peripheral compartments.

After induction, anesthetic-induced changes in blood flow distribution result in an increase in the size of the central

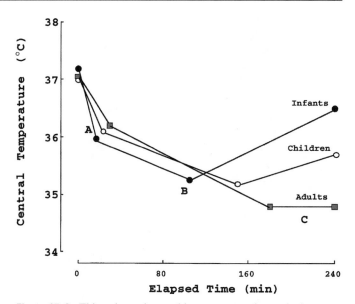

Figure 27–3. This schematic graphic represents the typical pattern of hypothermia during anesthesia, which occurs in three distinct phases during anesthesia for infants (closed circles), children (open circles), and adults (squares): (A) internal redistribution of heat, (B) heat loss to the environment, and (C) thermal steady-state or rewarming. It must be noted that the slopes of each phase vary as a function of the age groups. (From Bissonnette B: Thermoregulation and pediatric anesthesia. Curr Opin Anesthesiol 1993;6:537–542.

compartment, thus causing a redistribution of the central core's heat within a larger volume and an increase in the peripheral and skin compartment temperatures. The decrease in metabolic heat production caused by anesthetic agents further reduces the amount of energy available to compensate for the enlargement of this compartment. Internal redistribution of heat occurs even in the absence of heat loss, with the environment causing a measurable decrease in central temperature.

Thermal Imbalance

Anesthetic-induced thermal imbalance results from a reduction in heat production and an increase in heat loss to the environment. During this second phase, lasting 2 to 3 hours, the heat loss to the environment leads to an approximately linear decrease in mean body temperature (typically 0.5–1.0°C/hour). Anesthesia contributes to a decrease in heat production by limiting muscular activity, reducing metabolic rate, and diminishing the work of breathing.[28, 41, 42] Heat loss from the patient to the environment is a function of the temperature difference between the body surface and ambient structures. Heat loss decreases passively as patients become increasingly hypothermic and therefore become closer to the environmental temperature.

Conduction, evaporation, convection, and radiation contribute to heat loss from the patient to the environment during anesthesia and surgery. Conductive heat transfer depends on the temperature difference and the surface in contact between the two objects, such as the patient and operating room table and the conductance between them. The conductance is a property of the material the patient is in

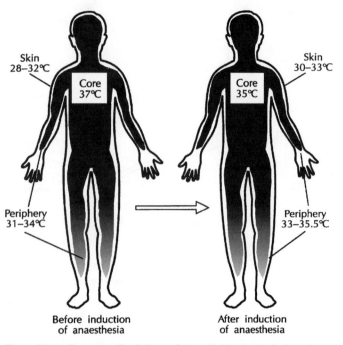

Before induction
of anaesthesia

After induction
of anaesthesia

Figure 27–4. Conceptually, it is useful to divide the body into three compartments. The central (core) and peripheral compartments are surrounded by the skin, which represents the envelope or the "shell." In the awake individual, the central core temperature is generally higher than that of peripheral tissues. After induction of anaesthesia, the vasodilatation induced by the anesthetic agents modifies the thermal balance between the compartments. (From Bissonnette B: Thermoregulation and pediatric anesthesia. Curr Opin Anesthesiol 1993;6:537–542.)

contact with or the interface between the patient and the object, such as a blanket or layers of blanket with air in between. Care should also be taken to ensure that the patient's skin is not in contact with metallic surfaces (high conductance).

Conductance determines the rate of heat transfer per unit area per unit temperature difference. Relatively little heat is lost during surgery via conduction to the environment because patients are well insulated from surrounding objects. However, the energy needed to warm irrigation solutions and intravenous fluids can have a profound impact either up or down on body temperature. Thus cold irrigation solutions may produce rapid heat loss, but conversely irrigation with warm solutions can increase the core temperature. *Evaporative* losses include several components: (1) sweating; (2) insensible water loss from the skin, respiratory tract, and open surgical wounds; and (3) evaporation of liquids applied to the skin such as antibacterial solutions. When water evaporates from a surface, energy is absorbed during transition from the liquid to the gaseous state. This energy is termed the latent heat of vaporization and in the case of evaporation of sweat it has a value of 2500 x 10^3 J/kg. This figure emphasizes the extraordinary power of the human sweating mechanism as a heat loss pathway. In environments in which the air temperature is the same or higher than skin temperature, sweating is the sole means available for dissipating metabolic heat production. In such situations, anything that limits evaporation, such as high ambient humidity or impermeable clothing, will readily lead to heat storage and a rise

in body temperature, hence the effectiveness of plastic wrap in maintaining a child's temperature intraoperatively.[43] Heat loss by evaporation depends on the water vapor pressure gradient between the skin surface and the ambient air.[44] As with convection, evaporation is determined by the vapor pressure gradient between the exposed body surface and the ambient air and the rate of air flow across the surface; alcohol-containing preparation solutions are therefore worse in terms of heat loss than water-based preparations.[44] This emphasizes the importance of keeping the patient well covered during transport to and from the operating room.[45–48]

Normally, evaporative losses from the skin surface are negligible except during sweating. Newborn infants will sweat in an effort to prevent overheating only when the environmental temperature exceeds 35°C and the rectal temperature is above 37°C.[49] Infants born at less than 30 weeks of gestation appear to have immature sweat glands resulting in defective sweat mechanisms.[15, 48, 50] A small amount of heat is lost when dry inspired respiratory gases are humidified by water evaporating from tracheobronchial epithelium. In adults, respiratory losses account for only 5 to 10% of total heat loss during anesthesia and surgery.[51] Insensible water loss accounts for approximately 25% of the total heat dissipated. Because minute ventilation on a per kilogram basis is higher in infants and children than in adults, respiratory losses represent about one third of this total heat loss. Heat loss from the respiratory tract increases if one breathes cool dry gas as opposed to warm, moisturized gas, hence the importance of heated humidifiers or artificial noses in maintaining body temperature of infants and small children during anesthesia.[4, 52] Finally, heat lost from evaporation inside large surgical incisions may equal all other sources of intraoperative loss combined.[53] Both conduction and evaporation account for about 15% of the total heat lost during surgical procedures. Hypothermia is more likely to occur if the patient is wet or in contact with wet drapes because of increased evaporative heat loss.

When a fluid (liquid or gas) at one temperature flows over a surface at a different temperature, heat is gained or lost by *convection*. In the case of naked humans, the rate and direction of convective exchange depends on the temperature difference between the air and the skin surface. The situation is more complicated in a clothed individual; convective losses increase in proportion to the temperature difference between the body surface and the surrounding fluid (liquid or gas). Convective losses are experienced outdoors as the "wind chill factor."

Exchange of heat by *radiation* between two surfaces depends on the difference in the fourth powers of the absolute temperature of the two surfaces (in this case, the body surface and the walls and other solid objects in the operating room). It is independent of atmospheric conditions in a manner similar to light passing through a vacuum. A patient in an operating room will warm up walls and solid objects by exchanging radiant energy.[54–56] At 22°C, 70% of the total heat loss is via radiation.[57] Both convection and radiation losses are dramatically reduced by even a single covering layer. Thus, a thin shirt (providing negligible insulation) considerably increases thermal comfort. Heat transfer by radiation depends principally on the temperature of the two surfaces concerned and is unaffected by air movement or the distance between the surfaces. Convection and radiation together contribute to 85% of the heat loss.

Thermal Steady-State (Plateau or Rewarming)

The third phase of the hypothermic response to anesthesia consists of a thermal steady-state in which metabolic heat production equals environmental heat loss and the core temperature therefore remains constant. In this situation, patients must either increase heat production or decrease heat loss, or both, to prevent further hypothermia. A study in adults undergoing isoflurane anesthesia[58] showed that the effect of cutaneous vasoconstriction decreases heat loss by only 10 to 15%, which is relatively small compared with the fall in metabolic rate from anesthesia and the increase in evaporative heat loss from the surgical wounds. It is presumed that this happens because heat loss to the environment is determined principally by capillary blood flow in large areas of skin covering the limbs and the trunk. These capillaries cannot constrict as much as peripheral arteriovenous shunts. Thus it is possible that vasoconstriction contributes to the thermal plateau by re-establishing the balance between the central and the peripheral compartments. The metabolic heat produced in the body core is distributed to a smaller central compartment and maintains the temperature of this compartment at a constant level. Consistent with this theory of compartmental size, the use of a limb tourniquet during surgery induces hyperthermia; this response is probably due to the reduction of the size of the peripheral compartment and the containment of metabolic heat within the central thermal compartment.[59]

Infants and children differ from adults because a rewarming phase occurs rather than the third (plateau) phase reported in adults (see Fig. 27–3). Despite the fact that general anesthesia decreases heat production by inhibiting muscular activity and reducing metabolic rate, there is a simultaneous increase in oxygen consumption, carbon dioxide production, and systemic noradrenaline levels in infants anesthetized with isoflurane and paralyzed with vecuronium. These observations are consistent with the increased role of non-shivering thermogenesis observed in unanesthetized infants. Although the only possible explanation initially suggested for this rewarming phase was the occurrence of non-shivering thermogenesis under anesthesia, other studies have reported in infants that halothane anesthesia blocks non-shivering thermogenesis.[28, 29, 60] Non-shivering thermogenesis does not appear to be functional in anesthetized adults. This can be supported by the fact that oxygen consumption does not increase when adults are vasoconstricted.[61] Infants differ from adults in that intraoperative thermoregulatory responses are sufficiently effective to increase central temperature despite constant ambient temperatures.

Effects of Anesthetic Medications on Thermoregulation

General anesthesia decreases the thermoregulatory threshold temperature triggering response to hypothermia by approximately 2.5°C and increases the threshold temperature initiating responses to hyperthermia to a lesser degree (approximately 1.3°C) (see Fig. 27–2).[31, 39] Anesthesia-induced expansion of the inter-threshold range results in a broad temperature range over which active thermoregulatory responses are absent. Within this range, patients are poikilothermic, and body temperature changes passively in proportion to the difference between metabolic heat production and heat loss to the environment. Vasoconstriction and non-shivering thermogenesis are the only thermoregulatory responses available to anesthetized, paralyzed, hypothermic patients. Patients who become sufficiently hypothermic during surgery (e.g., central body temperatures approximately 34.5°C) demonstrate profound peripheral vasoconstriction.[30, 61] The temperature at which vasoconstriction and non-shivering thermogenesis occur identifies the thermoregulatory threshold for the anesthetic agent and dose administered. The thermoregulatory threshold in healthy, adult patients given 1.0% halothane in oxygen for elective surgical procedures is approximately 34.4 ± 0.2°C.[61] The potent vasodilatory effect of isoflurane has been shown; the effect of isoflurane on the thermoregulatory threshold is inversely proportional to the inhaled concentration and is equal to approximately 3°C per percentage point of end-tidal concentration.[42]

The vasoconstriction threshold in infants and children anesthetized with isoflurane differs little from that of adults.[62] Thus the percentage increase in regulatory thermogenesis is similar in infants and adults. The thermoregulatory threshold for vasoconstriction in pediatric patients anesthetized with 1 minimum alveolar concentration (MAC) of halothane in 70% nitrous oxide (35.8 ± 0.5°C) is slightly higher than adults anesthetized with approximately 1.3 MAC and oxygen instead of nitrous oxide. Thermoregulatory inhibition is likely therefore to be similar for adults or children anesthetized with equipotent doses of halothane. The high surface area to mass ratio in infants, which allows rapid loss of heat to the environment, is largely offset by an intrinsically high metabolic rate. Environmental heat loss is further minimized by well-developed thermoregulatory vasoconstriction.[62] Although there is a trend toward decreased inhibition in smaller infants and children given similar isoflurane concentrations, differences between the groups were not statistically significant and spanned only approximately 0.3°C. This indicates that inhibition of thermoregulatory vasoconstriction is similar in anesthetized infants and children and therefore relatively independent of body weight.[62] Relatively constant thermoregulatory inhibition in infants and children of different ages is in marked contrast to the minimum alveolar concentration of isoflurane, which increases to approximately 1.5 times the adult requirement in infants 1 to 6 months of age. Thus inhibition of thermoregulatory vasoconstriction in infants and children is greater than in adults when administered anesthetic concentrations are adjusted for age.[62]

The influence of narcotics on thermoregulation remains controversial because their effects in animals differ from those in humans. Ketamine in anesthetized adults appears to cause less thermoregulatory suppression than other anesthetics.[63]

Central thermoregulation remains intact during regional anesthesia and therefore provides some protection against hypothermia. However, anesthetic interference with regional thermal sensation, increased heat loss to the environment, and regional depression of vasoconstriction and shivering may contribute to intraoperative hypothermia. The administration of a regional anesthetic technique reduces the risk of hypothermia, especially during surgery in which a small incision is made and the patient is kept well insulated beneath layered draping. In contrast, with large surgical incisions, hypothermia can be quite severe and recovery to normal body temperature may be prolonged.

Perioperative Hyperthermia

Physiologic Considerations

Because most operating rooms are equipped with air conditioning systems, perioperative hypothermia is typically the most commonly observed thermal disturbance in anesthetized patients. However, the observation that induced hyperthermia could be clinically useful in anesthesiology and surgery has revived interest in this topic. As previously mentioned, the thermal regulatory system responds to hypothermia and hyperthermia according to an engineering model of threshold and gains. The threshold represents the central temperature for which a particular regulatory effector becomes active, whereas the gain quantifies the intensity of the response (see Fig. 27–2). The effector mechanisms during hyperthermia are well preserved as central temperature increases during anesthesia. Studies concerning controlled hyperthermia (increased central temperature) have demonstrated that the expected efferent responses in an unanesthetized individual are preserved in the anesthetized subject.[31] However, similar to hypothermia, the efferent response thresholds are displaced to the right, creating a greater hyperthermic inter-threshold range (see Fig. 27–2). This inter-threshold range corresponds to the difference between the normal central temperature (approximately 37°C) and the first efferent response triggered by the hypothalamus in response to hyperthermia. In the normal unanesthetized person, the variability of the system is only 0.4°C. The range for hypothalamic response to hyperthermia (1.0 to 1.4°C) is considerably narrower under anesthesia compared with the range of response to hypothermia (2.5 to 3.5°C) under anesthesia[31]; this suggests that humans respond more aggressively to the consequences of hyperthermia than to hypothermia.

The efferent responses during hyperthermic stress under anesthesia are limited to two mechanisms: vasodilation and sweating. Active *vasodilation* (not simply the absence of active vasoconstriction) is triggered in response to warm stress.[64, 65] *Sweating* is an extremely effective process because of the relatively high heat of vaporization of water. This mechanism can allow up to a fivefold increase in heat loss to the environment, making it proportionately more effective than the combined defenses against cold.[66] In infants and children weighing less than 15 kg, sweating under anesthesia does not seem as effective as observed in older children and adults (Bissonnette and Sessler, unpublished data).[67–69] However, the observation of an active cutaneous vasodilation, although difficult to quantify (skin flushing), suggests that the thermoregulatory response to hyperthermia may be preserved in infants.

Clinical Implications

Hyperthermia can increase the blood flow of the forearm by three- to fourfold during exercise.[65] Because it is known that muscle blood flow does not increase significantly during heat stress, this observation suggests that skin blood flow must increase substantially more than three- to fourfold. The benefits provided by induced hyperthermia may be desirable during peripheral microvascular surgery when an increase in regional blood flow is important. One of the clinical limitations of the utilization of induced hyperthermia with the purpose of increasing cutaneous blood flow is the efficiency of the sweating mechanism. Although shivering can double heat production, sweating can lose up to five times the patient's central heat production.[14, 31]

Malignant Hyperthermia

Malignant hyperthermia (MH) is a genetically transmitted syndrome associated with abnormal muscle physiology related to calcium transport and homeostasis that results in uncontrolled increased metabolic activity in skeletal muscle.[70–72] This in turn results in increased oxygen consumption, increased carbon dioxide production, outstripping of oxygen delivery with oxygen demand, and resultant combined respiratory and metabolic acidosis. The diagnosis generally occurs with the clinical presentation of tachycardia, tachypnea, hypercarbia (which does not respond to the usual increase in minute ventilation), oxygen desaturation, cardiac arrhythmias, and frequently total body rigidity (occasionally just isolated masseter muscle tetany).

In the years since the first report of MH, dramatic advances have been made in understanding and treating this syndrome. Its genetic keys are slowly being discovered. This work is being assisted by the Human Genome Project which has unraveled the human genetic code in its entirety.[73, 74] The mechanism of the biochemical abnormalities with MH has been clarified for skeletal muscle, but the abnormalities in other tissues need further investigation. Early clinical diagnosis has been aided by the routine use of pulse oximetry and capnography monitoring.[75–78] Testing has been codified and the specificity and sensitivity of the diagnostic criteria improved.[79–82] Therapy with dantrolene sodium has reduced the mortality to less than 10%.[83–86] The establishment of the Malignant Hyperthermia Association of the United States (MHAUS) has given patients a strong support group.

Incidence

Malignant hyperthermia is a relatively rare disorder that is estimated to occur in 1 in 50,000 to 1 in 100,000 adult patients undergoing general anesthesia; in children, its incidence is reported to be 1 in 3000 to 1 in 15,000.[87, 88] The apparent higher incidence in children may reflect the retrospective nature of the literature, the age at which most operations are performed, and in the past, the common combined use of halothane or other potent inhalation agents and succinylcholine in children.[89–91] Between 1990 and 1994, the Malignant Hyperthermia Hotline received 2874 calls, of which 985 were consultations about clinical cases. Twenty-four percent of the cases (n = 235) were during otorhinolaryngologic procedures.[92] One hundred ninety-one of these cases were in children 0 to 10 years of age. The presenting symptoms were jaw rigidity (n = 133), temperature elevation (n = 77), tachycardia (n = 74), increased expired carbon dioxide (n = 42), arrhythmia (n = 25), myoglobinuria (n = 18), body rigidity (n = 16), tachypnea (n = 13), and decreased oxygen saturation (n = 10). Laboratory abnormalities included increased creatine phosphokinase levels (n = 106), respiratory acidosis (n = 49), myoglobinuria (n = 39), metabolic acidosis (n = 35), hyperkalemia (n = 7), and hypoxemia (n = 5). Sixty-six percent of cases occurred during induction, 13% during the procedure, and the remainder postoperatively. Fifty-four cases were not felt to represent an MH episode. The diagnoses made by the consultants included masseter muscle rigidity (n = 95; 40%), suspected mild MH (n = 34; 15%), masseter muscle rigidity and acute MH (n = 22; 9%), neuromuscular disease (n = 19; 8%), acute MH (n = 11; 5%), and not MH (n = 54; 23%). Halothane was used in 69% of cases and succinylcholine in 75% of cases. Six patients suffered cardiac arrest, two died, and 19 suffered morbidity. The most common clinical presentation of cases judged to be non-MH was an isolated increase in temperature in the postoperative period.[92] The take-home message of these reports is the high association of MH with the use of halothane and succinylcholine. *Succinylcholine should not be routinely used in children, particularly male children below the age of 10 years, but is indicated for treatment of laryngospasm, emergency airway management, or intramuscularly when a "suitable vein is not available."*[93, 94]

Although death due to high fever has been a known complication of general anesthesia, the initial descriptions of MH did not recognize it as a separate entity until the syndrome was accurately characterized by Denborough and Lovell in 1960.[95] At that time, the mortality rate approached 90%. With increased awareness of the syndrome and improved symptomatic management, the mortality rate decreased to 60%. However, the major breakthrough in the management occurred in 1979 with the Food and Drug Administration's (FDA) approval of dantrolene. The specific effectiveness of dantrolene sodium in the prevention and treatment of MH was recognized by Harrison 4 years earlier.[86, 96] MHAUS statistics suggest a current mortality rate of 2 in 137 possible episodes in children undergoing otorhinolaryngologic procedures.[92]

Genetics

Malignant hyperthermia is an inherited metabolic defect best described as autosomal dominant with reduced penetrance and variable expressivity.[70–72, 97–99] Reduced penetrance implies that fewer offspring are affected than would be predicted by a totally dominant pattern. Variable expressivity implies differing susceptibility between families, with little variation within the same family. However, not all patterns of inheritance fit this description; consequently, it is likely that the genetic abnormality of MH can be transmitted by more than one gene and more than one allele. The most commonly associated genetic abnormality associated with MH relates to the ryanodine receptor (RYR1) located on chromosome 19 (Fig. 27–5).[100–103] The ryanodine receptor is the major component of the ionized calcium release pathway between the sarcoplasmic reticulum and the sarcolemma.[104]

A German study reported 24% of MH-susceptible patients as having mutations of the RYR1 gene (the sole genetic defect in swine).[105] A Swedish study sought three specific RYR1 mutations and found 3 in 41 families to have a single

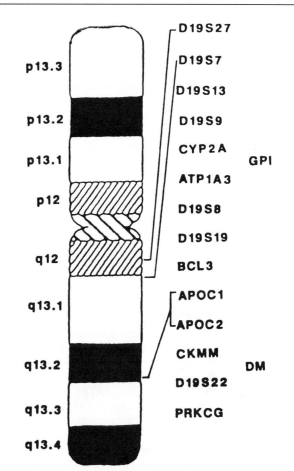

Figure 27–5. The location of malignant hyperthermia susceptibility to DNA markers from the 19q12-13.2 region of human chromosome 19 as reported by McCarthy et al. has a maximum likelihood of 450,000:1, favoring linkage of susceptibility to the cytochrome P-450 (CYP2A) locus. The location of DNA marker for Duchenne muscular dystrophy is shown by DMD. (From McCarthy TV, Healy JM, Heffron JJ, et al.: Localization of the malignant hyperthermia susceptibility locus to human chromosome 19q12-13.2. Nature 1990;343:562–564.)

RYR1 mutation.[106] A subsequent study of 48 Danish and 41 Swedish families found only 1 in 89 to have the specific mutation RYR1 G1021 A, which had previously been reported to account for 10% of MH-susceptible patients.[107] Quane et al.[103] described another specific mutation at amino acid position 614 in the ryanodine receptor. Up to 50% of MH patients have genetic mutations of the RYR1 gene; 16 mutations of this gene have been found in one Irish family.[107] It should be noted that these mutations do not always relate to a positive in vitro contracture test to halothane. This relationship varies from family to family. No clinical correlation exists between the clinical presentation and the genetic mutation observed.[108] Malignant hyperthermia in humans is not a single disease as in the pig, but a syndrome with multiple sites of causation and multiple mutations at these sites.

Pathophysiology

Episodes of both human and porcine MH syndromes demonstrate the same biochemical changes: hypercarbia, oxygen desaturation, tachycardia, tachypnea, cyanosis, mottling, cardiac arrhythmias, rigidity of muscles, fever, rhabdomyolysis, and eventually shock. Consequently, some porcine pedigrees particularly susceptible to MH have been identified (e.g., Landrace, Pietrain, Poland-China); these strains provide a model for the study of the human syndrome.[109–112] Much of our knowledge of the pathophysiology of this syndrome and the eventual identification of the specific treatment of MH are based on studies of this animal model.[113, 114] Most of the investigative work on the pathophysiology of MH has been performed on pigs. Swine breeders and veterinarians have long known that certain strains of pigs, when exposed to stresses related to slaughter, accelerate their metabolism; the muscle from these pigs deteriorates into pale, soft, exudative pork.[115] Further observations led to the conclusion that porcine stress syndrome and MH are practically the same genetic disease.[116]

The pathogenesis of MH involves defects in the release and reuptake of calcium from the sarcoplasmic reticulum. The physiology of normal muscle contraction is related to the release of ionized calcium into the sarcolemma after discharge from the sarcoplasmic reticulum (Fig. 27–6). The rapid increase in the intracellular ionized calcium concentration initiates muscle contraction; reuptake of ionized calcium into the sarcoplasmic reticulum causes muscle relaxation and requires adenosine triphosphate (ATP). The increase in intracellular calcium in MH is thought to be due to two mechanisms. The first is the marked increase in the amount of calcium released into the sarcolemma rather than the usual small aliquot. The second postulated defect is in ionized calcium reuptake by the sarcoplasmic reticulum that further adds to the high intracellular ionized calcium level.

This abnormality of intracellular ionized calcium homeostasis causes muscle to respond with a marked increase in energy production in an attempt to return ionized calcium to the sarcoplasmic reticulum. If unchecked, marked hypermetabolism and muscle contractures (rigidity) result. Dantrolene is thought to block the release of ionized calcium from the sarcoplasmic reticulum; this allows ionized calcium within the sarcolemma to fall, thus restoring the balance. This in turn reduces and finally stops the hypermetabolism caused by the marked need for ATP to restore ionized calcium to the sarcoplasmic reticulum.

The main defect lies in the inability of the sarcoplasmic reticulum to release the normal minute quantities of calcium upon stimulation.[117] This is evidenced by an increase in myoplasmic free ionized calcium.[118] At resting levels, the ionized calcium levels are three to four times normal[119]; triggering an MH episode increases the intracellular ionized calcium as much as 17 times.[120]

The elevated myoplasmic ionized calcium level causes (1) activation of adenosine triphosphatase (ATPase), thus accelerating the hydrolysis of ATP to adenosine diphosphate; (2) inhibition of troponin, thus permitting a biochemical contraction to occur; and (3) activation of phosphorylase kinase and glycogenolysis, with resulting production of ATP and heat. As the ionized calcium levels further increase, ionized calcium diffuses into a secondary storage site, the mitochondria. The infusion of ionized calcium into mitochondria stimulates aerobic activity within this organelle, as well as the sarcolemma. The ATP is rapidly diminished by this furious enzymatic activity; therefore, the supply of high-energy bonds diminishes, and the hypermetabolic muscles are unable to cope completely with the energy demands

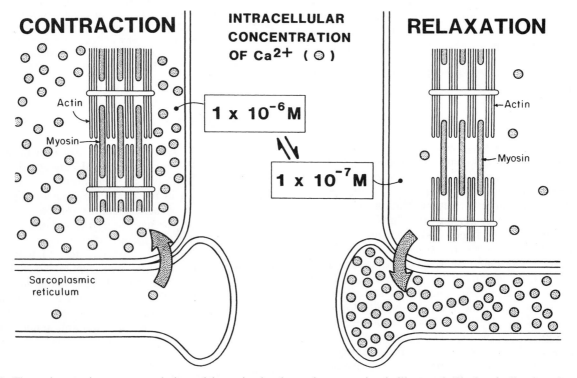

Figure 27–6. The actin myosin movement during calcium-stimulated muscle contraction is illustrated. Biochemically, the relaxation phase is the energy-utilizing process, and contraction is a more passive event. It is the failure of lowering myoplasmic calcium, which occurs normally during the relaxation phase, that leads to the development of malignant hyperthermia in a patient.

by means of aerobic metabolism. Consequently, the muscle resorts to anaerobic metabolism and lactic acid accumulates. As a result, the metabolic rate is accelerated, causing a high rate of oxygen consumption and CO_2 production, as well as generation of heat. Possibly adding to heat production is the report of significantly increased mitochondrial exo-NADH oxidase activity in MH pigs.[121]

The normal circulatory responses may allow heat dissipation early in this sequence, but soon, in an effort to supply the increased demands for oxygen to the muscles, peripheral vasoconstriction occurs, blood is shunted away from the skin, and the body temperature may rise dramatically. The venous blood is oxygen desaturated because of the marked increase in the oxygen uptake of muscle cells and has a high CO_2 concentration (respiratory acidosis) because of the enhanced intracellular metabolism; lactic acidosis (metabolic acidosis) results when oxygen demands outstrip oxygen delivery. The clinical importance is that the earliest change in the fulminant hypermetabolic state is mirrored on the venous side of the circulation as respiratory acidosis and markedly reduced venous oxygen values.

It is therefore very helpful to obtain a peripheral venous blood sample draining skeletal muscle tissues when seeking a diagnosis of possible MH; combined metabolic and respiratory acidosis with venous desaturation are consistent with a hypermetabolic state. A central venous sample would also likely demonstrate low venous oxygen content due to increased oxygen consumption. End-tidal CO_2 ($ETCO_2$) monitoring serves a similar purpose and provides an early warning.[78] The $ETCO_2$ monitor is the most sensitive and useful monitor for the early diagnosis of a hypermetabolic event[122]; the $ETCO_2$ is elevated before any clinically evident change in pulse or respirations.[116, 123–126] Pulse oximetry may also be of value; unanticipated desaturation occurs at intermediate and lower inspired oxygen concentrations during anesthesia as a result of marked oxygen extraction.[92] Both these monitors are useful in the continued post-treatment monitoring of an MH episode.

The continued uncontrolled contraction of large groups of muscles may lead to clinically observed muscle rigidity.[127–129] This most often occurs soon after administration of succinylcholine, but it may also be observed later. In the late stages of a full-blown MH episode, development of rigidity is attributable to the temperature rise within the muscle cells.[130] The actomyosin ATPase enzyme system ends skeletal muscle contraction. In the event of an enzyme malfunction, continued contraction leads to rigidity. Our laboratory (JFR) has noted a relationship between the clinical "rigid" form of MH and markedly lowered function of actomyosin ATPase. The presence or absence of rigidity may well be related to the level of free intracellular ionized calcium. In studies of animals, free intracellular ionized calcium concentrations that did not quite reach the threshold for muscle contraction (i.e., 1 μM) did not result in rigidity, although the hypermetabolic aspects of the syndrome were present.[131]

Another mechanism that may contribute to increased intracellular ionized calcium is elevated inositol polyphosphate concentrations; inositol receptors are another means of modulating calcium channel release. Halothane increases these concentrations in MH swine and dantrolene decreases intracellular inositol levels.[132, 133] Although there is a difference in muscle concentrations of inositol in patients with MH

compared with those without MH, there is no difference in blood concentrations, thus making a simple blood test unreliable.[134] The hormone-sensitive lipase is an enzyme system that mobilizes free fatty acids from triglycerides. Skeletal muscle free fatty acid metabolism is abnormal in MH patients; the source of the elevated free fatty acid appears to be triglycerides. The elevated free fatty acid may in part be responsible for the increased ionized calcium release and decreased sarcoplasmic reticulum ionized calcium uptake.[118–120, 122, 132, 135–141]

Skeletal muscles are the main tissues involved in this syndrome; a full-blown episode may be attended by rhabdomyolysis, massive swelling of the muscles, and a clinically important leak of intracellular potassium and calcium outside the cells into the circulation. The rapid increase in serum potassium can result in arrhythmias that rapidly progress to cardiac arrest. Hyperkalemia is the major cause of mortality early in an MH episode. It is important, however, to differentiate the hyperkalemia caused by acute succinylcholine-induced rhabdomyolysis and that caused by MH. Generally, acute rhabdomyolysis due to succinylcholine presents as sudden unexpected cardiac arrest shortly after induction of anesthesia and following the administration of succinylcholine.[94] This is most common in male children with undiagnosed muscular dystrophy under the age of 10 years.[94] The hyperkalemia from acute rhabdomyolysis is generally profound, is highly resistant to standard cardiopulmonary resuscitation measures, and will require extensive therapy in the form of calcium chloride, hyperventilation, administration of sodium bicarbonate, glucose, and insulin, and chelating agents. It is important to continue cardiopulmonary resuscitation (several hours may be required) because these patients are salvageable.[94] The hyperkalemia associated with malignant hyperthermia is generally slower in onset and is reversible once treatment with dantrolene has been instituted. If cardiac arrhythmias occur with an episode of MH, exogenous calcium may be administered with caution if indicated for the treatment of hyperkalemia-induced arrhythmias.

In general, however, the cardiac arrhythmias observed in MH are nonspecific. Several factors contribute to their occurrence: hyperkalemia, fever, acidosis, hypoxemia, and autonomic hyperactivity. It is also possible that the syndrome directly affects cardiac muscle. Calcium channel blockers have a profound interaction with dantrolene; fatal, evanescent rises in serum potassium levels in swine have been demonstrated. *Calcium channel blockers are contraindicated in the therapy of MH.*[142, 143] With adequate treatment of MH with dantrolene, these electrolyte abnormalities reverse spontaneously. Tissues other than muscle show various defects.[144]

If a patient survives the initial event, other complications may occur, including hemolysis, myoglobinemia, and myoglobinuria; the last may lead to renal failure. Disseminated intravascular coagulopathy can occur; early dantrolene therapy may prevent this complication. The cause of death in this syndrome is variable and is temporally related. In the initial few hours, it is most probably due to hyperkalemia-induced ventricular fibrillation. Death several hours after the initial MH episode or after a prolonged attempt at resuscitation may be due to pulmonary edema, coagulopathy, and acid-base or electrolyte imbalance. Before the discovery that dantrolene was an effective treatment, recovery with supportive therapy was generally accompanied by a transient but sharp *decrease* in plasma potassium concentrations. This intracellular redistribution was attributed to a return of plasma pH toward normal and therefore a return of potassium to its intracellular location. In the following 6 to 8 hours following this nadir, a slow increase in plasma potassium usually occurred. This hypokalemia was extremely sensitive to intravenous potassium supplementation. Deaths that occur days after an MH episode are likely to result from multiple organ failure, brain damage, or renal decompensation.

The height of the fever associated with MH has no specific predictive effect on outcome. My (JFR) first patient with MH had a temperature elevation greater than 43.8°C (110.8°F), cardiac arrest, and a plasma potassium level of 14.9 mEq/L, all occurring within an 18-minute period.[145] Approximately 2 hours later, this patient was attempting to vocalize her desire to be extubated. Despite this markedly elevated temperature, no brain damage ensued, and she eventually made a complete recovery. This example contrasts with the widely held view that brain damage inevitably occurs at these extreme temperature elevations.[146]

Diagnosis

Because the first systemic effect of MH is increased metabolism (increased oxygen consumption and CO_2 production),

the cardiovascular and respiratory systems respond to this increased oxygen demand by increasing cardiac output and respiratory rate. Therefore, the first clinically evident signs and symptoms of this syndrome in a spontaneously breathing patient are tachycardia and tachypnea (Table 27–1). However, an increased ETCO$_2$ value precedes these signs and symptoms and is generally evident in the patient either breathing spontaneously or on controlled ventilation (Fig. 27–7).[78, 122, 123, 125] Sudden unexpected cardiac arrest, especially during induction of anesthesia, is not a common presentation of an MH episode and generally suggests another cause, such as acute rhabdomyolysis following succinylcholine and resultant hyperkalemia.[94, 147]

A patient's response to surgery under "light" anesthesia is often tachycardia. However, in a healthy child of 7 years, an increase from 120 to 180 beats per minute (or an increase from 70 to 120 beats per minute in an adult) is usually a sign of pathology; not all tachycardia or tachypnea is attributable to light anesthesia. It is reasonable to deepen anesthesia, but it is also essential to immediately rule in or out other mechanical factors (e.g., endobronchial intubation, hypoventilation, or circuit problems). *Rapid increases in inspired desflurane or isoflurane concentrations can cause tachycardia and have been associated with delay in diagnosis.*[148, 149] If none of these factors appear to be causative, and a brief trial of deepened anesthesia fails to slow the heart rate, then a simultaneous venous and arterial blood sample should

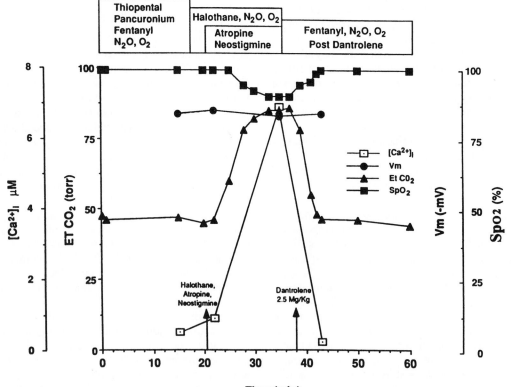

Figure 27–7. During the three study periods, the time course in minutes for four variables is displayed. Membrane potentials (V_m) are depicted as closed circles. Free intracellular concentrations ($[Ca^{++}]_i$) are open squares. End-tidal carbon dioxide (ETCO$_2$) values are in closed triangles, and oxygen saturation measurements (SPO$_2$) are detailed as closed squares. ETCO$_2$ and SPO$_2$ were measured continuously, whereas V_m and $[Ca^{++}]_i$ were measured only at the four specific time points. Data are presented as the mean of the four animals studied. (From Ryan JF, Lopez JR, Sanchez VB, et al.: Myoplasmic calcium changes precede metabolic and clinical signs of porcine malignant hyperthermia. Anesth Analg 1994;79:1007–1011.)

Table 27–1. Signs and Symptoms of Malignant Hyperthermia

Specific for Malignant Hyperthermia	Less Specific for Malignant Hyperthermia
Generalized muscle rigidity	Tachycardia
Rapidly increasing expired carbon dioxide	Tachypnea
	Arrhythmia
Rapidly developing fever (late sign)	Hypotension
Cola-colored urine (myoglobinemia) (late sign)	Hypertension
	Cyanosis
Increased serum creatine phosphate (late sign)	Metabolic acidosis
	Hyperkalemia
	Coagulopathy

determine the presence or absence of a hypermetabolic state. In this respect, an $ETCO_2$ monitor is particularly valuable. In hypermetabolic states, the $ETCO_2$ is high, especially during MH. In this condition, it becomes extremely difficult to bring the $ETCO_2$ level within the normal range, even with vigorous hyperventilation. Conversely, with airway obstruction, the recorded CO_2 levels are elevated; however, once the defect has been corrected, $ETCO_2$ rapidly returns to its normal value with mild to moderate hyperventilation.

Malignant hyperthermia can also initially present as ventricular ectopy in otherwise healthy patients; this manifestation is especially common during induction of anesthesia. In the absence of airway instrumentation, hypercarbia, hypoxia, or some other stimulus to explain the arrhythmia, MH becomes suspect.[150] Electrocardiographic investigation must also be carried out, as well as serial measurements of myoglobin and creatine phosphokinase (CPK) levels. If the electrocardiographic findings are normal and the CPK and myoglobin levels are elevated, one can make a tentative diagnosis of MH.[72] It should be noted, however, that CPK alterations after an MH episode not associated with the use of succinylcholine with or without dantrolene have been measured in the same range as expected from the procedure itself.[151]

Differential Diagnosis

A moderate but gradual temperature elevation may occur in patients excessively draped, those with air mattress warming devices, and patients covered with plastic occlusive wrap. However, the sudden onset of high fever must be more thoroughly investigated and may be due to sepsis, neurologic injury, thyroid storm,[152] metastatic carcinoid, cystinosis,[153] and pheochromocytoma.[154] At the Massachusetts General Hospital from 1974 to 1979, eight patients developed intraoperative temperatures greater than 108°F. These patients all had sepsis or prior neurologic trauma. The acid-base status remained normal in all these cases. Thyroid storm has not been associated with severe acid-base abnormalities.[93] Examination of the patient's neck for thyroid nodules or enlargement may be helpful in the differential diagnosis of this entity. Thyrotoxicosis factitia during anesthesia has also been reported.[152] In goats with thyroid storm, the elevation of $ETCO_2$ is delayed and gradual. Muscle rigidity distinguishes MH from thyroid storm. In patients presenting with metastatic carcinoid or pheochromocytoma, the initial symptoms resemble MH, but marked cardiovascular instability persists

after dantrolene therapy.[154] The serotonin syndrome and neuroleptic malignant syndrome cause symptoms similar to MH, but they have not been reported during general anesthesia; acute baclofen withdrawal may also be confused with MH.[99, 155–158] Acute cocaine intoxication and general anesthesia can produce an MH-type picture that is not responsive to dantrolene therapy (Table 27–2).[159, 160]

Masseter Spasm, Masseter Muscle Rigidity, Masseter Tetany

In the 1970s, masseter spasm following succinylcholine administration was recognized as a marker for the possible occurrence of MH.[161] If this tetany of the jaw muscles was appreciated by the anesthesiologist, the procedure, if elective, was usually immediately terminated. A strong correlation between succinylcholine-induced masseter spasm and MH has been described.[159, 161–163] In some patients, however, no cause was elicited.[164] The reports by van der Spek and colleagues upset this apparent relationship of masseter spasm with MH susceptibility.[165–167] These investigators found routinely increased tension in the muscles of mastication after intravenous administration of succinylcholine. At present, there is no physiologic explanation for this phenomenon. How can a depolarizing muscle relaxant that induces paralysis in all skeletal muscles produce increased tension in subsets of skeletal muscles at the same time? Does some intracellular action of succinylcholine in the muscles of mastication and possibly in the eye muscles override the neuromuscular junctional effect of the drug? The van der Spek investigations may in fact explain in part the inconsistent relationship between masseter spasm (also called masseter muscle rigidity) and MH. The administration of succinylcholine is always followed by a transient increase in

Table 27–2. Differential Diagnosis of Malignant Hyperthermia (MH)

Diagnosis	Distinguishing Traits
Hyperthyroidism	Symptoms and physical findings often present, blood gas abnormalities rise gradually
Sepsis	Usually normal blood gases
Pheochromocytoma	Similar to MH except marked blood pressure swings
Metastatic carcinoid	Same as pheochromocytoma
Cocaine intoxication	Fever, rigidity, rhabdomyolysis similar to malignant neurolept syndrome
Heat stroke	Similar to MH except that the patient is outside the operating room
Masseter spasm (MMR)	May progress to MH, total body spasm more likely than isolated MMR
Malignant neurolept syndrome	Similar to MH, usually associated with the use of antidepressants
Serotogenic syndrome	Similar to MH and malignant neurolept syndrome, associated with the administration of mood-elevating drugs

MMR, masseter muscle rigidity.

masseter muscle tone. However, this generally relaxes over a matter of seconds.

How should we now interpret masseter spasm? Is it a normal phenomenon, a normal or abnormal variant, or a developmental occurrence, or should we still consider increased tension as pathologic? It would appear that there may be an extreme variant of masseter spasm that we could now call masseter muscle tetany that may in fact be the response that is associated with MH (Fig. 27–8). At present, we have no definitive answers to these questions.

The inability to open the mouth of a heavily sedated patient after the administration of succinylcholine is a subjective judgment. The patient can be slightly resistant, or active tetany can be present. Inability to open the mouth despite loss of the train of four is highly suggestive of masseter tetany. Further succinylcholine administration does not result in paralysis of the masseter muscles. The increased masseter muscle tension may last from a few minutes to half an hour. *It is vital to appreciate that the majority of patients can be ventilated with a face mask despite the rigidity and the inability to open the mouth, because the chest wall and the glottis are relaxed. Simple bag and mask ventilation therefore sustains oxygenation until the masseter muscles relax.*

The relationship of succinylcholine-induced masseter spasm or tetany and a positive muscle biopsy specimen (more than half the patients studied have tested positive) needs to be carefully re-examined. The masseter muscles examined in one study have a predominant type I content.[168] A second report found that only 31% of patients with masseter spasm tested positive. In this study, there was no difference in CPK levels between patients who received dantrolene (n = 10) and those who did not (n = 72); therefore, rhabdomyolysis still occurred.[169] Myoglobinemia after succinylcholine has been noted to be more frequent in childhood

after halothane (40%) than after thiopental (20%).[170] Puberty lowers the frequency of myoglobinemia after both drugs to approximately 3%. Several retrospective pediatric studies described the incidence of masseter muscle rigidity following succinylcholine (as determined subjectively) and reported that approximately 1% of patients induced with halothane[163, 171, 172] had this clinical response; this incidence was 3% if strabismus was present.[172] However, this high incidence of clinical masseter spasm does not correlate with the experience of masseter muscle tetany and the incidence of positive muscle biopsies. Reports to the MH Hotline of cases of masseter spasm and cardiac arrest in children have declined. This may well be due to the decreased use of succinylcholine in anesthesia for pediatric patients.[173]

How should one respond to increased jaw tension following succinylcholine administration? A retrospective analysis of 68 patients recommends proceeding with the anesthetic procedure as though the event had not occurred.[173] Previous studies recommended discontinuation of anesthesia.[163, 164] Because we do not have the physiologic data to make a sound judgment based on scientific proof, caution is a sensible refuge. After discontinuing all trigger agents and observing the patient for 15 to 20 minutes to be certain that the symptoms and signs of a MH episode do not occur, one may continue the anesthetic using a non-triggering technique.[174] Another option is to stop the procedure and postpone the surgery if the surgery is elective. This decision is generally made concurrently by the anesthesiologist, the surgeon, and the family. If any of the three parties is not confident about proceeding, then the conservative approach (i.e., cancellation of surgery) seems appropriate. With any decision, patients should be carefully monitored, remain in the hospital overnight, have a CPK level assessed at 12 and 24 hours postoperatively, have all urine samples tested for myoglobin during the first postoperative day, and have a formal neurologic examination with electromyography to establish a baseline. The focus should be on determining the presence or absence of neuromuscular disease. As our knowledge increases, the management of patients with masseter spasm will become more rational.

Muscle Biopsy Testing

The diagnosis of MH is primarily determined by clinical responses. Once even a "weak" set of symptoms has been diagnosed as MH, the patient and the family are thereafter usually considered "positive" by all physicians. This may seem unjustified in some circumstances and perhaps medically incorrect, but it is the reality of present-day medicine. It is interesting to note that in a population referred to us (JFR), 50% of family members of known MH-susceptible patients may themselves be susceptible to MH, an observation that is consistent with the autosomal dominant mode of inheritance. This finding supports the need for caution when administering anesthesia to members of a family in which one person is known to be susceptible.

Muscle biopsy specimens have been used to determine the presence or absence of a consistent marker in muscle function associated with MH. The test that has gained acceptance is quantitation of the forces of muscle contracture after exposure of the muscle biopsy sample to halothane, caffeine,

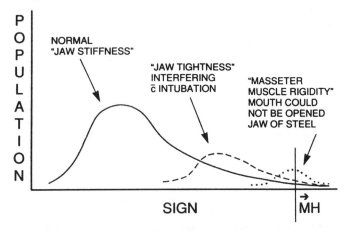

Figure 27–8. The spectrum of masseter muscle responses to succinylcholine varies from a slight jaw stiffness that does not interfere with endotracheal intubation to the extreme "jaws of steel," which is masseter muscle tetany not allowing the mouth to be opened. It is likely the latter response that is highly associated with malignant hyperthermia (MH). It should be noted that even with the inability to open the mouth, the patient should still be able to be ventilated by bag and mask, since all other muscles are relaxed. (From Kaplan RF: Malignant Hyperthermia, Annual Refresher Course Lectures. Washington DC: American Society of Anesthesiologists, 1993.)

Table 27–3. Caffeine Halothane Contracture Testing: Indications

Clinical history suspicious for malignant hyperthermia
The patient is a first-degree relative of a patient with documented
  malignant hyperthermia
Masseter muscle rigidity

or both.[82] The basis for halothane-caffeine contracture testing is an "abnormal" response by freshly excised skeletal muscle to halothane or caffeine or both (Table 27–3). The excised muscle is placed on stretch in a physiologic bath at 37°C. After optimal length tension has been determined, halothane or caffeine or both are added to the bath, the muscle is stimulated supramaximally, and the contracture amplitude is measured.[164, 175] Lack of response to twitch stimulation has been discounted as evidence of non-viability.[82, 176] Response to 32 mM caffeine is a better guide to viability.[177] The resting membrane potential is critical in the response to caffeine.[177] A vigorous in vitro contracture of a skeletal muscle specimen to halothane and a reduced contracture threshold to caffeine can identify the donor as MH susceptible. The response to 2 mmol of caffeine and to less than 2% halothane were the only tests that unequivocally discriminated between susceptible and normal control subjects.[178] However, simultaneous exposure to both halothane and caffeine produces considerable overlap between normal and known MH-susceptible patients, indicating that the combined test is too sensitive. In Europe, all testing follows a similar protocol.[175] Testing defines patients as positive (two tests positive), equivocal (one test positive), or negative. Approximately 15% of patients studied are "equivocal"; this diagnostic category has been questioned.[179] In North America, each laboratory and its own experience determine interpretive criteria for making the diagnosis of MH.[82] The patient needs to be physically present at the center performing the testing in North America.

In an attempt to unify current methods of testing, Larach and Landis reported the results of 176 "normal" muscle biopsy specimens studied in 11 North American laboratories.[81, 82] Using a "common" definition of normal, the incidence of a false-positive diagnosis in these 176 patients ranged from 10 to 70% with a mean of 38%. Recent standardization efforts in North America have led to findings overall of a sensitivity of 92% with a specificity of 78%. This is comparative to the use of creatine kinase levels as the sole diagnostic criterion for the possibility of myocardial infarction in patients with chest pain.[82] Outcome data comparing European and North American diagnostic protocols show an 87% concordance. A comparison of both protocols is outlined in Table 27–4.[180]

This conclusion is controversial depending on the laboratory involved. Any widely sensitive test to confirm an unequivocal diagnosis as either positive or negative has a gray zone. Some new markers for MH have been suggested, such as in vitro ^{31}P-magnetic resonance spectroscopy using glycerophosphorylcholine as the marker of impaired phospholipid metabolism.[181] Ryanodine, especially in low concentrations, (i.e., 0.5 μM) has been useful diagnostically.[182, 183]

How should one approach the anesthetic management of clinically positive patients who test unequivocally negative? This wide spectrum of MH susceptibility has been observed in both humans and pigs.[178] Therefore, most laboratories tend to take the conservative approach, favoring the diagnosis on the positive side (false positive) because the consequences of a false-negative result are much more serious than for a false-positive. It is better to treat patients as if they are susceptible to MH and avoid all triggering agents than to assume they are negative and confront catastrophic complications. The need for the patient to be present at the testing site may be mitigated by the finding that cold preservation of the muscle biopsy tissue for 24 hours does not affect the results.[184]

Table 27–4. Comparison of Protocols According to the European Malignant Hypothermia Group (EMHG) and the North American Malignant Hyperthermia Group (NAMHG)

Protocol	Halothane Administration	Caffeine Administration	Muscle Strips In Each Test	Accepted Muscles	Diagnostic Criteria	Optional Tests
EMHG	Incremental administration of halothane 0.5%, 1%, 2%	Incremental administration of caffeine 0.5, 1, 1.5, 2, 3, 4, 32 mM	Duplicate	M. vastus	Contracture halothane ≥0.2 g Contracture caffeine ≥0.2 g	Ryanodine; chlorcresol not used for diagnostic purposes
NAMHG	Single bolus administration of halothane 3%	Incremental administration of caffeine 0.5, 1, 2, 4, (8), 32 mM	Triplicate	Preferably m. vastus; if not possible, m. rectus abdominis or other muscles	Contracture halothane ≥0.7 g (≥0.5, <0.7 g equivocal) (earlier MHS >0.2–0.7 g) Contracture caffeine ≥0.3 g (≥0.2, <0.3 g equivocal) (earlier MHS ≥ 0.2 g)	Caffeine-specific concentration; 7% increase in baseline tension at 2 mM caffeine compared with maximal contracture; combined halothane and caffeine test

From Islander G, Twetman ER: Anesth Analg 1999; 88:1155–1160.
  MHS, malignant hyperthermia susceptible.

Patients with Malignant Hyperthermia Susceptibility

Most of the time, MH occurs in situations in which it is least suspected. With a careful history, however, information can be obtained to indicate that one of the patient's relatives has had a complicated anesthetic history. Some disorders have an inconstant association with MH.[185] These diseases include muscular dystrophies, and of these, the Duchenne type seems to be the one most commonly associated with MH.[137, 186, 187] Other associated diseases may include central core disease and hyperkalemic periodic paralysis.[188–190] Neuroleptic malignant syndrome has not been described clinically in a patient who has experienced an episode of MH. Additionally, biopsy studies have presented conflicting results when attempting to relate these two syndromes.[157, 158, 191–195]

Although patients with ptosis, squint, and skeletal deformities such as scoliosis or kyphosis have been suggested as possibly MH susceptible, historical associations have not been corroborative. The literature[196–198] and our own experience (JFR) in history taking demonstrate that the only helpful question in a medical history relates to previous difficulty or death in the family during anesthesia.

It has also been suggested that the sympathetic nervous system is abnormal in patients with MH; however, using norepinephrine turnover as an index of peripheral sympathetic nerve function, investigators noted no difference between age-matched controls and MH-susceptible patients.[199] Other case reports implicate Becker syndrome, motor neuron disease, Freeman-Sheldon syndrome, and centronuclear myopathy.[176, 200–204]

Management of a Malignant Hyperthermia Crisis

When a full-blown episode of MH is diagnosed, immediate aggressive therapy is indicated. Table 27–5 describes the standard treatment regimen and Table 27–6 details the suggested useful contents of a pediatric malignant hyperthermia treatment kit. The cornerstone of this approach is immediate cessation of triggering agents, delivery of 100% oxygen, hyperventilation, and treatment with dantrolene sodium.[143] This drug has been shown to be effective at a dose of 2.5 mg/kg IV without major adverse side effects. If administered early during the episode it blocks the abnormal cellular

Table 27–5. Standard Treatment Regimen

Stop triggering drugs immediately and terminate surgery if possible
Hyperventilate with 100% oxygen
Administer dantrolene (Dantrium), 2.5–3.0 mg/kg IV as soon as possible*
Initiate cooling
Correct acidosis
Secure monitoring lines: arterial pressure, central venous pressure
Insert urinary catheter
Maintain urine output
Monitor patient until danger of subsequent episodes is past (48–72 hr)
Administer additional dantrolene if symptoms recur

*See text for details.

Table 27–6. Pediatric Malignant Hyperthermia Emergency Box

Fluids

2000 mL D_5 0.2 NaCl 500 mL IV bottles
3000 mL   0.9 NaCl 500 mL IV bottles
   1   Regular insulin 100 Units/mL 10 mL vial
   4   Ice Packs

Drugs

Number	Drug	Dose	Vessel
10	Lasix	10 mg/mL	4 mL ampule
4	Mannitol 25%	12.5 g/50 mL	50 mL vial
4	Sodium bicarbonate	1 mEq/mL	50 mL vial
1	Sodium bicarbonate	1 mEq/mL	50 mL syringe
1	50% dextrose	500 mg/mL	50 mL/vial
10	Sterile injection NaCl		10 mL/vial
10	Dantrium IV	20 mg (dilute with 60 mL sterile water)	
10	100 mL sterile injectable water **for Dantrium use only** (red label)		
10	20- and 22-gauge IV catheters		
10	18-gauge and 20-gauge		
8	Syringes: TB, 6 mL, 12 mL, 20 mL, and 60 mL		

To rapidly mix dantrolene, use 18-gauge needles on 60 mL syringes to rapidly transfer sterile water to dantrolene vials. Have a colleague vigorously shake while diluting the next dantrolene vial to ensure adequate dissolution and reduce the time of preparation. Final concentration is 0.33 mg/mL. Administer 7.5–10 mL/kg. Note: for larger patients, several individuals may be needed to vigorously shake the multiple dantrolene vials.

IV, intravenous; TB, tuberculosis.

metabolism from abnormal calcium transport and in turn this reverses the biochemical changes of MH.[86, 205] Thus, the combined metabolic and respiratory acidosis as well as the hyperkalemia should gradually resolve following dantrolene administration. Although dantrolene is the key to successful outcome, the other supportive measures are essential. Active cooling, treating the associated acidosis, and correcting the electrolyte imbalance can make the difference between a borderline and a complete recovery.

Dantrolene has probably been responsible for the dramatic decrease in the mortality due to MH since its intravenous use was introduced (Fig. 27–9). The drug instructions recommend an initial dose of 1 mg/kg IV. However, a small number of patients do not respond to this dose. We strongly suggest an initial bolus dose of 2.5 to 3.0 mg/kg IV, followed in 45 minutes by a bolus dose of 10 mg/kg IV if all signs and symptoms of the syndrome have not resolved; no major side effects occur after a large intravenous dose. Higher

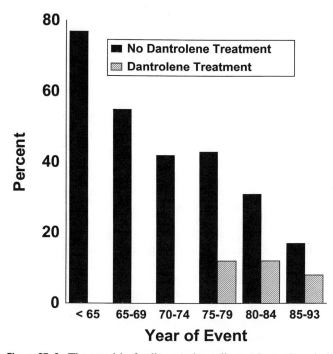

Figure 27–9. The trend in fatality rate in malignant hyperthermia is shown over time. The solid bars represent data from 361 patients and the hatched bars represent data from 142 patients. Note the marked improvement in mortality with dantrolene treatment. (Modified from Strazis KP, Fox AW: Malignant hyperthermia: A review of published cases. Anesth Analg 1993;77:297–304.)

doses have been used if indicated.[129] The complete cessation of (1) tachycardia, (2) tachypnea, (3) all muscle rigidity, (4) decreased urinary output, (5) altered consciousness, (6) blood gas abnormalities,[206] and (7) electrolyte disturbances should be attained. If initial therapy does not produce these results, a repeated higher dose of dantrolene should be administered or an alternative diagnosis for the problem should be sought.

Two experiences exemplify the reasons for this recommendation. A 19-year-old patient who developed MH was treated with dantrolene at a dose of 1 mg/kg IV. Twelve hours postoperatively, all signs of MH were absent except tachycardia (180 beats per minute) and marked hypertension (240/150 mm Hg) despite aggressive treatment with nitroprusside, nitroglycerin, and hydralazine. After intravenous dantrolene in a dose of 3 mg/kg, a brief improvement of the cardiovascular aberrations followed. Subsequent to 10 mg/kg IV of dantrolene, all parameters dramatically returned to normal values.

The second patient developed full-blown MH and 20 hours later was still unconscious, with marked left gastrocnemius muscle rigidity. He was receiving 1 mg/kg IV of dantrolene every 8 hours as a maintenance dose to prevent recurrence of MH; 30 minutes after the administration of dantrolene in a dose of 10 mg/kg IV, the patient was awake and the muscle rigidity relieved.

In our clinical and laboratory experience, the response to dantrolene takes 6 to 20 minutes (see Fig. 27–7). The $ETCO_2$ begins to decrease in about 6 minutes, and monitored arterial blood gas analysis demonstrates significant restoration toward normal within 20 minutes. *The important factor is that*

by 45 minutes, the patient should be completely normal. If not, intensive therapy should be pursued. Inadequate therapy can lead to a disastrous complication in a small number of patients when they redevelop the MH syndrome. This usually occurs 4 to 8 hours after the initial episode and has been noted as late as 36 hours after initial therapy. Characteristically, patients "smolder" along with modified symptoms until a triggering event ignites a renewed full-blown episode.[207] Table 27–7 outlines the signs and symptoms of a continuing subclinical episode of MH.

Patients with recrudescence have died as a result of a change in muscle cellular permeability. Such patients require enormous volume infusions to maintain intravascular volume. Muscles immediately take up this volume and swell dramatically. The two patients described in the report cited gained 24 kg in 18 hours and 15 kg in 36 hours, respectively.

Once the initial episode has been successfully treated, patients in the past have been given 1 mg/kg IV of dantrolene every 6 hours for 24 hours or by mouth for an additional 48 to 72 hours. There are no data to substantiate this therapy.

Actions of Dantrolene

Dantrolene's action has been identified as being specific for skeletal muscles.[143, 208] It does not affect neuromuscular transmission or have measurable effects on the electrically excitable surface membrane. It does, however, produce muscle weakness (reduced grip strength) with measurable twitch depression (up to 85%) and may markedly potentiate nondepolarizing neuromuscular blocking agents. Pulmonary functions such as vital capacity, $ETCO_2$, respiratory rate, and peak expiratory flow rate are not affected.[209] Dantrolene can also cause minor central nervous system effects such as dizziness, light headedness, or a feeling of dysequilibrium.[209] Evidence suggests that the site of action of dantrolene sodium is within the muscle itself and is related to the caffeine-sensitive calcium stores.[140, 210, 211] It is suggested that dantrolene sodium prevents the release of calcium from the sarcoplasmic reticulum, or antagonizes calcium effects at the actin-myosin-troponin-tropomyosin level, or both.[209, 212, 213] Such actions are proposed as explanations for the clinically observed skeletal muscle relaxant activity. A recent study did not identify the ryanodine receptor as the site of dantrolene action; this may implicate an intermediary role of this receptor site.[214]

Properties of dantrolene include the following:

1. At doses from 5 to 15 mg/kg IV, it produces a significant degree of muscle relaxation and in some patients even oral dantrolene can cause a feeling of weakness.[215–217] Common sense dictates that patients receiving dantrolene preoperatively or intraoperatively require a smaller dose of muscle relaxant.

Table 27–7. Signs and Symptoms of Continuing Malignant Hyperthermia Episode

Continued hyperkalemia
Residual muscle rigidity still present
Massive fluid requirements
Oliguria proceeding to anuria

2. At intravenous doses up to 15 mg/kg, it has no significant action on the cardiovascular system.
3. At intravenous doses up to 30 mg/kg, it does not depress respirations.
4. There is no indication of toxicity when the drug is administered intravenously on an acute basis.

Common side effects and drug interactions are presented in Table 27–8. Dantrolene normalizes all functions associated with muscle hypermetabolism in MH by reducing muscle rigidity and restoring normal muscle function. As cellular metabolism returns to aerobic processes and respiration normalizes, acid-base disorders are also corrected (see Fig. 27–7). One important effect is the rapid reduction in serum potassium; because the acidosis from MH is reversed, potassium is restored to cells. This effect helps normalize MH induced cardiac dysfunction. Thus, although dantrolene acts primarily on skeletal muscles, its beneficial effects are far reaching.

Subsequent Anesthetic Procedures

The common practice at present is to not "routinely" pretreat patients with dantrolene preoperatively.[218–221] The muscle weakness and nausea frequently associated with pretreatment in adults are thus eliminated.[209, 216, 222] In 237 MH biopsy negative patients, 17 anesthetic procedures with triggering drugs were uneventful.[194] Carr et al.[223] reported their experience with 2214 patients who underwent muscle biopsy for the possible diagnosis of MH without dantrolene pretreatment. A total of 2147 patients received nontriggering general anesthesia and the remainder regional anesthesia techniques; 1084 patients proved biopsy positive by the halothane/caffeine contracture test. Only 5 patients developed MH, and these reactions all occurred in the recovery room. All patients recovered from their MH reaction and the authors concluded that the incidence of MH reactions in patients who receive a trigger-free anesthetic is approximately 0.46% (95% CI, 0.015–1.07%). It would appear that pretreatment is not necessary for minor surgical procedures. If, however, a surgical procedure is planned in a known MH-susceptible patient and pretreatment with dantrolene sodium is desired because of the severity of the previous episode of MH or because of the patient's or anesthesiologist's concern, then dantrolene can be administered orally or intravenously.[209, 224] The recommended oral dosage is 4.8 mg/kg /day PO in three to four divided doses for 48 hours before anesthesia. A single intravenous dose of dantrolene (2.5 mg/kg) administered just before beginning anesthesia has been suggested as effective; this achieves a steady-state blood level of 3.6 μg/mL for approximately 6 hours, then slowly declines.[209] Patients have been reported as "triggering" despite preoperative adminis-

tration of oral[225] or intravenous[226] dantrolene. Since absorption of oral dantrolene is erratic, and since the patient side effects are so prominent, the intravenous route just prior to induction would appear to be the most reliable and patient-acceptable method of pretreatment.

Other measures useful in avoiding triggering MH in susceptible patients include the following: (1) moderate to heavy premedication with tranquilizers (no phenothiazines). Barbiturates, benzodiazepines and opiates may be used for premedication; in infants and young children, rectal methohexital is a good choice, since this provides an induction rather than just sedation).[227] (2) A balanced anesthetic technique (nitrous oxide-oxygen, barbiturate, opioid, and any nondepolarizing muscle relaxant). Ketamine[228] and propofol[229, 230] have not been reported as triggering drugs, but desflurane[149, 231] and sevoflurane[232–234] have been associated with the development of MH, as have *all potent inhalation anesthetic drugs*.[89] Propofol's safety might be related to its lack of effect on the RYR1 receptor.[154] Careful monitoring is the most important aspect of management. All changes in heart rate should be carefully monitored, and an ETCO$_2$ analyzer, a pulse oximeter, and a temperature monitor should be used. All local anesthetic drugs, whether amides or esters, may be used in patients suspected of having MH or in MH-susceptible patients.[235, 236] Immediate availability of dantrolene is mandatory. Although caffeine induces contracture responses in vitro, it seems that these effects do not apply to related compounds, such as theophylline or aminophylline.[237]

The Family

Caring for the family of an MH patient becomes a major challenge for the anesthesiologist in the period after a possible MH episode. Most importantly, the family needs information and support. The stunning effect of this complication frequently deters the anesthesiologist from close contact with the family. However, the psychological and legal consequences of such inaction, for both the family and physician, can be catastrophic, even with a good outcome of the MH episode.[238]

The advent of genetic testing may replace muscle testing as the laboratory determinant of MH susceptibility. Until a uniform genetic test is available, it seems reasonable to document the episode by muscle biopsy at an appropriate interval after the event (see Table 27–3). It is then necessary to determine which branch of the family is susceptible. Once these two goals have been accomplished, further testing within the family can be performed. A biopsy on other family members should be attempted only after they are informed that the test is not a medical necessity—all anesthesiologists will treat the entire family as positive regardless of test results—but that this is a personal choice based on the need for peace of mind. Obtaining a muscle biopsy specimen during incidental surgery in family members makes eminent sense. The only restriction is to withhold dantrolene sodium and droperidol before excising the muscle specimen. These two drugs have been shown to "normalize" abnormal responses of the muscle specimens in MH-susceptible individuals.[185]

A common practice in planning anesthesia for members of a family known to have MH is to request muscle testing separately before the procedure. In most instances, because

---

Table 27–8. Dantrolene: Adverse Effects and Drug Reactions

Adverse Effects

Most common: dizziness, light-headedness, drowsiness
Most serious: hepatic dysfunction—chronic, oral administration

Drug Interactions

Verapamil: myocardial depressant

a balanced technique will be used whether the results are normal or positive, it seems easier and less expensive for patients to have a muscle biopsy specimen taken at the time of the planned elective operation. Obviously, dantrolene will be available in the operating room, and the anesthesiologist's level of vigilance and awareness will be at a peak for these patients because of the family history.

The long-term relationship of the anesthesiologist with the family of an MH survivor, continued education of the family, and easy accessibility to the anesthesiologist by the family are important factors. The family needs literature and needs to have their questions answered. They need to be directed to the MHAUS support group; this organization maintains a hot-line number (1-800-98MHAUS or 607-674-7901) for physicians, for information during emergency situations, for follow-up advice, and for families with MH. It is staffed 24 hours a day. It is vital that anesthesiologists be aware that MH can occur even in very young infants, newborns, and the elderly.[239-241] With constant vigilance, it can be avoided or treated with a successful outcome. If neglected, undiagnosed, or mistreated, it can lead to disastrous consequences.

Temperature Monitoring

Temperature is usually expressed in degrees centigrade (°C) using the scale described by Celsius in 1742.

Indications for Temperature Monitoring

Perioperative measurement of body temperature is necessary in infants and children to detect both hypothermia and hyperthermia. Central temperature monitoring is preferable in children to determine the severity of heat loss. Since a rise in $ETCO_2$ is the earliest indicator of hypermetabolism, temperature monitoring is less likely to be useful in making the diagnosis of MH but rather has its best use as a guide to the adequacy of therapy.

Thermometers

Recorded temperatures may deviate from actual temperature because (1) the thermometer is inaccurate; (2) the temperature of the probe differs from that of surrounding tissue because of inadequate placement or contact with other devices that alter the temperature locally.[242] All thermometers provide temperature readings with reasonable accuracy. There are many different thermometers available, such as mercury-in-glass, thermistors, thermocouples, infrared thermometers, temperature-sensitive liquid crystals, and so on. Thermocouples (which measure a temperature-dependent bimetal electrical potential) are by far the most commonly used in anesthetic practice. Temperature-sensitive liquid crystals can be used for skin-surface thermometry. Although easy and convenient to use in pediatric anesthesia and relatively inexpensive, these devices generally do not have the range or accuracy necessary for clinical use.[243-245]

Temperature Monitoring Sites

Although it is suggested that the tympanic membrane is the ideal temperature monitoring site, there is no physiologic evidence to suggest that hypothalamic temperature represents central temperature precisely. The correct approach to temperature monitoring is to recognize that different tissues may have different temperatures but that the physiologic and practical significance of such differences varies (Fig. 27-10).

Temperature measurement sites may be central (core) or peripheral. In unanesthetized humans, tympanic membrane, pulmonary artery, rectal, nasopharyngeal and esophageal temperatures are similar.[246] Oral temperature is less accurate.[247] Temperatures at these central sites are similar in anesthetized children and infants undergoing non-cardiac surgery.[242]

Axillary temperature is useful only when the thermometer is carefully placed over the artery and the arm is adducted.[242] Axillary temperature was reported to be as accurate in measuring central temperature as tympanic membrane, esophageal, and rectal temperature sites.[242] It is the most commonly used site for temperature measurement in infants and children and it is the most convenient for short surgical procedures.

Nasopharyngeal temperature is measured by positioning the probe in the nasopharynx posterior to the soft palate. It should provide an estimate of the hypothalamic temperature. With the use of uncuffed endotracheal tubes, this site of temperature measurement is affected by leakage of air around the endotracheal tube and may occasionally provide inaccurate readings.

Esophageal temperature probes are usually incorporated into disposable esophageal stethoscopes. This system will measure central temperature reliably when the probe is

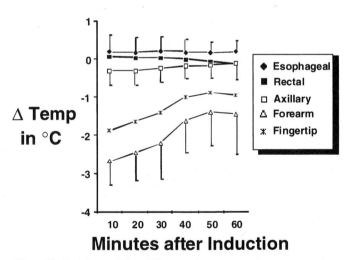

Figure 27-10. The average difference between temperatures at five different measurement sites and tympanic membrane temperature in 20 children weighing 5 to 30 kg. The central sites (esophagus, rectum, and axilla) did not differ significantly, whereas the peripheral skin-surface temperatures (forearm and fingertip) were significantly lower than the central temperatures. Vertical bars illustrate the standard deviation. The standard deviations of the rectal temperatures (omitted for clarity) were similar to those of the esophageal and axillary temperatures. The standard deviations of fingertip temperatures (also omitted for clarity) were similar to those of the forearm temperatures. (From Bissonnette B, Sessler DI, LaFlamme P: Intraoperative temperature monitoring sites in infants and children and the effect of inspired gas warming on esophageal temperature. Anesth Analg 1989; 69:192-196.)

placed in the distal third of the esophagus at the point where maximum heart sounds are heard.[42, 242] Infants and children have minimal thermal insulation between the tracheobronchial tree and the esophagus. Thus, the effects of respiratory gas temperature on esophageal temperature may produce an artifactual measurement.[242]

Rectal temperature probes have been used as a measure of core temperature despite problems such as insulation by feces, cool blood returning from the legs, and the influence of an open abdominal cavity. It has been shown that the rectal temperature in infants and children is similar to other sites of central temperature measurement.[242]

A *bladder temperature* probe has been suggested as one of the most accurate means of measuring central temperature. It has been demonstrated that bladder temperature is identical to pulmonary artery temperature when urine flow is high.[248] It is not clinically useful in patients whose urine output is at or below normal levels.

Tympanic membrane or aural canal thermistors provide a reasonable approximation of hypothalamic temperature. Early reports described tympanic membrane perforation by aural thermistors. However, currently available probes are so soft and flexible that even vigorous insertion is unlikely to damage the ear. After insertion of the probe it is necessary to block the aural canal with cotton wool, which will prevent cooling of the probe by environmental air movement.

Skin-surface temperatures do not correlate well with central temperatures and therefore should not be considered as a substitute for other central temperature monitoring sites.[243–245] Skin-surface temperatures are significantly lower than central temperatures and the difference between them does not remain constant[242, 245, 249]; simply adding a constant correcting value (e.g., 2.2°C) to an arbitrary skin temperature such as the forehead is unlikely to provide a reliable indication of central temperature.[243–245, 250] It is unlikely that skin temperature correlates with central temperature during the early phase of MH because circulating catecholamine concentrations increase to 20 times normal.[251, 252]

Prevention of Hypothermia

Mild postoperative hypothermia (central temperature 34–36°C) is a common occurrence following surgery. Mild hypothermia does not impair postanesthetic recovery in infants and children undergoing surgical procedures lasting less than 3 hours.[253] Mild hypothermia may, however, impede immune responses to perioperative wound infections.[254] Moderate to severe hypothermia is known to cause other complications, including prolonged drug effect,[255] hampered blood coagulation,[256] and thermal discomfort.[257] In contrast, 1° to 3°C of central hypothermia may provide significant protection against global and regional ischemia,[258] and hypoxemia[259] and malignant hyperthermia.[260] It is important to understand that thermal management, like any other therapies, must be given a thoughtful risk-benefit analysis and appropriate intraoperative cost-benefit consideration in each patient.[253] Careful attention to preventing or correcting hypothermia is vital to patient homeostasis.

Preventing Redistribution Hypothermia

As previously discussed, the initial reduction in core temperature (0.5–1.5°C) is difficult to prevent because it results from redistribution of compartmental heat from the central thermal compartment to cooler peripheral compartments (see Fig. 27–4). Therefore, the most effective clinical warming devices will not generally prevent hypothermia during the first hour of anesthesia. The transfer of heat, even from active skin-surface warming and even in the patient who is peripherally vasodilated following induction of anesthesia, will not improve core temperature because the central-to-peripheral flow of heat is massive.

Although redistribution of heat cannot be effectively treated, it can be prevented. Skin-surface warming before the induction of anesthesia will not significantly alter core temperature but will increase the temperature of the peripheral compartment and therefore reduce the gradient with the central compartment.

Operating Room Temperature

Since cutaneous heat loss is the primary determinant of heat balance, operating room temperature is the most important factor that will determine heat loss during surgery.[261] At an operating room temperature greater than 21°C, most adult patients will remain normothermic[262, 263]; premature infants and small children may require ambient temperatures higher than 26°C to maintain normothermia.[261]

Warming Devices

Thermal comfort determines behavioral reaction to heat loss. Thermal comfort is determined by skin-surface temperature, not by tissue heat content, cutaneous heat flux, or central temperature.[251] The utilization of skin-surface warming devices in adults prior to induction of anesthesia can prevent the hypothermic response resulting from the internal redistribution of heat within the body.[264] Aggressive skin-surface warming will cause peripheral vasodilatation and favorably increase the temperature of the peripheral compartment to values approaching those of the central compartment. The net result will be an increase in mean body temperature because skin-surface warming will reduce the amount of energy transferred from the central compartment to the peripheral compartment after induction of anesthesia.[265] A variety of passive and active skin-surface warmers are available, including circulating hot water blankets,[266] infrared radiant heaters,[263, 267] and convection heaters, which circulate warm air through disposable blankets and raise the effective ambient temperature around the patient.[268–270] Convective forced-air warmers are more effective than radiant infrared devices and as effective as circulating-water blankets when heat transfer across the entire skin surface is considered.[251] *The most important aspect about active surface warming is the amount of skin covered rather than the body surface insulated.* The popular perception that a large fraction of metabolic heat is lost from the head is false in adults; however, in infants and children, heat loss from the head can be substantial and the use of head caps during anesthesia can be useful to reduce heat loss.[271–273]

Passive insulators are commonly used to prevent cutaneous heat loss. Insulating covers may be chosen on the basis of cost and convenience. A single layer of any material reduces the heat loss approximately 30%. It is likely, however, that the amount of skin surface covered is more important than the choice of skin region covered or the choice of insulating material (Fig. 27–11).[270, 274]

The most effective perianesthetic warming system is forced air convection. The efficiency of this system is based on its ability to actively transfer heat to the patient. The best forced-air system can transfer up to 50 W across the skin surface, rapidly increasing mean body temperature (Fig. 27–12).[268, 269, 275]

Airway Humidification

Airway humidification in intubated patients prevents tracheal damage from dry inspired gases,[276] increases tracheal mucus flow,[277] and minimizes respiratory heat loss.[278, 279] Heat and humidity can be added to inspired gases actively by evaporative or ultrasonic humidifiers, or passively by heat and moisture exchangers ("artificial noses").[280, 281] Although airway humidification contributes minimally to the maintenance of normothermia in adult anesthesia, there is considerable evidence that a relative humidity of at least 50% maintains normal cilia function in the trachea and helps prevent bronchospasm.[277, 282, 283] Humidification of 50% is easily obtained with heat and moisture exchange filters and is desirable during prolonged procedures. The role of active airway heating devices with the current availability of surface warm air devices is now limited to patients with nonrebreathing anesthesia circuits to both heat and humidify the cool inspiratory gases.

Passive airway humidification is considerably more effective in pediatric patients than in adults because of the higher minute ventilation per kilogram body weight.[4] Additional advantages include the avoidance of over-humidification, which can be seen with ultrasonic devices, and the elimination of the danger of airway burns.[284, 285] The addition of an artificial nose with a dead space of approximately 1 mL

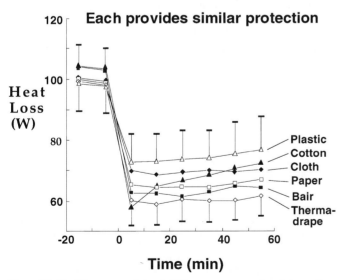

Figure 27–11. There are minimal differences among insulators. Covers act by trapping a small amount of air between them and the skin surface. There are few clinical important differences among the thermal barriers. Insulating covers should be chosen on the basis of cost and convenience. (From Sessler DI, McGuire J, Sessler SM: Perioperative thermal insulation. Anesthesiology 1991;74:875–879.)

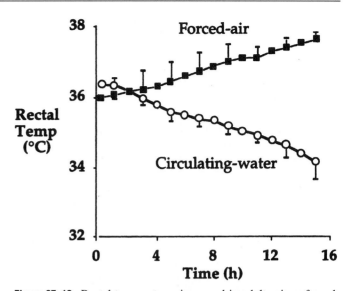

Figure 27–12. Rectal temperatures increased in adults given forced-air warming and decreased in those warmed with circulating water placed under the patient. (From Kurz A, Kurz M, Poeschl G, et al.: Forced-air warming maintains intraoperative normothermia better than circulating water mattresses. Anesth Analg 1993;77: 89–95.)

introduces trivial airway resistance and can be safely used with the smallest infants on a short-term basis.[286, 287] Differences in efficiencies among heat and moisture exchangers are small.[288, 289] It should be noted that the use of an artificial nose with a heated humidifier is not indicated and may result in airway occlusion.[290]

Intravenous Fluid Warming

The use of a fluid warmer in pediatric anesthesia is determined by the magnitude of the procedure and the anticipated fluid requirements. Heat loss due to cold intravenous fluids becomes clinically important only when large amounts of crystalloid solution or blood are administered rapidly. If the rate of infusion of the intravenous solutions is slow, fluid warmers become inefficient because the room air cools the fluid in the intravenous tubing again before it reaches the patient. The utilization of a fluid warmer close to the intravenous site improves the performance (see Chapter 12).

Conclusions

Temperature derangements frequently occur during and following anesthesia; hypothermia is the most common derangement. This transient dysfunction of the thermoregulatory system can, in certain instances, lead to potentially serious complications of surgery and anesthesia. A better understanding of the physiology of the temperature regulation system during anesthesia has improved intraoperative management. The concept that temperature is a "drug" that can be controlled and regulated according to the needs of a given patient undergoing a surgical procedure is a reality.

REFERENCES

1. Shanks CA: Mean skin temperature during anaesthesia: An assessment of formulae in the supine surgical patient. Br J Anaesth 1975;47:871–875.

2. Sessler DI, Olofsson CI, Rubinstein EH: The thermoregulatory threshold in humans during nitrous oxide–fentanyl anesthesia. Anesthesiology 1988;69:357–364.

3. Bissonnette B, Sessler DI: Thermoregulatory thresholds for vasoconstriction in pediatric patients anesthetized with halothane or halothane and caudal bupivacaine. Anesthesiology 1992;76:387–392.

4. Bissonnette B, Sessler DI, LaFlamme P: Passive and active inspired gas humidification in infants and children. Anesthesiology 1989;71:350–354.

5. Pierau FK, Wurster RD: Primary afferent input from cutaneous thermoreceptors. Fed Proc 1981;40:2819–2824.

6. Poulos DA: Central processing of cutaneous temperature information. Fed Proc 1981;40:2825–2829.

7. Hellon RF: Neurophysiology of temperature regulation: Problems and perspectives. Fed Proc 1981;40:2804–2807.

8. Hynson JM, Sessler DI, Glosten B, et al: Thermal balance and tremor patterns during epidural anesthesia. Anesthesiology 1991;74:680–690.

9. Sessler DI, Rubinstein EH, Eger EI 2d: Core temperature changes during N₂O fentanyl and halothane/O₂ anesthesia. Anesthesiology 1987;67:137–139.

10. Hillman PE, Scott NR, van Tienhoven A: Vasomotion in chicken foot: Dual innervation of arteriovenous anastomoses. Am J Physiol 1982;242:R582–590.

11. Hales J: Skin arteriovenous anastomoses, their control and role in thermoregulation. In: Johanse K, Burggren W, eds: Cardiovascular Shunts: Phylogenetic, Ontogenetic, and Clinical Aspects. Copenhagen: Munksgaard; 1984:433.

12. Sessler DI, Ponte J: Disparity between thermal comfort and physiological thermoregulatory responses during epidural anesthesia. Anesthesiology 1989;71:A682.

13. Coffman JD, Cohen AS: Total and capillary fingertip blood flow in Raynaud's phenomenon. N Engl J Med 1971;285:259–263.

14. Sessler DI: Sweating threshold during isoflurane anesthesia in humans. Anesth Analg 1991;73:300–303.

15. Bolton DP, Nelson EA, Taylor BJ, et al: Thermal balance in infants. J Appl Physiol 1996;80:2234–2242.

16. Jessen K: An assessment of human regulatory nonshivering thermogenesis. Acta Anaesthesiol Scand 1980;24:138–143.

17. Jahnukainen T, van Ravenswaaij-Arts C, Jalonen J, et al: Dynamics of vasomotor thermoregulation of the skin in term and preterm neonates. Early Hum Dev 1993;33:133–143.

18. Hurgoiu V: Thermal regulation in preterm infants. Early Hum Dev 1992;28:1–5.

19. Dawkins MJ, Scopes JW: Non-shivering thermogenesis and brown adipose tissue in the human new-born infant. Nature 1965;206:201–202.

20. Himms-Hagen J: Cellular thermogenesis. Annu Rev Physiol 1976;38:315–351.

21. Karlberg P, Moore RE, Oliver TK: Thermogenic and cardiovascular responses of the newborn baby to noradrenaline. Acta Paediatr Scand 1965;54:225–238.

22. Astrup A, Bulow J, Madsen J, et al: Contribution of BAT and skeletal muscle to thermogenesis induced by ephedrine in man. Am J Physiol 1985;248:E507–E515.

23. Schiff D, Stern L, Leduc J: Chemical thermogenesis in newborn infants: Catecholamine excretion and the plasma non-esterified fatty acid response to cold exposure. Pediatrics 1966;37:577–582.

24. Gale CC: Neuroendocrine aspects of thermoregulation. Annu Rev Physiol 1973;35:391–430.

25. Silva JE: Thyroid hormone control of thermogenesis and energy balance. Thyroid 1995;5:481–492.

26. Stern L, Lees MH, Leduc J: Environmental temperature, oxygen consumption, and catecholamine excretion in newborn infants. Pediatrics 1965;36:367–373.

27. Shibata M, Iriki M, Arita J, et al: Procaine microinjection into the lower midbrain increases brown fat and body temperatures in anesthetized rats. Brain Res 1996;716:171–179.

28. Dicker A, Ohlson KB, Johnson L, et al: Halothane selectively inhibits nonshivering thermogenesis: Possible implications for thermoregulation during anesthesia of infants. Anesthesiology 1995;82:491–501.

29. Ohlson KB, Mohell N, Cannon B, et al: Thermogenesis in brown adipocytes is inhibited by volatile anesthetic agents: A factor contributing to hypothermia in infants? Anesthesiology 1994;81:176–183.

30. Stuart D, Ott K, Ishikawa K, et al: The rhythm of shivering: 3. Central contributions. Am J Phys Med 1966;45:91–104.

31. Sessler DI: Perianesthetic thermoregulation and heat balance in humans. FASEB J 1993;7:638–644.

32. Hissa R: Central control of body temperature: A review. Arctic Med Res 1990;49:3–15.

33. Hemingway A, Price WM: The autonomic nervous system and regulation of body temperature. Anesthesiology 1968;29:693–701.

34. Hemingway A: Shivering. Physiol Rev 1963;43:397–422.

35. Frank SM, Higgins MS, Fleisher LA, et al: Adrenergic, respiratory, and cardiovascular effects of core cooling in humans. Am J Physiol 1997;272:R557–R562.

36. Benzinger TH: Heat regulation: Homeostasis of central temperature in man. Physiol Rev 1969;49:671–759.

37. Roe CF, Goldberg MJ, Blair CS, et al: The influence of body temperature on early postoperative oxygen consumption. Surgery 1966;60:85–92.

38. Adamsons K Jr, Gandy GM, James LS: The influence of thermal factors upon oxygen consumption of the newborn human infant. J Pediatr 1965;66:495–508.

39. Sessler DI: Perioperative thermoregulation and heat balance. Ann N Y Acad Sci 1997;813:757–777.

40. Just B, Delva E, Camus Y, et al: Oxygen uptake during recovery following naloxone: Relationship with intraoperative heat loss. Anesthesiology 1992;76:60–64.

41. Washington DE, Sessler DI, McGuire J, et al: Painful stimulation minimally increases the thermoregulatory threshold for vasoconstriction during enflurane anesthesia in humans. Anesthesiology 1992;77:286–290.

42. Stoen R, Sessler DI: The thermoregulatory threshold is inversely proportional to isoflurane concentration. Anesthesiology 1990;72:822–827.

43. Deacock S, Holdcroft A: Heat retention using passive systems during anaesthesia: Comparison of two plastic wraps, one with reflective properties. Br J Anaesth 1997;79:766–769.

44. Sessler DI, Sessler AM, Hudson S, et al: Heat loss during surgical skin preparation. Anesthesiology 1993;78:1055–1064.

45. Borse N, Deodhar J, Pandit AN: Effects of thermal environment on neonatal thermoregulation. Indian Pediatr 1997;34:718–720.

46. Telliez F, Bach V, Krim G, et al: Consequences of a small decrease of air temperature from thermal equilibrium on thermoregulation in sleeping neonates. Med Biol Eng Comput 1997;35:516–520.

47. Stern L: The newborn infant and his thermal environment. Curr Probl Pediatr 1970;1:1–29.

48. Heiser MS, Downes JJ: Temperature regulation in the pediatric patient. Semin Anesth 1984;3:37–42.

49. Hey EN, Katz G: Evaporative water loss in the new-born baby. J Physiol (Lond) 1969;200:605–619.

50. Harpin VA, Rutter N: Sweating in preterm babies. J Pediatr 1982;100:614–619.

51. Bickler PE, Sessler DI: Efficiency of airway heat and moisture exchangers in anesthetized humans. Anesth Analg 1990;71:415–418.

52. Bissonnette B, Sessler DI: Passive or active inspired gas humidification increases thermal steady-state temperatures in anesthetized infants. Anesth Analg 1989;69:783–787.

53. Roe CF: Effect of bowel exposure on body temperature during surgical operations. Am J Surg 1971;122:13–15.

54. Hammarlund K, Stromberg B, Sedin G: Heat loss from the skin of preterm and full term newborn infants during the first weeks after birth. Biol Neonate 1986;50:1–10.

55. Hammarlund K, Nilsson GE, Oberg PA, et al: Transepidermal water loss in newborn infants. V. Evaporation from the skin and heat exchange during the first hours of life. Acta Paediatr Scand 1980;69:385–392.

56. Bell EF, Gray JC, Weinstein MR, et al: The effects of thermal environment on heat balance and insensible water loss in low-birthweight infants. J Pediatr 1980;96:452–459.

57. Hardy JD, Milhorat AT, DuBois EF: Basal metabolism and heat loss of young women at temperatures from 22°C to 35°C. J Nutr 1941;21:383–404.

58. Sessler DI, McGuire J, Hynson J, et al: Thermoregulatory vasoconstriction during isoflurane anesthesia minimally decreases cutaneous heat loss. Anesthesiology 1992;76:670–675.

59. Bloch EC, Ginsberg B, Binner RA Jr, et al: Limb tourniquets and central temperature in anesthetized children. Anesth Analg 1992;74:486–489.

60. Ohlson KB, Lindahl SG, Cannon B, et al: Analysis of the cellular

mechanism for halothane inhibition of brown adipose tissue thermogenesis. Ann N Y Acad Sci 1997;813:718–721.

61. Sessler DI, Olofsson CI, Rubinstein EH, et al: The thermoregulatory threshold in humans during halothane anesthesia. Anesthesiology 1988;68:836–842.

62. Bissonnette B, Sessler DI: The thermoregulatory threshold in infants and children anesthetized with isoflurane and caudal bupivacaine. Anesthesiology 1990;73:1114–1118.

63. Hunter WS, Holmes KR, Elizondo RS: Thermal balance in ketamine-anesthetized rhesus monkey *Macaca mulatta*. Am J Physiol 1981;241:R301–R306.

64. Detry JM, Brengelmann GL, Rowell LB, et al: Skin and muscle components of forearm blood flow in directly heated resting man. J Appl Physiol 1972;32:506–511.

65. Tankersley CG, Smolander J, Kenney WL, et al: Sweating and skin blood flow during exercise: Effects of age and maximal oxygen uptake. J Appl Physiol 1991;71:236–242.

66. Fusi L, Steer PJ, Maresh MJ, et al: Maternal pyrexia associated with the use of epidural analgesia in labour. Lancet 1989;1:1250–1252.

67. Taylor BJ, Williams SM, Mitchell EA, et al: Symptoms, sweating and reactivity of infants who die of SIDS compared with community controls. New Zealand National Cot Death Study Group. J Paediatr Child Health 1996;32:316–322.

68. Sedin G, Hammarlund K, Nilsson GE, et al: Measurements of transepidermal water loss in newborn infants. Clin Perinatol 1985;12:79–99.

69. Harpin VA, Chellappah G, Rutter N: Responses of the newborn infant to overheating. Biol Neonate 1983;44:65–75.

70. Johnson C, Edleman KJ: Malignant hyperthermia: A review. J Perinatol 1992;12:61–71.

71. Harriman DG: Malignant hyperthermia myopathy: A critical review. Br J Anaesth 1988;60:309–316.

72. Denborough M: Malignant hyperthermia. Lancet 1998;352:1131–1136.

73. Rossiter BJ, Caskey CT: Impact of the human genome project on medical practice. Ann Surg Oncol 1995;2:14–25.

74. Sawicki MP, Samara G, Hurwitz M, et al: Human Genome Project. Am J Surg 1993;165:258–264.

75. Bacon AK: Pulse oximetry in malignant hyperthermia. Anaesth Intensive Care 1989;17:208–210.

76. Urwyler A, Hartung E: Malignant hyperthermia. [in German.] Anaesthesist 1994;43:557–569.

77. Williamson JA, Webb RK, Cockings J, et al: The Australian Incident Monitoring Study. The capnograph: Applications and limitations—an analysis of 2000 incident reports. Anaesth Intensive Care 1993;21:551–557.

78. Baudendistel L, Goudsouzian N, Coté CJ, et al: End-tidal CO_2 monitoring. Its use in the diagnosis and management of malignant hyperthermia. Anaesthesia 1984;39:1000–1003.

79. Larach MG, Localio AR, Allen GC, et al: A clinical grading scale to predict malignant hyperthermia susceptibility. Anesthesiology 1994;80:771–779.

80. Larach MG: Standardization of the caffeine halothane muscle contracture test. North American Malignant Hyperthermia Group. Anesth Analg 1989;69:511–515.

81. Allen GC, Larach MG, Kunselman AR: The sensitivity and specificity of the caffeine-halothane contracture test: A report from the North American Malignant Hyperthermia Registry. The North American Malignant Hyperthermia Registry of MHAUS. Anesthesiology 1998;88:579–588.

82. Larach MG, Landis JR, Bunn JS, et al: Prediction of malignant hyperthermia susceptibility in low-risk subjects: An epidemiologic investigation of caffeine halothane contracture responses. The North American Malignant Hyperthermia Registry. Anesthesiology 1992;76:16–27.

83. Ward A, Chaffman MO, Sorkin EM: Dantrolene: A review of its pharmacodynamic and pharmacokinetic properties and therapeutic use in malignant hyperthermia, the neuroleptic malignant syndrome and an update of its use in muscle spasticity. Drugs 1986;32:130–168.

84. McCoy EP, Maddineni VR, Elliott P, et al: Haemodynamic effects of rocuronium during fentanyl anaesthesia: Comparison with vecuronium. Can J Anaesth 1993;40:703–708.

85. Strazis KP, Fox AW: Malignant hyperthermia: A review of published cases. Anesth Analg 1993;77:297–304.

86. Kolb ME, Horne ML, Martz R: Dantrolene in human malignant hyperthermia. Anesthesiology 1982;56:254–262.

87. Britt BA: Recent advances in malignant hyperthermia. Anesth Analg 1972;51:841–850.

88. Relton JE, Britt BA, Steward DJ: Malignant hyperpyrexia. Br J Anaesth 1973;45:269–275.

89. Britt BA, Kalow W: Malignant hyperthermia: A statistical review. Can Anaesth Soc J 1970;17:293–315.

90. Pan TH, Wollack AR, DeMarco JA: Malignant hyperthermia associated with enflurane anesthesia: A case report. Anesth Analg 1975;54:47–49.

91. Boheler J, Hamrick JC Jr, McKnight RL, et al: Isoflurane and malignant hyperthermia. Anesth Analg 1982;61:712–713.

92. Greenberg CP, Hall SL, Karan SM, et al: MH during outpatient pediatric ENT surgery: An anesthesia concern. Anesthesiology 1995;83:A1002–A1004.

93. Bruton NH, Maree SM: A case approach: the pathophysiology of thyroid storm. AANA J 1983;51:295–301.

94. Larach MG, Rosenberg H, Gronert GA, et al: Hyperkalemic cardiac arrest during anesthesia in infants and children with occult myopathies. Clin Pediatr (Phila) 1997;36:9–16.

95. Denborough M, Lovell R: Anesthetic deaths in a family. Lancet 1960;2:45–46.

96. Harrison GG: Control of the malignant hyperpyrexic syndrome in MHS swine by dantrolene sodium. Br J Anaesth 1975;47:62–65.

97. Britt BA, Gordon RA: Three cases of malignant hyperthermia with special consideration of management. Can Anaesth Soc J 1969;16:99–105.

98. Kelstrup J, Haase J, Jorni J, et al: Malignant hyperthermia in a family. Acta Anaesthesiol Scand 1973;17:283–284.

99. Chan TC, Evans SD, Clark RF: Drug-induced hyperthermia. Crit Care Clin 1997;13:785–808.

100. Censier K, Urwyler A, Zorzato F, et al: Intracellular calcium homeostasis in human primary muscle cells from malignant hyperthermia-susceptible and normal individuals: Effect of overexpression of recombinant wild-type and Arg163Cys mutated ryanodine receptors. J Clin Invest 1998;101:1233–1242.

101. Manning BM, Quane KA, Lynch PJ, et al: Novel mutations at a CpG dinucleotide in the ryanodine receptor in malignant hyperthermia. Hum Mutat 1998;11:45–50.

102. Manning BM, Quane KA, Ording H, et al: Identification of novel mutations in the ryanodine-receptor gene (RYR1) in malignant hyperthermia: genotype-phenotype correlation. Am J Hum Genet 1998;62:599–609.

103. Quane KA, Ording H, Keating KE, et al: Detection of a novel mutation at amino acid position 614 in the ryanodine receptor in malignant hyperthermia. Br J Anaesth 1997;79:332–337.

104. Pessah IN, Lynch C 3d, Gronert GA: Complex pharmacology of malignant hyperthermia. Anesthesiology 1996;84:1275–1279.

105. Steinfath M, Singh S, Scholz J, et al: C1840-T mutation in the human skeletal muscle ryanodine receptor gene: Frequency in northern German families susceptible to malignant hyperthermia and the relationship to in vitro contracture response. J Mol Med 1995;73:35–40.

106. Hartung E, Anetseder M, Engelhardt W, et al: The ryanodine test might be helpful to solve discordances between phenotypes and genotypes in malignant hyperthermia families. Anesthesiology 1996;85:A306.

107. Fagerlund TH, Islander G, Twetman ER, et al: A search for three known RYR1 gene mutations in 41 Swedish families with predisposition to malignant hyperthermia. Clin Genet 1995;48:12–16.

108. Krivosic-Horber R, Reyford H, Adnet P, et al: Does the type of malignant hyperthermia mutation influence the clinical expression of malignant hyperthermia? Anesthesiology 1996;85:A301.

109. Mickelson JR, Knudson CM, Kennedy CF, et al: Structural and functional correlates of a mutation in the malignant hyperthermia-susceptible pig ryanodine receptor. FEBS Lett 1992;301:49–52.

110. Otsu K, Phillips MS, Khanna VK, et al: Refinement of diagnostic assays for a probable causal mutation for porcine and human malignant hyperthermia. Genomics 1992;13:835–837.

111. Otsu K, Khanna VK, Archibald AL, et al: Cosegregation of porcine malignant hyperthermia and a probable causal mutation in the skeletal muscle ryanodine receptor gene in backcross families. Genomics 1991;11:744–750.

112. Fujii J, Otsu K, Zorzato F, et al: Identification of a mutation in porcine ryanodine receptor associated with malignant hyperthermia. Science 1991;253:448–451.

113. Gronert GA, Milde JH, Theye RA: Dantrolene in porcine malignant hyperthermia. Anesthesiology 1976;44:488–495.

114. Gronert GA, Theye RA: Halothane-induced porcine malignant hyperthermia: Metabolic and hemodynamic changes. Anesthesiology 1976;44:36–43.

115. Eikelnboom G, Minkema D: Prediction of pale, soft, exudative muscle with a non-lethal test for the halothane-induced porcine malignant hyperthermia syndrome. Netherlands J Veterin Sci 1974;99:421–426.

116. Rutberg H, Henriksson KG, Jorfeldt L, et al: Metabolic changes in a case of malignant hyperthermia. Br J Anaesth 1983;55:461–467.

117. Knudson CM, Mickelson JR, Louis CF, et al: Distinct immunopeptide maps of the sarcoplasmic reticulum Ca²⁺ release channel in malignant hyperthermia. J Biol Chem 1990;265:2421–2424.

118. Britt BA: Etiology and pathophysiology of malignant hyperthermia. Fed Proc 1979;38:44–48.

119. Lopez JR, Allen PD, Alamo L, et al: Myoplasmic free [Ca²⁺] during a malignant hyperthermia episode in swine. Muscle Nerve 1988;11:82–88.

120. Kim DH, Sreter FA, Ohnishi ST, et al: Kinetic studies of Ca²⁺ release from sarcoplasmic reticulum of normal and malignant hyperthermia susceptible pig muscles. Biochim Biophys Acta 1984;775:320–327.

121. Rasmussen UF, Rasmussen HN, Andersen AJ, et al: Characterization of mitochondria from pig muscle: Higher activity of exo-NADH oxidase in animals suffering from malignant hyperthermia. Biochem J 1996;315:659–663.

122. Ryan JF, Lopez JR, Sanchez VB, et al: Myoplasmic calcium changes precede metabolic and clinical signs of porcine malignant hyperthermia. Anesth Analg 1994;79:1007–1011.

123. Lucke JN, Hall GM, Lister D: Porcine malignant hyperthermia. I: Metabolic and physiological changes. Br J Anaesth 1976;48:297–304.

124. Liebenschutz F, Mai C, Pickerodt VW: Increased carbon dioxide production in two patients with malignant hyperpyrexia and its control by dantrolene. Br J Anaesth 1979;51:899–903.

125. Triner L, Sherman J: Potential value of expiratory carbon dioxide measurement in patients considered to be susceptible to malignant hyperthermia. Anesthesiology 1981;55:482.

126. Dunn CM, Maltry DE, Eggers GW Jr: Value of mass spectrometry in early diagnosis of malignant hyperthermia. Anesthesiology 1985;63:333.

127. Cody JR: Muscle rigidity following administration of succinylcholine. Anesthesiology 1968;29:159–162.

128. MacLennan DH, Phillips MS: Malignant hyperthermia. Science 1992;256:789–794.

129. Blank JW, Boggs SD: Successful treatment of an episode of malignant hyperthermia using a large dose of dantrolene. J Clin Anesth 1993;5:69–72.

130. Fuchs F: Thermal inactivation of the calcium regulatory mechanism of human skeletal muscle actomyosin: A possible contributing factor in the rigidity of malignant hyperthermia. Anesthesiology 1975;42:584–589.

131. Lopez JR, Sanchez V, Lopez I, et al: The effects of extracellular magnesium on myoplasmic [Ca²⁺] in malignant hyperthermia susceptible swine. Anesthesiology 1990;73:109–117.

132. Lopez JR, Perez C, Linares N, et al: Hypersensitive response of malignant hyperthermia-susceptible skeletal muscle to inositol 1,4,5-triphosphate induced release of calcium. Naunyn Schmiedebergs Arch Pharmacol 1995;352:442–446.

133. Tonner PH, Scholz J, Richter A, et al: Alterations of inositol polyphosphates in skeletal muscle during porcine malignant hyperthermia. Br J Anaesth 1995;75:467–471.

134. Wappler F, Scholz J, Kochling A, et al: Inositol 1,4,5-trisphosphate in blood and skeletal muscle in human malignant hyperthermia. Br J Anaesth 1997;78:541–547.

135. Fletcher JE, Mayerberger S, Tripolitis L, et al: Fatty acids markedly lower the threshold for halothane-induced calcium release from the terminal cisternae in human and porcine normal and malignant hyperthermia susceptible skeletal muscle. Life Sci 1991;49:1651–1657.

136. Fletcher JE, Tripolitis L, Erwin K, et al: Fatty acids modulate calcium-induced calcium release from skeletal muscle heavy sarcoplasmic reticulum fractions: Implications for malignant hyperthermia. Biochem Cell Biol 1990;68:1195–1201.

137. Gronert GA: Malignant hyperthermia. Anesthesiology 1980;53:395–423.

138. Jardon OM: Physiologic stress, heat stroke, malignant hyperthermia: A perspective. Mil Med 1982;147:8–14.

139. Ohnishi ST, Taylor S, Gronert GA: Calcium-induced Ca²⁺ release from sarcoplasmic reticulum of pigs susceptible to malignant hyper-

thermia: The effects of halothane and dantrolene. FEBS Lett 1983;161:103–107.

140. Lopez JR, Medina P, Alamo L: Dantrolene sodium is able to reduce the resting ionic [Ca²⁺]i in muscle from humans with malignant hyperthermia. Muscle Nerve 1987;10:77–79.

141. Tregear RT, Marston SB: The crossbridge theory. Annu Rev Physiol 1979;41:723–736.

142. Saltzman LS, Kates RA, Corke BC, et al: Hyperkalemia and cardiovascular collapse after verapamil and dantrolene administration in swine. Anesth Analg 1984;63:473–478.

143. Harrison GG: Malignant hyperthermia. Dantrolene: Dynamics and kinetics. Br J Anaesth 1988;60:279–286.

144. Mickelson JR, Louis CF: Malignant hyperthermia: excitation-contraction coupling, Ca²⁺ release channel, and cell Ca²⁺ regulation defects. Physiol Rev 1996;76:537–592.

145. Ryan JF, Papper EM: Malignant fever during and following anesthesia. Anesthesiology 1970;32:196–201.

146. Cabral R, Prior PF, Scott DF, et al: Reversible profound depression of cerebral electrical activity in hyperthermia. Electroencephalogr Clin Neurophysiol 1977;42:697–701.

147. Mehler J, Bachour H, Simons F, et al: Cardiac arrest during anesthesia induction with halothane and succinylcholine in an infant. Massive hyperkalemia and rhabdomyolysis in suspected myopathy and/or malignant hyperthermia. [in German.] Anaesthesist 1991;40:497–501.

148. Weiskopf RB, Moore MA, Eger EI 2d, et al: Rapid increase in desflurane concentration is associated with greater transient cardiovascular stimulation than with rapid increase in isoflurane concentration in humans. Anesthesiology 1994;80:1035–1045.

149. Fu ES, Scharf JE, Mangar D, et al: Malignant hyperthermia involving the administration of desflurane. Can J Anaesth 1996;43:687–690.

150. Rolf N, Coté CJ: Persistent cardiac arrhythmias in pediatric patients: Effects of age, expired carbon dioxide values, depth of anesthesia, and airway management. Anesth Analg 1991;73:720–724.

151. Antognini JF: Creatine kinase alterations after acute malignant hyperthermia episodes and common surgical procedures. Anesth Analg 1995;81:1039–1042.

152. Bennett MH, Wainwright AP: Acute thyroid crisis on induction of anaesthesia. Anaesthesia 1989;44:28–30.

153. Purday JP, Montgomery CJ, Blackstock D: Intraoperative hyperthermia in a paediatric patient with cystinosis. Pediatr Anaesth 1995;5:389–392.

154. Crowley KJ, Cunningham AJ, Conroy B, et al: Phaeochromocytoma: A presentation mimicking malignant hyperthermia. Anaesthesia 1988;43:1031–1032.

155. Reeves RK, Stolp-Smith KA, Christopherson MW: Hyperthermia, rhabdomyolysis, and disseminated intravascular coagulation associated with baclofen pump catheter failure. Arch Phys Med Rehabil 1998;79:353–356.

156. Bertorini TE: Myoglobinuria, malignant hyperthermia, neuroleptic malignant syndrome and serotonin syndrome. Neurol Clin 1997;15:649–671.

157. Miyatake R, Iwahashi K, Matsushita M, et al: No association between the neuroleptic malignant syndrome and mutations in the RYR1 gene associated malignant hyperthermia. J Neurol Sci 1996;143:161–165.

158. Keck PEJ, Caroff SN, McElroy SL: Neuroleptic malignant syndrome and malignant hyperthermia: End of a controversy? J Neuropsychiatry Clin Neurosci 1995;7:135–144.

159. Daras M, Kakkouras L, Tuchman AJ, et al: Rhabdomyolysis and hyperthermia after cocaine abuse: A variant of the neuroleptic malignant syndrome? Acta Neurol Scand 1995;92:161–165.

160. Sato N, Brum JM, Mitsumoto H, et al: Effect of cocaine on the contracture response to 1% halothane in patients undergoing diagnostic muscle biopsy for malignant hyperthermia. Can J Anaesth 1995;42:158–162.

161. Donlon JV, Newfield P, Sreter F, et al: Implications of masseter spasm after succinylcholine. Anesthesiology 1978;49:298–301.

162. Ellis FR, Halsall PJ: Suxamethonium spasm: A differential diagnostic conundrum. Br J Anaesth 1984;56:381–384.

163. Schwartz L, Rockoff MA, Koka BV: Masseter spasm with anesthesia: Incidence and implications. Anesthesiology 1984;61:772–775.

164. Rosenberg H, Reed S: In vitro contracture tests for susceptibility to malignant hyperthermia. Anesth Analg 1983;62:415–420.

165. van der Spek AF, Fang WB, Ashton-Miller JA, et al: Increased masticatory muscle stiffness during limb muscle flaccidity associated with succinylcholine administration. Anesthesiology 1988;69:11–16.

166. van der Spek AF, Reynolds PI, Fang WB, et al: Changes in resistance to mouth opening induced by depolarizing and non-depolarizing neuromuscular relaxants. Br J Anaesth 1990;64:21–27.

167. van der Spek AF, Fang WB, Ashton-Miller JA, et al: The effects of succinylcholine on mouth opening. Anesthesiology 1987;67:459–465.

168. Butler-Browne GS, Eriksson PO, Laurent C, et al: Adult human masseter muscle fibers express myosin isozymes characteristic of development. Muscle Nerve 1988;11:610–620.

169. Larach MG, Allen GC, Kunselman AR, et al: Do patients who experience masseter muscle rigidity as part of a malignant hyperthermia episode differ from patients with isolated masseter muscle rigidity? Anesthesiology 1996;85:A1057.

170. Ryan JF, Kagen LJ, Hyman AI: Myoglobinemia after a single dose of succinylcholine. N Engl J Med 1971;285:824–827.

171. Kosko JR, Brandom BW, Chan KH: Masseter spasm and malignant hyperthermia: A retrospective review of a hospital-based pediatric otolaryngology practice. Int J Pediatr Otorhinolaryngol 1992;23:45–50.

172. Carroll JB: Increased incidence of masseter spasm in children with strabismus anesthetized with halothane and succinylcholine. Anesthesiology 1987;67:559–561.

173. Littleford JA, Patel LR, Bose D, et al: Masseter muscle spasm in children: Implications of continuing the triggering anesthetic. Anesth Analg 1991;72:151–160.

174. O'Flynn RP, Shutack JG, Rosenberg H, et al: Masseter muscle rigidity and malignant hyperthermia susceptibility in pediatric patients: An update on management and diagnosis. Anesthesiology 1994;80:1228–1233.

175. Anonymous: A protocol for the investigation of malignant hyperpyrexia (MH) susceptibility: The European Malignant Hyperpyrexia Group. Br J Anaesth 1984;56:1267–1269.

176. Fricker R, Musat J, Sipos E, et al: High-purity ryanodine contracture test for in vitro diagnosis of malignant hyperthermia susceptibility. Anesthesiology 1996;85:A977.

177. Adnet PJ, Krivosic-Horber RM, Adamantidis MM, et al: Is resting membrane potential a possible indicator of viability of muscle bundles used in the in vitro caffeine contracture test? Anesth Analg 1992;74:105–111.

178. Nelson TE, Flewellen EH, Gloyna DF: Spectrum of susceptibility to malignant hyperthermia: Diagnostic dilemma. Anesth Analg 1983;62:545–552.

179. Britt BA: Comparison of the North American and European protocols for the caffeine halothane (CHC) contracture test. J Neurol Sci 1990;98:522.

180. Islander G, Twetman ER: Comparison between the European and North American protocols for diagnosis of malignant hyperthermia susceptibility in humans. Anesth Analg 1999;88:1155–1160.

181. Payen JF, Fouilhe N, Sam-Lai E, et al: In vitro ^{31}P-magnetic resonance spectroscopy of muscle extracts in malignant hyperthermia-susceptible patients. Anesthesiology 1996;84:1077–1082.

182. Sudo RT, Nelson TE: Ryanodine contractures in human single, skinned skeletal muscle fibers are rapid in onset and offset. Anesthesiology 1996;85:A304.

183. Sudo RT, Nelson TE: MH diagnostic test: Effect of stimulus frequency on ryanodine contracture in MHS and normal dog skeletal muscle. Anesthesiology 1996;85:A305.

184. Kreul JF, Sufit RL, Helmer PR: Effects of cold storage on muscle biopsy contracture studies. J Neurol Sci 1990;98:523.

185. Gronert GA: Controversies in malignant hyperthermia. Anesthesiology 1983;59:273–274.

186. Brownell AK, Paasuke RT, Elash A, et al: Malignant hyperthermia in Duchenne muscular dystrophy. Anesthesiology 1983;58:180–182.

187. Miller ED Jr, Sanders DB, Rowlingson JC, et al: Anesthesia-induced rhabdomyolysis in a patient with Duchenne's muscular dystrophy. Anesthesiology 1978;48:146–148.

188. Frank JP, Harati Y, Butler IJ, et al: Central core disease and malignant hyperthermia syndrome. Ann Neurol 1980;7:11–17.

189. Denborough MA, Galloway GJ, Hopkinson KC: Malignant hyperpyrexia and sudden infant death. Lancet 1982;2:1068–1069.

190. Dallman JH: Neuroleptic malignant syndrome: a review. Mil Med 1984;149:471–473.

191. Lopez JR, Sanchez V, Lopez MJ: Sarcoplasmic ionic calcium concentration in neuroleptic malignant syndrome. Cell Calcium 1989;10:223–233.

192. Wedel DJ: Malignant hyperthermia and neuromuscular disease. Neuromuscul Disord 1992;2:157–164.

193. Iaizzo PA, Lehmann-Horn F: Anesthetic complications in muscle disorders. Anesthesiology 1995;82:1093–1096.

194. Islander G, Ranklev-Twetman E: Evaluation of anaesthesias in malignant hyperthermia negative patients. Acta Anaesthesiol Scand 1995;39:819–821.

195. Bello N, Adnet P, Saulnier F, et al: Lack of sensitivity to per-anesthetic malignant hyperthermia in 32 patients who developed neuroleptic malignant syndrome. [in French.] Ann Fr Anesth Reanim 1994;13:663–668.

196. Ellis FR, Halsall PJ, Christian AS: Clinical presentation of suspected malignant hyperthermia during anaesthesia in 402 probands. Anaesthesia 1990;45:838–841.

197. Hopkins PM, Halsall PJ, Ellis FR: Diagnosing malignant hyperthermia susceptibility. Anaesthesia 1994;49:373–375.

198. Hackl W, Mauritz W, Schemper M, et al: Prediction of malignant hyperthermia susceptibility: Statistical evaluation of clinical signs. Br J Anaesth 1990;64:425–429.

199. Muldoon SM, Boggs S, Bray J, et al: Sympathetic nervous system (SNS) function in malignant hyperthermia susceptible (MHS) subjects. J Neurol Sci 1990;98:521.

200. Ohkoshi N, Yoshizawa T, Mizusawa H, et al: Malignant hyperthermia in a patient with Becker muscular dystrophy: Dystrophin analysis and caffeine contracture study. Neuromuscul Disord 1995;5:53–58.

201. Monsieurs KG, Van Broeckhoven C, Martin JJ, et al: Malignant hyperthermia susceptibility in a patient with concomitant motor neuron disease. J Neurol Sci 1996;142:36–38.

202. Price SR, Currie J: Anaesthesia for a child with centronuclear myopathy. Pediatr Anaesth 1995;5:267–268.

203. Pennington GP, Joeris L: Malignant hyperthermia in a 3-month-old infant: A case report. J Med Assoc Ga 1996;85:162–163.

204. Jones R, Dolcourt JL: Muscle rigidity following halothane anesthesia in two patients with Freeman-Sheldon syndrome. Anesthesiology 1992;77:599–600.

205. Lopez JR, Allen P, Alamo L, et al: Dantrolene prevents the malignant hyperthermic syndrome by reducing free intracellular calcium concentration in skeletal muscle of susceptible swine. Cell Calcium 1987;8:385–396.

206. Kochs E, Hoffman WE, Schulte am Esch J: Improvement of brain electrical activity during treatment of porcine malignant hyperthermia with dantrolene. Br J Anaesth 1993;71:881–884.

207. Mathieu A, Bogosian AJ, Ryan JF, et al: Recrudescence after survival of an initial episode of malignant hyperthermia. Anesthesiology 1979;51:454–455.

208. Dykes MH: Evaluation of a muscle relaxant: dantrolene sodium (Dantrium). JAMA 1975;231:862–864.

209. Flewellen EH, Nelson TE, Jones WP, et al: Dantrolene dose response in awake man: Implications for management of malignant hyperthermia. Anesthesiology 1983;59:275–280.

210. Saito S, Harada M, Yamamoto M, et al: Muscle relaxant action of dantrolene sodium in rats. Res Commun Chem Pathol Pharmacol 1993;81:345–354.

211. Ellis KO, Butterfield JL, Wessels FL, et al: A comparison of skeletal, cardiac, and smooth muscle actions of dantrolene sodium: A skeletal muscle relaxant. Arch Int Pharmacodyn Ther 1976;224:118–132.

212. Fruen BR, Mickelson JR, Louis CF: Dantrolene inhibition of sarcoplasmic reticulum Ca^{2+} release by direct and specific action at skeletal muscle ryanodine receptors. J Biol Chem 1997;272:26965–26971.

213. Van Winkle WB: Calcium release from skeletal muscle sarcoplasmic reticulum: Site of action of dantrolene sodium. Science 1976;193:1130–1131.

214. Parness J, Palnitkar S, Herman K, et al: Synthesis of [^{3}H]azidodantrolene: identification of the putative skeletal muscle dantrolene receptor. Anesthesiology 1999;89:A491.

215. Wedel DJ, Quinlan JG, Iaizzo PA: Clinical effects of intravenously administered dantrolene. Mayo Clin Proc 1995;70:241–246.

216. Allen GC, Cattran CB, Peterson RG, et al: Plasma levels of dantrolene following oral administration in malignant hyperthermia-susceptible patients. Anesthesiology 1988;69:900–904.

217. Pandit SK, Kothary SP, Cohen PJ: Orally administered dantrolene for prophylaxis of malignant hyperthermia. Anesthesiology 1979;50:156–158.

218. Hackl W, Mauritz W, Winkler M, et al: Anaesthesia in malignant hyperthermia–susceptible patients without dantrolene prophylaxis: A report of 30 cases. Acta Anaesthesiol Scand 1990;34:534–537.

219. Dubrow TJ, Wackym PA, Abdul-Rasool IH, et al: Malignant hyper-

thermia: Experience in the prospective management of eight children. J Pediatr Surg 1989;24:163–166.

220. Ording H, Hedengran AM, Skovgaard LT: Evaluation of 119 anaesthetics received after investigation for susceptibility to malignant hyperthermia. Acta Anaesthesiol Scand 1991;35:711–716.

221. Allen GC, Rosenberg H, Fletcher JE: Safety of general anesthesia in patients previously tested negative for malignant hyperthermia susceptibility. Anesthesiology 1990;72:619–622.

222. Watson CB, Reierson N, Norfleet EA: Clinically significant muscle weakness induced by oral dantrolene sodium prophylaxis for malignant hyperthermia. Anesthesiology 1986;65:312–314.

223. Carr AS, Lerman J, Cunliffe M, et al: Incidence of malignant hyperthermia reactions in 2,214 patients undergoing muscle biopsy. Can J Anaesth 1995;42:281–286.

224. Flewellen EH, Nelson TE: Dantrolene dose response in malignant hyperthermia-susceptible (MHS) swine: Method to obtain prophylaxis and therapeusis. Anesthesiology 1980;52:303–308.

225. Fitzgibbons DC: Malignant hyperthermia following preoperative oral administration of dantrolene. Anesthesiology 1981;54:73–75.

226. Ruhland G, Hinkle AJ: Malignant hyperthermia after oral and intravenous pretreatment with dantrolene in a patient susceptible to malignant hyperthermia. Anesthesiology 1984;60:159–160.

227. Liu LMP, Goudsouzian NG, Liu P: Rectal methohexital premedication in children: A dose comparison study. Anesthesiology 1980;53:343–345.

228. Dershwitz M, Sreter FA, Ryan JF: Ketamine does not trigger malignant hyperthermia in susceptible swine. Anesth Analg 1989;69:501–503.

229. Gallen JS: Propofol does not trigger malignant hyperthermia. Anesth Analg 1991;72:413–414.

230. Raff M, Harrison GG: The screening of propofol in MHS swine. Anesth Analg 1989;68:750–751.

231. Wedel DJ, Iaizzo PA, Milde JH: Desflurane is a trigger of malignant hyperthermia in susceptible swine. Anesthesiology 1991;74:508–512.

232. Ducart A, Adnet P, Renaud B, et al: Malignant hyperthermia during sevoflurane administration. Anesth Analg 1995;80:609–611.

233. Ochiai R, Toyoda Y, Nishio I, et al: Possible association of malignant hyperthermia with sevoflurane anesthesia. Anesth Analg 1992;74:616–618.

234. Otsuka H, Komura Y, Mayumi T, et al: Malignant hyperthermia during sevoflurane anesthesia in a child with central core disease. Anesthesiology 1991;75:699–701.

235. Dershwitz M, Ryan JF, Guralnick W: Safety of amide local anesthetics in patients susceptible to malignant hyperthermia. J Am Dent Assoc 1989;118:276.

236. Maccani RM, Wedel DJ, Melton A, et al: Femoral and lateral femoral cutaneous nerve block for muscle biopsies in children. Pediatr Anaesth 1995;5:223–227.

237. Flewellen EH, Nelson TE: Is theophylline, aminophylline, or caffeine (methylxanthines) contraindicated in malignant hyperthermia susceptible patients? Anesth Analg 1983;62:115–118.

238. Gronert GA: Puzzles in malignant hyperthermia. Anesthesiology 1981;54:1–2.

239. Wiswell TE, Bent RC, Solenberger R: Malignant hyperthermia in infancy. South Med J 1989;82:1451–1452.

240. Sewall K, Flowerdew RM, Bromberger P: Severe muscular rigidity at birth: Malignant hyperthermia syndrome? Can Anaesth Soc J 1980;27:279–282.

241. Mayhew JF, Rudolph J, Tobey RE: Malignant hyperthermia in a six-month old infant: A case report. Anesth Analg 1978;57:262–264.

242. Bissonnette B, Sessler DI, LaFlamme P: Intraoperative temperature monitoring sites in infants and children and the effect of inspired gas warming on esophageal temperature. Anesth Analg 1989;69:192–196.

243. Reisinger KS, Kao J, Grant DM: Inaccuracy of the Clinitemp skin thermometer. Pediatrics 1979;64:4–6.

244. MacKenzie R, Asbury AJ: Clinical evaluation of liquid crystal skin thermometers. Br J Anaesth 1994;72:246–249.

245. Leon JE, Bissonnette B, Lerman J: Liquid crystalline temperature monitoring: Does it estimate core temperature in anaesthetized paediatric patients? Can J Anaesth 1990;37:S98.

246. Cork RC, Vaughan RW, Humphrey LS: Precision and accuracy of intraoperative temperature monitoring. Anesth Analg 1983;62:211–214.

247. Tandberg D, Sklar D: Effect of tachypnea on the estimation of body temperature by an oral thermometer. N Engl J Med 1983;308:945–946.

248. Horrow JC, Rosenberg H: Does urinary catheter temperature reflect core temperature during cardiac surgery? Anesthesiology 1988;69:986–989.

249. Lacoumenta S, Hall GM: Liquid crystal thermometry during anaesthesia. Anaesthesia 1984;39:54–56.

250. Burgess GE 3d, Cooper JR, Marino RJ, et al: Continuous monitoring of skin temperature using a liquid-crystal thermometer during anesthesia. South Med J 1978;71:516–518.

251. Sessler DI: Malignant hyperthermia. J Pediatr 1986;109:9–14.

252. Sessler DI, Moayeri A: Skin-surface warming: Heat flux and central temperature. Anesthesiology 1990;73:218–224.

253. Bissonnette B, Sessler DI: Mild hypothermia does not impair postanesthetic recovery in infants and children. Anesth Analg 1993;76:168–172.

254. Kurz A, Sessler DI, Lenhardt R: Perioperative normothermia to reduce the incidence of surgical-wound infection and shorten hospitalization. Study of Wound Infection and Temperature Group. N Engl J Med 1996;334:1209–1215.

255. Heier T, Caldwell JE, Sessler DI, et al: Mild intraoperative hypothermia increases duration of action and spontaneous recovery of vecuronium blockade during nitrous oxide–isoflurane anesthesia in humans. Anesthesiology 1991;74:815–819.

256. Valeri CR, Feingold H, Cassidy G, et al: Hypothermia-induced reversible platelet dysfunction. Ann Surg 1987;205:175–181.

257. Sessler DI, Rubinstein EH, Moayeri A: Physiologic responses to mild perianesthetic hypothermia in humans. Anesthesiology 1991;75:594–610.

258. Jurkovich GJ, Pitt RM, Curreri PW, et al: Hypothermia prevents increased capillary permeability following ischemia-reperfusion injury. J Surg Res 1988;44:514–521.

259. Artru AA, Michenfelder JD: Influence of hypothermia or hyperthermia alone or in combination with pentobarbital or phenytoin on survival time in hypoxic mice. Anesth Analg 1981;60:867–870.

260. Nelson TE: Porcine malignant hyperthermia: critical temperatures for in vivo and in vitro responses. Anesthesiology 1990;73:449–454.

261. Bennett EJ, Patel KP, Grundy EM: Neonatal temperature and surgery. Anesthesiology 1977;46:303–304.

262. Morris RH: Influence of ambient temperature on patient temperature during intraabdominal surgery. Ann Surg 1971;173:230–233.

263. Morris RH: Operating room temperature and the anesthetized, paralyzed patient. Arch Surg 1971;102:95–97.

264. Glosten B, Hynson J, Sessler DI, et al: Preanesthetic skin-surface warming reduces redistribution hypothermia caused by epidural block. Anesth Analg 1993;77:488–493.

265. Vale RJ, Lunn HF: Heat balance in anaesthetized surgical patients. Proc R Soc Med 1969;62:1017–1018.

266. Stephen CR, Dent SJ, Hall KD, et al: Body temperature regulation during anesthesia in infants and children: Constant monitoring of body temperature helps to prevent complications associated with hypothermia and hyperthermia. JAMA 1960;174:1579–1585.

267. Goldblat A, Miller R: Prevention of incidental hypothermia in neurosurgical patients. Anesth Analg 1972;51:536–543.

268. Ciufo D, Dice S, Coles C: Rewarming hypothermic postanesthesia patients: A comparison between a water coil warming blanket and a forced-air warming blanket. J Post Anesth Nurs 1995;10:155–158.

269. Giesbrecht GG, Ducharme MB, McGuire JP: Comparison of forced-air patient warming systems for perioperative use. Anesthesiology 1994;80:671–679.

270. Sessler DI, McGuire J, Sessler AM: Perioperative thermal insulation. Anesthesiology 1991;74:875–879.

271. Simbruner G, Weninger M, Popow C, et al: Regional heat loss in newborn infants. Part I. Heat loss in healthy newborns at various environmental temperatures. S Afr Med J 1985;68:940–944.

272. Rowe MI, Weinberg G, Andrews W: Reduction of neonatal heat loss by an insulated head cover. J Pediatr Surg 1983;18:909–913.

273. Stothers JK: Head insulation and heat loss in the newborn. Arch Dis Child 1981;56:530–534.

274. Erickson RS, Yount ST: Effect of aluminized covers on body temperature in patients having abdominal surgery. Heart Lung 1991;20:255–264.

275. Kurz A, Kurz M, Poeschl G, et al: Forced-air warming maintains intraoperative normothermia better than circulating-water mattresses. Anesth Analg 1993;77:89–95.

276. Chalon J, Patel C, Ali M, et al: Humidity and the anesthetized patient. Anesthesiology 1979;50:195–198.

277. Forbes AR: Temperature, humidity and mucus flow in the intubated trachea. Br J Anaesth 1974;46:29–34.

278. Berry FA Jr, Hughes-Davies DI, DiFazio CA: A system for minimizing respiratory heat loss in infants during operation. Anesth Analg 1973;52:170–175.

279. Tollofsrud SG, Gundersen Y, Andersen R: Peroperative hypothermia. Acta Anaesthesiol Scand 1984;28:511–515.

280. Chalon J, Markham JP, Ali MM, et al: The pall ultipor breathing circuit filter: An efficient heat and moisture exchanger. Anesth Analg 1984;63:566–570.

281. Newton DE: Proceedings: The effect of anaesthetic gas humidification on body temperature. Br J Anaesth 1975;47:1026.

282. Mercke U: The influence of varying air humidity on mucociliary activity. Acta Otolaryngol (Stockh) 1975;79:133–139.

283. Chalon J, Loew DA, Malebranche J: Effects of dry anesthetic gases on tracheobronchial ciliated epithelium. Anesthesiology 1972;37:338–343.

284. Smith HS, Allen R: Another hazard of heated water humidifiers. Anaesthesia 1986;41:215–216.

285. Shroff PK, Skerman JH: Humidifier malfunction: A cause of anesthesia circuit occlusion. Anesth Analg 1988;67:710–711.

286. Wilkinson KA, Cranston A, Hatch DJ, et al: Assessment of a hygroscopic heat and moisture exchanger for paediatric use. Anaesthesia 1991;46:296–299.

287. Steward DJ: A disposable condenser humidifier for use during anaesthesia. Can Anaesth Soc J 1976;23:191–195.

288. Eckerbom B, Lindholm CE: Heat and moisture exchangers and the body temperature: A peroperative study. Acta Anaesthesiol Scand 1990;34:538–542.

289. Baumgarten RK: Humidifiers are unjustified in adult anesthesia. Anesth Analg 1985;64:1224–1225.

290. Barnes SD, Normoyle DA: Failure of ventilation in an infant due to increased resistance of a disposable heat and moisture exchanger. Anesth Analg 1996;83:193.

28 Pediatric Regional Anesthesia

David M. Polaner, Santhanam Suresh, *and* Charles J. Coté

Pharmacology and Pharmacokinetics of Local Anesthetics

    Amides

    Esters

    Toxicity of Local Anesthetics

    Prevention of Toxicity

    Treatment of Toxic Reactions

    Hypersensitivity to Local Anesthetics

Specific Procedures

    Central Neuraxial Blocks

    Peripheral Nerve Blocks

Summary

The use of regional anesthesia techniques in children has increased dramatically.[1,2] Regional anesthesia is most commonly used in conjunction with general anesthesia, although in certain circumstances a regional anesthetic alone may be the technique of choice. There has been a generalized increase in the use and acceptance of combined regional and general anesthetic techniques because supplementing a general anesthetic with a nerve block results in a pain-free awakening and postoperative analgesia without the potentially deleterious side effects that may occur with the parenteral administration of opioids (see Chapter 29).[3] This benefit may be of particular importance to neonates, ex-premature infants, and children with cystic fibrosis and other conditions.[4] There is also evidence to suggest that regional anesthesia may improve pulmonary function in some patients who have undergone thoracic or upper abdominal surgery.[5–7] Lastly, the greatly increased number of "same day surgery" cases in recent years has made the advantages of regional anesthesia, especially the rapid awakening, enhanced postoperative analgesia with no sedation or altered sensorium, and lack of opioid-induced nausea or vomiting, even more apparent. The safe and effective use of these techniques in children, however, requires an understanding of both the developmental anatomy of the region to be blocked and the developmental pharmacology of local anesthetics.

Pharmacology and Pharmacokinetics of Local Anesthetics

Clinically useful local anesthetics are represented by two classes of compounds, the amino-amides (amides) and the amino-esters (esters) (Table 28–1). The amides undergo enzymatic degradation in the liver, whereas the esters are hydrolyzed primarily in the plasma by plasma cholinesterases.[8,9] These metabolic pathways are important because they account for some of the differences in distribution and metabolism of local anesthetics in pediatric patients, particularly in neonates, as compared with adults.

Amides

Amide local anesthetics commonly used in pediatric anesthesia practice include lidocaine, bupivacaine, and a newer agent, ropivacaine. The choice of agent is mostly dependent on the desired speed of onset and duration of action of the block, but in small infants and children issues of potential toxicity also play an important role. Compared with an adult's, the neonatal liver has limited enzymatic activity to metabolize and biotransform drugs (see Chapter 8). The ability to oxidize and to reduce drugs, in particular, is diminished.[10–22] Despite differences in the oxidative activity of the neonatal liver, the rates of plasma decay of single doses of both lidocaine and bupivacaine are similar in adults and neonates, although there are conflicting data. Neonatal metabolism of mepivacaine is virtually nonexistent, with most of the drug being excreted unchanged in the urine.[23,24] Conjugation reactions are severely limited at birth and do not reach adult levels until approximately 3 months of age.[13–16,20]

Table 28–1. Commonly Used Local Anesthetics

Esters	Amides
Procaine	Lidocaine
Tetracaine	Mepivacaine
2-Chloroprocaine	Bupivacaine
	Etidocaine
	Prilocaine

Older children also differ from adults with respect to the pharmacokinetics of local anesthetics. Children achieve peak plasma concentrations of amide local anesthetics more rapidly than adults after intercostal nerve blocks but at similar times after caudal epidural blocks.[25–27] After caudal epidural administration of lidocaine and bupivacaine, peak plasma levels are achieved at about 30 minutes in both children and adults.[25–27] Ilioinguinal nerve blocks in children under 15 kg may produce blood levels of bupivacaine in the toxic range if more than 1.25 mg/kg are administered.[28] The steady-state volume of distribution (Vd_{ss}) for amides is increased in children compared with adults; clearances (Cl), however, are similar.[27, 29, 30] Since the elimination half-life ($t_{1/2}$) is related to the volume of distribution and clearance as follows:

$$t_{1/2} = (0.693 \times Vd_{ss})/Cl,$$

the result of a larger steady-state volume of distribution is a prolongation of the elimination half-life. This prolongation of the half-life is probably of little clinical importance for single-dose administration but may have profound consequences for continuous administration; that is, the drug may accumulate over several days, resulting in toxicity. The risk of drug accumulation with repeated doses as well as continuous infusions appears to be significantly increased in infants and children.[31, 32]

Bupivacaine

Bupivacaine is the commonly used agent for regional blockade in pediatric patients. It has an analgesic duration of action in the epidural space of about 4 to 6 hours, although the duration appears to be somewhat shorter in small infants. The concentration used for regional anesthetic techniques depends on the site of injection, the desired density of blockade, consideration of the toxic threshold of the drug, and the concomitant administration of other local anesthetics, such as local infiltration by the surgeon or intravenous administration of lidocaine. The most commonly used concentration for peripheral nerve blocks is 0.25%, with lower concentrations of 0.1 to 0.125% used for continuous epidural administration. The 0.5% concentration is less commonly used in children, although it may be employed at times for peripheral nerve blocks in cases in which subsequent doses and drug accumulation are not of concern.

Bupivacaine is bound to plasma proteins, particularly to α-1-acid glycoprotein. It is a racemic mixture of the levo- and dextro-enantiomers; the levo isoform is the bioactive one with regard to clinical effect, but the dextro isoform contributes more to toxicity. Levobupivacaine has been introduced into clinical practice. Its major advantage over the racemic preparation is the potential to reduce cardiac and central nervous system toxicity. Levobupivacaine retains similar efficacy and duration of blockade as the racemic formulation; retention of efficacy has been demonstrated in both an ovine model and in human adult volunteers.[33, 34] The use of this agent, when available, could reduce many of the risks of toxicity currently associated with bupivacaine.

A new experimental preparation of bupivacaine has the potential to offer dramatically prolonged analgesia with a low potential for toxicity. This formulation consists of bioerodable encapsulated bupivacaine-dexamethasone microspheres that can be administered for peripheral neural blockade.[35] The release of local anesthetic occurs over several days, producing very prolonged analgesia.[36] The addition of dexamethasone to the microspheres prolonged the effect of the blockade up to 13-fold, and plasma bupivacaine levels were far below the limits of toxicity.[37] No adverse local reactions were noted. If this formulation becomes available for the clinician, it may be particularly useful for patients who cannot tolerate a catheter technique but still require prolonged neural blockade for analgesia. Potential applications are intercostal blockade for patients with rib fractures and postoperative analgesia for ambulatory surgery, and for patients in whom an indwelling epidural catheter poses an excessive infection risk.[38]

Ropivacaine

Ropivacaine is a new amide local anesthetic. Like levobupivacaine, it is a levo-enantiomer and has a higher threshold for cardiac and neurologic toxicity than bupivacaine.[39] The lethal dose in 50% of animals (LD_{50}) appears to be higher than bupivacaine. Rats of different maturity were found to have a threefold higher tolerance to equipotent doses of ropivacaine than to bupivacaine when administered for a femoral nerve block.[40] Ropivacaine is also reputed to have a lesser degree of motor blockade for equianalgesic potency, but there are conflicting data in this regard. Some studies have found that there is a greater sparing of motor function, whereas others have found no difference in motor and sensory blockade. Ropivacaine has been reported to produce denser blockade of the A delta and C fibers than bupivacaine when low concentrations are used, lending mechanistic credence to the idea of differential blockade.[41] Much of the infant animal data, however, do not support the existence of a greater sensory-motor differential block than that following bupivacaine. The few clinical studies in infants and children available at this time also do not report a detectable motor-sensory differential.[40, 42] Several clinical studies in infants and children report a longer duration of analgesia with ropivacaine, despite the use of a lower potency solution.[42–44] Although there are still only limited data available in pediatric patients, the decreased potential for toxicity makes ropivacaine an attractive agent for use in infants and children. Most reports in the literature have used a 0.2% solution (2 mg/mL). The volume of drug injected was similar to that of bupivacaine and depended on the type of block and size of the child.

Esters

The pharmacokinetics of the ester local anesthetics are also affected by the quantitative and qualitative difference in plasma proteins. Plasma pseudocholinesterase activity in infants is decreased compared with adults[45]; thus, the plasma half-life of the ester local anesthetics may be prolonged. Despite a longer half-life in infants, 2,3-chloroprocaine has been suggested as a particularly useful agent for neonatal regional blockade for techniques such as epidural blockade.[46, 47] Limited data suggest that 2,3-chloroprocaine may be safe in this setting and that undue accumulation may not occur with use over the time period of several days using a 1.5% concentration.

Another enzymatic system with decreased activity in neonates is methemoglobin reductase, which is responsible for maintaining hemoglobin in a reduced valence state, capable of binding and transporting oxygen. Hepatic metabolism of prilocaine results in the production of o-toluidine, which can induce the production of methemoglobinemia, rendering red blood cells incapable of carrying oxygen.[48] The decreased activity of methemoglobin reductase and the increased susceptibility of fetal hemoglobin to oxidization make prilocaine an unsuitable local anesthetic for use in neonates. Although prilocaine is no longer in general use in the United States as an injected local anesthetic, it is one of the components of EMLA (eutectic mixture of local anesthetics) cream, a commonly employed transdermal local anesthetic. The total dose and surface area for EMLA application is therefore limited in neonates, since methemoglobinemia has been reported in this age group.[49] Other local anesthetics, particularly topical agents such as benzocaine, are potentially dangerous in infants because of the risk of methemoglobinemia by this same mechanism.[50] EMLA cream should be applied only to normal intact skin in appropriate doses[51] (< 10 kg body weight, apply to a maximum of approximately 100 cm² surface area [SA]; 10–20 kg, apply to a maximum of approximately 600 cm² SA; > 20 kg, apply to a maximum of approximately 2000 cm² SA). The duration of action is 1 to 2 hours after the cream is removed. Adverse reactions include skin blanching, erythema, itching, rash, and methemoglobinemia. It is contraindicated in children less than 1 month of age, in patients with congenital or idiopathic methemoglobinemia, and in infants receiving methemoglobinemia-inducing drugs, such as phenytoin, phenobarbital, acetaminophen, and sulfonamides.

Toxicity of Local Anesthetics

With the exception of uncommon effects such as the production of methemoglobinemia, the major toxic effects of local anesthetics are on the cardiovascular and central nervous systems (CNS). Local anesthetics readily cross the blood-brain barrier to cause alterations in CNS function. A consistent sequence of symptoms can be observed as plasma local anesthetic concentrations progressively increase, although this may not be readily apparent in infants and small children. Because of the lower threshold for cardiac toxicity with bupivacaine, cardiac toxicity and neurotoxicity may occur virtually simultaneously in pediatric patients, or cardiac toxicity may even precede neurotoxicity. During the intraoperative use of bupivacaine, the risk of cardiac toxicity may be increased by the concomitant use of volatile anesthetics, and the CNS effects of the general anesthetic may obscure any signs of neurotoxicity until devastating cardiovascular effects are apparent.[52]

In adults, the earliest symptom reported is circumoral paresthesia, which is due to the high tissue concentrations of local anesthetic rather than CNS effects. The development of circumoral paresthesias is followed by the prodromal CNS symptoms of lightheadedness and dizziness, which progress to both visual and auditory disturbances such as difficulty in focusing and tinnitus. Objective signs of CNS toxicity during this time are shivering, slurred speech, and muscle twitching. As plasma levels of local anesthetic continue to rise, CNS excitation occurs, resulting in generalized seizures. With additional increases in plasma local anesthetic levels, CNS depression occurs; respiratory depression leads to respiratory arrest. In adults, cardiovascular toxicity usually follows CNS toxicity; the systemic blood pressure is decreased because of peripheral vasodilation and direct myocardial depression, and progressive bradycardia ensues. These combined effects ultimately produce cardiac arrest. Bupivacaine in high doses may also produce ventricular dysrhythmias, including ventricular tachycardia, and ST segment changes suggestive of myocardial ischemia, especially when epinephrine-containing solutions are used. Bupivacaine appears to have particular affinity for the fast sodium channels and perhaps also for the calcium and the slow potassium channels in the myocardium, explaining why it is frequently so difficult to resuscitate patients after the administration of a toxic dose of that drug.[53–55]

With an intravascular injection of bupivacaine with epinephrine, characteristic electrocardiographic changes can be seen without any observable symptoms of CNS toxicity. Figure 28–1 shows an electrocardiogram tracing obtained

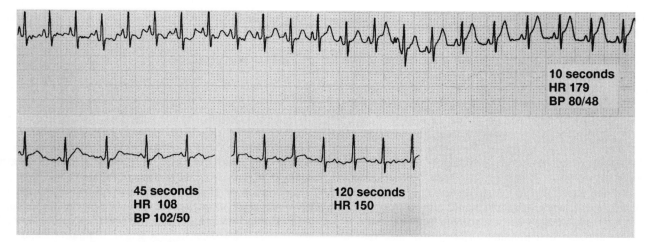

Figure 28–1. Electrocardiographic changes associated with the intravenous injection of bupivacaine and epinephrine 1:200,000. Note the marked increase in the height of the T wave. (From Freid EB, Bailey AG, Valley RD. Electrocardiographic and hemodynamic changes associated with unintentional intravascular injection of bupivacaine with epinephrine in children. Anesthesiology 1993;79:394–398.

during an intravenous injection of bupivacaine with and without epinephrine. Even a small intravenous dose of 1 to 2 μg/kg of epinephrine in a 1:200,000 solution with 0.25% bupivacaine will produce elevation of the T waves on the electrocardiogram, particularly in the lateral chest leads.[56–58] As opposed to the serious risk of ischemia and dysrhythmias with larger unintended doses of bupivacaine with epinephrine, the use of small test doses produces only brief transient changes in the electrocardiogram and may therefore be useful in the detection of an intravascular catheter or needle placement. These data suggest that careful observation of the electrocardiogram during test dose administration may be a sensitive indicator of unintended intravascular injection of bupivacaine in the child anesthetized with halothane (see Technique of Administration). The V5 lead appears to be the most sensitive in detecting these changes. The electrocardiographic changes seen with the epinephrine-containing test dose appear to be the result of the combination of the two drugs and not what would occur with either drug alone.

Plasma protein binding is the most important pharmacologic factor in determining the toxicity of local anesthetics, particularly for the amides, since it is the free (unbound) fraction of the drug that produces toxicity. Lower plasma protein concentrations cause more drug to remain in the unbound active form with greater potential for toxicity (see Chapter 8). Concentrations of both albumin and α-1-acid glycoprotein are lower in neonates, producing clinically crucial differences in the pharmacokinetics of amide local anesthetics between neonates, older children, and adults.[59] The significantly higher levels of free lidocaine and bupivacaine that result in infants are due primarily to the decreased level of α-1-acid glycoprotein, which is the primary binding protein of these drugs.[31, 60–63] Current data suggest that the plasma level of free drug may be expected to be approximately 30% higher in infants under 6 months of age, and possibly higher in premature infants. α-1-Acid glycoprotein is an acute phase reactant; the levels of this protein have been shown to rise following surgery. Levels were lower in infants undergoing elective surgery than in those having emergency operations.[64] It is not known whether these increased α-1-acid glycoprotein levels are sufficient to afford any protective effect on the risk of toxicity from bupivacaine accumulation in the perioperative period.

In addition to the differences in free drug levels, there may be differences in the susceptibility of the neonate to the toxic effects. Plasma levels of lidocaine that produce cardiovascular and respiratory depression are about half of those causing toxicity in adults.[65] In contrast, one study found that 2-day-old guinea pigs were less susceptible to the toxic effects of bupivacaine than those 2 weeks or 2 months of age, even though the blood levels achieved in those animals were higher.[52] Similar data were reported in infant versus adolescent versus adult rats for both bupivacaine and ropivacaine.[40] Young dogs, however, are reported to have a decreased threshold to both seizure and cardiac toxicity caused by excessive doses of bupivacaine.[66] Since species differences are known to be important, it is difficult to predict which study is more representative of the human neonate.[67] No data exist in humans regarding age-dependent differences in the toxic threshold of bupivacaine at a given blood level. Seizures and cardiovascular collapse have been reported in human infants at normal adult bupivacaine levels.

Although data from some animal studies suggest that the greater volume of distribution of amides in younger patients may afford some degree of protection against bupivacaine toxicity, retrospective analyses of large databases of infants who have received epidural infusions indicate that these findings may not be applicable to the human infant, particularly during continuous infusions or with repeated dosing. Current data on the pharmacokinetic and pharmacodynamic differences associated with early infancy suggest that caution should be exercised in the use of local anesthetics in infants. Several reports in the literature document that infants and children may develop signs of systemic toxicity, including dysrhythmias, seizures, and cardiovascular compromise from accumulation of epidural infusions of bupivacaine.[31, 68–71] Meticulous attention must be paid to total dose, rate of administration, site of injection, and the use of vasoconstrictors to diminish the rate of uptake. This is particularly important when a continuous regional anesthetic technique is to be utilized in the postoperative period, or during a long operative procedure when repeated doses of local anesthetic are administered.

We recommend that both the bolus and infusion doses of bupivacaine and lidocaine be reduced by 30% for infants under 6 months of age to decrease the risk for toxicity. This would result in a maximal hourly rate of not more than 0.25 mg/kg of bupivacaine.[32] These recommendations are particularly applicable to the use of continuous bupivacaine infusions for postoperative analgesia, but the same caveats must be borne in mind for large single injections, repeated injections, and continuous infusions of local anesthetics during long surgical procedures.

The d-stereoisomer of local anesthetics may also be a primary factor in the risk for both cardiac and central nervous system toxicity.[55] Both ropivacaine and levobupivacaine are levo enantiomers and have been demonstrated in adults and experimental animals to have decreased toxicity compared with bupivacaine, a racemic mixture.[72] This may be at least partly due to the reduced affinity of cardiac and central nervous system tissues for the l-enantiomer.[39] The introduction of levobupivacaine and ropivacaine into the clinical armamentarium may prove beneficial in decreasing toxicity.

Prevention of Toxicity

There are few data correlating anesthetic block, blood level, and dose for pediatric patients; most dosage guidelines have been derived from data extrapolated from studies of adults. Table 28–2 lists the maximum recommended doses of local anesthetics as well as their approximate durations of action. To avoid overdose and the possibility of toxic effects, it is important to remain within these guidelines until further pediatric studies have clarified the pharmacokinetics and pharmacodynamics of different local anesthetic agents with specific nerve blocks. As discussed earlier, all of these doses, particularly amides, should be reduced by 30% in infants under 6 months of age.

Toxic reactions from the administration of local anesthetics are a function of (1) the total dose administered, (2) the site of administration, (3) the rate of uptake, (4) pharmacologic alterations in toxic threshold, (5) the technique of administration, (6) the rate of degradation, metabolism, and

Table 28–2. Maximum Recommended Doses and Approximate Duration of Action of Commonly Used Local Anesthetics

Local Anesthetic	Maximum Dose (mg/kg)*	Duration of Action (min)†
Procaine	10	60–90
2-Chloroprocaine	20	30–60
Tetracaine	1.5	180–600
Lidocaine	7	90–200
Mepivacaine	7	120–240
Bupivacaine	3	180–600
Ropivacaine	2	180–600

*These are maximum doses of local anesthetics. Doses of amides should be decreased by 30% in infants less than 6 months of age. When lidocaine is being administered intravascularly (e.g., during intravenous regional anesthesia), the dose should be decreased to 3 to 5 mg/kg; there is no need to administer long-acting local anesthetic agents for intravenous regional anesthesia, and such a practice is potentially dangerous.
†Duration of action is dependent on concentration, total dose, site of administration, and the patient's age.

excretion of local anesthetic, and (7) the acid-base status of a patient.[73–78]

Total Drug Dose

The dose of local anesthetic should be determined according to a patient's age, physical status, and weight according to lean body mass, and the area to be anesthetized. A severely ill child who is in congestive heart failure, for example, has decreased metabolism of amide local anesthetics as a result of reduced cardiac output and hepatic blood flow. Similarly, a markedly obese child must not be given a higher dose simply on the basis of increased weight. If a large volume of local anesthetic is required for a particular procedure, a lower concentration should be used to avoid exceeding maximal safe dosage recommendations. Dosages are calculated based on the body weight of the child; for instance, a 20 kg child could receive up to 50 mg of bupivacaine. An easy approximation is 1 mL/kg of 0.25% bupivacaine, reduced by approximately one third for children less than 6 months of age.

Site of Injection

Injection of local anesthetics in highly vascular areas results in higher blood levels than the same dose injected into a less vascular area. The highest plasma concentrations of local anesthetics are achieved in adults with the following blocks (in order of highest to lowest): (1) intercostal nerve blocks, (2) caudal blocks, (3) epidural blocks, and (4) brachial plexus and femoral-sciatic nerve blocks.[79] An easy way to remember this is the mnemonic **ICE B**lock: **I** = intercostal, **C** = caudal, **E** = epidural, **B**lock = peripheral nerve blocks. Careful pediatric studies are required to determine whether this holds true for children. Very high levels, about twice those achieved in larger children, have been reported in children weighing less than 15 kg after ilioinguinal nerve block for herniorrhaphy using only 1.25 mg/kg of 0.5% bupivacaine without epinephrine, which is half the usual recommended maximal dose.[28] However, the fascia iliaca block in older children produced levels of bupivacaine well within the acceptable safe range.[80] Local infiltration of the

wound in herniorrhaphy has not been associated with elevated levels,[81] but scalp infiltration during neurosurgery may produce relatively high levels if higher concentrations of local anesthetic are used.[82] As would be expected, spinal anesthesia results in very low blood levels, even in newborns.[63]

Rate of Uptake

The rate of uptake of a local anesthetic is dependent on the vascularity of the site of injection; increased perfusion results in increased uptake, whereas decreased perfusion results in decreased uptake.[83] The rate of uptake in pediatric patients is usually more rapid than in adults; in general, the use of a vasoconstrictor reduces the rate of uptake and prolongs the duration of blockade. In adults, the dose of epinephrine is usually limited when used in conjunction with potent inhalation agents because of the risk of inducing cardiac arrhythmias. When using halothane, 1.0 to 1.5 μg/kg of epinephrine is the maximal recommended dose in adults; however, higher doses of epinephrine may be safe in children.[84–86] We have used as much as 10 μg/kg of epinephrine in pediatric patients, with a maximal dose of 250 μg, during halothane anesthesia without evidence of ventricular irritability. An epinephrine concentration of 1:100,000 should not be exceeded, and 1:200,000 or less is generally used. A quick reference for converting local anesthetic concentrations and the amount of epinephrine in various dilutions is presented in Tables 28–3 and 28–4. Epinephrine is contraindicated in blocks in which vasoconstriction of an end-artery could lead to tissue necrosis, such as for digital and penile blocks.

Alteration in Toxic Threshold

The pharmacologic alteration of CNS toxic threshold through the use of CNS depressants, such as diazepam or midazolam, can be a valuable adjunct to regional anesthesia. Virtually all of the benzodiazepines increase the seizure threshold. Premedication with diazepam (0.15–0.3 mg/kg) may not only decrease a patient's anxiety but also offers some degree of protection from toxic CNS effects of local anesthetic overdose.[87] Although diazepam is no longer in common clinical use in children in the perioperative period, evidence in animal models and considerable clinical experience suggest that midazolam is also effective in terminating seizure activity.[88] Animal data, however, suggest that the concomitant use of diazepam and bupivacaine decreases the elimination of bupivacaine from serum and cardiac tissue in mice.[89] This effect does not appear to be due to changes in protein binding.[90] It is not known whether this is true for all benzodiazepines or whether this is also the case in humans. One must keep in mind, however, that although premedica-

Table 28–3. Epinephrine Dilution and Conversion to μg/mL

Epinephrine Dilution	μg/mL
1:100,000	10
1:200,000	5
1:400,000	2.5
1:800,000	1.25

Table 28–4. Local Anesthetic Concentration and its Conversion to mg/mL

Concentration (%)	mg/mL
3.0	30
2.5	25
2.0	20
1.0	10
0.5	5
0.25	2.5
0.125	1.25

tion with a benzodiazepine prevents manifestations of CNS toxicity, the threshold for cardiovascular toxicity is unchanged.[91] Thus, after premedication with a benzodiazepine, cardiovascular collapse may occur without any warning, since the symptoms of CNS toxicity may be blunted.

Technique of Administration

A needle or catheter must always be aspirated before a local anesthetic is injected to determine the absence of vascular access. The inability to aspirate blood is not, however, an absolute indication that the needle or catheter is not in a blood vessel. This is especially true in small vessels such as the epidural venous plexus, where negative pressure in the vessel lumen from aspiration of the catheter may impede flow by pulling the vessel walls toward the catheter or needle orifice. For this reason, a test dose with a marker for intravascular injection such as epinephrine in a concentration of 1:200,000, is employed whenever possible. Data from awake adults indicate that this will result in an increase in heart rate within 1 minute of intravascular administration.[92] When the drugs are administered during a general anesthetic procedure, however, the efficacy of the test dose in detecting intravascular injection may be greatly reduced. Only 73% of children had increased heart rate after an intravenous injection of 0.5 μg/kg of epinephrine during halothane anesthesia, indicating that this marker for intravascular injection is not completely reliable.[93] Administration of atropine several minutes prior to the injection of the test dose increased the rate of positive responders to 92%, suggesting that vagal tone and the anesthetic's blunting of the sympathetic reflexes are responsible for the lower sensitivity of the test dose. Test doses during isoflurane anesthesia appear to have the same limitations.[94] With sevoflurane, positive results were obtained in all patients if the threshold for a positive response was set at an increase of 10 beats per minute (bpm) for heart rate and a dose of greater than 0.5 μg/kg of epinephrine was used; positive results were obtained in 85% of the children receiving 0.25 μg/kg of epinephrine.[95] In all patients, a change in the T wave amplitude was an effective indicator of intravascular injection with both doses of epinephrine. Patients in all groups were pretreated with atropine. It is not known whether increasing the dose of epinephrine to 1.0 μg/kg or increasing the concentration of epinephrine in the test dose solution to 1:100,000 during general anesthesia would increase the sensitivity of the heart rate response test without atropine. These investigators found, however, that the systolic blood pressure increased by more than 10%

within 60 seconds of the injection, suggesting that blood pressure elevation may be a more sensitive indicator of intravascular injection than heart rate changes during inhalation anesthesia. ST segment and T wave changes appear to be a sensitive indicator of intravascular injection of local anesthetic. Careful observation of the electrocardiogram, particularly the V5 lead, is highly sensitive in detecting an intravascular injection of bupivacaine with epinephrine; electrocardiographic alterations were found in 97% of infants and children receiving an intravenous dose of bupivacaine and epinephrine.[57] These investigators did not confirm the efficacy of pretreatment with atropine on heart rate response. Isoproterenol, 0.075 to 0.1 μg/kg, has been reported to increase heart rate in 90 to 100% of children receiving general anesthesia with halothane[96, 97]; isoproterenol also increases the heart rate in adults during isoflurane and sevoflurane anesthesia, but this agent has not been extensively studied.[98–100] Until more data are available, it would appear most prudent to utilize an epinephrine-containing test dose prior to the administration of the therapeutic dose of local anesthetic for neural blockade.[95] The test dose should be repeated prior to any subsequent bolus injections through a catheter, such as may occur during a long surgical procedure. If the child is receiving a general inhalation anesthetic, both blood pressure and the ST segment configuration, particularly in lead V5 if available, in addition to the heart rate, should be carefully and frequently monitored after injection of the test dose. Pretreatment with atropine may increase the rate of detection of unintended intravascular injection. In addition, the rate of injection may also be a factor in the development of toxicity. If injection is partially or completely intravascular, slow injection may not exceed the toxic threshold, whereas rapid injection might. Repeated injections within a brief period may also result in toxic reactions. Thus, slow incremental injection of the therapeutic blocking dose of local anesthetic (over several minutes) may further increase the safety of regional blockade.

Treatment of Toxic Reactions

Treatment of toxic reactions to local anesthetic overdose requires knowledge of the signs and symptoms previously described. Toxicity from high concentrations of bupivacaine, especially cardiac toxicity, is particularly difficult to treat, and it must be recognized that the signs of local anesthetic toxicity, with the exception of the catastrophic cardiovascular events, are all masked by general anesthesia. Indeed, inhaled anesthetics may actually raise the threshold for seizures and thereby delay the detection of toxicity until cardiovascular collapse occurs. Even in the nonanesthetized child, the progression from prodromal signs to frank cardiovascular collapse may be very rapid, and the initial definitive therapy in some cases may need to be directed at re-establishing circulation and normal cardiac rhythm. As always, initial management should consist of establishing and maintaining a patent airway and providing supplemental oxygen. The timely administration of a CNS depressant that alters the seizure threshold may prevent seizures. The agents midazolam (0.05–0.2 mg/kg IV), thiopental (2–3 mg/kg IV), and propofol (1–3 mg/kg) are efficacious in preventing or terminating seizure activity. If seizure activity is present, the use of succinylcholine by itself may facilitate orotracheal intubation but does not block CNS seizure activity. It should be remembered, however, that the acute morbidity from seizure activity is largely due to airway complications (hypoxia and aspiration) and that securing the airway takes precedence over the actual control of the electrical activity of the seizure. CNS excitability is exacerbated in the presence of hypercarbia; it is therefore important to mildly hyperventilate patients having seizures.

Because the initial stage of cardiovascular toxicity consists of peripheral vasodilation, treatment should consist of intravenous fluid loading (10–20 mL/kg of lactated Ringer's or 0.9% saline) and, if necessary, titration of a peripheral vasoconstrictor such as phenylephrine (initial rate of 0.1 μg/kg/min) to maintain vascular tone and systemic blood pressure at acceptable limits. As toxicity progresses to cardiovascular collapse, profound decreases in myocardial contractility occur, followed by dysrhythmias. In dogs, echocardiography showed that decreased systolic function always preceded the development of dysrhythmias. An investigation in rats demonstrated considerably increased efficacy when norepinephrine was used to treat bupivacaine cardiac toxicity compared with epinephrine, dopamine, isoproterenol, or amrinone.[101] In the event of bupivacaine toxicity refractory to norepinephrine, bretylium has been reported to be useful in restoring normal cardiac rhythm and perfusion.[102, 103] A report in infants found that phenytoin (5 mg/kg slow intravenous infusion) was particularly effective, even when all other agents, including bretylium, had failed.[104] Many toxic reactions are self-limited because the local anesthetic agents redistribute throughout the body and plasma levels rapidly decrease. Excretion of local anesthetic agents is hastened by hydration and alkalization of the urine by intravenous administration of sodium bicarbonate.[105, 106] Successful resuscitation of bupivacaine-induced cardiac toxicity has been carried out by placing the patient on cardiopulmonary bypass.[107]

Hypersensitivity to Local Anesthetics

Hypersensitivity reactions to local anesthetics are rare. Ester local anesthetics are metabolized to para-aminobenzoic acid, which is usually responsible for allergic reactions in this group. However, these agents may cause allergic phenomena in patients who are sensitive to sulfonamides, sulfites, or thiazide diuretics.[108, 109] Among the amide local anesthetics, only one case of a true allergic reaction has been documented; however, these agents sometimes contain methylparaben as a preservative, which may produce allergic reactions in patients sensitive to para-aminobenzoic acid.[109, 110] When in doubt, however, local anesthetic allergy must be ruled out. Detailed protocols are described elsewhere.[111–114]

Specific Procedures

Central Neuraxial Blockade

Anatomic and Physiologic Considerations

Several anatomic and physiologic differences between adults and children affect the performance of regional anesthetic techniques. The conus medullaris (the spinal cord's terminus) in neonates and infants is located at the L3 vertebra, which

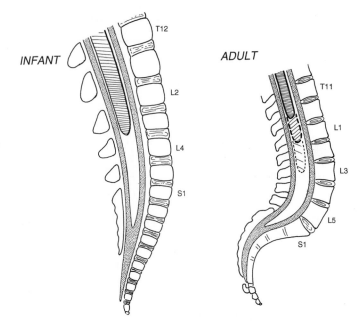

Figure 28–2. Anatomic differences between adults and children that affect the performance of spinal and epidural anesthesia; an infant's sacrum (left) is flatter and narrower than an adult's (right). Note that the tip of the spinal cord in a neonate ends at L3 and does not achieve the normal adult position (L1–2) until approximately 1 year of age.

is more caudal than in adults, and it does not reach its adult position at L1 until approximately 1 year of age (Fig. 28–2) because of the difference in the rates of growth between the spinal cord and the bony vertebral column. Thus, lumbar puncture for subarachnoid block in neonates and infants should be performed at the L4-5 or L5-S1 interspace to avoid needle injury to the spinal cord. The vertebral laminae are poorly calcified at this age, so a midline approach is preferable to a paramedian one in which the needle is "walked off" the laminae. Another anatomic difference is noted in the sacrum. In neonates, the sacrum is narrower and flatter than in adults (see Fig. 28–2). The approach to the subarachnoid space from the caudal canal is much more direct in neonates than in adults, making dural puncture more likely.[115] It should be noted that the presence of a sacral dimple may be associated with spina bifida occulta, which would make dural puncture highly probable. Thus a caudal block may not be indicated in these patients.

The distance from the skin to the subarachnoid space is very short in neonates (approximately 1.4 cm) and progressively increases with age (Fig. 28–3).[116] The ligamentum flavum is much thinner and less dense in infants and children, which makes the engagement of the epidural needle more difficult to detect, and unintended dural puncture during epidural catheter placement may be a greater risk for the infrequent operator. Cerebrospinal fluid (CSF) volume as a percentage of body weight is greater in infants and young children than in adults (Fig. 28–4), although studies of this are limited.[117–121] This finding may account in large part for the comparatively higher doses of local anesthetics required to produce surgical anesthesia with subarachnoid block in infants and young children. The CSF turnover rate is also considerably higher, perhaps in part accounting for the much

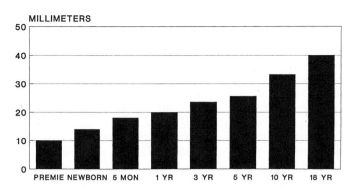

Figure 28–3. Distance from the skin to the subarachnoid space as a function of age. (Data from Bonadia et al: 1988; Kosaka et al: 1974; Lau: 1989.)

shorter duration of subarachnoid block with any given agent, as compared with adults. Obviously, these anatomic differences necessitate meticulous attention to detail to achieve successful and uncomplicated spinal or epidural anesthesia.

In contrast to older children and adults, subarachnoid block in infants and small children is characterized by remarkable hemodynamic stability, even when the level of the block reaches the high thoracic dermatomes.[122, 123] Although heart rate variability, as determined by spectral analysis, is less, the heart rate is preserved, as the parasympathetic activity modulating heart rate appears to be diminished in infants receiving spinal anesthesia.[124] This diminished vagal tone allows the heart rate to compensate for any alterations in peripheral vascular tone. This appears to be a greater factor in the preservation of hemodynamic stability than other contributing factors such as the relatively small venous capacitance in the lower extremities in infants and the relative lack of resting sympathetic peripheral vascular tone.[125]

Central neuraxial blockade can produce alterations in the respiratory mechanics of the chest wall and diaphragm by virtue of the diminution of intercostal muscle activity. This may be particularly relevant in infants and young children, whose chest walls are very compliant owing to limited ossification of the ribs.[126] Infants have a greater reliance on the diaphragm for the maintenance of tidal volume. One can easily observe the manifestations of diaphragmatic breathing

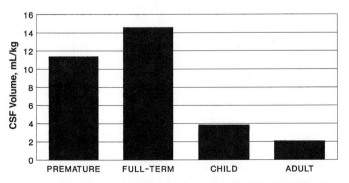

Figure 28–4. Approximate volume of cerebrospinal fluid (CSF) relative to weight and age. Note that premature and full-term infants have a much greater CSF volume relative to weight than a child or adult; this may account in part for the increased dose (mg/kg) of local anesthetic required in infants to produce a successful subarachnoid block. (Data from Lups et al: 1954; Cutler et al: 1968; Otila: 1948; Kruse: 1930; Samson: 1930.)

in the chest wall and abdomen of a sleeping infant; the abdomen rises and falls as the diaphragm descends and relaxes in an exaggerated fashion as compared with that of an older child. One may also observe some chest wall paradox—that is, inward displacement of the lower edge of the rib cage in infants during deep sleep even in the absence of airway obstruction. Studies of infants during sleep have demonstrated that during rapid eye movement (REM) and deep sleep, paradoxical chest wall motion occurs commonly, and increases as the force of diaphragmatic excursion increases.[127] In a similar fashion, suppression of intercostal muscle activity, leading to decreased rib cage contribution to ventilation, has also been measured during spontaneous breathing in infants undergoing halothane anesthesia.[128] One study used respiratory inductance plethysmography to study rib cage and diaphragmatic contributions to breathing in seven former premature infants who underwent spinal anesthesia for herniorrhaphy.[126] When high (T2–T4) levels of motor blockade were achieved, outward motion of the lower rib cage was decreased, and paradoxical motion of the lower rib cage was noted in over half of the infants. The diaphragmatic contribution to respiration, as estimated by abdominal displacement, was increased in all infants. This suggests a shift of respiratory workload from rib cage to diaphragm in compensation for the loss of the intercostal muscle's contribution to breathing. Other factors, such as the alteration of the conformation of the diaphragm relative to the chest wall, with concomitant changes in the size of the zone of apposition (the portion of the anterior diaphragm that lies against the lower rib cage) may also be a factor. These measurements were compared to each child's measurements in the control state, prior to the administration of the spinal anesthetic, but it is not known whether these findings are different than would be measured in unanesthetized infants during deep sleep. It is likely that these effects are well tolerated, and that the ability of the diaphragm to compensate for loss of the rib cage's contribution to breathing is adequate in the vast majority of infants.

Upper abdominal and thoracic surgery induces changes in respiration in the postoperative period that have been attributed to neural inhibition of diaphragmatic function.[129–131] The afferent pathways causing this inhibition are presumed to arise in the chest and abdominal walls, and perhaps in the diaphragm itself, although they have not been conclusively identified.[132] Contrary to popular belief, pain itself is not a major contributor to postoperative respiratory dysfunction, as numerous studies have shown that opioids, administered either parenterally or in the central neuraxis, have little effect on postoperative respiratory function.[133–135] Regional blockade, on the other hand, has been shown to improve several measures of postoperative respiratory function.[7, 130, 136] These data suggest that regional anesthesia has an important role to play in the amelioration of postoperative diaphragmatic dysfunction. Although the mechanism for this improvement has been postulated to be blockade of the putative inhibitory neural pathways, data suggest that alterations in respiratory mechanics, in particular the increase of the diaphragm's resting length to approximate its control value, and the shift of the workload from rib cage to diaphragm, may play a greater role.[6] These data also suggest that the beneficial effects of regional anesthesia on postoperative respiratory function may be in part related to the degree of motor blockade. It is not known whether the preoperative administration of regional blockade results in enhanced respiratory function compared with postoperative application of the blockade, as has been postulated to occur with "preemptive analgesia."

Spinal Anesthesia

Spinal anesthesia has been successfully performed in children since the turn of the 20th century.[137–140] The observation of postanesthetic apnea in former premature infants has led to a resurgence in the use of spinal anesthesia in infants, particularly for herniorrhaphy.[141, 142] Spinal anesthesia has also been used for myelomeningocele repair.[143] Spinal anesthesia was administered by direct injection of tetracaine into the sac and supplemented when needed by direct application of tetracaine by the surgeon. There were no complications in this study. It has also been used with success for a variety of other surgical procedures performed on infants.[143–146] It has been recognized since the early 1980s that premature infants are at significant risk for developing apnea after undergoing general anesthesia.[147, 148] Although the apneic events are most likely to occur either upon emergence or soon after emergence, apnea may occur at any time in the 24-hour period after the anesthetic, thus mandating admission and overnight cardiorespiratory monitoring. Apneic events can range from self-limited but prolonged periodic breathing to full life-threatening apneic and bradycardic events, and occur in 15 to 30% of infants at risk. The reason for this postanesthetic apnea is not well understood. It is not known whether the exposure to an anesthetic or sedative hypnotic agent transiently disrupts the brainstem's control of breathing, whether the agents produce a temporary alteration in the infant's ventilatory response to hypercarbia and hypoxia, or whether minute residual concentrations of the anesthetic agents are at fault. Sedation as well as general anesthesia can produce the same response. Ketamine, when used to supplement spinal anesthesia, was found to increase the incidence of postoperative apnea even more than general anesthesia.[149] An analysis of a number of prospective studies of this problem concluded that the statistical risk for apnea in infants born at less than 32 weeks of gestational age would not fall to less than 1% until 56 weeks of post-conceptual age; for those born at 35 weeks of gestational age, the risk would not fall to less than 1% until 54 weeks of post-conceptual age.[150]

In addition to several retrospective reports, prospective analyses of infants undergoing spinal anesthesia compared with those undergoing general anesthesia have found that spinal anesthesia produced fewer or no episodes of postanesthetic apnea.[142,149] Although most of these studies were potentially confounded by the lack of preoperative and postoperative pneumograms to control for baseline apnea and bradycardia, a prospective investigation addressed that study design flaw and confirmed that neonates receiving subarachnoid block had no alteration in heart rate or oxygen saturation when preoperative and postoperative pneumograms were compared.[151] The infants in the general anesthesia group, however, had episodes of lower saturation and heart rate in the postoperative period, and these episodes were more severe than those seen preoperatively. These events were not consistently associated with central apnea, which

was defined as a cessation of respirations lasting more than 10 seconds with no demonstrable chest wall movement. Although these data suggest that the several case reports of apnea after subarachnoid block may have occurred even in the absence of the anesthesia and surgery, one cannot entirely discount that they may indeed have been caused by the anesthetic agent or, perhaps, the stress of surgery itself. Although the data from this study are persuasive, we are still cautious and do not alter the routine postoperative monitoring standards in these patients. Until studies with greater numbers can distinguish which criteria would define a group with low apnea risk, all former preterm infants of less than approximately 55 weeks of post-conceptual age should be treated the same, regardless of the anesthetic technique.[152–154] We believe, however, that the best data available at this time suggest that regional anesthesia is the preferable anesthetic technique in premature infants for whom it would provide adequate operating conditions. It should be noted that the use of epidural anesthesia has also been reported for lower extremity and abdominal surgery in former premature infants. Continuous spinal and epidural anesthesia for surgical procedures outlasting the duration of a "single shot" subarachnoid block have been reported.[154–160]

TECHNIQUE. After routine monitoring devices (electrocardiogram, blood pressure cuff, pulse oximeter, and precordial stethoscope) are affixed, the patient is placed in a sitting or lateral decubitus position. In neonates and infants, care must be taken not to flex the neck as is done in adults, because this position may obstruct the airway (Fig. 28–5A).[161, 162] The sitting position may aid in recognizing successful dural puncture by increasing CSF hydrostatic pressure and therefore increasing flow through the spinal needle. The skin is infiltrated with a minute quantity of 1% lidocaine (less than 0.25 mL should be sufficient; we use a 30-gauge needle on an insulin syringe), or a small amount of EMLA cream is applied to the infant's lumbar area at least 1 hour prior to arrival in the operating room. The lumbar puncture is performed using a midline approach with a 22-gauge 1.5-inch styletted spinal needle (Fig. 28–5B&C). We do not routinely use a 25-gauge spinal needle because the time from entrance into the subarachnoid space until appearance of CSF in the needle hub is unduly long; this delay may result in difficulty in recognizing that the subarachnoid space has been entered. Whitaker, Sprotte, and other "pencil point" needles are now becoming available in pediatric sizes, and we expect that they will come into more common use, much as they have in adult practice.[163, 164] Lumbar puncture is performed only at the L4-5 or L5-S1 interspaces for reasons previously described. The subarachnoid space in infants less than 60 weeks of post-conceptual age is approximately 1.5 cm from the skin (see Fig. 28–3); care must be taken not to pass the needle too deeply, passing beyond the subarachnoid space.[116] When the subarachnoid space is located, the local anesthetic is slowly administered and the patient immediately placed flat in the supine position. After subarachnoid administration of local anesthetic, the patient's legs must not be elevated above the level of the head, particularly when the electrocautery pad is applied, because this has resulted in "total" spinal anesthesia (Fig. 28–6A&B).[165] The grounding pad can be safely placed by lifting the entire infant, keeping the body in the horizontal plane, or the pad can be affixed to the

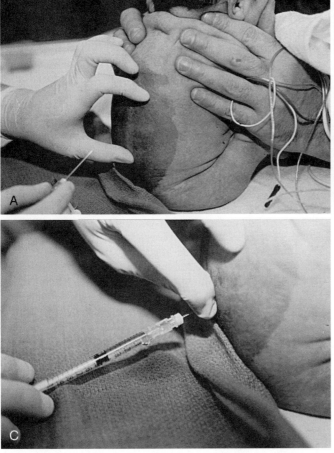

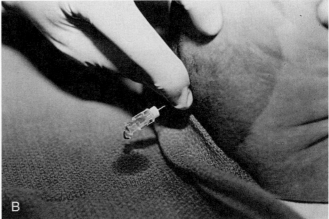

Figure 28–5. (A) Lumbar puncture in a neonate or infant is generally performed in the sitting position. Note that the head is maintained in the neutral position to prevent airway obstruction. (B) After local infiltration of 1% lidocaine with a 25- to 27-gauge needle, lumbar puncture is performed with a 22-gauge 1.5-inch styletted needle at the L4–5 or L5-S1 interspace. Entrance into the subarachnoid space is confirmed by free flow of cerebrospinal fluid. (C) Local anesthetic is injected with a tuberculin syringe. Care must be taken not to inject rapidly, or a high level of blockade might result.

anterior thigh if enough space and muscle mass is available there.

Because of the hemodynamic stability seen in infants with spinal anesthesia, some pediatric anesthesiologists have advocated that, in a patient who is not volume depleted, intravenous access may be established after the onset of lower extremity analgesia. Although this may be relatively safe in this setting, there is some potentially added safety in

the availability of intravenous access before the block is inserted, should a "total spinal" anesthesia develop and instrumentation of the airway become necessary. In addition, should intravenous access prove difficult, valuable operating time during a block of relatively short duration will have been lost while the anesthesiologist searches for a suitable vein. We have found that applying the pulse oximeter to a toe of one lower extremity and the blood pressure cuff to

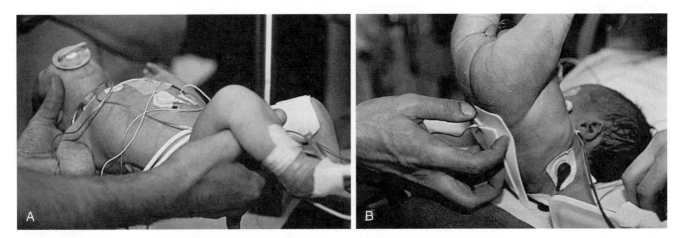

Figure 28–6. (A) The proper method of applying an electrocautery pad; the infant's entire body is elevated while maintaining the horizontal position to avoid excessively high spread of subarachnoid blockade. (B) Improper method of applying an electrocautery pad in a neonate after subarachnoid administration of local anesthetic; the legs should never be elevated.

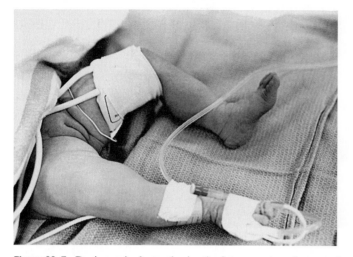

Figure 28–7. During spinal anesthesia, the intravenous catheter and oximeter probe are placed on one leg and the blood pressure cuff is applied to the other. The infant is thus allowed to remain undisturbed.

the thigh of the other leg allows a neonate to remain undisturbed during the surgical procedure, such as inguinal herniorrhaphy (Fig. 28–7).

Because the addition of sedating agents has been associated with postanesthetic apnea with an incidence at least as high as that of general anesthesia, we try to avoid any systemic sedating agents, especially ketamine.[149] Many, if not most, neonates will fall asleep once the block has set in, probably in large part because of the lack of afferent input through the infant's largest sensory organ, the skin. A pacifier dipped in 50% dextrose will also encourage the child to be quiet and still. Gentle restraint is necessary in some cases. It is particularly important for the child to be still and not bear down when the hernia sac is being dissected to avoid the extrusion of abdominal contents through the open hernia.

Selection of Drug

NEONATES AND INFANTS. The proportional dose of local anesthetic required for subarachnoid block in neonates is much higher than that required for adults. When calculated on a mg per kilogram basis, there is a nearly 10-fold increase in drug requirement to reach a similar dermatomal distribution. In addition, the relatively larger dose lasts only about one third to one half as long as in the adult. As discussed previously, this appears to be at least in part due to the greater volume of CSF per kilogram, and to the more rapid turnover of CSF in this age group. The drugs that have commonly been used for spinal anesthesia in neonates and infants include tetracaine, bupivacaine, and lidocaine.[117, 166–170] Reported doses of tetracaine range from 0.22 to 1.0 mg/kg, and most pediatric anesthesiologists currently use the higher dose to achieve adequate height and duration of blockade. We use hyperbaric tetracaine (0.75–1.0 mg/kg [equal volumes of tetracaine 1.0% and 10% dextrose]) with the addition of 0.01 mL/kg of epinephrine (1:100,000). Epinephrine has been shown to prolong the duration of block by more than 30%.[171] Our usual technique is to draw a 1:1000 epinephrine solution into a tuberculin or glass syringe

and expel the contents in the manner of heparinizing a blood-gas syringe. This leaves only a residual epinephrine "wash" in the hub of the needle. The tetracaine dose (and dextrose, if they are packaged separately) is then drawn into the syringe. This dose usually provides adequate analgesia for inguinal hernia repair with a duration of motor block of approximately 90 to 120 minutes and a dermatome height in the middle to upper thoracic region. For procedures on a lower extremity of limited duration we use lower doses (0.5–0.6 mg/kg). Both isobaric and hyperbaric bupivacaine have been used in neonates and infants, with a reported duration similar to that of tetracaine, although the isobaric solution lasts slightly longer than the hyperbaric solution.[169, 170, 172] Lidocaine at a dose of 2 mg/kg may be useful if a block of short duration is required, such as for incision and drainage of a perirectal abscess, but one can expect only about 30 minutes of useful blockade with this agent. Considering the recent concerns regarding lidocaine in the subarachnoid space, we no longer recommend this agent for use in infants.[173–175] A summary of doses for commonly used local anesthetics for subarachnoid block in neonates and infants is provided in Table 28–5.

CHILDREN. There is little information on the doses of local anesthetics for spinal anesthesia in children, and subarachnoid block is much less commonly used outside of the neonatal period. In most cases when a regional technique is desirable in these patients, it is more common to use epidural or caudal administration in conjunction with a "light" general anesthetic. One study described the use of 0.3 to 0.5 mg/kg of bupivacaine (5 mg/mL concentration) for children 2 months to 12 years of age.[164] Doses of 0.3 to 0.4 mg/kg of hyperbaric tetracaine have been used for subarachnoid block in patients aged 12 weeks to 2 years and 0.2 to 0.3 mg/kg in patients older than 2 years.[176–178] Based on more current data and practice, we would suspect that the doses in these studies for the younger infants were relatively low, *but it is apparent from these limited data that the dose requirement decreases with increasing age.* Because few data are available on drug doses and the height of anesthetic block produced in this age group, it is prudent to use these values as an appropriate reference point and to revise the dose as dictated by clinical experience.

COMPLICATIONS. Complications following spinal anesthesia include total spinal anesthesia, post–dural puncture headache, backache, neurologic sequelae, and the risk of lumbar epidermoid tumors if nonstyletted needles are used for subarachnoid puncture.[163–165, 179–185]

Total spinal anesthesia has been reported in neonates; it is manifested by apnea with no change in systemic blood

Table 28–5. Local Anesthetics for Spinal Anesthesia in Neonates and Infants

Anesthetic Drug	Dose (mg/kg)
1.0% Tetracaine in 5% dextrose	0.6–1.0
0.5% Bupivacaine (isobaric)	0.80–0.86[167]
0.75% Bupivacaine in 8.25% dextrose	0.6[168]
5.0% Lidocaine in 7.5% dextrose	1–3

pressure.[165] It can occur after a dose of as little as 0.6 mg/kg of tetracaine.[165] Alteration in patient position, particularly elevating the lower body above the level of the head or thorax, may be the most common predisposing factor in producing excessively high levels of blockade. Although the rate of administration has been reported not to alter the level of spinal anesthesia in adults, no such studies have been carried out in neonates or infants.[186] It is possible that factors such as the use of a relatively large bore needle (22-gauge) and a tuberculin syringe, providing the means for injecting with high pressure, along with the small distance between vertebrae, combine to make the rate of injection an important consideration in neonates and infants by producing unintended barbotage. We have also observed this complication with rapid drug administration. Management consists of assisted or controlled ventilation until the return of spontaneous respiratory function.

The incidence of post–dural puncture headache appears to be low in pediatric patients, although the incidence in preverbal children is, of course, unknown. An early study reported an incidence of spinal headache of approximately 2% when 20- to 22-gauge needles were used in patients 2 to 17 years of age.[178] However, no details were provided about the distribution of headache with respect to age. More recent studies have found an incidence of 5% in a group of 100 patients ranging from 2 months to nearly 10 years of age, but again, no age distribution is cited.[163, 164] A prospective study of pediatric oncology patients undergoing diagnostic or therapeutic lumbar puncture with a 20-gauge needle found that post–dural puncture headache was relatively rare in children less than 13 years of age compared with older children.[180] In most instances, the headaches were mild and resolved spontaneously. It is not entirely clear why young children should have a very low incidence of post–dural puncture headache. One author speculated that the lower CSF pressure in children protects them from prolonged CSF leakage through the puncture site and thus from post–dural puncture headache.[181] Alternatively, hormonal changes with age have been proposed as another explanation.[180] It is also possible that the increased rate of CSF production may be a factor. As more pediatric regional anesthesia equipment becomes readily available, we expect that the use of Whitaker or Sprotte needles will become more commonplace and reduce this low incidence even further.

Backache is a frequent postoperative complaint after both general and regional anesthesia in adults. It is thought to occur because of flattening of the normal lordotic lumbar curve secondary to muscle and ligament relaxation that occurs with spinal anesthesia. Its incidence in the pediatric population is unknown. Neurologic sequelae following spinal anesthesia are exceedingly rare. There are no reports in the literature of permanent neurologic injury due to subarachnoid block, but good data in children are lacking. There have been no cases detected in over 1000 consecutive spinal anesthetic procedures at the University of Vermont Medical Center (C. Abajian, personal communication).

Epidural Anesthesia

Epidural anesthesia administered by the caudal, lumbar, or thoracic route can be used for the same types of surgical procedures and indications as spinal anesthesia. Our most common indication, however, is for augmentation of general anesthesia and for postoperative pain management.

CAUDAL EPIDURAL ANESTHESIA. Caudal epidural anesthesia is the regional technique that is used with the greatest frequency in children, although this may decline as familiarity with lumbar and thoracic epidural techniques grows. Although its use was first described in 1933,[187] it was not until the early 1960s that caudal anesthesia gained any degree of popularity.[188–203] Improvements in catheter material and the availability of small diameter needles and catheters have resulted in increased interest in this technique for use in pediatric patients.

Technique. The patient is placed either in the lateral decubitus position or prone with a small roll beneath the anterior iliac crests. The cornuae of the sacral hiatus are most easily palpated as two bony ridges, about 0.5 to 1 cm apart, when the examiner moves his or her finger in a medial to lateral direction (Fig. 28–8A). It may prove easier to locate the space by palpating the L4-5 intervertebral space in the midline, and then palpating in a caudal direction until the sacral hiatus is reached. Since the space between the sacrum and coccyx may be mistaken for the sacral hiatus, the latter technique may make identification of the landmarks easier. The proper location is often, but not always, just at the beginning of the crease of the buttocks. A short bevel styletted needle, 22-gauge, should be used, as a long bevel needle may increase the risk of intravascular injection.[204] Some practitioners believe that a styletted needle avoids the possibility of introducing a dermal plug into the caudal space. Others suggest the use of a 22-gauge intravenous catheter, inserted with the bevel facing downward, because once it is in place, easy advancement of the intravenous catheter off the needle strongly suggests that the caudal canal has been entered and may reduce the risk of intravascular placement. The needle is initially directed cephalad at a 45- to 75-degree angle to the skin until it "pops" through the sacrococcygeal ligament (Fig. 28–8B) into the caudal canal, which is contiguous with the epidural space. If bone is encountered before the sacrococcygeal ligament, the needle should be withdrawn several millimeters, the angle with the skin decreased to approximately 30 degrees, and then the needle again advanced in a cephalad direction until the sacrococcygeal ligament is pierced (Fig. 28–8C). As the needle is advanced slightly further, bone (the anterior table of the sacrum) is encountered, and the needle should be leveled in orientation prior to further advancement, so that it is nearly parallel to the plane of the patient's back. Once the caudal-epidural space has been entered, the needle is advanced several millimeters. Further advancement with a needle should not be attempted, since in infants the dural sac lies relatively low, and it is possible to easily enter the subarachnoid space by this route.[115, 205] Negative aspiration for both blood and CSF is confirmed, and a test dose of local anesthetic is administered. If no cardiovascular or electrocardiographic changes are seen after the test dose, the remainder of the dose of local anesthetic for a single shot caudal administration is slowly injected in an incremental fashion over several minutes. We strongly recommend the use of a test dose, even with "single shot" caudal procedures. Although it is likely that the risk of intravascular

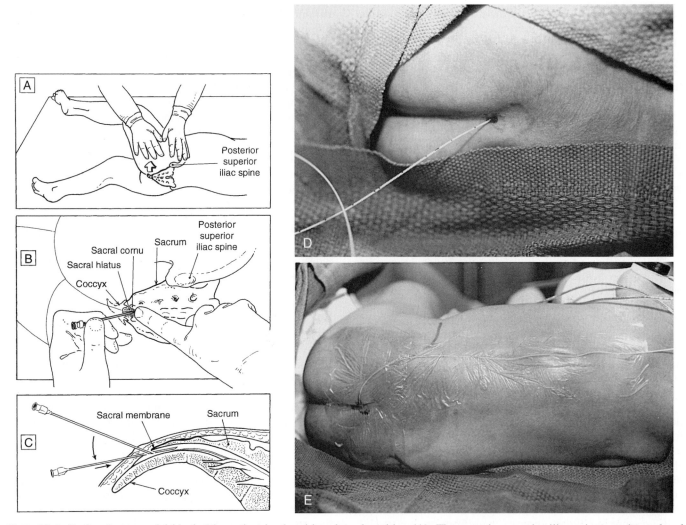

Figure 28–8. Performing a caudal block. The patient is placed in a lateral position (A). The posterior superior iliac spines are located and the sacral cornu palpated; an intravenous needle, an intravenous catheter, or a Crawford needle of appropriate size is advanced at an angle of approximately 45 degrees until a distinct "pop" is felt as the needle pierces the sacrococcygeal ligament (B). The angle of the needle with the skin is reduced parallel to the sacrum, and the needle or intravenous catheter is advanced into the caudal canal (C). If a continuous technique is used, the caudal catheter is advanced to the mid-level of the surgical incision (it usually readily passes in children less than 5 years of age), and the introducing needle or catheter is withdrawn (D). The catheter is secured with benzoin and an occlusive dressing (E).

injection may be lower with caudal blockade, it is more likely that the needle could be misplaced in the intramedullary cavity of the sacrum. Intraosseous injection of drugs into the bone marrow results in very rapid uptake, similar to direct intravenous injection. We are aware of at least one case of cardiovascular collapse that occurred from this complication when a test dose was not employed. The block may be placed prior to the onset of surgery without a significant decrement in duration of postoperative analgesia for short surgical procedures.[206] This has the advantage of reducing the amount of general anesthesia needed, resulting in a more rapid recovery. In addition, there is adequate time for the block to "set up," improving the chances of a pain-free awakening.

Catheter insertion for a continuous technique follows a similar procedure. First, one should determine the length to insert the catheter by measuring from the sacral hiatus to the desired site where the catheter tip will be positioned. Instead of a small-gauge needle or catheter, a 16- to 18-gauge

intravenous catheter[207] or an 18-gauge Crawford needle is used to enter the epidural space. Alternatively, a 20-gauge intravenous catheter or a 20-gauge Crawford needle may be used in smaller patients with a 24-gauge epidural catheter (Fig. 28–8D&E). Once the epidural space has been entered, the intravenous catheter and needle are advanced several millimeters. The catheter is then advanced off the needle for a distance of approximately 1 to 2 cm. Localization of the intravenous catheter tip in the epidural space is confirmed by lack of resistance to the injection of saline. During the injection, the area of the back overlying the intravenous catheter tip is palpated; crepitance on injection indicates subcutaneous rather than epidural placement of the catheter. Once the intravenous catheter is properly placed, the epidural catheter may then be advanced through the intravenous catheter, and the intravenous catheter is withdrawn. After confirming that no blood or CSF is withdrawn with aspiration, a test dose of local anesthetic containing 1:200,000 epinephrine is administered (see earlier). Test doses should be repeated each time a catheter is reinjected with a bolus dose of local anesthetic.

In patients younger than 5 years, the catheter can usually be advanced to any level desired without exiting a dural sleeve or becoming tangled or knotted.[158] For infants weighing less than 5 kg, successful catheter advancement may be less reliable, and an injection of 0.25 mL of a nonionic contrast agent, which is known to not be neurotoxic, may be needed to confirm proper placement of the catheter tip if the catheter is not radiopaque.[208] We usually advance the catheter tip to a level near or at the midpoint of the dermatomes encompassing the surgical incision. This position allows a more specific site of administration for both intraoperative anesthesia and continuous infusions for postoperative pain management, with the attendant advantage of being able to use a lower dose of medication. If the catheter does not pass easily to the desired level, it should be withdrawn several millimeters and left in place at a lower level. Because caudal catheters are at increased risk of contamination from fecal soiling in children who are not yet continent of stool, meticulous attention to the dressing is necessary. Our practice is to use Mastisol (Ferndale Labs, Ferndale, MI) or tincture of benzoin, and to secure the catheter with several layers of an adherent clear dressing such as Tegaderm (3M Health Care, St. Paul, MN) or OpSite (Smith & Nephew Richards, Memphis, TN). One must pay particular attention to affixing the dressing in the crease of the buttocks. A piece of single adhesive edged plastic drape (Steri-Drape 1010, 3M Health Care, St. Paul, MN) is affixed just caudad to the lower edge of the dressing in a similar manner, and prevents direct soiling of the dressing. If there is any question of contamination, the catheter should be promptly removed.

It is frequently preferable to place epidural catheters at a lumbar or thoracic interspace. Advantages include exclusion of the insertion site from the diaper area, with less risk of contamination by stool and urine; closer proximity to the desired tip location; lower volume of drug required for a higher dermatomal level (if the caudal catheter is not threaded cephalad). Experience has shown that both lumbar and thoracic epidural catheters may be safely placed in anesthetized infants and children by experienced anesthesiologists.[209] Although there are theoretically increased risks of neural injury in an unconscious patient, all of the longitudinal studies published to date have not shown this to be the case in practice, and have confirmed the safety of these techniques when performed by experienced and trained pediatric anesthesiologists. Indeed, many of the arguments against regional anesthesia in the unconscious patient are of speculative validity, especially when one considers as the alternative a moving and uncooperative child.[209]

The technique for both lumbar and thoracic epidural catheter placement is similar to that in adults, with certain important exceptions. The midline approach is most commonly used, for the same reasons cited above regarding subarachnoid block. The ligamentum flavum is considerably thinner and less dense in infants than in older children and adults. This makes recognition of engagement in the ligament more difficult and requires both extra care and slower, more deliberate passage of the needle to avoid subarachnoid puncture. It takes experience to perceive the more subtle differences in "feel" that are characteristic of the tissue

planes in small children. The angle of approach to the epidural space is slightly more perpendicular to the plane of the back than in older children and adults, owing to the orientation of the spinous processes in infants and small children. The loss of resistance technique should be used, but only with saline, not air. There are several reports of venous air embolism in infants and children when air was used to test for loss of resistance.[210-212] We use a short (5 cm) 18-gauge Tuohy needle and a 20- or 21-gauge catheter in infants and children. We have found that these catheters have fewer problems than the 24-gauge variety, and the needle is still of a small enough caliber to be used even in small infants. The shorter length offers much better control than an adult-length (10 cm) needle. Several manufacturers make epidural kits specifically for pediatric patients. Another method for identifying the epidural space is to attach an intravenous infusion chamber with a mini-drip to the epidural needle; commencement of dripping identifies entry into the epidural space.[213, 214]

Selection of Drug. The amount of drug needed to provide blockade to a given dermatomal level is primarily dependent on volume, not concentration, and the capacity of the epidural space may change with age. Numerous studies discuss doses of local anesthetic drugs used for caudal anesthesia in pediatric patients.[188, 190-192, 194, 195, 197-203] The volumes of local anesthetic that would be used in a 10 kg child to produce blocks with approximately a T4 to a T10 dermatome level span a fivefold range. In our experience, the formula of Takasaki et al.[195] has best approximated good clinical results:

Volume (mL) = 0.05 mL/kg/dermatome to be blocked

Thus, in a 10 kg child in whom we wish to produce a T10 dermatome level, we would use a volume of (0.05 mL/kg/dermatome) × (10 kg) × (12 dermatomes) = 6 mL.

Because the block level is dependent on drug volume, the concentration of local anesthetic must be chosen not only based on the desired density of the block (less dense for postoperative analgesia, more dense for intraoperative anesthesia), but also based on the considerations for potential toxicity described earlier. Another simple method is to administer 1 mL/kg (up to 20 mL) of 0.125% bupivacaine with 1:200,000 epinephrine; this generally provides a sensory block with minimal motor block up to the T4-T6 level.

Continuous Infusions. Although intermittent doses of local anesthetic are often used to maintain epidural anesthesia during a long surgical procedure, it is also common practice to use continuous infusions of local anesthetics in place of intermittent injections during surgery. Continuous infusions permit the block to be maintained at a constant level, assuming that the proper rate is chosen, and eliminate the need for repetitive test dosing. Fewer entries into the catheter may reduce the risk of infection and the risk of accidental injection of the wrong drug into the epidural catheter. Just as with intermittent injections and as with the postoperative use of local anesthetic infusions, strict attention must be paid to drug concentration and infusion rate so as to avoid the administration of potentially toxic doses of drug. We recommend that the same dosing guidelines for postoperative infusion rates be followed intraoperatively: *a maximum of 0.4* *mg/kg/h of bupivacaine following the initial establishment of the block, with this dose reduced by 30% for infants under 6 months of age.*[32] The concentration of local anesthetic solution that can be used will depend on the extent of the surgical procedure and the area that needs to be blocked, the age of the patient, and variation of surgical stimulus. When a more dense block is desired in a small infant, it may be beneficial to use 2,3-chloroprocaine, since it undergoes ester hydrolysis and has a much lower risk of accumulation than does bupivacaine; a denser block with a more concentrated solution may then be achieved. The advent of newer amides with lower toxic potential, such as ropivacaine and levobupivacaine, may also successfully address these issues, and allow the administration of more concentrated agents to produce denser blockade with less potential for adverse effects.

EPIDURAL OPIOIDS. Epidural opiates can be safely used to augment intraoperative anesthesia in pediatric patients, as well as to provide postoperative analgesia. Their use is discussed in detail in Chapter 29. If the patient is expected to be extubated at the end of the surgical procedure, one must take into account both the systemic and the central neuraxial opioid dose to avoid excessive respiratory depression.

Complications. Complications following epidural anesthesia or analgesia include intravascular or intraosseous injection, hematoma, neural injury, and infection. Figure 28–9 illustrates sites of unintended needle placement during the performance of a caudal epidural block. Injection of local anesthetic into an epidural blood vessel or intraosseous injection into the marrow cavity may result in a rapid rise in blood levels and a toxic reaction. Signs, symptoms, and treatment were discussed previously. It is also possible to pass the needle completely through the sacrum and instill local anesthetic into the pelvis, particularly in infants in whom ossification of the sacrum is not complete.

Infection is of grave concern when it occurs in either the subarachnoid or the epidural space.[215] A study of 1620 pediatric patients over a 6-year period found a zero incidence of epidural abscess.[216] Catheters were left in a mean of 2 days and as long as 8 days. The adult literature also suggests that infection is an uncommon complication.[217, 218] There are, however, several case reports and retrospective studies suggesting that both superficial and deep abscesses may rarely

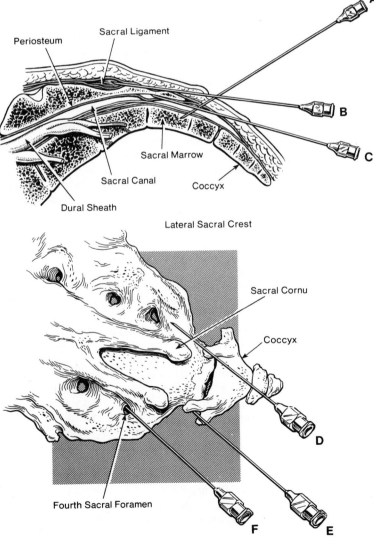

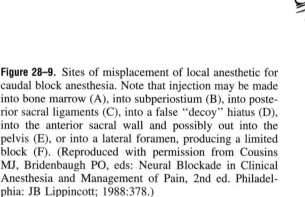

Figure 28–9. Sites of misplacement of local anesthetic for caudal block anesthesia. Note that injection may be made into bone marrow (A), into subperiostium (B), into posterior sacral ligaments (C), into a false "decoy" hiatus (D), into the anterior sacral wall and possibly out into the pelvis (E), or into a lateral foramen, producing a limited block (F). (Reproduced with permission from Cousins MJ, Bridenbaugh PO, eds: Neural Blockade in Clinical Anesthesia and Management of Pain, 2nd ed. Philadelphia: JB Lippincott; 1988:378.)

occur, particularly in patients with immunodeficiency syndromes and cancer on long-term infusions.[219] Epidural abscess, the most potentially serious complication, and meningitis have also been reported in adults.[215, 220] Of particular note is the report of infections that developed at the catheter insertion site that became apparent only days after the removal of the catheter. Whether these infections developed while the catheter was in place, or because the bacteria tracked through the open site in the skin after the catheter was removed and less care was paid to the site is unknown. In infants and toddlers who are in diapers, one must be particularly vigilant and meticulous in the management of these catheters and of their insertion site. A mild erythema occasionally occurs at the site of catheter insertion when patients have indwelling catheters in place for several days, and this must be distinguished from a cellulitis; if there is any doubt, the catheter should be removed. A prospective study of 210 children with 170 caudal catheters (age 3 ± 1 years) and 40 lumbar epidural catheters (age 11 ± 3 years) found no serious systemic infection.[221] Catheters were left in place for 3 ± 1 days; 35% were found to have bacterial colonization. This rate of colonization was similar with both approaches (caudal 25% vs. lumbar epidural 23%). It is also common for there to be leakage of edema fluid from the insertion site, especially in the child who has developed presacral edema in the perioperative period. In a child who has an indwelling epidural for postoperative pain management, we consider a fever of unknown origin a cause for removal of the catheter (see Chapter 29). The development of an epidural abscess is obviously a surgical emergency and can lead to compromise of neural function. The signs and symptoms (Table 28–6) are the same as for epidural hematoma, but fever, elevated erythrocyte sedimentation rate, and elevated leukocyte count with a leftward shift are also often present. Surgical drainage may be necessary.

Epidural hematoma is also a rare complication following epidural blockade. Optimal outcome depends on rapid diagnosis and prompt treatment and decompression. Signs and symptoms are presented in Table 28–6. The presence of clinically important coagulopathy or thrombocytopenia presents an unacceptable risk for hematoma and is a contraindication to central neuraxial blockade.

Urinary retention in the postoperative period has been anecdotally associated with both epidural and spinal anesthesia. In this regard, it is important to distinguish between local anesthetics and central neuraxial opioids. There are no data to support the contention that regional anesthesia with local anesthetics causes urinary retention, and indeed, there are data to the contrary. One prospective study examined 82 infants and children who underwent inguinal herniorrhaphy or orchidopexy. Patients were randomized to receive either caudal blockade or ilioinguinal-iliohypogastric nerve block by the surgeon, or to a control group receiving caudal injection of 1:200,000 epinephrine (no local anesthetic).[222] There were no differences in the mean time to void between the groups. A retrospective study analyzed the postoperative courses of 326 children undergoing inguinal herniorrhaphy and urologic surgery, 237 of whom had received caudal blockade and 66 of whom had received local anesthesia by the surgeon; the incidence of urinary retention was no different. The type of surgery was the primary influence on urinary retention.[223]

The epidural and subarachnoid use of opioids, however, is associated with an increased incidence of urinary retention. One paper reported an incidence of 50% in their series using epidural morphine at a dose of 70 μg/kg, a dose that would now be considered relatively high.[224] Of those that had urinary retention, 70% required treatment. Another study reported an incidence of 27%, but most of the patients had urinary catheters, precluding statistical analysis between different doses of caudal morphine that ranged from 33 to 100 μg/kg.[225] Another study reported an incidence of 11% of 150 patients, using a dose of 50 μg/kg of diamorphine.[226]

Data suggest that it is possible that the incidence of *neuronal injury* after epidural blockade may be higher than previously appreciated. A prospective study of more than 2500 infants and children failed to show any neurologic complications of significance, but another retrospective analysis found that 1 in 5000 infants under 3 months of age had neurologic complications with magnetic resonance imaging evidence of spinal cord ischemia.[70, 227] An in vivo study in young rabbits, using colored microspheres to assess spinal cord and organ blood flow, found that a fall in blood pressure, when accompanied by epidural anesthesia with lidocaine, resulted in a decrease in spinal cord blood flow.[228] The addition of epinephrine to the local anesthetic solution did not appear to result in an increased incidence of ischemia. These studies suggest that it may be particularly important to maintain adequate systemic blood flow during "combined technique" anesthesia in infants and children, and to treat hypotension promptly. Since blood pressure changes are uncommon in infants and children, hypotension is likely to be due to other causes, and should prompt an assessment of intravascular filling pressures, inotropic state, and the depth of general anesthesia.

Peripheral Nerve Blocks

Peripheral nerve blocks are useful adjuvants to general anesthesia. These blocks are also useful as a means for providing postoperative pain relief. Peripheral nerve blocks differ from central neuraxial blocks in several respects:

1. Generally only a targeted area is anesthetized.
2. There may be minimal side effects such as weakness of extremities.
3. A lower amount of local anesthetic is used.
4. There is no risk of an unintended spinal anesthetic.

Table 28–6. Signs and Symptoms of Epidural Hematoma and Abscess

Abscess	Hematoma
Fever	Afebrile
Localized back pain	Localized back pain
Radicular pain	Radicular pain
Paraplegia	Paraplegia
Sensory loss	Sensory loss
Urinary and fecal retention	Urinary and fecal retention
Incontinence	Incontinence
Local tenderness	Local tenderness
Defect on myelography	Defect on myelography
Localized lesion on magnetic resonance imaging	Localized lesion on magnetic resonance imaging

5. There is no potential for urinary retention.
6. It can be used in areas where a central neuraxial block is not possible, such as the face and scalp.
7. There are many peripheral nerve blocks that can be used in the practice of pediatric anesthesia (Table 28–7).

Selecting a Local Anesthetic for Peripheral Nerve Blocks

Local anesthetics commonly used for peripheral blocks include lidocaine, mepivacaine, and bupivacaine. More recently, levobupivacaine and ropivacaine have been used for regional anesthetic blocks in children.[42, 44, 229] Longer acting agents have a greater role in peripheral blocks than shorter acting agents because of the increased duration of postoperative analgesia. Lidocaine can sometimes be combined with bupivacaine to provide both a rapid onset and a long duration of action. We usually use a mixture of lidocaine and bupivacaine, particularly if the patient is having the procedure performed with a local block under sedation. The addition of sodium bicarbonate (1 mEq/10 mL of local anesthetic) can enhance the speed of onset and reduce the pain of injection of the block by raising the pH of the solution.[230–233] This alters the pKa of the solution, thus making the local anesthetic solution more available in the active cationic form.[234] Bicarbonate is generally added just prior to drug administration, since epinephrine degradation may occur.[234] Care should also be taken not to exceed the recommended upper limit (mg/kg) dose of local anesthetic (see Table 28–2). The addition of epinephrine (1:200,000) may decrease vascular absorption and the potential for toxicity; for some local anesthetics, the addition of epinephrine will also extend the duration of the block. The exact dose of local anesthetic in terms of volume or concentration needed for most peripheral blocks in children has not been adequately studied. Most blocks performed in children are based on adult experience.

Table 28–7. Peripheral Nerve Blocks

Region	Block
Head and neck	Supraorbital and supratrochlear
	Infraorbital nerve
	Greater occipital nerve
	Great auricular nerve
Chest wall	Intercostal
Upper extremity	Brachial plexus
	Elbow (ulnar, radial, and median nerves)
	Wrist (ulnar, radial, and median nerves)
	Digital
Abdomen and genitals	Ilioinguinal nerve
	Penile
Lower extremity	Femoral nerve
	Lateral femoral cutaneous
	Fascia iliaca
	Sciatic nerve
	Classic approach
	Lateral approach popliteal fossa
	Ankle
	Digital

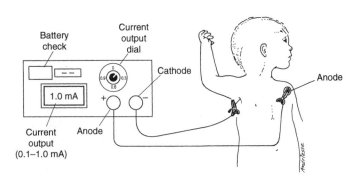

Figure 28–10. A nerve stimulator should be used to locate a nerve in a child who is anesthetized and in the awake, sedated child to avoid the need to seek a sensory paresthesia. In this example, the brachial plexus is sought in the axilla.

Use of a Nerve Stimulator

Since it is most common to perform peripheral nerve blocks in sedated or anesthetized infants and children, the use of a peripheral nerve stimulator is a safe and efficacious method for locating the nerve to be blocked. A nerve stimulator is not a substitute for anatomic knowledge but is a useful adjunct that allows the performance of the block in an unconscious or uncooperative, heavily sedated patient. It avoids the need to seek sensory paresthesias or to rely on anatomic landmarks alone, and it may diminish the potential for injury caused by needle impingement of a nerve. The tiny amount of current flowing from the uninsulated needle tip stimulates the nerve and produces a motor response when the needle is in close proximity to the nerve. The nerve stimulator is connected to a patient as shown in Figure 28–10. The cathode (negative pole) cable must be attached to the low output terminal of the nerve stimulator. The cathode is attached by means of a sterile alligator clip to the proximal (uninsulated) shaft of a Teflon-insulated needle or to the plug-in lead of a specially designed block needle, and the anode (positive lead) is connected to the patient by means of an electrocardiographic electrode, well distant from the block site.[235, 236] The needle is advanced in the appropriate anatomic direction, and when it is thought to be in the correct position, the nerve stimulator is turned on to generate approximately 0.5 mA of electric current with repetitive single pulse output at 1-second intervals. Local muscle contraction should be minimal at this setting, although direct muscle stimulation can occur and must be distinguished from neural stimulation. The area innervated by the nerves to be blocked is observed for the appropriate muscle contractions. As the uninsulated needle tip approaches the nerve, the muscle contractions will increase in intensity, and become less strong as it passes away from the nerve. One should be able to decrease the current to approximately 0.2 mA or less with continued elicitation of easily perceptible muscle contraction to be sure that the needle tip is correctly positioned. It should be noted that the injection of even a very small volume of local anesthetic will ablate or dramatically attenuate responses produced by the low current of the nerve stimulator, so the needle position should be optimized before injection. The responses to stimulation of the radial, median, ulnar, and musculocutaneous nerves are shown in Figure 28–11.

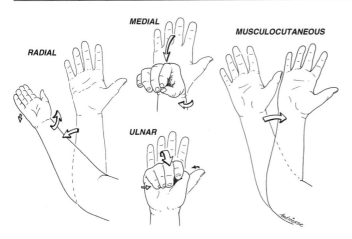

Figure 28-11. Characteristic movements of the fingers, wrist, and elbow in response to nerve stimulation. Note that the appropriate muscle response to nerve stimulation is elicited at 0.5 mA current and should continue to respond with 0.2 mA current. (Modified with permission from Cousins MJ, Bridenbaugh PO, eds: Neural Blockade in Clinical Anesthesia and Management of Pain, 2nd ed. Philadelphia: JB Lippincott; 1988:406.)

Head and Neck Blocks

Peripheral nerve blocks for postoperative pain relief for the head and neck can be performed with the patient under general anesthesia. These blocks can also be utilized for the provision of pain relief in patients with chronic painful problems such as headaches. Anatomically, two major nerves, the ophthalmic division (V1) of the trigeminal nerve

and the branches of the cervical root (C2) supply the sensory innervation of the face and scalp (Fig. 28-12).

SUPRAORBITAL AND SUPRATROCHLEAR NERVE BLOCK

Anatomy. These are the end branches of the ophthalmic division (V1) of the trigeminal nerve. The supraorbital nerve, the terminal branch of V1 exits the supraorbital foramen to supply the scalp anterior to the coronal suture (Fig. 28-13). The supratrochlear nerve leaves the orbit between the trochlea and the supraorbital foramen and innervates the lower part of the forehead (see Figs. 28-12, 28-13). We use this combined block to provide pain relief in patients undergoing frontal craniotomies and in patients undergoing frontal ventriculoperitoneal shunt revisions.

Technique. The patient is placed supine with the head in neutral position. The supraorbital notch is palpated by running a finger from the midline laterally along the eyebrow (the supraorbital notch is usually located in line with the pupil with the eye in the midline position). The skin is prepared with povidone iodine, with care taken to avoid spilling the solution into the eye. A 27-gauge needle is inserted into the supraorbital notch perpendicularly; 1 mL of bupivacaine (0.25% with epinephrine 1:200,000) is injected into the space after careful aspiration to prevent intravascular placement. To block the supratrochlear nerve, the needle is withdrawn to the skin level and then directed and advanced several millimeters medially toward the apex of the nose; 1 mL of bupivacaine (0.25% with epinephrine 1:200,000) is injected.

Complications. Because of the loose alveolar tissue of the eyelid, gentle pressure should be applied to the supraorbital

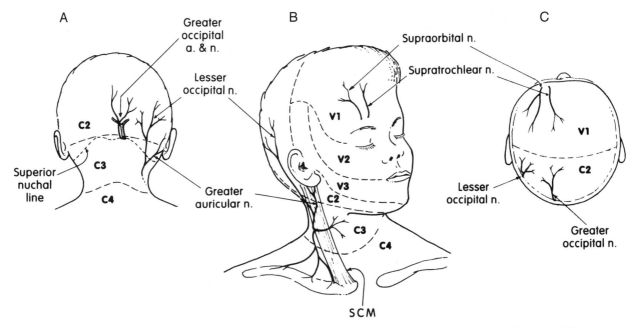

Figure 28-12. Dermatomal innervation of head and neck: sensory and dermatomal innervation of greater and lesser occipital nerves and the innervation of the anterior head by the first division of the trigeminal nerve. Note the sensory innervation anterior to the coronal suture is from the first division of the trigeminal nerve (supraorbital and supratrochlear nerves) and posterior to the coronal suture is from branches of C2 (greater and lesser occipital nerves). These nerves can be blocked individually and in combination to provide postoperative analgesia for a wide variety of procedures; see text for details. (A) Posterior view; (B) anterolateral view; (C) top view. (Modified with permission from Brown DL, Wong GY: Occipital nerve block. In: Waldman S, Winnie AP, eds: Interventional Pain Management. Philadelphia: WB Saunders; 1996:227.)

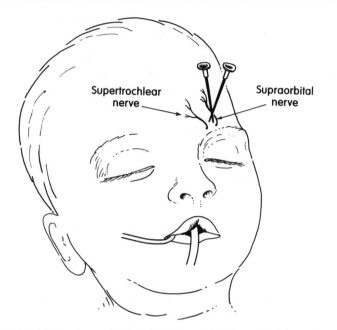

Figure 28–13. Supraorbital and supratrochlear nerve block: the supraorbital notch is palpated by running a finger from the midline laterally along the eyebrow. A 27-gauge needle is inserted into the supraorbital notch perpendicularly; 1 mL of bupivacaine (0.25% with epinephrine 1:200,000) is injected into the space after careful aspiration. To block the supratrochlear nerve, the needle is withdrawn to skin level and then directed medially several millimeters toward the apex of the nose. A dose of 1 mL of bupivacaine (0.25% with 1:200,000 epinephrine) is injected. This block provides postoperative pain relief for patients undergoing frontal craniotomies or frontal ventriculoperitoneal shunt insertion.

area; this prevents the dissection of the local anesthetic into the eyelid and supraorbital tissue and may reduce the potential for ecchymosis and hematoma.

GREATER OCCIPITAL NERVE BLOCK. The greater occipital nerve block is used to diagnose and treat occipital pain. If this technique is used for the diagnosis of occipital neuralgia, a careful history is taken and a physical examination is performed to rule out other pathologic causes of headaches, including posterior fossa tumors and Arnold-Chiari malformation. It can also be used for treating postoperative pain associated with surgery in the posterior fossa and in patients undergoing posterior ventriculoperitoneal shunt revisions.

Anatomy. The innervation of the posterior head and neck is from the cervical spinal nerves. The dorsal rami of C2 end in the greater occipital nerve, which provides the cutaneous innervation to the major portion of the posterior scalp (see Figs. 28–12, 28–14). The nerve becomes subcutaneous slightly inferior to the superior nuchal line by passing above the aponeurotic sling; here it is in close proximity and medial to the occipital artery (Fig. 28–14).

Technique. With the patient supine and with the head turned to one side or with the patient prone, the occipital artery is palpated at the level of the superior nuchal line. The occipital artery is usually located at approximately one third of the distance from the external occipital protuberance to the mastoid process on the superior nuchal line. A total volume of

2 mL of bupivacaine (0.25% with 1:200,000 epinephrine) is injected subcutaneously.

Complications. It is rare to see complications with this block because of the superficial location of the nerve. One has to bear in mind the close proximity to the spinal canal, particularly in patients who have had surgery in the area; thus the needle must remain just beneath the skin during injection of local anesthetic. Intravascular injection may be avoided with incremental injection with frequent withdrawal.

INFRAORBITAL NERVE BLOCK

Anatomy. The infraorbital nerve is the termination of the second division of the trigeminal nerve. The maxillary or second division of the trigeminal nerve is entirely sensory. It leaves the skull through the foramen rotundum and enters into the pterygopalatine fossa. It then enters the infraorbital groove and passes through the infraorbital canal. It is the terminal part of the maxillary nerve. The nerve emerges in front of the maxilla through the infraorbital foramen and then divides into four branches: the inferior palpebral, the external nasal, the internal nasal, and the superior labial. These branches innervate the lower eyelid, the lateral inferior portion of the nose and its vestibule, the upper lip, the mucosa along the upper lip, and the vermilion. This block can be effectively used for the provision of postoperative

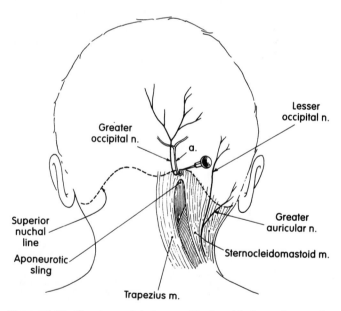

Figure 28–14. Greater occipital nerve block: with the patient supine and with the head turned to one side or with the patient prone, the occipital artery is palpated at the level of the superior nuchal line. The occipital artery is located about one third of the distance from the external occipital protuberance (broken line) to the mastoid process on the superior nuchal line. A total volume of 2 mL of bupivacaine (0.25% with 1:200,000 epinephrine) is injected subcutaneously to form a skin wheal. Frequent withdrawal and incremental injection may avoid intravascular injection. This block is used to diagnose occipital neuralgia as well as a means for providing postoperative pain relief for patients undergoing posterior fossa tumor resection or posterior ventriculoperitoneal shunt insertion. (Modified with permission from Brown DL, Wong GY: Occipital nerve block. In: Waldman S, Winnie AP, eds: Interventional Pain Management. Philadelphia: WB Saunders; 1996:228.)

analgesia to the upper lip and the vermilion after a cleft lip repair,[237, 238] reconstructive procedures on the nose including septal reconstruction and rhinoplasty,[239] and in patients undergoing endoscopic sinus surgery. There are two approaches to the infraorbital nerve: intraoral and extraoral.

Technique

Intraoral Approach. This is the technique we commonly use in our practice. The infraorbital foramen is located by palpation of the infraorbital notch. After folding back the upper lip, the practitioner inserts a 27-gauge needle through the buccal mucosa approximately parallel to the maxillary second molar and passed subcutaneously with the tip of the needle directed toward the infraorbital foramen. It is important to place a finger over the infraorbital foramen so as to palpate progress of the needle beneath the skin and prevent unintended passage of the needle into the orbit. With the tip of the needle at the level of the infraorbital foramen and after careful aspiration, 0.5 to 1.0 mL of local anesthetic is injected (Fig. 28–15). Use of bupivacaine (0.25% with epinephrine 1:200,000) provides prolonged postoperative analgesia.

Extraoral Approach. The infraorbital ridge of the maxillary bone should be identified and the infraorbital foramen

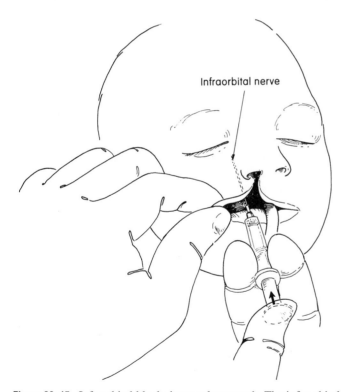

Infraorbital nerve

Figure 28–15. Infraorbital block: intraoral approach. The infraorbital foramen is located by palpation of the infraorbital notch. The lip is folded back and a 27-gauge needle is inserted through the buccal mucosa approximately parallel to the maxillary second molar. The tip of the needle is directed toward the infraorbital foramen. A finger is placed over the infraorbital foramen to avoid accidental placement of the needle into the orbit. After careful aspiration to avoid intravascular injection, 0.5 mL to 1 mL of bupivacaine (0.25% with 1:200,000 epinephrine) is injected. This block is used to provide postoperative pain relief for patients undergoing upper lip or cleft lip repair, reconstructive procedures of the nose (e.g., rhinoplasty), and endoscopic sinus surgery.

is palpated. A 27-gauge needle is advanced toward the foramen at a 45-degree angle to the maxilla. After careful aspiration, 0.5 to 1.0 mL of bupivacaine (0.25% with epinephrine 1:200,000) is injected.

Complications. Because of the loose adventitious tissue, patients can develop ecchymosis and swelling. Pressure applied to the infraorbital area ensures that the solution remains in the infraorbital foramen, prevents dissection of the local anesthetic into the periorbital area, and reduces the potential for the formation of a hematoma or ecchymosis. Care should be taken to avoid direct injection into the orbit or eye. Intravascular injection may be avoided with incremental injection with frequent withdrawal.

GREAT AURICULAR NERVE BLOCK. The great auricular nerve supplies the sensory innervation to the mastoid area and the external ear. It is a branch of the superficial cervical plexus. Cervical plexus blocks were first performed by Halstead in 1884.[240] This block has been used to provide postoperative analgesia in patients undergoing otoplasty repair[241] as well as in tympanomastoid surgery.[242] In our study we found that use of a great auricular nerve block decreases the incidence of nausea and vomiting, which is a major morbidity outcome associated with tympanomastoid surgery.[242] This block provides surface analgesia but not muscle relaxation and hence can be used despite the need for facial nerve monitoring in patients undergoing tympanomastoid procedures.

Anatomy. The cervical plexus is formed by the anterior primary division of the anterior and posterior roots of cervical nerves C2–C4. The great auricular nerve is derived from C3. It has been described by McKinney and the anatomic location of the nerve for blockade has been described as McKinney's point.[243] The great auricular nerve wraps around the belly of the sternocleidomastoid muscle at the level of the cricoid cartilage and emerges to supply the area of the mastoid and external ear (Fig. 28–16).

Technique. After induction of general anesthesia, the cricoid cartilage is identified. A line is drawn from the superior margin of the cricoid cartilage laterally to the posterior border of the sternocleidomastoid muscle (McKinney's point); 2 to 3 mL of bupivacaine (0.25% with epinephrine 1:200,000) is injected superficially at this point (Fig. 28–16).

Complications. Deep rather than superficial injection can result in a deep cervical plexus block and the potential for Horner's syndrome, phrenic nerve block, or unintended central neuraxial blockade. A small erythematous area may be seen at the site of injection. Intravascular injection may be avoided with incremental injection with frequent withdrawal.

Intercostal Nerve Block

Intercostal blocks following thoracotomy are useful in reducing opioid requirements, optimizing respiratory mechanics, and encouraging early ambulation.[244–246] Their major disadvantage is the limited duration of analgesia. Currently, we more commonly employ epidural blockade for this purpose. The development of degradable bupivacaine microspheres, which produce dramatically prolonged duration of analgesia, may change this in the future.[36, 37] There are, however, still

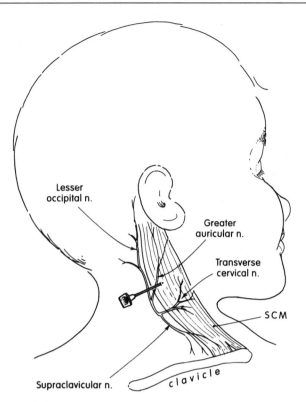

Figure 28–16. Great auricular nerve block: identify the cricoid cartilage. A line drawn from the superior border of the cricoid cartilage laterally to the posterior border of the sternocleidomastoid (McKinney's point) is identified. A dose of 2 to 3 mL of bupivacaine (0.25% with 1:200,000 epinephrine) is injected subcutaneously at this point. Gentle massage after the injection allows spread of the local anesthetic in the injected site. This block is used to provide postoperative analgesia for patients undergoing tympanomastoid surgery or otoplasty. (Modified with permission from Brown DL, ed: Atlas of Regional Anesthesia. Philadelphia: WB Saunders; 1999:185.)

situations in which intercostal blocks are useful, particularly in patients who cannot have a catheter placed.

Plasma concentrations of local anesthetics are higher after intercostal blocks than after any other regional technique, and plasma concentrations in children rise more rapidly than in adults.[25, 247] For this reason, epinephrine (1:200,000) is added to reduce the absorption of local anesthetic. We commonly use 0.25% bupivacaine with epinephrine in a dose of 1 to 5 mL for each nerve being blocked, depending on the size of the patient and the number of ribs to be blocked. A maximum of 2 mg/kg of bupivacaine is utilized, and this amount should be reduced for infants under 6 months of age. The concentration of bupivacaine may need to be decreased to avoid the risk of systemic toxicity while providing adequate volume for the desired number of intercostal blocks.

ANATOMY. The intercostal nerves are derived from the ventral rami of the first through twelfth thoracic nerves. There are four branches; the first is the gray rami communicans, which goes to the sympathetic ganglion; the second branch arises as the posterior cutaneous branch, which supplies the skin in the paravertebral area; the third branch, the lateral cutaneous branch, arises anterior to the midaxillary line and sends

subcutaneous branches both anteriorly and posteriorly; the final branch provides cutaneous innervation to the midline of the chest and abdomen. The dura mater and the arachnoid membrane fuse with the epineurium as they exit the vertebral foramen. This could lead to subarachnoid block if the posterior paravertebral approach is used.

TECHNIQUE. The site of injection may be either paravertebral or in the midaxillary line. The lower rib margin is located, and the skin is retracted cephalad (Fig. 28–17A); the needle is inserted perpendicular to the skin over the rib and advanced until the rib is encountered (Fig. 28–17B). The skin through which the needle is passed is allowed to retract caudally, and the needle is then walked off the edge of the rib a distance of 2 to 3 mm (Fig. 28–17C). This method may reduce the potential for pneumothorax, because the needle strikes the rib and is not advanced more than one half the thickness of the rib. A distinct "pop" may be felt as the needle enters the neurovascular sheath. After negative aspiration for blood, an appropriate volume of anesthetic is injected.

COMPLICATIONS. Pneumothorax has been reported with intercostal blocks; an analysis of 17,000 adult patients reported an incidence of pneumothorax of 0.082%.[248] The majority of blocks were performed by residents in training. Reabsorption of a small pneumothorax can be assisted with the use of oxygen. Placement of a chest tube is only indicated if there is respiratory embarrassment. Another complication that is far more common is the toxic effect from the absorbed local anesthetic drugs; as mentioned previously, an intercostal nerve block has a very high incidence of toxicity compared with other regional techniques.[79] Using smaller volumes of more dilute local anesthetic may reduce this undesired side effect. A third complication is high subarachnoid block, usually associated with the posterior paravertebral approach. Intravascular injection may be avoided with incremental injection with frequent withdrawal.

Inguinal Block (Ilioinguinal and Iliohypogastric Nerves)

Inguinal block, supplemented by wound infiltration, is sometimes used in adult patients for inguinal hernia repair. In the pediatric population, however, it is used almost exclusively for postoperative pain management and as an adjunct to general anesthesia. It is reported to be as effective as caudal anesthesia for inguinal operations.[249–253] Blockade of the ilioinguinal and iliohypogastric nerves is very successful for this purpose and has few associated complications, although injection into the femoral vessels is a possibility. The risks of toxicity from excessive drug dosage may be higher than previously recognized, as was discussed earlier. This block may be (and commonly is) performed in conjunction with infiltration of the wound.

ANATOMY. The inguinal area is innervated by the subcostal nerve (T12) and iliohypogastric and ilioinguinal nerves (derived from L1). These nerves lie in close proximity to each other medial and superior to the anterior superior iliac spine. After piercing the internal oblique aponeurosis approximately 2 to 3 cm medial to the anterior superior iliac spine,

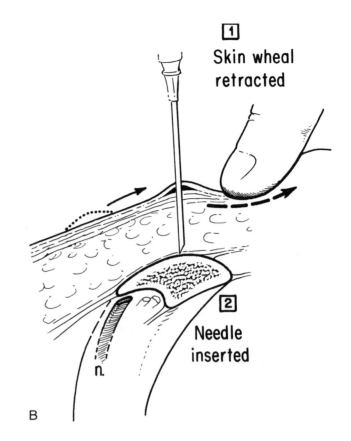

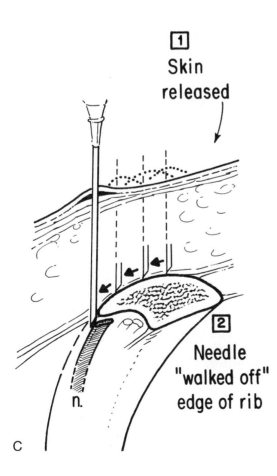

Figure 28–17. Intercostal block. A skin wheal is inserted on the lower rib margin (A). The skin wheal is retracted over the body of the rib, and a needle is inserted until contact is made with the rib (B). The skin is released, and the needle is carefully "walked" off the edge of the rib margin (C). After negative aspiration for blood, the appropriate volume of drug is injected. This block is used for postoperative analgesia for thoracotomy or chest tube insertion.

the nerve then travels between the internal oblique and the external oblique aponeurosis. Here it accompanies the spermatic cord to the genital area.

TECHNIQUE. The block may be performed either at the beginning of surgery or shortly before the end of general anesthesia. If bupivacaine is used, a minimum of 15 minutes is usually required from the completion of the block until maximal analgesia is obtained. Thus, blocks placed at the beginning of the surgical procedure (our preference) are usually more efficacious than those performed at the completion of the procedure. Blocks performed prior to incision may also have the advantage of providing "pre-emptive analgesia." This is one of the few blocks that has been proven to provide pre-emptive analgesia.[254] Duration of postoperative analgesia does not appear to be affected by placement of the block at the beginning of the procedure, assuming that the surgical procedure is not of more than 1.5 hours' duration. A short-bevel 27-gauge needle is inserted at a 45-degree angle at a point one-quarter of the way toward the midline along a line drawn from the anterior superior iliac spine to the umbilicus (approximately 1 to 1.5 cm cephalad and toward the midline from the anterior superior iliac spine in a 10 to 15 kg child). As the needle is advanced through the external and internal oblique muscles (Fig. 28–18), two "pops" are elicited and provide useful indications of proper needle placement. Negative aspiration should be confirmed several times during the incremental injection of anesthetic during this block. A volume of 0.3 mL/kg of local anesthetic is injected in a fan-like fashion, cephalad toward the umbilicus, caudad toward the groin, and medially. Before removal of the needle from the skin, an additional 0.5 to 1.0 mL of local anesthetic is injected subcutaneously to block the iliohypogastric nerve. Care must be taken to avoid entering the peritoneum. For inguinal herniorrhaphy, orchidopexy, or other inguinal procedures, local anesthetic poured directly onto the wound site before closure has also proved effective as an adjunct for postoperative analgesia.[255] The volume of drug used in this manner, like the volume of drug used for wound infiltration, must be accounted for when one calculates the maximal dose of local anesthetic that can be used for the block.

COMPLICATIONS. Complications are rare. Care should be taken not to enter the peritoneal cavity. Intravascular injection may be avoided with incremental injection with frequent withdrawal.

Penile Block

A penile block is used for anesthesia and postoperative analgesia for circumcision, urethral dilatation, and hypospadias repair. Caudal anesthesia is superior for proximal shaft or penoscrotal hypospadias repair because a penile block provides analgesia only for the distal two thirds of the penis.[199, 256–259] The block is easily performed and has a high success rate. Bupivacaine, levobupivacaine, and ropivacaine are the most useful agents because of their long duration of action. *Epinephrine must never be used because the dorsal artery of the penis is an end artery and vasospasm caused by epinephrine could cause necrosis.*

ANATOMY. The nerve supply of the penis is from the pudendal nerve and the pelvic plexus. Along the dorsal artery to the penis are two dorsal nerves that separate at the level of the symphysis pubis; these supply the sensory innervation to the penis.

TECHNIQUE. There are two commonly used techniques for penile block: (1) a ring block and (2) blockade of the dorsal nerve. One investigation compared the efficacy of these techniques and concluded that the ring block provided better results, and both techniques provided superior analgesia to EMLA cream.[260] The ring block is performed by inserting a 27-gauge needle at the base of the penis and, after negative aspiration, injecting the local anesthetic without epinephrine in a ring-shaped pattern around the base of the penile shaft. The needle can be inserted once in the midline and then redirected to each side (Fig. 28–19). The dorsal nerve block is performed with a 27-gauge needle, inserted 1 cm above the symphysis pubis, in the midline, at a 30-degree angle and directed caudally (Fig. 28–19). The needle is advanced 1 cm after it pierces the penile fascia. After negative aspiration for blood, 1 to 4 mL of local anesthetic *without epinephrine* is injected slowly. There is a small risk of injury to the adjacent neurovascular structures.

COMPLICATIONS. The major complication is compromise of organ blood flow. *Vasoconstrictors such as epinephrine must*

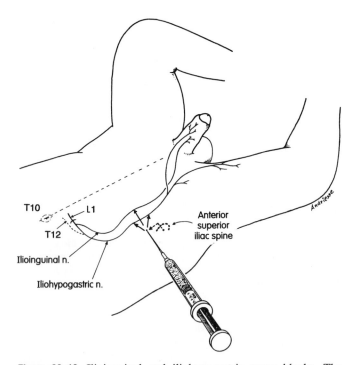

Figure 28–18. Ilioinguinal and iliohypogastric nerve blocks. The anterior superior iliac spine is palpated, and a point 1.0 to 1.5 cm cephalad and toward the midline is located (broken arrow). A 22-gauge needle is passed through the external and internal oblique muscles, and 1 to 5 mL of local anesthetic is deposited in a fan-like fashion cephalad toward the umbilicus, medially, and caudad toward the groin (solid arrows). Just before removal from the skin, another 0.5 to 1.0 mL of local anesthetic is injected subcutaneously to block the iliohypogastric nerve. Blockade of these nerves provide postoperative analgesia for inguinal hernia and orchidopexy procedures.

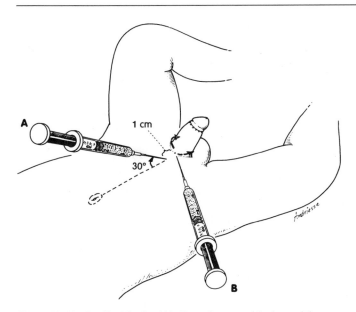

Figure 28–19. Penile block. (A) Dorsal nerve block: a 25-gauge needle is inserted in the midline, 1 cm above the symphysis pubis at an angle of 30 degrees and directed caudad. After piercing the penile fascia (0.5–1.0 cm) and negative aspiration for blood, 1 to 4 mL of local anesthetic without epinephrine is injected. (B) Ring block: a 25-gauge needle is inserted at the base of the penis at a 45 degree angle, and a ring of local anesthetic deposited. This may be done through a single needle placement by redirecting the needle. This block may be used in patients in whom a caudal block is contraindicated.

never be used for this block. Applying pressure after the injection may minimize hematoma formation. Intravascular injection may be avoided with incremental injection with frequent withdrawal.

Upper Extremity Block

BRACHIAL PLEXUS BLOCK. Of the three techniques used to block the brachial plexus (axillary, supraclavicular, and interscalene), the axillary approach is commonly used in pediatric practice.[261–263] Advantages include ease of insertion, a high rate of success in experienced hands, and low morbidity. The block is also well suited for orthopedic or plastic surgical repairs on the hand or forearm in a child with a full stomach. It must be recognized that in that situation, deeper levels of sedation place the patient at risk for aspiration of gastric contents. In addition, the consequences of intravascular injection or drug overdose may also place the child at risk for aspiration injury. Since it is unnecessary to elicit a sensory paresthesia, the block can also be performed in an anesthetized patient for postoperative pain management. Toxicity is avoided if the maximal dose of bupivacaine is 3 mg/kg or less.[264]

Supraclavicular and interscalene blocks are not as frequently used as the axillary block in pediatric patients. Unintentional block of the phrenic and recurrent laryngeal nerves is much more common in young patients because these nerves are closer to the site of injection. Data suggest that some degree of phrenic nerve blockade is present in all patients receiving interscalene blocks.[250, 265–268] Phrenic nerve blockade may cause respiratory failure in very young pa-

tients who are almost totally dependent on the diaphragm, whereas block of the recurrent laryngeal nerve may cause increased airway resistance due to vocal cord paralysis.[269] The risk of pneumothorax is greater because the apex of the lung is situated higher in infants and small children. Total spinal anesthesia is also more likely with the interscalene approach to axillary plexus blockade.[270, 271]

Anatomy. The brachial plexus arises in the neck from spinal nerves C5, C6, C7, C8, and T1, passes between the clavicle and first rib, and extends into the axilla. At that point, the axillary artery is surrounded by a narrow fascial sheath that contains the median nerve anteriorly, the ulnar nerve posteriorly, and the radial nerve on the posterolateral aspect (Fig. 28–20). In children, the axillary artery and at times the axillary sheath itself is easily palpable.

Technique. Several techniques can be used to establish that the needle is within the axillary sheath. The first is by eliciting a sensory paresthesia with the needle, but this has little application in pediatric practice, particularly in young patients. The use of a nerve stimulator allows precise placement of the needle in the neurovascular sheath without either the cooperation of the patient or the need for painful sensory paresthesias. In thin patients, the sheath can often be palpated as a cord-like structure inferior to the coracobrachialis muscle, allowing the placement of the needle in the sheath by "feel." A transarterial approach can also be used. With all techniques, it is useful to attach a short piece of extension tubing between the needle and syringe to facilitate precise handling of the apparatus during needle placement, aspiration, and drug injection.

The axillary approach to the brachial plexus is best accomplished by abducting the arm to 90 degrees. Care should be taken not to hyperabduct the arm, obscuring the axillary pulse. The artery is palpated in the axilla, and a short beveled needle is advanced toward it. When using a nerve stimulator, a distal motor response is elicited in the distribution of the

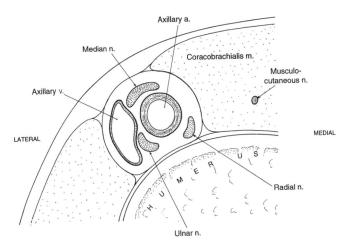

Figure 28–20. The anatomic relationships of the brachial plexus are presented. Note that the fascial sheath envelops the nerves and the axillary artery and vein; the musculocutaneous nerve lies within the body of the coracobrachialis muscle. Local anesthetic injected within the sheath (on either side of the axillary artery) produces a satisfactory block. There may be septation within the sheath in some individuals (not pictured).

radial, ulnar, or median nerves at a threshold of less than 0.2 mA (see Fig. 28–11). If one is not using a nerve stimulator, the needle is advanced until a distinct "pop" is felt as the needle pierces the axillary sheath. The axillary sheath may be divided into fascial compartments for each nerve, and these may limit the spread of local anesthetic within the axillary sheath.[272, 273] Although distinct paresthesias to the distribution of all three nerves can be elicited with the nerve stimulator, and divided doses of anesthetic administered to each of those locations, in practice it becomes extremely difficult to find the second and third motor paresthesia after the administration of even a very small amount of local anesthetic with the first injection. Alternatively, the transarterial technique, which involves direct puncture of the axillary artery, allows deposition of local anesthetic in two sites within the sheath. The needle is aimed directly toward the axillary pulse. Once blood is aspirated, the needle is advanced through the posterior wall of the artery; once blood can no longer be aspirated, half of the dose of local anesthetic is deposited posterior to the artery. The needle is withdrawn through the anterior wall of the artery, and the remainder of the dose is deposited anterior to the artery after reconfirming a negative aspiration for blood. Regardless of technique, aspiration must be performed to confirm that the needle is not within a blood vessel, and the local anesthetic is administered in incremental quantities with intermittent aspiration to confirm that the needle is not within a blood vessel. Some practitioners advocate applying a tourniquet distal to the site where the block is to be performed. It is sometimes difficult to block the musculocutaneous nerve, which carries sensory fibers to the radial aspect of the forearm, because it leaves the brachial plexus high in the axillary fossa. Applying a tourniquet may promote proximal spread of local anesthetic and enhance the chances of a successful block of this nerve.[274] Alternatively, the musculocutaneous nerve may be blocked by infiltrating 1 to several milliliters (proportional to the size of the child) of local anesthetic into the body of the coracobrachialis muscle. Regardless of the technique chosen, an additional 1 to 3 mL of local anesthetic is deposited as a subcutaneous cuff to block the intercostobrachial nerve and its communications with the musculocutaneous nerve. These additional quantities of local anesthetic must be taken into consideration when calculating the total drug dose for the block.

Selection of Drug. Local anesthetics commonly used in our practice include lidocaine and bupivacaine. As with other regional techniques that involve larger volumes of local anesthetic, the addition of both levobupivacaine and ropivacaine to the armamentarium is likely to prove beneficial in reducing the risk of toxicity from local anesthetics. Since it is desirable to have a prolonged duration of postoperative analgesia, longer acting agents are usually used in place of lidocaine. To help ensure block of the musculocutaneous nerve, we use large volumes, diluting the concentration of local anesthetic with normal saline as needed to avoid toxicity. When using 0.2 to 0.4% bupivacaine, we inject a slightly smaller volume (0.6 mL/kg). Care must always be taken not to exceed the maximal allowable doses of bupivacaine on a milligram per kilogram body weight basis (2–3 mg/kg).[264] Adding epinephrine (1:200,000) may decrease vascular absorption and the potential for toxicity. Sodium bicarbonate (1 mEq/10 mL of local anesthetic) may be added to the local anesthetic to speed the onset of blockade by raising the pH of the solution; this is particularly the case with the premixed anesthetic-epinephrine formulations that have a lower pH.

Complications. All of the nerves of the brachial plexus occupy a neurovascular bundle and hence are prone to unintended injection into a blood vessel. Resuscitation equipment should be available whenever these blocks are performed. A hematoma may form at the site of injection; if large enough, the hematoma may compress the neurovascular bundle, rendering the limb ischemic. Hence it is important to know the patient's coagulation status prior to attempting a brachial plexus block. Intravascular injection may be avoided with incremental injection with frequent withdrawal. Intraneural injection may be minimized by use of a nerve stimulator.

INTRAVENOUS REGIONAL ANESTHESIA. Intravenous regional anesthesia was first described in 1908 by August Bier and is frequently referred to as the Bier block.[275] This technique has been advocated for upper extremity procedures of 30 to 60 minutes' duration in children because of its rapid onset of anesthesia and its ease of performance.[276–279] Only dilute lidocaine (0.25 or 0.5%) can be used because of the risk of local anesthetic toxicity. No residual blockade persists after the tourniquet is released to provide postoperative analgesia; therefore, some other means for providing analgesia must be considered, such as intravenous opioids. This can be a useful block for upper extremity fracture reduction or suture of a large laceration in patients with a full stomach.[278] The exsanguination and manipulation of the limb before administering the local anesthetic may prove to be unduly painful for patients with a fracture, and many children may not tolerate the discomfort of the tourniquet without significant sedation. Another disadvantage is the possibility of toxic reactions in the event of tourniquet failure. Strict attention to detail—elevation or exsanguination of the extremity to be blocked, proper application of a double pneumatic cuff, careful attention to anesthetic dose, and care not to deflate the tourniquet until 30 minutes after injection of the local anesthetic—are important to avoid serious complications and provide a successful block. This block is unsuitable for patients under 1 year of age because of the risk of toxic reactions in infants. This technique may also be contraindicated for patients in whom the prolonged use of a tourniquet is inadvisable.

Technique. A small-gauge intravenous cannula is inserted in a vein on the dorsum of the hand. Exsanguination of the arm may be accomplished either by wrapping the limb with an Esmarch bandage or by elevation if wrapping is painful. The proximal compartment of a double tourniquet is inflated to a pressure of 200 to 250 mm Hg, although some have recommended that it be inflated to 150 mm Hg above the patient's systolic blood pressure.[280–282] If tourniquet pain develops during the course of the procedure, the distal cuff may be inflated, followed by deflation of the proximal cuff. The tourniquet must remain inflated for a minimum of 30 minutes to prevent a rapid intravenous infusion of lidocaine. It is best to deflate the tourniquet incrementally. Either local wound infiltration or systemic analgesics must be used to provide analgesia if postoperative pain is anticipated.

Selection of Drug. Only *preservative-free* 0.25 to 0.5% lidocaine without epinephrine (1 mL/kg) should be used for this block, but because the duration of the block is limited by tourniquet time, there is no need to use any agent with a longer duration of action. Deaths have been reported when the Bier block was performed with bupivacaine.[283, 284] A very low dose of a nondepolarizing neuromuscular blocking agent, such as rocuronium (0.03 mg/kg), may improve the quality of the motor blockade.

Complications. Unintended deflation of the tourniquet results in release of drug into the intravascular compartment; therefore, only a short acting local anesthetic such as lidocaine should be used. Bupivacaine should not be used for this technique because of its cardiotoxicity.

Peripheral Blocks at the Elbow

There is usually no great advantage to blocking the peripheral nerves at the elbow compared with blocking them at the wrist for analgesia or anesthesia of the hand, since the forearm is supplied by cutaneous branches that originate in the upper arm.[285] On some occasions, however, such as to avoid injections into surgical fields or areas of infection, anesthesia of the hand may be achieved by blocking the appropriate nerves at the elbow, since the cutaneous nerve supply to the hand arises at the elbow level.

RADIAL NERVE
Anatomy. The radial nerve supplies the radial side of the dorsum of the hand and the proximal parts of the radial three and a half digits. Block at the elbow is useful for the provision of anesthesia for an arteriovenous fistula. It is also useful to supplement an inadequate brachial plexus block at the axillary level. The radial nerve passes over the anterior aspect of the lateral epicondyle.

Technique. The intercondylar line is marked. After identification of the biceps tendon, a 27-gauge needle is inserted directly toward the bone of the lateral epicondyle toward the lateral margin, and 2 to 5 mL (depending on the patient's weight) of bupivacaine (0.25% with epinephrine 1:200,000) is injected into the area.

Complications. Intravascular injection and intraneural injection are potential complications. The use of a nerve stimulator can prevent unintended intraneural injection. Intravascular injection can be avoided with incremental injection with frequent withdrawal.

MEDIAN NERVE
Anatomy. This nerve supplies the radial side of the palm and the three and a half digits of the palmar aspect. It accompanies the brachial artery in its course down the arm. It is initially lateral and then crosses the ventral side of the artery and eventually lies medial to the artery at the bend of the elbow. It is deep to the bicipital fascia and superficial to the brachialis muscle.

Technique. The arm is abducted and the forearm supinated. After marking the intercondylar line between the medial and the lateral epicondyle of the humerus, the practitioner palpates the brachial artery. A 27-gauge needle is inserted just medial to the artery and directed perpendicular to the skin; 2 to 5 mL (depending upon the patient's weight) of bupivacaine (0.25% with epinephrine 1:200,000) is injected to the site. Caution must be exercised to avoid the artery, since it is in close proximity to the nerve.

Complications. Intravascular injection and intraneural injections are potential complications. The use of a nerve stimulator can prevent the unintended intraneural injection. Intravascular injection can be avoided with incremental injection with frequent withdrawal.

ULNAR NERVE
Anatomy. The ulnar nerve is the superficial nerve to the arm and the ulnar side of the forearm and the hand. It is the terminal continuation of the medial cord of the brachial plexus. At the elbow, it pierces the medial intermuscular septum and follows along the medial head of the triceps to the groove between the olecranon and the medial epicondyle of the humerus. It is only covered by skin and fascia and can be easily palpated and blocked at this level.

Technique. With the patient supine, the elbow is flexed. The medial epicondyle and the ulnar groove are palpated. A 27-gauge needle is advanced perpendicular to the skin along the line of the nerve; 2 to 3 mL (depending upon the size of the patient) of bupivacaine (0.25% with epinephrine 1:200,000) is injected in the area.

Complications. Intravascular injection and intraneural injections are potential complications. Since this is a very superficial nerve, injection just after the skin is pierced in the area of the ulnar nerve usually produces a good block. Intravascular injection may be avoided with incremental injection with frequent withdrawal.

Wrist Blocks

Blocking of the median, radial, and ulnar nerves at the wrist can be easily achieved. These blocks provide very good analgesia and, since they are easy to perform, they generally have a predictable, successful outcome.

RADIAL NERVE.
This nerve is also easy to block at the wrist. Its cutaneous branches supply the radial side of the dorsum of the hand and the proximal parts of the radial three and a half digits.

Anatomy. The superficial branch of the radial nerve runs along the lateral border of the forearm under the brachioradialis muscle. In the distal third of the forearm, it angles dorsally under the tendon of the brachioradialis toward the dorsum of the wrist. It pierces the deep fascia and divides into two branches: (1) the lateral branch, which supplies the radial side and the tip of the thumb; and (2) the medial branch, which communicates with the dorsal branch of the ulnar nerve. This then divides into the four digital nerves that supply the ulnar side of the thumb, the radial side of the index finger, the space between the index finger and thumb. A communicating branch with the ulnar nerve supplies the adjacent sides of the middle and ring finger.

Technique. This is essentially a field block of the superficial terminal branches. An attempt to make the "anatomic snuffbox" prominent by extension of the thumb prior to anesthesia is desirable. The extensor pollicis and brevis tendons are marked. A 27-gauge needle is inserted close to the dorsal radial tubercle over the extensor longus tendon and 2 mL of bupivacaine (0.25% with epinephrine 1:200,000) is injected subcutaneously. An attempt to fan the local anesthetic in the "anatomic snuffbox" helps distribute the local anesthetic over the radial nerve (Fig. 28–21).

Complications. Intravascular injection can be avoided with incremental injection with frequent withdrawal. Post–nerve block dysesthesia has been reported with radial nerve block. This is usually self-limited. However, if it persists, it can be treated with serial stellate ganglion blocks.

MEDIAN NERVE
Anatomy. In the palm of the hand, the median nerve is very superficial and is covered only by skin and the palmar aponeurosis and rests on the tendons of the flexor muscles. It emerges from under the retinaculum and splits into muscular and digital branches. The muscular division of the median nerve supplies the muscles of the thenar eminence. The palmar digital nerve supplies the thumb, the index finger, the middle finger, and the ring finger. These also supply the lumbricals.

Technique. The palmaris tendon is identified. This may be done prior to general anesthesia by asking the patient to flex the wrist against resistance. The radial border of the tendon is identified. Cutaneous landmarks include both distal wrist skin creases. A 27-gauge needle is inserted at the level of the second skin crease (approximately 1 to 1.5 cm proximal to the distal crease in teenagers) perpendicular to the skin. The nerve is at a depth of less than 1 cm in the teenager and less in younger children; 1 to 2 mL of bupivacaine (0.25% with epinephrine 1:200,000) is injected in the area.

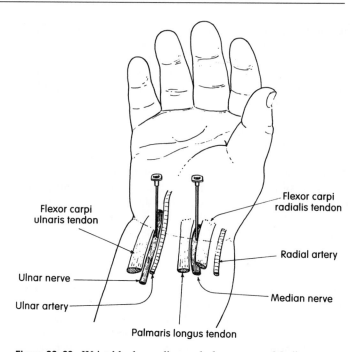

Figure 28–22. Wrist block: median and ulnar nerves. Median nerve: identify the palmaris tendon by asking awake cooperative patients to flex the wrist against resistance. Distal skin creases are identified. A 27-gauge needle is inserted at the level of the distal skin crease perpendicular to the skin. The nerve is at a depth of less than 1 cm in teenagers and less than that in younger children. A dose of 1 to 2 mL of bupivacaine (0.25% with 1:200,000 epinephrine) is injected in the area. If the patient is awake, it is better to elicit paresthesias, since the needle may be anterior to the neurovascular bundle and can be missed altogether. Ulnar nerve: identify the flexor carpi ulnaris tendon, which lies proximal to the pisiform bone. A 27-gauge needle is inserted just proximal to the pisiform bone and directed radially a distance of approximately 0.5 cm. A dose of 2 mL of bupivacaine (0.25% with epinephrine 1:200,000) is injected. (Modified with permission from Raj P, Pai U: Techniques of nerve blocking. In: Raj P, ed: Handbook of Regional Anesthesia. New York: Churchill Livingstone; 1985:185.)

If the patient is awake, it is better to elicit paresthesias, since the needle may be anterior to the neurovascular bundle and the nerve could be missed altogether (Fig. 28–22).

Complications. Intravascular placement should be avoided by repeated withdrawal prior to injection. Post-block dysesthesia may accompany median nerve block at the wrist; this may be treated with serial stellate ganglion blocks.

ULNAR NERVE
Anatomy. The palmar cutaneous branch of the ulnar nerve arises near the middle of the forearm and accompanies the ulnar artery into the hand. It then perforates the flexor retinaculum and ends in the skin of the palm communicating with the palmar branch of the median nerve. There are two dorsal digital nerves and a metacarpal communicating branch. The more medial digital nerve supplies the ulnar side of the little finger and the digital branch supplies the adjacent sides of the little and ring finger. The palmar or the terminal portion of the ulnar nerve crosses the ulnar border of the wrist in company with the ulnar artery.

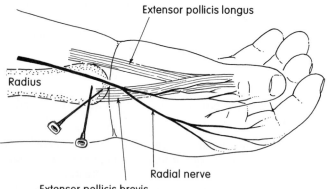

Figure 28–21. Wrist block: radial nerve. This is a superficial block of the terminal branches of the radial nerve. An attempt to make the "anatomical snuffbox" prominent by extension of the thumb prior to anesthesia is desirable. The extensor pollicis and brevis tendons are marked. A 27-gauge needle is inserted close to the dorsal radial tubercle over the extensor longus tendon. A dose of 2 mL of bupivacaine (0.25% with 1:200,000 epinephrine) is injected subcutaneously. Fanning the local anesthetic in the "anatomical snuffbox" helps to distribute the local anesthetic over the radial nerve. (Modified with permission from Raj P, Pai U: Techniques of nerve blocking. In: Raj P, ed: Handbook of Regional Anesthesia. New York: Churchill Livingstone; 1985:185.)

Technique. Blocking the ulnar nerve at the wrist is easier than at the elbow. The nerve is blocked at the wrist, where it lies under cover of the flexor carpi ulnaris tendon just proximal to the pisiform bone. The best way to access the nerve is to approach it from the ulnar side of the tendon. A 27-gauge needle is inserted just proximal to the pisiform bone and directed radially a distance of approximately 0.5 cm; 2 to 3 mL of bupivacaine (0.25% with epinephrine 1:200,000) is injected (see Fig. 28–22).

Complications. The ulnar artery runs in close proximity to the ulnar nerve; every possible effort should be made to avoid intravascular placement. Intravascular injection can be avoided with incremental injection with frequent withdrawal. Post-block dysesthesia may accompany median nerve block at the wrist; this can be treated with serial stellate ganglion blocks.

Digital Nerve Blocks: Hand

Digital nerve blocks are useful for providing pain relief to patients undergoing procedures to individual fingers. These are useful for postoperative analgesia in procedures such as trigger finger release and also for the provision of pain relief in patients undergoing laser therapy for warts on their fingers.[286]

Anatomy. The common digital nerves are derived from the median and ulnar nerves and divide in the palm to volar digital nerves that supply the fingers. All digital nerves are accompanied by digital vessels. There are three digital nerves derived from the median nerve: the first divides into three palmar digital nerves that supply the sides of the thumb; the second common digital nerve supplies the web between the index and middle finger; the third common palmar digital nerve communicates with a branch of the ulnar nerve and supplies the web between the middle and ring fingers. These common digital nerves then become the proper digital nerves (digital collaterals) that supply the skin of the palmar surface and the dorsal side of the terminal phalanx of their respective digits. All digital nerves ultimately terminate in two branches: (i) ramifies in the skin of the finger tips and (ii) in the pulp under the nail. Smaller digital nerves are derived from the radial and ulnar nerves and supply the back of the fingers. These tend to lie on the dorsolateral aspect of the finger. There are four dorsal digital nerves: (1) ulnar side of the thumb; (2) radial side of the index finger; (3) adjacent sides of index and middle fingers; and (4) communication to the adjacent sides of middle and ring finger.

Technique. There are two techniques for blockade of the digital nerves:

1. Blockade at the base of the thumb (Fig. 28–23A&B): With the thumb extended, on the palmar surface of the hand, one inserts a 27-gauge needle into the web space between the index finger and thumb. The needle is advanced to the junction of the web space and the palmar

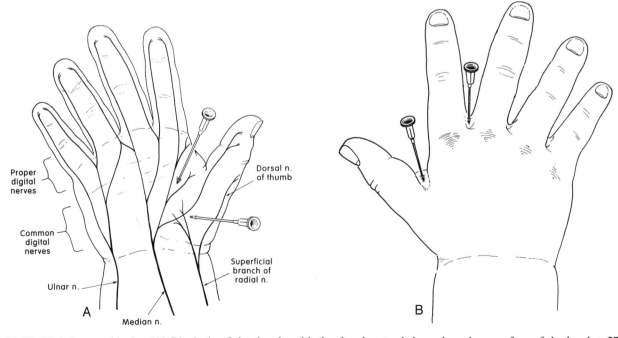

Figure 28–23. Digital nerve blocks. (A) Blockade of the thumb: with the thumb extended, on the palmar surface of the hand, a 27-gauge needle is inserted into the web space between the index finger and thumb. The needle is advanced to the junction of the web space and the palmar skin of the hand a distance of about 1 cm; 0.5 mL of bupivacaine *without epinephrine* is injected. A second needle is inserted into the thenar eminence on the radial aspect of the thumb. A dose of 1 mL of bupivacaine *without epinephrine* is injected. Caution has to be exercised if the patient has collagen vascular disease, since this may precipitate acute vascular spasm that may not be relieved. (B) Blockade of other digits: blockade of the other fingers is accomplished at the bifurcation between the metacarpal heads. With the fingers widely extended, a 27-gauge needle is inserted into the web about 3 mm proximal to the junction between the web and the palmar skin; 1 to 2 mL of bupivacaine *without epinephrine* is injected. This can be performed either from a dorsal approach or a volar approach. The web on either side will have to be blocked to provide analgesia for each finger to be anesthetized.

skin of the hand a distance of about 1 cm; 0.5 mL of bupivacaine *without epinephrine* is injected. A second needle is inserted into the thenar eminence on the radial aspect of the thumb. A dose of 1 mL of bupivacaine *without epinephrine* is injected. Caution has to be exercised if the patient has collagen vascular disease, since this may precipitate acute vascular spasm that may not be relieved.

2. Blockade of the other fingers is accomplished at the bifurcation between the metacarpal heads (Fig. 28–23B). With the fingers extended, a 27-gauge needle is inserted into the web about 3 mm proximal to the junction between the web and the palmar skin; 1 to 2 mL of bupivacaine *without epinephrine* is injected. This can be performed either from a dorsal approach or a volar approach.

Caution: *Vasoconstrictors are to be avoided, since these are end vessels and acute vasospasm due to epinephrine can lead to permanent damage or necrosis of the digits.*

COMPLICATIONS. Large volumes of local anesthetic are contraindicated because they may cause pressure and vascular compromise. Vasoconstrictors should be avoided, as they may cause necrosis of the digit. Intravascular injection can be avoided with incremental injection with frequent withdrawal.

Lower Extremity Blocks

The major use of nerve blocks of the lower extremity in pediatric patients is for managing postoperative pain and as an adjunct to general anesthesia. When considering the sensory and cutaneous innervation of the lower extremity (Fig. 28–24A&B), it is not surprising that few surgical procedures can be accomplished under single nerve blocks. However, combinations of sciatic, femoral, and lateral femoral cutaneous blockade can provide both excellent postoperative analgesia and surgical anesthesia for selected operations; the fascia iliaca block produces anesthesia of multiple nerves with a single injection.

SCIATIC NERVE BLOCK

Anatomy. The sciatic nerve arises from the L4 through S3 roots of the sacral plexus, passes through the pelvis, and becomes superficial at the lower margin of the gluteus maximus muscle. It then descends into the lower extremity in the posterior aspect of the thigh, supplying sensory innervation to the posterior thigh as well as to the entire leg and foot below the level of the knee except for the medial aspect, which is supplied by the femoral nerve (see Fig. 28–24A). Although a sciatic nerve block alone is useful for few surgical procedures, it can be combined with a femoral nerve block (see Fig. 28–24B) for operations below the knee and for postoperative pain relief.[236, 287] There are three approaches to the sciatic nerve. All blocks are performed with the aid of a nerve stimulator to elicit a motor paresthesia in the foot, and, if the block is performed in a lightly sedated trauma victim, the approach that places the patient in a greater position of comfort should be chosen. A newer approach to the sciatic nerve using a lateral approach to the popliteal fossa has been described.[288] This offers the additional advantage of being able to provide the block in a supine patient.

Approach of Labat (Posterior Approach)
Technique. The patient is placed in the lateral decubitus position, lying on the nonoperative leg. The leg to be blocked is flexed and the lower leg is extended. (Fig. 28–25A). A line is drawn from the posterior superior iliac spine to the greater trochanter of the femur. Another line is drawn from the greater trochanter to the coccyx. The first line is bisected, and a perpendicular line is drawn from that point to the second line; the point at which it intersects the second line is the site of needle insertion (Fig. 28–25B). A 22-gauge insulated needle is advanced in the perpendicular plane until it strikes bone (Fig. 28–25C). It is possible for the needle to

FEMORAL AND OBTURATOR DISTRIBUTION

SCIATIC DISTRIBUTION

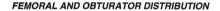

BACK   FRONT   MEDIAL   LATERAL

BACK   FRONT   MEDIAL   LATERAL

Figure 28–24. The sensory innervation of the lower extremity is presented. Note that anesthesia of the lower extremity requires block of the femoral nerve (A) (and its branches) as well as the sciatic nerve (B).

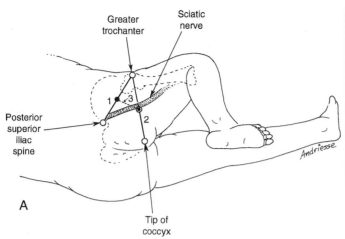

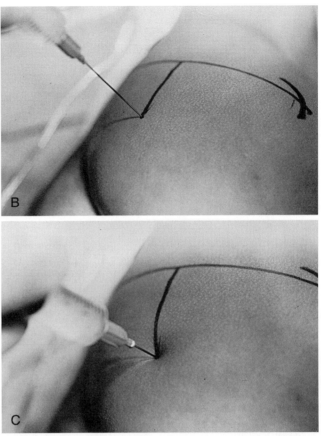

Figure 28–25. (A) Sciatic nerve block (approach of Labat). The patient is placed in a lateral position with the lower leg extended and the upper leg, the one to be blocked, flexed; a line is drawn from the greater trochanter of the femur to the posterior superior iliac spine (line 1). A second line is drawn from the greater trochanter to the coccyx (line 2). Line 1 is bisected, and a perpendicular line is drawn from that point to line 2 (broken line 3); the point at which the perpendicular broken line intersects line 2 (circle with dot) is the point of needle insertion. (B and C) A 22-gauge needle is advanced perpendicular to the skin until it strikes bone or, if the patient is awake, a paresthesia is elicited.

pass through the sciatic notch without either encountering bone or causing a paresthesia. In that case, the needle is redirected in a cephalad direction until bone is encountered. A motor paresthesia is then sought using an organized grid-like approach, fanning medially to laterally.[289]

Anterior Approach

Anatomy. As the sciatic nerve emerges from the lower border of the gluteus maximus to extend down the thigh, it passes medial and deep to the lesser trochanter of the femur (Fig. 28–26A).

Technique. With the patient in the supine position, a line is drawn from the anterior superior iliac spine to the pubic tuberosity. The greater trochanter is then located, and another line is drawn parallel to the first line (Fig. 28–26B); at the medial one third of the first line, a perpendicular line is dropped to the second line. The point of intersection with the line originating at the greater trochanter marks the point of needle entry. The needle is inserted in a perpendicular plane until bone is encountered (Fig. 28–26C). It is then partially withdrawn and redirected medially. When the needle is posterior to the posterior margin of the femur, ease of injection is determined after negative aspiration for blood (Fig. 28–26D). This approach carries a greater risk of unintended puncture of the femoral vessels, and repeated negative aspirations must precede incremental injection. If the needle is in muscle or a fascial bundle, resistance to injection will be felt. In this case, the needle is advanced until minimal resistance to injection is felt. Motor paresthesia is a helpful indicator.

For these two techniques, 0.5 mL/kg of bupivacaine (0.25% with epinephrine 1:200,000) is the dose usually administered for children older than 6 months of age. If the sciatic nerve block is used in conjunction with a femoral nerve block, consideration should be given to diluting the local anesthetic concentration further to limit the total combined injected dose to 2 to 3 mg/kg of bupivacaine.

Lateral Popliteal Sciatic Nerve Block. This approach to the sciatic nerve can be performed with the patient in the supine position.[290–293] This block provides postoperative analgesia in patients undergoing surgery to the foot and knee,[288] such as club foot repair or triple arthrodesis, and in patients who have knee surgery, particularly when combined with a femoral nerve block.[288, 294–296] This block has the advantage of preserving hamstring function and allows early ambulation with crutches.[296]

Anatomy. The popliteal fossa is a diamond-shaped area located behind the knee. It is bordered by the biceps femoris laterally, medially by the tendons of the semitendinosus and semimembranosus muscles, and inferiorly by the heads of the gastrocnemius muscle. The sciatic nerve, after its formation from the L4 through S5, innervates all areas of the leg and foot below the knee except the anteromedial cutaneous area of the leg and foot, which are supplied by the femoral nerve. The sciatic nerve divides into two branches, the larger tibial nerve located medially and the common peroneal nerve located laterally. The nerves are together at the apex of the popliteal fossa where they are in close proximity to each other and are enclosed in a connective tissue sheath for a

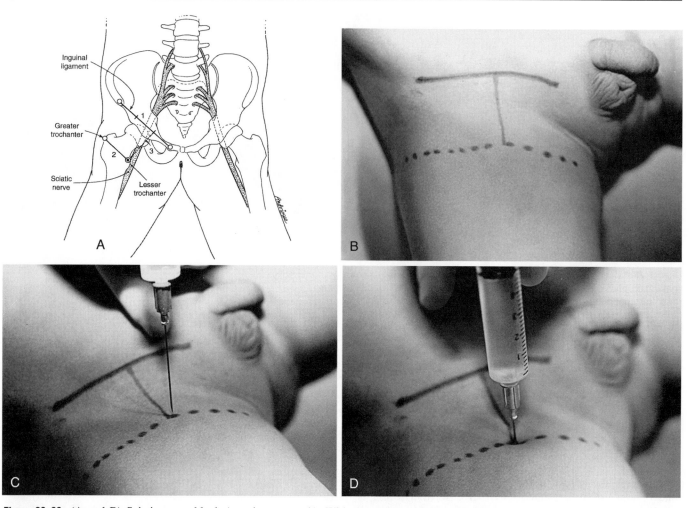

Figure 28–26. (A and B) Sciatic nerve block (anterior approach). With the patient in a supine position, a line is drawn from the anterior iliac spine to the pubic tuberosity (line 1). The greater trochanter is located, and another line is drawn parallel to the first (line 2). A perpendicular line is dropped from line 1 at a point one third the distance laterally from the pubic tuberosity to the anterior iliac spine (broken line 3). (C and D) A needle is inserted at the intersection of line 2 and the perpendicular line (in part A, circle with dot) until bone is encountered. The needle is redirected off the edge of the femur to the approximate posterior margin of the femur (see part A), and after negative aspiration for blood, ease of injection is ascertained. Resistance to injection indicates that the needle is within muscle or fascial bundle; the needle should be advanced until there is minimal resistance to injection or until a paresthesia is elicited.

few more centimeters before dividing into the component nerves (Fig. 28–27).

Technique. After induction of general anesthesia, the lower leg is elevated on a pillow. The biceps femoris tendon is palpated. The tendon is then traced upwards for about 3 to 5 cm. A 22-gauge insulated needle is inserted anterior to the tendon in a horizontal plane with a cephalad angulation (see Fig. 28–27). A nerve stimulator is attached to the sheathed needle, and with low voltage stimulation (0.2 to 0.5 mV), the foot is observed for plantar or dorsiflexion. On injection of a test dose of 1 mL bupivacaine (0.25% with epinephrine 1:200,000), the twitching is abolished. This confirms the correct placement of the needle; 5 to 10 mL of additional local anesthetic are then injected. In adult studies, it has been shown that the sciatic nerve block is longer lasting than an ankle block or subcutaneous infiltration and provides excellent postoperative analgesia.[288, 296]

Complications. Intraneural injection must be avoided. Use of a low-voltage nerve stimulator ensures the proper place-

ment of the needle. It is rare to see intravascular placement of the needle with this approach. Intravascular injection can be avoided with incremental injection with frequent withdrawal.

FEMORAL NERVE BLOCK. A femoral nerve block is particularly useful in patients with a fractured femoral shaft so that transport, radiography, and other manipulations are not painful.[297] This block provides analgesia and relieves muscle spasms around the fracture site.

Anatomy. The femoral nerve is located immediately lateral to the femoral artery and deep to both the fascia lata and fascia iliaca (Fig. 28–28).

Technique. A blunt 22-gauge b-bevel needle is advanced lateral to the pulsation of the femoral artery. Two fascial planes can be located by the distinct "pop" that is felt as the needle traverses these fascial tissues. The nerve is blocked by depositing an appropriate volume (5–10 mL) of local anesthetic lateral to the femoral pulse and deep to the fascia

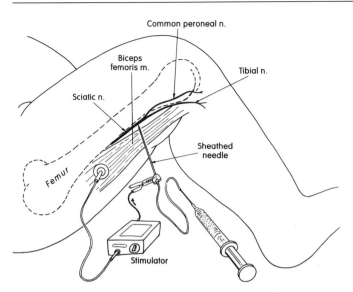

Figure 28-27. Lateral popliteal sciatic nerve block.– The lower leg is elevated on a pillow and the biceps femoris tendon is palpated. The tendon is traced proximally for about 3 to 5 cm. A 22-gauge insulated needle is inserted anterior to the tendon in a horizontal plane with a cephalad angulation. A nerve stimulator is attached to the needle and with low voltage stimulation (0.2 mV to 0.5 mV), the foot is observed for plantar or dorsiflexion. With injection of the test dose of 1 mL of bupivacaine (0.25% with 1:200,000 epinephrine), the twitching is abolished. This confirms the correct placement of the needle. A dose of 5 to 10 mL of additional local anesthetic is injected.

iliaca. The needle is advanced in a perpendicular plane. It is not necessary to elicit a motor paresthesia, provided that the two fascial planes are penetrated.[298] Performance of this block may on occasion produce a fascia iliaca block. Repeated aspiration and incremental injection should be used to avoid injection into the femoral artery.

Complications. It may be preferable to avoid this technique in patients who are on anticoagulants or who may have blood dyscrasias because of the close proximity of the nerve to the femoral artery. Intravascular injection can be avoided with incremental injection with frequent withdrawal.

LATERAL FEMORAL CUTANEOUS NERVE

Anatomy. The lateral femoral cutaneous nerve arises from the L2 and L3 roots of the lumbar plexus. It emerges from the lateral border of the psoas muscle and passes obliquely under the fascia iliaca to enter the thigh 1 to 2 cm medial to the anterior superior iliac crest (see Fig. 28–28). The nerve innervates the lateral aspect of the thigh. One of its anterior branches forms part of the patellar plexus; thus it must be blocked for regional anesthesia of the knee. Blockade is also indicated for supplementation of femoral and sciatic nerve blocks to provide relief of tourniquet pain. It is also suitable for anesthetizing the lateral aspect of the thigh as a donor site for small skin grafts, fascia iliaca grafts, or muscle biopsy for muscular disorders. In most cases, a fascia iliaca block will block this nerve along with the femoral and obturator nerves, thus obviating the need for performing an isolated lateral femoral cutaneous block.

Technique. A point approximately 2 cm caudal and 2 cm medial to the anterior superior iliac spine is located. A needle is then advanced through the skin and then through the fascia lata. A distinct "pop" is felt at this point. Two to 10 mL of local anesthetic, depending on the size of the child, is deposited in a fan-like fashion.

Complications. It is rare to see any complications associated with a lateral femoral cutaneous nerve block. However, care must be taken to avoid an intraneural placement of the local anesthetic solution. Intravascular injection can be avoided with incremental injection with frequent withdrawal.

FASCIA ILIACA BLOCK. This block is particularly useful in children to provide unilateral anesthesia or analgesia of the lower extremity.[299] The block has been reported to be less reliable in adults than in children.[300] It produces blockade of the femoral, lateral femoral cutaneous, and obturator nerves with a single injection of local anesthetic.

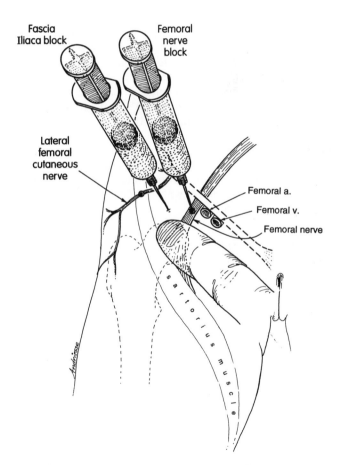

Figure 28-28. Femoral nerve block and fascia iliaca compartment block. Note that the femoral nerve lies lateral to the femoral artery. The appropriate dose of local anesthetic is administered while maintaining pressure on the nerve sheath distal to the site of injection just below the inguinal ligament; local anesthetic is thus forced proximally. For the femoral nerve block, the point of injection is lateral to the pulse, over the site of the nerve. For the fascia iliaca block, the point of injection is just lateral to the site depicted for the femoral nerve block, 1 cm inferior to the lateral and middle thirds of the inguinal ligament. An injection at this location will bathe all three nerves in the compartment, resulting in blockade with a single injection.

Anatomy. The compartment is bounded superficially by the fascia iliaca and iliacus muscle, superiorly by the iliac crest, and deeply by the psoas muscle. It has the advantage of producing blockade without requiring the needle to be in the close proximity to any major nerves or blood vessels. The authors[299] reported a greater than 90% success rate with this block and found it far superior in children to the "3 in 1" block described by Winnie.[301]

Technique. The injection is made approximately 1 cm inferior to the junction of the outer and middle thirds of the inguinal ligament. As the needle is inserted in a perpendicular angle of about 75 degrees to the skin, two characteristic "pops" are felt as the needle pierces the fascia lata and then the fascia iliaca. Slight pressure on a fluid-filled syringe attached to the needle may aid in placement of the block by producing a subtle loss of resistance when the fascia iliaca compartment is entered. The angle of needle is decreased and directed cephalad, and the local anesthetic is incrementally injected. One should feel little resistance to injection. Digital pressure is exerted distally to the site during the injection and for a short time afterwards, and the swelling produced in the groin by the volume of local anesthetic is massaged to promote proximal flow of the drug. Long-acting local anesthetics such as bupivacaine, ropivacaine, or levobupivacaine are usually chosen so that postoperative blockade can provide prolonged analgesia. A volume of 0.3 to 0.5 mL/kg is sufficient in most cases (see Fig. 28–28).

Complications. Owing to the larger volume that is required to provide an adequate block, care must be taken not to exceed the maximum dosage of the local anesthetic. Intravascular injection can be avoided with incremental injection with frequent withdrawal.

Ankle Block

Block of the nerves of the foot at the ankle is a technique that is valuable to produce both surgical anesthesia and postoperative analgesia for procedures on the foot. If a tourniquet is being used, one can use an Esmarch at the level of the ankle rather than the standard thigh or calf tourniquet.[274]

Anatomy. Three nerves can be blocked from the dorsal aspect of the foot. The deep peroneal nerve (L4, L5, S1, S2) innervates the web space between the great and second toes. This nerve extends down the anterior aspect of the leg medial to the extensor hallucis longus and lateral to both the anterior tibial muscle and the anterior tibial artery. It is blocked at the level of the ankle crease in the lower part of the leg, by insertion of a 25-gauge needle through the skin until it contacts the tibia (Fig. 28–29A). Several milliliters of local anesthetic are injected and then an additional amount as the needle is being withdrawn. The superficial peroneal nerve (L4, L5, S1, S2) innervates the medial and lateral aspects of the dorsum of the foot. Its anatomic course passes through the crural fascia on the anterior aspect of the distal two thirds of the leg and subcutaneously along the lateral aspect of the foot. It is blocked immediately above the talocrural joint. It can be blocked by subcutaneous infiltration of local anesthetic from the anterior border of the tibia to the lateral malleolus. The last nerve that lies on the dorsal aspect of the foot is the saphenous nerve, which innervates the skin over the medial malleolus. It is blocked by subcutaneous infiltration around the great saphenous vein at the level of the medial malleolus. The tibial and the sural nerves are blocked using a posterior approach. The tibial nerve (L4, L5, S1, S2, S3) lies posterior to the posterior tibial artery and divides into the medial and lateral plantar branches, which innervate their respective aspects of the sole of the foot. It is blocked at the level of the medial malleolus.

Technique. It is not necessary to elicit paresthesias, and an ankle block can be satisfactorily performed in sedated patients without the use of a nerve stimulator. Five principal nerves must be blocked to provide analgesia to the entire foot: (1) the deep and (2) superficial peroneal, (3) saphenous, (4) tibial, and (5) sural nerves. The technique is the same as in the adult. It should be noted that there might be some variation in the precise distribution of distal innervation from patient to patient. A 25-gauge needle is inserted at a 90-degree angle to the posterior aspect of the tibia and is

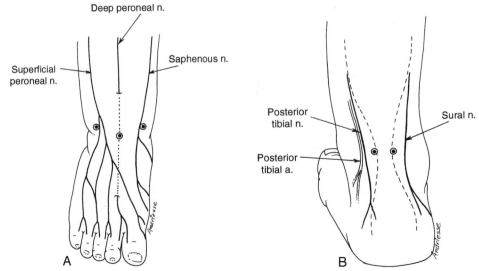

Figure 28–29. Ankle block. Block of the ankle generally requires five separate nerves to be blocked. Three nerves can be blocked from the dorsal aspect of the foot (A) and two on either side of the Achilles tendon (B). (Sites of injection are indicated by the circles with dots.)

directed lateral to the posterior tibial artery until the tibia is contacted. Several milliliters of local anesthetic are deposited at this level, and several more as the needle is withdrawn. The sural nerve innervates the heel. It is blocked by subcutaneous infiltration of local anesthetic from the Achilles tendon to the lateral malleolus (see Fig. 28–29A&B).

Complications. It is very rare to see complications from an ankle block. However, the use of vasoconstrictors can cause necrosis of the toes. Care should be taken to avoid the use of an ankle block in patients who may have compromised blood flow to the lower extremity.

Digital Nerve Blocks: Foot

This is an easy block to perform and is useful for surgeries that include trauma to the nails and toes, ingrown toenail surgery, and for laser treatment of warts.[286]

Anatomy. The digital nerves of the foot are derived from the plantar cutaneous branches of the tibial nerve. The proper digital nerve of the great toe pierces the plantar aponeurosis posterior to the tarsomedial joint and supplies the medial side of the great toe. The three common digital nerves pass between the divisions of the plantar aponeurosis and split into two proper digital nerves each. The first supplies the adjacent areas of the great and second toes; the second supplies the adjacent sides of the second and third toes; the third supplies the adjacent sides of the third and fourth toes. Each proper digital nerve gives off cutaneous and articular filaments that terminate in the tip of the toe. The superficial peroneal nerve gives off branches that supply the dorsum of the foot. They are derived from two nerves: (1) the dorsal cutaneous that divides into two branches, a medial that supplies the great toe and a lateral that supplies the adjacent sides of the second and third toes; and (2) the intermediate dorsal cutaneous nerve that passes along the lateral part of the foot supplying the lateral part of the dorsum of the foot and communicating with the sural nerve. It terminates by dividing into two dorsal digital branches, one of which supplies the adjacent sides of the third and fourth toes and another one that supplies the adjacent sides of the fourth and little toes.

Technique. Digital blocks of the foot can be difficult because of the thickness of the overlying skin. We prefer using an approach by which we access the nerve from the web space or at the dorsolateral aspect of the toe. A dose of 1 to 2 mL of bupivacaine *without epinephrine* is injected after aspiration to rule out intravascular placement. These blocks should be avoided in patients with already compromised blood flow to the toes.

Complications. Large volumes of local anesthetic are contraindicated, since they may cause pressure and vascular compromise. Vasoconstrictors should be avoided, as they may cause necrosis of the digit. Intravascular injection can be avoided with incremental injection with frequent withdrawal.

SUMMARY

Most regional techniques that are suitable for adults can be used in pediatric patients. Although in most cases, sedation or general anesthesia is necessary in addition to the regional anesthetic, in certain neonates, regional anesthesia is often used as the sole technique and may reduce the incidence of postanesthetic apnea in former premature infants. In addition to the intraoperative benefits, regional anesthesia may improve postoperative analgesia and may offer some improvement to postoperative respiratory function in selected patients. Regional anesthesia is particularly useful in outpatient surgery, providing postoperative analgesia with rapid emergence and a low incidence of side effects. It is important to realize, however, that anatomic, physiologic, and pharmacologic factors that are unique to pediatric patients can affect the performance and safety of regional anesthetic techniques. Once these differences are understood, regional anesthesia can be safely and efficaciously used either as the sole anesthetic or as a supplement to general anesthesia to provide a smooth intraoperative course and pain-free awakening.

REFERENCES

1. Yaster M, Maxwell LG: Pediatric regional anesthesia. Anesthesiology 1989;70:324–338.
2. Dalens B: Regional anesthesia in children. Anesth Analg 1989; 68:654–672.
3. Giaufre E, Dalens B, Gombert A: Epidemiology and morbidity of regional anesthesia in children: A one-year prospective survey of the French-Language Society of Pediatric Anesthesiologists. Anesth Analg 1996;83:904-912.
4. Ravilly S, Robinson W, Suresh S, et al.: Chronic pain in cystic fibrosis. Pediatrics 1996;98:741–777.
5. Fratacci MD, Kimball WR, Wain JC, et al.: Diaphragmatic shortening after thoracic surgery in humans: Effects of mechanical ventilation and thoracic epidural anesthesia. Anesthesiology 1993;79:654-665.
6. Polaner DM, Kimball WR, Fratacci MD, et al.: Thoracic epidural anesthesia increases diaphragmatic shortening after thoracotomy in the awake lamb. Anesthesiology 1993;79:808–816.
7. Manikian B, Cantineau JP, Bertrand M, et al.: Improvement of diaphragmatic function by a thoracic extradural block after upper abdominal surgery. Anesthesiology 1988;68:379–386.
8. Sung C-Y, Truant AP: The physiological disposition of lidocaine and its comparison in some respects with procaine. J Pharmacol Exp Ther 1954;112:432–443.
9. Brodie BB, Lief PA, Poet R: The fate of procaine in man following its intravenous administration and methods for the estimation of procaine and diethylaminoethanol. J Pharmacol Exp Ther 1948;94:359–366.
10. Treluyer JM, Gueret G, Cheron G, et al: Developmental expression of CYP2C and CYP2C-dependent activities in the human liver: invivo/in-vitro correlation and inducibility. Pharmacogenetics 1997;7:441–452.
11. Ward RM: Pharmacologic principles and practicalities. In: Taeusch HW, Ballard RA, eds: Avery's Diseases of the Newborn, 7th ed. Philadelphia: WB Saunders; 1998:404–412.
12. Ward RM, Lugo RA: Drug therapy in the newborn. In: Avery GBN, Fletcher MA, MacDonald M, eds: Neonatology: Pathophysiology and Management of the Newborn, 5th ed. Philadelphia: Lippincott-Williams & Wilkins; 1999:1363–1406.
13. Besunder JB, Reed MD, Blumer JL: Principles of drug biodisposition in the neonate: A critical evaluation of the pharmacokinetic-pharmacodynamic interface, Part I. Clin Pharmacokinet 1988;14:189–216.
14. Besunder JB, Reed MD, Blumer JL: Principles of drug biodisposition in the neonate: A critical evaluation of the pharmacokinetic-pharmacodynamic interface (Part II). Clin Pharmacokinet 1988;14:261–286.
15. Levy G: Pharmacokinetics of fetal and neonatal exposure to drugs. Obstet Gynecol 1981;58(Suppl):9S–16S.
16. Rane A, Sjoqvist F: Drug metabolism in the human fetus and newborn infant. Pediatr Clin North Am 1972;19:37–49.
17. Ward RM, Mirkin BL: Perinatal/neonatal pharmacology. In: Brody TM, Larner J, Minneman KP, eds: Human Pharmacology: Molecular-to-Clinical, 3rd ed. St Louis: Mosby–Year Book; 1998:873–883.

18. Cook DR: Paediatric anaesthesia: pharmacological considerations. Drugs 1976;12:212–221.

19. Cook DR, Marcy JH: Neonatal Anesthesia, 1st ed. Pasedena, California: Appleton Davies; 1988.

20. Brown AK, Zuelzer WW, Burnett HH: Studies on the neonatal development of the glucuronide conjugating system. J Clin Invest 1958;37:332–340.

21. Shnider SM, Way EL: The kinetics of transfer of lidocaine (Xylocaine) across the human placenta. Anesthesiology 1968;29:944–950.

22. Magno R, Berlin A, Karlsson K, et al.: Anesthesia for cesarean section IV: Placental transfer and neonatal elimination of bupivacaine following epidural analgesia for elective cesarean section. Acta Anaesthesiol Scand 1976;20:141–146.

23. Brown WU, Bell GC, Lurie AO, et al.: Newborn blood levels of lidocaine and mepivacaine in the first postnatal day following maternal epidural anesthesia. Anesthesiology 1975;42:698–707.

24. Meffin P, Long GJ, Thomas J: Clearance and metabolism of mepivacaine in the human neonate. Clin Pharmacol Ther 1973;14:218–225.

25. Rothstein P, Arthur GR, Feldman HS, et al.: Bupivacaine for intercostal nerve blocks in children: Blood concentrations and pharmacokinetics. Anesth Analg 1986;65:625–632.

26. Ecoffey C, Desparmet J, Berdeaux A, et al.: Pharmacokinetics of lignocaine in children following caudal anaesthesia. Br J Anaesth 1984;56:1399–1402.

27. Ecoffey C, Desparmet J, Maury M, et al.: Bupivacaine in children: Pharmacokinetics following caudal anesthesia. Anesthesiology 1985;63:447–448.

28. Smith T, Moratin P, Wulf H: Smaller children have greater bupivacaine plasma concentrations after ilioinguinal block. Br J Anaesth 1996;76:452–455.

29. Mather LE, Tucker GT: Pharmacokinetics and biotransformation of local anesthetics. Int Anesthesiol Clin 1978;16:23–51.

30. Murat I, Montay G, Delleur MM, et al.: Bupivacaine pharmacokinetics during epidural anaesthesia in children. Eur J Anaesthesiol 1988;5:113–120.

31. Luz G, Innerhofer P, Bachmann B, et al.: Bupivacaine plasma concentrations during continuous epidural anesthesia in infants and children. Anesth Analg 1996;82:231–234.

32. Berde CB: Convulsions associated with pediatric regional anesthesia. Anesth Analg 1992;75:164–166.

33. Huang YF, Pryor ME, Mather LE, et al.: Cardiovascular and central nervous system effects of intravenous levobupivacaine and bupivacaine in sheep. Anesth Analg 1998;86:797–804.

34. Bardsley H, Gristwood R, Baker H, et al.: A comparison of the cardiovascular effects of levobupivacaine and rac-bupivacaine following intravenous administration to healthy volunteers. Br J Clin Pharmacol 1998;46:245–249.

35. Masters DB, Berde CB, Dutta SK, et al: Prolonged regional nerve blockade by controlled release of local anesthetic from a biodegradable polymer matrix. Anesthesiology 1993;79:340–346.

36. Curley J, Castillo J, Hotz J, et al.: Prolonged regional nerve blockade: Injectable biodegradable bupivacaine/polyester microspheres. Anesthesiology 1996;84:1401–1410.

37. Castillo J, Curley J, Hotz J, et al.: Glucocorticoids prolong rat sciatic nerve blockade in vivo from bupivacaine microspheres. Anesthesiology 1996;85:1157–1166.

38. Drager C, Benziger D, Gao F, et al.: Prolonged intercostal nerve blockade in sheep using controlled-release of bupivacaine and dexamethasone from polymer microspheres. Anesthesiology 1998;89:969–979.

39. Thomas JM, Schug SA: Recent advances in the pharmacokinetics of local anaesthetics: Long-acting amide enantiomers and continuous infusions. Clin Pharmacokinet 1999;36:67–83.

40. Kohane DS, Sankar WN, Shubina M, et al.: Sciatic nerve blockade in infant, adolescent, and adult rats: A comparison of ropivacaine with bupivacaine. Anesthesiology 1998;89:1199–1208.

41. Markham A, Faulds D: Ropivacaine: A review of its pharmacology and therapeutic use in regional anaesthesia. Drugs 1996;52:429–449.

42. Ivani G, Lampugnani E, Torre M, et al.: Comparison of ropivacaine with bupivacaine for paediatric caudal block. Br J Anaesth 1998;81:247–248.

43. Ivani G, Mereto N, Lampugnani E, et al.: Ropivacaine in paediatric surgery: Preliminary results. Paediatr Anaesth 1998;8:127–129.

44. Ivani G, Mazzarello G, Lampugnani E, et al.: Ropivacaine for central blocks in children. Anaesthesia 1998;53:74–76.

45. Zsigmond EK, Downs JR: Plasma cholinesterase activity in newborns and infants. Can Anaesth Soc J 1971;18:278–285.

46. Tobias JD, Rasmussen GE, Holcomb GW III, et al.: Continuous caudal anaesthesia with chloroprocaine as an adjunct to general anaesthesia in neonates. Can J Anaesth 1996;43:69–72.

47. Henderson K, Sethna NF, Berde CB: Continuous caudal anesthesia for inguinal hernia repair in former preterm infants. J Clin Anesth 1993;5:129–133.

48. Duncan PG, Kobrinsky N: Prilocaine-induced methemoglobinemia in a newborn infant. Anesthesiology 1983;59:75–76.

49. Gourrier E, Karoubi P, el Hanache A, et al.: Use of EMLA cream in a department of neonatology. Pain 1996;68:431–434.

50. Engberg G, Danielson K, Henneberg S, et al.: Plasma concentrations of prilocaine and lidocaine and methaemoglobin formation in infants after epicutaneous application of a 5% lidocaine-prilocaine (EMLA). Acta Anaesthesiol Scand 1987;31:624–628.

51. Coté CJ, Strafford MA: The Principles of Pediatric Sedation. Boston: Tufts University School of Medicine; 1998.

52. Badgwell JM, Heavner JE, Kytta J: Bupivacaine toxicity in young pigs is age-dependent and is affected by volatile anesthetics. Anesthesiology 1990;73:297–303.

53. Clarkson CW, Hondeghem LM: Mechanism for bupivacaine depression of cardiac conduction: Fast block of sodium channels during the action potential with slow recovery from block during diastole. Anesthesiology 1985;62:396–405.

54. Tallman RD Jr, Rosenblatt RM, Weaver JM, et al.: Verapamil increases the toxicity of local anesthetics. J Clin Pharmacol 1988;28:317–321.

55. Valenzuela C, Snyders DJ, Bennett PB, et al.: Stereoselective block of cardiac sodium channels by bupivacaine in guinea pig ventricular myocytes. Circulation 1995;92:3014–3024.

56. Zavisca FG, Kytta J, Heavner JE, et al.: A rodent model for studying four well defined toxic endpoints during bupivacaine infusion. Reg Anesth 1991;16:223–227.

57. Fisher QA, Shaffner DH, Yaster M: Detection of intravascular injection of regional anaesthetics in children. Can J Anaesth 1997;44:592–598.

58. Freid EB, Bailey AG, Valley RD: Electrocardiographic and hemodynamic changes associated with unintentional intravascular injection of bupivacaine with epinephrine in infants. Anesthesiology 1993;79:394–398.

59. Ehrnebo M, Agurell S, Jalling B, et al.: Age differences in drug binding by plasma proteins: Studies in human foetuses, neonates, and adults. Eur J Clin Pharmacol 1971;3:189–193.

60. Morselli PL, Franco-Morselli R, Bossi L: Clinical pharmacokinetics in newborns and infants: Age-related differences and therapeutic implications. Clin Pharmacokinet 1980;5:485–527.

61. Mazoit JX, Denson DD, Samii K: Pharmacokinetics of bupivacaine following caudal anesthesia in infants. Anesthesiology 1988;68:387–391.

62. Tucker GT, Mather LE: Clinical pharmacokinetics of local anaesthetics. Clin Pharmacokinet 1979;4:241–278.

63. Beauvoir C, Rochette A, Desch G, et al: Spinal anaesthesia in newborns: Total and free bupivacaine plasma concentration. Paediatr Anaesth 1996;6:195–199.

64. Booker PD, Taylor C, Saba G: Perioperative changes in alpha 1-acid glycoprotein concentrations in infants undergoing major surgery. Br J Anaesth 1996;76:365–368.

65. Mirkin BL: Developmental pharmacology. Annu Rev Pharmacol 1970;10:255–272.

66. Riquelme CM, Bell B, Edwards J, et al.: The influence of age on the cardiovascular toxicity of intravenous bupivacaine in young dogs. Anaesth Intensive Care 1987;15:436–439.

67. Kasten GW, Martin ST: Comparison of resuscitation of sheep and dogs after bupivacaine-induced cardiovascular collapse. Anesth Analg 1986;65:1029–1032.

68. McCloskey JJ, Haun SE, Deshpande JK: Bupivacaine toxicity secondary to continuous caudal epidural infusion in children. Anesth Analg 1992;75:287–290.

69. Luz G, Ladner E, Innerhofer P, et al.: Accidents following extradural analgesia in children: The results of a retrospective study. Paediatr Anaesth 1995;5:273.

70. Flandin-Blety C, Barrier G: Accidents following extradural analgesia in children: The results of a retrospective study. Paediatr Anaesth 1995;5:41–46.

71. Goldman LJ: Complications in regional anaesthesia. Paediatr Anaesth 1995;5:3–9.

72. Nau C, Vogel W, Hempelmann G, et al.: Stereoselectivity of bupivacaine in local anesthetic-sensitive ion channels of peripheral nerve. Anesthesiology 1999;91:786–795.

73. De Jong RH, Heavner JE: Local anesthetic seizure prevention: Diazepam versus pentobarbital. Anesthesiology 1972;36:449–457.

74. Reidenberg MM, James M, Dring LG: The rate of procaine hydrolysis in serum of normal subjects and diseased patients. Clin Pharmacol Ther 1972;13:279–284.

75. Selden R, Sasahara AA: Central nervous system toxicity induced by lidocaine: Report of a case in a patient with liver disease. JAMA 1967;202:908–909.

76. Thomson PD, Melmon KL, Richardson JA, et al.: Lidocaine pharmacokinetics in advanced heart failure, liver disease, and renal failure in humans. Ann Intern Med 1973;78:499–508.

77. Englesson S: The influence of acid-base changes on central nervous system toxicity of local anaesthetic agents: I. An experimental study in cats. Acta Anaesthesiol Scand 1974;18:79–87.

78. Englesson S, Grevsten S: The influence of acid-base changes on central nervous system toxicity of local anaesthetic agents: II. Acta Anaesthesiol Scand 1974;18:88–103.

79. Covino BG, Vassallo HG: Local Anesthetics: Mechanisms of Action and Clinical Use, 1 ed. New York: Grune & Stratton; 1976.

80. Doyle E, Morton NS, McNicol LR: Plasma bupivacaine levels after fascia iliaca compartment block with and without adrenaline. Paediatr Anaesth 1997;7:121–124.

81. Mobley KA, Wandless JG, Fell D, et al.: Serum bupivacaine concentration following wound infiltration in children undergoing inguinal herniotomy. Anaesthesia 1991;46:500–501.

82. Hartley EJ, Bissonnette B, St Louis P, et al.: Scalp infiltration with bupivacaine in pediatric brain surgery. Anesth Analg 1991;73:29–32.

83. Morikawa KI, Bonica JJ, Tucker GT, et al.: Effect of acute hypovolaemia on lignocaine absorption and cardiovascular response following epidural block in dogs. Br J Anaesth 1974;46:631–635.

84. Melgrave AP: The use of epinephrine in the presence of halothane in children. Can Anaesth Soc J 1970;17:256–260.

85. Karl HW, Swedlow DB, Lee KW, et al.: Epinephrine-halothane interactions in children. Anesthesiology 1983;58:142–145.

86. Ueda W, Hirakawa M, Mae O: Appraisal of epinephrine administration to patients under halothane anesthesia for closure of cleft palate. Anesthesiology 1983;58:574–576.

87. Moore DC, Balfour RI, Fitzgibbons D: Convulsive arterial plasma levels of bupivacaine and the response to diazepam therapy. Anesthesiology 1979;50:454–456.

88. Raines A, Henderson TR, Swinyard EA, et al.: Comparison of midazolam and diazepam by the intramuscular route for the control of seizures in a mouse model of status epilepticus. Epilepsia 1990;31:313–317.

89. Bruguerolle B, Merland V, Prat M: Bupivacaine kinetics in serum, cardiac and brain tissues: Effect of diazepam pretreatment in mice. Life Sci 1991;48:569–574.

90. Bruguerolle B, Giaufre E, Morisson-Lacombe G, et al.: Bupivacaine free plasma levels in children after caudal anaesthesia: Influence of pretreatment with diazepam? Fund Clin Pharmacol 1990;4:159–161.

91. Bernards CM, Carpenter RL, Rupp SM, et al.: Effect of midazolam and diazepam premedication on central nervous system and cardiovascular toxicity of bupivacaine in pigs. Anesthesiology 1989;70:318–323.

92. Moore DC, Batra MS: The components of an effective test dose prior to epidural block. Anesthesiology 1981;55:693–696.

93. Desparmet J, Mateo J, Ecoffey C, et al.: Efficacy of an epidural test dose in children anesthetized with halothane. Anesthesiology 1990;72:249–251.

94. Liu SS: Hemodynamic responses to an epinephrine test dose in adults during epidural or combined epidural-general anesthesia. Anesth Analg 1996;83:97–101.

95. Tanaka M, Nishikawa T: The efficacy of a simulated intravascular test dose in sevoflurane-anesthetized children: A dose-response study. Anesth Analg 1999;89:632–637.

96. Perillo M, Sethna NF, Berde CB: Intravenous isoproterenol as a marker for epidural test-dosing in children. Anesth Analg 1993;76:178–181.

97. Kozek-Langenecker S, Chiari A, Semsroth M: Simulation of an epidural test dose with intravenous isoproterenol in awake and in halothane-anesthetized children. Anesthesiology 1996;85:277–280.

98. Tanaka M: Epidural test dose: isoproterenol is a reliable marker for intravascular injection in anesthetized adults. Anesth Analg 1996;82:1056–1059.

99. Tanaka M: Simulation of an epidural test dose with intravenous isoproterenol in isoflurane-anesthetized adults. Anesth Analg 1997;85:639–643.

100. Tanaka M, Nishikawa T: The combination of epinephrine and isoproterenol as a simulated epidural test dose in isoflurane-anesthetized adults. Anesth Analg 1998;86:1312–1317.

101. Heavner JE, Pitkanen MT, Shi B, et al.: Resuscitation from bupivacaine-induced asystole in rats: Comparison of different cardioactive drugs. Anesth Analg 1995;80:1134–1139.

102. Kasten GW, Martin ST: Bupivacaine cardiovascular toxicity: Comparison of treatment with bretylium and lidocaine. Anesth Analg 1985;64:911–916.

103. Feldman HS, Arthur GR, Pitkanen M, et al.: Treatment of acute systemic toxicity after the rapid intravenous injection of ropivacaine and bupivacaine in the conscious dog. Anesth Analg 1991;73:373–384.

104. Maxwell LG, Martin LD, Yaster M: Bupivacaine-induced cardiac toxicity in neonates: successful treatment with intravenous phenytoin. Anesthesiology 1994;80:682–686.

105. Covino BG: Local anesthesia. 1. N Engl J Med 1972;286:975–983.

106. Covino BG: Local anesthesia. 2. N Engl J Med 1972;286:1035–1042.

107. Long WB, Rosenblum S, Grady IP: Successful resuscitation of bupivacaine-induced cardiac arrest using cardiopulmonary bypass. Anesth Analg 1989;69:403–406.

108. Schwartz HJ, Sher TH: Bisulfite sensitivity manifesting as allergy to local dental anesthesia. J Allergy Clin Immunol 1985;75:525–527.

109. Klein CE, Gall H: Type IV allergy to amide-type local anesthetics. Contact Dermatitis 1991;25:45–48.

110. Bircher AJ, Messmer SL, Surber C, et al.: Delayed-type hypersensitivity to subcutaneous lidocaine with tolerance to articaine: confirmation by in vivo and in vitro tests. Contact Dermatitis 1996;34:387–389.

111. Sindel LJ, deShazo RD: Accidents resulting from local anesthetics. True or false allergy? Clin Rev Allergy 1991;9:379–395.

112. Glinert RJ, Zachary CB: Local anesthetic allergy: Its recognition and avoidance. J Dermatol Surg Oncol 1991;17:491–496.

113. Ruzicka T, Gerstmeier M, Przybilla B, et al.: Allergy to local anesthetics: Comparison of patch test with prick and intradermal test results. J Am Acad Dermatol 1987;16:1202–1208.

114. Chandler MJ, Grammer LC, Patterson R: Provocative challenge with local anesthetics in patients with a prior history of reaction. J Allergy Clin Immunol 1987;79:883–886.

115. Desparmet JF: Total spinal anesthesia after caudal anesthesia in an infant. Anesth Analg 1990;70:665–667.

116. Kosaka Y, Sato K, Kawaguchi R: Distance from the skin to the epidural space in children. [in Japanese]. Masui 1974;23:874–875.

117. Lups S, Haan AMFH, Bailey P: The Cerebrospinal Fluid. Amsterdam: Elsevier Publishing Company; 1954.

118. Cutler RWP, Spertell RB: Formation and absorption of cerebrospinal fluid in man. Brain 1968;91:707–720.

119. Otila E: Studies on the cerebrospinal fluid of premature infants. Acta Paediatr Scand 1948;35:3–100.

120. Kruse F: Cerebrale Krankheiten des Kindesalters in typischen Encephalogrammen. Ergeb Inn Med Kinderheilkd 1930;37:333–464.

121. Samson K: Der normale Liquor cerebrospinalis im ersten Lebenstrimenon. Gesamte Neurol Psychiat 1930;128:494–503.

122. Dohi S, Naito H, Takahashi T: Age-related changes in blood pressure and duration of motor block in spinal anesthesia. Anesthesiology 1979;50:319–323.

123. Tsuji MH, Horigome H, Yamashita M: Left ventricular functions are not impaired after lumbar epidural anaesthesia in young children. Paediatr Anaesth 1996;6:405–409.

124. Oberlander TF, Berde CB, Lam KH, et al.: Infants tolerate spinal anesthesia with minimal overall autonomic changes: Analysis of heart rate variability in former premature infants undergoing hernia repair. Anesth Analg 1995;80:20–27.

125. Payen D, Ecoffey C, Carli P, et al.: Pulsed Doppler ascending aortic, carotid, brachial, and femoral artery blood flows during caudal anesthesia in infants. Anesthesiology 1987;67:681–685.

126. Pascucci RC, Hershenson MB, Sethna NF, et al.: Chest wall motion of infants during spinal anesthesia. J Appl Physiol 1990;68:2087–2091.

127. Warren RH, Horan SM, Robertson PK: Chest wall motion in preterm infants using respiratory inductive plethysmography. Eur Respir J 1997;10:2295–2300.

128. Tusiewicz K, Bryan AC, Froese AB: Contributions of changing rib cage–diaphragm interactions to the ventilatory depression of halothane anesthesia. Anesthesiology 1977;47:327–337.

129. Easton PA, Fitting JW, Arnoux R, et al.: Recovery of diaphragm function after laparotomy and chronic sonomicrometer implantation. J Appl Physiol 1989;66:613–621.

130. Dureuil B, Viires N, Cantineau JP, et al.: Diaphragmatic contractility after upper abdominal surgery. J Appl Physiol 1986;61:1775–1780.

131. Torres A, Kimball WR, Qvist J, et al.: Sonomicrometric regional diaphragmatic shortening in awake sheep after thoracic surgery. J Appl Physiol 1989;67:2357–2368.

132. Road JD, Burgess KR, Whitelaw WA, et al.: Diaphragm function and respiratory response after upper abdominal surgery in dogs. J Appl Physiol 1984;57:576–582.

133. Bromage P: Spirometry in the assessment of analgesia after abdominal surgery. Br Med J 1955;2:589–593.

134. Spence AA, Smith G: Postoperative analgesia and lung function: A comparison of morphine with extradural block. Br J Anaesth 1971;43:144–148.

135. Simonneau G, Vivien A, Sartene R, et al.: Diaphragm dysfunction induced by upper abdominal surgery: Role of postoperative pain. Am Rev Respir Dis 1983;128:899–903.

136. Ballantyne JC, Carr DB, deFerranti S, et al.: The comparative effects of postoperative analgesic therapies on pulmonary outcome: Cumulative meta-analyses of randomized, controlled trials. Anesth Analg 1998;86:598–612.

137. Bainbridge WS: Analgesia in children by spinal injection, with a report of a new method of sterilization of the injection fluid. Medical Record 1900;58:937–940.

138. Gray HT: A study of spinal anaesthesia in children and infants: From a series of 200 cases, Part I. Lancet 1909;2:913–917.

139. Gray HT: A study of spinal anaesthesia in children and infants: From a series of 200 cases, Part II. A study of the second series of 100 cases. Lancet 1909;2:991–996.

140. Gray HT: A further study of spinal anaesthesia in children and infants. Lancet 1910;1:1611–1616.

141. Williams RK, McBride WJ, Abajian JC: Combined spinal and epidural anaesthesia for major abdominal surgery in infants. Can J Anaesth 1997;44:511–514.

142. Sartorelli KH, Abajian JC, Kreutz JM, et al.: Improved outcome utilizing spinal anesthesia in high-risk infants. J Pediatr Surg 1992;27:1022–1025.

143. Viscomi CM, Abajian JC, Wald SL, et al.: Spinal anesthesia for repair of meningomyelocele in neonates. Anesth Analg 1995;81:492–495.

144. Williams RK, Abajian JC: High spinal anaesthesia for repair of patent ductus arteriosus in neonates. Paediatr Anaesth 1997;7:205–209.

145. Aronsson DD, Gemery JM, Abajian JC: Spinal anesthesia for spine and lower extremity surgery in infants. J Pediatr Orthop 1996;16:259–263.

146. Vane DW, Abajian JC, Hong AR: Spinal anesthesia for primary repair of gastroschisis: A new and safe technique for selected patients. J Pediatr Surg 1994;29:1234–1235.

147. Liu LM, Coté CJ, Goudsouzian NG, et al.: Life-threatening apnea in infants recovering from anesthesia. Anesthesiology 1983;59:506–510.

148. Kurth CD, Spitzer AR, Broennle AM, et al.: Postoperative apnea in preterm infants. Anesthesiology 1987;66:483–488.

149. Welborn LG, Rice LJ, Hannallah RS, et al.: Postoperative apnea in former preterm infants: Prospective comparison of spinal and general anesthesia. Anesthesiology 1990;72:838–842.

150. Coté CJ, Zaslavsky A, Downes JJ, et al.: Postoperative apnea in former preterm infants after inguinal herniorrhaphy: A combined analysis. Anesthesiology 1995;82:809–822.

151. Krane EJ, Haberkern CM, Jacobson LE: Postoperative apnea, bradycardia, and oxygen desaturation in formerly premature infants: prospective comparison of spinal and general anesthesia. Anesth Analg 1995;80:7–13.

152. Wright TE, Orr RJ, Haberkern CM, et al.: Complications during spinal anesthesia in infants: High spinal blockade. Anesthesiology 1990;73:1290–1292.

153. Watcha MF, Thach BT, Gunter JB: Postoperative apnea after caudal anesthesia in an ex-premature infant. Anesthesiology 1989;71:613–615.

154. Cox RG, Goresky GV: Life-threatening apnea following spinal anesthesia in former premature infants. Anesthesiology 1990;73:345–347.

155. Tobias JD, Flannagan J: Regional anesthesia in the preterm neonate. Clin Pediatr (Phila) 1992;31:668–671.

156. Tobias JD, Flannagan J, Brock J, et al.: Neonatal regional anesthesia:

157. Welborn LG, Greenspun JC: Anesthesia and apnea: Perioperative considerations in the former preterm infant. Pediatr Clin North Am 1994;41:181–198.

158. Bosenberg AT, Bland BA, Schulte-Steinberg O, et al.: Thoracic epidural anesthesia via caudal route in infants. Anesthesiology 1988;69:265–269.

159. Gingrich BK: Spinal anesthesia for a former premature infant undergoing upper abdominal surgery. Anesthesiology 1993;79:189–190.

160. Spear RM, Deshpande JK, Maxwell LG: Caudal anesthesia in the awake, high-risk infant. Anesthesiology 1988;69:407–409.

161. Gleason CA, Martin RJ, Anderson JV, et al.: Optimal position for a spinal tap in preterm infants. Pediatrics 1983;71:31–35.

162. Weisman LE, Merenstein GB, Steenbarger JR: The effect of lumbar puncture position in sick neonates. Am J Dis Child 1983;137:1077–1079.

163. Kokki H, Salonvaara M, Herrgard E, et al.: Postdural puncture headache is not an age-related symptom in children: A prospective, open-randomized, parallel group study comparing a 22-gauge Quincke with a 22-gauge Whitacre needle. Paediatr Anaesth 1999;9:429–434.

164. Kokki H, Hendolin H, Turunen M: Postdural puncture headache and transient neurologic symptoms in children after spinal anaesthesia using cutting and pencil point paediatric spinal needles. Acta Anaesthesiol Scand 1998;42:1076–1082.

165. Bailey A, Valley R, Bigler R: High spinal anesthesia in an infant. Anesthesiology 1989;70:560.

166. Abajian JC, Mellish RW, Browne AF, et al.: Spinal anesthesia for surgery in the high-risk infant. Anesth Analg 1984;63:359–362.

167. Harnik EV, Hoy GR, Potolicchio S, et al.: Spinal anesthesia in premature infants recovering from respiratory distress syndrome. Anesthesiology 1986;64:95–99.

168. Blaise G, Roy WL: Spinal anesthesia in children. Anesth Analg 1984;63:1140–1141.

169. Mahe V, Ecoffey C: Spinal anesthesia with isobaric bupivacaine in infants. Anesthesiology 1988;68:601–603.

170. Parkinson SK, Little WL, Mueller JB, et al.: Duration of spinal anesthesia using hyperbaric bupivacaine with epinephrine in infants. Anesthesiology 1989;71.

171. Rice LJ, DeMars PD, Whalen TV, et al.: Duration of spinal anesthesia in infants less than one year of age. Comparison of three hyperbaric techniques. Reg Anesth 1994;19:325–329.

172. Kokki H, Tuovinen K, Hendolin H: Spinal anaesthesia for paediatric day-case surgery: A double-blind, randomized, parallel group, prospective comparison of isobaric and hyperbaric bupivacaine. Br J Anaesth 1998;81:502–506.

173. Hodgson PS, Neal JM, Pollock JE, et al.: The neurotoxicity of drugs given intrathecally (spinal). Anesth Analg 1999;88:797–809.

174. Severinghaus JW: Intrathecally, Caine may dis-Able. Reflections on lidocaine for spinal anesthesia. Acta Anaesthesiol Scand Suppl 1998;113:3–7.

175. Beardsley D, Holman S, Gantt R, et al.: Transient neurologic deficit after spinal anesthesia: Local anesthetic maldistribution with pencil point needles? Anesth Analg 1995;81:314–320.

176. Blaise GA, Roy WL: Spinal anaesthesia for minor paediatric surgery. Can Anaesth Soc J 1986;33:227–230.

177. Berkowitz S, Greene BA: Spinal anesthesia in children: report based on 350 patients under 13 years of age. Anesthesiology 1951;12:376–387.

178. Slater HM, Stephen CR: Hypobaric pontocaine spinal anaesthesia in children. Anesthesiology 1950;11:709–715.

179. Vereanu D: Spinalni anestezie v pediatricke chirurgii. Cas Lek Csek 1962;101:1206–1209.

180. Bolder PM: Postlumbar puncture headache in pediatric oncology patients. Anesthesiology 1986;65:696–698.

181. Purtock RV, Buhl JL, Abram SE: Epidural blood patch in a nine-year-old boy. Reg Anesth 1984;9:154–155.

182. Lund PC, Seldon TH: Principles and Practice of Spinal Anesthesia, 1 ed. Springfield: Charles C. Thomas; 1971.

183. Blockey NJ, Schorstein J: Intraspinal epidermoid tumours in the lumbar region of children. J Bone Joint Surg 1961;43B:556–562.

184. Choremis C, Economos D, Papatos C, et al.: Intraspinal epidermoid tumours (cholesteatomas) in patients treated for tuberculous meningitis. Lancet 1956;2:437–439.

185. Manno NJ, Uihlein A, Kernohan JW: Intraspinal epidermoids. J Neuro Surg 1962;19:754–765.

186. Stienstra R, Van Poorten F: Speed of injection does not affect sub-

Alternative to general anesthesia for urologic surgery. Urology 1993;41:362–365.

arachnoid distribution of plain bupivacaine 0.5%. Reg Anesth 1990;15:208–210.

187. Campbell MF: Caudal anesthesia in children. J Urol 1933;30:245–249.

188. Spiegel P: Caudal anesthesia in pediatric surgery: A preliminary report. Anesth Analg 1962;41:218–221.

189. Ruston FG: Epidural anaesthesia in paediatric surgery: Present status in the Hamilton General Hospital. Can Anaesth Soc J 1961;11:12–34.

190. Fortuna A: Caudal analgesia: A simple and safe technique in paediatric surgery. Br J Anaesth 1967;39:165–170.

191. Melman E, Penuelas JA, Marrufo J: Regional anesthesia in children. Anesth Analg 1975;54:387–390.

192. Jensen BH: Caudal block for post-operative pain relief in children after genital operations. A comparison between bupivacaine and morphine. Acta Anaesthesiol Scand 1981;25:373–375.

193. Lunn JN: Postoperative analgesia after circumcision: A randomized comparison between caudal analgesia and intramuscular morphine in boys. Anaesthesia 1979;34:552–554.

194. McGown RG: Caudal analgesia in children: Five hundred cases for procedures below the diaphragm. Anaesthesia 1982;37:806–818.

195. Takasaki M, Dohi S, Kawabata Y, et al.: Dosage of lidocaine for caudal anesthesia in infants and children. Anesthesiology 1977; 47:527–529.

196. Melman E, Arenas JA, Tandazo WE: Caudal anesthesia for pediatric surgery: an easy and safe method for calculating dose requirements. Anesthesiology 1985;63:A463–A463.

197. Schulte-Steinberg O, Rahlfs VW: Caudal anaesthesia in children and spread of 1 per cent lignocaine: A statistical study. Br J Anaesth 1970;42:1093–1099.

198. Hassan SZ: Caudal anesthesia in infants. Anesth Analg 1977;56:686–689.

199. Blaise G, Roy WL: Postoperative pain relief after hypospadias repair in pediatric patients: Regional analgesia versus systemic analgesics. Anesthesiology 1986;65:84–86.

200. Satoyoshi M, Kamiyama Y: Caudal anaesthesia for upper abdominal surgery in infants and children: A simple calculation of the volume of local anaesthetic. Acta Anaesthesiol Scand 1984;28:57–60.

201. Hain WR: Anaesthetic doses for extradural anaesthesia in children. Br J Anaesth 1978;50:303.

202. Armitage EN: Caudal block in children. Anaesthesia 1979;34:396–396.

203. Lourey CJ, McDonald IH: Caudal anaesthesia in infants and children. Anaesth Intens Care 1973;1:547–548.

204. Dalens B, Hasnaoui A: Caudal anesthesia in pediatric surgery: Success rate and adverse effects in 750 consecutive patients. Anesth Analg 1989;68:83–89.

205. Afshan G, Khan FA: Total spinal anaesthesia following caudal block with bupivacaine and buprenorphine. Paediatr Anaesth 1996;6:239–242.

206. Rice LJ, Pudimat MA, Hannallah RS: Timing of caudal block placement in relation to surgery does not affect duration of postoperative analgesia in paediatric ambulatory patients. Can Anaesth Soc J 1990;37:429–431.

207. Owens WD, Slater EM, Battit GE: A new technique of caudal anesthesia. Anesthesiology 1973;39:451–453.

208. van Niekerk J, Bax-Vermeire BM, Geurts JW, et al.: Epidurography in premature infants. Anaesthesia 1990;45:722–725.

209. Krane EJ, Dalens BJ, Murat I, et al.: The safety of epidurals placed during general anesthesia. Reg Anesth Pain Med 1998;23:433–438.

210. Saberski LR, Kondamuri S, Osinubi OY: Identification of the epidural space: Is loss of resistance to air a safe technique? A review of the complications related to the use of air. Reg Anesth 1997;22:3–15.

211. Schwartz N, Eisenkraft JB: Probable venous air embolism during epidural placement in an infant. Anesth Analg 1993;76:1136–1138.

212. Sethna NF, Berde CB: Venous air embolism during identification of the epidural space in children. Anesth Analg 1993;76:925–927.

213. Kumagai M, Yamashita M: Sacral intervertebral approach for epidural anaesthesia in infants and children: Application of "drip and tube" method. Anaesth Intens Care 1995;23:469–471.

214. Yamashita M, Tsuji M: Identification of the epidural space in children: The application of a micro-drip infusion set. Anaesthesia 1991; 46:872–874.

215. Pegues DA, Carr DB, Hopkins CC: Infectious complications associated with temporary epidural catheters. Clin Infect Dis 1994;19:970–972.

216. Strafford MA, Wilder RT, Berde CB: The risk of infection from epidural analgesia in children: A review of 1620 cases. Anesth Analg 1995;80:234–238.

217. Kilpatrick ME, Girgis NI: Meningitis: A complication of spinal anesthesia. Anesth Analg 1983;62:513–515.

218. Usubiaga JE: Neurological complications following epidural anesthesia. Int Anesthesiol Clin 1975;13:1–153.

219. Smitt PS, Tsafka A, Teng-van de Zande F, et al.: Outcome and complications of epidural analgesia in patients with chronic cancer pain. Cancer 1998;83:2015–2022.

220. Holt HM, Andersen SS, Andersen O, et al.: Infections following epidural catheterization. J Hosp Infect 1995;30:253–260.

221. Kost-Byerly S, Tobin JR, Greenberg RS, et al.: Bacterial colonization and infection rate of continuous epidural catheters in children. Anesth Analg 1998;86:712–716.

222. Fisher QA, McComiskey CM, Hill JL, et al.: Postoperative voiding interval and duration of analgesia following peripheral or caudal nerve blocks in children. Anesth Analg 1993;76:173–177.

223. Pappas AL, Sukhani R, Hatch D: Caudal anesthesia and urinary retention in ambulatory surgery. Anesth Analg 1997;85:706.

224. Valley RD, Bailey AG: Caudal morphine for postoperative analgesia in infants and children: A report of 138 cases. Anesth Analg 1991;72:120–124.

225. Krane EJ, Tyler DC, Jacobson LE: The dose response of caudal morphine in children. Anesthesiology 1989;71:48–52.

226. Wilson PT, Lloyd-Thomas AR: An audit of extradural infusion analgesia in children using bupivacaine and diamorphine. Anaesthesia 1993;48:718–723.

227. Dalens BJ, Mazoit JX: Adverse effects of regional anaesthesia in children. Drug Saf 1998;19:251-268.

228. Bouaziz H, Okubo N, Malinovsky JM, et al.: The age-related effects of epidural lidocaine, with and without epinephrine, on spinal cord blood flow in anesthetized rabbits. Anesth Analg 1999;88:1302–1307.

229. Ivani G, Lampugnani E, De Negri P, et al.: Ropivacaine vs bupivacaine in major surgery in infants. Can J Anaesth 1999;46:467–469.

230. Nuttall GA, Barnett MR, Smith RL II, et al.: Establishing intravenous access: A study of local anesthetic efficacy. Anesth Analg 1993;770:950–953.

231. Palmon SC, Lloyd AT, Kirsch JR: The effect of needle gauge and lidocaine pH on pain during intradermal injection. Anesth Analg 1998;86:379–381.

232. Curatolo M, Petersen-Felix S, Arendt-Nielsen L, et al.: Adding sodium bicarbonate to lidocaine enhances the depth of epidural blockade. Anesth Analg 1998;86:341–347.

233. Scarfone RJ, Jasani M, Gracely EJ: Pain of local anesthetics: Rate of administration and buffering. Ann Emerg Med 1998;31:36–40.

234. Wong K, Strichartz GR, Raymond SA: On the mechanisms of potentiation of local anesthetics by bicarbonate buffer: Drug structure-activity studies on isolated peripheral nerve. Anesth Analg 1993;76:131–143.

235. Smith BE, Allison A: Use of a low-power nerve stimulator during sciatic nerve block. Anaesthesia 1987;42:296–298.

236. Bosenberg AT: Lower limb nerve blocks in children using unsheathed needles and a nerve stimulator. Anaesthesia 1995;50:206–210.

237. Prabhu KP, Wig J, Grewal S: Bilateral infraorbital nerve block is superior to peri-incisional infiltration for analgesia after repair of cleft lip. Scand J Plast Reconstr Surg Hand Surg 1999;33:83–87.

238. Bosenberg AT, Kimble FW: Infraorbital nerve block in neonates for cleft lip repair: Anatomical study and clinical application. Br J Anaesth 1995;74:506–508.

239. Molliex S, Navez M, Baylot D, et al.: Regional anaesthesia for outpatient nasal surgery. Br J Anaesth 1996;76:151–153.

240. Wertheim HM, Rovenstein EA: Cervical plexus block. N Y State J Med 1939;39:1311–1315.

241. Cregg N, Conway F, Casey W: Analgesia after otoplasty: regional nerve blockade vs local anaesthetic infiltration of the ear. Can J Anaesth 1996;43:141–147.

242. Suresh S, Barcelona SL, Young N, et al.: Postoperative pain management in children undergoing tympanomastoid surgery: Is a local block better than intravenous opioid? Anesthesiology 1999;91:A1281.

243. McKinney P, Gottlieb J: The relationship of the great auricular nerve to the superficial musculoaponeurotic system. Ann Plast Surg 1985;14:310–314.

244. Bridenbaugh PO, Bridenbaugh LD, Moore DC, et al.: The role of intercostal block and three general anesthetic agents as predisposing factors to postoperative pulmonary problems. Anesth Analg 1972;51:638–644.

245. Fleming WH, Sarafian LB: Kindness pays dividends: The medical benefits of intercostal nerve block following thoracotomy. J Thorac Cardiovasc Surg 1977;74:273–274.

246. Crawford ED, Skinner DG, Capparell DB: Intercostal nerve block with thoracoabdominal incision. J Urol 1979;121:290–291.

247. Bricker SR, Telford RJ, Booker PD: Pharmacokinetics of bupivacaine following intraoperative intercostal nerve block in neonates and in infants aged less than 6 months. Anesthesiology 1989;70:942–947.

248. Moore DC, Bridenbaugh LD: Pneumothorax: Its incidence following intercostal nerve blocks. JAMA 1960;174:842–847.

249. Hannallah RS, Broadman LM, Belman AB, et al.: Comparison of caudal and ilioinguinal/iliohypogastric nerve blocks for control of post-orchiopexy pain in pediatric ambulatory surgery. Anesthesiology 1987;66:832–834.

250. Arthur DS, McNicol LR: Local anaesthetic techniques in paediatric surgery. Br J Anaesth 1986;58:760–778.

251. Shandling B, Steward DJ: Regional analgesia for postoperative pain in pediatric outpatient surgery. J Pediatr Surg 1980;15:477–480.

252. Cross GD, Barrett RF: Comparison of two regional techniques for postoperative analgesia in children following herniotomy and orchido-pexy. Anaesthesia 1987;42:845–849.

253. Trotter C, Martin P, Youngson G, et al.: A comparison between ilioinguinal-iliohypogastric nerve block performed by anaesthetist or surgeon for postoperative analgesia following groin surgery in children. Paediatr Anaesth 1995;5:363–367.

254. Dierking GW, Dahl JB, Kanstrup J, et al: Effect of pre- vs postoperative inguinal field block on postoperative pain after herniorrhaphy. Br J Anaesth 1992;68:344–348.

255. Casey WF, Rice LJ, Hannallah RS, et al.: A comparison between bupivacaine instillation versus ilioinguinal/iliohypogastric nerve block for postoperative analgesia following inguinal herniorrhaphy in children. Anesthesiology 1990;72:637–639.

256. Soliman MG, Tremblay NA: Nerve block of the penis for postoperative pain relief in children. Anesth Analg 1978;57:495–498.

257. Kirya C, Werthmann MWJ: Neonatal circumcision and penile dorsal nerve block: A painless procedure. J Pediatr 1978;92:998–1000.

258. Serour F, Cohen A, Mandelberg A, et al.: Dorsal penile nerve block in children undergoing circumcision in a day-care surgery. Can J Anaesth 1996;43:954–958.

259. Chhibber AK, Perkins FM, Rabinowitz R, et al.: Penile block timing for postoperative analgesia of hypospadias repair in children. J Urol 1997;158:1156–1159.

260. Lander J, Brady-Fryer B, Metcalfe JB, et al.: Comparison of ring block, dorsal penile nerve block, and topical anesthesia for neonatal circumcision: A randomized controlled trial. JAMA 1997;278:2157–2162.

261. Clayton ML, Turner DA: Upper arm block anesthesia in children with fractures. JAMA 1959;169:327–329.

262. Small GA: Brachial plexus block in children. JAMA 1951;147:1648–1651.

263. Fisher WJ, Bingham RM, Hall R: Axillary brachial plexus block for perioperative analgesia in 250 children. Paediatr Anaesth 1999;9:435–438.

264. Campbell RJ, Ilett KF, Dusci L: Plasma bupivacaine concentrations after axillary block in children. Anaesth Intens Care 1986;14:343–346.

265. Urmey WF, Talts KH, Sharrock NE: One hundred percent incidence of hemidiaphragmatic paresis associated with interscalene brachial plexus anesthesia as diagnosed by ultrasonography. Anesth Analg 1991;72:498–503.

266. Neal JM, Moore JM, Kopacz DJ, et al.: Quantitative analysis of respiratory, motor, and sensory function after supraclavicular block. Anesth Analg 1998;86:1239–1244.

267. al Kaisy AA, Chan VW, Perlas A: Respiratory effects of low-dose bupivacaine interscalene block. Br J Anaesth 1999;82:217–220.

268. Bennani SE, Vandenabele-Teneur F, Nyarwaya JB, et al.: An attempt to prevent spread of local anaesthetic to the phrenic nerve by compression above the injection site during the interscalene brachial plexus block. Eur J Anaesthesiol 1998;15:453–456.

269. Arthur DS: Local anaesthetic techniques in paediatric surgery. In: Henderson JJ, Nimmo WS, eds: Practical Regional Anaesthesia. Oxford: Blackwell Scientific Publications; 1983.

270. Iocolano CF: Total spinal anesthesia after an interscalene block. J Perianesth Nurs 1997;12:163–168.

271. Norris D, Klahsen A, Milne B: Delayed bilateral spinal anaesthesia following interscalene brachial plexus block. Can J Anaesth 1996;43:303–305.

272. Thompson GE, Rorie DK: Functional anatomy of the brachial plexus sheaths. Anesthesiology 1983;59:117–122.

273. De Jong RH: Axillary block of the brachial plexus. Anesthesiology 1961;22:215–225.

274. Eriksson E, Doberl A, Goldman V, et al.: Illustrated Handbook of Local Anaesthesia, 2nd ed. Philadelphia: W. B. Saunders Company; 1980.

275. Bier A: Ueber einen neuen Weg Localanasthesie an den Gliedmaasen zu erzeugen. Verh Dtsch Ges Chir 1908;37:204–213.

276. FitzGerald B: Intravenous regional anaesthesia in children. Br J Anaesth 1976;48:485–486.

277. Bolte RG, Stevens PM, Scott SM, et al: Mini-dose Bier block intravenous regional anesthesia in the emergency department treatment of pediatric upper-extremity injuries. J Pediatr Orthop 1994;14:534–537.

278. Blasier RD, White R: Intravenous regional anesthesia for management of children's extremity fractures in the emergency department. Pediatr Emerg Care 1996;12:404–406.

279. Hilgenhurst G: The Bier block after 80 years: A historical review. Reg Anesth 1990;15:2–5.

280. Fleming SA: Safety and usefulness of intravenous regional anaesthesia. Acta Anaesthesiol Scand Suppl 1969;36:21–25.

281. Mazze RI, Dunbar RW: Intravenous regional anesthesia: Report of 497 cases with toxicity study. Acta Anaesthesiol Scand Suppl 1969;36:27–34.

282. Finegan BA, Bukht MD: Venous pressures in the isolated upper limb during saline injection. Can Anaesth Soc J 1984;31:364–367.

283. Heath ML: Deaths after intravenous regional anaesthesia. Br Med J (Clin Res Ed) 1982;285:913–914.

284. Moore DC: Bupivacaine toxicity and Bier block: The drug, the technique, or the anesthetist. Anesthesiology 1984;61:782.

285. Bridenbaugh LD: The upper extremity: Somatic blockade. In: Cousins MJ, Bridenbaugh PO, eds: Neural Blockade in Clinical Anesthesia and Management of Pain, 2nd ed. Philadelphia: J.B. Lippincott; 1988:387–416.

286. Wagner AM, Suresh S: Peripheral nerve blocks for warts: Taking the cry out of cryotherapy and laser. Pediatr Dermatol 1998;15:238–241.

287. McNicol LR: Sciatic nerve block for children: Sciatic nerve block by the anterior approach for postoperative pain relief. Anaesthesia 1985;40:410–414.

288. McLeod DH, Wong DH, Claridge RJ, et al.: Lateral popliteal sciatic nerve block compared with subcutaneous infiltration for analgesia following foot surgery. Can J Anaesth 1994;41:673–676.

289. Dalens B, Tanguy A, Vanneuville G: Sciatic nerve blocks in children: Comparison of the posterior, anterior, and lateral approaches in 180 pediatric patients. Anesth Analg 1990;70:131–137.

290. Vloka JD, Hadzic A, Koorn R, et al.: Supine approach to the sciatic nerve in the popliteal fossa. Can J Anaesth 1996;43:964–967.

291. Zetlaoui PJ, Bouaziz H: Lateral approach to the sciatic nerve in the popliteal fossa. Anesth Analg 1998;87:79–82.

292. Hadzic A, Vloka JD: A comparison of the posterior versus lateral approaches to the block of the sciatic nerve in the popliteal fossa. Anesthesiology 1998;88:1480–1486.

293. Vloka JD, Hadzic A, Kitain E, et al.: Anatomic considerations for sciatic nerve block in the popliteal fossa through the lateral approach. Reg Anesth 1996;21:414–418.

294. Cappellino A, Jokl P, Ruwe PA: Regional anesthesia in knee arthroscopy: A new technique involving femoral and sciatic nerve blocks in knee arthroscopy. Arthroscopy 1996;12:120–123.

295. Greengrass RA, Klein SM, D'Ercole FJ, et al.: Lumbar plexus and sciatic nerve block for knee arthroplasty: comparison of ropivacaine and bupivacaine. Can J Anaesth 1998;45:1094–1096.

296. McLeod DH, Wong DH, Vaghadia H, et al.: Lateral popliteal sciatic nerve block compared with ankle block for analgesia following foot surgery. Can J Anaesth 1995;42:765–769.

297. Ronchi L, Rosenbaum D, Athouel A, et al.: Femoral nerve blockade in children using bupivacaine. Anesthesiology 1989;70:622–624.

298. Khoo ST, Brown TC: Femoral nerve block–the anatomical basis for a single injection technique. Anaesth Intens Care 1983;11:40–42.

299. Dalens B, Vanneuville G, Tanguy A: Comparison of the fascia iliaca compartment block with the 3-in-1 block in children. Anesth Analg 1989;69:705–713.

300. Capdevila X, Biboulet P, Bouregba M, et al.: Comparison of the three-in-one and fascia iliaca compartment blocks in adults: Clinical and radiographic analysis. Anesth Analg 1998;86:1039–1044.

301. Winnie AP: The "3-in-1 block": Is it really 4-in-1 or 2-in-1? [letter]. Reg Anesth 1992;17:176–179.

29 Postoperative Pain Management

Maurice S. Zwass, David M. Polaner, *and* Charles B. Berde

Assessment of Pain in Children

Pain Management Strategies

    Planning Postoperative Analgesia

    Preoperative Preparation of the Patient and Family

    Intraoperative Management and Postoperative Analgesia

Regional Blockade and Analgesia

The practice of pediatric anesthesia has evolved over recent years to include and incorporate the evaluation, treatment, and study of pain in infants and children. This enthusiasm of interest has resulted in an enormous expansion of the breadth of techniques that are currently employed as well as those being evaluated for perioperative pain management in the pediatric population. Clinicians who care for children are becoming skilled at techniques of assessment of pain and discomfort in the highly varied pediatric population. Healthcare professionals caring for all patients, and in particular children, are also evaluating the effectiveness of the pain management methods with respect to pain relief, incidence of side effects, and cost effectiveness.[1] Pain management techniques and their utilization in the pediatric postsurgical population has increased dramatically over recent years.[2] Anesthesiologists have the skills and knowledge that are particularly suited for the selection and application of safe and effective pain management techniques such as regional blockade and central neuraxis and parenteral opioid infusions. The recognition, study, and treatment of pain in infants and children are now an integral part of pediatric anesthetic practice.

Historically, postoperative analgesia was utilized sparingly, if administered at all, to pediatric patients. The common misconceptions were that neonates were physiologically unable to perceive pain, that children required primarily behavioral treatment for pain, and that all children were at excessive risk for respiratory depression after administration of opioids. These misconceptions led to limited use of analgesics in children. Studies comparing postoperative analgesic administration in children versus adults have repeatedly demonstrated under-dosing of children after surgery.[2] Agents such as acetaminophen were given in place of more potent drugs, and when opioids were used, only minimal amounts were administered. A limited understanding of the pharmacokinetics and pharmacodynamics of opioids in infancy and childhood raised concerns about the safety of their use, especially with regard to the risk of respiratory depression. With greater understanding of developmental physiology and pharmacology, there is no reason why any infant or child should be denied adequate analgesia. Indeed, mounting evidence suggests that inadequate analgesia may have detrimental consequences beyond the obvious concern for compassionate care.[3–6] Neuroendocrine responses, tissue catabolism, and postoperative pulmonary function are favorably altered by various techniques that provide postoperative analgesia.[7–10]

Assessment of Pain in Children

Although children 7 years of age and older can often use a visual analogue scale or numeric rating scale, assessing pain and the adequacy of therapy in younger children presents a challenge. Because pain is a subjective experience, a self-assessment scale is preferable to an observer's objective assessment and should be used whenever possible. Use of self-assessment ratings can help optimize analgesic therapy by avoiding overdoses and providing better analgesia during periods of greater pain. Younger school-aged children can often use a numeric rating scale. However, variations of traditional scales can improve the ability of a young patient's utilization of these measures. For example, a verbal self-assessment rating may prove to be easier to explain if the scores are reversed; because children associate high scores with good grades in school and thus a desirable outcome, a score of 10 is better interpreted as "no pain" and 0 as "the worst pain imaginable." Those not able to use numeric scales may be taught to use one of the visual scales such as the Oucher or Faces Pain Rating Scale. Presenting these to children in the preoperative period helps to familiarize them with the concept of rating pain and enables them to use the pain scale better after surgery. This teaching may be performed as a standard part of preoperative preparation of patients by the nursing staff and can help reassure children and parents that needs for pain relief will be attended to. If it is not possible to provide for thorough preoperative teaching of an assessment technique, hospital staff can provide this teaching early in the recovery period.

An objective observer must assess pain in preverbal children; there is no ideal assessment technique for pain for these patients. All objective rating systems rely on physical signs of sympathetic activity coupled with behavioral assessments; there is always some difficulty in separating behavior associated with pain from that caused by hunger, need for parents, and fear. Indeed, behavioral measurement scales, such as the Children's Hospital of Eastern Ontario Pain Scale,[11] may overestimate distress due to fear but may underestimate pain relative to measurements by self-reporting scales.[12] In general, if one believes that pharmacologic management has been adequate, an attempt should be made to comfort the child with behavioral interventions. If these measures are not successful, then additional analgesia should be provided. The opinion of a parent is often valuable in making these assessments, although some parents lose objectivity in such a situation. Similarly, older children with significant developmental delay may be best assessed by a regular caregiver. It should be remembered that fear and anxiety, especially in the intensive care unit setting, may also require treatment, and that sedation may be a desirable goal in some circumstances.[13]

Pain Management Strategies

Planning Postoperative Analgesia

The method by which one is to provide postoperative analgesia is an integral part of the anesthetic plan. Ideally, an analgesic plan should be clarified before induction of anesthesia, because of the need to obtain consent for certain procedures. Some analgesic techniques may also benefit from preoperative teaching of patients for the technique to be used optimally, such as patient-controlled analgesia (PCA).[14, 15] Other techniques will alter intraoperative anesthetic management. Some require the proper budgeting of induction time to avoid delaying the commencement of surgery. Consultation with the surgeon often provides information about the scope and requirements of the surgical procedure and particular postoperative care requirements that may further alter the anesthetic prescription for postoperative pain management. The clinician providing the perioperative anesthetic care for a patient should make it possible for patients to emerge from anesthesia in reasonable comfort. It is easier to maintain analgesia in a pain-free patient than to achieve analgesia in a patient experiencing severe pain.[16]

Developmental Considerations

When planning postoperative analgesia, it is prudent to consider both the chronologic and neurodevelopmental age of a patient. Older children with significant developmental delay may require a management technique that fits their developmental age rather than their chronologic age, although in most cases the pharmacologic actions of the drugs are not altered.

PREMATURE OR YOUNG INFANTS. Premature or very young infants who may have problems with central respiratory drive

may best benefit from a technique that minimizes use of opioids and central respiratory depressants.[17, 18] Infiltration of the wound edges with local anesthetics, peripheral nerve blocks, or regional blockade are especially useful in patients who are not mechanically ventilated. Regional blockade can be achieved by "single-shot" or continuous catheter techniques using low-concentration local anesthetics, which cause little motor blockade. Acetaminophen can be a useful adjunct because it has a large therapeutic window with few untoward effects (see later). Opioids are not contraindicated, but careful observation and monitoring are necessary to detect respiratory depression, especially in premature infants or term infants less than 1 month of age.[19] If opioids are administered to infants less than 6 months of age, they should be observed in either an intensive care setting or on a ward in which respiratory monitoring is available.

OLDER INFANTS AND TODDLERS. Older infants and toddlers can benefit from the same techniques described for younger infants. Continuous opioid infusions are appropriate in this age group, as are central neuraxis opioids in low to moderate doses. Behavioral techniques such as play therapy and the presence of a comforting parent can do much to augment whatever pharmacologic modalities are used. A painless and non-threatening induction technique and the presence of a parent or familiar adult during induction[20] and emergence can alleviate much of the anxiety and fear that may accompany the immediate postoperative period.[21]

PRESCHOOL- AND SCHOOL-AGED CHILDREN. Preschool- and school-aged children have both greater fears and better understanding of the postoperative experience than their younger counterparts. They need to be reassured that postoperative pain is of limited duration and that it will be treated effectively. Intellectually normal children older than approximately 7 years are often able to understand the concept of PCA, which may be very helpful in giving a sense of control back to the child during a period in which all other aspects of control are removed.[22] Regional techniques are, as in all age-groups, an excellent method of providing analgesia, especially for children who are easily nauseated or disturbed by the dysphoria that may accompany opioid administration.

ADOLESCENTS. Adolescents can be managed with any of the techniques described, although the issues of control and dependency assume even greater importance. Allowing them to participate in decision-making will contribute to the success of any analgesic technique.[22]

Surgical Considerations

The type of surgical procedure is often the deciding factor in choosing a particular technique for management of postoperative pain.[23–31] For example, with certain procedures, an epidural catheter may intrude into the surgical field, or access to the catheter site in the postoperative period may be obscured by a cast or dressing; in this circumstance, the catheter may be tunneled subcutaneously away from the surgical field. Urologic surgery, which is often associated with painful bladder spasms in the postoperative period, may be most advantageously managed with regional blockade, such as continuous lumbar or caudal analgesia with local anesthetics with or without epidural opioids. Preliminary evidence suggests that the incidence and severity of bladder spasms may be markedly reduced if regional blockade is administered for such procedures.[23, 24] There is some evidence that epidural blockade may favorably alter diaphragmatic mechanics after thoracotomy and upper abdominal surgery. Preliminary research suggests that this improvement may be a result of the motor blockade of the intercostal muscles and alteration in the resting length of the diaphragm, and not solely a result of actual reversal of diaphragmatic inhibition.[32–35] Most investigations do not support the contention that analgesia alone, achieved by either systemic or central neuraxis opioids, is of value in either diminishing postoperative diaphragmatic inhibition or significantly improving postoperative pulmonary function.[36, 37] Analgesia may, however, improve patient compliance with other measures, such as deep breathing and early mobilization, which are thought to reduce the incidence of postoperative complications.[25]

Anatomic Considerations

Certain techniques are not feasible in some patients because of anatomic anomalies. Most patients with myelodysplasia are not managed with an epidural catheter, although its use in these patients has been reported.[38] Patients with airway anomalies that may cause airway obstruction should not receive agents that cause excessive sedation. Patients who may have difficulty in operating the PCA pump control need a different analgesic technique. A patient with an anatomic contraindication to one technique, however, may be an excellent candidate for an alternative. Patients with airway anomalies causing a predisposition to obstruction, for example, may be ideally managed with regional blockade. Thus, the availability of various resources allows the anesthesia and surgical team to provide the best possible postoperative care for a wide variety of patients.

Preoperative Preparation of the Patient and Family

All patients benefit from a preoperative discussion with the anesthesiologist, but this is especially crucial with children. In pediatrics, one deals as much with the family as with the patient, and this time provides an opportunity to alleviate the fears of both the parents and the child regarding the postoperative period. This discussion can be reassuring to siblings as well, who often have fears and disturbing fantasies about their brother's or sister's operative experience. Psychological preparation of patients has long been known to favorably modify the amount of discomfort and anxiety experienced. The child and parents should be informed that every effort will be made to have the child as free of pain as possible and that although some discomfort is inevitable, it will be minimized. Patients who are to receive regional anesthesia and analgesia can benefit from an age-appropriate discussion of the temporary sensory and motor blockade that may be experienced postoperatively. Guided imagery and other relaxation techniques can be useful adjuncts to teach older children in the preoperative period.[39] Play therapy, both as a preoperative teaching tool and as a postoperative distracter, is also very helpful; a child life specialist is often enlisted by the pediatric service for this purpose.[40]

Intraoperative Management and Postoperative Analgesia

Neither the anesthetic plan nor the method of postoperative analgesia can be considered independently of each other. The analgesic technique must be instituted before emergence from anesthesia to allow patients to awaken from an anesthetic pain free. Thus, if a patient is to receive PCA, he or she should receive a loading dose of opioid before awakening. Likewise, if a patient is to receive a regional technique, the block should be placed while he or she is still anesthetized. On the other hand, if a patient is to receive a nerve block for postoperative analgesia, intraoperative opioids should not be required, unless they will fulfill another goal of the anesthetic plan. The next logical step in this line of reasoning is to incorporate the method of postoperative analgesia into the anesthetic plan as part of the anesthetic itself. When a continuous regional technique is to be used postoperatively, the catheter can be placed immediately after induction of general anesthesia and used as an adjunct to intraoperative anesthesia, thereby reducing the amount of general anesthetic agents required. If a single injection block is to be used, it too can be placed after induction and "topped up" with another injection of a long-acting agent at the end of the procedure. This technique has the advantage of a more rapid recovery time from general anesthesia, as well as the possibility of improved analgesia.[41] Experimental and clinical evidence suggest that preventing the transmission of painful nociceptive impulses to the central nervous system by using regional blockade before the surgical stimulus may result in improved analgesia in the postoperative period. Similarly, if PCA is to be used postoperatively, intraoperative use of opioids will reduce the requirement for volatile agents during surgery.

Techniques

NONOPIOID ANALGESICS. Acetaminophen is the nonopioid analgesic most commonly used in pediatrics. It should be regarded as the first-line agent in preference to aspirin because of aspirin's greater frequency of side effects, such as gastritis and platelet dysfunction as well as the rare but significant statistical association of aspirin with Reye syndrome. Acetaminophen is quite safe even in newborns[42]; in fact, immaturity of hepatic metabolism systems confers some degree of safety by decreasing the production of the toxic metabolite.[43] The traditionally recommended acetaminophen dose has probably been too conservative. A previous study showed that rectal dosage of 20 mg/kg in children after surgery resulted in inadequate levels.[44] Currently, the maximum oral dosage of acetaminophen is 15 mg/kg PO every 4 hours or a rectal loading dose of 30 to 40 mg/kg followed by 15 to 20 mg/kg PR or PO every 6 hours.[45, 46] Total daily dosing by either route should not exceed 100 mg/kg/day in children and, provisionally, 60 mg/kg/day in neonates.[47–49] Suppositories should not be cut, since the drug is not evenly distributed throughout the suppository; however, multiple suppository combinations can be used to obtain the desired dose. It should be noted that the absorption of rectal acetaminophen is quite irregular and delayed, with peak blood levels occurring at 60 to 180 minutes following administration.[47] In addition, the rectal dosage recommendations we make are manufacturer specific[50, 51] (FeverAll, Upsher-Smith Laboratories, distributed by Ascent Pediatrics, Inc., Wilmington, MA), since other manufacturers have different formulations that have not had extensive examination.[50, 51]

Several nonsteroidal anti-inflammatory drugs such as ibuprofen, indomethacin, and ketorolac have been studied in children. Perioperative intravenous administration of indomethacin reduces opioid requirements.[52] One report suggests that for children with arthritis, ibuprofen is as efficacious as aspirin and causes fewer side effects.[53] Although the intravenous formulation of ibuprofen is not approved for this indication in the United States, a rectal preparation that is available is a convenient alternative in patients unable to take oral medications. Short-course use of ketorolac is safe and efficacious when administered intravenously at a dosage of 0.5 mg/kg every 6 hours.[54–56] Ketorolac has been found to be useful in several situations, including (1) children who have cystic fibrosis and rib fractures, (2) children who experience bothersome opioid side effects postoperatively, and (3) children with sickle cell painful crisis and a narrow therapeutic margin for opioids.[57] Ketorolac can affect bleeding time[58] and can cause a degree of renovascular constriction; it therefore is of limited value in certain clinical situations, such as after tonsillectomy.[59] Another concern is the reports of impaired bone healing following spinal fusion; until further information is available, it may be reasonable to avoid ketorolac in this population.[60] Generally ketorolac is only administered following establishment of hemostasis.

A current area of research has been the study and development of NSAID-type agents of the cox-2 antagonist subtype.[61] These oral agents have the characteristic of analgesia with minimal effects on gastric mucosa and platelet function.[61–64] The currently available agents celecoxib (Celebrex) and rofecoxib (Vioxx) are approved for treatment of osteoarthritis and rheumatoid arthritis pain in adult patients. At this time there are no controlled studies evaluating the effects of these agents for treatment of pain in the pediatric population in the United States, although several preliminary studies from Italy suggest that cox-2 antagonists may be useful to treat pediatric patients, particularly those at increased risk for bleeding or gastritis.[65, 66]

OPIOIDS. Opioids are generally considered the first line of systemic therapy for moderate to severe postoperative pain. They can be safely and effectively administered without fear of oversedation and respiratory depression, provided the blood level of the opioid is maintained within a therapeutic range. Below this range, pain will resume, and above it, respiratory depression and other untoward effects can occur. Both the dose and the technique by which the opioid is delivered determine how well one is able to keep within this therapeutic window and avoid unwanted side effects.

Intramuscular and Subcutaneous Injections. These techniques have historically been the routine and most common routes of opioid administration in children, but they have significant disadvantages. Injections are frightening, unpleasant procedures for children and are often perceived as worse than the pain for which they are administered.[67] It is very common for a child in obvious pain to refuse or not request an injection of opioid because the continuous postsurgical pain is preferable to the fear and pain associated with needles.

Injections have the additional pharmacokinetic disadvantage of unpredictable and erratic uptake if regional blood flow is impaired and may produce pronounced peaks and valleys in blood concentration. The goal of maintaining an even level of analgesia is thus nearly impossible to achieve with this route of administration. This method also creates a situation in which patients must be perceived as having recurrence of pain to receive the next injection. More rational and compassionate methods of administration should relegate this route of administration to less frequent use.

Continuous subcutaneous administration of opioids may be one nonintravenous technique that will continue to have a place in postoperative pain management. Continuous-infusion opioids can be administered through a 25-gauge "butterfly" needle placed subcutaneously and secured with a clear bio-occlusive dressing. In patients who have adequate and consistent skin blood flow (no alterations of temperature or significant edema), this route may provide comparable blood levels to the intravenous route on a similar dosage schedule. A low rate of infusion (< 2–3 mL/hr) using concentrated opioid solutions and a highly accurate infusion pump are necessary. This technique can be particularly useful in patients with limited or difficult intravenous access, especially those with cancer pain or acquired immunodeficiency syndrome.[68, 69]

Intermittent Intravenous Injections. Although the use of an intravenous line eliminates the pain and fear of injections, intermittent intravenous injections with opioids of short or moderate duration do not achieve a stable blood level and predispose to periods of excessive sedation alternating with periods of inadequate analgesia. One solution to this problem is the use of methadone on a "sliding scale." Methadone has a much longer half-life than morphine, averaging approximately 19 hours, in children from 1 year of age through adolescence, although there is wide individual variation in clearance.[70–72] It provides much longer and more even periods of analgesia than that achieved with shorter-acting opioids, approaching the efficacy of continuous infusions. After adequate initial analgesia is achieved, children can receive intravenous doses of methadone as needed and titrated to their analgesic requirements. Mild pain can be treated with 0.03 mg/kg of methadone, moderate pain with 0.05 to 0.06 mg/kg, and severe pain with 0.07 to 0.08 mg/kg.[70, 73, 74] Children should be frequently assessed and the next dose administered before the recurrence of moderate to severe pain. A "reverse-PRN" schedule, in which the medication is offered but a patient can choose to refuse it, should be encouraged. The peak of respiratory depression and sedation occurs within 20 to 30 minutes of administration; the dose range should be decreased by 50% and the interval between injections increased if oversedation occurs.

Continuous Intravenous Infusion. In children who have moderate to severe pain and who are unable to take oral medications, opioids may be administered with great efficacy by continuous intravenous infusion. Once a therapeutic blood level is achieved, an infusion rate can be chosen to maintain that level. It is still necessary to observe patients on continuous infusions closely, because if excessive drug accumulates, respiratory depression will ensue. Many hours may elapse before this occurs, because the administered dose per hour in a continuous infusion is small and the rate of increase in the blood opioid level will be slow. In patients not receiving mechanical respiratory support and less than 1 year of age, respiratory monitoring and frequent nursing assessment are necessary safety measures. These patients, especially those younger than 1 month, may have immature ventilatory responses to hypoxia and hypercarbia and may be at greater risk for respiratory depression than older children.

Choice of Opioid for Intravenous Infusion. Morphine is the opioid most frequently used for postoperative analgesia. It has been extensively studied in all pediatric age groups. Preterm infants have extreme patient-to-patient variability in the terminal elimination half-life that is inversely related to postconceptual age; that is, the lower the post-conceptual age, the longer the elimination half-life.[75] In full-term infants less than 1 month of age, morphine clearance is about one third of that in older children and one half of that in adults. The elimination half-life is correspondingly prolonged, about three times that in adults.[19] Serum levels of 10 to 25 ng/mL are analgesic.[76] This level is usually achieved with an infusion rate of 5 to 15 μg/kg/hr after a loading dose of 0.025 to 0.075 mg/kg (25–75 μg/kg). In two neonates, seizures were reported during morphine infusions when the serum level exceeded 60 ng/mL, but a clear relationship between seizures and high serum morphine concentrations has not been firmly established.[77, 78]

It has long been assumed that infants are more likely to have respiratory depression due to opioids than older children on a pharmacodynamic basis, but this may not be the case. Although the data obtained from studies of rats suggest that neonates have increased brain concentrations of opioids for equal serum levels,[79] these findings may not be able to be extrapolated to humans. Newborn rats have a relatively immature brain and a far more permeable blood-brain barrier than do human infants, and thus this animal model may not accurately depict the human condition.[80] It appears that the "increased sensitivity" is related at least in part to pharmacokinetic variables, perhaps in some measure as a result of a neonate's decreased liver blood flow and conjugating ability. With appropriate doses and infusion rates, opioids can be safely, albeit cautiously, used in these patients. Hepatic disease, whether overt, as in neonatal hepatitis, or less obvious, as in impairment to hepatic blood flow after omphalocele repair, must be taken into account when choosing the dose of morphine. Vigilance in monitoring is, of course, mandatory in younger patients, and they need to be admitted to an appropriate unit where such nursing care is available.

After the age of 1 month and continuing throughout adolescence, morphine clearance is actually greater than in adults, primarily because of the metabolic pathways used for elimination and their relatively great hepatic blood flow. Although the ability of children to metabolize morphine with glucuronidase (the primary route of metabolism in adults) is deficient, the sulfation pathway is apparently more efficient and, in patients with normal renal excretion of the sulfated compound, leads to a higher clearance.[81] These children require a loading dose of 0.05 to 0.1 mg/kg and an initial infusion rate of 10 to 30 μg/kg/hr to maintain a morphine blood level in the analgesic range of 12 to 25 ng/mL. This provides adequate analgesia in most patients without hypercarbia due to respiratory depression (arterial carbon dioxide tension [$PaCO_2$] < 45 mm Hg). In cases in which higher infusion rates have been used and untoward effects occurred, sedation always preceded respiratory depression. *The onset of sedation is an important clinical index of incipient overdose and should alert the nursing staff and physicians to decrease the infusion rate and observe the patient more carefully.* Serum concentrations may vary considerably between patients; therefore, even at the lower rates of infusion, clinical vigilance is mandatory. Some children may require 40 to 50 μg/kg/hr, but infusions should generally be started at the lower to middle dosage range and titrated incrementally upward to avoid overdosage.

Hydromorphone has a spectrum of action similar to that of morphine and is roughly five times as potent with repeated systemic administration.[82] It may be a reasonable alternative to morphine as a means of avoiding morphine associated side effects. It should be noted that its potency in the epidural space is only two to three times that of morphine.

Fentanyl may be a useful substitute for morphine in patients who have hemodynamic instability and in whom any decrease in peripheral vascular tone is undesirable. This drug is also a good choice for patients who cannot tolerate the histamine release caused by morphine. In newborns, fentanyl, like morphine, has a prolonged elimination half-life, nearly twice that in adults. Neonates thus may be at greater risk for accumulation of drug than older infants. As with morphine, any impairment of hepatic blood flow further decreases the ability to conjugate fentanyl in these very young infants. Pharmacokinetic studies performed during steady-state infusions are lacking, but infants older than 3 months and less than 1 year of age have been reported to have lower plasma concentrations of fentanyl for a given administered bolus dose than older children and adults.[83] This finding is in keeping with the almost twofold greater clearance of fentanyl in these patients. They are also reported to have less respiratory depression (based on transcutaneous $PaCO_2$ measurements and the incidence of apnea) for a given plasma fentanyl concentration, although only two infants less than 6 months of age were studied.[84] Children older than 1 year have similar clearance to adults, but those less than 5 years of age also may have less respiratory depression than adults. Infusion rates of 1 to 4 μg/kg/hr are usually required for analgesia in children (born at term) over 3 months of age. Chest wall rigidity is exceedingly rare during these slow infusion rates.

Meperidine is an opioid that has been used clinically for many years.[85–87] Potency is approximately one tenth that of morphine. Meperidine has an active metabolite, normeperidine, which has central nervous system stimulant properties (some patients may describe euphoria) and can promote seizures in predisposed individuals.[88] Normeperidine has a relatively long half-life and levels can become quite elevated with prolonged administration and produce seizures.[88, 89] Normeperidine is renally excreted and can accumulate in patients with renal disease. This is not generally a drug of first choice for PCA and should be administered with caution if an infusion is to last for more than 36 hours because of the potential for normeperidine-induced seizures.

Patient-Controlled Analgesia. The major advantage of PCA is that an opioid blood level titrated to a patient's analgesic needs can be achieved by allowing the patient to self-administer small incremental intravenous boluses using a microprocessor-controlled pump. The patient is the one person best able to respond to the changing intensity of pain. He or she may activate the pump to deliver an additional amount of drug during physiotherapy, for example, and may use less drug during periods of rest and sleep. A safety mechanism is also inherent in PCA. Because the patient is the only one who administers the drug, he or she will fall asleep when oversedation occurs and is thus unlikely to self-administer an overdose. PCA requires, of course, that the pump settings be optimized for a patient's size and clinical status and that the administration of other potentially sedating agents such as antiemetics be considered when choosing the opioid dose and interval. The net result is a patient with an opioid blood level that is self-regulated within the therapeutic range. Most patients choose a dosage regimen that strikes a balance between sedation or other fairly minor side effects and adequate comfort.[90] Morphine is the usual drug of choice for PCA (Table 29–1).

Patient training is a necessary part of PCA, because successful use of PCA requires that both the child and family understand how it works.[15] They should be instructed that the pump should be activated whenever the child feels pain, that the child should not wait for severe pain to activate the pump, and that a dose can also be given in anticipation of painful stimuli such as ambulation or chest physiotherapy. Most children over 7 years of age can be taught to use the system properly,[91] but it is also essential that the parents understand that only the child should decide when to push the button for a dose of medication. The ability to give the child a sense of control over analgesic management is one of the most attractive features of PCA and makes it an especially useful mode of therapy for adolescents.

Most PCA pumps have four settings to adjust.

- A *loading dose* of opioid must be administered and, as with any morphine infusion, should total 0.025 to 0.1 mg/kg (25–100 µg/kg) divided into incremental doses. Further increments of 0.02 mg/kg can be added at 5- to 10-minute intervals until comfort is achieved. Optimal effectiveness with PCA necessitates that the patient is not in severe pain when therapy is turned over to him or her, since patient doses with this technique are generally small. If a patient is comfortable when he or she starts PCA, it will be easier to maintain comfort with the technique. It is necessary to provide a sufficient interval between incremental doses to allow the morphine to reach peak effect and thereby avoid overdose. If PCA is started in the postanesthesia recovery unit and the patient has awakened in comfort, a loading dose is not necessary. Similarly, if a nerve block was performed, the patient

may not begin to use the PCA demand boluses until the block begins to recede. In this case, the loading bolus increments can be administered as needed when the block begins to recede.

- A *patient bolus dose*, that is, the dose that will be administered with each patient activation of the pump, must be set. These small boluses are usually in the range of 0.01 to 0.025 mg/kg (10–25 µg/kg).
- A *lockout interval*, usually 6 to 12 minutes, must be set. This prevents a patient from activating the pump until the effect from the previous bolus is achieved, and it corresponds to the time from intravenous injection to the peak effect of the drug.
- A *maximum hourly dose* must be chosen. The physician can set a limit on the cumulative amount of drug a patient may administer, often ranging from 0.05 to 0.1 mg/kg/hr (50–100 µg/kg/hr). This amount may be chosen based on the average hourly use of morphine during the past 24 hours or, in patients started on PCA immediately after surgery, at the lower range of the dosage scale. Once this limit is reached, the patient is unable to activate the pump until the hour has passed. Many pumps have a 4-hour limit setting that allows for increased flexibility in dosing over longer periods of time and pain intensity.

In addition to self-activation of the pump, many devices have a basal infusion feature. This can be useful in providing background analgesia at night so that the patient is not awakened from sleep by the need to self-administer bolus doses. It also can be used to provide a low-rate (i.e., 10–15 µg/kg/hr of morphine) continuous infusion at all times to decrease the frequency with which a patient needs to activate the device.[92–97] One study suggests that the use of this basal infusion is advantageous, especially in the first 2 days after surgery.[98] There exists some controversy regarding routine basal infusion rates. Many surgical procedures result in postoperative pain that is not continuous, and the routine use of basal infusions has a potential for an increased incidence of minor side effects, such as pruritus and nausea without a large change in analgesic level.[92–94] Individual considerations are important, since some conditions or procedures are more likely to have continuous or larger degrees of discomfort. The use of a standing order form facilitates communication with the nursing staff and avoids confusion and errors in drug dosage. It also allows for a standardized approach to the treatment of complications (Fig. 29–1).

Variations of traditional PCA such as *parent*-controlled analgesia or *nurse*-controlled analgesia are used in several centers with reportedly good results.[97, 99] Nurse-controlled analgesia is especially flexible for titrating postoperative analgesia for infants and for children with developmental disabilities. Anecdotally, there have been several critical

Table 29–1. Patient-Controlled Analgesia (PCA) Dosage Guidelines (Morphine)*

Initial Bolus	PCA Dose	Basal Rate	Four-Hourly Maximum	Lockout Time
0.02 mg/kg (20 µg/kg) increments every 10 minutes until comfortable (see text)	0.01–0.025 mg/kg (10–25 µg/kg)	When used, 0.01–0.02 mg/kg/hr (10–20 µg/kg/hr); start immediately or after bolus (see text)	0.3 mg/kg (300 µg/kg)	6–12 min

*Recommendations apply to opioid naive subjects and may be modified further according to clinical need.

incidents with parent-controlled analgesia. We use it widely in the setting of palliative care, but are quite restrictive in its use for opioid-naïve children in the postoperative setting. These techniques require careful education of the individual in control of the medication administration. Some centers have found good results with these techniques by using a different philosophy regarding the orders for the pump. For example, with traditional PCA, small doses of opioid that can be administered frequently with a brief lockout interval, such as 6 minutes, are common. With nurse-controlled or parent-controlled techniques, the dosage lockout interval is usually longer, such as 10 to 15 minutes, but the dose of opioid may be slightly greater. This facilitates the parent's or nurse's not being required to push the button with great frequency. Careful selection of patients for nurse- or parent-controlled analgesia, monitoring of the patients, observing for side effects, and recognition of adequacy of pain control are critical with these techniques. In some centers, these variations of PCA may be offered to selected patients and families with significant experience within the hospital such as oncology patients.[82, 100, 101] This allows for administration of these techniques in somewhat younger patients than traditional PCA.

Side effects that may occur with any opioid administration technique include oversedation and respiratory depression, nausea, pruritus, dysphoria, and constipation. Titration to effect should avoid severe manifestations of these problems, although some patients are quite sensitive to the nausea that may accompany opioid use. In adults, scopolamine patches have been effective in treating opioid-induced nausea.[102] Droperidol (0.01 to 0.02 mg/kg; 10–20 μg/kg IV) or metoclopramide (0.10 to 0.15 mg/kg; 100–150 μg/kg IV) can both be effective, but these agents have potential for sedation and other side effects such as dystonia. The newer serotonin receptor antagonist antiemetics such as ondansetron and dolasetron have the advantage of virtually eliminating the risk of dystonic or oculogyric reactions seen with phenothiazines, butyrophenones, and metoclopramide, but headaches may be observed (see Fig 29–1).

Regional Blockade and Analgesia

The use of local anesthetics, both with and without the addition of central neuraxis opioids, offers many advantages in the postoperative setting. Blockade with long-acting local anesthetics can provide postoperative analgesia for outpatient surgery so that a child can be discharged home in comfort. Reducing or eliminating the need for systemic analgesics diminishes the potential for side effects associated with their use. Regional blockade affords the ability to provide high-quality analgesia to patients who might otherwise not tolerate larger amounts of opioids. This group includes some neonates, especially premature or former premature infants who are at risk for apnea; children with problems of central ventilatory control; patients with precarious airways, who risk obstruction with sedation; and those with respiratory disease.

There are few absolute contraindications to regional blockade. Anatomic anomalies, such as myelodysplasia, sacral dysgenesis, and other abnormalities either disrupting the epidural space or making access to it impossible, may pre-

vent the performance of a caudal or epidural block. A report of epidural analgesia in patients with myelodysplasia, however, suggests that catheters may be used safely in these patients when placed at a level above the anatomic neural abnormality.[38] A block should never be placed through an infected area or in proximity to it. Patients with burn injury may be candidates for continuous epidural techniques, provided the burned area is clearly distant from the catheter placement site, but we do not believe the benefits of regional analgesia outweigh the potential risks inherent in inserting catheters through burned tissue or close to it. We have limited our use of catheters in burned patients to those having burns on less than 30% of body surface area and having no burned areas contiguous with the catheter insertion site. Patients with sepsis present a similar problem; in general, we do not place caudal or epidural catheters in septic patients for fear of seeding the epidural space during a period of bacteremia. Axillary or intrapleural catheters may pose less of a problem, but no data regarding this issue exist. Coagulopathy and thrombocytopenia are relative contraindications to regional anesthesia, but milder abnormalities in hemostasis do not necessarily preclude a block. When a surgical procedure on an extremity has involved a nerve repair or revision, some surgeons may wish to assess motor or sensory function postoperatively. In these cases, consultation with the surgeon should precede a plan for postoperative regional analgesia. If the surgery involved the legs, a caudal or lumbar epidural catheter can be used with opioids rather than local anesthetics.

Opinions about whether a block should be placed at the beginning or end of the surgical procedure differ, but increasing evidence suggests that placing a block before the onset of surgery offers several advantages. Initial studies of adults demonstrated a dramatic decrease in the incidence of phantom limb pain when epidural blockade is administered before amputation; however, not all subsequent studies have confirmed this observation.[41, 103–108] Similarly, patients who receive intraoperative neural blockade may experience less postoperative pain than those managed with general anesthesia alone, with the duration of analgesia in some cases lasting beyond the pharmacologic action of the block.[109] It is theorized that interruption of nociceptive impulses at the spinal cord level prevents imprinting of painful stimuli on the sensory cortex or forestalls the development of spinal cord hyperexcitability, thereby reducing the neural input producing prolonged postoperative pain.[108, 110–112] Further evidence suggests that local anesthetic infiltration of the incision site, especially when performed in conjunction with a regional anesthetic technique, may be an effective means of providing prolonged analgesia after surgery.[113] Local infiltration of the incision site with local anesthetic solution alone is extremely effective in relieving postoperative pain.[114] This simple and effective adjunct can be used before virtually any surgical procedure. A major limitation of peripheral nerve blocks and wound infiltration with currently available local anesthetics is that the duration of analgesia is commonly only 4 to 6 hours. Since postoperative pain commonly persists for several days, it would be more useful to have local anesthetics that could provide analgesia for 2 to 4 days. One method currently under investigation to achieve prolonged analgesia involves injection of a suspension of microspheres containing bupivacaine, tiny amounts of dexa-

HYPOTHETICAL HOSPITAL ORDERS	USE PLATE OR PRINT
IMPORTANT: Pain service orders should be both institutional and practice specific; these orders are meant for illustration only.	PT. NAME _____ LAST FIRST MEDICAL REC. NO. _____

COMPLETE SECTION IF Admit OR Rewrite Orders
Weight _____ kg   Diagnosis _____
Allergies / adverse drug reactions _____

Date/Time	

PCA ORDER SHEETS – Page 1

1. Medication and Dosing:

    A. No other systemic analgesics or sedatives other than acetaminophen are to be administered unless approved by a pain service physician.

    B. Loading Dose (choose one, cross out others):
        If patient is alert and in pain give:

Morphine	0.03 mg/kg	× _____ kg =	_____ mg
Hydromorphone	0.006 mg/kg	× _____ kg =	_____ mg
Fentanyl	0.3 mCg/kg	× _____ kg =	_____ mg

        If comfortable or somnolence do not give loading dose.

    C. Mode (choose one, cross out others):
        _____ PCA   _____ continuous   _____ PCA and continuous

    D. PCA Settings: ♣♣ (Doses should be adjusted according to clinical circumstances.)

PCA dose **Morphine (1 mg/ml)**	0.025 mg/kg × _____ kg =	_____ mg
Lockout interval	(usual range 6–12 minutes)	_____ minutes
Continuous Morphine start at	0.015 mg/kg × _____ kg =	_____ mg/hr
4 hour limit Morphine	0.3 mg/kg × _____ kg =	_____ mg
PCA dose **Hydromorphone (0.5 mg/ml)**	0.005 mg/kg × _____ kg =	_____ mg
Lockout interval	(usual range 7–12 minutes	_____ minutes
Continuous Hydromorphone start at	0.003 mg/kg × _____ kg =	_____ mg/hr
4 hour limit Hydromorphone	0.06 mg/kg × _____ kg =	_____ mg
PCA dose **Fentanyl (50 mCg/ml)**	0.25 mCg/kg × _____ kg =	_____ mCg
Lockout interval	(usual range 7–12 minutes	_____ minutes
Continuous Fentanyl start at	0.15 mCg/kg × _____ kg =	_____ mCg/hr
4 hour limit Fentanyl	4 mCg/kg × _____ kg =	_____ mCg

♣♣Note that some PCA pumps will not allow exact settings and will require some slight increase or decrease compared with the desired setting.

2. Monitoring and Equipment:

	YES	NO
A. Continuous pulse oximetry	☐	☐
B. Ambu bag, O$_2$ tubing, face mask and suction at bedside	☐	☐
C. Ampule naloxone (Narcan®) immediately available	☐	☐
D. Impedance apnea monitor	☐	☐

Figure 29–1. *See legend on opposite page*

HYPOTHETICAL HOSPITAL ORDERS **IMPORTANT:** Pain service orders should be both institutional and practice specific; these orders are meant for illustration only.	USE PLATE OR PRINT PT. NAME _____ 　　　　　　　　LAST　　　　　　　　FIRST MEDICAL REC. NO. _____

COMPLETE SECTION IF Admit OR Rewrite Orders
Weight _____ kg　　　　　Diagnosis _____
Allergies / adverse drug reactions _____

Date/Time	
	PCA ORDER SHEETS – Page 2

3. Side Effects Management:

  A. Respiratory Management

      1. In the event of severe somnolence or RR < 12, stimulate, apply oxygen, disconnect PCA pump and notify pain service and primary service.

      2. If patient is cyanotic, severely unresponsive, RR < 8 or apnea, BP systolic < 65, stimulate, apply oxygen, disconnect PCA pump.
          Stat page "anesthesia-stat beeper," pain service physician, primary service
          Draw up naloxone (Narcan®) as follows. Dilute 1 ml of (0.4 mg) with 9 mL of normal saline to make 0.04 mg/mL (circle dose)

Age	Incremental Dose (mg)	Incremental Dose (mL)
< 1 year of age	0.02 mg	0.5 mL
≥ 1 year < 12 yrs	0.04 mg	1 mL
≥ 12 years	0.08 mg	2 mL

  B. For nausea (choose one, cross out the others):

    _____   1. Perphenazine (Trilafon) 0.015–0.025 mg/kg × _____ kg = _____ mg IV over 20 minutes q 6 hr prn; hold for somnolence

    _____   2. Prochlorperazine (Compazine) _____ mg PO PR IM (Circle one) q 6 h prn

    _____   3. Droperidol 0.010–0.025 mg/kg × _____ kg = _____ mg IV q 6 hr

    _____   4. Metoclopramide 0.1–0.2 mg/kg × _____ kg = _____ mg IV (max 1 mg) q 6 hr

    _____   5. Ondansetron (0.1–0.15 mg/kg) × _____ kg = _____ mg (4 mg max) q 6 h

    _____   6. Dolasetron 0.35 mg/kg × _____ kg = _____ mg (max 12.5 mg) ×1

  C. Urinary Retention: Assess for bladder distention and hypovolemia; if no urination for 8 hours, may straight cath PRN after notification of the primary service.

  D. Pruritus:

    Diphenhydramine (Benadryl)* 0.5 mg/kg　　× _____ kg = _____ mg
    IV over 20 minutes q 6h PRN pruritus, hold for somnolence.

    *PCA machine must be turned off 15 minutes prior to and during infusion of diphenhydramine and other sedating medications.

4. Non-Opioid Analgesia:
  Acetaminophen 10–15 mg/kg × _____ kg = _____ mg PO q 4 h PRN pain
  (10–15 mg/kg q 4 h with a maximum of 5 doses within 24 hours).
  Avoid PR route in patients with neutropenia and bleeding risk.

Ordered by _____ M.D.
Pain Service Physician

Figure 29–1. A typical standing order sheet for patient-controlled analgesia in children. Note that contingency orders for untoward effects are clearly spelled out and that physician backup is available at all times.

methasone, and a biodegradable polymer. Following injection, these microspheres release bupivacaine in a controlled manner to provide blockade of peripheral nerves for periods of 2 to 6 days, depending on dose, formulation, and site of injection.[115, 116]

Placing a single injection block before incision does not appear to shorten the duration of postoperative analgesia after brief surgical procedures; no difference was found in the time from awakening until the first request for analgesics whether a caudal block was placed before incision or after surgery for inguinal herniorrhaphy.[117] These data were for procedures of less than 1 hour in duration. For longer procedures, the block may be topped up with a second caudal injection before emergence. A volume of one half of the original injection is usually sufficient if less than 3 hours have elapsed. If a catheter technique is to be used for postoperative analgesia, it is preferable to place the catheter before surgery and use it as part of a "combined" anesthetic technique.

SINGLE INJECTION BLOCKS. When the duration of pain after surgery is not expected to be prolonged or the pain is not expected to be severe, a single-shot nerve block technique may be chosen. Both peripheral nerve blocks and central neuraxis blocks (caudal or lumbar epidural) may be used. This therapy is particularly valuable for outpatient surgery. Dilute long-acting local anesthetics are used, 0.1% or 0.125% bupivacaine being the most common. This agent has the dual advantages of long duration and minimal motor blockade. Epinephrine (1:200,000) is often added to decrease systemic absorption and increase duration of action but *must be omitted when a digital or penile block is performed because of the risk of inducing ischemia by direct vasoconstriction.* The duration of sensory blockade and quality of analgesia with 0.25% and 0.125% bupivacaine for caudal block have been found to be similar, although the patients receiving the 0.125% solution had significantly less motor blockade.[118] More concentrated solutions of bupivacaine (0.25%) may be used to block a nerve when motor function is not a concern, such as for an ilioinguinal-iliohypogastric nerve block after herniorrhaphy. There is no advantage in the use of bupivacaine 0.5% solutions in most settings, and use of several different solution concentrations may increase the risk of erroneous dose calculations, leading to potential overdosage. It is the impression of some clinicians that a better quality block results with the more concentrated solutions, although this has not been subjected to controlled investigation. The maximum allowable dose of bupivacaine is 2.5 to 3.0 mg/kg, and this dose may be a limiting factor when using the more concentrated solutions.

Other agents have been added to the local anesthetic in caudal blocks to attempt to improve the duration of the sensory block with local anesthetics. Clonidine, in a dose of 0.5 to 2 μg/kg seems to increase the duration of analgesia of bupivacaine in caudal blocks with insignificant hemodynamic effects, mild sedation, and no delay in recovery times.[119–124] Clonidine is an attractive additive, since it appears to produce much less nausea, itching, ileus, urinary retention, or respiratory depression than opioids. We discourage the addition of opioids to caudal blocks for outpatients because of their increased risk for these side effects.

Preservative-free ketamine has also been used as an agent in caudal blocks, both alone and in combination with bupivacaine. Doses of 0.5 mg/kg appeared to be adequate and no behavioral findings were noted with this dose; when used in combination with bupivacaine, duration of analgesia approached 24 hours. *It should be noted that only preservative-free ketamine should be used.*[125, 126] In the United States, no preservative-free formulation of ketamine is available.[121, 127]

Ropivacaine is a relatively recent addition to the choice of local anesthetic agents available for use. In adult studies, it may offer anesthesia and analgesia duration similar to bupivacaine with more selective sensory blockade and less cardiotoxicity than bupivacaine.[128–132] There is clinical experience in pediatric patients showing effectiveness of ropivacaine, but it has been difficult to demonstrate a clear advantage of this agent in pediatric patients with respect to sensory versus motor selectivity.[130, 132–137] There are presently no studies in infants and children showing a safety benefit to the use of ropivacaine. Neurologic toxicity such as seizures can occur with this compound.[138, 139] Should studies show an advantage with regard to patient safety, ropivacaine would become quite a popular agent for use in pediatric patients.[134–137]

Another local anesthetic agent undergoing clinical trials at the present time is levobupivacaine (the levo-isomer of bupivacaine). This agent may possess clinical properties similar to bupivacaine with a modest reduction of the toxicity risks inherent to bupivacaine.[140–142] Studies with this agent are ongoing.[143]

When performing a regional block, the total safe dose of local anesthetic should be calculated first, and the volume and concentration of the solution should be adjusted if necessary to avoid exposing patients to potentially toxic quantities. A valuable consideration is that since many pediatric patients will undergo regional blockade in combination with general anesthesia, surgical concentrations of local anesthetics are not necessary, and dilute agents can still provide excellent analgesia. This is particularly important when performing blocks in infants. For example, a 2 kg infant has a maximal allowable dose of 5 mg of bupivacaine; if a 0.25% solution (2.5 mg/mL) were to be administered, the total volume would have to be limited to only 2 mL.

Inguinal herniorrhaphy is frequently performed in children, and the placement of an ilioinguinal-iliohypogastric nerve block provides excellent postoperative analgesia. It appears similar in efficacy to a caudal block and has a duration of at least 4 hours when bupivacaine with epinephrine is used. For orchiopexy, ilioinguinal nerve block has been found to be as effective as caudal blockade to the T10 level in a randomized and blinded investigation.[144] In our experience, however, postoperative analgesia for procedures that involve considerable manipulation and traction on the spermatic cord and testis may be better managed with caudal blockade. Penile block is effective for both circumcision and distal, simple hypospadias repair; more extensive procedures on the penis, especially repair of penile-scrotal hypospadias, require a caudal block.[145]

Nerve blocks of the lower extremity can be used instead of caudal blockade. They provide a more limited field of analgesia, are of long duration, and eliminate some of the potential undesirable effects of central neuraxis blockade, such as urinary retention, widespread motor blockade, and the occasionally unpleasant sensation of numbness that can accompany a denser sensory block. The fascia iliaca block has been described in children and appears to offer an excellent alternative for postoperative analgesia of a lower extremity.[146] Blockade of the femoral nerve and the nerves of the ankle are easily performed in children, using similar landmarks as in adults (see Chapter 28). The femoral nerve is quite superficial, and the use of a nerve stimulator and Teflon-coated needle makes its identification much easier in an anesthetized child, while reducing the risk of injury to adjacent structures. The upper extremity may be approached by an axillary block or by blocks to the individual nerves of the arm or hand. Intercostal nerve blocks are commonly used after thoracic or upper abdominal surgery. This block may be particularly well suited for procedures of limited scope, such as open lung biopsy or thoracostomy for drainage. More extensive surgery can be anticipated to cause postoperative pain of longer duration and may be best managed with a catheter technique.

CATHETER TECHNIQUES. A catheter placed in the epidural space affords an anesthesiologist the ability to provide continuous uninterrupted analgesia for long periods after surgery. These catheters are usually left in place for about 3 days but can be used for as long as 7 days; if they are tunneled, even longer use may be possible with proper care. Catheters can also be placed in intrapleural or extrapleural/retropleural locations to provide analgesia after thoracic surgery and in the axillary sheath for upper extremity surgery. In our experience, intrapleural analgesia reduces, but does not eliminate, the need for systemic opioids. Continuous regional blockade is remarkably effective and safe, although, as with any technique, monitoring for untoward effects is necessary to prevent complications. A number of agents, alone or in combination, can be infused to optimize care for a particular patient (Table 29–2).

CAUDAL AND EPIDURAL CATHETERS. For practitioners who are less experienced with lumbar epidural catheterization in young children, the caudal route is recommended for patients younger than 6 years. With experience and proper equipment, the lumbar route is feasible at any age, but specific expertise is required for infants and toddlers. In infants and children up to about 6 years of age, some reports suggest

Table 29–2. Suggested Epidural Infusion Solutions

Common Epidural Infusion Solutions for Older Children

Bupivacaine 0.1% plain (no other medications)
Bupivacaine 0.1% with fentanyl, 1–3 μg/mL (0.001–0.003 mg/mL)
Bupivacaine 0.1% with fentanyl 1–3 μg/mL (0.001–0.003 mg/mL) and with clonidine 1 μg/mL (0.001 mg/mL)
Bupivacaine 0.1% with just clonidine 1 μg/mL (0.001 mg/mL)
Bupivacaine 0.1% with just hydromorphone 10 μg/mL (0.01 mg/mL)
Bupivacaine 0.1% with just morphine 20 μg/mL (0.02 mg/mL)

Epidural Infusion Solutions for Neonates

Chloroprocaine 1.5% plain (no other additives)
Chloroprocaine 1.5% with fentanyl, 0.4 μg/mL (0.0004 mg/mL)*
Chloroprocaine 1.5% with clonidine 0.2 μg/mL (0.0002 mg/mL)*

*Note that lower concentrations of fentanyl or clonidine are used in neonates because of the higher infusion rate used with chloroprocaine.

that catheters may be advanced freely from the caudal canal cephalad to lower thoracic levels with excellent success.[147] However, other authors describe less reliability with caudal-to-thoracic advancement of catheters in patients larger than 10 kg.[148] If specific dermatomal placement of a catheter is important, it may be wise to obtain an imaging study to confirm location of a catheter. The rationale for threading the caudal catheter up the epidural space is that these patients have a less developed vascular plexus and more compact and globular fat than in older children and adults, usually allowing the catheter to pass unimpeded.[147, 149] The distance from the sacral hiatus to the desired vertebral body is simply measured on the back and the catheter passed the appropriate distance. A standard 20-gauge epidural catheter can be passed through a 16- or 18-gauge (depending on the brand of epidural catheter used) intravenous cannula or a Crawford needle placed in the caudal space in most children weighing more than about 6 kg. In smaller infants and premature infants, 21- or 24-gauge "pediatric" epidural catheters allow the use of much smaller (19- or 20-gauge) introducer needles or cannulas. These small catheters also allow the use of a lumbar or thoracic approach with a Tuohy needle in any small child, should anatomic or surgical considerations require it. However, many practitioners prefer to use standard epidural kits with shorter introducer needles that accept the standard epidural catheters. Catheters made of nylon or polyamide may be less likely to kink beneath the skin and seem to thread more easily than those made of Teflon or other materials. The catheter should never be advanced if resistance is felt. It has been reported that in neonates weighing less than 3.5 kg, unlike in older infants and young children, one may not be able to pass catheters to higher levels without some risk of the catheter looping back, kinking, or puncturing the dura.[150] In that series of 20 premature infants, epidurography revealed misplaced catheters in three.

Threading catheters cephalad also appears less reliable in older children, probably because of the more mature composition of the epidural space. With age, the epidural fat appears to lose the spongy gelatinous character noted in infants, and the spaces between the fat globules become less distinct.[147, 149] Because the volume of local anesthetic solution required is directly related to the distance of the catheter tip from the innervation of the operative site, a caudal or low lumbar catheter may not provide adequate analgesia for upper abdominal or thoracic surgery unless a very high infusion rate is used. Even then, it may be difficult to maintain an adequate height of blockade if a patient is not fully recumbent. This is also true to some extent for the highly lipophilic opioids, such as sufentanil and fentanyl. In this circumstance, there are several alternative choices for upper abdominal or thoracic surgery.

■ Hydrophilic opioids, such as morphine or hydromorphone, can be administered through lumbar or caudal catheters. With these agents, a wider range of dermatomes can be covered after caudal or lumbar catheter placement, and only small increases in dose are required for a surgical site distant from the catheter tip. This same characteristic, unfortunately, also appears to increase the risk for side effects, including respiratory depression, as a result of rostral spread of morphine in the cerebrospinal fluid to the central respiratory center in the brainstem. Hydromorphone may also offer some advantages because there is less rostral spread when administered by the epidural route and slightly less itching than morphine, but it provides more rostral spread than fentanyl.[151, 152] Lumbar administration spreads sufficiently to provide thoracic analgesia.[153] It should be noted that the potency of hydromorphone in the epidural space is less than when it is administered systemically (2–3:1 epidural vs 5:1 systemic).[154]

■ A thoracic epidural catheter can be inserted in a sedated, awake patient. With the catheter tip located at a thoracic dermatomal level, local anesthetic-lipophilic opioid infusions, such as bupivacaine-fentanyl, may be chosen, as described later.

■ One accepts the calculated risk associated with thoracic catheter placement in an anesthetized patient. Some clinicians are hesitant to perform thoracic epidural puncture in anesthetized patients because of the inability to use patient reports (paresthesia, lancinating pain) as an indicator of improper catheter or needle placement. Although clinical series have reported successful and safe thoracic catheter placement in children,[155 156] this technique should be applied only by experienced practitioners who are mindful of the risk-to-benefit ratio of the technique.[157, 158]

It is extremely important to secure the catheter to the skin with a clear occlusive dressing so that the caudal catheter does not become contaminated or dislodged and the catheter site can be inspected daily. In addition, tincture of benzoin or other adhesive solution reduces the incidence of catheter and dressing displacement. The use of an adhesive-edged plastic drape, covering the area from the gluteal crease over the dressing, also helps prevent soiling of the dressing by children who are in diapers. We have not experienced any episodes of insertion site contamination or infection using these methods. The use of lumbar catheters removes the insertion site from the diaper area and thereby further reduces the potential for contamination of the catheter and the insertion site.

Management of patients with an epidural catheter involves nursing management and monitoring and medical management of drug selection and dosing. It is important to recognize that comprehensive treatment of these patients can be successful only if the medical and nursing services coordinate care in all areas. As with PCA or continuous-infusion opioids, the orders should be standardized and written in consultation with the nursing staff so that misinterpretations are less likely to occur (Fig. 29–2). Because the single most sensitive monitor of patients receiving epidural opioids is the nurse, not any mechanical or electronic device, education of the nursing staff is of paramount importance in ensuring safety. Nursing staff can also assess the adequacy of analgesia and thereby help titrate the drug dose. Catheter insertion sites should be inspected daily, both for the integrity of the dressing and for any evidence of erythema or skin infection. When continuous infusions are used, to preclude unintended epidural administration of drugs intended for intravenous use, the tubing connecting the infusion pump to the catheter should not have any injection ports and it should be clearly labeled as an epidural catheter.

A variation of traditional epidural analgesia and PCA that is being employed by some centers is the technique of patient-controlled epidural analgesia.[159] With this variation of traditional PCA, patients are generally maintained with an infusion of epidural analgesics (frequently opiate alone or an opiate–local anesthetic mixture), and have the capability of self-administering supplemental doses when needed.[160, 161] With this technique, the background infusion is used to provide the majority of the analgesia and the patient can add to this when needed. It is useful to realize that the time needed for a bolus dose to effect a change is somewhat longer with epidural administration compared with intravenous agents. Therefore with patient-controlled epidural anesthesia, lockout intervals are longer (often 15–30 minutes).[160, 161] The considerations one would employ for choosing this technique include the same patient monitoring factors for intravenous PCA and epidural analgesia.

SELECTION OF DRUGS AND DOSES. Many drugs and combinations have been administered via the epidural space to provide postoperative analgesia. The most common choices involve mixtures of local anesthetics and opioids, such as bupivacaine and fentanyl, although increasingly, clonidine is being used as well (see Table 29–2). The choice of drug is based on several factors: the age and size of the patient and the underlying medical conditions that may decrease the margin of safety of one of the agents. Epidural opioids should be used with great caution or at considerably reduced doses in patients with high risk for apnea or hypoventilation, such as premature infants or patients with chronic respiratory failure. Since it is often difficult to provide sufficient analgesia with bupivacaine alone at any safe infusion rate in the neonate, we commonly use epidural chloroprocaine infusions in neonates.[162] Epidural blockade in infants and young children is characterized by remarkable hemodynamic stability. They develop little or no hypotension in response to the sympathectomy caused by even high levels of thoracic blockade. This phenomenon has been attributed to their lack of significant resting sympathetic vascular tone, as demonstrated by Doppler studies of the lower extremities during caudal anesthesia.[163, 164]

For lower abdominal or lower extremity surgery in children, and lumbar epidural or caudal catheters with the tip in a lumbar position, one can recommend local anesthetic-opioid combined infusions, for example, 0.1% bupivacaine with fentanyl, 2 to 3 μg/mL, at starting infusion rates of 0.1 to 0.2 mL/kg/hr, ranging up to 0.4 mL/kg/hr. This regimen provides adequate analgesia in a majority of cases. When a block is not previously established in the operating room, it is useful to dose catheters with local anesthetic (without narcotics) at a volume of 0.05 mL/kg per spinal segment, not to exceed 5 mg/kg of lidocaine or 2.5 mg/kg of bupivacaine. We caution against administering bupivacaine chronically at infusion rates in excess of 0.4 mg/kg/hr (equaling 0.4 mL/kg/hr for 0.1% bupivacaine) for children, because toxicity may result.[165] Similarly, starting epidural fentanyl infusion rates should not exceed 1 μg/kg/hr; the upper limits of epidural fentanyl dosage are determined by clinical effect. If epidural local anesthetic infusions are begun without either opioids or clonidine (e.g., 0.1% bupivacaine), and inadequate analgesia occurs at infusion rates of 0.4 mL/kg/hr (a dosage of 0.4 mg/kg/hr), further increases in local anesthetic infusion rate or concentration should be avoided. Instead, the placement of the catheter should be confirmed, such as with a chloroprocaine test. If the catheter is properly located, an epidural opioid or clonidine should be added to the local anesthetic in the infusion. In our view, it is imperative to confirm that an epidural is properly functioning immediately after an infant or child arrives in the postanesthesia care unit or if there is any question of its proper location later. If lidocaine or bupivacaine has been given during surgery or postoperatively, for example, with an initial bolus and then a continuous infusion, then use of a repeat bolus dose of either of these amino-amides will result in a "staircasing" of plasma concentrations, with a risk of systemic toxicity. Although administration of epidural or systemic opioids may provide analgesia, they may not clarify the site of the epidural catheter. For this reason, we have chosen to use a standardized "chloroprocaine test," both to provide rapid analgesia and to confirm the site of placement. A chloroprocaine test is presented in Table 29–3.

Neonates have risk factors such as decreased protein binding of local anesthetic drugs (a problem with bolus administration resulting in increased free-unbound drug availability), and perhaps a less-developed metabolism (leading to drug accumulation) of these agents, which place them at risk for earlier potential toxicity. The symptomatic manifestations of toxicity in infants and neonates may be more difficult to recognize. Hence, a maximum infusion dose for bupivacaine of 0.2 mg/kg/hr is likely to be safe in the neonatal population.[166–168] In general, lower concentrations of bupivacaine than 0.05% to 0.1% may not consistently provide adequate analgesia, and concentrations greater than 0.125% may cause excessive motor blockade and increase the administered dose of drug. Because the volume of solution required to fill the epidural space on a milliliter per kilogram basis appears to decrease with age, older children and adolescents may require less volume than infants and young children based on weight (Table 29–4). Although the amino-amide local anesthetics have slow clearance in newborns and younger infants, the amino-ester chloroprocaine is cleared extremely rapidly even in premature infants, with elimination half-lives of at most a few minutes. This permits large doses and infusion rates with a reduced risk of systemic toxicity. Some previous concerns regarding chloroprocaine involved a succession of formulations with preservatives, including metabisulfite, methylparaben, and ethylene-diamine-tetra-acetic acid. A current formulation is truly preservative free.

If the catheter tip can be placed at thoracic dermatomes, similar bupivacaine-fentanyl[24, 25, 28, 29, 169, 170] or ropivacaine-fentanyl infusion solutions and rates may be used for thoracic and upper abdominal surgery.[171] If this is not possible, other agents may be administered through lumbar or caudal catheters as follows. For morphine, epidural bolus doses of 0.03 to 0.05 mg/kg (30–50 µg/kg) may be administered every 6 to 12 hours as needed.[172] Because the time to onset of analgesia is between 30 and 90 minutes, the doses must be administered at the earliest sign of return of pain. Alternatively, an epidural morphine infusion may be administered at a rate of 0.005 mg/kg/hr (5µg/kg; doses usually range from 4–8 µg/kg/hr) after a small initial bolus. Hydromorphone may be used either by bolus or infusion; studies of adults would suggest a 3:1 to 5:1 epidural potency ratio to morphine.[153] Lumbar epidural hydromorphone is commonly administered at epidural infusion rates of 0.001 to 0.003 mg/kg/hr (1 to 3 µg/kg/hr) for thoracic surgery. Hydrophilic opioids, especially when administered by infusion, require prolonged careful observation, as outlined later. *If somnolence or shallow breathing occur, infusions must be stopped,*

Table 29–3. Procedure for the Chloroprocaine Test

An anesthesiologist is present for the procedure, with use of standard monitors and supplies for providing respiratory or hemodynamic support.

1. A loading dose of chloroprocaine 3% is divided in five equal increments, each given at 1- to 2-minute intervals (over 5–10 minutes total) according to age approximately as follows (doses may be adjusted according to clinical circumstances):

Weight Group	Incremental Volume	Total Volume
0–10 kg	0.125 mL/kg	0.7 mL/kg
10–20 kg	0.1 mL/kg	0.5 mL/kg
20–35 kg	2.5 mL (fixed volume)	12.5 mL (fixed volume)
35–60 kg	3 mL (fixed volume)	15 mL (fixed volume)
≥ 60 kg	3.5 mL (fixed volume)	17.5 mL (fixed volume)

2. Incremental dosing is stopped before giving the full dose if there are clear signs of bilateral lower extremity sensory or motor block, or a very definite reduction in heart rate (e.g., 30 beats per minute) and blood pressure (e.g., 25 mm Hg drop in systolic pressure). In most cases, since you are performing this test because of signs of pain, there is some tachycardia and hypertension relative to baseline values at the start of the test. Transient cessation of crying in an infant or toddler is not a sufficiently specific positive response to warrant interruption of the test.
3. A catheter positioned in the *thoracic* epidural space will generally not show lower extremity sensory or motor block with the chloroprocaine test, but should give a very clear drop in heart rate and blood pressure, as well as a clear and persistent reduction in pain reports or pain behaviors.
4. If the chloroprocaine test is positive (i.e., confirms epidural placement), this implies that a stronger or different epidural solution is needed for steady-state pain relief. Since hydromorphone is sufficiently hydrophilic to spread from lumbar to thoracic spinal levels, *switching the solution from bupivacaine-fentanyl to bupivacaine-hydromorphone will provide good steady-state pain relief in more than 90% of these cases.* A typical loading dose of hydromorphone of 2 µg/kg (0.002 mg/kg) will provide analgesia within 30 minutes in most cases.
5. If the chloroprocaine test fails to confirm epidural placement, the catheter is either removed or replaced according to clinical circumstances.

HYPOTHETICAL HOSPITAL ORDERS	USE PLATE OR PRINT
IMPORTANT: Pain service orders should be both institutional and practice specific; these orders are meant for illustration only.	PT. NAME _____ LAST FIRST MEDICAL REC. NO. _____

COMPLETE SECTION IF Admit OR Rewrite Orders
Weight _____ kg
Allergies / adverse drug reactions

Date/Time	

EPIDURAL ANALGESIA ORDER SHEETS – Page 1

1. **Medication and Dosing:**
    A. No other systemic analgesics or sedatives other than acetaminophen are to be administered unless approved by a pain service physician.
    B. Patient has received bolus epidural ☐ or intrathecal ☐ opioid (check one) drug _____ dose _____, date & time _____. <u>Cross out if no bolus dose of epidural or intrathecal opioid.</u>
♣♣C. Epidural solution (50 ml syringes) check one and cross out others:
    _____ bupivacaine 0.1%
    _____ bupivacaine 0.1% with clonidine 1 μg/mL
    _____ bupivacaine 0.1% with fentanyl 2 μg/mL
    _____ bupivacaine 0.1% with fentanyl 2 μg/mL and clonidine 1 μg/mL
    _____ chloroprocaine 1.5% alone:*
    _____ chloroprocaine 1.5% with clonidine 0.2 μg/mL*
    _____ chloroprocaine 1.5% with fentanyl 0.4 μg/mL*
    _____ chloroprocaine 1.5% with clonidine 0.2 μg/mL and fentanyl 0.4 μg/mL*
    _____ bupivacaine 0.1% with hydromorphone 10 μg/mL
    _____ bupivacaine 0.1% with morphine 20 μg/mL
    _____ Other (specify) _____
    *Note that chloroprocaine may be administered at rates from 0.3 mL/kg/hr up to 1.2 mL/kg/hr; **the dose of clonidine and fentanyl must be proportionally reduced.**

    D. Epidural infusion rate: _____ mL/hr (usual rates are 0.1–0.4 mL/kg/hr).
    E. If the patient has no bladder catheter, may straight cath pm for urinary retention greater than _____ hours.

2. **Monitoring and Equipment:**

		YES	NO
A.	Continuous pulse oximetry	☐	☐
B.	Ambu bag, O$_2$ tubing, face mask, and suction at bedside	☐	☐
C.	If narcotics included in infusion, naloxone (Narcan®) ampule immediately available	☐	☐
D.	Continuous (impedance apnea monitor, pneumography).	☐	☐

3. **Patient Assessments:**

    A. HR, BP, assessment of analgesia (OPS 0-10 scale, ages < 7 years, VAS 0-10 scale, ages ≥ 7 years) and level of blockade q 4 hr. For patients > 12 years, check for orthostatic changes upon first morning ambulation; if patient dizzy or for > 20 mm Hg fall in BP or 20 beats per min increase in heart rate, call HO or pain service to evaluate patient.
    B. Monitor, assess, and document respiratory rate (RR) and depth q 1 h while asleep & q 2 h while alert. A stethoscope is to be used for this assessment.
    C. In this case, electronic monitoring (A & D above) is generally indicated because of (check only if indicated; otherwise, cross out):
    _____   1. Age less than 6 months
    _____   2. Somnolence
    _____   3. Lung disease
    _____   4. All patients receiving epidural morphine or hydromorphone (Dilaudid). Lower-limit apnea alarms are to be set as follows: RR 12 (ages 8 and above); RR 14 (ages below 8).
    D. Turn patient from side to side q 4 h and elevate heels off bed.
    E. For patients who received single dose intrathecal or epidural opioid only, continue above monitoring for 24 hours.

Figure 29–2. *See legend on opposite page*

HYPOTHETICAL HOSPITAL ORDERS

IMPORTANT: Pain service orders should be both institutional and practice specific; these orders are meant for illustration only.

USE PLATE OR PRINT

PT. NAME _____

         LAST   FIRST

MEDICAL REC. NO. _____

COMPLETE SECTION IF Admit OR Rewrite Orders
Weight _____ kg
Allergies / adverse drug reactions

Date/Time	

EPIDURAL ANALGESIA ORDER SHEETS – Page 2

4. **Side Effects Management:**
   A. Discontinue infusion and page pain service if:
      i. Patient is somnolent
      ii. RR less than 12 (ages 8 and above)
         RR less than 14 (ages below 8)
      iii. BP systolic less than 80 (ages below 12 months)
         BP systolic less than 90 (ages above 12 months)
      iv. no movement in toes or ankles

   B. Stat page "Anesthesia Stat Beeper," "code blue" (airway response team), pain service, and primary services.

   C. Apply oxygen, stimulate, and turn off infusion if:
      i. cyanosis
      ii. severe unresponsiveness
      iii. RR less than 8 or apnea
      iv. BP systolic less than 65
      v. Draw up naloxone (Narcan®) as follows. Dilute 1 mL of (0.4 mg) with 9 mL of normal saline to make 0.04 mg/mL (circle dose)

Age	Incremental Dose (mg)	Incremental Dose (mL)
< 1 year of age	0.02 mg	0.5 mL
≥ 1 year ≤ 12	0.04 mg	1 mL
yrs	0.08 mg	2 mL
≥ 12 years		

      vi. _____ Other (specify) _____

   ♣♣D. For pruritus (choose one, cross out the other):

   _____ 1. Diphenhydramine (Benadryl) 0.5 mg/kg × _____ kg = _____ mg IV over 20 minutes q 2 hr pm; hold for somnolence
   _____ 2. Naloxone (Narcan®) 0.002 mg/kg × _____ kg _____ mg IV over 20 minutes q 2 h pm (for use with epidural opioids only)
   _____ 3. Nalbuphine 0.04 mg/kg × _____ kg = _____ mg q 6 h pm

   ♣♣E. For nausea (choose one, cross out the others):

   _____ 1. Perphenazine (Trilafon) 0.015 − 0.025 mg/kg × _____ kg = _____ mg IV over 20 minutes q 6 hr pm; hold for somnolence
   _____ 2. Naloxone (Narcan®) 0.002 mg/kg × _____ kg = _____ mg IV over 20 minutes q 2 h pm (for use with epidural opioids only)
   _____ 3. Nalbuphine 0.04 mg/kg × _____ kg × _____ mg q 6 h pm
   _____ 4. Prochlorperazine (Compazine) _____ mg PO PR IM (Circle one) q 6 h pm
   _____ 5. Droperidol 0.010–0.025 mg/kg × _____ kg = _____ mg IV q 6 hr
   _____ 6. Metoclopramide 0.1–0.2 mg/kg × _____ kg = _____ mg IV (max 1 mg) q 6 hr
   _____ 7. Ondansetron (0.1–0.15 mg/kg) × _____ kg = _____ mg (4 mg max) q 6 h
   _____ 8. Dolasetron 0.35 mg/kg × _____ kg = _____ mg (max 12.5 mg) × 1

Ordered by _____ M.D.
Pain Service Physician

♣♣Note: Many options are provided for illustrative purposes; it is suggested that a smaller number of options be selected per institution so as to minimize the potential for confusion.

Figure 29–2. A typical standing order sheet for epidural analgesia in children. Note the different choices for infusion solutions particularly for neonates (see text for details).

Table 29–4. Suggested Doses for Epidural Analgesia with Local Anesthetic/Opioid Solutions at Different Ages

Age	Initial Bolus (mL/kg/segment)*	Infusion Rate (mL/kg/hr)*
Infants < 6 months	0.04–0.05	0.1–0.2 (max 1.2 mL/kg/hr)
Children > 6 months	0.03–0.04 (max 20 mL)	0.1–0.4 (max 20 mL/hr)

*Use lower infusion rates for epidural morphine or hydromorphone infusions. Chloroprocaine 1.5% solutions may be titrated upward to 1.2 mL/kg/hr in infants.

not simply decreased, until these effects subside, and appropriate therapy must be instituted (Table 29–5).

In very young infants, epidural infusions of both opioids and local anesthetics require increased surveillance and perhaps reduced initial infusion rates. This is because (1) drug clearance may be reduced, (2) decreased protein binding may increase free serum drug concentrations, and (3) titration to clinical end points, such as pain scoring, is less precise. At some centers, application of epidural infusions, especially with opioids, for children less than 3 to 6 months of age is restricted to intensive care areas. Acetaminophen can be administered orally or rectally if additional adjunctive analgesia is needed. Examples of epidural infusions and alternative modalities in clinical settings are provided in Table 29–6.

The sympathetic blockade that may occur in older children as a result of local anesthetic blockade may also be used advantageously to provide postoperative vasodilation in patients undergoing replantation of extremities. A similar technique using axillary sheath catheters can be used in the upper extremity.

Risks and Untoward Effects. Side effects associated with regional analgesia can be divided into those caused by local anesthetics and those caused by opioids. In addition, complications related to the catheter itself are possible.

Local anesthetics in the dilute concentrations used for postoperative analgesia have a very low incidence of untoward effects. Motor blockade occurs uncommonly but has been observed even with dilute bupivacaine (0.1%). As discussed earlier, patients with neuromuscular disorders causing motor weakness should be observed carefully for this complication. *Rapid onset of more profound motor block should raise immediate concerns about erosion of the catheter through the dura into the subarachnoid space.* The pharmacokinetics of bupivacaine have been studied in infants and children in both single injection doses[173] and during continuous infusion.[24, 28, 174, 175] Data suggest that in children younger than 6 months, a lower fraction of bupivacaine circulating in the plasma is protein bound, leading to the potential for higher serum levels and resultant toxicity.[176] Neonates or infants with impaired hepatic blood flow may be at particular risk for bupivacaine accumulation. Seizures and cardiac arrest have been reported when high doses of bupivacaine have been administered, usually following excessive infusion rates or unintended intravascular injection. Little information

Table 29–5. Treatment of Untoward Effects of Epidural Opioids

Side Effect	Treatment	Infusion Rate
Pruritus	Naloxone, 2 μg/kg IV q 2 h OR Nalbuphine 0.04 mg/kg q 6 h PRN OR Diphenhydramine, 0.5 mg/kg IV every 6 h; observe for sedation	Decrease by 10–20% or decrease opioid concentration
Nausea and vomiting	NPO for 24 h Naloxone, 2 μg/kg IV q 2 h PRN OR Metoclopramide, 0.1–0.15 mg/kg IV q 6–8 h PRN OR Droperidol, 0.01–0.025 mg/kg IV q 6 h PRN OR Ondansetron 0.1–0.15 mg/kg IV q 6 h PRN	Decrease by 10–20% or decrease opioid concentration
Urinary retention	Bladder catheterization (one time) Naloxone, 0.5 μg/kg IV Indwelling urinary catheter	Decrease opioid concentration
Oversedation; reduced respiratory rate or depth but patient arousable and responsive	Naloxone, 2 μg/kg IV	Decrease by 20–50%* Decrease opioid concentration
Respiratory depression; patient unarousable, hypoxemic, hypercarbic, or apneic	Oxygen by mask; assisted ventilation if needed Naloxone, 5–10 μg/kg IV Transfer patient to monitored setting until episode is fully resolved Consider naloxone infusion (5 μg/kg/hr)	Discontinue infusion Consider possibility of intrathecal catheter migration (check by aspirating)

*Stop infusion until patient is alert if using morphine or hydromorphone.

Table 29–6. Clinical Examples of Postoperative Analgesic Management Strategy

Considerations	Alternatives
	CASE 1: 2-Year-Old ASA 1 for Inguinal Hernia Repair, Weight 15 kg
• Mildly painful surgery • Outpatient setting—avoidance of nausea and oversedation is helpful	• Ilio-inguinal nerve block bupivacaine 0.25% with epinephrine 1 : 200,000, 0.5 mL/kg × 15 kg = 7.5 mL (3.75 mL on each side) • Wound infiltration with bupivacaine 0.25% with epinephrine 1 : 200,000, 0.5 mL/kg × 15 kg = 7.5 mL (3.75 mL on each side) • Caudal block using bupivacaine 0.25% with epinephrine 1 : 200,000, 0.5–0.6 mL/kg × 15 kg = 8–9 mL • Add acetaminophen, 10–15 mg/kg (oral) as needed at home
	CASE 2: 6-Month-Old, 6 kg Child, ASA 1, for Ureteral Reimplantation

• Moderately painful surgery, bladder spasms
• Urinary retention is not an issue
• Some difficulty with pain assessment
	1. *Inhalation general anesthesia with*
	  • Bupivacaine 0.1% with fentanyl 2–3 μg/mL, starting at 0.2 mL/kg/h × 6 kg = 1.2 mL/h
	  • Need to cover approximately 10 dermatomes (5 sacral, 5 lumbar); initial bolus, 10 × 0.05 mL/kg/dermatome × 6 kg = 3.0 mL
	  • Apnea monitoring (if opioid is used) and frequent observation
	  • Add acetaminophen as needed, 15–20 mg/kg every 4 h (oral) or 20–30 mg/kg every 4 h (rectal)
	2. *Continuous intravenous morphine infusion*
	  • Loading dose of up to 0.075–0.1 mg/kg × 6 kg = 0.45–0.6 mg in incremental doses if needed
	  • Infusion starting at 0.02 mg/kg/h (20 μg/kg/h) × 6 kg = 0.12 mg/h
	  • Apnea monitoring and frequent observation
	  • Add acetaminophen as needed

	CASE 3: 3-Year-Old for Thoracoabdominal Excision of Neuroblastoma, ASA 2, Weight 18 kg

• Major painful surgery
• Major impairment of respiration
• Bladder catheter warranted
• Many dermatomes involved
	1. *Continuous thoracic epidural infusion* (via caudal, lumbar, or thoracic entry) with bupivacaine 0.1% with fentanyl 2-3 μg/mL; catheter tip at T8–T9.
	  • Need to cover approximately 10 dermatomes: Initial bolus, 10 × 0.05 ml/kg/dermatome × 18 kg = 9.0 mL.
	  • Infusion rate to begin at 0.3 mL/kg/h × 18 kg = 5.4 mL/h
	  • Delivered drug doses: bupivacaine 5.4 mg/h = 0.3 mg/kg/h; fentanyl 10.8–16.2 μg/h = 0.6–0.9 μg/kg/h (starting doses less than 1 μg/kg/h)
	  • If ineffective then clonidine (1 μg/mL) could be added to the above solution
	  • If ineffective bupivacaine (0.1%) with hydromorphone (10 μg/mL) could be substituted
	2. *Lumbar or caudal epidural opioid*
	  • By bolus: preservative-free morphine, 0.03–0.05 mg/kg × 18 kg = 0.54–0.9 mg every 6–10 h
	  • By infusion: morphine, 0.005 mg/kg/h × 18 kg = 0.09 mg/h, or hydromorphone, 0.001 mg/kg/h (1 μg/kg/h) × 18 kg = 0.018 mg/h)
	  • If ineffective bupivacaine (0.1%) with hydromorphone (10 μg/mL) could be substituted
	  • Apnea monitoring and frequent observation
	3. *Continuous intravenous morphine infusion*
	  • Loading dose of up to 0.075–0.1 mg/kg × 18 kg = 1.3–1.8 mg in incremental doses if needed
	  • 0.03 mg/kg/h (30 μg/kg/h) × 18 kg = 0.54 mg/h

	CASE 4: 6-Week-Old, 3 kg Child, ASA III, for Thoracoabdominal Excision of a Wilms Tumor

• Painful surgery
• Difficulty in pain assessment
• Major impairment of respiration
• Many dermatomes involved
• Bladder catheter warranted
	1. *A continuous epidural infusion* (catheter inserted through the caudal approach and threaded to the mid-portion of the surgical incision)
	  • Need to cover approximately 16 dermatomes (5 sacral, 5 lumbar, 6 thoracic): Initial bolus 16 × 0.05 mL/kg/dermatome × 3 kg = 2.4 mL loading dose. The infusion could be:
	    • chloroprocaine 1.5% with fentanyl 0.4 μg/mL (0.0004 mg/mL) to be infused at a starting rate of 0.3 mL/kg/h up to 1.2 mL/kg/h
	    • Chloroprocaine 1.5% with clonidine 0.2 μg/mL. Also to be started at a rate of 0.3 mL/kg/h up to 1.2 ml/kg/h. **Note that the concentration of clonidine and fentanyl per mL of local anesthetic solution is reduced compared with that which would be used with older children because of the more rapid epidural infusion rate used in order to take maximal advantage of the local anesthetic.**
	2. *Continuous intravenous fentanyl.* A loading dose of 5–10 μg/kg (**at the beginning of anesthesia**) or 0.5 μg/kg (in an unintubated patient) followed by 0.15 μg/kg/h with a 4-hour limit of 4 μg/kg.

about more extended administration over days is available, but the use of low-concentration solutions (and therefore low total doses) reduces the potential for toxicity. Tachyphylaxis during prolonged administration of local anesthetics is a theoretic problem, although no systematic studies have addressed this phenomenon in children. Co-administration of opioids appears to reduce the incidence of tachyphylaxis. As discussed previously, hemodynamic stability exists in children less than 6 years of age during spinal or epidural blockade, even with relatively high degrees of sympathetic blockade. In infants, this extreme lack of hemodynamic response has been attributed to the lack of dependence of systemic vascular resistance on sympathetic outflow. As children approach school age, however, rapid position changes may produce hemodynamic responses after extensive sympathetic blockade.

Central neuraxis opioids have several potential side effects, the most worrisome being respiratory depression. The lipophilic agents (fentanyl and sufentanil) appear to have the widest therapeutic index in this regard, because less rostral spread of the drug occurs because of greater binding with receptors in the substantia gelatinosa of the spinal cord adjacent to the area of drug administration. Despite the fact that use of morphine poses a greater risk for respiratory depression, the incidence remains low. Reports in the pediatric literature of respiratory depression after epidural morphine administration demonstrate that vigilance in monitoring is mandatory.[177-179] The incidence of complications with caudal morphine is reduced if a dose of 0.033 mg/kg (33 μg/kg) is used in children older than 1 year.[155] The adequacy of analgesia at this dose was virtually unchanged from 0.1 mg/kg (100 μg/kg), with the exception of a prolongation of action with the higher dose. *The hallmark of impending overdose of central neuraxis opioids is increasing sedation and decreasing depth of respiration. It is important to recognize that the depth of respiration must be assessed, not just the rate, because patients frequently develop decreased tidal volume before the respiratory rate decreases, leading to alveolar hypoventilation and the potential for hypercarbia and hypoxemia.*[180]

In addition to clinical assessment, quantitative capnography and pulse oximetry, although not required, can be valuable monitors for these patients and provide more useful information than impedance-type respirometers, which count only respiratory rate. Impedance respiratory monitors may continue to register breathing efforts when significant airway obstruction exists, as long as the chest wall is still moving, thereby delaying the recognition of respiratory depression. *It again must be emphasized that no monitor can replace vigilant, frequent clinical assessment.* In our opinion, it is highly desirable to use monitors that are configured to ring at the nurses' station and in the hallways; monitors that ring only in the patient's room can easily be ignored. Oversedation, diminished respiratory depth, and slowing of the respiratory rate are treated, when lipophilic opioids such as fentanyl are used, by decreasing the rate of opioid administration and, if necessary, administering small incremental doses of naloxone. It is only necessary to administer naloxone in small incremental intravenous doses (0.5–1.0 μg/kg) every few minutes until reversal of the side effects is achieved. Untoward effects can thus be reversed without affecting analgesia. More profound respiratory depression,

including inability to arouse the patient and apnea, must be treated more vigorously. In this circumstance, the infusion should be discontinued, oxygen administered (by positive pressure if respirations are very slow, shallow, or absent), and 5 to 10 μg/kg of naloxone administered intravenously. *The new development of respiratory depression in a patient receiving what appears to be an appropriate opioid dose should always raise the question of catheter migration into the subarachnoid space.* The effective intrathecal dose of opioid is roughly one tenth that of the epidural dose, and the duration of action, especially with morphine, is significantly prolonged. Should this occur, observation in a monitored setting must be continued for 24 hours or until no further evidence of respiratory compromise exists without the use of naloxone. *Whenever central neuraxis opioids are administered, facilities must be immediately available at the patient's bedside for resuscitation in the unlikely event of an airway emergency.* Many centers utilize the policy to have oxygen, a bag-valve device and appropriate sizes of masks and airways, and suction at the bedside. All patients receiving continuous regional analgesia should also have an intravenous line (a heparin lock is adequate in those patients not requiring intravenous fluids), and naloxone must be immediately available.

Pruritus is common with epidural opioids, occurring in as many as 30% of patients. It is not usually severe enough to warrant intervention beyond a small dose of naloxone (0.5–1.0 μg/kg IV). Antihistamines are also effective, although one should use caution in prescribing drugs that may potentiate sedation. Nalbuphine is used in some centers to antagonize pruritus and pediatric studies are in progress. Nausea and vomiting may also occur and may be more common with morphine than fentanyl. Children who are not fed during the first 24 hours after surgery do not vomit excessively even when given caudal morphine.[181] As with all other opioid side effects, nausea and vomiting respond to the previously mentioned doses of naloxone. Antiemetics, like agents used to treat pruritus, may be sedating and should be used with caution. Metoclopramide in doses of 0.1 to 0.15 mg/kg (100–150 μg/kg) or droperidol in doses of 0.01 to 0.02 mg/kg (10–20 μg/kg) IV every 6 to 8 hours appears to provide adequate relief with low degrees of sedation. Serotonin receptor antagonists such as ondansetron (0.1–0.15 mg/kg; maximum, 4 mg) or dolasetron (0.35 mg/kg; maximum 12.5 mg) seem to have no sedative effects.[104] It is prudent to decrease the infusion rate when these untoward effects require treatment; if additional analgesia is required, acetaminophen or ketorolac can be added. Untoward effects of epidural opioids and their treatment are summarized in Table 29–5.

Catheter-related complications were mentioned in the previous sections. The potential for a catheter to migrate should always be borne in mind when unexpected changes occur in the course of postoperative analgesia management. In addition to subarachnoid migration, catheters may penetrate epidural blood vessels. When slowly administered, small intravenous doses of local anesthetics are unlikely to produce symptoms. A loss of analgesia may be noted or an increase in sedation may occur if opioids are being used. Catheters may also migrate through a spinal foramen, producing a unilateral one-dermatome band of analgesia. In this case, simply withdrawing the catheter 1 or 2 cm may allow proper repositioning within the epidural space. The existence of a median raphe in the epidural space has been postulated and may be the cause of unilateral multidermatome blockade.[182]

On occasion, a collection of fluid may be found, originating from the skin insertion site and pooling under the dressing. Experience and direct measurement suggest that in most cases this is not, as one may fear, cerebrospinal fluid, but rather edema fluid leaking through a hole in the skin from the subcutaneous tissues. It usually requires no special treatment except reinforcing the dressing. It subsides as the edema and third-space fluids are mobilized in the first days after surgery. If troublesome and persistent leakage occurs, a drop of collodion over the skin site may be effective in sealing the hole.

The catheter site should be inspected daily to ensure that the dressing is intact and to look for any signs of local infection. Infections are exceedingly rare, perhaps in part because of the bactericidal properties of the local anesthetics themselves.[183] Catheter-related infections of the deep tissues, including epidural abscess, appear to have their origin in local skin infections that track along the catheter's path. *Any sign of local infection is cause for immediate catheter removal.* Patients who develop fever or sepsis need to be evaluated on an individual basis, and there are no published guidelines to follow. If a clear source for the fever is found, it is acceptable to leave the catheter in place, but we generally elect to remove it if a patient is overtly septic or if the situation is unclear.

INTRAPLEURAL CATHETERS. Continuous intrapleural analgesia has been used in children after thoracic, upper abdominal, and retroperitoneal surgery.[184–186] Although specialized kits for this technique are appearing on the market, a standard epidural catheter may be used. The intrapleural space is entered in the same fashion as for a thoracentesis, over the *upper* margin of the rib to avoid the neurovascular structures. The catheter is threaded several centimeters and affixed with a clear occlusive dressing. Anchoring the catheter with a suture at the skin site is reported to help prevent its migration. Infusing 0.25% bupivacaine with epinephrine (1:200,000) at 0.5 mL/kg/hr is reported to provide excellent analgesia.[184] Because the local anesthetic solution flows with gravity, the position of the patient is important in determining the efficacy of analgesia achieved with this technique. Several risks are associated with it as well. The pleura forms a very large and efficient absorptive surface for the uptake of drug into the circulation. Although none of the patients in the initial reports of this technique in children had signs of clinical toxicity, total blood concentrations of bupivacaine (bound and unbound) reached the toxic range of 4 µg/mL 24 hours into therapy in some patients. Convulsions have been reported anecdotally with intrapleural analgesia in children. Given these concerns, *hourly bupivacaine infusion rates greater than 0.5 mg/kg/hr are not recommended.*[168] The potential also exists for paresis of the phrenic, recurrent laryngeal, and vagus nerves, as well as for direct effects on the diaphragm. Pneumothorax remains a risk with percutaneous placement through a closed chest. We have occasionally used prolonged intrapleural analgesia for sympathetic blockade for the upper extremity using bolus injections in a head-down, affected side–up position. In our experience, epidural analgesia is more effective and has a wider margin of safety than intrapleural analgesia for major thoracoabdominal surgery.

AXILLARY CATHETERS. Axillary sheath catheters can be used to provide continuous blockade of the brachial plexus.[187, 188] This technique is used relatively uncommonly, in part because of the very long duration of a single-injection axillary block. It may be useful for postoperative management of replantation of an arm or hand, however, because vasodilation produced by the block may aid in revascularization. Specialized kits for brachial plexus cannulation are commercially available, and the catheters are inserted in the same fashion as for placing an axillary block. After initial dosing, we infuse 0.125% bupivacaine at 0.25 mL/kg/hr.

Summary

Postoperative analgesia is an integral and essential component of any pediatric anesthetic plan. Contemporary knowledge of anatomy, physiology, pharmacokinetics, and pharmacodynamics in infancy and childhood permit the anesthesiologist to apply advanced anesthetic and analgesic techniques to all pediatric patients with a high degree of efficacy and safety. The optimal utilization of these techniques requires not only the understanding of the techniques outlined in this chapter, but also the integration of multiple medical and nursing disciplines in the assessment and care of these children. A well-organized pediatric pain service and an educated nursing staff are the key to the successful management of acute pain, which in turn can be expected to result in improved care for infants and children.[189]

REFERENCES

1. St. Lukes makes pain the fifth vital sign, cuts costs. Hosp Peer Rev 1996;21:54–59.
2. Mather L, Mackie J: The incidence of postoperative pain in children. Pain 1983;15:271–282.
3. Marshall TA, Deeder R, Pai S, et al: Physiologic changes associated with endotracheal intubation in preterm infants. Crit Care Med 1984;12:501–503.
4. Rawlings DJ, Miller PA, Engel RR: The effect of circumcision on transcutaneous PO_2 in term infants. Am J Dis Child 1980;134:676–678.
5. Talbert LM, Kraybill EN, Potter HD: Adrenal cortical response to circumcision in the neonate. Obstet Gynecol 1976;48:208–210.
6. Friesen RH, Honda AT, Thieme RE: Changes in anterior fontanel pressure in preterm neonates during tracheal intubation. Anesth Analg 1987;66:874–878.
7. Williamson PS, Williamson ML: Physiologic stress reduction by a local anesthetic during newborn circumcision. Pediatrics 1983;71:36–40.
8. Hickey PR, Hansen DD, Wessel DL, et al: Blunting of stress responses in the pulmonary circulation of infants by fentanyl. Anesth Analg 1985;64:1137–1142.
9. Anand KJ, Sippell WG, Aynsley-Green A: Randomized trial of fentanyl anaesthesia in preterm babies undergoing surgery: Effects on the stress response. Lancet 1987;1:62–66.
10. Anand KJ, Hickey PR: Pain and its effects in the human neonate and fetus. N Engl J Med 1987;317:1321–1329.
11. McGrath PJ, Johnson G, Goodman JT, et al: The CHEOPS: A behavioral scale to measure postoperative pain in children. In: Fields HW, Dubner R, Cervero F, eds: Advances in Pain Research and Therapy. New York: Raven Press; 1985:395–402.
12. Beyer JE, McGrath PJ, Berde CB: Discordance between self-report

and behavioral pain measures in children aged 3–7 years after surgery. J Pain Symptom Manage 1990;5:350–356.

13. Beyer JE, Wells N: The assessment of pain in children. Pediatr Clin North Am 1989;36:837–854.

14. Bender LH, Weaver K, Edwards K: Postoperative patient-controlled analgesia in children. Pediatr Nurs 1990;16:549–554.

15. Kotzer AM, Coy J, LeClaire AD: The effectiveness of a standardized educational program for children using patient-controlled analgesia. J Soc Pediatr Nurs 1998;3:117–126.

16. Woolf CJ, Wall PD: Morphine-sensitive and morphine-insensitive actions of C-fibre input on the rat spinal cord. Neurosci Lett 1986;64:221–225.

17. Welborn LG, Rice LJ, Hannallah RS, et al: Postoperative apnea in former preterm infants: Prospective comparison of spinal and general anesthesia. Anesthesiology 1990;72:838–842.

18. Krane EJ, Haberkern CM, Jacobson LE: Postoperative apnea, bradycardia, and oxygen desaturation in formerly premature infants: Prospective comparison of spinal and general anesthesia. Anesth Analg 1995;80:7–13.

19. Lynn AM, Slattery JT: Morphine pharmacokinetics in early infancy. Anesthesiology 1987;66:136–139.

20. Hannallah RS, Rosales JK: Experience with parents presence during anesthesia induction in children. Can Anaesth Soc J 1983;30:287–290.

21. Meyers EF, Muravchick S: Anesthesia induction techniques in pediatric patients: A controlled study of behavioral consequences. Anesth Analg 1977;56:538–542.

22. Hansen TG, Henneberg SW, Hole P: Age-related postoperative morphine requirements in children following major surgery: An assessment using patient-controlled analgesia (PCA). Eur J Pediatr Surg 1996;6:29–31.

23. Bires JA, McGregor DG: Continuous epidural infusion of 1/8% bupivacaine for postoperative pain relief in pediatric urology patients. Anesthesiology 1990;73:A1108.

24. Kart T, Walther-Larsen S, Svejborg TF, et al: Comparison of continuous epidural infusion of fentanyl and bupivacaine with intermittent epidural administration of morphine for postoperative pain management in children. Acta Anaesthesiol Scand 1997;41:461–465.

25. McBride WJ, Dicker R, Abajian JC, et al: Continuous thoracic epidural infusions for postoperative analgesia after pectus deformity repair. J Pediatr Surg 1996;31:105–107.

26. Luz G, Germann R, Innerhofer P, et al: Continuous caudal epidural bupivacaine infusions in children. Anesth Analg 1993;77:398.

27. Parkinson SK, Porter CT Jr, Little WL, et al: The use of continuous epidural morphine infusions in small children: A report of two cases. Reg Anesth 1989;14:152–154.

28. Scott DA, Beilby DS, McClymont C: Postoperative analgesia using epidural infusions of fentanyl with bupivacaine. A prospective analysis of 1,014 patients. Anesthesiology 1995;83:727–737.

29. Shaw BA, Watson TC, Merzel DI, et al: The safety of continuous epidural infusion for postoperative analgesia in pediatric spine surgery. J Pediatr Orthop 1996;16:374–377.

30. Shayevitz JR, Merkel S, O'Kelly SW, et al: Lumbar epidural morphine infusions for children undergoing cardiac surgery. J Cardiothorac Vasc Anesth 1996;10:217–224.

31. Bosenberg AT: Epidural analgesia for major neonatal surgery. Paediatr Anaesth 1998;8:479–483.

32. Manikian B, Cantineau JP, Bertrand M, et al: Improvement of diaphragmatic function by a thoracic extradural block after upper abdominal surgery. Anesthesiology 1988;68:379–386.

33. Wahba WM, Don HF, Craig DB: Post-operative epidural analgesia: effects on lung volumes. Can Anaesth Soc J 1975;22:519–527.

34. Fratacci MD, Kimball WR, Wain JC, et al: Diaphragmatic shortening after thoracic surgery in humans: Effects of mechanical ventilation and thoracic epidural anesthesia. Anesthesiology 1993;79:654–665.

35. Polaner DM, Kimball WR, Fratacci MD, et al: Thoracic epidural anesthesia increases diaphragmatic shortening after thoracotomy in the awake lamb. Anesthesiology 1993;79:808–816.

36. Simonneau G, Vivien A, Sartene R, et al: Diaphragm dysfunction induced by upper abdominal surgery: Role of postoperative pain. Am Rev Respir Dis 1983;128:899–903.

37. Bonnet F, Blery C, Zatan M, et al: Effect of epidural morphine on post-operative pulmonary dysfunction. Acta Anaesthesiol Scand 1984;28:147–151.

38. Cooper MG, Sethna NF: Epidural analgesia in patients with congenital lumbosacral spinal anomalies. Anesthesiology 1991;75:370–374.

39. Ellis JA, Spanos NP: Cognitive-behavioral interventions for children's distress during bone marrow aspirations and lumbar punctures: a critical review. J Pain Symptom Manage 1994;9:96–108.

40. Schechter NL: Pain and pain control in children. Curr Probl Pediatr 1985;15:1–67.

41. Kissin I: Preemptive analgesia: Why its effect is not always obvious. Anesthesiology 1996;84:1015–1019.

42. Lin YC, Sussman HH, Benitz WE: Plasma concentrations after rectal administration of acetaminophen in preterm neonates. Paediatr Anaesth 1997;7:457–459.

43. Tanaka E: In vivo age-related changes in hepatic drug-oxidizing capacity in humans. J Clin Pharm Ther 1998;23:247–255.

44. Gaudreault P, Guay J, Nicol O, et al: Pharmacokinetics and clinical efficacy of intrarectal solution of acetaminophen. Can J Anaesth 1988;35:149–152.

45. Houck CS, Sullivan LJ, Wilder RT, Rusy LM, Burrows FA: Pharmacokinetics of a higher dose of rectal acetaminophen in children. Anesthesiology 1995; 83:A1126.

46. Montgomery CJ, McCormack JP, Reichert CC, et al: Plasma concentrations after high-dose (45 mg.kg-1) rectal acetaminophen in children. Can J Anaesth 1995;42:982–986.

47. Birmingham PK, Tobin MJ, Henthorn TK, et al: Twenty-four-hour pharmacokinetics of rectal acetaminophen in children: An old drug with new recommendations. Anesthesiology 1997;87:244–252.

48. Rusy LM, Houck CS, Sullivan LJ, et al: A double-blind evaluation of ketorolac tromethamine versus acetaminophen in pediatric tonsillectomy: Analgesia and bleeding. Anesth Analg 1995;80:226–229.

49. Anderson BJ, Holford NH: Rectal paracetamol dosing regimens: Determination by computer simulation. Paediatr Anaesth 1997;7:451–455.

50. Anderson BJ, Monteleone J, Holford NH: Variability of concentrations after rectal paracetamol. Paediatr Anaesth 1998;8:274.

51. Anderson BJ, Holford NH: Rectal acetaminophen pharmacokinetics. Anesthesiology 1998;88:1131–1133.

52. Maunuksela EL, Olkkola KT, Korpela R: Does prophylactic intravenous infusion of indomethacin improve the management of postoperative pain in children? Can J Anaesth 1988;35:123–127.

53. Giannini EH, Brewer EJ, Miller ML, et al: Ibuprofen suspension in the treatment of juvenile rheumatoid arthritis. Pediatric Rheumatology Collaborative Study Group. J Pediatr 1990;117:645–652.

54. Olkkola KT, Maunuksela EL: The pharmacokinetics of postoperative intravenous ketorolac tromethamine in children. Br J Clin Pharmacol 1991;31:182–184.

55. Forrest JB, Heitlinger EL, Revell S: Ketorolac for postoperative pain management in children. Drug Saf 1997;16:309–329.

56. Dsida RM, Wheeler M, Birmingham PK, et al: Developmental pharmacokinetics of intravenous ketorolac in pediatric surgical patients. Anesthesiology 1997;87:A1055.

57. Gillis JC, Brogden RN: Ketorolac: A reappraisal of its pharmacodynamic and pharmacokinetic properties and therapeutic use in pain management. Drugs 1997;53:139–188.

58. Bean-Lijewski JD, Hunt RD: Effect of ketorolac on bleeding time and postoperative pain in children: A double-blind, placebo-controlled comparison with meperidine. J Clin Anesth 1996;8:25–30.

59. Gunter JB, Varughese AM, Harrington JF, et al: Recovery and complications after tonsillectomy in children: A comparison of ketorolac and morphine. Anesth Analg 1995;81:1136–1141.

60. Glassman SD, Rose SM, Dimar JR, et al: The effect of postoperative nonsteroidal anti-inflammatory drug administration on spinal fusion. Spine 1998;23:834–838.

61. Warner TD, Giuliano F, Vojnovic I, et al: Nonsteroid drug selectivities for cyclo-oxygenase-1 rather than cyclo-oxygenase-2 are associated with human gastrointestinal toxicity: A full in vitro analysis. Proc Natl Acad Sci U S A 1999;96:7563–7568.

62. Morrison BW, Christensen S, Yuan W, et al: Analgesic efficacy of the cyclooxygenase-2-specific inhibitor rofecoxib in post-dental surgery pain: A randomized, controlled trial. Clin Ther 1999;21:943–953.

63. Kaplan-Machlis B, Klostermeyer BS: The cyclooxygenase-2-inhibitors: Safety and effectiveness [In Process Citation]. Ann Pharmacother 1999;33:979–988.

64. Fung HB, Kirschenbaum HL: Selective cyclooxygenase-2 inhibitors for the treatment of arthritis. Clin Ther 1999;21:1131–1157.

65. Pasquale G, Scaricabarozzi I, D'Agostino R, et al: An assessment of the efficacy and tolerability of nimesulide vs paracetamol in children after adenotonsillectomy. Drugs 1993;46:234–237.

66. Facchini R, Selva G, Peretti G: Tolerability of nimesulide and ketoprofen in paediatric patients with traumatic or surgical fractures. Drugs 1993;46:238–241.

67. Eland JM, Anderson JE: The experience of pain in children. In: Jacox AK, ed: Pain: A Source Book for Nurses and Other Professionals. Boston: Little Brown & Co.; 1977:453–476.

68. Strafford M, Cahill C, Schwartz T, Yee J, Sethna N, Berde C: Recognition and treatment of pain in pediatric patients with AIDS. J Pain Symptom.Manage 1991; 6:146.

69. Miser AW, Davis DM, Hughes CS, et al: Continuous subcutaneous infusion of morphine in children with cancer. Am J Dis Child 1983;137:383–385.

70. Berde CB, Beyer JE, Bournaki MC, et al: Comparison of morphine and methadone for prevention of postoperative pain in 3- to 7-year-old children. J Pediatr 1991;119:136–141.

71. Shir Y, Shenkman Z, Shavelson V, et al: Oral methadone for the treatment of severe pain in hospitalized children: A report of five cases. Clin J Pain 1998;14:350–353.

72. Yaster M, Deshpande JK, Maxwell LG: The pharmacologic management of pain in children. Compr Ther 1989;15:14–26.

73. Birmingham PK: Recent advances in acute pain management. Curr Probl Pediatr 1995;25:99–112.

74. Berde CB: Pediatric postoperative pain management. Pediatr Clin North Am 1989;36:921–940.

75. Scott CS, Riggs KW, Ling EW, et al: Morphine pharmacokinetics and pain assessment in premature newborns. J Pediatr 1999;135:423–429.

76. Lynn AM, Opheim KE, Tyler DC: Morphine infusion after pediatric cardiac surgery. Crit Care Med 1984;123:863–866.

77. Koren G, Butt W, Pape K, et al: Morphine-induced seizures in newborn infants. Vet Hum Toxicol 1985;27:519–520.

78. Koren G, Butt W, Chinyanga H, et al: Postoperative morphine infusion in newborn infants: Assessment of disposition characteristics and safety. J Pediatr 1985;107:963–967.

79. Kupferberg HJ, Way HJ: Pharmacologic basis for the increased sensitivity of the newborn to morphine. J Pharmacol Exp Ther 1963;141:105–109.

80. Bradbury M: The blood-brain barrier during the development of the individual and the evolution of the phylum. In: Bradbury M, ed: The Concept of the Blood-Brain Barrier. New York: John Wiley & Sons; 1979:289–322.

81. Miller RP, Roberts RJ, Fischer LJ: Acetaminophen elimination kinetics in neonates, children and adults. Clin Pharmacol Ther 1976;19:284–294.

82. Collins JJ, Geake J, Grier HE, et al: Patient-controlled analgesia for mucositis pain in children: A three-period crossover study comparing morphine and hydromorphone. J Pediatr 1996;129:722–728.

83. Singleton MA, Rosen JI, Fisher DM: Plasma concentrations of fentanyl in infants, children and adults. Can J Anaesth 1987;34:152–155.

84. Hertzka RE, Gauntlett IS, Fisher DM, et al: Fentanyl-induced ventilatory depression: Effects of age. Anesthesiology 1989;70:213–218.

85. Joint Commission on Accreditation of Healthcare Organizations: Comprehensive Accreditation Manual for Hospitals. Oakbrook Terrace: 1999.

86. McDonald DD: Postoperative narcotic analgesic administration. Appl Nurs Res 1993;6:106–110.

87. Vetter TR: Pediatric patient-controlled analgesia with morphine versus meperidine. J Pain Symptom Manage 1992;7:204–208.

88. Kussman BD, Sethna NF: Pethidine-associated seizure in a healthy adolescent receiving pethidine for postoperative pain control. Paediatr Anaesth 1998;8:349–352.

89. Robieux IC, Kellner JD, Coppes MJ, et al: Analgesia in children with sickle cell crisis: Comparison of intermittent opioids vs. continuous intravenous infusion of morphine and placebo-controlled study of oxygen inhalation. Pediatr Hematol Oncol 1992;9:317–326.

90. Bennett RL, Batenhorst RL, Bivins BA, et al: Patient-controlled analgesia: A new concept of postoperative pain relief. Ann Surg 1982;195:700–705.

91. Berde CB, Lehn BM, Yee JD, et al: Patient-controlled analgesia in children and adolescents: A randomized, prospective comparison with intramuscular administration of morphine for postoperative analgesia. J Pediatr 1991;118:460–466.

92. Doyle E, Harper I, Morton NS: Patient-controlled analgesia with low dose background infusions after lower abdominal surgery in children. Br J Anaesth 1993;71:818–822.

93. Doyle E, Robinson D, Morton NS: Comparison of patient-controlled analgesia with and without a background infusion after lower abdominal surgery in children. Br J Anaesth 1993;71:670–673.

94. McNeely JK, Trentadue NC: Comparison of patient-controlled analgesia with and without nighttime morphine infusion following lower extremity surgery in children. J Pain Symptom Manage 1997;13:268–273.

95. Mackie AM, Coda BC, Hill HF: Adolescents use patient-controlled analgesia effectively for relief from prolonged oropharyngeal mucositis pain. Pain 1991;46:265–269.

96. Trentadue NO, Kachoyeanos MK, Lea G: A comparison of two regimens of patient-controlled analgesia for children with sickle cell disease. J Pediatr Nurs 1998;13:15–19.

97. Weldon BC, Connor M, White PF: Pediatric PCA: The role of concurrent opioid infusions and nurse-controlled analgesia. Clin J Pain 1993;9:26–33.

98. McKenzie R, Rudy T, Tantisira B: Comparison of PCA alone and PCA with continuous infusion on pain relief and quality of sleep. Anesthesiology 1990;73:A787.

99. Kanagasundaram SA, Cooper MG, Lane LJ: Nurse-controlled analgesia using a patient-controlled analgesia device: An alternative strategy in the management of severe cancer pain in children. J Paediatr Child Health 1997;33:352–355.

100. Gureno MA, Reisinger CL: Patient controlled analgesia for the young pediatric patient. Pediatr Nurs 1991;17:251–254.

101. Kerschbaum G, Altmeppen J, Funk W, et al: Patient-controlled analgesia. PCA in a three year old child after traumatic amputation. [in German]. Anaesthesist 1998;47:238–242.

102. Loper KA, Ready LB, Dorman BH: Prophylactic transdermal scopolamine patches reduce nausea in postoperative patients receiving epidural morphine. Anesth Analg 1989;68:144–146.

103. Bach S, Noreng MF, Tjellden NU: Phantom limb pain in amputees during the first 12 months following limb amputation, after preoperative lumbar epidural blockade. Pain 1988;33:297–301.

104. Dershwitz M, Di Biase PM, Rosow CE, et al: Ondansetron does not affect alfentanil-induced ventilatory depression or sedation. Anesthesiology 1992;77:447–452.

105. Nikolajsen L, Ilkjaer S, Jensen TS: Effect of preoperative extradural bupivacaine and morphine on stump sensation in lower limb amputees. Br J Anaesth 1998;81:348–354.

106. Pedersen JL, Crawford ME, Dahl JB, et al: Effect of preemptive nerve block on inflammation and hyperalgesia after human thermal injury. Anesthesiology 1996;84:1020–1026.

107. Kundra P, Deepalakshmi K, Ravishankar M: Preemptive caudal bupivacaine and morphine for postoperative analgesia in children. Anesth Analg 1998;87:52–56.

108. Ho JW, Khambatta HJ, Pang LM, et al: Preemptive analgesia in children. Does it exist? Reg Anesth 1997;22:125–130.

109. McQuay HJ, Carroll D, Moore RA: Postoperative orthopaedic pain: The effect of opiate premedication and local anaesthetic blocks. Pain 1988;33:291–295.

110. Wall PD: The prevention of postoperative pain. Pain 1988;33:289–290.

111. Berry FA: Preemptive analgesia for postop pain. Paediatr Anaesth 1998;8:187–188.

112. Litman RS: Recent trends in the management of acute pain in children. J Am Osteopath Assoc 1996;96:290–296.

113. Tverskoy M, Cozacov C, Ayache M, et al: Postoperative pain after inguinal herniorrhaphy with different types of anesthesia. Anesth Analg 1990;70:29–35.

114. Casey WF, Rice LJ, Hannallah RS, et al: A comparison between bupivacaine instillation versus ilioinguinal/iliohypogastric nerve block for postoperative analgesia following inguinal herniorrhaphy in children. Anesthesiology 1990;72:637–639.

115. Drager C, Benziger D, Gao F, et al: Prolonged intercostal nerve blockade in sheep using controlled-release of bupivacaine and dexamethasone from polymer microspheres. Anesthesiology 1998;89:969–979.

116. Masters DB, Berde CB, Dutta SK, et al: Prolonged regional nerve blockade by controlled release of local anesthetic from a biodegradable polymer matrix. Anesthesiology 1993;79:340–346.

117. Rice LJ, Pudimat MA, Hannallah RS: Timing of caudal block placement in relation to surgery does not affect duration of postoperative analgesia in paediatric ambulatory patients. Can Anaesth Soc J 1990;37:429–431.

118. Wolf AR, Valley RD, Fear DW, et al: Bupivacaine for caudal analgesia in infants and children: The optimal effective concentration. Anesthesiology 1988;69:102–106.

119. Constant I, Gall O, Gouyet L, et al: Addition of clonidine or fentanyl to local anaesthetics prolongs the duration of surgical analgesia after single shot caudal block in children. Br J Anaesth 1998;80:294–298.

120. Cook B, Grubb DJ, Aldridge LA, et al: Comparison of the effects of adrenaline, clonidine and ketamine on the duration of caudal analgesia produced by bupivacaine in children. Br J Anaesth 1995;75:698–701.

121. Cook B, Doyle E: The use of additives to local anaesthetic solutions for caudal epidural blockade. Paediatr Anaesth 1996;6:353–359.

122. Ivani G, Bergendahl HT, Lampugnani E, et al: Plasma levels of clonidine following epidural bolus injection in children. Acta Anaesthesiol Scand 1998;42:306–311.

123. Jamali S, Monin S, Begon C, et al: Clonidine in pediatric caudal anesthesia. Anesth Analg 1994;78:663–666.

124. Luz G, Innerhofer P, Oswald E, et al: Comparison of clonidine 1 microgram kg-1 with morphine 30 micrograms kg-1 for post-operative caudal analgesia in children. Eur J Anaesthesiol 1999;16:42–46.

125. Malinovsky JM, Cozian A, Lepage JY, et al: Ketamine and midazolam neurotoxicity in the rabbit. Anesthesiology 1991;75:91–97.

126. Malinovsky JM, Lepage JY, Cozian A, et al: Is ketamine or its preservative responsible for neurotoxicity in the rabbit? Anesthesiology 1993;78:109–115.

127. Findlow D, Aldridge LM, Doyle E: Comparison of caudal block using bupivacaine and ketamine with ilioinguinal nerve block for orchidopexy in children. Anaesthesia 1997;52:1110–1113.

128. Gaiser RR, Venkateswaren P, Cheek TG, et al: Comparison of 0.25% ropivacaine and bupivacaine for epidural analgesia for labor and vaginal delivery. J Clin Anesth 1997;9:564–568.

129. Da Conceicao MJ, Coelho L, Khalil M: Ropivacaine 0.25% compared with bupivacaine 0.25% by the caudal route. Paediatr Anaesth 1999;9:229–233.

130. Moriarty A: Postoperative extradural infusions in children: Preliminary data from a comparison of bupivacaine/diamorphine with plain ropivacaine. Paediatr Anaesth 1999;9:423–427.

131. Irestedt L, Ekblom A, Olofsson C, et al: Pharmacokinetics and clinical effect during continuous epidural infusion with ropivacaine 2.5 mg/ml or bupivacaine 2.5 mg/ml for labour pain relief. Acta Anaesthesiol Scand 1998;42:890–896.

132. Ivani G, Mereto N, Lampugnani E, et al: Ropivacaine in paediatric surgery: Preliminary results. Paediatr Anaesth 1998;8:127–129.

133. Ivani G, Lampugnani E, De Negri P, et al: Ropivacaine vs bupivacaine in major surgery in infants. Can J Anaesth 1999;46:467–469.

134. Ivani G, Lampugnani E, Torre M, et al: Comparison of ropivacaine with bupivacaine for paediatric caudal block. Br J Anaesth 1998;81:247–248.

135. Ivani G, Mazzarello G, Lampugnani E, et al: Ropivacaine for central blocks in children. Anaesthesia 1998;53:74–76.

136. Kohane DS, Sankar WN, Shubina M, et al: Sciatic nerve blockade in infant, adolescent, and adult rats: A comparison of ropivacaine with bupivacaine. Anesthesiology 1998;89:1199–1208.

137. Koinig H, Krenn CG, Glaser C, et al: The dose-response of caudal ropivacaine in children. Anesthesiology 1999;90:1339–1344.

138. Plowman AN, Bolsin S, Mather LE: Central nervous system toxicity attributable to epidural ropivacaine hydrochloride. Anaesth Intensive Care 1998;26:204–206.

139. Selander D, Sjovall J, Tucker G: CNS toxicity of ropivacaine. Anaesth Intensive Care 1999;27:320–321.

140. McClellan KJ, Spencer CM: Levobupivacaine. Drugs 1998;56:355–362.

141. Dyhre H, Lang M, Wallin R, et al: The duration of action of bupivacaine, levobupivacaine, ropivacaine and pethidine in peripheral nerve block in the rat. Acta Anaesthesiol Scand 1997;41:1346–1352.

142. Bay-Nielsen M, Klarskov B, Bech K, et al: Levobupivacaine vs bupivacaine as infiltration anaesthesia in inguinal herniorrhaphy. Br J Anaesth 1999;82:280–282.

143. Gunter JB, Gregg T, Varughese AM, et al: Levobupivacaine for ilioinguinal/iliohypogastric nerve block in children. Anesth Analg 1999;89:647–649.

144. Hannallah RS, Broadman LM, Belman AB, et al: Comparison of caudal and ilioinguinal/iliohypogastric nerve blocks for control of post-orchiopexy pain in pediatric ambulatory surgery. Anesthesiology 1987;66:832–834.

145. Blaise G, Roy WL: Postoperative pain relief after hypospadias repair in pediatric patients: Regional analgesia versus systemic analgesics. Anesthesiology 1986;65:84–86.

146. Dalens B, Vanneuville G, Tanguy A: Comparison of the fascia iliaca compartment block with the 3-in-1 block in children. Anesth Analg 1989;69:705–713.

147. Bosenberg AT, Bland BA, Schulte-Steinberg O, et al: Thoracic epidural anesthesia via caudal route in infants. Anesthesiology 1988;69:265–269.

148. Gunter JB, Eng C: Thoracic epidural anesthesia via the caudal approach in children. Anesthesiology 1992;76:935–938.

149. Tucker GT, Mather LE: Pharmacology of local anaesthetic agents: Pharmacokinetics of local anaesthetic agents. Br J Anaesth 1975;47:213–224.

150. van Niekerk J, Bax-Vermeire BM, Geurts JW, et al: Epidurography in premature infants. Anaesthesia 1990;45:722–725.

151. Chaplan SR, Duncan SR, Brodsky JB, et al: Morphine and hydromorphone epidural analgesia: A prospective, randomized comparison. Anesthesiology 1992;77:1090–1094.

152. Brose WG, Tanelian DL, Brodsky JB, et al: CSF and blood pharmacokinetics of hydromorphone and morphine following lumbar epidural administration. Pain 1991;45:11–15.

153. Shulman MS, Wakerlin G, Yamaguchi L, et al: Experience with epidural hydromorphone for post-thoracotomy pain relief. Anesth Analg 1987;66:1331–1333.

154. Brodsky JB, Chaplan SR, Brose WG, et al: Continuous epidural hydromorphone for postthoracotomy pain relief. Ann Thorac Surg 1990;50:888–893.

155. Ecoffey C, Dubousset AM, Samii K: Lumbar and thoracic epidural anesthesia for urologic and upper abdominal surgery in infants and children. Anesthesiology 1986;65:87–90.

156. Meignier M, Souron R, Le Neel JC: Postoperative dorsal epidural analgesia in the child with respiratory disabilities. Anesthesiology 1983;59:473–475.

157. Zipes DP, Fischer J, King RM, et al: Termination of ventricular fibrillation in dogs by depolarizing a critical amount of myocardium. Am J Cardiol 1975;36:37–44.

158. Krane EJ, Dalens BJ, Murat I, et al: The safety of epidurals placed during general anesthesia. Reg Anesth Pain Med 1998;23:433–438.

159. Birmingham PK, Wheeler M, Suresh S, et al.: Patient controlled epidural analgesia in children: Can they do it? Anesthesiology 1998;89:A1167.

160. Arms DM, Smith JT, Osteyee J, et al: Postoperative epidural analgesia for pediatric spine surgery. Orthopedics 1998;21:539–544.

161. Caudle CL, Freid EB, Bailey AG, et al: Epidural fentanyl infusion with patient-controlled epidural analgesia for postoperative analgesia in children. J Pediatr Surg 1993;28:554–558.

162. Henderson K, Sethna NF, Berde CB: Continuous caudal anesthesia for inguinal hernia repair in former preterm infants. J Clin Anesth 1993;5:129–133.

163. Payen D, Ecoffey C, Carli P, et al: Pulsed Doppler ascending aortic, carotid, brachial, and femoral artery blood flows during caudal anesthesia in infants. Anesthesiology 1987;67:681–685.

164. Oberlander TF, Berde CB, Lam KH, et al: Infants tolerate spinal anesthesia with minimal overall autonomic changes: Analysis of heart rate variability in former premature infants undergoing hernia repair. Anesth Analg 1995;80:20–27.

165. Wood CE, Goresky GV, Klassen KA, et al: Complications of continuous epidural infusions for postoperative analgesia in children. Can J Anaesth 1994;41:613–620.

166. Larsson BA, Lonnqvist PA, Olsson GL: Plasma concentrations of bupivacaine in neonates after continuous epidural infusion. Anesth Analg 1997;84:501–505.

167. McCloskey JJ, Haun SE, Deshpande JK: Bupivacaine toxicity secondary to continuous caudal epidural infusion in children. Anesth Analg 1992;75:287–290.

168. Berde CB: Convulsions associated with pediatric regional anesthesia. Anesth Analg 1992;75:164–166.

169. Brill JE: Control of pain. Crit Care Clin 1992;8:203–218.

170. Lin YC, Sentivany-Collins SK, Peterson KL, et al: Outcomes after single injection caudal epidural versus continuous infusion epidural via caudal approach for postoperative analgesia in infants and children undergoing patent ductus arteriosus ligation. Paediatr Anaesth 1999;9:139–143.

171. Scott DA, Blake D, Buckland M, et al: A comparison of epidural ropivacaine infusion alone and in combination with 1, 2, and 4 microg/mL fentanyl for seventy-two hours of postoperative analgesia after major abdominal surgery. Anesth Analg 1999;88:857–864.

172. Krane EJ, Tyler DC, Jacobson LE: The dose response of caudal morphine in children. Anesthesiology 1989;71:48–52.

173. Ecoffey C, Desparmet J, Maury M, et al: Bupivacaine in children: Pharmacokinetics following caudal anesthesia. Anesthesiology 1985;63:447–448.

174. Tobias JD, Oakes L, Rao B: Continuous epidural anesthesia for postoperative analgesia in the pediatric oncology patient. Am J Pediatr Hematol Oncol 1992;14:216–221.

175. Berde CB, Sethna NF, Yemen TA, et al.: Continuous epidural bupivacaine-fentanyl infusions in children following ureteral reimplantation. Anesthesiology 1990; 73:A1128.

176. Mazoit JX, Denson DD, Samii K: Pharmacokinetics of bupivacaine following caudal anesthesia in infants. Anesthesiology 1988;68:387–391.

177. Krane EJ: Delayed respiratory depression in a child after caudal morphine. Anesth Analg 1988;67:79–82.

178. Attia J, Ecoffey C, Sandouk P, et al: Epidural morphine in children: Pharmacokinetics and CO_2 sensitivity. Anesthesiology 1986;65:590–594.

179. Valley RD, Bailey AG: Caudal morphine for postoperative analgesia in infants and children: A report of 138 cases. Anesth Analg 1991;72:120–124.

180. Rawal N, Wattwil M: Respiratory depression after epidural morphine: An experimental and clinical study. Anesth Analg 1984;63:8–14.

181. Rasch DK, Webster DE, Pollard TG, et al: Lumbar and thoracic epidural analgesia via the caudal approach for postoperative pain relief in infants and children. Can J Anaesth 1990;37:359–362.

182. Blomberg R: The dorsomedian connective tissue band in the lumbar epidural space of humans: An anatomical study using epiduroscopy in autopsy cases. Anesth Analg 1986;65:747–752.

183. Noda H, Saionji K, Miyazaki T: Antibacterial activity of local anesthetics. Masui 1990;39:994–1001.

184. McIlvaine WB, Knox RF, Fennessey PV, et al: Continuous infusion of bupivacaine via intrapleural catheter for analgesia after thoracotomy in children. Anesthesiology 1988;69:261–264.

185. Semsroth M, Plattner O, Horcher E: Effective pain relief with continuous intrapleural bupivacaine after thoracotomy in infants and children. Paediatr Anaesth 1996;6:303–310.

186. Swinhoe CF, Pereira NH: Intrapleural analgesia in a child with a mediastinal tumour. Can J Anaesth 1994;41:427–430.

187. de la Linde CM, Polo A, Lopez-Andrade A: Continuous axillary plexus block in pediatrics. [in Spanish]. Rev Esp Anestesiol Reanim 1997;44:87–88.

188. Ebert B, Ganser J: Axillary plexus catheter block in childhood and adolescence. [in German]. Handchir Mikrochir Plast Chir 1997;29:303–306.

189. Miaskowski C, Crews J, Ready LB, et al: Anesthesia-based pain services improve the quality of postoperative pain management. Pain 1999;80:23–29.

Postanesthesia Care Unit

Alberto J. de Armendi *and* I. David Todres

Recovery from Anesthesia
  Indicators of Wakefulness
  Physicochemical Factors Governing Recovery from Inhalational Anesthesia
  Recovery of Respiratory Reflexes
  Recovery from Neuromuscular Blockade
  Recovery from Intravenous Opioids and Hypnotics
Procedural Aspects of Postanesthesia Care
  Endotracheal Extubation
  Transport to the Postanesthesia Care Unit
  Arrival in the Postanesthesia Care Unit
  Organization of the Postanesthesia Care Unit
  Discharge Criteria
Postanesthesia Care Unit Problems
  Anxiety and Agitation
  Respiratory Problems
  Dysrhythmias
  Pressure Control
  Pain
  Nausea and Vomiting
  Temperature Control
  Oliguria
  Neurologic Complications
Parents in the Postanesthesia Care Unit
Fast Track Recovery
Policies and Procedures

Unlike many other forms of central nervous system depression, general anesthesia can be reversed. It is not surprising that recovery of normal consciousness is not instantaneous; indeed, it is remarkable that recovery is so rapid. Postanesthesia care units (PACUs) became widespread after the realization that the period of emergence from anesthesia is associated with common and potentially catastrophic problems that can generally be obviated by an environment that facilitates close observation and rapid institution of rescue therapy. This chapter outlines general principles governing recovery from anesthesia, procedural and organizational issues in pediatric PACUs, and common clinical problems that arise in the care of children recovering from anesthesia.

Recovery From Anesthesia

Contemporary anesthetic practice frequently uses combinations of inhalation anesthetics, intravenous anesthetics, muscle relaxants, intravenous hypnotics and opioids, and regional techniques. We discuss each class separately, realizing that the effects of these agents in clinical practice can be synergistic and that the effects of such synergy on recovery have been poorly characterized in children.

Indicators of Wakefulness

Although complete recovery of mental acuity after an inhalation anesthetic may take 1 to 4 days, much of our concern in the PACU focuses on the more rapid return of the protective reflexes necessary for cardiorespiratory stability. These reflexes include the ability to prevent airway obstruction resulting from posterior displacement of the tongue, epiglottis, and soft palate or from secretions, the ability to expel tracheobronchial secretions by coughing, baroreceptor reflexes to support perfusion, and chemoreceptor reflexes to support respiration in response to hypercarbia or hypoxemia. The principles governing recovery from inhalation anesthesia are well summarized by Eger.[1] For inhalation anesthetics, 50% of patients have been shown to respond to a simple command such as "open your eyes" at 20% to 60% of the minimum alveolar concentration (MAC) of the anesthetic; such patients are said to be MAC-awake.[2-6] Achieving MAC-awake may also be confounded by interactions between potent anesthetic agents and other sedating medications.[7-9] A general clinical impression is that adults at MAC-awake levels of anesthesia (if unimpeded by other factors) are able to maintain and protect their airways. A similar impression in children recovering from anesthesia is that spontaneous eye opening predicts safe airway maintenance—that is, intact airway reflexes.

Physicochemical Factors Governing Recovery from Inhalation Anesthesia

When inhalation anesthesia is discontinued, the rate of decline of alveolar concentration of the gas is a function of alveolar ventilation, anesthetic solubility (blood/gas solubility coefficient, or λ), cardiac output, and the venous-to-alveolar partial pressure difference. Increased ventilation results in a more rapid decline in alveolar anesthetic concentration, which hastens recovery, provided that the arterial carbon dioxide pressure is not so low that it diminishes cerebral blood flow and the removal of anesthetic agent from the brain. The blood/gas solubility coefficient is an important determinant of recovery time. A MAC-awake state is generally reached within 2 minutes after the discontinuation of nitrous oxide; in contrast, reaching such a state may take several hours after discontinuation of a highly soluble agent such as ether. The λ, in order of decreasing solubility is ether (12), halothane (2.5), isoflurane (1.4), sevoflurane (0.65), nitrous oxide (0.47), and desflurane (0.45).[10] Thus for the potent inhalation agents currently used, the times required for patients to reach a MAC-awake state (when no other sedating medications have been administered) are generally intermediate between that for nitrous oxide and ether.

Maintenance of high anesthetic concentrations results in greater accumulation of the anesthetics in tissues and prolongs recovery time. The higher the λ, the more drug is taken up into body tissues and therefore the longer it takes for the drug to redistribute out of tissue upon discontinuing anesthesia. The duration of anesthesia therefore affects recovery, and this effect is more pronounced the more soluble the anesthetic agent. For example, maintenance of halothane anesthesia at 1.1 MAC for 15 minutes results in recovery to a MAC-awake state in approximately 4 minutes, whereas such recovery may take 15 minutes after 2 hours of anesthesia at the same MAC. A frequent rationale for the use of nitrous oxide and muscle relaxants is that they permit the use of lower concentrations of the more soluble inhalation agents and thus enable a more rapid recovery. Desflurane and sevoflurane are newer agents with low blood/gas partition coefficients, which result in more rapid elimination compared with the more soluble halothane and isoflurane.[11–18] For outpatient anesthesia, the use of desflurane (λ = 0.45) or sevoflurane (λ = 0.65) results in significantly shorter recovery times than the use of halothane (λ = 2.3) or isoflurane (λ = 1.4).[13–16, 19–24] Maintenance with desflurane may be particularly beneficial to neonates with a post-conceptual age of less than 60 weeks undergoing anesthesia for herniorrhaphy with a shorter recovery time when compared with halothane or sevoflurane.[17] However, despite an apparent shorter period for awakening with both sevoflurane and desflurane compared with halothane or isoflurane, this does not result in a more rapid discharge from the hospital or recovery room.[15, 16, 18, 21, 25] This may be a result of other factors such as local practice, emergence delirium, the need to treat pain, administration of other sedating medications, and nursing or parental issues unrelated to anesthetic management.[14, 16, 19, 20, 22, 26, 27]

Recovery of Respiratory Reflexes

Response to Carbon Dioxide

Although patients at MAC-awake levels of inhalation anesthesia may in general maintain airway patency, other reflexes may be variably depressed. There is a dose-related reduction in the ventilatory response to carbon dioxide; however, even at levels between 0.6 and 1.0 MAC, patients with patent airways and normal lungs do not generally become dangerously hypercarbic.[28–30] Patients with obstructive lung disease or other causes of increased work of breathing may become increasingly hypercarbic. The level of ventilation is also a function of the degree of painful stimulation; patients with a surgical stimulus will breathe more vigorously than less-stimulated patients, although if the act of breathing increases incisional pain, as is common for thoracic and upper abdominal surgery, they may have diminished tidal volumes. Patients in the PACU whose pain is well treated with a local anesthetic infiltration, regional nerve block, and opioid, may be at risk for resedation and hypercarbia once the stimulus of surgery has been removed.

Response to Oxygen

The effect of residual volatile anesthetic agents on the ventilatory response to hypoxemia is of potentially greater importance in a PACU than is the response to carbon dioxide.[31, 32] The responsiveness of the peripheral chemoreceptors, which govern the hypoxic drive in humans, is blunted by alveolar halothane concentrations as low as 0.1% and is abolished entirely at a concentration of 1.1%. Patients in a PACU are frequently predisposed to hypoxemia; the causes of this condition include airway obstruction, central hypoventilation (inhalation anesthetics, opioids), atelectasis with ventilation-perfusion imbalance, and diminished tidal volume as the result of pain, tight dressings, or casts. Because of the depressant effects of residual concentrations of inhalation anesthetics and interactions with other sedating medications such as opioids, patients may not struggle or hyperventilate and may lapse into unconsciousness. An important rationale for the routine administration of supplemental oxygen in a PACU is to prevent episodic hypoxemia, which may occur even after uneventful surgical procedures.[33, 34] Children recovering from or with an active upper respiratory tract infection (URI) are particularly likely to experience a prolonged period of oxygen requirement and episodes of oxygen desaturation compared with patients who do not have or are not recovering from a URI.[35, 36] In newborns, the ventilatory response to hypoxemia is attenuated even in the absence of anesthetic agents.[37–41] High concentrations of supplemental oxygen must be judiciously administered to premature infants; the potential risks of retinopathy of prematurity must be considered.[42–44] Although the arterial oxygen tension associated with retinopathy is unclear and many other factors are likely contributory,[45, 46] we administer oxygen to maintain an oxygen saturation of 93% to 95%.

Recovery from Neuromuscular Blockade

Recovery from neuromuscular blockade may be monitored by peripheral nerve stimulation and by clinical indices such as an inspiratory force greater than −20 cm H_2O, vital capacity greater than 15 to 20 mL/kg, and the ability to protrude the tongue and lift the head for longer than 5 seconds.[47] For small infants, who are unable to lift their heads, brisk flexion of hips and knees that lifts the feet off the table is associated with return of adequate muscular recovery.[48] Incomplete reversal of blockade may result in loss of airway patency and diminished ventilation and may be especially dangerous in combination with residual-inhalation anesthetics and opioids. Reversal by cholinesterase inhibitors and the addition of agents such as atropine to antagonize the muscarinic side effect has been well studied in infants and children; train-of-four monitoring can be performed in all age groups.[49–51] Intermediate-acting neuromuscular agents, such as rocuronium, may be preferable to the older long-acting agents, such as curare and pancuronium, because they are easily antagonized at the end of a short surgical procedure, but the older (less costly) agents are appropriate for procedures lasting longer than 45 minutes. The benzylisoquinolinium diester mivacurium is even more rapidly metabolized and may be administered by an infusion.[52–57] Mivacurium may need to be administered at an increased infusion rate in children compared with adults to maintain constant 90% to 95% blockade; this increased requirement correlates with the plasma cholinesterase activity. The requirement is reduced in the presence of potent inhalation agent.[58] Often such short-acting agents may not need to be antagonized at the end of a procedure, provided the patient demonstrates all signs of adequate recovery (see Chapter 10). Rarely, prolonged blockade with mivacurium (as with succinylcholine) may result from pseudocholinesterase deficiency.[59, 60] Lastly, rapacuronium is a new nondepolarizing neuromuscular blocking agent that is metabolized in a relatively short period of time and may be a future substitute for succinylcholine.[61–63] Thus, currently available muscle relaxants may improve the safety profile of recovery from residual neuromuscular blockade in children. Delayed recovery or residual neuromuscular blockade is manifest clinically by inadequate respiratory efforts, inability to maintain a patent airway, and weak uncoordinated movements of the extremities ("puppet-like" movements). Patients with such clinical manifestations should have their train-of-four tested[47, 51] for objective evidence of residual blockade and as a means of assessing the adequacy of treatment (reversal). Unusually long neuromuscular blockade is occasionally observed in patients who are hypothermic (delayed metabolism), in patients receiving medications known to potentiate the effect of neuromuscular blockade (e.g., some antibiotics), and in patients with metabolic abnormalities such as hypocalcemia or hypermagnesemia.[64–71]

Recovery from Intravenous Opioids and Hypnotics

Recovery from intravenous opioids and hypnotics may be more variable and difficult to quantify than recovery from inhalation and neuromuscular blocking agents.[72] Clearance of intravenous medications is characterized by a rapid redistribution phase and a slower elimination phase, caused by hepatic metabolism or renal excretion or both (see Chapter 8). Pharmacokinetic analysis may be misleading if one fails to consider the biologic activity of metabolites, for example, the prolonged action of diazepam metabolites.[73] The metabolism of some medications may be delayed, and the clinical effects of some medications therefore prolonged, due to inhibition of the cytochrome oxidase system.[74–78] The most likely pediatric example is the interaction between erythromycin and midazolam.[79, 80] In the case of other agents such as scopolamine and ketamine, biologic effects on memory and other cognitive functions are not easily accounted for

by plasma disappearance curves. The depressant effects of opioids and hypnotics on the ventilatory response to carbon dioxide are well known; it is worth noting that these intravenous anesthetics may depress the hypoxic drive as well. There is minimal pediatric information on the effects of various doses of opioids and hypnotics on the MAC-awake state for inhalation agents,[7, 9, 81, 82] as well as the effect of painful stimulation on the MAC-awake state.

Intravenous opioids and hypnotics are frequently given in combination with inhalation agents. A general impression is that combinations of such agents are commonly synergistic in their depression of respiratory and circulatory reflexes; this effect has been well described for combinations of opioids and benzodiazepines.[83, 84] Although opioid-induced depression is antagonized by naloxone (we would encourage use of this agent only for specific indications, e.g., severe hypoventilation), routine use of naloxone at the termination of an anesthetic can produce acute pain, anxiety, vomiting, and (rarely) pulmonary edema.[85, 86] Benzodiazepine-induced depression is antagonized by flumazenil.[87] Large or repeated doses of ketamine and droperidol are especially associated with prolongation of recovery time and may also result in an altered response to hypercarbia.[88]

Propofol has received considerable study for induction and maintenance of anesthesia. Pediatric studies suggest that propofol is associated with very rapid emergence and a low incidence of postoperative emesis.[89–94] Ketorolac has been shown to decrease the opioid use, suggesting beneficial effects for the treatment of pain while avoiding respiratory depression and nausea and vomiting.[95–103] These medications should be used with caution in patients with the potential for hemorrhage because of their effects on platelet function.[104–107] In general, it is safe to administer in the recovery room once hemostasis has been achieved. *Remifentanil is too short acting to provide any postoperative analgesia and has no role in the treatment of pediatric pain in the PACU. The fentanyl patch is only indicated in patients receiving chronic opioid therapy (chronic pain and cancer patients) and is contraindicated for the treatment of postoperative pain in narcotically naive patients, since several pediatric deaths have occurred due to prolonged and excessive drug absorbtion.*[108–112] There is minimal published pediatric experience with this formulation.[113] Studies with oral transmucosal fentanyl citrate as premedication compared with intravenous fentanyl provided equivalent postoperative analgesia and equivalent postoperative nausea and vomiting in children undergoing tonsillectomy.[114] This formulation may provide a painless means of administering additional opioid in patients who have pain but whose intravenous line has been removed or is no longer functioning.

Procedural Aspects of Postanesthesia Care

Recovery from anesthesia is a process of consecutive steps, as noted by Smith[115]:

Recovery begins as soon as the anesthesiologist stops active administration of anesthetic agents. It follows a definite progression, first in the operating room, where respiration is re-established and tracheal extubation is accomplished, then in the recovery room, where the patient regains full consciousness and cardiopulmonary stability (or in the PICU for prolonged support), and finally in the nursing division or ward, where the patient recovers his strength and becomes ambulatory and ready for discharge.

We would include the time of safe transport from the operating room to the PACU or pediatric intensive care unit (PICU) as an essential step in anesthesia care.

Endotracheal Extubation

Criteria for Extubation

In most cases, extubation may be safely performed in the operating room. However, a child's condition may necessitate delayed extubation at an appropriate time in the PACU or PICU. There is widespread agreement that children who have been anesthetized with a full stomach, children at risk for airway obstruction (including those whose jaws are wired shut and those with Pierre Robin syndrome, Treacher-Collins syndrome, hemifacial microsomia, or other syndromes associated with difficult airway maintenance, e.g., obstructive sleep apnea), premature infants, and other infants predisposed to apnea should be awake before extubation is attempted. Beyond this, the timing of extubation is a matter of individual judgment. For example, the practice at some institutions is to extubate when a patient is awake and demonstrating eye opening and other purposeful movement; the practice at others is to extubate while the patient is under a deep plane of inhalation anesthesia. Clinicians report only rare problems with either approach. Most clinicians would agree that either approach is preferable to extubation in a very light plane of anesthesia, when laryngospasm is a high probability and vomiting may occur while protective reflexes are impaired. Our approach is to extubate most children when they are awake with protective airway reflexes intact; exceptions include children with severe asthma, those with eye injuries, and those for whom severe coughing may jeopardize the surgical outcome. One study found fewer airway problems with halothane compared with isoflurane with deep extubation.[116] This finding is interesting but should be extrapolated with caution to anesthetics supplemented with opioids and muscle relaxants.

Procedure for Extubation

The stomach is routinely emptied before discontinuation of anesthesia; it is our practice to empty the stomach after induction or intubation. Extubation is preceded by pharyngeal suctioning and occurs with a full inspiration. Immediately after extubation, oxygen should be administered, and the child should be observed for adequate ventilation, satisfactory oxygen saturation, color of the mucous membranes, and the presence of laryngospasm or vomiting. Transport of patients should not be undertaken until the patency of the airway and the adequacy of oxygenation and ventilation have been confirmed, meaning stable, satisfactory oxygen saturation in room air. One study found a mean room air oxygen saturation of 95% at the end of surgery following anesthesia.[36] Therefore our criteria for transporting the patient from the operating room to PACU without oxygen is a stable oxygen saturation of 95% or greater in room air. If the patient cannot sustain this level of oxygen saturation, then either a longer time for recovery in the operating room is taken or the patient is transported with oxygen and a means for providing positive pressure ventilation.

Transport to the Postanesthesia Care Unit

Transport from the operating room to the PACU should be carried out under the direct supervision of the anesthesiologist, a Certified Registered Nurse Anesthetist (CRNA), or both. A check of the security and patency of the endotracheal tube (if a patient is to remain intubated) or laryngeal mask airway, all intravenous lines, the arterial line, chest tubes, drains, and the urinary catheter should be made before transport. It is reasonable and aesthetically proper to remove all blood and secretions from the surface of a patient's body and face before transport to the PACU or PICU. Children should be kept warm throughout transport to avoid the dangers of hypothermia. Unless patients are wide awake, with protective airway reflexes intact, or unless there is a specific contraindication, it is sensible to transport extubated patients in the lateral position, so that the tongue and secretions and possible vomitus are less likely to cause airway obstruction. A hand holding the chin up (extension at the atlanto-occipital junction) helps maintain a patient's airway and serves as a breath monitor; the exhaled breath can be felt on the hand. For sleepy children, continued use of the precordial stethoscope serves as a monitor of respiration and circulation; for screaming, crying, or otherwise highly active children, this means of monitoring may be unsatisfactory. Oxygen delivery via face mask may be indicated. We recommend that patients in a potentially unstable condition be transported with a battery-powered pulse oximeter, an electrocardiographic monitor, and a blood pressure cuff and aneroid manometer or a transduced arterial line. The monitoring lines, intravenous drips, infusion pumps, and other paraphernalia should be clearly sorted out and simplified before transport. For sick patients, intubated patients, and patients with potential airway difficulties, an appropriate resuscitation bag, face mask, oral airway, oxygen tanks (oxygen levels should be checked), functioning laryngoscopes, endotracheal tube, portable suction, and medications (including atropine and succinylcholine) should be carried en route to the PACU or PICU. A tackle box containing all of this paraphernalia is extremely helpful, especially when patients are transported to the PICU in an elevator. Patients receiving vasopressors or vasodilators require battery-powered infusion pumps so that these agents can be continuously administered at precise titrated levels.

Transport to the PACU or PICU is a time of potential danger. A patient often appears awake after the stimulation of extubation and transfer to the stretcher but may subsequently become more obtunded, and obstruction of the airway may occur during transit. Just as frequently, children may become restless during transit. Guardrails may be helpful, but most important is the anesthesiologist's constant observation of the patient. A gentle hand on the head may prevent bumping against the guardrails. As always, the cause of restlessness must be sought (especially if the cause is hypoxemia, discussed later).[117, 118]

Arrival in the Postanesthesia Care Unit

Attention is first directed to airway patency, the color of the lips and mucous membranes, oxygen saturation, and adequacy of ventilation, perfusion, and central nervous system function. Heart rate, blood pressure, oxygen saturation, respiratory rate, and temperature are recorded. The nurse-to-patient ratio is 1:1 for sick patients and 1:2 or 1:3 for routine cases. Supplemental oxygen is administered. In rare cases (preterm infants, late-stage cystic fibrosis), it may be necessary to regulate more precisely the inspired concentration of oxygen. Many children object to placement of an oxygen mask, and a funnel-type mask or open hose with high flow rates may be less objectionable (although less optimal). Thereafter, a report should be given to the nurses and physicians in attendance. This report should include, at a minimum, patient identification, age, preoperative vital signs, and specific circumstances, such as language barrier or developmental delay. The size and location of catheters, a description of the patient's current problem, past medical history, medications and allergies, operative procedure, and pertinent surgical problems should be outlined. The following should be described to the PACU team: the premedication and anesthetic agents used at induction and for maintenance, techniques used, reversal of neuromuscular blockade (adequacy of the train-of-four response), estimated blood loss, fluid replacement (including amount and type of solution), urine output, and vasoactive drugs, bronchodilators, and intraoperative medications (e.g., antibiotics) used. Regional anesthesia issues, such as epidural, location, drug, drug concentration and contents, effective level of analgesia, and infusion rate should be clearly transmitted. The administration of analgesics (time and dose, such as rectal acetaminophen), local blocks and wound infiltration with local anesthetics, problems with either surgery or anesthesia (difficult intravenous access, difficult intubation, intraoperative hemodynamic instability or cardiac changes), and potential problems in the PACU should be listed. Finally, the anesthesia team must remain with the patient until the patient is stable and the PACU team is ready to assume the care of the patient.

Organization of the Postanesthesia Care Unit

Organization of a PACU varies with the particular needs of each hospital and its surgical practice. In general, it is recommended that the PACU be located adjacent to the operating room to permit rapid transport of patients to and from the operating room, to allow ready access to surgeons and anesthesiologists, and to allow access to radiology and laboratory. On one hand, PACUs may function almost as PICUs, caring for critically ill patients, and on the other hand, PACUs for ambulatory surgery areas may receive only relatively healthy patients. Even in the latter case, it is essential that full facilities be available for resuscitation and that there be a protocol for transfer to an acute-care environment (in the same or a nearby hospital).

The number of beds required is largely a function of the volume and types of surgical procedures performed. Recommendations commonly include two PACU beds for each operating room; each bed space should include oxygen, suction, blood pressure cuffs, pulse oximetry, and the equipment listed in Table 30–1. Depending on the case mix, there should be a variable number of electrocardiographic monitors and pressure transducers for arterial and venous catheters, and so on. We recommend the use of portable

"crash carts," which can be moved to the bedside for acute airway management, resuscitation, or defibrillation. Medications should be readily accessible; a representative listing of necessary medications is included in Table 30–2.

The physical layout of a PACU is generally arranged to support optimal visibility of patients, so that events can be observed and treated rapidly; large, open rooms are usually used. Although such visibility is essential, large, noisy rooms can be frightening to children. When appropriate, curtains may be drawn to give a child some privacy, particularly if other patients are undergoing acute interventions. In all cases, but especially for adolescents, it is important to appreciate their modesty and their wish not to be unnecessarily exposed.

Patients awakening from anesthesia often complain of strange or loud noises, and increased noise may even in-

Table 30–1. Recovery Room Supplies

Essential Bedside Equipment

Oxygen supply with regulated flows
Oxygen face masks and face tents for spontaneous ventilation (various sizes)
Stethoscope
Resuscitation bags: self-inflating (Ambu) and Mapleson type
Anesthesia face masks for positive-pressure ventilation (pediatric sizes 0, 1, 2, 3, adult, small, medium, large)
Oral airways (sizes 00, 0, 1 to 5)
Nasal airways (sizes 12F to 36F)
Suction and appropriate suction catheters (sizes 6 1/2 to 12 French); tonsil-type (Yankauer) attachment
Needles, syringes, alcohol wipes, Betadine solution, gauze pads
Arterial blood gas kit
Gloves
Pulse oximeters and sensors
EKG pads and monitor
Manual and automated blood pressure device
All sizes of blood pressure cuffs

Emergency Supplies for "Crash Cart" or Central Location

Laryngoscopes with blades: Miller 0, 1, 2, 3; Macintosh 2, 3, 4; extra laryngoscope bulbs, batteries
Endotracheal tubes, sizes 2.5 mm ID (internal diameter) through 8 mm ID (cuffed and uncuffed tubes for all sizes)
Laryngeal Mask Airways, sizes 1, 1.5, 2, 2.5, 3, 4 and 5
Stylet appropriate for each endotracheal tube size
Syringe for endotracheal cuff inflation
Tape and liquid adhesive for endotracheal tube fixation
14-gauge catheter over needle (e.g., Medicut or Jelco), with 3-mm ID endotracheal tube adapter for emergency cricothyroidotomy
Backup resuscitation bags and masks, oral airways, as described above for each bedside
Nasogastric tubes
Intravenous infusion solutions, tubing, drip chambers
Supplies for intravenous cannulation catheter over needle sets sizes 24 to 14 gauge
Cutdown tray, tracheostomy, and suture sets
Central venous catheter insertion set
Tube thoracotomy set and system for suction and underwater seal
Defibrillator (adult, child paddles)
Electrocardiogram
Pressure transducer system and oscilloscope monitor
Sterile gowns, gloves, masks, towels, drapes
Urinary catheter
Bed board for cardiopulmonary resuscitation

Table 30-2. Recovery Room Medications

Emergency Medications on "Crash Cart"

Atropine
Epinephrine
Sodium bicarbonate
Dextrose
Calcium chloride or gluconate
Lidocaine (intravenous and topical)
Succinylcholine
Thiopental or methohexital
Diphenhydramine
Hydrocortisone, dexamethasone, methylprednisolone
Neostigmine, edrophonium
Physostigmine
Naloxone
Flumazenil
Aminophylline
Furosemide
Dopamine
Isoproterenol
Norepinephrine
Sodium nitroprusside
Heparin
Verapamil
Quinidine
Bretylium
Propranolol, atenolol, esmolol
Phenytoin
Mannitol
Racemic epinephrine (for inhalation)

Medications to Be Kept Under Lock

Fentanyl
Morphine
Meperidine
Ketamine
Midazolam (IV and PO)
Diazepam
Phenobarbital
Propofol

Other Medications for Central Location

Antibiotics
Acetaminophen (PO and PR)
Dantrolene
Digoxin
Pancuronium or other nondepolarizing relaxants
Antiemetics (e.g., ondansetron, dolansetron, droperidol,
    promethazine, metoclopramide)
Protamine
Insulin
Potassium chloride (KCl)

pediatric airway and circulatory problems, the pharmacology of anesthetic agents, opioids and other common medications administered to children, and the emotional and behavioral responses of children at various ages. Dedicated nursing considerations in pediatric PACUs are described elsewhere.[120] Physician coverage in a PACU also varies. In some hospitals, the anesthesiologist who administered the anesthetic remains responsible throughout the recovery period, whereas in others a separate physician is responsible for the PACU. Regardless of the system used, anesthesia personnel should be readily available for acute evaluation of patients and for necessary interventions. In accordance with the guidelines of the Joint Commission on Accreditation of Healthcare Organizations (JCAHO), we advise that an anesthesiologist supervise care in the PACU. It is also reasonable to use the PACU as a recovery area for children undergoing sedation and analgesia for procedures by nonanesthesiologists so as to provide the same level of recovery care for all sedated and anesthetized children. The American Academy of Pediatrics has published guidelines written by pediatric anesthesiologists for the perioperative environment that also describe desired PACU staffing, equipment, and medications.[121]

Discharge Criteria

Various criteria for readiness for discharge from PACUs have been established.[122] The modified Aldrete score is the most common system used to assess discharge readiness.[123] Although attempts have been made to use formal criteria to assess readiness for discharge, readiness for discharge is also a function of the situation (home environment) to which a patient is being discharged. For example, a patient with a slight degree of post-intubation croup might be readily discharged to a ward or a pediatric PICU where there are nurses and physicians skilled in assessing pediatric airways. However, it would not be appropriate to discharge a patient with an identical problem after outpatient surgery to the care of parents of questionable reliability who anticipate driving 70 miles to their home through a snowstorm. For inpatients not being transferred to a PICU, the general features or readiness for discharge are summarized in Table 30–3. For outpatients, these criteria hold and the additional criteria in Table 30–4 must generally be met before discharge. Many hospitals have a two-tier recovery, one for immediate recovery from general anesthesia and a second "step-down" area, which still provides observation and monitoring if indicated for an extended period but at a less intense and therefore lower cost. The issue of whether outpatients should not be

crease patients' discomfort.[119] Noise levels in PACUs commonly average between 50 and 70 decibels; these levels produce measurable autonomic changes suggestive of a stress reaction. Every effort should be made to diminish unnecessary noise and commotion in the PACU.

Staffing is also a function of the particular needs of the hospital. For patients who are not acutely ill, a nurse-to-patient ratio of 1:3 is generally deemed sufficient; for acutely ill patients, the ratio may be 1:1 or even 2:1. Ideally, nurses caring for pediatric patients should have specific training in

Table 30-3. Discharge Criteria (Inpatients)

1. Recovery of airway and respiratory reflexes adequate to support gas exchange and to protect against aspiration of secretions, vomitus, or bood
2. Stability of circulation and control of any surgical bleeding
3. Absence of anticipated instability in categories 1 and 2
4. Reasonable control of pain and vomiting
5. Appropriate duration of observation after narcotic or naloxone/ flumazenil administration (a minimum of 60 minutes after intravenous naloxone and up to 2 hours following flumazenil)

Table 30–4. Discharge Criteria (Outpatients)

All criteria in Table 30–3, *plus*
1. Cardiovascular function and airway patency are satisfactory and stable.
2. The patient is easily arousable, and protective reflexes are intact.
3. The patient can talk (if age appropriate).
4. The patient can sit up unaided (if age appropriate).
5. For a very young or handicapped child, incapable of the usually expected responses, the preanesthetic level of responsiveness or a level as close as possible to the normal level for that child should be achieved unless the child is to be transferred to another monitored location.
6. The state of hydration is adequate.
7. It may be permissible for parents to carry their children without full recovery of gait (parents must be advised that the child is at risk of injury if improperly supervised).
8. Control of pain to permit adequate analgesia via the oral route thereafter.
9. Control of nausea and vomiting to allow for oral hydration (see "Discharge Criteria" in text).

discharged until they can retain oral fluids must be addressed on a case-by-case basis. We no longer adhere to this rule before discharging a patient from the PACU. Pediatric outpatients, particularly small children and infants who are scheduled for later cases and have not been allowed oral intake for prolonged periods, are frequently deficient in fluids at the time of induction of anesthesia. We attempt to replace a greater fraction of the deficit intravenously in the operating room and in the PACU, so that even if these children drink very little fluid after the procedure, they will be less likely to become dehydrated. Attempts to force fluids often result in vomiting in the PACU or during the journey home.[124] In many cases, it may be more sensible to let a child go home and try to take fluids in a more comfortable environment if the parents are reliable, the deficit is small, and the likelihood of vomiting is slight. Before discharge, pain and nausea should be under control; patients should be easily aroused and oriented, hemodynamically stable, and normothermic; and patients should be able to protect their own airways and ventilate adequately. The new concept of "fast track" discharge is presented subsequently.

Postanesthesia Care Unit Problems

If pathophysiologic changes are carefully monitored, one can deal with the problem regardless of the nature of the surgical or anesthetic procedure. The incidence of complications varies with the severity of the conditions of the patient population. One paper describes a complication rate of approximately 13% for pediatric patients admitted to the PACU.[125]

Anxiety and Agitation

Infants and children in PACUs are frequently restless and agitated or may cry uncontrollably. Although these responses may be "normal" upon emergence from anesthesia in a strange and unfriendly environment, it is imperative that physicians and nurses first investigate whether they are seri-

ous signs of physiologic distress. Causes of such responses include the following:

1. Hypoxemia or hypercarbia resulting from upper airway obstruction (by the tongue, secretions, blood, or vomitus), lower airway obstruction (by bronchospasm or mucous plugs), or ventilation/perfusion imbalance (caused by atelectasis; poor inspiratory effort due to casts, bandages, or pain; pulmonary edema; pneumothorax)
2. Hypotension and inadequate perfusion (caused by hypovolemia, cardiac failure)
3. Metabolic disturbances, including hypoglycemia, hypocalcemia, sepsis, hyponatremia, hyperkalemia, and acid-base imbalance
4. Increased intracranial pressure or other primary central nervous system pathology, such as persistent effects of anesthesia or sedation, decreased cerebral perfusion, stroke, and thromboembolic or hemorrhagic phenomenon
5. Excitatory effects of drugs (such as scopolamine, ketamine, and the short-acting inhalation agents desflurane and sevoflurane)
6. "Pure" emergence delirium after inhalation anesthesia (especially following sevoflurane and desflurane) or excess atropine
7. Untreated or under-treated pain (look for unanticipated causes of pain, such as metal instruments left under patients; traction on nasogastric tubes, urinary catheters, or chest tubes; tight casts; and occlusive taping of intravenous boards; look for a distended bladder)
8. An awake child's behavioral reaction to threatening circumstances
9. Absence of parents

In many cases, consideration of the circumstances of the surgery and a brief examination, with attention to the adequacy of ventilation, and cardiovascular stability should suffice for ruling out the most important causes. When in doubt, arterial blood gases, electrolytes, and blood glucose levels should be measured as indicated. Oxygen should be administered in most cases.[126, 127] Because a tight mask may increase agitation, it may be necessary to use a funnel mask or an open hose. Opioids, physostigmine, or reassurance and cuddling should be used as indicated by the particular circumstances. Emergence delirium is exacerbated by emergence from inhalation anesthesia with untreated pain,[128] and we encourage the use of opioids intraoperatively or before emergence or regional nerve (caudal) blocks when appropriate. Emergence delirium occurs less commonly in children and adolescents when a predominantly nitrous oxide-opioid technique is used. Among the inhalation agents, isoflurane may be associated with a higher incidence of stormy emergence compared with halothane,[129] but sevoflurane and desflurane have the highest association with emergence delirium.[13, 14, 16, 18–20, 24, 26, 130]

Respiratory Problems

In the PACU, respiratory insufficiency may present with obvious signs of difficult breathing, but it may also present as anxiety, unresponsiveness, tachycardia, bradycardia, hypertension, arrhythmia, seizures, or cardiac arrest. When any of these other conditions are present, respiratory insufficiency must be considered as a cause until ruled out. Hypoxemia, hypoventilation, and upper airway obstruction are the three most common respiratory events for pediatric patients in the PACU.

Hypoxemia

Hypoxemia may be caused by hypoventilation, diffusion hypoxia, upper airway obstruction, bronchospasm, aspiration of gastric contents, pulmonary edema, pneumothorax, atelectasis, or, rarely, pulmonary embolism. General anesthesia inhibits the hypoxic and hypercapneic ventilatory drive, reduces functional residual capacity, and alters hypoxic pulmonary vasoconstriction of all patients. Postoperative desaturation is more common in children with an active URI or those recovering from a URI.[35, 131] In addition, oxygen saturation has been correlated with recovery scores in some studies but not in others.[34, 132–134]

Hypoventilation

A decrease in minute ventilation is caused by a decrease in the tidal volume, the respiratory rate, or both. Hypoventilation causes hypercarbia and promotes alveolar collapse. Severe hypoventilation results in respiratory acidosis, hypoxemia, carbon dioxide narcosis, and apnea. Hypoventilation may be caused by a decrease in the ventilatory drive, insufficiency of the muscular system, or both. Causes of decreased ventilatory drive include agents that depress the ventilatory drive, such as halogenated agents, opioids, benzodiazepines, and other sedating medications; other causes of hypoventilation include central nervous system insults such as head injury, strokes, and intracranial surgery. Muscular insufficiency may be caused by pre-existent muscular disease (obstructive or restrictive disease), inadequate reversal of neuromuscular blockade (with special considerations to myasthenia gravis, myasthenic syndrome, pseudocholinesterase deficiency, succinylcholine-induced phase II block, and anticholinesterase overdose), upper airway obstruction, inadequate analgesia leading to splinting with breathing, bronchospasm, and pneumothorax.

Airway Obstruction

Initially, the patency of the airway is checked, and, when necessary, stimulation of the patient, positioning, mandibular displacement, placement of oral or nasal airways, and suctioning of secretions may be used to open and clear the upper airway. In many cases, respiration improves with these measures alone (improved oxygen saturation). If these measures fail, however, one must consider the patency of the laryngeal inlet and the lower airway—that is, whether gas exchange is being compromised by laryngospasm, subglottic narrowing as the result of edema, bronchospasm, or tracheal secretions. Laryngospasm may require administration of oxygen under positive pressure by mask or, in rare cases, administration of succinylcholine. Postintubation croup or subglottic edema has been associated with a number of factors, including traumatic intubation, tight-fitting endotracheal tubes, coughing on the endotracheal tube, the presence of a URI, a change in the patient's position during surgery, prolonged duration of intubation, surgery of the head and neck, and in patients with a prior history of croup.[135] For

reasons that have not been adequately explained, postintubation croup is less common among infants younger than 3 months than among older infants and toddlers. Treatment initially consists of inhalation of cool mist. If the symptoms are sufficiently severe, inhalation of racemic epinephrine is generally effective, although its effects are temporary and its use may be followed by rebound edema. In general, a decision to use racemic epinephrine implies that prolonged observation of the patient will continue thereafter. For outpatients, this implies that the child will be admitted to the hospital overnight or observed for an extended period. Incomplete recovery from general anesthesia or neuromuscular blockade, wound hematoma, and vocal cord paralysis may also cause upper airway obstruction.

Respiratory Effort

If the airway is patent, attention turns to the adequacy of ventilatory effort. Residual neuromuscular blockade can be diagnosed by peripheral nerve stimulation.[47] Depending on the severity and the clinical situation, this condition may be treated with either additional doses of reversal agents or ventilatory assistance. If the signs of opioid overdose are present, naloxone will have an immediate effect. Administration of naloxone in small incremental doses (0.002 mg/kg), if the situation permits, may prevent precipitation of acute anxiety, pain, or pulmonary edema.[85, 86] Residual sedation from benzodiazepines may also be antagonized with flumazenil.[87, 136–139]

Patients may have an adequate airway and the potential for adequate ventilatory effort but may have difficulty breathing because of pain, restriction from bandages or casts, abdominal distension, pneumothorax, atelectasis, aspiration pneumonitis, or cardiogenic pulmonary edema. In most cases, the history and physical examination will focus the differential diagnosis, and, when necessary, chest radiographs, blood gas analysis, and possibly invasive hemodynamic monitoring will further guide diagnosis and treatment.

Several studies have disclosed a significant tendency toward postoperative apnea in preterm and, rarely, full-term infants.[140–146] We recommend overnight monitoring for the development of apnea in former preterm infants. Impedance pneumography, oxygen saturation, and other means of monitoring respirations are indicated for preterm infants 55 weeks or less of post-conceptual age, those who experience an episode of apnea in the PACU, and those older than 55 weeks of post-conceptual age who are anemic (hematocrit < 30%) (see Chapter 4).[146] Outpatient procedures are not recommended for these patients (see Chapter 2). A PICU should be immediately available in facilities in which elective surgery is undertaken in this population. In many cases, spells of periodic breathing or apnea can be terminated by stimulation alone; in others, assisted ventilation with a bag and mask and, occasionally, intubation and ventilation are required. For full-term infants, the onset of periodic breathing (usually typical for preterm infants but not full-term infants) may indicate an immaturity of the respiratory system (see Fig. 2–5).[144]

Dysrhythmias
Bradycardia

Bradycardia is the most common dysrhythmia in the pediatric patient and requires immediate attention because of its association with a decrease in cardiac output. *Bradycardia in the PACU most commonly reflects hypoxemia.* It may also reflect vagal responses to a number of stimuli, such as passage of a nasogastric tube. Medications such as neostigmine and opioids such as morphine and fentanyl may also induce bradycardia. In neurosurgical cases, bradycardia may accompany increased intracranial pressure; in this population, this warrants immediate evaluation by a neurosurgeon. High neuraxial anesthetic block and beta-adrenergic block are also possible causes of bradycardia. Treatment is directed at correcting the underlying cause, as in administration of oxygen, ensuring a clear or patent airway, administration of atropine, or reduction of intracranial pressure. Bradycardia should be immediately treated with oxygen and, if necessary, with ventilation and should never be initially treated with a vagolytic until the underlying cause is clarified.

Tachycardia

Tachycardia is an important postoperative sign signifying an attempt by the body's compensatory mechanism to maintain adequate cardiac output or oxygen delivery, or a response of the body to reflex stimuli (pain) or drugs (epinephrine, atropine). In addition, tachycardia may be due to hypoxemia, hypercarbia, hypovolemia, emergence delirium, anxiety, sepsis (fever), hypervolemia, or heart failure. Treatment is directed at correcting the underlying cause, for example, correcting hypovolemia with fluid administration, anemia with packed red blood cells, or pain with opioids or other analgesics. Occasionally, some children present with a sustained tachycardia; this may warrant consultation with a cardiologist to rule out an aberrant conduction system.

Other Arrhythmias

Development of premature ventricular beats or premature atrial beats may first occur in the PACU. Multifocal premature ventricular beats may represent the hallmark of malignant hyperthermia (see Chapter 27), acute rhabdomyolysis with hyperkalemia, inadequately treated pain, a congenital conduction defect, or the presence of a structural cardiac defect. In this circumstance, a careful physical examination will reveal pain or a structural cardiac defect (murmur), but a full 12-lead electrocardiogram and consultation with a cardiologist is usually warranted. Arterial blood gases and electrolytes are obtained as indicated.

Blood Pressure Control

Hypotension

In assessing hypotension, the anesthesiologist should be familiar with the normal blood pressure ranges of infants and children (see Chapter 2). The measurement should be obtained with an appropriately sized blood pressure cuff (two-thirds the length of the upper arm). An improperly sized cuff will give spurious readings. Small cuffs will yield a high reading while a large cuff may yield a spuriously low reading. Proper placement of the cuff is essential if errors in interpretation are to be avoided.

The most common cause of hypotension in children is hypovolemia, which may result from inadequate replacement of blood and fluids lost during the surgical procedure or ongoing blood loss. Any factor that interferes with venous return will result in hypotension; such factors include positive-pressure ventilation, auto–positive end-expiratory pressure, tension pneumothorax, inadequate venous return from hemorrhage, pericardial tamponade, and compression of the inferior vena cava.

High doses of inhalation and local anesthetic agents and opioids, as well as interactions between benzodiazepines and opioids, may produce hypotension through vasodilation (relative hypovolemia) and direct myocardial depression[147, 148]; these factors are rarely contributory in the care of children in the PACU. Other rare causes may include anaphylaxis, transfusion reaction, adrenal insufficiency, systemic inflammation, infection, severe liver failure, and the administration of antihypertensive, antidysrhythmic, and anticonvulsant medications. Increased body temperature causes vasodilation and a relative hypovolemia. In addition, the increased metabolic demands of fever may compromise an already stressed myocardium.

The vasodilation caused by sympathetic blockade when regional anesthesia is used will occasionally cause hypotension, especially if it is a high blockade and the patient's fluid intake is restricted. This is generally only a problem in children older than 6 years of age. Owing to the developmental changes in the sympathetic nervous system, most children under 6 are relatively peripherally vasodilated and therefore do not have much of a response to further vasodilation with a regional block.[149]

Decreased inotropy (caused by myocardial ischemia), dysrhythmia, calcium channel blockers, sepsis, hypothyroidism, malignant hyperthermia, negative inotropic agents, and congestive heart failure are other rare causes of hypotension. Treatment is directed at the underlying cause, such as correcting hypovolemia with volume loading, treating the allergic reaction, or treating the sepsis. Decreased cardiac contractility may be treated by the administration of inotropic agents, drugs that decrease the afterload and diuresis.

Hypertension

Postoperative hypertension in children is less common than hypotension. A blood pressure cuff that is too small may give a spuriously high blood pressure reading. Other causative factors include pain, hypervolemia, pre-existing hypertension, distended bladder, hypercarbia, hypoxemia, rapid central nervous system awakening, increased intracranial pressure, and exogenous vasoactive drugs (e.g., epinephrine). Pheochromocytoma and other vasoactive secreting tumors may rarely present as a cause of hypertension in PACU, but this is extremely rare. Therapy for hypertension includes treatment of pain, drainage of the bladder, treatment of intracranial pressure, antihypertensive medications and beta-adrenergic blockers, calcium channel blockers, hydralazine, nitrates, and alpha-adrenergic blockers, depending on the cause.

Pain

Besides being a problem in its own right, pain may precipitate several of the other signs discussed here, including tachycardia, arrhythmias, hypertension, nausea, vomiting, agitation, and anxiety. Untreated pain appears to exacerbate emergence delirium. Untreated pain is unacceptable. Every child should leave the PACU with a pain score of less than 2 on a scale with a maximum of 10. Pain scores should be part of the vital signs—the so-called fifth vital sign—recorded in the PACU and elsewhere in the hospital.[150-158]

Although we believe in prompt and vigorous treatment of pain, a patient's pain must be assessed, and the presence of pain that is inappropriate for a patient's condition may be of diagnostic significance. For example, severe limb pain after a limb procedure may suggest a compartment syndrome; shoulder pain after cystoscopy may suggest bladder perforation and peritoneal or diaphragmatic irritation.

Several generalizations apply to the treatment of pain in pediatric postoperative patients:

1. As with adults, children who are old enough to understand should be given preoperative encouragement and instruction, which will diminish the experience of pain. Pain is exacerbated by anxiety and a feeling of helplessness and uncertainty about what will happen.
2. When possible, long-acting local anesthetics, such as bupivacaine, should be administered intraoperatively to diminish postoperative pain; for example, infiltration of the spermatic cord and incision can make hernia repair much less painful and intercostal nerve blocks can diminish the pain of thoracotomy (see Chapters 28 and 29). In addition, patient-controlled and continuous epidural anesthesia should be started in the operating room and continued in the PACU. The combination of long-acting anesthetics and opioids produces a very useful synergistic benefit.
3. Distraction and reuniting the child with parents or other familiar persons are helpful; teddy bears, dolls, or other favorite personal objects that make a child feel more secure should be brought to the PACU when appropriate.
4. Nonsteroidal anti-inflammatory drugs complement opioids, but these drugs may cause platelet dysfunction and nephrotoxicity. Rectal administration of acetaminophen, administered right after induction of anesthesia and before surgery, is effective for mild pain and potentiates the alleviation of pain by opioids. Rectal dosing of 10 to 15 mg/kg results in inadequate plasma concentrations[159-161]; an initial dose of approximately 40 mg/kg results in a peak plasma value between 60 and 180 minutes.[160] Subsequent doses of 20 mg/kg may be administered at 6-hour intervals for 24 hours (see Chapters 8 and 9; Figure 9–6).[162]
5. For moderate and severe pain, intravenous opioids are the mainstay of treatment.

Incremental doses of fentanyl (0.00025 to 0.0005 mg/kg [0.25–0.5 μg/kg]), morphine (0.05–0.1 mg/kg) or meperidine (0.5–1.0 mg/kg) should be titrated to effect, with recognition of the following qualifiers. Opioids should be given with great caution to patients whose airways are compromised or to those whose hemodynamic condition is unstable. If an opioid is required, small doses should be gradually titrated to effect. In general, fentanyl should be used to treat short-term pain but because of the duration of action, a longer acting opioid such as morphine is preferred. Although it may be convenient to administer fentanyl so as to have a rapid onset and pain-free patient ready for discharge, that may not be in the patient's best interest when pain returns shortly after discharge from PACU. However, the maximum central

nervous system and respiratory effects of intravenous morphine may not be reached for 10 minutes; therefore, observation must continue for an appropriate period of time. This may delay discharge from PACU but improve patient care and patient and parent satisfaction.

Respiratory rate is a reasonable guide to opioid effect; it is unlikely that a tachypneic patient has received too much opioid, even though the dose may seem to be relatively high. In the PACU, opioids should be administered intravenously when possible rather than intramuscularly because the onset of action is more rapid (pain is more easily controlled before it becomes severe) and because peak effects occur while the patient is readily observed. The reaction to an intramuscular dose may not peak until a patient has left the PACU, when observation may be less than optimal. Most PACUs require that a patient who has received opioids remain there for approximately 30 minutes after the last dose; when there is any doubt, it is prudent to observe patients for longer periods.

In some cases, it is not possible to remove pain entirely, but it should be possible to attenuate the pain enough to make it tolerable. It is probable that errors in undertreatment are more common than errors in overtreatment because of preconceptions about the diminished experience or memory of pain in infants and children and because of inordinate fears of respiratory depression by opioids. Respiratory depression should rarely occur with step-by-step administration of opioids, titration to desired effect, and observation. Should respiratory depression occur, however, a child must receive assisted ventilation until opioid antagonists, such as naloxone, take effect. Further details of pain management are outlined in Chapters 28 and 29.

Nausea and Vomiting

Although rarely life-threatening (except when vomiting occurs in patients unable to protect themselves from aspiration), nausea and vomiting are important causes of unpleasant experiences and recollection for anesthetized children. We have drawn the following conclusions from a review of the literature and our own experience:

1. Although the reported incidence varies from less than 1% to more than 80%, nausea and vomiting are clearly very common problems. We suggest that the lower figures represent either underreporting or overly strict inclusion criteria.
2. Although the variation in incidence may be related to the individual patient, the operative procedure, and the anesthetic agents used, there is little basis for choosing one anesthetic regimen over another in this regard.
3. Emptying the stomach before emergence should be encouraged, thereby diminishing the quantity of potential vomitus, relieving stomach distension, which may trigger vomiting, and possibly removing blood clots after oral or pharyngeal surgery because they can be a chemical irritant stimulus for vomiting.
4. Patients who report a serious tendency for motion sickness are more likely to vomit.
5. Specific procedures in particular are associated with an especially high incidence of nausea and vomiting, such as tonsillectomy, strabismus repair, and mastoid surgery.

The use of antiemetics both prophylactically and after vomiting has started is the source of great debate, especially regarding cost/benefit ratios.[163–165] A number of studies of adults and children have shown that phenothiazines and butyrophenones, most notably droperidol (50–75 µg/kg), are effective in diminishing the incidence and the severity of postoperative vomiting.[166] Many studies include patients who have undergone several different types of surgical procedures and anesthetics, and the effects may be obscured by uncontrolled variables. Several points are noteworthy; some patients will experience extrapyramidal reactions and others will have a prolonged recovery time. In most cases, however, droperidol will not delay discharge or cause extrapyramidal reactions, especially if lower doses (10–30 µg/kg) are utilized.[167, 168]

At present, no treatment is guaranteed to be completely effective for postoperative nausea and vomiting, although virtually all antiemetics reduce the incidence and severity of these problems. The serotonin antagonists appear to be superior to droperidol.[169–176] Several studies have demonstrated that Decadron (0.15 mg/kg, maximum 8 mg) is an excellent antiemetic whose effect lasts longer than those of ondansetron[177, 178]; this treatment warrants investigation for other procedures because of the very low cost and because of the prolonged beneficial effects (beyond 6–8 hours).

The fluid and electrolytes lost because of vomiting should be replaced, and maintenance fluids should be given in the PACU and on the postoperative ward, especially to infants and small children, since excesive vomiting may require admission to avoid dehydration.

A review showed that approximately one third of adult respiratory complications due to perioperative pulmonary aspiration occurred in the PACU.[179] Therefore, patients considered to be at increased risk for this complication preoperatively—infants, children who have undergone previous esophageal surgery, or trauma patients—must also be considered to be at increased risk for pulmonary aspiration postoperatively.[180, 181] Therefore, although this potentially fatal complication is extremely rare in the pediatric population (1 in 40,000),[182] such patients require increased vigilance.

Temperature Control

Hypothermia

Hypothermia is a serious postoperative problem in infants. The response to hypothermia is to increase body temperature by shivering; this response is not well developed during the first few weeks of life. When shivering occurs, oxygen consumption increases, and this increased oxygen consumption causes potentially life-threatening stress; oxygen demand may outstrip oxygen delivery. In addition, the body attempts to diminish heat loss by a vasoconstrictor response, resulting in metabolic acidosis as the result of intense peripheral vasoconstriction and inadequate perfusion.[126] A warm blanket placed on the patient shortly after awakening can blunt this normal vasoconstrictor response following anesthesia.[183] Hypothermia affects platelet function, cardiac repolarization, and the metabolism of drugs. Problems of thermal balance are especially severe for premature infants. Thermal blankets and the infusion of warm fluids are frequently used to treat hypothermia in the PACU. Plastic wraps or bags are occasionally used in the operating room to avoid hypothermia when operative procedures are of long duration and also in the PACU. Forced air warming blankets are the most effective in treating hypothermia (see Chapter 27).

Hyperthermia

Elevation of body temperature may be the result of causes that are simple to treat, such as overheating, but it may be of serious importance when its origin is malignant hyperthermia syndrome (see Chapter 27). Other causes are viral or bacterial sepsis, dehydration, pyrogenic reaction to the infusion of fluids, drugs, and blood, hyperthyroidism, and neuroleptic malignant syndrome. Suspicion of sepsis necessitates a complete examination to localize the source. Routinely, uncovering the patient is enough to decrease the temperature, although acetaminophen and cooling blankets are occasionally used.

Oliguria

Oliguria is defined as urine output of less than 0.5 mL/kg/hour. The cause may simply be a blocked catheter. If a catheter is not in place, it may be advisable to insert one to confirm the diagnosis. Oliguria is often caused by hypovolemia; urine output is also a valuable indicator of adequacy of cardiac output. Another cause of oliguria is acute tubular necrosis, which usually has its origin in intraoperative or preoperative ischemia. Oliguria may occur with intraoperative manipulation of the kidneys or the aorta (even when the aorta is cross-clamped infrarenally).

The treatment of oliguric patients begins with assessment of the clinical signs of adequacy of perfusion and with appropriate treatment of circulatory insufficiency by expanding the intravascular volume with fluids (fluid challenge) and administrating inotropic agents and agents that promote renal blood flow (dopamine) as needed. Diuretics should be administered only when clinical or physiologic evidence demonstrates intravascular volume overload, not merely to treat inadequate urine output. Conversely, it should be realized that in pediatric patients who have had an adequate blood pressure preoperatively and intraoperatively without the support of alpha-adrenergic agents, renal failure is extraordinarily rare in the postoperative period, and one can err in too strict adherence to numeric guidelines for urine output in otherwise physiologically stable patients.

Neurologic Complications

Seizures

Seizures may occur in the PACU as the result of hypoxemia or metabolic imbalance (hypoglycemia, hyponatremia, hypocalcemia). On occasion, patients receiving anticonvulsant drugs may have missed a necessary dose. Every effort should be made to maintain therapeutic levels of anticonvulsant drugs, either by oral administration on the day of surgery or by intravenous administration at the time of surgery. Treatment of seizure consists of establishing a clear airway, providing adequate oxygenation and ventilation, seeking the underlying cause, and treating the cause, for example, by administration of glucose, calcium, or additional anticonvulsant drug as indicated.

Unresponsiveness

After a surgical procedure, a child's slow awakening may cause concern. Factors frequently involved in unresponsiveness include the following:

Hypoxemia

Hypercarbia (carbon dioxide narcosis)

Hypovolemia (inadequate cerebral perfusion)

Hypoglycemia

Residual anesthetic, opioid, or hypnotic effect (relative drug overdose)

Residual neuromuscular blockade

Increased intracranial pressure or other intracranial pathology, e.g., hemorrhage, tumor

Water and electrolyte imbalance (hyponatremia)

Postictal state

The treatment of a patient who is slow to awaken begins with a brief examination and review of the pertinent history, including pre-existing conditions and the anesthetic record. In many cases, it is easy to include or rule out conditions on the basis of the history and physical examination alone. For example, not all somnolent patients need blood gas determinations to rule out ventilatory disturbance or serum electrolyte values to rule out metabolic derangement. Pupillary signs, patterns and frequency of respiration, and the smell of a volatile agent on a patient's breath may provide clues to the presence of excessive opioid or residual anesthetic effect. If there is any doubt, the burden of proof lies on the physician to perform tests (blood gases, blood glucose, or others) to rule out life-threatening causes of unresponsiveness, most of which can be readily treated.

Parents in the Postanesthesia Care Unit

There has been a healthy trend toward allowing parents in the PACU.[184] Whether parents can be permitted at their child's bedside is a judgment that depends on the child's clinical status. A child awakening in strange surroundings can derive significant emotional benefit from the presence of his or her parents. This emotional benefit is also shared by the parents, who feel quite helpless when cut off from their child at this stage. The parents may be especially helpful in dealing with a handicapped child. Researchers using the State-Trait Anxiety Inventory to assess parental anxiety during the recovery phase found no significant increase in anxiety, and satisfaction was high.[185] In general, parents feel that they and their child benefit from their presence in PACU.[186, 187] However, it should be appreciated that flexibility in this arrangement is necessary and that allowing parents in the PACU must be evaluated on a case-by-case basis.

Fast Track Recovery

The rapidly escalating costs of health-care are an ever-present reality that will continue to face us in the future. Patients do not want to stay in the hospital any longer than is necessary. Recent innovations have aided in the rapid recovery of patients. New, shorter-acting drugs are allowing a more rapid awakening from anesthesia, which may allow the patient to bypass the traditional PACU and bring patients directly to a post-recovery lounge or step-down unit—that is, "fast track recovery."[188–191] Less time spent in the PACU may mean increased patient satisfaction and does usually mean lower costs.[192–196] Most of the savings as a result of using the "new" drugs are brought about not by the reduction in anesthesia time or the cost of anesthesiology-related drugs (usually higher than older drugs) but rather by reduced use of the operating room and the PACU. Anesthesiologists, CRNAs, nurses, surgeons, pharmacists, and administrators must be involved in the evaluation of the benefits of the "fast track." The protocol redesign needs to be understood and accepted by all involved so as to remove any bottleneck areas that threaten the success of the implementation of the fast-track program. Patients of all ages undergoing a wide variety of procedures have participated in the fast track. Newer monitoring tools, such as the Bispectral Index (only studied in adults), which is the only monitor of consciousness approved by the Food and Drug Administration, suggest that the patient can be more alert and awake than after a standard anesthetic procedure conducted on clinical signs without the Bispectral Index.[197] This costly item of equipment (for the monitoring strip) and costly new drugs are purchased in the context of what they may add and the value that they may bring to the fast-track system. The reduction in operating room and PACU time may be a more important consideration in the evaluation of new technology or drugs than the cost of the equipment or drug itself. The role of Bispectral Index monitoring is yet to be proven in children.

The clinical criteria for bypassing the PACU after anesthesia include no pain, no vomiting, minimal nausea, deep breathing, oxygen saturation greater than 95% or return to baseline on room air, movement of all extremities on command, hemodynamic stability, and orientation to name and place (Table 30–5). Complications that most frequently disrupt the fast track and increase cost and patient dissatisfaction include postoperative nausea and vomiting, pain, bleeding, and hypothermia.

Logistically, the step-down unit must be close to the operating room to facilitate ready access to the unit by the anesthesiologist or the CRNA. The nurse-to-patient ratio should be 1:3 and or less if ancillary personnel are available. Cross-training of nurses to float where needed is essential, especially in smaller hospital settings. The operating room nurse should be able to float from the preoperative area to the PACU and to the step-down unit.

The fast track cannot be implemented without education of the staff, the patient, and the family. Because in the past hospital stays have been much longer, the public at large expects a long hospital stay. The surgeon, the anesthesia team, and the recovery room staff need to take an active role to educate the patient and the family about the issues surrounding the fast track. Proposed criteria for bypassing the PACU are outlined in Table 30–5.[198]

Policies and Procedures

The hospital's Policy and Procedure Manual should contain a Patient Rights and Responsibilities. The policy should state

Table 30–5. Discharge Criteria for Fast Track

	Score
Level of consciousness	
Aware and oriented	2
Arousable with minimal stimulation	1
Responsive only to tactile stimulation	0
Physical activity	
Able to move all extremities on command	2
Some weakness in movement of extremities	1
Unable to voluntarily move extremities	0
Hemodynamic stability	
Blood pressure <15% of baseline MAP value	2
Blood pressure 15%–30% of baseline MAP value	1
Blood pressure >30% of baseline MAP value	0
Respiratory stability	
Able to breathe deeply	2
Tachypneic with good cough	1
Dyspneic with weak cough	0
Oxygen saturation status	
Maintains value >95% on room air	2
Requires supplemental oxygen (nasal prongs)	1
Saturation <90% with supplemental oxygen	0
Postoperative pain assessment	
None, or mild discomfort	2
Moderate to severe pain controlled with I.V. analgesics	1
Persistent, severe pain	0
Postoperative emetic symptoms	
None, or mild nausea with no active vomiting	2
Transient vomiting or retching	1
Persistent moderate to severe nausea and vomiting	0
Total*	14

MAP, mean arterial pressure.

*Pediatric patients must score 14 to bypass the Phase 1 (PACU) recovery unit to be admitted to the "step-down" unit.

From White PF, Song D: New criteria for fast-tracking after outpatient anesthesia: a comparison with the modified Aldrete's scoring system. Anesth Analg 1998; 88:1069–1072.

that the patient's chart should contain documentation of the discussion leading to informed consent for the procedure administered by the anesthesiologist, CRNA, or other Licensed Independent Practitioner, the requirements for the informed consent, and the authorization for and consent to surgery or special diagnostic or therapeutic procedures. The policy should outline the procedure for photographing the patient and for obtaining consent for photographs. A policy for "Do Not Resuscitate" orders should be easily available.

Specific guidelines and admission protocols should be readily available. Specific notes should address the reassessment of the patient with a condition whose scope and intensity demand more than routine attention. A PACU admission policy for admitting the patient from the operating room and a policy for receiving the report from the anesthesiologist, CRNA, or registered nurse, for patients receiving only local anesthesia, sedation, or analgesia should be included in the PACU policy and procedure manual. The Aldrete PACU scoring system is an example of a scoring system that can show readiness for discharge. A discharge policy to go into effect after the patient has recovered from anesthesia should also be available. Each patient's chart should contain a sheet with the PACU scoring guidelines. The PACU policy manual should contain criteria for notifying the anesthesiologist re-

garding recovery problems, and all PACU registered nurses should be familiar with the policy.

The postoperative nursing care plan should describe the actions taken to achieve the goals of safe PACU care. The plan should be developed and implemented by the registered nurses to optimize patient outcome and should follow written policies and guidelines for nursing interventions that are consistent with state licensure and facility policies. The perioperative nursing care plan sheet should be filled out by the PACU nurse, and the nursing interventions should be continually evaluated. The same standards of care should apply to any other area in the hospital in which patients recover from anesthesia or sedation and analgesia. The postanesthesia care of patients in the other areas of the hospital should be similar to the care rendered in the PACU next to the operating room, such as PACU care given to patients undergoing radiation therapy, magnetic resonance imaging, computed tomographic scans, fluoroscopic examinations, audiology examinations, and bone scans should be similar to the care rendered in the regular PACU. The policy and procedure manual should also outline the physician's responsibilities in the PACU, including the writing of postoperative orders. An emergency crash cart with emergency drugs and supplies should be immediately available for each patient care unit or service area. The security and accountability of the crash cart should be maintained by the nursing personnel and the pharmacy, in accordance with JCAHO guidelines (a crash cart/defibrillator checklist signature form is filled out every shift). Postanesthesia orders should be filled out for every patient. Concerns for the special pediatric patient (e.g., premature infants, those with ventricular septal defect, or those with developmental delay) should also be documented. Detailed uniform methods for the administration of pain medication should include patient-controlled analgesia, nurse-controlled analgesia, epidural anesthesia, patient-controlled epidural anesthesia, spinal anesthesia, and the administration of medications for break-through pain. PACU personnel should know how to administer oxygen via nasal cannula or face mask, initiate respiratory therapy for the intubated patient or the patient with an artificial airway, suction the endotracheal tube, insert and suction oral or nasopharyngeal airways, perform bag and mask ventilation, and manage the initial responses of a "Code Blue."

The care in the PACU should be evaluated on an ongoing basis to improve the quality of the care that patients receive. The objective is to ensure that the quality of patient care is optimally maintained to deliver the highest level of quality in an efficient and safe manner. Areas that can be evaluated are patient safety, equipment, nursing procedures, nosocomial infections, incomplete forms, cardiopulmonary arrests, unplanned admissions or transfers, unexpected outcomes, sensory or vascular deficit, system failure, incorrect controlled substance count, security, altered medical record, pain intervention, education (patient or family), patient outcomes, risk management, and so on. Concerns about the transfer of surgical patients to special units should be clearly outlined so that the quality of care in that area will be equal to that previously available in the PACU. The transfer of the patient to the new area should include all relevant patient care information transmitted from the PACU nurse to the licensed nurse or physician receiving the patient. Instructions for discharge after all types of outpatient sedation or surgical procedures, along with preprinted physician orders, should be available to all the patients and their families in a clear and comprehensible form.

REFERENCES

1. Eger EI II: Recovery from anesthesia. In: Eger EI II, ed: Anesthetic Uptake and Action. Baltimore: Williams & Wilkins; 1974:228–248.
2. Stoelting RK, Longnecker DE, Eger EI: Minimum alveolar concentrations in man on awakening from methoxyflurane, halothane, ether and fluroxene anesthesia: MAC awake. Anesthesiology 1970;33:5–9.
3. Chortkoff BS, Eger EI, Crankshaw DP, et al: Concentrations of desflurane and propofol that suppress response to command in humans. Anesth Analg 1995;81:737–743.
4. Tabo E, Ohkuma Y, Sakuragi Y, et al: MAC-awake and wake-up time of isoflurane and sevoflurane with reference to the concentration of gas, duration of inhalation and patient's age and obesity. [in Japanese]. Masui 1995;44:188–192.
5. Katoh T, Suguro Y, Kimura T, et al: Cerebral awakening concentration of sevoflurane and isoflurane predicted during slow and fast alveolar washout. Anesth Analg 1993;77:1012–1017.
6. Gaumann DM, Mustaki JP, Tassonyi E: MAC-awake of isoflurane, enflurane and halothane evaluated by slow and fast alveolar washout. Br J Anaesth 1992;68:81–84.
7. Glass PS, Gan TJ, Howell S, et al: Drug interactions: Volatile anesthetics and opioids. J Clin Anesth 1997;9:18S–22S.
8. Inagaki Y, Mashimo T, Kuzukawa A, et al: Epidural lidocaine delays arousal from isoflurane anesthesia. Anesth Analg 1994;79:368–372.
9. Katoh T, Uchiyama T, Ikeda K: Effect of fentanyl on awakening concentration of sevoflurane. Br J Anaesth 1994;73:322–325.
10. Eger EI II: Uptake and distribution. In: Miller RD, ed: Anesthesia, 5th ed. Philadelphia: Churchill Livingstone; 2000:74–95.
11. Miller EDJ, Greene NM: Waking up to desflurane: The anesthetic for the '90s? Anesth Analg 1990;70:1–2.
12. Zwass MS, Fisher DM, Welborn LG, et al: Induction and maintenance characteristics of anesthesia with desflurane and nitrous oxide in infants and children. Anesthesiology 1992;76:373–378.
13. Epstein RH, Mendel HG, Guarnieri KM, et al: Sevoflurane versus halothane for general anesthesia in pediatric patients: A comparative study of vital signs, induction, and emergence. J Clin Anesth 1995;7:237–244.
14. Lapin SL, Auden SM, Goldsmith LJ, et al: Effects of sevoflurane anaesthesia on recovery in children: A comparison with halothane. Paediatr Anaesth 1999;9:299–304.
15. Lerman J, Davis PJ, Welborn LG, et al: Induction, recovery, and safety characteristics of sevoflurane in children undergoing ambulatory surgery: A comparison with halothane. Anesthesiology 1996;84:1332–1340.
16. Welborn LG, Hannallah RS, Norden JM, et al: Comparison of emergence and recovery characteristics of sevoflurane, desflurane, and halothane in pediatric ambulatory patients. Anesth Analg 1996;83:917–920.
17. O'Brien K, Robinson DN, Morton NS: Induction and emergence in infants less than 60 weeks post-conceptual age: Comparison of thiopental, halothane, sevoflurane and desflurane. Br J Anaesth 1998;80:456–459.
18. Sury MR, Black A, Hemington L, et al: A comparison of the recovery characteristics of sevoflurane and halothane in children. Anaesthesia 1996;51:543–546.
19. Aono J, Ueda W, Mamiya K, et al: Greater incidence of delirium during recovery from sevoflurane anesthesia in preschool boys. Anesthesiology 1997;87:1298–1300.
20. Beskow A, Westrin P: Sevoflurane causes more postoperative agitation in children than does halothane. Acta Anaesthesiol Scand 1999;43:536–541.
21. Greenspun JC, Hannallah RS, Welborn LG, et al: Comparison of sevoflurane and halothane anesthesia in children undergoing outpatient ear, nose, and throat surgery. J Clin Anesth 1995;7:398–402.
22. Hobbhahn J, Funk W: Sevoflurane in pediatric anesthesia. [in German]. Anaesthesist 1996;45:S22–S27.
23. Kataria B, Epstein R, Bailey A, et al: A comparison of sevoflurane to halothane in paediatric surgical patients: Results of a multicentre international study. Pediatr Anaesth 1996;6:283–292.
24. Davis PJ, Cohen IT, McGowan FXJ, et al: Recovery characteristics of

25. Michalek-Sauberer A, Wildling E, Pusch F, et al: Sevoflurane anaesthesia in paediatric patients: Better than halothane? Eur J Anaesthesiol 1998;15:280–286.
26. Mazurek AJ, Przybylo HJ, Martini DR, DeMille A, Coté CJ: Emergence patterns following sevoflurane and halothane anesthesia in children. Anesthesiology 1999;91:A1299.
27. Patel N, Smith CE, Pinchak AC, et al: Desflurane is not associated with faster operating room exit times in outpatients. J Clin Anesth 1996;8:130–135.
28. Warner DO, Warner MA: Human chest wall function while awake and during halothane anesthesia. II. Carbon dioxide rebreathing. Anesthesiology 1995;82:20–31.
29. Stuth EA, Tonkovic-Capin M, Kampine JP, et al: Dose-dependent effects of halothane on the carbon dioxide responses of expiratory and inspiratory bulbospinal neurons and the phrenic nerve activities in dogs. Anesthesiology 1994;81:1470–1483.
30. Izumi Y, Kochi T, Mizuguchi T: An analysis of the ventilatory response to carbon dioxide during halothane, isoflurane, or enflurane anesthesia in humans. [in Japanese]. Masui 1991;40:1222–1227.
31. Knill RL, Gelb AW: Ventilatory responses to hypoxia and hypercapnia during halothane sedation and anesthesia in man. Anesthesiology 1978;49:244–251.
32. Dahan A, van den Elsen MJ, Berkenbosch A, et al: Influence of a subanesthetic concentration of halothane on the ventilatory response to step changes into and out of sustained isocapnic hypoxia in healthy volunteers. Anesthesiology 1994;81:850–859.
33. Motoyama EK, Glazener CH: Hypoxemia after general anesthesia in children. Anesth Analg 1986;65:267–272.
34. Soliman IE, Patel RI, Ehrenpreis MB, et al: Recovery scores do not correlate with postoperative hypoxemia in children. Anesth Analg 1988;67:53–56.
35. Levy L, Pandit UA, Randel GI, et al: Upper respiratory tract infections and general anaesthesia in children. Anaesthesia 1992;47:678–682.
36. Coté CJ, Rolf N, Liu LM, et al: A single-blind study of combined pulse oximetry and capnography in children. Anesthesiology 1991;74:980–987.
37. Cross KW, Oppé TE: The effect of inhalation of high and low concentrations of oxygen on the respiration of the premature infant. J Physiol 1952;117:38–55.
38. Rigatto H, Brady JP, De La Torre Verduzco R: Chemoreceptor reflexes in preterm infants: I. The effect of gestational and postnatal age on the ventilatory response to inhalation of 100% and 15% oxygen. Pediatrics 1975;55:604–613.
39. Rigatto H, De La Torre Verduzco R, Gates DB: Effects of O_2 on the ventilatory response to CO_2 in preterm infants. J Appl Physiol 1975;39:896–899.
40. Gerhardt T, Bancalari E: Apnea of prematurity: I. Lung function and regulation of breathing. Pediatrics 1984;74:58–62.
41. Gerhardt T, Bancalari E: Apnea of prematurity: II. Respiratory reflexes. Pediatrics 1984;74:63–66.
42. Flynn JT, O'Grady GE, Herrera J, et al: Retrolental fibroplasia: I. Clinical observations. Arch Ophthalmol 1977;95:217–223.
43. Kinsey VE, Arnold HJ, Kalina RE, et al: PaO_2 levels and retrolental fibroplasia: A report of the cooperative study. Pediatrics 1977;60:655–668.
44. Betts EK, Downes JJ, Schaffer DB, et al: Retrolental fibroplasia and oxygen administration during general anesthesia. Anesthesiology 1977;47:518–520.
45. Merritt JC, Sprague DH, Merritt WE, et al: Retrolental fibroplasia: a multifactorial disease. Anesth Analg 1981;60:109–111.
46. Phelps DL: Retinopathy of prematurity. Pediatr Clin North Am 1993;40:705–714.
47. Ali HH, Savarese JJ: Monitoring of neuromuscular function. Anesthesiology 1976;45:216–249.
48. Mason LJ, Betts EK: Leg lift and maximum inspiratory force, clinical signs of neuromuscular blockade reversal in neonates and infants. Anesthesiology 1980;52:441–442.
49. Meakin G, Sweet PT, Bevan JC, et al: Neostigmine and edrophonium as antagonists of pancuronium in infants and children. Anesthesiology 1983;59:316–321.
50. Fisher DM, Cronnelly R, Miller RD, et al: The neuromuscular pharmacology of neostigmine in infants and children. Anesthesiology 1983;59:220–225.

51. Goudsouzian NG: Maturation of neuromuscular transmission in the infant. Br J Anaesth 1980;52:205–214.

52. Alifimoff JK, Goudsouzian NG: Continuous infusion of mivacurium in children. Br J Anaesth 1989;63:520–524.

53. Goudsouzian NG, Alifimoff JK, Eberly C, et al: Neuromuscular and cardiovascular effects of mivacurium in children. Anesthesiology 1989;70:237–242.

54. Goudsouzian NG, Denman W, Schwartz A, et al: Pharmacodynamic and hemodynamic effects of mivacurium in infants anesthetized with halothane and nitrous oxide. Anesthesiology 1993;79:919–925.

55. Brandom BW, Woelfel SK, Cook DR, et al: Comparison of mivacurium and suxamethonium administered by bolus and infusion. Br J Anaesth 1989;62:488–493.

56. Gronert BJ, Brandom BW: Neuromuscular blocking drugs in infants and children. Pediatr Clin North Am 1994;41:73–91.

57. Woelfel SK, Brandom BW, McGowan FX Jr, et al: Clinical pharmacology of mivacurium in pediatric patients less than two years old during nitrous oxide-halothane anesthesia. Anesth Analg 1993;77:713–720.

58. Bevan JC, Reimer EJ, Smith MF, et al: Decreased mivacurium requirements and delayed neuromuscular recovery during sevoflurane anesthesia in children and adults. Anesth Analg 1998;87:772–778.

59. Bevan DR: Prolonged mivacurium-induced neuromuscular block. Anesth Analg 1993;77:4–6.

60. Goudsouzian NG, d'Hollander AA, Viby-Mogensen J: Prolonged neuromuscular block from mivacurium in two patients with cholinesterase deficiency. Anesth Analg 1993;77:183–185.

61. Goulden MR, Hunter JM: Rapacuronium (Org 9487): Do we have a replacement for succinylcholine? Br J Anaesth 1999;82:489–492.

62. Sparr HJ, Mellinghoff H, Blobner M, et al: Comparison of intubating conditions after rapacuronium (Org 9487) and succinylcholine following rapid sequence induction in adult patients. Br J Anaesth 1999;82:537–541.

63. Reynolds LM, Infosino A, Brown R, et al: Intramuscular rapacuronium in infants and children. Anesthesiology 1999;91:1285–1292.

64. Heier T, Caldwell JE, Sessler DI, et al: Mild intraoperative hypothermia increases duration of action and spontaneous recovery of vecuronium blockade during nitrous oxide-isoflurane anesthesia in humans. Anesthesiology 1991;74:815–819.

65. Booij LH: Neuromuscular transmission and its pharmacological blockade. Part 2: Pharmacology of neuromuscular blocking agents. Pharm World Sci 1997;19:13–34.

66. Hasfurther DL, Bailey PL: Failure of neuromuscular blockade reversal after rocuronium in a patient who received oral neomycin. Can J Anaesth 1996;43:617–620.

67. de Gouw NE, Crul JF, Vandermeersch E, et al: Interaction of antibiotics on pipecuronium-induced neuromuscular blockade. J Clin Anesth 1993;5:212–215.

68. Dehpour AR, Samadian T, Roushanzamir F: Interaction of aminoglycoside antibiotics and lithium at the neuromuscular junctions. Drugs Exp Clin Res 1992;18:383–387.

69. Okamoto T: Effects of magnesium and calcium on muscle contractility and neuromuscular blockade produced by muscle relaxants and aminoglycoside. [in Japanese]. Masui 1992;41:1910–1922.

70. Ostergaard D, Engbaek J, Viby-Mogensen J: Adverse reactions and interactions of the neuromuscular blocking drugs. Med Toxicol Adverse Drug Exp 1989;4:351–368.

71. Paradelis AG, Triantaphyllidis CJ, Mironidou M, et al: Interaction of aminoglycoside antibiotics and calcium channel blockers at the neuromuscular junctions. Methods Find Exp Clin Pharmacol 1988;10:687–690.

72. Stanley TH, Webster LR: Anesthetic requirements and cardiovascular effects of fentanyl-oxygen and fentanyl-diazepam-oxygen anesthesia in man. Anesth Analg 1978;57:411–416.

73. Mandelli M, Tognoni G, Garattini S: Clinical pharmacokinetics of diazepam. Clin Pharmacokinet 1978;3:72–91.

74. Leeder JS, Kearns GL: Pharmacogenetics in pediatrics: Implications for practice. Pediatr Clin North Am 1997;44:55–77.

75. Wood M, Uetrecht J, Phythyon JM, et al: The effect of cimetidine on anesthetic metabolism and toxicity. Anesth Analg 1986;65:481–488.

76. Weinberger MM, Smith G, Milavetz G, et al: Decreased clearance of theophylline due to cimetidine. N Engl J Med 1981;304:672.

77. Krishna DR, Klotz U: Newer H$_2$-receptor antagonists. Clinical pharmacokinetics and drug interaction potential. Clin Pharmacokinet 1988;15:205–215.

78. Klotz U, Reimann I: Delayed clearance of diazepam due to cimetidine. N Engl J Med 1980;302:1012–1014.

79. Olkkola KT, Aranko K, Luurila H, et al: A potentially hazardous interaction between erythromycin and midazolam. Clin Pharmacol Ther 1993;53:298–305.

80. Hiller A, Olkkola KT, Isohanni P, et al: Unconsciousness associated with midazolam and erythromycin. Br J Anaesth 1994;65:826–828.

81. Gross JB, Alexander CM: Awakening concentrations of isoflurane are not affected by analgesic doses of morphine. Anesth Analg 1988;67:27–30.

82. Katoh T, Ikeda K: The effects of fentanyl on sevoflurane requirements for loss of consciousness and skin incision. Anesthesiology 1998;88:18–24.

83. Alexander CM, Gross JB: Sedative doses of midazolam depress hypoxic ventilatory responses in humans. Anesth Analg 1988;67:377–382.

84. Gross JB, Zebrowski ME, Carel WD, et al: Time course of ventilatory depression after thiopental and midazolam in normal subjects and in patients with chronic obstructive pulmonary disease. Anesthesiology 1983;58:540–544.

85. Partridge BL, Ward CF: Pulmonary edema following low-dose naloxone administration. Anesthesiology 1986;65:709–710.

86. Prough DS, Roy R, Bumgarner J, et al: Acute pulmonary edema in healthy teenagers following conservative doses of intravenous naloxone. Anesthesiology 1984;60:485–486.

87. Gross JB, Weller RS, Conard P: Flumazenil antagonism of midazolam-induced ventilatory depression. Anesthesiology 1991;75:179–185.

88. Hamza J, Ecoffey C, Gross JB: Ventilatory response to CO$_2$ following intravenous ketamine in children. Anesthesiology 1989;70:422–425.

89. Watcha MF, Simeon RM, White PF, et al: Effect of propofol on the incidence of postoperative vomiting after strabismus surgery in pediatric outpatients. Anesthesiology 1991;75:204–209.

90. Aun CS, Short SM, Leung DH, et al: Induction dose-response of propofol in unpremedicated children. Br J Anaesth 1992;68:64–67.

91. Aun CS, Short TG, O'Meara ME, et al: Recovery after propofol infusion anaesthesia in children: comparison with propofol, thiopentone or halothane induction followed by halothane maintenance. Br J Anaesth 1994;72:554–558.

92. Barst SM, Markowitz A, Yossefy Y, et al: Propofol reduces the incidence of vomiting after tonsillectomy in children. Pediatr Anaesth 1995;5:249–252.

93. Martin TM, Nicolson SC, Bargas MS: Propofol anesthesia reduces emesis and airway obstruction in pediatric outpatients. Anesth Analg 1993;76:144–148.

94. Runcie CJ, Mackenzie SJ, Arthur DS, et al: Comparison of recovery from anaesthesia induced in children with either propofol or thiopentone. Br J Anaesth 1993;70:192–195.

95. Buck ML: Clinical experience with ketorolac in children. Ann Pharmacother 1994;28:1009–1013.

96. Dsida RM, Wheeler M, Birmingham PK, et al: Developmental pharmacokinetics of intravenous ketorolac in pediatric surgical patients. Anesthesiology 1997;87:A1055.

97. Forrest JB, Heitlinger EL, Revell S: Ketorolac for postoperative pain management in children. Drug Saf 1997;16:309–329.

98. Gonzalez A, Smith DP: Minimizing hospital length of stay in children undergoing ureteroneocystostomy. Urology 1998;52:501–504.

99. Hamunen K, Maunuksela EL: Ketorolac does not depress ventilation in children. Paediatr Anaesth 1996;6:79.

100. Maunuksela EL, Kokki H, Bullingham RE: Comparison of intravenous ketorolac with morphine for postoperative pain in children. Clin Pharmacol Ther 1992;52:436–443.

101. Munro HM, Riegger LQ, Reynolds PI, et al: Comparison of the analgesic and emetic properties of ketorolac and morphine for paediatric outpatient strabismus surgery. Br J Anaesth 1994;72:624–628.

102. Picard P, Bazin JE, Conio N, et al: Ketorolac potentiates morphine in postoperative patient-controlled analgesia. Pain 1997;73:401–406.

103. Vetter TR, Heiner EJ: Intravenous ketorolac as an adjuvant to pediatric patient-controlled analgesia with morphine. J Clin Anesth 1994;6:110–113.

104. Agrawal A, Gerson CR, Seligman I, et al: Postoperative hemorrhage after tonsillectomy: Use of ketorolac tromethamine. Otolaryngol Head Neck Surg 1999;120:335–339.

105. Bailey R, Sinha C, Burgess LP: Ketorolac tromethamine and hemorrhage in tonsillectomy: A prospective, randomized, double-blind study. Laryngoscope 1997;107:166–169.

106. Gunter JB, Varughese AM, Harrington JF, et al: Recovery and complications after tonsillectomy in children: A comparison of ketorolac and morphine. Anesth Analg 1995;81:1136–1141.

107. Bean-Lijewski JD, Hunt RD: Effect of ketorolac on bleeding time and postoperative pain in children: A double-blind, placebo-controlled comparison with meperidine. J Clin Anesth 1996;8:25–30.

108. Safety of novel fentanyl dosage forms questioned; several deaths attributed to misuse of patch. Am J Hosp Pharm 1994;51:870.

109. Hardwick WE Jr, King WD, Palmisano PA: Respiratory depression in a child unintentionally exposed to transdermal fentanyl patch. So Med J 1997;90:962–964.

110. Payne R, Chandler S, Einhaus M: Guidelines for the clinical use of transdermal fentanyl. Anti-Cancer Drugs 1995;6(Suppl 3):50–53.

111. Lehmann KA, Zech D: Transdermal fentanyl: Clinical pharmacology. J Pain Symptom Manage 1992;7:S8–S16.

112. Varvel JR, Shafer SL, Hwang SS, et al: Absorption characteristics of transdermally administered Fentanyl. Anesthesiology 1989;70:928–934.

113. Committee on Drugs American Academy of Pediatrics: Alternate routes of drug administration: Advantages and disadvantages. Pediatrics 1997;100:143–152.

114. Dsida RM, Wheeler M, Birmingham PK, et al: Premedication of pediatric tonsillectomy patients with oral transmucosal fentanyl citrate. Anesth Analg 1998;86:66–70.

115. Smith RM: Anesthesia for Infants and Children, 4th ed. St. Louis: CV Mosby; 1980.

116. Pounder DR, Blackstock D, Steward DJ: Tracheal extubation in children: Halothane versus isoflurane, anesthetized versus awake. Anesthesiology 1991;74:653–655.

117. Pullerits J, Burrows FA, Roy WL: Arterial desaturation in healthy children during transfer to the recovery room. Can J Anaesth 1987;34:470–473.

118. Patel R, Norden J, Hannallah RS: Oxygen administration prevents hypoxemia during post-anesthetic transport in children. Anesthesiology 1988;69:616–618.

119. Falk SA, Woods NF: Hospital noise: Levels and potential health hazards. N Engl J Med 1973;289:774–781.

120. Luczan ME: Tender loving care: Meeting the special needs of the pediatric patient. In: Luczan ME, ed: Postanesthesia Nursing. Rockville, MD: Aspen Publications; 1984:169–185.

121. Hackel A, Badgwell JM, Binding RR, et al: Guidelines for the pediatric perioperative anesthesia environment. American Academy of Pediatrics. Section on Anesthesiology. Pediatrics 1999;103:512–515.

122. Hartwell PW: Discharge criteria. Int Anesthesiol Clin 1983;21:107–114.

123. Aldrete JA, Kroulik D: A postanaesthetic recovery score. Anesth Analg 1970;49:924–934.

124. Schreiner MS, Nicolson SC, Martin T, et al: Should children drink before discharge from day surgery? Anesthesiology 1992;76:528–533.

125. Cohen MM, Cameron CB, Duncan PG: Pediatric anesthesia morbidity and mortality in the perioperative period. Anesth Analg 1990;70:160–167.

126. Gabrielczyk MR, Buist RJ: Pulse oximetry and postoperative hypothermia: An evaluation of the Nellcor N-100 in a cardiac surgical intensive care unit. Anaesthesia 1988;43:402–404.

127. Smith DC, Canning JJ, Crul JF: Pulse oximetry in the recovery room. Anaesthesia 1989;44:345–348.

128. Davis PJ, Greenberg JA, Gendelman M, et al: Recovery characteristics of sevoflurane and halothane in preschool-aged children undergoing bilateral myringotomy and pressure equalization tube insertion. Anesth Analg 1999;88:34–38.

129. Steward DJ: A trial of enflurane for paediatric out-patient anaesthesia. Can Anaesth Soc J 1977;24:603–608.

130. Wells LT, Rasch DK: Emergence "delirium" after sevoflurane anesthesia: A paranoid delusion? Anesth Analg 1999;88:1308–1310.

131. Rolf N, Coté CJ: Frequency and severity of desaturation events during general anesthesia in children with and without upper respiratory infections. J Clin Anesth 1992;4:200–203.

132. Xue FS, Tong SY, Liao X, et al: Observation of the correlation of postanaesthesia recovery scores with early postoperative hypoxaemia in children. Paediatr Anaesth 1999;9:145–151.

133. Xue FS, Huang YG, Luo LK, et al: Observation of early postoperative hypoxaemia in children undergoing elective plastic surgery. Paediatr Anaesth 1996;6:21–28.

134. Xue FS, Huang YG, Tong SY, et al: A comparative study of early postoperative hypoxemia in infants, children, and adults undergoing elective plastic surgery. Anesth Analg 1996;83:709–715.

135. Koka BV, Jeon IS, Andre JM, et al: Postintubation croup in children. Anesth Analg 1977;56:501–505.

136. Flogel CM, Ward DS, Wada DR, et al: The effects of large-dose flumazenil on midazolam-induced ventilatory depression. Anesth Analg 1993;77:1207–1214.

137. Flumazenil Study Group: Reversal of central nervous system effects by flumazenil after intravenous conscious sedation with midazolam: Report of a multicenter study. Clin Ther 1992;14:861–877.

138. Gross JB, Blouin RT, Zandsberg S, et al: Effect of flumazenil on ventilatory drive during sedation with midazolam and alfentanil. Anesthesiology 1996;85:713–720.

139. Sugarman JM, Paul RI: Flumazenil: A review. Pediatr Emerg Care 1994;10:37–43.

140. Steward DJ: Preterm infants are more prone to complications following minor surgery than are term infants. Anesthesiology 1982;56:304–306.

141. Liu LM, Coté CJ, Goudsouzian NG, et al: Life-threatening apnea in infants recovering from anesthesia. Anesthesiology 1983;59:506–510.

142. Kurth CD, Spitzer AR, Broennle AM, et al: Postoperative apnea in preterm infants. Anesthesiology 1987;66:483–488.

143. Welborn LG, Ramirez N, Oh TH, et al: Postanesthetic apnea and periodic breathing in infants. Anesthesiology 1986;65:658–661.

144. Coté CJ, Kelly DH: Postoperative apnea in a full-term infant with a demonstrable respiratory pattern abnormality. Anesthesiology 1990;72:559–561.

145. Tetzlaff JE, Annand DW, Pudimat MA, et al: Postoperative apnea in a full-term infant. Anesthesiology 1988;69:426–428.

146. Coté CJ, Zaslavsky A, Downes JJ, et al: Postoperative apnea in former preterm infants after inguinal herniorrhaphy: A combined analysis. Anesthesiology 1995;82:809–822.

147. Burtin P, Daoud P, Jacqz-Aigrain E, et al: Hypotension with midazolam and fentanyl in the newborn. Lancet 1991;337:1545–1546.

148. Jacqz-Aigrain E, Burtin P: Clinical pharmacokinetics of sedatives in neonates. Clin Pharmacokinet 1996;31:423–443.

149. Dohi S, Naito H, Takahashi T: Age-related changes in blood pressure and duration of motor block in spinal anesthesia. Anesthesiology 1979;50:319–323.

150. Beyer JE, Wells N: The assessment of pain in children. Pediatr Clin North Am 1989;36:837–854.

151. Buchholz M, Karl HW, Pomietto M, et al: Pain scores in infants: A modified infant pain scale versus visual analogue. J Pain Symptom Manage 1998;15:117–124.

152. Krechel SW, Bildner J: CRIES: a new neonatal postoperative pain measurement score. Initial testing of validity and reliability. Paediatr Anaesth 1995;5:53–61.

153. Taddio A, Nulman I, Koren BS, et al: A revised measure of acute pain in infants. J Pain Symptom Manage 1995;10:456–463.

154. Tarbell SE, Cohen IT, Marsh JL: The Toddler-Preschooler Postoperative Pain Scale: An observational scale for measuring postoperative pain in children aged 1–5. Preliminary report. Pain 1992;50:273–280.

155. Wilson GA, Doyle E: Validation of three paediatric pain scores for use by parents. Anaesthesia 1996;51:1005–1007.

156. Berde CB: Pediatric postoperative pain management. Pediatr Clin North Am 1989;36:921–940.

157. Andersen R, Krohg K: Pain as a major cause of postoperative nausea. Can Anaesth Soc J 1976;23:366–369.

158. Egbert LD, Battit GE, Welch CE, et al: Reduction of postoperative pain by encouragement and instruction of patients. N Engl J Med 1964;270:825–827.

159. Montgomery CJ, McCormack JP, Reichert CC, et al: Plasma concentrations after high-dose (45 mg·kg-1) rectal acetaminophen in children. Can J Anaesth 1995;42:982–986.

160. Birmingham PK, Tobin MJ, Henthorn TK, et al: Twenty-four-hour pharmacokinetics of rectal acetaminophen in children: An old drug with new recommendations. Anesthesiology 1997;87:244–252.

161. Houck CS, Sullivan LJ, Wilder RT, et al.: Pharmacokinetics of a higher dose of rectal acetaminophen in children. Anesthesiology 1995;83:A1126.

162. Birmingham PK, Tobin MJ, Henthorn TK, et al: "Loading" and subsequent dosing of rectal acetaminophen in children: A 24 hour pharmacokinetic study of new dosing recommendations. Anesthesiology 1996;85:A1105.

163. Fisher DM: Surrogate end points. Are they meaningful? Anesthesiology 1994;81:795–796.

164. Watcha MF, Smith I: Cost-effectiveness analysis of antiemetic therapy for ambulatory surgery. J Clin Anesth 1994;6:370–377.
165. Watcha MF, White PF: Economics of anesthetic practice. Anesthesiology 1997;86:1170–1196.
166. Abramowitz MD, Elder PT, Friendly DS, et al: Antiemetic effectiveness of intraoperatively administered droperidol in pediatric strabismus outpatient surgery: Preliminary report of a controlled study. J Pediatr Ophthalmol Strabismus 1981;18:22–27.
167. Patton CM Jr: Rapid induction of acute dyskinesia by droperidol. Anesthesiology 1975;43:126–127.
168. Dupre LJ, Stieglitz P: Extrapyramidal syndromes after premedication with droperidol in children. Br J Anaesth 1980;52:831–833.
169. Adams VR, Valley AW: Granisetron: the second serotonin-receptor antagonist. Ann Pharmacother 1995;29:1240–1251.
170. Bach-Styles T, Martin-Sheridan D, Hughes C, et al: Comparison of ondansetron, metoclopramide, and placebo in the prevention of postoperative emesis in children undergoing ophthalmic surgery. CRNA 1997;8:152–156.
171. Cieslak GD, Watcha MF, Phillips MB, et al: The dose-response relation and cost-effectiveness of granisetron for the prophylaxis of pediatric postoperative emesis. Anesthesiology 1996;85:1076–1085.
172. Davis A, Krige S, Moyes D: A double-blind randomized prospective study comparing ondansetron with droperidol in the prevention of emesis following strabismus surgery. Anaesth Intensive Care 1995;23:438–443.
173. Furst SR, Rodarte A: Prophylactic antiemetic treatment with ondansetron in children undergoing tonsillectomy. Anesthesiology 1994; 81:799–803.
174. Hamid SK, Selby IR, Sikich N, et al: Vomiting after adenotonsillectomy in children: A comparison of ondansetron, dimenhydrinate, and placebo. Anesth Analg 1998;86:496–500.
175. Morton NS, Camu F, Dorman T, et al: Ondansetron reduces nausea and vomiting after paediatric adenotonsillectomy. Paediatr Anaesth 1997;7:37–45.
176. Paxton D, Taylor RH, Gallagher TM, et al: Postoperative emesis following otoplasty in children. Anaesthesia 1995;50:1083–1085.
177. Splinter WM, Rhine EJ: Low-dose ondansetron with dexamethasone more effectively decreases vomiting after strabismus surgery in children than does high-dose ondansetron. Anesthesiology 1998;88:72–75.
178. Splinter WM, Roberts DJ: Dexamethasone decreases vomiting by children after tonsillectomy. Anesth Analg 1996;83:913–916.
179. Warner MA, Warner ME, Weber JG: Clinical significance of pulmonary aspiration during the perioperative period. Anesthesiology 1993;78:56–62.
180. Coté CJ: Aspiration: An overrated risk in elective patients. Advances Anesthesia 1992;9:1–26.
181. Coté CJ: NPO guidelines: Children and adults. In: McGoldrick KE, ed: Ambulatory Anesthesia: A Problem-Oriented Approach. Baltimore: Williams & Wilkins; 1995:20–32.
182. Tiret L, Desmonts JM, Hatton F, et al: Complications associated with anaesthesia: A prospective survey in France. Can Anaesth Soc J 1986;33:336–344.
183. Sessler DI, Moayeri A: Skin-surface warming: Heat flux and central temperature. Anesthesiology 1990;73:218–224.
184. McConachie IW, Day A, Morris P: Recovery from anaesthesia in children. Anaesthesia 1989;44:986–990.
185. Blesch P, Fisher ML: The impact of parental presence on parental anxiety and satisfaction. AORN J 1996;63:761–768.
186. Turner P: Establishing a protocol for parental presence in recovery. Br J Nurs 1997;6:794–799.
187. Hall PA, Payne JF, Stack CG, et al: Parents in the recovery room: Survey of parental and staff attitudes. Br Med J 1995;310:163–164.
188. Youngs EJ, Shafer SL: Pharmacokinetic parameters relevant to recovery from opioids. Anesthesiology 1994;81:833–842.
189. Cartwright DP, Kvalsvik O, Cassuto J, et al: A randomized, blind comparison of remifentanil and alfentanil during anesthesia for outpatient surgery. Anesth Analg 1997;85:1014–1019.
190. Ebert TJ, Robinson BJ, Uhrich TD, et al: Recovery from sevoflurane anesthesia: A comparison to isoflurane and propofol anesthesia. Anesthesiology 1998;89:1524–1531.
191. Song D, Joshi GP, White PF: Fast-track eligibility after ambulatory anesthesia: A comparison of desflurane, sevoflurane, and propofol. Anesth Analg 1998;86:267–273.
192. Chung F: Discharge criteria: A new trend. Can J Anaesth 1995;42:1056–1058.
193. Chung F: Are discharge criteria changing? J Clin Anesth 1993;5:64S–68S.
194. Tang J, Chen L, White PF, et al: Recovery profile, costs, and patient satisfaction with propofol and sevoflurane for fast-track office-based anesthesia. Anesthesiology 1999;91:253–261.
195. Lubarsky DA: Fast track in the postanesthesia care unit: unlimited possibilities? J Clin Anesth 1996;8:70S–72S.
196. Suttner S, Boldt J, Schmidt C, et al: Cost analysis of target-controlled infusion-based anesthesia compared with standard anesthesia regimens. Anesth Analg 1999;88:77–82.
197. Song D, van Vlymen J, White PF: Is the bispectral index useful in predicting fast-track eligibility after ambulatory anesthesia with propofol and desflurane? Anesth Analg 1998;87:1245–1248.
198. White PF, Song D: New criteria for fast-tracking after outpatient anesthesia: A comparison with the modified Aldrete's scoring system. Anesth Analg 1999;88:1069–1072.

31 Pediatric Equipment

Charles J. Coté

Heating and Cooling Systems
Suction Apparatus
Operating Table
Warming Devices
  Radiant Warmers
  Warming Blankets
  Warm Air Devices
  Passive Heat and Moisturizer Exchangers, "Artificial Nose"
  Fluid Warmers
  Heated Humidifiers
  Wrapping
Intravenous Therapy
Airway Apparatus
  Masks
  Oral Airways
  Nasopharyngeal Airways
  Laryngeal Mask Airway
  Endotracheal Tubes
Intubation Equipment
  Routine Equipment
  Special Equipment
Anesthesia Machine and Appendages
  Anesthesia Machine
  Scavenger
  Circuits
  Humidifiers
  Anesthesia Ventilators
Equipment Cart
Defibrillator and External Pacemakers
Monitoring Equipment
  Anesthesia Record
  Precordial/Esophageal Stethoscope
  Blood Pressure Devices
  Electrocardiograph
  Oxygen Monitors
  Temperature Monitors

Pulse Oximetry
Carbon Dioxide Analyzers
Anesthetic Agent Analyzers
Blood Loss Monitoring
Neuromuscular Transmission Monitoring
Bispectral Analysis
Disconnect/Apnea Alarms
Apnea Monitors
Volume Meter/Spirometer
Inspiratory Pressure Gauge
Urinary Catheter
Invasive Blood Pressure Monitors
Transcutaneous Oxygen/Carbon Dioxide Monitors
Intracranial Pressure Monitoring
Echocardiography
Electrocautery
Transport Apparatus
Purchasing Anesthesia Equipment

Heating and Cooling Systems

The operating room provides the physical environment for the conduct of anesthesia and may be compared to a large infant incubator. Readily controlled heating and cooling systems are crucial for thermal stability—that is, control of the external environment. Temperature regulation is a greater problem in a child than in an adult because of the higher ratio of body surface area to body mass. A neonate or small infant requires a warmer room temperature than an adult (see Chapters 14 and 27); the temperature may be reduced once a patient is prepared and draped. Exposure during anesthetic induction and surgical preparation before draping causes significant thermal stress.

Suction Apparatus

A functioning suction apparatus must be available before beginning any anesthetic procedure. The device should be capable of regulated pressures; suctioning the oropharynx requires a higher vacuum level than that necessary for endotracheal suction. Special circumstances, such as a full stomach, may require the availability of a second suction line. Additional vacuum equipment is needed for scavenging waste anesthetic agents. Several sizes of suction catheters are helpful, depending on the indication, that is, tracheal or gastric/oropharyngeal suction. A 6 French suction catheter with a thumb-control side port is useful for small endotracheal tubes, whereas 8 and 14 French catheters are useful for larger endotracheal tubes. Routine suction of stomach contents after induction of anesthesia may reduce the potential for serious pulmonary aspiration of gastric contents; in larger patients, vented catheters (e.g., Salem Sump, Sherwood Medical, St Louis, MO) may be more efficacious than unvented catheters. Suctioning the stomach with the patient supine and in left and right lateral positions has been shown to be most efficient in evacuation of stomach contents.[1]

Operating Table

The operating table is a vital piece of anesthesia equipment. The table should provide the full range of positioning including Trendelenburg controls in case of either regurgitation or the need to increase venous return. It must have appropriate padding to prevent patient contact with metal structures. The ability to remove the head support and to lower the foot section can provide a smaller table for infants. For extremely long procedures, an alternating-pressure air mattress placed between the patient and the operating table may help guard against decubitus injuries. Periodically changing the patient's head position may be important in preventing bald spots as a result of prolonged contact pressure in one location.[2]

Warming Devices

Hypothermia may cause the infant to become acidotic and apneic, alter the kinetics of medications, pose problems with reversal of neuromuscular blocking drugs, and increase oxygen consumption with shivering.[3] It cannot be overemphasized that the operating room itself is an important factor in temperature regulation for all patients.

Radiant Warmers

Overhead radiant heating units with servomechanism temperature control are useful; however, because of the risk of skin burn, the servomechanism control sensor must be applied to the warmed skin and should not measure body core temperature.[4] A maximum skin temperature of 37°C should preclude surface burns. The radiant warmer is used during the anesthetic induction and surgical preparation; it should be used once again as the drapes are removed at the end of the procedure. If infrared light bulbs are used, care must be taken to ensure that the heat lamp is an appropriate distance from the patient to avoid causing thermal injury[5]; their red cast may also make accurate evaluation of a patient's color difficult.

Warming Blankets

Circulating water mattresses are useful in maintaining normothermia in patients with body surface area of 0.5 m² (approximately 10 kg of body weight or less).[6] Above this weight, the decreasing ratio of body surface area to body mass generally makes heat transfer at safe temperatures inefficient enough to minimize the benefit. To avoid surface burns, the fluid temperature should never exceed 39°C and must be monitored[7]; several layers of material should be interposed between the patient and the warming blanket to avoid direct contact.

Warm Air Devices

The most useful devices for keeping pediatric patients warm are warm air mattresses that can be wrapped around the head or upper or lower torso.[8-12] These devices rely on the combination of convection with warm air and plastic wrap, which also serves to reduce evaporative heat losses. These devices are the single most effective means for warming patients and they are effective even when only a portion of the body can be covered.[8, 10] The major issue with these devices is the cost per patient, since the air mattress is a disposable item. One report suggests that simple delivery of warm air beneath bed sheets without the use of the plastic blanket can be effective.[8] In extreme cases of hypothermia, a blanket can be placed beneath and on top of a patient to speed the warming process. Our experience is that this is an extremely effective means for rewarming post–cardiac surgical patients and maintaining temperature in patients undergoing liver transplantation or other procedures involving prolonged exposure of viscera.

Passive Heat and Moisturizer Exchangers, "Artificial Nose"

Heat-moisture exchangers are reasonably effective in preserving body heat.[13-15] There is concern, however, with the resistance to breathing with spontaneous respirations and clogging with humidity over time.[16-18]

Fluid Warmers

The effectiveness of standard fluid warmers is dependent on the time that intravenous fluids or blood products are in contact with the warmer. Hemolysis of red blood cells may occur with excessive heating.[19] With slow intravenous fluid therapy, the fluid warmer does not contribute significant heat transfer because heat is lost along the length of the intravenous tubing between the warmer and the patient before the fluid enters the patient's body. Warming intravenous fluid during maintenance therapy is virtually useless for temperature regulation.

The new generation of warming devices is far superior to water bath warmers and use countercurrent heat exchange as a means of rapidly warming fluid along the length of the column of fluid.[20] The choice of device depends on the size of the patient, the anticipated rate of blood loss, and the cost. The rate of infusion with these devices is also limited by the length of the intravenous tubing and the diameter of the intravenous catheter. An example of the lowest capacity device with this design is the Hot Line (Level 1 Technologies, Inc., Rockland, MA), which is extremely effective at rates up to 75 mL/min.[21] The manufacturer's data suggest that approximately 90 mL/min of refrigerated blood products can be warmed to 35°C. A more complex and higher capacity system is the Level 1 System 1000 (Level 1 Technologies, Inc., Rockland, MA), which uses the same countercurrent warming technology but combined with the capacity to infuse fluid, blood, or plasma in bags under pressure. *Because this device infuses bags of fluid under pressure, it is important to eliminate all air from any bags so as to avoid the possibility of air embolization.* This system is capable of warming fluids at rates up to approximately 500 mL/min.[22] The level I device is capable of warming blood starting at 5°C to 6°C to at least 33°C at rates as high as 250 mL/min.[20] The manufacturer's data suggest that up to 600 mL/min of red cells diluted to a hematocrit of 60% can be delivered through a 14-gauge IV catheter and 750 mL/min through an 8.5 French introducer sheath. An example of a high capacity system is the Rapid Infusion System (Haemonetics Corporation, Braintree, MA), which combines the countercurrent warming technology with a large reservoir and infusion with roller pumps. The system allows blood or fluid to be infused at 100, 200, or 300 mm Hg pressure with bolus options of 100 or 500 mL, at an infusion rate of up to 1500 mL/min (through a 10-gauge intravenous line). This device also has an automatic slowing of the roller pump if the in-line fluid or blood temperature drops below 34°C. This latter device is very expensive as an initial purchase, as is the infusion kit for each use, but it certainly offers the most control and highest capacity possible. In general, the Hotline appears most suited for low-volume, relatively slow blood loss. The Level 1 system seems most appropriate for children who weigh approximately 40 kg or less with expected rapid and massive blood loss and the Rapid Infusion System for larger patients with expected massive and rapid blood loss. It should be noted that the Rapid Infusion System has its main advantage with large-bore catheters such as 5.5 French or greater in diameter; with standard intravenous catheters, the flow characteristics are similar to the Level 1.

Heated Humidifiers

Airstream warming and humidification devices are useful for maintaining body temperature.[23–25] If a humidifier is used, the anesthesiologist should be familiar with the potential hazards: overheating, leaks, "rain out," changes in compression volume, and obstruction if connected in reverse. Humidifiers with servomechanism-controlled temperature regulation may prevent overheating. Anesthesia circuits with heating elements within them may further reduce the rainout problem and minimize the risk of overheating; these advantages must be weighed against increased expense. With the advent of warm air mattresses, there appears to be less of a need for in-line humidification as a means of warming patients; rather, their main indication is to prevent drying of secretions when using nonrebreathing circuits.

Wrapping

Any form of wrapping can reduce radiant and convective heat losses; plastic wrap used for food is particularly effective and low cost. Covering an infant's head is of greatest value because the head represents such a large proportion of the body surface area. As with any warming device, there are hazards; the plastic drapes not only reduce conductive losses but also eliminate sweating as a mechanism of thermal regulation so that hyperthermia may result.[26] "Space" blankets with reflective aluminized Mylar layers are very effective in preventing heat loss.[27]

Intravenous Therapy

It is necessary to have available the appropriate range of intravenous equipment for the patient population being anesthetized. In general, it is most safe to establish intravenous access in all anesthetized patients. The only exception to this practice is a very short, noninvasive procedure such as myringotomy; in this situation, an intravenous line is set up and ready for use should it be needed.

The volume of the infusion fluid container should not exceed the patient's estimated fluid deficit unless a volume-limiting device is interposed between the intravenous container and the patient. Generally an intravenous set with a microdrop outlet (60 drops/mL) is most practical for children weighing less than 50 kg. The intravenous setup should include easily accessible injection ports; intravenous extension tubings are often required when lines are started in the foot. Infusion sets should be purged of all air bubbles, especially at each injection port, before use on patients.[28] In children with known intracardiac defects or an arteriovenous malformation or in neonates, the potential for paradoxic air emboli is always present. In these circumstances, intravenous air traps may reduce this risk.[29] In the smallest patients, a T-connector placed at the hub of the intravenous catheter allows direct injection of drugs with minimal fluid dead space.

When carefully metered transfusion of colloid or blood is necessary, a multiple-stopcock manifold, preferably with Luer locks to avoid disconnections, added to the infusion line allows the main line to continue infusing maintenance fluid except during the actual administration of either blood or colloid (Fig. 31–1). This arrangement provides an outlet

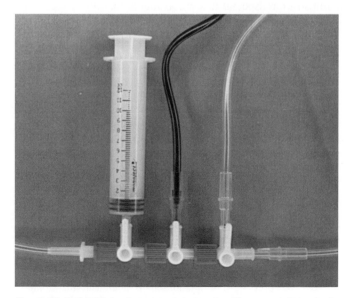

Figure 31–1. Multiple three-way stopcocks allow a syringe to be used precisely to administer blood, plasma, albumin, multiple vasopressors, or other fluids and medications.

for blood administration, another for colloid administration, and a third for a metering syringe. Careful titration of infusion rates may be facilitated by the use of electronic pumps or intravenous rate controllers. The infusion pump chosen for a pediatric patient must suit the circumstances. In most situations, a device with precise volume limits and air bubble and pressure alarms is the safest. These manifolds are also useful to allow the administration of several medications (e.g., vasopressors) simultaneously; special narrow-bore tubing also reduces the dead space of such a setup, thus minimizing delays in response to changes in the vasopressors because of the reduced dead space of the system.

The flow of crystalloid is not a simple linear function of perfusion pressure; the relationship is highly nonlinear, best described as a quadratic model:

$$P = R_L F + R_T F^2$$

where P is pressure, F is flow, R_L is resistance for laminar flow, and R_T is resistance for turbulent flow; the parameters R_L and R_T show a linear increase with the length of the intravenous tubing. Additionally, elements of the intravenous system have isolated effects on one factor or another. For example, a 5-μm filter alters R_L and thereby increases resistance and reduces flow at all pressures; a check-valve significantly alters R_T and thereby increases resistance but reduces flow primarily at high flow rates.[30] A similar quadratic function describes the pressure/flow relationship of intravenous cannulas.[31] Studies of crystalloid solutions demonstrate steep rises in resistance with increasing pressure in a nonlinear manner as smaller cannulas are used (Fig. 31–2). The effects of the tubing set add to the effects of the cannula; connection of a large-diameter tubing to a catheter of smaller diameter limits flow according to the diameter of the catheter. In this situation, the catheter limits flow. In situations in which massive and rapid blood loss is anticipated, insertion of extra-large peripheral intravenous catheters such as 5, 6, 7, or 8 French pulmonary artery flow catheter introducers will provide the most efficient method for rapid volume administration. Special kits are available that allow the dilation of small veins. Initially, insertion of either a small

diameter needle followed by a Seldinger guide wire or a small intravenous catheter followed by a guide wire is accomplished. This then allows passage of a dilator and eventually placement of a large-diameter cannula.

Accelerating flow through an intravenous line is a concern in emergency situations; rapid transfusion devices are the best method for increasing flow rates.[20–22] These new devices have rapid-warming and rapid-administration features that far outperform routine transfusion methods; however, they also require special expensive tubing. It is reasonable for trauma centers and tertiary care hospitals to acquire such devices (see previous discussion). For bags of crystalloid, colloid, or blood components, a pressure infusion cuff is the second fastest but most readily available and lowest-cost method for rapidly administering large volumes.[32] Next in order of efficacy are in-line blood pumps or a stopcock and syringe arrangement; gravity is the slowest method of infusion. Because we often use the syringe technique in pediatrics (primarily for accurate measurement in infants), it is worth noting that it is similar in efficiency to the in-line blood pump. Intravenous tubing designed for administering blood has better flow characteristics than standard intravenous tubing.[33] Large-bore "resuscitation" tubing provides the best flow characteristics; however, the final common pathway, the lumen of the intravenous catheter itself, is the major limitation of flow capacity.[20, 30–35] Larger-diameter short catheters allow greater flow than long narrow-diameter catheters.[35] This factor is particularly important when rapid volume administration is required but the only intravenous access is through a central venous catheter; this problem is greatly magnified when multilumen catheters are used.[35, 36] *If rapid volume resuscitation is a significant potential problem, then one single-lumen large-bore peripheral intravenous line is of much greater value than a multilumen central venous catheter.*

The choice of fluid and its temperature also has effects on the rate of infusion, primarily because of differences in viscosity. Crystalloid passes most readily, followed by colloid, whole blood, and packed red blood cells. Dilution of packed red blood cells with normal saline markedly improves the flow rate and decreases hemolysis during rapid infusion.[37] Questions remain about the clinical importance of this hemolysis. It has been shown that even through a 26-gauge needle with a driving pressure of 300 mm Hg, the plasma hemoglobin level increases from the normal baseline of 22.3 mg/100 mL to only 32.1 mg/100 mL in 7-day-old blood.[38]

Airway Apparatus

Masks

The smaller the patient, the more important is the elimination of mechanical dead space. Rendell-Baker/Soucek masks, developed from molds of the facial contours of children, were designed to minimize mechanical dead space without the inflatable cuff or high dome of adult masks. Transparent disposable plastic models are preferable to the classic black conductive rubber because they allow observation of a patient's color and condensate from exhaled humidity with respiration. Plastic disposable masks with soft inflatable cuffs, although less anatomically correct, seem particularly

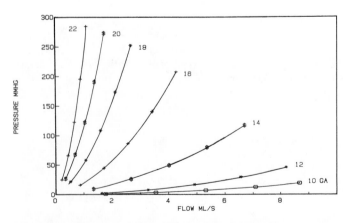

Figure 31–2. The pressure-flow relationship of intravenous catheters. Note that the pressure-flow relationship is nonlinear; the smaller the catheter diameter, the greater the resistance. (Data from Philip BK, Philip JH: Characteristics of flow in intravenous catheters. IEEE Trans Biomed Eng 1986;33:529–531.)

well suited for management of children with anatomic or mechanical problems that interfere with normal mask application. An especially useful mask has a built-in port that allows passage of an endotracheal tube over a fiberoptic scope, thus providing excellent fiberoptic intubation conditions while maintaining the patient's spontaneous respirations, oxygenation, and depth of anesthesia.[39]

Oral Airways

A complete selection of oral airways must be readily available. Infants have a relatively large tongue, which easily obstructs the airway once they lose consciousness. If too large an airway is inserted, damage to laryngeal structures (traumatic epiglottitis, uvular swelling) may result in postoperative airway obstruction.[40] Improperly inserted airways, by obstructing venous and lymphatic drainage, may also result in airway obstruction secondary to swelling of the tongue.[41, 42] A tongue blade is useful to help insert the airway without kinking the tongue or catching the tongue or lips between the airway and the teeth. The proper size oral airway may be estimated by comparing the artificial airway with the external anatomy of the patient (see Fig. 7–13); however, one study has shown a relationship with length of airway, age, and weight.[43] In that study, infants from 1 to 2 years of age would require a 7 cm airway, those 2 to 8 years an 8 cm airway, and those over 8 years a 9 cm airway. It should be noted that lower weight patients and female patients often required a shorter airway.

A new oral airway, the cuffed oropharyngeal airway (Mallinckrodt, Inc., St. Louis, MO) has been developed for use in adults and larger children. This device may offer an alternative to the laryngeal mask airway. Experience with adult patients suggests similarity with the laryngeal mask airway in terms of maintaining a clear airway and accuracy of measuring expired carbon dioxide when compared with an endotracheal tube.[44–46] There is some suggestion that insertion of the laryngeal mask airway is easier than the cuffed oropharyngeal airway.[44, 46]

Nasopharyngeal Airways

Nasopharyngeal airways are not as frequently used in pediatric patients because the internal diameter is often small, resulting in increased work of breathing. In addition, adenoid hypertrophy makes a child susceptible to bleeding after nasopharyngeal airway insertion. If such an airway is necessary, a well-lubricated endotracheal tube, cut to the appropriate length, may be used; however, it must be safely secured because it may accidentally pass into the nasopharynx.

Laryngeal Mask Airway

The laryngeal mask airway (LMA North America, Inc., San Diego, CA) has proven to be a great addition to the airway management of children. This device requires minimal practice to gain facility with insertion and in some circumstances can be life saving (see Chapter 7).[47–53] This device will generally provide a clear airway for maintaining spontaneous respirations; however, one must not rely on this device if controlled ventilation is required. Controlled ventilation has been described but carries the risk of gastric dilation.[54] It is my personal opinion that this device should be used primarily for spontaneous ventilation and used with great caution for controlled ventilation. This device is particularly useful in patients with anatomical airway abnormalities because it provides a clear airway while other measures are planned for successful endotracheal intubation or the performance of a tracheotomy.[53, 55] Fiberoptic intubation through the laryngeal mask airway is often used in children with midfacial hypoplasia syndromes and in patients with redundant airway tissue such as patients with mucopolysaccharidosis. Emergency placement of this device can also be life saving in patients who are difficult to ventilate with bag and mask with or without a nasal or oral airway.[56] Fiberoptic intubation is easier because the patient can be well oxygenated while using the fiberoptic scope to find the laryngeal inlet.

Endotracheal Tubes

A variety of endotracheal tubes (generally sizes 2.0 to 6.0 mm internal diameter [ID]) must be available with appropriate sizes of stylets. There may be considerable variations from one manufacturer to another in wall thickness, external diameter, kink resistance, and direction and angle of bevel, as well as differences in endotracheal tube cuff length and thickness of cuffed endotracheal tubes.[57] Despite these differences in endotracheal tube wall thickness, a first approximation for the correct endotracheal tube size for an average child older than 2 years is 4.5 mm ID plus the patient's age divided by 4.[58] A full-term neonate usually accepts an endotracheal tube of 3 mm ID, a normal 1-year-old 3.5 to 4.0 mm ID, and a 2-year-old 4.5 to 5.0 mm ID. Endotracheal tubes at least one half-size larger and smaller than estimated should always be kept at hand to accommodate airway size variability. The only true test for appropriate size selection is a leak between 20 and 40 cm H_2O peak inflation pressure. The leak may be easily assessed by closing the circuit pop-off valve and slowly increasing the pressure by gently squeezing the anesthesia bag while listening over the larynx with a stethoscope. This technique has been demonstrated to be a sensitive and accurate measure of fit between the tracheal lumen and the endotracheal tube.[59] If an infant has been intubated without the use of muscle relaxants, then one must wait until he or she is well anesthetized to assess the leak properly. If a child is coughing or has laryngospasm around the endotracheal tube, then the tube will appear to be too large because there may not be a leak. The relationship of age, endotracheal tube sizes, and peak inflation pressure leak is used to estimate laryngeal size (see Fig. 20–4).

It is important to remember that in a smaller child, the cricoid ring is narrower than the glottic opening. A snug-fitting endotracheal tube may cause edema formation and postoperative airway obstruction (postintubation croup). Uncuffed endotracheal tubes are generally used for elective cases until a 6 mm ID size is reached; uncuffed tubes are available down to 2.0 mm ID. Traditional teaching suggests that this is appropriate practice; however, it has not been confirmed on a scientific basis. The external diameter of a cuffed endotracheal tube is larger because of the cuff, so one must use a smaller-ID endotracheal tube for a given tracheal size. Cuffed endotracheal tubes as small as 3 mm ID are available and may be appropriate for use in patients with very noncompliant lungs, a full stomach, or hiatus hernia with reflux. If a cuffed endotracheal tube is used, the cuff is generally inflated just enough to provide a leak between 20 and 30 cm H_2O peak inflation pressure. One must be aware that the endotracheal tube cuff pressure will increase during a nitrous-oxide-supplemented anesthetic because of diffusion of nitrous oxide into the cuff.[60] This phenomenon may present a special additional hazard to children, in whom unanticipated cuff pressure may result in mucosal swelling at the level of the cricoid ring. One study has examined the use of cuffed endotracheal tubes and demonstrated fewer endotracheal tube changes due to improper size selection.[61] Their formula for size selection was (age ÷ 4) + 3. This study did not examine adequately the infants in the lowest age range, however. *I do not recommend the routine use of 3.0 mm ID cuffed endotracheal tubes in neonates because the potential for laryngeal or tracheal damage far outweighs the advantage of avoiding an extra laryngoscopy and intubation.*

Molded preformed endotracheal tubes are especially useful for head and neck surgery because they remove the anesthesia circuit connections from the surgical field.[62] Another special endotracheal tube has a built-in gas sampling port so that a true end-tidal gas sample can be obtained for carbon dioxide or anesthetic agent. This modification offers an advantage because no dead space is added to the system by an additional connector and there is one less connection to separate accidentally. However, secretions and water easily block the gas sample port, and the external diameter of the endotracheal tube is slightly larger when compared with standard endotracheal tubes.[63]

When excessive external pressure may be applied to the endotracheal tube or extreme flexion of the neck is likely to kink a standard endotracheal tube, an endotracheal tube with Tovell spiral wire reinforcement may be used. Its kink resistance is well known, but the additional wall thickness limits applicability in smaller patients. The spiral spring-like construction of this endotracheal tube has caused it to pop out of the airway; in addition, repeated improper sterilization may lead to bubble formation within the rubber, leading to airway obstruction when used with nitrous oxide.[64] The use of tapered Cole tubes should be abandoned.[65-67]

The CO_2 laser for the treatment of laryngeal polyposis and other airway lesions has introduced the problem of ignition of the endotracheal tube. Avoiding high levels of oxygen and nitrous oxide, which both support combustion, diminishes the risk of fire. Special stainless steel and metal implanted endotracheal tubes are available but quite expensive. Protecting the tube surface with aluminum or copper foil or wet sponges and using red rubber endotracheal tubes, which have a much lower ignition potential, may offer the greatest protection (see Chapter 20).[68-72] Electrocautery can ignite standard endotracheal tubes, esophageal stethoscopes, oral airways, and feeding tubes, if the correct circumstances combine.[73, 74]

The endotracheal tube itself creates significant resistance to airflow; this resistance is inversely proportional to the radius to the fourth power and directly proportional to the length. Therefore, the longer and narrower the endotracheal tube, the greater the resistance to gas flow; anything that increases turbulence may proportionally increase the resistance to gas flow. In practical terms, this means that when the respiratory rate is increased, turbulent flow results, de-

creasing the size of the delivered tidal volume.[75] Studies in our laboratory with in vivo models have shown that this effect is less pronounced with progressively larger endotracheal tubes but may result in reductions in delivered tidal volume when the respiratory rate is increased in patients who require a smaller than normal endotracheal tube (i.e., an increase in respiratory rate from 10 to 20 per minute does not double the delivered minute ventilation).[75, 76] The data from these studies suggest that in patients with poorly compliant lungs, lung compliance seems to be the most important factor even with very small endotracheal tubes (Fig. 31–3).[75] The implications of these observations are that accurate measurement of end-expired CO_2 or arterial blood gases is the only way to be certain of the effectiveness of ventilation. In patients with severe pulmonary disease with ventilation/perfusion mismatch, only arterial blood gases or transcutaneous carbon dioxide monitoring will provide the needed information.

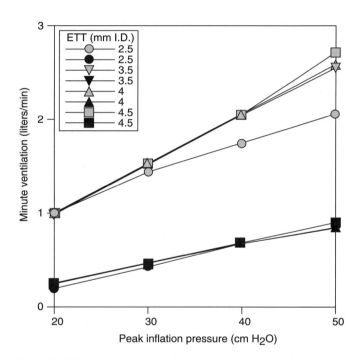

Figure 31–3. Delivered minute ventilation at various peak inflation pressures and with various endotracheal tube (ETT) sizes using an adult circle circuit and an in vitro lung model. Open symbols represent delivered minute ventilation obtained with normal lung compliance settings. Closed symbols represent delivered ventilation obtained at low lung compliance settings. Note that the delivered ventilation with all four endotracheal tubes in the *low lung compliance* model is nearly superimposed. The 2.5 mm ID endotracheal tube (but not the 3.5, 4.0, or 4.5 mm ID endotracheal tubes) decreased delivered ventilation in the *normal lung compliance* model when peak inflation pressure exceeded 20 cm H_2O and on the low compliance lung model at 50 cm H_2O. The clinical point is that with low lung compliance it would appear that the lungs are the main determinate of delivered ventilation whereas with normal compliance lungs, the endotracheal tube size does affect delivered ventilation. (From Stevenson GW, Tobin MJ, Horn BJ, et al: The effect of circuit compliance on delivered ventilation with use of an adult circle system for time cycled volume controlled ventilation using an infant lung model. Paediatr Anaesth 1998;8:139–144.)

Intubation Equipment

Routine Equipment

Intubation equipment must suit pediatric patients of all sizes. Magill forceps are available in two pediatric sizes. Laryngoscopes are available with lightweight small handles and a full range of blades. Generally, a straight blade design is better in smaller children, infants, and neonates because of the higher position of the larynx within the neck (see Chapter 7). A straight blade may be used in children as one would use a curved blade in an adult, that is, displacing the epiglottis by lifting the base of the tongue at the vallecula rather than by directly picking up the epiglottis with the tip of the blade. A special laryngoscope (Oxyscope, Forreger, Inc., Langhorne, PA), which incorporates a small-bore oxygen delivery tube, reduces the incidence of cyanosis and bradycardia in spontaneously breathing neonates should laryngoscopy be prolonged (see Fig. 7–26).[77]

Special Equipment

Occasionally, difficult airways may require special intubation equipment. Flexible and rigid fiberoptic laryngoscopes and bronchoscopes are available for the pediatric population. The flexible laryngoscope is used as an "optical stylet" over which an endotracheal tube may be passed under direct vision. Flexible fiberoptic laryngoscopes are available down to 1.8 mm external diameter; these are suitable for passage of a 2.5 mm ID diameter endotracheal tube.[78] The small scope is limited because there are no suction capabilities. Fiberoptic endoscopic skills should be developed during routine elective surgical cases so that the operator is sufficiently experienced to use these skills in emergency cases or for children with abnormal airway anatomy (see Chapter 7).[78]

The Bullard laryngoscope, which uses a combination of mirrors and fiberoptics, appears to provide a unique approach to anatomic airway problems. It is reported that proficiency with this instrument is rapidly acquired.[79] Lighted stylets also provide an alternate technique for management of a difficult airway (see Chapter 7).[80–83]

Anesthesia Machine and Appendages

Anesthesia Machine

All pediatric patients can be anesthetized with standard adult machinery as long as one is aware of the pitfalls and limitations. Anesthesia machines customized for pediatric use are of great value but not necessary. If one wishes to use special circuits, a Mapleson D system may be permanently mounted, allowing the choice of either a circle or open system. In addition, a cylinder yoke and a flow meter for air may offer particular advantages in circumstances in which nitrous oxide or a high inspired oxygen concentration is contraindicated (avoiding hyperoxia in a premature infant or nitrous oxide in a patient with bowel distension).[84, 85] An in-line oxygen analyzer and pulse oximetry are indicated to use an air-oxygen blend safely. The anesthesia machine should also be equipped with an alternate means of providing oxygen and positive pressure ventilation. An oxygen flow meter with anesthesia bag and pop-off valve always at the ready is helpful should an equipment failure with the machine occur.

Scavenger

The waste anesthetic gas scavenging system must be designed to eliminate applying either negative or positive pressure to a patient. Unless the system is able to open to the atmosphere by either a "tube within a tube" or a negative-pressure relief valve design, the wall suction may remove vital oxygen and anesthetic gases from the circuit and patient.[86, 87]

Circuits

A full spectrum of anesthetic circuits has been used in pediatric patients.[88] Adolescents and older children may be anesthetized with a standard adult semiclosed circle absorber system, perhaps with the substitution of a smaller rebreathing bag. Younger children may be anesthetized with the circuit modified by replacing the hoses with small-diameter "pediatric" tubing and by substituting a smaller rebreathing bag. In the past, most infants and neonates (10 kg or less) were anesthetized with nonrebreathing systems, such as the Mapleson D variety.

Mapleson D systems do not have directional valves or a CO_2 absorber, thus eliminating the resistance intrinsic to the opening pressure of circuit valves and to turbulent flow through soda lime.[89] This may be an advantage in spontaneously breathing neonates during induction before intubation. The main disadvantage of open systems is the need for relatively high fresh gas flows and waste of expensive anesthetic agents as well as unnecessary pollution of the environment. The work of breathing may be important for spontaneously breathing infants, so most pediatric circuits and masks are designed to eliminate both dead space and resistance. The classic example of this type of system is the Ayre T-piece; this circuit includes no valves or reservoir bags (Fig. 31–4).[90] Later modifications included changes of the T-piece and expiratory limb.[91] The Jackson-Rees modification involves the addition of a respiratory reservoir (bag) to the expiratory limb.[92] The most popular system is the Magill and its various modifications, Mapleson A–E (Fig. 31–5).[93]

These systems each consist of a source of fresh gas flow into the circuit, a reservoir bag, a pressure-relief (pop-off) valve, tubing of various lengths connecting all of these parts, and an adapter for the mask or endotracheal tube. Each of these has advantages and disadvantages, which are well reviewed elsewhere.[88, 94–96] The Mapleson D variety is the most commonly used because of its safety and versatility with both controlled and spontaneous ventilation.[96] The pop-off valve is at the end of the expiratory limb, just before the reservoir bag; thus, fresh gas washes alveolar gas out of the expiratory limb during expiration. The efficiency of this washout (to prevent rebreathing) is dependent on the volume of the expiratory limb, the fresh gas flow, and the size of the tidal volume.[94] Larger patients (heavier than 15 kg) require higher fresh gas flow rates to prevent rebreathing during spontaneous ventilation.[96, 97] Fresh gas flow rates as low as one times minute ventilation may be used with controlled ventilation without an increase in expired CO_2 values.[98]

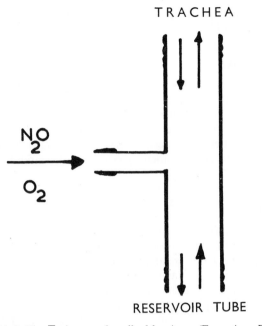

TRACHEA

N₂O

O₂

RESERVOIR TUBE

Figure 31–4. The T piece as described by Ayre. (From Ayre P: The T-piece technique. Br J Anaesth 1956;28:520–523.)

Rebreathing (an increase in inspired CO_2) can occur in patients with controlled ventilation when the respiratory rate increases above 20 breaths per minute. This apparent rebreathing can be diminished by using higher fresh gas flows and is markedly diminished when the respiratory rate is reduced below 20 breaths per minute (Fig. 31–6). The reason for this phenomenon may relate to inadequate washout of expired alveolar gas before the onset of the next breath. These phenomena may also represent an artifact of the sampling device, which is unable to sample gases at a sufficiently fast rate so as to separate breaths.[99] The clinical relevance of this observation remains to be evaluated. The advantages of minimal dead space and low resistance to flow with nonrebreathing circuits are counterbalanced by the disadvantages of heat and humidity lost to the anesthetic gases and significant waste of anesthetic agents because of the high flows required.[88, 96] A clinically important factor is that whenever a change in anesthetic gas concentration is made at the vaporizer, this change is immediately reflected at the airway. This allows a more rapid induction of anesthesia, which may be an advantage but also means a greater risk of producing an anesthetic overdose when compared with a circle system. With the increasing pressure for cost containment and the expense of the newer anesthetic agents it would seem that these circuits will fall into less common use and be of historical interest only.

The circle system can be safely used even in small infants and neonates and offers the advantage of using lower fresh gas flows and therefore cost savings and less pollution of the atmosphere with waste anesthetic gases.[100, 101] The use of the circle system in neonates and small infants generally requires assisted or controlled ventilation. The practitioner must be aware of the different pressure and volume characteristics of circle systems compared with nonrebreathing systems (Fig. 31–7). Since most pediatric anesthesiologists recommend controlled ventilation in this age group, there no longer seems to be a great need for special circuits. The

most important pitfall is if a practitioner selects a tidal volume based on weight rather than examining chest wall excursion, listening to breath sounds, observing the peak inflation pressure, and measuring end-tidal carbon dioxide values. Our in vitro studies have found that the main determinants of delivered tidal volume are peak inflation pressure and respiratory rate.[75, 76, 102] As long as attention is paid to this important observation, even tiny infants can be successfully ventilated with adult circuits and adult bellows with pressure limited ventilation (see further discussion). There is no difference between adult circle systems and a Bain (Mapleson D) type system if pressure-limited ventilation is used and the same peak inflation pressure is generated.[102] The most important factor is that tidal volume per kilogram will be very large with an adult circle system when compared with nonrebreathing systems, especially in infants. In my institution, we have eliminated all circuits except circle systems. This has simplified teaching and markedly reduced costs.

Humidifiers

A heated humidifier helps maintain body temperature and prevent drying of secretions whenever a nonrebreathing circuit is used.[103, 104] This effect may in turn lead to other problems, such as additional connections that may leak or become disconnected, "rain out" from humidified gas (re-

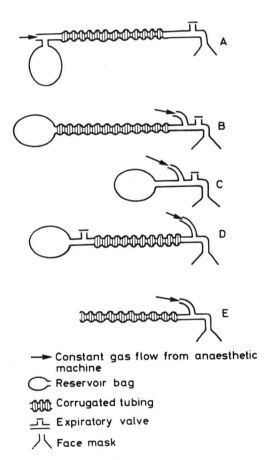

→ Constant gas flow from anaesthetic machine
⊂ Reservoir bag
▯▯▯ Corrugated tubing
⊥ Expiratory valve
∧ Face mask

Figure 31–5. The Mapleson categories of breathing circuits. The most commonly used circuit for infants is the Mapleson D configuration. (From Mapleson WW: The elimination of rebreathing in various semi-closed anaesthetic systems. Br J Anaesth 1954; 25:323–332.)

7 Kg infant

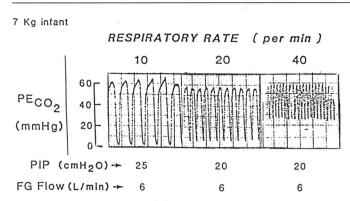

Figure 31–6. Note the marked increase in inspired carbon dioxide values during anesthesia in a 7-kg infant using a Mapleson D circuit with 3 L/min fresh gas flow when the respiratory rate is increased from 10 to 20 and 20 to 40 breaths per minute. This may result from inadequate washout of alveolar gases between breaths. Increasing fresh gas flow or decreasing respiratory rate improves washout of alveolar gases. FG, freshgas, PIP, peak inflation pressure. (Rolf N, Coté CJ: Previously unpublished data.)

sulting in water collection within the circuit or the endotracheal tube), added resistance to gas flow, and bubbling noises that distract from the ability to auscultate heart tones and breath sounds. Inhalation of excessively heated inspiratory gases may result in "hot pot tracheitis"; this can be avoided by monitoring inspired gas temperature proximal to the mask or endotracheal tube.[105] A heated humidifier also helps maintain body temperature with adult and pediatric circle systems.[23–25] Whenever a heated humidifier is added, the extra gas-containing volume of the tubing and humidifier increases the total volume of the anesthetic circuit,[106] in turn increasing both the volume of gas that can be compressed and the length of compliant tubing that can stretch during controlled positive-pressure ventilation. The result may be clinically important reductions in delivered minute ventilation, particularly if the humidifier is added after the anesthesia ventilator has been adjusted and no further compensation has been made for the increased compression volume and compliance losses (Fig. 31–8). The degree to which anesthetic circuit efficiency is affected depends on the gas-containing volume of the humidifier and the distensibility of the tubing used; highly compliant adult rubber tubing has greater adverse effects than wire-reinforced, small-diameter tubing (see Fig. 31–7).[106] These devices are now primarily limited to use with nonrebreathing systems.

Anesthesia Ventilators

Nearly any adult-volume ventilator may be used in pediatric patients by making appropriate adjustments in the respiratory rate, fresh gas flow, tidal volume, and inspiratory-to-expiratory time ratio. The use of adult ventilators in children, particularly neonates, requires meticulous attention to the settings prior to initiation of controlled respiration so as to avoid barotrauma. In old anesthesia machines, most volume ventilators could be converted to pressure ventilators by adjusting the pop-off valve to the desired peak inflation pressure. When this modification is made, one must pay special attention to the peak inflation pressure because a small turn of the pop-off valve in either direction could

result in excessively high or inadequate peak inflation pressure. New anesthesia machines, which have a switch at the CO_2 canister to change from manual to mechanical ventilation, do not allow adjustment of peak inflation pressure at the pop-off valve because in the mechanical ventilation mode the pop-off valve is out of the circuit. When such a configuration is used, the pop-off of the ventilator must be used to limit the peak inflation pressure. The excursion of the ventilator bellows may also be adjusted to limit the size of each tidal volume. Additionally, limiting the inflow of gas to the bellows will also in turn limit the bellows inflation. Studies in our laboratory have shown that any of three techniques for adjusting the excursion of adult bellows provides equal tidal volume as long as the anesthesiologist pays careful attention to peak inflation pressure.[75, 76, 102] Using the adult ventilator in pressure pop-off mode allows safe use even in neonates with a very small tidal volume. The following is a suggested means for setting up an adult ventilator for pediatric use in the pressure-controlled mode:

1. Set pop-off limit on ventilator to 20 cm H_2O.
2. Set rate to age appropriate.
3. Set inspiratory to expiratory ratio to 1:2.
4. Set gas flow to the middle range.
5. Set tidal volume to a minimum of 200 mL/kg/min.
6. Turn lever to ventilator mode (new systems) or attach ventilator hose to replace bag (old system).

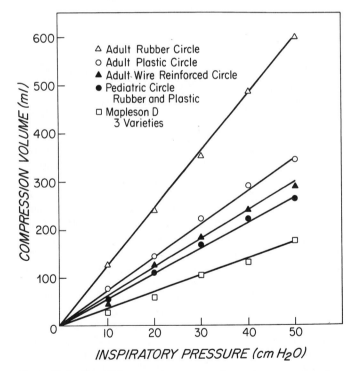

Figure 31–7. The differences in compression volumes among five anesthetic circuits. The Mapleson D systems are the most efficient with the lowest compression volume, whereas the adult rubber circle system has the highest compression volume and is the least efficient circuit. (From Coté CJ, Petkau AJ, Ryan JF, Welch JP: Wasted ventilation measured in vitro with eight anesthetic circuits with and without in-line humidification. Anesthesiology 1983; 59:442–446.)

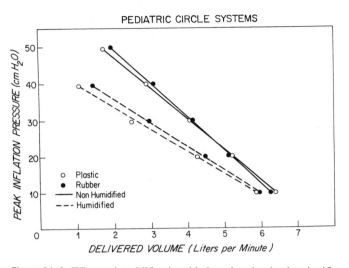

Figure 31–8. When a humidifier is added to the circuit, the significant reduction in delivered minute ventilation secondary to increased compression volume must be compensated with increased minute ventilation. (From Coté CJ, Petkau AJ, Ryan JF, Welch JP: Wasted ventilation measured in vitro with eight anesthetic circuits with and without in-line humidification. Anesthesiology 1983; 59:443–446.)

7. Observe peak inflation pressure to be certain that it is 20 cm H₂O or less. If the peak inflation pressure is less than 20 cm H₂O, then recheck pressure pop-off limit to make sure it is set at 20 cm H₂O and if correctly set slowly increase the size of the tidal volume until 20 cm H₂O is achieved.
8. Auscultate both lungs; observe chest excursion and end-tidal CO_2.
9. Make certain that there is adequate fresh gas flow to maintain bellows at full capacity.
10. Reassess the entire process based on step 8.
11. For non-compliant lungs, a very high peak inflation pressure may be required.[75, 76, 102]

It is my personal bias that manual bag ventilation provides immediate feedback about a patient's lung compliance or problems with the circuit (e.g., kinked tube, disconnections, and bronchospasm). However, under specific circumstances, the use of a ventilator provides valuable assistance by freeing the anesthesiologist's hands for other tasks. Whenever the immediate hand-bag feedback is given up for the convenience of a mechanical ventilator, a disconnect/apnea/peak inflation pressure alarm system is helpful to aid vigilance. One must be aware that these alarms are not perfect, particularly if the low-pressure alarm is located upstream from the endotracheal tube; with the correct combination of fresh gas flows and circuit resistance, resistance may not diminish enough to trigger the alarm.[107] A CO_2 detector can also rapidly diagnose this problem.

The user must understand what effects alterations in fresh gas flow may have on delivered tidal volume during volume-controlled ventilation.[108] For most ventilators used in the operating room, fresh gas flow into the circuit is added to the ventilator output during the inspiratory time; this augmentation effect may result in potentially serious errors in calculating delivered minute ventilation (V̇E), during volume controlled ventilation. *This is not a factor with pressure-*

controlled ventilation, since any added tidal volume is released through the pop-off valve. The following examples illustrate this situation in volume controlled ventilation:

An adult patient has a V̇E of 7 L/min, I:E ratio of 1:2, and fresh gas flow of 6 L/min. If there were no compliance or compression volume losses, the patient would receive 7 L/min + (1/3 × 6 L/min) = 9 L/min. If the fresh gas flow were reduced to 3 L/min, the patient would receive 7 L/min + (1/3 × 3 L/min) = 8 L/min. This is a change of about 11%.

A pediatric patient has a V̇E of 2 L/min, I:E ratio of 1:2, and fresh gas flow of 6 L/min. Again, assuming no compression or compliance volume losses, the patient would receive 2 L/min + (1/3 × 6 L/min) = 4 L/min. If the fresh gas flow were now reduced to 3 L/min, the patient would receive 2 L/min + (1/3 × 3 L/min) = 3 L/min. This is a 25% change in delivered minute ventilation (Fig. 31–9).

This effect has been compared in a group of infants and older children; simple changes in fresh gas flow during volume-controlled ventilation result in changes in delivered V̇E for all patients. The potential for clinically important effects on ventilation is greater in smaller patients; for example, several of our study patients were found to have a 40% difference in V̇E when fresh gas flow was changed from 1.5 L/min to 6.0 L/min without any change in the ventilator settings.[109] *When using volume-controlled ventilation, if a change is made in fresh gas flow for any circuit used in children, the adequacy of chest expansion, breath sounds, and peak inspiratory pressure must be re-evaluated.* Studies in our laboratory have shown that the next generation of operating room ventilators, which have built in sensors, eliminate this phenomenon by compensating for changes made in fresh gas flow.[110] *This effect does not occur during pressure controlled ventilation since excess flow is simply diverted out through the pop-off valve; however, if fresh gas flows were reduced such that the tidal volume fell below the peak pressure setting, then a reduced tidal volume delivered to the patient could result.*

6 Kg infant

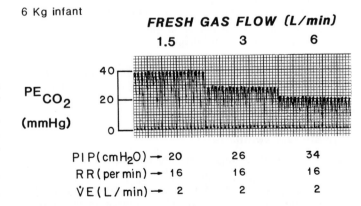

Figure 31–9. Changes in delivered minute ventilation using a pediatric circle system, as reflected by end-tidal carbon dioxide (CO_2) measurement, in a 6-kg child during volume controlled (not pressure controlled) ventilation. The only change made was in fresh gas flow. Note the near halving of end-expired CO_2 when fresh gas flow was increased from 1.5 L/min to 6 L/min. Whenever a change is made in fresh gas flow during volume controlled ventilation, new ventilatory settings must be determined. PIP, peak inflation pressure; RR, respiratory rate; VE, minute ventilation.

In some situations in children with very poor lung compliance, it has been suggested that ventilators used in the intensive care unit may be of greater value when compared with standard operating room ventilators.[100] Another study in our laboratory has shown that there is virtually no clinically important difference between several commonly used intensive care unit ventilators when compared with standard operating room ventilators when using pressure-controlled ventilation in infant lungs with low compliance[111] However, we have not yet examined other modes of ventilation such as volume-limited ventilation. It would appear that there is no advantage to using intensive care unit ventilators in pressure-limited ventilation and there may even be a disadvantage because the anesthesiologist may not be as familiar with these intensive care unit devices, thus leading to the potential for errors in ventilator adjustments.

Equipment Cart

It is advantageous to use mobile multi-drawer carts to stock the wide range and sizes of items necessary to care for the full spectrum of pediatric patients. The various drawers should be organized for ease of use: airway equipment, drugs, intravenous supplies, monitoring equipment, circuits, suction catheters, and so forth, may be separated into appropriately labeled drawers. Because pediatric anesthesia is often administered outside of the operating room suite (e.g., in radiology, radiation therapy, cardiac catheterization laboratory), these mobile carts simplify the safe practice of anesthesia for children and guarantee the availability of all necessary equipment even outside of the operating room (Table 31–1).

Defibrillator and External Pacemakers

Every operating room facility should be equipped with a direct-current defibrillator. It is not necessary to have a unit specifically for pediatrics, as long as the energy range may be adjusted to the appropriate levels (2 watt-sec/kg) and pediatric paddles are kept with the device. Ideally, the design should incorporate all controls in the paddles, facilitating use without leaving a patient. A desirable feature is a sensing circuit, providing the capacity for synchronous defibrillation should it be needed. External defibrillators with disposable pads applied to the front and back or right chest and left lateral chest of the patient have improved the rapidity of response in some circumstances. These can be placed on high-risk patients (those with cardiac surgery, cardiomyopathy, conduction defects) prior to anesthetic induction.[112–114] Similar devices that allow for external cardiac pacing are also a major new advance for high-risk patients.[115]

Monitoring Equipment

Anesthesia Record

In addition to its obvious role as a medical-legal document, the anesthetic record can be a very important monitor. Proper recording of a patient's status on arrival in the operating room encourages evaluation of the effects of any premedica-

Table 31–1. Suggested Pediatric Equipment Cart Inventory

Drawer 1
  Laryngoscope handles (functioning)
  Laryngoscope blades (functioning)

Miller	Macintosh	Wis-Hipple
0 (1)	1 (2)	1½ (2)
1 (2)	2 (2)	
2 (2)	3 (1)	
3 (1)		

  Magill forceps: 1 pediatric, 1 adult; 1″ tape (4); ½″ waterproof tape (4); 4 each ¾″ and ¼″ (tourniquets of non-latex material); scissors; flashlight.
Drawer 2
  Masks: neonate (3), infant (3), toddler (3), child (3), medium adult (3), large adult (3)
  Airways: 3.5 cm (5), 5.0 cm (5), 6.0 cm (5), 7.0 cm (5), 8.0 cm (5), 9.0 cm (5).
Drawer 3
  Gauze sponges (sterile and nonsterile), double-stick disks, rubber bands, adhesive bandages, alcohol swabs, antibiotic ointment, water-soluble surgical lubricant, lidocaine ointment 5%, bulldog clips, safety pins, corneal lubricant, pediatric blood tubes (blue, red, purple, and green), eye patches.
Drawer 4
  Adult sodium bicarbonate (2), pediatric sodium bicarbonate 8.4% (2), infant sodium bicarbonate 4.2% (2), cardiac lidocaine 100 mg (2), dextrose 50% (1), mannitol 25% (1), diphenhydramine 50 mg (2), potassium chloride 20 mEq (1), hydrocortisone 100 mg (2), calcium chloride 10% (4), sterile water, methohexital sodium 500 mg (8), lidocaine 1% (5), phenylephrine (5), prostigmine 1:2000 (10), ephedrine (5), atropine (10), isoproterenol (23), furosemide (3), epinephrine 1:1000 (10), succinylcholine (1), rocuronium (1), dexamethasone 4 mg/mL (2), dopamine (2).
Drawer 5
  Pediatric uncuffed endotracheal tubes: #2.5 (6), #3.0 (6), #3.5 (5), #4.0 (6), #4.5 (6), #5.0 (6), #6.0 (6). Pediatric cuffed endotracheal tubes #5.0 (3), #5.5 (3). Adult cuffed endotracheal tubes: 2 each of #6.0, #6.5, #7.0, stylets in various appropriate sizes.
Drawer 6
  Pediatric and adult esophageal stethoscopes (6), adult electrocardiography pads (10), pediatric electrocardiography pads (10), 6.5 F suction catheters (6), 10 of each size 8 F and 14 F.
Drawer 7
  Syringes: 12 mL (10) 6 mL (10), 3 mL 22 gauge (20), 3 mL 25 gauge (20), 1 mL 27 gauge (20).
  Needles: 15 gauge 1½″, 18 gauge 1½″, 20 gauge 1½″, 25 gauge ⅝″.
  Butterfly: 23 gauge, 25 gauge (10).
Drawer 8
  Intravenous catheters: 24 gauge, 22 gauge, 20 gauge, 18 gauge, 16 gauge, 14 gauge.
  Pediatric intravenous boards—2 sizes (4), T connector, 3-way stopcocks.
Drawer 9
  Pediatric intravenous sets (6); pediatric metriset (2); intravenous extension sets (2); 250 mL D$_5$L (10); lactated Ringer solution 250 mL (10); 250 mL 0.9 NS (5); air trap filters (6); head strap; blood pressure cuffs (2 each size), 1 adult size with stethoscope; oximeter sensors for infants and children.

tion, confirmation of NPO status, allergies, current medications, and assessment of weight and fluid balance. Careful logging of intraoperative fluid administration and losses allows assessment of a patient's replacement needs. Concurrent charting of a patient's vital signs and anesthetic drug administration allows correlations to be made and encourages trend analysis. Many changes that are too subtle to interpret on a moment-to-moment basis become obvious when plotted out over time. In addition, a numbering system correlating events with time on the anesthesia record documents the sequence of anesthetic management and may prove very useful should a medicolegal issue arise. Automated anesthesia records will eventually replace hand-recorded records and likely improve the accuracy of the data collection.[116, 117]

Precordial/Esophageal Stethoscope

In infants, neonates, and small children, an experienced ear can easily diagnose arrhythmias, assess cardiac output, and estimate the adequacy of blood pressure in the absence of interference from electrocautery or other electrical artifacts that can confound other electronic monitors. In addition, one can auscultate for pulmonary gas exchange. The precordial stethoscope may be stabilized with a double adhesive disk. For specialized needs, such as bronchography, angiography, or magnetic resonance imaging, a plastic stethoscope that is not radiopaque or ferromagnetic may be used. The optimal site where both heart tones and breath sounds can be heard is usually at the apex of the heart, but occasionally the suprasternal notch provides better listening conditions. The latter position may be more advantageous during induction and emergence, because airway information is more readily obtained. The stethoscope can provide early indications of developing airway obstruction and/or laryngospasm, allowing the practitioner to take corrective action (positive end-expiratory pressure) (see Fig. 15–1) before a full-blown episode of laryngospasm develops.

Whenever a patient has been intubated, the precordial stethoscope may be exchanged for an esophageal stethoscope. The pediatric size may be introduced atraumatically even in newborns. The less expensive adult variety is often usable in children age 6 years or older. Some disposable esophageal stethoscopes incorporate a thermistor, allowing the introduction of two monitors at once. One possible relative contraindication to esophageal stethoscopes is during performance of a pediatric tracheostomy. Misidentification of an esophageal stethoscope as an endotracheal tube has resulted in the surgeon opening the esophagus. During a pediatric tracheostomy, either the stethoscope should not be used or the surgeon should be informed that two stiff tubes pass through the neck structures, because this complication has occurred even in the hands of very experienced surgeons.[118]

The major drawback of a stethoscope as a monitor is that it provides information only when it is connected to the anesthesiologist. Custom-molded ear pieces, which better exclude room noises, are much more effective and more comfortable to wear than the conventional binaural stethoscope. These ear pieces have the added advantage of leaving the other ear open for communication with the surgeon and ancillary personnel. Even with pulse oximetry and capnography, the stethoscope can provide great reassurance that the patient has an adequate blood pressure and cardiac output. If the noninvasive blood pressure monitor fails and the oximeter fails but the patient has strong heart tones, then likely a technical problem exists. However, if the other monitors fail and the heart tones are very weak, then a serious problem with cardiac output has developed and one can immediately address that issue rather than wasting time trying to determine whether the problem is with the patient or the monitor.

Blood Pressure Devices

Blood pressure must be monitored in every patient. An appropriately sized blood pressure cuff, covering approximately two thirds of the length of the upper arm or thigh, must be applied.[119, 120] The cuff bladder should rest over the artery; in older children a stethoscope may be secured over the artery to listen for Korotkoff sounds. In smaller children, one may use the flicker of the needle in an aneroid sphygmomanometer dial as an indicator of systolic pressure.[121] When this flicker is not clearly readable, a distal pulse sensor is needed. This can be either a photoelectric plethysmograph over a digit, looking for return of the signal as the cuff is deflated, or a Doppler flow detector positioned over a distal artery.[122] Electronic oscillometer units (e.g., Dinamap) are capable of repeated, frequent, and accurate measurements.[123–126] If an automatic noninvasive blood pressure device is used, it is important that proper application, function, and adequate deflation time be assured; venous stasis, petechiae, and nerve compression damage are possible.[127] Most automated noninvasive blood pressure machines have specific cuff sizes for infants, neonates, and premature infants, and these must be matched with the appropriate tubing connecting the cuff with the monitor. If cuffs are improperly matched with the tubing, then the built-in algorithm will be "fooled," resulting in factitious data.[128] It appears that these devices offer reasonable accuracy for systolic blood pressure but may be less accurate for diastolic blood pressure.[129, 130] Noninvasive blood pressure monitors, when appropriately applied, provide very useful information during induction of anesthesia, particularly important during that period before establishing intravenous access. One study has demonstrated greater consistency and accuracy with these devices than with standard auscultatory methods.[126] One common practice is to place the cuff on the calf of infants as a substitute for upper extremity measurements. There is poor correlation between arm and calf blood pressures (systolic, diastolic, mean, r = 0.39–0.53); because of this variability, one should not simply substitute one measure for the other.[131] Another study has examined the use of loss of the pulse oximeter wave form with systolic arterial pressure and found a high correlation in children weighing less than 15 kg.[132]

Electrocardiograph

Although many arrhythmias may be diagnosed by careful attention to the heart sounds conducted through the precordial or esophageal stethoscope, the electrocardiogram (ECG) is still a mandatory monitor. In a healthy child, lead placement may differ from that selected for adults, because the principal need is for diagnosis and resolution of arrhythmias rather than detection of ischemia. One report has emphasized that pediatric patients undergoing cardiac surgery or patients with severe anemia may develop ST segment depression consistent with ischemia, although it occurs only rarely.[133] With the greater right heart predominance in the younger ages, a cross-chest lead generally provides the optimal combination of atrial and ventricular voltage signals. A QRS detector with a beeper is a useful accessory, particularly when vagal stresses are applied to a patient. The ECG heart rate is used for comparison with the pulse oximeter heart rate to confirm appropriate application and function of the pulse oximeter. A built-in lead fault detector is also useful to check the cables and a patient's leads when a poor signal is obtained. Cleaning, gently abrading, and defatting the skin with alcohol can improve the contact. Tincture of benzoin may also help to maintain secure adhesion in areas near surgical preparation solutions. Care must be taken not to allow the leads to become wet with preparation solutions and to isolate the leads from the electrocautery dispersive electrode to avoid electrical burns.[134]

Oxygen Monitor

Assessment of the inspired oxygen concentration is one aspect of the monitoring guidelines published by the American Society of Anesthesiologists (ASA) and the Harvard Medical School.[135, 136] In neonates, especially the premature, one must be alert to the possible ocular toxicity of high arterial oxygen tension (Pao_2) resulting from high inspired oxygen concentrations.[137] An oxygen monitor allows easy blending of air and oxygen to achieve the desired inspired oxygen concentration. In all patients, oxygen monitoring can help prevent hypoxemia. The standard, so-called fail-safe device built into most anesthesia machines is keyed only to pressure in the oxygen line; should the oxygen flow be turned off, a patient may receive a hypoxic mixture (air plus anesthetic agent, especially sevoflurane or desflurane) without warning from the fail-safe alarm. An oxygen monitor on the inspiratory limb would show the oxygen decline and provide an accurate alarm. With the more frequent use of closed-circuit anesthesia and air-oxygen blends, oxygen monitoring assumes even greater importance. Newer anesthesia machines provide an interlock system that always delivers minimal oxygen flows and prevents the delivery of hypoxic mixtures of nitrous oxide and oxygen; there is no interlock when air and oxygen are combined. A high alarm device is also desirable; this may detect when an air tank has run out. The oxygen analyzer should be calibrated and alarm limits set before anesthetic induction; a narrow band of alarm limits allows early detection of changes in gas flow ratio.

Temperature Monitors

Although there is medicolegal pressure to monitor temperature in every patient because of the potential danger of malignant hyperthermia, in reality temperature monitoring is mandated by other needs for patient care. Hypothermia is much more common in the operating room than hyperthermia and may be associated with acidosis, myocardial irritability, respiratory depression, prolonged neuromuscular

blockade, greater absorption of inhalation agents, and delayed emergence from anesthesia.[138–141]

The choice of monitoring site depends on the anesthetic and surgical procedure. Most mask anesthetics are monitored either with axillary or rectal probes; tympanic probes are rarely used. The axillary temperature monitor reflects core temperature measurement if the thermistor is carefully placed in proximity to the artery.[142] A well-placed axillary thermistor (positioned high in the axilla with the arm adducted, preferably an arm without an intravenous line) tracks the body temperature, except in severe shock states, when it trails by about 1°C to 1.5°C below true core temperature.[143] A rectal probe is subject to cooling during urologic or major peritoneal surgical procedures. A tympanic probe accurately reflects core temperature but if improperly inserted may injure the tympanic membrane.[144, 145]

When patients have been intubated, an esophageal or a nasopharyngeal probe is convenient and accurate. An esophageal probe may be influenced by the gas stream in the trachea; for greater accuracy, it must be placed near the great vessels of the heart (two-thirds the length of the esophagus).[142] A nasopharyngeal probe nearly reflects core temperature but may induce epistaxis when inserted. Skin surface thermocouples are only useful as a trend monitor and may be inadequate for intraoperative monitoring (see Chapter 27).[142]

Pulse Oximetry

Perhaps nothing has changed our anesthetic practice more than the introduction of routine pulse oximetry. This monitor determines the oxygen saturation of hemoglobin by spectrophotoelectric oximetric techniques. Measuring the amount of light transmitted through tissue between a two-wavelength light source (930 and 660 nm) and a detector allows continuous calculation of arterial oxygen saturation.[146] The use of two frequencies helps to eliminate interfering absorption by other molecules; however, intravenous dyes (indocyanine green, methylene blue) and colored nail polish may interfere with normal sensor function and fool the oximeter into reading a factitiously low oxygen saturation value.[147–149] Additionally, dyshemoglobinopathies such as carboxyhemoglobinemia and methemoglobinemia may result in significant artifact. Carboxyhemoglobinemia causes an overestimation of oxygen saturation because the photodetector is fooled into interpreting carboxyhemoglobin as oxyhemoglobin; this artifactual change is roughly proportional to the concentration of carboxyhemoglobin.[150] Methemoglobinemia results in desaturation, but the saturation recorded tends to read higher than the actual saturation; at high levels of methemoglobin, during episodes of desaturation, this disparity becomes greater.[151] Fetal hemoglobin, hyperbilirubinemia, and sickle cell disease have minimal effect on pulse oximetry.[152–156] This monitor is easy to use, noninvasive, and reasonably accurate although not perfect.[157, 158] There is some variability between manufacturers and accuracy declines with lower saturation values.[159]

The clinical efficacy of this monitor was demonstrated in a prospective single-blind study of pediatric patients; 50% of the cases were conducted with the saturation data and alarms made available to the anesthesia team, whereas in the remainder, the data were blinded and the alarms silenced. Several observations were made: (1) Twice as many "ma-

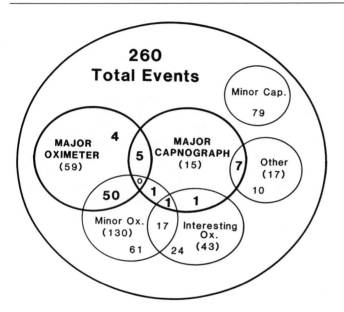

Figure 31–10. Two-hundred sixty problems were observed in 153 of 402 patients studied. Major desaturation events (SpO$_2$ $\leq$ 85 for $\geq$ 30 sec) and major capnograph events (esophageal intubation, kinked endotracheal tube, circuit disconnect, accidental extubation) are within the bold circles. Minor desaturation (SpO$_2$ $\leq$ 95% $\geq$ 60 sec) and interesting events (SpO$_2$ $\leq$ 85% $\geq$ 30 sec) are also presented. Minor capnographic problems were simple hypercarbia (PECO$_2$ $\geq$ 60 mm Hg $\geq$ 60 sec) or hypocarbia (PECO$_2$ $\leq$ 25 mm Hg $\geq$ 60 sec). The total number of events that fulfilled the criteria for each category is in parentheses. Note that some events fulfilled criteria in two or more categories. PECO$_2$, expired carbon dioxide; SpO$_2$, oxygen saturation. (From Coté CJ, Rolf N, Liu LM, et al: A single-blind study of combined pulse oximetry and capnography in children. Anesthesiology 1991;74:980–987.)

jor" desaturation events (defined as a saturation $\leq$ 85% for $\geq$ 30 sec) occurred in the blinded group. (2) The oximeter detected a greater number of desaturation events before clinical recognition by the anesthesiologist. (3) Major desaturation events were not accompanied by changes in vital signs in most cases (i.e., in only 4 of 19 such events was change in blood pressure, heart rate, or respiratory rate noted). (4) The incidence of these events in ASA physical status 3 and 4 patients was five times greater than in ASA 1 and 2

patients. (5) Desaturation events occurred with experienced as well as inexperienced anesthesia personnel. (6) Correlation between the observation of cyanosis and true desaturation was poor. (7) Desaturation events were as likely in brief as in prolonged procedures.[160]

In a subsequent study, the efficacy of combined pulse oximetry and capnography was examined to determine whether patient safety was improved with the addition of capnography.[161] Two hundred sixty problems were observed in 153 pediatric patients (Fig. 31–10). The study confirmed that pulse oximetry was superior to the human eye in diagnosing desaturation. Approximately a threefold greater incidence of major desaturation events occurred when oximeter data and alarms were blinded (Fig. 31–11). Capnography was not as helpful in diagnosing the majority of events leading to desaturation (Fig. 31–12). This is consistent with the Australia anesthesia incident study in which oximetry was felt to have helped in 85% of events.[162] Fifteen problems fulfilled the criteria of a major capnograph event—problems that posed a threat to life (kinked endotracheal tube, circuit disconnect, esophageal intubation, accidental extubation) and would be expected to be immediately detected by a capnograph. However, eight were diagnosed initially by the pulse oximeter (see Fig. 31–10). Capnography may have helped initially to diagnose the seven remaining events; however, pulse oximetry would have diagnosed these events as desaturation developed, though approximately 30 seconds later. This observation is also consistent with the Australia incident study.[163] We also examined the incidence of "minor" capnograph events, defined as an abnormality of ventilation that was not a threat to a patient's life (hypercarbia, hypocarbia). A significantly higher incidence of both hypercarbia and hypocarbia occurred in patients whose anesthesiologist was blinded from the capnographic data and alarms.

Infants 6 months of age or younger are at greatest risk for experiencing at least one major desaturation event (Fig. 31–13) or a major capnograph event. The number of patients with multiple problems was twice as great in the group in which neither pulse oximetry nor capnography data were available to the anesthesia team compared with those in which both were available. An interesting observation was the relatively high incidence of clinically unrecognized endobronchial intubation that manifested as a persistent though minor desaturation (93 to 95%).[164]

Figure 31–11. The number of patients with major desaturation events (black boxes) and the number of events (gray boxes) both were significantly higher when oximeter data were unavailable to the anesthesia team (P = 0.003). When capnography data were unavailable, there was no significant effect on the incidence of events leading to desaturation. (From Coté CJ, Rolf N, Liu LM, et al: A single-blind study of combined pulse oximetry and capnography in children. Anesthesiology 1991;74:980–987.)

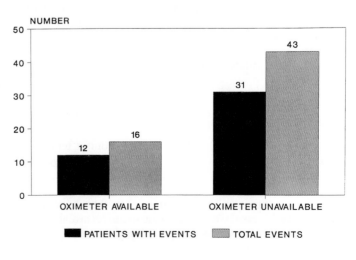

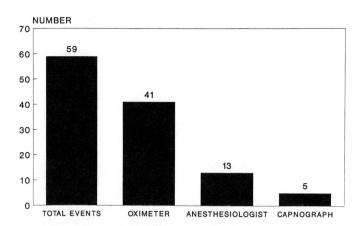

Figure 31–12. Fifty-nine major desaturation events were observed. Nearly 70% were first diagnosed by the oximeter, 22% by the anesthesiologist, and only 8% diagnosed by the capnograph. Pulse oximetry is by far the more sensitive monitor in providing an early warning of developing desaturation. (From Coté CJ, Rolf N, Liu LM, et al: A single-blind study of combined pulse oximetry and capnography in children. Anesthesiology 1991;74:980–987.)

These studies confirm that the pulse oximeter provides an early warning of developing desaturation well before a clinician is able to detect it clinically. This is easily explained by the fact that approximately 5 g of desaturated hemoglobin is required to detect cyanosis; if a patient has a hemoglobin level of 15 g, then saturation would have to decrease to 66% before cyanosis would be clearly evident. The pulse oximeter detects developing desaturation well before this value is achieved. The accuracy of oxygen saturation monitoring decreases with most oximeters with saturations below 70%; the degree of inaccuracy is a function of many variables.[152, 165, 166] Pulse oximeters are therefore reliable for the majority of patients free of cyanotic congenital heart disease.

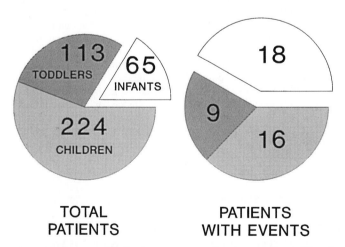

Figure 31–13. Age distribution versus major desaturations. The pie figure on the left presents the age distribution of the 402 patients studied, and the pie on the right presents the number of patients in each category with a major desaturation event. Note that infants had a significantly higher incidence than did toddlers or children ($P = 0.001$). (Data abstracted from Coté CJ, Rolf N, Liu LM, et al: A single-blind study of combined pulse oximetry and capnography in children. Anesthesiology 1991;74:980–987.)

Pulse oximetry provides additional information other than oxygen saturation values, including blood pressure.[132] Pulsus paradoxus may be observed in hypovolemic patients. Loss of the peripheral pulse by the oximeter probe sensor may accompany hypovolemia, vasoconstriction due to hypothermia, or inadequate cardiac output as a result of hypovolemia, allergic reaction, or anesthetic overdose.[167, 168]

The pulse oximeter is useful as a noninvasive trend monitor in individuals with anatomic or physiologic shunts, because the effects of anesthetic agents and positive-pressure ventilation are difficult to predict.[169–171] The pulse oximeter can be helpful to prevent hyperoxia in premature infants by maintaining the oxygen saturation between 93 and 95%.[172]

A number of common operating room events can affect oximeter sensor function: electrocautery, flickering operating room lights, movement, blood pressure cuff inflation, bright light, vasoconstriction, and injected dyes. Falsely high oxygen saturation measurements have been observed despite severe desaturation when there is interference with the oximeter sensor; therefore, this monitor is not foolproof.[173] A number of these problems in critically ill children and those with thermal injuries can be overcome by using a modified oximeter probe and applying it to the tongue.[174, 175] The tongue provides a rich blood supply unaffected by vasoconstriction, and electrocautery interference is less. If the tongue moves, the sensor may dislodge or record a false heart rate.

Thermal injury secondary to the interface of incompatible sensor probes and cables (equipment from more than one manufacturer) has been reported, as has pressure necrosis due to too tight application.[176, 177]

Movement artifact is the main cause of false alarms in sedated or awake patients requiring monitoring. This artifact may be eliminated with the next generation of pulse oximeters.[178, 179] This improvement hopefully will result in improved utilization in nonoperating room and noncritical care venues where patients are not under the effects of muscle relaxants, such as the emergency room, the recovery room, and the intensive care unit, and in patients receiving opioids on regular patient floors.

Carbon Dioxide Analyzers

The most commonly used gas analyzer is the expired CO_2 analyzer. It is particularly useful in teaching ventilation and airway management, provided the response time of the instrument is rapid enough to accurately reflect end-expired CO_2 tension.[180, 181] These monitors are made in two configurations: (1) with the expired gas suctioned from the anesthesia circuit (side-stream sampler) or (2) as a mainstream airway cuvette optical sensor. Both are infrared analyzers. Side-stream samplers, although less cumbersome, may become obstructed with water or secretions; the mainstream type is free of problems with obstruction but is heavy and leads to kinking of the endotracheal tube in smaller patients.[181] The latter type requires a large inventory of cuvettes, which must be sterilized between patients. Most operating room monitors now use side-stream sampling.

Measurement of expired CO_2 tension may be helpful in surgical patients in whom air embolism may occur. Clinically important air embolism causes a transient but marked reduction in CO_2 excretion because the lungs are ventilated but not perfused. Quantitative measurement may allow detection of change in circuit flows, disconnections, endotracheal tube kinking, or accidental extubations.[163, 182-184] This method also permits early diagnosis of malignant hyperpyrexia and evaluation of the adequacy of its therapy.[185] In critically ill neonates or hypermetabolic children with thermal injuries, ventilatory requirements may be as high as four times normal; therefore, a simple means of assessing adequacy of ventilation is extremely helpful.[186]

A capnograph with recorder or a display is most valuable because the CO_2 waveform may help in diagnosing other types of respiratory events (Fig. 31–14). The diagnosis of bronchospasm and its response to treatment is readily made by changes in the CO_2 waveform (see Fig. 15–6). There are some data to suggest that the shape of the CO_2 waveform changes with growth and achieves the normal adult configuration in the teenage years.[187] A slow-speed recorder also allows trending, which we have found particularly useful in diagnosing small circuit leaks, partially kinked endotracheal tubes, and rebreathing. It is important to have the proper sampling rate; sampling flows of 150 mL/min are required with many capnographs to produce CO_2 waveforms that reflect true events.[188] These sampling rates do not have clinically important effects on delivered minute ventilation. The next generation of capnographs will use technology that allows lower sampling rates and quantitates the expired CO_2 values with greater accuracy.

In children free from pulmonary shunts, the arterial and alveolar CO_2 values ($Paco_2$ and $Paco_2$ [as reflected by a true end-expired sample]) should be within 2 to 3 mm Hg. The severity of a shunt or the diagnosis of a shunt may be made if this difference is greater than 5 mm Hg and if the CO_2 sensor is properly calibrated. Patients with a variety of pulmonary problems may have significant differences between arterial and expired CO_2 values. In such patients, expired CO_2 monitoring may only be used for trending and as a disconnect alarm.[189, 190] Special endotracheal tubes that have a built-in sampling port at the distal end can provide a true end-expired sample even in infants ventilated with a nonrebreathing system; unfortunately, as currently designed, these sample ports readily obstruct with secretions and water.[191] Accurate CO_2 determinations may also be obtained by a needle inserted through the side of the endotracheal tube several centimeters below the 15 mm connector; this alternative may be used when a more distal port becomes obstructed or when using nonrebreathing circuits.[192] The accuracy of measurement of expired CO_2 is very important because samples obtained at the elbow with nonrebreathing circuits may result in false information so that the capnograph becomes a CO_2 sensor only (i.e., CO_2 is produced with each breath, but because the sample is diluted with inspiratory fresh gas flow, a valid interpretation cannot be made).[191]

This monitor is of great value in assessing the adequacy of ventilation in intubated patients but of less value in children managed by mask, when it is difficult to obtain an accurate end-expired sample.[161, 182] The accuracy of end tidal CO_2 monitoring is slightly more accurate with an LMA than with a face mask.[193]

No monitoring device is perfect, and it is possible to develop a false sense of security when monitoring the ECG, oxygen saturation, and expired CO_2 values. Anesthesiologists must not abandon stethoscopes and the powers of observation, because the practitioner is the ultimate monitor.

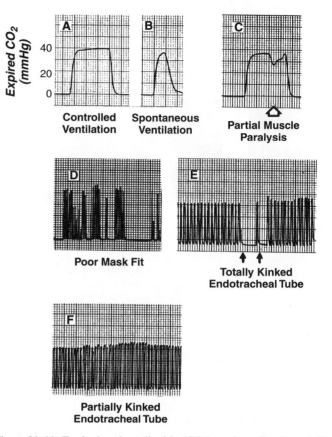

Figure 31–14. Expired carbon dioxide (CO_2) tracings (A, B, and C are rapid recording; D, E, and F are trend recording). (A) Normal waveform with a long alveolar plateau indicating good alveolar gas sampling during controlled ventilation. (B) Spontaneous ventilation with rapid respiratory rate; minimal alveolar plateau. (C) Patient with partial muscle paralysis: note change in carbon dioxide (CO_2) waveform (open arrow) during inspiration, which took place during the ventilator expiration. (D) Poor mask fit with many periods when no CO_2 was detected; this also results in many false alarms. (E) A totally kinked endotracheal tube was detected by the absence of a CO_2 waveform (between arrows); a similar trace could result with a circuit disconnect, esophageal intubation, or a simple pause in respiration. (F) A partially kinked endotracheal tube may result in a slow change in peak expired CO_2; a similar change could be noted with an unrecognized endobronchial intubation, change in pulmonary compliance, circuit leak, or increase in metabolic rate. The reverse would occur with air embolism, hypothermia (decreased metabolic rate), improved compliance, or increased fresh gas flow without compensatory change in ventilator settings. (From Coté CJ, Liu LM, Szyfelbein SK, et al: Intraoperative events diagnosed by expired carbon dioxide monitoring in children. Can Anaesth Soc J 1986;33:315–320.)

It is our powers of observation and clinical judgment, our ability to synthesize the data provided by the monitoring devices, and our clinical observations that determine the appropriate course of action. The following case is an example: An 8 kg infant with a 45% scald burn was anesthetized, her trachea was intubated, and she was placed in the prone position. The child was monitored with an ECG, a temperature probe, an esophageal stethoscope, an expired CO_2 mainstream sampler, a pulse oximeter, and an arterial line. The arterial line malfunctioned, and it took approximately 45 minutes to replace it. An arterial blood gas sample was obtained, and at that time, the oxygen saturation was 100% and the expired CO_2 was 43 mm Hg (mainstream device, no wave form, and circle system); there had been no noticeable changes in vital signs. The blood gas results were pH, 6.96; PaO_2, 214 mm Hg; and $PaCO_2$, 103 mm Hg. This child had a partially kinked endotracheal tube and a large shunt, both of which contributed to the false data from the capnograph. Although this is an extreme example, it emphasizes that even with highly sophisticated equipment, things can still go awry.

Anesthetic Agent Analyzers

Most anesthetic agent analyzers are based on ultraviolet or infrared monochromatic (only one agent detected) or polychromatic (more than one agent detected) absorption or on mass spectroscopy and provide a rapid time response.[194, 195] Polychromatic infrared analyzers are most useful because they can detect erroneously selected anesthetic agents.[196] Careful assessment of the end-expired vapor tensions may provide some indication of a patient's anesthetic depth, but each patient must be assessed on an individual basis. Vaporizer malfunctions and miss-fills may also be diagnosed. Mass spectroscopy may be particularly valuable in providing an early warning of air embolism (after a patient has been denitrogenated), because the sudden appearance of expired nitrogen would not be normal (entrainment of room air into the circuit and release of nitrogen from extremities with a tourniquet may also provide a source of nitrogen).[197] The purported advantages of less waste of anesthetic gases and a more rapid awakening are effects that have not been proven; however, the ability to use low flows offers the potential for significant cost savings in the form of less waste of anesthetic agent and less pollution of the atmosphere.[198] The report of accumulation of methane with closed circuit anesthesia and the inaccuracy of agent analysis (methane additive to the agent used) is worrisome but can be reversed with simple periodic flushing of the system.[199, 200]

Blood Loss Monitoring

Although close observation of the surgical field is the best single monitor, two ancillary devices may help. A small-volume trap on the suction line before the major evacuation trap is arranged so that the outlet leading to the large suction bottle is at the top, allowing emptying into the main container by inverting the mini-trap. This arrangement is particularly useful for small children and cases involving a fluid-filled organ, such as the bladder, because it can be "rezeroed" by dumping the mini-trap. Routinely weighing surgical sponges on a dietary scale, making the approximation that 1 g of weight is equivalent to 1 mL of blood, is also helpful. Greatest accuracy is obtained by immediate weighing as the sponges come off the surgical field, thus minimizing evaporative losses; the ultimate determinant of blood loss is a patient's physiologic status.

Neuromuscular Transmission Monitoring

Measuring the indirectly elicited twitch response is indicated when neuromuscular blocking agents are used. The most helpful clinical monitor during the use of nondepolarizing

competitive blockers is the train-of-four instrument. The train-of-four does not require recording capability or baseline measurement, because it works strictly by comparison with its own internal standard, the first twitch.[201, 202] The unit may also be used with depolarizing relaxants, monitoring only the first twitch amplitude. A significant decrement (greater than 50%) between the first and fourth twitch in this context suggests phase-two blockade (see Chapter 10).[203]

Needle electrodes are hazardous because they may cause bleeding, infection, burns, or nerve injury. Current density may be very high because of the limited contact surface and the resistance of surrounding skin. Self-adhesive electrodes designed specifically for twitch monitors are available, but they are unnecessary and expensive and tend to be too large for infants and small children. A reasonable alternative is a pair of infant-size ECG electrodes.

The choice of monitoring location depends on the nature of the surgery. One may choose any site where a motor nerve is close to the body surface and its associated muscle group is available for observation. The most common stimulation site is the ulnar nerve in the forearm, observing the thumb (adductor pollicis brevis); this is the standard site for most research reports. Using the facial nerve may result in false-positive responses, because the muscles may easily be stimulated directly. The power should be off between readings to avoid possible injury secondary to prolonged, repetitious exposure to electric current.

Bispectral Analysis

Bispectral analysis (BIS, Aspect Medical Systems, Inc., Natick, MA) is a value (0–100) derived from processed electroencephalographic data.[204–206] Because of the nature of the data collection in the awake patient, artifacts may occur due to eye movement, blinking, and so on, at baseline if the device is applied prior to induction. In a number of very well controlled studies in adults examining the effects of a broad spectrum of medications, this device was apparently able to monitor the effects of anesthetic drugs on awareness and patient responsiveness to painful and nonpainful stimuli.[207–213] However, BIS technology does not monitor the adequacy of anesthesia or analgesia. The effects on BIS appear to be more predictable with propofol or inhalation-based anesthesia than with opioid-based anesthesia.[207, 208, 214] There is little information currently available on the use of the BIS in pediatric patients. One issue unique to children is the threatening nature of applying any monitor. In some children, even the application of a pulse oximeter will frighten them. Thus the BIS monitor will in most cases be applied after anesthetic induction. Another disadvantage for children is that so many procedures involve the head (e.g., strabismus, tonsillectomy, dental), which may preclude the use of this monitor in nearly half the pediatric cases. It is hoped that well-controlled studies in children will better define the role of BIS monitoring in terms of rapidity of awakening or predicting movement in procedures in which muscle relaxants are not utilized.

Disconnect/Apnea Alarms

Whenever a ventilator is used, the tactile feedback from the breathing bag is lost. A disconnect alarm is especially useful in the absence of an in-line capnograph. Most anesthesia ventilators incorporate such a disconnect alarm, but it may be bought as a separate add-on for older designs. These alarms generally sense time cycling of pressure events. Most of these alarms can detect complete ventilator disconnects but may not be sensitive enough to detect extubations with small endotracheal tubes or partial circuit disconnects because of the continued presence of flow resistance. Other types of alarms, such as heat-sensing devices or capnographs, can provide more reliable means of detecting inadequate ventilation, accidental extubation, or disconnect.

Besides the sensing of pressure cycles, many newer monitors include high-pressure, continuous positive-pressure, and negative-pressure alarms. Some products include automatic switch-on when shifting from hand to machine ventilation, thereby avoiding failure to monitor.

Apnea Monitors

Apnea monitors, whether based on transthoracic impedance, motion, or other patient parameters, are helpful in the perioperative and recovery room phases for any prematurely born infant of less than 60 weeks of postconceptual age.[215] Infants with a history of apnea spells and any child with ongoing apnea spells are much more likely to develop apnea in the postoperative period. Even if a patient has had a period of some months with a normal respiratory pattern at home, the anesthetic state may bring about a temporary return of apnea spells (see Chapters 2, 4, and 14).

Volume Meter/Spirometer

In some instances, it may be desirable to monitor a patient's respiratory gas exchange. A Wright turbine respirometer, Drager positive displacement spirometer, and newer designs based on either the pneumotachograph operating principle, vortex detectors, or thermistor flow meters are available. Some devices allow measure of flow-volume loops, which can be very useful in both diagnosing and correcting ventilatory issues such as bronchospasm, airway compression, and one-lung ventilation.[216–221]

Inspiratory Pressure Gauge

In patients requiring ventilatory assistance, a pressure gauge applied at the airway allows delivery of precise pressures and thus helps to minimize barotrauma. When using the adult circle absorber system or a ventilator, the gauges built into these devices are remote from the airway and may be somewhat inaccurate. When infants are treated with positive end-expiratory pressure and continuous positive airway pressure, airway pressures are best measured as close to the airway as possible. Such a device is useful in accurately determining leaks around an endotracheal tube used to determine the size of the larynx.[222]

Urinary Catheter

Aseptically inserted, a catheter in the bladder connected to a closed drainage system is of little risk to a patient. Urine output is a very useful indicator of volume and perfusion status; the presence of hematuria or hemoglobinuria can aid in the diagnosis of surgical trauma to the urinary system, a bleeding dyscrasia, or a transfusion reaction. Indications for a urinary catheter include massive fluid shifts, prolonged radiologic procedures with large doses of contrast material, prolonged surgery, neurosurgery with osmotic diuretic therapy, and urinary reconstructive procedures. In infants, standard urinary catheters might be difficult to insert; a feeding tube provides an excellent substitute. Because the urine output in infants is scant, connecting a feeding tube to a syringe barrel provides an adequate system for measurement.

Invasive Blood Pressure Monitors

When clinically indicated, arterial, central venous, or pulmonary artery pressure monitoring cannulas should be inserted. Percutaneous arterial cannulation is performed with a 22- to 24-gauge catheter-over-needle device in infants and neonates, with a 20-gauge device in older children (see Chapter 32).[223, 224] Central venous and pulmonary artery cannulation are usually achieved using the Seldinger technique.[225, 226] The proper reference location for all pressure transducers is usually the level of the patient's right atrium. If intracranial pressure monitoring is also used, many practitioners prefer to use a reference zero position at some easily reproducible cranial site (e.g., the external ear canal) to facilitate the estimation of cerebral perfusion pressure. In cases with moderate blood loss or small circulatory alterations, an oscilloscopic display is adequate. In more difficult cases, the addition of a multichannel recording polygraph capable of slow paper speed assists in trend analysis.

Placement of any of these invasive monitors provides additional benefits other than direct hemodynamic monitoring. Serial pH and arterial blood gas tension measurements from an arterial line or determination of serial chemistries, ionized calcium, glucose levels, hematocrit, coagulation profiles, and osmolality through either an arterial, venous, or pulmonary artery line allows continual assessment of a complex case. Mixed venous sampling from the pulmonary arterial catheter yields a measure of oxygen extraction. Cardiac output may be determined by Fick, thermodilution, or dye dilution techniques with appropriate catheters. Furthermore, in operations performed in the sitting position, a right atrial catheter provides an approach to therapy for air embolism (see Chapter 22).

To withdraw a valid blood sample, an adequate volume of blood must be aspirated; two to three times the dead space (the point of aspiration to the tip of the catheter) usually accomplishes this.[227] In infants, these systems must be flushed with small volumes at slow rates. In infant arterial lines, this amount is 0.5 mL/5 sec, to avoid dangerous fluctuations in blood pressure and retrograde flow.[228]

Transcutaneous Oxygen/Carbon Dioxide Monitors

Serial sampling of arterial blood gases tensions through an indwelling cannula is unfortunately an episodic monitor. Continuous monitoring of oxygen and CO_2 tensions is possible by means of electrodes mounted on the skin. The area underlying the electrode is warmed, "arterializing" the region. Response time depends on the thickness of the skin and the temperature of the electrode and is faster in small infants and neonates.[229] Correlation with arterial levels in the clinical range is generally good, but variations in perfusion can alter the readings, particularly for oxygen.[229–231] Transcutaneous CO_2 monitoring may more closely approximate Pa_{CO_2} in patients who have large ventilation/perfusion mismatch.[232–234] Transcutaneous CO_2 monitoring may have a role in anesthetized patients with severe pulmonary disease or other pathology that prevents accurate end-tidal CO_2 measurement.

Intracranial Pressure Monitoring

In patients with increased intracranial pressure, direct monitoring of intracranial pressure may be helpful. Measurement may be accomplished by transduced pressures through either a ventricular cannula placed through a burr hole or by a subarachnoid bolt or equivalent. Measurement can also be performed noninvasively in infants with an open anterior fontanelle (see Chapter 22).

Echocardiography

A number of reports have examined the usefulness of transesophageal echocardiography as a means of continuously monitoring cardiac output and the cardiac response to surgery and anesthetic agents. This equipment is very expensive and requires a great deal of skill and experience to take full advantage of its capacity. The practicality of this device in pediatric patients appears to be primarily limited to those patients undergoing corrective cardiac surgery (see Chapters 17 and 18).[235–241]

Electrocautery

Although anesthesiologists are not directly responsible for electrocautery devices, they should have a basic knowledge of how they function and the necessary precautions to prevent burn injury. The most important means of preventing injury is to ensure that an appropriately sized grounding pad has been applied and that no blood, urine, or preparation solutions have been allowed to pool around or under the grounding pad. Additionally, the electrocautery can ignite any flammable implements, drapes, and an oxygen-rich environment. Severe injuries and deaths have occurred when high concentrations of oxygen have been allowed to build up beneath drapes (supplemental oxygen in awake or sedated patients) and have been ignited by the spark of the electrocautery on the other side of the surgical drape.[242]

Transport Apparatus

Because transport environments (particularly outside the hospital in ambulances, helicopters, and fixed-wing aircraft) are exceedingly noisy, we depend on electronic monitoring for the heart rate more than we would in an operating theater (where we could use a stethoscope). The monitor must have battery-mode capability and if possible aircraft and ambulance power (direct current), as well as routine hospital power (alternating current). If the monitor incorporates a QRS beeper, it should be capable of high volume to compete with the noisy transport environment. The oscilloscopic display must have bright phosphors to allow arterial and ECG waveforms to be observed. A pulse oximeter and a means of measuring expired carbon dioxide should also be incorporated into the transport unit.

Purchasing Anesthesia Equipment

With the increasing sophistication of monitoring and life support equipment, purchasing decisions can no longer be intuitive. A complete grounding in the underlying engineering concepts would probably require an advanced degree in engineering, but a good working knowledge of the operating principles, advantages, and special hazards of the various types of apparatus is relatively easy to obtain. Although vendors are pleased to promote a product, the manufacturer's information literature should be obtained from an unbiased source such as the equipment periodical *Health Devices*, published by ECRI (formerly Emergency Care Research Institute) of Plymouth Meeting, PA. The safety office of each hospital usually subscribes to this periodical.

Another useful source of information is the specialty pediatric hospital. Whether through inquiry at medical meetings or by direct solicitation, practitioners at these unique resource institutions are often willing to share their special expertise.

The following are useful principles for any equipment purchase:

1. New purchases should interface with equipment that is already present. Considerable cost savings can occur if the same equipment is used in the operating room and the intensive care unit.
2. Recognize that the sales person is inherently biased.
3. Always test proposed equipment in the environment in which it will be used, with the personnel who will be using it. What appears attractive in a display may not function well in practice.
4. Do not use equipment for any purpose other than that for which it has been designed.
5. Have your hospital safety office check for electrical leakage and take other safety measures.
6. Spend as much on maintenance as on the product. Consider a maintenance contract, if available. Ask that the company ensure the future availability of parts and the compatibility of subsequent modifications or design evolutions with your equipment.
7. If two products are comparable but one has local service facilities, that one may be the better choice.
8. If areas of special needs have been recognized, be as detailed with specifications as possible. For example, if a monitor is to be used strictly in the operating room, it may be reasonable to operate it from wall power. Conversely, if the monitor is to serve in the operating room and for transport between the operating theater and the recovery room or intensive care unit, it must have internal battery backup.

The more precisely one can define needs, the more accurate will be the comparisons between the bids of rival vendors. Note that any given piece of equipment will occasionally be out of service, whether for regular preventive maintenance or for some unanticipated repair; although it is difficult in this era of cost containment to convince the hospital administration, this fact dictates a need for additional spare units.

REFERENCES

1. Cook-Sather SD, Liacouras CA, Previte JP, et al: Gastric fluid measurement by blind aspiration in paediatric patients: A gastroscopic evaluation. Can J Anaesth 1997;44:168–172.
2. Patel KD, Henschel EO: Postoperative alopecia. Anesth Analg 1980;59:311–313.
3. Leslie K, Sessler DI, Bjorksten AR, et al: Mild hypothermia alters propofol pharmacokinetics and increases the duration of action of atracurium. Anesth Analg 1995;80:1007–1014.
4. Levison H, Linsao L, Swyer PR: A comparison of infra-red and convective heating for newborn infants. Lancet 1966;2:1346–1348.
5. Zukowski ML, Lord JL, Ash K: Precautions in warming light therapy as an adjuvant to postoperative flap care. Burns 1998;24:374–377.
6. Goudsouzian NG, Morris RH, Ryan JF: The effects of a warming blanket on the maintenance of body temperatures in anesthetized infants and children. Anesthesiology 1973;39:351–353.
7. Crino MH, Nagel EL: Thermal burns caused by warming blankets in the operating room. Anesthesiology 1968;29:149–150.
8. Kempen PM: Full body forced air warming: commercial blanket vs air delivery beneath bed sheets. Can J Anaesth 1996;43:1168–1174.
9. Russell SH, Freeman JW: Prevention of hypothermia during orthotopic liver transplantation: comparison of three different intraoperative warming methods. Br J Anaesth 1995;74:415–418.
10. Murat I, Berniere J, Constant I: Evaluation of the efficacy of a forced-air warmer (Bair Hugger) during spinal surgery in children. J Clin Anesth 1994;6:425–429.
11. Borms SF, Engelen SL, Himpe DG, et al: Bair hugger forced-air warming maintains normothermia more effectively than thermo-lite insulation. J Clin Anesth 1994;6:303–307.
12. Camus Y, Delva E, Just B, et al: Leg warming minimizes core hypothermia during abdominal surgery. Anesth Analg 1993;77:995–999.
13. Bissonnette B, Sessler DI: Passive or active inspired gas humidification increases thermal steady-state temperatures in anesthetized infants. Anesth Analg 1989;69:783–787.
14. Bissonnette B, Sessler DI, LaFlamme P: Passive and active inspired gas humidification in infants and children. Anesthesiology 1989;71:350–354.
15. Schiffmann H, Rathgeber J, Singer D, et al: Airway humidification in mechanically ventilated neonates and infants: A comparative study of a heat and moisture exchanger vs. a heated humidifier using a new fast-response capacitive humidity sensor. Crit Care Med 1997;25:1755–1760.
16. Barnes SD, Normoyle DA: Failure of ventilation in an infant due to increased resistance of a disposable heat and moisture exchanger. Anesth Analg 1996;83:193.
17. Jerwood DC, Jones SE: HME filter and Ayre's T piece. Anaesthesia 1995;50:915–916.
18. Warmington A, Peck D: HME plus heated humidifier danger. Anaesth Intensive Care 1995;23:125.
19. Russell WJ: A review of blood warmers for massive transfusion. Anaesth Intensive Care 1974;2:109–130.
20. Presson RG Jr, Haselby KA, Bezruczko AP, et al: Evaluation of a new high-efficiency blood warmer for children. Anesthesiology 1990;73:173–176.
21. Smallman JM, Morgan M: Evaluation of the Level 1 Hotline blood warmer. Anaesthesia 1992;47:869–871.
22. Arndt M, Hofmockel R, Benad G: LEVEL 1—a new blood warming device [in German]. Anaesthesiol Reanim 1994;19:78–79.
23. Chalon J, Patel C, Ramanathan S, et al: Humidification of the circle absorber system. Anesthesiology 1978;48:142–146.
24. Tausk HC, Miller R, Roberts RB: Maintenance of body temperature by heated humidification. Anesth Analg 1976;55:719–723.
25. Berry FA Jr, Hughes-Davies DI: Methods of increasing the humidity and temperature of the inspired gases in the infant circle system. Anesthesiology 1972;37:456–462.
26. Bacon C, Scott D, Jones P: Heatstroke in well-wrapped infants. Lancet 1979;1:422–425.
27. Baum JD, Scopes JW: The silver swaddler: Device for preventing hypothermia in the newborn. Lancet 1968;1:672–673.
28. Petty C: Needle venting of air from intravenous tubing. Anesth Analg 1974;53:1016–1017.
29. Gronert GA, Messick JM Jr, Cucchiara RF, et al: Paradoxical air embolism from a patent foramen ovale. Anesthesiology 1979;50:548–549.
30. Philip BK, Philip JH: Characterization of flow in intravenous infusion systems. IEEE Trans Biomed Eng 1983;30:702–707.
31. Philip BK, Philip JH: Characterization of flow in intravenous catheters. IEEE Trans Biomed Eng 1986;33:529–531.
32. Dula DJ, Muller HA, Donovan JW: Flow rate variance of commonly used IV infusion techniques. J Trauma 1981;21:480–482.
33. Dutky PA, Stevens SL, Maull KI: Factors affecting rapid fluid resuscitation with large-bore introducer catheters. J Trauma 1989;29:856–860.
34. Krivchenia A, Knauf MA, Iserson KV: Flow characteristics of admixed erythrocytes through medex tubing with a pall filter. J Emerg Med 1988;6:269–271.
35. Hodge D 3d, Fleisher G: Pediatric catheter flow rates. Am J Emerg Med 1985;3:403–407.
36. Ikeda S, Schweiss JF: Maximum infusion rates and CVP accuracy during high-flow delivery through multilumen catheters. Crit Care Med 1985;13:586–588.
37. Calkins JM, Vaughan RW, Cork RC, et al: Effects of dilution, pressure, and apparatus on hemolysis and flow rate in transfusion of packed erythrocytes. Anesth Analg 1982;61:776–780.
38. Eurenius S, Smith RM: Hemolysis in blood infused under pressure. Anesthesiology 1973;39:650–651.
39. Frei FJ, Ummenhofer W: A special mask for teaching fiber-optic intubation in pediatric patients. Anesth Analg 1993;76:458.
40. Haselby KA, McNiece WL: Respiratory obstruction from uvular edema in a pediatric patient. Anesth Analg 1983;62:1127–1128.
41. Bennett RL, Lee TS, Wright BD: Airway-obstructing supraglottic edema following anesthesia with the head positioned in forced flexion. Anesthesiology 1981;54:78–80.
42. Moore MW, Rauscher LA: A complication of oropharyngeal airway placement. Anesthesiology 1977;47:526.
43. Greenberg RS, Zahurak M, Belden C, et al: Assessment of oropharyngeal distance in children using magnetic resonance imaging. Anesth Analg 1998;87:1048–1051.
44. Brimacombe JR, Brimacombe JC, Berry AM, et al: A comparison of the laryngeal mask airway and cuffed oropharyngeal airway in anesthetized adult patients. Anesth Analg 1998;87:147–152.
45. Nakata Y, Goto T, Uezono S, et al: Relationship between end-tidal and arterial carbon dioxide partial pressure using a cuffed oropharyngeal airway and a tracheal tube. Br J Anaesth 1998;80:253–254.
46. Greenberg RS, Brimacombe J, Berry A, et al: A randomized controlled trial comparing the cuffed oropharyngeal airway and the laryngeal mask airway in spontaneously breathing anesthetized adults. Anesthesiology 1998;88:970–977.
47. Lopez-Gil M, Brimacombe J, Alvarez M: Safety and efficacy of the laryngeal mask airway: A prospective survey of 1400 children. Anaesthesia 1996;51:969–972.
48. O'Neil B, Templeton JJ, Caramico L, et al: The laryngeal mask airway in pediatric patients: Factors affecting ease of use during insertion and emergence. Anesth Analg 1994;78:659–662.
49. Brain AI: The laryngeal mask: A new concept in airway management. Br J Anaesth 1983;55:801–805.
50. Badr A, Tobias JD, Rasmussen GE, et al: Bronchoscopic airway evaluation facilitated by the laryngeal mask airway in pediatric patients. Pediatr Pulmonol 1996;21:57–61.
51. Bandla HP, Smith DE, Kiernan MP: Laryngeal mask airway facilitated fibreoptic bronchoscopy in infants. Can J Anaesth 1997;44:1242–1247.
52. Ferrari LR, Goudsouzian NG: The use of the laryngeal mask airway in children with bronchopulmonary dysplasia. Anesth Analg 1995;81:310–313.
53. King CJ, Davey AJ, Chandradeva K: Emergency use of the laryngeal mask airway in severe upper airway obstruction caused by supraglottic oedema. Br J Anaesth 1995;75:785–786.
54. Gursoy F, Algren JT, Skjonsby BS: Positive pressure ventilation with the laryngeal mask airway in children. Anesth Analg 1996;82:33–38.
55. Holmstrom A, Akeson J: Fibreoptic laryngotracheoscopy via the laryngeal mask airway in children. Acta Anaesthesiol Scand 1997;41:239–241.

56. The use of the laryngeal mask airway by nurses during cardiopulmonary resuscitation. Results of a multicentre trial. Anaesthesia 1994;49:3–7.

57. Bernhard WN, Yost L, Turndorf H, et al: Cuffed tracheal tubes: Physical and behavioral characteristics. Anesth Analg 1982;61:36–41.

58. Corfield HMC: Orotracheal tubes and the metric system. Br J Anaesth 1963;35:34.

59. Finholt DA, Audenaert SM, Stirt JA, et al: Endotracheal tube leak pressure and tracheal lumen size in swine. Anesth Analg 1986;65:667–671.

60. Munson ES, Stevens DS, Redfern RE: Endotracheal tube obstruction by nitrous oxide. Anesthesiology 1980;52:275–276.

61. Khine HH, Corddry DH, Kettrick RG, et al: Comparison of cuffed and uncuffed endotracheal tubes in young children during general anesthesia. Anesthesiology 1997;86:627–631.

62. Ring WH, Adair JC, Elwyn RA: A new pediatric endotracheal tube. Anesth Analg 1975;54:273–274.

63. Miller BR: Problems associated with endotracheal tubes with monitoring lumens in pediatric patients. Anesthesiology 1987;67:1018–1019.

64. Ohn KC, Wu W: Another complication of armored endotracheal tubes. Anesth Analg 1980;59:215–216.

65. Brandstater B: Dilatation of the larynx with cole tubes. Anesthesiology 1969;31:378–379.

66. Hatch DJ: Tracheal tubes and connectors used in neonates: Dimensions and resistance to breathing. Br J Anaesth 1978;50:959–964.

67. Glauser EM, Cook CD, Bougas TP: Pressure-flow characteristics and dead spaces of endotracheal tubes used in infants. Anesthesiology 1961;22:339–341.

68. Patel KF, Hicks JN: Prevention of fire hazards associated with use of carbon dioxide lasers. Anesth Analg 1981;60:885–888.

69. Paes ML: General anaesthesia for carbon dioxide laser surgery within the airway: A review. Br J Anaesth 1987;59:1610–1620.

70. Sosis MB: What is the safest endotracheal tube for Nd-YAG laser surgery? A comparative study. Anesth Analg 1989;69:802–804.

71. Sosis MB, Braverman B: Prevention of cautery-induced airway fires with special endotracheal tubes. Anesth Analg 1993;77:846–847.

72. van der Spek AF, Spargo PM, Norton ML: The physics of lasers and implications for their use during airway surgery. Br J Anaesth 1988;60:709–729.

73. Simpson JI, Wolf GL: Flammability of esophageal stethoscopes, nasogastric tubes, feeding tubes, and nasopharyngeal airways in oxygen- and nitrous oxide-enriched atmospheres. Anesth Analg 1988;67:1093–1095.

74. Wolf GL, Simpson JI: Flammability of endotracheal tubes in oxygen and nitrous oxide enriched atmosphere. Anesthesiology 1987;67:236–239.

75. Tobin MJ, Stevenson GW, Horn BJ, et al: A comparison of three modes of ventilation with the use of an adult circle system in an infant lung model. Anesth Analg 1998;87:766–771.

76. Stevenson GW, Tobin MJ, Horn BJ, et al: The effect of circuit compliance on delivered ventilation with use of an adult circle system for time cycled volume controlled ventilation using an infant lung model. Paediatr Anaesth 1998;8:139–144.

77. Todres ID, Crone RK: Experience with a modified laryngoscope in sick infants. Crit Care Med 1981;9:544–545.

78. Roth AG, Wheeler M, Stevenson GW, et al: Comparison of a rigid laryngoscope with the ultrathin fibreoptic laryngoscope for tracheal intubation in infants. Can J Anaesth 1994;41:1069–1073.

79. Borland LM, Casselbrant M: The Bullard laryngoscope: A new indirect oral laryngoscope (pediatric version). Anesth Analg 1990;70:105–108.

80. Holzman RS, Nargozian CD, Florence FB: Lightwand intubation in children with abnormal upper airways. Anesthesiology 1988;69:784–787.

81. Ellis DG, Jakymec A, Kaplan RM, et al: Guided orotracheal intubation in the operating room using a lighted stylet: A comparison with direct laryngoscopic technique. Anesthesiology 1986;64:823–826.

82. Ellis DG, Stewart RD, Kaplan RM, et al: Success rates of blind orotracheal intubation using a transillumination technique with a lighted stylet. Ann Emerg Med 1986;15:138–142.

83. Rehman MA, Schreiner MS: Oral and nasotracheal light wand guided intubation after failed fibreoptic bronchoscopy. Pediatr Anaesth 1997;7:349–351.

84. Eger EI II, Saidman LJ: Hazards of nitrous oxide anesthesia in bowel obstruction and pneumothorax. Anesthesiology 1965;26:61–66.

85. Lucey JF, Dangman B: A reexamination of the role of oxygen in retrolental fibroplasia. Pediatrics 1984;73:82–96.

86. Mazze RI: Waste anesthetic gases and the regulatory agencies. Anesthesiology 1980;52:248–256.

87. Patel KD, Dalal FY: A potential hazard of the Drager Scavenging Interface System for Wall Suction. Anesth Analg 1979;58:327–328.

88. Coté CJ: Pediatric breathing circuits and anesthesia machines. Int Anesthesiol Clin 1992;30:51–61.

89. Bain JA, Spoerel WE: A streamlined anaesthetic system. Can Anaesth Soc J 1972;19:426–435.

90. Ayre P: The T-piece technique. Br J Anaesth 1956;28:520–523.

91. Harrison GA: Ayer's T-piece: A review of its modifications. Br J Anaesth 1964;36:115–120.

92. Jackson-Rees GJ: Anaesthesia in the newborn. Br Med J 1950;2:1419–1422.

93. Mapleson WW: The elimination of rebreathing in various semi-closed anaesthetic systems. Br J Anaesth 1954;26:323–332.

94. Dorsch JA, Dorsch SE: Understanding Anesthesia Equipment: Construction, Care and Complications. Baltimore: Williams & Wilkins; 1994.

95. Lin YC, Brock-Utne JG: Paediatric anaesthetic breathing systems. Paediatr Anaesth 1996;6:1–5.

96. Miller DM: Breathing systems for use in anaesthesia: Evaluation using a physical lung model and classification. Br J Anaesth 1988;60:555–564.

97. Bain JA, Spoerel WE: Carbon dioxide output and elimination in children under anaesthesia. Can Anaesth Soc J 1977;24:533–539.

98. Badgwell JM, Wolf AR, McEvedy BA, et al: Fresh gas formulae do not accurately predict end-tidal P_{CO_2} in paediatric patients. Can J Anaesth 1988;35:581–586.

99. Badgwell JM, Kleinman SE, Heavner JE: Respiratory frequency and artifact affect the capnographic baseline in infants. Anesth Analg 1993;77:708–712.

100. Badgwell JM, Swan J, Foster AC: Volume-controlled ventilation is made possible in infants by using compliant breathing circuits with large compression volume. Anesth Analg 1996;82:719–723.

101. Peters JW, Bezstarosti-van EJ, Erdmann W, et al: Safety and efficacy of semi-closed circle ventilation in small infants. Pediatr Anaesth 1998;8:299–304.

102. Stevenson GW, Tobin M, Horn B, et al: An adult system vs. a Bain system: Comparative ability to deliver minute ventilation to an infant lung model with pressure limited ventilation. Anesth Analg 1999;88:527–530.

103. Chalon J, Loew DA, Malebranche J: Effects of dry anesthetic gases on tracheobronchial ciliated epithelium. Anesthesiology 1972;37:338–343.

104. Weeks DB: Provision of endogenous and exogenous humidity for the Bain breathing circuit. Can Anaesth Soc J 1976;23:185–190.

105. Klein EF Jr, Graves SA: "Hot pot" tracheitis. Chest 1974;65:225–226.

106. Coté CJ, Petkau AJ, Ryan JF, et al: Wasted ventilation measured in vitro with eight anesthetic circuits with and without inline humidification. Anesthesiology 1983;59:442–446.

107. Slee TA, Pavlin EG: Failure of low pressure alarm associated with the use of a humidifier. Anesthesiology 1988;69:791–793.

108. Ghani GA: Fresh gas flow affects minute volume during mechanical ventilation. Anesth Analg 1984;63:619.

109. Moynihan R, Coté CJ: Fresh gas flow changes during controlled mechanical ventilation with the circle system have significantly greater effects on the ventilatory parameters of toddlers compared with children. Paediatr Anaesth 1992;2:211–215.

110. Rothschiller JL, Uejima T, Dsida RM, et al: Evaluation of a new operating room ventilator with volume controlled ventilation: the Ohmeda 7900. Anesth Analg 1999;88:39–42.

111. Stevenson GW, Horn B, Tobin M, et al: Pressure limited ventilation of infants with low compliance lungs: Efficacy of an adult circle system vs. two freestanding ICU ventilators systems using an in vitro model. Anesth Analg 1999;89:638–641.

112. Thies WR, Breymann T, Kleikamp G, et al: Early rhythm disorders after arterial switch and intraatrial repair in infants with simple transposition of the great arteries. Thorac Cardiovasc Surg 1991;39(Suppl 2):190–193.

113. Stewart JT, McKenna WJ: Management of arrhythmias in hypertrophic cardiomyopathy. Cardiovasc Drugs Ther 1994;8:95–99.

114. Villain E: Pediatric arrhythmias. Curr Opin Cardiol 1994;9:114–120.

115. Grubb BP, Samoil D, Temesy-Armos P, et al: The use of external,

noninvasive pacing for the termination of supraventricular tachycardia in the emergency department setting. Ann Emerg Med 1993;22:714–717.

116. Bicker AA, Gage JS, Poppers PJ: An evolutionary solution to anesthesia automated record keeping. J Clin Monit Comput 1998;14:421–424.

117. Lubarsky DA, Sanderson IC, Gilbert WC, et al: Using an anesthesia information management system as a cost containment tool. Description and validation. Anesthesiology 1997;86:1161–1169.

118. Schwartz AJ, Downes JJ: Hazards of a simple monitoring device, the esophageal stethoscope. Anesthesiology 1977;47:64–65.

119. Gomez-Marin O, Prineas RJ, Rastam L: Cuff bladder width and blood pressure measurement in children and adolescents. J Hypertens 1992;10:1235–1241.

120. Jenner DA, Vandongen R, Beilin LJ: Blood pressure and body composition in children: Importance of allowing for cuff size. J Hum Hypertens 1994;5:367–374.

121. Van Bergen FH, Weatherhead DS, Treloar AE, et al: Circulation 1954;10:481–490.

122. Poppers PJ: Controlled evaluation of ultrasonic measurement of systolic and diastolic blood pressures in pediatric patients. Anesthesiology 1973;38:187–191.

123. Yelderman M, Ream AK: Indirect measurement of mean blood pressure in the anesthetized patient. Anesthesiology 1979;50:253–256.

124. Friesen RH, Lichtor JL: Indirect measurement of blood pressure in neonates and infants utilizing an automatic noninvasive oscillometric monitor. Anesth Analg 1981;60:742–745.

125. Kimble KJ, Darnall RA Jr, Yelderman M, et al: An automated oscillometric technique for estimating mean arterial pressure in critically ill newborns. Anesthesiology 1981;54:423–425.

126. Park MK, Menard SM: Accuracy of blood pressure measurement by the Dinamap monitor in infants and children. Pediatrics 1987;79:907–914.

127. Sy WP: Ulnar nerve palsy possibly related to use of automatically cycled blood pressure cuff. Anesth Analg 1981;60:687–688.

128. Peterson CA: A note of caution when using different cuffs with the DINAMAP. Anesthesiology 1987;67:607–608.

129. Wattigney WA, Webber LS, Lawrence MD, et al: Utility of an automatic instrument for blood pressure measurement in children. The Bogalusa Heart Study. Am J Hypertens 1996;9:256–262.

130. Triedman JK, Saul JP: Comparison of intraarterial with continuous noninvasive blood pressure measurement in postoperative pediatric patients. J Clin Monit 1994;10:11–20.

131. Crapanzano MS, Strong WB, Newman IR, et al: Calf blood pressure: Clinical implications and correlations with arm blood pressure in infants and young children. Pediatrics 1996;97:220–224.

132. Movius AJ, Bratton SL, Sorensen GK: Use of pulse oximetry for blood pressure measurement after cardiac surgery. Arch Dis Child 1998;78:457–460.

133. Bell C, Rimar S, Barash P: Intraoperative ST-segment changes consistent with myocardial ischemia in the neonate: A report of three cases. Anesthesiology 1989;71:601–604.

134. Chandra P: Severe skin damage from EKG electrodes. Anesthesiology 1982;56:157–158.

135. Eichhorn JH, Cooper JB, Cullen DJ, et al: Standards for patient monitoring during anesthesia at Harvard Medical School. JAMA 1986;256:1017–1020.

136. Standards for Basic Intra-operative Monitoring. Chicago, IL, American Society of Anesthesiologists, 1991.

137. Merritt JC, Sprague DH, Merritt WE, et al: Retrolental fibroplasia: a multifactorial disease. Anesth Analg 1981;60:109–111.

138. Bennett EJ, Patel KP, Grundy EM: Neonatal temperature and surgery. Anesthesiology 1977;46:303–304.

139. Farman JV: Heat losses in infants undergoing surgery in air-conditioned theatres. Br J Anaesth 1962;34:543–557.

140. Munson ES, Eger EI 2d: The effects of hyperthermia and hypothermia on the rate of induction of anesthesia: Calculations using a mathematical model. Anesthesiology 1970;33:515–519.

141. Dundee JW, Clark RS: Pharmacology of hypothermia. Int Anesthesiol Clin 1964;2:857–872.

142. Bissonnette B, Sessler DI, LaFlamme P: Intraoperative temperature monitoring sites in infants and children and the effect of inspired gas warming on esophageal temperature. Anesth Analg 1989;69:192–196.

143. Kuzucu EY: Measurement of temperature. Int Anesthesiol Clin 1965;3:435–449.

144. Wallace CT, Marks WE Jr, Adkins WY, et al: Perforation of the tympanic membrane, a complication of tympanic thermometry during anesthesia. Anesthesiology 1974;41:290–291.

145. Benzinger M: Tympanic thermometry in surgery and anesthesia. JAMA 1969;209:1207–1211.

146. Yelderman M, New W Jr: Evaluation of pulse oximetry. Anesthesiology 1983;59:349–352.

147. Kessler MR, Eide T, Humayun B, et al: Spurious pulse oximeter desaturation with methylene blue injection [published erratum appears in Anesthesiology 1987 May; 66(5):701]. Anesthesiology 1986;65:435–436.

148. Coté CJ, Goldstein EA, Fuchsman WH, et al: The effect of nail polish on pulse oximetry. Anesth Analg 1988;67:683–686.

149. Gorman ES, Shnider MR: Effect of methylene blue on the absorbance of solutions of haemoglobin. Br J Anaesth 1988;60:439–444.

150. Barker SJ, Tremper KK: The effect of carbon monoxide inhalation on pulse oximetry and transcutaneous P_{O_2}. Anesthesiology 1987;66:677–679.

151. Barker SJ, Tremper KK, Hyatt J: Effects of methemoglobinemia on pulse oximetry and mixed venous oximetry. Anesthesiology 1989;70:112–117.

152. Tremper KK, Barker SJ: Pulse oximetry. Anesthesiology 1989;70:98–108.

153. Veyckemans F, Baele P, Guillaume JE, et al: Hyperbilirubinemia does not interfere with hemoglobin saturation measured by pulse oximetry. Anesthesiology 1989;70:118–122.

154. Pianosi P, Charge TD, Esseltine DW, et al: Pulse oximetry in sickle cell disease. Arch Dis Child 1993;68:735–738.

155. Rackoff WR, Kunkel N, Silber JH, et al: Pulse oximetry and factors associated with hemoglobin oxygen desaturation in children with sickle cell disease. Blood 1993;81:3422–3427.

156. Weston Smith SG, Glass UH, Acharya J, et al: Pulse oximetry in sickle cell disease. Clin Lab Haemat 1989;11:185–188.

157. Severinghaus JW, Naifeh KH: Accuracy of response of six pulse oximeters to profound hypoxia. Anesthesiology 1987;67:551–558.

158. Taylor MB, Whitwam JG: The accuracy of pulse oximeters: A comparative clinical evaluation of five pulse oximeters. Anaesthesia 1988;43:229–232

159. Severinghaus JW, Naifeh KH, Koh SO: Errors in 14 pulse oximeters during profound hypoxia. J Clin Monit 1989;5:72–81.

160. Coté CJ, Goldstein EA, Coté MA, et al: A single-blind study of pulse oximetry in children. Anesthesiology 1988;68:184–188.

161. Coté CJ, Rolf N, Liu LM, et al: A single-blind study of combined pulse oximetry and capnography in children. Anesthesiology 1991;74:980–987.

162. Runciman WB, Webb RK, Barker L, et al: The Australian Incident Monitoring Study. The pulse oximeter: Applications and limitations—an analysis of 2000 incident reports. Anaesth Intensive Care 1993;21:543–550.

163. Williamson JA, Webb RK, Cockings J, et al: The Australian Incident Monitoring Study. The capnograph: Applications and limitations—an analysis of 2000 incident reports. Anaesth Intensive Care 1993;21:551–557.

164. Rolf N, Coté CJ: Diagnosis of clinically unrecognized endobronchial intubation in paediatric anaesthesia: Which is more sensitive, pulse oximetry or capnography? Paediatr Anaesth 1992;2:31–35.

165. Fanconi S: Pulse oximetry for hypoxemia: A warning to users and manufacturers. Intensive Care Med 1989;15:540–542.

166. Fanconi S: Reliability of pulse oximetry in hypoxic infants. J Pediatr 1988;112:424–427.

167. Partridge BL: Use of pulse oximetry as a noninvasive indicator of intravascular volume status. J Clin Monit 1987;3:263–268.

168. Wallace CT, Baker JD 3d, Alpert CC, et al: Comparison of blood pressure measurement by Doppler and by pulse oximetry techniques. Anesth Analg 1987;66:1018–1019.

169. Ramanathan R, Durand M, Larrazabal C: Pulse oximetry in very low birth weight infants with acute and chronic lung disease. Pediatrics 1987;79:612–617.

170. Jennis MS, Peabody JL: Pulse oximetry: an alternative method for the assessment of oxygenation in newborn infants. Pediatrics 1987;79:524–528.

171. Pearlman SA, Maisels MJ: Preductal and postductal transcutaneous oxygen tension measurements in premature newborns with hyaline membrane disease. Pediatrics 1989;83:98–100.

172. Bucher HU, Fanconi S, Baeckert P, et al: Hyperoxemia in newborn infants: Detection by pulse oximetry. Pediatrics 1989;84:226–230.

173. Costarino AT, Davis DA, Keon TP: Falsely normal saturation reading with the pulse oximeter. Anesthesiology 1987;67:830–831.

174. Jobes DR, Nicolson SC: Monitoring of arterial hemoglobin oxygen saturation using a tongue sensor. Anesth Analg 1988;67:186–188.

175. Coté CJ, Daniels AL, Connolly M, et al: Tongue oximetry in children with extensive thermal injury: Comparison with peripheral oximetry. Can J Anaesth 1992;39:454–457.

176. Miyasaka K, Ohata J: Burn, erosion, and "sun" tan with the use of pulse oximetry in infants. Anesthesiology 1987;67:1008–1009.

177. Murphy KG, Secunda JA, Rockoff MA: Severe burns from a pulse oximeter. Anesthesiology 1990;73:350–352.

178. Dumas C, Wahr JA, Tremper KK: Clinical evaluation of a prototype motion artifact resistant pulse oximeter in the recovery room. Anesth Analg 1996;83:269–272.

179. Barker SJ, Shah NK: The effects of motion on the performance of pulse oximeters in volunteers (revised publication). Anesthesiology 1997;86:101–108.

180. From RP, Scamman FL: Ventilatory frequency influences accuracy of end-tidal CO_2 measurements. Analysis of seven capnometers. Anesth Analg 1988;67:884–886.

181. Kinsella SM: Assessment of the Hewlett-Packard HP47210A capnometer. Br J Anaesth 1985;57:919–923.

182. Coté CJ, Liu LM, Szyfelbein SK, et al: Intraoperative events diagnosed by expired carbon dioxide monitoring in children. Can Anaesth Soc J 1986;33:315–320.

183. Morray JP, Geiduschek JM, Caplan RA, et al: A comparison of pediatric and adult anesthesia closed malpractice claims. Anesthesiology 1993;78:461–467.

184. Caplan RA, Vistica MF, Posner KL, et al: Adverse anesthetic outcomes arising from gas delivery equipment: A closed claims analysis. Anesthesiology 1997;87:741–748.

185. Baudendistel L, Goudsouzian N, Coté CJ, et al: End-tidal CO_2 monitoring: Its use in the diagnosis and management of malignant hyperthermia. Anaesthesia 1984;39:1000–1003.

186. Epstein RA, Hyman AI: Ventilatory requirements of critically ill neonates. Anesthesiology 1980;53:379–384.

187. Ream RS, Schreiner MS, Neff JD, et al: Volumetric capnography in children: Influence of growth on the alveolar plateau slope. Anesthesiology 1995;82:64–73.

188. Gravenstein N: Capnometry in infants should not be done at lower sampling flow rates. J Clin Monit 1989;5:63–64.

189. Lindahl SG, Yates AP, Hatch DJ: Relationship between invasive and noninvasive measurements of gas exchange in anesthetized infants and children. Anesthesiology 1987;66:168–175.

190. McEvedy BA, McLeod ME, Mulera M, et al: End-tidal, transcutaneous, and arterial pCO_2 measurements in critically ill neonates: A comparative study. Anesthesiology 1988;69:112–116.

191. Badgwell JM, McLeod ME, Lerman J, et al: End-tidal PCO_2 measurements sampled at the distal and proximal ends of the endotracheal tube in infants and children. Anesth Analg 1987;66:959–964.

192. Rich GF, Sullivan MP, Adams JM: Is distal sampling of end-tidal CO_2 necessary in small subjects? Anesthesiology 1990;73:265–268.

193. Chhibber AK, Fickling K, Kolano JW, et al: Comparison of end-tidal and arterial carbon dioxide in infants using laryngeal mask airway and endotracheal tube. Anesth Analg 1997;84:51–53.

194. Gillbe CE, Heneghan CP, Branthwaite MA: Respiratory mass spectrometry during general anaesthesia. Br J Anaesth 1981;53:103–109.

195. Whitcher C, Piziali R: Monitoring occupational exposure to inhalation anesthetics. Anesth Analg 1977;56:778–785.

196. Walder B, Lauber R, Zbinden AM: Accuracy and cross-sensitivity of 10 different anesthetic gas monitors. J Clin Monit 1993;9:364–373.

197. Lanier WL: Intraoperative air entrainment with Ohio Modulus anesthesia machine. Anesthesiology 1986;64:266–268.

198. Logan M, Farmer JG: Anaesthesia and the ozone layer. Br J Anaesth 1989;63:645–647.

199. Mortier E, Rolly G, Versichelen L: Methane influences infrared technique anesthetic agent monitors. J Clin Monit Comput 1998;14:85–88.

200. Rolly G, Versichelen LF, Mortier E: Methane accumulation during closed-circuit anesthesia. Anesth Analg 1994;79:545–547.

201. Ali HH, Savarese JJ: Monitoring of neuromuscular function. Anesthesiology 1976;45:216–249.

202. Goudsouzian NG, Liu LM, Coté CJ: Comparison of equipotent doses of non-depolarizing muscle relaxants in children. Anesth Analg 1981;60:862–866.

203. Churchill-Davidson HC, Katz RL: Dual, phase II, or desensitization block? Anesthesiology 1966;27:536–538.

204. Schneider G, Sebel PS: Monitoring depth of anaesthesia. Eur J Anaesthesiol Suppl 1997;15:21–28.

205. Rampil IJ: A primer for EEG signal processing in anesthesia. Anesthesiology 1998;89:980–1002.

206. Todd MM: EEGs, EEG processing, and the bispectral index. Anesthesiology 1998;89:815–817.

207. Kearse LAJ, Rosow C, Zaslavsky A, et al: Bispectral analysis of the electroencephalogram predicts conscious processing of information during propofol sedation and hypnosis. Anesthesiology 1998;88:25–34.

208. Glass PS, Bloom M, Kearse L, et al: Bispectral analysis measures sedation and memory effects of propofol, midazolam, isoflurane, and alfentanil in healthy volunteers. Anesthesiology 1997;86:836–847.

209. Billard V, Gambus PL, Chamoun N, et al: A comparison of spectral edge, delta power, and bispectral index as EEG measures of alfentanil, propofol, and midazolam drug effect. Clin Pharmacol Ther 1997;61:45–58.

210. Liu J, Singh H, White PF: Electroencephalogram bispectral analysis predicts the depth of midazolam-induced sedation. Anesthesiology 1996;84:64–69.

211. Sebel PS, Bowles SM, Saini V, et al: EEG bispectrum predicts movement during thiopental/isoflurane anesthesia. J Clin Monit 1995;11:83–91.

212. Vernon JM, Lang E, Sebel PS, et al: Prediction of movement using bispectral electroencephalographic analysis during propofol/alfentanil or isoflurane/alfentanil anesthesia. Anesth Analg 1995;80:780–785.

213. Kearse LAJ, Manberg P, Chamoun N, et al: Bispectral analysis of the electroencephalogram correlates with patient movement to skin incision during propofol/nitrous oxide anesthesia. Anesthesiology 1994;81:1365–1370.

214. Sebel PS, Lang E, Rampil IJ, et al: A multicenter study of bispectral electroencephalogram analysis for monitoring anesthetic effect. Anesth Analg 1997;84:891–899.

215. Coté CJ, Zaslavsky A, Downes JJ, et al: Postoperative apnea in former preterm infants after inguinal herniorrhaphy: A combined analysis. Anesthesiology 1995;82:809–822.

216. Bardoczky GI, Engelman E, d'Hollander A: Continuous spirometry: an aid to monitoring ventilation during operation. Br J Anaesth 1993;71:747–751.

217. Bardoczky GI, Engelman E, Levarlet M, et al: Ventilatory effects of pneumoperitoneum monitored with continuous spirometry. Anaesthesia 1993;48:309–311.

218. Govindarajan N, Meiyappan S, Prakash O: Real-time respiratory monitoring workstation: Software and hardware engineering aspects. Int J Clin Monit Comput 1992;9:141–148.

219. Wensley DF, Noonan P, Seear MD, et al: Pilot study for the development of a monitoring device for ventilated children. Pediatr Pulmonol 1991;11:272–279.

220. Breen PH, Serina ER, Barker SJ: Exhaled flow monitoring can detect bronchial flap-valve obstruction in a mechanical lung model. Anesth Analg 1995;81:292–296.

221. Hoffstein V, Zamel N, McClean P, et al: Changes in pulmonary function and cross-sectional area of trachea and bronchi in asthmatics following inhalation of procaterol hydrochloride and ipratropium bromide. Am J Respir Crit Care Med 1994;149:81–85.

222. Myer CM 3d, O'Connor DM, Cotton RT: Proposed grading system for subglottic stenosis based on endotracheal tube sizes. Ann Otol Rhinol Laryngol 1994;103:319–323.

223. Todres ID, Rogers MC, Shannon DC, et al: Percutaneous catheterization of the radial artery in the critically ill neonate. J Pediatr 1975;87:273–275.

224. Cole FS, Todres ID, Shannon DC: Technique for percutaneous cannulation of the radial artery in the newborn infant. J Pediatr 1978;92:105–107.

225. Todres ID, Crone RK, Rogers MC, et al: Swan-Ganz catheterization in the critically ill newborn. Crit Care Med 1979;7:330–334.

226. Coté CJ, Jobes DR, Schwartz AJ, et al: Two approaches to cannulation of a child's internal jugular vein. Anesthesiology 1979;50:371–373.

227. Clapham MC, Willis N, Mapleson WW: Minimum volume of discard for valid blood sampling from indwelling arterial cannulae. Br J Anaesth 1987;59:232–235.

228. Butt WW, Gow R, Whyte H, et al: Complications resulting from use of arterial catheters: Retrograde flow and rapid elevation in blood pressure. Pediatrics 1985;76:250–254.

229. Rooth G, Huch A, Huch R: Transcutaneous oxygen monitors are

reliable indicators of arterial oxygen tension (if used correctly). Pediatrics 1987;79:283–286.

230. Gothgen I, Jacobsen E: Transcutaneous oxygen tension measurement II. The influence of halothane and hypotension. Acta Anaesthesiol Scand Suppl 1978;67:71–75.

231. Lanigan C, Ponte J, Moxham J: Performance of transcutaneous PO_2 and PCO_2 dual electrodes in adults. Br J Anaesth 1988;60:736–742.

232. Bucher HU, Fanconi S, Fallenstein F, et al: Transcutaneous carbon dioxide tension in newborn infants: Reliability and safety of continuous 24-hour measurement at 42 degrees C. Pediatrics 1986;78:631–635.

233. Dennhardt R, Fricke M, Mahal S, et al: Transcutaneous PO_2 monitoring in anaesthesia. Eur J Intensive Care Med 1976;2:29–33.

234. Rafferty TD, Marrero O, Nardi D, et al: Transcutaneous PO_2 as a trend indicator of arterial PO_2 in normal anesthetized adults. Anesth Analg 1982;61:252–255.

235. Nomura M, Hillel Z, Shih H, et al: The association between Doppler transmitral flow variables measured by transesophageal echocardiography and pulmonary capillary wedge pressure. Anesth Analg 1997;84:491–496.

236. Thys DM, Hillel Z: Left ventricular performance indices by transesophageal Doppler. Anesthesiology 1988;69:728–737.

237. Abel MD, Nishimura RA, Callahan MJ, et al: Evaluation of intraoperative transesophageal two-dimensional echocardiography. Anesthesiology 1987;66:64–68.

238. Vieli A: Doppler flow determination. Br J Anaesth 1988;60(Suppl 1):107S–112S.

239. Cahalan MK, Lurz FC, Schiller NB: Transoesophageal two-dimensional echocardiographic evaluation of anaesthetic effects on left ventricular function. Br J Anaesth 1988;60(Suppl 1):99S–106S.

240. Abrams JH, Weber RE, Holmen KD: Continuous cardiac output determination using transtracheal Doppler: Initial results in humans. Anesthesiology 1989;71:11–15.

241. Abrams JH, Weber RE, Holmen KD: Transtracheal Doppler: A new procedure for continuous cardiac output measurement. Anesthesiology 1989;70:134–138.

242. Bowdle TA, Glenn M, Colston H, et al: Fire following use of electrocautery during emergency percutaneous transtracheal ventilation. Anesthesiology 1987;66:697–698.

32 Procedures

I. David Todres *and* Charles J. Coté

Venous Cannulation
  Peripheral Intravenous Cannulation
  Central Venous Catheterization
  Intraosseous Infusion
  Pulmonary Artery Catheterization
  Umbilical Vein Catheterization
Arterial Cannulation
  Umbilical Artery Catheterization
  Radial Artery Catheterization
  Temporal Artery Catheterization
  Femoral Artery Catheterization
  Dorsalis Pedis and Posterior Tibial Artery
  Catheterization

Vascular cannulation is an important procedure in the anesthetic and intensive care management of children. It ranges from a simple intravenous line to more sophisticated pulmonary artery catheterization. The indications for the insertion of these devices in children are the same as in adults—namely, to provide a route for fluid and drug administration and monitoring of cardiopulmonary function. However, the materials used, insertion techniques, and complications are often specifically modified according to the age of a child. Although the technique of insertion may be extremely difficult in a young infant, no child should be denied an indicated procedure because of an operator's inexperience; appropriate consultation should be sought. The anesthesiologist should wear gloves to maintain sterility and to protect from exposure to blood.[1-3]

Venous Cannulation

Peripheral Intravenous Cannulation

Percutaneous

Indications. Ideally, percutaneous intravenous cannulation should be used in all anesthetized patients for the following purposes:

1. To provide access for administering drugs, fluid and electrolytes, glucose, and blood products.
2. To have access to the circulation for administering resuscitation drugs and fluids.

3. To provide a route for immediate postoperative pain relief.

Equipment and Practical Suggestions

1. If the patient is awake, establish a cooperative patient/anesthesiologist interaction.
2. Secure the extremity for an intravenous site, preferably one in close proximity to the anesthesiologist.
3. Insert a scalp vein needle (Butterfly) for induction, followed by an appropriately sized catheter under anesthesia or a vascular catheter inserted after injection of a local anesthetic drug with a small needle (25- to 27-gauge).
4. A T-connector (Abbott Hospitals, Inc., Chicago IL) is used to minimize the fluids necessary to flush drugs administered through the intravenous line; this is especially important for infants.
5. Clear plastic dressing (Tegaderm, 3M Medical-Surgical Division, St. Paul, MN) and tape should be available.
6. A calibrated burette is used to limit the total infusion and provide a means to titrate fluids accurately.
7. A flow-limiting infusion pump is used for infants and neonates.

Complications

1. Hematoma—usually of no serious consequence.
2. Infection/thrombosis—may be limited by aseptic technique.[4-6]
3. Skin sloughing—usually caused by subcutaneous infiltration of calcium, potassium, or hypertonic solutions; may be avoided by frequent inspection, such as checking intravenous function before injecting medications.[7] The risk of subcutaneous infiltration when using an infusion pump, however, is not related to the use of calcium, potassium, or infusion pumps.[8]

Establishing a Large Intravenous Catheter in Small Patients

Indications. Any small patient with the potential for massive, rapid hemorrhage (trauma, tumor excision, liver transplant) should receive an intravenous catheter.

1. The appropriate area is prepared and draped using standard sterile techniques.
2. Perform a standard intravenous cannulation of an antecubital, saphenous, or external jugular vein with a small (22- or 20-gauge) intravenous catheter.

3. Pass a small, flexible guide wire (0.18 mm) through the intravenous catheter, remove the catheter, and with a number 11 blade make a small incision at the entry point of the wire at the skin.
4. Pass the next larger size intravenous catheter over the wire to dilate the vein and leave in place; stiff intravenous catheters are more effective than soft ones. An alternative is to use a small dilator from a pulmonary artery catheter introducer and leave the introducer in place. The wire is removed, and the next larger size wire is inserted (0.25 mm). The catheter (or introducer) is removed, leaving this larger wire within the vein.
5. Pass the next larger size intravenous catheter over the wire (usually 18-gauge) several times and then pass the next larger size catheter (usually 16-gauge); remove the guide wire, leaving the intravenous catheter within the vein.
6. Pass the next larger flexible guide wire (0.35 mm) into the vein, remove the 16-gauge intravenous catheter, and insert a 14-gauge catheter. An alternative is to leave progressively larger pulmonary artery introducers in the vein; both techniques provide a reasonably rapid method of establishing a large-bore intravenous infusion site.
7. A similar technique may be used to insert a pulmonary artery catheter introducer sheath.

Intravenous Cutdown

Indications
1. Any patient in whom percutaneous cannulation is unsuccessful.
2. Any patient in whom percutaneous cannulation is tenuous.
3. If the catheter in place is inadequate for the planned surgical procedure.

The most common sites for insertion are the saphenous vein at the ankle (medial malleolus) and the brachiocephalic vein in the arm (antecubital fossa).

Complications. Intravenous cutdown has a higher incidence of infection and therefore should be used only on a short-term basis.

Central Venous Catheterization

Indications
1. To provide a secure means for administration of fluid and blood when major shifts in intravascular volume are anticipated (e.g., multiple trauma, intestinal obstruction, burns).
2. To monitor cardiac filling pressures.
3. For infusion of drugs and fluids that are sclerosing to peripheral veins (e.g., antibiotics, vasopressors, and hyperalimentation fluids).
4. Measurement of mixed venous acid-base balance or estimation of cardiac output (Fick principle).
5. Measurement of cardiac output (dye dilution).
6. Route for aspiration of air emboli.

The common sites for central venous cannulation are the external and internal jugular, the subclavian and brachiocephalic, the femoral, and the umbilical vein in neonates. The more invasive approaches (internal jugular and subclavian) should be used with extreme caution in the presence of a bleeding diathesis.

In our experience, the percutaneous approach to central venous cannulation is most successful using modified Seldinger techniques.[9, 10] This approach is demonstrated in Figure 32–1. The advantages of this technique are that it avoids the need for a cutdown, only one venipuncture is made with a thin-walled small-gauge needle, a guide wire directs the catheter within the blood vessel, introducing a large catheter through the small venipuncture site minimizes the chances of significant hematoma formation even after systemic heparinization, and the procedure can often be accomplished in an emergency situation in less than 1 minute.

Alternative techniques include locating the vein with a small-gauge needle, followed by venipuncture with a large needle (Intracath, Deseret, Sandy UT) through which the catheter is threaded. This technique is successful in the hands of experienced operators but has the disadvantage of requiring several venipunctures, and the larger needle may cause hematoma formation or may damage surrounding tissues (Horner syndrome).[11]

Whenever a central line is inserted, care must be taken to ensure that the catheter tip is not inserted against the wall of a major blood vessel, deep in the right atrium, or in a ventricular position, because these positions have been associated with perforation of large vessels and the myocardium.[12]

External Jugular Vein Catheterization

1. The patient is placed in Trendelenburg position with the head turned 45 degrees away from the side of cannulation.
2. A pillow or rolled sheet is placed under the shoulders to extend the head and allow complete access to the neck.
3. Under aseptic conditions, venipuncture and catheter insertion are completed according to the techniques shown in Figure 32–1. A J-wire is usually more useful to circumvent the plexus of veins at the clavicle.[13, 14]
4. Apply antibiotic ointment, suture or tape appropriately, and cover with an occlusive dressing. A significant number of catheters will not pass beyond the clavicle or will pass into the axillary vein; the right side is generally more successful.[15, 16] If a shorter catheter is used, infusion and pressure monitoring are very position dependent.[17] Continuous free-flowing infusion is maintained when the head is turned away from the side of catheter insertion.

Internal Jugular Vein Catheterization

Numerous approaches and techniques are used for internal jugular vein cannulation.[18-21] We have had the most success with a high approach using the apex of a triangle formed by the two bellies of the sternocleidomastoid muscle and the clavicle as a landmark for insertion (Fig. 32–2). Using the Seldinger technique, our success rate, even in neonates, approaches 75% on the first attempt and 90 to 95% on the second attempt.[9] Cannulation of the right side virtually ensures a central location, because the internal jugular vein, the superior vena cava, and the right atrium are in a straight line (see Fig. 32–2). Left-sided cannulation risks injury to the thoracic duct and possible pneumothorax, because the

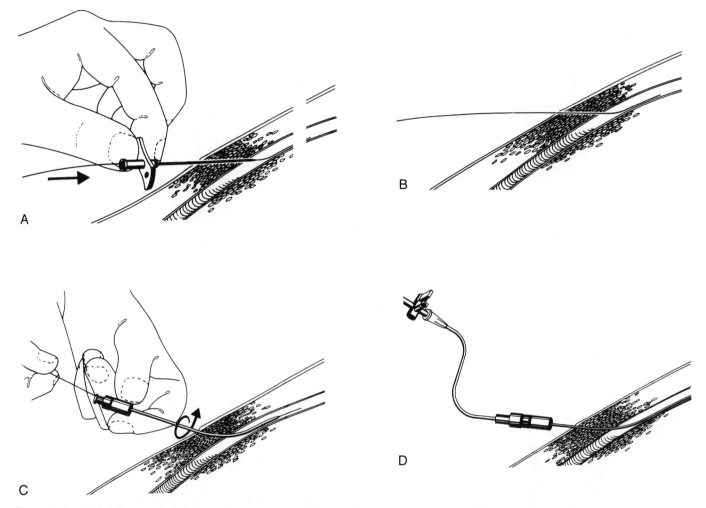

Figure 32–1. (A) Seldinger technique for catheter placement. The needle is inserted into the target vessel, and the flexible end of the guide wire is passed freely into the vessel. (B) The needle is then removed, leaving the guide wire in place. (C) The catheter is advanced with a twisting motion into the vessel. (D) The wire is removed, and the catheter is connected to an appropriate infusion or monitoring device. (From Schwartz AJ, Coté CJ, Jobes DR et al: Central venous catheterization in pediatrics. Scientific Exhibit, American Society of Anesthesiologists, New Orleans, 1977.)

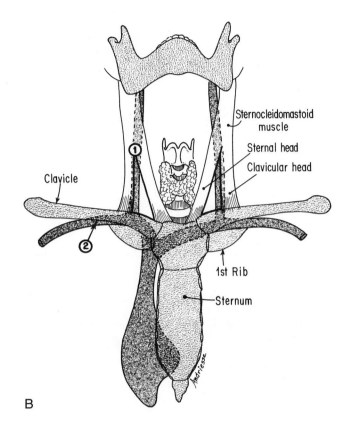

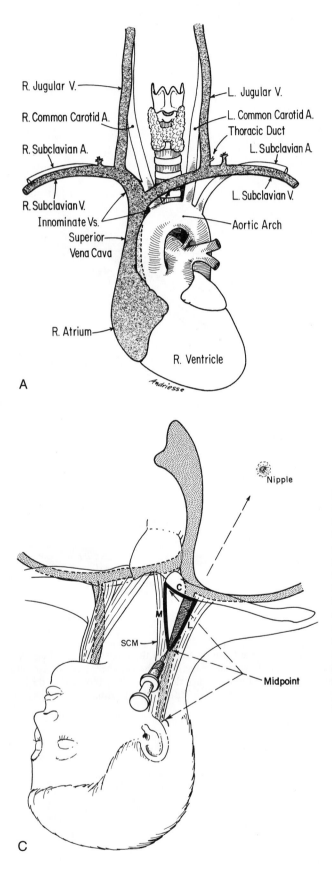

Figure 32–2. (A) The anatomic relationships of major chest and neck structures. Note how the internal jugular vein is in close proximity to the carotid artery. Also note that a nearly straight line is formed by the internal jugular vein, innominate vein, superior vena cava, and right atrium; thus it is rare for a right internal jugular catheter to migrate anywhere but to the right atrium. (B) The relationship of external anatomic landmarks to the anatomy in part A. Note the triangle formed by the two bellies of the sternocleidomastoid muscle and the clavicle. 1, The preferred point of needle insertion at the apex of this triangle for internal jugular vein puncture. 2, The point of needle insertion for subclavian vein puncture. (C) The anatomic landmarks as they would appear to an anesthesiologist. Note that the needle is introduced at the apex of the triangle outlined in part C and is directed at an angle of 30 degrees to the skin toward the ipsilateral nipple. This point of entry is half the distance between the mastoid process and the clavicle. C, clavicle; SCM, sternocleidomastoid muscle; M and L, medial and lateral bellies of the SCM.

apex of the lung is higher on the left. In addition, if a catheter inserted on the left is too short, it is not unusual for the tip to rest against the wall of the superior vena cava, be position dependent, and possibly erode through the wall of the vessel (Fig. 32–3). The principal advantage of the high approach is that the most common complication (arterial puncture, approximately 10%) is easily recognized and usually treated uneventfully. A lower approach risks life-threatening complications (pneumothorax, hemothorax), which may go unrecognized.[31, 74]

Technique

1. The patient is positioned as for external jugular vein cannulation (see Fig. 32–2).
2. The apex of a triangle formed by the two bellies of the sternocleidomastoid muscle is located. This point is usually where the external jugular vein crosses the sternocleidomastoid muscle or the midpoint between the mastoid process and the sternal notch.
3. The carotid artery is palpated, and the needle is introduced just lateral to it at an angle of 30 degrees to the skin surface. In some children, the internal jugular vein is superficial, in which case even a less acute angle may be indicated. While continuously aspirating, advance the needle toward the ipsilateral nipple a distance of no more than 2.5 cm. If no blood is freely obtained, slowly withdraw the needle while maintaining aspiration. The needle often kinks the vessel upon entry, and it unkinks during withdrawal, allowing free aspiration of blood.
4. Once venipuncture is accomplished, the syringe is carefully removed and the end of the needle occluded (to prevent air embolism) until a flexible guide wire is inserted (see Fig. 32–1).[10] The wire should advance with almost no resistance. However, if the wire cannot be advanced, the needle has passed out of the vessel lumen or its tip rests against the vessel wall. In this situation, the wire and needle should be withdrawn simultaneously to avoid shearing the wire. If the wire passes easily, then cannulation proceeds as demonstrated in Figure 32–1. Catheter tip location should be confirmed radiologically and repositioned if necessary (see Fig. 32–3).
5. Generally the catheter site is covered with antibiotic ointment, sutured, and protected with an occlusive dressing.

Contraindications

1. A bleeding diathesis is a relative contraindication; in life-threatening emergencies, the benefit may outweigh the risk.
2. Contralateral pneumothorax.
3. Raised intracranial pressure (Trendelenburg position as well as venous occlusion by the catheter may increase intracranial pressure).
4. Aberrant vessels (e.g., cervical aortic arch).

Subclavian Vein Catheterization

The subclavian vein is a site frequently used for central vein cannulation.[22, 23] The advantages include fixed landmarks, ease of securing the line to patients for long-term management, and patient comfort. Disadvantages include potential life-threatening complications (e.g., pneumothorax, hemothorax). If this site is chosen preoperatively, we routinely obtain a chest radiograph after the catheter is inserted and

before surgery commences to circumvent the danger of an unrecognized intraoperative tension pneumothorax. The use of the Seldinger technique (our preference) may reduce the incidence of damage to intrathoracic structures compared with other techniques. As with left-sided internal jugular vein cannulation, if a left subclavian catheter tip rests against the wall of the superior vena cava, it can erode through, resulting in hemothorax or hydrothorax.

Technique

1. The patient is prepared and positioned as previously described for external jugular vein puncture.
2. A needle is inserted immediately inferior to the clavicle at a point one-half to two-thirds its length from the sternoclavicular junction; while "hugging" the undersurface of the clavicle, the needle is directed toward the suprasternal notch while continuously aspirating.
3. As soon as free blood flow is obtained, proceed as in Figure 32–1A–D. If the Seldinger technique is not used, then first locating the subclavian vein with a small-gauge needle is recommended.
4. The catheter insertion site is covered with antibiotic ointment, the catheter is sutured in place, and an occlusive dressing is applied.

The anesthesiologist may be of great help in avoiding complications by momentarily ceasing ventilation when the surgeon is probing for the subclavian vein; the apex of the lung is thus kept away from the needle. Once successful venipuncture has been achieved, maintaining positive end-expiratory pressure reduces the possibility of air embolization.

Contraindications. Contraindications are the same as for internal jugular vein catheterization.

Brachiocephalic Vein Catheterization

The brachiocephalic vein offers the advantage of being far removed from vital intrathoracic structures.[24] The main disadvantage is that a significant number of catheters introduced at this site do not pass centrally—that is, they are caught up in the axilla or pass up the jugular vein (internal or external).[25, 26] Other disadvantages include significant catheter migration with movement of the arm and possibly an increased incidence of infection. This approach is commonly used by radiologists for placement of peripherally inserted central (PIC) lines, which can be used on a long-term basis.[27, 28] These catheters often markedly improve patient care and the quality of life for the child because of the reduced need for venous access and the reduced number of venipunctures for blood testing.

Technique

1. The arm is aseptically prepared and draped.
2. The brachiocephalic vein is cannulated either using the modified Seldinger technique (special long catheters and wires for this purpose) or by passing a standard catheter through a needle (Intracath). If the catheter cannot be threaded once the vein is entered, initiating rapid intravenous fluid administration, cephalad positioning of the arm, and anterior displacement of the shoulder may assist advancement.

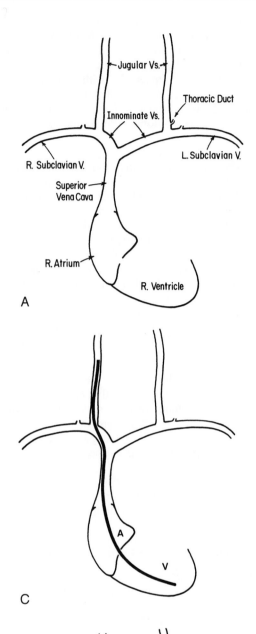

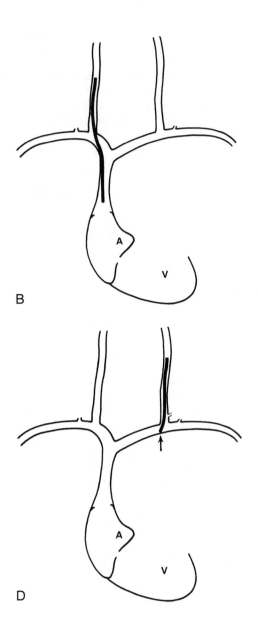

A

Jugular Vs.

Thoracic Duct

Innominate Vs.

R. Subclavian V.

L. Subclavian V.

Superior
Vena Cava

R. Atrium

R. Ventricle

B

C

D

E

Figure 32–3. Proper and improper central venous pressure catheter placement. (A) Normal vascular anatomy. (B) Proper location for right internal jugular catheter (i.e., high right atrium or superior vena cava). (C) Ventricular location of any catheter is dangerous and contraindicated. (D) A short left-sided internal jugular catheter may erode through the innominate vein. (E) A left-sided internal jugular catheter striking the lateral wall of the superior vena cava may erode through and must be partially withdrawn or advanced.

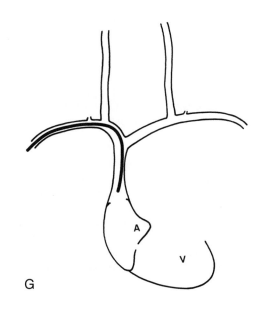

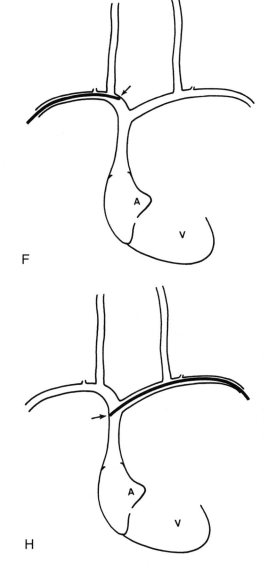

Figure 32–3 *Continued.* (F) A short right subclavian catheter may strike the lateral wall of the innominate vein and erode through; this catheter should be advanced or withdrawn. (G) Proper location for a right subclavian line. (H) A short left subclavian line may erode through the superior vena cava; this catheter should be advanced or withdrawn.

If percutaneous techniques are not possible, direct venous cutdown may be performed or a PIC line inserted by a radiologist.

Femoral Vein Catheterization

The femoral vein may also be used for access to the central circulation.[29] However, the catheter must pass into the thorax to provide accurate cardiac filling pressure measurements. One advantage is that the vein is large and presents easy access distant from vital intrathoracic structures. Disadvantages include difficulty in securing the catheter to the patient, kinking of the catheter with leg flexion, and problems in keeping the site of catheter insertion sterile. Short-term catheterization can provide a large venous access for the duration of a procedure with expected large and rapid blood loss if other veins are not accessible. Generally the catheter is removed after the procedure and hemostasis is assured.

Technique
1. The groin is prepared and draped with aseptic technique.
2. The femoral artery is palpated at a point midway between the pubic tubercle and the anterior superior iliac spine.
3. Using the Seldinger technique, the vein is entered at a point just medial to the femoral artery and 1 to 2 cm below the inguinal ligament. A catheter is inserted as in Figure 32–1. As for the brachiocephalic vein, special long catheters and wires are needed to achieve a central location.
4. The catheter insertion site is protected as previously described (see Internal Jugular Vein Catheterization). If an alternative technique is used (e.g., catheter through the needle), compression of the cannulation site should be maintained until hemostasis is ensured. The saphenous vein may be cannulated by direct venous cutdown at its junction with the femoral vein if percutaneous techniques are unsuccessful.

Intraosseous Infusion

The administration of intravenous fluid into the medullary cavity of long bones is a proven method for volume resuscitation in a hypovolemic child.[30–33] This method has been demonstrated to deliver drugs to the central circulation as quickly as using peripheral intravenous infusion sites.[34] It may therefore be a particularly valuable emergency route of drug administration even in the hands of emergency medical technicians.[35–37] Complications such as cellulitis, abscess, and osteomyelitis have been reported in less than 1% of cases and this technique does not appear to affect later growth of the tibia.[38] These complications relate in part to duration of infusion and to the underlying medical conditions. The major difficulties with this technique are due to failure to adhere to proper landmarks and bending and clotting of the needle. This technique is used in an emergency situation if attempts at peripheral or central venous cannulation have failed (usually after three attempts or 90 seconds).[39] Intraosseous infusions are discontinued once an alternative intravenous infusion site has been secured. This technique has been successfully used for resuscitation of burn victims.[40, 41]

Technique
1. The tibial tuberosity is palpated.
2. A point on the medial surface of the tibia 1 to 2 cm below and medial to the tibial tuberosity is the site of needle puncture because the mantle of the tibia is thin at this location (Fig. 32–4A).
3. A special short needle with a stylet is used to puncture the mantle of the tibia at a 75-degree angle directed toward the feet to avoid the epiphyseal plate (Fig. 32–4B–C). A styletted spinal needle may also be used.
4. The appropriate position is readily achieved with the loss of resistance; care must be taken to avoid advancing the needle too far (i.e., out the opposite side or against the opposite mantle of the tibia). The needle is usually quite stable if properly positioned.
5. Standard intravenous infusion equipment is attached, and fluid should flow freely without extravasation (Fig. 32–4D).

Pulmonary Artery Catheterization

Measurement of pulmonary artery occlusion pressure has become increasingly important for operative and intensive care management of selected pediatric patients.[42–47] The catheters are available in various sizes (2 to 7 French) with many capabilities, including pressure monitoring, thermodilution measurement of cardiac output, continuous measurement of mixed venous oxygen tension and saturation, and cardiac pacing.[48, 49] These catheters can be used in children of all ages, including newborns.[47]

Indications
1. Measurement of left- and right-sided cardiac filling pressures (hypovolemia versus congestive heart failure).
2. Pulmonary artery hypertension.
3. Measurement of cardiac output.
4. Measurement of mixed venous oxygen tension and saturation.
5. Cardiac pacing.
6. Diagnosing and treating air emboli.

Technique
1. The patient is prepared, draped, and positioned as for central venous catheterization.
2. The Seldinger technique is used to gain access to a large vein (internal jugular, subclavian, femoral, or brachiocephalic).
3. Instead of a catheter introduced over a wire, a dilator and sheath of appropriate size are inserted (Fig. 32–5A–G).
4. All air is flushed from the pulmonary artery catheter, which is then attached to a calibrated pressure transducer.
5. The catheter is slowly advanced until a central venous (right atrial) tracing is obtained (Fig. 32–6A). The balloon tip is then inflated with a measured amount of air (carbon dioxide for children with possible intracardiac shunts).
6. The catheter is advanced farther until a right ventricular tracing appears (Fig. 32–6B). Once this is obtained, further advance of 2 to 3 cm usually results in successful pulmonary artery cannulation. Note: There must be a step-up in diastolic pressure signaling the crossover from right ventricle to pulmonary artery (Fig. 32–6C).

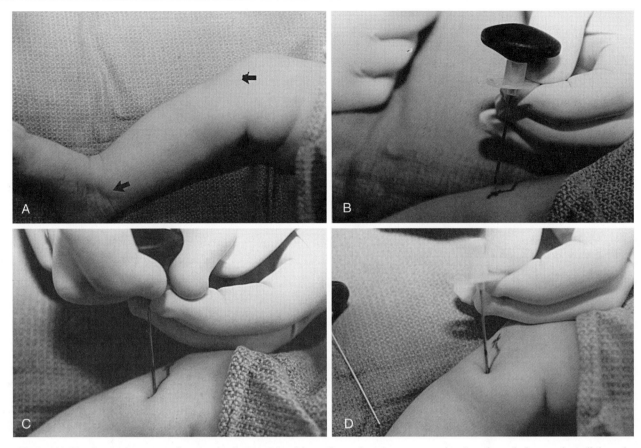

Figure 32–4. (A) The intraosseous needle may be inserted in either of two locations: at a point 1 to 2 cm below and medial to the tibial tuberosity or at the medial malleolus (arrows). (B, C) The leg is prepared, and the intraosseous needle punctures the skin (note the two X marks connecting the tibial tuberosity with the point of needle insertion); the needle is advanced with a twisting motion in a caudal direction. (D) The stylet is removed, and the selected solution is infused.

7. The catheter is advanced farther until a wedge tracing is obtained (Fig. 32–6D). A return of the pulmonary artery tracing should occur with deflation of the balloon. Wedge pressure should return with *gentle* reinflation of the balloon. Confirmation of wedge position should be made by radiograph and pressure waveform and by obtaining blood gas analysis both with and without the balloon inflated. With the balloon inflated, arterialized blood should be obtained; if not, then the catheter is against the wall of the vessel, the balloon has herniated over the tip of the catheter, giving a false impression of occlusion position, or the catheter is wedged into the wall of the heart chamber, usually the right ventricle.

8. The introducer sheath is withdrawn so that only the distal portion remains within the superior vena cava. The sheath site is then covered with antibiotic ointment, and the catheter sutured in place and covered with an occlusive dressing.

Complications. The complications associated with pulmonary artery cannulation are similar to those of central venous cannulation—hematoma, arterial puncture, pneumothorax, hemothorax, arrhythmias, and air emboli.[42, 50] Pulmonary infarction, rupture of the pulmonary artery, thrombocytopenia, and altered pulmonary blood flow are additional significant risks.[51–54] These latter complications may be minimized by avoiding prolonged measurement of pulmonary

artery occlusion pressure and not overinflating the balloon. One method of achieving this is to continuously transduce the pulmonary artery tracing to immediately diagnose catheter migration. Another is to determine how much air results in successful occlusion. Once the latter is achieved, holes punctured in the air syringe at the desired volume may prevent accidental overinflation (Fig. 32–7).[55]

Umbilical Vein Catheterization

Indications. The umbilical vein provides convenient access to the central circulation of a newborn infant for restoration of blood volume and for administration of glucose and drugs.[56] It provides a route for the procedure of exchange transfusion and for measuring central venous pressure.

Materials

Umbilical artery catheter sizes 3 1/2 and 5 French

Scalpel and blade

Fine curved forceps

Mosquito hemostats

Umbilical tape

Scissors

Sutures with needle (3-0 silk)

Antiseptic solutions (povidone-iodine and alcohol)

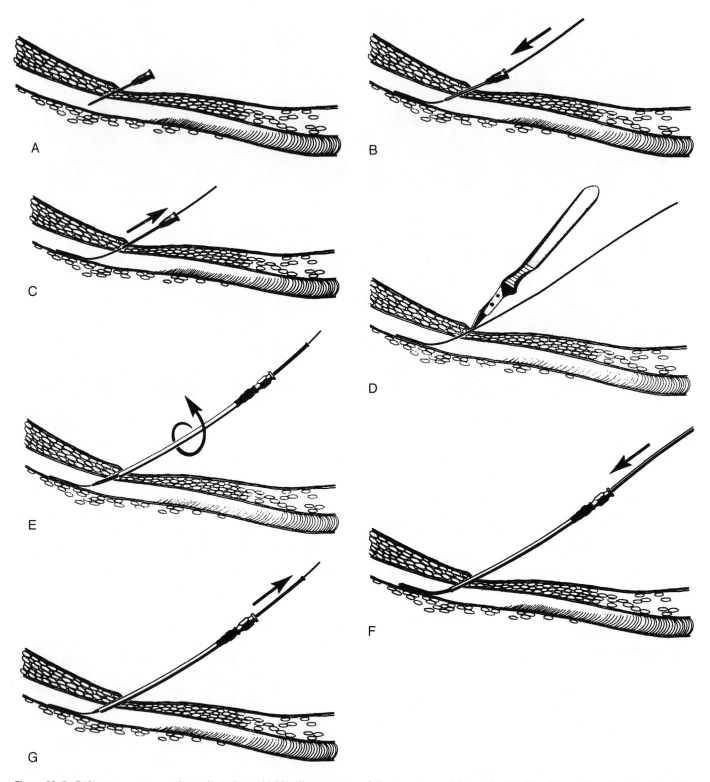

Figure 32–5. Pulmonary artery catheter insertion. (A) Needle puncture of the target vessel is made. (B) Flexible guide wire should easily pass into the vessel. (C) Needle is withdrawn, leaving wire in vessel. (D) Skin incision made with scalpel blade. (E) With a twisting motion, the introducer follows the wire into the vessel. (F) Sheath and introducer further advanced as a unit into the vessel. (G) Guide wire and introducer are removed, leaving the sheath in place. (From Conahan TJ III: Air embolization during percutaneous Swan-Ganz catheter placement. JAMA 237:447. Copyright 1977, American Medical Association.)

PULMONARY ARTERY CATHETERIZATION

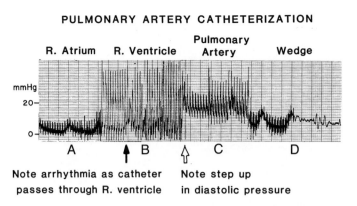

Note arrhythmia as catheter passes through R. ventricle   Note step up in diastolic pressure

Figure 32–6. Pulmonary artery catheterization. (A) Right artical tracing. (B) Right ventricular tracing; note arrhythmia when the catheter tip strikes ventricular tissue (solid arrow). (C) Pulmonary artery tracing; note the step up in diastolic pressure that is the hallmark of the catheter in the pulmonary artery (open arrow). (D) Wedge location; note the loss of pulmonary artery tracing and that the tracing pattern is very similar to right artial.

Three-way stopcocks

10 mL syringe

Infusion solution of 10% dextrose in water, with 2 units of heparin per milliliter

Calibrated transducer/monitoring system if used for central venous pressure measurement

Technique. After preparing and draping the umbilicus, cut the cord approximately 1 cm above the umbilicus. The umbilical vein orifice is more patulous and thin walled (Fig. 32–8). Holding the catheter filled with heparinized solution 2 cm from the tip, gently introduce it into the vein. In some situations, forceps can aid in directing the catheter. Traction of the umbilical stump *caudally* may facilitate the catheter's advance (see Fig. 32–8). The catheter is passed a distance that approximates the length between the umbilical stump and the right atrium. Blood should freely aspirate into a syringe. Inability to withdraw blood may occur if the tip of the catheter is resting against a vessel wall or if a clot is

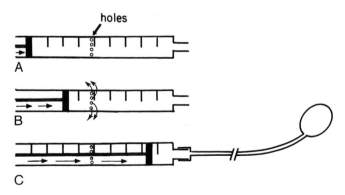

Figure 32–7. (A) To prevent accidental overinflation of a pulmonary artery catheter balloon, the inflation syringe is punctured several times at the appropriate volume. (B) As the plunger is depressed, air vents out the puncture holes. (C) Only the volume distal to the puncture holes is transmitted to the balloon. (From Coté CJ: A simple technique to avoid over distension of flow directed catheters. Anesthesiology 1978;49:154.)

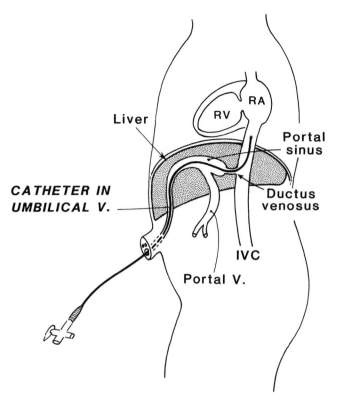

Figure 32–8. Umbilical vein catheterization. The umbilical vein is thin walled and patulous, whereas umbilical arteries are thicker walled and of smaller diameter. *Caudal* traction on the umbilical stump may facilitate catheter advancement. The catheter should be advanced through the liver into the central circulation before administration of any medications.

present within the catheter lumen. *It is important that the tip of the catheter be placed in the proper position—that is, at the junction of the inferior vena cava and right atrium.* A radiograph confirms proper catheter position. At times, the catheter may fail to traverse the ductus venosus and may become wedged in the liver. This position is potentially dangerous should hyperosmolar or sclerosing solutions be injected (calcium, sodium bicarbonate, 25% to 50% glucose), because portal necrosis and subsequent cirrhosis may result. The catheter is sutured in place, its insertion site is covered with antibiotic ointment, and it is taped to the abdominal wall. The catheter is then connected to a constant-infusion system and should be removed as soon as the indications for its insertion have passed. Complications appear to relate in part to the duration of insertion.[57]

Complications
1. Thrombosis of portal or mesenteric veins[58]
2. Infection (septicemia)
3. Endocarditis
4. Pulmonary infarction (misplacement of the catheter into the pulmonary vein through a patent foramen ovale)
5. Portal cirrhosis and esophageal varices later in life[59–62]
6. Cardiac tamponade[63]

Arterial Cannulation

Umbilical Artery Catheterization

The umbilical artery in a neonate is a convenient site for monitoring arterial blood pressure, blood gases, and pH. It

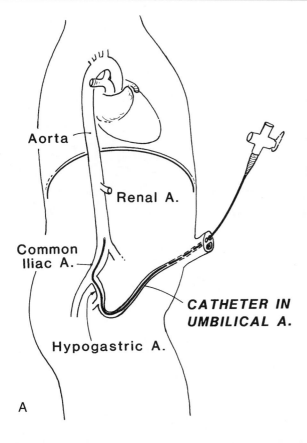

Aorta

Renal A.

Common
Iliac A.

Hypogastric A.

CATHETER IN
UMBILICAL A.

A

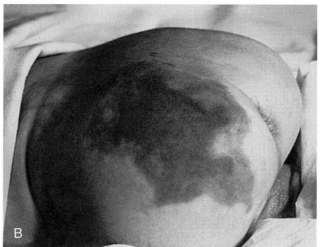

B

Figure 32–9. Umbilical artery catheterization. (A) *Cephalad* traction on the umbilical stump may facilitate catheter advancement. The catheter tip at L3-4 just above the aortic bifurcation is the ideal position. An alternative accepted location is at the level of the diaphragm. (B) An area of necrosis resulting from a catheter migrating into the internal iliac vessel, occluding one of its branches.

provides emergency access to an infant's circulation for restoration of blood volume and for administration of glucose and drugs.[64–66] Continuous monitoring of arterial oxygen saturation is also possible.[67]

Materials. The materials used for cannulation are identical to those described for umbilical venous catheterization. Equipment is required for continuous monitoring of blood pressure.

Technique. After preparing and draping, cut the umbilical cord approximately 1 cm above the umbilicus. The two umbilical arteries are identified (Fig. 32–9). The cut vessel ends have thicker walls and are smaller than the vein and are usually in spasm. The artery is entered in the manner described for umbilical vein catheterization, except that *cephalad* traction is applied to the umbilical stump (Fig. 32–9A). The catheter courses through the umbilical artery into the iliohypogastric artery and then into the descending aorta. Proper positioning of the catheter tip is crucial. If the catheter is advanced too far up the aorta, it may pass through the ductus arteriosus and into the pulmonary artery. If this situation is not recognized, blood pressure and blood gas measurements may be misleading. Care should also be taken to ensure the placement of the catheter in the descending aorta proximal (level of diaphragm) or distal (bifurcation of aorta) to the origin of the renal arteries (L1) and visceral branches of the aorta (Fig. 32–9B). The catheter should be positioned just above the bifurcation of the descending aorta—that is, at L3-4 (see Fig. 32–9A). This position can be difficult to maintain, and if the catheter tip slips into one of the iliac arteries, tissue ischemia can result (see Fig. 32–9B). The alternative ac-

cepted placement, at the level of the diaphragm, is easier to maintain but predisposes the infant to the increased risk of embolization to renal or mesenteric vessels.[68–71] Correct positioning is confirmed radiologically. Once the catheter is properly positioned, the system is connected to a constant-infusion pump and heparinized fluids (10% dextrose in water or normal saline) are infused. The catheter is sutured and taped, and antibiotic ointment is applied as for umbilical vein catheters.

Complications. Complications may be minimized by using the umbilical artery as a source for blood pressure monitoring and blood gas analysis only and reserving alternative sites for glucose and drug administration. Changes in cerebral blood flow are associated with intraventricular hemorrhage and have been documented to occur with umbilical artery blood sampling; there are fewer changes in cerebral blood flow with low positioned catheters.[72] The incidence of documented intraventricular hemorrhage appears to have a stronger relationship with age than with catheter position.[73] Complications include

1. Accidental disconnection of stopcocks and catheters, which can lead to potentially dangerous exsanguination.
2. Embolization of blood clot or air.[74] Blood clots may embolize retrograde or, more likely, distally, leading to ischemia or infarction of the infant's gut, kidneys, or lower limbs (Fig. 32–9B).
3. Vascular spasm, usually transitory, which may be resolved by withdrawal of the catheter. Several cases of flaccid paraplegia have been reported due to either spasm or embolic phenomena.[75]

4. Sepsis. The infant is always at risk for sepsis; therefore, clear indications for the insertion of this catheter are mandatory. The catheter should be removed at the earliest possible time.
5. Hypertension as a result of renal artery emboli causing ischemia and infarction of the kidney.[71, 76]
6. Aortic thrombosis.

Radial Artery Catheterization

Radial artery cannulation is a reasonable alternative to umbilical artery cannulation in a neonate and is the primary site of arterial cannulation in infants and children in our institution. Percutaneous radial artery cannulation is widely practiced with minimal morbidity.[77–81] Failure to cannulate the artery percutaneously may be followed successfully by direct arterial cutdown.

Indications. Indications for radial artery cannulation include monitoring of arterial blood pressure, gases, and pH. The right radial artery is preferred in neonates because it is representative of preductal blood flow.

Technique. Adequacy of ulnar artery collateral flow is confirmed by the modified Allen test (Fig. 32–10). The color of the hand is noted. The hand is passively clenched, and the radial and ulnar arteries are simultaneously compressed at the wrist. The ulnar artery is then released, and flushing (reperfusion) of the blanched hand is noted. If the entire hand is well perfused while the radial artery remains occluded, indicating adequate collateral flow, catheterization of the radial artery is performed. The hand is secured on an arm board with slight extension of the wrist to avoid excessive median nerve stretching. The fingertips should be left exposed when the hand is taped down so that any peripheral ischemic changes due to spasm, clot, or air can be observed.

The course of the radial artery may be observed in a neonate with the aid of a fiberoptic light source directed toward the lateral side or dorsal aspect of the wrist. Use of a Doppler device may also be of some value.[77, 82, 83] A 20-gauge needle is used to make a small skin puncture over the maximal pulsation of the radial artery, usually at the second proximal wrist crease. This step eases passage of the cannula by reducing resistance offered by the skin. Cannulation is accomplished either on direct entry of the artery at an angle of 15 to 20 degrees or on withdrawing the cannula after transfixion of the artery (Fig. 32–11A–C). The catheter is then firmly attached to a T-connector to permit continuous infusion of heparinized isotonic saline (1 U/mL) at the rate of 1 to 2 mL/hr via a constant-infusion pump (Fig. 32–11D). Antibiotic ointment is applied, the surrounding skin is coated with tincture of benzoin, and the catheter is securely taped in place (Fig. 32–11E–F). A pressure transducer is connected to allow continuous arterial pressure monitoring. To ensure accurate blood pressure measurement, it is essential that the transducer be calibrated with mercury to the patient's heart level, that all air bubbles be removed from the system, and that no more than 3 feet of tubing be used between the patient and the transducer to minimize artifacts caused by the monitoring tubing.[84]

Blood samples are obtained by clamping off the distal end of the T-connector, cleaning the injection port of the T-connector with povidone-iodine, introducing a 22-gauge needle, and allowing three to four drops of blood to flow out (Fig. 32–11G). A sample of blood is obtained by use of

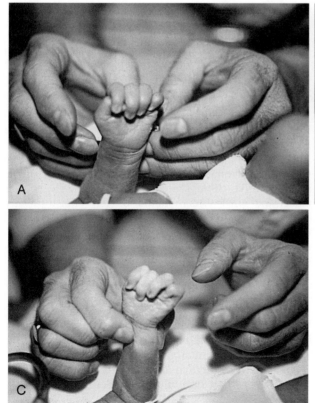

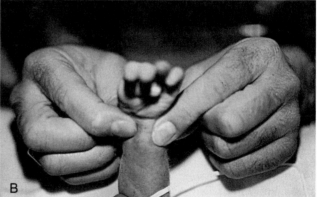

Figure 32–10. Modified Allen's test. (A) Color and perfusion of the hand are noted. (B) The hand is first passively clenched, and then both radial and ulnar vessels are occluded. (C) The ulnar artery is released while the radial artery remains occluded. If flow through the ulnar artery is adequate, then the color and perfusion should rapidly return.

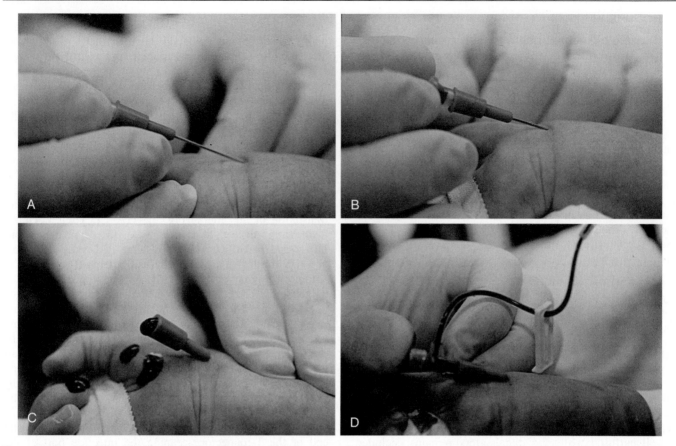

Figure 32–11. (A) After adequate collateral circulation has been assured, the radial artery is palpated and the appropriate catheter advanced into the vessel. (B) After blood return is noted, the catheter is threaded over the needle and into the artery. (C) Pulsatile back-bleeding confirms intra-arterial position. (D) A T-connector with appropriate flush solution is connected; the catheter is aspirated to clear air bubbles and then gently flushed. Antibiotic ointment and benzoin are applied. (E) A strip of tape is wrapped around the catheter and T-connector. (F) A second piece of tape is torn down the center; one half is applied and wrapped around the catheter and T-connector, and the other half is wrapped from the opposite direction.

a heparinized syringe, with minimal blood loss and minimal manipulation of the system (Fig. 32–11H).[77, 85] After sampling, the clamp is released and continuous infusion is resumed. This method of sampling avoids the use of stopcocks, which are potential sources of infection. Bolus flushes are avoided, an important consideration because bolus flushing has been associated with retrograde blood flow to the brain. Disastrous results may occur if an air bubble or blood clot should accompany a bolus flush.[86] Only heparinized normal or half-normal saline is infused to avoid arterial damage and thrombosis. *All arterial lines must be clearly identified (red tape) to avoid accidental infusion of hypertonic solutions and sclerosing medications.*

Complications

1. Infection at the site of the catheter insertion, with possible septicemia.
2. Arterial thrombus formation. This is dependent on the size of catheter inserted, the material of which it is constructed, the technique of insertion, and duration of cannulation.
3. Emboli. A blood clot or air may embolize to the digits, resulting in arteriolar spasm or more serious ischemic necrosis.
4. Disconnection of the catheter from the infusion system. Blood loss may be life-threatening, especially in an infant.
5. Ischemia. The radial artery cannula should be withdrawn if ischemic changes develop.

The previous method described is the traditional percutaneous radial artery cannulation at the ventral aspect of the wrist. The radial artery on the dorsal aspect of the wrist within the anatomic snuff box may be used as an alternative site.[87] Once an attempt at cannulation of the radial artery is made, the ulnar artery should be left uninstrumented to ensure adequate perfusion of the entire hand. Strict indications for inserting radial artery catheters are necessary, and their removal must be considered at the earliest possible time.[88–91]

Temporal Artery Catheterization

When the radial artery has been previously cannulated or is inaccessible, the temporal artery may be used.[92] The complication of cerebral infarction has been described with this technique. The infarction appears to be related to retrograde embolization of air or a blood clot.[93]

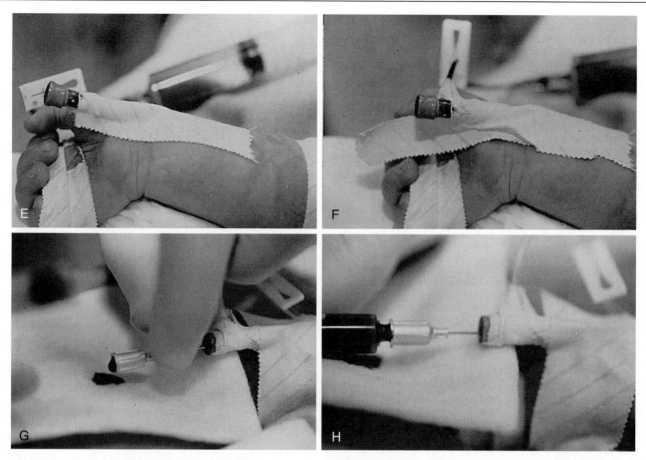

Figure 32–11 *Continued.* (G) Blood gas samples are obtained by occluding the T-connector, passing a small-gauge needle into the injection port and allowing several drops of blood to be drained, thus clearing the catheter of flush solution. (H) A dry heparinized syringe is attached to the needle hub, and the sample is aspirated. The T-connector occlusion is freed, and the system is gently flushed.

An advantage of this sampling site is that it provides preductal blood gas values. However, in our experience, the tortuous course of the artery and the resultant apposition of the distal tip of the catheter and the arterial wall have caused difficulties in freely drawing blood samples.

Femoral Artery Catheterization

The femoral artery is more commonly used in adults. In situations in which peripheral arterial cannulation is impossible (e.g., in burned patients), the femoral artery may be used.[94] This site should not be the first choice for arterial cannulation if other more peripheral sites are available.

Technique. The femoral artery is located by palpation at the groin. Anatomically, it is situated midway between the anterior superior iliac spine and the pubic tubercle.

After sterile preparation of the skin, a catheter of appropriate size is inserted into the femoral artery using the Seldinger technique. The artery is entered at the point of maximal pulsation, approximately 1 cm below the line joining the anterior superior iliac spine and the pubic tubercle. After cannulation, the catheter is connected to a continuous-flow system and pressure transducer. The catheter is sutured in place, the insertion site is covered with antibiotic ointment, and an occlusive dressing is applied. The likelihood

of fecal and urinary contamination makes this last step particularly important.

Complications
1. Infection.
2. Emboli of clot and air, leading to ischemic necrosis of the lower limb.
3. Poor arterial puncture technique leading to osteoarthritis of the hip joint. Severe trauma to the femoral artery has resulted in gangrene of the lower limb, retroperitoneal hemorrhage, and arteriovenous fistula formation.[95–97]

Dorsalis Pedis and Posterior Tibial Artery Catheterization

The dorsalis pedis and posterior tibial arteries are additional useful sites for arterial cannulation in children when more desirable locations are inaccessible. Collateral circulation should always be checked. If one cannulates or attempts to cannulate one artery in the foot, the other should always be left uninstrumented to ensure adequate collateral blood flow.

Technique. The artery is cannulated in the same manner as the radial artery. The cannulation is attempted at a point of maximal pulsation. One should have a clear picture of the anatomy of the dorsalis pedis and posterior tibial arteries before attempting this procedure. If percutaneous cannulation is impossible, then the cutdown technique should be carried out to ensure successful cannulation.

REFERENCES

1. American Association of Colleges of Nursing: Policy and guidelines for prevention and management of human immunodeficiency virus and hepatitis B virus infection in the nursing education community. J Prof Nurs 1997;13:325–328.
2. Moore S, Goodwin H, Grossberg R, et al: Compliance with universal precautions among pediatric residents. Arch Pediatr Adolesc Med 1998;152:554–557.
3. Tait AR, Tuttle DB: Preventing perioperative transmission of infection: A survey of anesthesiology practice. Anesth Analg 1995;80:764–769.
4. Collins RN, Braun PA, Zinner SH, et al: Risk of local and systemic infection with polyethylene intravenous catheters: A prospective study of 213 catheterizations. N Engl J Med 1968;279:340–343.
5. Duma RJ, Warner JF, Dalton HP: Septicemia from intravenous infusions. N Engl J Med 1971;284:257–260.
6. Smits H, Freedman LR: Prolonged venous catheterization as a cause of sepsis. N Engl J Med 1967;276:1229–1233.
7. Yosowitz P, Ekland DA, Shaw RC, et al: Peripheral intravenous infiltration necrosis. Ann Surg 1975;182:553–556.
8. Phelps SJ, Helms RA: Risk factors affecting infiltration of peripheral venous lines in infants. J Pediatr 1987;111:384–389.
9. Coté CJ, Jobes DR, Schwartz AJ, et al: Two approaches to cannulation of a child's internal jugular vein. Anesthesiology 1979;50:371–373.
10. Seldinger SI: Catheter replacement of the needle in percutaneous arteriography. Acta Radiol 1953;39:368–376.
11. Prince SR, Sullivan RL, Hackel A: Percutaneous catheterization of the internal jugular vein in infants and children. Anesthesiology 1976;44:170–174.
12. Jay AW, Kehler CH: Heart perforation by central venous catheters. Can J Anaesth 1987;34:333–335.
13. Blitt CD, Wright WA, Petty WC, et al: Central venous catheterization via the external jugular vein. A technique employing the J-WIRE. JAMA 1974;229:817–818.
14. Schwartz AJ, Jobes DR, Levy WJ, et al: Intrathoracic vascular catheterization via the external jugular vein. Anesthesiology 1982;56:400–402.
15. Belani KG, Buckley JJ, Gordon JR, et al: Percutaneous cervical central venous line placement: A comparison of the internal and external jugular vein routes. Anesth Analg 1980;59:40–44.
16. Blitt CD, Carlson GL, Wright WA, et al: J-wire versus straight wire for central venous system cannulation via the external jugular vein. Anesth Analg 1982;61:536–537.
17. Stoelting RK: Evaluation of external jugular venous pressure as a reflection of right atrial pressure. Anesthesiology 1973;38:291–294.
18. Boulanger M, Delva E, Mailleet, et al: A new way of access into the internal jugular vein. [in French]. Can Anaesth Soc J 1976;23:609–615.
19. Civetta JM, Gabel JC, Gemer M: Internal-jugular-vein puncture with a margin of safety. Anesthesiology 1972;36:622–623.
20. Hayashi Y, Maruyama K, Takaki O, et al: Optimal placement of CVP catheter in paediatric cardiac patients. Can J Anaesth 1995;42:479–482.
21. Rao TL, Wong AY, Salem MR: A new approach to percutaneous catheterization of the internal jugular vein. Anesthesiology 1977;46:362–364.
22. Casado-Flores J, Valdivielso-Serna A, Perez-Jurado L, et al: Subclavian vein catheterization in critically ill children: Analysis of 322 cannulations. Intensive Care Med 1991;17:350–354.
23. Cogliati AA, Dell'Utri D, Picardi A, et al: Central venous catheterization in pediatric patients affected by hematological malignancies. Haematologica 1995;80:448–450.
24. Klein MD, Rudd M: Successful central venous catheter placement from peripheral subcutaneous veins in children. Anesthesiology 1980;52:447–448.
25. Kuramoto T, Sakabe T: Comparison of success in jugular versus basilic vein technics for central venous pressure catheter positioning. Anesth Analg 1975;54:696–697.
26. Webre DR, Arens JF: Use of cephalic and basilic veins for introduction of central venous catheters. Anesthesiology 1973;38:389–392.
27. Donaldson JS, Morello FP, Junewick JJ, et al: Peripherally inserted central venous catheters: US-guided vascular access in pediatric patients. Radiology 1995;197:542–544.
28. Stovroff MC, Totten M, Glick PL: PIC lines save money and hasten discharge in the care of children with ruptured appendicitis. J Pediatr Surg 1994;29:245–247.
29. Celermajer DS, Robinson JT, Taylor JF: Vascular access in previously catheterized children and adolescents: a prospective study of 131 consecutive cases. Br Heart J 1993;70:554–557.
30. Cilley RE: Intraosseous infusion in infants and children. Semin Pediatr Surg 1992;1:202–207.
31. Driggers DA, Johnson R, Steiner JF, et al: Emergency resuscitation in children: The role of intraosseous infusion. Postgrad Med 1991;89:129–132.
32. Evans RJ, McCabe M, Thomas R: Intraosseous infusion. Br J Hosp Med 1994;51:161–164.
33. Guy J, Haley K, Zuspan SJ: Use of intraosseous infusion in the pediatric trauma patient. J Pediatr Surg 1993;28:158–161.
34. Bilello JF, O'Hair KC, Kirby WC, et al: Intraosseous infusion of dobutamine and isoproterenol. Am J Dis Child 1991;145:165–167.
35. Glaeser PW, Hellmich TR, Szewczuga D, et al: Five-year experience in prehospital intraosseous infusions in children and adults. Ann Emerg Med 1993;22:1119–1124.
36. Losek JD, Szewczuga D, Glaeser PW: Improved prehospital pediatric ALS care after an EMT-paramedic clinical training course. Am J Emerg Med 1994;12:429–432.
37. Seigler RS, Tecklenburg FW, Shealy R: Prehospital intraosseous infusion by emergency medical services personnel: A prospective study. Pediatrics 1989;84:173–177.
38. Fiser RT, Walker WM, Seibert JJ, et al: Tibial length following intraosseous infusion: A prospective, radiographic analysis. Pediatr Emerg Care 1997;13:186–188.
39. Emergency Cardiac Care Committee and Subcommittees, American Heart Association: Guidelines for cardiopulmonary resuscitation and emergency cardiac care. Part VI. Pediatric advanced life support. JAMA 1992;268:2262–2275.
40. Goldstein B, Doody D, Briggs S: Emergency intraosseous infusion in severely burned children. Pediatr Emerg Care 1990;6:195–197.
41. Hurren JS, Dunn KW: Intraosseous infusion for burns resuscitation. Burns 1995;21:285–287.
42. Cardwell ME, Winter B: Pericardial placement of a pulmonary artery catheter. Anaesthesia 1998;53:290–292.
43. Ceneviva G, Paschall JA, Maffei F, et al: Hemodynamic support in fluid-refractory pediatric septic shock. Pediatrics 1998;102:e19.
44. Forrester JS, Ganz W, Diamond G, et al: Thermodilution cardiac output determination with a single flow-directed catheter. Am Heart J 1972;83:306–311.
45. Swan HJ, Ganz W, Forrester J, et al: Catheterization of the heart in man with use of a flow-directed balloon-tipped catheter. N Engl J Med 1970;283:447–451.
46. Thompson AE: Pulmonary artery catheterization in children. New Horiz 1997;5:244–250.
47. Todres ID, Crone RK, Rogers MC, et al: Swan-Ganz catheterization in the critically ill newborn. Crit Care Med 1979;7:330–334.
48. Vedrinne C, Bastien O, De Varax R, et al: Predictive factors for usefulness of fiberoptic pulmonary artery catheter for continuous oxygen saturation in mixed venous blood monitoring in cardiac surgery. Anesth Analg 1997;85:2–10.
49. Vender JS: Clinical utilization of pulmonary artery catheter monitoring. Int Anesthesiol Clin 1993;31:57–85.
50. Kelso LA: Complications associated with pulmonary artery catheterization. New Horiz 1997;5:259–263.
51. Berry AJ, Geer RT, Marshall BE: Alteration of pulmonary blood flow by pulmonary-artery occluded pressure measurement. Anesthesiology 1979;51:164–166.
52. Chun GM, Ellestad MH: Perforation of the pulmonary artery by a Swan-Ganz catheter. N Engl J Med 1971;284:1041–1042.
53. Foote GA, Schabel SI, Hodges M: Pulmonary complications of the flow-directed balloon-tipped catheter. N Engl J Med 1974;290:927–931.
54. Kim YL, Richman KA, Marshall BE: Thrombocytopenia associated with Swan-Ganz catheterization in patients. Anesthesiology 1980;53:261–262.
55. Coté CJ: A simple technique to prevent overdistention of flow-directed catheters. Anesthesiology 1978;49:154.
56. Kitterman JA, Phibbs RH, Tooley WH: Catheterization of umbilical vessels in newborn infants. Pediatr Clin North Am 1970;17:895–912.
57. Guimaraes H, Castelo L, Guimaraes J, et al: Does umbilical vein catheterization to exchange transfusion lead to portal vein thrombosis? Eur J Pediatr 1998;157:461–463.

58. Rehan VK, Cronin CM, Bowman JM: Neonatal portal vein thrombosis successfully treated by regional streptokinase infusion. Eur J Pediatr 1994;153:456–459.

59. Brans YW, Ceballos R, Cassady G: Umbilical catheters and hepatic abscesses. Pediatrics 1974;53:264–266.

60. Fey D, Perrotta L: Peritoneal perforation resulting from umbilical vein catheterization: An unusual pattern. J Pediatr 1973;83:501.

61. Orloff MJ, Orloff MS, Rambotti M: Treatment of bleeding esophagogastric varices due to extrahepatic portal hypertension: Results of portal-systemic shunts during 35 years. J Pediatr Surg 1994;29:142–151.

62. Vos LJ, Potocky V, Broker FH, et al: Splenic vein thrombosis with oesophageal varices: A late complication of umbilical vein catheterization. Ann Surg 1974;180:152–156.

63. Van Niekerk M, Kalis NN, Van der Merwe PL: Cardiac tamponade following umbilical vein catheterization in a neonate. S Afr Med J 1998;88:Suppl-90.

64. Cole AF, Rolbin SH: A technique for rapid catheterization of the umbilical artery. Anesthesiology 1980;53:254–255.

65. Kanarek KS, Kuznicki MB, Blair RC: Infusion of total parenteral nutrition via the umbilical artery. JPEN J Parenter Enteral Nutr 1991;15:71–74.

66. Sherman NJ: Umbilical artery cutdown. J Pediatr Surg 1977;12:723–724.

67. Cohen RS, Ramachandran P, Kim EH, et al: Retrospective analysis of risks associated with an umbilical artery catheter system for continuous monitoring of arterial oxygen tension. J Perinatol 1995;15:195–198.

68. Adelman RD, Karlowicz MG: What is the appropriate workup and treatment for an infant with an umbilical artery catheter-related thrombosis? Semin Nephrol 1998;18:362–364.

69. Fletcher MA, Brown DR, Landers S, et al: Umbilical arterial catheter use: Report of an audit conducted by the Study Group for Complications of Perinatal Care. Am J Perinatol 1994;11:94–99.

70. Ford KT, Teplick SK, Clark RE: Renal artery embolism causing neonatal hypertension: A complication of umbilical artery catheterization. Radiology 1974;113:169–170.

71. Plumer LB, Kaplan GW, Mendoza SA: Hypertension in infants: A complication of umbilical arterial catheterization. J Pediatr 1976;89:802–805.

72. Lott JW, Conner GK, Phillips JB: Umbilical artery catheter blood sampling alters cerebral blood flow velocity in preterm infants. J Perinatol 1996;16:341–345.

73. Umbilical Artery Catheter Trial Study Group: Relationship of intraventricular hemorrhage or death with the level of umbilical artery catheter placement: A multicenter randomized clinical trial.. Pediatrics 1992;90:881–887.

74. Rudolph N, Wang HH, Dragutsky D: Gangrene of the buttock: A complication of umbilical artery catheterization. Pediatrics 1974;53:106–109.

75. Munoz ME, Roche C, Escriba R, et al: Flaccid paraplegia as complication of umbilical artery catheterization. Pediatr Neurol 1993;9:401–403.

76. Bauer SB, Feldman SM, Gellis SS, et al: Neonatal hypertension: A complication of umbilical-artery catheterization. N Engl J Med 1975;293:1032–1033.

77. Cole FS, Todres ID, Shannon DC: Technique for percutaneous cannulation of the radial artery in the newborn infant. J Pediatr 1978;92:105–107.

78. Ducharme FM, Gauthier M, Lacroix J, et al: Incidence of infection related to arterial catheterization in children: A prospective study. Crit Care Med 1988;16:272–276.

79. Furfaro S, Gauthier M, Lacroix J, et al: Arterial catheter-related infections in children: A 1-year cohort analysis. Am J Dis Child 1991;145:1037–1043.

80. Sellden H, Nilsson K, Larsson LE, et al: Radial arterial catheters in children and neonates: A prospective study. Crit Care Med 1987;15:1106–1109.

81. Todres ID, Rogers MC, Shannon DC, et al: Percutaneous catheterization of the radial artery in the critically ill neonate. J Pediatr 1975;87:273–275.

82. Buakham C, Kim JM: Cannulation of a nonpalpable artery with the aid of a Doppler monitor. Anesth Analg 1977;56:125–126.

83. Morray JP, Brandford HG, Barnes LF, et al: Doppler-assisted radial artery cannulation in infants and children. Anesth Analg 1984;63:346–348.

84. Shinozaki T, Deane RS, Mazuzan JE: The dynamic responses of liquid-filled catheter systems for direct measurements of blood pressure. Anesthesiology 1980;53:498–504.

85. Galvis AG, Donahoo JS, White JJ: An improved technique for prolonged arterial catheterization in infants and children. Crit Care Med 1976;4:166–169.

86. Lowenstein E, Little JW, Lo HH: Prevention of cerebral embolization from flushing radial-artery cannulas. N Engl J Med 1971;285:1414–1415.

87. Amato JJ, Solod E, Cleveland RJ: A "second" radial artery for monitoring the perioperative pediatric cardiac patient. J Pediatr Surg 1977;12:715–717.

88. Bedford RF: Radial arterial function following percutaneous cannulation with 18- and 20-gauge catheters. Anesthesiology 1977;47:37–39.

89. Hager DL, Wilson JN: Gangrene of the hand following intra-arterial injection. Arch Surg 1967;94:86–89.

90. Katz AM, Birnbaum M, Moylan J, et al: Gangrene of the hand and forearm: A complication of radial artery cannulation. Crit Care Med 1974;2:270–272.

91. Miyasaka K, Edmonds JF, Conn AW: Complications of radial artery lines in the paediatric patient. Can Anaesth Soc J 1976;23:9–14.

92. Gauderer M, Holgersen LO: Peripheral arterial line insertion in neonates and infants: A simplified method of temporal artery cannulation. J Pediatr Surg 1974;9:875–877.

93. Prian GW, Wright GB, Rumack CM, et al: Apparent cerebral embolization after temporal artery catheterization. J Pediatr 1978;93:115–118.

94. Park MK, Guntheroth WG: Direct blood pressure measurements in brachial and femoral arteries in children. Circulation 1970;41:231–237.

95. Bogart DB, Bogart MA, Miller JT, et al: Femoral artery catheterization complications: a study of 503 consecutive patients. Cathet Cardiovasc Diagn 1995;34:8–13.

96. Riker AI, Gamelli RL: Vascular complications after femoral artery catheterization in burn patients. J Trauma 1996;41:904–905.

97. Taylor LMJ, Troutman R, Feliciano P, et al: Late complications after femoral artery catheterization in children less than five years of age. J Vasc Surg 1990;11:297–304.

Index

Note: Page numbers in *italics* refer to illustrations; page numbers followed by t refer to tables.

Abdomen, trauma to, blunt, 343
  evaluation of, 342–343
Abdominal surgery, postoperative analgesia for, catheter
    techniques for, 685–686
  epidural, 686–687, 687t
Abscess, epidural, with caudal epidural anesthesia,
    650–651, 651t
  peritonsillar, *465*, 465–466
  retropharyngeal, *465*, 465–466
Abuse, child. See *Child abuse.*
Acetaminophen (Tylenol), 152
  for postoperative analgesia, 181, *181–182*, 467, 677–
    678
    dose of, 677
  in outpatients, 61
  glucuronidation of, in neonates, 127
  in myringotomy, 474
  oral and rectal administration of, 181, *181–182*, 707
  pharmacokinetics and pharmacodynamics of, 152
Acetazolamide, for glaucoma therapy, systemic effects
    of, 486
Achondroplasia, airway difficulties with, 117t
Acid aspiration prophylaxis, 42, 183, 184t, 580
α-1-Acid glycoprotein, in children vs. adults, toxicity of
    local anesthetics and, 639
Acid-base balance, dehydration and, 229, *229*
  in congenital diaphragmatic hernia, 304
  in liver transplantation, 556
  in malignant hyperthermia, 619
  in massive blood transfusion, 245–246
Acidosis, metabolic and respiratory, in malignant
    hyperthermia, 619
Acinus, development of, 9
Acquired immunodeficiency syndrome (AIDS), blood
    transfusions and, 235
  informed consent issues with, 75
Actinomyosin ATPase enzyme system, in muscle
    rigidity, in malignant hyperthermia, 619
Acupressure, for nausea after strabismus surgery, 488
Acute respiratory distress syndrome, liver
    transplantation and, 552
Adductor pollicis, evoked tension of, 196, *197*
Adenoidectomy, as outpatient surgery, 56–57
  discharge after, 467
  indications for, 461, 461t
Adenosine, doses and cardiac effects of, 376t, 379
  for supraventricular tachycardia, 285–286
Adenotonsillectomy. See also *Adenoidectomy;*
    Tonsillectomy.
  as outpatient surgery, 56–57
Adenyl cyclase, expression of, in newborn, 366
Admissions, unplanned, after outpatient surgery, 64, 64t
Adolescents, anxiety of, 172
  as emancipated minors, informed consent by, 71, 72
  confidentiality for, 74
  postoperative analgesic technique and, 676
  pregnant, abortions in, informed consent and, 71
  requiring emergency care, 72
Adrenergic drugs, beta agonists as, for treatment of
    hyperkalemia, 231

Adrenergic drugs *(Continued)*
  beta blockers as, doses and cardiac effects of, 371t,
    372, 377–378
    in controlled hypotension, 251
  for asthma, 324t
  for cardiopulmonary resuscitation, 277–278
  for glaucoma therapy, systemic effects of, 486
  for premedication, 180
Adrenergic receptors, beta-, in newborn, 366
Advanced Trauma Life Support, 336
Afterload, in cardiac transplantation, 546
Age. See also *Adolescents; Gestational age; Growth
    and development; Neonates.*
  and parental separation, 173
  facial growth and, 8
  fine motor and adaptive milestones and, 21, 21t
  personal/social milestones and, 21, 21t
  total body water and, 7, 8t
  weight and, 7, 8t
Agitation, emergence. See also *Emergence.*
  halothane vs. sevoflurane use in, 139–140
    in outpatient anesthesia, 60
  in postanesthesia care unit, causes of, 704
  with midazolam, 175
  with parental separation, 25–27, 173, 499. See also
    Parents.
Air, entrainment of, 504
  in central venous catheterization, 550
  in retinal detachment surgery, 487
Air breathing, transition to, 10–11
Air embolism, expired carbon dioxide tension
    measurement and, 729
  monitoring modalities for, *505*
  venous, in neurosurgical procedures, 504–506, *505*
    incidence of, 504
    management of, 504–505, *505*
    in repair of craniosynostosis, 515
    in surgery for brain tumors, 510
    nitrous oxide and, in surgery for congenital heart
      disease, 398
Airflow, resistance to, by endotracheal tubes, 720
Airway(s), 79–116. See also *Breathing; Respiratory
    system; Ventilation.*
  abnormalities of, emergency neonatal surgery for,
    301–304
  access to, with stereotactic head frames, 510, *511*
  anatomy of, developmental, 81–82
    larynx in, 79–81, *80*
    neonatal vs. adult, 81–82
  artificial, glottic aperture seal, 96
    laryngeal mask. See *Laryngeal mask airway.*
    nasopharyngeal, 89–90
      properties of, 719
    oral, in fiberoptic laryngoscopy, 105
      properties of, 719
    oropharyngeal, 89, *90*
      cuffed, 96, *96*, 719
  burn injury of, 523
  collapse of, 267
    in infants, 84–85, *86*

Airway(s) *(Continued)*
  difficult. See also *Airway(s), management of.*
  awake approach to, 98
  cervical spine anomalies causing, 97t, 509
  documentation of, 99
  equipment needed for, 97t, 337, 718–720
  extubation of, 100–101
  intubation of, 103–109. See also *Endotracheal intu-
    bation; Intubation.*
    Bullard laryngoscope for, 107, *108*, 721
    combined techniques of, 108–109
    fiberoptic laryngoscopy for, 105–107, *106*, 721
    laryngeal mask airway as conduit for, 108
    lighted stylet for, 107
    retrograde wire-guided, 107–108
      with flexible fiberoptic scope, 108
    rigid laryngoscopy for, 103–105, *104–105*
      with flexible fiberoptic scope, 108
    sight wands for, 108
  pediatric syndromes and conditions causing, 96–97,
    97t, 117t–120t
  principles of management of, 97–101
  spontaneous ventilation with, 98, *99*
  unexpected, preparation for, 99–100, *100*
  ventilation of. See also *Ventilation.*
    special techniques of, 101–103
  edema of, in infant and adult, 82, *85*
    in prone position, 501–502
  emergency management of, 315–316, *318, 323*
  evaluation of, 87–89, *88*
  gestational and postnatal development of, 9–10
  humidification of, for prevention of heat loss, 614,
    629, 722–723, *724*
  imaging of, 89
  in cardiopulmonary resuscitation, 266–267
  in initial survey of trauma victim, 336–338
  in status epilepticus, 326–327
  laser procedures on, 469–472
  management of, equipment needed for, 97t, 337,
    718–720
    in neurosurgical procedures, 499–500
    normal, 89–96
      laryngeal mask airway for, 94–96, *95*, 95t. See
        also *Laryngeal mask airway.*
      mask ventilation of, 89–90, 101, *101*, 267, 718–
        719
    other airway devices for, 96, 718–720
    tracheal intubation of, 90–94, *91*, 92t, 93t, *93–
      94.* See also *Endotracheal intubation; Intu-
      bation.*
  obstructed, assessment of after rigid bronchoscopy,
    469, *470*
    by hypertrophied tonsils, 463, *464*, 466
    during anesthesia, 87
    dynamics of, 84–85, *86*, 87
    in burn injuries, 523, 524, 526–527, *527*
    in postanesthesia care unit, 704, 705
    initial response to, 317
    lower, emergency management of, 322–325, *323*
    signs of, 317

Airway(s) *(Continued)*
  upper, emergency management of, 319–322
  uptake and distribution of inhalation agents and, 134
  physical examination of, *88,* 88–89
  resistance in, in infants and adults, 13, 87
  surgical, 103
  topical anesthesia of, 98
Albumin, loss of, in burn injuries, 522–523
Alfentanil (Alfenta), pharmacokinetics and pharmacodynamics of, 149
Allergic rhinitis, vs. upper respiratory infection, 43
Allergies, history of, and reactions to contrast agents, 497
  latex, 497
    myelodysplasia and, 516–517
Alveolar hypoventilation, hypertrophied tonsils and, 462, *463*
Alveolar-arterial oxygen difference, in infants and adults, 14
Alveoli, development and growth of, 9
ε-Aminocaproic acid, impaired hemostasis and, on separation from bypass, 401–402
Amiodarone, doses and cardiac effects of, 376t, 378
  in cardiopulmonary resuscitation, 285
Amrinone, doses and cardiac effects of, 366t, 369–370
Analgesia, epidural. See *Epidural analgesia.*
  in burn patients, 536–537
  nonopioid, for premedication, 181–182
  postoperative, 677–678
  patient-controlled, 679–681
    basal infusion feature of, 680
    dosage guidelines for, 680, 680t
    patient training for, 680
    pump settings for, 680
    side effects of, 681
    standing order form for, 680, *682–683*
    variations in, 680–681
  patient-controlled epidural, 686
  postoperative, 61–62
    for tonsillectomy, 61–62
    in emergencies, 317
    intraoperative management of, 677–681
    nonopioid analgesics for, 677–678
    opioid analgesics for, 678–681. See also names of specific drugs, e.g., *Fentanyl.*
    in outpatients, 61
    preoperative planning for, 676–677
      anatomic aspects of, 677
      patient age and, 676
      surgical procedure and, 676–677
    preparation of patient and family for, 677
    regional blockade for, 681–693. See also names of specific blocks, e.g., *Axillary block; Regional blockade.*
    techniques of, 677–681
Anaphylactic shock, 326
Anemia, in end-stage renal failure, 560
  in preoperative evaluation, 42–43
  liver transplantation and, 552
  of prematurity, 20
Anesthesia, in non-operating room location, 571–583. See also specific procedures, e.g., *Computed tomography.*
  equipment for, 572
  facilities evaluation for, 571–572
  goals of, 572–573
  monitoring for, 572
  patient evaluation for, 571
  post-study care of, 580
Anesthesia machine, circuits of, 721–722, *722*
  circle system in, 300, 301t, 722, *723*
  in MRI studies, 578
  Mapleson D system of, 721–722, *722*
  uptake and distribution in, 134–135

Anesthesia machine *(Continued)*
  components of, 721–725
  gas scavenging system of, 721
  humidifiers of, 722–723, *724*
  properties of, 721–725
  ventilator(s) of, 723–725
    intensive care unit types vs. operating room types of, 725
    pediatric use of adult units, 723–724
    volume-controlled vs. pressure-controlled, 724, *724*
Anesthesia record, 725–726
Anesthesia team, 4
Anesthesiologist(s), in consultation with surgeon or health professional, 4
  before sedation, 588, 591
  family/patient interaction with, 1, 37–38, 57–58
  infectious disease precautions for, 248
  postoperative visit of, 4
  production pressure on, 75–76
  radiation protection of, 580
  roles of, 1
  safety of MRI and, 576
Anesthetic agents, analyzers of, 731
  electrophysiologic effects of, 408
  for sedation. See under *Sedation.*
  in status epilepticus, 327
  in surgery for congenital heart disease, 397–399
  inhalation, 133–143. See also names of specific drugs, e.g., *Halothane (Fluothane).*
    avoidance of, with malignant hyperthermia, 626
    ideal, 141
    in neurosurgical procedures, 502–503, 503t
    in renal transplantation, 563
    uptake and distribution of, 134–135
  intravenous, 143–146. See also *Intravenous anesthesia;* names of specific drugs, e.g., *Propofol (Diprivan).*
  minimum alveolar concentration of, with vaporizers in neonates, 138, *138*
  neurophysiologic effects of, 503t
  postoperative apnea and, 47, *48*
  thermoregulatory effects of, 615–616
  topical, 98, 485, 597
  volatile, intraocular pressure and, 481
Aneurysms, intracranial, 511–512
Angiography, anesthesia for, 574–575
Angioplasty, 451
Angiotensin-converting enzyme inhibitors, doses and cardiac effects of, 374
Ankle block, *668,* 668–669
  for postoperative analgesia, 685
Antacids, for premedication, 42, 183, 184t, 580
Anterior commissure scope, for ventilation of difficult airway, 103
Anterior fontanelle, palpation of, 8
Antiarrhythmic agents, doses and cardiac effects of, 375–379, 376t
Antibiotics, for premedication, 183
  in cardiac catheterization, 408
  muscle relaxant action and, 209
Anticholinergic drugs, 155
  for glaucoma therapy, systemic effects of, 486
  for induction in ophthalmologic procedures, 484
  for premedication, 180
Anticonvulsants, for epilepsy, 512
  in status epilepticus, 327
Antidiuretic hormone, in regulation of serum osmolality, 217, *219*
Antiemetic agents, 708. See also names of specific agents; *Nausea and vomiting.*
  after neurosurgical procedures, 506
  after strabismus surgery, 488
  after tonsillectomy, 62, 465, 466
  for premedication, 182–183
Antihistamines, 154–155

Antihistamines *(Continued)*
  for premedication, 180
Antihypertensives, doses and cardiac effects of, 371t, 372
Antisialogogues, in difficult airway managment, 98
Anxiety, age and, 172–173
  behavioral changes with, 25
  in burn patients, 536
  in emergencies, 317
  in postanesthesia care unit, causes of, 704
  parental, in behavioral preoperative programs for children, 29
    in preoperative interview, *30,* 30–31, 37–38
  preoperative, intervention(s) for, behavioral, 28–31
    pharmacologic, 31–32, 172–173
    preoperative interview as, 30–31
    preoperative preparation programs as, 28–29
  outcomes of, 32–34
  postoperative recovery and, 32–34, *33*
  risk factors for, *27,* 27t, 27–28
  separation, 25–26, 173. See also *Parents.*
Anxiolytics, for sedation, 598t–602t, 598–603
Aorta, coarctation of. See *Coarctation of aorta.*
  gestational development of, 10
Aortic valve, stenosis of, cardiac catheterization for, 450
Apert syndrome, airway difficulties with, 117t
Apnea, in cerebral angiography, 575
  in infants, functional residual capacity and, 12–13
  preterm, 45–48
    vs. periodic breathing, 14–15, *14–15*
  types of, 294–295, 295t
  in laser surgery on airway, 471–472
  in trauma cases, 335
  monitoring devices for, 732
  postoperative, 294–295, 295t
    age and, 45–46, *46,* 644
    caffeine and, 47, *47*
    causes of, 47, *47–48*
    in postanesthesia care unit, 705
    preoperative evaluation and, 45–48
    regional anesthesia and, vs. general anesthesia, 47–48, 644
    risk of, 15, 46, *46*
      in former preterm infants, 45–48, 55–56
    with ophthalmologic procedures, 484
    with tonsillectomy, 57
  sleep, abnormalities with, 462, 462t, *463*
    diagnosis of, 462
    presentation of, 462t
    tonsillar hyperplasia and, 461–462
Aprotonin, impaired hemostasis on separation from bypass and, 401–402
Aqueous humor, intraocular pressure and, 479, *480*
Aqueous vasopressin, for diabetes insipidus, after neurosurgical procedures, 507
Arfonad (trimethaphan), in controlled hypotension, 250–252
Arginine vasopressin, in regulation of serum osmolality, 217, *219*
Arrhythmias, atrial septal defect repair and, 427
  drug treatment of, 375–379, 376t
  in brain tumor surgery, 510
  in cardiac transplantation, 546
  in long-term Fontan procedure patients, 449
  in malignant hyperthermia, 619
  in patients with Mustard and Senning procedure repairs, 441
  in postanesthesia care unit, causes of, 705–706
  in tetralogy of Fallot repair, 435–437
  oculocardiac reflex and, 480
  preoperative, cardiac repair and, 418, 419t–421t
  radiofrequency ablation for, 379–380
  succinylcholine use and, 200
  ventricular, with tetralogy of Fallot repair, 437

Arrhythmias *(Continued)*
ventricular septal defect repair and, 430
Arterial blood gases, in burn patients, 533
in controlled hypotension, 254
in pediatric trauma cases, 341
in surgery for congenital heart disease, 395
Arterial pressure, intraocular pressure and, 480
regulation of, 216–218, *219*
Arterial puncture site, in angiographic procedures, care of, 575
Arterial switch operation, for repair of transposition of great arteries, 442t, 442–444, 443t, *443–444*
residua and sequelae with, 362, *363,* 442–444, 443t
risk factors with, 442t, 443t
Arteriovenous malformation, 510–511
angiography for, anesthetic technique for, 574–575
surgery for, complications with, 511–512
Arteriovenous shunts, in hands and feet, in thermoregulatory response, 612
liver transplantation and, 552
Artery(ies), bleeding from, embolization of, 575–576
catheterization of, of dorsalis pedis artery, 753–754
of femoral artery, 753
of posterior tibial artery, 753–754
of radial artery, 751–752, *751–753*
of temporal artery, 752–753
of umbilical artery, 749–751, *750*
techniques of, 749–754
coronary, after arterial switch procedure, 443–444
great, transposition of. See *Transposition of great arteries.*
nonmuscular, pulmonary, 10
partially muscular, pulmonary, 10
percutaneous cannulation of, for blood pressure monitoring, 732
pulmonary. See *Pulmonary artery.*
wall structure of, development of, 10
in fetus and adults, 10
Arthrogryposis multiplex congenita, airway difficulties with, 117t
Artificial nose, for operating room, 614, 629, 716
Asthma, airway obstruction with, emergency management of, 323t–324t, 323–325
anesthesia in, 324–325
in outpatient surgery, 56
in preoperative evaluation, 49–50
Atenolol, doses and cardiac effects of, 372, 378
Atracurium, for intubation, with open eye injury, 489
in renal transplantation, 563
pharmacokinetics of, *202,* 203–204
Atrial communications, opening of, with cardiac catheterization, 451
Atrial septal defect, 426–428
repair of, 427
preoperative factors influencing, 427
residua of, 427–428
sequelae of, 427–428
surgery for, 403–404
types of, *426,* 426–427
Atrial switch procedure, for repair of transposition of great arteries, 438–442, *440–441*
residua and sequelae of, 439–442
Atrioventricular septal defect, 431–433
abnormalities in, 431, *431–433*
repair of, 432
complications with, 433
preoperative factors influencing, 431–432
residua and sequelae of, 432–433
Atropine, 155
for cardiac arrest, 269
for management of oculocardiac reflex, 480
for ophthalmologic procedures, systemic effects of, 485
for premedication, 180
in cardiopulmonary resuscitation, 279

Atropine *(Continued)*
in emergencies, 318
with succinylcholine, for neurosurgical procedures, 500
in rapid-sequence induction, 316
with test dose of local anesthetic, 641
Automobile accidents, blunt trauma with, 343
Axilla, temperature of, 627, *627*
monitoring of, 727
Axillary block, for postoperative pain, 685, 693
Ayre T-piece, of anesthesia circuit, 721, *722*

Baby Doe regulations, 70
Backache, with spinal anesthesia, 647
Bag-valve-mask devices, for ventilation, 267–268
Barbiturates, 143–144
for induction in neurosurgical procedures, 499
for premedication, 176–177
for surgery for congenital heart disease, 400
intraocular pressure and, 481
rectal, for neurosurgical procedures, 498, 499
Basic life support, in trauma cases, 335
Basilar skull fractures, 508
Beckwith-Wiedemann syndrome, airway difficulties with, 117t
Behavioral changes, perioperative anxiety and, 25
Behavioral preoperative programs, for psychological preparation for surgery, 28–29
Benadryl (diphenhydramine), 154
Benzodiazepines, for premedication, 174–176
for sedation, 98, 599, 599t–600t
intraocular pressure and, 481
recovery from, 700
with local anesthetics, 640–641
with opioids for sedation, in difficult airway management, 98
Benzyl alcohol, diazepam administration and, 153
Betaxolol, for glaucoma therapy, systemic effects of, 486
Bier block, 660–661
Bile ducts, growth and development of, 17–18
Bilirubin, in neonates, 17t, 17–18
Bioprosthetic valves, stenosis of, cardiac catheterization treatment for, 450
Biotransformation, drug changes in, 125
Birth weight, and retinopathy of prematurity, 488
and subsequent growth, 7, 8t
classification of, 6, 6t
gestational age and, 38
neonatal problems associated with, 6, 6t
Bispectral Index, for monitoring consciousness, 709, 731
Bladder, temperature of, 628
Blalock-Taussig shunt, for hypoplastic left heart syndrome, 445, *446*
Bleeding. See also *Blood loss.*
arterial, embolization of, 575–576
fibrinolytic, with separation from bypass, 401–402
risk of, ketorolac use and, 152
tests of, coagulopathy diagnosis and, 241
unexpected, in neurosurgical procedures, 504
with adenotonsillectomy or tonsillectomy, 56–57, 466
Bleeding profile, in preoperative evaluation, 41
Blood, autologous donation of, presurgical, 249
autotransfusion of (intraoperative blood scavenging), 249
directed donor, 238, 249
oxygenated to deoxygenated proportions in, hypoxemia with, in congenital heart disease, 360
swallowed, after tonsillectomy, 466
whole, citrated, composition of, 238t
ionized calcium monitoring with, 395
compatibilities of, 237t
dilutional thrombocytopenia and, 242

Blood *(Continued)*
massive transfusion of, hyperkalemia with, 242–244
hypocalcemia with, 244–245
normal, composition of, 238t
transfusion of, after separation from cardiopulmonary bypass, 401
Blood factors, clotting. See *Coagulation factors.*
Blood flow, anesthesia-induced changes in, 613, *614*
cerebral. See *Cerebral blood flow.*
gestational development of, 10
hepatic, drug metabolism and excretion and, 123–124
in shock, 325, 325t
mechanisms of, 270–274
cardiac pump, 270, *272*
thoracic pump, 270, 271, *272, 273*
myocardial, regulation of, in cardiac transplantation, 546
pulmonary, after birth, 10
vs. systemic, in neonates with congenital heart disease, 367–368
Blood loss. See also *Bleeding.*
in burn excision, 534, *534,* 534t
in craniofacial reconstruction, 516
in craniosynostosis repair, 515
in neurosurgical procedures, 503
in surgery for intracranial aneurysms, 511
massive. See also *Blood transfusion, massive.*
with arterial bleeding, 575–576
maximum allowable for red cell transfusion, estimation of, 236
monitors for, 236, 237t, 731
Blood pressure, cerebral blood flow and, 496, *496*
developmental changes in, 16, 16t
in postanesthesia care unit, 706
in surgery for brain tumors, 510
measuring devices for, 726
monitoring of, in MRI studies, 578
invasive, 732
propofol and, 144
with test dose of local anesthetic, 641
Blood product(s), 237–240. See also *Red blood cells.*
compatibilities of, 237t
composition of, 238t
cryoprecipitate as, 239
desmopressin as, 240
factor concentrates as, 239–240
fresh frozen plasma as, 238. See also *Fresh frozen plasma.*
clinical uses of, 238
compatibility of, 237t
composition of, 238t
in trauma cases, 341
platelets as, 237t, 238–239. See also *Platelets.*
rapid administration of, through central lines, 535
reduced patient exposure to, 248–256
by autotransfusion (blood scavenging), 249
by controlled hypotension, 249–254
by directed donation, 249
by hemodilution, 254–256
by presurgical autologous donation, 249
by recombinant erythropoietin, 248–249
warming devices for, 717
whole blood as, 237–238
Blood transfusion, blood volume estimation and, 236–237
in craniosynostosis repair, 515
in neurosurgical procedures, 503–504
in pediatric emergencies, 316
in postoperative care after cardiac surgery, 406
in renal transplantation, 564
in sickle cell disease, 45
massive, 240–248
coagulopathy of, 240–242
factor deficiency with, 240–241, *241*

Blood transfusion (Continued)
  hyperkalemia with, 242–244
  hypocalcemia and, 244–245
  miscellaneous complications of, 247
  monitoring during, 247–248, 248
  side effects of, in liver transplantation, 557–558
  risk with, 235
  screening process for, 235, 236t
  serum citrate levels with, in liver transplantation, 556
  with whole blood, after separation from cardiopulmonary bypass, 401
    hyperkalemia with, 242–244
    hypocalcemia and, 244–245
Blood viscosity, in burn injuries, 525
  in intentional hemodilution, 255
Blood volume, cerebral, and intracranial pressure, 495–496
  circulating, 219, 221t
  estimation of, 236–237
  in neonates, 19–20
Blood-brain barrier, cerebral edema with, in neurosurgical procedures, 503
  damage to, and brain development, 21
  in cardiopulmonary resuscitation, 278
Body compartments, fluid, composition of, 218–219, 221, 221t
  thermal imbalance in, anesthesia-induced, 613–615, 614
Body composition, drug volume of distribution and, 122–123
  in infants with growth, 9
Body water, losses of, normal, 223t
  regulation of, 218–219, 220
  total, 7, 8t, 9, 298
Bone marrow, transplantation of, 564–567
  anesthetic management in, 566–567
  classification of, 565t
  indications for, 565t
  operative procedure for, 565–566
  postoperative care for, 567
  recipient preparation for, 565
  rejection of, 567, 567t
Bowel, blunt trauma to, 343
  large, obstruction of, emergency surgery for, 310
Brachial plexus block, 659, 659–660
Bradycardia, atropine for, 180, 500
  in postanesthesia care unit, 705–706
  in rapid-sequence induction, 316
  oculocardiac reflex and, 480
  postoperative care for, after ophthalmologic procedures, 484
  with succinylcholine, prevention of, 500
Brain, injury of, evaluation of, in trauma patients, 342
  ischemia of, cerebral blood flow and, pathophysiology of, 494, 494
  normal development of, 21
  protection of, after neurosurgical procedures, 506t, 506–507
Brain tumors, craniotomy for, 509–510
Breathing. See also Airway(s); Respiratory function; Ventilation.
  in infants, normal parameters of, 15, 295
    obligate nasal, 82–84
    vs. adults, regulation of, 14–15
  in preterm infants, periodic, vs. apnea, 14–15, 14–15
  in trauma cases, 338, 340
  mechanics of, 11–13
  work of, 85, 87, 87, 295
Bretylium, doses and cardiac effects of, 376t, 378
  in cardiopulmonary resuscitation, 284–285
  toxic reactions to local anesthetics and, 642
Bronchiolitis, airway obstruction with, emergency management of, 322–323
Bronchodilator therapy, for asthma, 324–325
Bronchogenic cysts, congenital, emergency surgery for, 305

Bronchopulmonary dysplasia, in neonates, 295–296
  in preoperative evaluation, 48
Bronchoscopy, anesthesia for, 468–469
  fiberoptic, 105
  in obstructed airway, 319
  rigid, uses and technique of, 103, 468–469
  size of scope vs. endotracheal tube, 468, 469t
Bronchospasm, emergency surgery and, 49–50
  upper respiratory infection and, 44
Bronchus, burn injury of, 523–524, 524
  function of, in infants, 84–85, 86, 87
Brown fat, metabolism of, in non-shivering thermogenesis, 612
Bullard laryngoscope, 721
  in difficult airways, 107, 108
Buphthalmos, in congenital glaucoma, 487
Bupivacaine, cardiac toxicity of, 638
  dose of, in neonates, 639, 687
  for postoperative analgesia, following tonsillectomy, 62
    risks of, 690
  for regional nerve block, in brachial plexus block, 660
    in caudal epidural anesthesia, 650
    in outpatients, 61
    in subarachnoid block, 646, 646t
  pharmacokinetics of, 637
  topical administration of, 598
  with dexamethasone, microspheres of, for long-lasting analgesia, 637, 681, 684
  with epinephrine, for intercostal nerve block, 656
    for neurosurgical procedures, 502
    for postoperative analgesia, 684
Burn injuries, anesthetic management of, 530–536
  awakening in, 536
  drug responses in, 535
  endotracheal tube size in, 536
  general principles of, 530–535
  hyperalimentation in, 536
  methemoglobinemia in, 535–536
  calcium homeostasis in, 526, 526
  cardiac effects of, 523
  circumferential, 529, 529–530
  cutaneous effects of, 525
  drug effects in, 526
  electrical, 530
    from ECG wires in MRI studies, 578
  excision of burn in, blood-conserving techniques in, 534
  gastrointestinal effects of, 525
  heat loss in, minimization of, 531
  hematologic effects of, 525
  hepatic effects of, 524–525
  in children vs. adults, 522, 523
  intravascular volume correction in, 531
  metabolic effects of, 525–526
  monitoring of, 531
  muscle relaxants and, 210
  neurologic effects of, 525
  pathophysiology of, 522–526
  psychological support in, 531
  pulmonary effects of, 523–524
  regional blockade and, 681
  renal effects of, 524
  resuscitation and initial evaluation of, 526–530
    of airway, 526–527
    of associated injuries, 529
    of carbon monoxide poisoning, 527–528, 528
    of circulation, 528–529
    of circumferential burns, 529–530
    of electrical burns, 530
    of oxygenation, 526–527
  sedation and pain control for, 531
  systemic effects of, 530t
Butorphanol (Stadol), 151

Butorphanol (Stadol) (Continued)
  for premedication, 178–179
Butyrophenones, for premedication, 176

Caffeine, postoperative apnea and, 47, 47
Caffeine-halothane muscle contracture testing, indications for, 623, 623t
Calcium, for ionized hypocalcemia, 244, 245
  homeostasis of, in burn injuries, 299, 526, 526
  in cardiopulmonary resuscitation, 281
  ionized, in liver transplantation, 556
    in muscle contraction, in malignant hyperthermia, 618, 618, 619
    in myocardial function, 370
    loss of, in burn injuries, 526, 526, 534–535
      in neonates, 299
    monitoring of, in surgery for congenital heart disease, 395
Calcium channel blockers, in malignant hyperthermia, 619
Calcium chloride, 366t
  doses and cardiac effects of, 366t, 370–372
Calcium gluconate, doses and cardiac effects of, 366t
Calcium-sensitizing agents, doses and cardiac effects of, 372
Cancer. See also Tumors.
  bone marrow transplantation for, 565
Cannulation. See also Catheterization.
  arterial, techniques of, 749–754
  venous, central, 740–746
    intravenous cutdown, 740
    peripheral intravenous, 739–740
    techniques of, 739–749
Capnography, for emergency neonatal surgery, 300, 301t
  in expired carbon dioxide measurements, 730, 730
  vs. pulse oximetry, 728, 728–729
Captopril, doses and cardiac effects of, 374
Carbicarb, in cardiopulmonary resuscitation, 280
Carbon dioxide, analyzers of, 729–731
  end-expired monitoring of, 720, 729–731, 730
    in burn patients, 533–534
    in MRI studies, 578
  end-tidal concentration of, in cardiopulmonary resuscitation, 268, 280
    in malignant hyperthermia, 619–621, 620
    monitoring of, for diagnosis of venous air emboli, 505, 505
      in surgery for moyamoya disease, 512
  expired concentrations of, measurement of, 143
  partial pressure of, arterial, cerebral blood flow and, 497
    normal values of, age-related changes in, 15
  transcutaneous monitors of, 732–733
  ventilatory response to, after inhalation anesthesia, 699
Carbon monoxide poisoning, hyperbaric oxygen and, 537
  in burn injuries, 526–528, 528
Carbon octofluorine, in retinal detachment surgery, 487
Carbonic anhydrase inhibitors, for glaucoma therapy, systemic effects of, 486
Carboxyhemoglobin, in carbon monoxide poisoning, 527
  pulse oximetry and, 727
Cardiac. See also Heart.
Cardiac arrest, perioperative, algorithm for, 271
  bradycardia and, 269–270
  causes of, 268–269
  chest geometry and, 273–274
  incidence of, 268
  rate and duty cycle in, 273
  witnessed, excorporeal membrane oxygenation for, 381
Cardiac catheterization, anesthesia for, 407–409, 579

Cardiac catheterization (Continued)
  data from, in preanesthetic evaluation, 392
  for congenital heart disease, 449–452, 450t
  general rules for, 407
  patient management in, 407–408
  postcatheterization management in, 408–409
  procedures performed during, 407t
  repairs with, 417
Cardiac output, assessment of, by pulsed Doppler
      methods, 16
    in surgery for congenital heart disease, 396
  developmental changes in, 16
  in burn injuries, 523
  in intentional hemodilution, 255
  in neonates, 296, 356, 357–358
  in single-ventricle physiology, 367
  liver transplantation and, 551–552
Cardiac tamponade, during transport to intensive care,
      406
Cardiogenic shock, 325, 326
Cardiomyopathy, 381t, 381–384
  dilated, 381t, 381–382
    causes of, 381, 382
    management of, 382
    prognosis for, 381–382
  hypertrophic, 382–383
    anesthetic management of, 383
Cardiopulmonary bypass, in cardiac transplantation, 546
  in cardiopulmonary resuscitation, 275
  in lung transplantation, 550, 551
  in surgery for congenital heart disease, 399–401
  in ventricular septal defect repair, 404–405
  separation from, 400–401
    impaired hemostasis with, 393, 401–402
    management of, 400–401
  stress response to, 402–403
Cardiopulmonary function, neonatal, 294–297
Cardiopulmonary resuscitation, 265–293
  cardiac pump mechanisms in, 270, 272
  chest compressions in, 273, 273t
  chest geometry in, 273–274
  epidemiology of, 266
  fluid administration during, 276–277
  historical background of, 265–266
  in perioperative cardiac arrest, 268–282
    blood flow mechanisms and, 270–274
  in supraventricular tachycardia, 285–286
  in ventricular fibrillation, 282–285
  management of, 266–268
  monitoring during, 275–276
  newer techniques of, 274–277
    abdominal binding, 274
    abdominal compression, 274–275
    active compression-decompression, 274
    cardiopulmonary bypass, 275
    open chest, 275
    simultaneous compression and ventilation, 274
  outcome of, 266
  pharmacology of, 277–282
  pulseless electrical activity and, 286
  thoracic pump mechanisms in, 270, 271, 272, 273
  vascular access during, 276
  ventilatory rate in, 273, 273t
Cardiovascular function, desflurane use and, 140
  drugs affecting, 365–379
    antiarrhythmic agents as, 375–379, 376t
    local anesthetics as, 638, 641, 642
    vasoactive, 365–375, 366t
  fetal circulation and, 353–354, 354–355
  growth and development of, 15–16
  halothane use and, 135
  in congenital diaphragmatic hernia, 304
  in liver transplantation, 555–556
  in neonates, 353–357
  invasive monitoring equipment for, 3, 732

Cardiovascular function (Continued)
    sevoflurane use and, 137–138
    transitional circulation and, 354–356, 355t
Cartilage, laryngeal, 79, 80
Cataracts, congenital, surgery for, 487
Catecholamines, in stress response to cardiac surgery,
      402
  isoflurane use and, 137
Catheter(s), arterial, for neurosurgical procedures,
      498–499
    in congenital heart disease surgery, 395–396
    in massive blood transfusion, 247, 248
  axillary, for administration of postoperative analgesia,
      693
  caudal. See Caudal epidural anesthesia.
  central venous. See Catheterization, central venous.
  epidural. See also Epidural analgesia; Epidural anes-
      thesia.
    insertion of, 648–649
      chloroprocaine test for, 687, 687t
      infection with, 651
      thoracic, 686
    techniques with, for regional blockade, 685–693
      infusion solutions for, 685t
  for fluid administration, 224
  intraosseous, 224
  intrapleural, for administration of postoperative anal-
      gesia, 693
  intravascular, in neurosurgical procedures, 500–501
  intravenous, insertion of, in children, 739–740
    large diameter vs. small diameter, 718
    pressure-flow relationship of, 718, 718
  migration of, into subarachnoid space, 692–693
  pulmonary artery, for monitoring, 732
    in lung transplantation, 549
    in massive blood transfusion, 248
    technique of insertion of, 746–747, 748–749
  suction, for operating room, 716
  techniques with, approach used with, 685
    for pulmonary artery catheterization, 746–747,
      748–749
    for regional blockade, 685–693
    for upper abdominal or thoracic surgery, 685–686
    nursing management of, 686, 688–689, 693
    size of catheter for, 685
  umbilical, in neonates, 298
  urinary, 732
    in massive blood transfusion, 247
  ventricular, for monitoring intracranial pressure, 495
Catheterization. See also Catheter(s).
  cardiac. See Cardiac catheterization.
  central venous, for blood pressure monitoring, 732
    in neurosurgical procedures, 499, 505
    in surgery for congenital heart disease, 396
    indications for, 740
    of brachiocephalic vein, 743, 746
    of external jugular vein, 740
    of femoral vein, 746
    of internal jugular vein, 740, 742, 743, 744–745
    of subclavian vein, 743
    percutaneous approach to, 740, 741–742
    Seldinger (percutaneous) approach to, 740, 741–
      742
    techniques of, 740–746
  pressure in, in lung transplantation, 550
    in massive blood transfusion, 247–248
  pulmonary artery, 746–747, 748–749
  umbilical vein, 747, 749, 749
Caudal block, for postoperative analgesia, agents used
      for, 684
  in outpatients, 61
Caudal epidural anesthesia, 647–650
  complications with, 650, 650–651, 651t
  continuous infusion with, 649–650
  drug selection for, 649

Caudal epidural anesthesia (Continued)
  opioids with, 650, 651. See also Opioids, epidural.
  technique of, 647–649, 648, 650, 685
Celebrex (celecoxib), for postoperative analgesia, 678
Celecoxib (Celebrex), for postoperative analgesia, 678
Central nervous system, congenital anomalies of, 516,
      516–517
  drug effects on, 132–133
  dysfunction of, sleep apnea and, 462
  in burn injuries, 525
  in controlled hypotension, 249–250
  in mitochondrial disorders, 383
  local anesthetic toxicity of, signs of, 638
  neonatal development of, 299
  pathophysiology of, 493–497
    intracranial compartments in, 493–494
Central neuraxial blockade, vs. peripheral nerve blocks,
      651–652
Central venous lines. See Catheterization, central
      venous.
Cerebral angiography, anesthetic technique for, 574–575
Cerebral blood flow, blood pressure and, 496, 496
  brain ischemia and, 494, 494
  carbon dioxide and, 497
  cerebrovascular autoregulation of, 496–497
  halothane use and, 135
  in cardiopulmonary resuscitation, 278
  in controlled hypotension, 249–250
  intracranial pressure and, 495–496
  isoflurane use and, 137
  normal, 496
  oxygenation and, 496–497
Cerebral blood volume, and intracranial pressure,
      495–496
Cerebral edema, prevention of, in neurosurgical
      procedures, 503–504
Cerebral hemispheres, tumors of, 510
Cerebral metabolic rate for oxygen (CMRO$_2$), and
      cerebral blood flow, 496
  in controlled hypotension, 249
Cerebral perfusion pressure, and brain ischemia, 494,
      494
  and intracranial pressure, 496
  in trauma patients, 342
Cerebrospinal fluid (CSF), and intracranial pressure,
      493–494
  in hydrocephalus, 514
  production and absorption of, 493–494
  translocation of, 494
  volume of, local anesthetics and, 642, 643
Cerebrovascular autoregulation, 496–497
Cervical spine, conditions of, causing airway
      difficulties, 97t
  in infants and adults, central nerve blocks and, 642,
      642
  injury of, 508–509
    airway control in, for cardiopulmonary resuscita-
      tion, 266
    in trauma cases, 336, 338, 342
CHARGE association, emergency neonatal surgery for,
      301
Chemical effects, of burn injuries, 523
Cherubism, airway difficulties with, 117t
Chest wall, in infants, in central neuraxial blockade,
      643
  in newborns, respiratory function and, 11
Chiari malformation, myelodysplasia and, 517, 517,
      517t
  types of, 517, 517t
Child abuse, in trauma cases, 329
  signs of, 345, 346
  suspicion of, 75
Child life specialists, in behavioral preoperative
      programs for children, 28
  preoperative preparation by, for outpatient surgery,
      57–58

Children, deceased, procedures practiced on, informed consent for, 75
Chloral hydrate, 154
  for premedication, 177
    for sedation, 598t, 598–599
      for CT scans, 574
  pharmacokinetics and pharmacodynamics of, 154
Chloramphenicol, in neonates, 125
Chloroprocaine, for postoperative analgesia, in infants, 687
  with epidural catheter, 686, 687, 687t
  in caudal epidural anesthesia, 650
  in neonatal regional blockade, 637
Choanal atresia and stenosis, emergency neonatal surgery for, 301
Cholinergic drugs, for glaucoma therapy, systemic effects of, 486
Chronic lung disease, in neonates, 295–296
Cimetidine (Tagamet), 154–155
  for premedication, 42, 184, 184t
Circuits, of anesthesia machine. See *Anesthesia machine, circuits of.*
Circulation, fetal, 353–354, *354–355,* 357
  in burn patients, 528–529
  in neonates, 296–297
  in status epilepticus, 327
  in transposition of great arteries, 437, *438–439*
  in trauma cases, 340
  mechanical support devices for, 380–381
  problems with, emergency management of, 325t, 325–326
  systemic and pulmonary balance of, in neonates with congenital heart disease, 367–368
  transitional, 354–356, 355t
    conditions prolonging, 359t
Circulatory arrest, hypothermic, in repair of neonatal cardiac defects, 400
Circumcision, dorsal nerve block for, 61
Cisatracurium, pharmacokinetics of, 204
Citrate, in blood products, 235t
  hyperkalemia with, 242–244
  hypocalcemia and, 244–245
  in liver transplantation, 556
  ionized calcium monitoring with, 395
Clonidine, for nausea after strabismus surgery, 488
  for postoperative analgesia, in caudal block, 684
  for premedication, 180
Coagulation, evaluation of, by thromboelastography, 555, *555*
  in newborn, 20
Coagulation factors, after bypass in congenital heart disease, 394
  concentrates of, 239–240
  factor VIII, 239–241
Coagulopathy, in liver transplantation, 552, 556–557
  regional blockade and, 681
  with massive blood transfusion, 240–242, *241*
Coarctation of aorta, 424–426
  associated defects with, 424
  complications of, 426
  infantile and adult forms of, 424, *424*
  natural history of, after repair, 425
  recurrent, balloon angioplasty for, 451
  repair of, 424–425, *425*
  residua of, 425
  sequelae of, 425–426
  surgery for, 405–406
Cocaine hydrochloride, for ophthalmologic procedures, systemic effects of, 485
Collagen vascular diseases, inflammatory, cardiac pathophysiology with, 365
Colloid solutions, in trauma cases, 341
Complement, impaired hemostasis on separation from bypass and, 401
Computed tomography, anesthesia for, *573,* 573–574

Conductance, in heat transfer during anesthesia, 614
Congenital abnormalities, in preoperative evaluation, 39
  of central nervous system, *516,* 516–517
Congenital dystrophica myotonica, 210
Congenital heart disease, 353. See also specific types, e.g., *Patent ductus arteriosus.*
  anesthetic management of, 394–397
    agents used in, 397–399
    cardiopulmonary bypass in, 399–401
    control of vascular resistance during, 397, 397t
    impaired hemostasis after bypass in, 401–402
    in specific defects, 403–406
    induction in, 396–397
    maintenance in, 397
    monitoring in, 395–396
    planning for, 394–395
    preanesthetic evaluation for, 392–393
    premedication in, 395
    specific problems in, 393–394
  arrhythmias in, 419t–421t
  cardiac catheterization for, 449–452, 450t
  clinical signs of, 359
  cyanotic, 393
  history of, 392
  hypoxemia in, 359–360
  incidence and terminology of, 415–416, 416t
  laboratory evaluation for, 392–393
  outcome of, 409
  outpatient surgery and, 56
  physical examination for, 392
  physiologic categories of, 358–360, *360*
  pressure loading in, 359, *360*
  prevalence of, 357–358, 359t
  repaired, 415–460
    arrhythmias in, 419t–421t
    complications of, 417
    definitive, 416–417
    endocarditis risk in, 421, 421t–423t
    evaluation of, 452, 452t
    interventional (cardiac catheterization), 417
    monitoring in, 419
    noncardiac defects in, 419, 421
    outcome after, 417–418
      preoperative factors influencing, 417–419
    palliative, 417
    perioperative considerations in, 360–362, *361*
    psychosocial concerns in, 419, 421
    residua of, 417
    risks with, 419, 421, 452
    sequelae of, 417
  shunts with, 393t, 393–394. See also *Shunt(s), intracardiac.*
  single ventricle. See *Ventricle(s), single.*
  surgery for, postoperative care in, 406–407
    procedures performed for, 403t
    stress response to, 402–403
  systemic vs. pulmonary blood flow in, drug treatment for, 367–368
  unrepaired, arrhythmias in, 419t
  volume loading in, 358–359, *360*
Congestive heart failure, in atrioventricular septal defect patients, 432
  preoperative, cardiac repair and, 418
Continuous positive airway pressure, in emergencies, 318, *318*
Contrast agents, for radiologic or angiographic studies, 575
  low- and high-osmolality types of, 575
  reactions to, 497
Convection, in heat transfer during anesthesia, 614
Cooley's anemia (thalassemia major), airway difficulties with, 120t
Cor pulmonale, hypertrophied tonsils and, 462, *463*
Cornelia de Lange syndrome, airway difficulties with, 117t

Coronary arteries, after arterial switch procedure, 443–444
Corpus callostomy, for seizures, 513
Corticosteroids, for asthma, 324t
  for premedication, 183
  for spine injury, 509
  topical, for glaucoma therapy, systemic effects of, 487
Costs, in choice of drugs for postoperative nausea and vomiting, 63
  of diagnostic procedures outside operating room, 584–585
Cox-2 antagonists, for postoperative analgesia, 678
Craniofacial dysostosis (Crouzon's syndrome), airway difficulties with, 117t
Craniofacial reconstruction, 515–516
Craniopharyngioma, 510
Craniosynostosis, 8, 514–515
Craniotomy, "awake," 513
  for brain tumors, 509–510
Crash cart, in operating room, 725, 725t
  in postanesthesia care unit, 702t, 703t, 710
Creatine kinase, serum, succinylcholine use and, 201
Cricoid pressure, in bag-valve-mask ventilation, 267
  in emergencies, 318
  in manual hyperventilation, 500
  in rapid-sequence induction, 42, 188, 316, 337, 339t, 554
Cricothyroid angle, during phonation, 81
Cricothyrotomy, in trauma cases, 338
  percutaneous dilation, for ventilation, 101–102, *103*
  percutaneous needle, for ventilation, 101–102, *102–103*
    vs. laryngeal mask airway, 102–103
  with spinal injury, 509
Croup, after outpatient surgery, 64
  emergency management of, 320–321, *321*
  postintubation, 93
  in postanesthesia care unit, 705
Crouzon's syndrome (craniofacial dysostosis), airway difficulties with, 117t
Cryoprecipitate, 239
  for impaired hemostasis on separation from bypass, 401
Cryotherapy, for retinopathy of prematurity, 489
Crystalloid solutions, flow of in intravenous catheters, 718, *718*
  in burn patients, 528
  in neurosurgical procedures, 504
  in trauma cases, 341
CSF. See *Cerebrospinal fluid (CSF).*
Curare, metabolism of, renal function and, 128
Cyanide poisoning, in burned patients, 527
Cyanosis, in burn patients, methemoglobinemia and, 535
  in repair of tetralogy of Fallot, 405
  in repair of ventricular septal defect, 404
  preoperative, cardiac repair and, 418
Cyclocryotherapy, for repair of infantile glaucoma, 487
Cyclopentolate hydrochloride, for ophthalmologic procedures, systemic effects of, 485
Cycloplegics, for ophthalmologic procedures, systemic effects of, 485
Cysts, pulmonary and bronchogenic congenital, emergency surgery for, 305
Cytochrome P450 system, developmental changes in, 125, 126t
  phase I drug metabolism and, 125, 126t
Cytokines, impaired hemostasis on separation from bypass and, 401

Damus-Stansel-Kaye operation, for relief of systemic outflow obstruction, 445, *447*
Dantrolene, for malignant hyperthermia, 617, 619, 624–625, *625*

Dantrolene *(Continued)*
    actions of, 625–626, 626t
    dose of, 624–625
    effects of, on intracellular calcium, 618
    pretreatment with, 626
    properties of, 625–626
    response to, 625
    side effects of, 626, 626t
    signs and symptoms of continuing episode with, 625t
DDAVP (desmopressin), clinical uses of, 240
Death, sudden, with tetralogy of Fallot repair, 436
Decadron, for postoperative vomiting, 708
Defibrillators, for operating room, 725
Dehydration, acid-base imbalance and, 229, *229*
    after tonsillectomy, 466
    management of, 227–230. See also *Fluid(s), management of.*
    osmolar disturbance and, 228–229
    potassium homeostasis and, 229
    renal function impairment and, 229
    signs and symptoms of, 228t
    volume deficit and, 228
    with diuretics, in neurosurgical procedures, 504
Demerol. See *Meperidine (Demerol).*
Dental mirror, for aid in rigid laryngoscopy, 104
Dental procedures, endocarditis prophylaxis with, 422t
Denver developmental screening test, for assessing mental milestones, 21, 21t
Desflurane (Suprane), 140t, 140–141, *141*
    cardiovascular effects of, 140
    concerns with, 141
    in outpatient anesthesia, 60
    in rigid bronchoscopy, 468
    recovery time from, 699
Dexamethasone, for bronchopulmonary dysplasia in neonates, 296
    for postoperative analgesia following tonsillectomy, 62
    for premedication, 183
    with bupivacaine microspheres, for long-lasting analgesia, 637, 681, 684
Diabetes insipidus, 232
    postoperative, after neurosurgical procedures, 507
        treatment of, 510
    with craniopharyngioma, 510
Diabetes mellitus, maternal, effects on infant of, 6, 19
    outpatient surgery and, 56
    preoperative evaluation of, 48–49
Diagnostic studies, sedation and anesthesia for, 584–585
Dialysis, before renal transplantation, 561–562
Diamox (acetazolamide), for glaucoma therapy, systemic effects of, 486
Diaphragm, in breathing, in central neuraxial blockade, 643
    in epidural anesthesia, 677
Diaphragmatic hernia, congenital, emergency surgery for, *304,* 304–305
    survival from, 305
Diazepam (Valium), 152–153
    electroencephalographic effect of, vs. midazolam, *176*
    for premedication, 175, 640
    for sedation, 599, 599t
    pharmacokinetics and pharmacodynamics of, 152–153, *153*
Dichloroacetate, in cardiopulmonary resuscitation, 280
Digital block, for postoperative analgesia, epinephrine and, 684
    of fingers, *663,* 663–664
    of foot, 669
Digoxin, doses and cardiac effects of, 366t, 370, 376t, 379
    toxicity of, 379
Dimenhydrinate, for premedication, 183
    for postoperative nausea and vomiting, in outpatients, 62

Diphenhydramine (Benadryl), 154
    for premedication, 180
2,3-Diphosphoglycerate, oxygen-hemoglobin dissociation and, 246–247, 247t
Diprivan. See *Propofol (Diprivan).*
Discharge criteria, after outpatient surgery, 63–64
    fast track, 65
    from postanesthesia care unit, 703t, 703–704, 704t
    fast track, 709, 710t
Disseminated intravascular coagulopathy, vs. dilutional coagulopathy, in massive blood loss, 245
    with massive blood transfusion, 245
Diuretics, in neurosurgical procedures, 504
DNA markers, for malignant hyperthermia, 617, *617*
Dobutamine, doses and cardiac effects of, 366t, 368–369
Donors, of bone marrow transplants, preparation and presentation of, 566
Do-not-resuscitate (DNR) orders, in operating room, informed consent and, 72–73
Dopamine, doses and cardiac effects of, 366t, 368
    in cardiac transplantation, 547
Doppler ultrasonography, precordial, for venous air emboli, 504–505, *505*
Dorsalis pedis artery, catheterization of, 753–754
Dorzolamide, for glaucoma therapy, systemic effects of, 486
Down syndrome (trisomy 21), airway difficulties with, 120t
    congenital heart disease with, 362
Doxacurium, pharmacokinetics of, 207–208
DPT. See *Lytic cocktail (DPT).*
Dreaming, perioperative, succinylcholine use and, 201
Droperidol (Inapsine), 146
    advantages and disadvantages of, 146
    for postoperative nausea and vomiting, 708
        after strabismus surgery, 488
        after tonsillectomy, 466
        in outpatients, 62
    for premedication, 176, 182–183
Drugs. See also names of specific drugs and classes of drugs, e.g., *Narcotics; Midazolam (Versed).*
    anesthetic. See *Anesthetic agents.*
    approval process for, 133
    distribution of, 122–123
        apparent volume of, 131–132
        body composition and, 122–123
        protein binding of, 122, *122*
        volume of, in infants vs. adults, 122–123, *123*
    dosing of, lethal in 50%, 132
        loading, 132
        repetitive, and drug accumulation, 132
    effects of, in burn injuries, 526, 535
        on central nervous system, 132–133
    for crash cart, in operating room, 725, 725t
    in postanesthesia care unit, 703t
    for glaucoma therapy, systemic effects of, 485–487
    for premedication, 174–184. See also *Premedication.*
    inotropic. See *Inotropic drugs.*
    labeling and studies of, FDA approval of, 133, 202, 597
    metabolism of, 124–127, 126t, 127t
        cytochrome P450 system in, 125, 126t
        hepatic blood flow and, 123–124
        phase I reactions in, 124–125, 126t
        phase II (conjugation) reactions in, 125, 127
    package insert for, 133
    pharmacokinetic principles of, 131–132
        Michaelis-Menton kinetics and, 131, *131*
    pharmacologic principles of, 128–132
        first-order kinetics of, 128
            multicompartment, 129–130, *130*
            single-compartment, 129
        half-life of, 128–129, *129,* 637
        loading dose in, 132

Drugs *(Continued)*
    repetitive dosing and drug accumulation in, 132
        steady state in, 132
        zero-order kinetics of, 130–131, *131*
    renal excretion of, 127–128, *127–128*
    shorter-acting, and fast track recovery, 709
    unapproved use vs. improper use of, 133
    vasoactive. See *Vasoactive drugs.*
Dubowitz scoring system, of gestational age, 6
Duchenne muscular dystrophy, muscle relaxants for, 209–210
Duodenal atresia, congenital, emergency surgery for, *307,* 307–308
Dysrhythmias. See *Arrhythmias.*
Dystrophin, in Duchenne muscular dystrophy, 209

Ear, middle, 475
    surgery on, 473–475
        for myringotomy and tube insertion, 473–475
Echocardiography, 733
    in preanesthetic evaluation, 392–393
    in surgery for congenital heart disease, 396
    transesophageal, in surgery for congenital heart disease, 396
Echothiophate iodide, for glaucoma therapy, systemic effects of, 486
ECMO, for mechanical circulatory support, 380–381
Edema, airway, in infants and adults, 82, *85*
    in prone position, 501–502
    cerebral, in neurosurgical procedures, 503–504
    differential diagnosis of, 228t
    in burn patients, escharotomy for, 529, *529*
        fluid replacement and, 528
        management of, 227
    pulmonary, after tonsillectomy, 466
Edrophonium, for reversal of muscle relaxants, 208
Elastic recoil, of lungs, closing capacity and, 13
    development of, 11–12
    functional residual capacity and, 12
Elbow, peripheral nerve blocks at, 661
Electrical burns, 530
    from electrocardiographic wires, in MRI studies, 578
Electrocardiographic leads, in burn patients, 534
Electrocardiographic studies, 726–727
    age-related changes in, 16
    in cardiac transplantation, 546
    in MRI, hazards of, 578
    of bupivacaine combined with epinephrine, *638,* 638–639
    of local anesthetics, 639, 641
Electrocautery, 733
Electrocorticography, during seizure surgery, 513, *513*
Electroencephalographic studies, bispectral analysis of, 709, 731
    in seizure surgery, 513
Electrolytes. See also *Fluid and electrolyte status.*
    distribution of, 219, *221*
    regulation of, 216–218, *218*
        in emergencies, 316
    requirements for, 222–223, 223t
Electromechanical dissociation (pulseless electrical activity), 286
Embolization procedures, anesthesia for, 575–576
    for arteriovenous malformations, 511
    in neuroradiologic procedures, 518
Emergence, agitation with, halothane vs. sevoflurane use and, 139–140
    in outpatients, 60
    delirium with, in postanesthesia care unit, 704
    in neurosurgical procedures, 506t, 506–507, 511
    in ophthalmologic procedures, 484
Emergencies, equipment in, for "crash cart," 702t, 710, 725, 725t
    in neonates, 294–314

Emergency medical technicians, response of, in trauma cases, 335
Emergency room, anesthesia in, 579–580
  care of surgical patients in, *328,* 328–329
  care of trauma victims in, 335–336
    equipment needed for, 335t
    team approach to, 336
  procedures in, sedation for, 586–587
Emergency surgery, 315–333
  airway management in, 317–325
  anesthesia for, 315–317
  circulation in, and shock, 325–326
  emergency room management in, *328,* 328–329
  in neonates, for gastrointestinal problems, 305–310
    for respiratory problems, 300–305
  operating room management in, 329–330
  pain management in, 317
  poisoning in, 327
  status epilepticus in, 326–327
  trauma in, 328
Emesis. See *Nausea and vomiting.*
EMLA cream (eutectic mixture of local anesthetics), for neurosurgical procedures, 498
  for outpatient anesthesia, 60
  for premedication for ophthalmologic procedures, 483
  in neonates, 638
  topical administration and doses of, 597
Emphysema, congenital lobar, emergency surgery for, 305
Enalapril, doses and cardiac effects of, 371t, 374
Encephalocele, 516, *516*
Endocarditis, cardiac pathophysiology with, 365
  risk of, in repaired congenital heart disease, 421, 421t–423t
Endoscopy, gastrointestinal, sedation for, 586–587
  masks for, 105
Endotracheal intubation. See also *Intubation.*
  in cardiopulmonary resuscitation, access for, 276–277
    airway control in, 266–267
  in congenital diaphragmatic hernia, 304
  in emergency cases, by nonanesthesiologists, 335, 337
  in epiglottitis, 319
  in infants and adults, 82
  in infants with tracheoesophageal fistula, 303
  in MRI studies, 579
  in neurosurgical procedures, 499–500
  in ophthalmologic procedures, 484
  in rigid bronchoscopy, 468, 469, 469t, *470*
  in tonsillectomy, 463
    vs. laryngeal mask airway, 464
  in trauma cases, 338, *340*
    on site, 335
  intraocular pressure and, 482
  technique of, 90–94, *91,* 92t, 93t, *93–94*
    blind, 98, *99*
    distance for, 92–93, *93,* 93t
    in infants and adults, 82
  upper respiratory infection and, 44
  with bag-valve-mask devices for ventilation, 268
Endotracheal tubes, airflow resistance by, 720, *720*
  complications of, 93–94, *94*
  cuffed and uncuffed, in burn patients, 527
    in laser surgery, 471, *471*
    in operating room, 719–720
    in ophthalmologic procedures, 484
  drug administration through, in neonates, 298
  for operating room, ignition of, 720
    molded preformed, 720
    plastic vs. metal, 471, 471t
    selection of, 92, 92t
    sizes and types of, 719–720
    with Tovell spiral wire reinforcement, 720
  in asthmatic patients, 49, 56
  in burn patients, 527, 534, 536

Endotracheal tubes *(Continued)*
  in fiberoptic laryngoscopy, 106–107
  in laser surgery, 471, *471,* 471t
  in lung transplantation, 550
  injuries from, pathogenesis of, 94, *94*
Enflurane, intraocular pressure and, 481
Enoximone, doses and cardiac effects of, 370
Enteral feeding, in burn patients, 525
Epidermolysis bullosa, airway difficulties with, 118t
Epidural analgesia, 685–693
  adverse effects of, 690, 692–693
    treatment of, 690t
  catheter migration in, 692–693
  clinical examples of, 691t
  for thoracic or upper abdominal surgery, doses of, 687, 690, 690t
  order sheets for, *688–689*
Epidural anesthesia, caudal, 647–650
  complications with, *650,* 650–651, 651t
  continuous infusions with, 649–650
  drug selection for, 649
  opioids with, 650
  technique of, 647–649, *648, 650*
  diaphragmatic mechanics and, 677
  technique of, for regional blockade, 685, 685t, 693
Epidural hematoma, surgery for, 508
Epidural monitors, for monitoring intracranial pressure, 495
Epiglottis, in infant and adult, 82, *84–85*
Epiglottitis, airway obstruction with, emergency management of, 319–320, *320*
Epilepsy, surgery for, 512–513
  temporal lobe, methohexital-induced seizures and, 573
Epinephrine, as marker for intravascular injection, in test dose of local anesthetic, 641
  doses and cardiac effects of, 366t, 369
  in burn excision, for prevention of blood loss, 534
  in cardiac arrest, 269
  in cardiopulmonary resuscitation, 277–279
  in glaucoma therapy, systemic effects of, 486
  in halothane anesthesia, in children vs. adults, 135
  with bupivacaine, for neurosurgical procedures, 502
    for postoperative analgesia, 684
    in intercostal nerve block, 656
  with local anesthetics, calculations for, 640, 640t–641t
    in peripheral nerve blocks, 652
Equipment, for airway management, 97t, *99,* 104, 337, 718–720, 721
  for anesthesia in non-operating room location, 572
  for anesthesia in operating room, 715–738
  for anesthesia machine, 721–725
  for "crash cart," in operating room, 725, 725t
    in PACU, 702t, 703t, 710
  for echocardiography, 733
  for electrocautery, 733
  for emergency neonatal surgery, 300, 301t
  for fiberoptic laryngoscopy, 105
  for heating and cooling systems in OR, 715
  for intravenous therapy, *717,* 717–718
  for lung transplantation, 549
  for monitoring, 725–733
  for operating table, 716
  for suction apparatus, 715–716
  for trauma room, 335t, 335–336
  for warming devices, 716–717
  purchase of, 733–734
Erythropoiesis, in newborns and infants, 20
Erythropoietin, recombinant, before renal transplantation, 561
  uses of, 248–249
Escharotomy, in burn patients, 529, *529*
Esmolol, doses and cardiac effects of, 371t, 372, 376t, 378

Esophageal atresia, 18
  emergency neonatal surgery for, 302–304, *303*
Esophagus, procedures on, endocarditis prophylaxis with, 422t
  temperature of, *627,* 627–628
Ethics, 68–78
  acquired immunodeficiency syndrome in children and, 75
  confidentiality for adolescents and, 74
  consultation service for, 76
  forgoing life-sustaining treatment and, 72–73
  informed consent and, 68–72
  pain management and, 73–74
  pediatric research in, special requirements for, 74
  procedures on deceased children and, 75
  production pressure on anesthesiologists and, 75–76
  suspicion of child abuse and, 75
Etomidate, for induction, 187, 187t
  in neurosurgical procedures, 499
  in trauma cases, 345
  intraocular pressure and, 481
Evaporation, in heat transfer during anesthesia, 614
Evoked response, for evaluation of neuromuscular function, 186, *197*
Expiration, airway obstruction during, in infants, *86*
  laryngeal function during, 81
  normal, in infants, *86*
Extracellular volume, in infants, 9
Extracorporeal membrane oxygenation, for mechanical circulatory support, 380–381
Extraocular muscles, traction on, oculocardiac reflex with, 480, *481*
Extremity(ies), lower, postoperative analgesia for, 686–687, 687t
    via peripheral nerve blocks, 664–669
    via regional blockade, 684–685
  sensory innervation of, *664*
  upper, nerve block(s) of, Bier block as, 660–661
    brachial plexus block as, *659,* 659–660
Extubation, 100–101
  after cardiac surgery, 406
  after neurosurgical procedures, 506–507
  after ophthalmologic procedures, 484
  procedure for, 701
  timing of, 701
Eyes, intraocular pressure in. See *Intraocular pressure.*
  laser surgery hazards and, 469–470
  pathophysiology of, 479–482
  surgery on, anesthesia for, 482–484
    drugs for, systemic effects of, 484–485
    for congenital cataracts, 487
    for glaucoma, 487–488
    for open eye injury with full stomach, 489–490
    for retinopathy of prematurity, 488–489
    for strabismus, 488

Face, growth of, 8
Face masks, for endoscopy, 105
  for ventilation, in bag-valve-mask devices, 267
    multihanded techniques with, 101, *101*
    of normal airway, 89–90
  in premedication for ophthalmologic procedures, 483
  pediatric, 718–719
Facial burns, 527, *527*
Failure to thrive, causes of, 8t
Family history, of anesthesia complications, 39
Faraday cage, 576
Fascia iliaca block, *667,* 667–668
  for postoperative analgesia, vs. caudal blockade, 684–685
Fasciculations, succinylcholine use and, 201
Fast track recovery, 65, 709, 710t
Fasting, before sedation, guidelines for, 588t
  fluid recommendations for, 225t, 225–226
  in emergency room patients, 580

Fasting (Continued)
  in emergency surgery, gastric residual volume and, 42, 43, 316
  in outpatient surgery, 57
  preoperative evaluation of, 41, 41–42
Fat, drug volume of distribution and, in infants vs. adults, 123, 124
Fatty acid metabolism, of skeletal muscle, in malignant hyperthermia, 619
Fear, of diagnostic and therapeutic procedures, 584
Femoral artery, catheterization of, 753
Femoral nerve block, 666–667, 667
  for postoperative analgesia, 685
  of lateral femoral cutaneous nerve, 667, 667
Fentanyl (Sublimaze), for premedication, 149
  for sedation, 602, 602t
  high-dose, in postoperative care after cardiac surgery, 406
    stress response and, 403
  in burn patients, 532
  in cardiac transplantation, 546
  in neurosurgical procedures, 503, 503t
    before extubation, 506
    for induction, 499
  in postanesthesia care unit, 406, 707
  in postoperative analgesia, 679
    in outpatients, 61
  in renal transplantation, 563
  midazolam administration and, 148, 153
  patch form of, 149, 700
  pharmacokinetics of, 148–149
Fentanyl Oralet, for premedication, 149, 178, 179
  for sedation in children, 602, 602t
Fetal circulation, 353–354, 354–355
  persistent, 357
Fetal shunts, and transition to air breathing, 11
Fever, in preoperative evaluation, 44
FFP. See Fresh frozen plasma (FFP).
Fibrinolytic system, impaired hemostasis on separation from bypass and, 401–402
Fibrous dysplasia of jaw (cherubism), airway difficulties with, 117t
Final rule legislation, for drug labeling, 133
Fingers, digital nerve block of, 663, 663–664
Fistula, tracheoesophageal, 18
  emergency neonatal surgery for, 302–304, 303
Flecainide, doses and cardiac effects of, 377
Fluid(s), body, composition of, 227, 227t
  homeostatic mechanisms governing, 219, 221–222
  maturation of fluid compartments and, 218–222, 220–221, 221t
    circulating blood volume in, 219, 221t
    regulatory mechanisms of, 216–219, 217–220, 221–222
  requirements for, 222–223, 223, 223t
  clear, preoperative, in outpatient surgery, 57
  hyperalimentation, 49
  maintenance, 222–223, 223t
  management of, 4, 216–234
    crystalloid solutions for, 341
    discharge from postanesthesia care unit and, 704
    in bone marrow transplant recipients, 566–567
    in burn patients, 522, 528t, 528–529
    in cardiopulmonary resuscitation, 276–277
    in emergencies, 316
    in lung transplantation, 551
    in neonates, 223–224, 298
    in neurosurgical procedures, 503–504, 507
    in pathophysiologic state(s), 227–232
      dehydration, 227–230, 228t, 229
      diabetes insipidus, 232
      disorders of potassium homeostasis, 231, 231–232
      fluid overload, 227, 228t
      hypernatremia, 230–231

Fluid(s) (Continued)
  hyponatremia, 230–231
    SIADH, 232
  in renal transplantation, 563–564
  in trauma cases, 340, 341
  intraoperative, 224–226
    blood transfusions in, 341
    choice and composition of fluids for, 224–225, 225t
    devices for, 224
    fasting and, 225, 225t
    in outpatient surgery, 60–61
    intravascular volume assessment and, 226, 236, 237
    intravenous access for, 224
    ongoing losses and third-spacing and, 226
    warming of, 341, 614, 629, 716–717
  monitoring of, 528
  Parkland and Brooke formulas for, 528, 528t
  postoperative, 226–227
    general approach to, 226–227
    hypertonic, in trauma, 341
    hyponatremia and, 227
    isotonic vs. hypotonic fluids and, 224, 227, 341
    pulmonary edema and, 227
    preoperative fasting and, 1, 41, 41–42, 57, 225t, 225–226, 580
    third space accumulation and, 226
    with open eye injury, 489
  toxic reactions to local anesthetics and, 642
  warming of, 341, 614, 629, 716–717
Fluid and electrolyte status, liver transplantation and, 552
  renal transplantation and, 562
  requirements for, 222, 222–223
Fluid overload, differential diagnosis of, 228t
  management of, 227
Flumazenil, for reversal of benzodiazepine effects, 599–600
Fluothane. See Halothane (Fluothane).
Follow-up, after outpatient surgery, 64t, 64–65
Fontan procedure, 417, 444–449, 445–449
  completion (lateral tunnel), 447, 448
  hemi-Fontan operation and, 447, 448
  historical development of, 444
  modifications of, 445, 446–448, 447
  original repair of, 445
  repaired, sequelae with, 362, 364
  residua and sequelae of, 447, 449
  with fenestration of intra-atrial baffle, 447, 449
Food, preoperative abstinence from, 1
Food and Drug Administration (FDA), approval of pediatric drugs by, 597
Foot, digital nerves of, blocks of, 669
Forane. See Isoflurane (Forane).
Forced air convection, 629, 629
Foreign bodies, aspiration of, airway obstruction with, emergency management of, 321–322, 321–322
  metallic, in magnetic resonance imaging, 576
Fracture, basilar skull, 508
  cervical, intubation with, 336, 338
  skull, 507–508
Freeman-Sheldon syndrome (whistling face), airway difficulties with, 118t
Frei endoscopy mask, 105, 106
Fresh frozen plasma (FFP), administration of, calcium loss with, 535
  compatibilities of, 237t
  for blood transfusion, 244–245, 246
    indications and timing of, 241, 242t
    rapid administration of, 535
    vs. citrated whole blood, 244
Functional residual capacity, in infants and adults, 12–13, 13

Gas exchange, age-related changes in, 14–15

Gas exchange (Continued)
  in neonates, 294–296
  monitoring devices for, 732
Gastric acid, aspiration of, prophylaxis of, 183, 184t, 580
  in burn injuries, 525
Gastric residual volume, and fasting before surgery, 41–42. See also Fasting.
  and preoperative anxiety, 25
  in emergency room patients, 580
  with full stomach, in emergency surgery, 42, 43, 316
Gastroesophageal reflux, in newborns, 18–19
Gastrointestinal endoscopy, sedation for, 586–587
Gastrointestinal motility, drugs for, for premedication, 183, 184t
Gastrointestinal system, developmental anomalies of, 18
  emergency surgery on, in neonates, 305–310
  function of, in burn injuries, 525
    in neonates, 299
  growth and development of, 18–19
  procedures on, endocarditis prophylaxis with, 422t, 423t
Gastroschisis, 18
  in neonates, emergency surgery for, 309, 309t, 309–310
General anesthesia, in non-operating room location, 573
  masking toxic reaction of, to local anesthetic, 641
Genetic factors, in malignant hyperthermia, 616, 617, 617
  in mitochondrial disorders, 383
Genetic testing, of family, in malignant hyperthermia, 626
Genitourinary tract, procedures on, endocarditis prophylaxis with, 422t, 423t
Gestational age, and retinopathy of prematurity, 488
  assessment of, 6, 7t
  birth weight and, 38
  head circumference and, 8, 8t
  weight and, 5, 6t
GFR. See Glomerular filtration rate (GFR).
Glasgow Coma Scale, 328, 337t
  modifications of, for children, 339
Glaucoma, drug therapy for, systemic effects of, 485–487
  surgery for, 487–488
Glenn shunt, bidirectional and classic, in Fontan repair, 445, 447, 447
Gliomas, of optic pathways, with neurofibromatosis, 510
Glomerular filtration rate (GFR), in burn injuries, 526
  in neonates, 17, 127–128, 127–128, 297–298
Glottic aperture seal airway, 96
Glottic closure, during swallowing, 81
  forced, laryngeal function during, 81
Glucose, administration of, in cardiopulmonary resuscitation, 281–282
  in neurosurgical procedures, 504
  in trauma cases, 341
  intraoperative, 225
  blood, in controlled hypotension, 254
  intraoperative monitoring of, in diabetics, 48
  metabolism of, abnormal, liver transplantation and, 552
Glucose homeostasis, neonatal, 223, 298–299
  intolerance in, 19
  normal levels of, 19
Glucuronidation, in neonates and adults, 125, 127
Glucuronosyltransferase, conjugation by, in neonates, 125
Glycerophosphorylcholine, as marker for malignant hyperthermia, 623
Glycopyrrolate (Robinul), 155
  for management of oculocardiac reflex, 480
  for premedication, 180
Goldenhar syndrome, airway difficulties with, 118t

Graft-versus-host disease, in bone marrow transplant recipients, 567
Granisetron, for postoperative nausea and vomiting, in outpatients, 62–63
    in strabismus surgery, 488
    for premedication, 182
Gray Baby syndrome, 125
Great auricular nerve block, 655, *656*
Greater occipital nerve block, 654, *654*
Growth and development, 5–22
    infant, terminology used in, 5–6
    neurologic, 21t, 21–22
    normal and abnormal, 5–9
    of airway dynamics, 13
    of breathing mechanics, 11–13
    of cardiovascular system, 15–16
    of gas exchange, 14–15
    of gastrointestinal system, 18–19
    of hematopoietic system, 19–20
    of hepatic system, 17–18
    of organ systems, 9–11
    of pancreas, 19
    of renal system, 16–17
    prenatal, infant weight and, 5–6, 6t
Guedel airway, 105

H₂-antagonists, for premedication, 183, 184t
Haemophilus influenzae, epiglottitis with, 319
Half-life, of diazepam, in children vs. adults, 153, *153*
    of drugs, determination of, 128–129, *129*
    of local anesthetics, in children vs. adults, 637
Hallerman-Streiff syndrome, airway difficulties with, 118t
Halogenated agents, for neurosurgical procedures, 503, 503t
Halothane (Fluothane), *134,* 135–136
    advantages of, 135
    as induction agent, 59
        vs. sevoflurane, 59
        with desflurane maintenance, 60
    cardiovascular dysfunction with, 135, 535
    cerebral blood flow and, 135
    hepatic toxicity and, 135–136
    in emergencies, 318
    in rigid bronchoscopy, 468
    in surgery for congenital heart disease, 398
    intraocular pressure and, 481
    malignant hyperthermia and, 617
    minimum alveolar concentration of, age and, 133–134, *134*
    recovery time from, 699
    thermoregulatory threshold for, 615
    uses of, 135
    vs. other anesthetic agents, 136
    vs. sevoflurane, 59, 138–140, 140t
Hand, digital nerve block of, *663,* 663–664
Head, circumference of, gestational age and, 8, 8t
    heat loss from, 628
    in infants, assessment of, 8
    positioning of, for neurosurgical procedures, 500, *501*
        in prone position, 501
Head and neck, dermatomal innervation of, *653*
    great auricular nerve block of, 655, *656*
    greater occipital nerve block of, 654, *654*
    infraorbital nerve block of, 654–655, *655*
    peripheral nerve blocks of, 653–655
    supraorbital nerve block of, 653–654, *654*
    supratrochlear nerve block of, 653–654, *654*
Head frames, airway accessibility and, 510, *511*
    cerebellar, 500, 501
    in neuroradiologic procedures, 518
Head injuries, hypertonic solutions and, 341
    in trauma cases, 329, 336, 342
    surgery for, 507

Headache, post–dural puncture, with spinal anesthesia, 647
Heart. See also *Cardiac entries.*
    damage to, in Duchenne muscular dystrophy, 209
    function of, in burn injuries, 523
        in hyperkalemia, 231, *231*
        in perioperative cardiac arrest, 268–274, *271*
    physiology of, in controlled hypotension, 250–251
        in neonates, 356–357
    transplantation of, anesthesia for, 544–547
        cardiopulmonary bypass with, 546
        contraindications to, 545
        demographics for, 544–545
        donor selection for, 545, 545t
        dysrhythmias with, 546
        indications for, 544–545
        induction techniques in, 546
        monitoring devices for, 546
        outcome of, 547
        postoperative management of, 547
        preoperative evaluation for, 545
        rejection with, 547
        surgical technique of, 545
Heart disease, acquired, pathophysiology of, 362, 365
    congenital. See *Congenital heart disease.*
Heart rate, developmental changes in, 15–16, 16t
Heart valves, stenosis of, cardiac catheterization for, 450–451
Heart-lung transplantation, 547–551
    complications of, 551
    vs. lung transplantation, 547–548
Heat. See also *Temperature; Thermoregulation.*
    internal redistribution of, anesthesia-induced, 613
Heat loss, anesthesia-induced, 613–614
    cutaneous, insulators and, 628–629, *629*
    from head, in infants and children, 628
    in burn patients, 529, 531
    in neonates, 297
    in thermoregulation, 612
    in trauma patients, 341–342
Heating and cooling systems, in operating room, 715
Heat-moisture exchangers, in operating room, 716
Hemangioma, subglottic, emergency neonatal surgery for, 302, *302*
Hematocrit, minimum values of, 42–43
    for blood transfusion, 236
Hematologic function, in burn injuries, 525
    outpatient surgery and, 56
Hematoma, epidural, 508
    signs and symptoms of, 651t
    intracerebral, 508
    subdural, 508
Hematopoietic system, growth and development of, 19–20
    in burn injuries, 525
Hemispherectomy, for seizures, 513
Hemodialysis, before renal transplantation, 561–562
Hemodilution, advantages of, 256
    complications of, 256
    for reduction of exposure to blood transfusion, 254–256
    in cardiopulmonary bypass in congenital heart disease surgery, 400
    indications for and contraindications to, 256
    physiologic data for, 255
    technique of, 255–256
Hemodynamic changes, in cervical spine injury, 509
    in reperfusion syndrome, in liver transplantation, 556
Hemodynamic stability, in emergence, surgery for intracranial aneurysms and, 511
    in infants, with spinal anesthesia, 692
    in subarachnoid block, in children vs. adults, 643
Hemofiltration, for impaired hemostasis on separation from bypass, 401
Hemoglobin, in controlled hypotension, 254

Hemoglobin *(Continued)*
    in newborns and infants, 20
    preoperative determination of, 40–41
Hemoglobin SC, in sickle cell disease, 45
Hemophilia, treatment of, 239–240
Hemorrhage. See *Bleeding; Blood loss.*
Hemostasis, impaired, after bypass in congenital heart disease, 394
Heparin, in flush solutions, in angiographic procedures, 575
Hepatic system. See also *Liver.*
    growth and development of, 17–18
    physiology of, in controlled hypotension, 251
Hepatic toxicity, halothane use and, 135–136
    sevoflurane use and, 139
Hering-Breuer reflex, in infants, 14
Hernia, congenital diaphragmatic, emergency surgery for, *304,* 304–305
    survival from, 305
    infantile, emergency surgery for, 308
Herniation syndromes, intracranial pressure and, 494
Herniorrhaphy, inguinal, regional nerve block with, for postoperative analgesia, 684
Hirschsprung disease, 18, 19
    in neonates, emergency surgery for, 310
Histamine release, with meperidine vs. morphine, 147
History. See *Medical history.*
HIV. See *Human immunodeficiency virus (HIV).*
Hospitalization, previous, in behavioral preoperative programs for children, 28–29
Hot Line, for warming fluids, 716–717
Human immunodeficiency virus (HIV), blood transfusions and, 235
    informed consent issues with, 75
    precautions against by anesthesiologists, 248
Humidifiers, artificial nose and, 614, 629, 716
    during anesthesia, heat transfer and, 614, 629
    heated, for operating room, 717
    of anesthesia machine, 722–723, *724*
Hunter syndrome, airway difficulties with, 119t
Hurler's syndrome, airway difficulties with, 118t
Hurler-Scheie syndrome, airway difficulties with, 119t
Hyaline membrane disease, in neonates, 296
    in preterm infants, bronchopulmonary dysplasia and, 48
Hydralazine, doses and cardiac effects of, 371t, 374
Hydration, in sickle cell disease, 45
Hydration therapy, 222–223. See also *Fluid(s), management of.*
Hydrocephalus, 513–514, *515*
Hydromorphone, epidural, for thoracic or upper abdominal surgery, 687
    for postoperative pain, 679, 687
Hydroxyzine, for premedication, 180
Hyperalimentation, in burn patients, 536
    in preoperative evaluation, 49
Hyperbaric oxygenation, in carbon monoxide poisoning, in burned patients, 527
Hyperbilirubinemia, in neonates, 17t, 17–18
Hypercapnia, intraocular pressure and, 482
Hypercarbia, hypertrophied tonsils and, 462, *463*
Hypercholesterolemia, liver transplantation and, 552
Hyperglycemia, in liver transplantation, 552, 556, *556*
    in newborns, 19
    stress-induced, neurologic outcome of cardiac surgery and, 403
Hyperkalemia, in malignant hyperthermia, 619
        vs. succinylcholine-induced rhabdomyolysis, 619
    in preterm infants, 17
    management of, 231, *231*
    renal transplantation induction and, 563
    succinylcholine use and, 200–202, 619
    with massive blood transfusion, 242–244
Hypernatremia, fluid imbalance and, 230
Hyperosmolar hyperglycemic nonketotic coma, in burn patients, 528

Hyperoxia, retinopathy of prematurity and, 143, 300
in low birth weight infants, 45
Hyperreflexia, autonomic, spine injury and, 509
Hypertension, before renal transplantation, 562
in postanesthesia care unit, 706
in rapid-sequence induction, 316
in surgery for intracranial aneurysms, 511
intracranial, with hydrocephalus, 514
malignant, expired carbon dioxide tension measurement and, 730
pulmonary. See *Pulmonary hypertension.*
with repaired coarctation of aorta, 426
Hyperthermia, in postanesthesia care unit, 708
inter-threshold range in, anesthesia-induced, 616
malignant, 616–627
animal models of, 618
avoidance of, 626
definition of, 616
diagnosis of, 616, 620, *620,* 621t
differential diagnosis of, 621, 621t
genetics of, 616, 617, *617*
incidence of, 616–617
management of, 624t–625t, 624–625, *625*
masseter spasm and tetany in, 621–622, *622*
muscle biopsy testing for, 622–623, 623t
muscle relaxants and, 209
outpatient surgery and, 56
pathophysiology of, 617–620, *618*
succinylcholine use and, 200
susceptibility to, 624
therapy of, 616
perioperative, 616
Hypertonic solutions, for glaucoma therapy, systemic effects of, 487
in trauma cases, 341
Hypertrophic pyloric stenosis, in neonates, emergency surgery for, 306–307, *307*
Hyperventilation, controlled, for neurosurgical procedures, 502, 503
for reduction of intracranial pressure, 497
risk of, in surgery for moyamoya disease, 512
Hypnotics, recovery from, 700
Hypocalcemia, 244–245. See also *Calcium* entries.
ionized, in burn injuries, 526, *526,* 534–535
in neonates, 299
Hypoglycemia, definition of, in full-term neonates, 19
in fasting before surgery, 41
in infants of diabetic mothers, 19
in newborns, 19
liver transplantation and, 552
Hypokalemia, management of, 231–232
Hypomagnesemia, with hypocalcemia, in infants, 299
Hyponatremia, fluid imbalance and, 230–231
Hypoplastic left heart syndrome, Fontan procedure for repair of, 444, 445, *446*
Hypotension, controlled, anesthetic management of, 253
contraindications to, 254
for reduction of intraoperative blood loss, 249–254
general concepts of, 253–254
in surgery for intracranial aneurysms, 511
laboratory parameters for, 254
monitoring of, 253–254
patient position for, 254
pharmacology of, 252–253
physiology of, 249–252
premedication for, 253
in liver transplantation, 555
in postanesthesia care unit, 704, 706
in rapid-sequence induction, 316
in renal transplantation, 564
in trauma patients, 342
midazolam administration and, 153
physiologic responses to, 218, *219*
Hypothalamus, role in thermoregulation, *611,* 611–612
Hypothermia. See also *Thermoregulation.*

Hypothermia *(Continued)*
circulatory arrest with, in cardiac transplantation, 546
during anesthesia, physiologic modifications with, *613–614,* 613–615
in liver transplantation, 557, *558*
in newborns and infants, thermoregulation and, 612–613
in postanesthesia care unit, 708
in repair of neonatal cardiac defects, 400
induced, in neurosurgical procedures, 504
muscle relaxant action and, 209
postoperative, prevention of, 628–629
redistribution, prevention of, 628
with massive blood loss, 246
Hypothyroidism, congenital, airway difficulties with, 117t
Hypoventilation, alveolar, hypertrophied tonsils and, 462, *463*
in postanesthesia care unit, 705
Hypovolemia, hypotension with, in postanesthesia care unit, 706
in pediatric emergencies, 316
Hypovolemic shock, 325, 325t, 326
Hypoxemia, bradycardia with, in postanesthesia care unit, 706
hypertrophied tonsils and, 462, *463*
in burn injuries, 524
in congenital heart disease, 359–360
in liver transplantation, 552
in postanesthesia care unit, 705
ventilatory response to, after inhalation anesthesia, 699
Hypoxia, in infants, 14
intraocular pressure and, 482

Ibuprofen, for postoperative analgesia, 678
for premedication, 181
Ibutilide, doses and cardiac effects of, 378–379
Identification bracelet, 2
Ileal obstruction, congenital, emergency surgery for, 307–308
Iliohypogastric nerve block, 656, 658, *658*
Ilioinguinal nerve block, 656, 658, *658*
Ilioinguinal-iliohypogastric nerve block, for inguinal herniorrhaphy, for postoperative analgesia, 684
Immobilization, in MRI studies, 576
in spinal injury, 509
in trauma cases, 336
in-line, in trauma cases, 336, *338*
Imperforate anus, emergency surgery for, 308
Implants, surgical, in magnetic resonance imaging, 576
Inappropriate secretion of antidiuretic hormone, after neurosurgical procedures, 507
Inapsine. See *Droperidol (Inapsine).*
Incision site, heat loss from, during anesthesia, 614
local anesthetics in, postoperative analgesia and, 681
Indomethacin, for postoperative analgesia, 678
Induction, 3, 184–189, 188
for neurosurgical procedures, 499
for ophthalmologic procedures, 484
halothane vs. sevoflurane use in, 139, 140t
hypnotic, 185–186
in burn patients, 531–532
in cardiac transplantation, 546
in lung transplantation, 550
in pediatric trauma cases, 345
inhalation, 184–186
in congenital heart disease surgery, 396–397
choice of agents for, 397–399
techniques of, 184–186. See also specific agents, e.g., *Sevoflurane (Ultane).*
by face mask, 184–185
distraction for, 185
in outpatient surgery, 59–60
scented mask for, 185

Induction *(Continued)*
intramuscular, 188
in congenital heart disease surgery, choice of agents for, 399
intravenous, 186–188
drugs for, 187t, 187–188
in congenital heart disease surgery, 396
choice of drugs for, 396, 399
in outpatient surgery, 60
in renal transplantation, 563
rapid, with full stomach, 42
technique of, 186–188
modified single-breath technique of, 186
parental presence during, 188–189
in behavioral preoperative programs, *29,* 29–30
in emergencies, 318
in outpatient surgery, 59
with mentally handicapped child, 45
preinduction techniques for, in outpatient surgery, 59
rapid-sequence, 188
in emergency cases, 337, 339t
in liver transplantation, 554
with full stomach, 42, 316
rectal, 188
Infants, anesthetic requirements in, vs. adults, 133–134
anxiety and separation from parents and, 172
body composition of, drug distribution and, 122–123, *123–124*
fluid resuscitation formulas in, 528
large for gestational age, problems with, 5t, 6
low birth weight, 6
cholestatic jaundice in, 18
hyperglycemia in, 19
oxygen therapy for, retinopathy of prematurity and, 45, 142–143, 300
stool passage in, 19
newborn. See *Neonates.*
non-shivering thermogenesis in, 612
of diabetic mothers, 19
physiologic acidemia in, 17
postoperative analgesic technique and, 676
postoperative apnea in, 45–48, 294–295, 295t. See also under *Apnea.*
in former preterm infants, 45–48, 55–56
in postanesthesia care unit, 705
postterm, definition of, 6
preterm, classification of, 6
definition of, 5
former, as candidates for outpatient surgery, 55–56
hernia repair in, 308
postoperative apnea in, 45–48, *46–48,* 55–56, 644
postoperative care for, after ophthalmologic procedures, 484
hyperkalemia in, 17
periodic breathing in, vs. apnea, 14–15, *14–15*
postoperative analgesic technique and, 676
total body water in, 7, 8t
weight gain in, 7–8
rewarming phase in, during anesthesia, 615
small for gestational age, problems with, 6, 6t, 19
subarachnoid block in, drugs used for, 646
technique of, 644–646, *645–646*
term, definition of, 5–6
toxicity of local anesthetics in, 639
weight of, neonatal problems associated with, 6, 6t
Infection, regional blockade and, 681
with caudal epidural anesthesia, 650–651
Inflammatory collagen vascular diseases, cardiac pathophysiology with, 365
Informed consent, Baby Doe regulations and, 70
before sedation, 588
components of, 68, 68t
concept of futility in, 73
consent and assent in, 68, 68t, 70

Informed consent *(Continued)*
do-not-resuscitate (DNR) orders in operating room and, 72–73
emancipated minor status in, 71
for pediatric patients, 69–70
in adolescents, 71
in children of Jehovah's Witnesses, 71–72
in children requiring emergency care, 72
informed permission of parents and, 69–70
informed refusal and, 70–71
interview for, parental anxiety about, *30,* 30–31
legal standards for, 69
mature minor doctrine in, 71
preoperative presentation of, 2
relevant risks in, 69
unacceptable and acceptable treatment and, 70
withdrawing and withholding care and, 73
Infraorbital nerve block, 654–655, *655*
Infusion, intraosseous, technique of, 746, *747*
Infusion pump, 718
Inguinal block, 656, 658, *658*
Inhalation anesthesia, 184–186. See also *Anesthetic agents, inhalation.*
recovery from, physicochemical factors in, 698–699
Inhalation injury, in burned patients, 524, 526–527
Inositol polyphosphide, in muscle rigidity, in malignant hyperthermia, 619
Inotropic drugs. See also *Vasoactive drugs.*
doses and cardiac effects of, 366t
during transport to intensive care after cardiac surgery, 406
practical considerations with, 365–367, 366t
Inspiration, during airway obstruction, in infants, *86*
laryngeal function during, 81
normal, in infants, *86*
pressure, monitoring devices for, 732
Insulators, for prevention of heat loss, 628–629, *629*
Insulin, for premedication, 183, *183*
intraoperative, in diabetics, 48–49
Intensive care, preoperative planning for, 2
Intercostal muscle, activity of, in infants, in central neuraxial blockade, 643
Intercostal nerve block, 655–656, *657*
uses of, 655–656
for postoperative analgesia, 685
Interscalene block, 659
Intestinal atresia, 18
congenital, emergency surgery for, *307,* 307–308
Intestines, duplication and diverticula of, 18
Intracerebral hematoma, surgery for, 508
Intracranial compliance, 495, *495*
with hydrocephalus, 514
Intracranial pressure, brain injury and, pathophysiology of, 494–495
cerebrospinal fluid and, 493–494
hydrocephalus and, 514
in induction for neurosurgical procedures, 499
in surgery for brain tumors, 510
increased, signs of, 495
intracranial compliance and, 495, *495*
ketamine use and, 145–146
monitoring of, 495, 733
normal values of, 495
Intramuscular anesthesia, 188
Intraocular gases, in retinal detachment surgery, 487
Intraocular pressure, aqueous humor and, 479, *480*
arterial pressure and, 480
effects of anesthesia on, 480–482
normal range of, 479
pathophysiology of, 479–482
succinylcholine use and, 201
for intubation with open eye injury, 489
Intraosseous access, in cardiopulmonary resuscitation, 276
in trauma cases, 337, *338,* 340

Intrapleural analgesia, for postoperative pain, 693
Intravascular volume, in burn patients, 531
in emergencies, 316
intraoperative assessment of, 226
ongoing losses of, 226
Intravenous access, 224
in cardiopulmonary resuscitation, 276
in emergencies, 317
in methohexital-sedated patient for CT scans, 574
in open eye injury, 489
in ophthalmologic procedures, 484
in status epilepticus, 327
neonatal, 298
Intravenous anesthesia, 186–188. See also specific agents, e.g., *Propofol (Diprivan).*
agents used for, 143–146
equipment for, *717,* 717–718
in outpatient surgery, 60
induction in, in ophthalmologic procedures, 483
Intubation. See also *Endotracheal intubation; Endotracheal tubes.*
awake, in emergencies, 315
in trauma cases, 336–337
equipment for, 721
guides for, *99,* 104
inhalational, in emergencies, 315–316
minimum alveolar concentration for, age and, 134
nasotracheal, for neurosurgical procedures, 500
placement of tube for, in prone position, 501
oral, in neurosurgical procedures, 499–500
prophylactic, in facial burn injuries, 527, *527*
retrograde, in spinal injury, 509
special technique(s) of, Bullard laryngoscope for, 107, *108*
combination techniques for, 108–109
fiberoptic laryngoscopy for, 105–107, *106*
laryngeal mask airway used as conduit for, 108
lighted stylet for, 107
retrograde wire-guided, 107–108
rigid laryngoscopy for, 103–105, *104–105*
sight wands for, 108
with cervical fracture, in trauma cases, 336, *338,* 342
Isoflurane (Forane), *136,* 136–137
advantages of, 137
adverse side effects of, 137
for induction, 185
in congenital heart disease surgery, 398
in liver transplantation, 554
in neurosurgical procedures, 503, 503t
intraocular pressure and, 481
minimum alveolar concentration of, 136, *136*
thermoregulatory threshold for, 615
uses of, 137
vs. halothane, 136–137
Isoproterenol, doses and cardiac effects of, 366t, 369
in cardiac transplantation, 546–547
Isotonic solutions, in trauma cases, 341

Jackson-Rees anesthesia circuit, 721
Jaundice, pathologic causes of, in neonates, 18, 18t
physiologic, in neonates, 17t, 17–18
Jaw stiffness, succinylcholine use and, 200
Jet ventilation, in laser surgery on airway, 472
Sanders, in rigid bronchoscopy, 469
Jet-Ventilation Catheter, for percutaneous needle cricothyrotomy, 101, *103*

Kawasaki disease, cardiac pathophysiology with, 365
Kernicterus, in newborn, 18
Ketamine (Ketalar), 145–146
adverse side effects of, 145–146
doses of, 145
effects of, 145
for induction, 187t, 187–188, 345, 499

Ketamine (Ketalar) *(Continued)*
intramuscular, 188
rapid intravenous, 42
for premedication, 179
for sedation in non-operating room location, 574, 603, 603t–604t
in burn patients, 531–533
in cardiac catheterization, 408
in congenital heart disease surgery, 399
in difficult airway management, 98
in hypovolemia, in emergencies, 316
in outpatient surgery, as preinduction technique, 59
in radiation therapy, disadvantages of, 572
indications and contraindications for, 145–146
intraocular pressure and, 481–482
postanesthetic apnea in infants and, 644
preservative-free, for postoperative analgesia in caudal block, 684
routes of administration of, 145
Ketoacidosis, correction of, 49
Ketorolac (Toradol), 151–152
for postoperative analgesia, 62, 467, 678
in outpatients, 61
for premedication, 181–182
pharmacokinetics and pharmacodynamics of, 151–152
recovery from, 700
side effects of, 61
Kidney(s). See also *Renal* entries.
blunt trauma to, 343
development of, 16–17
failure of, causes of, 560, 560t
pathophysiologic changes with, 560t
transplantation of, 559–564
anesthetic management in, 562–564
operative technique for, 562
postoperative management of, 564
preoperative considerations with, 560–562
with living related donor organ, 562

Labetalol, before extubation, after neurosurgical procedures, 506
doses and cardiac effects of, 371t, 372
Laboratory studies, in preoperative evaluation, 40–41
for neurosurgical procedures, 498
for outpatient surgery, 57
of congenital heart disease, 392–393
Language milestones, and age, 21, 21t
Laryngeal braking, 12
Laryngeal mask airway, 94–96, *95,* 95t
advantages of, 94–95
as conduit for intubation of difficult airway, 108
in adenotonsillectomy, 463–465
in bag-valve-mask devices for ventilation, 268
in ophthalmologic procedures, 484
in patients with asthma, 49
in patients with bronchopulmonary dysplasia, 48
indications and uses of, 95
injuries and mistakes with, 96
insertion of, 95–96
modification of for children, 96
removal of, 96
size of, *95,* 95t
uses of, 101, 719
vs. percutaneous cricothyrotomy and transtracheal jet ventilation, 102–103
Laryngeal obstruction, emergency neonatal surgery for, 301
Laryngeal papilloma, airway difficulties with, 119t
laser surgery for, 472, *472*
Laryngeal webs, emergency neonatal surgery for, 301–302, *302*
Laryngomalacia, stridor with, 467–468
Laryngoscope, Bullard, 107, *108,* 721
flexible pediatric, 721

Laryngoscope *(Continued)*
  rigid pediatric, 721
  suspension, in laser surgery on airway, 472, *472*
Laryngoscopy, fiberoptic, advantages and disadvantages
    of, 107
  retrograde, 108–109
  rigid, 108
  technique of, 105–107, *106*
    with retrograde wire-guided intubation, 108
  grading system for laryngeal visualization in, *99*
  in epiglottitis, 319
  in poisoning cases, 327
  rigid, alternative approaches to, 104–105, *105*
    technique of, 103–105, *104–105*
    with flexible fiberoptic scope, 108
  selection of blade for, 92, 92t
  technique of, 91–92
  with airway obstruction, *318,* 318–319
Laryngospasm, laryngeal function during, 81
  upper respiratory infection and, 44
Laryngotracheal stenosis, 93–94
Laryngotracheobronchitis, airway obstruction with,
    emergency management of, 320–321, *321*
Larynx, anatomy of, 79–81, *80*
  in infant, 81–82, *82–83*
  location of, in airway evaluation, *88, 89, 99*
  structure and function of, 79–81, *80*
  visualization of, grading system for, *99*
Laser surgery, anesthetic techniques of, 471–472, *472*
  carbon dioxide, anesthesia for, 470–471
    hazards of, 469–470
    uses of, 469
  endoscopic, 469–472
  for laryngeal papilloma, 472, *472*
  indications for, 472
Latex allergy, history of, 497
  myelodysplasia and, 516–517
Legal problems, with parental presence during
    anesthesia induction, 30
Legs, peripheral nerve blocks of, 664–669
  sensory innervation of, *664*
Leukemia, bone marrow transplantation for, 565
Level 1 System, for warming fluids, 717
Levobupivacaine, for postoperative analgesia, 684
  pharmacokinetics of, 637
Lidocaine, dose, and cardiac effects of, 375, 376t, 377
    in neonates, 639
  for nausea after strabismus surgery, 488
  in anesthesia of vocal cords, 468
  in brachial plexus block, 660
  in cardiopulmonary resuscitation, 283–284
  in neurosurgical procedures, 499, 506
  in subarachnoid block in neonates and infants, 646,
    646t
  in topical anesthesia, in difficult airway management,
    98
  intraocular pressure and, 482
  prilocaine cream of, for premedication for ophthalmo-
    logic procedures, 483
Light wand, in difficult airways, 107
Lighted stylet, in difficult airways, 107
Limb tourniquet, in anesthesia, hyperthermia and, 615
Liquids, clear, in fasting before surgery, *41,* 41–42
Liver. See also *Hepatic* entries.
  blood flow in, drug metabolism and excretion and,
    123–124
  blunt trauma to, 343
  first-pass effect in, 124
  growth and development of, 17–18
  in burn injuries, 524–525
  neonatal, drug metabolism in, 636
  penetrating injuries of, 342
Liver disease, end-stage, pathophysiologic changes
    with, 551–552, 552t
Liver transplantation, 551–559

Liver transplantation *(Continued)*
  anesthetic management in, 554–555, *555*
    induction and maintenance in, 554
    intravenous access in, 555
    monitoring in, 555
    patient positioning in, 555
  cardiovascular issues in, 551–552
  hematologic and coagulation issues in, 552
  indications for, 551
  intraoperative problems in, cardiovascular instability
      in, 555–556
    coagulation defects in, 556–557
    hypothermia in, 557
    massive blood transfusion in, side effects of, 557–
      558
    metabolic abnormalities in, 556
    operative technique in, 552–554, *553–554*
    renal insufficiency in, 557
  living related donors for, partial grafts from, 554
  outcome of, 558–559, *558–560*
  reduced-size cadaveric livers in, 553, *554*
  renal and metabolic issues in, 552
  respiratory issues in, 551–552
  split-liver grafts in, 553–554
Lobar emphysema, congenital, emergency surgery for,
    305
Lobectomy, for seizures, 513
Local anesthetics. See also *Regional anesthesia.*
  amide, pharmacokinetics of, in children vs. adults,
    636–637
    pharmacology of, 636t, 636–637
  doses of, calculation of, 640, 640t
    maximum, and duration of action, 597t, 640t
    test of, 639, 641
  d-stereoisomer of, and toxicity, 639
  electrocardiographic monitoring of test doses of, 639
  epidural, with opioids, for postoperative analgesia,
    686–687, 687t, 690, 690t, 691t, 692–693, 707
  epinephrine with, calculations for, 640, 640t–641t
    in peripheral nerve blocks, 652
  ester, pharmacokinetics of, in children vs. adults,
    636t, 637–638
  for sedation, 597t, 597–598
  hypersensitivity to, 642
  in neurosurgical procedures, 502
  in peripheral nerve blocks, 652
  in postoperative analgesia, 681–693. See also *Re-
      gional blockade, for postoperative analgesia.*
    epidural, 686–687, 687t, *688–689,* 690, 690t, 691t,
      692–693
    risks and adverse effects of, 690, 692
  opioids with, for postoperative analgesia, 686–687,
    687t, 690, 690t, 691t, 692–693, 707
  pharmacology and pharmacokinetics of, 636–642
  rate of uptake of, 640
  site of injection of, 640
  technique of administration of, 641
  test dose of, 639, 641
  topical, 597
  toxicity of, *638,* 638–639
    causes of, 639–640
    in infants and neonates, 639
    prevention of, 639–641, 640t
    treatment of, 641–642
Lorazepam, for premedication, 175–176
Lumbar puncture, in infants and adults, 642, *642*
Lung(s). See also *Pulmonary; Respiratory* entries.
  closing capacity in, in infants and adults, 13
  compliance of, specific, changes in, 11
    ventilation effectiveness and, 720, *720*
  development of, gestational, 9–10
    postnatal, 10
    principles of, 9
  diffusing capacity of, 14
  elasticity of, 11–12

Lung(s) *(Continued)*
  embryology of, 9
  function of, in burn injuries, 523–524
  functional residual capacity of, in infants and adults,
    12–13, *13*
  physiology of, in controlled hypotension, 251
  total capacity of, in infants and adults, 12
Lung parenchyma, in infants, surgery on, general
      principles of, 304
  in emergencies, 304–305
Lung transplantation, 547–551
  anesthesia management in, 549–551
  bridge to transplant devices for, 548
  complications of, 551
  donor evaluation for, 549, 549t
  indications for, in children, 547, 547t
  lobar transplantation from living related donors, 548
  operative technique for, 549
  postoperative care in, 551
  recipient selection criteria for, 548t, 548–549
  single vs. double, 548, *548*
    operative technique of, 549
  vs. heart-lung transplantation, 547–548
  xenotransplantation for, 548
Lung volumes, static, in adults and children, 12, *12,* 12t
Lung water, in intentional hemodilution, 255
Lytic cocktail (DPT), 586
  for sedation in children, 601–602

MAC. See *Minimum alveolar concentration (MAC)*
Magill anesthesia circuit, 721
Magnesium sulfate, doses and cardiac effects of, 376t
Magnetic resonance imaging (MRI), anesthesia for,
    576–579, *577–578*
  hazards with, 576
  scanner for, floor plan and organization of facilities
    for, *577,* 577–578
  therapy unit for, 518, *518*
Malrotation, in neonates, emergency surgery for, 310
Managed care, production pressure on anesthesiologists
    and, 75–76
Mandible, configuration of, in airway evaluation, *88, 89*
Mandibular hypoplasia, laryngeal position in, 82, *83*
Mannitol, for glaucoma therapy, systemic effects of,
    487
Mapleson D circuit system, of anesthesia machine,
    721–722, *722–723*
Marfan syndrome, airway difficulties with, 118t
  cardiac pathophysiology with, 362
Masks. See *Face masks.*
Masseter muscle, spasm and tetany of, in malignant
    hyperthermia, 621–622, *622*
  stiffness of, succinylcholine use and, 200
Mastoidectomy, anesthesia for, 475
Maximum allowable blood loss, for red cell transfusion,
    236
Meconium, in newborns, 19
Meconium ileus, emergency surgery for, 307–308
Median nerve, elbow block of, 661
  wrist block of, 662, *662*
Medic Alert registry, documentation of difficult airway
    problems in, 99
Medical history, before sedation, guidelines for, 588
  in pediatric emergencies, 315
  in preoperative evaluation, 39, 497
  of congenital heart disease, 392
Medical record, documentation of difficult airway
      problems in, 99
  in mentally handicapped child, 45
  of anesthetic procedure, 4
Mendelson syndrome (pulmonary acid aspiration
      syndrome), 41–42
  premedication for, 183–184, 184t
Meningomyelocele, 516
  Arnold-Chiari malformation and, 517, *517,* 517t

Mental handicaps, anesthesia for patients with, 580
  causes of, 22t
  in preoperative evaluation, 45
  signs of, 21–22
Meperidine (Demerol), 147–148
  for postoperative analgesia, 679
    in outpatients, 61
  for premedication, 178
  for sedation in children, 601
  in renal transplantation, 563
  vs. morphine, 147–148
Metabolic abnormalities, in burn injuries, 525–526
  in liver transplantation, 556, 556
  in stress response, 403
Metabolic rate, in malignant hyperthermia, 619
  increased, as thermoregulatory response, 612
Methadone, for postoperative analgesia, 678
Methemoglobin reductase, in neonates, prilocaine
    metabolism and, 638
Methemoglobinemia, in burn patients, 535–536
  pulse oximetry and, 727
Methohexital, for induction, 187, 187t
    intramuscular, 188
  for premedication, 176–177, 177
  for sedation in non-operating room location, 573, 604
  intraocular pressure and, 481
  rectal, 143
    for outpatient surgery, 59
    for premedication, 177
      for ophthalmologic procedures, 483
    for sedation for CT scans, 573
Methoxamine, for cardiopulmonary resuscitation, 278
Methylprednisolone, for spine injury, 509
Metoclopramide (Reglan), 155
  for postoperative nausea and vomiting, in outpatients,
    62
    in strabismus surgery, 488
    in tonsillectomy, 466
  for premedication, 42, 184, 184t
Metocurine, pharmacokinetics of, 207, 207
Midazolam (Versed), doses of, 154, 154t
  electroencephalographic effect of, 176
  fentanyl use and, 148
  for premedication, 174–175
    in neurosurgical procedures, 498
    in ophthalmologic procedures, 483
    in outpatient surgery, 58–59
    with local anesthetics, 640–641
  for sedation, 599, 600t
    in non-operating room location, 574
  in difficult airway management, 98
  pharmacokinetics and pharmacodynamics of, 153,
    153–154
  rectal, as preinduction technique, 59
  route of administration of, 154, 154t, 174–175
Midgut volvulus, in neonates, emergency surgery for,
  310
Milrinone, doses and cardiac effects of, 366t, 370
Minimum alveolar concentration (MAC), for intubation,
    age and, 134
  of anesthetic agents, allowed by vaporizers, 138, 138
    inhalation, age and, 133–134, 134
    of desflurane, by age, 140t, 140–141, 141
    of halothane, 133–134, 134
    of isoflurane, 136, 136
    of sevoflurane, by age, 138, 138
Mitochondrial myopathy, 383–384
Mitral valve, regurgitation with, atrioventricular septal
    defect repair and, 432
  stenosis of, cardiac catheterization treatment for, 450
Mivacurium, recovery from, 700
  uses and complications of, 202, 202–203
Monitoring, device(s) used for, 2–3, 725–733
    and MRI scanner, 576
    anesthesia record as, 725–726

Monitoring (Continued)
    blood pressure measuring, 726
    capnography as. See Capnography
    electrocardiograph as, 726–727
    oxygen monitors as, 727
    pulse oximeters as, 727–729, 728–729
    sequence of application of, 3
    stethoscope as, 726
    temperature monitors as, 727
  during transport to postanesthesia care unit, 701
  epidural, for intracranial pressure, 495
  for air emboli, modalities of, 505
  for diagnosis of malignant hyperthermia, 626
  for opioid-induced respiratory depression, 692
  for postoperative apnea in former preterm infants, 48
  in burn patients, 531
  in cardiac catheterization, 407
  in cardiac transplantation, 546
  in congenital heart disease patients, 395–396
  in controlled hypotension, 253–254
  in liver transplantation, 555
  in lung transplantation, 549
  in massive blood transfusion, 247–248, 248
  in neurosurgical procedures, 498–499
  in ophthalmologic procedures, 483–484
  in renal transplantation, 562
  methods of, in neonates, 298
  of intracranial pressure, 495
Morphine, 146–147, 147
  clearance of, 146–147, 147
  dose of, epidural, in thoracic or upper abdominal sur-
    gery, 687
    in children, 679
  for postoperative analgesia, 679
  for premedication, 178
  for sedation, 601
  in burn patients, slow-release, 536
    tolerance to, 537, 538
  in infants and neonates, 679
    glucuronidation of, 125
    respiratory depression and, 147
  in patient-controlled analgesia, dosage for, 680t
  in postanesthesia care unit, 707
  in renal transplantation, 563
Morquio syndrome, airway difficulties with, 119t
Motor blockade, with bupivacaine, 690
Motor milestones, and age, 21, 21t
Motor vehicle accidents, blunt trauma with, 343
  surgery for, 507
Mouth opening, in examination of airway, 88
Moyamoya disease, 512, 512
Mucopolysaccharidoses, airway difficulties with,
    118t–119t
Mucosa, nasal, and cribriform plate interface, drug
    administration and, 175, 175
    oral, 79–80
Muscle(s), biopsy of, in malignant hyperthermia,
    622–623, 626
  diaphragm and intercostal, fiber composition of, 87,
    87
  drug volume of distribution in, in infants vs. adults,
    123, 124
  physiology of, in controlled hypotension, 251–252
  respiratory, in newborns, mechanics of breathing and,
    11
  smooth, of pulmonary arteries, development of, 10
  voluntary and involuntary activity of, in thermoregula-
    tion, 612
Muscle relaxant(s), 196–215
  antagonism of, 208–209
  depolarizing, 199–202
    succinylcholine as, 199–202
      controversies in use of, 201–202
      doses for, 199t, 199–200
      duration of action of, 200

Muscle relaxant(s) (Continued)
    routes of administration of, 200
    side effects of, 200–201
    uses of, 201
  effects of intentional hemodilution on, 255
  in burn injuries, 210–211
  in myasthenia gravis, 210
  in myotonia, 210
  in neurosurgical procedures, 500
  in progressive muscular dystrophy, 209–210
  in status epilepticus, 327
  in surgery for congenital heart disease, 399
  in tracheal intubation, in emergencies, 318
    with open eye injury, 489
  intraocular pressure and, 482
  neuromuscular transmission monitors for, 731
  nondepolarizing, disadvantages of, 206
    in burn patients, 532
    in neurosurgical procedures, 500
    in rapid-sequence induction, 316
    intermediate-acting, 203–206
      clinical implications of, 206
    long-acting, 206–208
    short-acting, 202–203
      clinical implications of, 206
  with nitrous oxide, recovery time from, 699
Muscle rigidity, in malignant hyperthermia, 619
Muscle tone, of pharyngeal structures, in airway
    obstruction during anesthesia, 87
Muscular dystrophy, progressive, muscle relaxants for,
    209–210
Muscularization, of pulmonary arteries, development of,
    10
Mustard procedure, for transposition of great arteries,
    439–440, 441
  long-term sequelae of, 362, 363, 439
Myasthenia gravis, muscle relaxants for, 210
Mydriatics, for ophthalmologic procedures, systemic
    effects of, 485
Myelodysplasia, 516, 516
  Chiari malformation with, 517, 517, 517t
  latex allergy and, 516-517
Myelography, anesthesia for, 574
Myocardium, physiology of, in controlled hypotension,
    250–251
Myoglobinemia, succinylcholine use and, 201
Myopathy, mitochondrial, 383–384
Myotonia, muscle relaxants for, 210
Myringotomy, for drainage in otitis media, 473–475,
    474

Nager's syndrome, airway difficulties with, 119t
Nalbuphine (Nubain), 151
  for reversal of opioid-induced pruritus, 692
Nalmefene, for reversal of narcotics, 602
Naloxone (Narcan), for reversal of narcotics, 602, 692
Naropin. See Ropivacaine (Naropin)
Narcotics, 146–151. See also Opioids.
  for postoperative analgesia in outpatients, 61
  in burn patients, 536–537
  in neurosurgical procedures, 503, 503t
  thermoregulatory effects of, 615
Nasal mucosa, and cribriform plate interface, drug
    administration and, 175, 175
  vasoconstrictors in, 500
Nasal suctioning, traumatic, functional choanal atresia
    with, emergency neonatal surgery for, 301
Nasolacrimal duct, drug absorption through, 485
Nasopharyngitis, outpatient surgery and, 56
Nasopharynx, temperature of, 627, 627
Nasotracheal intubation, for neurosurgical procedures,
    500
Nasotracheal tube, positioning of, in prone position, 501
Nausea and vomiting, in postanesthesia care unit,
    707–708

Nausea and vomiting (Continued)
  postoperative, after neurosurgical procedures, 506
    after strabismus surgery, prophylaxis for, 488
    after tonsillectomy, 62, 465, 466
    in outpatient surgery, 62–63
  with epidural opioids, 692
Necrotizing enterocolitis (NEC), in neonates, emergency surgery for, 308, 308–309
Nembutal (pentobarbital), for sedation, 600, 601t
Neonates. See also Infants.
  airway of, vs. adult, 81–82, 82–83
  apnea in, 45–48, 55–56, 294–295, 295t
  blood transfusion in, with whole blood, hyperkalemia and, 244
  bupivacaine in, maximum infusion dose of, 687
    toxicity of, 690
  calcium homeostasis in, 299
  cardiopulmonary function in, 294–297
  cardiovascular physiology in, 353–357
  chest compressions in, in CPR, 270, 272
  emergencies in, 294–314
  EMLA cream in, 638
  fluid management in, 223–224, 298
  gastrointestinal function in, 299
  glucose homeostasis in, 298–299
  growth and development of, blood pressure in, 16
    blood values in, 20
    blood volume in, 19–20
    body composition in, 9
    breathing and gas exchange in, 14–15
    cardiac output in, 16
    coagulation in, 20
    drug metabolism in, 124–125, 126t, 127t
    electrocardiographic findings in, 16
    facial growth in, 8
    gastrointestinal system development in, 18–19
    head circumference in, 8
    heart rate in, 15–16
    hematopoietic system development in, 19–20
    hepatic system function in, 17
    hyperbilirubinemia in, 17t, 17–18
    hyperglycemia in, 19
    hypoglycemia in, 19
    lung development in, 9–11
    maternal history and, 38, 39t
    normal respiratory parameters in, 15
    pancreatic development in, 19
    protein binding of drugs in, 122
    pulmonary ventilation in, 10–11
    renal system in, 16–17
    teeth in, 9
    thermoregulation in, 612–613
    weight assessment in, 5–8, 6t, 7, 8t
  hepatic function in, 299
    metabolism of drugs by, 636
  HIV testing in, informed consent of mother for, 75
  intravenous access in, 298
  local anesthetic toxicity in, 639
    precautions for, 687, 690t
  methemoglobin reductase in, prilocaine metabolism and, 638
  monitoring in, 298
  morphine half-life in, 679
  muscle relaxants in, 208
  neurologic development in, 299–300
  physiology of, 294–300
  pulmonary hypertension in, persistent, 10, 297
    inhaled nitric oxide for, 305
  renal function in, 297–298
  stress response in, 403
  subarachnoid block in, drugs used for, 646
    technique of, 644–646, 645–646
  surgery in, emergency, 300–310
    for gastrointestinal problems, 305–310
    for respiratory problems, 300–305

Neonates (Continued)
    preparation for, 300
  temperature regulation in, 297
  transitional circulation in, 354–356, 355t, 359t
Neostigmine, for reversal of muscle relaxants, 208
Neo-Synephrine (phenylephrine), 278, 366t, 369, 485, 500
Nephrotoxicity, of sevoflurane, 138–139
Nerve(s), recurrent laryngeal, 80
  superior laryngeal, 80
Nerve block(s), caudal, in outpatients, 61
    in postoperative analgesia, 684
  central, anatomic and physiologic aspects of, 642–643, 642–644
    epidural anesthesia and, 647–651
    spinal anesthesia and, 644–647, 645–646
  for postoperative analgesia. See Regional blockade.
  ilioinguinal and iliohypogastric, in outpatients, 61
  in sedated children, 597
  peripheral, 651–669
    ankle, 668, 668–669
    digital, of foot, 669
      of hand, 663, 663–664
    elbow, 661
    head and neck, 653–655, 653–656
    inguinal, 656, 658, 658
    intercostal, 655–656, 657
    lower extremity, 664–667, 664–668
    nerve stimulator use with, 652–653, 652–653
    penile, 658–659, 659
      for postoperative analgesia, 684
      in outpatients, 61
    selection of local anesthetic for, 652
    types of, 652t
    upper extremity, 659, 659–661
    vs. central neuraxial blockade, 651–652
    wrist, 661–663, 662
  recovery from after inhalation anesthesia, 699–700
  reversal of by cholinesterase inhibitors, 700
  sites of, and toxicity of local anesthetics, 640
Nerve stimulator, use with peripheral nerve blocks, 652–653, 652–653
Nervous system, development of, 21t, 21–22
  in neonates, 299–300
  local anesthetic toxicity affecting, 638, 641, 642
Neuroendocrine response, to cardiac surgery, opioids for, 403
Neurofibromatosis, 510
Neurologic disease, pathophysiology of, 493–497
Neurologic function, evaluation of, 196–199
    frequency of stimulation for, 196–199, 197–198
    types of stimulation in, 196–199, 197–198
      in peripheral nerve blocks, 652–653, 652–653
  in postanesthesia care unit, 708–709
  in trauma patients, 340
  problems with, in burn patients, hyperbaric oxygen for, 537–538
Neuromuscular transmission, monitors for, 731
Neuronal injury, with caudal epidural anesthesia, 651
Neuroradiologic procedures, 517–518
Neurosurgical procedure(s), anesthetic management in, 497–507
  craniofacial reconstruction as, 515–516
  craniosynostosis and, 514–515
  craniotomy as, 509–513
  for congenital anomalies, 516–517
  hydrocephalus and, 513–514
  trauma as, 507–509
Nitric oxide, 141–142, 142t
  inhaled, cardiac effects of, 374, 375
    for pulmonary hypertension, 305, 374, 375
    for pulmonary vasodilation, in separation from cardiopulmonary bypass, 401
    in congenital heart disease, 375
    in postoperative care after cardiac surgery, 406

Nitroglycerin, doses and cardiac effects of, 371t, 373
  in controlled hypotension, 250–253
    dosage of, 252
    toxicity of, 253
Nitrous oxide, contraindications to, 142
  general properties of, 141–142
  in neurosurgical procedures, 503, 503t
  in sedation in non-operating room location, 604–605, 606t
  in subsequent seizure surgery, 513
  in surgery for congenital heart disease, 398–399
  inhaled, in middle ear surgery, 475
  with muscle relaxants, recovery time from, 699
Nonsteroidal anti-inflammatory drugs (NSAIDs), 151–152
  for postoperative analgesia, 467, 678, 707
  in outpatients, 61
Noonan syndrome (Turner syndrome), airway difficulties with, 120t
Norepinephrine, brown fat metabolism and, in thermoregulation, 612
  in arteriovenous shunt blood flow, in thermoregulation, 612
  with toxic reactions to local anesthetics, 642
Norwood procedure, for hypoplastic left heart syndrome, 445, 446
Nose, artificial, for perioperative airway humidification, 614, 629, 716
NSAIDs. See Nonsteroidal anti-inflammatory drugs (NSAIDs).
Nubain (nalbuphine), 151
Nursing care, in postanesthesia care unit, 710
  role in sedation, 596

Obesity, with sleep apnea, 462
Occipital pain, greater occipital nerve block for, 654, 654
Oculoauriculovertebral syndrome (Goldenhar syndrome), airway difficulties with, 118t
Oculocardiac reflex, 480, 481
  management of, 480
Oculomandibulodyscephaly (Hallerman-Streif syndrome), airway difficulties with, 118t
Oliguria, in postanesthesia care unit, 708
Omphalocele, 18
  in neonates, emergency surgery for, 309, 309t, 309–310
Ondansetron (Zofran), 155
  for postoperative nausea and vomiting, after strabismus surgery, 488
    after tonsillectomy, 466
    in outpatients, 62
  for premedication, 182
Operating room, for trauma cases, set-up of, 344–345
  monitoring equipment in, 2–3
  supply cart in, 725, 725t
  temperature of, 628
Operating table, properties of, 716
Ophthalmologic procedures, anesthesia for, 482–484
  drugs for, systemic effects of, 484–485
  for congenital cataracts, 487
  for glaucoma, 487–488
  for open eye injury with full stomach, 489–490
  for retinopathy of prematurity, 488–489
  for strabismus, 488
  induction and intubation for, 484
  monitoring for, 483–484
  premedication for, 483
  preoperative evaluation for, 482–483
Opioids, antagonists of, for reversal of narcotics, 602
  central neuraxial, risks of, 692
  effect on stress response, 403
  epidural, 650
    urinary retention and, 651

Opioids *(Continued)*
  with local anesthetics, for postoperative analgesia,
      686–687, 687t, 690, 690t, 691t, 692–693, 707
  for postoperative analgesia, 678–681
    choice of drug in, 679
    continuous intravenous, 678–679
    hydrophilic, catheter administration of, 685–686
    intermittent intravenous, 678
    intramuscular, 678
    patient-controlled, 679–681
    risks and adverse effects of, 692, 693
    subcutaneous, 678
    with local anesthetics, 686–687, 687t, 690, 690t,
        691t, 692–693, 707
  for premedication, 177–179
  for sedation in children, 600
  hydrophilic, for postoperative analgesia, 685–686
    for thoracic or upper abdominal surgery, 687, 690
  in pediatric emergencies, 317
  in postanesthesia care unit, 707
  in surgery for congenital heart disease, 399
  intraocular pressure and, 481
  intravenous, for postoperative analgesia, 678
  recovery from, 700
Optimal external laryngeal manipulation (OELM), 104
Oral procedures, endocarditis prophylaxis with, 422t
Oralet (fentanyl), for premedication, 149, 178, *179*
  for sedation in children, 602, 602t
Orchiopexy, ilioinguinal nerve block with, for
    postoperative analgesia, 684
Organ systems, development of, 9–11
Osmolality, regulation of, 216–218, *218*
Osmolar disturbances, dehydration and, 228–229
Otitis media, myringotomy for, 473–475
Otorhinolaryngology procedures, anesthesia for,
    461–477
Outpatient surgery, 55–67
  anesthetic agents and techniques used in, 59–61
  choice of procedure for, 56–57
  complications and admissions in, 64–65
  patient selection criteria for, 55–57
  postoperative analgesia in, 61–62
  postoperative nausea and vomiting in, 62–63
  pre-anesthetic management in, 58–59
  preoperative requirements for, 57–58
  recovery and discharge in, 63–64
  screening for, 58
  staff and facility issues in, 57
Oxygen, 142–143
  after inhalation anesthesia, 699
  cerebral blood flow and, 496–497
  for bronchiolitis, 322
  in rapid-sequence induction, 188
  operating room monitors for, 727
  partial pressure of, normal values of, age-related
      changes in, 15
  retinopathy of prematurity and, 45, 142–143, 300,
      488–489
  supplemental, on arrival in postanesthesia care unit,
      702
  transcutaneous monitors of, 732–733
  uptake and delivery of, in neonates, 296–297
  venous, in malignant hyperthermia, 619
Oxygen consumption, in burn patients, 536
  in neonates, 294, 295t
    environmental temperature and, 613
  in thermoregulatory response, 612
Oxygen saturation, in burn patients, 533
  pulse oximetry monitoring of, 727–729
Oxygenation, in burn injuries, 526–527
  hyperbaric, 537–538
  tissue, in intentional hemodilution, 255
Oxygen-hemoglobin dissociation, in carbon monoxide
    poisoning, 527, *528*
  with massive blood loss, 246–247, *247*, 247t

Oxyscope, 104, *104*

Pacemakers, external, 725
    properties of, 725
  in magnetic resonance imaging, 576
  transcutaneous, in cardiopulmonary resuscitation, 277
PACU. See *Postanesthesia care unit (PACU)*
Pain. See also *Analgesia.*
  in children, assessment of, 675–676
    management of, 73–74
  in diagnostic procedures in non-operating room loca-
      tion, sedation for, 584
  in postanesthesia care unit, 704, 706–707
  management of, general principles of, 73–74, 707
    in burn patients, 531, 536–537, 537t
    in pediatric emergencies, 317
  postoperative, 676–681. See also *Analgesia, postoper-
      ative.*
    after neurosurgical procedures, 507
    after tonsillectomy, 466–467
  scales of, 675–676
  self-assessment ratings of, 675
PALS (Pediatric Advanced Life-Support), 336
Pancreas, blunt trauma to, 343
  development of, 19
Pancuronium, for anesthesia maintenance, in cardiac
    transplantation, 546
  in neurosurgical procedures, 500
  in postoperative care after cardiac surgery, 406
  in surgery for congenital heart disease, 399
  pharmacokinetics of, 207, *207*
Papillomas, choroid plexus, 510
Papillomatosis, laryngeal, airway difficulties with, 119t
  laser surgery for, 472, *472*
Paramyotonia, 210
Parents, anxiety of, and preoperative anxiety in
    children, 28
  in behavioral preoperative programs for children,
      29
  in preoperative interview, *30*, 30–31, 37–38
    for outpatient surgery, 57
  informed consent and, *30*, 30–31
  care of, in malignant hyperthermia episode, 626
  in anesthesia induction, in mentally handicapped
      child, 45
  in emergency neonatal surgery, 300
  in postanesthesia care unit, 63, 709
  preparation of, for postoperative pain, 677
  presence during induction, 188–189
    in ophthalmologic procedures, 483
    in outpatient surgery, 59
    in pediatric emergencies, 318
  separation anxiety in children and, 25–27, 173
Partial thromboplastin time, coagulopathy with, 241
Patent ductus arteriosus, 421–424
  complications of, 424
  in neonates, 296–297
  repair of, 422–423, *423*
  residua of, 423
  sequelae of, 423–424
  surgery for, 406
Patient-controlled analgesia (PCA), 679–681
  basal infusion feature of, 680
  dosage guidelines for, 680, 680t
  patient training for, 680
  pump settings for, 680
  side effects of, 681
  standing order form for, 680, *682–683*
  variations of, 680–681
Patient-controlled epidural analgesia (PCEA), 686
Patil-Syracuse endoscopy mask, 105
PCA. See *Patient-controlled analgesia (PCA)*
Pediatric Advanced Life Support (PALS), 336
Pediatric research, federal classifications of, 74t
  informed consent for, 74

Pediatric syndromes and conditions, causing airway
    difficulties, 117t–120t
Penile block, 658–659, *659*
  for postoperative analgesia, 684
  in outpatients, 61
Pentobarbital, for premedication, 176
  for sedation, 600, 601t
Peripheral vascular resistance, in transition to air
    breathing, 11
Peritoneal bands, 18
Peroneal nerve, deep and superficial, block of, 668, *668*
Perphenazine, for premedication, 183
Persistent pulmonary hypertension of newborn, 10, 297
pH, normal values of, age-related changes in, 15
Pharyngeal structures, muscle tone of, in airway
    obstruction during anesthesia, 87
Phenothiazines, for premedication, 176
Phenoxybenzamine, doses and cardiac effects of, 373
Phentolamine, doses and cardiac effects of, 371t, 373
Phenylephrine (Neo-Synephrine), doses and cardiac
    effects of, 366t, 369
  for cardiopulmonary resuscitation, 278
  for ophthalmologic procedures, systemic effects of,
      485
  in nasal mucosa, 500
Phenytoin, doses and cardiac effects of, 376t, 377
Phonation, laryngeal function during, 81
Phosphodiesterase inhibitors, doses and cardiac effects
    of, 369
Phrenic nerve blockade, with upper extremity blocks,
    659
Physical examination, before sedation, guidelines for,
    588
  in airway evaluation, *88*, 88–89
  in congenital heart disease, 392
  in neurosurgical procedures, 497–498
  in pediatric emergencies, 315
  in preoperative evaluation, 39–40
Physiologic acidemia of infancy, 17
Pierre Robin syndrome, airway difficulties with, 119t
  laryngeal position in, 82, *82*
Pilocarpine, for glaucoma therapy, systemic effects of,
    486
Pipecuronium, pharmacokinetics of, 208
Plasma cholinesterase, deficiency of, neuromuscular
    blockade and, 203
  succinylcholine action and, 200
Plasminogen, impaired hemostasis on separation from
    bypass and, 401–402
Plastic wrap, during anesthesia, for reducing heat loss,
    614, 717
Platelets, compatibilities of, 237t
  dilutional thrombocytopenia and, 242, *242–243*
  doses of, 239
  indications for, 238–239
  ketorolac use and, 152
  transfusion of, for impaired hemostasis on separation
      from bypass, 394, 401
  units and storage of, 239
Pneumothorax, with intercostal nerve block, 656
Poisoning, emergency management of, 327
Polycythemia, neonatal, 20
  preoperative, cardiac repair and, 418
Polytomography, anesthesia for, 574
Pompe disease, airway difficulties with, 119t
Position(ing), for neurosurgical procedures, modified
    lateral, 502
  prone, *501*, 501–502
  sitting, 502, *502*
  in cardiac catheterization, 408
  in liver transplantation, 555
  in lung transplantation, 550
  in renal transplantation, 563
  sitting, venous air emboli and, 504
Positive end-expiratory pressure, with airway
    obstruction, 318, *318*

Postanesthesia care unit (PACU), 698–714
  arrival in, 701–702
  crash cart in, 702t, 703t, 710
  discharge from, 703t, 703–704, 704t
  documentation in, 710
  endotracheal extubation in, 701
  fast-track recovery in, 65, 709, 710t
  in outpatient surgery, 63
  nursing care in, 710
  organization of, 702t, 702–703, 703t
  parents in, 63, 709
  policies and procedures in, 709–711
  problems in, 704–709
  procedural aspects of, 700–704
  size and physical layout of, 702
  staffing of, 703
  transport to, 701
Post-dural puncture headache, with spinal anesthesia,
      647
Post-tetanic count and facilitation, in evaluation of
      neuromuscular function, 198, 199
Potassium, homeostasis of, dehydration and, 229
  disorders of, 231–232
  in renal transplantation, 564
  serum, in malignant hyperthermia, 619
Potter syndrome, 16
Premature ventricular arrhythmias, in postanesthesia
      care unit, 706
  with tetralogy of Fallot repair, 436
Premedication, 172–184
  drugs for, 174t, 174–184
    factors influencing, 172
    ideal, 173
    in outpatient surgery, 58–59
    for reducing anxiety, 31–32, 31–32
      vs. behavioral interventions, 31–32, 32
  general principles of, 172–174
  in cardiac transplantation, 546
  in congenital heart disease patients, 395
  in controlled hypotension, 253
  in neurosurgical procedures, 498
  in ophthalmologic procedures, 483
  in pediatric emergencies, 316–317
  objectives of, 172
  preoperative consideration of, 2
  route of administration of, 173–174
  types of, 31, 32
Preoperative period, anxiety in, interventions for,
      behavioral, 28–31
    pharmacologic, 31–32
  outcomes of, 32–34
  risk factors for, 27, 27t, 27–28
  evaluation in, 1–2, 37–54
    anemia in, 42–43
    asthma and reactive airway disease in, 49–50
    bronchopulmonary dysplasia in, 48
    diabetic children in, 48–49
    fasting in, 41, 41–42
    fever in, 44
    for neurosurgical procedures, 497–498
    full stomach in, 42. See also Fasting.
    hyperalimentation in, 49
    laboratory data in, 40–41
    medical history in, 38–39, 39t
    mentally handicapped children in, 45
    physical examination in, 39–40
    postoperative apnea in. See Apnea, postoperative.
    retinopathy of prematurity in, 45. See also Retinop-
      athy of prematurity.
    seizure disorders in, 49
    sickle cell disease in, 44–45
    upper respiratory tract infection in, 43–44
  interview in, 37–38
    in behavioral preoperative program, 30, 30–31
  patient monitoring in, 2

Preoperative period (Continued)
    preparation programs in, for outpatient surgery,
      57–58
    risks in, 1–2
Prilocaine, metabolism of, in neonates, 638
  topical administration and doses of, 597
Procainamide, doses and cardiac effects of, 375, 376t
Progressive muscular dystrophy, muscle relaxants for,
      209–210
Promethazine, for premedication, 176
Propafenone, doses and cardiac effects of, 377
Proparacaine, for ophthalmologic procedures, systemic
      effects of, 485
Propofol (Diprivan), 144–145
  advantages of, 144
  for avoidance of malignant hyperthermia, 626
  for induction, 187, 187t
    in neurosurgical procedures, 499
    in outpatient anesthesia, 60
    rapid intravenous, 42
  for nausea after strabismus surgery, 488
  for sedation in non-operating room location, 603–
      604, 605t
  for toxic reactions to local anesthetics, 641
  in cardiac catheterization, 408
  in critical care medicine, 144–145
  in surgery for congenital heart disease, 399
  intraocular pressure and, 481
  recovery from, 700
Propranolol, doses and cardiac effects of, 371t, 372,
      376t, 377–378
Prostacyclin, cardiac effects of, 375
Prostaglandin E₁, doses and cardiac effects of, 371t, 374
Protamine, in separation from cardiopulmonary bypass,
      401
Protein binding, drug distribution and, 122–123
Prothrombin time, coagulopathy with, 241
Pruritus, with epidural opioids, 692
Pseudocholinesterase deficiency, 700
Psychological preparation, for postoperative pain, 677
  for surgery, 37–38
    behavioral preoperative programs for, 28–29
Psychological support, for burn patients, 531
Pulmonary. See also Lung(s).
Pulmonary acid aspiration syndrome (Mendelson
      syndrome), 41–42
  premedication for, 183–184, 184t
Pulmonary artery, blood flow in, in congenital heart
      disease, 360
  catheterization of, for blood pressure monitoring, 732
    in lung transplantation, 549
    in massive blood transfusion, 248
    technique of, 746–747, 748–749
  clamping of before pneumonectomy, in lung trans-
      plantation, 550–551
  development of, 9–10
    neonatal, 358
  nonmuscular, 10
  partially muscular, 10
  pressure in, in lung transplantation, 550–551
  stenosis of, balloon angioplasty for, 451
  thermodilution lines in, in congenital heart disease
      surgery, 396
Pulmonary cysts, congenital, emergency surgery for,
      305
Pulmonary edema, after tonsillectomy, 466
Pulmonary gas exchange, age-related changes in, 14–15
  in neonates, 294–296
  monitoring devices for, 732
Pulmonary hypertension, after cardiac surgery,
      prevention of, 406
  in atrial septal defect, 427
  in atrioventricular septal defect, 432
  in congenital heart disease, separation from cardiopul-
      monary bypass and, 401

Pulmonary hypertension (Continued)
  in newborns, inhaled nitric oxide for, 305
    persistent, 10, 297
  in ventricular septal defect, 428–429, 430
  inhaled nitric oxide for, 305, 374, 375
  liver transplantation and, 552
  persistent, of newborn, 10, 297
  preoperative, cardiac repair and, 419
  primary, cardiac pathophysiology with, 365
Pulmonary regurgitation, with tetralogy of Fallot repair,
      435
Pulmonary valve, stenosis of, cardiac catheterization
      treatment for, 450
Pulmonary vascular obstructive disease, in atrial septal
      defect, 427
  in atrioventricular septal defect, 432
  in ventricular septal defect, 428–429
  with transposition of great arteries, 439
Pulmonary vascular resistance (PVR), and separation
      from cardiopulmonary bypass, 401
  in atrial septal defect, 427
  in cardiac transplantation, 546
  in congenital heart disease surgery, 394, 395, 397,
      397t
    nitrous oxide and, 398
  in intracardiac shunts, 393–394
  in neonates, 296–297, 356–357, 359t
  in transition to air breathing, 11
  in ventricular septal defect repair, 404
Pulmonary vessels, gestational development of, 9–10
  neonatal development of, 356, 358
Pulse oximetry, 727–729, 728–729
  clinical efficacy of, 727–728
  function of, 729
  in burn patients, 533, 533
  in malignant hyperthermia, 619
  in MRI studies, 578–579
  in pediatric emergencies, 300, 317
  in sickle cell disease, 45
  in surgery for congenital heart disease, 395
  vs. capnography, 728, 728–729
Pulseless electrical activity, 286
Pulselessness, in trauma cases, 335
Pyloric stenosis, hypertrophic, neonatal, emergency
      surgery for, 306–307, 307

Quinsy tonsil, 465, 465–466

Radial artery, catheterization of, 751–752, 751–753
Radial nerve, elbow block of, 661
  wrist block of, 661–662, 662
Radiant warmers, for operating room, 614, 716
Radiation, protection against by anesthesiologist, 580
Radiofrequency ablation, anesthetic management
      during, 408
  for arrhythmias, 379–380
Radiologic procedures, anesthesia for, 574–575, 579
  equipment for, for trauma victims, 344
  in evaluation for neurosurgical procedures, 498
  sedation for, 586–587
Ranitidine (Zantac), 154–155
  for premedication, 184, 184t
Rapacuronium (Raplon), recovery from, 700
  uses and complications of, 203
Rapid Infusion System, for warming fluids, 717
Reactive airway disease, in preoperative evaluation,
      49–50
Recovery from anesthesia, 698–700
  fast track, 65, 709
    discharge criteria for, 710t
  from inhalation anesthetics, 698–699
  from outpatient surgery, 63, 65
  in 23-hour unit, 65
  intravenous opioids and hypnotics in, 700

Recovery from anesthesia (Continued)
  neuromuscular blockade in, 699–700
  physicochemical factors in, 698–699
  respiratory reflexes in, 699
  signs of, 698
Recovery room, 4
Rectal administration, of methohexital, for induction, 143
  for outpatient surgery, 59
  for premedication, 177, 483
  for sedation for CT scans, 573
Rectal temperature, 627, 628
Recurrent laryngeal nerve, blockade of, with interscalene block, 659
Red blood cells, blood products containing, 237t, 237–238, 238t
  irradiated, potassium values of, 244
  packed, citrated, 238t
    clinical uses of, 238
    compatibilities of, 237t
    frozen, 238t
    transfusion of, clotting factor deficiency with, 241
Regional anesthesia, 636–674. See also Local anesthetics.
  advantages of, 636
  central neuraxial blockade in, 642–651. See also Nerve block(s), central.
  for postoperative analgesia, in outpatient surgery, 61
  in bone marrow transplant recipients, 566
  intravenous (Bier block), 660–661
  peripheral nerve blocks in, 651–669. See also Nerve block(s), peripheral.
  thermoregulation in, 615–616
  vs. general anesthesia, and postoperative apnea, 47–48
Regional blockade. See also Nerve block(s).
  for postoperative analgesia, 681–693
    catheter techniques of, 685–693
    contraindications to, 681
    drug selection for, 686–687, 687t, 690, 690t, 691t, 692–693
    limitations of, 681, 684
    single-injection technique of, 684–685
    timing of, 681
  in emergencies, 317
Reglan. See Metoclopramide (Reglan).
Rehydration, rapid, in emergencies, 318
Remifentanil (Ultiva), 150–151
  for sedation in children, 600–601
  in postanesthesia care unit, 700
  pharmacokinetics and pharmacodynamics of, 150–151, 151
Renal. See also Kidney(s).
Renal function, dehydration and, 229
  growth and development of, 16–17
  in liver transplantation, 557
  in neonates, 127–128, 127–128
  physiology of, in controlled hypotension, 251
  sevoflurane use and, 138–139
Renal output curve, 218, 219
Reperfusion syndrome, in liver transplantation, 556
Respiration, muscles of, in newborn, 11
  normal parameters of, in infants and adults, 15
Respiratory depression, with meperidine, vs. morphine, 148
  with midazolam, 154
  with morphine, in children, 147
    in neonates, 679
  with opioids, 692
  with sedatives combined with narcotics, 599, 600
Respiratory distress syndrome, in neonates, 296
Respiratory function. See also Breathing; Ventilation.
  cervical spine injury and, 509
  problems with, emergency surgery for, in neonates, 300–305

Respiratory function (Continued)
  in congenital diaphragmatic hernia, 304
  in postanesthesia care unit, 704–705
  recovery after inhalation anesthesia, 699
  with central neuraxial blockade, in infants, 643
  postoperative, 643
Respiratory system, physiology of, 82–87
  obligate nasal breathing in, 82–84
  tracheal and bronchial function in, 84–86, 86
  work of breathing in, 85, 87
  procedures on, endocarditis prophylaxis with, 422t
  upper, infection of, 474, 475t
Resuscitation, in pediatric emergencies, 315
  drug dosages in, 316t
Retinopathy of prematurity, causes of, 45
  correction of, anesthesia for, 484
  factors influencing, 142
  in preoperative evaluation, 45
  oxygen use and, 45, 142–143, 300, 488–489
  surgery for, 488–489
Retrolental fibroplasia. See Retinopathy of prematurity.
Revex (nalmefene), for reversal of narcotics, 602
Rhabdomyolysis, succinylcholine use and, 202
Rheumatic heart disease, cardiac pathophysiology with, 365
Rheumatoid arthritis, airway difficulties with, 119t
Rhinitis, runny nose with, outpatient surgery and, 56
Ribavirin, for bronchiolitis, 323
Right ventricular outflow tract obstruction, with tetralogy of Fallot repair, 435
Risk management, preoperative, 1–2, 38
  role in implementing sedation guidelines, 596
Robinul (glycopyrrolate), 155
Rocuronium (Zemuron), in neurosurgical procedures, 500
  in pediatric trauma, 337, 345
  in rapid intravenous induction, 42, 345
  intramuscular, 206
  intraocular pressure and, 482
  pharmacokinetics of, 205–206
  recovery from, 700
Rofecoxib (Vioxx), for postoperative analgesia, 678
Ropivacaine (Naropin), for postoperative analgesia in caudal block, 684
  pharmacokinetics of, 637
Rubenstein-Taybi syndrome, airway difficulties with, 120t
Runny nose, outpatient surgery and, 56
Ryanodine, in malignant hyperthermia, 617, 617, 623

Salbutamol, for treatment of hyperkalemia, 231
Sanfillipo syndrome, airway difficulties with, 119t
Saphenous nerve, block of, 668, 668
Scalp, injuries of, surgery for, 507
  local anesthesia in, for neurosurgical procedures, 502
Scheie syndrome, airway difficulties with, 119t
Sciatic nerve block, 664–665, 665–666
  lateral popliteal, 665–666, 667
SCIWORA (spinal cord injury without radiological abnormalities), 509
Scleral buckling procedure, for retinopathy of prematurity, 489
Scleroderma, airway difficulties with, 120t
Scopolamine, 155
  for premedication, 180
Secobarbital, for premedication, 176
Sedation, assessment of, 585, 585
  definition of, 585, 585–576
  discharge criteria for patients with, 599
  drugs used for, 152–154, 153
    anxiolytic, 598t–602t, 598–603
    local anesthetic, 597t, 597–598
    nonbarbiturate, for premedication, 177
    systemic anesthetic, 603t–606t, 603–605
  for anesthesia in non-operating room location, 573

Sedation (Continued)
  for CT scans, 573, 573–574
  goals of, 576
  guidelines for, 587–595
    after sedation, 591, 594, 594–595
    before sedation, 588, 589–590, 591
    during sedation, 591, 591t, 592–593
    implementation of, 596–597
  in burn patients, 531
  in cardiac catheterization, 408
  in difficult airway intubation, 98
  in emergency room patients, 580
  in non-operating room location, 584–609
  in postoperative care after cardiac surgery, 406
  morphine overdose and, 679
  of mentally handicapped child, 45
  opioid-induced respiratory depression with, 692
  preoperative, for neurosurgical procedures, 498
  recommended intensity and documentation for, 591, 591t, 592–593
  risks and complications of, 576–587, 586, 587t
  service for, establishment of, 605–606
  specific techniques of, 597–605
  treatment plan for, 597
Seizures, in postanesthesia care unit, 708–709
  in preoperative evaluation, 49
  in status epilepticus, emergency management of, 326–327
  methohexital-induced, with temporal lobe epilepsy, 573
  surgery for, 512–513
    awake craniotomy for, 513
  threshold for, benzodiazepine premedicaton and, with local anesthetics, 640–641
  toxicity of local anesthetics and, 641
Senning procedure, for transposition of great arteries, 439–440, 440
  long-term sequelae of, 439
  sequelae with, 362, 363
Separation anxiety, in children, 25–26. See also under Parents.
Sepsis, regional blockade and, 681
Septic shock, 326
Serotonin antagonists, for postoperative vomiting, 708
Sevoflurane (Ultane), 137–140, 138, 138t, 140t
  cardiovascular effects of, 137–138
  for induction, 59–60, 185
    for neurosurgical procedures, 499
  in emergencies, 318
  in rigid bronchoscopy, 468–469
  in surgery for congenital heart disease, 398
  nephrotoxicity of, 138–139
  recovery time from, 699
  vs. halothane, 59–60, 138–140, 140t
Shaken baby syndrome, 508
Shivering, in thermoregulation, 612
  meperidine use and, 148
Shock, anaphylactic, 326
  cardiogenic, 325, 326
  emergency management of, 325t, 325–326, 328
  hypovolemic, 325, 325t, 326
  septic, 326
Shunt(s), arteriovenous, liver transplantation and, 552
  of hands and feet, in thermoregulatory response, 612
  Blalock-Taussig, for hypoplastic left heart syndrome, 445, 446
  extracranial, for hydrocephalus, 514, 515
    precautions with, 514
  Glenn, in Fontan repair, 445, 447, 447
  intracardiac, dependent, 393t, 393–394
    during anesthesia, 394
    in neonates, 296, 297
    in repair of ventricular septal defect, 404
    left-to-right, in atrial septal defect, 427

Shunt(s) *(Continued)*
   in congenital heart disease, 359
   in ventricular septal defect, 404, 428–429
     systemic blood flow in, vs. pulmonary blood
      flow, 367
     vascular resistance and, during anesthesia, 394,
      395, 397
     nitrous oxide and, in congenital heart disease sur-
      gery, 398
     obligatory, 393t, 393–394
     restrictive, 393t, 394
     right-to-left, hypoxemia with, in congenital heart
      disease, 359–360
     in congenital heart disease, 359–360
     in newborns, 11
     vascular resistance and, during anesthesia, 394,
      395, 397
   venous admixture and, in infants, 14
Sickle cell disease, in preoperative evaluation, 44–45
Sight wands, for intubation, 108
Skeletal muscle, fatty acid metabolism of, in malignant
   hyperthermia, 619
Skin, in burn injuries, 525
   physiology of, in controlled hypotension, 251–252
Skull, defects in, herniation through, 494
   fractures of, 507–508
   intracranial compartments in, pathophysiology of,
    493–494
Slit ventricle syndrome, 514, *515*
Smith-Lemli-Opitz syndrome, airway difficulties with,
   120t
Smoke inhalation injury, 524, 526–527
   carbon monoxide poisoning with, 527
Sodium bicarbonate, in cardiopulmonary resuscitation,
   279–280
   with local anesthetic, in peripheral nerve blocks, 652
Sodium nitroprusside, doses and cardiac effects of,
   371t, 373
   in controlled hypotension, 250–252
    dosage of, 252
   toxicity of, 252
Sodium thiopental, for premedication, 176–177
   intraocular pressure and, 481
Somnolence, in postanesthesia care unit, 709
Sotalol, doses and cardiac effects of, 378
   in cardiopulmonary resuscitation, 285
Spinal anesthesia, 644–647, *645–646*
   complications of, 646–647
   selection of drug for, 646
   technique of, 644–646, *645–646*
   uses of, 644
Spinal cord, injury of, 508–509
    airway control in, in cardiopulmonary resuscitation,
    266
    without radiologic abnormalities, 509
   tethered, 517
Spine, cervical. See also *Cervical spine.*
   defects of, miscellaneous, 517
   injury of, surgery for, 508–509
Spleen, blunt trauma to, 343
Stadol (butorphanol), 151
Status asthmaticus, airway obstruction with, emergency
   management of, 323t–324t, 323–325
   anesthesia in, 324–325
   nebulized drugs for, 323t
   parenteral drug therapy for, 324t
Status epilepticus, emergency management of, 326–327
Stenosis, laryngotracheal (subglottic), 93–94
Stents, cardiovascular, for prevention of restenosis, 451
Stethoscope, esophageal, 726
   precordial, 726
   for monitoring, 3
Stevens-Johnson syndrome, airway difficulties with,
   120t
Strabismus, surgery for, 488

Strabismus *(Continued)*
   oculocardiac reflex and, 480
Stress response, behavioral, 25–36
   in children, 25–36
   to cardiac surgery, 402–403
Stridor, 467t, 467–468
   causes of, 467, 467t
   signs and symptoms of, 468t
Stroke volume, in neonates, 356, *357–358*
Subarachnoid block, complications with, 646–647
   drugs used for, 646
   hemodynamic stability in, in children vs. adults, 643
   technique of, 644–646, *645–646*
Subarachnoid bolts, for monitoring intracranial pressure,
   495
Subarachnoid space, distance from skin to, 642, *643*
Subdural hematoma, surgery for, 508
Subglottic hemangioma, emergency neonatal surgery
   for, 302, *302*
Subglottic stenosis, 93–94
   congenital, emergency neonatal surgery for, 302
Subglottis, in infant and adult, 82, *85*
Sublimaze. See *Fentanyl (Sublimaze).*
Succinylcholine, contraindications to, 500
   for induction in trauma cases, 345
   for intubation with open eye injury, 489
   in burn patients, 211, 532
   in neurosurgical procedures, 500
   in pediatric trauma, 337
   in rapid intravenous induction, 42
   in rapid-sequence induction, 316
   in renal transplantation, 563
   intraocular pressure rise and, 482
   malignant hyperthermia and, 617, 619
   masseter muscle response to, 621–622, *622*
   rhabdomyolysis induced by, vs. hyperkalemia in ma-
    lignant hyperthermia, 619
   routine use of, in children, 209–210
   toxic reactions to local anesthetics and, 641–642
Suction apparatus, properties of, 715–716
Suctioning, nasal, traumatic, functional choanal atresia
   with, 301
   of blood, after tonsillectomy, 465, 466
Sufentanil (Sufenta), 149–150, *150*
   for premedication, 178
   in cardiac transplantation, 546
   pharmacokinetics and pharmacodynamics of, 149–
    150, *150*
Sulfur hexafluoride, in retinal detachment surgery, 487
Supraclavicular block, 659
Suprane. See *Desflurane (Suprane).*
Supraorbital nerve block, 653–654, *654*
Supratrochlear nerve block, 653–654, *654*
Supraventricular tachycardia, 285–286
Sural nerve block, 668, *668*
Surfactant, production of, 9
Surgery, emergency. See *Emergency surgery.*
Swallowing, development of, 18
   laryngeal function during, 81
Sweating, in anesthesia-induced hyperthermia, 616
Syndrome of inappropriate antidiuretic hormone
   secretion, 232
System review, in preoperative evaluation, anesthetic
   implications of, 38, 40t
Systemic vascular resistance, in anesthesia for surgery
   for congenital heart disease, 394, 395, 397, 397t
   in intracardiac shunts, 393–394
   in repair of ventricular septal defect, 404
Systemic venous obstruction, balloon angioplasty for,
   451

TAC (tetracaine/adrenalin/cocaine), topical
   administration and doses of, 597–598
Tachycardia, in malignant hyperthermia, 620, *620*
   in postanesthesia care unit, 706

Tachycardia *(Continued)*
   succinylcholine use and, 200
Tachyphylaxis, with local anesthetics, 692
Tagamet (cimetidine), 42, 154–155, 184, 184t
TAL (tetracaine/adrenalin/lidocaine), 598
Teeth, abnormalities of, 9
   examination of, in airway evaluation, *88, 89*
   growth of, 9
Temperament, separation anxiety and, 27
Temperature, axillary, 627, *627*
   monitors for, 727
   bladder, 628
   control of, in neurosurgical procedures, 504
    in postanesthesia care unit, 708
   esophageal, 627, *627*
    monitors for, 727
   in cardiopulmonary bypass, 400
   maintenance of, in trauma cases, 330
   mean body, 611–612
    anesthesia-induced changes in, 613
   monitoring of, 627–628
    in surgery for congenital heart disease, 395
    indications for, 627
    sites of, *627*, 627–628, 727
    thermometers used for, 627
   nasopharyngeal, 627, *627*
    monitors for, 727
   of central core, anesthesia-induced cooling of, 613,
    614
   rectal, *627*, 628
   regulation of. See *Thermoregulation.*
   skin-surface, 628
    and prevention of hypothermia, 628–629, *629*
   tympanic membrane, 628
Temporal artery, catheterization of, 752–753
Tetanic stimulation, for measurement of neuromuscular
   function, 197–198, *197–198*
Tethered spinal cords, 517
Tetracaine, for subarachnoid block in neonates and
   infants, 646, 646t
Tetracaine/adrenalin/cocaine (TAC), 597–598
Tetracaine/adrenalin/lidocaine (TAL), 598
Tetralogy of Fallot, 433–437
   abnormalities in, 433–434, *435*
   repair of, 405, 434–435, *436*
    complications of, 437
    preoperative factors influencing, 434
    residua and sequelae of, 361–362, 435–437
Thalassemia major (Cooley's anemia), airway
   difficulties with, 120t
Theophylline, postoperative apnea and, 47
Thermal imbalance, anesthesia-induced, 613–615
Thermogenesis, non-shivering, during anesthesia, effects
   of anesthetic drugs on, 615
   in infants, rewarming phase in, 615
   in thermoregulation, 612
Thermometers, 627
Thermoregulation, in burn patients, 529, *529*
   neutral thermal environment in, 613
   normal, afferent sensing in, 611
    central regulation in, *611*, 611–612
    efferent responses to, 612
    physiologic mechanisms of, 610–612, *611*
    thermoregulatory thresholds in, *611*, 611–612
    effects of anesthetic drugs on, 615–616
Thiamylal, for induction, 187, 187t
Thiopental, for control of intracranial hypertension, 144
   for induction, 144, 187, 187t
    in neurosurgical procedures, 499
    in outpatients, 60
   for sedation for CT scans, 573, 574
   for toxic reactions to local anesthetics, 641
   in burn patients, 531, *531*
   in rapid intravenous induction, 42
   in surgery for congenital heart disease, 399

Thiopental *(Continued)*
  metabolism of, hepatic maturity and, 124, *124*
Thomsen disease, 210
Thoracic surgery, postoperative analgesia for, catheter
        techniques for, 685–686
  epidural, 687, 690
Thorax, trauma to, blunt, 343
  evaluation of, 342–343
Thrombocytopenia, dilutional, with massive blood
        transfusion, 242, *242–243*
  in burn injuries, 525
  in newborn, 20
  regional blockade and, 681
Thromboelastography, in liver transplantation, 555, *555,
        556, 557*
  in massive blood transfusion, 248
Thrombosis, with antifibrinolytic therapy, on separation
        from bypass, 402
Thumb, digital nerve block of, *663,* 663–664
Thyroid disorders, in malignant hyperthermia, 621, 621t
  with craniopharyngioma, 510
Tibial artery, posterior, catheterization of, 753–754
Tibial nerve, block of, 668, *668*
Timolol, for glaucoma therapy, systemic effects of, 486
Toes, nerve blocks of, 669
Tongue, infant's, 81
Tonsil(s), quinsy, *465,* 465–466
  size of, classification of, 463, *464*
Tonsillectomy, analgesia following, 61–62
  and adenoidectomy, anesthesia for, 461–467
        intraoperative management of, 463–465
  discharge after, 467
  indications for, 461t
  postoperative care for, 57, 466–467
  postoperative emesis with, 62, 465, 466
  preoperative evaluation for, 462–463, *464*
Topical anesthetics, for ophthalmologic procedures,
        systemic effects of, 485
  in difficult airway management, 98
  in sedated child, 597
Topical corticosteroids, for glaucoma therapy, systemic
        effects of, 487
Toradol. See *Ketorolac (Toradol).*
Total body water, and age, 7, 8t
  in infants, 9
  in neonates, 298
  losses of, 223t
  regulation of, 218–219, *220*
Trabeculotomy, for glaucoma, 488
Trachea, compliance of, in newborns vs. adults, 13
  function of, in infants, 84–85, *86*
  intubation of. See *Endotracheal intubation.*
  upper, obstruction of, emergency neonatal surgery
        for, 301
  webs of, emergency neonatal surgery for, 301–302
Tracheoesophageal fistula, 18
  emergency neonatal surgery for, 302–304, *303*
Tracheostomy, "awake," 473
  elective, 473
  emergency, with spinal injury, 509
  in burn patients, 527
  insertion of tube in, 473, *474*
Train-of-four testing, in evaluation of neuromuscular
        function, 196–197, *197–199*
  in recovery from neuromuscular blockade, 700
  monitors of, 731
Tramadol (Ultram), 151
Tranexamic acid, impaired hemostasis on separation
        from bypass and, 401–402
Tranquilizers, for premedication, 174–176
Transcutaneous cardiac pacing, in cardiopulmonary
        resuscitation, 277
Transient tachypnea of newborn, 11
Transplantation. See also under anatomy for detail, e.g.,
        Liver transplantation.

Transplantation *(Continued)*
  anesthesia for, 544–569
  bone marrow, 564–567
  cardiac, 544–547
  heart-lung, 547–551
  liver, 551–559
  lung, 547–551
  renal, 559–564
Transport, after cardiothoracic surgery, 406
  equipment needed for, 733
  of trauma cases, in-hospital, 344
        interhospital, 344
  to and from operating room, heat transfer and, 614
  to postanesthesia care unit, 701
Transposition of great arteries, 437–449
  abnormalities in, 437, *438–439*
  arterial switch repair of, preoperative factors influenc-
        ing, 442t, 442–444, 443t, *443–444*
  atrial switch repair of, preoperative factors influenc-
        ing, 438–442, *440–441*
  Fontan procedure for, 444–449, *445–449*
  management milestones in, 437–438, 438t
  repaired, sequelae with, 362, *363*
Transtracheal catheter ventilation, 268, *269–270*
Trauma, 334–352
  blunt vs. penetrating, 342–343
  child abuse and, 345
        cutaneous signs of, *346*
  diagnostic procedures for, 344
  emergency management of, 328
  emergency room care for, *328,* 328–329, 329t, 335–
        336
  in children, time pattern of, 334
        types of, 334
        vs. trauma in adults, 334
  initial assessment for, airway in, 336–338
        breathing in, 338, 340
        circulation in, 340
        disability in, 340
        exposure in, 340
        scoring systems for, 336, 336t–337t, 339t
  initial resuscitation for, 328
  operating room management of, 329–330
  operative procedures for, 507–509
        preparation for, 344–345
  prehospital care for, 334–335
  secondary survey for, 329, 342–343
  temperature maintenance in, 341–342
  transport for, in-hospital, 344
        interhospital, 344
  vascular access and, 340–341
Treacher-Collins syndrome, airway difficulties with,
        120t
Trigeminal nerve, ophthalmic division of, peripheral
        nerve block of, 653–654, *654*
Trimethamine, in cardiopulmonary resuscitation,
        280–281
Trimethaphan (Arfonad), in controlled hypotension,
        250–252
Trisomy 21 (Down syndrome), airway difficulties with,
        120t
Tropicamide, for ophthalmologic procedures, systemic
        effects of, 485
Tubocurarine, in burn patients, 532, *532*
  intraocular pressure and, 482
  pharmacokinetics of, 206–207, *207*
  side effects of, 207
Tumors. See also *Cancer.*
  brain, craniotomy for, 509–510
  midbrain, 510
  posterior fossa, 509
Turner syndrome (Noonan syndrome), airway
        difficulties with, 120t
Twitch tension measurement, monitors of, 731
Tylenol (acetaminophen), 152

Tympanic membrane, temperature of, 628
Tympanoplasty, anesthesia for, 475

Ulnar nerve, elbow block of, 661
  wrist block of, *662,* 662–663
Ultane. See *Sevoflurane (Ultane).*
Ultiva (remifentanil), 150–151, *151,* 600–601, 700
Ultrafiltration, modified, for impaired hemostasis on
        separation from bypass, 401
Ultrasonography, Doppler precordial, for venous air
        emboli, 504–505, *505*
Umbilical artery, catheterization of, 749–751, *750*
Umbilical catheter, in neonates, 298
Umbilical vein, catheterization of, 747, 749, *749*
Unresponsiveness, in postanesthesia care unit, causes
        of, 709
Upper respiratory infection, criteria for, myringotomy
        and, 474, 475t
  hypoxemia with, after inhalation anesthesia, 699
  in preoperative evaluation, 43–44
  outpatient surgery and, 56
  vs. allergic rhinitis, 43
Uridine diphosphoglucuronosyltransferase, conjugation
        by, in neonates, 125
Urinary retention, with caudal epidural anesthesia, 651
Urine output, in burn patients, fluid replacement and,
        528
  invasive monitoring equipment for, 3

VACTERL association, imperforate anus with,
        emergency surgery for, 308
Vagal nerve stimulator, for seizure treatment, 513
Valium (diazepam), 152–153. See also *Diazepam.*
Valsalva maneuver, laryngeal function during, 81
Valvuloplasty, with cardiac catheterization, 450–451
Variance reports, in implementing sedation guidelines,
        596–597
Vascular access. See also *Intravenous access.*
  in trauma patients, 340–341
Vascular anomalies, 510–512
Vascular communications, closing of, with cardiac
        catheterization, 451
Vasoactive drugs, practical considerations with,
        365–367, 366t
  rational use of, 365
Vasoconstriction, cutaneous, as thermoregulatory
        response, 612
  during anesthesia, anesthetic drug effects on, 615
  in thermal steady-state, 615
Vasoconstrictors, in nasal mucosa, 500
  with toxic reactions to local anesthetics, 642
Vasodilation, in anesthesia-induced hyperthermia, 616
Vasodilators, doses and cardiac effects of, 371t, 372
  in congenital diaphragmatic hernia, 304–305
Vasopressin, aqueous, for diabetes insipidus after
        neurosurgical procedures, 507
  arginine, in regulation of serum osmolality, 217, *219*
VATER association, emergency neonatal surgery for,
        302
Vecuronium, for intubation, with open eye injury, 489
  in burn patients, 532, *532*
  long-term administration of, 205
  pharmacokinetics of, *202,* 204–205
Veins, pulmonary, gestational development of, 9–10
Venous air emboli, in repair of craniosynostosis, 515
  in surgery for brain tumors, 510
Veno-veno bypass, during liver transplantation, 555–556
Ventilating stylet, for use in extubation, 100
Ventilation. See also *Airway(s); Breathing.*
  bag-valve-mask devices for, 267–268
  by face mask, 89–90
        multihanded techniques for, 101, *101*

Ventilation *(Continued)*
  controlled, in neonates and infants, anesthesia machine circuits and, 722
  difficulty with, in postanesthesia care unit, 705
  expired carbon dioxide measurements and, 730
  in cardiopulmonary resuscitation, 267–268
    devices for, 267–268
  in laser surgery on airway, 472
  in rigid bronchoscopy, 469
  in status epilepticus, 326
  mechanical, effect on congenital heart disease patients, 368
  monitoring of, 267
    during anesthesia, 4
  mouth-to-mask, 267
  mouth-to-mouth, 267
  special techniques of, anterior commissure scope for, 103
    multihanded mask techniques of, 101, *101*
    percutaneous dilation cricothyrotomy for, 101–102, *103*
    percutaneous needle cricothyrotomy for, 101–102, *102*
    rigid ventilating bronchoscope for, 103
    surgical airway for, 103
    with laryngeal mask airway, 101. See also *Laryngeal mask airway.*
  spontaneous, in difficult airway management, 98
  transtracheal catheter, 268, *269–270*
Ventilation-perfusion imbalance, in infants, 14
  in postanesthesia care unit, 704
Ventilators, disconnect-apnea alarms for, 731–732
  in MRI studies, 578
  inspiratory pressure gauges for, 732
  of anesthesia machine, 723–725
Ventricle(s), compliance of, in neonates, 356, *356*
  outflow obstruction to, drug treatment for, 367

Ventricle(s) *(Continued)*
  right, after Mustard and Senning procedure repairs, 441–442
    afterload increases in, in lung transplantation, 549–551
  single, abnormalities with, 445
    Fontan operation for, 444–449, *445–449*
      sequelae with, 362, *364*
    in congenital heart disease, hypoxemia with, 360
    palliative repair and, 417
    systemic blood flow in, vs. pulmonary blood flow, 367
Ventricular assist devices, for mechanical circulatory support, 380
Ventricular ectopy, in malignant hyperthermia, 621
Ventricular fibrillation, defibrillation for, automated external, 283
  in children, 282–283
  open chest, 283
  drugs for, 283–285
    bretylium, 284–285
    lidocaine, 283–284
  electric countershock for, 282
  in cardiac arrest, 282–285
Ventricular septal defect, 428–431
  location of, 428, *428–429*
  repair of, 429t, 429–430
    complications with, 431
    preoperative factors influencing, 428–429
    sequelae with, 361, *361,* 430–431
  residual, 404, 430
    with tetralogy of Fallot repair, 435
  surgery for, 404–405, 428, 429–430
Ventriculostomy, for hydrocephalus, 514
Ventriculotomy, right, with tetralogy of Fallot repair, 435
Verapamil, doses and cardiac effects of, 376t, 379

Versed. See *Midazolam (Versed).*
Vessels, intraacinar, postnatal growth of, 10
Vioxx (rofecoxib), for postoperative analgesia, 678
Vitamin K, neonatal deficiency of, 20
Vitrectomy, for retinopathy of prematurity, 489
Vocal cords, anesthesia on, in bronchoscopy, 468
  oral mucosa and, 80
Vocal folds, in infant and adult, 82
  in phonation, 81
Volatile anesthetics, intraocular pressure and, 481

Warming devices, 628–629
  for fluids, 629, 716–717
  for operating room, 716
  properties of, 716–717
Weight. See also *Birth weight.*
  age and, 7–8, 8t
  gestational age and, 5, 6t
  growth assessment and, 6–8, *7,* 8t
  in preterm infants, 7–8
Wheezing, causes of, 323t
Whistling face, airway difficulties with, 118t
White blood cells, in newborns and infants, 20
Wound infiltration, with local anesthetics, postoperative analgesia and, 681
Wrapping, for reducing heat loss, 614, 717
Wrist, peripheral nerve blocks at, 661–663, *662*

Xanthines, for asthma, 324t

Zantac (ranitidine), 154–155, 184, 184t
Zemuron. See *Rocuronium (Zemuron).*
Zofran (ondansetron), 62, 155, 182, 466, 488